SAUNDERS

COMPREHENSIVE REVIEW FOR THE NCLEX-RN® EXAMINATION

8 EDITION

Linda Anne Silvestri, PhD, RN
Instructor of Nursing, Salve Regina University
Newport, Rhode Island
Part-Time Instructor, University of Nevada, Las Vegas, Las Vegas, Nevada
President, Nursing Reviews, Inc. and Professional Nursing Seminars, Inc.
Henderson, Nevada
Elsevier Consultant, HESI NCLEX-RN® and NCLEX-PN® Live Review Courses

Angela E. Silvestri, PhD, APRN, FNP-BC, CNE
Assistant Professor & BSN Program Director, University of Nevada, Las Vegas, Las Vegas, Nevada
Registered Nurse, Henderson Hospital Medical Center, Henderson, Nevada
Consultant, Nursing Reviews, Inc., Henderson, Nevada

Associate Editor

Katherine M. Silvestri, BSN, RN
Consultant, Nursing Reviews, Inc., Henderson, Nevada

ELSEVIER

Elsevier
3251 Riverport Lane
St. Louis, Missouri 63043

SAUNDERS COMPREHENSIVE REVIEW FOR THE NCLEX-RN® EXAMINATION
EIGHTH EDITION

ISBN: 978-0-323-35841-5

Library of Congress Control Number: 2019946366

Senior Content Strategist: Jamie Blum
Senior Content Development Specialist: Laura Goodrich
Publishing Services Manager: Julie Eddy
Senior Project Manager: Cindy Thoms
Senior Book Designer: Amy Buxton

Printed in Canada

Last digit is the print number: 9 8 7 6 5 4 3

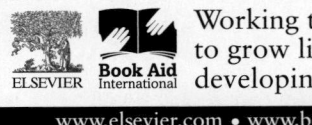

Contents

In loving memory of my parents—

To my mother, ***Frances Mary****, and my father,* ***Arnold Lawrence****, who taught me to always love, care, and be the best that I could be. My memories of their love, support, and words of encouragement will remain in my heart forever!*

Linda Anne Silvestri

To my parents, ***Mary Elizabeth*** *and* ***Lawrence Peter****, who have instilled in me the values of working hard and being selfless, and who have been my support system as I pursue my professional goals and life aspirations. My success thus far would not have been possible without them. From the bottom of my heart, thank you, Mom & Dad!*

Angela E. Silvestri

To All Future Registered Nurses,

Congratulations to you!

You should be very proud and pleased with yourself on your most recent well-deserved accomplishment of completing your nursing program to become a registered nurse. We know that you have worked very hard to become successful and that you have proven to yourself that indeed you can achieve your goals.

In our opinion, you are about to enter the most wonderful and rewarding profession that exists. Your willingness, desire, and ability to assist those who need nursing care will bring great satisfaction to your life. In the profession of nursing, your learning will be a lifelong process. This aspect of the profession makes it stimulating and dynamic. Your learning process will continue to expand and grow as the profession continues to evolve. Your next very important endeavor will be the learning process involved to achieve success in your examination to become a registered nurse.

We are excited and pleased to be able to provide you with the Saunders *Pyramid to Success* products, which will help you prepare for your next important professional goal, becoming a registered nurse. We want to thank all of our former and current nursing students whom we have assisted in their studies for the NCLEX-RN® examination for their willingness to offer ideas regarding their needs in preparing for licensure. Student ideas have certainly added a special uniqueness to all of the products available in the Saunders *Pyramid to Success.*

Saunders *Pyramid to Success* products provide you with everything that you need to ready yourself for the NCLEX-RN examination. These products include material that is required for the NCLEX-RN examination for all nursing students regardless of educational background, specific strengths, areas in need of improvement, or clinical experience during the nursing program.

So let's get started and begin our journey through the Saunders *Pyramid to Success,* and welcome to the wonderful profession of nursing!

Sincerely,
Dr. Linda Anne Silvestri and Dr. Angela E. Silvestri

About the Authors

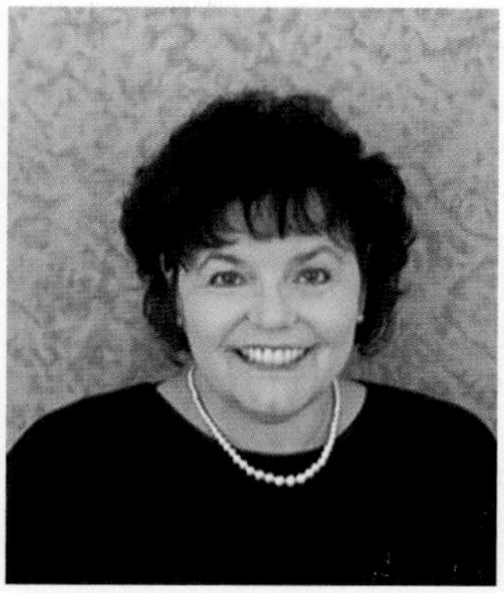

Linda Anne Silvestri, PhD, RN

(Photo by Laurent W. Valliere.)

As a child, I always dreamed of becoming either a nurse or a teacher. Initially I chose to become a nurse because I really wanted to help others, especially those who were ill. Then I realized that both of my dreams could come true; I could be both a nurse and a teacher. So I pursued my dreams.

I received my diploma in nursing at Cooley Dickinson Hospital School of Nursing in Northampton, Massachusetts. Afterward, I worked at Baystate Medical Center in Springfield, Massachusetts, where I cared for clients in acute medical-surgical units, the intensive care unit, the emergency department, pediatric units, and other acute care units. Later I received an associate degree from Holyoke Community College in Holyoke, Massachusetts; my BSN from American International College in Springfield, Massachusetts; and my MSN from Anna Maria College in Paxton, Massachusetts, with a dual major in Nursing Management and Patient Education. I received my PhD in Nursing from the University of Nevada, Las Vegas, and conducted research on self-efficacy and the predictors of NCLEX® success. I am also a member of the Honor Society of Nursing, Sigma Theta Tau International, Phi Kappa Phi, the American Nurses Association, the National League for Nursing, the Western Institute of Nursing, the Eastern Nursing Research Society, and the Golden Key International Honour Society. In addition, I received the 2012 Alumna of the Year/Nurse of the Year Award from the University of Nevada, Las Vegas, School of Nursing. I was selected for Fellowship in the American Academy of Nursing and will be inducted in October, 2019.

As a native of Springfield, Massachusetts, I began my teaching career as an instructor of medical-surgical nursing and leadership-management nursing in 1981 at Baystate Medical Center School of Nursing. In 1989, I relocated to Rhode Island and began teaching advanced medical-surgical nursing and mental health nursing to RN and LPN students at the Community College of Rhode Island. While teaching there, a group of students approached me for assistance in preparing for the NCLEX examination. I have always had a very special interest in test success for nursing students because of my own personal experiences with testing. Taking tests was never easy for me, and as a student I needed to find methods and strategies that would bring success. My own difficult experiences, desire, and dedication to assist nursing students to overcome the obstacles associated with testing inspired me to develop and write the many products that would foster success with testing. My experiences as a student, nursing educator, and item writer for the NCLEX examinations aided me as I developed a comprehensive review course to prepare nursing graduates for the NCLEX examination.

Later, in 1994, I began teaching medical-surgical nursing at Salve Regina University in Newport, Rhode Island, and I remain there as an adjunct faculty member preparing senior nursing students for the NCLEX-RN examination. Also, I am currently a part-time instructor at the University of Nevada, Las Vegas.

I established Professional Nursing Seminars, Inc. in 1991 and Nursing Reviews, Inc. in 2000. These companies are located in Henderson, Nevada. Both companies are dedicated to helping nursing graduates achieve their goals of becoming registered nurses, licensed practical/vocational nurses, or both.

Today, I am the successful author of numerous review products. Also, I serve as an Elsevier consultant for HESI Live Reviews, the review courses for the NCLEX examinations conducted throughout the country. I am so pleased that you have decided to join me on your journey to success in testing for nursing examinations and for the NCLEX-RN examination!

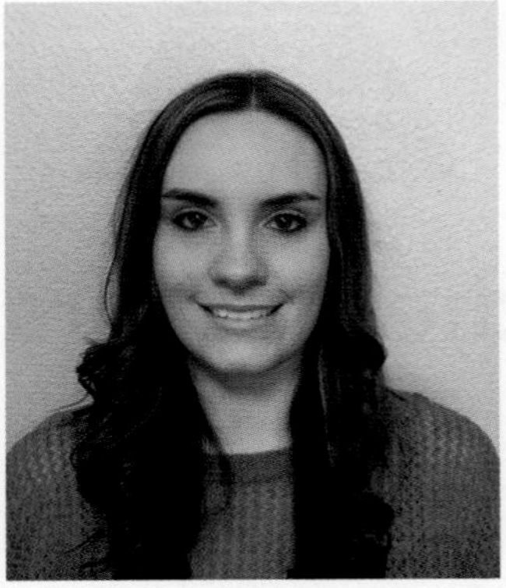

Angela E. Silvestri, PhD, APRN, FNP-BC, CNE

(Photo by Brent A. Elmore)

Being a nurse is one of the most enriching aspects of my life. It is a career that is multifaceted and complex, and allows me to be challenged scientifically, technically, and spiritually. As a nurse educator, I feel honored to impart my knowledge and experience to others who are hoping to serve in this selfless, caring profession. As a nurse scientist, I aim to make an impact on health care delivery methods, quality of care provided, and overall health care outcomes.

I earned my baccalaureate of science in nursing at Salve Regina University in Newport, Rhode Island. Upon graduation, I worked in long-term care, subacute care, rehabilitation, and acute care settings. I continue to work as a bedside nurse to maintain my technical skills set and to remain apprised of the changes reflected in health care today. I had the opportunity to serve as a preceptor for new graduate RNs while working in these areas. With the desire to become an educator, I pursued my Master of Science in nursing with a focus in education from the University of Nevada, Las Vegas, and began my teaching career. I continued my studies in the Doctor of Philosophy program at the University of Nevada, Las Vegas, focusing on beginning my research program as a nurse scientist. I completed my postgraduate certificate in advanced practice recently and am looking forward to serving in the role of the advanced practice nurse.

Throughout the years, I have worked extensively in the development of NCLEX review products, as well as with students in live review courses for the NCLEX. I am very excited at the prospect of helping graduates take the final step in becoming a licensed nurse. Thank you for your dedication to the profession of nursing, and I hope you find this resource useful as you move forward in your journey in becoming a licensed nurse. If you don't already know, nursing is an amazing profession!

Contributors

Consultants

Dianne E. Fiorentino
Research Coordinator
Nursing Reviews, Inc.
Henderson, Nevada

James J. Guilbault, PharmD, BS
Pharmacy Manager
Walgreens Pharmacy
Palmer, Massachusetts

Clinical Staff Pharmacist
Mercy Medical Center
Springfield, Massachusetts

Nicholas L. Silvestri, BA
Editorial and Communications Analyst
Nursing Reviews, Inc.
Henderson, Nevada

Contributors

Carmen George, DNP, MSN, BSN, APRN, WHNP-C
Women's Health Associates of Southern Nevada
Las Vegas, Nevada

Eileen H. Gray, DNP, RN, CPNP
Adjunct Professor, Nursing
Salve Regina University, Newport, Rhode, Island

Debra Hagler, PhD, RN, ACNS-BC, CNE, CHSE, ANEF, FAAN
Clinical Professor
College of Nursing and Health Innovation
Arizona State University, Phoenix
Phoenix, Arizona

Lisa Nicholas, MSN, RN
Clinical Instructor/Lecturer
School of Nursing
University of Nevada, Las Vegas

Registered Nurse
Sunrise Hospital Medical Center
Las Vegas, Nevada

Paula Richards, BA
Counsellor
Behaviorial Health
Baystate Medical Center
Springfield, Massachusetts

Katherine M. Silvestri, BSN, RN
Associate Editor
Consultant, Nursing Reviews, Inc.,
Henderson, Nevada

Jane Tyerman, RN, MScN, PhD
Professor, Nursing
Trent/Fleming School of Nursing, Peterborough
Ontario, Canada

Laurent W. Valliere, BS, DD
Vice President
Professional Nursing Seminars, Inc.
Marketing
Nursing Reviews, Inc.
Henderson, Nevada

Reviewers

Amber Ballard, MSN, RN
Registered Nurse
Emergency Department
Sparrow Health System
Lansing, Michigan

Brenda A. Battle, RN, BSN, MBA
Vice President, Urban Health Initiative and Chief Diversity, Inclusion and Equity Officer Administration,
The Office of Community Affairs and Diversity, Inclusion and Equity
The University of Chicago Medicine
Chicago, Illinois

Dawn Carpenter, DNP, ACNP-BC, CCRN
Assistant Professor
Coordinator, Adult Gerontology Acute Care Nurse Practitioner track
University of Massachusetts Medical School
Worcester, Massachusetts

Mary Carrico, MSN, RN
Associate Professor of Nursing
West Kentucky Community and Technical College
Paducah, Kentucky

Debra A. Cherubini, PhD, RN
Assistant Professor
Chair, Department of Nursing
Salve Regina University
Newport, Rhode, Island

Kim Clevenger, EdD, MSN, RN, BC
Associate Professor of Nursing
Morehead State University
Morehead, Kentucky

Christine R. Durbin, PhD, JD, RN
Associate Professor and Chair, Primary Care & Health Systems
Southern Illinois University Edwardsville School of Nursing
Edwardsville, Illinois

Janine Eagon, RNC, MS, CNS Certified Inpatient Obstetrics
Professor
Nursing Faculty
Bryant & Stratton College
Wauwatosa, Wisconsin

Alena Grewal, MSN, APRN, FNP-BC
Clinical Instructor
University of Nevada, Las Vegas School of Nursing
Las Vegas, Nevada

Jessica Leanne Grimm, DNP, APRN, ACNP-BC, CNE
Assistant Professor
College of Nursing
Touro University Nevada
Henderson, Nevada

Brad Harrell, DNP, APRN, ACNP-BC
Assistant Professor, Director of MSN and TNeCampus Programs
Loewenberg College of Nursing
University of Memphis
Memphis, Tennessee

Kimberly Head, BA, BS, DC
Director, Healthcare Programs
Collin College
Plano, Texas

Tiffany Jakubowski, BSN, RN, CMSRN, ONC
Clinical Nurse III
Ortho/Neuro
Longmont United Hospital
Longmont, Colorado

Ronald Jolley, MSN, RN
Registered Nurse
Adult Health Medical-Surgical
Henderson Hospital
Henderson, Nevada

Clinical Instructor
Chamberlain College of Nursing
Las Vegas, Nevada

Donna E. McCabe, DNP, APRN-BC, GNP
Clinical Assistant Professor
New York University Rory Meyers College of Nursing
New York, New York

Janis Longfield McMillan, MSN, RN, CNE
Associate Clinical Professor
School of Nursing
Northern Arizona University
Flagstaff, Arizona

Lisa Nicholas, MSN, RN
Clinical Instructor/Lecturer
School of Nursing
University of Nevada, Las Vegas

Registered Nurse
Sunrise Hospital Medical Center
Las Vegas, Nevada

David Petersen, MSN-Ed, RN
Adjunct Faculty
Paradise Valley Community College
Phoenix, Arizona

Karen Petersen, MSN-L, RN
Adjunct Faculty
Maricopa Community College District
Phoenix, Arizona

Misty Britt Stone, MSN RN
Clinical Assistant Professor
Nursing
The University of North Carolina at Pembroke
Pembroke, North Carolina

Jane Tyerman, RN, MScN, PhD
Professor, Nursing
Trent/Fleming School of Nursing
Peterborough,
Ontario, Canada

Joanna Van Sant, MSN, RN
RN Team Coordinator
Pain Management
Sentara Princess Anne Hospital
Virginia Beach, Virginia

Veronica Vital, PhD, RN
Clinical Assistant Professor
University of Arizona—College of Nursing
Tucson, Arizona

Student and Graduate Reviewers

Lea Adams, Graduate Nurse
Salve Regina University
Newport, Rhode, Island

Margaret Adams, Student Nurse
Salve Regina University
Newport, Rhode, Island

Emily Besaw, Student Nurse
Salve Regina University
Newport, Rhode, Island

Megan Bosetti, Student Nurse
Salve Regina University
Newport, Rhode, Island

Jenna Lynn Boyle, Student Nurse
Salve Regina University
Newport, Rhode, Island

Isabella Buda, Graduate Nurse
Salve Regina University
Newport, Rhode, Island

Monica Burritt, MAEd, BSN, RN
Graduate, Northern Arizona University
Flagstaff, Arizona

Morgan Cahill, Graduate Nurse
Salve Regina University
Newport, Rhode, Island

Hayley Cambrola, Graduate Nurse
Salve Regina University
Newport, Rhode, Island

Jennifer Carlson, RN, BSN
Graduate, Chamberlain College of Nursing
Phoenix, Arizona

Mary Cugini, Student Nurse
Salve Regina University
Newport, Rhode, Island

Kirsten Cunneen, Graduate Nurse
Salve Regina University
Newport, Rhode, Island

Stefanie Dias, Graduate Nurse
Salve Regina University
Newport, Rhode, Island

Caitlin Ecsedy, Graduate Nurse
Salve Regina University
Newport, Rhode, Island

Kelly Feola, Student Nurse
Salve Regina University
Newport, Rhode, Island

Megan Gilmore, Student Nurse
Salve Regina University
Newport, Rhode, Island

Megan Guest, Student Nurse
Salve Regina University
Newport, Rhode, Island

Ashley Haskell, Student Nurse
Salve Regina University
Newport, Rhode, Island

Kristen Hickey, Graduate Nurse
Salve Regina University
Newport, Rhode, Island

Valerie Huard, Student Nurse
Salve Regina University
Newport, Rhode, Island

Ariana Incorvati, Student Nurse
Salve Regina University
Newport, Rhode, Island

Hathaithip Keophakdy, Student Nurse
Salve Regina University
Newport, Rhode, Island

Michaela Lacerra, Student Nurse
Salve Regina University
Newport, Rhode, Island

Brianna Machnacz, Student Nurse
Salve Regina University
Newport, Rhode, Island

Elizabeth Maher, Student Nurse
Salve Regina University
Newport, Rhode, Island

Kara Merryfield, Graduate Nurse
Salve Regina University
Newport, Rhode, Island

Emma Murray, Student Nurse
Salve Regina University
Newport, Rhode, Island

Hien Nguyen, Student Nurse
Salve Regina University
Newport, Rhode, Island

Serena O'Hara, Graduate Nurse
Salve Regina University
Newport, Rhode, Island

Baleigh Payne, Graduate Nurse
Salve Regina University
Newport, Rhode, Island

Ashley Polson, Student Nurse
Salve Regina University
Newport, Rhode, Island

Isabelle Rella, Graduate Nurse
Salve Regina University
Newport, Rhode, Island

Jeff Risano, RN, BSN
Graduate, Chamberlain College of Nursing
Phoenix, Arizona

Melissa Rocchio, Student Nurse
Salve Regina University
Newport, Rhode, Island

Samantha Rudnik, Student Nurse
Salve Regina University
Newport, Rhode, Island

Jenny Scheer, Student Nurse
Salve Regina University
Newport, Rhode, Island

Mallory Tassone, Graduate Nurse
Salve Regina University
Newport, Rhode, Island

Brianna Wilcox, Graduate Nurse
Salve Regina University,
Newport, Rhode, Island

Contributors to Previous Edition

The author and publisher would also like to acknowledge the following individuals for contributions to the previous edition of this book:

Marilee Aufdenkamp, BSN, MS
Assistant Professor, School of Nursing, Creighton University, Omaha, Nebraska

Jaskaranjeet Bhullar, RN
Graduate, School of Nursing, Touro University Nevada, Henderson, Nevada

Jean Burt, BS, BSN, MSN
Instructor, Nursing, City Colleges of Chicago, Chicago, Illinois

Reitha Cabaniss, EdD, MSN
Nursing Director, Bevill State Community College, Jasper, Alabama

Barbara Callahan, MEd, RN, NCC, CHSE
Retired, Lenoir Community College, Kinston, North Carolina

Nancy Curry, BSN, MSN
Assistant Professor, Nursing, Northwestern State University College of Nursing and School of Allied Health, Shreveport, Louisiana

Mattie Davis, DNP, MSN, RN
Nursing Instructor, Health Sciences, J.F. Drake State Technical College, Huntsville, Alabama

Margie Francisco, EdD, MSN, RN
Nursing Professor, Health Division, Illinois Valley Community College, Oglesby, Illinois

Marilyn Greer, MS, RN
Associate Professor of Nursing, Rockford College, Rockford, Illinois

Joyce Hammer, RN, MSN
Adjunct Faculty, Nursing, Monroe County Community College, Monroe, Michigan

Donna Russo, MSN, CCRN, CNE
Nursing Instructor, ARIA Health School of Nursing, Philadelphia, Pennsylvania

Mary Scheid, RN, MSN
NCMC Breast Center, North, Colorado Medical Center, Greeley, Colorado

Laurent W. Valliere, BS, DD
Vice President of Nursing Reviews, Inc., Professional Nursing Seminars, Inc., Henderson, Nevada

Donna Wilsker, MSN, BSN
Assistant Professor, Dishman Department of Nursing, Lamar University, Beaumont, Texas

Item Writer and Section Editor

Donna Russo, MSN, CCRN, CNE
Nursing Instructor, ARIA Health School of Nursing, Philadelphia, Pennsylvania

Item Writers

Amber Ballard, MSN, RN
Registered Nurse, Emergency Department, Sparrow Health System, Lansing, Michigan

Betty Cheng, MSN
Assistant Professor, School of Nursing, MCPHS University, Boston, Massachusetts

Christina Keller, MSN, RN
Instructor, School of Nursing, Radford University, Radford, Virginia

Heidi Monroe, MSN, RN-BC, CAPA
Assistant Professor of Nursing, NCLEX-RN® Coordinator, Bellin College, Green Bay, Wisconsin

Bethany Hawes Sykes, EdD, RN, CEN, CCRN
Adjunct Faculty, Department of Nursing, Salve Regina University, Newport, Rhode, Island

Emergency Department RN, St Luke's Hospital, New Bedford, Massachusetts

Linda Turchin, RN, MSN, CNE
Assistant Professor, Nursing, Fairmont State University, Fairmont, West Virginia

Olga Van Dyke, PhD (c), CAGS, MSN
Assistant Professor, School of Nursing, MCPHS University, Boston, Massachusetts

Donna Wilsker, MSN, BSN
Assistant Professor, Dishman Department of Nursing, Lamar University, Beaumont, Texas

Preface

Linda Anne Silvestri, PhD, RN

"To laugh often and much, to appreciate beauty, to find the best in others, to leave the world a bit better, to know that even one life has breathed easier because you have lived, this is to have succeeded."

—Ralph Waldo Emerson

Angela Elizabeth Silvestri PhD, APRN, FNP-BC, CNE

"Success is never an accident. To be successful is to have been perseverant, to have sacrificed, and to have loved what you are cultivating to become successful."

Welcome to Saunders *Pyramid to Success!*

An Essential Resource for Test Success

Saunders Comprehensive Review for the NCLEX-RN® Examination is one in a series of products designed to assist you in achieving your goal of becoming a registered nurse. This text will provide you with a comprehensive review of all nursing content areas specifically related to the new 2019 test plan for the NCLEX-RN examination, which is implemented by the National Council of State Boards of Nursing. This resource will help you achieve success on your nursing examinations during nursing school and on the NCLEX-RN examination.

Organization

This book contains 20 units and 70 chapters. The chapters are designed to identify specific components of nursing content. They contain practice questions, both multiple-choice and alternate item formats, that reflect the chapter content and the 2019 test plan for the NCLEX-RN examination. The final unit, Chapter 70, contains a 75-question Comprehensive Test. All questions in the book and on the Evolve site are presented in NCLEX-style format.

The new test plan identifies a framework based on *Client Needs*. These Client Needs categories include Safe and Effective Care Environment, Health Promotion and Maintenance, Psychosocial Integrity, and Physiological Integrity. *Integrated Processes* are also identified as a component of the test plan. These include Caring, Communication and Documentation, Culture and Spirituality, Nursing Process, and Teaching and Learning. All chapters address the components of the test plan framework.

Special Features of the Book

Pyramid Terms

Pyramid Terms are important to the discussion of the content in the chapters in each unit. Therefore, they are in bold **green** type throughout the content section of each chapter. Definitions can be reviewed in the Audio Glossary on the Evolve site.

Pyramid to Success

The *Pyramid to Success,* a featured part of each unit introduction, provides you with an overview, guidance, and direction regarding the focus of review in the particular content area, as well as the content area's relative importance to the 2019 test plan for the NCLEX-RN examination. The *Pyramid to Success* reviews the Client Needs and provides learning objectives as they pertain to the content in that unit. These learning objectives identify the specific components to keep in mind as you review each chapter.

Priority Concepts

Each chapter identifies two *Priority Concepts* reflective of its content. These *Priority Concepts* will assist you to focus on the important aspects of the content and associated nursing interventions.

Pyramid Points

Pyramid Points (▲) are placed next to specific content throughout the chapters. The *Pyramid Points* highlight content that is important for preparing for the NCLEX-RN examination and identify content that is likely to appear on the NCLEX-RN examination.

Pyramid Alerts

Pyramid Alerts are the red text found throughout the chapters that alert you to important information about nursing concepts. These alerts identify content that typically appears on the NCLEX-RN examination.

Special Features Found on Evolve

Pretest and Study Calendar

The accompanying Evolve site contains a 75-question pretest that provides you with feedback on your strengths and weaknesses. The results of your pretest will generate an individualized study calendar to guide you in your preparation for the NCLEX-RN examination.

Heart, Lung, and Bowel Sound Questions

The accompanying Evolve site contains *Audio Questions* representative of content addressed in the 2019 test plan for the NCLEX-RN examination. Each question presents an audio clip as a component of the question.

Video Questions

The accompanying Evolve site contains *Video Questions* representative of content addressed in the 2019 test plan for the NCLEX-RN examination. Each question presents a video clip as a component of the question.

Case Study (Testlet) Questions

The accompanying Evolve site contains case study questions. These question types include a client scenario and several accompanying practice questions that relate to the content of the scenario.

Audio Review Summaries

The companion Evolve site includes three *Audio Review Summaries* that cover challenging subject areas addressed in the 2019 test plan for the NCLEX-RN examination, including *Pharmacology*, *Acid-Base Balance*, and *Fluids and Electrolytes*.

Practice Questions

While preparing for the NCLEX-RN examination, it is crucial for students to practice taking test questions. This book contains 945 NCLEX-style multiple-choice and alternate item format questions. The accompanying software includes all questions from the book plus additional Evolve questions for a total of more than 5200 questions.

Multiple-Choice and Alternate Item Format Questions

Starting with Unit II, each chapter is followed by a practice test. Each practice test contains several questions reflective of the content in the chapter and those presented on the NCLEX-RN examination. These questions provide you with practice in prioritizing, decision-making, critical thinking, and clinical judgment skills. Chapter 1 of this book provides a description of each question type. Sample questions of the Next Generation NCLEX (NGN) are also provided in this chapter.

The answer section for each practice question throughout the chapters and on the Evolve site provides the correct answer, the rationale for the correct and incorrect options, and a specific test-taking strategy that will assist you in answering the question correctly. The specific test-taking strategy is highlighted in bold **blue** type. This highlighting will provide you with guidance and direction for further remediation in the *Saunders Strategies for Test Success: Passing Nursing School and the NCLEX® Exam*.

The categories identified in each practice question include Level of Cognitive Ability, Client Needs, Integrated Process, the specific nursing Content Area, the Health Problem, and Priority Concepts. Every question on the accompanying Evolve site is organized by these question codes, so you can customize your study session to be as specific or as generic as you need. Additionally, a link to view normal laboratory reference intervals are provided with each practice question.

Pharmacology and Medication Calculations Review

Students consistently state that pharmacology is an area with which they need assistance. The 2019 NCLEX-RN test plan continues to incorporate pharmacology in the examination, but only the generic drug names will be included. Therefore, pharmacology chapters have been included for your review and practice. This book includes 13 pharmacology chapters, a medication and intravenous prescriptions calculation chapter, and a pediatric medication administration and calculation chapter. Each of these chapters is followed by a practice test that uses the same question format described earlier. This book contains numerous pharmacology questions. Additionally, more than 950 pharmacology questions can be found on the accompanying Evolve site.

Next Generation NCLEX (NGN) Questions

The NCSBN is currently piloting research questions for a project known as the "Next Generation NCLEX." An NCLEX candidate may encounter these questions once they complete their examination, and they will have the option to answer these questions as part of NCSBN's research on these new item types. The NCSBN is aiming to launch the NGN questions on the examination sometime during the years 2022-2023, and these item types are designed to test the candidate's ability to make safe and competent clinical judgments. This resource incudes 25 NGN item types, and although it is not live on the NCLEX now, practicing these items will assist the current candidate in preparing for the NCLEX examination. The NGN questions are located on the Evolve site.

How to Use This Book

Saunders Comprehensive Review for the NCLEX-RN® Examination is especially designed to help you with your successful journey to the peak of the Saunders *Pyramid to Success*: becoming a registered nurse! As you begin your journey through this book, you will be introduced to all of the important points regarding the 2019 NCLEX-RN examination, the process of testing, and unique and special tips regarding how to prepare yourself for this very important examination.

You should begin your process through the Saunders *Pyramid to Success* by reading all of Unit I in this book and becoming familiar with the central points regarding the NCLEX-RN examination. Be sure to read Chapter 3, written by a nursing graduate who recently passed the examination, and note what she has to say about the testing experience. Chapter 4 will provide you with the critical testing strategies that will guide you in selecting the correct option or assist you in selecting an answer to a question if you must guess. Keep these strategies in mind as you proceed through this book. Continue by studying the specific content areas addressed in Units II through XIX. Review the definitions of the *Pyramid Terms* located in each chapter, and the *Pyramid to Success* notes, and the Client Needs and Learning Objectives located in each unit introduction. Read through the chapters and focus on the *Pyramid Points* and *Pyramid Alerts* that identify the areas most likely to be tested on the NCLEX-RN examination. Pay particular attention to the *Priority Nursing Actions* boxes because they provide information about the steps you will take in clinical situations requiring clinical judgment and prioritization.

As you read each chapter, identify your areas of strength and those in need of further review. Highlight these areas and test your abilities by taking all practice tests provided at the end of the chapters. Be sure to review all rationales and test-taking strategies.

After reviewing all chapters in the book, turn to Unit XX, Chapter 70, the Comprehensive Test. Take this examination and then review each question, answer, and rationale. Identify any areas requiring further review; then take the time to review those areas in both the book and the companion Evolve site. In preparation for the NCLEX-RN examination, be sure to take the pretest and generate your study calendar. Follow the calendar for your review because the calendar represents your pretest results and the best study path to follow based on your strong and weak content areas. Also, be sure to access the *Case Studies* and the *Audio Review Summaries* as part of your preparation for the NCLEX-RN examination.

Climbing the Pyramid to Success

The purpose of this book is to provide a **comprehensive review** of the nursing content you will be tested on during the NCLEX-RN examination. However, *Saunders Comprehensive Review for the NCLEX-RN® Examination* is intended to do more than simply prepare you for the rigors of the NCLEX-RN examination; this book is also meant to serve as a valuable study tool that you can refer to throughout your nursing program, with specific customizable Evolve site selections to help identify and reinforce key content areas and prepare you for your nursing exams.

After using this book for comprehensive content review, your next step in the *Pyramid to Success* is to get additional practice with the **Q&A review** product. *Saunders Q&A Review for the NCLEX-RN® Examination* offers more than 6000 unique practice questions in the book and on the companion Evolve site. The questions are focused on the Client Needs and Integrated Processes of the NCLEX-RN test plan, making it easy to access your study area of choice. For on-the-go Q&A review, you can pick up *Saunders Q&A Review Cards for the NCLEX-RN® Examination*.

Your final step on the *Pyramid to Success* is to master the **online review**. *Saunders Online Review for the NCLEX-RN® Examination* provides an interactive and individualized platform to get you ready for your NCLEX exam. This online course provides 10 high-level content modules, supplemented with instructional videos, animations, audio, illustrations, case studies, and several subject matter exams. End-of-module practice tests are provided along with several *Crossing the Finish Line* practice tests. In addition, you can assess your progress with a *Pretest, Test Yourself quizzes*, and a *Comprehensive Exam* in a computerized environment that prepares you for the actual NCLEX-RN examination.

At the base of the *Pyramid to Success* are our **test-taking strategies**, which provide a foundation for understanding and unpacking the complexities of NCLEX-RN examination questions, including alternate item formats. *Saunders Strategies for Test Success: Passing Nursing School and the NCLEX® Exam* takes a detailed look at all of the test-taking strategies you will need to know in order to pass any nursing examination, including the NCLEX-RN. Special tips are integrated for nursing students, and there are more than 1200 practice questions included so you can apply the testing strategies. NGN questions are included on the Evolve site.

Good luck with your journey through the Saunders *Pyramid to Success*. We wish you continued success throughout your new career as a registered nurse!

Acknowledgments

A Few Words From Linda

There are many individuals who in their own ways have contributed to my success in making my professional dreams become a reality. My sincere appreciation and warmest thanks are extended to all of them.

First, I want to acknowledge my parents, who opened my door of opportunity in education. I thank my mother, Frances Mary, for all of her love, support, and assistance as I continuously worked to achieve my professional goals. I thank my father, Arnold Lawrence, who always provided insightful words of encouragement. My memories of their love and support will always remain in my heart. I am certain that they are very proud of my professional accomplishments.

I also thank my best friend and love of my life, my husband, Larry; my sister, Dianne Elodia, and her husband, Lawrence; my brother, Lawrence Peter, and my sister-in-law, Mary Elizabeth; my cousin Paula; and my nieces and nephews, Angela, Gina, Karen, Katie, Brianna, and Nicholas, who were continuously supportive, giving, and helpful during my research and preparation of this publication. They were always there and by my side whenever I needed them.

I want to thank my nursing students at the Community College of Rhode Island who approached me in 1991 and persuaded me to assist them in preparing to take the NCLEX-RN examination. Their enthusiasm and inspiration led to the commencement of my professional endeavors in conducting review courses for the NCLEX-RN examination for nursing students. I also thank the numerous nursing students who have attended my review courses for their willingness to share their needs and ideas. Their input has certainly added a special uniqueness to this publication.

I also wish to acknowledge all of the nursing faculty who taught in my review courses for the NCLEX-RN examination. Their commitment, dedication, and expertise have certainly assisted nursing students in achieving success with the NCLEX-RN examination. I also want to extend a very special thank you to my niece, Angela, for joining me in preparing and authoring these NCLEX resources. Angela is wonderful to work with. Her tremendous theoretical and clinical knowledge and expertise and her consistent ideas and input certainly added to the excellent quality of this product. She is very dedicated to promoting and ensuring student success. Thank you, Angela!

A special thank you goes to Loren Wilson, former Senior Vice President, for her years of expert guidance and continuous support for all of the products in the *Pyramid to Success*.

I would also like to acknowledge Patricia Mieg, former educational sales representative, who encouraged me to submit my ideas and initial work for the first edition of this book to the W.B. Saunders Company.

I also need to thank Salve Regina University for the opportunity to educate nursing students in the baccalaureate nursing program and for its support during my research and writing of this publication. I would like to especially acknowledge my colleague Dr. Eileen Gray for all of her encouragement and support and dedication to my professional endeavors.

I wish to acknowledge the Community College of Rhode Island, which provided me with the opportunity to educate nursing students in the Associate Degree of Nursing Program. A special thank you goes to Patricia Miller, MSN, RN, and Michelina McClellan, MS, RN, from Baystate Medical Center, School of Nursing, in Springfield, Massachusetts, who were my first mentors in nursing education.

And finally, a very sincere and special acknowledgment to my husband, Laurent (Larry) W. Valliere, for his contribution to this publication, for teaching in my review courses for the NCLEX-RN examination, and for his commitment and dedication in assisting my nursing students to prepare for the examination from a nonacademic point of view. I thank him for all of his continuous support; he was so loyal and loving to me each and every moment as I worked to achieve my professional goals. Larry, you are my "rock of support!" Thank you so much!

A Few Words From Angela

There are many people who contributed to my success in my work on this product. I am very grateful for their continued support in all of my endeavors.

First and foremost, I would like to thank my husband, Brent, for his light-hearted and positive attitude. He always knows how to make me laugh, especially when I'm stressed. All of this would not be possible without him!

I would also like to thank my parents, Mary and Larry, for their continued support throughout the years. Their words of encouragement and wisdom have been tremendously important to my success. I also don't know what I would do without their support in caring for my kids!

I would like to thank my sister Katie, who is a wonderful nurse. Her ambitions as a nursing student were so inspiring and reminded me about why I'm so passionate about being an educator. Thank you to my brother, Nick, who always is positive and encouraging about my work. His wit and sarcasm are always a great way to lift your mood at the end of the day. I would also like to thank my friends Jessica, Alena, and Lisa for their continued support, encouragement, and camaraderie throughout my professional endeavors.

Finally, I want to extend a special thank you to Linda for her collaboration, guidance, and expertise. Without her, I would not be where I am today. Thank you, Linda!

A Few Words From Both Linda and Angela

First and foremost, we want to thank our associate editor, Katie Silvestri, for all of her dedicated and hard work in editing and preparing manuscript for this edition. Her expertise and close attention to details have certainly added to the quality of this resource. In addition, we sincerely thank Katie for writing a chapter for this book about her experiences with preparing for and taking the NCLEX-RN examination. Katie, thank you so much!

We also want to acknowledge and thank Laurent W. Valliere for writing a chapter addressing those important nonacademic test preparation issues.

A very special thank you and acknowledgment goes to all of the reviewers, contributors, and item writers who updated and provided many of the practice questions and all of the previous contributors who provided contributions to this book.

Additionally, we want to thank Paula Richards for her expertice and input in creating our new chapter, titled Care of Special Populations. Thank you, Paula!

We wish to offer a very special acknowledgment and thank you to Jane Tyerman for reviewing many sections of this book, including the Mental Health section, to ensure that it included Canadian nursing practice and standards. Thank you, Jane!

We would also like to thank other reviewers and contributors who spent so much of their own time reviewing and/or contributing to the new chapters of the book and the specialty sections of this book. Their expertise has certainly added to the quality of this book. Thank you, Jessica Grimm and David Peterson, for your expertise in reviewing the new Complex Care chapter. Thank you, Lisa Nicholas, for your expertise in reviewing and updating developmental stages. Thank you, Eileen Gray, for your updates in Pediatrics; and thank you, Carmen George, for your updates in Maternity. Finally, thank you, Debra Hagler, for your expertise in updating the cardiovascular section of this edition. In addition, a special thank you to both, Veronica Vital and Kimberly Head, for reviewing our new Special Populations chapter.

We thank Dianne E. Fiorentino for her continuous support and dedication to our work and in her reference support and other secretarial responsibilities for the eight editions of this book. We thank Jimmy Guibault for providing medication research support, and Nick Silvestri for his communication and proofreading skills as he reviewed the manuscript. And we thank Mary and Larry Silvestri for their assistance with all of the tasks and projects we needed completed. A special thank you to all of you!

We thank all of our student and graduate reviewers who read all of the practice questions in this book and provided input on their quality. And we sincerely extend a very special thank you to Kristen Hickey, a nursing graduate, who edited and coded all of our practice questions on the Evolve site.

We sincerely acknowledge and thank some very important and special people from Elsevier. We thank Jamie Blum, Senior Content Strategist, and Laurie Gower, Director of Development, for their continuous support, enthusiasm, and expert professional guidance throughout the preparation of this edition. And a very special thank you goes to Laura Goodrich, Senior Content Development Specialist, for her tremendous amount of support and assistance, for prioritizing for us to keep us on track, for her ideas for the product, and for her professional and expert skills in organizing and maintaining an enormous amount of manuscript for production. We could not have completed this project without Laura—thank you, Laura!

We want to acknowledge all of the staff at Elsevier for their tremendous help throughout the preparation and production of this publication. A special thanks to all of them. We thank Julie Eddy, Publishing Services Manager and Amy Buxton, Designer. You have all played such significant roles in finalizing this publication. We need to especially acknowledge Cindy Thoms, Senior Project Manager, who took over when Laura was on maternity leave. Cindy, you were so supportive and so awesome to work with. Your attention to the many details to ensure and maintain the quality of this book was so greatly appreciated. We thank you so much!

Lastly, a very special thank you to all our nursing students: past, present, and future. All of you light up our life! Your love and dedication to the profession of nursing and your commitment to provide health care will bring never-ending rewards!

UNIT I

NCLEX-RN® Exam Preparation

CHAPTER 1

Clinical Judgment and the NCLEX-RN® Examination

The Pyramid to Success

Saunders Comprehensive Review for the NCLEX-RN® Examination

About This Resource and the NCLEX-RN® Examination

Welcome to the *Pyramid to Success* and *Saunders Comprehensive Review for the NCLEX-RN® Examination.* This resource is specially designed to help you begin your successful journey to the peak of the pyramid, becoming a registered nurse. As you begin your journey, you will be introduced to all of the important points regarding the NCLEX-RN examination and the process of testing, and to unique and special tips regarding how to prepare yourself for this important examination. You will read what a nursing graduate who recently passed the NCLEX-RN examination has to say about the test. Important test-taking strategies are detailed. These details will guide you in selecting the correct option or assist you in making an educated guess if you are not entirely sure about the correct answer. Each unit in this book begins with the Pyramid to Success. The Pyramid to Success addresses specific points related to the NCLEX-RN examination. Client Needs as identified in the test plan framework for the examination are listed, as are learning objectives for the unit. Pyramid Terms are key words that are defined in the glossary located in Evolve and set in color throughout each chapter to direct your attention to significant points for the examination.

This resource provides you with nursing content review, including the content identified in the current NCLEX test plan, and practice questions. Throughout each chapter, you will find Pyramid Point bullets that identify areas most likely to be tested on the NCLEX-RN examination. Read each chapter, and identify your strengths and areas that are in need of further review.

The book contains 945 NCLEX-style questions. The Evolve site accompanying this book contains all of the questions from the book plus additional Evolve questions for a total of more than 5200 practice questions. The types of practice questions include multiple choice; fill-in-the-blank; multiple-response; ordered-response (also known as drag and drop); questions that contain a figure, chart/exhibit, or graphic option item; audio or video item formats; and case studies. In addition, the new Next Generation NCLEX® (NGN) question types are also provided on the accompanying Evolve site. Examples of question types can be located throughout this chapter.

Test your strengths and abilities by taking all practice tests provided in this book and on the accompanying Evolve site. Be sure to read all rationales and test-taking strategies. The rationale provides you with significant information regarding the correct and incorrect options. The test-taking strategy provides you with the logical path to selecting the correct option. reference source and page number are provided so that you can easily find information you need to review in another Elsevier text. You may also review in the content review sections of this book. Each question in the book and on the accompanying Evolve site is coded on the basis of the Level of Cognitive Ability, the Client Needs category, the Integrated Process, Content Area being tested, and a Health Problem, if applicable. The Health Problem code allows you to filter and select questions based on a disease process. For example, if heart failure is the area of interest, you can select "Adult Health, Cardiovascular, Heart Failure" on the Evolve site. In addition, two Priority Concepts that relate to the content of the question are identified. This code is helpful for students specifically whose curriculum is concept-based. Additionally, information about all of the special features of this resource and the question types is located in the preface of this book.

Other Resources in the Saunders Pyramid to Success

There are several other resources in the Saunders Pyramid to Success program. These include the following: *The Saunders Q&A Review for the NCLEX-RN® Examination, The HESI/Saunders Online Review for the NCLEX-RN® Examination, Saunders Strategies for Test Success: Passing Nursing School and the NCLEX® Exam, Saunders Q&A Review Cards for the NCLEX-RN® Exam,* and *Saunders RNtertainment for the NCLEX-RN® Exam.*

All of these resources in the Saunders Pyramid to Success are described in the preface of this book and can be obtained online by visiting http://elsevierhealth.com or by calling 800-545-2522.

Let's begin our journey through the Pyramid to Success.

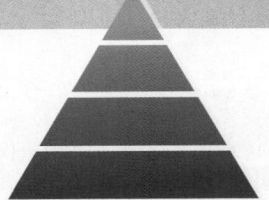

Examination Process

An important step in the Pyramid to Success is to become as familiar as possible with the examination process. Candidates facing the challenge of this examination can experience significant anxiety. Knowing what the examination is all about and knowing what you will encounter during the process of testing will assist in alleviating fear and anxiety. The information contained in this chapter was obtained from the NCSBN Web site (www.ncsbn.org) and from the NCSBN 2019 test plan for the NCLEX-RN and includes some procedures related to registering for the exam, testing procedures, and the answers to the questions most commonly asked by nursing students and graduates preparing to take the NCLEX. You can obtain additional information regarding the test and its development by accessing the NCSBN Web site and clicking on the NCLEX Exam tab or by writing to the National Council of State Boards of Nursing, 111 East Wacker Drive, Suite 2900, Chicago, IL 60601. You are encouraged to access the NCSBN Web site, because this site provides you with the most up-to-date and valuable information about the NCLEX and other resources available to an NCLEX candidate. You are also encouraged to access the most up-to-date *Candidate Bulletin.* This document provides you with everything you need to know about registration procedures and scheduling a test date.

Computer Adaptive Testing

The acronym *CAT* stands for computer adaptive test, which means that the examination is created as the test-taker answers each question. All the test questions are categorized on the basis of the test plan structure and the level of difficulty of the question. As you answer a question, the computer determines your competency based on the answer you selected. If you selected a correct answer, the computer scans the question bank and selects a more difficult question. If you selected an incorrect answer, the computer scans the question bank and selects an easier question. This process continues until all test plan requirements are met and a reliable pass-or-fail decision is made.

When taking a CAT, once an answer is recorded, all subsequent questions administered depend, to an extent, on the answer selected for that question. Skipping and returning to earlier questions are not compatible with the logical methodology of a CAT. The inability to skip questions or go back to change previous answers will not be a disadvantage to you; you will not fall into that "trap" of changing a correct answer to an incorrect one with the CAT system.

If you are faced with a question that contains unfamiliar content, you may need to guess at the answer. There is no penalty for guessing, but you need to make an educated guess. With most of the questions, the answer will be right there in front of you. If you need to guess, use your nursing knowledge and clinical experiences to their fullest extent and all of the test-taking strategies you have practiced in this review program.

You do not need any computer experience to take this examination. A keyboard tutorial is provided and administered to all test-takers at the start of the examination. The tutorial will instruct you on the use of the on-screen optional calculator, the use of the mouse, and how to record an answer. The tutorial provides instructions on how to respond to all question types on this examination. This tutorial is also provided on the NCSBN Web site, and you are encouraged to view the tutorial when you are preparing for the NCLEX examination. In addition, at the testing site, a test administrator is present to assist in explaining the use of the computer to ensure your full understanding of how to proceed.

Development of the Test Plan

The test plan for the NCLEX-RN examination is developed by the NCSBN. The examination is a national examination; the NCSBN considers the legal scope of nursing practice as governed by state laws and regulations, including the Nurse Practice Act, and uses these laws to define the areas on the examination that will assess the competence of the test-taker for licensure.

The NCSBN also conducts an important study every 3 years, known as a *practice analysis study,* that is conducted to link the examination to nursing practice. The results of this study determine the framework for the test plan for the examination. The participants in this study include newly licensed registered nurses from all types of generalist nursing education programs. From a list of nursing care activities (activity statements) provided, the participants are asked about the applicability, frequency, and importance of performing these activities in relation to client safety. A panel of content experts at the NCSBN analyzes the results of the study and makes decisions regarding the test plan framework. The results of this recently conducted study provided the structure for the test plan implemented in April 2019.

Test Plan

The content of the NCLEX-RN examination reflects the activities identified in the practice analysis study conducted by the NCSBN. The questions are written to address Level of Cognitive Ability, Client Needs, and Integrated Processes as identified in the test plan developed by the NCSBN.

Level of Cognitive Ability

Levels of cognitive ability include knowledge, understanding, applying, analyzing, synthesizing, evaluating, and creating. The practice of nursing requires complex thought processing and critical thinking in decision making. Therefore, you will not encounter any knowledge or understanding questions on the NCLEX. Questions on this examination are written at the applying level or at higher levels of cognitive ability. Table 1-1 provides descriptions and examples of each level of cognitive ability. Box 1-1 presents an example of a question that requires you to apply data.

Client Needs

The NCSBN identifies a test plan framework based on Client Needs, which includes 4 major categories. Some of these categories are divided further into subcategories. The Client Needs categories are Safe and Effective Care Environment, Health Promotion and Maintenance, Psychosocial Integrity, and Physiological Integrity (Table 1-2).

Safe and Effective Care Environment

The Safe and Effective Care Environment category includes 2 subcategories: Management of Care, and Safety and Infection Control. According to the NCSBN, Management of Care addresses prioritizing care and providing and directing nursing care that will ensure a safe care delivery setting to protect clients and health care personnel. The NCSBN indicates that Safety and Infection Control addresses content that will protect clients and health care personnel from health and environmental hazards within health care facilities and in community settings. Box 1-2 presents examples of questions that address these 2 subcategories.

Health Promotion and Maintenance

The Health Promotion and Maintenance category addresses the principles related to growth and development. According to the NCSBN, this Client Needs category also addresses content required to assist the individual to prevent health problems; to recognize alterations in health; and to develop health practices that promote and support optimal wellness. See Box 1-3 for an example of a question in this Client Needs category.

Psychosocial Integrity

The Psychosocial Integrity category addresses content required to promote and support the ability of the client to cope, adapt, and problem-solve during stressful events. The NCSBN also indicates that this Client Needs category addresses the emotional, mental, and social well-being of the client experiencing stressful events

TABLE 1-1 Levels of Cognitive Ability: Descriptions and Examples

Level	Description and Example
Knowledge	Recalling information from memorizing. Example: A normal blood glucose level is 70 to 99 mg/dL (3.9 to 5.5 mmol/L).
Understanding	Recognizing the meaning of information. Example: A blood glucose level of 60 mg/dL (3.34 mmol/L) is lower than the normal reference range.
Applying	Carrying out an appropriate action based on information. Example: Administering 10 to 15 g of carbohydrate such as a ½ glass of fruit juice to treat mild hypoglycemia.
Analyzing	Examining a broad concept and breaking it down into smaller parts. Example: The broad concept is mild hypoglycemia and the smaller concepts are the signs and symptoms of mild hypoglycemia, such as hunger, irritability, weakness, headache, or blood glucose level lower than 70 mg/dL (3.9 mmol/L). So, for example, the question may present information that you need to interpret as mild hypoglycemia. Then, the question asks you to select the option(s) that identify the appropriate nursing action(s) to correct hypoglycemia.
Synthesizing	Examining smaller parts or information and determining the broad concept. Example: The smaller concepts are manifestations such as polyuria, polydipsia, polyphagia, vomiting, abdominal pain, weakness, confusion, and Kussmaul respirations. The broad concept is diabetic ketoacidosis (DKA). So, for example, the question may provide specific information about the manifestations of DKA. You need to interpret these manifestations as DKA. Then, the question asks you to select the option(s) that identify the appropriate nursing action(s), based on your interpretation that the client is experiencing DKA.
Evaluating	Making judgments, conclusions, or validations based on evidence. Example: Determining that treatment for mild hypoglycemia was effective if the blood glucose level returned to a normal level between 70 to 99 mg/dL (3.9 to 5.5 mmol/L) after a specified time period.
Creating	Generating or producing a new outcome or plan by putting parts of information together. Example: Designing a safe and individualized plan of care with the interprofessional health care team for a client with diabetes mellitus that meets the client's physiological, psychosocial, and health maintenance needs.

Adapted from *Understanding Bloom's (and Anderson and Krathwohl's) taxonomy, 2015*, ProEdit, Inc. http://www.proedit.com/understanding-blooms-and-anderson-and-krathwohls-taxonomy/
Reference: Ignatavicius, Workman (2018), pp. 1331-1333.

BOX 1-1 Level of Cognitive Ability: Applying

The nurse notes blanching, coolness, and edema at the peripheral intravenous (IV) site. On the basis of these findings, the nurse would implement which action?

1. Remove the IV.
2. Apply a warm compress.
3. Check for a blood return.
4. Measure the area of infiltration.

***Answer:* 1**

This question requires that you focus on the data in the question and determine that the client is experiencing an infiltration. Next, you need to consider the harmful effects of infiltration and determine the action to implement. Because infiltration can be damaging to the surrounding tissue, the appropriate action is to remove the IV to prevent any further damage. Once the IV is removed, further action would be taken depending on the medication infusing at the time of infiltration based on agency protocol, but may include aspiration of the fluid from the site, injection of an antidote, application of warm or cool compresses for specified time intervals, and elevation of the extremity.

TABLE 1-2 Client Needs Categories and Percentage of Questions on the NCLEX-RN Examination

Client Needs Category and Subcategory	Percentage of Questions
Safe and Effective Care Environment	
Management of Care	17-23
Safety and Infection Control	9-15
Health Promotion and Maintenance	6-12
Psychosocial Integrity	6-12
Physiological Integrity	
Basic Care and Comfort	6-12
Pharmacological and Parenteral Therapies	12-18
Reduction of Risk Potential	9-15
Physiological Adaptation	11-17

From National Council of State Boards of Nursing: *2019 NCLEX-RN® examination: Test plan for the National Council Licensure Examination for Registered Nurses*Chicago, 2018, National Council of State Boards of Nursing.

BOX 1-2 Safe and Effective Care Environment

Management of Care

The nurse has received the client assignment for the day. Which client would the nurse assess **first**?

1. The client who needs to receive subcutaneous insulin before breakfast
2. The client who has a nasogastric tube attached to intermittent suction
3. The client who is 2 days postoperative and is complaining of incisional pain
4. The client who has a blood glucose level of 50 mg/dL (2.8 mmol/L) and complaints of blurred vision

***Answer:* 4**

This question addresses the subcategory Management of Care in the Client Needs category Safe and Effective Care Environment. Note the strategic word, *first,* so you need to establish priorities by comparing the needs of each client and deciding which need is urgent. The client described in the correct option has a low blood glucose level and symptoms reflective of hypoglycemia. This client would be assessed first so that treatment can be implemented. Although the clients in options 1, 2, and 3 have needs that require assessment, their assessments can wait until the client in the correct option is stabilized.

Safety and Infection Control

The nurse prepares to care for a client on contact precautions who has a hospital-acquired infection caused by methicillin-resistant *Staphylococcus aureus* (MRSA). The client has an abdominal wound that requires irrigation and has a tracheostomy attached to a mechanical ventilator, which requires frequent suctioning. The nurse would assemble which necessary protective items before entering the client's room?

1. Gloves and gown
2. Gloves and face shield
3. Gloves, gown, and face shield
4. Gloves, gown, and shoe protectors

***Answer:* 3**

This question addresses the subcategory Safety and Infection Control in the Client Needs category Safe and Effective Care Environment. It addresses content related to protecting oneself from contracting an infection and requires that you consider the methods of possible transmission of infection, based on the client's condition. Note the data in the question. Because of the potential for splashes of infective material occurring during the wound irrigation or suctioning of the tracheostomy, option 3 is correct.

and care for the client with an acute or chronic mental illness. See Box 1-4 for an example of a question in this Client Needs category.

Physiological Integrity

The Physiological Integrity category includes 4 subcategories: Basic Care and Comfort, Pharmacological and Parenteral Therapies, Reduction of Risk Potential, and Physiological Adaptation. The NCSBN describes these subcategories as follows. Basic Care and Comfort addresses content for providing comfort and assistance to the client in the performance of activities of daily living. Pharmacological and Parenteral Therapies addresses content for administering medications and parenteral therapies, such as intravenous therapies and parenteral nutrition, and administering blood and

BOX 1-3 Health Promotion and Maintenance

The nurse is choosing age-appropriate toys for a toddler. Which toy is the **best** choice for this age?

1. Puzzle
2. Toy soldiers
3. Large stacking blocks
4. A card game with large pictures

Answer: *3*

This question addresses the Client Needs category Health Promotion and Maintenance and specifically relates to the principles of growth and development of a toddler. Note the strategic word, *best.* Toddlers like to master activities independently, such as stacking blocks. Because toddlers do not have the developmental ability to determine what could be harmful, toys that are safe need to be provided. A puzzle and toy soldiers provide objects that can be placed in the mouth and may be harmful for a toddler. A card game with large pictures may require cooperative play, which is more appropriate for a school-age child.

BOX 1-4 Psychosocial Integrity

A client with end-stage chronic obstructive pulmonary disease has selected guided imagery to help cope with psychological stress. Which client statement indicates an understanding of this stress-reduction measure?

1. "This will help only if I play music at the same time."
2. "This will work for me only if I am alone in a quiet area."
3. "I need to do this only when I lie down in case I fall asleep."
4. "The best thing about this is that I can use it anywhere, anytime."

Answer: *4*

This question addresses the Client Needs category Psychosocial Integrity and the content addresses coping mechanisms. Focus on the subject, a characteristic of guided imagery. Guided imagery involves the client creating an image in the mind, concentrating on the image, and gradually becoming less aware of the offending stimulus. It can be done anytime and anywhere; some clients may use other relaxation techniques or play music with it.

blood products. Reduction of Risk Potential addresses content for preventing complications or health problems related to the client's condition or any prescribed treatments or procedures. Physiological Adaptation addresses content for managing and providing care to clients with acute, chronic, or life-threatening conditions. See Box 1-5 for examples of questions in this Client Needs category.

Integrated Processes

The NCSBN identifies five processes in the test plan that are fundamental to the practice of nursing. These processes are incorporated throughout the major categories of Client Needs. The Integrated Process subcategories are Caring, Communication and Documentation, Nursing Process (Assessment, Analysis, Planning, Implementation, and Evaluation),

BOX 1-5 Physiological Integrity

Basic Care and Comfort

A client with Parkinson's disease develops akinesia while ambulating, increasing the risk for falls. Which suggestion would the nurse provide to the client to alleviate this problem?

1. Use a wheelchair to move around.
2. Stand erect and use a cane to ambulate.
3. Keep the feet close together while ambulating and use a walker.
4. Consciously think about walking over imaginary lines on the floor.

Answer: *4*

This question addresses the subcategory Basic Care and Comfort in the Client Needs category Physiological Integrity and addresses client mobility and promoting assistance in an activity of daily living to maintain safety. Focus on the subject, akinesia. Clients with Parkinson's disease can develop bradykinesia (slow movement) or akinesia (freezing or no movement). Having these clients imagine lines on the floor to walk over can keep them moving forward while remaining safe.

Pharmacological and Parenteral Therapies

The nurse monitors a client receiving digoxin for which **early** manifestation of digoxin toxicity?

1. Anorexia
2. Facial pain
3. Photophobia
4. Yellow color perception

Answer: *1*

This question addresses the subcategory Pharmacological and Parenteral Therapies in the Client Needs category Physiological Integrity. Note the strategic word, *early.* Digoxin is a cardiac glycoside that is used to manage and treat heart failure and to control ventricular rates in clients with atrial fibrillation. The most common early manifestations of toxicity include gastrointestinal disturbances such as anorexia, nausea, and vomiting. Neurological abnormalities can also occur early and include fatigue, headache, depression, weakness, drowsiness, confusion, and nightmares. Facial pain, personality changes, and ocular disturbances

BOX 1-5 Physiological Integrity—cont'd

(photophobia, diplopia, light flashes, halos around bright objects, yellow or green color perception) are also signs of toxicity, but are not early signs.

Reduction of Risk Potential

A magnetic resonance imaging (MRI) study is prescribed for a client with a suspected brain tumor. The nurse would implement which action to prepare the client for this test?

1. Shave the groin for insertion of a femoral catheter.
2. Remove all metal-containing objects from the client.
3. Keep the client NPO (nothing by mouth) for 6 hours before the test.
4. Instruct the client in inhalation techniques for the administration of the radioisotope.

***Answer:* 2**

This question addresses the subcategory Reduction of Risk Potential in the Client Needs category Physiological Integrity, and the nurse's responsibilities in preparing the client for the diagnostic test. Focus on the **subject**, preparing a client for an MRI. In an MRI study, radiofrequency pulses in a magnetic field are converted into pictures. All metal objects, such as rings, bracelets, hairpins, and watches, should be removed. In addition, a history should be taken to ascertain whether the client has any internal metallic devices, such as orthopedic hardware, pacemakers, or shrapnel. A femoral catheter is not used for this diagnostic test. An intravenous (IV) catheter may be inserted if a contrast agent is prescribed. Additionally, shaving is not a common practice because of the risk for microabrasions and infection. If needed, hair may be clipped away from a surgical or insertion site. NPO status is not necessary for an MRI study of the head. Inhalation of the radioisotope may be prescribed with other types of scans but is not a part of the procedures for an MRI.

Physiological Adaptation

A client with renal insufficiency has a magnesium level of 3.5 mEq/L (1.44 mmol/L). On the basis of this laboratory result, the nurse interprets which sign as significant?

1. Hyperpnea
2. Drowsiness
3. Hypertension
4. Physical hyperactivity

***Answer:* 2**

This question addresses the subcategory Physiological Adaptation in the Client Needs category Physiological Integrity. It addresses an alteration in body systems. Focus on the **data in the question**. The normal magnesium level is 1.8 to 2.6 mEq/L (0.74 to 1.07 mmol/L). A magnesium level of 3.5 mEq/L (1.44 mmol/L). indicates hypermagnesemia. Neurological manifestations begin to occur when magnesium levels are elevated and are noted as symptoms of neurological depression, such as drowsiness, sedation, lethargy, respiratory depression, muscle weakness, and areflexia. Bradycardia and hypotension also occur.

Culture and Spirituality, and Teaching and Learning. See Box 1-6 for an example of a question that incorporates the Integrated Process of Caring.

Types of Questions on the Examination

The types of questions that may be administered on the examination include multiple-choice; fill-in-the-blank; multiple-response; ordered-response (also known as drag and drop); image (hot spot) questions; figure, chart/exhibit, or graphic option items; and audio formats. You may also be administered some Next Generation NCLEX® (NGN) questions, which may be a part of the NCSBN research study. A pilot study on NGN questions is being conducted by the NCSBN, and results demonstrate that there is an asymmetrical relationship between knowledge and clinical judgment; thus, recall of learned material is not translating to safety and efficacy in practice. This is the impetus behind these new item types. Research on these new item types is still being conducted. The candidate will be informed if the questions are research items and will be given the option to answer them or to decline. Regardless, you need to focus and use critical thinking and clinical judgment skills to answer these correctly.

BOX 1-6 Integrated Processes

A client is scheduled for angioplasty. The client says to the nurse, "I'm so afraid that it will hurt and will make me worse off than I am." Which response by the nurse is therapeutic?

1. "Can you tell me what you understand about the procedure?"
2. "Your fears are a sign that you really should have this procedure."
3. "Those are very normal fears, but please be assured that everything will be okay."
4. "Try not to worry. This is a well-known and easy procedure for the cardiologist."

***Answer:* 1**

This question addresses the subcategory Caring in the category of Integrated Processes. The correct option utilizes a **therapeutic communication technique** that explores the client's feelings, determines the level of client understanding about the procedure, and displays caring. Option 2 demeans the client and does not encourage further sharing by the client. Option 3 does not address the client's fears, provides false reassurance, and puts the client's feelings on hold. Option 4 diminishes the client's feelings by directing attention away from the client and toward the health care provider's importance.

These NGN question types will be accompanied by a single episode or unfolding case study and include extended multiple response, extended drag and drop, cloze (drop-down) enhanced hot spot (highlighting), and matrix/grid. These new item types are intended to evaluate a candidate's ability to utilize the dynamic skill of clinical judgment, rather than knowledge or recall alone.

Some questions may require you to use the mouse and cursor on the computer. For example, you may be presented with a picture that displays the arterial vessels of an adult client. In this picture, you may be asked to "point and click" (using the mouse) on the area (hot spot) where the dorsalis pedis pulse could be felt.

In all types of questions, the answer is scored as either right or wrong. Credit is not given for a partially correct answer. In addition, all question types may include pictures, graphics, tables, charts, or sound. The NCSBN provides specific directions for you to follow with all question types to guide you in your process of testing. Be sure to read these directions as they appear on the computer screen. Examples of some of these types of questions are noted in this chapter. All question types are provided in this book and on the accompanying Evolve site.

Multiple-Choice Questions

Many of the questions that you will be asked to answer will be in the multiple-choice format. These questions provide you with data about a client situation and four answers, or options.

Fill-in-the-Blank Questions

Fill-in-the-blank questions may ask you to perform a medication calculation, determine an intravenous flow rate, or calculate an intake or output record on a client. You will need to type only a number (your answer) in the answer box. If the question requires rounding the answer, this needs to be performed at the end of the calculation. The rules for rounding an answer are described in the tutorial provided by the NCSBN and are also provided in the specific question on the computer screen. In addition, you must type in a decimal point if necessary. See Box 1-7 for an example.

Multiple-Response Questions

For a multiple-response question, you will be asked to select or check all of the options, such as nursing interventions, that relate to the information in the question. In these question types, there may be 1 correct answer, there may be more than 1 correct answer, or all answers could be correct. No partial credit is given for correct selections. You need to do exactly as the question asks, which will be to select all of the options that apply. See Box 1-8 for an example.

BOX 1-7 Fill-in-the-Blank Question

A prescription reads: acetaminophen liquid, 650 mg orally every 4 hours PRN for pain. The medication label reads: 500 mg/15 mL. The nurse prepares how many milliliters to administer one dose? **Fill in the blank. Record your answer using one decimal place.**

***Answer:* 19.5 mL**

Formula:

$$\frac{Desired}{Available} \times volume = mL$$

$$\frac{650\,mg}{500\,mg} \times 15\,mL = 19.5\,mL$$

In this question, you need to focus on the **subject**, mL per dose, and use the formula for calculating a medication dose. When the dose is determined, you will need to type your numeric answer in the answer box. Always follow the specific directions noted on the computer screen. Also, remember that there will be an on-screen calculator on the computer for your use.

BOX 1-8 Multiple-Response Question

The emergency department nurse is caring for a child suspected of acute epiglottitis. Which interventions apply in the care of the child? **Select all that apply.**

- ☐ 1. Obtain a throat culture.
- ☑ 2. Auscultate lung sounds.
- ☑ 3. Prepare the child for a chest x-ray.
- ☐ 4. Maintain the child in a supine position.
- ☑ 5. Obtain a pediatric-size tracheostomy tray.
- ☑ 6. Place the child on an oxygen saturation monitor.

In a multiple-response question, you will be asked to select or check all of the options, such as interventions, that relate to the information in the question. Focus on the **subject**, interventions for the child with suspected acute epiglottitis. To answer this question, recall that acute epiglottitis is a serious obstructive inflammatory process that requires immediate intervention and that airway patency is a priority. Auscultating lung sounds allows the nurse to obtain information about airway patency without causing further airway compromise by examining the throat. Examination of the throat with a tongue depressor or attempting to obtain a throat culture is contraindicated because the examination can precipitate further obstruction. A lateral neck and chest x-ray is obtained to determine the degree of obstruction, if present. To reduce respiratory distress, the child should sit upright. The child is placed on an oxygen saturation monitor to monitor oxygenation status. Tracheostomy and intubation may be necessary if respiratory distress is severe. Remember to follow the specific directions given on the computer screen.

Ordered-Response Questions

In this type of question, you will be asked to use the computer mouse to drag and drop your nursing actions in order of priority. Information will be presented in a question and, based on the data, you need to determine what you will do first, second, third, and so forth. The unordered options will be located in boxes on the left side of the screen, and you need to move all options in order of priority to ordered-response boxes to the right side of the screen. Specific directions for moving the options are provided with the question. See Figure 1-1 for an example. These type of practice questions are located on the accompanying Evolve site.

Figure or Hot Spot Questions

A question with a picture or graphic will ask you to answer the question based on the picture or graphic. The question could contain a chart, a table, or a figure or illustration. You also may be asked to use the computer mouse to point and click on a specific area in the visual. A chart, table, figure, or illustration may appear in any type of question, including a multiple-choice question. See Box 1-9 for an example.

Chart/Exhibit Questions

In this type of question, you will be presented with a problem and a chart or exhibit. You will be provided with tabs or buttons that you need to click to obtain the information needed to answer the question. A prompt or message will appear that will indicate the need to click on a tab or button. See Box 1-10 for an example.

Graphic Item Option Questions

In this type of question, the option selections will be pictures rather than text. You will need to use the computer mouse to click on the option that represents your answer choice. See Box 1-11 for an example.

Audio Questions

Audio questions will require listening to a sound to answer the question. These questions will prompt you to use the headset provided and to click on the sound icon. You will be able to click on the volume button to adjust the volume to your comfort level, and you will be able to listen to the sound as many times as necessary. Content examples include, but are not limited to, various lung sounds, heart sounds, or bowel sounds. Examples of this question type are located on the accompanying Evolve site (Fig. 1-2).

Clinical Judgment and Next Generation NCLEX (NGN) Item Types

Clinical judgment is the observed outcome of critical thinking and decision-making (Dickison, Haerling, & Lasater, 2019). There is heightened attention being paid to clinical judgment as a means of teaching,

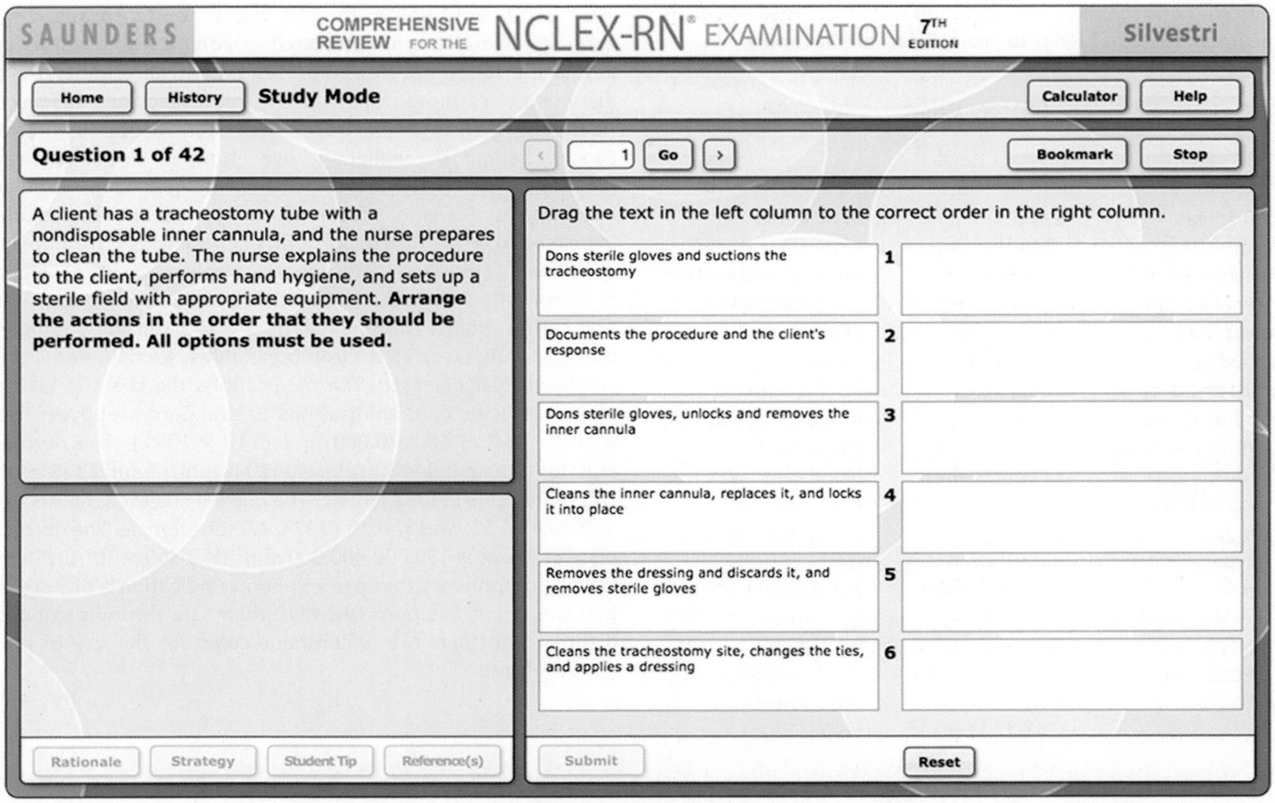

FIG. 1-1 Example of an ordered-response question.

BOX 1-9 Figure Question

A client who experienced a myocardial infarction is being monitored via cardiac telemetry. The nurse notes the sudden onset of this cardiac rhythm on the monitor **(refer to figure)** and **immediately** takes which action?

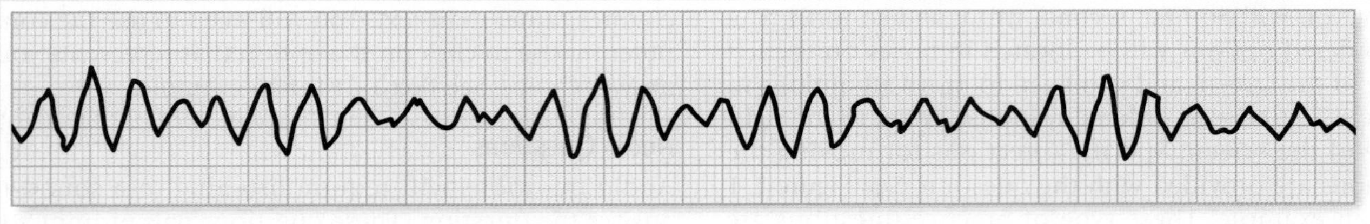

1. Takes the client's blood pressure
2. Initiates cardiopulmonary resuscitation (CPR)
3. Places a nitroglycerin tablet under the client's tongue
4. Continues to monitor the client and then contacts the cardiologist

***Answer:* 2**

This question requires you to identify the cardiac rhythm, and then determine the priority nursing action. Note the **strategic word**, *immediately*. This cardiac rhythm identifies a coarse ventricular fibrillation (VF). The goals of treatment are to terminate VF promptly and to convert it to an organized rhythm. The primary health care provider, cardiologist, or an Advanced Cardiac Life Support (ACLS)–qualified nurse must immediately defibrillate the client. If a defibrillator is not readily available, CPR is initiated until the defibrillator arrives. Options 1, 3, and 4 are incorrect actions and delay lifesaving treatment.

BOX 1-10 Chart/Exhibit Question

The nurse reviews the history and physical examination documented in the medical record of a client requesting a prescription for oral contraceptives. The nurse determines that oral contraceptives are contraindicated because of which documented items? **Refer to chart. Select all that apply.**

Client's Chart

History and Physical	Medications	Diagnostic Results
Item 1: Has admitting diagnosis of renal calculi	*Item 6:* Multivitamin orally daily	*Item 10:* Renal ultrasound shows no hydronephrosis, low probability of renal artery stenosis
Item 2: Past medical history: deep vein thrombosis with associated thrombophlebitis	*Item 7:* Lisinopril 40 mg orally daily	*Item 11:* Complete blood cell (CBC) shows white blood cells (WBC) 13,000 mm^3 ($13 \times 10^9/L$), hemoglobin (Hgb) 16 g/dL (60 mmol/L), hematocrit (Hct) 47% (0.47), platelets 490,000 mm^3 ($490 \times 10^9/L$)
Item 3: Hypertension	*Item 8:* Atorvastatin 10 mg orally daily	
Item 4: Hyperlipidemia	*Item 9:* Metformin 500 mg orally twice daily	
Item 5: Prediabetes		

***Answer:* Items 2, 3, 4, 11**

This chart/exhibit question provides you with data from the client's medical record. Focus on the **subject**, the item(s) that are a contraindication to the use of oral contraceptives. Oral contraceptives are contraindicated in women with a history of any of the following: thrombophlebitis and thromboembolic disorders, cardiovascular or cerebrovascular diseases (including stroke), any estrogen-dependent cancer or breast cancer, benign or malignant liver tumors, impaired liver function, hypertension, and diabetes mellitus with vascular involvement. Adverse effects of oral contraceptives include increased risk of superficial and deep venous thrombosis, pulmonary embolism, thrombotic stroke (or other types of strokes), myocardial infarction, and accelerations of preexisting breast tumors. Item 2 is a thromboembolic disorder with associated thrombophlebitis. Items 3 and 4 are cardiovascular diseases. The medications the client is taking are not specific contraindications to oral contraceptives. The normal WBC is 5000-10,000 mm^3 ($5\text{-}10 \times 10^9/L$). The normal Hgb for a male is 14-18 g/dL (140-180 mmol/L) and 12-16 g/dL (120-160 mmol/L) for a female. The normal Hct for a male is 42-52% (0.42-0.52) and 37-47% (0.37-0.47) for a female. The normal platelet count is 150,000-400,000 mm^3 ($150\text{-}400 \times 10^9/L$). Item 11 has components that present contraindications; of note is that this client has polycythemia, which is a thromboembolic disorder and therefore is contraindicated for the use of oral contraceptives.

BOX 1-11 Graphic Item Option Question

The nurse would place the client in which position to administer an enema? **(Refer to the figures in 1 to 4.)**

1. 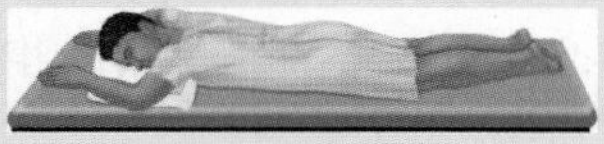

2. 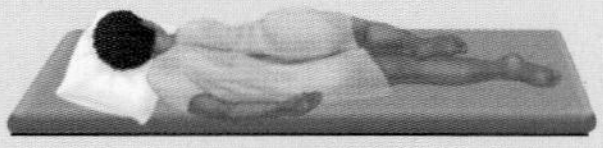

3. 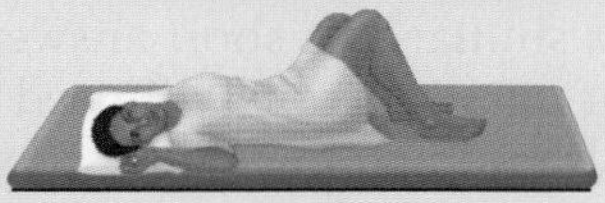

4. 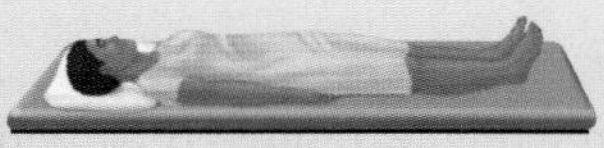

***Answer:* 2**

This question requires you to select the picture that represents your answer choice. Focus on the **subject**, the position for administering an enema. To administer an enema, the nurse assists the client into the left side-lying (Sims') position with the right knee flexed. This position allows the enema solution to flow downward by gravity along the natural curve of the sigmoid colon and rectum, improving the retention of solution. Option 1 is a prone position. Option 3 is a dorsal recumbent position. Option 4 is a supine position.

learning, assessment, and testing. The NCLEX-RN examination requires candidates to demonstrate the ability to use clinical judgment in the delivery of client care. Clinical judgment would also be used as a test-taking strategy to answer test questions (Refer to Chapter 4). The National Council of State Boards of Nursing (NCSBN) has created a Clinical Judgment Measurement Model (CJMM) that consists of applying 6 cognitive skills or processes. These include: (1) recognizing cues; (2) analyzing cues; (3) prioritizing hypotheses; (4) generating solutions; (5) taking action; and (6) evaluating outcomes (Dickison et al., 2019). See Table 1-3. This model also serves as a guide for the NCSBN to create Next Generation NCLEX (NGN) questions. The CJMM continues to evolve as may the NGN item types that will be presented in the exam. Currently, the test items that will be used are extended multiple response, extended drag and drop, cloze (drop-down), enhanced hot spot (highlighting), and matrix/grid. It is expected that the NGN test items will be scored items in the new test plan implemented in 2023. Some of these NGN item types can be found on the Evolve site accompanying this book. We highly encourage you to frequently access the NCSBN website at HYPERLINK "http://www.ncsbn.org" www.ncsbn.org for updates.

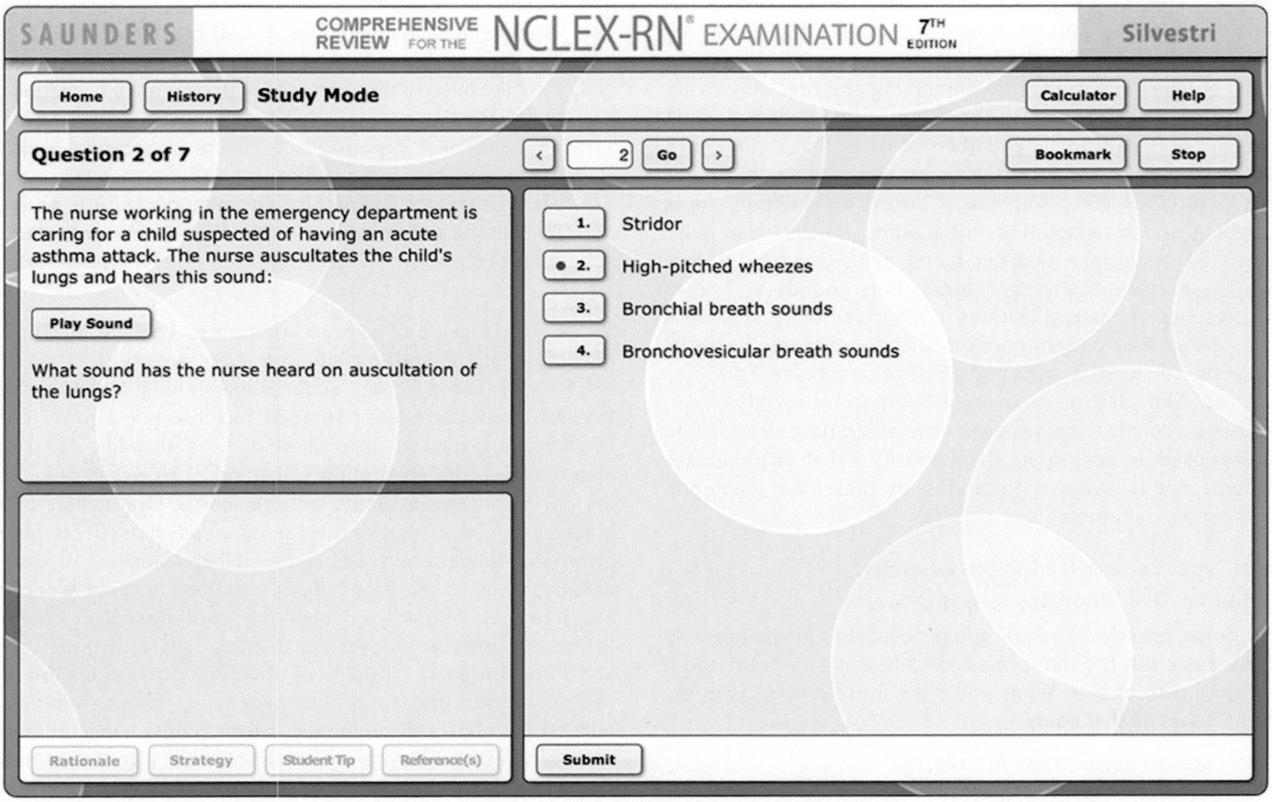

FIG. 1-2 Example of an audio question.

TABLE 1-3 Cognitive Skills/Processes and Descriptions

Cognitive Skill/ Process	Description
Recognize cues	Identifying significant data; data can be from many sources (assessment)
Analyze cues	Connecting data to the client's clinical presentation—determining is the data is expected? Unexpected? (analysis)
Prioritize hypotheses	Ranking hypotheses; what are the concerns or client needs/problems and their priority? (analysis)
Generate solutions	Using hypotheses to determine interventions for an expected outcome (planning)
Take action	Implementing the generated solutions addressing the highest priorities or hypotheses (implementation)
Evaluate outcomes	Comparing observed outcomes with expected ones (evaluation)

From Dickison, P., Haerling, K. A., & Lasater, K. (2019). Integrating the National Council of State Boards of Nursing Clinical Judgment Model into Nursing Educational Frameworks. *Journal of Nursing Education, 58*(2), 72–78.

Extended Multiple Response

This type is similar to a multiple response question in that it allows more than one option to be chosen. The difference is that an extended multiple-response question presents more options, from 7 to 10 options. An example of one way they may be presented can be located in Box 1-12.

CLOZE Item

The CLOZE item type is similar to a short-answer type question. In this type of question, you will need to select a response from a drop-down menu. See Box 1-12 for an example.

Extended Drag and Drop

There are various ways in which extended drag and drop question types will be presented. An extended drag and drop question will provide you with several pieces of specific information and will ask you to order that information into the correct order of action or placement. See Box 1-13 for an example.

BOX 1-12 NGN Items: Case Study With Extended Multiple Response and CLOZE Item

Victoria Machane, 76 years old, is brought to the emergency department by her son, Michael. Michael tells the nurse that Victoria has not been able to tolerate any physical activity and that when she tries to do something she tires very easily. Victoria began to experience shortness of breath and a cough that started this morning, and Michael states that his mother's skin looked pale and gray. On assessment, the nurse notes that Victoria exhibits shortness of breath on exertion; she is coughing and expectorating frothy white mucus. Her pulse rate is 102 beats/min, and her blood pressure is 164/98 mm Hg. The nurse auscultates Victoria's lung sounds and notes the presence of bilateral crackles in the lower lobes. Victoria is hospitalized. Her current home medications include betaxolol hydrochloride for glaucoma and glimepiride for type 2 diabetes mellitus. She also takes over-the-counter hydroxyaluminum sodium carbonate to help prevent acid indigestion. Heart failure is diagnosed. In addition to the medication that Victoria takes at home, the following medications are prescribed: captopril, furosemide, metoprolol, and digoxin.

Item Type: **Extended Multiple Response**
Cognitive Skill: **Prioritize Hypotheses**

The nurse reviews Victoria's admission data and prepares to collaborate with the interprofessional health care team about Victoria's plan of care. What would the nurse discuss with the team? **Select all that apply.**

1. Victoria's age as a risk for falls.
2. The need for respiratory treatments.
3. Victoria's inability to tolerate activity.
4. That the antacid could affect the absorption of digoxin.
5. That metoprolol may mask symptoms of hypoglycemia.
6. That the antacid must be used with caution in clients with glaucoma.
7. That potential systemic side effects of betaxolol hydrochloride include heart failure.
8. That betaxolol hydrochloride may contribute to hypertension when taken with the newly prescribed medications.

Answer: ***1, 2, 3, 4, 5, 7***

Victoria is 76 years of age. In addition to her age, her poor respiratory status and inability to tolerate activity place her at risk for falls. These factors require implementing a plan of care that will meet her needs. Antacids increase the digoxin level by increasing digoxin absorption or bioavailability. Antacids also decrease the absorption of captopril. However, antacids are not a concern in clients with glaucoma. Ophthalmic beta blockers can have additive therapeutic or adverse effects when given with systemically administered beta blockers or other cardiovascular medications. Toxic reactions to beta blockers are rare but primarily involve the cardiovascular system. Symptoms include bradycardia, cardiac failure, hypotension, and bronchospasm. Treatment involves discontinuation of the medication and supportive care (e.g., administration of adrenergic and anticholinergic medications). In addition, the nonselective beta blockers can interfere with the normal responses to hypoglycemia, such as tremor, tachycardia, and

BOX 1-12 NGN Items: Case Study With Extended Multiple Response and CLOZE Item—cont'd

nervousness, in essence masking the signs and symptoms of hypoglycemia. Hypotension is more likely than hypertension in clients taking beta-blocker medications.

On the following morning (day 2 of hospitalization), the nurse checks Victoria's vital signs and notes a blood pressure (BP) of 98/64 mm Hg and a heart rate of 62 beats per minute. On review of the laboratory data, the nurse notes the following:

Hemoglobin 14 g/dL (140 g/L)
Hematocrit 41% (0.41)
White blood cell count 7,000 mm^3 (7×10^9/L)
Sodium 145 mEq/L (145 mmol/L)
Potassium 3.6 mEq/L (3.6 mmol/L)
Blood urea nitrogen 20 mg/dL (7.1 mmol/L)
Creatinine 1.1 mg/dL (97 mcmol/L)
Blood glucose 99 mg/dL (5.5 mmol/L)

***Item Type:* CLOZE**

***Cognitive Skill:* Analyze Cues**

Which medication would be of **most** concern and require clarification prior to administration? **Complete the following sentences by choosing from the dropdown lists.**

The nurse should not administer the **(Select one)**

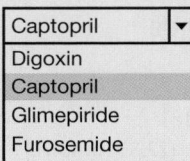

Captopril ▾
Digoxin
Captopril
Glimepiride
Furosemide

Because **(Select one)**

The BP is low ▾
The BP is low
The pulse is low
The blood glucose is low
The potassium level is low

Captopril is an angiotensin-converting enzyme (ACE) inhibitor. The main side/adverse effects of this medication are cough, hypotension, hyperkalemia, and tachycardia. Other side effects associated with ACE inhibitors include headache, dizziness, fatigue, insomnia, and weight loss. Victoria's BP is low at 98/64 mm Hg. Digoxin is a cardiac glycoside and would require clarification about administration if the pulse were below 60 beats per minute or if she were showing signs of toxicity. Victoria's pulse rate is 62 beats per minute. Glimepiride is used to manage blood glucose levels and would require clarification about administration if the blood glucose was low. Victoria's blood glucose is normal (normal level is 70 - 99 mg/dL [3.9 - 5.5 mmol/L]). Furosemide is a diuretic. Although the nurse would monitor for a drop in BP in the client receiving furosemide, the primary concern is hypokalemia. Victoria's potassium level is normal (normal level is 3.5-5.0 mEq/L [3.5-5.0 mmol/L]).

BOX 1-13 NGN Item: Extended Drag and Drop; Cognitive Skill: Generate Solutions

The nurse is preparing assignments for the day for the eight clients below and needs to assign clients to a registered nurse (RN), a licensed practical nurse (LPN), and an assistive personnel (AP). Drag each client to the **most appropriate** health care provider.

Clients

A client requiring a platelet transfusion.
A client requiring a colostomy irrigation.
A client receiving continuous tube feedings.
A client with respiratory failure on a mechanical ventilator.
A client who requires frequent ambulation and has a steady gait.
A client who requires a bed bath and range of motion exercises.
A client who requires hourly pulse and blood pressure measurements.
A client requiring abdominal wound irrigations and dressing changes every 3 hours.

Answer

RN Assignment	LPN Assignment	AP Assignment
A client requiring a platelet transfusion.	A client requiring a colostomy irrigation.	A client who requires frequent ambulation and has a steady gait.
A client with respiratory failure on a mechanical ventilator.	A client receiving continuous tube feedings.	A client who requires a bed bath and range-of-motion exercises.
	A client requiring abdominal wound irrigations and dressing changes every 3 hours.	A client who requires hourly pulse and blood pressure measurements.

The nurse must determine the most appropriate assignment based on the education and skills of the health care provider and the needs of the client. *In general,* noninvasive interventions,

BOX 1-13 NGN Item: Extended Drag and Drop; Cognitive Skill: Generate Solutions—cont'd

such as skin care, range-of-motion exercises, ambulation, grooming, and hygiene measures, can be assigned to the AP. *In general*, a LPN or vocational nurse (VN) can perform not only the tasks that a AP can perform but also certain invasive tasks, such as dressing changes, wound irrigations, tube feedings, colostomy irrigations, suctioning, urinary catheterization, and medication administration (oral, subcutaneous, intramuscular, and selected piggyback medications), according to the education and job description of the LPN or VN. The LPN or VN can also review with the client teaching plans that were initiated by the registered nurse. A registered nurse can perform the tasks that an LPN or VN can perform and is responsible for assessment and planning care, initiating teaching, and administering medications intravenously.

Enhanced Hot Spot (Highlighting)

These items present data pertinent to a client case, and asks the student to highlight the information that requires follow-up. See Box 1-14 for an example.

Matrix Items

These items present data regarding a client, and may ask the student to select actions that are essential, nonessential, and contraindicated. See Box 1-15 for an example.

BOX 1-14 NGN Item: Enhanced Hot Spot (Highlighting); Cognitive Skill: Recognize Cues

The nurse is assessing a male client admitted 1 day ago for newly diagnosed type 2 diabetes mellitus. Clinical findings are noted below.

	Current	12 hours ago	24 hours ago
Blood pressure	122/68 mmHg	128/70 mmHg	130/70 mmHg
Pulse	122 beats per minute (bpm)	110 bpm	108 bpm
Respirations	24 breaths per minute (bpm)	22 bpm	22 bpm
Oral temperature	36.2C (97.1F)	36.4C (97.5F)	36.2C (97.1F)
Capillary glucose	410 mg/dL (23.4 mmol/L)	360 mg/dL (20.57 mmol/L)	400 mg/dL (22.85 mmol/L)
Serum glucose	425 mg/dL(25.2 mmol/L)	360 mg/dL (20.57 mmol/L)	410 mg/dL(23.4 mmol/L)
Serum potassium	2.8 mEq/L (2.8 mmol/L)	3.2 mEq/L (3.2 mmol/L)	3.6 mEq/L (3.6 mmol/L)
Urine output	23 mL/hr	30 mL/hr	40 mL/hr

Which of the current findings requires ***immediate*** follow-up?

Click on the current findings that require immediate follow-up to highlight it. Highlight only findings that require follow-up. To deselect, click the finding again.

Answer:

	Current	12 hours ago	24 hours ago
Blood pressure	122/68 mmHg	128/70 mmHg	130/70 mmHg
Pulse	**122 bpm**	110 bpm	108 bpm
Respirations	**24 bpm**	22 bpm	22 bpm
Oral temperature	36.2C (97.1F)	36.4C (97.5F)	36.2C (97.1F)
Capillary glucose	**410 mg/dL(22.8 mmol/L)**	360 mg/dL(20.0 mmol/L)	400 mg/dL (22.3 mmol/L)
Serum glucose	**425 mg/dL(23.7 mmol/L)**	360 mg/dL(20.0 mmol/L)	410 mg/dL(22.8 mmol/L)
Serum potassium	**2.8mEq/L(2.8 mmol/L)**	3.2mEq/L(3.2 mmol/L)	3.6mEq/L(3.6 mmol/L)
Urine output	**23mL/hr**	36mL/hr	40mL/hr

With newly diagnosed type 2 diabetes mellitus, the client is at risk for diabetic ketoacidosis or hyperglycemic hyperosmolar nonketotic syndrome, both of which can lead to hypovolemia and shock. The blood pressure has remained stable for this client but is declining. At this time, it does not require further follow-up. The pulse rate has increased significantly since admission, and is a sign of hypovolemia, which is a finding that should be addressed. The respiratory rate is slightly elevated and should be addressed early on because this is a sensitive indicator of fluid status. The capillary glucose and serum glucose levels at each of the timepoints has been elevated, and an intervention is required to address this abnormality. The serum potassium level was within the normal range initially but has decreased since admission and is now at a critical level. This could be due to the client's treatment, which likely involves insulin. This requires follow-up because of the risks associated with hypokalemia. The urine output has steadily decreased and could be an indicator of hypovolemia, and therefore requires follow-up. The temperature is normal and does not require follow-up.

BOX 1-15 NGN Item: Matrix Item; Cognitive Skill: Take Action

The nurse notes that there has been an increase in the number of central-line–associated blood stream infections (CLABSIs) that developed in the clients being cared for on the nursing unit. How would the nurse proceed to implement a quality improvement program? **For each action below, click or mark with an X to specify whether the action would be:**

Indicated: An action that the nurse would take to resolve the problem
Nonessential: An action that the nurse could take without harming the client, but the action would not be likely to address the problem
Contraindicated: An action that could harm the client and would not be taken

Action	Indicated	Nonessential	Contraindicated
1 Collect identifying client information			X
2 Note the mental status of the client		X	
3 Note primary and secondary diagnoses of client's affected	X		
4 Note the type and location of IV catheter used	X		
5 Note the type of IV dressings being used	X		
6 Note the medication types being infused		X	
7 Note frequency of assessments of IV sites	X		
8 Note the expected duration of the IV site		X	
9 Note care procedures to the IV site	X		
10 Note frequency of changing IV sites	X		

Quality improvement, also known as performance improvement, focuses on processes or systems that significantly contribute to client safety and effective client care outcomes; criteria are used to monitor outcomes of care and to determine the need for change to improve the quality of care. If the nurse notes a particular problem, such as an increase in the CLABSIs, the nurse should collect data about the problem. This should include information such as the primary and secondary diagnoses of the clients developing the infection, the type and location of IV catheters being used, the site of the catheter, IV site dressings being used, frequency of assessment and methods of care to the IV site, and length of time that the IV catheter was inserted. Once these data are collected and analyzed, the nurse should examine evidence-based practice protocols to identify the best practices for care to IV sites to prevent infection. These practices can then be implemented and followed by evaluation of results based on the evidence-based practice protocols used. Collecting identifying client information is contraindicated because of client confidentiality and is unnecessary in this quality improvement effort. Noting the mental status of the client can be done but is not likely to address the problem. Noting the types of medications being infused can also be done but will not address the problem of IV site infection. Although it is helpful to know the expected duration of the IV site, this information does not change infection control practices in managing the IV site and is therefore considered a nonessential action.

Case Studies (Testlets) and NGN Items

Case Studies and NGN Item Types are included in this resource and can be located in the Evolve site accompanying this book. These are specially designed to simulate the NCLEX experience of testing for these Next Generation NCLEX (NGN) Item Types. Refer to the Evolve site for practice with these question types.

The NCSBN Practice Test Questions for the NCLEX

The NCSBN provides a practice test for candidates that is composed of previously used NCLEX questions that are no longer a part of the NCLEX. This exam simulates the look of the real exam and provides the candidate with practice for the NCLEX. This practice test can be purchased through the NCSBN at www.ncsbn.org

Registering to Take the Examination

It is important to obtain an NCLEX Examination Candidate Bulletin from the NCSBN Web site at www.ncsbn.org, because this bulletin provides all of the information you need to register for and schedule your examination. It also provides you with Web site and telephone information for NCLEX examination contacts. The initial step in the registration process is to submit an application to the state board of nursing in the state in which you intend to obtain licensure. You need to obtain information from the board of nursing regarding the specific registration process, because the process may vary from state to state. Then, use the NCLEX Examination Candidate Bulletin as your guide to complete the registration process.

Following the registration instructions and completing the registration forms precisely and accurately are important. Registration forms not properly completed or not accompanied by the proper fees in the required method of payment will be returned to you and will delay testing. You must pay a fee for taking the examination; you also may have to pay additional fees to the board of nursing in the state in which you are applying.

Authorization to Test Form and Scheduling an Appointment

Once you are eligible to test, you will receive an Authorization to Test (ATT) form. You cannot make an appointment until you receive an ATT form. Note the validity dates on the ATT form, and schedule a testing date and time before the expiration date on the ATT form. The NCLEX Examination Candidate Bulletin provides you with the directions for scheduling an appointment; you do not have to take the examination in the same state in which you are seeking licensure.

The ATT form contains important information, including your test authorization number, candidate identification number, and validity date. You need to take your ATT form to the testing center on the day of your examination. You will not be admitted to the examination if you do not have it.

Changing Your Appointment

If for any reason you need to change your appointment to test, you can make the change on the candidate Web site or by calling candidate services. Refer to the NCLEX Examination Candidate Bulletin for this contact information and other important procedures for canceling and changing an appointment. If you fail to arrive for the examination or fail to cancel your appointment to test without providing appropriate notice, you will forfeit your examination fee and your ATT form will be invalidated. This information will be reported to the board of nursing in the state in which you have applied for licensure, and you will be required to register and pay the testing fees again.

Day of the Examination

It is important that you arrive at the testing center at least 30 minutes before the test is scheduled. If you arrive late for the scheduled testing appointment, you may be required to forfeit your examination appointment. If it is necessary to forfeit your appointment, you will need to reregister for the examination and pay an additional fee. The board of nursing will be notified that you did not take the test. A few days before your scheduled date of testing, take the time to drive to the testing center to determine its exact location, the length of time required to arrive at that destination, and any potential obstacles that might delay you, such as road construction, traffic, or parking sites.

In addition to the ATT form, you must have proper identification (ID) such as a U.S. driver's license, passport, U.S. state ID, or U.S. military ID to be admitted to take the examination. All acceptable identification must be valid and not expired and contain a photograph and signature (in English). In addition, the first and last names on the ID must match the ATT form. According to the NCSBN guidelines, any name discrepancies require legal documentation, such as a marriage license, divorce decree, or court action legal name change. Refer to the NCLEX Examination Candidate Bulletin for acceptable forms of identification.

Testing Accommodations

If you require testing accommodations, you should contact the board of nursing before submitting a registration form. The board of nursing will provide the procedures for the request. The board of nursing must authorize testing accommodations. Following board of nursing approval, the NCSBN reviews the requested accommodations and must approve the request. If the request is approved, the candidate will be notified and provided the procedure for registering for and scheduling the examination.

Testing Center

The testing center is designed to ensure complete security of the testing process. Strict candidate identification requirements have been established. You may be required to wear a mask and follow other safety and social distancing guidelines and will also be asked to read the rules related to testing. A digital fingerprint and palm vein print will be taken. A digital signature and photograph will also be taken at the testing center. These identity confirmations will accompany the NCLEX exam results. In addition, if you leave the testing room for any reason, you may be required to perform these identity confirmation procedures again to be readmitted to the room.

Personal belongings are not allowed in the testing room; all electronic devices must be placed in a sealable bag provided by the test administrator and kept in a locker. Any evidence of tampering with the bag could result in the need to report the incident and test cancellation. A locker and locker key will be provided for you; however, storage space is limited, so you must plan accordingly. In addition, the testing center will not assume responsibility for your personal belongings. The testing waiting areas are generally small; friends or family members who accompany you are not permitted to wait in the testing center while you are taking the examination.

Once you have completed the admission process, the test administrator will escort you to the assigned computer. You will be seated at an individual workspace area that includes computer equipment, appropriate lighting, an erasable note board, and a marker. No items, including unauthorized scratch paper, are allowed into the testing room. Eating, drinking, or the use of tobacco is not allowed in the testing room. You will be observed at all times by the test administrator while taking the examination. In addition, video and audio recordings of all test sessions are made. The testing center has no control over the sounds made by typing on the computer by others. If these sounds are distracting, raise your hand to summon the test administrator. Earplugs are available on request.

You must follow the directions given by the testing center staff and must remain seated during the test except when authorized to leave. If you think that you have a problem with the computer, need a clean note board, need to take a break, or need the test administrator for any reason, you must raise your hand. You are also encouraged to access the NCSBN candidate Web site to obtain additional information about the physical environment of the testing center and to view a virtual tour of the testing center.

Testing Time

The maximum testing time is 6 hours; this period includes the tutorial, the sample items, all breaks, and the examination. All breaks are optional. The first optional break will be offered after 2 hours of testing. The second optional break is offered after 3.5 hours of testing. Remember that all breaks count against testing time. If you take a break, you must leave the testing room, and when you return you may be required to perform identity confirmation procedures to be readmitted. Note that modifications in testing time may be made due to the COVID-19 pandemic.

Length of the Examination

The minimum number of questions that you will need to answer is 75. Of these 75 questions, 60 will be operational (scored) questions and 15 will be pretest (unscored) questions. The maximum number of questions in the test is 265.

The pretest questions are questions that may be presented as scored questions on future examinations. These pretest questions are not identified as such. In other words, you do not know which questions are the pretest (unscored) questions; however, these pretest (unscored) questions will be administered among the first 75 questions in the test. Note that modifications in the exam length may be made due to the COVID-19 pandemic; modifications do not make the test harder or affect reliability or validity in determining your competence.

Pass-or-Fail Decisions

All examination questions are categorized by test plan area and level of difficulty. This is an important point to keep in mind when you consider how the computer makes a pass-or-fail decision, because a pass-or-fail decision is not based on a percentage of correctly answered questions.

The NCSBN indicates that a pass-or-fail decision is governed by three different scenarios. The first scenario is the 95% Confidence Interval Rule, in which the computer stops administering test questions when it is 95% certain that the test-taker's ability is clearly above the passing standard or clearly below the passing standard. The second scenario is known as the Maximum-Length Exam, in which the final ability estimate of the test-taker is considered. If the final ability estimate is above the passing standard, the test-taker passes; if it is below the passing standard, the test-taker fails.

The third scenario is the Run-Out-Of-Time (R.O.O.T) Rule. If the examination ends because the test-taker ran out of time, the computer may not have enough information with 95% certainty to make a clear pass-or-fail decision. If this is the case, the computer will review the test-taker's performance during testing. If the test-taker has not answered the minimum number of required questions, the test-taker fails. If the test-taker's ability estimate was consistently above the passing standard on the last 60 questions, the test-taker passes. If the test-taker's ability estimate falls below the passing standard, even once, the test-taker fails. Additional information about pass-or-fail decisions can be found in the NCLEX Examination Candidate Bulletin located at www.ncsbn.org.

Completing the Examination

When the examination has ended, you will complete a brief computer-delivered questionnaire about your testing experience. After you complete this questionnaire, you need to raise your hand to summon the test administrator. The test administrator will collect and inventory all note boards and then permit you to leave.

Processing Results

Every computerized examination is scored twice, once by the computer at the testing center and again after the examination is transmitted to the test scoring center. No results are released at the testing center; testing center staff do not have access to examination results. The board of nursing receives your result, and your result will be mailed to you approximately 6 weeks after you take the examination. In some states, an unofficial result can be obtained via the Quick Results Service 2 business days after taking the examination. There is a fee for this service, and information about obtaining your NCLEX result by this method can be obtained on the NCSBN Web site under candidate services.

Candidate Performance Report

A candidate performance report is provided to a test-taker who failed the examination. This report provides the test-taker with information about her or his strengths and weaknesses in relation to the test plan framework and provides a guide for studying and retaking the examination. If a retake is necessary, the candidate must wait 45 days between examination administration, depending on state procedures. Test-takers should refer to the state board of nursing in the state in which licensure is sought for procedures regarding when the examination can be taken again.

Interstate Endorsement and Nurse Licensure Compact

Because the NCLEX-RN examination is a national examination, you can apply to take the examination in any state. When licensure is received, you can apply for interstate endorsement, which is obtaining another license in another state to practice nursing in that state. The procedures and requirements for interstate endorsement may vary from state to state, and these procedures can be obtained from the state board of nursing in the state in which endorsement is sought. It may be possible to practice nursing in another state under the mutual recognition model of nursing licensure if the state has enacted a Nurse Licensure Compact. To obtain information about the Nurse Licensure Compact and the states that are part of this interstate compact, access the NCSBN Web site at www.ncsbn.org.

The Foreign-Educated Nurse

An important first step in the process of obtaining information about becoming a registered nurse in the United States is to access the NCSBN Web site at www.ncsbn.org and obtain information provided for international nurses in the NCLEX Web site link. The NCSBN provides information about some of the documents you need to obtain as an international nurse seeking licensure in the United States and about credentialing agencies. Refer to Box 1-16 for a listing of some of these documents. The NCSBN also provides information regarding the requirements for education and English proficiency, and immigration requirements such as visas and VisaScreen. You are encouraged to access the NCSBN Web site to obtain the most current information about seeking licensure as a registered nurse in the United States.

An important factor to consider as you pursue this process is that some requirements may vary from state to state. You need to contact the board of nursing in the state in which you are planning to obtain licensure to determine the specific requirements and documents that you need to submit.

Boards of nursing can decide either to use a credentialing agency to evaluate your documents or to review your documents at the specific state board, known as in-house evaluation. When you contact the board of nursing in the state in which you intend to work as a nurse, inform them that you were educated

BOX 1-16 Foreign-Educated Nurse: Some Documents Needed to Obtain Licensure

1. Proof of citizenship or lawful alien status
2. Work visa
3. VisaScreen certificate
4. Commission on Graduates of Foreign Nursing Schools (CGFNS) certificate
5. Criminal background check documents
6. Official transcripts of educational credentials sent directly to credentialing agency or board of nursing from home country school of nursing
7. Validation of a comparable nursing education as that provided in U.S. nursing programs; this may include theoretical instruction and clinical practice in a variety of nursing areas including, but not limited to, medical nursing, surgical nursing, pediatric nursing, maternity and newborn nursing, community and public health nursing, and mental health nursing
8. Validation of safe professional nursing practice in home country
9. Copy of nursing license or diploma or both
10. Proof of proficiency in the English language
11. Photograph(s)
12. Social Security number
13. Application and fees

outside of the United States and ask that they send you an application to apply for licensure by examination. Be sure to specify that you are applying for registered nurse (RN) licensure. You should also ask about the specific documents needed to become eligible to take the NCLEX exam. You can obtain contact information for each state board of nursing through the NCSBN Web site at www.ncsbn.org. In addition, you can write to the NCSBN regarding the NCLEX exam. The address is 111 East Wacker Drive, Suite 2900, Chicago, IL 60601. The telephone number for the NCSBN is 1-866-293-9600; international telephone is 011 1 312 525 3600; the fax number is 1-312-279-1032.

CHAPTER 2

Pathways to Success

Laurent W. Valliere, BS, DD

The Pyramid to Success

Preparing to take the NCLEX-RN® examination can produce a great deal of anxiety. You may be thinking that this exam is the most important test you will ever have to take and that it reflects the culmination of everything you have worked so hard for. This is an important examination because receiving your nursing license means that you can begin your career as a registered nurse. Your success on this exam involves freeing yourself of all thoughts that allow this examination to appear overwhelming and intimidating. Such thoughts can take complete control over your destiny. A strong positive attitude, a structured plan for preparation, and maintaining control in your pathway to success ensure reaching the peak of the Pyramid to Success (Fig. 2-1).

Pathways to Success (Box 2-1)

Foundation

The foundation of pathways to success begins with a strong positive attitude, the belief that you will achieve success, and developing self-control. It also includes developing a list of your personal short-term and long-term goals and a plan for preparation. Without these components, your pathway to success leads to nowhere and has no endpoint. You will expend energy and valuable time in your journey, lack control over where you are heading, and experience exhaustion without any accomplishment.

Where do you start? To begin, find a location that offers solitude. Sit or lie in a comfortable position, close your eyes, relax, inhale deeply, hold your breath to a count of 4, exhale slowly, and, again, relax. Repeat this breathing exercise several times until you feel relaxed, free from anxiety, and in control of your destiny. Allow your mind to become void of all mind chatter; now you are in control and your mind's eye can see for miles. Next, reflect on all that you have accomplished and the path that brought you to where you are today. Keep a journal of your reflections as you plan the order of your journey through the Pyramid to Success.

List

It is time to create the "List." The List is your set of short-term and long-term goals. Begin by developing the goals that you wish to accomplish today, tomorrow, over the next month, and in the future. Allow yourself the opportunity to list all that is flowing from your mind. Write your goals in your personal journal. When the List is complete, put it away for 2 or 3 days. After that time, retrieve and review the List and begin the process of planning to prepare for the NCLEX-RN exam.

Plan for Preparation

Now that you have the List in order, look at the goals that relate to studying for the licensing exam. The first task is to decide what study pattern works best for you. Think about what has worked most successfully for you in the past. Questions that must be addressed to develop your plan for study are listed in Box 2-2.

The plan must include a schedule. Use a calendar to plan and document the daily times and nursing content areas for your study sessions. Establish a realistic schedule that includes your daily, weekly, and future goals, and stick to your plan of study. This consistency will provide advantages to you and the people supporting you. You will develop a rhythm that can enhance your retention and positive momentum. The people who are supporting you will share this rhythm and be able to schedule their activities and lives better when you are consistent with your study schedule.

The length of the study session depends on your ability to focus and concentrate. You need to think about quality rather than quantity when you are deciding on a realistic amount of time for each session. Plan to schedule at least 2 hours of quality study time daily. If you can spend more than 2 hours, by all means do so.

You may ask, "What do you mean by quality study time?" Quality study time means spending uninterrupted quiet time at your study session. This may mean that you have to isolate yourself for these study sessions. Think again about what has worked for you during nursing school when you studied for examinations; select a study place that has worked for you in the past.

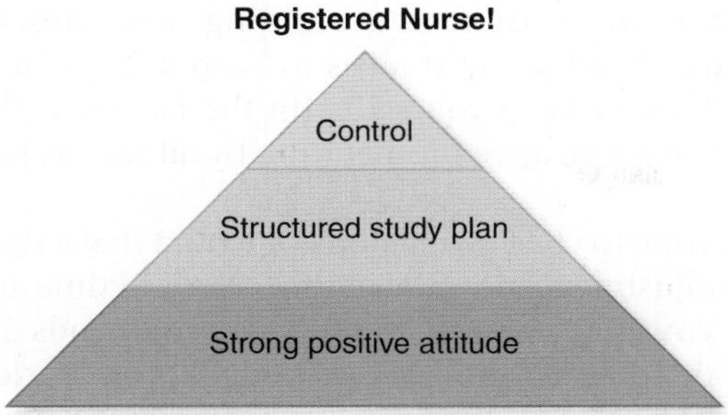

FIG. 2-1 Pyramid to Success.

BOX 2-1 Pathways to Success

Foundation
Maintaining a strong positive attitude
Thinking about short-term and long-term realistic goals
Developing a plan for preparation
Maintaining control

List
Writing short-term and long-term realistic goals in a journal

Plan for Preparation
Developing a study plan and schedule
Deciding on the place to study
Balancing personal and work obligations with the study schedule
Sharing the study schedule and personal needs with others
Implementing the study plan

Positive Pampering
Planning time for exercise and fun activities
Establishing healthy eating habits
Including activities in the schedule that provide positive mental stimulation

Final Preparation
Reviewing and identifying goals achieved
Remaining focused to complete the plan of study
Writing down the date and time of the examination and posting it next to your name with the letters "RN" following, and the word "YES!"
Planning a test drive to the testing center
Engaging in relaxing activities on the day before the examination

Day of the Examination
Grooming yourself for success
Eating a nutritious breakfast
Maintaining a confident and positive attitude
Maintaining control—breathe and focus
Meeting the challenges of the day
Reaching the peak of the Pyramid to Success

If you have a special study room at home that you have always used, plan your study sessions in that special room. If you have always studied at a library, plan your study sessions at the library. Sometimes it is difficult to balance your study time with your family obligations and possibly a work schedule, but, if you can, plan your study time when you know that you will be at home alone. Try to eliminate anything that may be distracting during your study time. Silence your cellphone appropriately so that you will not be disturbed. If you have small children, plan your study time during their nap time or during their school hours.

BOX 2-2 Developing a Plan for Study

Do I work better alone or in a study group?
If I work best in a group, how many study partners should I have?
Who are these study partners?
How long should my study sessions last?
Does the time of day that I study make a difference? Do I retain more if I study in the morning?
How does my work schedule affect my study pattern?
How do I balance my family obligations with my need to study?
Do I have a comfortable study area at home or should I find another environment that is conducive to my study needs?

Your plan must include how you will manage your study needs with your other obligations. Your family and friends are key players in your life and are going to become part of your Pyramid to Success. After you have established your study needs, communicate your needs and the importance of your study plan to your family and friends.

A difficult part of the plan may be how to deal with family members and friends who choose not to participate in your plan for success. For example, what do you do if a friend asks you to go to a movie and it is your scheduled study time? Your friend may say, "Take some time off. You have plenty of time to study. Study later when we get back!" You are faced with a decision. You must weigh all factors carefully. You must keep your goals in mind and remember that your need for positive momentum is critical. Your decision may not be an easy one, but it must be one that will ensure that your goal of becoming a registered nurse is achieved.

Positive Pampering

Positive pampering means that you must continue to care for yourself holistically. Positive momentum can be maintained only if you are properly balanced. Proper exercise, diet, and positive mental stimulation are crucial to achieving your goal of becoming a registered nurse. Just as you have developed a schedule for study, you should have a schedule that includes fun and physical activity. It is your choice—aerobics, walking, weight lifting, bowling, or whatever makes you feel good about yourself. Time spent away from the hard study schedule and devoted to some fun and physical exercise pays you back a hundredfold. You will be more energetic with a schedule that includes these activities.

Establish healthy eating habits. Be sure to drink plenty of water, which will flush and clean your body cells. Stay away from fatty foods because they slow you down. Eat lighter meals and eat more frequently. Include complex carbohydrates such as oatmeal or whole grain foods in your diet for energy, and be careful not to include too much caffeine in your daily diet.

Take the time to pamper yourself with activities that make you feel even better about who you are. Make dinner reservations at your favorite restaurant with someone who is special and is supporting your goal. Take walks in a place that has a particular tranquility that enables you to reflect on the positive momentum that you have achieved and maintained. Whatever it is, wherever it takes you, allow yourself the time to do some positive pampering.

Final Preparation

You have established the foundation of your Pyramid to Success. You have developed your list of goals and your study plan, and you have maintained your positive momentum. You are moving forward, and in control. When you receive your date and time for the NCLEX-RN examination, you may immediately think, "I am not ready!" Stop! Reflect on all you have achieved. Think about your goal achievement and the organization of the positive life momentum with which you have surrounded yourself. Think about all of the people who love and support your effort to become a registered nurse. Believe that the challenge that awaits you is one that you have successfully prepared for and will lead you to your goal of becoming a registered nurse.

Take a deep breath and organize the remaining days so that they support your educational and personal needs. Support your positive momentum with a visual technique. Write your name in large letters, and write the letters "RN" after it. Post 1 or more of these visual reinforcements in areas that you frequent. This is a visual motivational technique that works for many nursing graduates preparing for this examination.

It is imperative that you not fall into the trap of expecting too much of yourself. The idea of perfection must not drive you to a point that causes your positive momentum to falter. You must believe and stay focused on your goal. The date and time are at hand. Write the date and time, and underneath write the word "YES!" Post this next to your name plus "RN."

Ensure that you have command over how to get to the testing center. A test run is a must. Time the drive, and allow for road construction or other factors that might occur to slow traffic down. On the test run, when you arrive at the test facility, walk into it and become familiar with the lobby and the surroundings. This may help alleviate some of the peripheral nervousness associated with entering an unknown building. Remember that you must do whatever it takes to keep yourself in control. If familiarizing yourself with the facility will help you maintain positive momentum, by all means be sure to do so.

It is time to check your study plan and make the necessary adjustments now that a firm date and time are set. Adjust your review so that your study plan ends 2 days before the examination. The mind is like a muscle. If it is overworked, it has no strength or stamina. Your strategy is to rest the body and mind on the day before the examination. Your strategy is to stay in control and allow yourself the opportunity to be absolutely fresh and attentive on the day of the examination. This will help you control the nervousness that is natural, achieve the clear thought processes required, and feel confident that you have done all that is necessary to prepare for and conquer this challenge. The day before the examination is to be one of pleasure. Treat yourself to what you enjoy the most.

Relax! Take a deep breath, hold to a count of 4, and exhale slowly. You have prepared yourself well for the challenge of tomorrow. Allow yourself a restful night's sleep, and wake up on the day of the examination knowing that you are absolutely prepared to succeed. Look at your name with "RN" after it and the word "YES!"

Day of the Examination (Box 2-3)

Wake up believing in yourself and that all you have accomplished is about to propel you to the professional level of registered nurse. Allow yourself plenty of time, eat a nutritious breakfast, and groom yourself for success. You are ready to meet the challenges of the day and overcome any obstacle that may face you. Today will soon be history, and tomorrow will bring you the envelope on which you read your name with the words "Registered Nurse" after it.

Be proud and confident of your achievements. You have worked hard to achieve your goal of becoming a registered nurse. If you believe in yourself and your goals, no one person or obstacle can move you off the pathway that leads to success! Congratulations, and I wish you the very best in your career as a registered nurse!

BOX 2-3 Day of the Examination

Breathe: Inhale deeply, hold your breath to a count of 4, exhale slowly.
Believe: Have positive thoughts today and keep those thoughts focused on your achievements.
Control: You are in command.
Believe: This is your day.
Visualize: "RN" with your name.

This Is Not a Test

1. What are the factors needed to ensure a productive study environment? **Select all that apply.**
   1. Secure a location that offers solitude.
   2. Plan breaks during your study session.
   3. Establish a realistic study schedule that includes your goals.
   4. Continue with the study pattern that has worked best for you.

Answer: 1, 2, 3, 4
Rationale: A location of solitude helps to ensure concentration. Taking breaks during your study session helps to clear your mind and increase your ability to concentrate and focus. Establishing a realistic study pattern will keep you in control. Do not vary your study pattern. It has been successful for you, so why change now?

2. What are key factors in your final preparation? **Select all that apply.**
   1. Remain focused on the study plan.
   2. Visualize the "RN" after your name.
   3. Avoid studying on the day before the exam and relax.
   4. Know where the testing center is and how long it takes to get there.

Answers: 1, 2, 3, 4
Rationale: Focus on your plan of study and success will follow. Enact positive reinforcement: Write your name in large letters on a piece of paper with "RN" after your name and post it where you will see it often. Allow yourself a day of pampering before the test. Wake up on the day of the test refreshed and ready to succeed. Ensure that you know where the testing center is; map out your route and the average time it takes to arrive.

3. What key points do the "Pathways to Success" emphasize to help ensure your success? **Select all that apply.**
   1. A strong positive attitude
   2. Believing in your ability to succeed
   3. Being proud and confident in your achievements
   4. Maintaining control of your mind, surrounding environment, and physical being

Answers: 1, 2, 3, 4
Rationale: A strong *positive attitude* leads to success. *Believe* in who you are and the goals you have set for yourself. Be *"proud and confident."* If you believe in yourself, you will achieve success. *Maintain control,* and all of your goals are attainable.

Your grade: A+
Continue to "Believe" and you will succeed.
RN belongs to you!

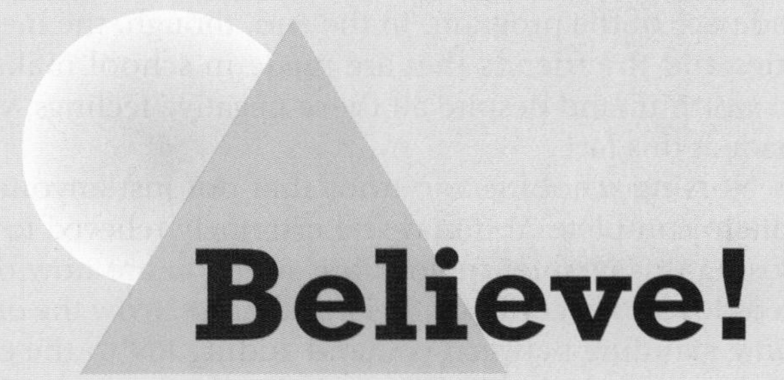

CHAPTER 3

The NCLEX-RN® Examination: From a Graduate's Perspective

Katherine M. Silvestri, BSN, RN

Congrats new grad! You made it through nursing school…that place where you can get a question on an exam wrong even if your answer is correct, *BUT* just not the most correct. You have more than likely endured several trying challenges during the program with moments of intense self-doubt due to the difficult content and pace of the program. In the end, though, the memories and the friends that are made in school make it all worth it, and despite all those negative feelings, you made it this far!

Nursing school is a journey that not just anyone is able to complete. You may feel extremely relieved to be closing this chapter in your life, and you are now one step closer to becoming a registered nurse. Now the only thing standing between you and adding RN to the end of your name is the NCLEX. Spending late nights studying and stressing over tests and sterile technique has become the new norm during your nursing program; however, the NCLEX is an exam in its own league. It is important to remember that nursing school has been preparing you to take this test throughout its entirety. Taking the NCLEX can be a less stressful experience by preparing yourself throughout nursing school and not just once you schedule a testing date.

While in my nursing program, I strongly disliked studying for exams by going back through chapters I had already read for lecture. My mind would always wander, and I would get distracted because that study method does not engage my mind to think about material in a different way. I would prepare for my lecture exams, and also for my standardized exams, by doing practice questions from the *Saunders RN-Q&A Review for the NCLEX-RN®*, paying close attention to the rationales while taking down succinct notes. By looking at the content area codes I was also able to organize my notes into different sections, which was extremely helpful when I had an exam coming up on a certain subject. I also paid close attention to the test-taking strategy. I came to find if I happened upon a question that I was not sure on, I was able to use the strategies I learned to narrow down the options and arrive at the correct answer. Half the battle is figuring out what exactly a question is trying to ask you, and reading the test-taking strategy was helpful in allowing me to focus in on the subject of the question. I feel studying in this manner during my program made taking the NCLEX a much less stressful experience.

Applying to take the NCLEX is quite the process. I applied through the Nevada State Board of Nursing. I had to make an appointment to get my fingerprints taken at the state board office, which I was able to do while I was still in my nursing program. An application also has to be filled out and turned in, along with an application fee. Doing these two steps as early as possible is important, as getting the paperwork processed can take a few weeks to a few months. Then, once I graduated and received my degree, I sent in my official transcripts to the state board, as this must be done to receive your authorization to test (ATT) from a third-party testing administrator called Pearson Vue. Once you turn in your information to your state board, it will be sent to Pearson Vue, who will then contact you with your ATT once everything is verified. This requirement may vary from state to state. I remember waiting to get my ATT to be the most frustrating part of the application process. I would check my e-mail obsessively multiple times a day, refreshing it and hoping that magical e-mail with ATT in the subject line would pop up. At this point, it was early August, and the day I finally got my ATT I rushed home to look for the earliest available test date. The Las Vegas testing center was booked until the end of September. I had already been studying for several weeks doing at least 300 practice questions a day and I was frustrated. I did not want to wait more than a month to take the exam.

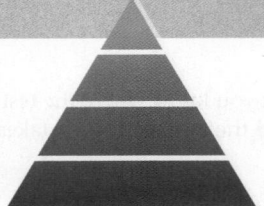

I then began the search for testing centers in neighboring states, including Arizona, Utah, and California. I even went so far as to look at testing centers in Washington state. No luck in Arizona, Utah, or Washington. I found a date in a testing center in California about 4.5 hours away. The testing appointment was for the next day. I called my sister to ask for her advice on signing up for it, and she told me to just go for it. I had been preparing for the exam for at least the past several weeks and I felt I was ready. I booked the appointment, hoping I had not just made a terrible mistake. My sister and cousin said they would ride with me and help me review on the way. The appointment was for 2:00 PM, so we made a plan to leave Las Vegas at 5:00 AM to make sure we had plenty of time. I packed a travel bag with a change of clothes and toiletries, as we planned to go to a workout class before the exam. We arrived near the testing center at about 9:30 AM and worked out for an hour and showered. I was dropped off at the testing center about an hour ahead of the scheduled exam time to give me ample time to check in. I remember three other people in the office when I had checked in. It was clear to me that not everyone was there for the NCLEX, and so I made it a point to not become anxious if I saw one or all of them get up and leave before me. The anxiety level in the room was tangible as we all sat and waited for our names to be called. I brought my driver's license and had to verify my ATT. My picture was taken, and I was told to put my belongings in a locker. A palm vein scan was done and then I was being brought into the testing room. I sat down at the computer with my heart racing. There was a camera beside the computer that was watching my every move. All the hard work I had put in the past 16 months had led me to this moment. I had to remind myself to take a deep breath and just relax. I clicked the button to begin the exam.

The hardest part for me during the exam was to not read each question too quickly because of my anxiety. Remember to slow down, take a deep breath, and recenter yourself, and say something positive in your head, then reapproach the question if you find yourself lost in what the question is asking or getting overwhelmed. I relied on the test-taking strategies I had learned while studying to help me analyze what the question was really asking. I felt the questions were getting harder and harder, and the one thought in my head was, "How am I getting this many select-all-that-apply questions?!" The computer shut down when I submitted question 75, and I did not know what to think. I spent the ride home thinking about all the questions I was not sure about and soon enough I was feeling anxiety about questions I thought I should have answered differently. However, I knew at the end of the day I did the best I could, and it was out of my hands now.

I took the NCLEX on Friday, and Sunday I had the option to view my exam results early on the National Council of State Boards of Nursing (NCSBN) website for a small fee. I remember entering my debit card information, and I had to have my sister click submit because I could not bring myself to do it. I shut my eyes while the screen loaded, and to my relief, it said I had passed! I was now a registered nurse. I could not believe it. All of my hard work had brought me to this point, and since I now had RN next to my name, the next task was to find a job to put my practice into play. I went to a career fair for "Experienced RNs" with my two nursing school friends, and all three of us got hired despite being new graduates. As a new graduate RN, I learn something new every day at work and love the nursing profession. Now that you are done, you will notice that even in regard to everyday matters, you will be thinking like a nurse and you might not realize it. I have caught myself doing it on multiple occasions and assessing random people I see in public.

A few important things to remember, both as a nursing student and as a new graduate RN: Do tasks in a way that works best for you and stick with it, do not be too hard on yourself, do not be afraid to ask questions (there is no stupid question), and do not give up. I have had days both in nursing school and in my career where I thought to myself, "Is this really worth it?" The answer is yes. You will grow immensely as a human being. I remember being scared to even turn a patient or give a bed bath in my fundamentals course, and now I have the strength to hold a deteriorating patient's hand and look in their eyes as they are rushed to the intensive care unit after I assessed the patient was in distress. As a nurse, you are in the position to care for sick people who will remember your face and the way you made them feel for the rest of their lives. The impact you have as a nurse is bigger than you realize. Nursing is not an easy profession, but your passion has brought you this far, and it will bring you farther than you can imagine. Congratulations on making it this far, and good luck on the NCLEX and your future career! As a nurse, you will make a difference wherever you go!

CHAPTER 4

Test-Taking Strategies

If you would like to read more about test-taking strategies after completing this chapter, *Saunders Strategies for Test Success: Passing Nursing School and the NCLEX® Exam* focuses on the test-taking strategies that will help you pass your nursing examinations while in nursing school and will prepare you for the NCLEX-RN® examination.

I. Clinical Judgment

Clinical judgment is the observed outcome of critical thinking and decision-making (Dickison et al., 2019). The NCLEX-RN examination requires candidates to demonstrate the ability to use clinical judgment in client care. Thus, clinical judgment skills along with other traditional test-taking strategies should be used to answer test questions. The National Council of State Boards of Nursing (NCSBN) has created a Clinical Judgment Measurement Model (CJMM) that consists of applying 6 cognitive skills or processes: (1) recognizing cues; (2) analyzing cues; (3) prioritizing hypotheses; (4) generating solutions; (5) taking action; and (6) evaluating outcomes. See Chapter 1, Table 1.1 for a description of these six cognitive skills/processes. Also see Box 4-24 for an example of how to apply the six cognitive skills/processes when answering test questions (from Dickison P, Haerling KA, Lasater K: Integrating the NCSBN Clinical Judgment Model into Nursing Educational Frameworks. *J Nurs Educ* 58[2]:72–78, 2019).

II. Key Test-Taking Strategies (Box 4-1)

III. How to Avoid Reading into the Question (Box 4-2)

A. Pyramid points

1. Avoid asking yourself the forbidden words, "Well, what if …?" because this will lead you to the "forbidden" area: reading into the question.
2. Focus only on the data in the question, read every word, and make a decision about what the question is asking. Recognize cues presented in the question. Reread the question more than one time; ask yourself, "What is this question asking?" and "What content is this question testing?"
3. Determine whether an abnormality exists. Look at data or information in the question and in the responses and decide what is significant. What

BOX 4-1 Key Test-Taking Strategies

The Question

- Focus on the data or information, read every word, recognize cues, and make a decision about what the question is asking.
- Note the subject and determine what content is being tested.
- Visualize the event; analyze cues and note if an abnormality exists in the data provided.
- Determine who "the client of the question" is.
- Look for the strategic words; strategic words make a difference regarding what the question is asking about and prioritizing hypotheses.
- Think about the client's presenting situation and needs to generate solutions and determine which actions to take.
- Determine whether the question presents a positive or negative event query; negative event queries are usually most associated with the skill of evaluating outcomes.
- Avoid asking yourself, "Well, what if …?" because this will lead you to reading into the question.
- Apply the Clinical Judgment Measurement Model (CJMM) and the 6 cognitive skills/processes alongside other test-taking strategies.

The Options

- Always use the process of elimination when choices or options are presented and read each option carefully; once you have eliminated options, reread the question before selecting your final choice or choices.
- Look for comparable or alike options and eliminate these.
- Determine whether there is an umbrella or encompassing option; if so, this could be the correct option.
- Identify any closed-ended words; if present, the option is likely incorrect.
- Use the ABCs—airway, breathing, and circulation—Maslow's Hierarchy of Needs, and the steps of the Nursing Process to answer questions that require prioritizing.
- Use therapeutic communication techniques to answer communication questions and remember to focus on the client's thoughts, feelings, concerns, anxieties, and fears.
- Use delegating and assignment-making guidelines to match the client's needs with the scope of practice of the health care provider.
- Use pharmacology guidelines to select the correct option if the question or options address a medication.

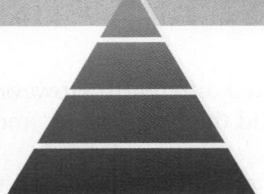

BOX 4-2 Practice Question: Avoiding the "What if ...?" Syndrome and Reading into the Question

The nurse is caring for a hospitalized client with a diagnosis of heart failure who suddenly complains of shortness of breath and dyspnea during activity. After assisting the client to bed and placing the client in high-Fowler's position, the nurse would take which **immediate** action?

1. Administer high-flow oxygen to the client.
2. Call the consulting cardiologist to report the findings.
3. Prepare to administer an additional dose of furosemide.
4. Obtain a set of vital signs and perform focused respiratory and cardiovascular assessments.

Answer: 4

Test-Taking Strategy: This question measures the cognitive skill, take action. You may immediately think that the client has developed pulmonary edema, a complication of heart failure, and needs additional diuresis. In pulmonary edema, you may see this as an emergency, and might think an action should be taken before further assessment, which may lead you to choose option 3. Although pulmonary edema is a complication of heart failure, the question does not specifically state that pulmonary edema has developed; the client could be experiencing shortness of breath or dyspnea as a symptom of heart failure exacerbation, which may be expected, particularly on exertion or during activity. This is why it is important to base your answer only on the information presented, without assuming something else could be occurring. Read the question carefully. Note the strategic word, *immediate*, and focus on the data in the question, the client's complaints. Use the nursing process, and note that vital signs and assessment data would be needed before administering oxygen, administering medications, or contacting the cardiologist. Although the cardiologist may need to be notified, this is not the immediate action. Because there are no data in the question that indicate the presence of pulmonary edema, option 4 is correct. Additionally, focus on what the question is asking. The question is asking you for a nursing action, so that is what you need to look for as you eliminate the incorrect options. Use nursing knowledge and test-taking strategies to assist in answering the question. Remember to focus on the data in the question, focus on what the question is asking, and avoid the "What if ...?" syndrome and reading into the question.

is abnormal data? Analyze the cues. Pay close attention to this information as you read the question and as you answer the question.

4. Focus on the client in the question. At times, there are other people discussed in the question who also impact how the question should be answered. Remember the concepts of client-centered and family-centered care.
5. Look for the strategic words in the question, such as *immediate, initial, first, priority, initial, best, need for follow-up,* and *need for further teaching;* strategic words make a difference regarding what the question is asking and will assist in prioritizing hypotheses.
6. Consider available resources as you generate solutions and answer the question. Remember that you will have all resources you need at the client's bedside to provide quality client care.
7. In multiple-choice questions, multiple-response questions, extended multiple response questions, matrix-type questions, CLOZE questions, or questions that require you to arrange nursing interventions or other data in order of priority (drag and drop or extended drag and drop), read every choice or option presented before answering.
8. *Always* use the process of elimination when choices or options are presented; after you have eliminated options, reread the question before selecting your final choice or choices. Focus on the data in both the question and the options to assist in the process of elimination and directing you to the correct answer. In taking action questions, think about the client's presentation and needs to answer correctly. In evaluating outcomes questions, read carefully especially if the question is asking which option indicates the need for further teaching or follow-up.
9. With questions that require you to fill in the blank or complete a sentence (CLOZE question), focus on the data in the question and determine what the question is asking; if the question requires you to calculate a medication dose, an intravenous flow rate, or intake and output amounts, recheck your work in calculating and always use the on-screen calculator to verify the answer.

B. Ingredients of a question (Box 4-3)

1. The ingredients of a question include the event, which is a client or clinical situation; the event query; and the options or answers.
2. The event provides you with the content about the client or clinical situation that you need to think about when answering the question.
3. The event query asks something specific about the content of the event.
4. The options are all of the answers provided with the question.
5. Traditional NCLEX® test questions
   - **a.** In a multiple-choice question, there will be 4 options and you must select 1; read every option carefully and think about the event and the event query as you use the process of elimination.
   - **b.** In a multiple-response question, there will be several options (up to 6) and you must select all options that apply to the event in the question. The correct answer could be

BOX 4-3 Ingredients of a Question: Event, Event Query, and Options

Event

The nurse is caring for a client with terminal cancer.

Event Query

The nurse would consider which factor when planning pain relief?

Options

1. Not all pain is real.
2. Opioid analgesics are highly addictive.
3. Opioid analgesics can cause tachycardia.
4. Around-the-clock dosing gives better pain relief than as-needed dosing.

Answer: 4

Test-Taking Strategy: Focus on **what the question is asking**, the factor to consider when planning pain relief, and consider the client's diagnosis of terminal cancer. Around-the-clock dosing provides increased pain relief and decreases stressors associated with pain, such as anxiety and fear. Pain is what the client describes it as, and any indication of pain should be perceived as real for the client. Opioid analgesics may be addictive, but this is not a concern for a client with terminal cancer. Not all opioid analgesics cause tachycardia. Remember to focus on **what the question is asking.**

only one of the options, *all* of the options, *or* any number of the total options provided. Visualize the event, and use your nursing knowledge and clinical experiences to answer the question.

c. In an ordered-response (prioritizing)/drag-and-drop question, you will be required to arrange in order of priority nursing actions or other data; visualize the event and use your nursing knowledge and clinical experiences to answer the question. These questions are usually related to nursing procedures.

d. A fill-in-the-blank question does not contain options, and some figure/illustration questions and audio item formats may or may not contain options. A graphic option item will contain options in the form of a picture or graphic.

e. A chart/exhibit question will most likely contain options; read the question carefully and all of the information in the chart or exhibit before selecting an answer. In this question type, there will be information in the chart/exhibit that is pertinent to how the question is answered, and there may also be information that is not pertinent. Read all of the information in the chart before answering. It is necessary to discern what information is important and what the "distractors" are.

6. Next Generation NCLEX® (NGN) Item Types

a. The NGN item types will use a case study approach and accompanying test questions will be designed to assess the six cognitive skills identified in the CJMM developed by the NCSBN.

b. There will be single episode case studies and unfolding case studies.

c. Single episode case studies will be accompanied by a test question that will most likely assess only 1 of the cognitive skills. Note that there may be some single episode case studies that will be accompanied by 2 test questions assessing 2 of the cognitive skills.

d. Unfolding case studies will be accompanied by six test questions in which all 6 cognitive skills are assessed.

e. It is important to read all of the data in the case study and look for abnormalities in the information presented before answering the accompanying questions.

f. Use nursing knowledge and clinical experiences to assist in answering the questions.

g. Currently, the NGN item types include enhanced hot spot (highlighting), extended multiple response, extended drag and drop, matrix, and cloze. Examples of these NGN item types can be located on the Evolve site accompanying this book.

IV. Strategic Words (Boxes 4-4 and 4-5)

A. Strategic words focus your attention on a critical point to consider when answering the question and will assist you in eliminating the incorrect options. These words can be located in either the event or the query of the question.

B. Some strategic words may indicate that all options are correct and that it will be necessary to prioritize to select the correct option; words that reflect the process of assessment or recognizing cues are also important to note (see Box 4-4). Words that reflect assessment usually indicate the need to look for an option that is a first step, since assessment is the first step in the nursing process.

C. As you read the question, look for the strategic words; strategic words make a difference regarding the focus of the question. Throughout this book, *strategic words* presented in the question, such as those that indicate the need to prioritize, are bolded. If the test-taking strategy is to focus on *strategic words,* then *strategic words* is highlighted in blue where it appears in the test-taking strategy.

BOX 4-4 Common Strategic Words: Words That Indicate the Need to Prioritize and Words That Reflect Assessment

Words That Indicate the Need to Prioritize

Best
Early or late
Essential
First
Highest priority
Immediate
Initial
Most
Most appropriate
Most important
Most likely
Next
Primary
Vital

Words That Reflect Assessment

Ascertain
Assess
Check
Collect
Determine
Find out
Gather
Identify
Monitor
Observe
Obtain information
Recognize

BOX 4-5 Practice Question: Strategic Words

The nurse is caring for a client who just returned from the recovery room after undergoing abdominal surgery. The nurse would monitor for which **early** sign of hypovolemic shock?

1. Sleepiness
2. Increased pulse rate
3. Increased depth of respiration
4. Increased orientation to surroundings

***Answer:* 2**

Test-Taking Strategy: Note the strategic word, *early*, in the query and the word *just* in the event. Think about the pathophysiology that occurs in hypovolemic shock to recognize cues. Restlessness is one of the earliest signs followed by cardiovascular changes (increased heart rate and a decrease in blood pressure). Sleepiness is expected in a client who has just returned from surgery. Although increased depth of respirations occurs in hypovolemic shock, it is not an early sign. Rather, it occurs as the shock progresses. This is why it is important to recognize the strategic word, *early*, when you read the question. It requires the ability to discern between early and late signs of impending shock. Increased orientation to surroundings is expected and will occur as the effects of anesthesia resolve. Remember to look for strategic words, in both the event and the query of the question.

BOX 4-6 Practice Question: Subject of the Question

The nurse is teaching a client in skeletal leg traction about measures to increase bed mobility. Which item would be **most** helpful for this client?

1. Television
2. Fracture bedpan
3. Overhead trapeze
4. Reading materials

***Answer:* 3**

Test-Taking Strategy: This question measures the cognitive skill, generate solutions. Focus on the subject, increasing bed mobility. Also note the strategic word, *most*. The use of an overhead trapeze is extremely helpful in assisting a client to move about in bed and to get on and off the bedpan. Television and reading materials are helpful in reducing boredom and providing distraction, and a fracture bedpan is useful in reducing discomfort with elimination; these items are helpful for a client in traction, but they are not directly related to the subject of the question. Remember to focus on the subject.

V. Subject of the Question (Box 4-6)

A. The subject of the question is the specific topic or what the question is asking about.

B. Identifying the subject of the question will assist in eliminating the incorrect options and direct you in selecting the correct option. Throughout this book, if the *subject* of the question is a specific strategy to use in answering the question correctly, it is highlighted in blue in the test-taking strategy.

C. The highlighting of the strategy will provide you with guidance on what strategies to review in *Saunders Strategies for Test Success: Passing Nursing School and the NCLEX® Exam*.

VI. Positive and Negative Event Queries (Boxes 4-7 and 4-8)

A. A positive event query uses strategic words that ask you to select an option that is correct; for example, the event query may read, "Which statement by a client *indicates an understanding* of the side effects of the prescribed medication?"

B. A negative event query uses strategic words that ask you to select an option that is an incorrect item or statement; for example, the event query may read, "Which statement by a client *indicates a need for further teaching* about the side effects of the prescribed medication?"

VII. Questions That Require Prioritizing

A. Many questions on the examination will require you to use the skill of prioritizing hypotheses or nursing actions.

B. Look for the strategic words in the question that indicate the need to prioritize (see Box 4-4).

BOX 4-7 Practice Question: Positive Event Query

The nurse provides medication instructions to a client about digoxin. Which statement by the client indicates an understanding of its adverse effects?

1. "Blurred vision is expected."
2. "If my pulse rate drops below 60 beats per minute, I should let my cardiologist know."
3. "This medication may cause headache and weakness but that is nothing to worry about."
4. "If I am nauseated or vomiting, I should stay on liquids and take some liquid antacids."

Answer: 2

Test-Taking Strategy: This question is an example of a positive event query question and measures the cognitive skill evaluate outcomes. Note the words *indicates an understanding*, and focus on the subject, adverse effects. Additionally, focus on the data provided in the options. Digoxin is a cardiac glycoside and works by increasing contractility of the heart. This medication has a narrow therapeutic range, and is a major concern is toxicity. Currently, it is considered second-line treatment for heart failure because of its narrow therapeutic range and potential for adverse effects. Adverse effects that indicate toxicity include gastrointestinal disturbances, neurological abnormalities, bradycardia or other cardiac irregularities, and ocular disturbances. If any of these occur, the cardiologist is notified. Additionally, the client should notify the cardiologist if the pulse rate drops below 60 beats per minute, because serious dysrhythmias are another potential adverse effect of digoxin therapy. Remember to focus on the data provided and note positive event queries.

BOX 4-8 Practice Question: Negative Event Query

The nurse has reinforced discharge instructions to a client who has undergone a right mastectomy with axillary lymph node dissection. Which statement by the client indicates a need for further teaching regarding home care measures?

1. "I should use a straight razor to shave under my arms."
2. "I need to be sure that I do not have blood pressures or blood drawn from my right arm."
3. "I should inform all of my other health care providers that I have had this surgical procedure."
4. "I need to be sure to wear thick mitt hand covers or use thick pot holders when I am cooking and touching hot pans."

Answer: 1

Test-Taking Strategy: This question is an example of a negative event query and measures the cognitive skill evaluate outcomes. Note the strategic words, *need for further teaching*. These strategic words indicate that you need to select an option that identifies an incorrect client statement. Recall that edema and infection are concerns with this client due to the removal of lymph nodes in the surgical area. Lymphadenopathy with associated lymphedema can result, and the client needs to be instructed in the measures that will avoid trauma to the affected arm. Recalling that trauma to the affected arm could potentially result in edema and/or infection will direct you to the correct option. Remember to watch for negative event queries.

C. Remember that when a question requires prioritization, all options may be correct and you need to determine the correct order of action.

D. Strategies to use to prioritize include the ABCs (airway–breathing–circulation), Maslow's Hierarchy of Needs theory, and the steps of the nursing process and the cognitive skills in he CJMM focusing on what the question is asking.

E. The ABCs (Box 4-9)

1. Use the ABCs—airway–breathing–circulation—when selecting an answer or determining the order of priority.
2. Remember the order of priority: airway–breathing–circulation.
3. Airway is always the first priority. Note that an exception occurs when cardiopulmonary resuscitation is performed; in this situation, the nurse follows the CAB (compressions/circulation–airway–breathing) guidelines.

F. Maslow's Hierarchy of Needs theory (Box 4-10; Fig. 4-1)

1. According to Maslow's Hierarchy of Needs theory, physiological needs are the priority, followed by

BOX 4-9 Practice Question: Use of the ABCs

A client with a diagnosis of cancer is receiving morphine sulfate for pain. The nurse would employ which **priority** action in the care of the client?

1. Monitor stools.
2. Monitor urine output.
3. Encourage fluid intake.
4. Encourage the client to cough and deep breathe.

Answer: 4

Test-Taking Strategy: This question measures the cognitive skill, take action. Use the ABCs—airway, breathing, circulation—as a guide to direct you to the correct option and note the strategic word, *priority*. Recall that morphine sulfate suppresses the cough reflex and the respiratory reflex, and a common adverse effect is respiratory depression. Coughing and deep breathing can assist with ensuring adequate oxygenation, since the number of respirations per minute can potentially be decreased in a client receiving this medication. Although options 1, 2, and 3 are components of the plan of care, the correct option addresses airway and breathing. Remember to use the ABCs—airway, breathing, circulation—to prioritize.

BOX 4-10 Practice Question: Maslow's Hierarchy of Needs Theory

The nurse caring for a client experiencing dystocia determines that the **priority** is which action?

1. Position changes and providing comfort measures
2. Explanations about what is happening to the client
3. Monitoring for changes in the condition of the mother and fetus
4. Reinforcement of breathing techniques learned in childbirth preparatory classes

***Answer:* 3**

Test-Taking Strategy: This question measures the cognitive skill, prioritizing hypotheses. All the options are correct and would be implemented during the care of this client. Note the strategic word, *priority*, and use Maslow's Hierarchy of Needs theory to prioritize, remembering that physiological needs come first. Also, the correct option is the only one that addresses both the mother and the fetus. Remember to use Maslow's Hierarchy of Needs theory to prioritize.

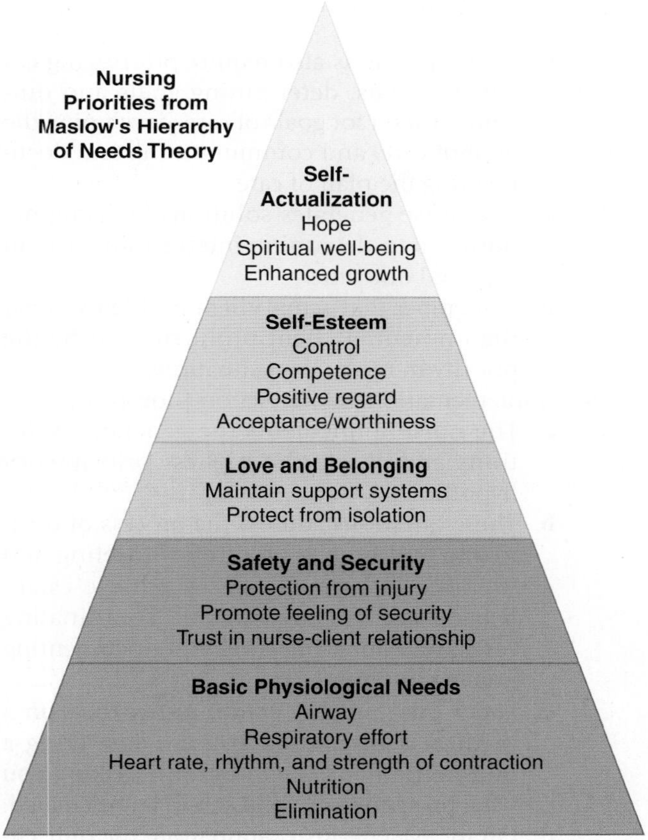

FIG. 4-1 Use Maslow's Hierarchy of Needs theory to establish priorities.

safety and security needs, love and belonging needs, self-esteem needs, and, finally, self-actualization needs; select the option or determine the order of priority by addressing physiological needs first.

2. When a physiological need is not addressed in the question or noted in one of the options, continue to use Maslow's Hierarchy of Needs theory sequentially as a guide and look for the option that addresses safety.

G. Steps of the nursing process and CJMM and Cognitive Skills

1. The steps of the nursing process include assessment, analysis, planning, implementation, and evaluation (AAPIE) and are followed in this order.
2. Assessment/Recognize Cues
   - **a.** The nurse recognizes cues by identifying significant data from many sources
   - **b.** These questions address the process of gathering subjective and objective data and cues relative to the client and the client's problem, confirming the data, and communicating and documenting the data.
   - **c.** Remember that assessment/recognizing cues is a first step.
   - **d.** When you are asked to select your first, immediate, or initial nursing action, assess and recognize cues *first* to prioritize when selecting the correct option.
   - **e.** Look for strategic words in the options that reflect data collection (assessment)/recognizing cues (see Box 4-4).
   - **f.** If an option contains the concept of assessment or the collection of client data, the best choice is to select that option. (Box 4-11)

BOX 4-11 Practice Question: The Nursing Process—Assessment

A client who had an application of a right arm cast complains of pain at the wrist when the arm is passively moved. What action would the nurse take **first?**

1. Elevate the arm.
2. Document the findings.
3. Medicate with an additional dose of an opioid.
4. Check for paresthesias and paralysis of the right arm.

***Answer:* 4**

Test-Taking Strategy: This question measures the cognitive skill, take action. Note the strategic word, *first*. Based on the data in the question, determine whether an abnormality exists. The question event indicates that the client complains of pain at the wrist when the arm is passively moved. This could indicate an abnormality; therefore, the nurse needs to take action and further assessment or intervention is required. Use the steps of the nursing process, remembering that assessment is the first step. The only option that addresses assessment is the correct option. Options 1, 2, and 3 address the implementation step of the nursing process. Also, these options are incorrect first actions. The arm in a cast should have already been elevated. The client may be experiencing compartment syndrome, a complication following trauma to the extremities and application of a cast. Additional data need to be collected to determine whether this complication is present. Remember that assessment is the first step in the nursing process.

g. Possible exception to the guideline—if the question presents an emergency situation, read carefully; in an emergency situation, an action may be the priority rather than taking the time to collect further data.

3. Analysis/Analyze Cues (Box 4-12)
   a. The nurse analyzes cues by connecting significant data to the client's clinical presentation and determining: is the data expected? Unexpected? What are the concerns?
   b. These questions are the most difficult questions because they require understanding of the principles of physiological responses and require interpretation of the data collected.
   c. They require critical thinking and decision-making and determining the rationale for therapeutic prescriptions or actions that may be addressed in the question.
   d. These questions may address the formulation of a hypothesis that identifies a client need or problem and may also include the communication and documentation of the results from the process of the analyzing cues.
4. Planning/Prioritizing Hypotheses and Generating Solutions (Box 4-13)
   a. These questions require the nurse to prioritize hypotheses (concerns, client needs) by ranking the hypotheses from highest to lowest priority

BOX 4-12 Practice Question: The Nursing Process—Analysis

The nurse reviews the arterial blood gas results of a client and notes the following: pH 7.45, Pco_2 30 mm Hg, and HCO_3 22 mEq/L (22 mmol/L). The nurse analyzes these results as indicating which condition?

1. Metabolic acidosis, compensated
2. Respiratory alkalosis, compensated
3. Metabolic alkalosis, uncompensated
4. Respiratory acidosis, uncompensated

***Answer:* 2**

Test-Taking Strategy: Use the steps of the nursing process and analyze cues, the blood gas values. The question does not require further assessment; therefore, it is appropriate to move to the next step in the nursing process, analysis. The normal pH is 7.35 to 7.45. In a respiratory condition, an opposite effect will be seen between the pH and the Pco_2. In this situation, the pH is at the high end of the normal value and the Pco_2 is low. So, you can eliminate options 1 and 3. In an alkalytic condition, the pH is elevated. The values identified indicate a respiratory alkalosis. Compensation occurs when the pH returns to a normal value. Because the pH is in the normal range at the high end, compensation has occurred. Remember that analysis is the second step in the nursing process.

BOX 4-13 Practice Question: The Nursing Process—Planning

The nurse developing a plan of care for a client with a cataract understands that which problem is the **priority?**

1. Concern about the loss of eyesight
2. Altered vision due to opacity of the ocular lens
3. Difficulty moving around because of the need for glasses
4. Becoming lonely because of decreased community immersion

***Answer:* 2**

Test-Taking Strategy: Note the strategic word, *priority*, and use the steps of the nursing process. This question relates to prioritizing hypotheses and planning nursing care and asks you to identify the priority problem. Use Maslow's Hierarchy of Needs theory to answer the question, remembering that physiological needs are the priority. Concern and becoming lonely are psychosocial needs and would be the last priorities. Note that the correct option directly addresses the client's problem. Remember that planning is the third step of the nursing process.

   b. These questions also require prioritizing client problems, determining goals and outcome criteria for goals of care, developing the plan of care, and communicating and documenting the plan of care.
   c. The nurse generates solutions by using hypotheses to determine interventions for an expected outcome.
   d. Remember that actual client problems rather than potential client problems will be the priority in most client situations.
5. Implementation/Taking Action (Box 4-14)
   a. The nurse implements the generated solutions addressing the highest priorities or hypotheses.
   b. These questions address the process of organizing and managing care, counseling and teaching, providing care to achieve established goals, supervising and coordinating care, and communicating and documenting nursing interventions.
   c. Focus on a nursing action rather than on a medical action when you are answering a question, unless the question is asking you what prescribed medical action is anticipated.
   d. On the NCLEX-RN examination, the only client whom you need to be concerned about is the client in the question that you are answering; avoid the "What if ...?" syndrome and remember that the client in the question on the computer screen is your only assigned client.
   e. Answer the question from a textbook and ideal point of view; remember that the nurse has all of the time and all of the equipment

BOX 4-14 Practice Question: The Nursing Process—Implementation

The nurse is caring for a hospitalized client with angina pectoris who begins to experience chest pain. The nurse administers a nitroglycerin tablet sublingually as prescribed, but the pain is unrelieved. The nurse would take which action **next?**

1. Reposition the client.
2. Call the client's family.
3. Contact the health care provider.
4. Administer another nitroglycerin tablet.

***Answer:* 4**

***Test-Taking Strategy*:** This question measures the cognitive skill, take action. Note the strategic word, *next*, and use the steps of the nursing process. Implementation questions address the process of organizing and managing care. This question also requires that you prioritize nursing actions. Additionally, focus on the data in the question to assist in avoiding reading into the question. You may think it is necessary to check the blood pressure before administering another tablet, which is correct. However, there are no data in the question indicating that the blood pressure is abnormal and could not sustain if another tablet were given. In addition, checking the blood pressure is not one of the options. Recalling that the nurse would administer 3 nitroglycerin tablets 5 minutes apart from each other to relieve chest pain in a hospitalized client will assist in directing you to the correct option. Remember that implementation is the fourth step of the nursing process.

needed to care for the client readily available at the bedside; remember that you do not need to run to the supply room to obtain, for example, sterile gloves because the sterile gloves will be at the client's bedside.

6. Evaluation/Evaluate Outcomes (Box 4-15)
   - **a.** The nurse compares observed outcomes with expected ones.
   - **b.** These questions focus on comparing the actual outcomes of care with the expected outcomes and on communicating and documenting findings.
   - **c.** They also focus on assisting in determining the client's response to care and identifying factors that may interfere with achieving expected outcomes.
   - **d.** In these question types, watch for negative event queries because they are frequently used.

H. Determine Whether an Abnormality Exists (Box 4-16)

1. In the event, the client scenario will be described. Use your nursing knowledge to determine whether any of the information presented is indicating an abnormality.
2. If an abnormality exists, either further assessment or further intervention will be required. Therefore, continuing to monitor or documenting will not be a correct answer; don't select these options if they are presented!

BOX 4-15 Practice Question: The Nursing Process—Evaluation

The nurse is evaluating the client's response to treatment of a pleural effusion with a chest tube. The nurse notes a respiratory rate of 20 breaths per minute, fluctuation of the fluid level in the water seal chamber, and a decrease in the amount of drainage by 30 mL since the previous shift. Based on this information, which interpretation would the nurse make?

1. The client is responding well to treatment.
2. Suction should be decreased to the system.
3. The system should be assessed for an air leak.
4. Water should be added to the water seal chamber.

***Answer:* 1**

***Test-Taking Strategy*:** Use the steps of the nursing process and note that the nurse needs to evaluate the client's response to treatment; therefore this question measures the cognitive skill, evaluate outcomes. Focus on the subject and the data in the question. Also, determine whether an abnormality exists based on these data. Remember that fluctuation in the water seal chamber is a normal and expected finding with a chest tube. Because the client is being treated for a pleural effusion, it can be determined that he or she is responding well to treatment if the amount of drainage is gradually decreasing because the fluid from the pleural effusion is being effectively removed. If the drainage were to stop suddenly, the chest tube should be assessed for a kink or blockage. There is no indication based on the data in the question to decrease suction to the system; in fact, it is unclear as to whether the client is on suction at all. There are also no data in the question indicating an air leak. Lastly, there are no data in the question indicating the need to add water to the water seal chamber; again, it is unclear as to whether the client has this type of chest tube versus a dry suction chest tube. Remember that evaluation is the fifth step of the nursing process.

VIII. Client Needs

A. Safe and Effective Care Environment

1. According to the National Council of State Boards of Nursing (NCSBN), these questions test the concepts of providing safe nursing care and collaborating with other health care team members to facilitate effective client care; these questions also focus on the protection of clients, significant others, and health care personnel from environmental hazards.
2. Focus on safety with these types of questions, and remember the importance of hand washing, call lights or bells, bed positioning, appropriate use of side rails, asepsis, use of standard and other precautions, triage, and emergency response planning.

B. Physiological Integrity

1. The NCSBN indicates that these questions test the concepts that the nurse provides care as it relates to comfort and assistance in the

BOX 4-16 Practice Question: Determine Whether an Abnormality Exists

The nurse is caring for a client being admitted to the emergency department with a chief complaint of anorexia, nausea, and vomiting. The nurse asks the client about the home medications being taken. The nurse would be **most** concerned if the client stated that which medication was being taken at home?

1. Digoxin
2. Captopril
3. Losartan
4. Furosemide

Answer: *1*

Test-Taking Strategy: This question measures the cognitive skill, analyzing cues. Note the strategic word, *most*. The first step in approaching the answer to this question is to determine whether an abnormality exists. The client is complaining of anorexia, nausea, and vomiting; therefore, an abnormality does exist. This tells you that this could be an adverse or toxic effect of one of the medications listed. Although gastrointestinal distress can occur as an expected side effect of many medications, anorexia, nausea, and vomiting are hallmark signs of digoxin toxicity. Therefore, the nurse would be most concerned with this medication if taken at home by the client. Remember to first determine whether an abnormality exists in the event before choosing the correct option.

performance of activities of daily living as well as care related to the administration of medications and parenteral therapies.

2. These questions also address the nurse's ability to reduce the client's potential for developing complications or health problems related to treatments, procedures, or existing conditions and to provide care to clients with acute, chronic, or life-threatening physical health conditions.
3. Focus on Maslow's Hierarchy of Needs theory in these types of questions and remember that physiological needs are a priority and are addressed first.
4. Use the ABCs—airway–breathing–circulation—and the steps of the nursing process when selecting an option addressing Physiological Integrity.

C. Psychosocial Integrity

1. The NCSBN notes that these questions test the concepts of nursing care that promote and support the emotional, mental, and social well-being of the client and significant others.
2. Content addressed in these questions relates to supporting and promoting the client's or significant others' ability to cope, adapt, or problem-solve in situations such as illnesses; disabilities; or stressful events including abuse, neglect, or violence.
3. In this Client Needs category, you may be asked communication-type questions that relate to how you would respond to a client, a client's family member or significant other, or other health care team members.
4. Use therapeutic communication techniques to answer communication questions because of their effectiveness in the communication process.
5. Remember to select the option that focuses on the thoughts, feelings, concerns, anxieties, or fears of the client, client's family member, or significant other (Box 4-17).

D. Health Promotion and Maintenance

1. According to the NCSBN, these questions test the concepts that the nurse provides and assists in directing nursing care to promote and maintain health.
2. Content addressed in these questions relates to assisting the client and significant others during the normal expected stages of growth and development, and providing client care related to the prevention and early detection of health problems.
3. Use the Teaching and Learning theory if the question addresses client teaching, remembering that the client's willingness, desire, and readiness to learn is the first priority.
4. Watch for negative event queries, because they are frequently used in questions that address Health Promotion and Maintenance and client education.

BOX 4-17 Practice Question: Communication

A client scheduled for surgery states to the nurse, "I'm not sure if I should have this surgery." Which response by the nurse is appropriate?

1. "It's your decision."
2. "Don't worry. Everything will be fine."
3. "Why don't you want to have this surgery?"
4. "Tell me what concerns you have about the surgery."

Answer: *4*

Test-Taking Strategy: This question measures the cognitive skill, take action. Use therapeutic communication techniques to answer communication questions and remember to focus on the client's thoughts, feelings, concerns, anxieties, and fears. The correct option is the only one that addresses the client's concern. Additionally, asking the client about what specific concerns he or she has about the surgery will allow for further decisions in the treatment process to be made. Option 1 is a blunt response and does not address the client's concern. Option 2 provides false reassurance. Option 3 can make the client feel defensive and uses the nontherapeutic communication technique of asking "why." Remember to use therapeutic communication techniques and focus on the client.

IX. Eliminate Comparable or Alike Options (Box 4-18)

A. When reading the options in multiple-choice or multiple-response questions, look for options that are comparable or alike.

B. Comparable or alike options can be eliminated as possible answers, because it is unlikely that both options will be correct.

X. Eliminate Options Containing Closed-Ended Words (Box 4-19)

A. Some closed-ended words are "all," "always," "every," "must," "none," "never," and "only."

B. Eliminate options that contain closed-ended words, because these words imply a fixed or extreme meaning; these types of options are usually incorrect.

C. Options that contain open-ended words, such as "may," "usually," "normally," "commonly," or "generally," should be considered as possible correct options.

XI. Look for the Umbrella Option (Box 4-20)

A. When answering a question, look for the umbrella option.

B. The umbrella option is one that is a broad or universal statement and that usually encompasses the concepts of the other options within it.

C. The umbrella option will be the correct answer.

XII. Use the Guidelines for Delegating and Assignment Making (Box 4-21)

A. You may be asked a question that will require you to decide how you will delegate a task or assign clients to other health care providers (HCPs).

B. Focus on the information in the question and what task or assignment is to be delegated and available HCPs.

C. When you have determined what task or assignment is to be delegated, consider the client's needs and match the client's needs with the scope of practice of the HCPs identified in the question.

D. The Nurse Practice Act and any practice limitations define which aspects of care can be delegated and which must be performed by a registered nurse. Use nursing scope of practice as a guide to assist in

BOX 4-18 Practice Question: Eliminate Comparable or Alike Options

The nurse is caring for a group of clients. On review of the clients' medical records, the nurse determines that which client is at risk for excess fluid volume?

1. The client taking diuretics
2. The client with an ileostomy
3. The client with kidney disease
4. The client undergoing gastrointestinal suctioning

Answer: *3*

Test-Taking Strategy: This question measures the cognitive skill, analyzing cues. Focus on the subject, the client at risk for excess fluid volume. Think about the pathophysiology associated with each condition identified in the options. The only client who retains fluid is the client with kidney disease. The client taking diuretics, the client with an ileostomy, and the client undergoing gastrointestinal suctioning all lose fluid; these are comparable or alike options. Remember to eliminate comparable or alike options.

BOX 4-19 Practice Question: Eliminate Options That Contain Closed-Ended Words

A client is to undergo a computed tomography (CT) scan of the abdomen with oral contrast, and the nurse provides preprocedure instructions. The nurse instructs the client to take which action in the preprocedure period?

1. Avoid eating or drinking for at least 3 hours before the test.
2. Limit self to only 2 cigarettes on the morning of the test.
3. Have a clear liquid breakfast only on the morning of the test.
4. Take all routine medications with a glass of water on the morning of the test.

Answer: *1*

Test-Taking Strategy: This question measures the cognitive skill, take action. Note the closed-ended words "only" in options 2 and 3 and "all" in option 4. Eliminate options that contain closed-ended words, because these options are usually incorrect. Also, note that options 2, 3, and 4 are comparable or alike options in that they all involve taking in something on the morning of the test. Remember to eliminate options that contain closed-ended words.

BOX 4-20 Practice Question: Look for the Umbrella Option

A client admitted to the hospital is diagnosed with a pressure injury on the coccyx with a wound vac. The wound culture results indicate *methicillin-resistant staphylococcus aureus* is present. The wound dressing and wound vac foam is due to be changed. The nurse would employ which protective precautions to prevent contraction of the infection during care?

1. Gown and gloves
2. Gloves and a mask
3. Contact precautions
4. Airborne precautions

Answer: *3*

Test-Taking Strategy: This question measures the cognitive skill, take action. Focus on the client's diagnosis and recall that this infection is through direct contact. Recall that contact precautions involves the use of gown and gloves for routine care, and the use of gown, gloves, and face shield if splashing is anticipated during care. Note that the correct option is the umbrella option. Remember to look for the umbrella option, a broad or universal option that includes the concepts of the other options in it.

BOX 4-21 Practice Question: Use Guidelines for Delegating and Assignment Making

The nurse in charge of a long-term care facility is planning the client assignments for the day. Which client would be assigned to the assistive personnel (AP)?

1. A client on strict bed rest
2. A client with dyspnea who is receiving oxygen therapy
3. A client scheduled for transfer to the hospital for surgery
4. A client with a gastrostomy tube who requires tube feedings every 4 hours

Answer: *1*

Test-Taking Strategy: This question measures the cognitive skill, generate solutions. Note the **subject** of the question, the assignment to be delegated to the AP. When asked questions about delegation, think about the role description and scope of practice of the employee and the needs of the client. A client with dyspnea who is receiving oxygen therapy, a client scheduled for transfer to the hospital for surgery, or a client with a gastrostomy tube who requires tube feedings every 4 hours has both physiological and psychosocial needs that require care by a licensed nurse. The AP has been trained to care for a client on bed rest. Remember to match the client's needs with the scope of practice of the health care provider.

BOX 4-22 Available Resources

The nurse is called to a client's room to assist the client who has a chest tube. The client states that it felt like the tube pulled out. The nurse assesses the client and finds that the tube has dislodged from the chest and is laying on the floor. What action would the nurse take **next**?

1. Obtain a pair of sterile gloves.
2. Contact the respiratory therapist for help.
3. Cover the insertion site with a sterile dressing.
4. Submerge the dislodged tube into sterile water.

Answer: *3*

Test-Taking Strategy: This question measures the cognitive skill, prioritize hypotheses. Note the **strategic word**, *next*. This question measures the cognitive skill, take action. Recognize cues in the question and analyze the cues for their significance to identify the action that needs to be taken. When providing care to a client, particularly in emergency situations, keep in mind that all of the resources needed to provide client care will be readily available at the client's bedside. Most students would eliminate option 4 first, knowing that this action is not necessary in this scenario since the tube has dislodged from the chest. From the remaining options, you may think, "I don't have sterile gloves or a sterile dressing with me, so let me call for help first." Remember, you have everything you need wherever and whenever you need it!

answering questions. Remember that the NCLEX is a national exam and national standards rather than agency-specific standards must be followed when delegating.

E. In general, noninvasive interventions, such as skin care, range-of-motion exercises, ambulation, grooming, and hygiene measures, can be assigned to an assistive personnel (AP).

F. A licensed practical nurse (LPN) can perform the tasks that a AP can perform and can usually perform certain invasive tasks, such as dressings, suctioning, urinary catheterization, and administering medications orally or by the subcutaneous or intramuscular route; some selected piggyback intravenous medications may also be administered.

G. A registered nurse can perform the tasks that an LPN can perform and is responsible for assessment and planning care, analyzing client data, implementing and evaluating client care, supervising care, initiating teaching, and administering medications intravenously.

XIII. Available Resources and Ideal Situations (Box 4-22)

A. When providing care to a client, particularly in emergency situations, keep in mind that all of the resources needed (i.e., blood pressure cuff, dressing supplies, gloves, masks) to provide client care will be readily available. Remember, you have everything you need wherever and whenever you need it!

B. Answer the question as if it were an ideal situation. Remember that NCLEX requires that you will answer questions based on textbook information.

XIV. Answering Pharmacology Questions (Box 4-23)

A. If you are familiar with the medication, use nursing knowledge to answer the question.

B. Remember that the question only will identify the generic name of the medication on most occasions.

C. If the question identifies a medical diagnosis, try to form a relationship between the medication and the diagnosis; for example, you can determine that cyclophosphamide is an antineoplastic medication if the question refers to a client with breast cancer who is taking this medication.

D. Try to determine the classification of the medication being addressed to assist in answering the question. Identifying the classification will assist in determining a medication's action or side effects or both.

E. Recognize the common side effects and adverse effects associated with each medication classification and relate the appropriate nursing interventions to each effect; for example, if a side effect is hypertension, the associated nursing intervention would be to monitor the blood pressure.

BOX 4-23 Practice Question: Answering Pharmacology Questions

Quinapril hydrochloride is prescribed as adjunctive therapy in the treatment of heart failure. After administering the first dose, the nurse would monitor which item as the **priority?**

1. Weight
2. Urine output
3. Lung sounds
4. Blood pressure

***Answer:* 4**

Test-Taking Strategy: Focus on the name of the medication and note the strategic word, *priority*. Recall that the medication names of most angiotensin-converting enzyme (ACE) inhibitors end with "*-pril*," and one of the indications for use of these medications is hypertension. Excessive hypotension ("first-dose syncope") can occur in clients with heart failure or in clients who are severely sodium-depleted or volume-depleted. Although weight, urine output, and lung sounds would be monitored, monitoring the blood pressure is the priority. Remember to use pharmacology guidelines to assist in answering questions about medications and note the strategic words.

F. Focus on what the question is asking or the subject of the question; for example: intended effect, side effect, adverse effect, or toxic effect. It is helpful to learn the most common side effects, adverse effects, and toxic effects by medication classification.

G. Learn medications that belong to a classification by commonalities in their medication names; for example, medications that act as beta blockers end with "*-lol*" (e.g., atenolol).

H. If the question requires a medication calculation, remember that a calculator is available on the computer; talk yourself through each step to be sure the answer makes sense, and recheck the calculation before answering the question, particularly if the answer seems like an unusual dosage.

I. Pharmacology: Pyramid Points to remember

1. In general, the client should not take an antacid with medication, because the antacid will affect the absorption of the medication, either increasing or decreasing the absorption.
2. Enteric-coated and sustained-release tablets should not be crushed; also, capsules should not be opened.
3. The client should never adjust or change a medication dose or abruptly stop taking a medication.
4. The nurse never adjusts or changes the client's medication dosage and never discontinues a medication.
5. The client needs to avoid taking any over-the-counter medications or any other medications, such as herbal preparations, unless they are approved for use by the primary health care provider.
6. The client needs to avoid consuming alcohol.
7. Medications are never administered if the prescription is difficult to read, is unclear, or identifies a medication dose that is not a normal one. It is safer if medications are prescribed electronically.
8. Additional strategies for answering pharmacology questions are presented in *Saunders Strategies for Test Success: Passing Nursing School and the NCLEX® Exam.*

XV. Using the CJMM and the 6 Cognitive Skills to Answer a Test Question (Box 4-24)

A. You may encounter questions on the NCLEX exam that present a single case study or an unfolding case study. A single case study will be accompanied by 1 or maybe 2 questions measuring selected cognitive skills. The unfolding case study will be accompanied by 6 questions that measure all 6 cognitive skills. Included in the scenario may be demographic information such as age and gender, chief concern, admitting diagnosis, history of present illness, past medical history, surgical history, family history, social history, allergies, and medications, which provides the situation and background for the case.

B. These case studies may also include data such as vital signs, physical assessment findings, laboratory and diagnostic test results, client prescriptions, and a medication administration record.

C. The candidate may be required to discern between important, relevant data to the clinical situation and data that, although it is important to be aware of, may not have any bearing, relevance, or effect on nursing interventions for the client and the current medical problems.

D. While reviewing the case, try to look at each piece of data in a step-by-step fashion and decide whether it has bearing, relevance, or a potential effect on nursing interventions for the client.

BOX 4-24 Using the Clinical Judgment Measurement Model and Cognitive Skills to Answer Test Questions

Case Study

A client in the emergency department has anorexia, nausea, vomiting, and visual problems. The nurse asks about medications the client takes at home and the client provides a list.

Medication List:
Amiodarone 400 mg orally daily
Digoxin 0.25 mg orally daily
Lisinopril 20 mg orally daily
Furosemide 40 mg orally daily
Metformin 1000 mg orally twice daily

Cognitive Skill: Recognize Cues

Question types that may be presented to measure your ability to recognize cues that are significant include enhanced hot spot (highlighting), cloze, extended multiple response, and extended drag and drop. Ask yourself: "What data matters the most?" Focus on the following to answer the question.

- Client observation cues: Anorexia, nausea, and vomiting, visual problems
- Environmental: Emergency department
- Medical record: Each medication taken by the client
- In this case, the client observation cues and medications are significant.

Cognitive Skill: Analyze Cues

Question types that may be presented to measure your ability to analyze cues include cloze, extended multiple response, matrix, and extended drag and drop. Ask yourself: "What does the significant assessment data mean?" Focus on the following to answer the question.

- Linking recognized cues with client data.
- What client conditions are consistent with the cues?
- Using knowledge of the medications and their adverse effects.
- In this case, make a determination that the client exhibits signs of digoxin toxicity.

Cognitive Skill: Prioritize Hypotheses

Question types that may be presented to measure your ability to prioritize hypotheses include cloze, extended multiple response, and extended drag and drop. Ask yourself: "What is happening to the client and what are the client needs?" Focus on the following to answer the question.

- Interpreting relevant data
- Considering all possibilities about what is happening and client needs
- Ranking the urgency of client needs with regard to planning care
- In this case, client needs can be ranked as 1) checking the digoxin level; 2) treating toxicity; 3) treating nausea and vomiting.

Cognitive Skill: Generate Solutions

Question types that may be presented to measure your ability to generate solutions include matrix, extended multiple response, and extended drag and drop. Ask yourself: "What must I do, what can I do, and what would I not do?" Focus on the following to answer the question.

- Identifying client goals and potential interventions
- Acceptable actual or potential evidence-based actions
- Actions that need to be avoided or are contraindicated
- In this case, goals are to 1) reduce the digoxin level—potential intervention is consider an antidote; 2) eliminate nausea and vomiting—potential intervention is consider an antiemetic

Cognitive Skill: Take Action

Question types that may be presented to measure your ability to take action include cloze, extended multiple response, matrix, and extended drag and drop. Ask yourself: "What will I do?" Focus on the following to answer the question.

- Actions to take
- Actions that address the highest priorities of care
- In this case, actions are to 1) withhold the digoxin; 2) monitor vital signs (VS) and the apical heart rate; 3) notify the PHCP for prescriptions to treat digoxin toxicity and the nausea and vomiting; 4) administer antidote and antiemetics

Cognitive Skill: Evaluate Outcomes

Question types that may be presented to measure your ability to evaluate outcomes include enhanced hot spot (highlighting), extended multiple response, matrix, and extended drag and drop. Ask yourself: "Did the action help?" Focus on the following to answer the question.

- Actions that resulted in improvement, a decline, or no change in the client's condition, or actions that were effective, ineffective, or were unrelated actions.
- In this case, to evaluate outcomes and determine effectiveness of actions the nurse would note 1) that the digoxin level is in the therapeutic range; 2) clinical symptoms are resolved; 3) vital signs and heart rate are stable

UNIT II

Professional Standards in Nursing

Pyramid to Success

Nurses often care for clients who come from ethnic, cultural, or religious backgrounds that are different from their own. Nurses are also in a primary and unique position to address the individualized needs and care for various special population groups. Awareness of and sensitivity to the unique health and illness beliefs and practices of people of different backgrounds and those of special population groups are essential for the delivery of safe and effective care. Acknowledgment and acceptance of personal, cultural, religious, and spiritual differences with a nonjudgmental attitude are essential to providing culturally sensitive care. The NCLEX-RN® exam test plan is unique and individualized to the client's personal and cultural beliefs. The nurse needs to avoid stereotyping and needs to be aware that there are several special population groups, subcultures within cultures, and there are several dialects within languages. In nursing practice, the nurse should assess the client's perceived needs before planning and implementing a plan of care.

Across all settings in the practice of nursing, nurses frequently are confronted with ethical and legal issues related to client care. The professional nurse has the responsibility to be aware of the ethical principles, laws, and guidelines related to providing safe and quality care to clients. In the Pyramid to Success, focus on ethical practices; the Nurse Practice Act and clients' rights, particularly confidentiality, information security, and informed consent; advocacy, documentation, and advance directives; and cultural, religious, and spiritual issues. Knowledgeable use of information technology, such as an electronic health record, is also an important role of the nurse.

The National Council of State Boards of Nursing (NCSBN) defines management of care as the nurse directing nursing care to enhance the care delivery setting to protect the client and health care personnel. As described in the NCLEX-RN exam test plan, a professional nurse needs to provide integrated, cost-effective care to clients by coordinating, supervising, and collaborating or consulting with members of the interprofessional health care team. A primary Pyramid Point focuses on the skills required to prioritize client care activities. Pyramid Points also focus on concepts of leadership and management, the process of delegation, emergency response planning, and triaging clients.

Client Needs: Learning Objectives

Safe and Effective Care Environment

Acting as a client advocate
Integrating advance directives into the plan of care
Becoming familiar with the emergency response plan
Delegating client care activities and providing continuity of care
Ensuring ethical practices are implemented
Ensuring informed consent has been obtained
Ensuring legal rights and responsibilities are maintained
Collaborating with interprofessional teams
Establishing priorities related to client care activities
Instituting quality improvement procedures
Integrating case management concepts
Maintaining confidentiality and information security issues related to the client's health care
Supervising the delivery of client care
Triaging clients
Upholding client rights
Using information technology in a confidential manner
Using leadership and management skills effectively

Health Promotion and Maintenance

Considering cultural, religious, and spiritual issues related to family systems and family planning

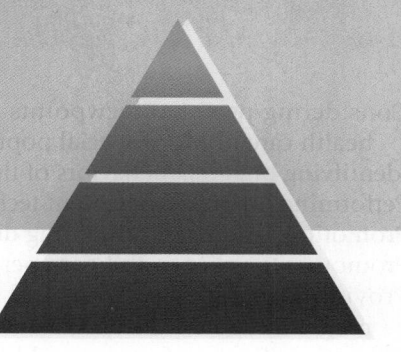

Considering personal viewpoints and individualized health care needs of special population groups
Identifying high-risk behaviors of the client
Performing physical assessment techniques
Promoting health and preventing disease
Promoting the client's ability to perform self-care
Providing health screening and health promotion programs
Respecting client preferences and lifestyle choices

Psychosocial Integrity

Addressing needs based on the client's preferences and beliefs
Assessing the use of effective coping mechanisms
Becoming aware of personal, cultural, religious, and spiritual preferences and incorporating these preferences when planning and implementing care
Identifying abuse and neglect issues
Identifying clients who do not speak or understand English and determining how language needs will be met by the use of agency-approved interpreters
Identifying family dynamics as they relate to the client
Identifying support systems for the client
Providing a therapeutic environment and building a relationship based on trust

Physiological Integrity

Ensuring that emergencies are handled using a prioritization procedure
Identifying client preferences for providing holistic client care
Implementing therapeutic procedures considering individual preferences
Providing nonpharmacological comfort interventions
Providing nutrition and oral hydration, considering client preferences
Monitoring for alterations in body systems or unexpected responses to therapy

CHAPTER 5

Care of Special Populations

PRIORITY CONCEPTS Caregiving, Health Disparities

I. Special Population Groups

A. Special population is a term that is generally used to refer to a disadvantaged group meaning those who are vulnerable to health care disparities. US Legal, https://definitions.uslegal.com/s/special-population/

B. The literature identifies numerous groups that may be designated as a special population group.

C. For this chapter, based on the literature, the authors have identified certain special groups most commonly cared for in the health care environment that require nursing's special attention, care, and sensitivity regarding their health care needs to ensure that their needs are met.

II. Health Care Disparities

A. Health disparities are differences in health care offered to different groups of people.

B. Some of the vulnerable groups that are at risk for health disparities include minority groups, those who are uninsured, those living in poverty or are homeless, those with chronic health problems and disabilities, immigrants, refugees, those with limited English proficiency, those who are incarcerated, and members of the LGBTQ (lesbian, gay, bisexual, transgender, queer or questioning) community.

C. Vulnerable groups experience greater risk factors, lack of necessary access to care, and increased morbidity and mortality as compared with the general population. (Joszt, L. [2018]. 5 Vulnerable populations in health care. *The American Journal of Managed Care [AJM]*. https://www.ajmc.com/view/5-vulnerable-populations-in-healthcare)

D. Nurses often care for clients who are vulnerable and are at risk for health disparities; nurses need to be aware that health care disparities exist and plan and provide care to prevent a disparity.

E. Nurses also need to be aware of the most prevalent chronic health problems and infectious diseases in the United States (U.S.) and their associated risk factors. This is important because on assessment, the nurse needs to screen for these health problems and infections, the associated risk factors, and determine necessary support services for the individual or family. Then, the nurse needs to plan appropriate educational strategies and teach about the measures that will either prevent or treat these health problems and infectious diseases and connect the client or family with identified support services. Box 5-1 identifies chronic health problems in the U.S. and associated risk factors. Box 5-2 identifies common infectious diseases.

III. Nursing Assessment

A. See Box 5-3 for a comprehensive nursing assessment tool written by the authors of this chapter, titled *Special Populations: Needs Assessment Tool*, that can be used to obtain information from the client about his or her special needs in order to plan care. This tool can be adapted, based on the individual or family group being cared for.

B. Nurses' self-awareness of their own culture, values, beliefs, ethics, personality, and communication style

BOX 5-1 Chronic Health Problems in the U.S. and Risk Factors

Chronic Health Problems
Heart disease
Cancer
Chronic lung disease
Stroke
Alzheimer's disease
Diabetes
Chronic kidney disease
Risk Factors
Tobacco use
Poor nutrition
Obesity
Lack of physical activity
Excessive alcohol use

Centers for Disease Control and Infections (2019). *Chronic diseases in America*. https://www.cdc.gov/chronicdisease/resources/infographic/chronic-diseases.htm file:///C:/Users/owner/Downloads/chronic-disease-H.pdf

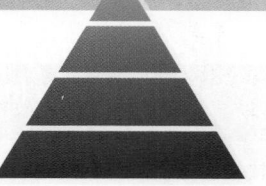

BOX 5-2 Common Infectious Diseases in the U.S.

COVID-19 (Coronavirus)
Sexually transmitted diseases (chlamydia, syphilis, gonorrhea)
Human immunodeficiency virus and acquired immunodeficiency syndrome
Influenza
Staphylococcus aureus
Escherichia coli (E. coli)
Herpes simplex 1, Herpes simplex 2
Shigellosis
Norovirus
Salmonella
Pneumonia
Hepatitis C

Data in part from John Hopkins Medicine (2020). *Infectious diseases*, at https://www.hopkinsmedicine.org/health/infectious-diseases

helps to promote optimal health outcomes for clients of diverse populations. Recognizing one's own biases and being respectful to all people despite differences can influence satisfaction of care.

An encounter with a client needs to elicit the client's unique perspectives based on their own preferences. This will allow the nurse to understand what health care treatments will be realistic and acceptable.

C. It is imperative for nurses to understand that special population groups may share dominant characteristics; however, all clients are individuals and stereotyping must be avoided.

D. It is also very important for nurses to be aware of the health problems that are common in a population group so that specific and special attention can be made when performing a comprehensive assessment.

BOX 5-3 Special Populations: Needs Assessment Tool

Not all questions listed in this assessment tool will need to be used for the assessment. The nurse needs to make a judgment on appropriate questions for each population and needs to ask questions within that list, if appropriate for the client, based on the *General Background Questions*. Use the *General Background Questions* as a guide to determine additional questions that should be included in the assessment.

Initial

- Introduce yourself and describe your role.
- Example: "I would like to ask you some questions so that we have information about your individualized needs. Do I have your permission to ask you some questions?"

General Background Questions

- Are you comfortable talking to me?
- What name would you like us to use to address you?
- What is your primary language spoken?
- Do you speak and understand English?
- In which language do you wish to communicate?
- Do you need an interpreter?
- Do you feel you are able to adequately answer questions regarding your health?
- What is your age?
- Is there a specific gender in which you identify with?
- What is your ethnicity?
- Do you have any cultural, religious, or spiritual preferences you would like us to consider in your plan of care?
- Do you have any dietary preferences that you would like us to include in your plan of care? Describe your eating patterns in a 24-hour period.
- Do you exercise? What do you do and how often?
- Do you use any remedies when you are sick?
- What do you do when you are sick?
- What is your living situation? Where do you live? Who do you live with? Do you have children?
- Do you have a support system?
- Would you like to name a support person or emergency contact person?
- Do you have access to financial resources needed to live?
- Do you have health insurance?
- Do you feel safe at home or where you live? Have you been abused within the last 12 months? Do you encounter crime or violence in your life? Is anyone hurting you, physically or emotionally or in any other way? Have you ever been or are you now being bullied?
- Do you smoke, drink alcohol, or use any type of drug?
- Do you have or need a health care proxy?
- Do you have an advance directive? If not, would you like more information about this?
- When was the last time you sought health care? For what reason?
- Do you have any fears about seeing your provider?
- Do you currently or have you ever had a communicable disease?
- Have you been exposed to anyone with a communicable disease? If so, how was this exposure treated?
- Have you ever been tested for COVID-19? Or, tested for immunity?
- Have you traveled outside of the country recently?
- Are you up-to-date on immunizations?
- When was your last influenza vaccine?
- Have you ever been vaccinated for pneumonia? If so, when?
- Do you have a history of mental illness?
- Have you ever had feelings of committing suicide? If so, do you have these feelings now? Do you have a plan?
- Are you a veteran or member of the military?
- Do you have any chronic illness, disability, or other past medical history?
- Have you ever been incarcerated?
- Are you an immigrant or refugee?

Further Questions Based on Living Situation

- Do you have a home? Do you live alone? Who do you live with at home?
- Do you drink alcohol? Any other type of drug use?
- Have you been exposed to environmental irritants?

BOX 5-3 **Special Populations: Needs Assessment Tool—cont'd**

- Have you had problems with asthma, anemia, lead exposure, ear infections, gastrointestinal illness, or mental illness?
- Are you willing to follow up on your health care recommendations if given the necessary resources?

Further Questions Based on Health Insurance Coverage

- What health insurance do you have?
- Do you have the financial means to pay for your health care?
- Are you willing to work with a social worker to seek health coverage?

Further Questions Based on Financial Status and Access to Resources

- What is your education level?
- What is your income?
- Do you have family you are in contact with?
- Is anyone in your immediate family disabled?
- Do you have a support system?
- Do you live in a safe community?
- Do you seek health care on a routine basis?
- Are you willing to work with a social worker to increase your access to community resources?

Further Questions Related to Abuse

- Do you have or have you had any bruises, sprains, broken bones, fatigue, shortness of breath, muscle tension, involuntary shaking, changes in eating or sleeping, sexual dysfunction, or fertility problems?
- Do you experience nightmares, anxiety, uncontrollable thoughts, depression, or low self-esteem?
- Do you have anxiety or depression? Have you felt suicidal? If so, do you have a plan?
- Do you ever feel hopeless, worthless, apprehensive, discouraged? Do you lack motivation or faith? Have you questioned your trust in others?
- For a child: do you have any problems at school? Are you bullied?

Further Questions Based on Racial/Ethnic Background

- Are there any resources you need to ensure your ability to follow up on your health care recommendations?
- Do you have any past medical history or family history of chronic diseases, such as diabetes mellitus, hypertension, heart disease, stroke, cancer, renal disease, injuries or accidents, depression, or anxiety?

Further Questions Based on Gender and Sexual Orientation

- Can you describe your sexual orientation preferences?
- Which pronoun would you like to be referred to by (he, she, other)?
- Do you seek regular and routine health care? When were you last seen?
- When was your last breast exam, mammogram, Pap smear, testicular exam, prostate exam?
- Do you do a breast self-examination or a testicular self-examination?
- Do you have any past medical history?
- Are you sexually active? If so, how many partners do you have? Do you employ safe sex practices?
- Do you smoke, drink alcohol, or use any other type of drug?
- Do you have any problems with depression or anxiety? Have you ever felt suicidal? If so, do you have a plan?
- Do you take hormone therapy?
- Are you up to date on your immunizations?
- Do you have children? If not, do you wish to or plan on having children?
- Do you feel you have access to necessary resources such as health care or other benefits?

Further Questions Related to Mental Illness

- Do you seek routine health care?
- Describe your eating habits in a 24-hour period.
- Describe your activity level.
- Do you have any past medical history?
- Do you take any medications? If so, what are they and do you experience any side effects?
- Do you smoke, drink, or use any other type of drug?
- Do you experience depression or anxiety? Have you ever had thoughts of suicide? If so, do you have a plan?
- Are you sexually active? If so, do you employ safe sex practices? How many partners do you have?

Further Questions Related to Veteran/Military Status

- Do you have any problems with mental illness, such as posttraumatic stress disorder, moral injury?
- Have you had any traumatic brain injuries?
- Have you had any other injuries?
- Describe your living situation.
- Are you interested in any community support groups?

Further Questions Related to Incarceration

- Have you ever been a victim of abuse or rape?
- Do you have any past medical history, particularly asthma, diabetes mellitus, hypertension, heart disease, mental illness, or communicable diseases?

Further Questions Related to Immigration

- Do you have problems with mental illness?
- Are you able to speak and understand English?
- Do you have access to resources such as housing, transportation, health care, and education services?
- Do you have any past medical history, such as accidents, injuries, hypothermia, gastrointestinal illness, heart problems, pregnancy complications, diabetes, hypertension, malnutrition, or infectious or communicable disease?

Further Questions Related to Chronic Illness

- Do you have access to a primary health care provider?
- Do you see a specialist on a regular basis?
- Are you able to follow up on the recommendations made by your primary health care provider and/or specialist?

Summary

- Is there anything else you would like to share regarding your ability to maintain your health or any other issue or concern?

Authors of the *Special Populations: Needs Assessment Tool:* Linda A. Silvestri, Angela E. Silvestri, and Paula Richards

IV. COVID-19 – Coronavirus

A. The COVID-19 pandemic is a serious global health threat and has caused severe illness and even death in some individuals.

B. It is considered a respiratory illness that is caused by a virus called SARS-CoV. Although the illness is a respiratory one, the virus also attacks and affects many different body systems.

C. Symptoms of the illness include but are not limited to cough, shortness of breath, fever, muscle pain, sore throat, loss of taste and/or smell.

D. COVID-19 is a highly contagious illness and controlling its spread is a primary goal.

E. There are special population groups that are at higher risk of contracting the infection and also at higher risk for dying because of the virus. Those at high risk include the elderly, those with a chronic health condition such as diabetes or respiratory disease, those who have cancer, those who are immunocompromised from chemotherapy or a disease, and minority groups. For additional information refer to: https://www.hopkinsmedicine.org/health/conditions-and-diseases/coronavirus/covid19-racial-disparities

F. Other special population groups at risk are those that are living in crowded conditions or are institutionalized, such as those in a nursing home or in a prison.

G. Working in essential fields such as health care environments, inconsistent access to health care, stress and a low immune response also plays a role in increasing the risk for this infection.

H. When performing an assessment on a client, the nurse must assess for any risk factors for COVID-19 and must institute safety measures for protecting and preventing that client from contracting the illness.

I. The nurse must be aware of the critical measures needed to protect oneself from contracting the virus and must be an advocate in educating the public about the measures to prevent spread. These primary measures are handwashing, wearing a mask and eye protection, social distancing (6 feet apart), avoiding crowded situations, avoiding close contact with people who are sick, covering your nose and mouth when coughing or sneezing, keeping the hands away from the eyes and face, and self-quarantine.

V. Minority Groups

A. Minority groups are more often affected by health care disparities than non-minority groups.

B. Some individuals in these groups may be less likely to have health insurance coverage or a regular source of health care. Center for American Progress (2010). *Fact sheet: Health disparities by race and ethnicity.* https://cdn.americanprogress.org/wp-content/uploads/issues/2010/12/pdf/disparities_factsheet.pdf

C. Obesity, diabetes mellitus, end-stage renal disease secondary to diabetes, and cervical cancer are more common among the Hispanic/Latino population.

D. The Native Hawaiians and other Pacific Islanders population is noted to have higher rates of smoking, alcohol consumption, obesity, and diabetes mellitus. Hepatitis B, human immunodeficiency virus (HIV) and acquired immunodeficiency syndrome (AIDS) and tuberculosis are more frequent diseases. Noted is that there is a high incidence of infant mortality and sudden infant death syndrome (SIDS) in this population.

E. In the Native American and Alaska Native populations, geographic isolation and income may be factors with regard to receiving health care. Inadequate water supply and sewage disposal can be a factor with infectious diseases. Smoking and alcohol use is more common and diabetes mellitus, cancer, stroke, heart disease, and accidents are a concern. Additional concerns include mental health alterations, suicide, infant mortality, sudden infant death syndrome (SIDS), teenage pregnancy, liver disease, and hepatitis.

F. Obesity, diabetes mellitus, hypertension, heart disease, asthma, and cancer occur more commonly among the black population with leading causes of death being heart disease, cancer, and stroke.

G. Cancer, tuberculosis, and hepatitis are more common health problems of Asian Americans with leading causes of death being cancer, heart disease, and stroke.

⚠ Some people in minority groups report hesitancy in seeking health care due to a language barrier. Ineffective communication between the nurse or other health care provider and the client can affect the client's health care and the client's ability to comply with follow-up care.

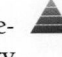

H. Health care considerations for minority groups
1. Cultural competence is critical in the effort to reduce health care disparity and is a necessary ability for health care professionals to acquire in order to provide care for a diverse population. This can help improve health outcomes and quality of care.
2. The nurse and other health care professionals need to be aware of health care variations and risk factors for various populations in order to facilitate appropriate care and access to needed health care services.
3. It is important for the nurse to examine his or her own values in order to competently care for someone of a differing population group; awareness is a useful tool in caring for these special populations.

4. Language barriers influence access to health care. It is important to remember that family members and friends must not be asked to be an interpreter for the client because of confidentiality, the potential for conflict of interest, and the risk associated with relaying inaccurate information; only specified individuals as designated by the health care agency need to be asked to interpret for a client.
5. Lack of access to preventative care needs to be addressed; lack of routine health care and delay in seeking health care for illness are common.
6. Some important education health topics include diet and meal planning, exercise, and other healthy lifestyle practices to prevent disease, including infectious and communicable diseases.
7. Return explanation and demonstration (teach-back) are of particular importance to ensure safety and mutual understanding.

VI. Lesbian, Gay, Bisexual, Transgender and Queer or Questioning Individuals

A. Commonly referred to as the "LGBTQ" community, this group is represented by a wide range of varying characteristics in terms of race, ethnicity, age, socioeconomic status, and identity.

B. There is often a lack of awareness and understanding among health care professionals in managing the health care needs of this population—providing access to health care to meet their needs is critical.

C. When performing an assessment, the nurse needs to individualize and take into account the characteristics in terms of race, ethnicity, age, and socioeconomic status; the assessment needs to focus on health concerns unique to each characteristic.

D. Some LGBTQ persons may be less likely to access health care than other population groups due to fear of stigmatization and being viewed as different.

E. Transgender individuals require special attention and care. They may be less likely than other groups to have certain screenings completed, such as mammograms, breast exams, cervical cancer screening, testicular cancer exams, and prostate screening. For additional information, refer to the GLAAD Media Reference Guide: Transgender at https://www.glaad.org/reference/transgender

F. Sexually transmitted infections are of concern in this population.

G. Breast cancer and cervical cancer are a concern likely a result of decreased screening and nulliparity.

H. Depression and suicide is a concern

I. Rejection from friends, family members, and social support systems may be a stressor. Teenage members of the LGBTQ population are more likely to be threatened, bullied, injured, raped, and victimized. For these reasons, school absenteeism can be a problem. LGBTQ youth are at risk for abuse by family members due to their sexual orientation.

J. Many same sex couples desire children; there may be some barriers to child-rearing for this population, such as the expenses associated with adoption, artificial insemination, and surrogacy.

Members of the LGBTQ population are less likely to have family members who can assist them with elder or disability care. Additionally, certain benefits may not be available to them, such as spousal death benefits, which could impact their ability to manage finances and expenses associated with health.

K. Health care considerations for the LGBTQ population
1. Health care professionals need to create a welcoming, nonjudgmental environment when caring for this population.
2. Using the preferred pronoun when addressing these clients is important in developing and maintaining a rapport.
3. Measures such as altering signage on paperwork and documents asking for gender identification will better serve the health needs of this population. In addition, the health care facility must develop institutional polices inclusive of all gender identities and preferences. Such measures will allow the primary health care provider to treat the client according to their preferences while also maintaining an understanding of their risk factors based on biological drivers of health.
4. Health promotion measures need to focus on screening for health concerns such as cancer, sexually transmitted infections, depression, suicide, and on educating on safe sex practices.
5. A careful sexual history and appropriate counseling is important for all members of the LGBTQ population.
6. Nonoccupational postexposure prophylaxis (nPEP) or the use of prophylactic antiretrovirals before and after potential HIV exposure needs to be considered.
7. Transgender persons taking hormone therapy need to be monitored at regular intervals; associated complications, such as polycythemia occurring with exogenous testosterone use, need to be detected and treated early.
8. Transgendered persons who have undergone sexual reassignment surgery must have the respective preventive screenings. For example, male-to-female need to have breast cancer screening by way of mammography if they are older than 50 years. Additionally, female-to-male would still have mammography routinely as indicated due to the risk for residual breast tissue to develop cancerous growth.

VII. Homeless

A. Affects men, women, children, and persons of all backgrounds, and family units can be affected as a whole.

B. There is a risk for early death related to health problems (Box 5-4).

C. Disability often results from illness and becomes a barrier to employment, which further augments the problem of homelessness.

D. Infants affected by homelessness often have low birth weights and are more likely to die within the first 12 months of life than in other population groups.

E. Children affected by homelessness are sick more often with illnesses such as asthma, iron deficiency, lead poisoning, ear infections, gastrointestinal illness, and behavioral and mental health problems.

F. Children may begin to act out or become less attentive in the classroom when basic needs are not met.

G. Youth experience health problems related to risk-taking behaviors such as alcohol and drug abuse, and depression and suicide are concerns. Unintended pregnancy and sexually transmitted infections (STIs), are a concern; physical and sexual abuse is also a concern.

H. Health care considerations for the homeless

1. Identification of those who are homeless needs to be accomplished through avenues such as outreach programs.
2. The initial health care visit and every visit thereafter needs to be done with a nonjudgmental, nonthreatening approach.

BOX 5-4 Links Between Homeless and Health and Common Problems in the Homeless

Links

Limited access to health care
Problems getting enough food
Difficulty staying safe
Violence
Stress
Unsanitary living conditions
Exposure to extremes in weather

Common Health Problems

Dental problems
Malnutrition
Sexually transmitted diseases including HIV and AIDS
Lung diseases including bronchitis, tuberculosis, and pneumonia
Infectious and communicable diseases
Mental health problems
Substance abuse problems
Wounds and skin infections

MedlinePlus (2020). *Homeless health concerns.* https://medlineplus.gov/homelesshealthconcerns.html

3. The nurse needs to focus on reported symptoms first—this will encourage adherence and follow-up.
4. Subsequent care would include health maintenance, attention to common problems and concerns, and establishing an emergency contact person if available.
5. Members of the homeless population may not adhere to medical treatment recommendations and therefore require close follow-up as much as possible.
6. This population tends to have longer hospital stays, and have poorer health outcomes.
7. Certain medications must be avoided in the homeless population due to the potential for abuse, and contraindications in chronic conditions; the nurse needs to ensure that any medication prescribed is safe for the person.
8. Multiple resources are available to increase access to health care for the homeless population and the nurse needs to establish connections for the client as appropriate.
9. See https://www.aafp.org/afp/2014/0415/p634.html for more information about the homeless population.

VIII. Socioeconomically Disadvantaged Individuals and Families

A. Disadvantage in the socioeconomic sense can correlate with poor health outcomes.

B. Education level, income, family, social support, and community safety are social determinants that can influence health and health outcomes.

C. In addition to healthy lifestyle and access to routine, quality care, the social determinants of health are equally as important in promoting positive health outcomes.

D. Individuals of low socioeconomic status (SES) are more likely to engage in risky health behaviors.

E. Due to limited financial resources, these individuals are at a higher risk for chronic disease and any diseases associated with primary prevention.

F. The health of children can be affected later in life due to risk factors.

G. Health care considerations for socioeconomically disadvantaged individuals and families

1. Social work services are helpful in connecting this population to needed health care services and resources to assist in paying for health care.
2. The nurse needs to carefully assess the client for at-risk behaviors and intervent appropriately including providing education.
3. The nurse also needs to initiate social service contacts to ensure adequate health care.

IX. Uninsured and Underinsured Individuals

A. Individuals with low incomes are most at risk for being uninsured or underinsured.
B. Those who are uninsured or underinsured are at increased risk for health complications due to lack of access to care and the likelihood that preventive care services and chronic disease management will not be sought.
C. Most individuals receive health insurance coverage through an employer. If the employer does not offer this coverage, the employee is at risk for being uninsured or underinsured.
D. Medicaid is an option for some low-income families who meet eligibility criteria. Commercial insurance is another option but may still be cost prohibitive depending on the individual circumstance. The client would be referred to social services or financial services to apply for Medicaid.
E. Risk factors: Refer to risk factors for socioeconomically disadvantaged individuals and families.
F. Health care considerations for uninsured and underinsured individuals: Refer to health care considerations for socioeconomically disadvantaged individuals and families.

X. Intellectually Disabled Individuals

A. Intellectually disabled individuals are at high risk for certain health disorders.
B. Often, these health disorders go untreated due to atypical symptom presentation, which leads to additional problems later in life.
C. Communication barriers between health care professionals and those with an intellectual disability presents a unique challenge in identifying and managing health care needs in this population.
D. These clients may have difficulty recalling their personal medical history, so it may be necessary to take more time to ask questions in a variety of different ways.
E. More common health conditions include motor deficits, epilepsy, allergies, otitis media, gastroesophageal reflux disease (GERD), dysmenorrhea, sleep problems, mental illness, vision and hearing impairments, constipation, and oral health problems.
F. These clients may tend to eat quickly and so should be assessed for risk of choking and aspiration.
G. Certain conditions can cause changes in behavior; for example, there may be eating disturbances due to GERD or self-injury due to the presence of an ear infection.
H. Health care considerations for intellectually disabled individuals
1. Safety is a priority; ensure a safe environment.
2. Functional behavioral assessment is important in identifying existing health problems.
3. Awareness of altered behavior as a manifestation of an illness is important in early identification and prevention of secondary problems.
4. Health interventions must be focused on treating a medical condition, followed by behavioral interventions to prevent continued behavioral response to an illness.

XI. Battered Individuals and Victims of Abuse or Neglect

Health care professionals are often the first point of contact for victims of abuse or neglect.

A. Abuse of the older client (refer to Chapter 19 and Chapter 67).
B. Child abuse: Consequences are long lasting, both impacting initial development and influencing adult health (refer to Chapter 67).
C. Females are affected more than men.
D. Some of the outcomes of abuse or neglect may include physical, somatic, psychological, behavioral, sexual, and pregnancy-related effects.
E. Children birth to 1 year of age are at risk of maltreatment—the majority are victims of neglect; maternal socioeconomic status and parental behavioral issues impact a child's risk.
F. Victims are prone to certain health effects as a result of the abuse or neglect; these effects can include bruises, sprains or broken bones, chronic fatigue, shortness of breath, muscle tension, involuntary shaking, changes in eating and sleeping patterns, sexual dysfunction, and fertility issues.
G. Mental health issues can arise, including posttraumatic stress disorder (PTSD), nightmares, anxiety, uncontrollable thoughts, depression, low self-esteem, and alcohol and drug abuse.
H. Feelings of hopelessness, lack of worth, apprehension, discouragement, inability to trust others, and lack of motivation are common.
I. Children who witness violence are prone to fearfulness, anxiety, depression, and problems in school.
J. Health care considerations for battered individuals and victims of abuse or neglect
1. Safety is a priority; provide a safe environment and ensure that the victim has a safe environment to live and has contact information for seeking a safe haven if necessary.
2. Treat victims with compassion and respect.
3. Acknowledge and respect the dignity of each person.
4. Nurses are mandated reporters of domestic violence and abuse incidents; it may be necessary to take photographs of injuries for legal reasons.
5. Cleaning and dressing wounds, administering pain medications, use of assistive devices such as for sprains or fractures, education for

self-management and seeking safety, and emotional support may be needed in the care of these victims.

6. Provide parental education and support programs; increase awareness of potential battering and abuse or neglect.

XII. Single Parents

A. The nurse should establish a therapeutic relationship with the client and encourage the single parent to express any concerns and needs about single-parenting; this information will assist the nurse in identifying appropriate resources for the client.

B. Initiating access to community organizations can assist in alleviating some burden and provide needed services such as child care, food security, health care including immunizations, and employment.

C. The nurse may need to assist single parents to address the child's sexual development, especially those with a child of the opposite sex.

D. Preventive screenings are important in this population due to risk factors and the negative effects of stress from single parenting.

XIII. Foster Children

A. Needs that often go unmet for children in foster care include physical, mental, behavioral, and dental health; this increases the risk for health problems later in life (Box 5-5).

B. Some children in foster care may have complex and chronic health conditions.

C. Health care considerations for foster children
1. Community resources are important for this population to facilitate the provision of health, safety, stability, and permanence.
2. Social workers must be included in the care of a foster child to facilitate access to community resources.
3. Medically equipped homes may be needed, as well as in-home nursing care services for those children with complex or chronic health conditions.
4. Frequent health visits may be needed for children transitioning to and from foster care.

BOX 5-5 Some Mental Health Concerns for Foster Children

Attention-deficit hyperactivity disorder
Anxiety disorder
Bipolar disorder
Depression
Posttraumatic stress disorder

From: Turney, K., & Wildeman, C. (2016). Mental and physical health of children in foster care. *Pediatrics, 138*(5), e20161118.

XIV. Individuals With Mental Illness

A. Lifestyle choices, chronic health problems, psychotropic medications, limitation in access to health care, and lack of preventive screening are concerns.

B. Side effects of psychotropic medications may contribute to an altered health state. Certain psychotropic medications can contribute to weight gain.

C. Lack of exercise and poor diet, as well as features of an illness, such as depression or disorganized thought processes, may contribute to health problem development.

D. Side effects from psychotropic medications, such as sedation, weight gain, and increased appetite contribute to the incidence of diabetes mellitus and metabolic syndrome in this population.

E. Due to the higher frequency of substance abuse, risky sexual behaviors, and lack of knowledge regarding risks, individuals with mental illness are at increased risk for sexually transmitted infections.

F. Sexual dysfunction can result from mental illness as well as the medication used to treat it.

G. Xerostomia from reduction in salivary gland flow due to medications can result in difficulty maintaining oral hygiene and overall health.

H. Health care considerations for individuals with mental illness
1. Individuals with mental illness have a difficult time accessing needed and available health care services.
2. Family and social service support are important for these individuals.
3. Governmental insurance has expanded to cover individuals in need of mental health care.
4. Mental health screenings must be completed regularly for all individuals, which allows for prompt and accurate treatment strategies to prevent further health complications.
5. Refer to the mental health chapters for additional information about this special population.

XV. Older Adults

A. Elder abuse is a concern for this population; health care providers are mandated to report if there is suspicion of elder abuse. The most common type of abuse is neglect.

B. There are many health problems that can occur in the older client (Box 5-6 lists some of these health problems).

C. See Chapter 19 for more information on common health conditions experienced by older adults and care of the older adult.

XVI. Military Veterans

A. This population is at increased risk for injury-related and stress-related health illnesses.

B. Mental health or behavioral adjustment disorders are common.

BOX 5-6 Some Health Problems That Occur in Older Adults

Alzheimer's disease
Arthritis
Dementia
Depression
Falls
Heart disease
Influenza
Obesity
Oral/dental health problems
Osteoporosis
Pneumonia
Poverty
Respiratory diseases
Shingles
Substance abuse

Healthy People 2020. (2020). *Older adults*. Retrieved from https://www.healthypeople.gov/2020/topics-objectives/topic/older-adults
Healthy West Orange. (n.d.). *15 common health concerns for seniors*. Retrieved from https://healthywestorange.org/15-senior-concerns/

C. Substance use disorders with tobacco, alcohol, or other drugs and suicide are more common.
D. PTSD and moral injury is common among this population.
E. Traumatic brain injury can occur as a result of external force injuries.
F. Limb amputations and disfigurement are more common.
G. Long-term health problems may result from exposure to chemicals and environmental irritants.
H. Military veterans can experience issues leading to homelessness.
I. Health care considerations for military veterans
  1. Identifying and treating mental health disorders assists in mitigating suicide risk.
  2. Treatment of comorbid conditions such as PTSD or moral injury may help to address substance use disorders.
  3. Use of screening tools in identifying substance use disorder will help to plan appropriate care.
  4. Veterans' Affairs Services can assist in managing some of the health issues experienced by these individuals.

XVII. Prisoners

The environment of a prison can predispose a person to different health conditions, such as tuberculosis, sexually transmitted diseases, or other infectious or communicable diseases.

A. Social determinants of poor health are often present in prisoners.
B. Health concerns are asthma, diabetes, hypertension, heart disease, and mental illness.
C. Infectious and communicable diseases are also a concern for this population
D. Health care considerations for prisoners
  1. The correctional facility is usually the sole provider of health care for this population.
  2. Screening protocols and procedures for individuals in this setting need to be thorough, consistent, and performed regularly.
  3. Educational and vocational programs may help mitigate the health problems associated with living in a prison.
  4. History of incarceration increases the risk of poor health due to limited opportunities to reform; inadequate housing, employment, and education; and lack of family stability.
  5. Failure to address mental health issues among this population may contribute to repeated crimes when released from prison; those who are in prison for life need adequate screening and health care as well.

XIX. Immigrants and Refugees

A. Challenges include learning to speak English (or the adopted language of their new country), citizenship, raising children, employment, housing, accessing health care, transportation, and overcoming cultural barriers.
B. Acculturation to the U.S. increases the risk for poor health. Poor health can be the result of eating a less healthy diet, increased risk-taking behaviors, and separation from family support networks.
C. There are many health concerns for this population. Many result from the process of migration and include infectious diseases such as tuberculosis, hepatitis, vector-borne disease, influenza, coronavirus, sexually transmitted diseases, childhood diseases such as measles, mumps, rubella, and polio; antimicrobial resistance is a concern.
D. For refugees, mental health issues due to war, violence, and rape occurring in camps is a concern.
E. Health care considerations for immigrants and refugees
  1. A process for offering services and treating immigrants and refugees must be available regardless of insurance status.
  2. Refugees may be eligible for short-term medical assistance in the United States but then may lack health care coverage due to ineligibility for state medical assistance or inability to afford private health insurance.

3. Nurses need to be aware of the limited access to health care resources and explore possible health care services for this population.
4. Vaccinations must be provided to prevent communicable diseases.

XX. Individuals With Chronic Illness

A. Individuals with multiple chronic illnesses need special attention.
B. Chronic illness is the leading cause of death and disability in the United States; the prevalence increases with age and is a major cause of disability.
C. Chronic illnesses include cardiovascular disease, cancer, respiratory disease, diabetes, mental disorders, vision and hearing impairment, oral diseases, bone and joint disorders, and genetic disorders.
D. Poor health outcomes and high health care costs are associated with chronic illness.
E. Optimal care for individuals with multiple chronic illnesses may be limited because of multiple health needs present.
F. Many health professionals do not feel adequately prepared to manage individuals with multiple chronic illnesses.
G. Individuals with one chronic illness are at risk for developing multiple chronic illnesses.
H. Modifiable factors include an unhealthy diet, physical inactivity, and tobacco use; nonmodifiable factors include age and genetics.
I. Health care considerations for individuals with chronic illness
   1. Follow-up care is important in promoting health for individuals with chronic illness.
   2. Focusing on a single illness does not effectively manage an individual with multiple chronic diseases—rather, the "big picture" needs to be understood in managing these clients.
   3. Interprofessional collaboration is important in safely managing individuals with chronic diseases.
   4. Nurses play a key role in facilitating interprofessional communication between providers and specialists.
   5. Inclusion of the client and support person(s) in health care decisions helps to increase adherence to a complex health care regimen.

PRACTICE QUESTIONS

1. Which teaching method is **most effective** when providing instruction to members of special populations?
1. Teach-back
2. Video instruction
3. Written materials
4. Verbal explanation

2. Which is **most appropriate** when communicating with a transgender person?
1. Using preferred pronouns
2. Using their first name to address them
3. Using pronouns associated with birth sex
4. Anticipating the client's needs and making suggestions

3. The nurse is volunteering with an outreach program to provide basic health care for homeless people. Which finding, if noted, must be addressed **first**?
1. Blood pressure 154/72 mm Hg
2. Visual acuity of 20/200 in both eyes
3. Random blood glucose level of 206 mg/dL (11.77 mmol/L)
4. Complaints of pain associated with numbness and tingling in both feet

4. The nurse is completing the admission assessment of a client who is intellectually disabled. Which part of the client encounter may require more time to complete?
1. The history
2. The physical assessment
3. The nursing plan of care
4. The readmission risk assessment

5. The nurse working in a correctional facility is caring for a new prisoner. The client asks about health risks associated with living in a prison. How would the nurse respond?
1. "Health care is very limited in the prison setting."
2. "Living in a prison isn't different than living at home."
3. "Living in a prison can predispose a person to different health conditions."
4. "Living in a prison is similar to living in a condominium complex or dormitory."

6. The nurse is caring for a female client in the emergency department who presents with a complaint of fatigue and shortness of breath. Which physical assessment findings, if noted by the nurse, warrant a **need for follow-up**?
1. Reddened sclera of the eyes
2. Dry flaking noted on the scalp
3. A reddish-purple mark on the neck
4. A scaly rash noted on the elbows and knees

7. The nurse working in a community outreach program for foster children plans care knows that which health conditions are common in this population? **Select all that apply.**
1. Asthma
2. Claustrophobia
3. Sleep problems
4. Bipolar disorder
5. Aggressive behavior
6. Attention-deficit hyperactivity disorder (ADHD)

8. The nurse planning care for a military veteran must **prioritize** nursing interventions targeted at managing which condition, if present, that commonly occurs in this population?
1. Hypertension
2. Hyperlipidemia
3. Substance abuse disorder
4. Post-traumatic stress disorder

9. The nurse caring for a refugee considers which health care need a **priority** for this client?
1. Access to housing
2. Access to clean water
3. Access to transportation
4. Access to mental health care services

10. Which action by the nurse will **best** facilitate adherence to the treatment regimen for a client with a chronic illness?
1. Arranging for home health care
2. Focusing on managing a single illness at a time
3. Communicating with one provider only to avoid confusion for the client
4. Allowing the client to teach a support person about their treatment regimen

ANSWERS

1. *Answer:* 1
Rationale: When providing education to members of special populations, return explanation and demonstration (teach-back) are of particular importance to ensure safety and mutual understanding. This method is the most reliable in confirming client understanding of the instructions. Video instruction, written materials, and verbal explanation are helpful and may be incorporated with the teach-back method.
Test-Taking Strategy: Note the strategic words, *most effective.* Note that the correct option—the teach-back method—is the umbrella option, which encompasses all other options. Recall that asking the client to perform a return demonstration is the best way to confirm his or her understanding.
Level of Cognitive Ability: Applying
Client Needs: Health Promotion and Maintenance
Integrated Process: Teaching and Learning
Content Area: Foundations of Care—Community Health
Health Problem: N/A
Priority Concepts: Client Education; Health Promotion
Reference: Russell, L. (2010). *Fact sheet: Health disparities by race and ethnicity.* Retrieved from https://cdn.americanprogress.org/wp-content/uploads/issues/2010/12/pdf/disparities_factsheet.pdf

2. *Answer:* 1
Rationale: The nurse needs to address the client with the name and pronouns that the client prefers, and the first name may not necessarily be their preference. For the transgender person, it is likely that they would like to be addressed using pronouns associated with the sex they identify with now, which typically is not their birth sex. Anticipating the client's needs and making suggestions may be seen as passing judgment, so the nurse should refrain from doing this.
Test-Taking Strategy: Note the strategic words, *most appropriate.* Recalling that clarification regarding name preference for any client will assist you in eliminating option 2. Recalling that use of pronouns associated with birth sex is inappropriate will assist you in eliminating option 3. Noting the word *making suggestions* in option 4 will assist you in eliminating this option.
Level of Cognitive Ability: Applying
Client Needs: Psychosocial Integrity
Integrated Process: Caring
Content Area: Foundations of Care—Community Health
Health Problem: N/A
Priority Concepts: Professional Identity; Safety
Reference: Ard, K. L. (n.d.). *Improving the health care of lesbian, gay, bisexual, and transgender people: Understanding and eliminating health disparities.* Retrieved from https://www.lgbthealtheducation.org/wp-content/uploads/Improving-the-Health-of-LGBT-People.pdf

3. *Answer:* 4
Rationale: The nurse needs to address the complaints of pain and numbness and tingling in both feet first with this population. If the client perceives value to the service provided and his or her complaint is addressed, they will be more likely to return for follow-up care. While the blood pressure, blood glucose, and vision results are concerning, the client's stated concern must be addressed first.
Test-Taking Strategy: Note the subject, the finding to be addressed, and focus on the strategic word, *first.* Recalling that adherence is a problem for this population will direct you to the correct option. Also note that the correct option is the only subjective finding.
Level of Cognitive Ability: Analyzing
Client Needs: Health Promotion and Maintenance
Integrated Process: Nursing Process—Assessment

Content Area: Foundations of Care—Community Health
Health Problem: N/A
Priority Concepts: Clinical Judgment; Health Promotion
Reference: Maness, D. L. & Khan, M. (2014). Care of the homeless: An overview. *American Family Physician, 89*(8), 634-640.

4. *Answer:* 1
Rationale: Intellectually disabled clients tend to have difficulty trying to remember their medical history. It may be necessary for the nurse to take more time to ask questions in a variety of different ways when collecting the history data. The physical assessment, nursing plan of care, and readmission risk assessment portions, although they rely on the history, take less time because they require less client questioning.
Test-Taking Strategy: Note the subject, conducting an admission assessment for an intellectually disabled client and the part that may take more time to complete. Recall that individuals in this special population group tend to have difficulty remembering their medical history. The use of questioning in a variety of ways may be necessary to obtain the necessary assessment data.
Level of Cognitive Ability: Applying
Client Needs: Psychosocial Integrity
Integrated Process: Nursing Process—Assessment
Content Area: Health Assessment/Physical Exam: Health History
Health Problem: N/A
Priority Concepts: Communication; Functional Ability
Reference: May, M. E. & Kennedy, C. H. (2010). Health and problem behavior among people with intellectual disabilities. *Behavioral Annals of Practice, 3*(2), 4-12.

5. *Answer:* 3
Rationale: The environment of a prison can predispose a person to different health conditions, such as tuberculosis, sexually transmitted infections, or other infectious diseases. Option 1 does not address the client's question. Options 2 and 4 convey incorrect information.
Test-Taking Strategy: Note the subject—health conditions associated with living in a prison. Remember that the prison is a confined environment, and a variety of health problems including infectious diseases are prevalent.
Level of Cognitive Ability: Applying
Client Needs: Safe and Effective Care Environment
Integrated Process: Teaching and Learning
Content Area: Foundations of Care—Communication
Health Problem: N/A
Priority Concepts: Communication; Health Promotion
Reference: Issues in Science and Technology. (n.d.). *Correctional health is community health.* Retrieved from http://issues.org/32-1/correctional-health-is-community-health/

6. *Answer:* 3
Rationale: The client in this question must be screened for abuse. Battered women experience bruises, particularly around the eyes, red or purple marks on the neck, sprained or broken wrists, chronic fatigue, shortness of breath, muscle tension, involuntary shaking, changes in eating and sleeping, sexual dysfunction, and fertility issues. Mental health issues can also arise, including posttraumatic stress disorder, nightmares, anxiety, uncontrollable thoughts, depression, low self-esteem, and alcohol and drug abuse. Reddened sclera, a dry rash on the elbows, and flaking of the scalp do not pose an indication of abuse.
Test-Taking Strategy: Note the strategic words, *need for follow-up.* Also focus on the data in the question and select the option that indicates the most concern and is indicative of abuse. Remember that battered women often present with bruising around the eyes or on the neck.
Level of Cognitive Ability: Analyzing
Client Needs: Safe and Effective Care Environment
Integrated Process: Nursing Process/Assessment
Content Area: Mental Health
Health Problem: Mental Health: Violence
Priority Concepts: Communication; Health Promotion
Reference: Bohn, D. K. & Holz, K. A. (1996). Sequelae of abuse: Health effects of childhood sexual abuse, domestic battering, and rape. *Journal of Midwifery & Women's Health, 41*(6), 442-456.

7. *Answer:* 3, 4, 5, 6
Rationale: Foster children are at risk for a variety of health conditions, including ADHD, aggressive behavior, anxiety disorder, bipolar disorder, depression, mood disorder, posttraumatic stress disorder, reactive detachment disorder, sleep problems, and personality disorder. Claustrophobia and asthma are not specifically associated with foster children.
Test-Taking Strategy: Note the subject—health concerns for foster children. Recall that mental health is a major concern for this population. This will assist in directing you to the correct options.
Level of Cognitive Ability: Applying
Client Needs: Health Promotion and Maintenance
Integrated Process: Nursing Process—Planning
Content Area: Foundations of Care—Community Health
Health Problem: N/A
Priority Concepts: Development; Health Promotion
Reference: American Academy of Pediatrics. (n.d.). *Healthy foster care America.* Retrieved from https://www.aap.org/en-us/advocacy-and-policy/aap-health-initiatives/healthy-foster-care-america/Documents/HFCAJudgesToolkit.pdf

8. *Answer:* 4
Rationale: Post-traumatic stress disorder (PTSD) is extremely common in this population. Identifying and treating mental health disorders assists in mitigating suicide risk. Treatment of comorbid conditions such as PTSD may also help to address any substance use disorder. Use of screening tools in identifying substance use disorder is helpful. Treatment of PTSD includes exposure therapy, psychotherapy, and family/group therapy. Hypertension and hyperlipidemia are important but are not the priority; the risk of suicide and other safety concerns associated with PTSD are the priority for this population.
Test-Taking Strategy: Note the strategic word, *prioritize.* This word indicates that although all options may be important, one option is a priority due to safety considerations. Also note

that options 1 and 2 are comparable or alike and therefore can be eliminated. Although substance abuse may be a concern, PTSD is the priority.
Level of Cognitive Ability: Applying
Client Needs: Health Promotion and Maintenance
Integrated Process: Nursing Process—Planning
Content Area: Mental Health
Health Problem: Mental Health: Post-Traumatic Stress Disorder
Priority Concepts: Health Promotion; Safety
Reference: US National Library of Medicine. (2017). *Veterans and military health.* Retrieved from https://medlineplus.gov/veteransandmilitaryhealth.html

9. *Answer:* 4
Rationale: Mental health problems are the primary issue for this population as a result of difficult events. While all other options are important for all clients, they do not address the specific needs of this special population.
Test-Taking Strategy: Note the strategic word, *priority.* This indicates that all options are important and are most likely correct. It is necessary to recall that due to the potential trauma experienced by refugees, mental health is a priority.
Level of Cognitive Ability: Applying
Client Needs: Psychosocial Integrity
Integrated Process: Nursing Process—Planning
Content Area: Foundations of Care—Community Health
Health Problem: N/A
Priority Concepts: Clinical Judgment; Health Promotion
Reference: Global Citizen. (2018). *The 7 biggest challenges facing refugees and immigrants in the US.* Retrieved from https://www.globalcitizen.org/en/content/the-7-biggest-challenges-facing-refugees-and-immig/

10. *Answer:* 1
Rationale: Nursing follow-up visits are important in promoting health for individuals with chronic illness; therefore, arranging for home health care is an important strategy. Focusing on a single illness does not effectively manage an individual with multiple chronic diseases—rather, the "big picture" needs to be understood in managing these clients. Interprofessional collaboration is important in safely managing individuals with chronic diseases and often involves consulting with specialist providers. Nurses play a key role in facilitating communication between providers and specialists. Inclusion of the client and support persons in health care decisions helps to increase adherence to a complex health care regimen. The nurse would be the facilitator of this communication.
Test-Taking Strategy: Note the strategic word, *best.* Recalling that these clients often have complex histories and health care needs will assist you in choosing the option that relates to nursing support services.
Level of Cognitive Ability: Applying
Client Needs: Health Promotion and Maintenance
Integrated Process: Nursing Process—Planning
Content Area: Foundations of Care—Community Health
Health Problem: N/A
Priority Concepts: Health Promotion; Safety
Reference: Benjamin, R. M. (2010). Multiple chronic conditions: A public health challenge. *Public Health Repository, 125*(5), 626-627.

CHAPTER 6

Ethical and Legal Issues

PRIORITY CONCEPTS **Ethics; Health Care Law**

I. Ethics

A. Description: The branch of philosophy concerned with the distinction between right and wrong on the basis of a body of knowledge, not only on the basis of opinions

B. **Morals:** Behavior in accordance with customs or tradition, usually reflecting personal or religious beliefs

C. **Ethical principles:** Codes that direct or govern nursing actions (Box 6-1)

D. Values: Beliefs and attitudes that may influence behavior and the process of decision making

E. Values clarification: Process of analyzing one's own values to understand oneself more completely regarding what is truly important

F. Ethical codes

1. Ethical codes provide broad principles for determining and evaluating client care.
2. These codes are not legally binding, but the board of nursing has authority in most states to reprimand nurses for unprofessional conduct that results from violation of the ethical codes.
3. Specific ethical codes are as follows:
    a. The Code of Ethics for Nurses developed by the International Council of Nurses; Web site: http://www.old.icn.ch/who-we-are/code-of-ethics-for-nurses/.
    b. The American Nurses Association Code of Ethics can be viewed on the American Nurses Association; Web site: http://www.nursingworld.org/codeofethics.

BOX 6-1 Ethical Principles

Autonomy: Respect for an individual's right to self-determination
Nonmaleficence: The obligation to do or cause no harm to another
Beneficence: The duty to do good to others and to maintain a balance between benefits and harms; paternalism is an undesirable outcome of beneficence, in which the health care provider decides what is best for the client and encourages the client to act against his or her own choices
Justice: The equitable distribution of potential benefits and tasks determining the order in which clients should be cared for
Veracity: The obligation to tell the truth
Fidelity: The duty to do what one has promised

G. Ethical dilemma

1. An ethical dilemma occurs when there is a conflict between two or more **ethical principles**.
2. No correct decision exists, and the nurse must make a choice between two alternatives that are equally unsatisfactory.
3. Such dilemmas may occur as a result of differences in cultural or religious beliefs.
4. Ethical reasoning is the process of thinking through what one should do in an orderly and systematic manner to provide justification for actions based on principles; the nurse should gather all information to determine whether an ethical dilemma exists, examine his or her own values, verbalize the problem, consider possible courses of action, negotiate the outcome, and evaluate the action taken.

H. Advocate

1. An advocate is a person who speaks up for or acts on the behalf of the client, protects the client's right to make his or her own decisions, and upholds the principle of **fidelity**.
2. An advocate represents the client's viewpoint to others.
3. An advocate avoids letting personal values influence **advocacy** for the client and supports the client's decision, even when it conflicts with the advocate's own preferences or choices.

I. Ethics committees

1. Ethics committees take an interprofessional approach to facilitate dialogue regarding ethical dilemmas.
2. These committees develop and establish policies and procedures to facilitate the prevention and resolution of dilemmas.

⚠ An important nursing responsibility is to act as a client advocate and protect the client's rights.

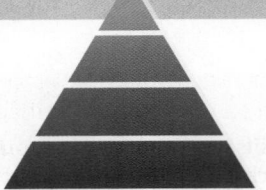

II. Regulation of Nursing Practice

A. Nurse Practice Act
1. A nurse practice act is a series of statutes that have been enacted by each state legislature to regulate the practice of nursing in that state.
2. Nurse practice acts set educational requirements for the nurse, distinguish between nursing practice and medical practice, and define the scope of nursing practice.
3. Additional issues covered by nurse practice acts include licensure requirements for protection of the public, grounds for disciplinary action, rights of the nurse licensee if a disciplinary action is taken, and related topics.
4. All nurses are responsible for knowing the provisions of the act of the state or province in which they work.

B. Standards of care
1. Standards of care are guidelines that identify what the client can expect to receive in terms of nursing care.
2. The guidelines determine whether nurses have performed duties in an appropriate manner.
3. If the nurse does not perform duties within accepted standards of care, the nurse may be in jeopardy of legal action.
4. If the nurse is named as a defendant in a **malpractice** lawsuit and proceedings show that the nurse followed neither the accepted standards of care outlined by the state or province nurse practice act nor the policies of the employing institution, the nurse's legal liability is clear; he or she is liable.

C. Employee guidelines
1. Respondeat superior: The employer is held liable for any negligent acts of an employee if the alleged negligent act occurred during the employment relationship and was within the scope of the employee's responsibilities.
2. Contracts
   a. Nurses are responsible for carrying out the terms of a contractual agreement with the employing agency and the client.
   b. The nurse–employee relationship is governed by established employee handbooks and client care policies and procedures that create obligations, rights, and duties between those parties.
3. Institutional policies
   a. Written policies and procedures of the employing institution detail how nurses are to perform their duties.
   b. Policies and procedures are usually specific and describe the expected behavior on the part of the nurse.
   c. Although policies are not laws, courts generally rule against nurses who violate policies.
   d. If the nurse practices nursing according to client care policies and procedures established by the employer, functions within the job responsibility, and provides care consistently in a nonnegligent manner, the nurse minimizes the potential for liability.

⚠ The nurse must follow the guidelines identified in the Nurse Practice Act and agency policies and procedures when delivering client care.

D. Hospital staffing
1. Charges of abandonment may be made against nurses who "walk out" when staffing is inadequate.
2. Nurses in short staffing situations are obligated to make a report to the nursing administration.

E. Floating
1. Floating is an acceptable practice used by health care facilities to alleviate understaffing and overstaffing.
2. Legally, the nurse cannot refuse to float unless a union contract guarantees that nurses can work only in a specified area or the nurse can prove lack of knowledge for the performance of assigned tasks.
3. Nurses in a floating situation must not assume responsibility beyond their level of experience or qualification.
4. Nurses who float should inform the supervisor of any lack of experience in caring for the type of clients on the new nursing unit.
5. A resource nurse who is skilled in the care of clients on the unit should also be assigned to the float nurse; in addition, the float nurse should be given an orientation of the unit and the standards of care for the unit should be reviewed (the float nurse should care for clients whose acuity level more closely match the nurses' experience).

F. Disciplinary action
1. Boards of nursing may deny, revoke, or suspend any license to practice as a registered nurse, according to their statutory authority.
2. Some causes for disciplinary action are as follows:
   a. Unprofessional conduct
   b. Conduct that could affect the health and welfare of the public adversely
   c. Breach of client **confidentiality**
   d. Failure to use sufficient knowledge, skills, or nursing judgment
   e. Physically or verbally abusing a client
   f. Assuming duties without sufficient preparation
   g. Knowingly delegating to unlicensed personnel nursing care that places the client at risk for injury
   h. Failure to maintain an accurate record for each client

- **i.** Falsifying a client's record
- **j.** Leaving a nursing assignment without properly notifying appropriate personnel

III. Legal Liability

A. Laws

1. Nurses are governed by civil and criminal law in roles as providers of services, employees of institutions, and private citizens.
2. The nurse has a personal and legal obligation to provide a standard of client care expected of a reasonably competent professional nurse.
3. Professional nurses are held responsible (liable) for harm resulting from their negligent acts or their failure to act.

B. Types of laws (Box 6-2; Fig. 6-1)

C. **Negligence** and **malpractice** (Box 6-3)

1. Negligence is conduct that falls below the standard of care.
2. Negligence can include acts of commission and acts of omission.
3. The nurse who does not meet appropriate standards of care may be held liable.
4. Malpractice is negligence on the part of the nurse.
5. Malpractice is determined if the nurse owed a duty to the client and did not carry out the duty and the client was injured because the nurse failed to perform the duty.
6. Proof of liability
   - **a.** Duty: At the time of injury, a duty existed between the plaintiff and the defendant.

BOX 6-2 Types of Law

Contract Law

Contract law is concerned with enforcement of agreements among private individuals.

Civil Law

Civil law is concerned with relationships among persons and the protection of a person's rights. Violation may cause harm to an individual or property, but no grave threat to society exists.

Criminal Law

Criminal law is concerned with relationships between individuals and governments, and with acts that threaten society and its order; a crime is an offense against society that violates a law and is defined as a misdemeanor (less serious nature) or felony (serious nature).

Tort Law

A tort is a civil wrong, other than a breach in contract, in which the law allows an injured person to seek damages from a person who caused the injury.

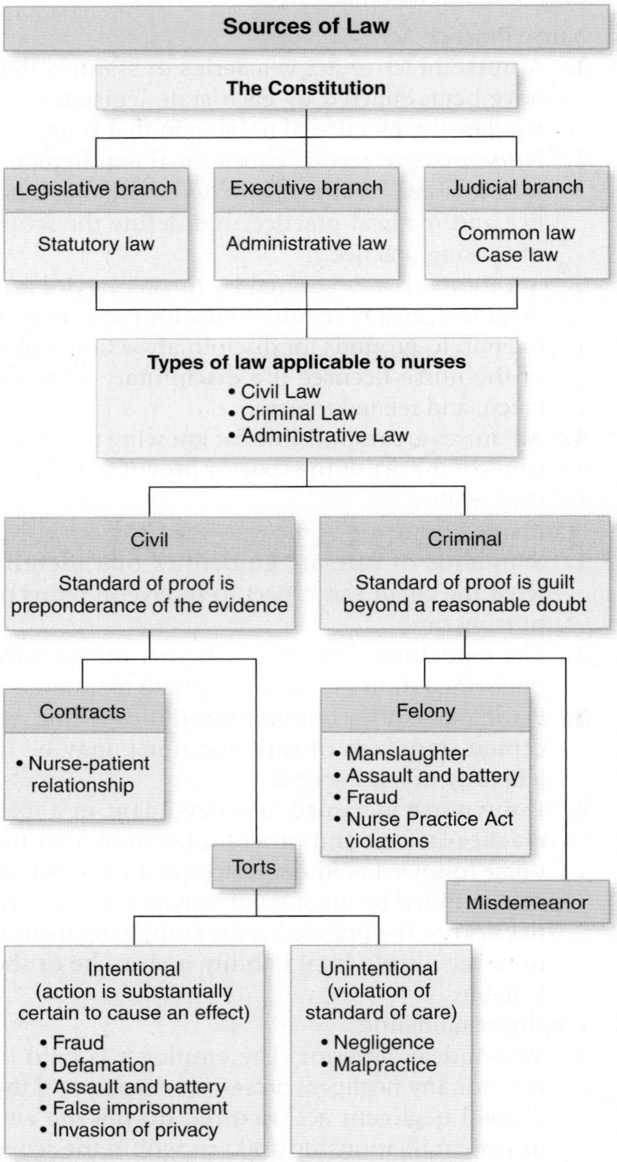

FIG. 6-1 Sources of law for nursing practice.

   - **b.** Breach of duty: The defendant breached duty of care to the plaintiff.
   - **c.** Proximate cause: The breach of the duty was the legal cause of injury to the client.
   - **d.** Damage or injury: The plaintiff experienced injury or damages or both and can be compensated by law.

⚠ The nurse must meet appropriate standards of care when delivering care to the client; otherwise the nurse would be held liable if the client is harmed.

D. Professional liability insurance

1. Nurses need their own liability insurance for protection against malpractice lawsuits.

BOX 6-3 Examples of Negligent Acts

- Medication errors that result in injury to the client
- Intravenous administration errors, such as incorrect flow rates, failure to monitor a flow rate that results in injury to the client, infiltration, or phlebitis
- Falls that occur as a result of failure to provide safety to the client
- Failure to use aseptic technique when indicated
- Failure to check equipment for proper functioning
- Burns sustained by the client as a result of failure to monitor bath temperature or equipment, protect the client from spills of hot liquids or foods
- Errors in sponge, instrument, or needle counts in surgical cases, meaning that an item was left in a client
- Failure to adequately monitor a client's condition
- Failure to report changes in the client's condition to the primary health care provider
- Failure to give a report or giving an incomplete report to the oncoming shift personnel

Adapted from Potter P, Perry A, Stockert P, Hall A: *Essentials for nursing practice*, ed 8, St. Louis, 2015, Mosby.

2. Having their own insurance provides nurses protection as individuals; this allows the nurse to have an attorney, who has only the nurse's interests in mind, present if necessary.

E. Good Samaritan laws
1. State legislatures pass Good Samaritan laws, which may vary from state to state.
2. These laws encourage health care professionals to assist in emergency situations and limit liability and offer legal immunity for persons helping in an emergency, provided that they give reasonable care.
3. Immunity from suit applies only when all conditions of the state law are met, such as that the health care provider (HCP) receives no compensation for the care provided and the care given is not intentionally negligent.

F. Controlled substances
1. The nurse should adhere to facility policies and procedures concerning administration of controlled substances, which are governed by federal and state laws.
2. Controlled substances must be kept locked securely, and only authorized personnel should have access to them.
3. Controlled substances must be properly signed out for administration and a correct inventory must be maintained.

IV. Collective Bargaining

A. Collective bargaining is a formalized decision-making process between representatives of management and representatives of labor to negotiate wages and conditions of employment.

B. When collective bargaining breaks down because the parties cannot reach an agreement, the employees may call a strike or take other work actions.

C. Striking presents a **moral** dilemma to many nurses, because nursing practice is a service to people.

V. Legal Risk Areas

A. Assault
1. Assault occurs when a person puts another person in fear of a harmful or offensive contact.
2. The victim fears and believes that harm will result because of the threat.

B. Battery is an intentional touching of another's body without the other's **consent**.

C. Invasion of privacy includes violating **confidentiality**, intruding on private client or family matters, and sharing client information with unauthorized persons.

D. False imprisonment
1. False imprisonment occurs when a client is not allowed to leave a health care facility when there is no legal justification to detain the client.
2. False imprisonment also occurs when restraining devices are used without an appropriate clinical need.
3. A client can sign an Against Medical Advice form when the client refuses care and is competent to make decisions.
4. The nurse should document circumstances in the medical record to avoid allegations by the client that cannot be defended.

E. Defamation is a false communication that causes damage to someone's reputation, either in writing (libel) or verbally (slander).

F. Fraud results from a deliberate deception intended to produce unlawful gains.

G. There may be exceptions to certain legal risks areas, such as assault, battery, and false imprisonment, when caring for a client with a mental health disorder experiencing acute distress who poses a risk to themself or others. In this situation, the nurse must assess the client to determine loss of control and intervene accordingly; the nurse should use the least restrictive methods initially, but then use interventions such as restraint if the client's behavior indicates the need for this intervention.

VI. Client's Rights

A. Description
1. The client's rights document, also called the **Client's (Patient's) Bill of Rights**, reflects acknowledgment of a client's right to participate in their health care with an emphasis on client autonomy.
2. The document provides a list of the rights of the client and responsibilities that the hospital cannot violate (Box 6-4).

BOX 6-4 Client's Rights When Hospitalized

- Right to considerate and respectful care
- Right to be informed about diagnosis, possible treatments, and likely outcome, and to discuss this information with the health care provider
- Right to know the names and roles of the persons who are involved in care
- Right to consent or refuse a treatment
- Right to have an advance directive
- Right to privacy
- Right to expect that medical records are confidential
- Right to review the medical record and to have information explained
- Right to expect that the hospital will provide necessary health services
- Right to know if the hospital has relationships with outside parties that may influence treatment or care
- Right to consent or refuse to take part in research
- Right to be told of realistic care alternatives when hospital care is no longer appropriate
- Right to know about hospital rules that affect treatment and about charges and payment methods

From Christensen B, Kockrow E: *Foundations of nursing*, ed 6, St. Louis, 2010, Mosby; and adapted from American Hospital Association: *The patient care partnership: understanding expectations, rights and responsibilities*. Available at www.aha.org/content/00-10/pcp_english_030730.pdf.

3. The Client's Bill of Rights protects the client's ability to determine the level and type of care received; all health care agencies are required to have a Client's Bill of Rights posted in a visible area.
4. Several laws and standards pertain to client's rights (Box 6-5).

B. Rights for the mentally ill (Box 6-6)

1. The Mental Health Systems Act created rights for mentally ill people.

BOX 6-5 Laws and Standards

American Hospital Association
Issued Patient's Bill of Rights

American Nurses Association
Developed the Code of Ethics for Nurses, which defines the nurse's responsibility for upholding client's rights

Mental Health Systems Act
Developed rights for mentally ill clients

The Joint Commission
Developed policy statements on the rights of mentally ill individuals

Americans With Disabilities Act
Prohibits discrimination against an individual with disabilities in all areas of public life

BOX 6-6 Rights for the Mentally Ill

- Right to be treated with dignity and respect
- Right to communicate with persons outside the hospital
- Right to keep clothing and personal effects with them
- Right to religious freedom
- Right to be employed
- Right to manage property
- Right to execute wills
- Right to enter into contractual agreements
- Right to make purchases
- Right to education
- Right to habeas corpus (written request for release from the hospital)
- Right to an independent psychiatric examination
- Right to civil service status, including the right to vote
- Right to retain licenses, privileges, or permits
- Right to sue or be sued
- Right to marry or divorce
- Right to treatment in the least restrictive setting
- Right not to be subject to unnecessary restraints
- Right to privacy and confidentiality
- Right to informed consent
- Right to treatment and to refuse treatment
- Right to refuse participation in experimental treatments or research

Adapted from Stuart G: *Principles and practice of psychiatric nursing*, ed 10, St. Louis, 2013, Mosby; Varcarolis, E: *Essentials of psychiatric mental health nursing: a communication approach to evidence-based care*, ed 3, St. Louis, 2017, Saunders.

2. The Joint Commission has developed policy statements on the rights of mentally ill people.
3. Psychiatric facilities are required to have a Client's Bill of Rights posted in a visible area.

C. Organ donation and transplantation

1. A client has the right to decide to become an organ donor and a right to refuse organ transplantation as a treatment option.
2. An individual who is at least 18 years old may indicate a wish to become a donor on their driver's license (state-specific) or in an **advance directive**.
3. The Uniform Anatomical Gift Act provides a list of individuals who can provide **informed consent** for the donation of a deceased individual's organs.
4. The United Network for Organ Sharing sets the criteria for organ donations.
5. Some organs, such as the heart, lungs, and liver, can be obtained only from a person who is on mechanical ventilation and has suffered brain death, whereas other organs or tissues can be removed several hours after death.
6. A donor must be free of infectious disease and cancer.
7. Requests to the deceased's family for organ donation usually are done by the primary health care provider (PHCP) or nurse specially trained for making such requests.

8. Donation of organs does not delay funeral arrangements; no obvious evidence that the organs were removed from the body shows when the body is dressed; and the family incurs no cost for removal of the organs donated.

D. Religious beliefs: Organ donation and transplantation
1. Catholic Church: Organ donation and transplants are acceptable.
2. Orthodox Church: Church usually discourages organ donation.
3. Islam (Muslim) beliefs: Body parts should not be removed or donated for transplantation.
4. Jehovah's Witness: An organ transplant may be accepted, but the organ must be cleansed with a nonblood solution before transplantation.
5. Orthodox Judaism
   a. All body parts removed during autopsy must be buried with the body because it is believed that the entire body must be returned to the earth; organ donation may not be considered by family members.
   b. Organ transplantation may be allowed with the rabbi's approval.
6. Refer to Chapter 18 for additional information regarding end-of-life care.

VII. Consents

A. Description
1. Consents, or releases, are legal documents that indicate the client's permission to perform surgery, perform a treatment or procedure, or give information to a third party.
2. There are different types of consents (Box 6-7).
3. Informed consent indicates the client's participation in the decision regarding health care. It is the client's approval (or that of the client's legal representative) to have their body touched by a specific individual.
4. The client must be informed, in understandable terms, of the risks and benefits of the surgery or treatment, what the consequences are for not having the surgery or procedure performed, treatment options, and the name of the HCP performing the surgery or procedure.
5. A client's questions about the surgery or procedure must be answered before signing the consent.
6. A consent must be signed freely by the client without threat or pressure and must be witnessed (the witness must be an adult).
7. A client who has been medicated with sedating medications or any other medications that can affect the client's cognitive abilities must not be asked to sign a consent.
8. Legally, the client must be mentally and emotionally competent to give consent.
9. If a client is declared mentally or emotionally incompetent, the next of kin, appointed guardian (appointed by the court), or durable power of attorney for health care has legal authority to give consent (Box 6-8).
10. A competent client 18 years of age or older must sign the consent.

BOX 6-7 Types of Consents

Admission Agreement

Admission agreements are obtained at the time of admission and identify the health care agency's responsibility to the client.

Immunization Consent

An immunization consent may be required before the administration of certain immunizations; the consent indicates that the client was informed of the benefits and risks of the immunization.

Blood Transfusion Consent

A blood transfusion consent indicates that the client was informed of the benefits and risks of the transfusion. Some clients hold religious beliefs that would prohibit them from receiving a blood transfusion, even in a life-threatening situation.

Surgical Consent

Surgical consent is obtained for all surgical or invasive procedures or diagnostic tests that are invasive. The primary health care provider, surgeon, or anesthesiologist who performs the operative or other procedure is responsible for explaining the procedure, its risks and benefits, and possible alternative options.

Research Consent

The research consent obtains permission from the client regarding participation in a research study. The consent informs the client about the possible risks, consequences, and benefits of the research.

Special Consents

Special consents are required for the use of restraints, photographing the client, disposal of body parts during surgery, donating organs after death, or performing an autopsy.

BOX 6-8 Mentally or Emotionally Incompetent Clients

- Declared incompetent
- Unconscious
- Under the influence of chemical agents such as alcohol or drugs
- Chronic dementia or other mental deficiency that impairs thought processes and ability to make decisions

11. In most states, when the nurse is involved in the informed consent process, the nurse is witnessing only the signature of the client on the informed consent form.
12. An informed consent can be waived for urgent medical or surgical intervention as long as institutional policy so indicates.
13. A client has the right to refuse information and waive the informed consent and undergo treatment, but this decision must be documented in the medical record.
14. A client may withdraw consent at any time.

An informed consent is a legal document, and the client must be informed by the PHCP (i.e., physician, surgeon), in understandable terms, of the risks and benefits of surgery, treatments, procedures, and plan of care. The client needs to be a participant in decisions regarding health care.

B. Minors
1. A minor is a client under legal age as defined by state statute (usually younger than 18 years).
2. A minor may not give legal consent, and consent must be obtained from a parent or the legal guardian; agreement by the minor is important because it allows for communication of the minor's thoughts and feelings.
3. Parental or guardian consent should be obtained before treatment is initiated for a minor except in the following cases: in an emergency; in situations in which the consent of the minor is sufficient, including treatment related to substance abuse, treatment of a sexually transmitted infection, human immunodeficiency virus (HIV) testing and acquired immunodeficiency syndrome (AIDS) treatment, birth control services, pregnancy, or psychiatric services; the minor is an emancipated minor; or a court order or other legal authorization has been obtained. Refer to the Guttmacher Report on Public Policy for additional information: http://www.guttmacher.org/pubs/tgr/03/4/gr030404.html.

C. Emancipated minor
1. An emancipated minor has established independence from his or her parents through marriage, pregnancy, or service in the armed forces, or by a court order.
2. An emancipated minor is considered legally capable of signing an informed consent.

VIII. Health Insurance Portability and Accountability Act

A. Description
1. The Health Insurance Portability and Accountability Act (HIPAA) describes how personal health information (PHI) may be used and how the client can obtain access to the information.
2. PHI includes individually identifiable information that relates to the client's past, present, or future health; treatment; and payment for health care services.
3. The act requires health care agencies to keep PHI private, provides information to the client about the legal responsibilities regarding privacy, and explains the client's rights with respect to PHI.
4. The client has various rights as a consumer of health care under HIPAA, and any client requests may need to be placed in writing; a fee may be attached to certain client requests.
5. The client may file a complaint if the client believes that privacy rights have been violated.

B. Client's rights include the right to do the following:
1. Inspect a copy of PHI.
2. Ask the health care agency to amend the PHI that is contained in a record if the PHI is inaccurate.
3. Request a list of disclosures made regarding the PHI as specified by HIPAA.
4. Request to restrict how the health care agency uses or discloses PHI regarding treatment, payment, or health care services, unless information is needed to provide emergency treatment.
5. Request that the health care agency communicate with the client in a certain way or at a certain location; the request must specify how or where the client wishes to be contacted.
6. Request a paper copy of the HIPAA notice.

C. Health care agency use and disclosure of PHI
1. The health care agency obtains PHI in the course of providing or administering health insurance benefits.
2. Use or disclosure of PHI may be done for the following:
   a. Health care payment purposes
   b. Health care operations purposes
   c. Treatment purposes
   d. Providing information about health care services
   e. Data aggregation purposes to make health care benefit decisions
   f. Administering health care benefits
3. There are additional uses or disclosures of PHI (Box 6-9).

IX. Confidentiality/Information Security

A. Description
1. In the health care system, **confidentiality/information security** refers to the protection of privacy of the client's PHI.
2. Clients have a right to privacy in the health care system.
3. A special relationship exists between the client and nurse, in which information discussed is not shared with a third party who is not directly involved in the client's care.

BOX 6-9 Uses or Disclosures of Personal Health Information

- Compliance with legal proceedings or for limited law enforcement purposes
- To a family member or significant other in a medical emergency
- To a personal representative appointed by the client or designated by law
- For research purposes in limited circumstances
- To a coroner, medical examiner, or funeral director about a deceased person
- To an organ procurement organization in limited circumstances
- To avert a serious threat to the client's health or safety or the health or safety of others
- To a governmental agency authorized to oversee the health care system or government programs
- To the Department of Health and Human Services for the investigation of compliance with the Health Insurance Portability and Accountability Act or to fulfill another lawful request
- To federal officials for lawful intelligence or national security purposes
- To protect health authorities for public health purposes
- To appropriate military authorities if a client is a member of the armed forces
- In accordance with a valid authorization signed by the client

Adapted from U.S. Department of Health and Human Services Office for Civil Rights: Health information privacy. Available at http://www.hhs.gov/ocr/privacy/.

4. Violations of privacy occur in various ways (Box 6-10).

B. Nurse's responsibility

1. Nurses are bound to protect client **confidentiality** by most nurse practice acts, by **ethical principles** and standards, and by institutional and agency policies and procedures.
2. Disclosure of confidential information exposes the nurse to liability for invasion of the client's privacy.
3. The nurse needs to protect the client from indiscriminate disclosure of health care information that may cause harm (Box 6-11).

C. Social networks and health care (Box 6-12)

D. Medical records

1. Medical records are confidential.
2. The client has the right to read the medical record and have copies of the record.
3. Only staff members directly involved in care have legitimate access to a client's record; these may include PHCPs and nurses caring for the client, technicians, therapists, social workers, unit secretaries, client advocates, and administrators (e.g., for statistical analysis, staffing, quality care review). Others must ask permission from the client to review a record.
4. Per health care facility procedures, the medical record is stored in the records or the health information department after discharge of the client from the facility.

BOX 6-10 Violations and Invasion of Client Privacy

- Taking photographs of the client
- Release of medical information to an unauthorized person, such as a member of the press, family, friend, or neighbor of the client, without the client's permission
- Use of the client's name or picture for the health care agency's sole advantage
- Intrusion by the health care agency regarding the client's affairs
- Publication of information about the client or photographs of the client, including on a social networking site
- Publication of embarrassing facts
- Public disclosure of private information
- Leaving the curtains or room door open while a treatment or procedure is being performed
- Allowing individuals to observe a treatment or procedure without the client's consent
- Leaving a confused or agitated client sitting in the nursing unit hallway
- Interviewing a client in a room with only a curtain between clients or where conversation can be overheard
- Accessing medical records when unauthorized to do so

BOX 6-11 Maintenance of Confidentiality

- Not discussing client issues with other clients or staff uninvolved in the client's care
- Not sharing health care information with others without the client's consent (includes family members or friends of the client and social networking sites)
- Keeping all information about a client private, and not revealing it to someone not directly involved in care
- Discussing client information only in private and secluded areas
- Protecting the medical record from all unauthorized readers

BOX 6-12 Social Networking and Health Care

- Specific social networking sites can be beneficial to health care providers (HCPs) and clients; misuse of social networking sites by the HCP can lead to Health Insurance Portability and Accountability Act (HIPAA) violations and subsequent termination of the employee.
- Nurses need to adhere to the code of ethics, confidentiality rules, and social media rules. Additional information about these codes and rules can be located at the American Nurses Association Web site at https://www.nursingworld.org/social/
- Standards of professionalism need to be maintained, and any information obtained through any nurse-client relationship cannot be shared in any way.
- The nurse is responsible for reporting any identified breach of privacy or confidentiality.

E. Information technology/computerized medical records
1. Health care employees should have access only to the client's records in the nursing unit or work area.
2. Confidentiality/information security can be protected by the use of special computer access codes to limit what employees have access to in computer systems.
3. The use of a password or identification code is needed to enter and sign off a computer system.
4. A password or identification code should never be shared with another person.
5. Personal passwords should be changed periodically to prevent unauthorized computer access.

F. When conducting research, any information provided by the client is not to be reported in any manner that identifies the client and is not to be made accessible to anyone outside the research team.

! The nurse must always protect client confidentiality.

X. Legal Safeguards

A. Risk management
1. Risk management is a planned method to identify, analyze, and evaluate risks, followed by a plan for reducing the frequency of accidents and injuries.
2. Programs are based on a systematic reporting system for unusual occurrences.

B. Occurrence reports (Box 6-13)
1. The occurrence report is used as a means of identifying risk situations and improving client care.
2. Follow specific documentation guidelines.
3. Fill out the report completely, accurately, and factually.
4. The report form should not be copied or placed in the client's record.
5. Make no reference to the occurrence report form in the client's record.
6. The report is not a substitute for a complete entry in the client's record regarding the occurrence.
7. If a client injury or error in care occurred, assess the client frequently.

C. The PHCP must be notified of the incident and the client's condition.

D. Safeguarding valuables
1. Client's valuables should be given to a family member or secured for safekeeping in a stored and locked designated location, such as the agency's safe; facility security may handle the safeguarding of valuables. The location of the client's valuables should be documented per agency policy.
2. Many health care agencies require a client to sign a release to free the agency of the responsibility for lost valuables.
3. A client's wedding band can be taped in place unless a risk exists for swelling of the hands or fingers.
4. Religious items, such as medals, may be pinned to the client's gown if allowed by agency policy.

E. PHCP's prescriptions
1. The nurse is obligated to carry out a PHCP's prescription except when the nurse believes a prescription to be inappropriate or inaccurate.
2. The nurse carrying out an inaccurate prescription may be legally responsible for any harm suffered by the client.
3. If no resolution occurs regarding the prescription in question, the nurse should contact the nurse manager or supervisor.
4. The nurse should follow specific guidelines for telephone prescriptions (Box 6-14).
5. The nurse should ensure that all components of a medication prescription are documented (Box 6-15).

BOX 6-13 Examples of Occurrences That Need to Be Reported

- Accidental omission of prescribed therapies
- Circumstances that led to injury or a risk for client injury
- Client falls
- Medication administration errors
- Needle-stick injuries
- Procedure-related or equipment-related accidents
- A visitor injury that occurred on the health care agency premises
- A visitor who exhibits symptoms of a communicable disease

BOX 6-14 Telephone Prescription Guidelines

- Date and time the entry.
- Repeat the prescription to the primary health care provider (PHCP), and record the prescription.
- Sign the prescription; begin with "t.o." (telephone order), write the PHCP's name, and sign the prescription.
- If another nurse witnessed the prescription, that nurse's signature follows.
- The PHCP needs to countersign the prescription within a time frame according to agency policy.

BOX 6-15 Components of a Medication Prescription

- Date and time prescription was written
- Medication name
- Medication dosage
- Route of administration
- Frequency of administration
- Primary health care provider's signature

The nurse should never carry out a prescription if it is unclear or inappropriate. The person who wrote the prescription should be contacted immediately.

F. Documentation
   1. Documentation is legally required by accrediting agencies, state licensing laws, and state nurse and medical practice acts.
   2. The nurse should follow agency guidelines and procedures (Box 6-16).
   3. Refer to The Joint Commission Web site for acceptable abbreviations and documentation guidelines: http://www.jointcommission.org/standards_information/npsgs.aspx.

G. Client and family teaching
   1. Provide complete instructions in a language that the client or family can understand.
   2. Document client and family teaching, what was taught, evaluation of understanding, and who was present during the teaching.
   3. Inform the client of what could happen if information shared during teaching is not followed.

XI. Advance Directives

A. Patient Self-Determination Act
   1. The Patient Self-Determination Act is a law that requires clients be provided with information about their right to have written directions about the care that they wish to receive in the event that they become incapacitated and are unable to make health care decisions.
   2. On admission to a health care facility, the client is asked about the existence of an advance directive, and if one exists, it must be documented and included as part of the medical record; if the client signs an advance directive at the time of admission, it must be documented in the client's medical record.
   3. The two basic types of advance directives include instructional directives and durable power of attorney for health care.
      a. Instructional directives: Lists the medical treatment that a client chooses to omit or refuse if the client becomes unable to make decisions and is terminally ill.
      b. Durable power of attorney for health care: Appoints a person (health care proxy) chosen by the client to make health care decisions on the client's behalf when the client can no longer make decisions.

B. Do not resuscitate (DNR) prescriptions
   1. The PHCP writes a DNR prescription if the client and PHCP have made the decision that the client's health is deteriorating and the client chooses not to undergo cardiopulmonary resuscitation if needed.
   2. The client or his or her legal representative must provide informed consent for the DNR status.
   3. The DNR prescription must be defined clearly so that other treatment, not refused by the client, will be continued.
   4. Some states offer DNR Comfort Care and DNR Comfort Care Arrest protocols; these protocols list specific actions that HCPs will take when providing cardiopulmonary resuscitation (CPR).
   5. All health care personnel must know whether a client has a DNR prescription; if a client does not have a DNR prescription, HCPs need to make every effort to revive the client.
   6. A DNR prescription needs to be reviewed regularly according to agency policy and may need to be changed if the client's status changes.
   7. DNR protocols may vary from state to state, and it is important for the nurse to know their state's protocols.

C. The nurse's role
   1. Discussing advance directives with the client opens the communication channel to establish what is important to the client and what the client may view as promoting life versus prolonging dying.
   2. The nurse needs to ensure that the client has been provided with information about the right to identify written directions about the care that the client wishes to receive.

BOX 6-16 Do's and Don'ts Documentation Guidelines: Narrative and Information Technology

- Date and time entries.
- Provide objective, factual, and complete documentation.
- Document care, medications, treatments, and procedures as soon as possible after completion.
- Document client responses to interventions.
- Document consent for or refusal of treatments.
- Document calls made to other primary health care providers.
- Use quotes as appropriate for subjective data.
- Use correct spelling, grammar, and punctuation.
- Sign and title each entry.
- Follow agency policies when an error is made.
- Follow agency guidelines regarding late entries.
- Use only the user identification code, name, or password for computerized documentation.
- Maintain privacy and confidentiality of documented information printed from the computer.
- Do not document for others or change documentation for other individuals.
- Do not use unacceptable abbreviations.
- Do not use judgmental or evaluative statements, such as "uncooperative client."
- Do not leave blank spaces on documentation forms.
- Do not lend access identification computer codes to another person; change password at regular intervals.

3. On admission to a health care facility, the nurse determines whether an advance directive exists and ensures that it is part of the medical record; the nurse also offers information about advance directives if the client indicates he or she wants more information.
4. The nurse ensures that the PHCP is aware of the presence of an advance directive.
5. All health care workers need to follow the directions of an advance directive to be safe from liability.
6. Some agencies have specific policies that prohibit the nurse from signing as a witness to a legal document, such as an instructional directive.
7. If allowed by the agency, when the nurse acts as a witness to a legal document, the nurse must document the event and the factual circumstances surrounding the signing in the medical record; documentation as a witness should include who was present, any significant comments by the client, and the nurse's observations of the client's conduct during this process.

XII. Reporting Responsibilities

A. Nurses are required to report certain communicable diseases or criminal activities such as child or elder abuse or domestic violence; dog bite or other animal bite, gunshot or stab wounds, assaults, and homicides; and suicides to the appropriate authorities.

B. Impaired nurse
1. If the nurse suspects that a coworker is abusing chemicals and potentially jeopardizing a client's safety, the nurse must report the individual to the nursing supervisor/nursing administration in a confidential manner. (Client safety is always the first priority.)
2. Nursing administration notifies the board of nursing regarding the nurse's behavior.
3. Many institutions have policies that allow for drug testing if impairment is suspected.

C. Occupational Safety and Health Act (OSHA)
1. OSHA requires that an employer provide a safe workplace for employees according to regulations.
2. Employees can confidentially report working conditions that violate regulations.
3. An employee who reports unsafe working conditions cannot be retaliated against by the employer.

D. Sexual harassment
1. Sexual harassment is prohibited by state and federal laws.
2. Sexual harassment includes unwelcome conduct of a sexual nature.
3. Follow agency policies and procedures to handle reporting a concern or complaint.

PRACTICE QUESTIONS

16. The nurse hears a client calling out for help, hurries down the hallway to the client's room, and finds the client lying on the floor. The nurse performs an assessment, assists the client back to bed, notifies the primary health care provider, and completes an occurrence report. Which statement should the nurse document on the occurrence report?
1. The client fell out of bed.
2. The client climbed over the side rails.
3. The client was found lying on the floor.
4. The client became restless and tried to get out of bed.

17. A client is brought to the emergency department by emergency medical services (EMS) after being hit by a car. The name of the client is unknown, and the client has sustained a severe head injury and multiple fractures and is unconscious. An emergency craniotomy is required. Regarding informed consent for the surgical procedure, which is the **best** action?
1. Obtain a court order for the surgical procedure.
2. Ask the EMS team to sign the informed consent.
3. Transport the victim to the operating room for surgery.
4. Call the police to identify the client and locate the family.

18. The nurse has just assisted a client back to bed after a fall. The nurse and primary health care provider have assessed the client and have determined that the client is not injured. After completing the occurrence report, the nurse should implement which action **next?**
1. Reassess the client.
2. Conduct a staff meeting to describe the fall.
3. Contact the nursing supervisor to update information regarding the fall.
4. Document in the nurse's notes that an occurrence report was completed.

19. The nurse arrives at work and is told to report (float) to the intensive care unit (ICU) for the day because the ICU is understaffed and needs additional nurses to care for the clients. The nurse has never worked in the ICU. The nurse should take which **best** action?
1. Refuse to float to the ICU based on lack of unit orientation.
2. Clarify the ICU client assignment with the team leader to ensure that it is a safe assignment.
3. Ask the nursing supervisor to review the hospital policy on floating.
4. Submit a written protest to nursing administration, and then call the hospital lawyer.

20. The nurse who works on the night shift enters the medication room and finds a coworker with a tourniquet wrapped around the upper arm. The coworker is about to insert a needle, attached to a syringe containing a clear liquid, into the antecubital area. Which is the **most appropriate** action by the nurse?
1. Call security.
2. Call the police.
3. Call the nursing supervisor.
4. Lock the coworker in the medication room until help is obtained.

21. A hospitalized client tells the nurse that an instructional directive is being prepared and that the lawyer will be bringing the document to the hospital today for witness signatures. The client asks the nurse for assistance in obtaining a witness to the will. Which is the **most appropriate** response to the client?
1. "I will sign as a witness to your signature."
2. "You will need to find a witness on your own."
3. "Whoever is available at the time will sign as a witness for you."
4. "I will call the nursing supervisor to seek assistance regarding your request."

22. The nurse has made an error in documentation of the dose administered of an opioid pain medication in the client's record. The nurse draws 1 mg from the vial and another registered nurse (RN) witnesses wasting of the remaining 1 mg. When scanning the medication, the nurse entered into the medication administration record (MAR) that 2 mg of hydromorphone was administered instead of the actual dose administered, which was 1 mg. The nurse should take which action(s) to correct the error in the MAR? **Select all that apply.**
- ❑ 1. Complete and file an occurrence report.
- ❑ 2. Right-click on the entry and modify it to reflect the correct information.
- ❑ 3. Document the correct information and end with the nurse's signature and title.
- ❑ 4. Obtain a cosignature from the RN who witnessed the waste of the remaining 1 mg.
- ❑ 5. Document in a nurse's note in the client's record detailing the corrected information.

23. Which identifies accurate nursing documentation notation(s)? **Select all that apply.**
- ❑ 1. The client slept through the night.
- ❑ 2. Abdominal wound dressing is dry and intact without drainage.
- ❑ 3. The client seemed angry when awakened for vital sign measurement.
- ❑ 4. The client appears to become anxious when it is time for respiratory treatments.
- ❑ 5. The client's left lower medial leg wound is 3 cm in length without redness, drainage, or edema.

24. A nursing instructor delivers a lecture to nursing students regarding the issue of clients' rights and asks a nursing student to identify a situation that represents an example of *invasion of client privacy*. Which situation, if identified by the student, indicates an understanding of a violation of this client right?
1. Performing a procedure without consent
2. Threatening to give a client a medication
3. Telling the client that he or she cannot leave the hospital
4. Observing care provided to the client without the client's permission

25. Nursing staff members are sitting in the lounge taking their morning break. An assistive personnel (AP) tells the group that she thinks that the unit secretary has acquired immunodeficiency syndrome (AIDS) and proceeds to tell the nursing staff that the secretary probably contracted the disease from her husband, who is supposedly a drug addict. The registered nurse should inform the AP that making this accusation has violated which legal tort?
1. Libel
2. Slander
3. Assault
4. Negligence

26. An older woman is brought to the emergency department for treatment of a fractured arm. On physical assessment, the nurse notes old and new ecchymotic areas on the client's chest and legs and asks the client how the bruises were sustained. The client, although reluctant, tells the nurse in confidence that her son frequently hits her if supper is not prepared on time when he arrives home from work. Which is the **most appropriate** nursing response?
1. "Oh, really? I will discuss this situation with your son."
2. "Let's talk about the ways you can manage your time to prevent this from happening."
3. "Do you have any friends who can help you out until you resolve these important issues with your son?"
4. "As a nurse, I am legally bound to report abuse. I will stay with you while you give the report and help find a safe place for you to stay."

27. The nurse calls the primary health care provider (PHCP) regarding a new medication prescription, because the dosage prescribed is higher than the recommended dosage. The nurse is unable to locate the PHCP, and the medication is due to be administered. Which action should the nurse take?
1. Contact the nursing supervisor.
2. Administer the dose prescribed.

3. Hold the medication until the PHCP can be contacted.
4. Administer the recommended dose until the PHCP can be located.

28. The nurse employed in a hospital is waiting to receive a report from the laboratory via the facsimile (fax) machine. The fax machine activates and the nurse expects the report, but instead receives a sexually oriented photograph. Which is the **most appropriate initial** nursing action?
1. Call the police.
2. Cut up the photograph and throw it away.
3. Call the nursing supervisor and report the occurrence.
4. Call the laboratory and ask for the name of the individual who sent the photograph.

ANSWERS

16. *Answer:* 3
Rationale: The occurrence report should contain a factual description of the occurrence, any injuries experienced by those involved, and the outcome of the situation. The correct option is the only one that describes the facts as observed by the nurse. Options 1, 2, and 4 are interpretations of the situation and are not factual information as observed by the nurse.
Test-Taking Strategy: Focus on the subject, documentation of events, and note the data in the question to select the correct option. Remember to focus on factual information when documenting, and avoid including interpretations. This will direct you to the correct option.
Level of Cognitive Ability: Applying
Client Needs: Safe and Effective Care Environment
Integrated Process: Communication and Documentation
Content Area: Leadership/Management: Ethical/Legal
Health Problem: N/A
Priority Concepts: Communication; Health Care Law
Reference: Potter et al. (2017), p. 367.

17. *Answer:* 3
Rationale: In general, there are two situations in which informed consent of an adult client is not needed. One is when an emergency is present and delaying treatment for the purpose of obtaining informed consent would result in injury or death to the client. The second is when the client waives the right to give informed consent. Option 1 will delay emergency treatment, and option 2 is inappropriate. Although option 4 may be pursued, it is not the best action because it delays necessary emergency treatment.
Test-Taking Strategy: Note the strategic word, *best.* Also note that an emergency is present. Recalling that a delay in treatment for the purpose of obtaining informed consent could result in injury or death will direct you to the correct option.
Level of Cognitive Ability: Applying
Client Needs: Safe and Effective Care Environment
Integrated Process: Nursing Process—Implementation
Content Area: Leadership/Management: Ethical/Legal
Health Problem: Adult Health: Neurological: Head Injury/Trauma
Priority Concepts: Ethics; Health Care Law
References: Potter et al. (2017), pp. 309-310.

18. *Answer:* 1
Rationale: After a client's fall, the nurse must frequently reassess the client, because potential complications do not always appear immediately after the fall. The client's fall should be treated as private information and shared on a "need to know" basis. Communication regarding the event should involve only the individuals participating in the client's care. An occurrence report is a problem-solving document; however, its completion is not documented in the nurse's notes. If the nursing supervisor has been made aware of the occurrence, the supervisor will contact the nurse if status update is necessary.
Test-Taking Strategy: Note the strategic word, *next.* Using the steps of the nursing process will direct you to the correct option. Remember that assessment is the first step. Additionally, use Maslow's Hierarchy of Needs theory, recalling that physiological needs are the priority. The correct option is the only option that addresses a potential physiological need of the client.
Level of Cognitive Ability: Applying
Client Needs: Safe and Effective Care Environment
Integrated Process: Nursing Process—Implementation
Content Area: Foundations of Care: Safety
Health Problem: N/A
Priority Concepts: Communication; Safety
References: Potter et al. (2017), pp. 312, 367.

19. *Answer:* 2
Rationale: Floating is an acceptable practice used by hospitals to solve understaffing problems. Legally, the nurse cannot refuse to float unless a union contract guarantees that nurses can work only in a specified area or the nurse can prove the lack of knowledge for the performance of assigned tasks. When encountering this situation, the nurse should set priorities and identify potential areas of harm to the client. That is why clarifying the client assignment with the team leader to ensure that it is a safe one is the best option. The nursing supervisor is called if the nurse is expected to perform tasks that he or she cannot safely perform. Submitting a written protest and calling the hospital lawyer is a premature action.
Test-Taking Strategy: Note the strategic word, *best.* Eliminate option 1 first because of the word *refuse.* Next, eliminate options 3 and 4 because they are premature actions.
Level of Cognitive Ability: Applying
Client Needs: Safe and Effective Care Environment

Integrated Process: Nursing Process—Implementation
Content Area: Leadership/Management: Ethical/Legal
Health Problem: N/A
Priority Concepts: Care Coordination; Professionalism
Reference: Potter et al. (2017), p. 311.

20. *Answer:* 3
Rationale: Nurse practice acts require reporting impaired nurses. The board of nursing has jurisdiction over the practice of nursing and may develop plans for treatment and supervision of the impaired nurse. This occurrence needs to be reported to the nursing supervisor, who will then report to the board of nursing and other authorities, such as the police, as required. The nurse may call security if a disturbance occurs, but no information in the question supports this need, and so this is not the appropriate action. Option 4 is an inappropriate and unsafe action.
Test-Taking Strategy: Note the strategic words, *most appropriate*. Eliminate option 4 first, because this is an inappropriate and unsafe action. Recall the lines of organizational structure to assist in directing you to the correct option.
Level of Cognitive Ability: Applying
Client Needs: Safe and Effective Care Environment
Integrated Process: Nursing Process—Implementation
Content Area: Leadership/Management: Ethical/Legal
Health Problem: Mental Health: Addictions
Priority Concepts: Ethics; Professionalism
References: Lewis et al. (2017), p. 125; www.americannursetoday.com/the-impaired-nurse-would-you-know-what-to-do-if-you-suspected-substance-abuse.

21. *Answer:* 4
Rationale: Instructional directives (living wills) are required to be in writing and signed by the client. The client's signature must be witnessed by specified individuals or notarized. Laws and guidelines regarding instructional directives vary from state to state, and it is the responsibility of the nurse to know the laws. Many states prohibit any employee, including the nurse of a facility where the client is receiving care, from being a witness. Option 2 is nontherapeutic and not a helpful response. The nurse should seek the assistance of the nursing supervisor.
Test-Taking Strategy: Note the strategic words, *most appropriate*. Options 1 and 3 are comparable or alike and should be eliminated first. Option 2 is eliminated because it is a nontherapeutic response.
Level of Cognitive Ability: Applying
Client Needs: Safe and Effective Care Environment
Integrated Process: Nursing Process—Implementation
Content Area: Leadership/Management: Ethical/Legal
Health Problem: N/A
Priority Concepts: Health Care Law; Professionalism
Reference: Ignatavicius, Workman, Rebar (2018), pp. 104, 106.

22. *Answer:* 2, 3, 4, 5
Rationale: Electronic health records (EHR) will have a time date stamp that indicates an amendment has been entered. If the nurse makes an error in the MAR, the nurse should follow agency policies to correct the error. In the MAR, the nurse can click on the entry (usually right-click) and modify it to reflect the corrected information. Since this is an opioid medication, the nurse should obtain a cosignature from the RN who witnessed the wasting of the excess medication, to validate that 1 mg, rather than 2 mg, was given. A nurse's note should be used to detail the event and the corrections made, and the nurse's name and title will be stamped on the entry in the EHR. An occurrence report is not necessary in this situation.
Test-Taking Strategy: Focus on the subject, correcting a documentation error, and use principles related to documentation. Recalling the purpose of an occurrence report will assist in eliminating option 1. From the remaining options, focusing on the subject of the question and using knowledge regarding the principles related to documentation will direct you to the correct options.
Level of Cognitive Ability: Applying
Client Needs: Safe and Effective Care Environment
Integrated Process: Communication and Documentation
Content Area: Leadership/Management: Ethical/Legal
Health Problem: N/A
Priority Concepts: Communication; Professionalism
References: Potter et al. (2017), p. 358.

23. *Answer:* 1, 2, 5
Rationale: Factual documentation contains descriptive, objective information about what the nurse sees, hears, feels, or smells. The use of inferences without supporting factual data is not acceptable, because it can be misunderstood. The use of vague terms, such as *seemed* or *appears*, is not acceptable because these words suggest that the nurse is stating an opinion.
Test-Taking Strategy: Focus on the subject, accurate documentation notations. Eliminate options 3 and 4 because they are comparable or alike and include vague terms (seemed, appears).
Level of Cognitive Ability: Applying
Client Needs: Safe and Effective Care Environment
Integrated Process: Communication and Documentation
Content Area: Leadership/Management: Ethical/Legal
Health Problem: N/A
Priority Concepts: Communication; Professionalism
Reference: Potter et al. (2017), pp. 361-362.

24. *Answer:* 4
Rationale: Invasion of privacy occurs with unreasonable intrusion into an individual's private affairs. Performing a procedure without consent is an example of battery. Threatening to give a client a medication constitutes assault. Telling the client that the client cannot leave the hospital constitutes false imprisonment.
Test-Taking Strategy: Focus on the subject, invasion of privacy. Noting the words *without the client's permission* will direct you to this option.
Level of Cognitive Ability: Evaluating
Client Needs: Safe and Effective Care Environment
Integrated Process: Teaching and Learning
Content Area: Leadership/Management: Ethical/Legal
Health Problem: N/A
Priority Concepts: Ethics; Professionalism
Reference: Potter et al. (2017), p. 308.

25. *Answer:* 2
Rationale: Defamation is a false communication or a careless disregard for the truth that causes damage to someone's

reputation, either in writing (libel) or verbally (slander). An assault occurs when a person puts another person in fear of a harmful or offensive contact. Negligence involves the actions of professionals that fall below the standard of care for a specific professional group.

Test-Taking Strategy: Note the subject, the legal tort that was violated. Focus on the data in the question and eliminate options 3 and 4 first because their definitions are unrelated to the data. Recalling that slander constitutes verbal defamation will direct you to the correct option from the remaining options.

Level of Cognitive Ability: Applying
Client Needs: Safe and Effective Care Environment
Integrated Process: Nursing Process—Implementation
Content Area: Leadership/Management: Ethical/Legal
Health Problem: N/A
Priority Concepts: Health Care Law; Professionalism
Reference: Potter et al. (2017), pp. 308-309.

26. *Answer:* 4

Rationale: The nurse must report situations related to child or elder abuse, gunshot wounds and other criminal acts, and certain infectious diseases. Confidential issues are not to be discussed with nonmedical personnel or the client's family or friends without the client's permission. Clients should be assured that information is kept confidential, unless it places the nurse under a legal obligation. Options 1, 2, and 3 do not address the legal implications of the situation and do not ensure a safe environment for the client.

Test-Taking Strategy: Note the strategic words, *most appropriate.* Focus on the data in the question and note that an older woman is receiving physical abuse by her son. Recall the nursing responsibilities related to client safety and reporting obligations. Options 1, 2, and 3 should be eliminated because they are comparable or alike in that they do not protect the client from injury.

Level of Cognitive Ability: Applying
Client Needs: Safe and Effective Care Environment
Integrated Process: Nursing Process—Implementation
Content Area: Leadership/Management: Ethical/Legal
Health Problem: Mental Health: Abusive Behaviors
Priority Concepts: Health Care Law; Interpersonal Violence
References: Potter et al. (2017), pp. 35, 188-189.

27. *Answer:* 1

Rationale: If the PHCP writes a prescription that requires clarification, the nurse's responsibility is to contact the PHCP. If there is no resolution regarding the prescription because the PHCP cannot be located or because the prescription remains as it was written after talking with the PHCP, the nurse should contact the nurse manager or nursing supervisor for further clarification as to what the next step should be. Under no circumstances should the nurse proceed to carry out the prescription until obtaining clarification.

Test-Taking Strategy: Eliminate options 2 and 4 first because they are comparable or alike and are unsafe actions. Holding the medication can result in client injury. The nurse needs to take action. The correct option clearly identifies the required action in this situation.

Level of Cognitive Ability: Applying
Client Needs: Safe and Effective Care Environment
Integrated Process: Nursing Process—Implementation
Content Area: Leadership/Management: Ethical/Legal
Health Problem: N/A
Priority Concepts: Clinical Judgment; Safety
Reference: Potter et al. (2017), pp. 624-625, 628.

28. *Answer:* 3

Rationale: Ensuring a safe workplace is a responsibility of an employing institution. Sexual harassment in the workplace is prohibited by state and federal laws. Sexually suggestive jokes, touching, pressuring a coworker for a date, and open displays of or transmitting sexually oriented photographs or posters are examples of conduct that could be considered sexual harassment by another worker and is an abusive behavior. If the nurse believes that he or she is being subjected to unwelcome sexual conduct, these concerns should be reported to the nursing supervisor immediately. Option 1 is unnecessary at this time. Options 2 and 4 are inappropriate initial actions.

Test-Taking Strategy: Note the strategic words, *most appropriate initial.* Remember that using the organizational channels of communication is best. This will assist in directing you to the correct option.

Level of Cognitive Ability: Applying
Client Needs: Safe and Effective Care Environment
Integrated Process: Nursing Process—Implementation
Content Area: Leadership/Management: Ethical/Legal
Health Problem: Mental Health: Abusive Behaviors
Priority Concepts: Health Care Law; Professionalism
Reference: Zerwekh, Zerwekh Garneau (2015), pp. 300-301.

CHAPTER 7

Prioritizing Client Care: Leadership, Delegation, and Emergency Response Planning

PRIORITY CONCEPTS **Leadership; Health Care Organizations**

I. Health Care Delivery Systems

A. Managed care

1. *Managed care* is a broad term used to describe strategies used in the health care delivery system that reduce the costs of health care.
2. Client care is outcome driven and is managed by a case management process.
3. Managed care emphasizes the promotion of health, client education and responsible self-care, early identification of disease, and the use of health care resources.

B. Case management

1. Case management is a health care delivery strategy that supports managed care; it uses an interprofessional health care delivery approach that provides comprehensive client care throughout the client's illness, using available resources to promote high-quality and cost-effective care.
2. Case management includes assessment and development of a plan of care, coordination of all services, referral, and follow-up.
3. Critical pathways are used, and variation analysis is conducted.
4. The core functions of case management are assessment, treatment planning, linking, advocacy, and monitoring.

Case management involves consultation and collaboration with an interprofessional health care team.

C. Case manager

1. A case manager is a professional nurse who assumes responsibility for coordinating the client's care at admission and after discharge.
2. The case manager establishes a plan of care with the client, coordinates any interprofessional consultations and referrals, and facilitates discharge.
3. A case manager is knowledgeable in various types of health insurance, which allows them to assist clients in navigating health care options covered by insurance.

D. Health Insurance

1. There are state and federal insurance plans.
2. An aim of the Affordable Care Act is to reduce the amount of uncompensated care the average U.S. family pays for by requiring everyone to have health insurance or pay a tax penalty. Its goals are to expand access to health insurance, reduce costs, and protect clients against arbitrary actions by insurance companies.
3. There are many insurance companies that provide state marketplace insurance; some include Aetna, Blue Cross Blue Shield, Cigna, Humana, Kaiser, United, and TriCare/Humana.
4. Types of insurance plans include health maintenance organizations (HMOs), preferred provider organizations (PPOs), exclusive provider organizations (EPOs), point-of-service (POS) plans, high-deductible health plans (HDHPs), and health savings accounts (HSAs); these offer varying options in terms of insurance coverage and out-of-pocket costs and premiums.
5. Medicare is a federal health insurance program for persons aged 65 or older, certain younger people with disabilities, and people with end-stage renal disease (ESRD) requiring dialysis or renal transplant. Certain premiums are attached to each part.
   a. Part A: covers hospital stays, skilled nursing facility stays, hospice care, and some home health care

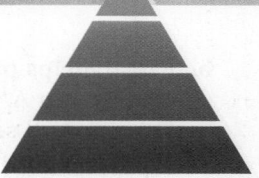

b. Part B: helps pay for some services not covered by Part A. Medicare usually covers 80% for approved services; remaining 20% is the client's responsibility and a supplemental insurance needs to be obtained
c. Part C: a health plan offered by a private insurance agency that contracts with Medicare to supplement coverage
d. Part D: covers prescription medication needs
6. Medicaid is a joint federal and state program that provides health benefits to eligible low-income adults, children, pregnant women, elderly individuals, and people with disabilities. A concern associated with these programs is fraud and abuse; a case manager needs to know how to complete insurance, state, and federal applications and be astute enough to know if an individual is reporting incorrect information.

E. Critical pathway
1. A critical pathway is a clinical management care plan for providing client-centered care and for planning and monitoring the client's progress within an established time frame; interprofessional collaboration and teamwork ensure shared decision making and quality client care.
2. Critical pathways are based on evidence-based practice and include evidence-based medical practice, budgetary, organizational, and systems-wide information.
3. Variation analysis is a continuous process that the case manager and other caregivers conduct by comparing the specific client outcomes with the expected outcomes described on the critical pathway.
4. The goal of a critical pathway is to anticipate and recognize negative variance (i.e., client problems) early so that appropriate action can be taken and positive client outcomes can result.
5. Critical pathways are used to ensure medical care is consistent within budget constraints and to allow providers to care for more complex clients. For example, some ambulatory practices have critical pathways for certain conditions such as blood pressure monitoring or urinary tract infections.

F. Nursing Care Plan
1. A nursing care plan is a written guideline and communication tool that identifies the client's pertinent assessment data, problems and nursing diagnoses, goals, interventions, and expected outcomes.
2. The plan enhances interprofessional continuity of care by identifying specific nursing actions necessary to achieve the goals of care.
3. The client and family are involved in developing the plan of care, and the plan identifies short-term and long-term goals.
4. Client problems, goals, interventions, and expected outcomes are documented in the care plan, which provides a framework for evaluation of the client's response to nursing actions. The care plan is modified as the client condition changes.

II. Nursing Delivery Systems

A. Functional nursing
1. Functional nursing involves a task approach to client care, with tasks being delegated by the charge nurse to individual members of the team.
2. This type of system is task-oriented, and the team member focuses on the delegated task rather than the total client; this results in fragmentation of care and lack of accountability by the team member.

B. Team nursing
1. The team generally is led by a registered nurse (team leader) who is responsible for assessing clients, analyzing client data, planning, and evaluating each client's plan of care.
2. The team leader determines the work assignment; each staff member works fully within the realm of his or her educational and clinical expertise and job description.
3. Each staff member is accountable for client care and outcomes of care delivered in accordance with the licensing and practice scope as determined by health care agency policy and state law.
4. Modular nursing is similar to team nursing but takes into account the structure of the unit; the unit is divided into modules, allowing nurses to care for a group of clients who are geographically close by.

C. Relationship-based practice (primary nursing)
1. Relationship-based practice (primary nursing) is concerned with keeping the nurse at the bedside, actively involved in client care, while planning goal-directed, individualized care.
2. One (primary) nurse is responsible for managing and coordinating the client's care while in the hospital and for discharge, and an associate nurse cares for the client when the primary nurse is off-duty.

D. Client-focused care
1. This is also known as the total care or case method; the registered nurse assumes total responsibility for planning and delivering care to a client.
2. The client may have different nurses assigned during a 24-hour period; the nurse provides all necessary care needed for the assigned time period.

III. Professional Responsibilities

A. Accountability
1. The process in which individuals have an obligation (or duty) to act and are answerable for their choices, decisions, and actions.
2. Involves assuming only the responsibilities that are within one's scope of practice and not assuming responsibility for activities in which competence has not been achieved.

3. Involves admitting mistakes rather than blaming others and evaluating the outcomes of one's own actions.
4. Includes a responsibility to the client to be competent and provide nursing care in accordance with standards of nursing practice while adhering to the professional ethics codes.

Accountability is the acceptance of responsibility for one's choices, decisions, and actions. The nurse is always responsible for their actions when providing care to a client.

B. Leadership and management
1. Leadership is the interpersonal process that involves influencing others (followers) to achieve goals.
2. Management is the accomplishment of tasks or goals by oneself or by directing others.

C. Theories of leadership and management (Box 7-1)

D. Leader and manager approaches
1. Authoritarian leadership
   a. The leader or manager is focused and maintains strong control, makes decisions, and addresses all problems.
   b. The leader or manager dominates the group and commands rather than seeks suggestions or input.
2. Democratic leadership
   a. This is also called *participative management*.
   b. It is based on the belief that every group member should have input into problem solving and the development of goals; leader obtains participation from group and then makes best decision for the organization, based on the input from group.
   c. The democratic style is a more "talk with the members" style and much less authoritarian than the autocratic style.
3. Laissez-faire leadership
   a. A laissez-faire leader or manager assumes a passive, nondirective, and inactive approach and relinquishes part or all of the responsibilities to the members of the group.
   b. Decision making is left to the group, with the laissez-faire leader or manager providing little, if any, guidance, support, or feedback.
4. Situational leadership
   a. Situational approach uses a combination of styles based on the current circumstances and events.
   b. Situational styles are assumed according to the needs of the group and the tasks to be achieved.
5. Bureaucratic leadership
   a. The leader or manager believes that individuals are motivated by external forces.
   b. The leader or manager relies on organizational policies and procedures for decision making.
6. Transformational leadership
   a. Focused on building relationships.
   b. Motivates staff members through a shared vision and mission.
   c. Encourages and praises staff members and inspires them to improve performance levels while earning staff respect and loyalty.
7. Servant leadership
   a. Servant leaders influence and motivate others by building relationships and developing the skills of individual team members.
   b. Servant leaders make sure to meet the needs of the individual team members and to give each person input in decisions.

E. Effective leader and manager behaviors and qualities (Box 7-2)

BOX 7-1 Theories of Leadership and Management

Charismatic: Based on personal beliefs and characteristics of influence
Quantum: Based on the concepts of chaos theory; maintaining a balance between tension and order prevents an unstable environment and promotes creativity
Relational: Based on collaboration and teamwork
Servant: Based on a desire to serve others; the leader emerges when another's needs assume priority
Shared: Based on the belief that several individuals share the responsibility for achieving the health care agency's goals
Transactional: Based on the principles of social exchange theory
Transformational: Based on the individual's commitment to the health care agency's vision; focuses on promoting change

BOX 7-2 Effective Leader and Manager Behaviors and Qualities

Behaviors

Treats followers as unique individuals
Inspires followers and stimulates critical thinking
Shows followers how to think about old problems in new ways and assists with adapting to change
Is visible to followers; is flexible; and provides guidance, assistance, and feedback
Communicates a vision, establishes trust, and empowers followers
Motivates followers to achieve goals

Qualities

Effective communicator; promotes interprofessional collaboration
Credible
Critical thinker
Initiator of action
Risk taker
Is persuasive and influences employees

Adapted from Huber D: *Leadership and nursing care management*, ed 5, Philadelphia, 2014, Saunders.

F. Functions of management (Box 7-3)
G. Problem-solving process and decision making
 1. Problem solving involves obtaining information and using it to reach an acceptable solution to a problem.
 2. Decision making involves identifying a problem and deciding which alternatives can best achieve objectives.
 3. Steps of the problem-solving process are similar to the steps of the nursing process (Table 7-1).
H. Types of managers
 1. Front-line manager
  a. Front-line managers function in supervisory roles of those involved with delivery of client care. Front-line managers may temporarily assume a client care role.
  b. Front-line roles usually include charge nurse, team leader, and client care coordinator.
  c. Front-line managers coordinate the activity of all staff who provide client care and supervise team members during the manager's period of accountability.
 2. Middle manager
  a. Middle manager roles usually include unit manager and supervisor.
  b. A middle manager's responsibilities may include supervising staff, preparing budgets, preparing work schedules, writing and implementing policies that guide client care and unit operations, and maintaining the quality of client services.
 3. Nurse executive
  a. The nurse executive is a top-level nurse manager and may be the director of nursing services or the vice president for client care services that assists with carrying out the mission of a health care organization.
  b. The nurse executive supervises numerous departments and works closely with the administrative team of the organization to ensure that nursing staff provide optimal client care.
  c. The nurse executive ensures that all client care provided by nurses is consistent with the objectives of the health care organization.

IV. Power

A. Power is the ability to influence others and control their actions to achieve desired results.
B. Powerful people are able to modify behavior and influence others to change, even when others are resistant to change.
C. Powerful people are change agents that lead or create positive change to support or maintain high-quality care and decrease adverse effects.
D. Effective nurse leaders use power to improve the delivery of care and to enhance the profession.
E. There are different types of power (Box 7-4).

V. Empowerment

A. Empowerment is an interpersonal process of enabling others to do for themselves.
B. Empowerment occurs when individuals are able to influence what happens to them more effectively.
C. Empowerment involves open communication, mutual goal setting, and shared decision making.
D. Nurses can empower clients and others through teaching and advocacy.

VI. Formal Organizations

A. An organization's mission statement communicates in broad terms its reason for existence and the attitudes, beliefs, and values by which the organization functions.

BOX 7-3 Functions of Management

Planning: Determining objectives and identifying methods that lead to achievement of objectives
Organizing: Using resources (human and material) to achieve predetermined outcomes
Directing: Guiding and motivating others to meet expected outcomes
Controlling: Using performance standards as criteria for measuring success and taking corrective action

TABLE 7-1 Similarities of the Problem-Solving Process and the Nursing Process

Problem-Solving Process	Nursing Process
Identifying a problem and collecting data about the problem	Assessment
Determining the exact nature of the problem	Analysis (Diagnosis)
Deciding on a plan of action	Planning
Carrying out the plan	Implementation
Evaluating the plan	Evaluation

BOX 7-4 Types of Power

Reward: Ability to provide incentives
Coercive: Ability to punish
Referent: Based on attraction, loyalty, and respect
Expert: Based on having an expert knowledge foundation and skill level
Legitimate: Based on a position in society
Personal: Derived from a high degree of self-confidence
Informational: When one person provides explanations why another should behave in a certain way

B. Goals and objectives are measurable activities specific to the development of designated services and programs of an organization.
C. The organizational chart depicts and communicates how activities are arranged, how authority relationships are defined, and how communication channels are established.
D. Policies, procedures, and protocols
 1. Policies are guidelines that define the organization's directives on courses of action.
 2. Procedures are based on policy and define methods for tasks.
 3. Protocols prescribe a specific course of action for a specific type of client or problem.
  a. Centralization is the making of decisions by a few individuals at the top of the organization or by managers of a department or unit, and decisions are communicated thereafter to the employees.
  b. Decentralization is the distribution of authority throughout the organization to allow for increased responsibility and **delegation** in decision making; decentralization tries to move the decision making as close to the client as possible.

The nurse must follow policies, procedures, and protocols of the health care agency in which he or she is employed.

VII. Evidence-Based Practice

A. Research is an important role of the professional nurse. Research provides a foundation for improvement in nursing practice.
B. Evidence-based practice is an approach to client care in which the nurse integrates the client's preferences, clinical expertise, and the best research evidence to deliver quality care.
C. Determining the client's personal, social, cultural, and religious preferences ensures individualization and is a component of implementing evidence-based practice.
D. The nurse needs to be an observer and identify and question situations that require change or result in a less than desirable outcome.
E. Use of information technology such as online resources, including research publications, provides current research findings related to areas of practice.
F. The nurse needs to follow evidence-based practice protocols developed by the institution and question the rationale for nursing approaches identified in the protocols as necessary. The nurse should use appropriate evaluation criteria when determining areas in need of research (Table 7-2).

TABLE 7-2 Evaluation Criteria for Evidence for Clinical Questions

Level	Definition
Level I	Evidence comes from a review of a number of randomized controlled trials (RCTs) or from clinical practice guidelines that are based on such a review.
Level II	Evidence comes from at least one well-designed RCT.
Level III	Evidence comes from well-designed controlled studies that are not randomized.
Level IV	Evidence comes from well-designed case-controlled and cohort studies.
Level V	Evidence comes from a number of descriptive or qualitative studies.
Level VI	Evidence comes from a single descriptive or qualitative study.
Level VII	Evidence comes from the opinion of authorities and/or reports of expert committees.

From Zerwekh J, Zerwekh Garneau A: *Nursing today: transition and trends*, ed 8, Philadelphia, 2015, Saunders. Data from Sackett D et al.: *Evidence-based medicine: how to practice and teach EBM*, London, 2000, Churchill Livingstone.

Evidence-based practice requires that the nurse base nursing practice on the best and most applicable evidence from clinical research studies. The nurse should also be alert to clinical issues that warrant investigation and develop a researchable question about the problem.

VIII. Quality Improvement

A. Also known as performance improvement, quality improvement focuses on processes or systems that significantly contribute to client safety and effective client care outcomes; criteria are used to monitor outcomes of care and to determine the need for change to improve the quality of care.
B. Quality improvement processes or systems may be named quality assurance, continuous quality management, or continuous quality improvement.
C. When quality improvement is part of the philosophy of a health care agency, every staff member becomes involved in ways to improve client care and outcomes.
D. A retrospective ("looking back") audit is an evaluation method used to inspect the medical record after the client's discharge for documentation of compliance with the standards.
E. A concurrent ("at the same time") audit is an evaluation method used to inspect compliance of nurses with predetermined standards and criteria while the nurses are providing care during the client's stay.
F. Peer review is a process in which nurses employed in an organization evaluate the quality of nursing care delivered to the client.

G. The quality improvement process is similar to the nursing process and involves an interprofessional approach.
H. An outcome describes the response to care; comparison of client responses with the expected outcomes indicates whether the interventions are effective, whether the client has progressed, how well standards are met, and whether changes are necessary.
I. The nurse is responsible for recognizing trends in nursing practice, identifying recurrent problems, and initiating opportunities to improve the quality of care.

⚠ Quality improvement processes improve the quality of care delivery to clients and the safety of health care agencies.

IX. Change Process

A. Change is a dynamic process that leads to an alteration in behavior.
B. A change agent can be used to effectively facilitate change. Change agents appropriately assess and manage the reactions of staff members. They can connect and balance all aspects of the organization that will be affected by change.
C. Leadership style influences the approach to initiating the change process.
D. Lewin's basic concept of the change process includes 3 elements for successful change: unfreezing, moving and changing, and refreezing (Fig. 7-1).
   1. Unfreezing is the first phase of the process, during which the problem is identified and individuals involved gather facts and evidence supporting a basis for change.
   2. During the moving and changing phase, change is planned and implemented.
   3. Refreezing is the last phase of the process, during which the change becomes stabilized.
E. Types of change
   1. Planned change: A deliberate effort to improve a situation
   2. Unplanned change: A reactive response that is required because of a disruption. The change is beneficial and may go unnoticed.
F. Resistance to change (Box 7-5)
   1. Resistance to change occurs when an individual rejects proposed new ideas without critically thinking about the proposal.
   2. Change requires energy.
   3. The change process does not guarantee positive outcomes.
G. Overcoming barriers
   1. Create a flexible and adaptable environment.
   2. Encourage the people involved to plan and set goals for change.
   3. Include all involved in the plan for change.
   4. Focus on the benefits of the change in relation to improvement of client care.
   5. Delineate the drawbacks from failing to make the change in relation to client care.
   6. Evaluate the change process on an ongoing basis and keep everyone informed of progress.
   7. Provide positive feedback to all involved.
   8. Commit to the time it takes to change.

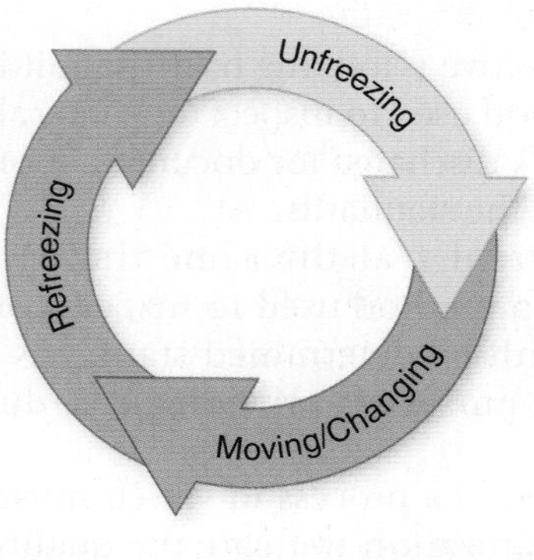

FIG. 7-1 Elements of a successful change.

BOX 7-5 Reasons for Resisting Change

Conformity
One goes along with others to avoid conflict.

Dissimilar Beliefs and Values
Differences can impede positive change.

Habit
Routine, set behaviors are often hard to change.

Secondary Gains
Benefits or payoff are present, so there is no incentive to change.

Threats to Satisfying Basic Needs
Change may be perceived as a threat to self-esteem, security, or survival.

Fear
One fears failure or has fear of the unknown.

X. Conflict

A. Conflict is an internal or external friction that arises from a perception of incompatibility or difference in beliefs, attitudes, values, goals, priorities, or decisions.
B. Types of conflict
   1. Intrapersonal: Occurs within a person
   2. Interpersonal: Occurs between and among clients, nurses, or other staff members
   3. Organizational: Occurs when an employee confronts the policies and procedures of the organization

C. Modes of conflict resolution
   1. Avoidance
      a. Avoiders are unassertive and uncooperative.
      b. Avoiders do not pursue their own needs, goals, or concerns, and they do not assist others to pursue theirs.
      c. Avoiders postpone dealing with the issue.
   2. Accommodation
      a. Accommodators neglect their own needs, goals, or concerns (unassertive) while trying to satisfy those of others.
      b. Accommodators obey and serve others and often feel resentment and disappointment because they "get nothing in return."
   3. Competition
      a. Competitors pursue their own needs and goals at the expense of others.
      b. Competitors also may stand up for rights and defend important principles.
   4. Compromise
      a. Compromisers are assertive and cooperative.
      b. Compromisers work creatively and openly to find the solution that most fully satisfies all important objectives and goals to be achieved.

XI. Roles of Health Care Team Members

A. Nurse roles are as follows:
   1. Promote health and prevent disease
   2. Provide comfort and care to clients
   3. Make decisions
   4. Act as client advocate
   5. Lead and manage the nursing team
   6. Serve as case manager
   7. Function as a rehabilitator
   8. Communicate effectively
   9. Educate clients, families, and communities and health care team members
   10. Act as a resource person
   11. Allocate resources in a cost-effective manner

B. Primary health care provider (PHCP): A PHCP or specialist diagnoses and treats disease.

C. Physician's assistant
   1. A physician's assistant (PA) acts to a limited extent in the role of the physician during the physician's absence.
   2. The PA conducts physical examinations, performs diagnostic procedures, assists in the operating room and emergency department, and performs treatments.
   3. Certified and licensed PAs in some states have prescriptive powers.

D. Nurse practitioner: an advanced practice registered nurse (APRN) who is educated to diagnose and treat acute illness and chronic conditions; health promotion and maintenance is a focus.
   1. An APRN may work in a variety of specialty areas including family practice, internal medicine, acute gerontology, women's health or obstetrics, acute care, pediatrics, or other specialty areas.
   2. APRNs have independent practice authority in most states.

E. Physical therapist: A physical therapist assists in examining, testing, and treating clients recuperating from injuries, illness, or surgery and physically disabled clients.

F. Occupational therapist: An occupational therapist develops adaptive devices that help chronically ill clients or clients with a disability perform activities of daily living.

G. Respiratory therapist: A respiratory therapist delivers treatments designed to improve the client's ventilation and oxygenation status.

H. Speech therapist: A speech therapist evaluates a client's ability to swallow safely and evaluates speech and communication ability. The speech therapist develops a plan to treat communication and swallowing disorders. These therapists also work to prevent, assess, diagnose, and treat speech, language, social communication, and cognitive communication in children and adults.

I. Nutritionist: A nutritionist or dietitian assists in planning dietary measures to improve or maintain a client's nutritional status.

J. Continuing care nurse: This nurse coordinates discharge plans for the client.

K. Assistive personnel, help the registered nurse with specified tasks and functions.

L. Pharmacist: A pharmacist formulates and dispenses medications.

M. Social worker: A social worker counsels clients and families about home care services and assists the continuing care nurse with planning and facilitating discharge.

N. Chaplain: A chaplain (or trained layperson) offers spiritual support and guidance to clients and families.

O. Administrative staff: Administrative or support staff members organize and schedule diagnostic tests and procedures and arrange for services needed by the client and family.

XII. Interprofessional Collaboration

A. Client care planning can be accomplished through referrals, consultations, or interprofessional collaborations with other health care specialists and through client care conferences, which involve members from all health care disciplines. This approach helps ensure continuity of care.

B. Reports
   1. Reports should be factual, accurate, current, complete, and organized.

2. Reports should include essential background information, subjective data, objective data, any changes in the client's status, client problems or nursing diagnoses as appropriate, treatments and procedures, medication administration, client teaching, discharge planning, family information, the client's response to treatments and procedures, and the client's priority needs.
3. Change-of-shift (handoff) report
   a. The report facilitates continuity of care among nurses who are responsible for a client.
   b. The report may be written, oral, audiotaped, or provided during walking rounds at the client's bedside.
   c. The report describes the client's health status and informs the nurse who assumes care about the client's needs and priorities for care.
   d. The report may be done at the client's bedside to allow the client to participate in care planning, as well as to establish the stability of the client before the oncoming nurse assumes care.
4. Telephone reports
   a. Purposes include informing a PHCP of a client's change in status, communicating information about a client's transfer to or from another unit or facility, and obtaining results of laboratory or diagnostic tests.
   b. The telephone report should be documented and should include when the call was made, who made the call, who was called, to whom information was given, what information was given, and what information was received.
5. Transfer reports
   a. Transferring nurse reports provide continuity of care and may be given by telephone or in person (Box 7-6).
   b. Receiving nurse should repeat transfer information to ensure client safety and ask questions to clarify information about the client's status.
6. Situation, Background, Assessment, Recommendation (SBAR)
   a. SBAR, a communication model, is a structured and standardized communication technique that improves communication among team members when sharing information on a client.
   b. SBAR includes up-to-date information about the client's situation, associated background information, assessment data, and recommendations for care, such as treatments, medications, or services needed.
   c. Refer to Chapter 12 for SOAP (subjective, objective, assessment, plan) notes

XIII. Interprofessional Consultation

A. Consultation is a process in which a specialist is sought to identify methods of care or treatment plans to meet the needs of a client.

B. Consultation is needed when the nurse encounters a problem that cannot be solved using nursing knowledge, skills, and available resources.

C. Consultation also is needed when the exact problem remains unclear; a consultant can objectively and more clearly assess and identify the exact nature of the problem.

D. Rapid-response teams are being developed within hospitals to provide nursing staff with internal consultative services provided by expert clinicians.

E. Rapid-response teams are used to assist nursing staff with early detection and resolution of client problems.

F. Rapid-response teams are also teams of health care providers that respond to hospitalized clients with early signs of deterioration on non-intensive care units to prevent respiratory or cardiac arrest.

G. Medication reconciliation includes collaboration among the client, PHCPs, nurses, and pharmacists to ensure medication accuracy when clients experience changes in health care settings or levels of care or are transferred from one care unit to another, and upon discharge (Box 7-7).

BOX 7-6 Transfer Reports

- Client's name, age, health care provider, and diagnoses
- Current health status and plan of care
- Client's needs and priorities for care
- Any assessments or interventions that need to be performed after transfer, such as laboratory tests, medication administration, or dressing changes
- Need for any special equipment
- Additional considerations such as allergies, resuscitation status, precautionary considerations, cultural or religious issues, or family issues

BOX 7-7 Process for Medication Reconciliation

1. Obtain a list of current medications from the client.
2. Develop an accurate list of newly prescribed medications.
3. Compare new medications to the list of current medications.
4. Identify and investigate any discrepancies and collaborate with the health care provider as necessary.
5. Communicate the finalized list with the client, caregivers, primary health care provider, and other team members.

From Potter P, Perry A, Stockert P, Hall A: *Fundamentals of nursing*, ed 8, St. Louis, 2013, Mosby.

XIV. Discharge Planning

A. Discharge planning begins when the client is admitted to the hospital or health care facility.

B. Discharge planning is an interprofessional process that ensures that the client has a plan for continuing care after leaving the health care facility and assists in the client's transition from one environment to another.

C. All caregivers need to be involved in discharge planning, and referrals to other PHCPs or agencies may be needed. A PHCP's prescription may be needed for the referral, and the referral needs to be approved by the client's health care insurer.

D. The nurse should anticipate the client's discharge needs and make the required referral as soon as possible (involving the client and family in the referral process).

E. The nurse needs to educate the client and family regarding care at home (Box 7-8).

XV. Delegation and Assignments

A. Delegation
1. Delegation is a process of transferring performance of a selected nursing task in a situation to an individual who is competent and has the authority to perform that specific task.
2. Delegation involves achieving outcomes and sharing activities with other individuals who have the authority to accomplish the task.
3. The nurse practice act and any practice limitations (institutional policies and procedures, and job descriptions of personnel provided by the institution) define which aspects of care can be delegated and which must be performed by a registered nurse.
4. Even though a task may be delegated to someone, the nurse who delegates maintains ultimate accountability for the task.
5. The nurse cannot delegate any activity that involves nursing judgment or critical decision making.
6. The 5 rights of delegation include the right task, right circumstances, right person, right direction/communication, and right supervision/evaluation.

BOX 7-8 Discharge Teaching

- How to administer prescribed medications
- Side and adverse effects of medications that need to be reported to the primary health care provider (PHCP)
- Prescribed dietary and activity measures
- Complications of the medical condition that need to be reported to the PHCP
- How to perform prescribed treatments
- How to use special equipment prescribed for the client
- Schedule for home care services that are planned
- How to access available community resources
- When to obtain follow-up care

⚠ The nurse delegates only tasks for which he or she is responsible. The nurse who delegates is accountable for the task; the person who assumes responsibility for the task is also accountable.

B. Principles and guidelines of delegating (Box 7-9)

C. Assignments
1. Assignment is the transfer of performance of client care activities to specific staff members.
2. Guidelines for client care assignments
   a. Always ensure client safety.
   b. Be aware of individual variations in work abilities.
   c. Determine which tasks can be delegated and to whom.
   d. Match the task to the delegatee on the basis of the nurse practice act and any practice limitations (institutional policies and procedures, and job descriptions of personnel provided by the institution).

BOX 7-9 Principles and Guidelines of Delegating

- Delegate the right task to the right delegatee. Be familiar with the experience of the delegatees, their scopes of practice, their job descriptions, agency policy and procedures, and the state nurse practice act.
- Provide clear directions about the task and ensure that the delegatee understands the expectations.
- Determine the degree of supervision that may be required.
- Provide the delegatee with the authority to complete the task; provide a deadline for completion of the task.
- Evaluate the outcome of care that has been delegated.
- Provide feedback to the delegatee regarding his or her performance.
- *In general,* noninvasive interventions, such as skin care, range-of-motion exercises, ambulation, grooming, and hygiene measures, can be assigned to the assistive personnel (AP).
- *In general,* a licensed practical nurse (LPN) or vocational nurse (VN) can perform not only the tasks that an AP can perform, but also certain invasive tasks, such as dressing changes, suctioning, urinary catheterization, and medication administration (oral, subcutaneous, intramuscular, and selected piggyback medications), according to the education and job description of the LPN or VN. The LPN or VN can data collect and also review with the client teaching plans that were initiated by the registered nurse.
- A registered nurse (RN) can perform the tasks that an LPN or VN can perform and is responsible for assessment and planning care, initiating teaching, and administering medications intravenously.
- An RN can care for stable and unstable clients.
- An LPN or VN cares for stable clients.
- An AP provides basic care that does not require any type of assessment; they can perform routine tasks in client care.

e. Provide directions that are clear, concise, accurate, and complete.
f. Validate the delegatee's understanding of the directions.
g. Communicate a feeling of confidence to the delegatee, and provide feedback promptly after the task is performed.
h. Maintain continuity of care as much as possible when assigning client care.

XVI. Time Management

A. Description
1. Time management is a technique designed to assist in completing tasks within a definite time period.
2. Learning how, when, and where to use one's time and establishing personal goals and time frames are part of time management.
3. Time management requires an ability to anticipate the day's activities, to combine activities when possible, and to not be interrupted by nonessential activities.
4. Time management involves efficiency in completing tasks as quickly as possible and effectiveness in deciding on the most important task to do (i.e., **prioritizing**) and doing it correctly.

B. Principles and guidelines
1. Identify tasks, obligations, and activities and write them down.
2. Organize the workday; identify which tasks must be completed in specified time frames.
3. Prioritize client needs according to importance.
4. Anticipate the needs of the day and provide time for unexpected and unplanned tasks that may arise.
5. Focus on beginning the daily tasks, working on the most important first while keeping goals in mind; look at the final goal for the day to help break down tasks into manageable parts.
6. Begin client rounds at the beginning of the shift, collecting data on each assigned client.
7. Delegate tasks when appropriate.
8. Keep a daily hour-by-hour log to assist in providing structure to the tasks that must be accomplished, and cross tasks off the list as they are accomplished.
9. Use health care agency resources wisely, anticipating resource needs, and gather the necessary supplies before beginning the task.
10. Organize paperwork and continuously document task completion and necessary client data throughout the day (i.e., documentation should be concurrent with completion of a task or observation of pertinent client data).
11. At the end of the day, evaluate the effectiveness of time management.

XVII. Prioritizing Care

A. Prioritizing is deciding which needs or problems require immediate action and which ones could tolerate a delay in response until a later time because they are not urgent.

B. Guidelines for prioritizing (Box 7-10)

C. Setting priorities for client teaching
1. Determine the client's immediate learning needs.
2. Identify the type of learning needs for the individual; for example, consider the client's age, cognitive age, language needs, and generational concerns.

BOX 7-10 Guidelines for Prioritizing

- The nurse and the client mutually rank the client's needs in order of importance based on the client's preferences and expectations, safety, and physical and psychological needs; what the client sees as his or her priority needs may be different from what the nurse sees as the priority needs.
- Priorities are classified as high, intermediate, or low.
- Client needs that are life-threatening or that could result in harm to the client if they are left untreated are high priorities.
- Nonemergency and non–life-threatening client needs are intermediate priorities.
- Client needs that are not related directly to the client's illness or prognosis are low priorities.
- The nurse can use the ABCs—airway, breathing, and circulation—as a guide when determining priorities; client needs related to maintaining a patent airway are always the priority.
- If cardiopulmonary resuscitation (CPR) is necessary, the order of priority is CAB—compressions, airway, and breathing—this is the exception to using the ABCs when determining priorities.
- When providing care, the nurse needs to decide which needs or problems require immediate action and which ones could be delayed until a later time because they are not urgent.
- The nurse considers client problems that involve actual or life-threatening concerns before potential health-threatening concerns.
- The nurse can use Maslow's Hierarchy of Needs theory as a guide to determine priorities and to identify the levels of physiological needs, safety, love and belonging, self-esteem, and self-actualization (basic needs are met before moving to other needs in the hierarchy).
- When prioritizing care, the nurse must consider time constraints and available resources.
- Problems identified as important by the client must be given high priority.
- The nurse can use the steps of the nursing process as a guide to determine priorities, remembering that assessment is the first step of the nursing process.
- Prioritization may be different in a disaster or emergency situation, where an action should be taken before gathering further information.

3. Review the learning objectives established for the client.
4. Determine what the client perceives as important.
5. Assess the client's anxiety level and the time available to teach.

D. Prioritizing when caring for a group of clients
1. Identify the problems of each client.
2. Review the problems and any nursing diagnoses.
3. Determine which client problems are most urgent based on basic needs, the client's changing or unstable status, and complexity of the client's problems.
4. Anticipate the time that it may take to care for the priority needs of the clients.
5. Combine activities, if possible, to resolve more than one problem at a time.
6. Involve the client in his or her care as much as possible (see Priority Nursing Actions).

PRIORITY NURSING ACTIONS

Assessing a Group of Clients in Order of Priority

The nurse is assigned to the following clients. The order of priority in assessing the clients is as follows:

1. A client with heart failure who has a 4-lb weight gain since yesterday and is experiencing shortness of breath
2. A 24-hour postoperative client who had a wedge resection of the lung and has a closed chest tube drainage system
3. A client admitted to the hospital for observation who has absent bowel sounds
4. A client who is undergoing surgery for a hysterectomy on the following day

References

Potter et al. (2017), pp. 284-285
Zerwekh, Zerwekh Garneau (2015), pp. 511, 514.

Use the ABCs—airway, breathing, and circulation—Maslow's Hierarchy of Needs theory, and the steps of the nursing process (assessment is first) to prioritize. Also consider the acuity level of clients when applying these guidelines. If cardiopulmonary resuscitation (CPR) needs to be initiated, use CAB—compressions, airway, breathing—as the priority guideline.

XVIII. Disasters and Emergency Response Planning

A. Description
1. A disaster is any human-made or natural event that causes destruction and devastation that cannot be alleviated without assistance (Box 7-11).
2. Internal disasters are disasters that occur within a health care agency (e.g., health care agency fire, structural collapse, radiation spill), whereas external disasters are disasters that occur outside the health care agency (e.g., mass transit accident that could send hundreds of victims to emergency departments).

BOX 7-11 Types of Disasters

Human-Made Disasters

Dam failures resulting in flooding
Hazardous substance accidents such as pollution, chemical spills, or toxic gas leaks
Accidents involving release of radioactive material
Resource shortages such as food, water, and electricity
Structural collapse, fire, or explosions
Terrorist attacks such as bombing, riots, and bioterrorism
Mass transportation accidents

Natural Disasters

Avalanches
Blizzards
Communicable disease epidemics
Cyclones
Droughts
Earthquakes
Floods
Forest fires
Hailstorms
Hurricanes
Landslides
Mudslides
Tidal waves
Tornadoes
Volcanic eruptions

3. A **multicasualty event** involves a limited number of victims or casualties and can be managed by a hospital with available resources; a **mass casualty event** involves a number of casualties that exceeds the resource capabilities of the hospital, and is also known as a disaster.
4. An emergency response plan is a formal plan of action for coordinating the response of the health care agency staff in the event of a disaster in the health care agency or surrounding community.

B. American Red Cross (ARC)
1. The ARC has been given authority by the federal government to provide disaster relief.
2. All ARC disaster relief assistance is free, and local offices are located across the United States.
3. The ARC participates with the government in developing and testing community disaster plans.
4. The ARC identifies and trains personnel for emergency response.
5. The ARC works with businesses and labor organizations to identify resources and individuals for disaster work.

6. The ARC educates the public about ways to prepare for a disaster.
7. The ARC operates shelters, provides assistance to meet immediate emergency needs, and provides disaster health services, including crisis counseling.
8. The ARC handles inquiries from family members.
9. The ARC coordinates relief activities with other agencies.
10. Nurses are involved directly with the ARC and assume functions such as managers, supervisors, and educators of first aid; they also participate in emergency response plans and disaster relief programs and provide services, such as blood collection drives and immunization programs.

C. HAZMAT (hazardous materials) team
1. HAZMAT teams are typically composed of emergency department health care providers and nursing staff, because they will be the first individuals to encounter the potential exposure.
2. Members of HAZMAT teams have been educated on how to recognize patterns of illness that may be indicative of nuclear, biological, and chemical exposure; protocols for pharmacological treatment of infectious disease agents; availability of decontamination facilities and personal protective gear; safety measures; and the methods of responding to an exposure.

D. Phases of disaster management
1. The Federal Emergency Management Agency (FEMA) identifies 4 disaster management phases: mitigation, preparedness, response, and recovery.
2. Mitigation encompasses the following:
   a. Actions or measures that can prevent the occurrence of a disaster or reduce the damaging effects of a disaster
   b. Determination of the community hazards and community risks (actual and potential threats) before a disaster occurs
   c. Awareness of available community resources and community health personnel to facilitate mobilization of activities and minimize chaos and confusion if a disaster occurs
   d. Determination of the resources available for care to infants, older adults, disabled individuals, and individuals with chronic health problems
3. Preparedness encompasses the following:
   a. Plans for rescue, evacuation, and caring for disaster victims
   b. Plans for training disaster personnel and gathering resources, equipment, and other materials needed for dealing with the disaster
   c. Identification of specific responsibilities for various emergency response personnel
   d. Establishment of a community emergency response plan and an effective public communication system
   e. Development of an emergency medical system and a plan for activation
   f. Verification of proper functioning of emergency equipment
   g. Collection of anticipatory provisions and creation of a location for providing food, water, clothing, shelter, other supplies, and needed medicine
   h. Inventory of supplies on a regular basis and replenishment of outdated supplies
   i. Practice of community emergency response plans (mock disaster drills)
4. Response encompasses the following:
   a. Putting disaster planning services into action and the actions taken to save lives and prevent further damage
   b. Primary concerns include safety and the physical and mental health of victims and members of the disaster response team
5. Recovery encompasses the following:
   a. Actions taken to return to a normal situation after the disaster
   b. Preventing debilitating effects and restoring personal, economic, and environmental health and stability to the community

E. Levels of disaster
1. FEMA identifies three levels of disaster with FEMA response (Box 7-12).
2. When a federal emergency has been declared, the federal response plan may take effect and activate emergency support functions.
3. The emergency support functions of the ARC include performing emergency first aid, sheltering, feeding, providing a disaster welfare information

BOX 7-12 Federal Emergency Management Agency (FEMA) Levels of Disaster

Level I Disaster

Massive disaster that involves significant damage and results in a presidential disaster declaration, with major federal involvement and full engagement of federal, regional, and national resources

Level II Disaster

Moderate disaster that is likely to result in a presidential declaration of an emergency, with moderate federal assistance

Level III Disaster

Minor disaster that involves a minimal level of damage but could result in a presidential declaration of an emergency

BOX 7-13 Emergency Plans and Supplies

- Plan a meeting place for family members.
- Identify where to go if an evacuation is necessary.
- Determine when and how to turn off water, gas, and electricity at main switches.
- Locate the safe spots in the home for each type of disaster.
- Replace stored water supply every 3 months and stored food supply every 6 months.
- Include the following supplies:
  - Backpack, clean clothing, sturdy footwear
  - Pocket knife or multi-tool
  - A 3-day supply of water (1 gallon per person per day)
  - A 3-day supply of nonperishable food
  - Blankets/sleeping bags/pillows
  - First-aid kit with over-the-counter medications and vitamins
  - Adequate supply of prescription medication
  - Battery-operated radio
  - Flashlight and batteries
  - Credit card, cash, or traveler's checks
  - Personal ID card, list of emergency contacts, allergies, medical information, list of credit card numbers and bank accounts (all sealed in a water-tight package)
  - Extra set of car keys and a full tank of gas in the car
  - Sanitation supplies for washing, toileting, and disposing of trash; hand sanitizer
  - Extra pair of eyeglasses/sunglasses
  - Special items for infants, older adults, or disabled individuals
  - Items needed for a pet such as food, water, and leash
  - Paper, pens, pencils, maps
  - Cell phone
  - Work gloves
  - Rain gear
  - Roll of duct tape and plastic sheeting
  - Radio and extra batteries
  - Toiletries (basic daily needs, sunscreen, insect repellent, toilet paper)
  - Plastic garbage bags and resealable bags
  - Household bleach for disinfection
  - Whistle
  - Matches in a waterproof container

From Ignatavicius D, Workman M: *Medical surgical nursing: patient-centered collaborative care*, ed 7, Philadelphia, 2013, Saunders.

system, and coordinating bulk distribution of emergency relief supplies.

4. Disaster medical assistant teams (teams of specially trained personnel) can be activated and sent to a disaster site to provide triage and medical care to victims until they can be evacuated to a hospital.

F. Nurse's role in disaster planning

1. Personal and professional preparedness

a. Make personal and family preparations (Box 7-13).

b. Be aware of the disaster plan at the place of employment and in the community.

c. Maintain certification in disaster training and in CPR.

d. Participate in mock disaster drills, including bomb threat and active shooter drills.

e. Prepare professional emergency response items, such as a copy of nursing license, personal health care equipment such as a stethoscope, cash, warm clothing, recordkeeping materials, and other nursing care supplies.

2. Disaster response

a. In the health care agency setting, if a disaster occurs, the agency disaster preparedness plan (emergency response plan) is activated immediately, and the nurse responds by following the directions identified in the plan.

b. In the community setting, if the nurse is the first responder to a disaster, the nurse cares for the victims by attending to the victims with life-threatening problems first; when rescue workers arrive at the scene, immediate plans for triage should begin.

In the event of a disaster, activate the emergency response plan immediately.

G. Triage

1. In a disaster or war, triage consists of a brief assessment of victims that allows the nurse to classify victims according to the severity of the injury, urgency of treatment, and place for treatment (see Priority Nursing Actions).

PRIORITY NURSING ACTIONS

Triaging Victims at the Site of an Accident

The nurse is the first responder at the scene of a school bus accident. The nurse triages the victims from highest to lowest priority as follows:

1. Confused child with bright red blood pulsating from a leg wound
2. Child with a closed head wound and multiple compound fractures of the arms and legs
3. Child with a simple fracture of the arm complaining of arm pain
4. Sobbing child with several minor lacerations on the face, arms, and legs

Reference

Ignatavicius. (2018). Workman, Rebar, 151–152.

2. Simple Triage and Rapid Treatment (START) is a strategy used to evaluate the severity of injury of each victim as quickly as possible and tag the victims in about 30 to 60 seconds.

3. In an emergency department, triage consists of a brief assessment of clients that allows the nurse to classify clients according to their need for care and establish priorities of care; the type of illness or injury, the severity of the problem, and the resources available govern the process.

H. Emergency department triage system
   1. A commonly used rating system in an emergency department is a 3-tier system that uses the categories of emergent, urgent, and nonurgent; these categories may be identified by color coding or numbers (Box 7-14).
   2. The nurse needs to be familiar with the triage system of the health care agency.
   3. When caring for a client who has died, the nurse needs to recognize the importance of family and cultural and religious rituals and provide support to loved ones.
   4. Organ donation procedures of the health care agency need to be addressed if appropriate.

Think survivability. If you are the first responder to a scene of a disaster, such as a train crash, a priority victim is one whose life can be saved.

I. Client assessment in the emergency department
   1. Primary assessment
      a. The purpose of primary assessment is to identify any client problem that poses an immediate or potential threat to life.
      b. The nurse gathers information primarily through objective data and, on finding any abnormalities, immediately initiates interventions.
      c. The nurse uses the ABCs—airway, breathing, and circulation—as a guide in assessing a client's needs and assesses a client who has sustained a traumatic injury for signs of a head injury or cervical spine injury. If CPR needs to be initiated, use CAB—compressions, airway, breathing—as the priority guideline.
      d. Agonal breathing does not provide effective respiration and ventilation and indicates a need for ventilatory support.
      e. Only central pulses, such as the carotid or femoral pulses, should be used to assess circulation; they should be checked for at least 5 seconds but no longer than 10 seconds so as to not delay chest compressions.
   2. Secondary assessment
      a. The nurse performs secondary assessment after the primary assessment and after treatment for any primary problems identified.
      b. Secondary assessment identifies any other life-threatening problems that a client might be experiencing.
      c. The nurse obtains subjective and objective data, including a history, general overview, vital sign measurements, neurological assessment, pain assessment, and complete or focused physical assessment.

BOX 7-14 Emergency Department Triage

Emergent (Red): Priority 1 (Highest)

This classification is assigned to clients who have life-threatening injuries and need immediate attention and continuous evaluation but have a high probability for survival when stabilized.

Such clients include trauma victims, clients with chest pain, clients with severe respiratory distress or cardiac arrest, clients with limb amputation, clients with acute neurological deficits, and clients who have sustained chemical splashes to the eyes.

Urgent (Yellow): Priority 2

This classification is assigned to clients who require treatment and whose injuries have complications that are not life-threatening, provided that they are treated within 30 minutes to 2 hours; these clients require continuous evaluation every 30 to 60 minutes thereafter.

Such clients include clients with an open fracture with a distal pulse and large wounds.

Nonurgent (Green): Priority 3

This classification is assigned to clients with local injuries who do not have immediate complications and who can wait at least 2 hours for medical treatment; these clients require evaluation every 1 to 2 hours thereafter.

Such clients include clients with conditions such as a closed fracture, minor lacerations, sprains, strains, or contusions.

Note: Some triage systems include tagging a client "Black" if the victim is dead or soon will be deceased because of severe injuries; these are victims that would not benefit from any care because of the severity of injuries.

From Ignatavicius D, Workman M: *Medical surgical nursing: patient-centered collaborative care*, ed 7, Philadelphia, 2013, Saunders.

PRACTICE QUESTIONS

29. The nurse is assigned to care for four clients. In planning client rounds, which client should the nurse assess **first?**
   1. A postoperative client preparing for discharge with a new medication
   2. A client requiring daily dressing changes of a recent surgical incision
   3. A client scheduled for a chest x-ray after insertion of a nasogastric tube
   4. A client with asthma who requested a breathing treatment during the previous shift

30. The nurse employed in an emergency department is assigned to triage clients coming to the emergency department for treatment on the evening shift. The nurse should assign **priority** to which client?
1. A client complaining of muscle aches, a headache, and history of seizures
2. A client who twisted her ankle when rollerblading and is requesting medication for pain
3. A client with a minor laceration on the index finger sustained while cutting an eggplant
4. A client with chest pain who states that he just ate pizza that was made with a very spicy sauce

31. A nursing graduate is attending an agency orientation regarding the nursing model of practice implemented in the health care facility. The nurse is told that the nursing model is a team nursing approach. The nurse determines that which scenario is characteristic of the team-based model of nursing practice?
1. Each staff member is assigned a specific task for a group of clients.
2. A staff member is assigned to determine the client's needs at home and begin discharge planning.
3. A single registered nurse (RN) is responsible for providing care to a group of 6 clients with the aid of an assistive personnel (AP).
4. An RN leads 2 licensed practical nurses (LPNs) and 3 APs in providing care to a group of 12 clients.

32. The nurse has received the assignment for the day shift. After making initial rounds and checking all of the assigned clients, which client should the nurse plan to care for **first?**
1. A client who is ambulatory demonstrating steady gait
2. A postoperative client who has just received an opioid pain medication
3. A client scheduled for physical therapy for the first crutch-walking session
4. A client with a white blood cell count of 14,000 mm^3 (14×10^9/L) and a temperature of 38.4° C

33. The nurse is giving a bed bath to an assigned client when an assistive personnel (AP) enters the client's room and tells the nurse that another assigned client is in pain and needs pain medication. Which is the **most appropriate** nursing action?
1. Finish the bed bath and then administer the pain medication to the other client.
2. Ask the AP to find out when the last pain medication was given to the client.
3. Ask the AP to tell the client in pain that medication will be administered as soon as the bed bath is complete.
4. Cover the client, raise the side rails, tell the client that you will return shortly, and administer the pain medication to the other client.

34. The nurse manager has implemented a change in the method of the nursing delivery system from functional to team nursing. An assistive personnel (AP) is resistant to the change and is not taking an active part in facilitating the process of change. Which is the **best** approach in dealing with the AP?
1. Ignore the resistance.
2. Exert coercion on the AP.
3. Provide a positive reward system for the AP.
4. Confront the AP to encourage verbalization of feelings regarding the change.

35. The registered nurse is planning the client assignments for the day. Which is the **most appropriate** assignment for an assistive personnel (AP)?
1. A client requiring a colostomy irrigation
2. A client receiving continuous tube feedings
3. A client who requires urine specimen collections
4. A client with difficulty swallowing food and fluids

36. The nurse manager is discussing the facility protocol in the event of a tornado with the staff. Which instructions should the nurse manager include in the discussion? **Select all that apply.**
- ❑ 1. Open doors to client rooms.
- ❑ 2. Move beds away from windows.
- ❑ 3. Close window shades and curtains.
- ❑ 4. Place blankets over clients who are confined to bed.
- ❑ 5. Relocate ambulatory clients from the hallways back into their rooms.

37. The nurse employed in a long-term care facility is planning assignments for the clients on a nursing unit. The nurse needs to assign four clients and has a licensed practical nurse and 3 assistive personnel (APs) on a nursing team. Which client would the nurse **most appropriately** assign to the licensed practical nurse?
1. A client who requires a bed bath
2. An older client requiring frequent ambulation
3. A client who requires hourly vital sign measurements
4. A client requiring abdominal wound irrigations and dressing changes every 3 hours

38. The charge nurse is planning the assignment for the day. Which factors should the nurse remain mindful of when planning the assignment? **Select all that apply.**
- ❑ 1. The acuity level of the clients
- ❑ 2. Specific requests from the staff
- ❑ 3. The clustering of the rooms on the unit
- ❑ 4. The number of anticipated client discharges
- ❑ 5. Client needs and workers' needs and abilities

ANSWERS

29. *Answer:* 4
Rationale: Airway is always the highest priority, and the nurse would attend to the client with asthma who requested a breathing treatment during the previous shift. This could indicate that the client was experiencing difficulty breathing. The clients described in options 1, 2, and 3 have needs that would be identified as intermediate priorities.
Test-Taking Strategy: Note the strategic word, *first.* Use the ABCs—airway, breathing, and circulation—to answer the question. Remember that airway is always the highest priority. This will direct you to the correct option.
Level of Cognitive Ability: Analyzing
Client Needs: Safe and Effective Care Environment
Integrated Process: Nursing Process—Planning
Content Area: Leadership/Management: Prioritizing
Health Problem: N/A
Priority Concepts: Care Coordination; Clinical Judgment
References: Potter et al. (2017), pp. 284-285, 1287.

30. *Answer:* 4
Rationale: In an emergency department, triage involves brief client assessment to classify clients according to their need for care and includes establishing priorities of care. The type of illness or injury, the severity of the problem, and the resources available govern the process. Clients with trauma, chest pain, severe respiratory distress or cardiac arrest, limb amputation, and acute neurological deficits and those who have sustained chemical splashes to the eyes are classified as emergent and are the highest priority. Clients with conditions such as a simple fracture, asthma without respiratory distress, fever, hypertension, abdominal pain, or a renal stone have urgent needs and are classified as a second priority. Clients with conditions such as a minor laceration, sprain, or cold symptoms are classified as nonurgent and are a third priority.
Test-Taking Strategy: Note the strategic word, *priority.* Use the ABCs—airway, breathing, and circulation—to direct you to the correct option. A client experiencing chest pain is always classified as priority 1 until a myocardial infarction has been ruled out.
Level of Cognitive Ability: Analyzing
Client Needs: Safe and Effective Care Environment
Integrated Process: Nursing Process—Assessment
Content Area: Leadership/Management: Prioritizing
Health Problem: N/A
Priority Concepts: Care Coordination; Clinical Judgment
Reference: Ignatavicius, Workman, Rebar (2018), pp. 123-124.

31. *Answer:* 4
Rationale: In team nursing, nursing personnel are led by a registered nurse leader in providing care to a group of clients. Option 1 identifies functional nursing. Option 2 identifies a component of case management. Option 3 identifies primary nursing (relationship-based practice).
Test-Taking Strategy: Focus on the subject, team nursing. Keep this subject in mind and select the option that best describes a team approach. The correct option is the only one that identifies the concept of a team approach.
Level of Cognitive Ability: Applying
Client Needs: Safe and Effective Care Environment
Integrated Process: Nursing Process—Planning
Content Area: Leadership/Management: Delegating/Supervising
Health Problem: N/A
Priority Concepts: Care Coordination; Collaboration
Reference: Yoder-Wise (2015), pp. 236-237.

32. *Answer:* 4
Rationale: The nurse should plan to care for the client who has an elevated white blood cell count and a fever first, because this client's needs are the priority. The client who is ambulatory with steady gait and the client scheduled for physical therapy for a crutch-walking session do not have priority needs. Waiting for pain medication to take effect before providing care to the postoperative client is best.
Test-Taking Strategy: Note the strategic word, *first,* and use principles related to prioritizing. Recalling the normal white blood cell count is 5000 to 10,000 mm^3 (5 to 10 × 10^9/L) and the normal temperature range 97.5° F to 98.6° F (36.4° C to 37° C) will direct you to the correct option.
Level of Cognitive Ability: Analyzing
Client Needs: Safe and Effective Care Environment
Integrated Process: Nursing Process—Planning
Content Area: Leadership/Management: Prioritizing
Health Problem: N/A
Priority Concepts: Care Coordination; Clinical Judgment
References: Potter et al. (2017), pp. 284-285.

33. *Answer:* 4
Rationale: The nurse is responsible for the care provided to assigned clients. The appropriate action in this situation is to provide safety to the client who is receiving the bed bath and prepare to administer the pain medication. Options 1 and 3 delay the administration of medication to the client in pain. Option 2 is not a responsibility of the AP.
Test-Taking Strategy: Note the strategic words, *most appropriate,* and use principles related to priorities of care. Options 1 and 3 are comparable or alike and delay the administration of pain medication, and option 2 is not a responsibility of the AP. The most appropriate action is to plan to administer the medication.
Level of Cognitive Ability: Applying
Client Needs: Safe and Effective Care Environment
Integrated Process: Nursing Process—Implementation
Content Area: Leadership/Management: Prioritizing
Health Problem: N/A
Priority Concepts: Care Coordination; Clinical Judgment
Reference: Potter et al. (2017), pp. 284-285, 382.

34. *Answer:* 4
Rationale: Confrontation is an important strategy to meet resistance head-on. Face-to-face meetings to confront the issue at hand will allow verbalization of feelings, identification of problems and issues, and development of strategies to solve the problem. Option 1 will not address the problem. Option 2 may produce additional resistance. Option 3 may provide a temporary solution to the resistance but will not address the concern specifically.
Test-Taking Strategy: Note the strategic word, *best.* Options 1 and 2 can be eliminated first because of the words *ignore* in option 1 and *coercion* in option 2. From the remaining options, select the correct option over option 3 because the correct option specifically addresses problem-solving measures.

Level of Cognitive Ability: Applying
Client Needs: Safe and Effective Care Environment
Integrated Process: Nursing Process—Implementation
Content Area: Leadership/Management: Ethical/Legal
Health Problem: N/A
Priority Concepts: Leadership; Professional Identity
Reference: Zerwekh, Zerwekh Garneau (2015), pp. 230, 233.

35. *Answer:* 3
Rationale: The nurse must determine the most appropriate assignment based on the skills of the staff member and the needs of the client. In this case, the most appropriate assignment for the AP would be to care for the client who requires urine specimen collections. The AP is skilled in this procedure. Colostomy irrigations and tube feedings are not performed by APs because these are invasive procedures. The client with difficulty swallowing food and fluids is at risk for aspiration.
Test-Taking Strategy: Note the strategic words, *most appropriate,* and note the subject, an assignment to the AP. Eliminate option 4 first because of the words *difficulty swallowing.* Next, eliminate options 1 and 2 because they are comparable or alike and are both invasive procedures and as such an AP cannot perform these procedures.
Level of Cognitive Ability: Creating
Client Needs: Safe and Effective Care Environment
Integrated Process: Nursing Process—Planning
Content Area: Leadership/Management: Delegating/Supervising
Health Problem: N/A
Priority Concepts: Care Coordination; Clinical Judgment
References: Ignatavicius, Workman, Rebar (2018), p. 6.

36. *Answer:* 2, 3, 4
Rationale: In this weather event, the appropriate nursing actions focus on protecting clients from flying debris or glass. The nurse should close doors to each client's room and move beds away from windows, and close window shades and curtains to protect clients, visitors, and staff from shattering glass and flying debris. Blankets should be placed over clients confined to bed. Ambulatory clients should be moved into the hallways from their rooms, away from windows.
Test-Taking Strategy: Focus on the subject, protecting the client in the event of a tornado. Visualize each of the actions in the options to determine whether these actions would assist in protecting the client and preventing an accident or injury.
Level of Cognitive Ability: Applying
Client Needs: Safe and Effective Care Environment
Integrated Process: Nursing Process—Implementation
Content Area: Leadership/Management: Management of Care
Health Problem: N/A
Priority Concepts: Leadership; Professional Identity
Reference: Potter et al. (2017), pp. 381, 394.

37. *Answer:* 4
Rationale: When delegating nursing assignments, the nurse needs to consider the skills and educational level of the nursing staff. Giving a bed bath, assisting with frequent ambulation, and taking vital signs can be provided most appropriately by an AP. The licensed practical nurse is skilled in wound irrigations and dressing changes and most appropriately would be assigned to the client who needs this care.
Test-Taking Strategy: Focus on the subject, assignment to a licensed practical nurse, and note the strategic words, *most appropriately.* Recall that education and job position as described by the nurse practice act and employee guidelines need to be considered when delegating activities and making assignments. Options 1, 2, and 3 can be eliminated because they are noninvasive tasks that the AP can perform.
Level of Cognitive Ability: Creating
Client Needs: Safe and Effective Care Environment
Integrated Process: Nursing Process—Planning
Content Area: Leadership/Management: Delegating/Supervising
Health Problem: N/A
Priority Concepts: Care Coordination; Clinical Judgment
Reference: Potter et al. (2017), pp. 287-288.

38. *Answer:* 1, 5
Rationale: There are guidelines that the nurse should use when delegating and planning assignments. These include the following: ensure client safety; be aware of individual variations in work abilities; determine which tasks can be delegated and to whom; match the task to the delegatee on the basis of the nurse practice act and appropriate position descriptions; provide directions that are clear, concise, accurate, and complete; validate the delegatee's understanding of the directions; communicate a feeling of confidence to the delegatee and provide feedback promptly after the task is performed; and maintain continuity of care as much as possible when assigning client care. Staff requests, convenience as in clustering client rooms, and anticipated changes in unit census are not specific guidelines to use when delegating and planning assignments.
Test-Taking Strategy: Focus on the subject, guidelines to use when delegating and planning assignments. Read each option carefully and use Maslow's Hierarchy of Needs theory. Note that the correct options directly relate to the client's needs and client safety.
Level of Cognitive Ability: Applying
Client Needs: Safe and Effective Care Environment
Integrated Process: Nursing Process—Planning
Content Area: Leadership/Management: Delegating/Supervising
Health Problem: N/A
Priority Concepts: Clinical Judgment; Professionalism
References: Potter et al. (2017), p. 288.

UNIT III

Foundations of Care

Pyramid to Success

Pyramid Points focus on fluids and electrolytes, acid–base balance, vital signs, laboratory reference intervals, and nutrition. Fluids and electrolytes and acid–base balance constitute a content area that is sometimes complex and difficult to understand. For a client who is experiencing these imbalances, it is important to remember that maintenance of a patent airway is a priority, and the nurse needs to monitor vital signs, physiological status, intake and output, laboratory reference intervals, and arterial blood gas values. Be certain to know the normal vital sign values and the baseline values for each client that you are caring for so that you are able to determine changes in the client status. Remember that pain is also a vital sign, and to assess each client for verbal and nonverbal signs of pain. It is also important to remember that normal laboratory reference levels may vary slightly, depending on the laboratory setting and equipment used in testing. If you are familiar with the normal reference intervals, you will be able to determine whether an abnormality exists when a laboratory value is presented in a question. The specific laboratory reference levels identified in the NCLEX® test plan that you need to know include arterial blood gases known as ABGs (pH, PO_2, Pco_2, SaO_2, HCO_3), blood urea nitrogen (BUN), cholesterol (total), glucose, hematocrit, hemoglobin, glycosylated hemoglobin (HgbA1C), platelets, potassium, sodium, white blood cell (WBC) count, creatinine, prothrombin time (PT), activated partial thromboplastin time (aPTT), and international normalized ratio (INR). The questions on the NCLEX-RN examination related to laboratory reference intervals will require you to identify whether the laboratory value is normal or abnormal, and then you will be required to think critically about the effects of the laboratory value in terms of the client. Note the disorder presented in the question and the associated body organ affected as a result of the disorder. This process will assist you in determining the correct answer.

Nutrition is a basic need that must be met for all clients. The NCLEX-RN examination addresses the dietary measures required for basic needs and for particular body system alterations. When presented with a question related to nutrition, consider the client's diagnosis and the particular requirement or restriction necessary for treatment of the disorder.

On the NCLEX-RN, safety and infection control concepts, including standard precautions and transmission-based precautions related to client care, are a priority focus. Medication or intravenous (IV) calculation questions are also a focus on the NCLEX-RN examination. Fill-in-the-blank questions may require that you calculate a medication dose or an IV flow rate. Use the on-screen calculator for these medications and IV problems, and then recheck the calculation before selecting an option or typing the answer.

The Pyramid to Success also focuses on the assessment techniques for a health and physical assessment of the adult client and collecting both subjective and objective data. Perioperative nursing care and monitoring for postoperative complications is also a priority. Client safety related to positioning and ambulation are important concepts addressed on the NCLEX. Because many surgical procedures are performed through ambulatory care units (1-day-stay units), Pyramid Points also focus on preparing the client for discharge, assisting with teaching related to the prescribed treatments and medications, follow-up care, and the mobilization of home care support services.

Client Needs: Learning Objectives

Safe and Effective Care Environment

Acting as an advocate regarding the client's wishes
Applying principles of infection control
Collaborating with interprofessional teams
Ensuring environmental, personal, and home safety
Ensuring that the client's rights, including informed consent, are upheld

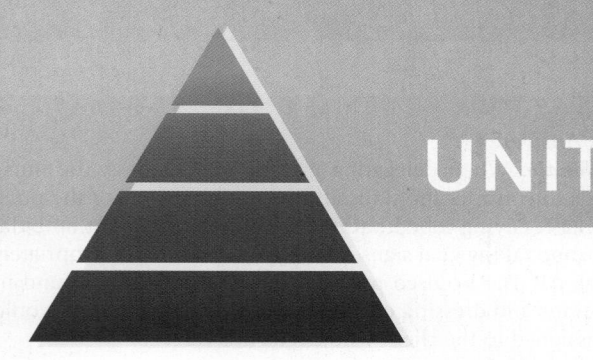

Establishing priorities of client assessment and interventions
Following advance directives regarding the client's documented requests
Following guidelines regarding the use of safety devices
Handling hazardous and infectious materials safely to prevent injury to health care personnel and others
Identifying the client with at least two identifiers (e.g., name and identification number)
Informing the client of the surgical process and ensuring that informed consent for a surgical procedure and other procedures has been obtained
Knowing the emergency response plan and actions to take for exposure to biological and chemical warfare agents
Maintaining confidentiality
Maintaining continuity of care and initiating referrals to home care and other support services
Maintaining asepsis and preventing infection in the client when samples for laboratory studies are obtained
Maintaining precautions to prevent errors, accidents, and injury
Positioning the client appropriately and safely
Preparing and administering medications, using the rights of medication administration
Preventing accidents and ensuring safety of the client when a fluid or electrolyte imbalance exists, particularly when changes in cardiovascular, respiratory, gastrointestinal, neuromuscular, renal, or central nervous systems occur, or when the client is at risk for complications such as seizures, respiratory depression, or dysrhythmias
Preventing a surgical infection
Protecting the medicated client from injury
Providing information to the client about community classes for nutrition education
Providing safety for the client during implementation of treatments
Using equipment such as electronic IV infusion devices safely
Using ergonomic principles and body mechanics when moving a client
Using special equipment safely
Upholding client rights
Using standard, transmission-based precautions, and surgical asepsis procedures to prevent infection and the transmission of infection to self and others

Health Promotion and Maintenance

Assessing the client's ability to perform self-care
Assisting clients and families to identify environmental hazards in the home
Assessing home safety and the need for modifications
Discussing high-risk behaviors and lifestyle choices
Evaluating the client's home environment for self-care modifications
Identifying clients at risk for an acid–base imbalance
Identifying community resources available for follow-up
Implementing health screening and monitoring for the potential risk for a fluid and electrolyte imbalance
Performing physical assessment techniques
Providing education related to medication and diet management
Providing education related to the potential risk for a fluid and electrolyte imbalance, measures to prevent an imbalance, signs and symptoms of an imbalance, and actions to take if signs and symptoms develop
Respecting lifestyle choices and health care beliefs and preferences
Teaching clients and families about accident prevention
Teaching clients and families about measures to be implemented in an emergency or disaster
Teaching clients and families about preventing the spread of infection and preventing diseases
Teaching the client and family about prevention, early detection, and treatment measures for health disorders
Teaching the client to monitor for signs and symptoms that indicate the need to notify the primary health care provider

Psychosocial Integrity

Assessing the client's emotional response to treatment
Considering cultural, religious, and spiritual preferences related to nutritional patterns and lifestyle choices and other factors influencing health
Promoting an environment that will allow the client to express concerns
Providing emotional support to the client during testing
Providing reassurance to the client who is experiencing a fluid or electrolyte imbalance
Providing support and continuously informing the client of the purposes for prescribed interventions

Physiological Integrity

Assessing for expected and unexpected responses to therapeutic interventions and documenting findings
Assessing the mobility level of the client
Assisting the client with activities of daily living
Assisting with obtaining an ABG specimen and analyzing the results
Calculating medication doses and IV flow rates
Handling medical or surgical emergencies
Identifying clients who are at risk for a fluid or electrolyte imbalance
Implementing priority nursing actions in an emergency or disaster
Initiating nursing interventions when surgical complications arise
Managing and providing care to clients with infectious diseases
Monitoring for changes in status and for complications; taking actions if a complication arises

Monitoring laboratory reference intervals; determining the significance of an abnormal laboratory value and the need to implement specific actions based on the laboratory results
Monitoring nutritional intake and oral hydration
Monitoring for surgical complications
Monitoring for wound infection
Preventing complications of immobility
Providing comfort and assistance to the client
Providing nutrition and oral intake
Providing interventions compatible with the client's age; cultural, religious, spiritual and health care beliefs; education level; and language
Providing personal hygiene as needed
Providing site care following arterial blood draw
Recognizing changes in the client's condition that indicate a potential complication and intervening appropriately
Reducing the likelihood that an acid–base imbalance will occur
Using assistive devices to prevent injury

CHAPTER 8

Fluids and Electrolytes

PRIORITY CONCEPTS **Cellular Regulation; Fluid and Electrolytes**

I. Concepts of Fluid and Electrolyte Balance

A. Electrolytes
1. Description: An electrolyte is a substance that, on dissolving in solution, ionizes; that is, some of its molecules split or dissociate into electrically charged atoms or ions (Box 8-1).
2. Measurement
   a. The metric system is used to measure volumes of fluids—liters (L) or milliliters (mL).
   b. The unit of measure that expresses the combining activity of an electrolyte is the milliequivalent (mEq).
   c. One milliequivalent (1 mEq) of any cation always reacts chemically with 1 mEq of an anion.
   d. Milliequivalents provide information about the number of anions or cations available to combine with other anions or cations.

B. Body fluid compartments (Fig. 8-1)
1. Description
   a. Fluid in each of the body compartments contains electrolytes.
   b. Each compartment has a particular composition of electrolytes, which differs from that of other compartments.
   c. To function normally, body cells must have fluids and electrolytes in the right compartments and in the right amounts.
   d. Whenever an electrolyte moves out of a cell, another electrolyte moves in to take its place.
   e. The numbers of cations and anions must be the same for homeostasis to exist.
   f. Compartments are separated by semipermeable membranes.
2. Intravascular compartment: Refers to fluid inside a blood vessel
3. Intracellular compartment
   a. The intracellular compartment refers to all fluid inside the cells.
   b. Most bodily fluids are inside the cells.
4. Extracellular compartment
   a. Refers to fluid outside the cells.
   b. The extracellular compartment includes the interstitial fluid, which is fluid between cells (sometimes called the *third space*), blood, lymph, bone, connective tissue, water, and transcellular fluid.

C. Third-spacing
1. Third-spacing is the accumulation and sequestration of trapped extracellular fluid in an actual or potential body space as a result of disease or injury.
2. The trapped fluid represents a volume loss and is unavailable for normal physiological processes.
3. Fluid may be trapped in body spaces such as the pericardial, pleural, peritoneal, or joint cavities; the bowel; the abdomen; or within soft tissues after trauma or burns.
4. Assessing the intravascular fluid loss caused by third-spacing is difficult. The loss may not be reflected in weight changes or intake and output records and may not become apparent until after organ malfunction occurs.

D. Edema
1. Edema is an excess accumulation of fluid in the interstitial space; it occurs as a result of alterations in oncotic pressure, hydrostatic pressure, capillary permeability, and lymphatic obstruction (see F. Body fluid transport, for descriptions).
2. Localized edema occurs as a result of traumatic injury from accidents or surgery, local inflammatory processes, or burns.
3. Generalized edema, also called *anasarca*, is an excessive accumulation of fluid in the interstitial space throughout the body and occurs as a result of conditions such as cardiac, renal, or liver failure.

E. Body fluid
1. Description
   a. Body fluids transport nutrients to the cells and carry waste products from the cells.
   b. Total body fluid (intracellular and extracellular) amounts to about 60% of body weight in the adult, 55% in the older adult, and 80% in the infant.

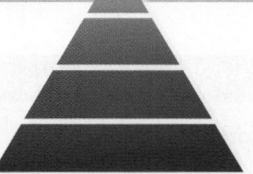

BOX 8-1 Properties of Electrolytes and Their Components

Atom

An atom is the smallest part of an element that still has the properties of the element.

The atom is composed of particles known as the *proton* (positive charge), *neutron* (neutral), and *electron* (negative charge).

Protons and neutrons are in the nucleus of the atom; therefore, the nucleus is positively charged.

Electrons carry a negative charge and revolve around the nucleus.

As long as the number of electrons is the same as the number of protons, the atom has no net charge; that is, it is neither positive nor negative.

Atoms that gain, lose, or share electrons are no longer neutral.

Molecule

A molecule is 2 or more atoms that combine to form a substance.

Ion

An ion is an atom that carries an electrical charge because it has gained or lost electrons.

Some ions carry a negative electrical charge and some carry a positive charge.

Cation

A cation is an ion that has given away or lost electrons and therefore carries a positive charge.

The result is fewer electrons than protons, and the result is a positive charge.

Anion

An anion is an ion that has gained electrons and therefore carries a negative charge.

When an ion has gained or taken on electrons, it assumes a negative charge and the result is a negatively charged ion.

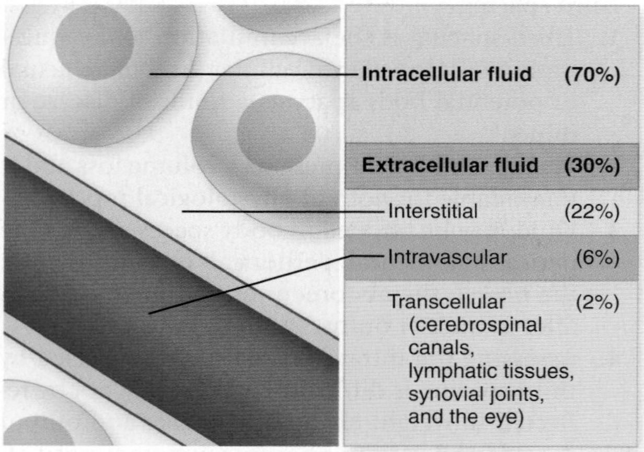

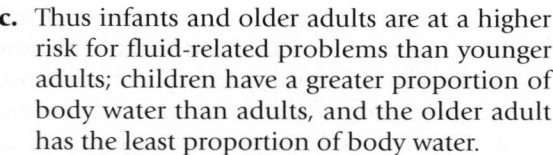

FIG. 8-1 Distribution of fluid by compartments in the average adult.

c. Thus infants and older adults are at a higher risk for fluid-related problems than younger adults; children have a greater proportion of body water than adults, and the older adult has the least proportion of body water.

2. Constituents of body fluids
   a. Body fluids consist of water and dissolved substances.
   b. The largest single fluid constituent of the body is water.
   c. Some substances, such as glucose, urea, and creatinine, do not dissociate in solution; that is, they do not separate from their complex forms into simpler substances when they are in solution.
   d. Other substances do dissociate; for example, when sodium chloride is in a solution, it dissociates, or separates, into 2 parts or elements.

⚠ Infants and older adults need to be monitored closely for fluid imbalances.

F. Body fluid transport
1. Diffusion
   a. Diffusion is the process whereby a solute (substance that is dissolved) may spread through a solution or solvent (solution in which the solute is dissolved).
   b. Diffusion of a solute spreads the molecules from an area of higher concentration to an area of lower concentration.
   c. A permeable membrane allows substances to pass through it without restriction.
   d. A selectively permeable membrane allows some solutes to pass through without restriction but prevents other solutes from passing freely.
   e. Diffusion occurs within fluid compartments and from one compartment to another if the barrier between the compartments is permeable to the diffusing substances.
2. Osmosis
   a. Osmosis is the movement of solvent molecules across a membrane in response to a concentration gradient, usually from a solution of lower to one of higher solute concentration.
   b. Osmotic pressure is the force that draws the solvent from a less concentrated solute through a selectively permeable membrane into a more concentrated solute, thus tending to equalize the concentration of the solvent.
   c. If a membrane is permeable to water but not to all solutes present, the membrane is a selective or semipermeable membrane.

d. When a more concentrated solution is on one side of a selectively permeable membrane and a less concentrated solution is on the other side, a pull called *osmotic pressure* draws the water through the membrane to the more concentrated side, or the side with more solute.

3. Filtration
   a. Filtration is the movement of solutes and solvents by hydrostatic pressure.
   b. The movement is from an area of higher pressure to an area of lower pressure.
4. Hydrostatic pressure
   a. Hydrostatic pressure is the force exerted by the weight of a solution.
   b. When a difference exists in the hydrostatic pressure on two sides of a membrane, water and diffusible solutes move out of the solution that has the higher hydrostatic pressure by the process of filtration.
   c. At the arterial end of the capillary, the hydrostatic pressure is higher than the osmotic pressure; therefore, fluids and diffusible solutes move out of the capillary.
   d. At the venous end, the osmotic pressure, or pull, is higher than the hydrostatic pressure, and fluids and some solutes move into the capillary.
   e. The excess fluid and solutes remaining in the interstitial spaces are returned to the intravascular compartment by the lymph channels.
5. Osmolality
   a. Osmolality refers to the number of osmotically active particles per kilogram of water; it is the concentration of a solution.
   b. In the body, osmotic pressure is measured in milliosmoles (mOsm).
   c. The normal osmolality of plasma is 275 to 295 mOsm/kg (275 to 295 mmol/kg).

G. Movement of body fluid

1. Description
   a. Cell membranes and capillary walls separate body compartments.
   b. Cell membranes are selectively permeable; that is, the cell membrane and the capillary wall allow water and some solutes free passage through them.
   c. Several forces affect the movement of water and solutes through the walls of cells and capillaries; for example, the greater the number of particles within the cell, the more pressure exists to force the water through the cell membrane out of the cell.
   d. If the body loses more electrolytes than fluids, as can happen in diarrhea, then the extracellular fluid contains fewer electrolytes or less solute than the intracellular fluid.
   e. Fluids and electrolytes must be kept in balance for health; when they remain out of balance, death can occur.
2. Isotonic solutions
   a. When the solutions on both sides of a selectively permeable membrane have established equilibrium or are equal in concentration, they are isotonic.
   b. Isotonic solutions are isotonic to human cells, and thus very little osmosis occurs; isotonic solutions have the same osmolality as body fluids.
   c. Refer to Chapter 69, Table 69-1, for a list of solutions, types, and uses.
3. Hypotonic solutions
   a. When a solution contains a lower concentration of salt or solute than another, more concentrated solution, it is considered hypotonic.
   b. A hypotonic solution has less salt or more water than an isotonic solution; these solutions have lower osmolality than body fluids.
   c. Hypotonic solutions are hypotonic to the cells; therefore, osmosis would continue in an attempt to bring about balance or equality.
   d. Refer to Chapter 69, Table 69-1, for a list of solutions, types, and uses.
4. Hypertonic solutions
   a. A solution that has a higher concentration of solutes than another, less concentrated solution is hypertonic; these solutions have a higher osmolality than body fluids.
   b. Refer to Chapter 69, Table 69-1, for a list of solutions, types, and uses.
5. Osmotic pressure
   a. The amount of osmotic pressure is determined by the concentration of solutes in solution.
   b. When the solutions on each side of a selectively permeable membrane are equal in concentration, they are isotonic.
   c. A hypotonic solution has less solute than an isotonic solution, whereas a hypertonic solution contains more solute.
6. Active transport
   a. If an ion is to move through a membrane from an area of lower concentration to an area of higher concentration, an active transport system is necessary.
   b. An active transport system moves molecules or ions against concentration and osmotic pressure.
   c. Metabolic processes in the cell supply the energy for active transport.
   d. Substances that are transported actively through the cell membrane include ions of sodium, potassium, calcium, iron, and hydrogen; some of the sugars; and the amino acids.

H. Body fluid intake and output (Fig. 8-2)

1. Body fluid intake

a. Water enters the body through 3 sources—orally ingested liquids, water in foods, and water formed by oxidation of foods.

b. About 10 mL of water is released by the **metabolism** of each 100 calories of fat, carbohydrates, or proteins.

2. Body fluid output

a. Water lost through the skin is called *insensible loss* (the individual is unaware of losing that water).

b. The amount of water lost by perspiration varies according to the temperature of the environment and of the body.

c. Water lost from the lungs is called *insensible loss* and is lost through expired air that is saturated with water vapor.

d. The amount of water lost from the lungs varies with the rate and the depth of respiration.

e. Large quantities of water are secreted into the gastrointestinal tract, but almost all of this fluid is reabsorbed.

f. A large volume of electrolyte-containing liquids moves into the gastrointestinal tract and then returns again to the extracellular fluid.

g. Severe diarrhea results in the loss of large quantities of fluids and electrolytes.

h. The kidneys play a major role in regulating fluid and electrolyte balance and excrete the largest quantity of fluid.

i. Normal kidneys can adjust the amount of water and electrolytes leaving the body.

j. The quantity of fluid excreted by the kidneys is determined by the amount of water ingested and the amount of waste and solutes excreted.

k. As long as all organs are functioning normally, the body is able to maintain balance in its fluid content.

Fluid intake	
Ingested water	1200-1500 mL
Ingested food	800-1100 mL
Metabolic oxidation	300 mL
TOTAL	2300-2900 mL

Fluid output	
Kidneys	1500 mL
Insensible loss through skin	600-800 mL
Insensible loss through lungs	400-600 mL
Gastrointestinal tract	100 mL
TOTAL	2600-3000 mL

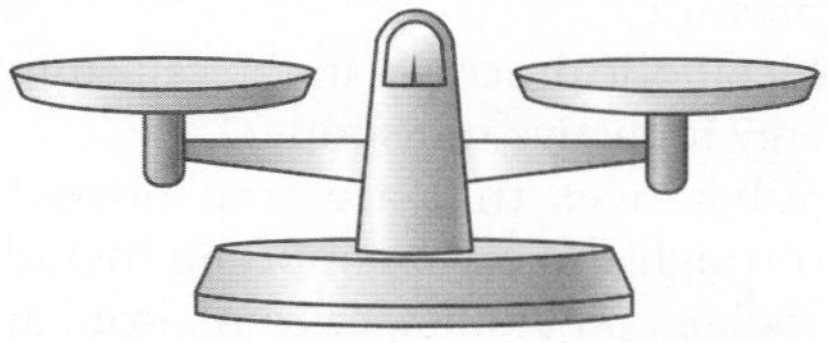

FIG. 8-2 Sources of fluid intake and fluid output (approximates).

The client with diarrhea is at high risk for a fluid and electrolyte imbalance.

II. Maintaining Fluid and Electrolyte Balance

A. Description

1. Homeostasis is a term that indicates the relative stability of the internal environment.

2. Concentration and composition of body fluids must be nearly constant.

3. When one of the substances in a client is deficient—either fluids or electrolytes—the substance must be replaced normally by the intake of food and water or by therapy such as intravenous (IV) solutions and medications.

4. When the client has an excess of fluid or electrolytes, therapy is directed toward assisting the body to eliminate the excess.

B. The kidneys play a major role in controlling balance in fluid and electrolytes.

C. The adrenal glands, through the secretion of aldosterone, also aid in controlling extracellular fluid volume by regulating the amount of sodium reabsorbed by the kidneys.

D. Antidiuretic hormone from the pituitary gland regulates the osmotic pressure of extracellular fluid by regulating the amount of water reabsorbed by the kidneys.

If the client has a fluid or an electrolyte imbalance, the nurse must closely monitor the client's cardiovascular, respiratory, neurological, musculoskeletal, renal, integumentary, and gastrointestinal status.

III. Fluid Volume Deficit

A. Description

1. Dehydration occurs when the fluid intake of the body is not sufficient to meet the fluid needs of the body.

2. The goal of treatment is to restore fluid volume, replace electrolytes as needed, and eliminate the cause of the fluid volume deficit.

B. Types of fluid volume deficits

1. Isotonic dehydration

a. Water and dissolved electrolytes are lost in equal proportions.

b. Known as *hypovolemia*, isotonic dehydration is the most common type of dehydration.

c. Isotonic dehydration results in decreased circulating blood volume and inadequate tissue perfusion.

2. Hypertonic dehydration

a. Water loss exceeds electrolyte loss.

b. The clinical problems that occur result from alterations in the concentrations of specific plasma electrolytes.

c. Fluid moves from the intracellular compartment into the plasma and interstitial fluid spaces, causing cellular dehydration and shrinkage.

3. Hypotonic dehydration
   a. Electrolyte loss exceeds water loss.
   b. The clinical problems that occur result from fluid shifts between compartments, causing a decrease in plasma volume.
   c. Fluid moves from the plasma and interstitial fluid spaces into the cells, causing a plasma volume deficit and causing the cells to swell.

C. Causes of fluid volume deficits
1. Isotonic dehydration
   a. Inadequate intake of fluids and solutes
   b. Fluid shifts between compartments
   c. Excessive losses of isotonic body fluids
2. Hypertonic dehydration—conditions that increase fluid loss, such as excessive perspiration, hyperventilation, ketoacidosis, prolonged fevers, diarrhea, early-stage kidney disease, and diabetes insipidus
3. Hypotonic dehydration
   a. Chronic illness
   b. Excessive fluid replacement (hypotonic)
   c. Kidney disease
   d. Chronic **malnutrition**

D. Assessment (Table 8-1)

E. Interventions
1. Prevent further fluid losses and increase fluid compartment volumes to normal ranges.
2. Provide oral rehydration therapy if possible and IV fluid replacement if the dehydration is severe; monitor intake and output.

TABLE 8-1 Assessment Findings: Fluid Volume Deficit and Fluid Volume Excess

Fluid Volume Deficit	Fluid Volume Excess
Cardiovascular	
■ Thready, increased pulse rate	■ Bounding, increased pulse rate
■ Decreased blood pressure and orthostatic (postural) hypotension	■ Elevated blood pressure
■ Flat neck and hand veins in dependent positions	■ Distended neck and hand veins
■ Diminished peripheral pulses	■ Elevated central venous pressure
■ Decreased central venous pressure	■ Dysrhythmias
■ Dysrhythmias	
Respiratory	
■ Increased rate and depth of respirations	■ Increased respiratory rate (shallow respirations)
■ Dyspnea	■ Dyspnea
	■ Moist crackles on auscultation
Neuromuscular	
■ Decreased central nervous system activity, from lethargy to coma	■ Altered level of consciousness
■ Fever, depending on the amount of fluid loss	■ Headache
■ Skeletal muscle weakness	■ Visual disturbances
	■ Skeletal muscle weakness
	■ Paresthesias
Renal	
■ Decreased urine output	■ Increased urine output if kidneys can compensate; decreased urine output if kidney damage is the cause
Integumentary	
■ Dry skin	■ Pitting edema in dependent areas
■ Poor turgor, tenting	■ Pale, cool skin
■ Dry mouth	
Gastrointestinal	
■ Decreased motility and diminished bowel sounds	■ Increased motility in the gastrointestinal tract
■ Constipation	■ Diarrhea
■ Thirst	■ Increased body weight
■ Decreased body weight	■ Liver enlargement
	■ Ascites
Laboratory Findings	
■ Increased serum osmolality	■ Decreased serum osmolality
■ Increased hematocrit	■ Decreased hematocrit
■ Increased blood urea nitrogen (BUN) level	■ Decreased BUN level
■ Increased serum sodium level	■ Decreased serum sodium level
■ Increased urinary specific gravity	■ Decreased urine specific gravity

3. In general, isotonic dehydration is treated with isotonic fluid solutions, hypertonic dehydration with hypotonic fluid solutions, and hypotonic dehydration with hypertonic fluid solutions.
4. Administer medications, such as antidiarrheal, antimicrobial, antiemetic, and antipyretic medications, as prescribed to correct the cause and treat any symptoms.
5. Monitor electrolyte values and prepare to administer medication to treat an imbalance, if present.

IV. Fluid Volume Excess

A. Description
1. Fluid intake or fluid retention exceeds the fluid needs of the body.
2. Fluid volume excess is also called *overhydration* or *fluid overload*.
3. The goal of treatment is to restore fluid balance, correct electrolyte imbalances if present, and eliminate or control the underlying cause of the overload.

B. Types
1. Isotonic overhydration
   - **a.** Known as *hypervolemia*, isotonic overhydration results from excessive fluid in the extracellular fluid compartment.
   - **b.** Only the extracellular fluid compartment is expanded, and fluid does not shift between the extracellular and intracellular compartments.
   - **c.** Isotonic overhydration causes **circulatory overload** and interstitial edema; when severe or when it occurs in a client with poor cardiac function, heart failure and pulmonary edema can result.
2. Hypertonic overhydration
   - **a.** The occurrence of hypertonic overhydration is rare and is caused by an excessive sodium intake.
   - **b.** Fluid is drawn from the intracellular fluid compartment; the extracellular fluid volume expands, and the intracellular fluid volume contracts.
3. Hypotonic overhydration
   - **a.** Hypotonic overhydration is known as *water intoxication*.
   - **b.** The excessive fluid moves into the intracellular space, and all body fluid compartments expand.
   - **c.** Electrolyte imbalances occur as a result of dilution.

C. Causes
1. Isotonic overhydration
   - **a.** Inadequately controlled IV therapy
   - **b.** Kidney disease
   - **c.** Long-term corticosteroid therapy
2. Hypertonic overhydration
   - **a.** Excessive sodium ingestion
   - **b.** Rapid infusion of hypertonic saline
   - **c.** Excessive sodium bicarbonate therapy
3. Hypotonic overhydration
   - **a.** Early kidney disease
   - **b.** Heart failure
   - **c.** Syndrome of inappropriate antidiuretic hormone secretion
   - **d.** Inadequately controlled IV therapy
   - **e.** Replacement of isotonic fluid loss with hypotonic fluids
   - **f.** Irrigation of wounds and body cavities with hypotonic fluids

D. Assessment (see Table 8-1)

⚠ A client with acute kidney injury, chronic kidney disease, and heart failure is at high risk for fluid volume excess.

E. Interventions
1. Prevent further fluid overload and restore normal fluid balance.
2. Administer diuretics; osmotic diuretics may be prescribed initially to prevent severe electrolyte imbalances.
3. Restrict fluid and sodium intake as prescribed.
4. Monitor intake and output; monitor weight.
5. Monitor electrolyte values and prepare to administer medication to treat an imbalance if present.

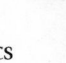

V. Hypokalemia

⚠ The normal potassium level is 3.5 to 5.0 mEq/L (3.5 to 5.0 mmol/L).

A. Description
1. Hypokalemia is a **serum potassium** level lower than 3.5 mEq/L (3.5 mmol/L)
2. Potassium deficit is potentially life-threatening because every body system is affected

B. Causes
1. Actual total body potassium loss
   - **a.** Excessive use of medications such as diuretics or corticosteroids
   - **b.** Increased secretion of aldosterone, such as in Cushing's syndrome
   - **c.** Vomiting, diarrhea
   - **d.** Wound drainage, particularly gastrointestinal
   - **e.** Prolonged nasogastric suction
   - **f.** Excessive diaphoresis
   - **g.** Kidney disease impairing reabsorption of potassium
2. Inadequate potassium intake: Fasting; nothing by mouth status
3. Movement of potassium from the extracellular fluid to the intracellular fluid
   - **a.** Alkalosis
   - **b.** Hyperinsulinism
4. Dilution of serum potassium
   - **a.** Water intoxication
   - **b.** IV therapy with potassium-deficient solutions

C. Assessment (Tables 8-2 and 8-3)

TABLE 8-2 Assessment Findings: Hypokalemia and Hyperkalemia

Hypokalemia	Hyperkalemia
Cardiovascular	
■ Thready, weak, irregular pulse ■ Weak peripheral pulses ■ Orthostatic hypotension ■ Dysrhythmias	■ Slow, weak, irregular heart rate ■ Decreased blood pressure ■ Dysrhythmias
Respiratory	
■ Shallow, ineffective respirations that result from profound weakness of the skeletal muscles of respiration ■ Diminished breath sounds	■ Profound weakness of the skeletal muscles leading to respiratory failure
Neuromuscular	
■ Anxiety, lethargy, confusion, coma ■ Skeletal muscle weakness, leg cramps ■ Loss of tactile discrimination ■ Paresthesias ■ Deep tendon hyporeflexia	■ *Early:* Muscle twitches, cramps, paresthesias (tingling and burning followed by numbness in the hands and feet and around the mouth) ■ *Late:* Profound weakness, ascending flaccid paralysis in the arms and legs (trunk, head, and respiratory muscles become affected when the serum potassium level reaches a lethal level)
Gastrointestinal	
■ Decreased motility, hypoactive to absent bowel sounds ■ Nausea, vomiting, constipation, abdominal distention ■ Paralytic ileus	■ Increased motility, hyperactive bowel sounds ■ Diarrhea
Laboratory Findings	
■ Serum potassium level lower than 3.5 mEq/L (3.5 mmol/L) ■ Electrocardiogram changes: ST depression; shallow, flat, or inverted T wave; and prominent U wave	■ Serum potassium level that exceeds 5.0 mEq/L (5.0 mmol/L) ■ Electrocardiographic changes: Tall peaked T waves, flat P waves, widened QRS complexes, and prolonged PR intervals

TABLE 8-3 Electrocardiographic Changes in Electrolyte Imbalances

Electrolyte Imbalance	Electrocardiographic Changes
Hypokalemia	ST depression Shallow, flat, or inverted T wave Prominent U wave
Hyperkalemia	Tall peaked T waves Flat P waves Widened QRS complexes Prolonged PR interval
Hypocalcemia	Prolonged ST segment Prolonged QT interval
Hypercalcemia	Shortened ST segment Widened T wave Heart block
Hypomagnesemia	Tall T waves Depressed ST segment
Hypermagnesemia	Prolonged PR interval Widened QRS complexes

D. Interventions
1. Monitor electrolyte values.
2. Administer potassium supplements orally or intravenously, as prescribed.
3. Oral potassium supplements
   a. Oral potassium supplements may cause nausea and vomiting and should not be taken on an empty stomach; if the client complains of abdominal pain, distention, nausea, vomiting, diarrhea, or gastrointestinal bleeding, the supplement may need to be discontinued.
   b. Liquid potassium chloride has an unpleasant taste and should be taken with juice or another liquid.
4. Intravenously administered potassium (Box 8-2)
5. Institute safety measures for the client experiencing muscle weakness.
6. If the client is taking a potassium-losing diuretic, it may be discontinued; a potassium-sparing (retaining) diuretic may be prescribed.
7. Instruct the client about foods that are high in potassium content (see Box 11-2).

⚠ Potassium is never administered by IV push, intramuscular, or subcutaneous routes. IV potassium is always diluted and administered using an infusion device!

VI. Hyperkalemia

A. Description
1. Hyperkalemia is a serum potassium level that exceeds 5.0 mEq/L (5.0 mmol/L)
2. Pseudohyperkalemia: a condition that can occur due to methods of blood specimen collection and cell lysis; if an increased serum value is obtained in the absence of clinical symptoms, the specimen should be redrawn and evaluated.

B. Causes
1. Excessive potassium intake
   a. Overingestion of potassium-containing foods or medications, such as potassium chloride or salt substitutes

BOX 8-2 Precautions With Intravenously Administered Potassium

- Potassium is never given by intravenous (IV) push or by the intramuscular or subcutaneous route.
- A dilution of no more than 1 mEq/10 mL (1 mmol/10 mL) of solution is recommended.
- Many health care agencies supply prepared IV solutions containing potassium; before administering and frequently during infusion of the IV solution, rotate and invert the bag to ensure that the potassium is distributed evenly throughout the IV solution.
- Ensure that the IV bag containing potassium is properly labeled.
- The maximum recommended infusion rate is 5 to 10 mEq/hr (5 to 10 mmol/hr), never to exceed 20 mEq/hr (20 mmol/hr) under any circumstances.
- A client receiving more than 10 mEq/hr (10 mmol/hr) should be placed on a cardiac monitor and monitored for cardiac changes, and the infusion should be controlled by an infusion device.
- Potassium infusion can cause phlebitis; therefore, the nurse should assess the IV site frequently for signs of phlebitis or infiltration. If either occurs, the infusion should be stopped immediately.
- The nurse should assess renal function before administering potassium and monitor intake and output during administration.

b. Rapid infusion of potassium-containing IV solutions

2. Decreased potassium excretion
   a. Potassium-sparing (retaining) diuretics
   b. Kidney disease
   c. Adrenal insufficiency, such as in Addison's disease
3. Movement of potassium from the intracellular fluid to the extracellular fluid
   a. Tissue damage
   b. Acidosis
   c. Hyperuricemia
   d. Hypercatabolism

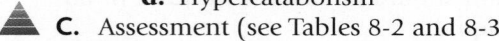

C. Assessment (see Tables 8-2 and 8-3)

Monitor the client closely for signs of a potassium imbalance. A potassium imbalance can cause cardiac dysrhythmias that can be life-threatening, leading to cardiac arrest!

D. Interventions

1. Discontinue IV potassium (keep the IV catheter patent) and withhold oral potassium supplements.
2. Initiate a potassium-restricted diet.
3. Prepare to administer potassium-excreting diuretics if renal function is not impaired.
4. If renal function is impaired, prepare to administer sodium polystyrene sulfonate (oral or rectal route), a cation-exchange resin that promotes gastrointestinal sodium absorption and potassium excretion.
5. Prepare the client for dialysis if potassium levels are critically high.
6. Prepare for the administration of IV calcium if hyperkalemia is severe, to avert myocardial excitability.
7. Prepare for the IV administration of hypertonic glucose with regular insulin to move excess potassium into the cells.
8. When blood transfusions are prescribed for a client with a potassium imbalance, the client should receive fresh blood, if possible; transfusions of stored blood may elevate the potassium level because the breakdown of older blood cells releases potassium.
9. Teach the client to avoid foods high in potassium (see Box 11-2).
10. Instruct the client to avoid the use of salt substitutes or other potassium-containing substances.
11. Monitor the serum potassium level closely when a client is receiving a potassium-sparing (retaining) diuretic.

VII. Hyponatremia

The normal sodium level is 135 to 145 mEq/L (135 to 145 mmol/L)

A. Description

1. Hyponatremia is a **serum sodium** level lower than 135 mEq/L (135 mmol/L).
2. Sodium imbalances usually are associated with fluid volume imbalances.

B. Causes

1. Increased sodium excretion
   a. Excessive diaphoresis
   b. Diuretics
   c. Vomiting
   d. Diarrhea
   e. Wound drainage, especially gastrointestinal
   f. Kidney disease
   g. Decreased secretion of aldosterone
2. Inadequate sodium intake
   a. Fasting; nothing by mouth status
   b. Low-salt diet
3. Dilution of serum sodium
   a. Excessive ingestion of hypotonic fluids or irrigation with hypotonic fluids
   b. Kidney disease
   c. Freshwater drowning
   d. Syndrome of inappropriate antidiuretic hormone secretion
   e. Hyperglycemia
   f. Heart failure

C. Assessment (Table 8-4)

TABLE 8-4 Assessment Findings: Hyponatremia and Hypernatremia

Hyponatremia	Hypernatremia
Cardiovascular	
▪ Symptoms vary with changes in vascular volume	▪ Heart rate and blood pressure respond to vascular volume status
▪ *Normovolemic:* Rapid pulse rate, normal blood pressure	
▪ *Hypovolemic:* Thready, weak, rapid pulse rate; hypotension; flat neck veins; normal or low central venous pressure	
▪ *Hypervolemic:* Rapid, bounding pulse; blood pressure normal or elevated; normal or elevated central venous pressure	
Respiratory	
▪ Shallow, ineffective respiratory movement is a late manifestation related to skeletal muscle weakness	▪ Pulmonary edema if hypervolemia is present
Neuromuscular	
▪ Generalized skeletal muscle weakness that is worse in the extremities	▪ *Early:* Spontaneous muscle twitches; irregular muscle contractions
▪ Diminished deep tendon reflexes	▪ *Late:* Skeletal muscle weakness; deep tendon reflexes diminished or absent
Central Nervous System	
▪ Headache	▪ Altered cerebral function is the most common manifestation of hypernatremia
▪ Personality changes	▪ *Normovolemia or hypovolemia:* Agitation, confusion, seizures
▪ Confusion	▪ *Hypervolemia:* Lethargy, stupor, coma
▪ Seizures	
▪ Coma	
Gastrointestinal	
▪ Increased motility and hyperactive bowel sounds	▪ Extreme thirst
▪ Nausea	
▪ Abdominal cramping and diarrhea	
Renal	
▪ Increased urinary output	▪ Decreased urinary output
Integumentary	
▪ Dry mucous membranes	▪ Dry and flushed skin
	▪ Dry and sticky tongue and mucous membranes
	▪ Presence or absence of edema, depending on fluid volume changes
Laboratory Findings	
▪ Serum sodium level less than 135 mEq/L (135 mmol/L)	▪ Serum sodium level that exceeds 145 mEq/L (145 mmol/L)
▪ Decreased urinary specific gravity	▪ Increased urinary specific gravity

D. Interventions
  1. If hyponatremia is accompanied by a fluid volume deficit (hypovolemia), IV sodium chloride infusions are administered to restore sodium content and fluid volume.
  2. If hyponatremia is accompanied by fluid volume excess (hypervolemia), osmotic diuretics may be prescribed to promote the excretion of water rather than sodium.
  3. If hyponatremia is caused by inappropriate or excessive secretion of antidiuretic hormone, medications that antagonize antidiuretic hormone may be administered.
  4. Instruct the client to increase oral sodium intake as prescribed and inform the client about the foods to include in the diet (see Box 11-2).
  5. If the client is taking lithium, monitor the lithium level, because hyponatremia can cause diminished lithium excretion, resulting in toxicity.

Hyponatremia precipitates lithium toxicity in a client taking this medication.

VIII. Hypernatremia

A. Description: Hypernatremia is a serum sodium level that exceeds 145 mEq/L (145 mmol/L).

B. Causes
  1. Decreased sodium excretion
    a. Corticosteroids
    b. Cushing's syndrome
    c. Kidney disease
    d. Hyperaldosteronism

2. Increased sodium intake: Excessive oral sodium ingestion or excessive administration of sodium-containing IV fluids
3. Decreased water intake: Fasting; nothing-by-mouth status
4. Increased water loss: Increased rate of metabolism, fever, hyperventilation, infection, excessive diaphoresis, watery diarrhea, diabetes insipidus

C. Assessment (see Table 8-4)

D. Interventions
1. If the cause is fluid loss, prepare to administer IV infusions.
2. If the cause is inadequate renal excretion of sodium, prepare to administer diuretics that promote sodium loss.
3. Restrict sodium and fluid intake as prescribed.

IX. Hypocalcemia

The normal calcium level is 9 to 10.5 mg/dL (2.25 to 2.75 mmol/L)

A. Description: Hypocalcemia is a **serum calcium** level lower than 9.0 mg/dL (2.25 mmol/L).

B. Causes
1. Inhibition of calcium absorption from the gastrointestinal tract
   a. Inadequate oral intake of calcium
   b. Lactose intolerance
   c. Malabsorption syndromes such as celiac sprue or Crohn's disease
   d. Inadequate intake of vitamin D
   e. End-stage kidney disease
2. Increased calcium excretion
   a. Kidney disease, polyuric phase
   b. Diarrhea
   c. Steatorrhea
   d. Wound drainage, especially gastrointestinal
3. Conditions that decrease the ionized fraction of calcium
   a. Hyperproteinemia
   b. Alkalosis
   c. Medications such as calcium chelators or binders
   d. Acute pancreatitis
   e. Hyperphosphatemia
   f. Removal or destruction of the parathyroid glands

C. Assessment (Table 8-5 and Fig. 8-3; also see Table 8-3)

D. Interventions
1. Administer calcium supplements orally or calcium intravenously.
2. When administering calcium intravenously, warm the injection solution to body temperature before administration and administer slowly; monitor for electrocardiographic changes, observe for **infiltration**, and monitor for hypercalcemia.
3. Administer medications that increase calcium absorption.
   a. Aluminum hydroxide reduces **phosphorus** levels, causing the countereffect of increasing calcium levels.
   b. Vitamin D aids in the absorption of calcium from the intestinal tract.
4. Provide a quiet environment to reduce environmental stimuli.
5. Initiate seizure precautions.
6. Move the client carefully, and monitor for signs of a pathological fracture.
7. Keep 10% calcium gluconate available for treatment of acute calcium deficit.
8. Instruct the client to consume foods high in calcium (see Box 11-2).

X. Hypercalcemia

A. Description: Hypercalcemia is a serum calcium level that exceeds 10.5 mg/dL (2.75 mmol/L).

B. Causes
1. Increased calcium absorption
   a. Excessive oral intake of calcium
   b. Excessive oral intake of vitamin D
2. Decreased calcium excretion
   a. Kidney disease
   b. Use of thiazide diuretics
3. Increased bone resorption of calcium
   a. Hyperparathyroidism
   b. Hyperthyroidism
   c. Malignancy (bone destruction from metastatic tumors)
   d. Immobility
4. Hemoconcentration
   a. Dehydration
   b. Use of lithium
   c. Adrenal insufficiency

C. Assessment (see Tables 8-3 and 8-5)

D. Interventions

A client with a calcium imbalance is at risk for a pathological fracture. Move the client carefully and slowly; assist the client with ambulation.

1. Discontinue IV infusions of solutions containing calcium and oral medications containing calcium or vitamin D.
2. Thiazide diuretics may be discontinued and replaced with diuretics that enhance the excretion of calcium.
3. Administer medications as prescribed that inhibit calcium resorption from the bone, such as phosphorus, calcitonin, bisphosphonates,

TABLE 8-5 Assessment Findings: Hypocalcemia and Hypercalcemia

Hypocalcemia	Hypercalcemia
Cardiovascular	
■ Decreased heart rate ■ Hypotension ■ Diminished peripheral pulses	■ Increased heart rate in the early phase; bradycardia that can lead to cardiac arrest in late phases ■ Increased blood pressure ■ Bounding, full peripheral pulses
Respiratory	
■ Not directly affected; however, respiratory failure or arrest can result from decreased respiratory movement because of muscle tetany or seizures	■ Ineffective respiratory movement as a result of profound skeletal muscle weakness
Neuromuscular	
■ Irritable skeletal muscles: Twitches, cramps, tetany, seizures ■ Painful muscle spasms in the calf or foot during periods of inactivity ■ Paresthesias followed by numbness that may affect the lips, nose, and ears in addition to the limbs ■ Positive Trousseau's and Chvostek's signs ■ Hyperactive deep tendon reflexes ■ Anxiety, irritability	■ Profound muscle weakness ■ Diminished or absent deep tendon reflexes ■ Disorientation, lethargy, coma
Renal	
■ Urinary output varies depending on the cause	■ Urinary output varies depending on the cause
Gastrointestinal	
■ Increased gastric motility; hyperactive bowel sounds ■ Cramping, diarrhea	■ Decreased motility and hypoactive bowel sounds ■ Anorexia, nausea, abdominal distention, constipation
Laboratory Findings	
■ Serum calcium level less than 9.0 mg/dL (2.25 mmol/L) ■ Electrocardiographic changes: Prolonged ST interval, prolonged QT interval	■ Serum calcium level that exceeds 10.5 mg/dL (2.75 mmol/L) ■ Electrocardiographic changes: Shortened ST segment, widened T wave, heart block

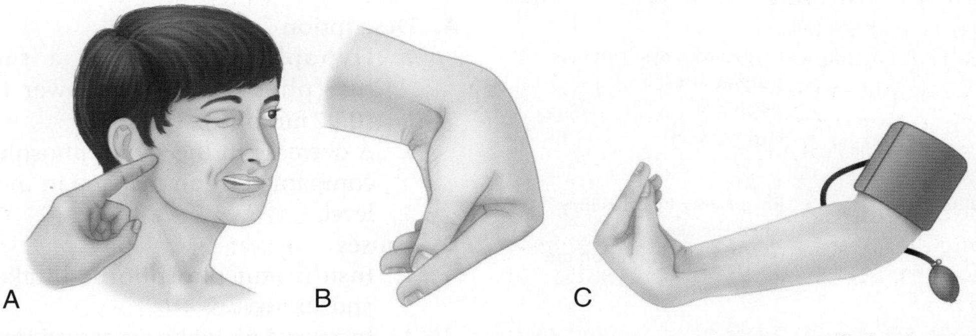

FIG. 8-3 Tests for hypocalcemia. **A**, Chvostek's sign is contraction of facial muscles in response to a light tap over the facial nerve in front of the ear. **B**, Trousseau's sign is a carpal spasm induced by inflating a blood pressure cuff **(C)** above the systolic pressure for a few minutes.

and prostaglandin synthesis inhibitors (acetylsalicylic acid, nonsteroidal antiinflammatory medications).

4. Prepare the client with severe hypercalcemia for dialysis if medications fail to reduce the serum calcium level.

5. Move the client carefully and monitor for signs of a pathological fracture.

6. Monitor for flank or abdominal pain, and strain the urine to check for the presence of urinary stones.

7. Instruct the client to avoid foods high in calcium (see Box 11-2).

XI. Hypomagnesemia

The normal magnesium level is 1.8 to 2.6 mEq/L (0.74 to 1.07 mmol/L).

A. Description: Hypomagnesemia is a **serum magnesium** level lower than 1.8 mEq/L (0.74 mmol/L).

B. Causes

1. Insufficient magnesium intake

a. Malnutrition and starvation

b. Vomiting or diarrhea

c. Malabsorption syndrome

d. Celiac disease

e. Crohn's disease
2. Increased magnesium excretion
 a. Medications such as diuretics
 b. Chronic alcoholism
3. Intracellular movement of magnesium
 a. Hyperglycemia
 b. Insulin administration
 c. Sepsis

C. Assessment (Table 8-6; also see Table 8-3)

D. Interventions
1. Because hypocalcemia frequently accompanies hypomagnesemia, interventions also aim to restore normal serum calcium levels.
2. Oral preparations of magnesium may cause diarrhea and increase magnesium loss.
3. Magnesium sulfate by the IV route may be prescribed in ill clients when the magnesium level is low (intramuscular injections cause pain and tissue damage); initiate seizure precautions, monitor serum magnesium levels frequently, and monitor for diminished deep tendon reflexes, suggesting hypermagnesemia, during the administration of magnesium.

TABLE 8-6 Assessment Findings: Hypomagnesemia and Hypermagnesemia

Hypomagnesemia	Hypermagnesemia
Cardiovascular	
▪ Tachycardia	▪ Bradycardia, dysrhythmias (cardiac arrest if severe)
▪ Hypertension	▪ Hypotension
Respiratory	
▪ Shallow respirations	▪ Respiratory insufficiency when the skeletal muscles of respiration are involved
Neuromuscular	
▪ Twitches, paresthesias ▪ Positive Trousseau's and Chvostek's signs ▪ Hyperreflexia ▪ Tetany, seizures	▪ Diminished or absent deep tendon reflexes ▪ Skeletal muscle weakness
Central Nervous System	
▪ Irritability ▪ Confusion	▪ Drowsiness and lethargy that progresses to coma
Laboratory Findings	
▪ Serum magnesium level less than 1.8 mEq/L (0.74 mmol/L)	▪ Serum magnesium level that exceeds 2.6 mEq/L (1.07 mmol/L)
▪ Electrocardiographic changes: Tall T waves, depressed ST segments	▪ Electrocardiographic changes: Prolonged PR interval, widened QRS complexes

4. Instruct the client to increase the intake of foods that contain magnesium (see Box 11-2).

XII. Hypermagnesemia

A. Description: Hypermagnesemia is a **serum magnesium** level that exceeds 2.6 mEq/L (1.07 mmol/L).

B. Causes
1. Increased magnesium intake
 a. Magnesium-containing antacids and laxatives
 b. Excessive administration of magnesium intravenously
2. Decreased renal excretion of magnesium as a result of renal insufficiency

C. Assessment (see Tables 8-3 and 8-6)

D. Interventions

⚠ Calcium gluconate is the antidote for magnesium overdose.

1. Diuretics are prescribed to increase renal excretion of magnesium.
2. Intravenously administered calcium chloride or calcium gluconate may be prescribed to reverse the effects of magnesium on cardiac muscle.
3. Instruct the client to restrict dietary intake of magnesium-containing foods (see Box 11-2).
4. Instruct the client to avoid the use of laxatives and antacids containing magnesium.

XIII. Hypophosphatemia

A. Description
1. Hypophosphatemia is a **serum phosphorus** (phosphate) level lower than 3.0 mg/dL (0.97 mmol/L).
2. A decrease in the serum phosphorus level is accompanied by an increase in the serum calcium level.

B. Causes
1. Insufficient phosphorus intake: Malnutrition and starvation
2. Increased phosphorus excretion
 a. Hyperparathyroidism
 b. Malignancy
 c. Use of **magnesium**-based or aluminum hydroxide–based antacids
3. Intracellular shift
 a. Hyperglycemia
 b. **Respiratory alkalosis**

C. Assessment
1. Cardiovascular
 a. Decreased contractility and cardiac output
 b. Slowed peripheral pulses
2. Respiratory: Shallow respirations
3. Neuromuscular
 a. Weakness
 b. Decreased deep tendon reflexes

c. Decreased bone density that can cause fractures and alterations in bone shape
d. Rhabdomyolysis
4. Central nervous system
a. Irritability
b. Confusion
c. Seizures
5. Hematological
a. Decreased platelet aggregation and increased bleeding
b. Immunosuppression

D. Interventions
1. Discontinue medications that contribute to hypophosphatemia.
2. Administer phosphorus orally along with a vitamin D supplement.
3. Prepare to administer phosphorus intravenously when serum phosphorus levels fall below 1 mg/dL and when the client experiences critical clinical manifestations; administer IV phosphorus slowly because of the risks associated with hyperphosphatemia.
4. Assess the renal system before administering phosphorus.
5. Move the client carefully, and monitor for signs of a pathological fracture.
6. Instruct the client to increase the intake of the phosphorus-containing foods while decreasing the intake of any calcium-containing foods (see Box 11-2).

A decrease in the serum phosphorus level is accompanied by an increase in the serum calcium level, and an increase in the serum phosphorus level is accompanied by a decrease in the serum calcium level. This is called a reciprocal relationship.

XIV. Hyperphosphatemia

A. Description
1. Hyperphosphatemia is a serum phosphorus level that exceeds 4.5 mg/dL (1.45 mmol/L).
2. Most body systems tolerate elevated serum phosphorus levels well.
3. An increase in the serum phosphorus level is accompanied by a decrease in the serum calcium level.
4. The problems that occur in hyperphosphatemia center on the hypocalcemia that results when serum phosphorus levels increase.

B. Causes
1. Decreased renal excretion resulting from renal insufficiency
2. Tumor lysis syndrome
3. Increased intake of phosphorus, including dietary intake or overuse of phosphate-containing laxatives or enemas
4. Hypoparathyroidism

C. Assessment: Refer to assessment of hypocalcemia.

D. Interventions
1. Interventions entail the management of hypocalcemia.
2. Administer phosphate-binding medications that increase fecal excretion of phosphorus by binding phosphorus from food in the gastrointestinal tract.
3. Instruct the client to avoid phosphate-containing medications, including laxatives and enemas.
4. Instruct the client to decrease the intake of food that is high in phosphorus (see Box 11-2).
5. Instruct the client in medication administration: Take phosphate-binding medications, emphasizing that they should be taken with meals or immediately after meals.

PRACTICE QUESTIONS

39. The nurse is caring for a client with heart failure. On assessment, the nurse notes that the client is dyspneic, and crackles are audible on auscultation. What additional manifestations would the nurse expect to note in this client if excess fluid volume is present?
1. Weight loss and dry skin
2. Flat neck and hand veins and decreased urinary output
3. An increase in blood pressure and increased respirations
4. Weakness and decreased central venous pressure (CVP)

40. The nurse reviews a client's record and determines that the client is at risk for developing a potassium deficit if which situation is documented?
1. Sustained tissue damage
2. Requires nasogastric suction
3. Has a history of Addison's disease
4. Uric acid level of 9.4 mg/dL (557 mcmol/L)

41. The nurse reviews a client's electrolyte laboratory report and notes that the potassium level is 2.5 mEq/L (2.5 mmol/L). Which patterns should the nurse watch for on the electrocardiogram (ECG) as a result of the laboratory value? **Select all that apply.**
1. U waves
2. Absent P waves
3. Inverted T waves
4. Depressed ST segment
5. Widened QRS complex

42. Potassium chloride intravenously is prescribed for a client with heart failure experiencing hypokalemia. Which actions should the nurse take to plan for preparation and administration of the potassium? **Select all that apply.**

1. Obtain an intravenous (IV) infusion pump.
2. Monitor urine output during administration.
3. Prepare the medication for bolus administration.
4. Monitor the IV site for signs of infiltration or phlebitis.
5. Ensure that the medication is diluted in the appropriate volume of fluid.
6. Ensure that the bag is labeled so that it reads the volume of potassium in the solution.

43. The nurse is assessing a client with a lactose intolerance disorder for a suspected diagnosis of hypocalcemia. Which clinical manifestation would the nurse expect to note in the client?
1. Twitching
2. Hypoactive bowel sounds
3. Negative Trousseau's sign
4. Hypoactive deep tendon reflexes

44. The nurse is caring for a client with Crohn's disease who has a calcium level of 8 mg/dL (2 mmol/L). Which patterns would the nurse watch for on the electrocardiogram? **Select all that apply.**
1. U waves
2. Widened T wave
3. Prominent U wave
4. Prolonged QT interval
5. Prolonged ST segment

45. The nurse reviews the electrolyte results of a client with chronic kidney disease and notes that the potassium level is 5.7 mEq/L (5.7 mmol/L). Which patterns would the nurse watch for on the cardiac monitor as a result of the laboratory value? **Select all that apply.**
1. ST depression
2. Prominent U wave
3. Tall peaked T waves
4. Prolonged ST segment
5. Widened QRS complexes

46. Which client is at risk for the development of a sodium level at 130 mEq/L (130 mmol/L)?
1. The client who is taking diuretics
2. The client with hyperaldosteronism
3. The client with Cushing's syndrome
4. The client who is taking corticosteroids

47. The nurse is caring for a client with heart failure who is receiving high doses of a diuretic. On assessment, the nurse notes that the client has flat neck veins, generalized muscle weakness, and diminished deep tendon reflexes. The nurse suspects hyponatremia. What additional signs would the nurse expect to note in a client with hyponatremia?
1. Muscle twitches
2. Decreased urinary output
3. Hyperactive bowel sounds
4. Increased specific gravity of the urine

48. The nurse reviews a client's laboratory report and notes that the client's serum phosphorus (phosphate) level is 1.8 mg/dL (0.58 mmol/L). Which condition **most likely** caused this serum phosphorus level?
1. Malnutrition
2. Renal insufficiency
3. Hypoparathyroidism
4. Tumor lysis syndrome

49. The nurse is reading a primary health care provider's (PHCP's) progress notes in the client's record and reads that the PHCP has documented "insensible fluid loss of approximately 800 mL daily." The nurse makes a notation that insensible fluid loss occurs through which type of excretion?
1. Urinary output
2. Wound drainage
3. Integumentary output
4. The gastrointestinal tract

50. The nurse is assigned to care for a group of clients. On review of the clients' medical records, the nurse determines that which client is **most likely** at risk for a fluid volume deficit?
1. A client with an ileostomy
2. A client with heart failure
3. A client on long-term corticosteroid therapy
4. A client receiving frequent wound irrigations

51. The nurse caring for a client who has been receiving intravenous (IV) diuretics suspects that the client is experiencing a fluid volume deficit. Which assessment finding would the nurse note in a client with this condition?
1. Weight loss and poor skin turgor
2. Lung congestion and increased heart rate
3. Decreased hematocrit and increased urine output
4. Increased respirations and increased blood pressure

52. On review of the clients' medical records, the nurse determines that which client is at risk for fluid volume excess?
1. The client taking diuretics who has tenting of the skin
2. The client with an ileostomy from a recent abdominal surgery
3. The client who requires intermittent gastrointestinal suctioning
4. The client with kidney disease and a 12-year history of diabetes mellitus

53. Which client is at risk for the development of a potassium level of 5.5 mEq/L (5.5 mmol/L)?
1. The client with colitis
2. The client with Cushing's syndrome
3. The client who has been overusing laxatives
4. The client who has sustained a traumatic burn

ANSWERS

39. *Answer:* 3

Rationale: A fluid volume excess is also known as *overhydration* or *fluid overload* and occurs when fluid intake or fluid retention exceeds the fluid needs of the body. Assessment findings associated with fluid volume excess include cough, dyspnea, crackles, tachypnea, tachycardia, elevated blood pressure, bounding pulse, elevated CVP, weight gain, edema, neck and hand vein distention, altered level of consciousness, and decreased hematocrit. Dry skin, flat neck and hand veins, decreased urinary output, and decreased CVP are noted in fluid volume deficit. Weakness can be present in either fluid volume excess or deficit.

Test-Taking Strategy: Focus on the subject, fluid volume excess. Remember that when there is more than one part to an option, all parts need to be correct in order for the option to be correct. Think about the pathophysiology associated with a fluid volume excess to assist in directing you to the correct option. Also, note that the incorrect options are comparable or alike in that each includes manifestations that reflect a decrease.

Level of Cognitive Ability: Synthesizing
Client Needs: Physiological Integrity
Integrated Process: Nursing Process—Assessment
Content Area: Foundations of Care: Fluids & Electrolytes
Health Problem: Adult Health: Cardiovascular: Heart Failure
Priority Concepts: Fluids and Electrolytes; Perfusion
References: Lewis et al. (2017), pp. 276-277.

40. *Answer:* 2

Rationale: The normal serum potassium level is 3.5 to 5.0 mEq/L (3.5 to 5.0 mmol/L). A potassium deficit is known as *hypokalemia*. Potassium-rich gastrointestinal fluids are lost through gastrointestinal suction, placing the client at risk for hypokalemia. The client with tissue damage or Addison's disease and the client with hyperuricemia are at risk for hyperkalemia. The normal uric acid level for a female is 2.7 to 7.3 mg/dL (160 to 430 mcmol/L) and for a male is 4.0 to 8.5 mg/dL (240 to 501 mcmol/L).

Test-Taking Strategy: Note the subject, causes of potassium deficit. First recall the normal uric acid levels and the causes of hyperkalemia to assist in eliminating option 4. For the remaining options, note that the correct option is the only one that identifies a loss of body fluid.

Level of Cognitive Ability: Analyzing
Client Needs: Physiological Integrity
Integrated Process: Nursing Process—Assessment
Content Area: Foundations of Care: Fluids & Electrolytes
Health Problem: N/A
Priority Concepts: Clinical Judgment; Fluids and Electrolytes
Reference: Ignatavicius, Workman, Rebar (2018), pp. 175, 331.

41. *Answer:* 1, 3, 4

Rationale: The normal serum potassium level is 3.5 to 5.0 mEq/L (3.5 to 5.0 mmol/L). A serum potassium level lower than 3.5 mEq/L (3.5 mmol/L) indicates hypokalemia. Potassium deficit is an electrolyte imbalance that can be potentially life-threatening. Electrocardiographic changes include shallow, flat, or inverted T waves; ST segment depression; and prominent U waves. Absent P waves are not a characteristic of hypokalemia but may be noted in a client with atrial fibrillation, junctional rhythms, or ventricular rhythms. A widened QRS complex may be noted in hyperkalemia and in hypermagnesemia.

Test-Taking Strategy: Focus on the subject, the ECG patterns that may be noted with a client with a potassium level of 2.5 mEq/L (2.5 mmol/L). From the information in the question, you need to determine that the client is experiencing severe hypokalemia. From this point, you must know the electrocardiographic changes that are expected when severe hypokalemia exists.

Level of Cognitive Ability: Analyzing
Client Needs: Physiological Integrity
Integrated Process: Nursing Process—Assessment
Content Area: Foundations of Care: Fluids & Electrolytes
Health Problem: N/A
Priority Concepts: Clinical Judgment; Fluid and Electrolytes
References: Ignatavicius, Workman, Rebar (2018), p. 176.

42. *Answer:* 1, 2, 4, 5, 6

Rationale: Potassium chloride administered intravenously must always be diluted in IV fluid and infused via an infusion pump. Potassium chloride is never given by bolus (IV push). Giving potassium chloride by IV push can result in cardiac arrest. The nurse should ensure that the potassium is diluted in the appropriate amount of diluent or fluid. The IV bag containing the potassium chloride should always be labeled with the volume of potassium it contains. The IV site is monitored closely, because potassium chloride is irritating to the veins and there is risk of phlebitis. In addition, the nurse should monitor for infiltration. The nurse monitors urinary output during administration and contacts the primary health care provider if the urinary output is less than 30 mL/hr.

Test-Taking Strategy: Focus on the subject, the preparation and administration of potassium chloride intravenously. Think about this procedure and the effects of potassium. Note the word *bolus* in option 3 to assist in eliminating this option.

Level of Cognitive Ability: Analyzing
Client Needs: Physiological Integrity
Integrated Process: Nursing Process—Implementation
Content Area: Pharmacology: Fluid and Electrolyte Balance: Electrolytes
Health Problem: Adult Health: Cardiovascular: Heart Failure
Priority Concepts: Clinical Judgment; Safety
References: Lewis et al. (2017), p. 282.

43. *Answer:* 1

Rationale: A client with lactose intolerance is at risk for developing hypocalcemia, because food products that contain calcium also contain lactose. The normal serum calcium level is 9 to 10.5 mg/dL (2.25 to 2.75 mmol/L). A serum calcium level lower than 9 mg/dL (2.25 mmol/L) indicates hypocalcemia. Signs of hypocalcemia include paresthesias followed by numbness, hyperactive deep tendon reflexes, and a positive Trousseau's or Chvostek's sign. Additional signs of hypocalcemia include increased neuromuscular excitability, muscle cramps, twitching, tetany, seizures, irritability, and anxiety. Gastrointestinal symptoms include increased gastric motility, hyperactive bowel sounds, abdominal cramping, and diarrhea.

Test-Taking Strategy: Note that the three incorrect options are comparable or alike in that they reflect a hypoactivity. The option that is different is the correct option.

Level of Cognitive Ability: Analyzing
Client Needs: Physiological Integrity
Integrated Process: Nursing Process—Assessment
Content Area: Foundations of Care: Fluids & Electrolytes
Health Problem: Adult Health: Gastrointestinal: Nutrition Problems
Priority Concepts: Clinical Judgment; Fluids and Electrolytes
Reference: Lewis et al. (2017), p. 284.

44. *Answer:* 4, 5
Rationale: A client with Crohn's disease is at risk for hypocalcemia. The normal serum calcium level is 9 to 10.5 mg/dL (2.25 to 2.75 mmol/L). A serum calcium level lower than 9 mg/dL (2.25 mmol/L) indicates hypocalcemia. Electrocardiographic changes that occur in a client with hypocalcemia include a prolonged QT interval and prolonged ST segment. A shortened ST segment and a widened T wave occur with hypercalcemia. ST depression and prominent U waves occur with hypokalemia.
Test-Taking Strategy: Focus on the **subject**, the electrocardiographic patterns that occur in a client with Crohn's disease who has a calcium level of 8 mg/dL (2 mmol/L). It is necessary to know this client is at risk for hypocalcemia and that a level of 8 mg/dL (2 mmol/L) is low. Then it is necessary to recall the electrocardiographic changes that occur in hypocalcemia. Remember that hypocalcemia causes a prolonged ST segment and prolonged QT interval.
Level of Cognitive Ability: Analyzing
Client Needs: Physiological Integrity
Integrated Process: Nursing Process—Assessment
Content Area: Foundations of Care: Fluids & Electrolytes
Health Problem: Adult Health: Gastrointestinal: Lower GI Disorders
Priority Concepts: Clinical Judgment; Fluids and Electrolytes
Reference: Lewis et al. (2017), p. 284.

45. *Answer:* 3, 5
Rationale: The client with chronic kidney disease is at risk for hyperkalemia. The normal potassium level is 3.5 to 5.0 mEq/L (3.5 to 5.0 mmol/L). A serum potassium level greater than 5.0 mEq/L (5.0 mmol/L) indicates hyperkalemia. Electrocardiographic changes associated with hyperkalemia include flat P waves, prolonged PR intervals, widened QRS complexes, and tall peaked T waves. ST depression and a prominent U wave occurs in hypokalemia. A prolonged ST segment occurs in hypocalcemia.
Test-Taking Strategy: Focus on the **subject**, a client with chronic kidney disease and the electrocardiographic changes that occur in a potassium imbalance. From the information in the question you need to determine that this condition is a hyperkalemic one. From this point, you must know the electrocardiographic changes that are expected when hyperkalemia exists. Remember that tall peaked T waves, flat P waves, widened QRS complexes, and prolonged PR interval are associated with hyperkalemia.
Level of Cognitive Ability: Analyzing
Client Needs: Physiological Integrity
Integrated Process: Nursing Process—Assessment
Content Area: Foundations of Care: Fluids & Electrolytes
Health Problem: Adult Health: Renal and Urinary: Chronic Kidney Disease
Priority Concepts: Clinical Judgment; Fluids and Electrolytes
Reference: Lewis et al. (2017), p. 281.

46. *Answer:* 1
Rationale: The normal serum sodium level is 135 to 145 mEq/L (135 to 145 mmol/L). A serum sodium level of 130 mEq/L (130 mmol/L) indicates hyponatremia. Hyponatremia can occur in the client taking diuretics. The client taking corticosteroids and the client with hyperaldosteronism or Cushing's syndrome are at risk for hypernatremia.
Test-Taking Strategy: Focus on the **subject**, the causes of a sodium level of 130 mEq/L (130 mmol/L). First, determine that the client is experiencing hyponatremia. Next, you must know the causes of hyponatremia to direct you to the correct option. Also, recall that when a client takes a diuretic, the client loses fluid and electrolytes.
Level of Cognitive Ability: Analyzing
Client Needs: Physiological Integrity
Integrated Process: Nursing Process—Assessment
Content Area: Foundations of Care: Fluids & Electrolytes
Health Problem: N/A
Priority Concepts: Clinical Judgment; Fluids and Electrolytes
Reference: Ignatavicius, Workman, Rebar (2018), pp. 173-174.

47. *Answer:* 3
Rationale: The normal serum sodium level is 135 to 145 mEq/L (135 to 145 mmol/L). Hyponatremia is evidenced by a serum sodium level lower than 135 mEq/L (135 mmol/L). Hyperactive bowel sounds indicate hyponatremia. The remaining options are signs of hypernatremia. In hyponatremia, muscle weakness, increased urinary output, and decreased specific gravity of the urine would be noted.
Test-Taking Strategy: Focus on the **data in the question** and the **subject** of the question, signs of hyponatremia. It is necessary to know the signs of hyponatremia to answer correctly. Also, think about the action and effects of sodium on the body to answer correctly. Remember that increased bowel motility and hyperactive bowel sounds indicate hyponatremia.
Level of Cognitive Ability: Analyzing
Client Needs: Physiological Integrity
Integrated Process: Nursing Process—Assessment
Content Area: Foundations of Care: Fluids & Electrolytes
Health Problem: N/A
Priority Concepts: Clinical Judgment; Fluids and Electrolytes
Reference: Lewis et al. (2017), p. 279.

48. *Answer:* 1
Rationale: The normal serum phosphorus (phosphate) level is 3.0 to 4.5 mg/dL (0.97 to 1.45 mmol/L). The client is experiencing hypophosphatemia. Causative factors relate to malnutrition or starvation and the use of aluminum hydroxide–based or magnesium-based antacids. Renal insufficiency, hypoparathyroidism, and tumor lysis syndrome are causative factors of hyperphosphatemia.
Test-Taking Strategy: Note the **strategic words**, *most likely.* Focus on the **subject**, a serum phosphorus level of 1.8 mg/dL (0.58 mmol/L). First, you must determine that the client is experiencing hypophosphatemia. From this point, think about the effects of phosphorus on the body and recall the causes of hypophosphatemia in order to answer correctly.
Level of Cognitive Ability: Analyzing
Client Needs: Physiological Integrity
Integrated Process: Nursing Process—Assessment
Content Area: Foundations of Care: Fluids & Electrolytes

Health Problem: N/A
Priority Concepts: Clinical Judgment; Fluids and Electrolytes
Reference: Lewis et al. (2017), pp. 285-286.

49. *Answer:* 3
Rationale: Insensible losses may occur without the person's awareness. Insensible losses occur daily through the skin and the lungs. Sensible losses are those of which the person is aware, such as through urination, wound drainage, and gastrointestinal tract losses.
Test-Taking Strategy: Note that the subject of the question is insensible fluid loss. Note that urination, wound drainage, and gastrointestinal tract losses are comparable or alike in that they can be measured for accurate output. Fluid loss through the skin cannot be measured accurately; it can only be approximated.
Level of Cognitive Ability: Applying
Client Needs: Physiological Integrity
Integrated Process: Communication and Documentation
Content Area: Foundations of Care: Fluids & Electrolytes
Health Problem: N/A
Priority Concepts: Clinical Judgment; Fluids and Electrolytes
References: Lewis et al. (2017), p. 274.

50. *Answer:* 1
Rationale: A fluid volume deficit occurs when the fluid intake is not sufficient to meet the fluid needs of the body. Causes of a fluid volume deficit include vomiting, diarrhea, conditions that cause increased respirations or increased urinary output, insufficient intravenous fluid replacement, draining fistulas, and the presence of an ileostomy or colostomy. A client with heart failure or on long-term corticosteroid therapy or a client receiving frequent wound irrigations is most at risk for fluid volume excess.
Test-Taking Strategy: Note the strategic words, *most likely.* Read the question carefully, noting the subject, the client at risk for a deficit. Read each option and think about the fluid imbalance that can occur in each. The clients with heart failure, on long-term corticosteroid therapy, and receiving frequent wound irrigations retain fluid. The only condition that can cause a deficit is the condition noted in the correct option.
Level of Cognitive Ability: Analyzing
Client Needs: Physiological Integrity
Integrated Process: Nursing Process—Assessment
Content Area: Foundations of Care: Fluids & Electrolytes
Health Problem: Adult Health: Gastrointestinal: Dehydration
Priority Concepts: Clinical Judgment; Fluids and Electrolytes
Reference: Lewis et al. (2017), p. 276.

51. *Answer:* 1
Rationale: A fluid volume deficit occurs when the fluid intake is not sufficient to meet the fluid needs of the body. Assessment findings in a client with a fluid volume deficit include increased respirations and heart rate, decreased central venous pressure (CVP), weight loss, poor skin turgor, dry mucous membranes, decreased urine volume, increased specific gravity of the urine, increased hematocrit, and altered level of consciousness. Lung congestion, increased urinary output, and increased blood pressure are all associated with fluid volume excess.
Test-Taking Strategy: Focus on the subject, assessment findings in a fluid volume deficit. Think about the pathophysiology for fluid volume deficit and fluid volume excess to answer correctly. Note that options 2, 3, and 4 are comparable or alike and are manifestations associated with fluid volume excess.
Level of Cognitive Ability: Analyzing
Client Needs: Physiological Integrity
Integrated Process: Nursing Process—Assessment
Content Area: Foundations of Care: Fluids & Electrolytes
Health Problem: N/A
Priority Concepts: Clinical Judgment; Fluids and Electrolytes
Reference: Lewis et al. (2017), p. 276.

52. *Answer:* 4
Rationale: A fluid volume excess is also known as *overhydration* or *fluid overload* and occurs when fluid intake or fluid retention exceeds the fluid needs of the body. The causes of fluid volume excess include decreased kidney function, heart failure, use of hypotonic fluids to replace isotonic fluid losses, excessive irrigation of wounds and body cavities, and excessive ingestion of sodium. The client taking diuretics, the client with an ileostomy, and the client who requires gastrointestinal suctioning are at risk for fluid volume deficit.
Test-Taking Strategy: Focus on the subject, fluid volume excess. Think about the pathophysiology associated with fluid volume excess. Read each option and think about the fluid imbalance that can occur in each. Clients taking diuretics or having ileostomies or gastrointestinal suctioning all lose fluid. The only condition that can cause an excess is the condition noted in the correct option.
Level of Cognitive Ability: Analyzing
Client Needs: Physiological Integrity
Integrated Process: Nursing Process—Assessment
Content Area: Foundations of Care: Fluids & Electrolytes
Health Problem: N/A
Priority Concepts: Clinical Judgment; Fluids and Electrolytes
Reference: Ignatavicius, Workman, Rebar (2018), pp. 171-172.

53. *Answer:* 4
Rationale: The normal potassium level is 3.5 to 5.0 mEq/L (3.5 to 5.0 mmol/L). A serum potassium level higher than 5.0 mEq/L (5.0 mmol/L) indicates hyperkalemia. Clients who experience cellular shifting of potassium in the early stages of massive cell destruction, such as with trauma, burns, sepsis, or metabolic or respiratory acidosis, are at risk for hyperkalemia. The client with Cushing's syndrome or colitis and the client who has been overusing laxatives are at risk for hypokalemia.
Test-Taking Strategy: Eliminate the client with colitis and the client overusing laxatives first, because they are comparable or alike, with both reflecting a gastrointestinal loss. From the remaining options, recalling that cell destruction causes potassium shifts will assist in directing you to the correct option. Also, remember that Cushing's syndrome presents a risk for hypokalemia and that Addison's disease presents a risk for hyperkalemia.
Level of Cognitive Ability: Analyzing
Client Needs: Physiological Integrity
Integrated Process: Nursing Process—Assessment
Content Area: Foundations of Care: Fluids & Electrolytes
Health Problem: N/A
Priority Concepts: Clinical Judgment; Fluids and Electrolytes
Reference: Ignatavicius, Workman, Rebar (2018), pp. 178-179.

CHAPTER 9

Acid-Base Balance

PRIORITY CONCEPTS **Acid-Base Balance; Oxygenation**

I. Hydrogen Ions, Acids, and Bases

A. Hydrogen ions
1. Vital to life because hydrogen ions determine the pH of the body, which must be maintained in a narrow range
2. Expressed as pH; the pH scale is determined by the number of hydrogen ions and goes from 1 to 14; 7 is considered neutral.
3. The number of hydrogen ions in the body fluid determines whether it is acid (acidosis), alkaline (alkalosis), or neutral.
4. The pH of body fluid is between 7.35 and 7.45.

B. Acids
1. Produced as end products of metabolism
2. Contain hydrogen ions
3. Are hydrogen ion donors; they give up hydrogen ions to neutralize or decrease the strength of an acid or to form a weaker base.

C. Bases
1. Contain no hydrogen ions
2. Are hydrogen ion acceptors; they accept hydrogen$^+$ ions from acids to neutralize or decrease the strength of a base or to form a weaker acid.
3. Normal serum levels of bicarbonate (HCO^{3-}) are 21 to 28 mEq/L (21 to 28 mmol/L).

II. Regulatory Systems for Hydrogen Ion Concentration in the Blood

A. Buffers
1. Buffers are the fastest-acting regulatory system.
2. Buffers provide immediate protection against changes in hydrogen ion concentration in the extracellular fluid.
3. Buffers are reactors that function only to keep the pH within the narrow limits of stability when too much acid or base is released into the system, and buffers absorb or release hydrogen ions as needed.
4. Buffers serve as a transport mechanism that carries excess hydrogen ions to the lungs.
5. Once the primary buffer systems react, they are consumed, leaving the body less able to withstand further stress until the buffers are replaced.

⚠ The underlying cause of an acid-base imbalance needs to be identified and the cause needs to be treated to resolve the imbalance.

B. Primary buffer systems in extracellular fluid
1. Hemoglobin system
a. System maintains acid-base balance by a process called *chloride shift*.
b. Chloride shifts in and out of the cells in response to the level of oxygen (O_2) in the blood.
c. For each chloride ion that leaves a red blood cell, a bicarbonate ion enters.
d. For each chloride ion that enters a red blood cell, a bicarbonate ion leaves.
2. Plasma protein system
a. The system functions along with the liver to vary the amount of hydrogen ions in the chemical structure of plasma proteins.
b. Plasma proteins have the ability to attract or release hydrogen ions.
3. Carbonic acid–bicarbonate system
a. Primary buffer system in the body
b. The system maintains a pH of 7.4 with a ratio of 20 parts bicarbonate (HCO_3^-) to 1 part carbonic acid (H_2CO_3) (Fig. 9-1).
c. This ratio (20:1) determines the hydrogen ion concentration of body fluid.
d. Carbonic acid concentration is controlled by the excretion of CO_2 by the lungs; the rate and depth of respiration change in response to changes in the CO_2.
e. The kidneys control the bicarbonate concentration and selectively retain or excrete bicarbonate in response to bodily needs.
4. Phosphate buffer system
a. System is present in cells and body fluids and is especially active in the kidneys.

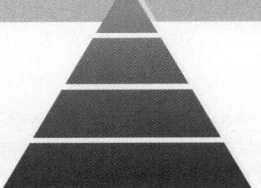

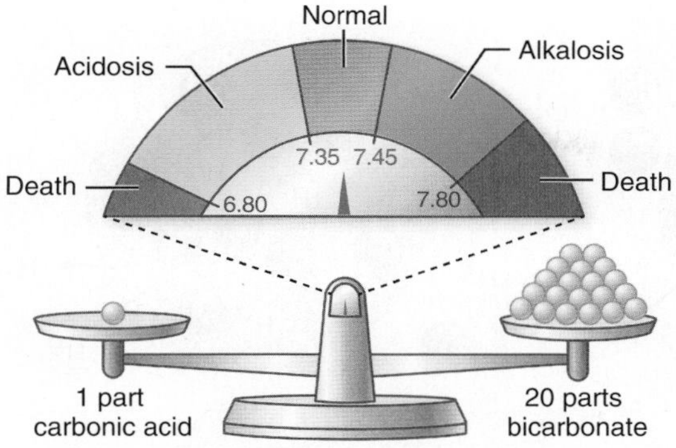

FIG. 9-1 Acid-base balance. In the healthy state, a ratio of 1 part carbonic acid to 20 parts bicarbonate provides a normal serum pH between 7.35 and 7.45. Any deviation to the left of 7.35 results in an acidotic state. Any deviation to the right of 7.45 results in an alkalotic state.

b. System acts like bicarbonate and neutralizes excess hydrogen ions.

C. Lungs

1. The lungs are the second defense of the body; they interact with the buffer system to maintain acid-base balance.
2. During acidosis, the pH decreases and the respiratory rate and depth increase in an attempt to exhale acids. The carbonic acid created by the neutralizing action of bicarbonate can be carried to the lungs, where it is reduced to CO_2 and water and is exhaled; thus, hydrogen ions are inactivated and exhaled.
3. During alkalosis, the pH increases and the respiratory rate and depth decrease; CO_2 is retained and carbonic acid increases to neutralize and decrease the strength of excess bicarbonate.
4. The action of the lungs is reversible in controlling an excess or deficit.
5. The lungs can hold hydrogen ions until the deficit is corrected or can inactivate hydrogen ions, changing the ions to water molecules to be exhaled along with CO_2, thus correcting the excess.
6. The process of correcting a deficit or excess takes 10 to 30 seconds to complete.
7. The lungs are capable of inactivating only hydrogen ions carried by carbonic acid; excess hydrogen ions created by other mechanisms must be excreted by the kidneys.

! Monitor the client's respiratory status closely. During acidosis, the respiratory rate and depth increase in an attempt to exhale acids. During alkalosis, the respiratory rate and depth decrease; CO_2 is retained to neutralize and decrease the strength of excess bicarbonate.

D. Kidneys

1. The kidneys provide a more inclusive corrective response to acid-base disturbances than other corrective mechanisms, even though the renal excretion of acids and alkalis occurs more slowly.
2. Compensation requires a few hours to several days; however, the compensation is more thorough and selective than that of other regulators, such as the buffer systems and lungs.
3. During acidosis, the pH decreases and excess hydrogen ions are secreted into the tubules and combine with buffers for excretion in the urine.
4. During alkalosis, the pH increases and excess bicarbonate ions move into the tubules, combine with sodium, and are excreted in the urine.
5. Selective regulation of bicarbonate occurs in the kidneys.
   - **a.** The kidneys restore bicarbonate by excreting hydrogen ions and retaining bicarbonate ions.
   - **b.** Excess hydrogen ions are excreted in the urine in the form of phosphoric acid.
   - **c.** The alteration of certain amino acids in the renal tubules results in a diffusion of ammonia into the kidneys; the ammonia combines with excess hydrogen ions and is excreted in the urine.

E. Potassium (K^+)

1. Potassium plays an exchange role in maintaining acid-base balance.
2. The body changes the potassium level by drawing hydrogen ions into the cells or by pushing them out of the cells (potassium movement across cell membranes is facilitated by transcellular shifting in response to acid-base patterns).
3. The potassium level changes to compensate for hydrogen ion level changes (Fig. 9-2).
   - **a.** During acidosis, the body protects itself from the acidic state by moving hydrogen ions into the cells. Therefore, potassium moves out to make room for hydrogen ions and the potassium level increases.
   - **b.** During alkalosis, the cells release hydrogen ions into the blood in an attempt to increase the acidity of the blood; this forces the potassium into the cells and potassium levels decrease.

! When the client experiences an acid-base imbalance, monitor the potassium level closely, because the potassium moves in or out of the cells in an attempt to maintain acid-base balance. The resulting hypokalemia or hyperkalemia predisposes the client to associated complications.

III. Respiratory Acidosis

A. Description: The total concentration of buffer base is lower than normal, with a relative increase in hydrogen ion concentration; thus, a greater number of hydrogen ions is circulating in the blood than can be absorbed by the buffer system.

B. Causes (Box 9-1)

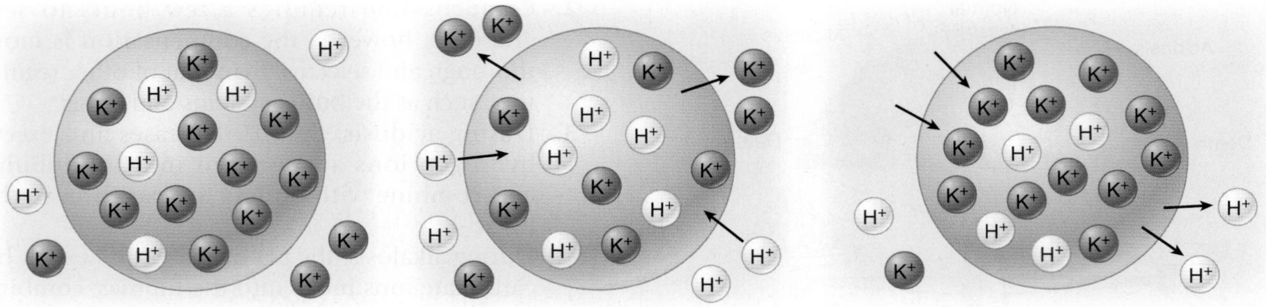

Under normal conditions, the intracellular potassium content is much greater than that of the extracellular fluid. The concentration of hydrogen ions is low in both compartments.

In acidosis, the extracellular hydrogen ion content increases, and the hydrogen ions move into the intracellular fluid. To keep the intracellular fluid electrically neutral, an equal number of potassium ions leave the cell, creating a relative hyperkalemia.

In alkalosis, more hydrogen ions are present in the intracellular fluid than in the extracellular fluid. Hydrogen ions move from the intracellular fluid into the extracellular fluid. To keep the intracellular fluid electrically neutral, potassium ions move from the extracellular fluid into the intracellular fluid, creating a relative hypokalemia.

FIG. 9-2 Movement of potassium in response to changes in the extracellular fluid hydrogen ion concentration.

BOX 9-1 Causes of Respiratory Acidosis

- Asthma: Spasms resulting from allergens, irritants, or emotions cause the smooth muscles of the bronchioles to constrict, resulting in ineffective gas exchange.
- Atelectasis: Excessive mucus collection, with the collapse of alveolar sacs caused by mucous plugs, infectious drainage, or anesthetic medications, results in ineffective gas exchange.
- Brain trauma: Excessive pressure on the respiratory center or medulla oblongata depresses respirations.
- Bronchiectasis: Bronchi become dilated as a result of inflammation, and destructive changes and weakness in the walls of the bronchi occur.
- Bronchitis: Inflammation causes airway obstruction, resulting in inadequate gas exchange.
- Central nervous system depressants: Depressants such as sedatives, opioids, and anesthetics depress the respiratory center, leading to hypoventilation (excessive sedation from medications may require reversal by opioid antagonist medications); carbon dioxide (CO_2) is retained and the hydrogen ion concentration increases.
- Emphysema and chronic obstructive pulmonary disease: Loss of elasticity of alveolar sacs restricts air flow in and out, primarily out, leading to an increased CO_2 level.
- Hypoventilation: CO_2 is retained and the hydrogen ion concentration increases, leading to the acidotic state; carbonic acid is retained and the pH decreases.
- Pneumonia: Excess mucus production and lung congestion cause airway obstruction, resulting in inadequate gas exchange.
- Pulmonary edema: Extracellular accumulation of fluid in pulmonary tissue causes disturbances in alveolar diffusion and perfusion.
- Pulmonary emboli: Emboli cause obstruction in a pulmonary artery resulting in airway obstruction and inadequate gas exchange.

1. Respiratory acidosis is caused by primary defects in the function of the lungs or changes in normal respiratory patterns.
2. Any condition that causes an obstruction of the airway leading to hypoventilation or depresses the respiratory system can cause respiratory acidosis.

C. Assessment (Table 9-1)

For any acid-base imbalance, it is important to closely monitor the client's level of consciousness, use protective measures to ensure safety, and monitor electrolyte levels and follow-up ABG test results.

D. Interventions

1. Monitor for signs of respiratory distress.
2. Administer O_2 as prescribed.
3. Place the client in a semi-Fowler's position.
4. Encourage and assist the client to turn, cough, and deep breathe.
5. Encourage hydration to thin secretions.
6. Reduce restlessness by improving ventilation rather than by administering tranquilizers, sedatives, or opioids, because these medications further depress respirations.
7. Prepare to administer respiratory treatments as prescribed; suction the client's airway, if necessary.
8. Prepare for endotracheal intubation and mechanical ventilation if CO_2 levels rise above 50 mm Hg and signs of acute respiratory distress are present.

If the client has a condition that causes an obstruction of the airway or depresses the respiratory system, monitor the client for respiratory acidosis.

IV. Respiratory Alkalosis

A. Description: A deficit of carbonic acid and a decrease in hydrogen ion concentration that results from the

TABLE 9-1 Clinical Manifestations of Acidosis

Respiratory (↓ pH, ↑ $Paco_2$)	Metabolic (↓ pH, ↓ HCO_3)
Neurological	
Lethargy	Lethargy
Confusion	Confusion
Dizziness	Dizziness
Headache	Headache
Coma	Coma
Cardiovascular	
Decreased blood pressure	Decreased blood pressure
Dysrhythmias (related to hyperkalemia from compensation)	Dysrhythmias (related to hyperkalemia from compensation)
Warm, flushed skin (related to peripheral vasodilation)	Cold, clammy skin
Gastrointestinal	
No significant findings	Nausea, vomiting, diarrhea, abdominal pain
Neuromuscular	
Seizures	Muscle weakness
Respiratory	
The respiratory rate and depth increase in an attempt to exhale acids. However, when there is a respiratory problem and the lungs are unable to compensate, hypoventilation with hypoxia occurs.	Deep, rapid respirations (compensatory action by the lungs); known as Kussmaul's respirations

Adapted from Lewis S, Bucher L, Heitkemper M, Harding, M, Kwong J, Roberts D: *Medical-surgical nursing: assessment and management of clinical problems*, ed 10, St. Louis, 2017, Mosby.

accumulation of base or from a loss of acid without a comparable loss of base in the body fluids.

B. Causes: Respiratory alkalosis results from conditions that cause overstimulation of the respiratory system (Box 9-2).

C. Assessment (Table 9-2)

D. Interventions

1. Monitor for signs of respiratory distress.
2. Provide emotional support and reassurance to the client.
3. Encourage appropriate breathing patterns.
4. Assist with breathing techniques and breathing aids if needed and as prescribed (voluntary holding of breath, using a rebreathing mask, CO_2 breaths with rebreathing into a paper bag).
5. Provide cautious care with ventilator clients so that they are not forced to take breaths too deeply or rapidly.
6. Prepare to administer calcium gluconate for tetany as prescribed.

BOX 9-2 Causes of Respiratory Alkalosis

- Fever: Causes increased metabolism, resulting in overstimulation of the respiratory system.
- Hyperventilation: Rapid respirations cause the blowing off of carbon dioxide (CO_2), leading to a decrease in carbonic acid.
- Hypoxia: Stimulates the respiratory center in the brainstem, which causes an increase in the respiratory rate in order to increase oxygen (O_2); this causes hyperventilation, which results in a decrease in the CO_2 level.
- Overventilation by mechanical ventilators: The administration of O_2 and the depletion of CO_2 can occur from mechanical ventilation, causing the client to be hyperventilated.
- Pain: Overstimulation of the respiratory center in the brainstem results in a carbonic acid deficit.
- Severe anxiety and hysteria: Often is neurogenic and related to a psychoneurosis; however, this condition leads to vigorous breathing and excessive exhaling of CO_2.

TABLE 9-2 Clinical Manifestations of Alkalosis

Respiratory (↑pH, ↓ $Paco_2$)	Metabolic (↑pH, ↑ HCO_3)
Neurological	
Dizziness	Lethargy
Lightheadedness	Irritability
Confusion	Confusion
Headache	Headache
Cardiovascular	
Low blood pressure	Low blood pressure
Tachycardia	Tachycardia
Dysrhythmias	Dysrhythmias
Gastrointestinal	
Nausea, vomiting, diarrhea	Anorexia
Epigastric pain	Nausea, vomiting
Neuromuscular	
Tetany	Tetany
Numbness	Tremors
Tingling of extremities	Tingling of extremities
Hyperreflexia	Muscle cramps, hypertonic muscles
Seizures	Seizures
Respiratory	
Respiratory rate and depth decrease as a compensatory action by the lungs. However, when there is a respiratory problem and lungs are unable to compensate, hyperventilation can occur.	Respiratory rate and depth decrease as a compensatory action by the lungs (hypoventilation)

Adapted from Lewis S, Bucher L, Heitkemper M, Harding, M, Kwong J, Roberts D: *Medical-surgical nursing: assessment and management of clinical problems*, ed 10, St. Louis, 2017, Mosby.

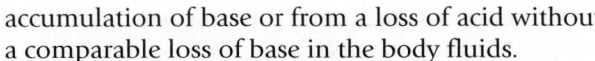

V. Metabolic Acidosis

A. Description: A total concentration of buffer base that is lower than normal, with a relative increase in the hydrogen ion concentration, resulting from loss of too much base and/or retention of too much acid.

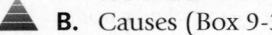

B. Causes (Box 9-3)

An insufficient supply of insulin in a client with diabetes mellitus can result in metabolic acidosis known as diabetic ketoacidosis.

C. Assessment (see Table 9-1)

D. Interventions
1. Monitor for signs of respiratory distress.
2. Monitor intake and output and assist with fluid and electrolyte replacement as prescribed.
3. Prepare to administer solutions intravenously as prescribed to increase the buffer base.
4. Initiate seizure precautions.

E. Interventions in diabetes mellitus and diabetic ketoacidosis
1. Give insulin as prescribed to hasten the movement of glucose into the cells, thereby decreasing the concurrent ketosis.
2. When glucose is being properly metabolized, the body will stop converting fats to glucose.
3. Monitor for circulatory collapse caused by polyuria, which may result from the hyperglycemic state; osmotic diuresis may lead to extracellular volume deficit.

Monitor the client experiencing severe diarrhea for manifestations of metabolic acidosis.

BOX 9-3 Causes of Metabolic Acidosis

- Diabetes mellitus or diabetic ketoacidosis: An insufficient supply of insulin causes increased fat metabolism, leading to an excess accumulation of ketones or other acids; the bicarbonate then ends up being depleted.
- Excessive ingestion of acetylsalicylic acid: Causes an increase in the hydrogen ion concentration.
- High-fat diet: Causes a much too rapid accumulation of the waste products of fat metabolism, leading to a buildup of ketones and acids.
- Insufficient metabolism of carbohydrates: When the oxygen supply is not sufficient for the metabolism of carbohydrates, lactic acid is produced and lactic acidosis results.
- Malnutrition: Improper metabolism of nutrients causes fat catabolism, leading to an excess buildup of ketones and acids.
- Renal insufficiency, acute kidney injury, or chronic kidney disease: Increased waste products of protein metabolism are retained; acids increase, and bicarbonate is unable to maintain acid-base balance.
- Severe diarrhea: Intestinal and pancreatic secretions are normally alkaline; therefore, excessive loss of base leads to acidosis.

F. Interventions in kidney disease
1. Dialysis may be necessary to remove protein and waste products, thereby lessening the acidotic state.
2. A diet low in protein and high in calories decreases the amount of protein waste products, which in turn lessens the acidosis.

VI. Metabolic Alkalosis

A. Description: A deficit of carbonic acid and a decrease in hydrogen ion concentration that results from the accumulation of base or from a loss of acid without a comparable loss of base in the body fluids.

B. Causes: Metabolic alkalosis results from a dysfunction of metabolism that causes an increased amount of available base solution in the blood or a decrease in available acids in the blood (Box 9-4).

C. Assessment (see Table 9-2)

Monitor the client experiencing excessive vomiting or the client with gastrointestinal suctioning for manifestations of metabolic alkalosis.

D. Interventions
1. Monitor for signs of respiratory distress.
2. Prepare to administer medications and intravenous fluids as prescribed to promote the kidney excretion of bicarbonate.
3. Prepare to replace potassium as prescribed.

VII. Arterial Blood Gases (ABGs) (Table 9-3)

A. Collection of an ABG specimen
1. Obtain vital signs.
2. Determine whether the client has an arterial line in place (allows for arterial blood sampling without further puncture to the client).
3. Perform the **Allen's test** to determine the presence of collateral circulation (see Priority Nursing Actions).
4. Assess factors that may affect the accuracy of the results, such as changes in the O_2 settings, suctioning within the past 20 minutes, and the client's activities.
5. Provide emotional support to the client.

BOX 9-4 Causes of Metabolic Alkalosis

- Diuretics: The loss of hydrogen ions and chloride from diuresis causes a compensatory increase in the amount of bicarbonate in the blood.
- Excessive vomiting or gastrointestinal suctioning: Leads to an excessive loss of hydrochloric acid.
- Hyperaldosteronism: Increased renal tubular reabsorption of sodium occurs, with the resultant loss of hydrogen ions.
- Ingestion of and/or infusion of excess sodium bicarbonate: Causes an increase in the amount of base in the blood.
- Massive transfusion of whole blood: The citrate anticoagulant used for the storage of blood is metabolized to bicarbonate.

TABLE 9-3 Normal Arterial Blood Gas Values

Laboratory Test	Normal Range	
	Conventional Units	SI Units
Arterial		
pH (arterial)	7.35-7.45	7.35-7.45
$Paco_2$	35-45 mm Hg	35-45 mm Hg
Bicarbonate (HCO_3^-)	21-28 mEq/L	21-28 mmol/L
Pao_2	80-100 mm Hg	80-100 mm Hg
Venous		
pH (venous)	7.31-7.41	7.31-7.41
$Pv\ o_2$	40-50 mm Hg	40-50 mm Hg

kPa, Kilopascal; *mmol*, millimole (10^{-3} mole); *$Paco_2$*, partial pressure of carbon dioxide in arterial blood; *Pao_2*, partial pressure of oxygen in arterial blood; *Pvo_2*, partial pressure of oxygen in venous blood. *Note:* Because arterial blood gases are influenced by altitude, the value for Pao_2 decreases as altitude increases.

6. Assist with the specimen draw; prepare a heparinized syringe (if not already prepackaged). After obtaining a specimen, prevent any air entering the syringe, because air can cause a blood gas analysis alteration.
7. Apply pressure immediately to the puncture site following the blood draw; maintain pressure for 5 minutes or for 10 minutes if the client is taking an anticoagulant to decrease the risk of hematoma. Reassess the radial pulse after removing the pressure.
8. Appropriately label the specimen and transport it on ice to the laboratory.
9. On the laboratory form, record the client's temperature and the type of supplemental O_2 that the client is receiving.

B. Respiratory acid-base imbalances (Table 9-4)

1. Remember that the respiratory function indicator is the $Paco_2$.
2. In a respiratory imbalance, you will find an opposite relationship between the pH and the $Paco_2$; in other words, the pH will be elevated with a decreased $Paco_2$ (alkalosis) or the pH will be decreased with an elevated $Paco_2$ (acidosis).
3. Look at the pH and the $Paco_2$ to determine whether the condition is a respiratory problem.
4. Respiratory acidosis: The pH is decreased; the $Paco_2$ is elevated.
5. Respiratory alkalosis: The pH is elevated; the $Paco_2$ is decreased.

C. Metabolic acid-base imbalances (see Table 9-4)

1. Remember, the metabolic function indicator is the bicarbonate ion (HCO_3^-).
2. In a metabolic imbalance, there is a corresponding relationship between the pH and the HCO_3^-; in other words, the pH will be elevated and HCO_3^- will be elevated (alkalosis), or the pH will be decreased and HCO_3^- will be decreased (acidosis).
3. Look at the pH and the HCO_3^- to determine whether the condition is a metabolic problem.
4. Metabolic acidosis: The pH is decreased; the HCO_3^- is decreased.
5. Metabolic alkalosis: The pH is elevated; the HCO_3^- is elevated.

TABLE 9-4 Acid-Base Imbalances: Usual Laboratory Value Changes

Imbalance	pH	HCO_3^-	Pao_2	$Paco_2$	K^+
Respiratory acidosis	U: Decreased PC: Decreased C: Normal	U: Normal PC: Increased C: Increased	Usually decreased	U: Increased PC: Increased C: Increased	Increased
Respiratory alkalosis	U: Increased PC: Increased C: Normal	U: Normal PC: Decreased C: Decreased	Usually normal but depends on other accompanying conditions	U: Decreased PC: Decreased C: Decreased	Decreased
Metabolic acidosis	U: Decreased PC: Decreased C: Normal	U: Decreased PC: Decreased C: Decreased	Usually normal but depends on other accompanying conditions	U: Normal PC: Decreased C: Decreased	Increased
Metabolic alkalosis	U: Increased PC: Increased C: Normal	U: Increased PC: Increased C: Increased	Usually normal but depends on other accompanying conditions	U: Normal PC: Increased C: Increased	Decreased

C, Compensated; *PC*, partially compensated; *U*, uncompensated.

In a respiratory imbalance, the ABG result indicates an opposite relationship between the pH and the $Paco_2$. In a metabolic imbalance, the ABG result indicates a corresponding relationship between the pH and the HCO_3^-.

D. Compensation (see Table 9-4)
 1. Compensation refers to the body processes that occur to counterbalance the acid-base disturbance.
 2. When full compensation has occurred, the pH is within normal limits.

E. Steps for analyzing ABG results (Box 9-5)

F. Mixed acid-base disorders
 1. Occurs when 2 or more disorders are present at the same time.
 2. The pH will depend on the type and severity of the disorders involved, including any compensatory mechanisms at work, e.g., respiratory acidosis combined with metabolic acidosis will result in a greater decrease in pH than either imbalance occurring alone.
 3. Example: Mixed alkalosis can occur if a client begins to hyperventilate due to postoperative pain (respiratory alkalosis) and is also losing acid due to gastric suctioning (metabolic alkalosis).

BOX 9-5 Analyzing Arterial Blood Gas Results

If you can remember the following Pyramid Points and Pyramid Steps, you will be able to analyze any blood gas report.

Pyramid Points

In acidosis, the pH is decreased.
In alkalosis, the pH is elevated.
The respiratory function indicator is the $Paco_2$.
The metabolic function indicator is the bicarbonate ion (HCO_3^-).

Pyramid Steps

Pyramid Step 1

Look at the arterial blood gas results. Look at the pH. Is the pH elevated or decreased? If the pH is elevated, it reflects alkalosis. If the pH is decreased, it reflects acidosis.

Pyramid Step 2

Look at the $Paco_2$. Is the $Paco_2$ elevated or decreased? If the $Paco_2$ reflects an opposite relationship to the pH, the condition is a respiratory imbalance. If the $Paco_2$ does not reflect an opposite relationship to the pH, go to Pyramid Step 3.

Pyramid Step 3

Look at the HCO_3^-. Does the HCO_3^- reflect a corresponding relationship with the pH? If it does, the condition is a metabolic imbalance.

Pyramid Step 4

Full compensation has occurred if the pH is in a normal range of 7.35 to 7.45. If the pH is not within normal range, look at the respiratory or metabolic function indicators.

If the condition is a respiratory imbalance, look at the HCO_3^- to determine the state of compensation.

If the condition is a metabolic imbalance, look at the $Paco_2$ to determine the state of compensation.

Refer to Table 9-4 for laboratory results in partially compensated and uncompensated conditions.

PRIORITY NURSING ACTIONS

Performing the Allen's Test Before Radial Artery Puncture

1. Explain the procedure to the client.
2. Apply pressure over the ulnar and radial arteries simultaneously.
3. Ask the client to open and close the hand repeatedly.
4. Release pressure from the ulnar artery while compressing the radial artery.
5. Assess the color of the extremity distal to the pressure point.
6. Document the findings.

Reference

Perry et al. (2018), pp. 207-208, 211.

PRACTICE QUESTIONS

54. The nurse reviews the arterial blood gas results of a client and notes the following: pH 7.45, $Paco_2$ of 30 mm Hg (30 mm Hg), and HCO_3^- of 20 mEq/L (20 mmol/L). The nurse analyzes these results as indicating which condition?
1. Metabolic acidosis, compensated
2. Respiratory alkalosis, compensated
3. Metabolic alkalosis, uncompensated
4. Respiratory acidosis, uncompensated

55. The nurse is caring for a client with a nasogastric tube that is attached to low suction. The nurse monitors the client for manifestations of which disorder that the client is at risk for?
1. Metabolic acidosis
2. Metabolic alkalosis
3. Respiratory acidosis
4. Respiratory alkalosis

56. A client with a 3-day history of nausea and vomiting presents to the emergency department. The client is hypoventilating and has a respiratory rate of 10 breaths per minute. The electrocardiogram (ECG) monitor displays tachycardia, with a heart rate of 120 beats per minute. Arterial blood gases are drawn and the nurse reviews the results, expecting to note which finding?
1. A decreased pH and an increased $Paco_2$
2. An increased pH and a decreased $Paco_2$
3. A decreased pH and a decreased HCO_3^-
4. An increased pH and an increased HCO_3^-

57. The nurse is caring for a client having respiratory distress related to an anxiety attack. Recent arterial blood gas values are pH = 7.53, Pao_2 = 72 mm Hg

(72 mm Hg), $Paco_2$ = 32 mm Hg (32 mm Hg), and HCO_3^- = 28 mEq/L (28 mmol/L). Which conclusion about the client should the nurse make?
1. The client has acidotic blood.
2. The client is probably overreacting.
3. The client is fluid volume overloaded.
4. The client is probably hyperventilating.

58. The nurse is caring for a client with diabetic ketoacidosis and documents that the client is experiencing Kussmaul's respirations. Which patterns did the nurse observe? **Select all that apply.**
- ☐ 1. Respirations that are shallow
- ☐ 2. Respirations that are increased in rate
- ☐ 3. Respirations that are abnormally slow
- ☐ 4. Respirations that are abnormally deep
- ☐ 5. Respirations that cease for several seconds

59. A client who is found unresponsive has arterial blood gases drawn and the results indicate the following: pH is 7.12, $Paco_2$ is 90 mm Hg (90 mm Hg), and HCO_3^- is 22 mEq/L (22 mmol/L). The nurse interprets the results as indicating which condition?
1. Metabolic acidosis with compensation
2. Respiratory acidosis with compensation
3. Metabolic acidosis without compensation
4. Respiratory acidosis without compensation

60. The nurse notes that a client's arterial blood gas (ABG) results reveal a pH of 7.50 and a $Paco_2$ of 30 mm Hg (30 mm Hg). The nurse monitors the client for which clinical manifestations associated with these ABG results? **Select all that apply.**
- ☐ 1. Nausea
- ☐ 2. Confusion
- ☐ 3. Bradypnea
- ☐ 4. Tachycardia
- ☐ 5. Hyperkalemia
- ☐ 6. Lightheadedness

61. The nurse reviews the blood gas results of a client with atelectasis. The nurse analyzes the results and determines that the client is experiencing respiratory acidosis. Which result validates the nurse's findings?
1. pH 7.25, $Paco_2$ 50 mm Hg (50 mm Hg)
2. pH 7.35, $Paco_2$ 40 mm Hg (40 mm Hg)
3. pH 7.50, $Paco_2$ 52 mm Hg (52 mm Hg)
4. pH 7.52, $Paco_2$ 28 mm Hg (28 mm Hg)

62. The nurse is caring for a client who is on a mechanical ventilator. Blood gas results indicate a pH of 7.50 and a $Paco_2$ of 30 mm Hg (30 mm Hg). The nurse has determined that the client is experiencing respiratory alkalosis. Which laboratory value would **most likely** be noted in this condition?
1. Sodium level of 145 mEq/L (145 mmol/L)
2. Potassium level of 3.0 mEq/L (3.0 mmol/L)
3. Magnesium level of 1.8 (0.74 mmol/L)
4. Phosphorus level of 3.0 mg/dL (0.97 mmol/L)

63. The nurse is caring for a client with several broken ribs. The client is **most likely** to experience what type of acid-base imbalance?
1. Respiratory acidosis from inadequate ventilation
2. Respiratory alkalosis from anxiety and hyperventilation
3. Metabolic acidosis from calcium loss due to broken bones
4. Metabolic alkalosis from taking analgesics containing base products

ANSWERS

54. *Answer:* 2

Rationale: The normal pH is 7.35 to 7.45. In a respiratory condition, an opposite effect will be seen between the pH and the $Paco_2$. In this situation, the pH is at the high end of the normal value and the Pco_2 is low. In an alkalotic condition, the pH is elevated. Therefore, the values identified in the question indicate a respiratory alkalosis that is compensated by the kidneys through the renal excretion of bicarbonate. Because the pH has returned to a normal value, compensation has occurred.

Test-Taking Strategy: Focus on the data in the question, noting the arterial blood gas results. Remember that in a respiratory imbalance you will find an opposite response between the pH and the Pco_2 as indicated in the question. Therefore, you can eliminate the options reflective of a primary metabolic problem. Also, remember that the pH increases in an alkalotic condition and compensation can be evidenced by a normal pH. The correct option reflects a respiratory alkalotic condition and compensation and describes the blood gas values as indicated in the question.

Level of Cognitive Ability: Analyzing
Client Needs: Physiological Integrity
Integrated Process: Nursing Process—Assessment
Content Area: Foundations of Care: Acid-Base
Health Problem: N/A
Priority Concepts: Acid-Base Balance; Clinical Judgment
Reference: Lewis et al. (2017), p. 288.

55. *Answer:* 2

Rationale: *Metabolic alkalosis* is defined as a deficit or loss of hydrogen ions or acids or an excess of base (bicarbonate) that results from the accumulation of base or from a loss of acid without a comparable loss of base in the body fluids. This occurs in conditions resulting in hypovolemia, the loss of gastric fluid, excessive bicarbonate intake, the massive transfusion of

whole blood, and hyperaldosteronism. Loss of gastric fluid via nasogastric suction or vomiting causes metabolic alkalosis as a result of the loss of hydrochloric acid. The remaining options are incorrect interpretations.
Test-Taking Strategy: Focus on the data in the question, a client with a nasogastric tube attached to suction. Remembering that a client receiving nasogastric suction loses hydrochloric acid will direct you to the option identifying an alkalotic condition. Because the question addresses a situation other than a respiratory one, the acid-base disorder would be a metabolic condition.
Level of Cognitive Ability: Analyzing
Client Needs: Physiological Integrity
Integrated Process: Nursing Process—Assessment
Content Area: Foundations of Care: Acid-Base
Health Problem: Adult Health: Gastrointestinal: Upper GI Disorder
Priority Concepts: Acid-Base Balance; Clinical Judgment
Reference: Ignatavicius, Workman, Rebar (2018), p. 196.

56. *Answer:* 4
Rationale: Clients experiencing nausea and vomiting would most likely present with metabolic alkalosis resulting from loss of gastric acid, thus causing the pH and HCO_3^- to increase. Symptoms experienced by the client would include a decrease in the respiratory rate and depth, and tachycardia. Option 1 reflects a respiratory acidotic condition. Option 2 reflects a respiratory alkalotic condition, and option 3 reflects a metabolic acidotic condition.
Test-Taking Strategy: Focus on the subject, expected arterial blood gas findings. Note the data in the question and that the client is vomiting. Recalling that vomiting most likely causes metabolic alkalosis will assist in directing you to the correct option.
Level of Cognitive Ability: Synthesizing
Client Needs: Physiological Integrity
Integrated Process: Nursing Process—Assessment
Content Area: Foundations of Care: Acid-Base
Health Problem: Adult Health: Gastrointestinal: Upper GI Disorder
Priority Concepts: Acid-Base Balance; Clinical Judgment
Reference: Lewis et al. (2017), p. 288.

57. *Answer:* 4
Rationale: The ABG values are abnormal, which supports a physiological problem. The ABGs indicate respiratory alkalosis as a result of hyperventilating, not acidosis. Concluding that the client is overreacting is an inaccurate analysis. No conclusion can be made about a client's fluid volume status from the information provided.
Test-Taking Strategy: Focus on the data in the question. Note the ABG values and use knowledge to interpret them. Note that the pH is elevated and the $Paco_2$ is decreased from normal. This will assist you in determining that the client is experiencing respiratory alkalosis. Next, think about the causes of respiratory alkalosis to answer correctly.
Level of Cognitive Ability: Analyzing
Client Needs: Physiological Integrity
Integrated Process: Nursing Process—Analysis
Content Area: Foundations of Care: Acid-Base
Health Problem: Mental Health: Anxiety Disorder
Priority Concepts: Acid-Base Balance; Clinical Judgment
Reference: Lewis et al. (2017), p. 288.

58. *Answer:* 2, 4
Rationale: Kussmaul's respirations are abnormally deep and increased in rate. These occur as a result of the compensatory action by the lungs. In bradypnea, respirations are regular but abnormally slow. Apnea is described as respirations that cease for several seconds.
Test-Taking Strategy: Focus on the subject, the characteristics of Kussmaul's respirations. Use knowledge of the description of Kussmaul's respirations. Recalling that this type of respiration occurs in diabetic ketoacidosis will assist you in answering correctly.
Level of Cognitive Ability: Applying
Client Needs: Physiological Integrity
Integrated Process: Nursing Process—Assessment
Content Area: Foundations of Care: Acid-Base
Health Problem: Adult Health: Endocrine: Diabetes Mellitus
Priority Concepts: Acid-Base Balance; Glucose Regulation
Reference: Lewis et al. (2017), pp. 467, 1144.

59. *Answer:* 4
Rationale: The acid-base disturbance is respiratory acidosis without compensation. The normal pH is 7.35 to 7.45. The normal $Paco_2$ is 35 to 45 mm Hg (35 to 45 mm Hg). In respiratory acidosis the pH is decreased and the Pco_2 is elevated. The normal bicarbonate HCO_3^-) level is 21 to 28 mEq/L (21 to 28 mmol/L). Because the bicarbonate is still within normal limits, the kidneys have not had time to adjust for this acid-base disturbance. In addition, the pH is not within normal limits. Therefore, the condition is without compensation. The remaining options are incorrect interpretations.
Test-Taking Strategy: Focus on the data in the question and the subject, interpretation of arterial blood gas results. Remember that in a respiratory imbalance you will find an opposite response between the pH and the $Paco_2$. Also, remember that the pH is decreased in an acidotic condition and that compensation is reflected by a normal pH.
Level of Cognitive Ability: Analyzing
Client Needs: Physiological Integrity
Integrated Process: Nursing Process—Assessment
Content Area: Foundations of Care: Acid-Base
Health Problem: N/A
Priority Concepts: Acid-Base Balance; Clinical Judgment
Reference: Lewis et al. (2017), pp. 291, 457.

60. *Answer:* 1, 2, 4, 6
Rationale: Respiratory alkalosis is defined as a deficit of carbonic acid or a decrease in hydrogen ion concentration that results from the accumulation of base or from a loss of acid without a comparable loss of base in the body fluids. This occurs in conditions that cause overstimulation of the respiratory system. Clinical manifestations of respiratory alkalosis include lethargy, lightheadedness, confusion, tachycardia, dysrhythmias related to hypokalemia, nausea, vomiting, epigastric pain, and numbness and tingling of the extremities. Hyperventilation (tachypnea) occurs. Bradypnea describes respirations that are regular but abnormally slow. Hyperkalemia is associated with acidosis.
Test-Taking Strategy: Focus on the subject, the interpretation of ABG values. Note the data in the question to determine that the client is experiencing respiratory alkalosis. Next, it is necessary to think about the pathophysiology that occurs in this acid-base condition and recall the manifestations that occur.
Level of Cognitive Ability: Analyzing

Client Needs: Physiological Integrity
Integrated Process: Nursing Process—Assessment
Content Area: Foundations of Care: Acid-Base
Health Problem: N/A
Priority Concepts: Acid-Base Balance; Clinical Judgment
Reference: Ignatavicius, Workman, Rebar (2018), pp. 196-197.

61. *Answer:* 1

Rationale: Atelectasis is a condition characterized by the collapse of alveoli, preventing the respiratory exchange of oxygen and carbon dioxide in a part of the lungs. The normal pH is 7.35 to 7.45. The normal $Paco_2$ is 35 to 45 mm Hg (35 to 45 mm Hg). In respiratory acidosis, the pH is decreased and the $Paco_2$ is elevated. Option 2 identifies normal values. Option 3 identifies an alkalotic condition, and option 4 identifies respiratory alkalosis.

Test-Taking Strategy: Focus on the **subject,** the arterial blood gas results in a client with atelectasis. Remember that in a respiratory imbalance you will find an opposite response between the pH and the $Paco_2$. Also, remember that the pH is decreased in an acidotic condition. First eliminate option 2 because it reflects a normal blood gas result. Options 3 and 4 identify an elevated pH, indicating an alkalotic condition. The correct option is the only one that reflects an acidotic condition.

Level of Cognitive Ability: Analyzing
Client Needs: Physiological Integrity
Integrated Process: Nursing Process—Assessment
Content Area: Foundations of Care: Acid-Base
Health Problem: N/A
Priority Concepts: Acid-Base Balance; Clinical Judgment
Reference: Lewis et al. (2017), p. 288.

62. *Answer:* 2

Rationale: Respiratory alkalosis is defined as a deficit of carbonic acid or a decrease in hydrogen ion concentration that results from the accumulation of base or from a loss of acid without a comparable loss of base in the body fluids. This occurs in conditions that cause overstimulation of the respiratory system. Some clinical manifestations of respiratory alkalosis include lightheadedness, confusion, tachycardia, dysrhythmias related to hypokalemia, nausea, vomiting, diarrhea, epigastric pain, and numbness and tingling of the extremities. All three incorrect options identify normal laboratory values. The correct option identifies the presence of hypokalemia.

Test-Taking Strategy: Note the **strategic words,** *most likely.* Focus on the **data in the question** and use knowledge about the interpretation of arterial blood gas values to determine that the client is experiencing respiratory alkalosis. Next, recall the manifestations that occur in this condition and the normal laboratory values. The only abnormal laboratory value is the potassium level, the correct option.

Level of Cognitive Ability: Analyzing
Client Needs: Physiological Integrity
Integrated Process: Nursing Process—Assessment
Content Area: Foundations of Care: Acid-Base
Health Problem: N/A
Priority Concepts: Acid-Base Balance; Clinical Judgment
Reference: Ignatavicius, Workman, Rebar (2018), pp. 195-196.

63. *Answer:* 1

Rationale: Respiratory acidosis is most often caused by hypoventilation. The client with broken ribs will have difficulty with breathing adequately and is at risk for hypoventilation and resultant respiratory acidosis. The remaining options are incorrect. Respiratory alkalosis is associated with hyperventilation. There are no data in the question that indicate calcium loss or that the client is taking analgesics containing base products.

Test-Taking Strategy: Note the **strategic words**, *most likely.* Focus on the **data in the question.** Think about the location of the ribs to determine that the client will have difficulty breathing adequately. This will assist in directing you to the correct option. Remembering that hypoventilation results in respiratory acidosis will direct you to the correct option.

Level of Cognitive Ability: Analyzing
Client Needs: Physiological Integrity
Integrated Process: Nursing Process—Assessment
Content Area: Foundations of Care: Acid-Base
Health Problem: Adult Health: Respiratory: Chest Injuries
Priority Concepts: Acid-Base Balance; Clinical Judgment
Reference: Lewis et al. (2017), p. 288.

CHAPTER 10

Vital Signs and Laboratory Reference Intervals

PRIORITY CONCEPTS Cellular Regulation; Perfusion

I. Vital Signs

A. Description: Vital signs include temperature, pulse, respirations, blood pressure (BP), oxygen saturation (pulse oximetry), and pain assessment.

B. Guidelines for measuring vital signs

1. Initial measurement of vital signs provides baseline data on a client's health status and is used to help identify changes in the client's health status.
2. Some vital sign measurements (temperature, pulse, respirations, BP, pulse oximetry) may be delegated to assistive personnel (AP), but the nurse is responsible for interpreting the findings.
3. The nurse collaborates with the primary health care provider (PHCP) in determining the frequency of vital sign assessment and also makes independent decisions regarding their frequency on the basis of the client's status.

The nurse ensures that vital sign measurements are documented correctly and always reports abnormal findings to the PHCP.

C. When vital signs are measured

1. On initial contact with a client (e.g., when a client is admitted to a health care facility)
2. During physical assessment of a client
3. Before and after an invasive diagnostic procedure or surgical procedure
4. During the administration of medication that affects the cardiac, respiratory, or temperature-controlling functions (e.g., in a client who has a fever); may be required before, during, and after administration of the medication
5. Before, during, and after a blood transfusion
6. Whenever a client's condition changes or the client verbalizes unusual feelings such as nonspecific symptoms of physical distress (i.e., feeling funny or different)
7. Whenever an intervention (e.g., ambulation) may affect a client's condition
8. When a fever or known infection is present (check vital signs every 2 to 4 hours)

II. Temperature

A. Description

1. Normal body temperature ranges from 36.4° to 37.5° Celsius (C) (97.5° to 99.5° Fahrenheit [F]); the average in a healthy young adult is 37.0° C (98.6° F).
2. Common measurement sites are the mouth, rectum (unless contraindicated), axilla, ear, and across the forehead (temporal artery site); various types of electronic measuring devices are commonly used to measure temperature.
3. Rectal temperatures are usually 1° F (0.5° C) higher and tympanic and axillary temperatures about 1° F (0.5° C) lower than the normal oral temperature.
4. Know how to convert a temperature to a Fahrenheit or Celsius value (Box 10-1).

B. Nursing considerations

1. Time of day
   a. Temperature is generally in the low-normal range at the time of awakening as a result of muscle inactivity.
   b. Afternoon body temperature may be high-normal as a result of the metabolic process, activity, and environmental temperature.
2. Environmental temperature: Body temperature is lower in cold weather and higher in warm weather.
3. Age: Temperature may fluctuate during the first year of life because the infant's heat-regulating mechanism is not fully developed.
4. Physical exercise: Use of the large muscles creates heat, causing an increase in body temperature.
5. Menstrual cycle: Temperature decreases slightly just before ovulation but may increase to 1° F above normal during ovulation.
6. Pregnancy: Body temperature may consistently stay at high-normal because of an increase in the woman's metabolic rate.

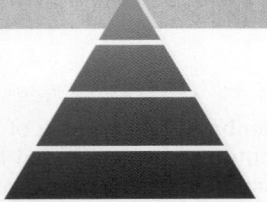

BOX 10-1 Body Temperature Conversion

To convert Fahrenheit to Celsius: Degrees Fahrenheit − 32 × 5/9 = Degrees Celsius
Example: 98.2° F − 32 × 5/9 = 36.7° C
To convert Celsius to Fahrenheit: Degrees Celsius × 9/5 + 32 = Degrees Fahrenheit
Example: 38.6° C × 9/5 + 32 = 101.5° F

7. Stress: Emotions increase hormonal secretion, leading to increased heat production and a higher temperature.
8. Illness: Infective agents and the inflammatory response may cause an increase in temperature.
9. The inability to obtain a temperature should not be ignored, because it could represent a condition of hypothermia, a life-threatening condition in very young and older clients.

C. Methods of measurement
1. Oral
   a. If the client has recently consumed hot or cold foods or liquids or has smoked or chewed gum, the nurse must wait 15 to 30 minutes before taking the temperature orally.
   b. The thermometer is placed under the tongue in one of the posterior sublingual pockets; ask the client to keep the tongue down and the lips closed and to not bite down on the thermometer.
2. Rectal
   a. Place the client in the Sims' position.
   b. The temperature is taken rectally when an accurate temperature cannot be obtained orally or via other methods including by an electronic method, or when the client has nasal congestion, has undergone nasal or oral surgery or had the jaws wired, has a nasogastric tube in place, is unable to keep the mouth closed, or is at risk for seizures.
   c. The thermometer is lubricated and inserted into the rectum, toward the umbilicus, about 1.5 inches (3.8 cm) (no more than 0.5 inch [1.25 cm] in an infant).

The temperature is not taken rectally in cardiac clients; the client who has undergone rectal surgery; or the client with diarrhea, fecal impaction, or rectal bleeding or who is at risk for bleeding.

3. Axillary
   a. This method of taking the temperature is used when the oral or other methods of temperature measurement are contraindicated.
   b. Axillary measurement is not as accurate as the oral, rectal, tympanic, or temporal artery method but is used when other methods of measurement are not possible.
   c. The thermometer is placed in the client's dry axilla, and the client is asked to hold the arm tightly against the chest, resting the arm on the chest; follow the instructions accompanying the measurement device for the amount of time the thermometer should remain in the axillary area.
4. Tympanic
   a. The auditory canal is checked for the presence of redness, swelling, discharge, or a foreign body before the probe is inserted; the probe should not be inserted if the client has an inflammatory condition of the auditory canal or if there is discharge from the ear.
   b. The reading may be affected by an ear infection or excessive wax blocking the ear canal.
5. Temporal artery
   a. Ensure that the client's forehead is dry.
   b. The thermometer probe is placed flush against the skin and slid across the forehead or placed in the area of the temporal artery and held in place.
   c. If the client is diaphoretic, the temporal artery thermometer probe may be placed on the neck, just behind the earlobe.

III. Pulse

A. Description
1. Pulse is a palpable bounding of blood flow in a peripheral artery; it is an indirect indicator of circulatory status.
2. The average adult pulse (heart) rate is 60 to 100 beats per minute.
3. Changes in pulse rate are used to evaluate the client's tolerance of interventions such as ambulation, bathing, dressing, and exercise.
4. Pedal pulses are checked to determine whether the circulation is blocked in the artery up to that pulse point.
5. When the pedal pulse is difficult to locate, a Doppler ultrasound stethoscope (ultrasonic stethoscope) may be needed to amplify the sounds of pulse waves.

B. Nursing considerations
1. The heart rate slows with age.
2. Exercise increases the heart rate.
3. Emotions stimulate the sympathetic nervous system, increasing the heart rate.
4. Pain increases the heart rate.
5. Increased body temperature causes the heart rate to increase.

6. Stimulant medications increase the heart rate; depressants and medications affecting the cardiac system slow it.
7. When the BP is low, the heart rate is usually increased.
8. Hemorrhage increases the heart rate.

C. Assessing pulse qualities
1. When the pulse is being counted, note the rate, rhythm, strength (force or amplitude), and equality.
2. Once you have checked these parameters, use the grading scale for pulses to assess the information you have elicited (Box 10-2).

D. Pulse points and locations
1. The temporal artery can be palpated anterior to or in the front of the ear.
2. The carotid artery is located in the groove between the trachea and the sternocleidomastoid muscle, medial to and alongside the muscle.
3. The apical pulse may be detected at the left midclavicular, fifth intercostal space.
4. The brachial pulse is located above the elbow at the antecubital fossa, between the biceps and triceps muscles.
5. The radial pulse is located in the groove along the radial or thumb side of the client's inner wrist.
6. The ulnar pulse is located on the medial side of the wrist (little finger side of the forearm at the wrist).
7. The femoral pulse is located below the inguinal ligament, midway between the symphysis pubis and the anterosuperior iliac spine.
8. The popliteal pulse is located behind the knee.
9. The posterior tibial pulse is located on the inner side of the ankle, behind and below the medial malleolus (ankle bone).
10. The dorsalis pedis pulse is located on the top of the foot, in line with the groove between the extensor tendons of the great and first toes.

⚠ The apical pulse is counted for 1 full minute and is assessed in clients with an irregular radial pulse or a heart condition, before the administration of cardiac medications such as digoxin and beta blockers, and in children younger than 2 years.

BOX 10-2 Grading Scale for Pulses

4 + = Strong and bounding
3 + = Full pulse, increased
2 + = Normal, easily palpable
1 + = Weak, barely palpable
0 = Absent, not palpable

E. Pulse deficit
1. In this condition, the peripheral pulse rate (radial pulse) is less than the ventricular contraction rate (apical pulse).
2. A pulse deficit indicates a lack of peripheral perfusion; it can be an indication of cardiac dysrhythmias.
3. One-examiner technique: Auscultate and count the apical pulse first and then immediately count the radial pulse.
4. Two-examiner technique: One person counts the apical pulse and the other counts the radial pulse simultaneously.
5. A pulse deficit indicates that cardiac contractions are ineffective, failing to send pulse waves to the periphery.
6. If a difference in pulse rate is noted, the PHCP is notified.

IV. Respirations

A. Description
1. Respiration is a mechanism the body uses to exchange gases between the atmosphere and the blood and between the blood and the cells.
2. Respiratory rates vary with age.
3. The normal adult respiratory rate is 12 to 20 breaths per minute.

B. Nursing considerations
1. Many of the factors that affect the pulse rate also affect the respiratory rate.
2. An increased level of carbon dioxide or a lower level of oxygen in the blood results in an increase in respiratory rate.
3. Head injury or increased intracranial pressure will depress the respiratory center in the brain, resulting in shallow respirations or slowed breathing.
4. Medications such as opioid analgesics depress respirations.
5. Additional factors that can affect the respiratory rate include exercise, pain, anxiety, smoking, and body position.

C. Assessing respiratory rate
1. Count the client's respirations after measuring the radial pulse. (Continue holding the client's wrist while counting the respirations or position the hand on the client's chest.)
2. One respiration includes both inspiration and expiration.
3. The rate, depth, pattern, and sounds are assessed.

⚠ The respiratory rate may be counted for 30 seconds and multiplied by 2, except in a client who is known to be very ill or is exhibiting irregular respirations, in which case respirations are counted for 1 full minute.

V. Blood Pressure

A. Description

1. Blood pressure (BP) is the force on the walls of an artery exerted by the pulsating blood under pressure from the heart.
2. The heart's contraction forces blood under high pressure into the aorta; the peak of maximum pressure when ejection occurs is the systolic pressure; the blood remaining in the arteries when the ventricles relax exerts a force known as the *diastolic pressure.*
3. The difference between the systolic and diastolic pressures is called the *pulse pressure.*
4. For an adult (age 18 years and older), a normal BP is a systolic pressure below 120 mm Hg and a diastolic pressure below 80 mm Hg.
5. Categories of hypertension (Box 10-3).

BOX 10-3 Hypertension Categories and Guidelines

Categories

Normal: Less than 120/80 mm Hg

Elevated: Systolic between 120-129 mm Hg *and* diastolic less than 80 mm Hg

Stage 1: Systolic between 130-139 mm Hg *or* diastolic between 80-89 mm Hg

Stage 2: Systolic at least 140 mm Hg *or* diastolic at least 90 mm Hg

Hypertensive crisis: Systolic over 180 mm Hg and/or diastolic over 120 mm Hg, with clients needing prompt changes in medication if there are no other indications of problems, or immediate hospitalization if there are signs of organ damage.

Guidelines

- Using proper technique to measure blood pressure.
- Use of home blood pressure monitoring using validated devices.
- Appropriate training of health care providers to reveal *white-coat hypertension.*
- Only prescribing medication for stage I hypertension if a client has already had a cardiovascular event such as a heart attack or stroke or is at high risk for heart attack or stroke based on age, the presence of diabetes mellitus, chronic kidney disease, or calculation of atherosclerotic risk (using the same risk calculator used in evaluating high cholesterol).
- Recognizing that many people will need two or more types of medications to control their blood pressure, and that people may take their pills more consistently if multiple medications are combined into a single pill.
- Identifying socioeconomic status and psychosocial stress as risk factors for high blood pressure that should be considered in a client's plan of care.

From American College of Cardiology, 2017, New ACC/AHA High Blood Pressure Guidelines Lower Definition of Hypertension. http://www.acc.org/latest-in-cardiology/articles/2017/11/08/11/47/mon-5pm-bp-guideline-aha-2017

6. In postural (orthostatic) hypotension, a normotensive client exhibits symptoms and low BP on rising to an upright position.
7. To obtain orthostatic vital sign measurements, check the BP and pulse with the client supine, sitting, and standing; readings are obtained 1 to 3 minutes after the client changes position.

B. Nursing considerations

1. Factors affecting BP
   - **a.** BP tends to increase as the aging process progresses.
   - **b.** Stress results in sympathetic stimulation that increases the BP.
   - **c.** The incidence of high BP is higher among African Americans than among Americans of European descent.
   - **d.** Antihypertensive medications and opioid analgesics can decrease BP.
   - **e.** BP is typically lowest in the early morning, gradually increases during the day, and peaks in the late afternoon and evening.
   - **f.** After puberty, males tend to have higher BP than females; after menopause, women tend to have higher BP than men of the same age.
   - **g.** Additional factors affecting the BP include smoking, activity, and body weight.
2. Guidelines for measuring BP
   - **a.** Determine the best site for assessment.
   - **b.** Avoid applying a cuff to an extremity into which intravenous (IV) fluids are infusing, where an arteriovenous shunt or fistula is present, on the side on which breast or axillary surgery has been performed, or on an extremity that has been traumatized or is diseased.
   - **c.** The leg may be used if the brachial artery is inaccessible; the cuff is wrapped around the thigh and the stethoscope is placed over the popliteal artery.
   - **d.** Ensure that the client has not smoked or exercised in the 30 minutes before measurement, because both activities can yield falsely high readings.
   - **e.** Have the client assume a sitting (with feet flat on floor) or lying position and then rest for 5 minutes before the measurement; ask the client not to speak during the measurement.
   - **f.** Ensure that the cuff is fully deflated, then wrap it evenly and snugly around the extremity.
   - **g.** Ensure that the stethoscope being used fits the examiner and does not impair hearing.
   - **h.** Document the first Korotkoff sound at phase 1 (heard as the blood pulsates through the vessel when air is released from the BP cuff and pressure on the artery is reduced) as the systolic pressure, and the beginning of the fifth Korotkoff sound at phase 5 as the diastolic pressure.

i. BP readings obtained electronically with a vital sign monitoring machine should be checked with a manual cuff if there is any concern about the accuracy of the reading.

When taking a BP, select the appropriate cuff size; a cuff that is too small will yield a falsely high reading, and a cuff that is too large will yield a falsely low one.

VI. Pulse Oximetry

A. Description

1. Pulse oximetry is a noninvasive test that registers the oxygen saturation of the client's hemoglobin.
2. The capillary oxygen saturation (Sao_2) is recorded as a percentage.
3. The normal value is 95% to 100%.
4. After a hypoxic client uses up the readily available oxygen (measured as the arterial oxygen pressure, Pao_2, on arterial blood gas [ABG] testing), the reserve oxygen—that is, oxygen attached to the hemoglobin (Sao_2)—is drawn on to provide oxygen to the tissues.
5. A pulse oximeter reading can alert the nurse to hypoxemia before clinical signs occur.
6. If pulse oximetry readings are below normal, instruct the client in deep breathing technique and recheck the pulse oximetry.

B. Nursing Considerations

1. A vascular, pulsatile area, such as the fingertip or earlobe, is needed to detect the degree of change in the transmitted light that measures the oxygenated and deoxygenated hemoglobin.
2. Factors that affect light transmission also affect the measurement of SpO_2.
3. Some factors that affect light transmission can include sensor movement, fingernail polish, hypotension, anemia, or peripheral vascular disorders.

C. Procedure

1. A sensor is placed on the client's finger, toe, nose, earlobe, or forehead to measure oxygen saturation, which then is displayed on a monitor.
2. Do not select an extremity with an impediment to blood flow.

A usual pulse oximetry reading is between 95% and 100%. A pulse oximetry reading lower than 90% necessitates PHCP notification; values below 90% are acceptable only in certain chronic conditions. Agency procedures and PHCP prescriptions are followed regarding actions to take for specific readings.

VII. Pain

A. Types of pain

1. Acute/transient pain: Usually associated with an injury, medical condition, or surgical procedure; lasts hours to a few days
2. Chronic/persistent noncancer pain: Usually associated with long-term or chronic illnesses or disorders; may continue for months or even years
3. Chronic/episodic pain: Occurs sporadically over an extended period of time. Pain episodes last for hours, days, or weeks. Examples are migraine headaches and pain related to sickle cell crisis.
4. Cancer pain: Not all people with cancer have pain. Some have acute and/or chronic pain. Cancer pain is usually caused by tumor progression and related pathological processes, invasive procedures, treatment toxicities, infection, and physical limitations.
5. Idiopathic pain: This is a chronic pain in the absence of an identifiable physical or psychological cause or pain perceived as excessive for the extent of an organic pathological condition.

B. Assessment

1. Pain is a highly individual experience.
2. Ask the client to describe pain in terms of timing, location, severity, quality, aggravating and precipitating factors, and relief measures.
3. Ask the client about the use of complementary and alternative therapies to alleviate pain.
4. Pain experienced by the older client may be manifested differently than pain experienced by members of other age groups (e.g., sleep disturbances, changes in gait and mobility, decreased socialization, depression).
5. Clients with cognitive disorders (e.g., a client with dementia, a comatose client) may not be able to describe their pain experiences.
6. The nurse should be alert to nonverbal indicators of pain (Box 10-4).
7. Ask the client to use a number-based pain scale (a picture-based scale may be used in children or clients who cannot verbally describe their pain) to rate the degree of pain (Fig. 10-1).
8. Evaluate client response to nonpharmacological interventions.

BOX 10-4 Nonverbal Indicators of Pain

- Moaning
- Crying
- Irritability
- Restlessness
- Grimacing or frowning
- Inability to sleep
- Rigid posture
- Increased blood pressure, heart rate, or respiratory rate
- Nausea
- Diaphoresis
- Use of the FLACC® (face, legs, activity, cry, consolability) scale or FACES® pain scale are appropriate in clients who cannot communicate their pain verbally.

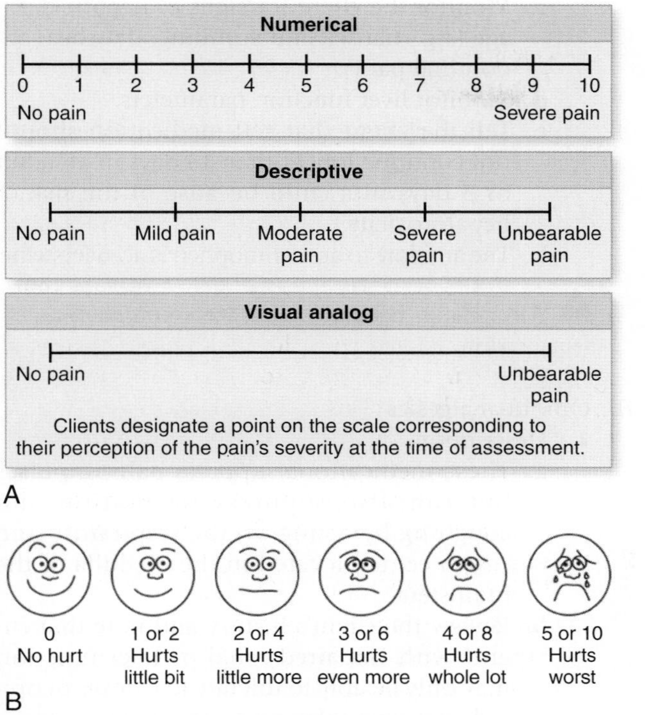

FIG. 10-1 Pain assessment scales. **A,** Numerical, descriptive, and visual analog scales. **B,** Wong-Baker FACES® Pain Rating Scale. (**B,** Copyright 1983, Wong-Baker FACES® Foundation, www.WongBakerFACES.org. Used with permission. Originally published in *Whaley & Wong's Nursing Care of Infants and Children*. ©Elsevier Inc.)

Consider the client's culture and spiritual and religious beliefs in assessing pain; some cultures frown on the outward expression of pain.

C. Conventional nonpharmacological interventions

1. Cutaneous stimulation

a. Techniques include heat, cold, and pressure and vibration. Therapeutic touch and massage are also cutaneous stimulation and may be considered complementary and alternative techniques.

b. Such treatments may require a PHCP's prescription.

2. Transcutaneous electrical nerve stimulation (TENS)

a. TENS is also referred to as *percutaneous electrical nerve stimulation (PENS)*.

b. This technique, which may require a PHCP's prescription, involves the application of a battery-operated device that delivers a low electrical current to the skin and underlying tissues to block pain (some similar units can be purchased without a prescription).

3. Binders, slings, and other supportive devices

a. Cloths or other materials or devices, wrapped around a limb or body part, can ease the pain of strains, sprains, and surgical incisions.

b. Some devices may require a PHCP's prescription.

c. Elevation of the affected body part is another intervention that can reduce swelling; supporting an extremity on a pillow may lessen discomfort.

4. Heat and cold

a. The application of heat and cold or alternating application of the two can soothe pain resulting from muscle strain; cold reduces swelling.

b. In some conditions, such treatment may require a PHCP's prescription.

c. Heat applications may include warm-water compresses, warm blankets, thermal pads, and tub and whirlpool baths.

d. The temperature of the application must be monitored carefully to help prevent burns; the skin of very young and older clients is extra sensitive to heat.

e. The client should be advised to remove the source of heat or cold if changes in sensation or discomfort occur. If the change in sensation or discomfort is not relieved after removal of the application, the PHCP should be notified.

Ice or heat should be applied with a towel or other barrier between the pack and the skin but should not be left in place for more than 15 to 30 minutes.

D. Complementary and alternative therapies

1. Description: Therapies are used in addition to conventional treatment to provide healing resources and focus on the mind-body connection (Box 10-5).

2. Nursing considerations

a. Some complementary and alternative therapies require a PHCP's prescription.

BOX 10-5 Complementary and Alternative Therapies

Acupuncture and acupressure
Biofeedback
Chiropractic manipulation
Distraction techniques
Guided imagery and meditation techniques
Herbal therapies
Hypnosis
Laughter and humor
Massage
Relaxation and repositioning techniques
Spiritual measures (e.g., prayer, use of a rosary or prayer beads, reading of scripture)
Therapeutic touch

b. Herbal remedies are considered pharmacological therapy by some PHCPs; because of the risk for interaction with prescription medications, it is important that the nurse ask the client about the use of such therapies.
c. If cultural or spiritual measures are to be employed, the nurse must elicit from the client the preferred forms of spiritual expression and learn when they are practiced so that they may be integrated into the plan of care.

VIII. Pharmacological Interventions

A. Nonopioid analgesics

1. Nonsteroidal antiinflammatory drugs (NSAIDs) and acetylsalicylic acid (aspirin) (Box 10-6)

a. These medication types are contraindicated if the client has gastric irritation or ulcer disease or an allergy to the medication.
b. Bleeding is a concern with the use of these medication types.
c. Instruct the client to take oral doses with milk or a snack to reduce gastric irritation.
d. NSAIDs can amplify the effects of anticoagulants.
e. Hypoglycemia may result for the client taking ibuprofen if the client is concurrently taking an oral antidiabetic agent.
f. A high risk of toxicity exists if the client is taking ibuprofen concurrently with a calcium channel blocker.

2. Acetaminophen

a. Acetaminophen, commonly known as Tylenol, is contraindicated in clients with hepatic or renal disease, alcoholism, or hypersensitivity.
b. Assess the client for a history of liver dysfunction.

BOX 10-6 Side and Adverse Effects of NSAIDs and Acetylsalicylic Acid

NSAIDs

- Gastric irritation
- Hypotension
- Sodium and water retention
- Blood dyscrasias
- Dizziness
- Tinnitus
- Pruritus

Acetylsalicylic Acid

- Gastric irritation
- Flushing
- Tinnitus
- Drowsiness
- Headaches
- Vision changes

c. Monitor the client for signs of hepatic damage (e.g., nausea and vomiting, diarrhea, abdominal pain).
d. Monitor liver function parameters.
e. Tell the client that self-medication should not continue longer than 10 days in an adult or 5 days in a child because of the risk of hepatotoxicity.
f. The antidote to acetaminophen is acetylcysteine.

⚠ The major concern with acetaminophen is hepatotoxicity.

B. Opioid analgesics

1. Description

a. These medications suppress pain impulses but can also suppress respiration and coughing by acting on the respiratory and cough center, located in the medulla of the brainstem.
b. Review the client's history and note that clients with impaired renal or liver function may only be able to tolerate low doses of opioid analgesics; also assess for allergy.
c. Intravenous route administration produces a faster effect than other routes, but the effect lasts shorter to relieve pain.
d. Opioids, which produce euphoria and sedation, can cause physical dependence.
e. Administer the medication 30 to 60 minutes before painful activities.
f. Monitor the respiratory rate; if it is slower than 12 breaths per minute in an adult, withhold the medication and notify the PHCP.
g. Monitor the pulse; if bradycardia develops, withhold the medication and notify the PHCP.
h. Monitor the BP for hypotension and assess before administering pain medications to decrease the risk of adverse effects.
i. Auscultate the lungs for normal breath sounds.
j. Encourage activities such as turning, deep breathing, and incentive spirometry to help prevent atelectasis and pneumonia.
k. Monitor the client's level of consciousness.
l. Initiate safety precautions.
m. Monitor intake and output and assess the client for urine retention; also constipation is common with opioid use.
n. Instruct the client to take oral doses with milk or a snack to reduce gastric irritation.
o. Instruct the client to avoid activities that require alertness.
p. Assess the effectiveness of the medication 30 minutes after administration.

q. Have an opioid antagonist (e.g., naloxone), oxygen, and resuscitation equipment available.
r. In many states, prescriptions for opioid analgesics can be given in only very specific circumstances, and a consent form needs to be obtained from the prescribing provider. Frequent collaboration between the nurse and the provider on continued need for this type of medication should be done.

! An electronic infusion device is always used for continuous or dose-demand IV infusion of opioid analgesics.

2. Codeine sulfate
   a. This medication is also used in low doses as a cough suppressant.
   b. It may cause constipation.
   c. Common medications in this class are hydrocodone and oxycodone (synthetic forms).
3. Hydromorphone
   a. The primary concern is respiration depression.
   b. Other effects include drowsiness, dizziness, and orthostatic hypotension.
   c. Monitor vital signs, especially the respiratory rate and BP.
4. Morphine sulfate
   a. Used to ease acute pain resulting from myocardial infarction or cancer, for dyspnea resulting from pulmonary edema, and as a preoperative medication.
   b. The major concern is respiratory depression, but postural hypotension, urine retention, constipation, and pupillary constriction may also occur; monitor the client for adverse effects.
   c. Morphine may cause nausea and vomiting by increasing vestibular sensitivity.
   d. It is contraindicated in severe respiratory disorders, head injuries, severe renal disease, or seizure activity and in the presence of increased intracranial pressure.
   e. Monitor the client for urine retention.
   f. Monitor bowel sounds for decreased peristalsis; constipation may occur.
   g. Monitor the pupil for changes; pinpoint pupils may indicate overdose.

IX. Laboratory Reference Intervals

For reference throughout the chapter, see Fig. 10-2.

A. Methods for drawing blood (Table 10-1)

B. Serum sodium
   1. A major cation of extracellular fluid
   2. Maintains osmotic pressure and acid-base balance, and assists in the transmission of nerve impulses
   3. Is absorbed from the small intestine and excreted in the urine in amounts dependent on dietary intake
   4. Normal reference interval: 135 to 145 mEq/L (135 to 145 mmol/L)
   5. Elevated values occur in the following: dehydration, impaired renal function, increased dietary or IV intake of sodium, primary aldosteronism, use of corticosteroid therapy

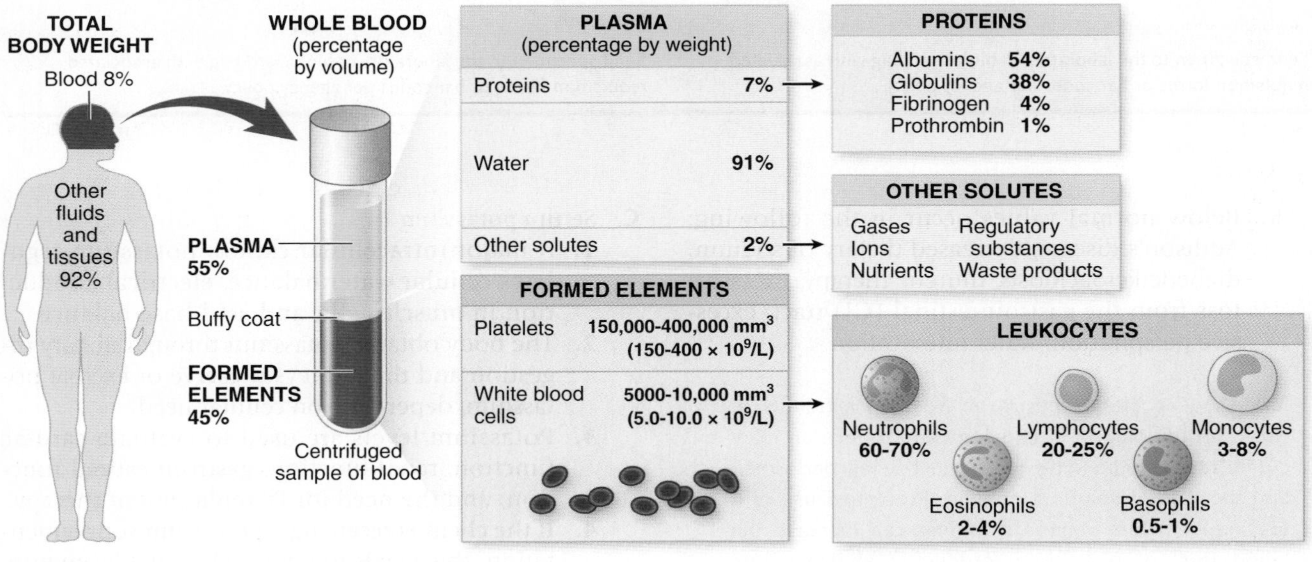

FIG. 10-2 Approximate values for the components of blood in a normal adult.

TABLE 10-1 Obtaining a Blood Sample

Peripheral Intravenous Line	Central Intravenous Line
Check PHCP's prescription. A blood sample may be drawn from a peripheral line on insertion, but typically not thereafter. Check the agency's policy on this practice.	Check PHCP's prescription.
Identify foods, medications, or other factors such as the type of solution infusing that may affect the procedure or results.	Identify foods, medications, or other factors such as the type of solution infusing that may affect the procedure or results.
Gather needed supplies, including gloves, tourniquet, transparent dressing or other type of dressing, tape, 2- by 2-inch gauze, antiseptic agent, extension set (optional), two 5- or 10-mL normal saline flushes, one empty 5- or 10-mL syringe (depending on the amount of blood needed), transfer/collection device per agency policy, specimen containers per agency policy, alcohol-impregnated intravenous (IV) line end caps, tube labels, biohazard bag, requisition form or bar code per agency policy.	Gather needed supplies, including gloves, transfer/collection device per agency policy, specimen containers per agency policy, two 5- or 10-mL normal saline flushes, one empty 5- or 10-mL syringe (depending on the amount of blood needed), antiseptic swabs, alcohol-impregnated IV line end caps, 2 masks, biohazard bag, requisition form or bar code per agency policy.
Perform hand hygiene. Identify the client with at least 2 accepted identifiers.	Perform hand hygiene. Identify the client with at least 2 accepted identifiers.
Explain the purpose of the test and procedure to the client.	Explain the purpose of the test and procedure to the client.
Prepare extension set if being used by priming with normal saline. Attach syringe to extension set. Place extension set within reach while maintaining aseptic technique and keeping it in the package.	Place mask on self and client or ask client to turn the head away. Stop any running infusions for at least 1 minute.
Apply tourniquet 10 to 15 cm above intravenous site.	Clamp all ports. Scrub port to be used with antiseptic swab.
Apply gloves. Scrub tubing insertion port with antiseptic solution or per agency policy.	Attach 5- or 10-mL normal saline flush and unclamp line. Flush line with appropriate amount per agency policy and withdraw 5-10 mL of blood to discard (per agency policy). Clamp line and detach flush syringe.
Attach 5- or 10-mL normal saline flush and unclamp line. Flush line with appropriate amount per agency policy and withdraw 5-10 mL of blood to discard (per agency policy). Clamp line and detach flush syringe.	Scrub port with antiseptic swab. Attach 5- or 10-mL syringe or transfer/collection device to port (depending on available equipment), unclamp line, and withdraw needed sample or attach specimen container to withdraw using vacuum system. Clamp line and detach syringe or transfer/collection device.
Scrub tubing insertion port. Attach 5- or 10-mL syringe, extension set, or transfer/collection device to port (depending on available equipment), unclamp line, and withdraw needed sample or attach specimen container to withdraw using vacuum system. Clamp line and detach syringe or transfer/collection device.	Scrub port with antiseptic swab. Attach a 5- or 10-mL normal saline flush. Unclamp line and flush with amount per agency policy. Clamp line, remove flush syringe, and place end cap on IV line. Remove masks.
Remove tourniquet and flush with normal saline to ensure patency.	Transfer specimen to collection device per agency policy and procedure.
Send specimen to the laboratory in biohazard bag with associated requisition forms or bar codes per agency policy.	Send specimen to the laboratory in biohazard bag with associated requisition forms or bar codes per agency policy.

6. Below normal values occur in the following: Addison's disease, decreased dietary of sodium, diabetic ketoacidosis, diuretic therapy, excessive loss from the gastrointestinal (GI) tract, excessive perspiration, water intoxication

⚠ Drawing blood specimens from an extremity in which an IV solution is infusing can produce an inaccurate result, depending on the test being performed and the type of solution infusing. Prolonged use of a tourniquet before venous sampling can increase the blood level of potassium, producing an inaccurate result.

C. Serum **potassium**

1. A major intracellular cation, potassium regulates cellular water balance, electrical conduction in muscle cells, and acid-base balance.
2. The body obtains potassium through dietary ingestion and the kidneys preserve or excrete potassium, depending on cellular need.
3. Potassium levels are used to evaluate cardiac function, renal function, gastrointestinal function, and the need for IV replacement therapy.
4. If the client is receiving a potassium supplementation, this needs to be noted on the laboratory form.

5. Normal reference interval: 3.5 to 5.0 mEq/L (3.5 to 5.0 mmol/L)
6. Elevated values occur in the following: acute kidney injury or chronic kidney disease, Addison's disease, dehydration, diabetic ketoacidosis, excessive dietary or IV intake of potassium, massive tissue destruction, metabolic acidosis
7. Below normal values occur in the following: Burns, Cushing's syndrome, deficient dietary intake of potassium, diarrhea (severe), diuretic therapy, GI fistula, insulin administration, pyloric obstruction, starvation, vomiting
8. Clients with elevated white blood cell (WBC) counts and platelet counts may have falsely elevated potassium levels.

D. Activated partial thromboplastin time (aPTT)
1. The aPTT evaluates how well the coagulation sequence (intrinsic clotting system) is functioning by measuring the amount of time it takes in seconds for recalcified citrated plasma to clot after partial thromboplastin is added to it.
2. The test screens for deficiencies and inhibitors of all factors, except factors VII and XIII.
3. Usually, the aPTT is used to monitor the effectiveness of heparin therapy and screen for coagulation disorders.
4. Normal reference interval: 30 to 40 seconds (conventional and SI units [International System of Units]), depending on the type of activator used.
5. If the client is receiving intermittent heparin therapy, draw the blood sample 1 hour before the next scheduled dose.
6. Do not draw samples from an arm into which heparin is infusing.
7. Transport specimen to the laboratory immediately.
8. Provide direct pressure to the venipuncture site for 3 to 5 minutes.
9. The aPTT should be between 1.5 and 2.5 times normal when the client is receiving heparin therapy.
10. Elevated values occur in the following: Deficiency of one or more of the following: factor I, II, V, or VIII; factors IX and X; factor XI; and factor XII; hemophilia; heparin therapy; liver disease

If the aPTT value is prolonged (longer than 100 seconds or per agency policy) in a client receiving IV heparin therapy or in any client at risk for thrombocytopenia, initiate bleeding precautions.

E. Prothrombin time (PT) and international normalized ratio (INR)
1. Prothrombin is a vitamin K–dependent glycoprotein produced by the liver that is necessary for fibrin clot formation.
2. Each laboratory establishes a normal or control value based on the method used to perform the PT test.
3. The PT measures the amount of time it takes in seconds for clot formation and is used to monitor response to warfarin sodium therapy or to screen for dysfunction of the extrinsic clotting system resulting from liver disease, vitamin K deficiency, or disseminated intravascular coagulation.
4. A PT value within 2 seconds (plus or minus) of the control is considered normal.
5. The INR is a frequently used test to measure the effects of some anticoagulants.
6. The INR standardizes the PT ratio and is calculated in the laboratory setting by raising the observed PT ratio to the power of the international sensitivity index specific to the thromboplastin reagent used.
7. If a PT is prescribed, baseline specimen should be drawn before anticoagulation therapy is started; note the time of collection on the laboratory form.
8. Provide direct pressure to the venipuncture site for 3 to 5 minutes.
9. Concurrent warfarin therapy with heparin therapy can lengthen the PT for up to 5 hours after dosing.
10. Diets high in green leafy vegetables can increase the absorption of vitamin K, which shortens the PT.
11. Orally administered anticoagulation therapy usually maintains the PT at 1.5 to 2 times the laboratory control value.
12. Normal reference intervals
    a. PT: 11 to 12.5 seconds (conventional and SI units)
    b. INR: 0.81 to 1.20 (conventional and SI units)
13. For both the PT and INR, elevated values occur in the following: deficiency of one or more of the following: factor I, II, V, VII, or X; liver disease; vitamin K deficiency; warfarin therapy

If the PT value is longer than 25 seconds and the INR is greater than 3.0 in a client receiving standard warfarin therapy (or per agency policy), initiate bleeding precautions.

F. Platelet count
1. Platelets function in hemostatic plug formation, clot retraction, and coagulation factor activation.
2. Platelets are produced by the bone marrow to function in hemostasis.
3. Normal reference interval: 150,000 to 400,000 mm^3 (150 to 400 × 10^9/L)
4. Elevated values occur in the following: acute infections, chronic granulocytic leukemia, chronic pancreatitis, cirrhosis, collagen disorders,

polycythemia, postsplenectomy; high altitudes and chronic cold weather can increase values.

5. Below normal values occur in the following: acute leukemia, chemotherapy, disseminated intravascular coagulation, hemorrhage, infection, systemic lupus erythematosus, thrombocytopenic purpura.
6. Monitor the venipuncture site for bleeding in clients with known thrombocytopenia.
7. Bleeding precautions should be instituted in clients when the platelet count falls sufficiently below the normal level; the specific value for implementing bleeding precautions usually is determined by agency policy.

Monitor the platelet count closely in clients receiving chemotherapy because of the risk for thrombocytopenia. In addition, any client who will be having an invasive procedure (such as a liver biopsy or thoracentesis) should have coagulation studies and platelet counts done before the procedure.

G. Hemoglobin and hematocrit

1. Hemoglobin is the main component of erythrocytes and serves as the vehicle for transporting oxygen and carbon dioxide.
2. Hematocrit represents red blood cell (RBC) mass and is an important measurement in the presence of anemia or polycythemia (Table 10-2).
3. Fasting is not required for this test.
4. Elevated values occur in the following:
   - **a.** Hemoglobin: chronic obstructive pulmonary disease, high altitudes, polycythemia
   - **b.** Hematocrit: dehydration, high altitudes, polycythemia
5. Below normal values occur in the following:
   - **a.** Hemoglobin: anemia, hemorrhage
   - **b.** Hematocrit: anemia, bone marrow failure, hemorrhage, leukemia, overhydration

H. Lipids

1. Blood lipids consist primarily of cholesterol, triglycerides, and phospholipids.
2. Lipid assessment includes total cholesterol, high-density lipoprotein (HDL), low-density lipoprotein (LDL), and triglycerides.
3. Cholesterol is present in all body tissues and is a major component of LDLs, brain and nerve cells, cell membranes, and some gallbladder stones.
4. Low-density lipoprotein (LDL) transports cholesterol from the liver to the tissues of the body.
5. Triglycerides are synthesized in the liver from fatty acids, protein, and glucose and are obtained from the diet.
6. Increased cholesterol levels, LDL levels, and triglyceride levels place the client at risk for coronary artery disease.
7. HDL helps protect against the risk of coronary artery disease.
8. Instruct the client to abstain from food and fluid, except for water, for 12 to 14 hours and from alcohol for 24 hours before the test.
9. Instruct the client to avoid consuming high-cholesterol foods with the evening meal before the test.
10. Normal reference intervals (Table 10-3).
11. Elevated values occur in the following:
    - **a.** Cholesterol, LDL: biliary obstruction, cirrhosis hyperlipidemia, hypothyroidism, idiopathic hypercholesterolemia, renal disease, uncontrolled diabetes, oral contraceptive use
    - **b.** Triglycerides: diabetes mellitus, hyperlipidemia, hypothyroidism, liver disease
12. Below normal values occur in the following:
    - **a.** Cholesterol, LDL: extensive liver disease, hyperthyroidism, malnutrition, use of corticosteroid therapy
    - **b.** Triglycerides: hyperthyroidism, malabsorption syndrome, malnutrition

TABLE 10-2 Hemoglobin and Hematocrit: Reference Intervals

Blood Component	Reference Interval
Hemoglobin (altitude dependent)	
Male adult	14-18 g/dL (140-180 mmol/L)
Female adult	12-16 g/dL (120-160 mmol/L)
Hematocrit (altitude dependent)	
Male adult	42%-52% (0.42-0.52)
Female adult	37%-47% (0.37-0.47)

TABLE 10-3 Lipids: Reference Intervals

Blood Component	Reference Interval
Cholesterol	<200 mg/dL (<5.0 mmol/L)
High-density lipoproteins (HDLs)	>60 mg/dL (>1.55 mmol/L)
Low-density lipoproteins (LDLs)	<100 mg/dL (<2.59 mmol/L)
Triglycerides	Male: 40-160 mg/dL (0.45-1.81 mmol/L) Female: 35-135 mg/dL (0.40-1.52 mmol/L)

I. Fasting blood glucose
1. Glucose is a monosaccharide found in fruits and is formed from the digestion of carbohydrates and the conversion of glycogen by the liver.
2. Glucose is the main source of cellular energy for the body and is essential for brain and erythrocyte function.
3. Fasting blood glucose levels are used to help diagnose diabetes mellitus and hypoglycemia.
4. Instruct the client to fast for 8 to 12 hours before the test.
5. Instruct a client with diabetes mellitus to withhold morning insulin or oral hypoglycemic medication until after the blood is drawn.
6. Normal reference interval: glucose (fasting) 70-99 mg/dL (3.9-5.5 mmol/L).
7. Elevated values occur in the following: acute stress, cerebral lesions, Cushing's syndrome, diabetes mellitus, hyperthyroidism, pancreatic insufficiency
8. Below normal values occur in the following: Addison's disease, hepatic disease, hypothyroidism, insulin overdosage, pancreatic tumor, pituitary hypofunction, postdumping syndrome

J. Glycosylated hemoglobin (HgbA1C)
1. HgbA1C is blood glucose bound to hemoglobin.
2. Hemoglobin A_{1c} (glycosylated hemoglobin A; HbA_{1c}) is a reflection of how well blood glucose levels have been controlled for the past 3 to 4 months.
3. Fasting is not required before the test.
4. Normal reference interval: <6% (adult without diabetes).
5. Elevated values occur in the following: nondiabetic hyperglycemia, poorly controlled diabetes mellitus
6. Below normal values occur in the following: chronic blood loss, chronic kidney disease, pregnancy, sickle cell anemia
7. HgbA1C and estimated average glucose (eAG) reference intervals (Table 10-4)

TABLE 10-4 Glycosylated Hemoglobin (HgbA1C) and Estimated Average Glucose (eAG)

HgbA1C %	eAG mg/dL	eAG mmol/L
4	65	3.62
5	100	5.57
6	135	7.52
7	170	9.47
8	205	11.42

Pagana KD, Pagana TJ, Pagana TN. *Mosby's Diagnostic and Laboratory Test Reference*, ed 13, Grafton, IL: Mosby; 450.

K. Renal function studies
1. Serum creatinine
a. Creatinine is a specific indicator of renal function.
b. Increased levels of creatinine indicate a slowing of the glomerular filtration rate.
c. Instruct the client to avoid excessive exercise for 8 hours and excessive red meat intake for 24 hours before the test.
d. Normal reference interval: Male: 0.6 to 1.2 mg/dL (53 to 106 mcmol/L); female: 0.5 to 1.1 mg/dL (44 to 97 mcmol/L)
e. Elevated values occur in severe renal disease.
f. Below normal values occur in diseases with decreased muscle mass such as muscular dystrophy and myasthenia gravis.
2. Blood urea nitrogen (BUN)
a. Urea nitrogen is the nitrogen portion of urea, a substance formed in the liver through an enzymatic protein breakdown process.
b. Urea is normally freely filtered through the renal glomeruli, with a small amount reabsorbed in the tubules and the remainder excreted in the urine.
c. BUN and creatinine ratios should be analyzed when renal function is evaluated.
d. Normal reference interval: 10 to 20 mg/dL (3.6 to 7.1 mmol/L)
e. Elevated levels indicate a slowing of the glomerular filtration rate.
f. Elevated values occur in the following: burns, dehydration, GI bleeding, increase in protein catabolism (fever, stress), renal disease, shock, urinary tract infection
g. Below normal values occur in the following: fluid overload, malnutrition, severe liver damage, syndrome of inappropriate antidiuretic hormone

L. White blood cell (WBC) count
1. WBCs function in the immune defense system of the body.
2. The WBC differential provides specific information on WBC types.
3. A "shift to the left" (in the differential) means that an increased number of immature neutrophils is present in the blood.
4. A low total WBC count with a left shift indicates a recovery from bone marrow depression or an infection of such intensity that the demand for neutrophils in the tissue is higher than the capacity of the bone marrow to release them into the circulation.
5. A high total WBC count with a left shift indicates an increased release of neutrophils by the bone marrow in response to an overwhelming infection or inflammation.

6. An increased neutrophil count with a left shift is usually associated with bacterial infection.
7. A "shift to the right" means that cells have more than the usual number of nuclear segments; found in liver disease, Down's syndrome, and megaloblastic and pernicious anemia.
8. Normal reference interval: 5000 to 10,000 mm^3 (5.0 to $10.0 \times 10^9/L$)
9. Elevated values occur in the following: inflammatory and infectious processes, leukemia
10. Below normal values occur in the following: aplastic anemia, autoimmune diseases, overwhelming infection, side effects of chemotherapy and irradiation

⚠ Monitor the WBC count and differential closely in clients receiving chemotherapy because of the risk for neutropenia; neutropenia places the client at risk for infection.

PRACTICE QUESTIONS

64. A client with atrial fibrillation who is receiving maintenance therapy of warfarin sodium has a prothrombin time (PT) of 35 seconds. On the basis of these laboratory values, the nurse anticipates which prescription?
1. Adding a dose of heparin sodium
2. Holding the next dose of warfarin
3. Increasing the next dose of warfarin
4. Administering the next dose of warfarin

65. A staff nurse is precepting a new graduate nurse and the new graduate is assigned to care for a client with chronic pain. Which statement, if made by the new graduate nurse, indicates the **need for further teaching** regarding pain management?
1. "I will be sure to ask my client what his pain level is on a scale of 0 to 10."
2. "I know that I should follow up after giving medication to make sure it is effective."
3. "I will be sure to cue in to any indicators that the client may be exaggerating their pain."
4. "I know that pain in the older client might manifest as sleep disturbances or depression."

66. A client has been admitted to the hospital for gastroenteritis and dehydration. The nurse determines that the client has received adequate volume replacement if the blood urea nitrogen (BUN) level drops to which value?
1. 3 mg/dL (1.08 mmol/L)
2. 15 mg/dL (5.4 mmol/L)
3. 29 mg/dL (10.44 mmol/L)
4. 35 mg/dL (12.6 mmol/L)

67. The nurse is explaining the appropriate methods for measuring an accurate temperature to an assistive personnel (AP). Which method, if noted by the UAP as being an appropriate method, indicates the **need for further teaching**?
1. Taking a rectal temperature for a client who has undergone nasal surgery
2. Taking an oral temperature for a client with a cough and nasal congestion
3. Taking an axillary temperature for a client who has just consumed hot coffee
4. Taking a temperature on the neck behind the ear using an electronic device for a client who is diaphoretic

68. A client is receiving a continuous intravenous infusion of heparin sodium to treat deep vein thrombosis. The client's activated partial thromboplastin time (aPTT) is 65 seconds. The nurse anticipates that which action is needed?
1. Discontinuing the heparin infusion
2. Increasing the rate of the heparin infusion
3. Decreasing the rate of the heparin infusion
4. Leaving the rate of the heparin infusion as is

69. A client with a history of heart failure is due for a morning dose of furosemide. Which serum potassium level, if noted in the client's laboratory report, should be reported before administering the dose of furosemide?
1. 3.2 mEq/L (3.2 mmol/L)
2. 3.8 mEq/L (3.8 mmol/L)
3. 4.2 mEq/L (4.2 mmol/L)
4. 4.8 mEq/L (4.8 mmol/L)

70. Several laboratory tests are prescribed for a client, and the nurse reviews the results of the tests. Which laboratory test results should the nurse report? **Select all that apply.**
- ☐ 1. Platelets 35,000 mm^3 ($35 \times 10^9/L$)
- ☐ 2. Sodium 150 mEq/L (150 mmol/L)
- ☐ 3. Potassium 5.0 mEq/L (5.0 mmol/L)
- ☐ 4. Segmented neutrophils 40% (0.40)
- ☐ 5. Serum creatinine, 1 mg/dL (88.3 mcmol/L)
- ☐ 6. White blood cells, 3000 mm^3 ($3.0 \times 10^9/L$)

71. The nurse is caring for a client who takes ibuprofen for pain. The nurse is gathering information on the client's medication history and determines it is necessary to contact the primary health care provider (PHCP) if the client is also taking which medications? **Select all that apply.**
- ☐ 1. Warfarin
- ☐ 2. Glimepiride
- ☐ 3. Amlodipine
- ☐ 4. Simvastatin
- ☐ 5. Atorvastatin

72. A client with diabetes mellitus has a glycosylated hemoglobin A_{1c} level of 8%. On the basis of this test result, the nurse plans to teach the client about the need for which measure?
1. Avoiding infection
2. Taking in adequate fluids
3. Preventing and recognizing hypoglycemia
4. Preventing and recognizing hyperglycemia

73. The nurse is caring for a client with a diagnosis of breast cancer who is immunosuppressed. The nurse would consider implementing neutropenic precautions if the client's white blood cell count was which value?
1. 2000 mm^3 (2.0×10^9/L)
2. 5800 mm^3 (5.8×10^9/L)
3. 8400 mm^3 (8.4×10^9/L)
4. 11,500 mm^3 (11.5×10^9/L)

74. A client brought to the emergency department states that he has accidentally been taking 2 times his prescribed dose of warfarin for the past week. After noting that the client has no evidence of obvious bleeding, the nurse plans to take which action?
1. Prepare to administer an antidote.
2. Draw a sample for type and crossmatch and transfuse the client.
3. Draw a sample for an activated partial thromboplastin time (aPTT) level.
4. Draw a sample for prothrombin time (PT) and international normalized ratio (INR).

75. The nurse is caring for a postoperative client who is receiving demand-dose hydromorphone via a patient-controlled analgesia (PCA) pump for pain control. The nurse enters the client's room and finds the client drowsy and records the following vital signs: temperature 97.2° F (36.2° C) orally, pulse 52 beats per minute, blood pressure 101/58 mm Hg, respiratory rate 11 breaths per minute, and SpO_2 of 93% on 3 liters of oxygen via nasal cannula. Which action should the nurse take **next**?
1. Document the findings.
2. Attempt to arouse the client.
3. Contact the primary health care provider (PHCP) immediately.
4. Check the medication administration history on the PCA pump.

76. An adult female client has a hemoglobin level of 10.8 g/dL (108 mmol/L). The nurse interprets that this result is **most likely** caused by which condition noted in the client's history?
1. Dehydration
2. Heart failure
3. Iron deficiency anemia
4. Chronic obstructive pulmonary disease

77. A client with a history of upper gastrointestinal bleeding has a platelet count of 300,000 mm^3 (300×10^9/L). The nurse should take which action after seeing the laboratory results?
1. Report the abnormally low count.
2. Report the abnormally high count.
3. Place the client on bleeding precautions.
4. Place the normal report in the client's medical record.

ANSWERS

64. ***Answer:* 2**
Rationale: The normal PT is 11 to 12.5 seconds (conventional therapy and SI units). A therapeutic PT level is 1.5 to 2 times higher than the normal level. Because the value of 35 seconds is high, the nurse should anticipate that the client would not receive further doses at this time. Therefore, the prescriptions noted in the remaining options are incorrect.
Test-Taking Strategy: Focus on the subject, a PT of 35 seconds. Recall the normal range for this value and remember that a PT greater than 25 seconds places the client at risk for bleeding; this will direct you to the correct option.
Level of Cognitive Ability: Analyzing
Client Needs: Physiological Integrity
Integrated Process: Nursing Process—Analysis
Content Area: Foundations of Care: Laboratory Tests
Health Problem: Adult Health: Cardiovascular: Dysrhythmias
Priority Concepts: Clinical Judgment; Clotting
Reference: Lewis et al. (2017), p. 601.

65. ***Answer:* 3**
Rationale: Pain is a highly individual experience, and the new graduate nurse should not assume that the client is exaggerating his pain. Rather, the nurse should frequently assess the pain and intervene accordingly through the use of both nonpharmacological and pharmacological interventions. The nurse should assess pain using a number-based scale or a picture-based scale for clients who cannot verbally describe their pain to rate the degree of pain. The nurse should follow up with the client after giving medication to ensure that the medication is effective in managing the pain. Pain experienced by the older client may be manifested differently than pain experienced by clients in other age groups, and they may have sleep disturbances, changes in gait and mobility, decreased socialization, and depression; the nurse should be aware of this attribute in this population.
Test-Taking Strategy: Note the strategic words, *need for further teaching*. These words indicate a negative event query and the need to select the incorrect statement as the answer. Recall that pain is a highly individual experience, and the nurse should not assume that the client is exaggerating pain.

Level of Cognitive Ability: Evaluating
Client Needs: Physiological Integrity
Integrated Process: Teaching and Learning
Content Area: Skills: Vital Signs
Health Problem: Adult Health: Neurological: Pain
Priority Concepts: Clinical Judgment; Pain
Reference: Lewis et al. (2017), pp. 110-111, 123.

66. *Answer:* 2
Rationale: The normal BUN level is 10 to 20 mg/dL (3.6 to 7.1 mmol/L). Values of 29 mg/dL (10.44 mmol/L) and 35 mg/dL (12.6 mmol/L) reflect continued dehydration. A value of 3 mg/dL (1.08 mmol/L) reflects a lower than normal value, which may occur with fluid volume overload, among other conditions.
Test-Taking Strategy: Focus on the **subject**, adequate fluid replacement and the normal BUN level. The correct option is the only option that identifies a normal value.
Level of Cognitive Ability: Evaluating
Client Needs: Physiological Integrity
Integrated Process: Nursing Process—Evaluation
Content Area: Foundations of Care: Laboratory Tests
Health Problem: Adult Health: Gastrointestinal: Dehydration
Priority Concepts: Fluids and Electrolytes; Leadership
Reference: Lewis et al. (2017), p. 1026.

67. *Answer:* 2
Rationale: An oral temperature should be avoided if the client has nasal congestion. One of the other methods of measuring the temperature should be used according to the equipment available. Taking a rectal temperature for a client who has undergone nasal surgery is appropriate. Other, less invasive measures should be used if available; if not available, a rectal temperature is acceptable. Taking an axillary temperature on a client who just consumed coffee is also acceptable; however, the axillary method of measurement is the least reliable, and other methods should be used if available. If electronic equipment is available and the client is diaphoretic, it is acceptable to measure the temperature on the neck behind the ear, avoiding the forehead.
Test-Taking Strategy: Note the **strategic words**, *need for further teaching*. These words indicate a **negative event query** and the need to select the incorrect action as the answer. Recall that nasal congestion is a reason to avoid taking an oral temperature, as the nasal congestion will cause problems with breathing while the temperature is being taken.
Level of Cognitive Ability: Evaluating
Client Needs: Safe and Effective Care Environment
Integrated Process: Teaching and Learning
Content Area: Skills: Vital Signs
Health Problem: N/A
Priority Concepts: Teaching and Learning; Thermoregulation
Reference: Perry et al. (2018), pp. 68-69.

68. *Answer:* 4
Rationale: The normal aPTT varies between 30 and 40 seconds (30 and 40 seconds), depending on the type of activator used in testing. The therapeutic dose of heparin for treatment of deep vein thrombosis is to keep the aPTT between 1.5 (45 to 60) and 2.5 (75 to 100) times normal. This means that the client's value should not be less than 45 seconds or greater than 100 seconds. Thus, the client's aPTT is within the therapeutic range and the dose should remain unchanged.
Test-Taking Strategy: Focus on the **subject**, the expected aPTT for a client receiving a heparin sodium infusion. Remember that the normal range is 30 to 40 seconds and that the aPTT should be between 1.5 and 2.5 times normal when the client is receiving heparin therapy. Simple multiplication of 1.5 and 2.5 by 30 and 40 will yield a range of 45 to 100 seconds. This client's value is 65 seconds.
Level of Cognitive Ability: Analyzing
Client Needs: Physiological Integrity
Integrated Process: Nursing Process—Analysis
Content Area: Foundations of Care: Laboratory Tests
Health Problem: Adult Health: Cardiovascular: Vascular Disorders
Priority Concepts: Clinical Judgment; Clotting
Reference: Lewis et al. (2017), p. 601.

69. *Answer:* 1
Rationale: The normal serum potassium level in the adult is 3.5 to 5.0 mEq/L (3.5 to 5.0 mmol/L). The correct option is the only value that falls below the therapeutic range. Administering furosemide to a client with a low potassium level and a history of cardiac problems could precipitate ventricular dysrhythmias. The remaining options are within the normal range.
Test-Taking Strategy: Note the **subject** of the question, the level that should be reported. This indicates that you are looking for an abnormal level. Remember, the normal serum potassium level in the adult is 3.5 to 5.0 mEq/L (3.5 to 5.0 mmol/L). This will direct you to the correct option.
Level of Cognitive Ability: Applying
Client Needs: Physiological Integrity
Integrated Process: Nursing Process—Implementation
Content Area: Foundations of Care: Laboratory Tests
Health Problem: Adult Health: Cardiovascular: Heart Failure
Priority Concepts: Clinical Judgment; Fluids and Electrolytes
Reference: Lewis et al. (2017), p. 280.

70. *Answer:* 1, 2, 4, 6
Rationale: The normal values include the following: platelets 150,000 to 400,000 mm^3 (150 to 400 × 10^9/L); sodium 135 to 145 mEq/L (135 to 145 mmol/L); potassium 3.5 to 5.0 mEq/L (3.5 to 5.0 mmol/L); segmented neutrophils 62% to 68% (0.62 to 0.68); serum creatinine male: 0.6 to 1.2 mg/dL (53 to 106 mcmol/L); female: 0.5 to 1.1 mg/dL (44 to 97 mcmol/L); and white blood cells 5000 to 10,000 mm^3 (5.0 to 10.0 × 10^9/L). The platelet level noted is low; the sodium level noted is high; the potassium level noted is normal; the segmented neutrophil level noted is low; the serum creatinine level noted is normal; and the white blood cell level is low.
Test-Taking Strategy: Focus on the **subject**, the abnormal laboratory values that need to be reported. Recalling the normal laboratory values for the blood studies identified in the options will assist in answering this question.
Level of Cognitive Ability: Analyzing
Client Needs: Physiological Integrity
Integrated Process: Nursing Process—Implementation
Content Area: Foundations of Care: Laboratory Tests
Health Problem: N/A
Priority Concepts: Clinical Judgment; Collaboration
Reference: Lewis et al. (2017), pp. 599-601, 1026.

71. *Answer:* 1, 2, 3

Rationale: Nonsteroidal antiinflammatory drugs (NSAIDs) can amplify the effects of anticoagulants; therefore, these medications should not be taken together. Hypoglycemia may result for the client taking ibuprofen if the client is concurrently taking an oral antidiabetic agent such as glimepiride; these medications should not be combined. A high risk of toxicity exists if the client is taking ibuprofen concurrently with a calcium channel blocker such as amlodipine; therefore, this combination should be avoided. There is no known interaction between ibuprofen and simvastatin or atorvastatin.

Test-Taking Strategy: Note the subject of the question, data provided by the client necessitating contacting the PHCP. Determining that ibuprofen is classified as an NSAID will help you determine that it should not be combined with anticoagulants. Also recalling that hypoglycemia can occur as an adverse effect if taken with antidiabetic agents will help you recall that these medications should not be combined. From the remaining options, it is necessary to remember that toxicity can result if NSAIDs are combined with calcium channel blockers. Also note that options 4 and 5 are comparable or alike and are antilipemic medications. This will assist in eliminating these options.

Level of Cognitive Ability: Analyzing
Client Needs: Physiological Integrity
Integrated Process: Nursing Process—Implementation
Content Area: Skills: Vital Signs
Health Problem: Adult Health: Neurological: Pain
Priority Concepts: Clinical Judgment; Safety
Reference: Lewis et al. (2017), p. 111.

72. *Answer:* 4

Rationale: The normal reference range for the glycosylated hemoglobin A_{1c} is less than 6.0%. This test measures the amount of glucose that has become permanently bound to the red blood cells from circulating glucose. Erythrocytes live for about 120 days, giving feedback about blood glucose for the past 120 days. Elevations in the blood glucose level will cause elevations in the amount of glycosylation. Thus, the test is useful in identifying clients who have periods of hyperglycemia that are undetected in other ways. The estimated average glucose for a glycosylated hemoglobin A_{1c} of 8% is 205 mg/dL (11.42 mmol/L). Elevations indicate continued need for teaching related to the prevention of hyperglycemic episodes.

Test-Taking Strategy: Focus on the subject, a glycosylated hemoglobin A_{1c} level of 8%. Recalling the normal value and that an elevated value indicates hyperglycemia will assist in directing you to the correct option.

Level of Cognitive Ability: Applying
Client Needs: Health Promotion and Maintenance
Integrated Process: Teaching and Learning
Content Area: Foundations of Care: Laboratory Tests
Health Problem: Adult Health: Endocrine: Diabetes Mellitus
Priority Concepts: Client Education; Glucose Regulation
Reference: Lewis et al. (2017), p. 1118.

73. *Answer:* 1

Rationale: The normal WBC count ranges from 5000 to 10,000 mm^3 (5 to 10 × 10^9/L). The client who has a decrease in the number of circulating WBCs is immunosuppressed. The nurse implements neutropenic precautions when the client's values fall sufficiently below the normal level. The specific value for implementing neutropenic precautions usually is determined by agency policy. The remaining options are normal values.

Test-Taking Strategy: Focus on the subject, the need to implement neutropenic precautions. Recalling that the normal WBC count is 5000 to 10,000 mm^3 (5 to 10 × 10^9/L) will direct you to the correct option.

Level of Cognitive Ability: Applying
Client Needs: Physiological Integrity
Integrated Process: Nursing Process—Planning
Content Area: Foundations of Care: Laboratory Tests
Health Problem: Adult Health: Cancer: Breast
Priority Concepts: Clinical Judgment; Infection
Reference: Potter et al. (2017), p. 451.

74. *Answer:* 4

Rationale: The action that the nurse should take is to draw a sample for PT and INR level to determine the client's anticoagulation status and risk for bleeding. These results will provide information as to how to best treat this client (e.g., if an antidote such as vitamin K or a blood transfusion is needed). The aPTT monitors the effects of heparin therapy.

Test-Taking Strategy: Focus on the subject, a client who has taken an excessive dose of warfarin. Eliminate the option with aPTT first because it is unrelated to warfarin therapy and relates to heparin therapy. Next, eliminate the options indicating to administer an antidote and to transfuse the client because these therapies would not be implemented unless the PT and INR levels were known.

Level of Cognitive Ability: Applying
Client Needs: Physiological Integrity
Integrated Process: Nursing Process—Planning
Content Area: Foundations of Care: Laboratory Tests
Health Problem: N/A
Priority Concepts: Clinical Judgment; Clotting
Reference: Ignatavicius, Workman, Rebar (2018), pp. 744-745.

75. *Answer:* 2

Rationale: The primary concern with opioid analgesics is respiratory depression and hypotension. Based on the assessment findings, the nurse should suspect opioid overdose. The nurse should first attempt to arouse the client and then reassess the vital signs. The vital signs may begin to normalize once the client is aroused, because sleep can also cause decreased heart rate, blood pressure, respiratory rate, and oxygen saturation. The nurse should also check to see how much medication has been taken via the PCA pump and should continue to monitor the client closely to determine whether further action is needed. The nurse should contact the PHCP and document the findings after all data are collected, after the client is stabilized, and if an abnormality still exists after arousing the client.

Test-Taking Strategy: First, note the strategic word, *next*. Focus on the data in the question and determine if an abnormality exists. It is clear that an abnormality exists because the client is drowsy and the vital signs are outside of the normal range. Recall that attempting to arouse the client should come before further assessment of the pump. The client should always be assessed before the equipment, before contacting the PHCP, and before documentation.

Level of Cognitive Ability: Synthesizing
Client Needs: Physiological Integrity
Integrated Process: Nursing Process—Implementation
Content Area: Skills: Vital Signs
Health Problem: Adult Health: Neurological: Pain
Priority Concepts: Clinical Judgment; Pain
Reference: Lewis et al. (2017), pp. 114-115, 152.

76. *Answer:* 3
Rationale: The normal hemoglobin level for an adult female client is 12 to 16 g/dL (120 to 160 mmol/L). Iron deficiency anemia can result in lower hemoglobin levels. Dehydration may increase the hemoglobin level by hemoconcentration. Heart failure and chronic obstructive pulmonary disease may increase the hemoglobin level as a result of the body's need for more oxygen-carrying capacity.
Test-Taking Strategy: Note the **strategic words,** *most likely.* Evaluate each of the conditions in the options in terms of their pathophysiology and whether each is likely to raise or lower the hemoglobin level. Also, note the relationship between hemoglobin level in the question and the correct option.
Level of Cognitive Ability: Analyzing
Client Needs: Physiological Integrity
Integrated Process: Nursing Process—Assessment
Content Area: Foundations of Care: Laboratory Tests
Health Problem: Adult Health: Hematological: Anemias
Priority Concepts: Clinical Judgment; Gas Exchange
Reference: Lewis et al. (2017), p. 600.

77. *Answer:* 4
Rationale: A normal platelet count ranges from 150,000 to 400,000 mm^3 (150 to 400 × 10^9/L). The nurse should place the report containing the normal laboratory value in the client's medical record. A platelet count of 300,000 mm^3 (300 × 10^9/L) is not an elevated count. The count also is not low; therefore, bleeding precautions are not needed.
Test-Taking Strategy: Focus on the **subject,** a platelet count of 300,000 mm^3 (300 × 10^9/L). Remember that options that are **comparable or alike** are not likely to be correct. With this in mind, eliminate options indicating to report the abnormally low count and placing the client on bleeding precautions first. From the remaining options, recalling the normal range for this laboratory test will direct you to the correct option.
Level of Cognitive Ability: Applying
Client Needs: Physiological Integrity
Integrated Process: Nursing Process—Implementation
Content Area: Foundations of Care: Laboratory Tests
Health Problem: Adult Health: Gastrointestinal: Upper GI Disorders
Priority Concepts: Clinical Judgment; Clotting
Reference: Lewis et al. (2017), p. 601.

CHAPTER 11

Nutrition

PRIORITY CONCEPTS Health Promotion; Nutrition

I. Nutrients

A. Carbohydrates
1. Carbohydrates are the preferred source of energy.
2. Sugars, starches, and cellulose provide 4 cal/g.
3. Carbohydrates promote normal fat **metabolism,** spare protein, and enhance lower gastrointestinal function.
4. Major food sources of carbohydrates include milk, grains, fruits, and vegetables.
5. Inadequate carbohydrate intake affects metabolism.

B. Fats
1. Fats provide a concentrated source and a stored form of energy.
2. Fats protect internal organs and maintain body temperature.
3. Fats enhance absorption of the fat-soluble vitamins.
4. Fats provide 9 cal/g.
5. Inadequate intake of essential fatty acids leads to clinical manifestations of sensitivity to cold, skin lesions, increased risk of infection, and amenorrhea in women.
6. Diets high in fat can lead to obesity and increase the risk of cardiovascular disease and some cancers.

C. Proteins
1. Amino acids, which make up proteins, are critical to all aspects of growth and development of body tissues and provide 4 cal/g.
2. Proteins build and repair body tissues, regulate fluid balance, maintain acid-base balance, produce antibodies, provide energy, and produce enzymes and hormones.
3. Essential amino acids are required in the diet because the body cannot manufacture them.
4. Complete proteins contain all essential amino acids; incomplete proteins lack some of the essential fatty acids.
5. Inadequate protein can cause protein energy **malnutrition** and severe wasting of fat and muscle tissue.

Major stages of the lifespan with specific nutritional needs are pregnancy, lactation, infancy, childhood, and adolescence. Adults and older adults may experience physiological aging changes, which influence individual nutritional needs.

D. Vitamins (Box 11-1)
1. Vitamins facilitate metabolism of proteins, fats, and carbohydrates and act as catalysts for metabolic functions.
2. Vitamins promote life and growth processes and maintain and regulate body functions.
3. Fat-soluble vitamins A, D, E, and K can be stored in the body, so an excess can cause toxicity.
4. The B vitamins and vitamin C are water-soluble vitamins, are not stored in the body, and can be excreted in the urine.

E. Minerals and electrolytes (Box 11-2)
1. Minerals are components of hormones, cells, tissues, and bones.
2. Minerals act as catalysts for chemical reactions and enhancers of cell function.
3. Almost all foods contain some form of minerals.
4. A deficiency of minerals can develop in chronically ill or hospitalized clients.
5. Electrolytes play a major role in osmolality and body water regulation, acid-base balance, enzyme reactions, and neuromuscular activity (see Chapter 8 for additional information regarding electrolytes).

F. Water
1. Critical for cell function.
2. Makes 60% to 70% of total body weight.
3. A person cannot survive without water for more than a few days.

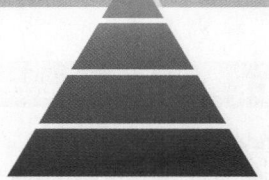

BOX 11-1 Food Sources of Vitamins

Water-Soluble Vitamins

Folic acid: Green leafy vegetables; liver, beef, and fish; legumes; grapefruit and oranges
Niacin: Meats, poultry, fish, beans, peanuts, grains
Vitamin B_1 (thiamine): Pork and nuts, whole-grain cereals, and legumes
Vitamin B_2 (riboflavin): Milk, lean meats, fish, grains
Vitamin B_6 (pyridoxine): Yeast, corn, meat, poultry, fish
Vitamin B_{12} (cobalamin): Meats, poultry, fish, shellfish, eggs, dairy products, citrus fruits, dried beans, green leafy vegetables, liver, nuts, brewer's yeast
Vitamin C (ascorbic acid): Citrus fruits, tomatoes, broccoli, cabbage

Fat-Soluble Vitamins

Vitamin A: Liver, egg yolk, whole milk, green or orange vegetables, fruits
Vitamin D: Fortified milk, fish oils, cereals
Vitamin E: Vegetable oils; green leafy vegetables; cereals; apricots, apples, and peaches
Vitamin K: Green leafy vegetables; cauliflower and cabbage

BOX 11-2 Food Sources of Minerals

Calcium
Cheese
Collard greens
Milk and soy milk
Rhubarb
Sardines
Tofu
Yogurt

Chloride
Salt

Iron
Breads and cereals
Dark green vegetables
Dried fruits
Egg yolk
Legumes
Liver
Meats

Magnesium
Almonds
Avocado
Canned white tuna
Cauliflower
Cooked rolled oats
Green leafy vegetables
Milk
Peanut butter
Peas
Pork, beef, chicken
Potatoes
Raisins
Soybeans
Yogurt

Phosphorus
Dairy products
Fish
Nuts
Pumpkin
Organ meats
Pork, beef, chicken
Squash
Whole-grain breads and cereals

Potassium
Avocado
Bananas
Cantaloupe
Carrots
Fish
Mushrooms
Oranges
Pork, beef, veal
Potatoes
Raisins
Spinach
Strawberries
Tomatoes

Sodium
Bacon
Butter
Canned food
Cheese
Cured pork
Hot dogs
Ketchup
Lunch meat
Milk
Mustard
Processed food
Snack food
Soy sauce
Table salt
White and whole-wheat bread

Zinc
Eggs
Leafy vegetables
Meats
Protein-rich foods

II. Malnutrition Laboratory Markers

A. Hematological studies and studies evaluating protein balance
1. Complete blood cell count with red blood cell indices and peripheral smear to differentiate between anemias and nutritional deficiencies
2. Long-term protein status can be determined by evaluating serum albumin levels.
3. Short-term protein status is best determined by evaluating retinol-binding protein, prealbumin, transferrin, creatinine, and blood urea nitrogen (BUN) levels.
4. Serum electrolytes (see Chapter 8).
5. Nitrogen balance is evaluated by measuring urea in the urine, which provides information regarding protein loss.

⚠ Always assess the client's ability to eat and swallow and promote independence in eating as much as is possible.

III. MyPlate (Fig. 11-1)

A. Provides a description of a balanced diet that includes grains, vegetables, fruits, dairy products, and protein foods (see http://www.choosemyplate.gov/).
B. A nutritionist should be consulted for individualized dietary recommendations (see Box 11-3 for nutrition throughout growth and development).
C. Guidelines
1. Avoid eating oversized portions of foods.
2. Fill half of the plate with fruits and vegetables.
3. Vary the type of vegetables and fruits eaten.
4. Select at least half of the grains as whole grains.
5. Ensure that foods from the dairy group are high in calcium.
6. Drink milk that is fat-free or low fat (1%).
7. Eat protein foods that are lean.
8. Select fresh foods over frozen or canned foods.
9. Drink water rather than liquids that contain sugar.

⚠ Always consider the client's cultural, spiritual, and personal choices when planning nutritional intake.

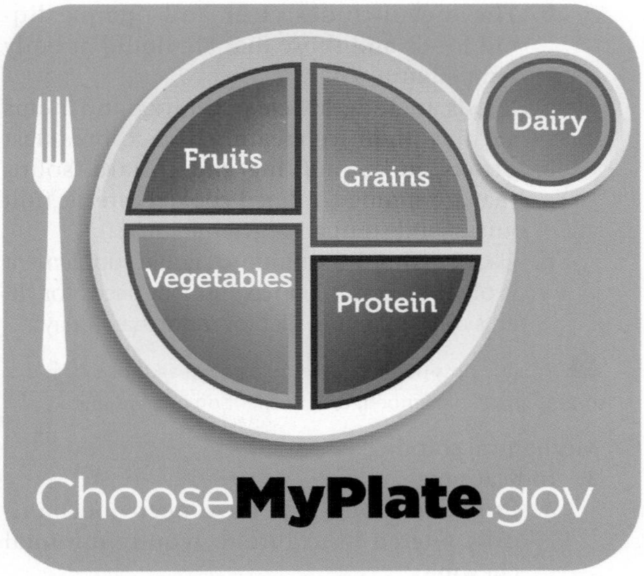

FIG. 11-1 MyPlate. (From U.S. Department of Agriculture. Available at http://www.choosemyplate.gov.)

IV. 2015-2020 Dietary Guidelines for Americans

A. Provides average daily consumption guidelines for the five food groups (see https://health.gov/dietaryguidelines/2015/guidelines/).

B. Guidelines

1. Maintain healthy body weight.
2. Increase physical activity and decrease sedentary activities.
3. Limit saturated fats and trans fats, with less than 10% of daily calories from saturated fats.
4. Limit added sugars so that less than 10% of daily calories are from added sugars.
5. Consume less than 2300 milligrams (mg) of sodium per day.
6. Consume low-sodium and potassium-rich foods.
7. Limit alcohol intake to moderate use (one drink daily for women and two drinks daily for men).
8. Use food-safety principles of Clean, Separate, Cook, and Chill.

BOX 11-3 Nutrition Throughout Growth and Development

Infant

The American Academy of Pediatrics recommends breastfeeding for the first 6 months of life and breastfeeding with additional foods from age 6 to 12 months.

Introduce new foods one at a time, 4-7 days apart, to identify allergies.

Infants should not have cow's milk before the age of 1 year.

Children under 1 year of age should not ingest honey or corn syrup products due to the risk of botulism toxin.

Toddlers and Preschoolers

Milk is a poor source of iron, and children who consume more than 24 ounces of milk per day are at risk for developing milk anemia. Whole milk should be consumed until 2 years of age to ensure adequate fatty acid intake.

Limit foods that pose choking hazards, such as hot dogs, candy, nuts, grapes, popcorn, and raw vegetables.

School-Age

Children in this age group have better appetites with a more varied intake. Assess for adequate intake of protein and vitamins A and C.

This age group is at risk for high intake of fats, sugar, and salt related to snack foods.

Promote healthy choices and encourage physical activity.

Adolescent

Energy needs increase to meet the increased metabolic needs of growth.

This age group has increased requirements of daily protein, calcium for bone growth, and iron to replace menstrual losses for girls and promote muscle development for boys.

Increased intake of iodine and B-complex vitamins are necessary to support thyroid development and metabolism.

Fast-food consumption is common and puts the adolescent at risk for malnutrition and obesity.

The onset of eating disorders commonly occurs during adolescence.

Young and Middle Adults

Energy needs decrease as the growth period ends. Lack of physical activity and access to certain foods increases the risk of obesity.

Pregnancy

During pregnancy, protein requirements increase to 60 g per day.

Calcium needs increase to promote fetal bone mineralization.

Iron supplements support increased blood volume.

Folic acid intake is required for DNA synthesis and red blood cell production.

Breastfeeding

For the breastfeeding mother, encourage intake of protein, calcium, and vitamins A, B, and C. Promote adequate fluid intake.

Breastfeeding mothers should consume an additional 500 kilocalories per day to support adequate production of breastmilk. Avoid alcohol, caffeine, and drugs, as these are absorbed into breast milk.

Older Adults

Energy needs are decreased due to slowed metabolic rate.

Age-related changes that affect nutrition include changes in teeth and saliva production, reduced taste and smell, decreased thirst sensation, and decreased gag reflex.

Ensure adequate calcium and vitamin D intake to prevent osteoporosis.

V. Therapeutic Diets

A. Clear liquid diet
1. Indications
a. Provides fluids and some electrolytes to prevent dehydration.
b. Used as an initial feeding after complete bowel rest.
c. Used initially to feed a malnourished person or a person who has not had any oral intake for some time.
d. Used for bowel preparation for surgery or diagnostic tests, as well as postoperatively and in clients with fever, vomiting, or diarrhea.
e. Used in gastroenteritis.
2. Nursing considerations
a. Clear liquid diet is deficient in energy (calories) and many **nutrients**.
b. Clear liquid diet is easily digested and absorbed.
c. Minimal residue is left in the gastrointestinal tract.
d. Clients may find a clear liquid diet unappetizing and boring.
e. As a transition diet, clear liquids are intended for short-term use.
f. Clear liquids and foods that are relatively transparent to light and are liquid at body temperature are considered "clear liquids," such as water, bouillon, clear broth, carbonated beverages, gelatin, hard candy, lemonade, ice pops, and regular or decaffeinated coffee or tea.
g. By limiting caffeine intake, an upset stomach and sleeplessness may be prevented.
h. The client may consume salt and sugar.
i. Dairy products and fruit juices with pulp are not clear liquids.
j. Instruct the client doing bowel preparation to avoid liquids that contain red or purple dye, which can mask the normal color of the lining of the colon.

Monitor the client's hydration status by assessing intake and output, assessing weight, monitoring for edema, and monitoring for signs of dehydration. Each kilogram (2.2 lb) of weight gained or lost is equal to 1 liter of fluid retained or lost.

B. Full liquid diet
1. Indication: May be used as a transition diet after clear liquids following surgery or for clients who have difficulty chewing, swallowing, or tolerating solid foods.
2. Nursing considerations
a. A full liquid diet is nutritionally deficient in energy (calories) and many nutrients.
b. The diet includes clear and opaque liquid foods and those that are liquid at body temperature.
c. Foods include all clear liquids and items such as plain ice cream, sherbet, breakfast drinks, milk, pudding and custard, soups that are strained, refined cooked cereals, fruit juices, and strained vegetable juices.
d. Use of a complete nutritional liquid supplement is often necessary to meet nutrient needs for clients on a full liquid diet for more than 3 days.

Provide nutritional supplements such as those high in protein, as prescribed, for the client on a liquid diet.

C. Mechanical soft diet
1. Indications
a. Provides foods that have been mechanically altered in texture to require minimal chewing.
b. Used for clients who have difficulty chewing but can tolerate more variety in texture than a liquid diet offers.
c. Used for clients who have dental problems, surgery of the head or neck, or dysphagia (requires swallowing evaluation and may require thickened liquids if the client has swallowing difficulties).
2. Nursing considerations
a. Degree of texture modification depends on individual need, including pureed, mashed, ground, or chopped.
b. Foods include those that are part of a clear and full liquid diet, with the addition of all cream soups, ground or diced meats, flaked fish, cottage cheese, rice, potatoes, pancakes, light breads, cooked vegetables, canned or cooked fruits, bananas, peanut butter, and nonfried eggs.
c. Foods to be avoided in mechanically altered diets include nuts; dried fruits; raw fruits and vegetables; fried foods; tough, smoked, or salted meats; and foods with coarse textures.

D. Soft diet
1. Indications
a. Used for clients who have difficulty chewing or swallowing.
b. Used for clients who have ulcerations of the mouth or gums, oral surgery, broken jaw, plastic surgery of the head or neck, or dysphagia, or for the client who has had a stroke.
2. Nursing considerations
a. Foods include easily digestible foods such as pastas, casseroles, tender meats, canned fruit, cooked vegetables, cakes, and cookies without nuts or coconut.

b. Clients with mouth sores should be served foods at cooler temperatures.
c. Clients who have difficulty chewing and swallowing because of dry mouth can increase salivary flow by sucking on sour candy.
d. Encourage the client to eat a variety of foods.
e. Provide plenty of fluids with meals to ease chewing and swallowing of foods.
f. Drinking fluids through a straw may be easier than drinking from a cup or glass; a straw may not be allowed for clients with dysphagia (because of the risk of aspiration).
g. All foods and seasonings are permitted; however, liquid, chopped, or pureed foods or regular foods with a soft consistency are tolerated best.
h. Foods that contain nuts or seeds, which easily can become trapped in the mouth and cause discomfort, should be avoided.
i. Raw fruits and vegetables, fried foods, and whole grains should be avoided.

! Consider the client's disease or illness and how it may affect nutritional status.

E. Low-fiber (low-residue) diet
1. Indications
a. Supplies foods that are least likely to form an obstruction when the intestinal tract is narrowed by inflammation or scarring or when gastrointestinal motility is slowed.
b. Used for inflammatory bowel disease, partial obstructions of the intestinal tract, gastroenteritis, diarrhea, or other gastrointestinal disorders.
2. Nursing considerations
a. Foods that are low in fiber include white bread, refined cooked cereals, cooked potatoes without skins, white rice, and refined pasta.
b. Foods to limit or avoid are raw fruits (except bananas), vegetables, nuts and seeds, plant fiber, and whole grains.
c. Dairy products should be limited to 2 servings a day.

F. High-fiber (high-residue) diet
1. Indication: Used for constipation, irritable bowel syndrome when the primary symptom is alternating constipation and diarrhea, and asymptomatic diverticular disease.
2. Nursing considerations
a. High-fiber diet provides 20 to 35 g of dietary fiber daily.
b. Volume and weight are added to the stool, speeding the movement of undigested materials through the intestine.
c. High-fiber foods are fruits and vegetables and whole-grain products.
d. Increase fiber gradually and provide adequate fluids to reduce possible undesirable side effects such as abdominal cramps, bloating, diarrhea, and dehydration.
e. Gas-forming foods should be limited (Box 11-4).

G. Cardiac diet (Box 11-5)
1. Indications
a. Indicated for atherosclerosis, diabetes mellitus, hyperlipidemia, hypertension, myocardial infarction, nephrotic syndrome, and renal failure.
b. Reduces the risk of heart disease.
c. **D**ietary **A**pproaches to **S**top **H**ypertension (DASH) diet: recommended to prevent and control hypertension, hypercholesterolemia, and obesity.
d. The DASH diet includes fruits, vegetables, whole grains, low-fat dairy foods, meat, fish, poultry, nuts, and beans; it is limited in sugar-sweetened foods and beverages, red meat, and added fats.
2. Nursing considerations
a. Restrict total amounts of fat, including saturated, trans, polyunsaturated, and monounsaturated; cholesterol; and **sodium**.
b. Teach the client about the DASH diet or other prescribed diet.

BOX 11-4 Gas-Forming Foods

Apples	Melons
Artichokes	Milk
Barley	Molasses
Beans	Nuts
Bran	Onions
Broccoli	Radishes
Brussels sprouts	Soybeans
Cabbage	Wheat
Celery	Yeast
Figs	

BOX 11-5 Sodium-Free Spices and Flavorings

Allspice	Ginger
Almond extract	Lemon extract
Bay leaves	Maple extract
Caraway seeds	Marjoram
Cinnamon	Mustard powder
Curry powder	Nutmeg
Garlic powder or garlic	

H. Fat-restricted diet
1. Indications
a. Used to reduce symptoms of abdominal pain, steatorrhea, flatulence, and diarrhea associated with high intakes of dietary fat and to decrease nutrient losses caused by ingestion of dietary fat in individuals with malabsorption disorders.
b. Used for clients with malabsorption disorders, pancreatitis, gallbladder disease, and gastroesophageal reflux.
2. Nursing considerations
a. Restrict total amount of fat, including saturated, trans, polyunsaturated, and monounsaturated.
b. Clients with malabsorption may also have difficulty tolerating fiber and lactose.
c. Vitamin and mineral deficiencies may occur in clients with diarrhea or steatorrhea.
d. A fecal fat test may be prescribed and indicates fat malabsorption with excretion of more than 6 to 8 g of fat (or more than 10% of fat consumed) per day during the 3 days of specimen collection.

I. High-calorie, high-protein diet
1. Indication: Used for severe stress, burns, wound healing, cancer, human immunodeficiency virus, acquired immunodeficiency syndrome, chronic obstructive pulmonary disease, respiratory failure, or any other type of debilitating disease.
2. Nursing considerations
a. Encourage nutrient-dense, high-calorie, high-protein foods such as whole milk and milk products, peanut butter, nuts and seeds, beef, chicken, fish, pork, and eggs.
b. Encourage snacks between meals, such as milkshakes, instant breakfasts, and nutritional supplements.

Calorie counts assist in determining the client's total nutritional intake and can identify a deficit or excess intake.

J. Carbohydrate-consistent diet
1. Indication: Used for clients with diabetes mellitus, hypoglycemia, hyperglycemia, and obesity.
2. Nursing considerations
a. The Exchange System for Meal Planning, developed by the Academy of Nutrition and Dietetics and the American Diabetes Association, is a food guide that may be recommended.
b. The Exchange System groups foods according to the amounts of carbohydrates, fats, and proteins they contain; major food groups include the carbohydrate, meat and meat substitute, and fat groups.
c. A carbohydrate-consistent diet focuses on maintaining a consistent amount of carbohydrate intake each day and with each meal; also known as "carb counting." For additional information, refer to: http://www.livestrong.com/article/436101-the-consistent-carbohydrate-diet-for-diabetics/
d. The MyPlate diet may also be recommended.

K. Sodium-restricted diet (see Box 11-5)
1. Indication: Used for hypertension, heart failure, renal disease, cardiac disease, and liver disease.
2. Nursing considerations
a. Individualized; can include 4 g of sodium daily (no-added-salt diet), 2 to 3 g of sodium daily (moderate restriction), 1 g of sodium daily (strict restriction), or 500 mg of sodium daily (severe restriction and seldom prescribed).
b. Encourage intake of fresh foods, rather than processed foods that contain higher amounts of sodium.
c. Canned, frozen, instant, smoked, pickled, and boxed foods usually contain higher amounts of sodium. Lunch meats, soy sauce, salad dressings, fast foods, soups, and snacks such as potato chips and pretzels also contain large amounts of sodium; teach clients to read nutritional facts on product packaging regarding sodium content per serving.
d. Certain medications contain significant amounts of sodium.
e. Salt substitutes may be used to improve palatability; most salt substitutes contain large amounts of potassium and should not be used by clients with renal disease.

L. Protein-restricted diet
1. Indication: Used for renal disease and end-stage liver disease.
2. The nutritional status of critically ill clients with protein-losing renal diseases, malabsorption syndromes, and continuous renal replacement therapy or dialysis should have their protein needs assessed by estimating the protein equivalent of nitrogen appearance (PNA); a nutritionist should be consulted.
3. Nursing considerations
a. Provide enough protein to maintain nutritional status but not an amount that will allow the buildup of waste products from protein metabolism (40 to 60 g of protein daily).
b. The less protein allowed, the more important it becomes that all protein in the diet be of high biological value (contain all essential amino acids in recommended proportions).
c. An adequate total energy intake from foods is critical for clients on protein-restricted

diets (protein will be used for energy rather than for protein synthesis).

d. Special low-protein products, such as pastas, bread, cookies, wafers, and gelatin made with wheat starch, can improve energy intake and add variety to the diet.

e. Carbohydrates in powdered or liquid forms can provide additional energy.

f. Vegetables and fruits contain some protein and, for very-low-protein diets, these foods must be calculated into the diet.

g. Foods are limited from the milk, meat, bread, and starch groups.

M. Gluten-free diet: A treatment for celiac disease and gluten sensitivity for clients needing the protein fraction "gluten" eliminated from their diet. See Chapter 33 for information on this diet.

Fluid restrictions may be prescribed for clients with hyponatremia, severe extracellular volume excess, and renal disorders. Ask specifically about client preferences regarding types of oral fluids and temperature preference of fluids.

N. Renal diet (see Box 11-2)

1. Indication: Used for the client with acute kidney injury or chronic kidney disease and those requiring hemodialysis or peritoneal dialysis

2. Nursing considerations

a. Controlled amounts of protein, sodium, **phosphorus,** calcium, potassium, and fluids may be prescribed; may also need modification in fiber, cholesterol, and fat based on individual requirements; clients on peritoneal dialysis usually have diets prescribed that are less restrictive with fluid and protein intake than those on hemodialysis.

b. Most clients receiving dialysis need to restrict fluids (Box 11-6).

c. Monitor weight daily as a priority, because weight is an important indicator of fluid status.

An initial assessment includes identifying allergies and food and medication interactions.

O. Potassium-modified diet (see Box 11-2)

1. Indications

a. Low-potassium diet is indicated for hyperkalemia, which may be caused by impaired renal function, hypoaldosteronism, Addison's disease, angiotensin-converting enzyme inhibitor medications, immunosuppressive medications, potassium-retaining diuretics, and chronic hyperkalemia.

b. High-potassium diet is indicated for hypokalemia, which may be caused by renal tubular acidosis, gastrointestinal losses (diarrhea, vomiting), intracellular shifts, potassium-losing diuretics, antibiotics, mineralocorticoid or glucocorticoid excess resulting from primary or secondary aldosteronism, Cushing's syndrome, or exogenous corticosteroid use.

2. Nursing considerations

a. Foods that are low in potassium include applesauce, green beans, cabbage, lettuce, peppers, grapes, blueberries, cooked summer squash, cooked turnip greens, pineapple, and raspberries.

b. Box 11-2 lists foods that are high in potassium.

P. High-calcium diet

1. Indication: Calcium is needed during bone growth and in adulthood to prevent osteoporosis and to facilitate vascular contraction, vasodilation, muscle contraction, and nerve transmission.

2. Nursing considerations

a. Primary dietary sources of calcium are dairy products (see Box 11-2 for food items high in calcium).

b. Lactose-intolerant clients should incorporate nondairy sources of calcium into their diet regularly.

Q. Low-purine diet

1. Indication: Used for gout, kidney stones, and elevated uric acid levels

2. Nursing considerations

a. Purine is a precursor for uric acid, which forms stones and crystals.

b. Foods to restrict include anchovies, herring, mackerel, sardines, scallops, organ meats, gravies, meat extracts, wild game, goose, and sweetbreads.

R. High-iron diet

1. Indication: Used for clients with anemia

2. Nursing considerations

a. The high-iron diet replaces iron deficit from inadequate intake or loss.

b. The diet includes organ meats, meat, egg yolks, whole-wheat products, dark green leafy vegetables, dried fruit, and legumes.

c. Inform the client that concurrent intake of vitamin C with iron foods enhances absorption of iron.

BOX 11-6 Measures to Relieve Thirst

- Chew gum or suck hard candy.
- Freeze fluids so they take longer to consume.
- Add lemon juice to water to make it more refreshing.
- Gargle with refrigerated mouthwash.

VI. Vegan and Vegetarian Diets

A. Vegan

1. Vegans follow a strict vegetarian diet and consume no animal foods.
2. Eat only foods of plant origin (e.g., whole or enriched grains, legumes, nuts, seeds, fruits, vegetables).
3. The use of soybeans, soy milk, soybean curd (tofu), and processed soy protein products enhance the nutritional value of the diet.

B. Lacto-vegetarian

1. Lacto-vegetarians eat milk, cheese, and dairy foods but avoid meat, fish, poultry, and eggs.
2. A diet of whole or enriched grains, legumes, nuts, seeds, fruits, and vegetables in sufficient quantities to meet energy needs provides a balanced diet.

C. Lacto-ovo-vegetarian

1. Lacto-ovo-vegetarians follow a food pattern that allows for the consumption of dairy products and eggs.
2. Consumption of adequate plant and animal food sources that excludes meat, poultry, pork, and fish poses no nutritional risks.

D. Ovo-vegetarians: The only animal foods that the ovo-vegetarian consumes are eggs, which are an excellent source of complete proteins.

E. Nursing considerations

1. Vegan and vegetarian diets are not usually prescribed but are a diet choice made by a client.
2. Ensure that the client eats a sufficient amount of varied foods to meet nutrient and energy needs.
3. Clients should be educated about consuming complementary proteins over the course of each day to ensure that all essential amino acids are provided.
4. Potential deficiencies in vegetarian diets include energy, protein, vitamin B_{12}, zinc, iron, calcium, omega-3 fatty acids, and vitamin D (if limited exposure to sunlight).
5. To enhance absorption of iron, vegetarians should consume a good source of iron and vitamin C with each meal.
6. Foods eaten may include tofu, tempeh, soy milk and soy products, meat analogs, legumes, nuts and seeds, sprouts, and a variety of fruits and vegetables.
7. Soy protein is considered equivalent in quality to animal protein.

Body mass index (BMI) can be calculated by dividing the client's weight in kilograms by height in meters squared. For example, a client who weighs 75 kg (165 pounds) and is 1.8 m (5 feet, 9 inches) tall has a BMI of 23.15 (75 divided by $1.8^2 = 23.15$). From: Potter et al. (2013), p. 1008.

VII. Enteral Nutrition

A. Description: Provides liquefied foods into the gastrointestinal tract via a tube

B. Indications

1. When the gastrointestinal tract is functional but oral intake is not meeting estimated nutrient needs
2. Used for clients with swallowing problems, burns, major trauma, liver or other organ failure, or severe **malnutrition**

C. Nursing considerations

1. Clients with lactose intolerance need to be placed on lactose-free formulas.
2. See Chapter 69 for information regarding the administration of gastrointestinal tube feedings and associated complications.

PRACTICE QUESTIONS

78. The nurse is teaching a client who has iron deficiency anemia about foods she should include in the diet. The nurse determines that the client understands the dietary modifications if which items are selected from the menu?

1. Nuts and milk
2. Coffee and tea
3. Cooked rolled oats and fish
4. Oranges and dark green leafy vegetables

79. The nurse is planning to teach a client with malabsorption syndrome about the necessity of following a low-fat diet. The nurse develops a list of high-fat foods to avoid and should include which food items on the list? **Select all that apply.**

- ☐ 1. Oranges
- ☐ 2. Broccoli
- ☐ 3. Margarine
- ☐ 4. Cream cheese
- ☐ 5. Luncheon meats
- ☐ 6. Broiled haddock

80. The nurse instructs a client with chronic kidney disease who is receiving hemodialysis about dietary modifications. The nurse determines that the client understands these dietary modifications if the client selects which items from the dietary menu?

1. Cream of wheat, blueberries, coffee
2. Sausage and eggs, banana, orange juice
3. Bacon, cantaloupe melon, tomato juice
4. Cured pork, grits, strawberries, orange juice

81. The nurse is conducting a dietary assessment on a client who is on a vegan diet. The nurse provides dietary teaching and should focus on foods high in which vitamin that may be lacking in a vegan diet?

1. Vitamin A
2. Vitamin B_{12}
3. Vitamin C
4. Vitamin E

82. A client with hypertension has been told to maintain a diet low in sodium. The nurse who is teaching this client about foods that are allowed should include which food item in a list provided to the client?
1. Tomato soup
2. Boiled shrimp
3. Instant oatmeal
4. Summer squash

83. A postoperative client has been placed on a clear liquid diet. The nurse should provide the client with which items that are allowed to be consumed on this diet? **Select all that apply.**
- ☐ 1. Broth
- ☐ 2. Coffee
- ☐ 3. Gelatin
- ☐ 4. Pudding
- ☐ 5. Vegetable juice
- ☐ 6. Pureed vegetables

84. The nurse is instructing a client with hypertension on the importance of choosing foods low in sodium. The nurse should teach the client to limit intake of which food?
1. Apples
2. Bananas
3. Smoked salami
4. Steamed vegetables

85. A client who is recovering from surgery has been advanced from a clear liquid diet to a full liquid diet. The client is looking forward to the diet change because he has been "bored" with the clear liquid diet. The nurse should offer which full liquid item to the client?
1. Tea
2. Gelatin
3. Custard
4. Ice pop

86. A client is recovering from abdominal surgery and has a large abdominal wound. The nurse should encourage the client to eat which food item that is naturally high in vitamin C to promote wound healing?
1. Milk
2. Oranges
3. Bananas
4. Chicken

87. The nurse is caring for a client with cirrhosis of the liver. To minimize the effects of the disorder, the nurse teaches the client about foods that are high in thiamine. The nurse determines that the client has the **best** understanding of the dietary measures to follow if the client states an intention to increase the intake of which food?
1. Milk
2. Chicken
3. Broccoli
4. Legumes

88. The nurse provides instructions to a client with a low potassium level about the foods that are high in potassium and tells the client to consume which foods? **Select all that apply.**
- ☐ 1. Peas
- ☐ 2. Raisins
- ☐ 3. Potatoes
- ☐ 4. Cantaloupe
- ☐ 5. Cauliflower
- ☐ 6. Strawberries

89. The nurse is reviewing laboratory results and notes that a client's serum sodium level is 150 mEq/L (150 mmol/L). The nurse reports the serum sodium level to the primary health care provider (PHCP), and the PHCP prescribes dietary instructions based on the sodium level. Which acceptable food items does the nurse instruct the client to consume? **Select all that apply.**
- ☐ 1. Peas
- ☐ 2. Nuts
- ☐ 3. Cheese
- ☐ 4. Cauliflower
- ☐ 5. Processed oat cereals

ANSWERS

78. *Answer:* 4
Rationale: Dark green leafy vegetables are a good source of iron, and oranges are a good source of vitamin C, which enhances iron absorption. All other options are not food sources that are high in iron and vitamin C.
Test-Taking Strategy: Focus on the subject, diet choices for a client with anemia. Think about the pathophysiology of anemia and determine that the client needs foods high in iron and recall that vitamin C enhances iron absorption. Use knowledge of foods high in iron and vitamin C. Remember that green leafy vegetables are high in iron and oranges are high in vitamin C.
Level of Cognitive Ability: Evaluating
Client Needs: Physiological Integrity
Integrated Process: Nursing Process—Evaluation
Content Area: Foundations of Care: Therapeutic Diets
Health Problem: Adult Health: Hematological: Anemias
Priority Concepts: Client Education; Nutrition
Reference: Lewis et al. (2017), p. 610.

79. *Answer:* 3, 4, 5
Rationale: Fruits and vegetables tend to be lower in fat because they do not come from animal sources. Broiled haddock is also naturally lower in fat. Margarine, cream cheese, and luncheon meats are high-fat foods.
Test-Taking Strategy: Focus on the subject of the question, the high-fat foods. Oranges and broccoli (fruit and vegetable) can be eliminated first. Next eliminate haddock because it is a broiled food. Remember that margarine, cheese, and luncheon meats are high in fat content.
Level of Cognitive Ability: Applying
Client Needs: Physiological Integrity
Integrated Process: Teaching and Learning
Content Area: Foundations of Care: Therapeutic Diets
Health Problem: Adult Health: Gastrointestinal: Nutrition Problems
Priority Concepts: Client Education; Nutrition
Reference: Nix (2017), p. 33.

80. *Answer:* 1
Rationale: The diet for a client with chronic kidney disease who is receiving hemodialysis should include controlled amounts of sodium, phosphorus, calcium, potassium, and fluids, which is indicated in the correct option. The food items in the remaining options are high in sodium, phosphorus, or potassium.
Test-Taking Strategy: Focus on the subject, dietary modification for a client with chronic kidney disease. Think about the pathophysiology of this disorder to recall that sodium needs to be limited. Noting the items sausage, bacon, and cured pork will assist in eliminating these options.
Level of Cognitive Ability: Evaluating
Client Needs: Physiological Integrity
Integrated Process: Nursing Process—Evaluation
Content Area: Foundations of Care: Therapeutic Diets
Health Problem: Adult Health: Renal and Urinary: Chronic kidney disease
Priority Concepts: Client Education; Nutrition
Reference: Lewis et al. (2017), p. 1083.

81. *Answer:* 2
Rationale: Vegans do not consume any animal products. Vitamin B_{12} is found in animal products and therefore would most likely be lacking in a vegan diet. Vitamins A, C, and E are found in fresh fruits and vegetables, which are consumed in a vegan diet.
Test-Taking Strategy: Focus on the subject, a vegan diet and the vitamin lacking in this diet. Recalling the food items eaten and restricted in this diet will direct you to the correct option. Remember that vegans do not consume any animal products and as a result may be deficient in vitamin B_{12}.
Level of Cognitive Ability: Applying
Client Needs: Physiological Integrity
Integrated Process: Teaching and Learning
Content Area: Foundations of Care: Therapeutic Diets
Health Problem: N/A
Priority Concepts: Health Promotion; Nutrition
Reference: Lewis et al. (2017), p. 856.

82. *Answer:* 4
Rationale: Foods that are lower in sodium include fruits and vegetables (summer squash) because they do not contain physiological saline. Highly processed or refined foods (tomato soup, instant oatmeal) are higher in sodium unless their food labels specifically state "low sodium." Saltwater fish and shellfish are high in sodium.
Test-Taking Strategy: Focus on the subject, foods low in sodium. Begin to answer this question by eliminating boiled shrimp, recalling that saltwater fish and shellfish are high in sodium. Next, eliminate tomato soup and instant oatmeal because they are processed foods.
Level of Cognitive Ability: Applying
Client Needs: Physiological Integrity
Integrated Process: Teaching and Learning
Content Area: Foundations of Care: Therapeutic Diets
Health Problem: Adult Health: Cardiovascular: Hypertension
Priority Concepts: Health Promotion; Nutrition
Reference: Lewis et al. (2017), p. 688.

83. *Answer:* 1, 2, 3
Rationale: A clear liquid diet consists of foods that are relatively transparent to light and are clear and liquid at room and body temperature. These foods include items such as water, bouillon, clear broth, carbonated beverages, gelatin, hard candy, lemonade, ice pops, and regular or decaffeinated coffee or tea. The incorrect food items are items that are allowed on a full liquid diet.
Test-Taking Strategy: Focus on the subject, a clear liquid diet. Recalling that a clear liquid diet consists of foods that are relatively transparent to light and are clear will assist in answering the question.
Level of Cognitive Ability: Applying
Client Needs: Physiological Integrity
Integrated Process: Nursing Process—Implementation
Content Area: Foundations of Care: Therapeutic Diets
Health Problem: N/A
Priority Concepts: Health Promotion; Nutrition
Reference: Potter et al. (2017), p. 1074.

84. *Answer:* 3
Rationale: Smoked foods are high in sodium, which is noted in the correct option. The remaining options are fruits and vegetables, which are low in sodium.
Test-Taking Strategy: Note the subject, the food item that is high in sodium. Remember that smoked foods are high in sodium. Also eliminate options 1, 2, and 4 because they are comparable or alike and are nonprocessed foods.
Level of Cognitive Ability: Applying
Client Needs: Physiological Integrity
Integrated Process: Teaching and Learning
Content Area: Foundations of Care: Therapeutic Diets
Health Problem: Adult Health: Cardiovascular: Hypertension
Priority Concepts: Health Promotion; Nutrition
Reference: Ignatavicius, Workman, Rebar (2018), p. 173.

85. *Answer:* 3
Rationale: Full liquid food items include items such as plain ice cream, sherbet, breakfast drinks, milk, pudding and custard, soups that are strained, refined cooked cereals, and strained vegetable juices. A clear liquid diet consists of foods that are relatively transparent. The food items in the incorrect options are clear liquids.
Test-Taking Strategy: Focus on the subject, a full liquid item. Remember that a clear liquid diet consists of foods that are relatively transparent. This will assist you in eliminating tea, gelatin, and ice pops; in addition, these are comparable or alike options.
Level of Cognitive Ability: Applying
Client Needs: Physiological Integrity
Integrated Process: Nursing Process—Implementation
Content Area: Foundations of Care: Therapeutic Diets
Health Problem: N/A
Priority Concepts: Health Promotion; Nutrition
Reference: Potter et al. (2017), p. 1074.

86. *Answer:* 2
Rationale: Citrus fruits and juices are especially high in vitamin C. Bananas are high in potassium. Meats and dairy products are two food groups that are high in the B vitamins.
Test-Taking Strategy: Note the subject, food items naturally high in vitamin C. It is necessary to recall that citrus fruits and juices are high in vitamin C; this will direct you to the correct option.
Level of Cognitive Ability: Applying
Client Needs: Physiological Integrity
Integrated Process: Nursing Process—Implementation
Content Area: Foundations of Care: Therapeutic Diets
Health Problem: Adult Health: Integumentary: Wounds
Priority Concepts: Nutrition; Tissue Integrity
Reference: Lewis et al. (2017), p. 610.

87. *Answer:* 4
Rationale: The client with cirrhosis needs to consume foods high in thiamine. Thiamine is present in a variety of foods of plant and animal origin. Legumes are especially rich in this vitamin. Other good food sources include nuts, whole-grain cereals, and pork. Milk contains vitamins A, D, and B_2. Poultry contains niacin. Broccoli contains vitamins C, E, and K and folic acid.
Test-Taking Strategy: Note the strategic word, *best.* This may indicate that more than one option may be a food that contains thiamine. Remembering that legumes are especially rich in thiamine will direct you to the correct option.
Level of Cognitive Ability: Evaluating
Client Needs: Physiological Integrity
Integrated Process: Nursing Process—Evaluation
Content Area: Foundations of Care: Therapeutic Diets
Health Problem: Adult Health: Gastrointestinal: GI Accessory Organs
Priority Concepts: Health Promotion; Nutrition
Reference: Nix (2017), p. 96.

88. *Answer:* 2, 3, 4, 6
Rationale: The normal potassium level is 3.5 to 5.0 mEq/L (3.5 to 5.0 mmol/L). Common food sources of potassium include avocado, bananas, cantaloupe, carrots, fish, mushrooms, oranges, potatoes, pork, beef, veal, raisins, spinach, strawberries, and tomatoes. Peas and cauliflower are high in magnesium.
Test-Taking Strategy: Focus on the subject, foods high in potassium. Read each food item and use knowledge about nutrition and components of food. Recall that peas and cauliflower are high in magnesium.
Level of Cognitive Ability: Applying
Client Needs: Physiological Integrity
Integrated Process: Teaching and Learning
Content Area: Foundations of Care: Therapeutic Diets
Health Problem: N/A
Priority Concepts: Client Education; Nutrition
Reference: Ignatavicius, Workman, Rebar (2018), p. 175.

89. *Answer:* 1, 2, 4
Rationale: The normal serum sodium level is 135 to 145 mEq/L (135 to 145 mmol/L). A serum sodium level of 150 mEq/L (150 mmol/L) indicates hypernatremia. On the basis of this finding, the nurse would instruct the client to avoid foods high in sodium. Peas, nuts, and cauliflower are good food sources of phosphorus and are not high in sodium (unless they are canned or labeled salted). Peas and cauliflower are also a good source of magnesium. Processed foods such as cheese and processed oat cereals are high in sodium content.
Test-Taking Strategy: Focus on the subject, foods acceptable to be consumed by a client with a sodium level of 150 mEq/L (150 mmol/L). First, you must determine that the client has hypernatremia. Select peas and cauliflower first because these are vegetables. From the remaining options, note the word *processed* in option 5 and recall that cheese is high in sodium. Remember that processed foods tend to be higher in sodium content.
Level of Cognitive Ability: Applying
Client Needs: Physiological Integrity
Integrated Process: Teaching and Learning
Content Area: Foundations of Care: Therapeutic Diets
Health Problem: N/A
Priority Concepts: Client Education; Nutrition
Reference: Ignatavicius, Workman, Rebar (2018), p. 173.

CHAPTER 12

Health and Physical Assessment of the Adult Client

PRIORITY CONCEPTS **Clinical Judgment; Health Promotion**

I. Environment/Setting

A. Establish a relationship and explain the procedure to the client.

B. Ensure privacy and make the client feel comfortable (comfortable room temperature, sufficient lighting, remove distractions such as noise or objects, and avoid interruptions).

C. Sit down for the interview (avoid barriers such as a desk), maintain an appropriate social distance, and maintain eye level.

D. Use therapeutic communication techniques and open-ended questions to obtain information about the client's symptoms and concerns; allow time for the client to ask questions.

E. Consider religious and cultural characteristics such as language (the need for an interpreter), values and beliefs, health practices, eye contact, and touch.

F. Keep note-taking to a minimum so the client is the focus of attention.

G. Types of health and physical assessments (Box 12-1)

H. SOAP (subjective, objective, assessment, plan) notes are a frequently used format for documenting client data including health history, physical examination, assessment or diagnosis, and plan of care. The nurse should be familiar with SOAP notes, how to interpret the initial history and physical (H&P) SOAP notes, and how to follow subsequent progress SOAP notes so as to maintain abreast of changes in the client's plan of care. See Table 12-1 for a detailed list of information contained in SOAP notes.

II. Health History (refer to section titled "Subjective" in Table 12-1)

A. General state of health: Body features and physical characteristics, body movements, body posture, level of consciousness, nutritional status, speech

B. Chief complaint and history of present illness (document direct client quotes) that leads the client to seek care

C. Family history: The health status of direct blood relatives as well as the client's spouse

D. Social history

1. Data about the client's lifestyle, with a focus on factors that may affect health
2. Information about alcohol, drug, and tobacco use; sexual practices; tattoos; body piercing; travel history; and work setting to identify occupational hazards

E. Domestic violence screening

1. Done to determine whether the client is experiencing any form of domestic violence
2. Conducted during a one-to-one interview with the client while obtaining the health history

III. Mental Status Exam

A. The mental status can be assessed while obtaining subjective data from the client during the health history interview.

B. Appearance

1. Note appearance, including posture, body movements, dress, and hygiene and grooming.
2. An inappropriate appearance and poor hygiene may be indicative of depression, manic disorder, dementia, organic brain disease, or another disorder.

BOX 12-1 Types of Health and Physical Assessments

Complete Assessment: Includes a complete health history and physical examination and forms a baseline database.

Focused Assessment: Focuses on a limited or short-term problem, such as the client's complaint.

Episodic/Follow-up Assessment: Focuses on evaluating a client's progress.

Emergency Assessment: Involves the rapid collection of data, often during the provision of lifesaving measures.

TABLE 12-1 SOAP Notes

Subjective	
Identifying client information	Name, date of birth, medical record number
Problems, allergies, medications, immunizations (PAMI) list	Ongoing list of medical problems, allergies with reactions, medications with dosages and directions, and past immunizations
General client information	Address, phone numbers, employer, work address and phone number, email address, gender, marital status, health insurance status and information
Chief complaint or reason for seeking care	Brief description of main problem; stated verbatim in quotation marks; duration is always included
History of present illness	Detailed description of all symptoms that may be related to the chief complaint Guided by "OLDCARTS" symptom analysis: (onset, location, duration, character, aggravating/associated factors, relieving factors, timing, severity)
Past medical history	Hospitalizations, surgeries, childhood illnesses, adult illnesses, injuries/accidents, immunizations, past and current medications, allergies, mental health, recent laboratory tests
Family history	Pedigree may be included Includes but not limited to major health or genetic disorders, such has hypertension, cancer, cardiac, respiratory, and thyroid disorders, allergies, hepatitis Age and health of spouse and children included
Personal and social history	Varies based on health influences Cultural background and practices, home environment, general life satisfaction, safety/abuse, stressors, religious preferences, occupation, exposure to heat/cold or toxins, exposure to contagious diseases, health habits such as diet, exercise, smoking, salt intake, obesity, alcohol intake, recreational drug use, caffeine use, sexual activity, concerns about cost of care
Review of systems (may include some objective data)	General or constitutional symptoms: fever, chills, malaise, night sweats, fatigue, unintentional weight loss or gain, overall behavior Skin, hair, nails: rash, itching, pigmentation change, sweating, abnormal hair or nail growth Head and neck: headache, dizziness, syncope, concussions, loss of consciousness Eyes: visual acuity, double vision, blurring, light sensitivity, glaucoma, use of glasses or contacts, use of eyedrops Ears: hearing loss, ear pain, tinnitus, vertigo Nose: smell, colds, nosebleeds, postnasal discharge, sinus pain Throat and mouth: hoarseness, change in voice, sore throat, gum bleeding or swelling, taste changes Lymphatics: enlargement, tenderness Chest and lungs: respiratory pain, dyspnea, wheezing, cyanosis, cough, sputum, hemoptysis, last chest x-ray Breasts: development, pain, tenderness, lumps, discharge, last mammogram Heart and circulation: chest pain, edema, history of hypertension, myocardial infarction, exercise tolerance, previous cardiac tests, claudication, bruising, thrombophlebitis Hematologic: anemia, blood cell disorder, bleeding Gastrointestinal: appetite, food intolerance, dysphagia, heartburn, nausea, vomiting, diarrhea, constipation, change in stool, dark urine, previous studies such as colonoscopy, diet recall Endocrine: thyroid enlargement, heat or cold intolerance, polyphagia, polydipsia, polyuria, changes in facial or body hair, striae Genitourinary: for males, puberty onset, testicular pain, libido, infertility; for females, menses onset, regularity, duration, dysmenorrhea, last period, itching, date of last Papanicolaou (Pap) smear/human papilloma virus (HPV) test, age at menopause, libido, sexual difficulties, pregnancy (GTPAL; refer to Chapter 21); for both, dysuria, flank pain, urgency, frequency, nocturia, dribbling, hematuria, incontinence Musculoskeletal: joint pain, stiffness, redness, swelling, restricted motion, deformities Neurological: syncope, seizures, weakness, paralysis, incoordination, tremors, cognition Mental health: mood changes, depression, anxiety, difficulty concentrating, suicidal thoughts, irritability, sleep disturbances
Objective	
General statement	Age, race, gender, general appearance, weight, height, body mass index, vital signs (including orthostatic if applicable)

TABLE 12-1 SOAP Notes—cont'd

Mental status	Physical appearance, behavior, facial expression and body language, appropriate eye contact, level of consciousness (alertness and awareness and ability to interact appropriately with the environment), response to questions, reasoning, emotion, speech and language
Skin	Color, texture, temperature, turgor, uniformity, hygiene, scars, tattoos, moisture, edema, odor, lesions, trauma, hair texture and distribution, nail configuration
Head	Size, contour, scalp, facial features, facies, edema, temporal arteries
Eyes	Acuity, visual fields, edema, conjunctiva and sclera, eyebrows, extraocular movements, corneal light reflex, cover-uncover test, nystagmus, pupils equal, round, react to light, accommodation (PERRLA) both direct and consensual, fundoscopic findings
Ears	Configuration, position, alignment, tenderness, nodules, hearing, otoscopic findings
Nose	Appearance, patency, discharge, polyps, turbinates, septum, sinus tenderness, odors
Throat and mouth	Teeth, lips, tongue, buccal and oral mucosa, floor of mouth, appearance of palate, tonsils, tonsil grade, gag reflex, phonation of "Ah," voice, taste
Neck	Fullness, mobility, strength, trachea, thyroid size, shape, nodules, tenderness, bruits, masses, lymphadenopathy
Chest	Size, shape, anterior and posterior (AP) and transverse diameter, respiration, tenderness on bones, retractions/accessory muscle use
Lungs	Respiration rate, depth, work of breathing, regularity, tactile fremitus, percussion notes, breath sounds, friction rub
Breasts	Size, symmetry, contour, lesions, masses, tenderness, retractions, dimpling, nipple discharge, nipple retraction
Heart	Apical impulse, pulsation, heart rate, rhythm, thrills, heaves, lifts, heart tones, murmurs, rubs, gallops
Vasculature	Pulses, jugular venous distention or pulsations, carotid, abdominal aortic, temporal, renal, iliac, femoral artery bruit, temperature, color, skin texture, hair distribution, edema, nailbeds, tenderness
Abdomen	Shape, contour, pulsations, bowel sounds, masses, organomegaly, tenderness, distention, costovertebral angle tenderness
Genitalia	Male: Symmetry, circumcision, color, urethral opening, discharge, lesions, hair distribution, palpation of penis, testes, epididymides, vasa deferentia, tenderness, masses, hernia, scrotal swelling, transillumination Female: Tenderness, discharge, inflammation, lesions, polyps, vaginal mucosa, cervix, discharge, odor, size and contour of uterus, mobility of cervix, adnexa, ovaries
Anus and rectum	Hemorrhoids, fissures, skin tags, inflammation, excoriation, sphincter tone and control, prostate size, contour, consistency, mobility, color and consistency of stool
Lymphatics	Presence of palpable lymph nodes, size, shape, warmth, tenderness, mobility, consistency
Musculoskeletal	Posture, alignment, symmetry, spasms, active and passive range of motion, deformities, tenderness, swelling, crepitus, muscle strength
Neurologic	Cranial nerves, gait, balance, coordination with rapid alternating movements, sensory function with pain, touch, fibration, superficial and deep tendon reflexes

Assessment

- Diagnosis with rationale
- Rationale derived from subjective and objective data
- Symptoms can be listed as diagnoses
- There may be a list of differential diagnoses, which are suspected diagnoses that are yet to be confirmed
- May include anticipated problems such as progression of disease or complications

Plan

- Typically denoted in the following order:
- Diagnostic tests, treatment plan with rationale
- Client education and counseling
- Referrals
- Follow-up or dates for re-evaluating results of plan

From Ball JW, Dains JE, Flynn JA, Solomon BS, Stewart RW: *Seidel's guide to physical examination,* ed 8, St. Louis, 2015, Elsevier.

BOX 12-2 The Mental Status Examination: Cognitive Level of Functioning

Orientation: Assess client's orientation to person, place, and time.
Attention Span: Assess client's ability to concentrate.
Recent Memory: Assessed by asking the client to recall a recent occurrence (e.g., the means of transportation used to get to the health care agency for the physical assessment).
Remote Memory: Assessed by asking the client about a verifiable past event (e.g., a vacation).
New Learning: Used to assess the client's ability to recall unrelated words identified by the nurse; the nurse selects four words and asks the client to recall the words 5, 10, and 30 minutes later.
Judgment: Determine whether the client's actions or decisions regarding discussions during the interview are realistic.
Thought Processes and Perceptions: The way the client thinks and what the client says should be logical, coherent, and relevant; the client should be consistently aware of reality.

C. Behavior
1. Level of consciousness: Assess alertness and awareness and the client's ability to interact appropriately with the environment.
2. Facial expression and body language: Check for appropriate eye contact and determine whether facial expression and body language are appropriate to the situation; this assessment also provides information regarding the client's mood and affect.
3. Speech: Assess speech pattern for articulation and appropriateness of conversation.

D. Cognitive level of functioning (Box 12-2)

IV. Physical Exam (refer to section titled "Objective" in Table 12-1)

A. Overview
1. Gather equipment needed for the examination.
2. Use the senses of sight, smell, touch, and hearing to collect data.
3. Assessment includes **inspection**, **palpation**, **percussion**, and **auscultation**; these skills are performed one at a time, in this order (except the abdominal assessment).

B. Assessment techniques
1. Inspection
   a. The first assessment technique, which uses vision and smell senses while observing the client
   b. Requires good lighting, adequate body exposure with draping, and possibly the use of certain instruments such as an otoscope or ophthalmoscope
2. Palpation
   a. Uses the sense of touch; warm the hands before touching the client.
   b. Identify tender areas and palpate them last.
   c. Start with light palpation to detect surface characteristics, and then perform deeper palpation.
   d. Light palpation is done with 1 hand by pressing the skin gently with the tips of 2 or 3 fingers held close together; deep palpation is done by placing 1 hand on top of the other and pressing down with the fingertips of both hands.
   e. Assess texture, temperature, and moisture of the skin, as well as organ location and size and symmetry if appropriate.
   f. Assess for swelling, vibration or pulsation, rigidity or spasticity, and crepitation.
   g. Assess for the presence of lumps or masses, as well as the presence of tenderness or pain.
3. Percussion
   a. Involves tapping the client's skin to assess underlying structures and to determine the presence of vibrations and sounds and, if present, their intensity, duration, pitch, quality, and location
   b. Provides information related to the presence of air, fluid, or solid masses as well as organ size, shape, and position
   c. Descriptions of findings include resonance, hyperresonance, tympany, dullness, or flatness.
4. Auscultation: Involves listening with a stethoscope to sounds produced by the body for presence and quality, such as heart, lung, or bowel sounds

C. Vital signs
1. Includes temperature, radial pulse (apical pulse may be measured during the cardiovascular assessment), respirations, blood pressure, pulse oximetry, and presence of pain (refer to Chapter 10 for information on vital signs, pulse oximetry, and pain)
2. Height, weight, and nutritional status are also assessed.

V. Body Systems Assessment

A. Integumentary system: Involves inspection and palpation of skin, hair, and nails.
1. **Subjective data:** Self-care behaviors, history of skin disease, medications being taken, environmental or occupational hazards and exposure to toxic substances, changes in skin color or pigmentation, change in a mole or a sore that does not heal
2. **Objective data:** Color, temperature (hypothermia or hyperthermia); excessive dryness or moisture; skin turgor; texture (smoothness, firmness); excessive bruising, itching, rash; hair loss (alopecia) or nail abnormalities such as pitting; lesions

(may be inspected with a magnifier and light or with the use of a Wood's light [ultraviolet light used in a darkened room]); scars or birthmarks; edema; capillary filling time (Boxes 12-3 and 12-4; Table 12-2)

3. Dark-skinned client
   a. Cyanosis: Check lips and tongue for a gray color; nailbeds, palms, and soles for a blue color; and conjunctivae for pallor.
   b. Jaundice: Check oral mucous membranes for a yellow color; check the sclera nearest to the iris for a yellow color.
   c. Bleeding: Look for skin swelling and darkening and compare the affected side with the unaffected side.
   d. Inflammation: Check for warmth or a shiny or taut and pitting skin area, and compare with the unaffected side.
4. Refer to Chapter 42 for diagnostic tests related to the integumentary system

⚠ To test skin turgor, pinch a large fold of skin and assess the ability of the skin to return to its place when released. Poor turgor occurs in severe dehydration or extreme weight loss.

BOX 12-3 Characteristics of Skin Color

Cyanosis: Mottled bluish coloration
Erythema: Redness
Pallor: Pale, whitish coloration
Jaundice: Yellow coloration

BOX 12-4 Assessing Capillary Filling Time

1. Depress the nailbed to produce blanching.
2. Release and observe for the return of color.
3. Color will return within 3 seconds if arterial capillary perfusion is normal.

5. Client teaching
   a. Provide information about factors that can be harmful to the skin, such as sun exposure.
   b. Encourage performing self-examination of the skin for lesions monthly using the ABCDE (asymmetry, border irregularity, color variance, diameter greater than 6 mm, evolving size, shape, and color) mnemonic.

B. Head, neck, and lymph nodes: Involves inspection, palpation, and auscultation of the head, neck, and lymph nodes
1. Ask the client about headaches; episodes of dizziness (lightheadedness) or vertigo (spinning sensation); history of head injury; loss of consciousness; seizures; episodes of neck pain; limitations of range of motion; numbness or tingling in the shoulders, arms, or hands; lumps or swelling in the neck; difficulty swallowing; medications being taken; and history of surgery in the head and neck region.
2. Head
   a. Inspect and palpate: Size, shape, masses or tenderness, and symmetry of the skull
   b. Palpate temporal arteries, located above the cheekbone between the eye and the top of the ear.
   c. Palpate frontal and maxillary sinuses for tenderness.
   d. Temporomandibular joint: Ask the client to open his or her mouth and move it from side to side; note any crepitation, tenderness, or limited range of motion. This tests cranial nerve V, the trigeminal nerve.
   e. Face: Inspect facial structures for shape, symmetry, involuntary movements, or swelling, such as periorbital edema (swelling around the eyes).
3. Neck
   a. Inspect for symmetry of accessory neck muscles.
   b. Assess range of motion.

TABLE 12-2 Pitting Edema Scale

Scale	Description	"Measurement"*
1+	A barely perceptible pit	2 mm ($\frac{3}{32}$ in)
2+	A deeper pit, rebounds in a few seconds	4 mm ($\frac{6}{32}$ in)
3+	A deep pit, rebounds in 10-20 sec	6 mm ($\frac{1}{4}$ in)
4+	A deeper pit, rebounds in >30 sec	8 mm ($\frac{5}{16}$ in)

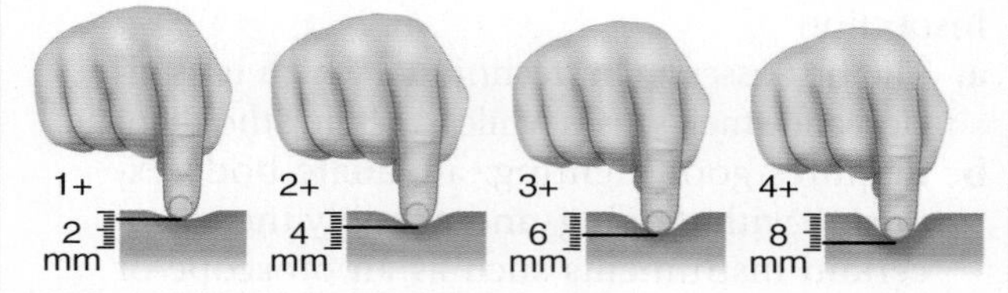

* "Measurement" is in quotation marks because depth of edema is rarely actually measured but is included as a frame of reference.
Data from Wilson AF, Giddens JF: *Health assessment for nursing practice*, ed 5, St. Louis, 2013, Mosby. Description column data from Kirton C: Assessing edema, *Nursing 96* 26(7):54, 1996.

c. Test cranial nerve XI (spinal accessory nerve) to assess muscle strength: Ask the client to push against resistance applied to the side of the chin (tests sternocleidomastoid muscle); also ask the client to shrug the shoulders against resistance (tests trapezius muscle).

d. Palpate the trachea: It should be midline, without any deviations.

e. Thyroid gland: Inspect the neck as the client takes a sip of water and swallows (thyroid tissue moves up with a swallow); palpate using an anterior-posterior approach (usually the normal adult thyroid cannot be palpated); if it is enlarged, auscultate for a bruit.

4. Lymph nodes

a. Palpate using a gentle pressure and a circular motion of the finger pads.

b. Begin with the preauricular lymph nodes (in front of the ear); move to the posterior auricular lymph nodes and then downward toward the supraclavicular lymph nodes. Lymph nodes in the head and neck area to be palpated include preauricular, postauricular, tonsillar, submandibular, submental, anterior cervical chain (superficial and deep), posterior cervical chain, supraclavicular, and infraclavicular.

c. Palpate with both hands, comparing the 2 sides for symmetry.

d. If nodes are palpated, note their size, shape, location, mobility, consistency, and tenderness.

5. Client teaching: Instruct the client to notify the primary health care provider (PHCP) if persistent headache, dizziness, or neck pain occurs; if swelling or lumps are noted in the head and neck region; or if a neck or head injury occurs.

! Neck movements are never performed if the client has sustained a neck injury or if a neck injury is suspected.

C. Eyes: Includes inspection, palpation, vision-testing procedures, and the use of an ophthalmoscope

1. Subjective data: Difficulty with vision (e.g., decreased acuity, double vision, blurring, blind spots); pain, redness, swelling, watery or other discharge from the eye; use of glasses or contact lenses; medications being taken; history of eye problems

2. Objective data

a. Inspect the external eye structures, including eyebrows, for symmetry; eyelashes for even distribution; eyelids for ptosis (drooping); eyeballs for exophthalmos (protrusion) or enophthalmos (recession into the orbit; sunken eye).

b. Inspect the conjunctiva (should be clear), sclera (should be white), and lacrimal apparatus (check for excessive tearing, redness, tenderness, or swelling); cornea and lens (should be smooth and clear); iris (should be flat, with a round regular shape and even coloration); eyelids; and pupils.

3. Snellen eye chart

a. The Snellen eye chart is a simple tool used to measure distance vision.

b. Position the client in a well-lit spot 20 feet (6 meters) from the chart, with the chart at eye level, and ask the client to read the smallest line that he or she can discern.

c. Instruct the client to leave on glasses or leave in contact lenses; if the glasses are for reading only, they are removed because they blur distance vision.

d. Test 1 eye at a time, cover the eye not being tested.

e. Record the result using the fraction at the end of the last line successfully read on the chart.

f. Normal visual acuity is 20/20 (distance in feet at which the client is standing from the chart/distance in feet at which a normal eye could have read that particular line).

g. This assessment tests cranial nerve II, the optic nerve.

4. Near vision

a. Use a handheld vision screener (held about 14 inches [35.5 cm] from the eye) that contains various sizes of print or ask the client to read from a magazine.

b. Test each eye separately with the client's glasses on or contact lenses in. Cover the eye not being tested.

c. Normal result is 14/14 (distance in inches at which the subject holds the card from the eye/distance in inches at which a normal eye could have read that particular line).

d. This assessment tests cranial nerve II, the optic nerve.

5. Confrontation test

a. A crude but rapid test used to measure peripheral vision and compare the client's peripheral vision with the nurse's (assuming that the nurse's peripheral vision is normal)

b. The client covers 1 eye and looks straight ahead; the nurse, positioned 2 feet away (60 cm), covers his or her eye opposite the client's covered eye.

c. The nurse advances a finger or other small object from the periphery from several directions; the client should see the object at the same time the nurse does.

d. Documented as the client's peripheral vision is equal to that of the examiner's.
e. This assessment tests cranial nerve II, the optic nerve.

6. Corneal light reflex
   a. Used to assess for parallel alignment of the axes of the eyes
   b. Client is asked to gaze straight ahead as the nurse holds a light about 12 inches (30 cm) from the client.
   c. The nurse looks for reflection of the light on the corneas in exactly the same spot in each eye.
7. Cover/uncover test
   a. Used to check for slight degrees of deviated alignment
   b. Each eye is tested separately.
   c. The nurse asks the client to gaze straight ahead and cover 1 eye.
   d. The nurse examines the uncovered eye, expecting to note a steady, fixed gaze.
8. Diagnostic positions test (6 cardinal positions of gaze) (Fig. 12-1)
   a. The 6 muscles that attach the eyeball to its orbit and serve to direct the eye to points of interest are tested.
   b. Client holds head still and is asked to move his or her eyes and follow a small object.
   c. The examiner notes any parallel movements of the eye or nystagmus, an involuntary, rhythmic, rapid twitching of the eyeballs.
   d. This assessment tests cranial nerves III, IV, and VI, oculomotor, trochlear, and abducens, respectively.
9. Color vision
   a. Tests for color vision involve the client picking numbers or letters out of a complex and colorful picture using what is known as the *Ishihara chart.*
   b. The test is sensitive for the diagnosis of red-green blindness but cannot detect discrimination of blue.

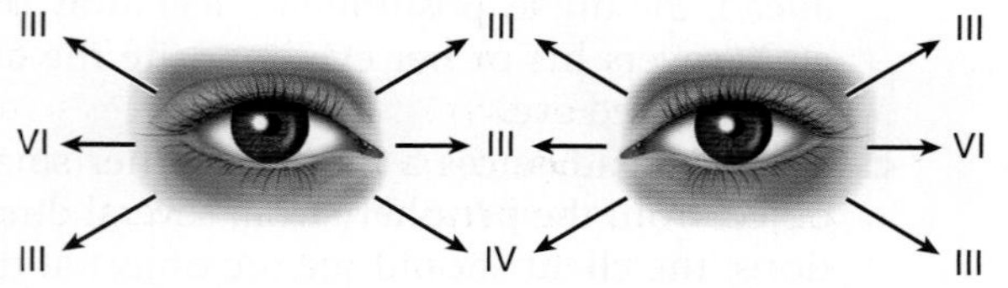

FIG. 12-1 Checking extraocular muscles in the 6 cardinal positions. This indicates the functioning of cranial nerves III, IV, and VI.

! The first slide on the Ishihara chart is one that everyone can discriminate; failure to identify numbers on this slide suggests a problem with performing the test, not a problem with color vision.

10. Pupils (Box 12-5)
    a. The pupils are round and of equal size.
    b. Increasing light causes pupillary constriction.
    c. Decreasing light causes pupillary dilation.
    d. Constriction of both pupils is a normal response to direct light. Constriction of the pupil in which the light is being shone is considered reaction to direct light, and constriction of the pupil in which the light is not being shone is considered reaction to consensual light.
11. Sclera and cornea
    a. Normal sclera color is white.
    b. A yellow color to the sclera may indicate jaundice or systemic problems.
    c. In a dark-skinned person, the sclera may normally appear yellow; pigmented dots may be present.
    d. The cornea is transparent, smooth, shiny, and bright.
    e. Cloudy areas or specks on the cornea may be the result of an accident or eye injury.

BOX 12-5 Assessing and Documenting Pupillary Responses

Pupillary Light Reflex

1. Darken the room (to dilate the client's pupils) and ask the client to look forward.
2. Test each eye.
3. Advance a light in from the side to note constriction of the same-side pupil (direct light reflex) and simultaneous constriction of the other pupil (consensual light reflex).

Accommodation

1. Ask the client to focus on a distant object (dilates the pupil).
2. Ask the client to shift gaze to a near object held about 3 inches (7.5 cm) from the nose.
3. Normal response includes pupillary constriction and convergence of the axes of the eyes.

Documenting Normal Findings: PERRLA

P = pupils
E = equal
R = round
RL = reactive to light (direct and consensual)
A = reactive to accommodation

12. Ophthalmoscopy or fundoscopy
- **a.** The ophthalmoscope, or funduscope, is an instrument used to examine the external structures and the interior of the eye.
- **b.** The room is darkened so that the pupil will dilate.
- **c.** The instrument is held with the right hand when examining the right eye and with the left hand when examining the left eye.
- **d.** The client is asked to look straight ahead at an object on the wall.
- **e.** The examiner should approach the client's eye from about 12 to 15 inches (30.5 to 38 cm) away and 15 degrees lateral to the client's line of vision.
- **f.** As the instrument is directed at the pupil, a red glare (red reflex) is seen in the pupil.
- **g.** The red reflex is the reflection of light on the vascular retina.
- **h.** Absence of the red reflex may indicate opacity of the lens.
- **i.** The optic disc, retinal vessels, general background, and macula can be examined.
- **j.** The optic disc should be creamy yellow-orange to pink, round or oval shape with distinct margins. Retinal vessels should be visible without nicking and engorgement. General background varies from light red to dark brown red, corresponding with the person's color.

13. Refer to Chapter 56 for diagnostic tests related to the eye.

14. Client teaching
- **a.** Instruct the client to notify the PHCP if alterations in vision occur or any redness, swelling, or drainage from the eye is noted.
- **b.** Inform the client of the importance of regular eye examinations.

D. Ears: Includes inspection, palpation, hearing tests, vestibular assessment, and the use of an otoscope

1. Subjective data: Difficulty hearing, earaches, drainage from the ears, dizziness, ringing in the ears, exposure to environmental noise, use of a hearing aid, medications being taken, history of ear problems or infections

2. Objective data
- **a.** Inspect and palpate the external ear, noting size, shape, symmetry, skin color, and the presence of pain.
- **b.** Inspect the external auditory meatus for size, swelling, redness, discharge, and foreign bodies; some cerumen (earwax) may be present.

3. Auditory assessment
- **a.** Sound is transmitted by air conduction and bone conduction.
- **b.** Air conduction takes 2 or 3 times longer than bone conduction.
- **c.** Hearing loss is categorized as conductive, sensorineural, or mixed conductive and sensorineural.
- **d.** Conductive hearing loss is caused by any physical obstruction to the transmission of sound waves.
- **e.** Sensorineural hearing loss is caused by a defect in the cochlea, eighth cranial nerve, or the brain itself.
- **f.** A mixed hearing loss is a combination of a conductive and sensorineural hearing loss; it results from problems in both the inner ear and the outer ear or middle ear.

4. Voice (Whisper) test
- **a.** Used to determine whether hearing loss has occurred
- **b.** One ear is tested at a time (the ear not being tested is occluded by the client).
- **c.** The nurse stands 1 to 2 feet (30 to 60 cm) from the client, covers his or her mouth so that the client cannot read the lips, exhales fully, and softly whispers 2-syllable words in the direction of the unoccluded ear; the client points a finger up during the test when the nurse's voice is heard (a ticking watch may also be used to test hearing acuity).
- **d.** Failure to hear the sounds could indicate possible fluid collection and/or consolidation, requiring further assessment.

5. Watch test
- **a.** A ticking watch is used to test for high-frequency sounds.
- **b.** The examiner holds a ticking watch about 5 inches (12.5 cm) from each ear and asks the client if the ticking is heard.

6. Tuning fork tests
- **a.** Used to measure hearing on the basis of air conduction or bone conduction; includes the Weber's and Rinne's tests. These tests are not commonly used because of their limited sensitivity to detect hearing loss.

7. Vestibular assessment (Box 12-6)

8. Otoscopic exam

⚠ Before performing an otoscopic exam and inserting the speculum, check the auditory canal for foreign bodies. Instruct the client not to move the head during the examination to avoid damage to the canal and tympanic membrane.

- **a.** The client's head is tilted slightly away and the otoscope is held upside down as if it were a large pen; this permits the examiner's hand to lay against the client's head for support.
- **b.** In an adult, pull the pinna up and back to straighten the external canal.
- **c.** Visualize the external canal while slowly inserting the speculum.

BOX 12-6 Vestibular Assessment

Test for Falling

1. The examiner asks the client to stand with the feet together, arms hanging loosely at the sides, and eyes closed.
2. The client normally remains erect, with only slight swaying.
3. A significant sway is a positive Romberg's sign.

Test for Past Pointing

1. The client sits in front of the examiner.
2. The client closes the eyes and extends the arms in front, pointing both index fingers at the examiner.
3. The examiner holds and touches his or her own extended index fingers under the client's extended index fingers to give the client a point of reference.
4. The client is instructed to raise both arms and then lower them, attempting to return to the examiner's extended index fingers.
5. The normal test response is that the client can easily return to the point of reference.
6. The client with a vestibular function problem lacks a normal sense of position and cannot return the extended fingers to the point of reference; instead, the fingers deviate to the right or left of the reference point.

Gaze Nystagmus Evaluation

1. The client's eyes are examined as the client looks straight ahead, 30 degrees to each side, upward and downward.
2. Any spontaneous nystagmus—an involuntary, rhythmic, rapid twitching of the eyeballs—represents a problem with the vestibular system.

Dix-Hallpike Maneuver

1. The client starts in a sitting position; the examiner lowers the client to the exam table and rather quickly turns the client's head to the 45-degree position.
2. If after about 30 seconds there is no nystagmus, the client is returned to a sitting position and the test is repeated on the other side.

d. The normal external canal is pink and intact, without lesions and with varying amounts of cerumen and fine little hairs.

e. Assess the tympanic membrane for intactness; the normal tympanic membrane is intact, without perforations, and should be free from lesions.

f. The tympanic membrane is transparent, opaque, pearly gray, and slightly concave. The cone of light reflex is noted at 5 o'clock on the right and 7 o'clock on the left, and there is positive mobility when the client swallows.

g. A fluid line or the presence of air bubbles is not normally visible.

h. If the tympanic membrane is bulging or retracting, the edges of the light reflex will be fuzzy (diffuse) and may spread over the tympanic membrane.

⚠ The otoscope is never introduced blindly into the external canal because of the risk of perforating the tympanic membrane.

9. Refer to Chapter 56 for diagnostic tests related to the ear.
10. Client teaching
    a. Instruct the client to notify the PHCP if an alteration in hearing or ear pain or ringing in the ears occurs, or if redness, swelling, or drainage from the ear is noted.
    b. Instruct the client in the proper method of cleaning the ear canal.
    c. The client should cleanse the ear canal with the corner of a moistened washcloth and should never insert sharp objects or cotton-tipped applicators into the ear canal.

E. Nose, mouth, and throat: Includes inspection and palpation

1. Subjective data
    a. Nose: Ask about discharge or nosebleed (epistaxis), facial or sinus pain, history of frequent colds, altered sense of smell, allergies, medications being taken, history of nose trauma, or surgery.
    b. Mouth and throat: Ask about the presence of sores or lesions; bleeding from the gums or elsewhere; altered sense of taste; toothaches; use of dentures or other appliances; tooth and mouth care hygiene habits; at-risk behaviors (e.g., smoking, alcohol consumption); and history of infection, trauma, or surgery.
2. Objective data
    a. External nose should be midline and in proportion to other facial features.
    b. Patency of the nostrils can be tested by pushing each nasal cavity closed and asking the client to sniff inward through the other nostril.
    c. A nasal speculum and penlight or a short, wide-tipped speculum attached to an otoscope head is used to inspect for redness, swelling, discharge, bleeding, or foreign bodies; the nasal septum is assessed for deviation.
    d. The nurse presses the frontal sinuses (located below the eyebrows) and over the maxillary sinuses (located below the cheekbones); the client should feel firm pressure but no pain.
    e. The external and inner surfaces of the lips are assessed for color, moisture, cracking, or lesions.
    f. The teeth are inspected for condition and number (should be white, spaced evenly, straight, and clean, free of debris and decay).

g. The alignment of the upper and lower jaws is assessed by having the client bite down.
h. The gums are inspected for swelling, bleeding, discoloration, and retraction of gingival margins (gums normally appear pink).
i. The tongue is inspected for color, surface characteristics, moisture, white patches, nodules, and ulcerations (dorsal surface is normally rough; ventral surface is smooth and glistening, with visible veins).
j. The nurse retracts the cheek with a tongue depressor to check the buccal mucosa for color and the presence of nodules or lesions; normal mucosa is glistening, pink, soft, moist, and smooth.
k. Using a penlight and tongue depressor, the nurse inspects the hard and soft palates for color, shape, texture, and defects; the hard palate (roof of the mouth), which is located anteriorly, should be white and dome-shaped, and the soft palate, which extends posteriorly, should be light pink and smooth.
l. The uvula is inspected for midline location; the nurse asks the client to say "ahhh" and watches for the soft palate and uvula to rise in the midline (this tests 1 function of cranial nerve X, the vagus nerve).
m. Using a penlight and tongue depressor, the nurse inspects the throat for color, presence of tonsils, and the presence of exudate or lesions; tonsils should be graded (0 is surgically removed; 1+ is tonsils hidden within pillars; 2+ is tonsils extending to the pillars, 3+ is tonsils extending beyond the pillars, 4+ is tonsils extending to the midline). One technique to test cranial nerve XII (the hypoglossal nerve) is asking the client to stick out the tongue (should protrude in the midline).
n. To test the gag reflex, touch the posterior pharynx with the end of a tongue blade; the client should gag momentarily (this tests the function of cranial nerve IX, the glossopharyngeal nerve).

3. Client teaching
   a. Emphasize the importance of hygiene and tooth care, as well as regular dental examinations and the use of fluoridated water or fluoride supplements.
   b. Encourage the client to avoid at-risk behaviors (e.g., smoking, alcohol consumption).
   c. Stress the importance of reporting pain or abnormal occurrence (e.g., nodules, lesions, signs of infection).

F. Lungs
1. Subjective data: Cough; expectoration of sputum; shortness of breath or dyspnea; chest pain on breathing; smoking history; environmental exposure to pollution or chemicals; medications being taken; history of respiratory disease or infection; last tuberculosis test, chest radiograph, pneumonia, and any influenza immunizations. Record the smoking history in pack-years (the number of packs per day times the number of years smoked). For example, a client who has smoked one-half pack a day for 20 years has a 10-pack/year smoking history.
2. Objective data: Includes inspection, palpation, percussion, and auscultation
3. Inspection of the anterior and posterior chest: Note skin color and condition and the rate and quality of respirations, look for lumps or lesions, note the shape and configuration of the chest wall, and note the position the client takes to breathe.
4. Palpation: Palpate the entire chest wall, noting skin temperature and moisture and looking for areas of tenderness and lumps, lesions, or masses; assess chest excursion and tactile or vocal fremitus (Box 12-7).
5. Percussion
   a. Starting at the apices, percuss across the top of the shoulders, moving to the interspaces, making a side-to-side comparison all the way down the lung area (Fig. 12-2).
   b. Determine the predominant note; resonance is noted in healthy lung tissue.
   c. Hyperresonance is noted when excessive air is present and a dull note indicates lung density.

BOX 12-7 Palpation of the Chest

Chest Excursion

Posterior: The nurse places the thumbs along the spinal processes at the 10th rib, with the palms in light contact with the posterolateral surfaces.

The nurse's thumbs should be about 2 inches (5 cm) apart, pointing toward the spine, with the fingers pointing laterally.

Anterior: The nurse places the hands on the anterolateral wall with the thumbs along the costal margins, pointing toward the xiphoid process.

The nurse instructs the client to take a deep breath after exhaling.

The nurse should note movement of the thumbs, and chest excursion should be symmetrical, separating the thumbs approximately 2 inches (5 cm).

Tactile or Vocal Fremitus

The nurse places the ball or lower palm of the hand over the chest, starting at the lung apices and palpating from side to side.

The nurse asks the client to repeat the words "ninety-nine." Symmetrical palpable vibration should be felt by the nurse.

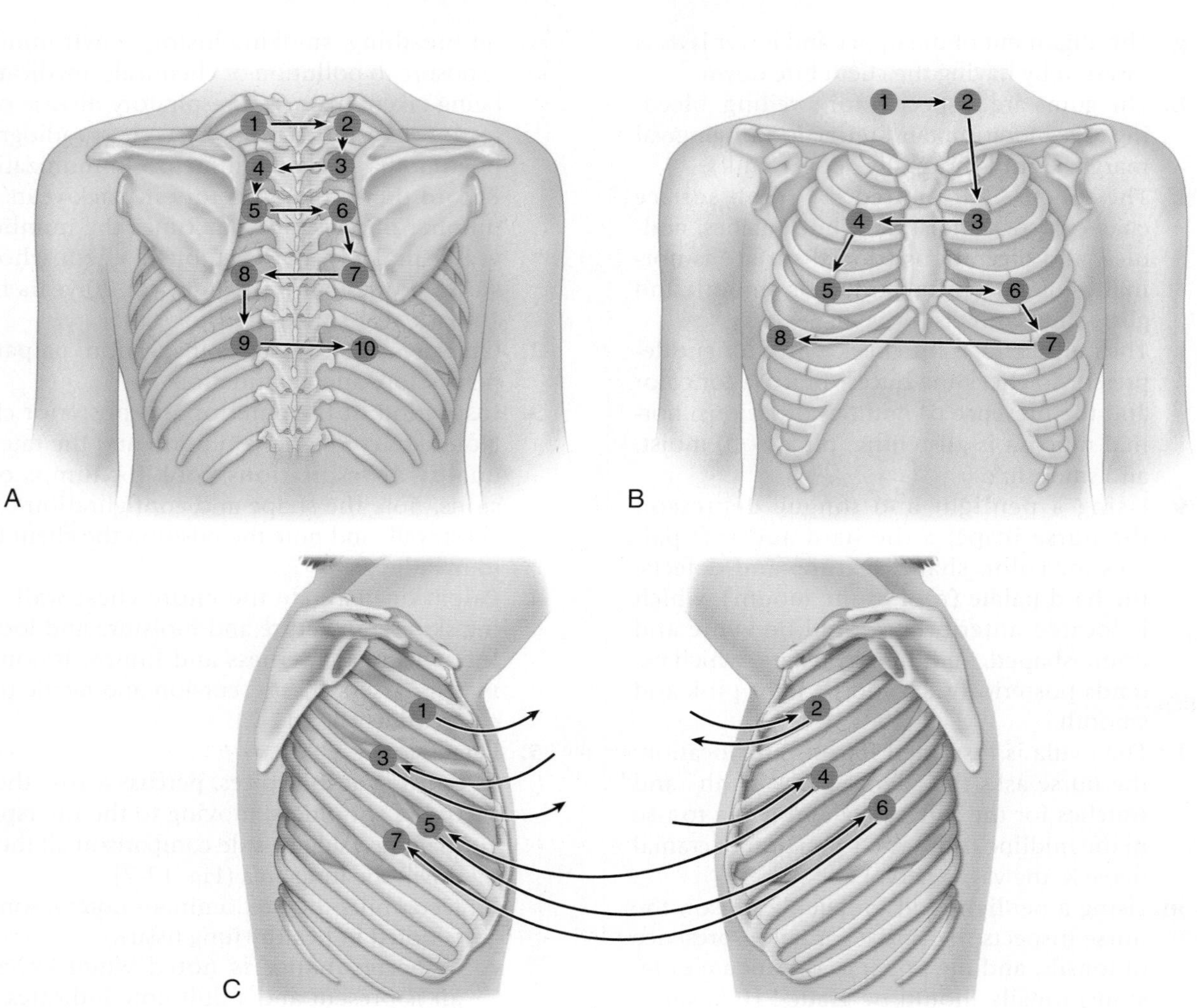

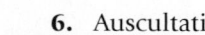

FIG. 12-2 Landmarks for chest auscultation and percussion. **A,** Posterior view. **B,** Anterior view. **C,** Lateral views.

6. Auscultation

a. Using the flat diaphragm endpiece of the stethoscope, hold it firmly against the chest wall and listen to at least 1 full respiration in each location (anterior, posterior, and lateral).

b. Posterior: Start at the apices and move side to side for comparison (see Fig. 12-2).

c. Anterior: Auscultate the lung fields from the apices in the supraclavicular area down to the 6th rib; avoid percussion and auscultation over female breast tissue (displace this tissue), because a dull sound will be produced (see Fig. 12-2).

d. Compare findings on each side.

7. Normal breath sounds: Three types of breath sounds are considered normal in certain parts of the thorax, including vesicular, bronchovesicular, and bronchial; breath sounds should be clear to auscultation (Fig. 12-3).

8. Abnormal breath sounds: Also known as *adventitious sounds* (Table 12-3)

9. Voice sounds (Box 12-8)

a. Performed when a pathological lung condition is suspected

b. Auscultate over the chest wall; the client is asked to vocalize words or a phrase while the nurse listens to the chest.

c. Normal voice transmission is soft and muffled; the nurse can hear the sound but is unable to distinguish exactly what is being said.

When auscultating breath sounds, instruct the client to breathe through the mouth and monitor the client for dizziness.

10. Refer to Chapter 50 for diagnostic tests related to the respiratory system.

11. Client teaching

a. Encourage the client to avoid exposure to environmental hazards, including smoking (discuss smoking cessation programs as appropriate).

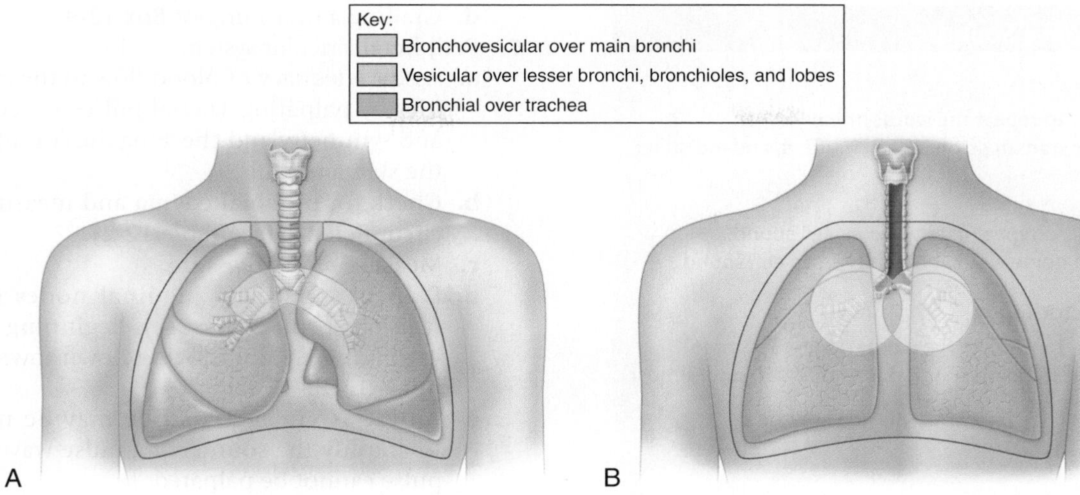

FIG. 12-3 Auscultatory sounds. **A,** Anterior thorax. **B,** Posterior thorax.

TABLE 12-3 Characteristics of Adventitious Sounds

Adventitious Sound	Characteristics	Clinical Examples
Fine crackles	High-pitched crackling and popping noises (discontinuous sounds) heard during the end of inspiration. Not cleared by cough.	May be heard in pneumonia, heart failure, asthma, and restrictive pulmonary diseases
Medium crackles	Medium-pitched, moist sound heard about halfway through inspiration. Not cleared by cough.	Same as above, but condition is worse
Coarse crackles	Low-pitched, bubbling or gurgling sounds that start early in inspiration and extend into the first part of expiration. Not cleared by cough.	Same as above, but condition is worse or may be heard in terminally ill clients with diminished gag reflex. Also heard in pulmonary edema and pulmonary fibrosis.
Wheeze (also called *sibilant* wheeze)	High-pitched, musical sound similar to a squeak. Heard more commonly during expiration, but may also be heard during inspiration. Occurs in small airways.	Heard in narrowed airway diseases such as asthma
Rhonchi (also called *sonorous* wheeze)	Low-pitched, coarse, loud, low snoring or moaning tone. Actually sounds like snoring. Heard primarily during expiration, but may also be heard during inspiration. Coughing may clear.	Heard in disorders causing obstruction of the trachea or bronchus, such as chronic bronchitis
Pleural friction rub	A superficial, low-pitched, coarse rubbing or grating sound. Sounds like 2 surfaces rubbing together. Heard throughout inspiration and expiration. Loudest over the lower anterolateral surface. Not cleared by cough.	Heard in individuals with pleurisy (inflammation of the pleural surfaces)

Data from Wilson AF, Giddens JF: *Health assessment for nursing practice*, ed 5, St. Louis, 2013, Mosby.

b. Client should undergo periodic examinations as prescribed (e.g., chest x-ray study, tuberculosis skin testing; refer to Chapter 50.

c. Encourage the client to obtain pneumonia and influenza immunizations.

d. PHCP should be notified if client experiences persistent cough, shortness of breath, or other respiratory symptoms.

G. Heart

1. Subjective data: Chest pain, dyspnea, cough, fatigue, edema, nocturia, leg pain or cramps (claudication), changes in skin color, obesity, medications being taken, cardiovascular risk factors, family history of cardiac or vascular problems, personal history of cardiac or vascular problems

2. Objective data: May include inspection, palpation, percussion, and auscultation

3. Inspection: Inspect the anterior chest for pulsations (apical impulse) created as the left ventricle rotates against the chest wall during systole; not always visible.

BOX 12-8 Voice Sounds

Bronchophony

1. Ask the client to repeat the words "ninety-nine."
2. Normal voice transmission is soft, muffled, and indistinct.

Egophony

1. Ask the client to repeat a long "ee-ee-ee" sound.
2. Normally the nurse would hear the "ee-ee-ee" sound.

Whispered Pectoriloquy

1. Ask the client to whisper the words "one, two, three."
2. Normal voice transmission is faint, muffled, and almost inaudible.

4. Palpation
   a. Palpate the apical impulse at the fourth or fifth interspace, or medial to the midclavicular line (not palpable in obese clients or clients with thick chest walls).
   b. Palpate the apex, left sternal border, and base for pulsations; normally none are present.
5. Percussion: May be performed to outline the heart's borders and to check for cardiac enlargement (denoted by resonance over the lung and dull notes over the heart).
6. Auscultation
   a. Areas of the heart (Fig. 12-4)
   b. Auscultate heart rate and rhythm; check for a pulse deficit (auscultate the apical heartbeat while palpating an artery) if an irregularity is noted.
   c. Assess S1 ("lub") and S2 ("dub") sounds, and listen for extra heart sounds, as well as the presence of murmurs (blowing or swooshing noise that can be faint or loud with a high, medium, or low pitch).

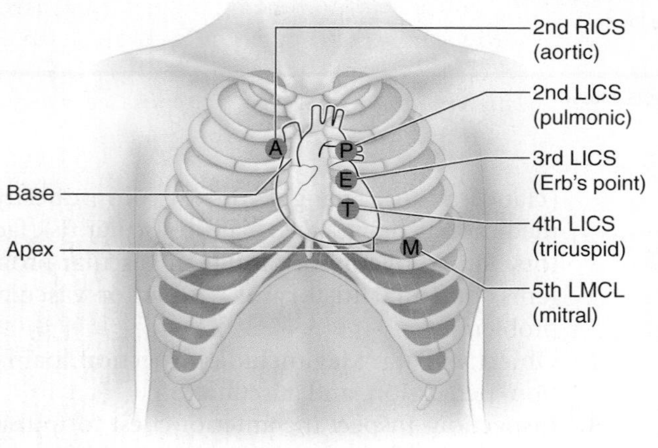

FIG. 12-4 Auscultation areas of the heart. *LICS*, Left intercostal space; *LMCL*, left midclavicular line; *RICS*, right intercostal space.

   d. Grading a murmur: See Box 12-9.
7. Peripheral vascular system
   a. Assess adequacy of blood flow to the extremities by palpating arterial pulses for equality and symmetry and checking the condition of the skin and nails.
   b. Check for pretibial edema and measure calf circumference (see Table 12-2).
   c. Measure blood pressure.
   d. Palpate superficial inguinal nodes (using firm but gentle pressure), beginning in the inguinal area and moving down toward the inner thigh.
   e. An ultrasonic stethoscope may be needed to amplify the sounds of a pulse wave if the pulse cannot be palpated.
   f. Carotid artery: Located in the groove between the trachea and sternocleidomastoid muscle, medial to and alongside the muscle
   g. Palpate 1 carotid artery at a time to avoid compromising blood flow to the brain.
   h. Auscultate each carotid artery for the presence of a bruit (a blowing, swishing, or buzzing, humming sound), which indicates blood flow turbulence; normally a bruit is not present.
   i. Palpate the arteries in the extremities (Box 12-10).
8. Refer to Chapter 52 for diagnostic tests related to the cardiovascular system.
9. Client teaching
   a. Advise client to modify lifestyle for risk factors associated with heart and vascular disease.
   b. Encourage the client to seek regular physical examinations.
   c. Client should seek medical assistance for signs of heart or vascular disease.

H. Breasts
1. Subjective data: Pain or tenderness, lumps or thickening, swollen axillary lymph nodes, nipple discharge, rash or swelling, medications being taken, personal or family history of breast disease, trauma or injury to the breasts, previous surgery on the breasts, breast self-examination (BSE) compliance, mammograms as prescribed
2. Objective data: Inspection and palpation

BOX 12-9 Grading a Murmur

Grade I: Barely audible
Grade II: Quiet but clearly audible
Grade III: Moderately loud
Grade IV: Loud, associated with a thrill
Grade V: Very loud, easily palpable thrill
Grade VI: Very loud, audible without using a stethoscope, thrill easily palpable and visible

BOX 12-10 Arterial Pulse Points and Grading the Force of Pulses

Arteries in the Arms and Hands

Radial Pulse: Located at the radial side of the forearm at the wrist

Ulnar Pulse: Located on the opposite side of the location of the radial pulse at the wrist

Brachial Pulse: Located above the elbow at the antecubital fossa, between the biceps and triceps muscles

Arteries in the Legs

Femoral Pulse: Located below the inguinal ligament, midway between the symphysis pubis and the anterosuperior iliac spine

Popliteal Pulse: Located behind the knee

Dorsalis Pedis Pulse: Located at the top of the foot, in line with the groove between the extensor tendons of the great and first toes

Posterior Tibial Pulse: Located on the inside of the ankle, behind and below the medial malleolus (ankle bone)

Grading the Force

4 + = Strong and bounding
3 + = Full pulse, increased
2 + = Normal, easily palpable
1 + = Weak, barely palpable

3. Inspection
   a. Performed with the client's arms raised above the head, the hands pressed against the hips, and the arms extended straight ahead while the client sits and leans forward
   b. Assess size and symmetry (1 breast is often larger than the other); masses, flattening, retraction, or dimpling; color and venous pattern; size, color, shape, and discharge in the nipple and areola; and the direction in which nipples point.
4. Palpation
   a. Client lies supine, with the arm on the side being examined behind the head and a small pillow under the shoulder.
   b. The nurse uses the pads of the first 3 fingers to compress the breast tissue gently against the chest wall, noting tissue consistency.
   c. Palpation is performed systematically, ensuring that the entire breast and tail are palpated.
   d. The nurse notes the consistency of the breast tissue, which normally feels dense, firm, and elastic.
   e. The nurse gently palpates the nipple and areola and compresses the nipple, noting any discharge.
   f. It is important to document lump or mass characteristics, which includes size, shape, consistency, movability, distinctness, nipple characteristics, skin findings over the lump, tenderness, and lymphadenopathy.
5. Axillary lymph nodes
   a. The nurse faces the client and stands on the side being examined, supporting the client's arm in a slightly flexed position, and abducts the arm away from the chest wall.
   b. The nurse places the free hand against the client's chest wall and high in the axillary hollow, then, with the fingertips, gently presses down, rolling soft tissue over the surface of the ribs and muscles.
   c. Lymph nodes are normally not palpable.
6. Client teaching
   a. Encourage and teach the client to perform BSE (refer to Chapter 44 for information on performing BSE).
   b. Client should report lumps or masses to the PHCP immediately.
   c. Regular physical examinations and mammograms should be obtained as prescribed.

I. Abdomen
1. Subjective data: Changes in appetite or weight, difficulty swallowing, dietary intake, intolerance to certain foods, nausea or vomiting, pain, bowel habits, medications currently being taken, history of abdominal problems or abdominal surgery
2. Objective data
   a. Ask the client to empty the bladder.
   b. Be sure to warm the hands and the endpiece of the stethoscope.
   c. Examine painful areas last.

When performing an abdominal assessment, the specific order for assessment techniques is inspection, auscultation, percussion, and palpation.

3. Inspection
   a. Contour: Look down at the abdomen and then across the abdomen from the rib margin to the pubic bone; describe as flat, rounded, concave, or protuberant.
   b. Symmetry: Note any bulging or masses.
   c. Umbilicus: Should be midline and inverted
   d. Skin surface: Should be smooth and even
   e. Pulsations from the aorta may be noted in the epigastric area, and peristaltic waves may be noted across the abdomen.
4. Auscultation
   a. Performed before percussion and palpation, which can increase peristalsis.
   b. Hold the stethoscope lightly against the skin and listen for bowel sounds in all 4 quadrants; begin in the right lower quadrant (bowel sounds are normally heard here).
   c. Note the character and frequency of normal bowel sounds: high-pitched gurgling sounds occurring irregularly from 5 to 30 times a minute.

d. Identify as normal, hypoactive, or hyperactive (borborygmus).
e. Absent sounds: Auscultate for 5 minutes before determining that sounds are absent.
f. Auscultate over the aorta, renal arteries, iliac arteries, and femoral arteries for vascular sounds or bruits with the bell of the stethoscope.

5. Percussion
a. All 4 quadrants are percussed lightly.
b. Borders of the liver and spleen are percussed and measured.
c. Tympany should predominate over the abdomen, with dullness over the liver and spleen.
d. Percussion over the kidney at the 12th rib (costovertebral angle) should produce no pain. This is also known as *costovertebral tenderness.*

6. Palpation
a. Begin with light palpation of all 4 quadrants, using the fingers to depress the skin about 1 cm; next perform deep palpation, depressing 5 to 8 cm.
b. Palpate the liver and spleen (spleen may not be palpable).
c. Palpate the aortic pulsation in the upper abdomen slightly to the left of midline; normally it pulsates in a forward direction (pulsation expands laterally if an aneurysm is present).

7. Refer to Chapter 48 for diagnostic tests related to the gastrointestinal system.

8. Client teaching
a. Encourage the client to consume a balanced diet; obesity needs to be prevented.
b. Substances that can cause gastric irritation should be avoided.
c. The regular use of laxatives is discouraged.
d. Lifestyle behaviors that can cause gastric irritation (e.g., spicy foods) should be modified.
e. Regular physical examinations are important.
f. The client should report gastrointestinal problems to the PHCP.

J. Musculoskeletal system

1. Subjective data: Joint pain or stiffness; redness, swelling, or warm joints; limited motion of joints; muscle pain, cramps, or weakness; bone pain; limitations in activities of daily living; exercise patterns; exposure to occupational hazards (e.g., heavy lifting, prolonged standing or sitting); medications being taken; history of joint, muscle, or bone injuries; history of surgery of the joints, muscles, or bones
2. Objective data: Inspection and palpation
3. Inspection: Inspect gait and posture, and for cervical, thoracic, and lumbar curves (Box 12-11).
4. Palpation: Palpate all bones, joints, and surrounding muscles.
5. Range of motion
a. Perform active and passive range-of-motion exercises of each major joint.
b. Check for pain, limited mobility, spastic movement, joint instability, stiffness, and contractures.
c. Normally joints are nontender, without swelling, and move freely.
6. Muscle tone and strength
a. Assess during measurement of range of motion.
b. Ask client to flex the muscle to be examined and then to resist while applying opposing force against the flexion.
c. Assess for increased tone (hypertonicity) or little tone (hypotonicity).
7. Grading muscle strength (Table 12-4)

BOX 12-11 Common Postural Abnormalities

Lordosis (Swayback): Increased lumbar curvature
Kyphosis (Hunchback): Exaggeration of the posterior curvature of the thoracic spine
Scoliosis: Lateral spinal curvature

TABLE 12-4 Criteria for Grading and Recording Muscle Strength

Functional Level	Lovett Scale	Grade	Percentage of Normal
No evidence of contractility	Zero (0)	0	0
Evidence of slight contractility	Trace (T)	1	10
Complete range of motion with gravity eliminated	Poor (P)	2	25
Complete range of motion with gravity	Fair (F)	3	50
Complete range of motion against gravity with some resistance	Good (G)	4	75
Complete range of motion against gravity with full resistance	Normal (N)	5	100

Data from Wilson AF, Giddens JF: *Health assessment for nursing practice*, ed 5, St. Louis, 2013, Mosby.

8. Refer to Chapter 60 for diagnostic tests related to the musculoskeletal system.
9. Client teaching
   a. The client should consume a balanced diet, including foods containing calcium and vitamin D.
   b. Activities that cause muscle strain or stress to the joints should be avoided.
   c. Encourage the client to maintain a normal weight.
   d. Participation in a regular exercise program is beneficial.
   e. The client should contact the PHCP if joint or muscle pain or problems occur or if limitations in range of motion or muscle strength develop.

K. Neurological system
1. Subjective data: Headaches, dizziness or vertigo, tremors, weakness, incoordination, numbness or tingling in any area of the body, difficulty speaking or swallowing, medications being taken, history of seizures, history of head injury or surgery, exposure to environmental or occupational hazards (e.g., chemicals, alcohol, drugs)
2. Objective data: Assessment of cranial nerves, level of consciousness, pupils, motor function, cerebellar function, coordination, sensory function, and reflexes
3. Note mental and emotional status, behavior and appearance, language ability, and intellectual functioning, including memory, knowledge, abstract thinking, association, and judgment.
4. Vital signs: Check temperature, pulse, respirations, and blood pressure; monitor for blood pressure or pulse changes, which may indicate increased intracranial pressure (see Chapter 50 for abnormal respiratory patterns).
5. Cranial nerves (Table 12-5)
6. Level of consciousness
   a. Assess the client's behavior to determine level of consciousness (e.g., alertness, confusion, delirium, unconsciousness, stupor, coma); assessment becomes increasingly invasive as the client is less responsive. Use the Glasgow Coma

TABLE 12-5 Assessment of the Cranial Nerves

Cranial Nerve	Test
Cranial Nerve I: Olfactory ▪ Sensory ▪ Controls the sense of smell	▪ Have the client close the eyes and occlude 1 nostril with a finger ▪ Ask the client to identify nonirritating and familiar odors (e.g., coffee, tea, cloves, soap, chewing gum, peppermint) ▪ Repeat the test on the other nostril
Cranial Nerve II: Optic ▪ Sensory ▪ Controls vision	▪ Assess visual acuity with a Snellen chart and perform an ophthalmoscopic exam ▪ Check peripheral vision by confrontation ▪ Check color vision
Cranial Nerves III, IV, and VI ***Cranial Nerve III: Oculomotor*** ▪ Motor ▪ Controls pupillary constriction, upper-eyelid elevation, and most eye movement	▪ The motor functions of cranial nerves III, IV, and VI overlap; therefore, they should be tested together ▪ Inspect the eyelids for ptosis (drooping); then assess ocular movements and note any eye deviation ▪ Test accommodation and direct and consensual light reflexes
Cranial Nerve IV: Trochlear ▪ Motor ▪ Controls downward and inward eye movement	
Cranial Nerve VI: Abducens ▪ Motor ▪ Controls lateral eye movement	
Cranial Nerve V: Trigeminal ▪ Sensory and motor ▪ Controls sensation in the cornea, nasal and oral mucosa, and facial skin, as well as mastication	▪ To test motor function, ask the client to clench the teeth and assess the muscles of mastication; then try to open the client's jaws after asking the client to keep them tightly closed ▪ The corneal reflex may be tested by the primary health care provider; this is done by lightly touching the client's cornea with a cotton wisp (this test may be omitted if the client is alert and blinking normally) ▪ Check sensory function by asking the client to close the eyes; lightly touch forehead, cheeks, and chin, noting whether the touch is felt equally on the 2 sides

TABLE 12-5 Assessment of the Cranial Nerves—cont'd

Cranial Nerve	Test
Cranial Nerve VII: Facial ▪ Sensory and motor ▪ Controls movement of the face and taste sensation	▪ Test taste perception on the anterior two-thirds of the tongue; the client should be able to taste salty and sweet tastes ▪ Have the client smile, frown, and show the teeth ▪ Ask the client to puff out the cheeks ▪ Attempt to close the client's eyes against resistance
Cranial Nerve VIII: Acoustic or Vestibulocochlear ▪ Sensory ▪ Controls hearing and vestibular function	▪ Assessing the client's ability to hear tests the cochlear portion ▪ Assessing the client's sense of equilibrium tests the vestibular portion ▪ Check the client's hearing, using acuity tests ▪ Observe the client's balance and watch for swaying when he or she is walking or standing ▪ Assessment of sensorineural hearing loss may be done with the Weber's or Rinne's tests
Cranial Nerves IX and X ***Cranial Nerve IX: Glossopharyngeal*** ▪ Sensory and motor ▪ Controls swallowing ability, sensation in the pharyngeal soft palate and tonsillar mucosa, taste perception on the posterior third of the tongue, and salivation	▪ Usually cranial nerves IX and X are tested together ▪ Test taste perception on the posterior one third of the tongue or pharynx; the client should be able to taste bitter and sour tastes ▪ Inspect the soft palate and watch for symmetrical elevation when the client says "aaah" ▪ Touch the posterior pharyngeal wall with a tongue depressor to elicit the gag reflex
Cranial Nerve X: Vagus ▪ Sensory and motor ▪ Controls swallowing and phonation, sensation in the exterior ear's posterior wall, and sensation behind the ear ▪ Controls sensation in the thoracic and abdominal viscera	
Cranial Nerve XI: Spinal Accessory ▪ Motor ▪ Controls strength of neck and shoulder muscles	▪ The nurse palpates and inspects the sternocleidomastoid muscle as the client pushes the chin against the nurse's hand ▪ The nurse palpates and inspects the trapezius muscle as the client shrugs the shoulders against the nurse's resistance
Cranial Nerve XII: Hypoglossal ▪ Motor ▪ Controls tongue movements involved in swallowing and speech	▪ Observe the tongue for asymmetry, atrophy, deviation to 1 side, and fasciculations (uncontrollable twitching); ask the client to stick out the tongue (tongue should be midline) ▪ Ask the client to push the tongue against a tongue depressor, and then have the client move the tongue rapidly in and out and from side to side

Scale as appropriate (eye opening, motor response, verbal response, graded on a scale). See Chapter 58 for a description of this scale.
   - **b.** Speak to client.
   - **c.** Assess appropriateness of behavior and conversation.
   - **d.** Lightly touch the client (as culturally appropriate).

7. Pupils
   - **a.** Assess size, equality, and reaction to light (brisk, slow, or fixed) and note any unusual eye movements (check direct light and consensual light reflex); refer to Chapter 58 for abnormal pupillary findings.
   - **b.** This component of the neurological examination may be performed during assessment of the eye.
8. Motor function
   - **a.** Assess muscle tone, including strength and equality.
   - **b.** Assess for voluntary and involuntary movements and purposeful and nonpurposeful movements.
   - **c.** This component of the neurological examination may be performed during assessment of the musculoskeletal system.
9. Cerebellar function
   - **a.** Monitor gait as the client walks in a straight line, heel to toe (tandem walking).
   - **b.** Romberg's test: Client is asked to stand with the feet together and the arms at the sides and to close the eyes and hold the position; normally the client can maintain posture and balance.

c. If appropriate, ask the client to perform a shallow knee bend or to hop in place on 1 leg and then the other.

10. Coordination
    a. Assess by asking the client to perform rapid alternating movements of the hands (e.g., turning the hands over and patting the knees continuously).
    b. The nurse asks the client to touch the nurse's finger, then his or her own nose; the client keeps the eyes open and the nurse moves the finger to different spots to ensure that the client's movements are smooth and accurate.
    c. Heel-to-shin test: Assist the client into a supine position, then ask the client to place the heel on the opposite knee and run it down the shin; normally the client moves the heel down the shin in a straight line.
11. Sensory function
    a. Pain: Assess by applying an object with a sharp point and one with a dull point to the client's body in random order; ask the client to identify the sharp and dull feelings.
    b. Light touch: Brush a piece of cotton over the client's skin at various locations in a random order and ask the client to say when the touch is felt.
    c. Position sense (kinesthesia): Move the client's finger or toe up or down and ask the client which way it has been moved; this tests the client's ability to perceive passive movement.
    d. Stereognosis: Tests the client's ability to recognize objects placed in his or her hand
    e. Graphesthesia: Tests the client's ability to identify a number traced on the client's hand
    f. Two-point discrimination: Tests the client's ability to discriminate 2 simultaneous pinpricks on the skin
12. Deep tendon reflexes
    a. Includes testing the following reflexes: biceps, triceps, brachioradialis, patella, Achilles
    b. Limb should be relaxed.
    c. The tendon is tapped quickly with a reflex hammer, which should cause contraction of muscle.
    d. Scoring deep tendon reflex activity (Box 12-12)
13. Plantar reflex
    a. A cutaneous (superficial) reflex is tested with a pointed but not sharp object.
    b. The sole of the client's foot is stroked from the heel, up the lateral side, and then across the ball of the foot to the medial side.
    c. The normal response is plantar flexion of all toes.

BOX 12-12 Scoring Deep Tendon Reflex Activity

0 = No response
1 + = Sluggish or diminished
2 + = Active or expected response
3 + = Slightly hyperactive, more brisk than normal; not necessarily pathological
4 + = Brisk, hyperactive with intermittent clonus associated with disease

Data from Wilson AF, Giddens JF: *Health assessment for nursing practice*, ed 5, St. Louis, 2013, Mosby.

⚠ Dorsiflexion of the great toe and fanning of the other toes (Babinski's sign) after firmly stroking the sole of the foot, is abnormal in anyone older than 2 years and indicates the presence of central nervous system disease.

14. Testing for meningeal irritation
    a. A positive Brudzinski's sign or Kernig's sign indicates meningeal irritation.
    b. Brudzinski's sign is tested with the client in the supine position. The nurse flexes the client's head (gently moves the head to the chest) and there should be no reports of pain or resistance to the neck flexion; a positive Brudzinski's sign is observed if the client passively flexes the hip and knee in response to neck flexion and reports pain in the vertebral column.
    c. Kernig's sign is positive when the client flexes the legs at the hip and knee and complains of pain along the vertebral column when the leg is extended.
15. Refer to Chapter 58 for additional neurological assessments and diagnostic tests.
16. Client teaching
    a. Client should avoid exposure to environmental hazards (e.g., insecticides, lead).
    b. High-risk behaviors that can result in head and spinal cord injuries should be avoided.
    c. Protective devices (e.g., a helmet, body pads) should be worn when participating in high-risk behaviors.
    d. Seat belts should always be worn.

L. Female genitalia and reproductive tract
1. Subjective data: Urinary difficulties or symptoms such as frequency, urgency, or burning; vaginal discharge; pain; menstrual and obstetrical histories; onset of menopause; medications being taken; sexual activity and the use of barrier and other contraceptives; history of sexually transmitted infections
2. Objective data
    a. Use a calm and relaxing approach; the examination is embarrassing for many clients and may be a difficult experience for an adolescent.

b. Consider the client's cultural background and their beliefs regarding examination of the genitalia.
c. Consider sexual orientation in these types of exams, such as a transgendered individual and the sensitivity required in caring for this special population.
d. A complete examination will include the external genitalia and a pelvic (speculum and bi-manual) examination.
e. The nurse's role is to prepare the client for the examination and to assist the PHCP or other practitioner.
f. The client is asked to empty her bladder before the examination.
g. The client is placed in the lithotomy position, and a drape is placed across the client.

3. External genitalia
   a. Quantity and distribution of hair
   b. Characteristics of labia majora and minora (make note of any inflammation, edema, lesions, or lacerations)
   c. Urethral orifice is observed for color and position.
   d. Vaginal orifice (introitus) is inspected for inflammation, edema, discoloration, discharge, and lesions.
   e. The examiner may check Skene's and Bartholin's glands for tenderness or discharge (if discharge is present, color, odor, and consistency are noted and a culture of the discharge is obtained).
   f. The client is assessed for the presence of a cystocele (in which a portion of the vaginal wall and bladder prolapse, or fall, into the orifice anteriorly) or a rectocele (bulging of the posterior wall of the vagina caused by prolapse of the rectum).
4. Speculum examination of the internal genitalia
   a. Performed by the PHCP or other practitioner
   b. Permits visualization of the cervix and vagina
   c. Papanicolaou (Pap) smear (test): A painless screening test for cervical cancer is done; the specimen is obtained during the speculum examination, and the nurse helps prepare the specimen for laboratory analysis. This test may or may not include screening for human papilloma virus (HPV).
5. Bimanual examination
   a. Performed by PHCP or other practitioner
   b. Internal examination of the structures of the female reproductive tract
   c. May reveal masses, nodules, growths, or tenderness
   d. The uterus is palpated for position, size, shape, contour, and mobility.
   e. The adnexa and ovaries are palpated for masses or tenderness.
   f. A rectovaginal examination may be done for further examination of the pelvic structures.
6. Client teaching
   a. Stress the importance of personal hygiene.
   b. Explain the purpose and recommended frequency of Pap tests.
   c. Explain the signs of sexually transmitted infections.
   d. Educate the client on measures to prevent a sexually transmitted infection.
   e. Inform the client with a sexually transmitted infection that she must inform her sexual partner(s) of the need for an examination.

M. Male genitalia
1. Subjective data: Urinary difficulty (e.g., frequency, urgency, hesitancy or straining, dysuria, nocturia); pain, lesions, or discharge on or from the penis; pain or lesions in the scrotum; medications being taken; sexual activity and the use of contraceptives; history of sexually transmitted infections
2. Objective data
   a. Includes assessment (inspection and palpation) of the external genitalia and inguinal ring and canal
   b. Client may stand or lie down for this examination.
   c. Genitalia are manipulated gently to avoid causing erection or discomfort.
   d. Sexual maturity is assessed by noting the size and shape of the penis and testes, the color and texture of the scrotal skin, and the character and distribution of pubic hair.
   e. The penis is checked for the presence of lesions or discharge; a culture is obtained if a discharge is present.
   f. The scrotum is inspected for size, shape, and symmetry (normally the left testicle hangs lower than the right) and is palpated for the presence of lumps.
   g. Inguinal ring and canal: inspection (asking the client to cough or bear down) and palpation are performed to assess for the presence of a hernia.
3. Client teaching
   a. Stress the importance of personal hygiene.
   b. Teach the client how to perform testicular self-examination (TSE); a day of the month is selected and the exam is performed on the same day each month after a shower or bath when the hands are warm and soapy and the

scrotum is warm. (Refer to Chapter 44 for information on performing TSE.)

c. Explain the signs of sexually transmitted infections.
d. Educate the client on measures to prevent sexually transmitted infections.
e. Inform the client with a sexually transmitted infection that he must inform his sexual partner(s) of the need for an examination.

N. Rectum and anus

1. Subjective data: Usual bowel pattern; any change in bowel habits; rectal pain, bleeding from the rectum, or black or tarry stools; dietary habits; problems with urination; previous screening for colorectal cancer; previous screening for prostate cancer; medications being taken; history of rectal or colon problems; family history of rectal or colon problems
2. Objective data
   a. Examination can detect colorectal cancer in its early stages; in men, the rectal examination can also detect prostate tumors.
   b. Women may be examined in the lithotomy position after examination of the genitalia.
   c. A man is best examined by having the client bend forward with his hips flexed and upper body resting over the examination table.
   d. A nonambulatory client may be examined in the left lateral (Sims') position.
   e. The external anus is inspected for lumps or lesions, rashes, inflammation or excoriation, scars, or hemorrhoids.
   f. Digital examination will most likely be performed by the PHCP or other practitioner.
   g. Digital examination is performed to assess sphincter tone; to check for tenderness, irregularities, polyps, masses, or nodules in the rectal wall; and to assess the prostate gland.
   h. The prostate gland is normally firm, without bogginess, tenderness, or nodules (hardness or nodules may indicate the presence of a cancerous lesion; bogginess or tenderness may indicate infection).
3. Client teaching
   a. Diet should include high-fiber and low-fat foods and plenty of liquids.
   b. The client should obtain regular digital examinations.
   c. The client should be able to identify the symptoms of colorectal cancer or prostatic cancer (men).
   d. The client should follow the American Cancer Society's guidelines for screening for colorectal cancer and prostate cancer.

VI. Documenting Health and Physical Assessment Findings

A. Documentation of findings may be either written or recorded electronically (depending on agency protocol).

B. Whether written or electronic, the documentation is a legal document and a permanent record of the client's health status.

C. Principles of documentation need to be followed and data need to be recorded accurately, concisely, completely, legibly, and objectively without bias or opinions; always follow agency protocol for documentation.

D. Documentation findings serve as a source of client information for other health care providers; procedures for maintaining confidentiality are always followed.

E. Record findings about the client's health history and physical examination as soon as possible after completion of the health assessment.

F. Refer to Chapter 6 for additional information about documentation guidelines.

PRACTICE QUESTIONS

90. A Spanish-speaking client arrives at the triage desk in the emergency department and states to the nurse that an interpreter is needed. Which is the **best** action for the nurse to take?

1. Have one of the client's family members interpret.
2. Have the Spanish-speaking triage receptionist interpret.
3. Page an interpreter from the hospital's interpreter services.
4. Obtain a Spanish-English dictionary and attempt to triage the client.

91. The nurse is performing a neurological assessment on a client and notes a positive Romberg's test. The nurse makes this determination based on which observation?

1. An involuntary rhythmic, rapid, twitching of the eyeballs
2. A dorsiflexion of the great toe with fanning of the other toes
3. A significant sway when the client stands erect with feet together, arms at the side, and the eyes closed
4. A lack of normal sense of position when the client is unable to return extended fingers to a point of reference

92. The nurse notes documentation that a client is exhibiting Cheyne-Stokes respirations. On assessment of the client, the nurse should expect to note which finding?

1. Rhythmic respirations with periods of apnea
2. Regular rapid and deep, sustained respirations

3. Totally irregular respiration in rhythm and depth
4. Irregular respirations with pauses at the end of inspiration and expiration

93. A client diagnosed with conductive hearing loss asks the nurse to explain the cause of the hearing problem. The nurse plans to explain to the client that this condition is caused by which problem?
1. A defect in the cochlea
2. A defect in cranial nerve VIII
3. A physical obstruction to the transmission of sound waves
4. A defect in the sensory fibers that lead to the cerebral cortex

94. While performing a cardiac assessment on a client with an incompetent heart valve, the nurse auscultates a murmur. The nurse documents the finding and describes the sound as which?
1. Lub-dub sounds
2. Scratchy, leathery heart noise
3. A blowing or swooshing noise
4. Abrupt, high-pitched snapping noise

95. The nurse is testing the extraocular movements in a client to assess for muscle weakness in the eyes. The nurse should implement which assessment technique to assess for muscle weakness in the eye?
1. Test the corneal reflexes.
2. Test the 6 cardinal positions of gaze.
3. Test visual acuity, using a Snellen eye chart.
4. Test sensory function by asking the client to close the eyes and then lightly touching the forehead, cheeks, and chin.

96. The nurse is instructing a client how to perform a testicular self-examination (TSE). The nurse should explain that which is the **best** time to perform this exam?
1. After a shower or bath
2. While standing to void
3. After having a bowel movement
4. While lying in bed before arising

97. The nurse is assessing a client suspected of having meningitis for meningeal irritation and elicits a positive Brudzinski's sign. Which finding did the nurse observe?
1. The client rigidly extends the arms with pronated forearms and plantar flexion of the feet.
2. The client flexes a leg at the hip and knee and reports pain in the vertebral column when the leg is extended.
3. The client passively flexes the hip and knee in response to neck flexion and reports pain in the vertebral column.
4. The client's upper arms are flexed and held tightly to the sides of the body and the legs are extended and internally rotated.

98. A client with a diagnosis of asthma is admitted to the hospital with respiratory distress. Which type of adventitious lung sounds should the nurse expect to hear when performing a respiratory assessment on this client?
1. Stridor
2. Crackles
3. Wheezes
4. Diminished

99. The clinic nurse prepares to perform a focused assessment on a client who is complaining of symptoms of a cold, a cough, and lung congestion. Which should the nurse include for this type of assessment? **Select all that apply.**
- ☐ 1. Auscultating lung sounds
- ☐ 2. Obtaining the client's temperature
- ☐ 3. Assessing the strength of peripheral pulses
- ☐ 4. Obtaining information about the client's respirations
- ☐ 5. Performing a musculoskeletal and neurological examination
- ☐ 6. Asking the client about a family history of any illness or disease

ANSWERS

90. Answer: 3

Rationale: The best action is to have a professional hospital-based interpreter translate for the client. English-speaking family members may not appropriately understand what is asked of them and may paraphrase what the client is actually saying. Also, client confidentiality as well as accurate information may be compromised when a family member or a non–health care provider acts as interpreter.

Test-Taking Strategy: Note the strategic word, *best*. Initially focus on what the client needs. In this case the client needs and asks for an interpreter. Next keep in mind the issue of confidentiality and making sure that information is obtained in the most efficient and accurate way. This will assist in eliminating options 1, 2, and 4.

Level of Cognitive Ability: Applying

Client Needs: Psychosocial Integrity

Integrated Process: Communication and Documentation

Content Area: Foundations of Care: Communication

Health Problem: N/A
Priority Concepts: Communication; Culture
Reference: Lewis et al. (2017), p. 31.

91. *Answer:* 3
Rationale: In Romberg's test, the client is asked to stand with the feet together and the arms at the sides, and to close the eyes and hold the position; normally the client can maintain posture and balance. A positive Romberg's sign is a vestibular neurological sign that is found when a client exhibits a loss of balance when closing the eyes. This may occur with cerebellar ataxia, loss of proprioception, and loss of vestibular function. A lack of normal sense of position coupled with an inability to return extended fingers to a point of reference is a finding that indicates a problem with coordination. A positive gaze nystagmus evaluation results in an involuntary rhythmic, rapid twitching of the eyeballs. A positive Babinski's test results in dorsiflexion of the great toe with fanning of the other toes; if this occurs in anyone older than 2 years it indicates the presence of central nervous system disease.
Test-Taking Strategy: Note the subject, Romberg's sign. You can easily answer this question if you can recall that the client's balance is tested in this test.
Level of Cognitive Ability: Analyzing
Client Needs: Physiological Integrity
Integrated Process: Nursing Process—Assessment
Content Area: Health Assessment/Physical Exam: Neurological
Health Problem: N/A
Priority Concepts: Clinical Judgment; Mobility
Reference: Ignatavicius, Workman, Rebar (2018), p. 850.

92. *Answer:* 1
Rationale: Cheyne-Stokes respirations are rhythmic respirations with periods of apnea and can indicate a metabolic dysfunction in the cerebral hemisphere or basal ganglia. Neurogenic hyperventilation is a regular, rapid and deep, sustained respiration that can indicate a dysfunction in the low midbrain and middle pons. Ataxic respirations are totally irregular in rhythm and depth and indicate a dysfunction in the medulla. Apneustic respirations are irregular respirations with pauses at the end of inspiration and expiration and can indicate a dysfunction in the middle or caudal pons.
Test-Taking Strategy: Focus on the subject, the characteristics of Cheyne-Stokes respirations. Recalling that periods of apnea occur with this type of respiration will help direct you to the correct answer.
Level of Cognitive Ability: Applying
Client Needs: Physiological Integrity
Integrated Process: Nursing Process—Assessment
Content Area: Health Assessment/Physical Exam: Thorax and Lungs
Health Problem: N/A
Priority Concepts: Clinical Judgment; Gas Exchange
Reference: Lewis et al. (2017), p. 1324.

93. *Answer:* 3
Rationale: A conductive hearing loss occurs as a result of a physical obstruction to the transmission of sound waves. A sensorineural hearing loss occurs as a result of a pathological process in the inner ear, a defect in cranial nerve VIII, or a defect of the sensory fibers that lead to the cerebral cortex.
Test-Taking Strategy: Focus on the subject, a conductive hearing loss. Noting the relationship of the word *conductive* in the question and *transmission* in the correct option will direct you to this option.
Level of Cognitive Ability: Applying
Client Needs: Physiological Integrity
Integrated Process: Teaching and Learning
Content Area: Health Assessment/Physical Exam: Ear, Nose, and Throat
Health Problem: Adult Health: Ear: Hearing Loss
Priority Concepts: Client Education; Sensory Perception
Reference: Ignatavicius, Workman, Rebar (2018), pp. 996-997.

94. *Answer:* 3
Rationale: A heart murmur is an abnormal heart sound and is described as a faint or loud blowing, swooshing sound with a high, medium, or low pitch. Lub-dub sounds are normal and represent the S1 (first) heart sound and S2 (second) heart sound, respectively. A pericardial friction rub is described as a scratchy, leathery heart sound. A click is described as an abrupt, high-pitched snapping sound.
Test-Taking Strategy: Focus on the subject, characteristics of a murmur. Eliminate option 1 because it describes normal heart sounds. Next recall that a murmur occurs as a result of the manner in which the blood is flowing through the cardiac chambers and valves. This will direct you to the correct option.
Level of Cognitive Ability: Applying
Client Needs: Physiological Integrity
Integrated Process: Communication and Documentation
Content Area: Health Assessment/Physical Exam: Heart and Peripheral Vascular
Health Problem: Adult Health: Cardiovascular: Inflammatory and Structural Heart Disorders
Priority Concepts: Clinical Judgment; Perfusion
Reference: Ignatavicius, Workman, Rebar (2018), p. 655.

95. *Answer:* 2
Rationale: Testing the 6 cardinal positions of gaze (diagnostic positions test) is done to assess for muscle weakness in the eyes. The client is asked to hold the head steady, and then to follow movement of an object through the positions of gaze. The client should follow the object in a parallel manner with the 2 eyes. A Snellen eye chart assesses visual acuity and cranial nerve II (optic). Testing sensory function by having the client close his or her eyes and then lightly touching areas of the face and testing the corneal reflexes assess cranial nerve V (trigeminal).
Test-Taking Strategy: Focus on the subject, assessing for muscle weakness in the eyes. Note the relationship between the words *extraocular movements* in the question and *positions of gaze* in the correct option.
Level of Cognitive Ability: Applying
Client Needs: Physiological Integrity
Integrated Process: Nursing Process—Assessment
Content Area: Health Assessment/Physical Exam: Ear, Nose, and Throat
Health Problem: N/A
Priority Concepts: Clinical Judgment; Sensory Perception
Reference: Ignatavicius, Workman, Rebar (2018), p. 964.

96. Answer: 1

Rationale: The nurse needs to teach the client how to perform a TSE. The nurse should instruct the client to perform the exam on the same day each month. The nurse should also instruct the client that the best time to perform a TSE is after a shower or bath when the hands are warm and soapy and the scrotum is warm. Palpation is easier and the client will be better able to identify any abnormalities. The client would stand to perform the exam, but it would be difficult to perform the exam while voiding. Having a bowel movement is unrelated to performing a TSE.

Test-Taking Strategy: Note the strategic word, *best.* Think about the purpose of this test and visualize this assessment technique to answer correctly.

Level of Cognitive Ability: Applying
Client Needs: Health Promotion and Maintenance
Integrated Process: Teaching and Learning
Content Area: Health Assessment/Physical Exam: Testicles
Health Problem: N/A
Priority Concepts: Client Education; Sexuality
Reference: Ignatavicius, Workman, Rebar (2018), p. 1486.

97. Answer: 3

Rationale: Brudzinski's sign is tested with the client in the supine position. The nurse flexes the client's head (gently moves the head to the chest), and there should be no reports of pain or resistance to the neck flexion. A positive Brudzinski's sign is observed if the client passively flexes the hip and knee in response to neck flexion and reports pain in the vertebral column. Kernig's sign also tests for meningeal irritation and is positive when the client flexes the legs at the hip and knee and complains of pain along the vertebral column when the leg is extended. Decorticate posturing is abnormal flexion and is noted when the client's upper arms are flexed and held tightly to the sides of the body and the legs are extended and internally rotated. Decerebrate posturing is abnormal extension and occurs when the arms are fully extended, forearms pronated, wrists and fingers flexed, jaws clenched, neck extended, and feet plantar-flexed.

Test-Taking Strategy: Focus on the subject, a positive Brudzinski's sign. Recalling that a positive sign is elicited if the client reports pain will assist in eliminating options 1 and 4. Next it is necessary to know that a positive Brudzinski's sign is observed if the client passively flexes the hip and knee in response to neck flexion and reports pain in the vertebral column.

Level of Cognitive Ability: Applying
Client Needs: Physiological Integrity
Integrated Process: Nursing Process—Assessment
Content Area: Health Assessment/Physical Exam: Neurological
Health Problem: Adult Health: Neurological: Inflammation/ Infections
Priority Concepts: Clinical Judgment; Intracranial Regulation
Reference: Jarvis (2016), p. 688.

98. Answer: 3

Rationale: Asthma is a respiratory disorder characterized by recurring episodes of dyspnea, constriction of the bronchi, and wheezing. Wheezes are described as high-pitched musical sounds heard when air passes through an obstructed or narrowed lumen of a respiratory passageway. Stridor is a harsh sound noted with an upper airway obstruction and often signals a life-threatening emergency. Crackles are produced by air passing over retained airway secretions or fluid, or the sudden opening of collapsed airways. Diminished lung sounds are heard over lung tissue where poor oxygen exchange is occurring.

Test-Taking Strategy: Note the subject, assessment of abnormal lung sounds. Note the client's diagnosis and think about the pathophysiology that occurs in this disorder. Recalling that bronchial constriction occurs will assist in directing you to the correct option. Also, thinking about the definition of each adventitious lung sound identified in the options will direct you to the correct option.

Level of Cognitive Ability: Analyzing
Client Needs: Physiological Integrity
Integrated Process: Nursing Process—Assessment
Content Area: Health Assessment/Physical Exam: Thorax and Lungs
Health Problem: Adult Health: Respiratory: Asthma
Priority Concepts: Clinical Judgment; Gas Exchange
Reference: Ignatavicius, Workman, Rebar (2018), pp. 519, 521.

99. Answer: 1, 2, 4

Rationale: A focused assessment focuses on a limited or short-term problem, such as the client's complaint. Because the client is complaining of symptoms of a cold, a cough, and lung congestion, the nurse would focus on the respiratory system and the presence of an infection. A complete assessment includes a complete health history and physical examination and forms a baseline database. Assessing the strength of peripheral pulses relates to a vascular assessment, which is not related to this client's complaints. A musculoskeletal and neurological examination also is not related to this client's complaints. However, strength of peripheral pulses and a musculoskeletal and neurological examination would be included in a complete assessment. Likewise, asking the client about a family history of any illness or disease would be included in a complete assessment.

Test-Taking Strategy: Focus on the subject and note the words *focused assessment.* Noting that the client's symptoms relate to the respiratory system and the presence of an infection will direct you to the correct options.

Level of Cognitive Ability: Analyzing
Client Needs: Health Promotion and Maintenance
Integrated Process: Nursing Process—Assessment
Content Area: Health Assessment/Physical Exam: Health History
Health Problem: N/A
Priority Concepts: Clinical Judgment; Gas Exchange
Reference: Lewis et al. (2017), pp. 40, 44.

CHAPTER 13

Provision of a Safe Environment

PRIORITY CONCEPTS Infection, Safety

I. Environmental Safety

A. Fire safety (see Priority Nursing Actions)
1. Keep open spaces free of clutter.
2. Clearly mark fire exits.
3. Know the locations of all fire alarms, exits, and extinguishers (Table 13-1; also see Priority Nursing Actions).

PRIORITY NURSING ACTIONS

Event of a Fire

Race
1. Rescue clients who are in immediate danger.
2. Activate the fire alarm.
3. Confine the fire.
4. Extinguish the fire.

Pass
5. Obtain the fire extinguisher.
6. Pull the pin on the fire extinguisher.
7. Aim at the base of the fire.
8. Squeeze the extinguisher handle.
9. Sweep the extinguisher from side to side to coat the area of the fire evenly.

Reference
Potter et al. (2017), pp. 392-393.

TABLE 13-1 Types of Fire Extinguishers

Type	Class of Fire
A	Wood, cloth, upholstery, paper, rubbish, plastic
B	Flammable liquids or gases, grease, tar, oil-based paint
C	Electrical equipment

4. Know the telephone number for reporting fires.
5. Know the fire drill and evacuation plan of the agency.
6. Never use the elevator in the event of a fire.
7. Turn off oxygen and appliances in the vicinity of the fire.
8. In the event of a fire, if a client is on life support, maintain respiratory status manually with an Ambu bag (resuscitation bag) until the client is moved away from the threat of the fire and can be placed back on life support.
9. In the event of a fire, ambulatory clients can be directed to walk by themselves to a safe area and, in some cases, may be able to assist in moving clients in wheelchairs.
10. Bedridden clients generally are moved from the scene of a fire by stretcher, their bed, or wheelchair.
11. If a client must be carried from the area of a fire, appropriate transfer techniques need to be used.
12. If fire department personnel are at the scene of the fire, they will help evacuate clients.

Remember the mnemonic RACE (Rescue clients, Activate the fire alarm, Confine the fire, Extinguish the fire) to set priorities in the event of a fire and the mnemonic PASS (Pull the pin, Aim at the base of the fire, Squeeze the handle, Sweep from side to side) to use a fire extinguisher.

B. Electrical safety
1. Electrical equipment must be maintained in good working order and should be grounded; otherwise, it presents a **physical hazard**; remove equipment that is not in proper working order and notify appropriate staff.
2. Use a 3-pronged electrical cord.
3. In a 3-pronged electrical cord, the third, longer prong of the cord is the ground; the other 2 prongs carry the power to the piece of electrical equipment.

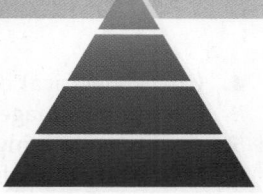

4. Check electrical cords and outlets for exposed, frayed, or damaged wires.
5. Avoid overloading any circuit.
6. Read warning labels on all equipment; never operate unfamiliar equipment.
7. Use safety extension cords only when absolutely necessary, and tape them to the floor with electrical tape.
8. Never run electrical wiring under carpets.
9. Never pull a plug by using the cord; always grasp the plug itself.
10. Never use electrical appliances near sinks, bathtubs, or other water sources.
11. Always disconnect a plug from the outlet before cleaning equipment or appliances.
12. If a client receives an electrical shock, turn off the electricity before touching the client.

! Any electrical equipment that the client brings into the health care facility must be inspected for safety before use.

C. Radiation safety (Refer to Chapter 44 for additional radiation safety measures)
   1. Know the protocols and guidelines of the health care agency.
   2. Label potentially radioactive material.
   3. To reduce exposure to radiation, do the following.
      a. Limit the time spent near the source.
      b. Make the distance from the source as great as possible.
      c. Use a shielding device such as a lead apron.
   4. Monitor radiation exposure with a film (dosimeter) badge.
   5. Place the client who has a radiation implant in a private room.
   6. Never touch dislodged radiation implants.
   7. Keep all linens in the client's room until the implant is removed.

D. Disposal of infectious wastes
   1. Handle all infectious materials as a hazard.
   2. Dispose of waste in designated areas only, using proper containers for disposal.
   3. Ensure that infectious material is labeled properly.
   4. Dispose of all sharps immediately after use in closed, puncture-resistant disposal containers that are leak-proof and labeled or color-coded.

! Needles (sharps) should not be recapped, bent, or broken because of the risk of accidental injury (needle stick).

E. Physiological changes in the older client that increase the risk of accidents (Box 13-1)

F. Risk for falls assessment
   1. Should be client-centered and include the use of a fall risk scale per agency procedures
   2. Include the client's own perceptions of their risk factors for falls and their method to adapt to these factors. Areas of concern may include gait stability, muscle strength and coordination, balance, and vision.
   3. Assess for any previous accidents.
   4. Assess with the client any concerns about their immediate environment, including stairs, use of throw rugs, grab bars, a raised toilet seat, or environmental lighting.
   5. Review/analyze the medications, both prescription and nonprescription, that the client is taking that could have side/adverse effects that could place the client at risk for a fall.
   6. Determine any scheduled procedures that pose risks to the client.

G. Measures to prevent falls (Box 13-2)

H. Measures to promote safety in ambulation for the client
   1. Gait belt may be used to keep the center of gravity midline.
      a. Place the belt on the client prior to ambulation.
      b. Encircle the client's waist with the belt.
      c. Hold on to the side or back of the belt so that the client does not lean to one side.
      d. Return the client to bed or a nearby chair if the client develops dizziness or becomes unsteady.
      e. When finished safely ambulating the client, remove belt and replace it in its appropriate storage area.

I. The Joint Commission: National Patient Safety Goals 2018

BOX 13-1 Physiological Changes in Older Clients That Increase the Risk of Accidents

Musculoskeletal Changes

Strength and function of muscles decrease.
Joints become less mobile and bones become brittle.
Postural changes and limited range of motion occur.

Nervous System Changes

Voluntary and autonomic reflexes become slower.
Decreased ability to respond to multiple stimuli occurs.
Decreased sensitivity to touch occurs.

Sensory Changes

Decreased vision and lens accommodation and cataracts develop.
Delayed transmission of hot and cold impulses occurs.
Impaired hearing develops, with high-frequency tones less perceptible.

Genitourinary Changes

Increased nocturia and occurrences of incontinence may occur.

Adapted from Potter A, Perry P, Stockert P, Hall A: *Fundamentals of nursing*, ed 8, St. Louis, 2013, Mosby; and Touhy T, Jett K: *Ebersole and Hess' toward healthy aging*, ed 8, St. Louis, 2012, Mosby.

BOX 13-2 Measures to Prevent Falls

- Assess the client's risk for falling; use agency fall risk assessment scale.
- Assign the client at risk for falling to a room near the nurses' station.
- Alert all personnel to the client's risk for falling; use agency fall risk alert procedures and methods as necessary.
- Assess the client frequently.
- Orient the client to physical surroundings.
- Instruct the client to seek assistance when getting up.
- Explain the use of the nurse call system.
- Use safety devices such as floor pads, and bed or chair alarms that alert health care personnel of the person getting out of bed or a chair.
- Keep the bed in the low position with side rails adjusted to a safe position (follow agency policy).
- Lock all beds, wheelchairs, and stretchers.
- Keep clients' personal items within their reach.
- Eliminate clutter and obstacles in the client's room.
- Provide adequate lighting.
- Reduce bathroom hazards.
- Maintain the client's toileting schedule throughout the day.

1. See Box 13-3 for a list of the National Patient Safety Goals
2. Refer to the following website for detailed information on these goals https://www.jointcommission.org/assets/1/6/NPSG_Chapter_HAP_Jan2018.pdf

J. Steps to prevent injury to the health care worker (Box 13-4)

K. Restraints (safety devices)
1. Restraints (safety devices) are protective devices used to limit the physical activity of a client or to immobilize a client or an extremity.
   a. The agency policy should be checked and followed when using side rails.
   b. The use of side rails is not considered a restraint when they are used to prevent a sedated client from falling out of bed.

BOX 13-3 The Joint Commission: 2018 National Patient Safety Goals

- Improve the accuracy of client identification.
- Improve the effectiveness of communication among caregivers
- Improve the safety of using medications
- Focus on the risk points related to medication reconciliation
- Reduce the harm associated with clinical alarm systems
- Reduce the risk of health care–associated infections
- Identify client safety risks
- Prevent mistakes in surgery

https://www.jointcommission.org/assets/1/6/NPSG_Chapter_HAP_Jan2018.pdf
https://www.jointcommission.org/assets/1/6/2018_HAP_NPSG_goals_final.pdf

BOX 13-4 Steps to Prevent Injury to the Health Care Worker When Moving a Client

- Use available safety equipment.
- Keep the weight to be lifted as close to the body as possible.
- Bend at the knees.
- Tighten abdominal muscles and tuck the pelvis.
- Maintain the trunk erect and knees bent so that multiple muscle groups work together in a coordinated manner.

Adapted from Potter A, Perry P, Stockert P, Hall A: *Fundamentals of nursing*, ed 8, St. Louis, 2013, Mosby.

   c. The client must be able to exit the bed easily in case of an emergency when using side rails. Only the top two side rails should be used.
   d. The bed must be kept in the lowest position.
2. *Physical restraints* restrict client movement through the application of a device.
3. *Chemical restraints* are medications given to inhibit a specific behavior or movement.
4. Interventions
   a. Use alternative devices, such as pressure-sensitive beds or chair pads with alarms or other types of bed or chair alarms, whenever possible.
   b. If restraints are necessary, the primary health care provider's (PHCP's) prescriptions should state the type of restraint, identify specific client behaviors for which restraints are to be used, and identify a limited time frame for use.
   c. The PHCP's prescriptions for restraints should be renewed within a specific time frame according to agency policy.
   d. Restraints are not to be prescribed PRN (as needed).
   e. The reason for the safety device should be given to the client and the family, and their permission should be sought and documented.
   f. Restraints should not interfere with any treatments or affect the client's health problem.
   g. Use a half-bow, a safety knot (quick release tie), or a restraint with a quick release buckle to secure the device to the bed frame or chair, not to a movable part of bed (including the side rails).
   h. Ensure that there is enough slack on the straps to allow some movement of the body part.
   i. Assess skin integrity and neurovascular and circulatory status every 30 minutes and remove the safety device at least every 2 hours to permit muscle exercise and to promote circulation (follow agency policies).

BOX 13-5 Documentation Points With Use of a Safety Device (Restraint)

- Reason for safety device
- Method of use for safety device
- Date and time of application of safety device
- Duration of use of safety device and client's response
- Release from safety device with periodic exercise and circulatory, neurovascular, and skin assessment
- Assessment of continued need for safety device
- Evaluation of client's response

j. Continually assess and document the need for safety devices (Box 13-5).
k. Offer fluids if clinically indicated at least every 2 hours.
l. Offer bedpan or toileting every 2 hours.

⚠ An PHCP's prescription for use of a safety device (restraint) is needed. Alternative measures for safety devices should always be used first.

5. Alternatives to safety devices for a client with confusion
   a. Orient the client and family to the surroundings with every interaction and identify the client by their name.
   b. Explain all procedures and treatments to the client and family.
   c. Encourage family and friends to stay with the client, and use sitters for clients who need supervision.
   d. Assign confused and disoriented clients to rooms near the nurses' station.
   e. Provide appropriate visual and auditory stimuli, such as a night light, clocks, calendars, television, and a radio, to the client; leave the client's room door open.
   f. Place familiar items, such as family pictures, near the client's bedside.
   g. Maintain toileting routines.
   h. Eliminate bothersome treatments, such as nasogastric tube feedings, as soon as possible.
   i. Evaluate all medications that the client is receiving.
   j. Use relaxation techniques with the client.
   k. Institute exercise and ambulation schedules as the client's condition allows.
   l. Collaborate with the PHCP to evaluate oxygenation status, vital signs, electrolyte/laboratory values, and other pertinent assessment findings that may provide information about the cause of the client's confusion.

L. Poisons
1. A poison is any substance that impairs health or destroys life when ingested, inhaled, or otherwise absorbed by the body.
2. Specific antidotes or treatments are available only for some types of poisons.
3. The capacity of body tissue to recover from a poison determines the reversibility of the effect.
4. Poison can impair the respiratory, circulatory, central nervous, hepatic, gastrointestinal, and renal systems of the body.
5. The infant, toddler, the preschooler, and the young school-age child must be protected from accidental poisoning.
6. In older adults, diminished eyesight and impaired memory may result in accidental ingestion of poisonous substances or an overdose of prescribed medications.
7. A Poison Control Center phone number should be visible on the telephone in homes with small children; in all cases of suspected poisoning, the number should be called immediately.
8. Interventions
   a. Remove any obvious materials from the mouth, eyes, or body area immediately.
   b. Identify the type and amount of substance ingested.
   c. Call the Poison Control Center before attempting an intervention.
   d. If the victim vomits or vomiting is induced, save the vomitus if requested to do so, and deliver it to the Poison Control Center.
   e. If instructed by the Poison Control Center to take the person to the emergency department, call an ambulance.
   f. Never induce vomiting following ingestion of lye, household cleaners, grease, or petroleum products.
   g. Never induce vomiting in an unconscious victim.

⚠ The Poison Control Center should be called first before attempting an intervention.

II. Health Care–Associated (Nosocomial) Infections

A. Health care–associated (nosocomial) infections also are referred to as *hospital-acquired infections*.
B. These infections are acquired in a hospital or other health care facility and were not present or incubating at the time of a client's admission.
C. *Clostridium difficile* is spread mainly by hand-to-hand contact in a health care setting. Clients taking multiple antibiotics for a prolonged period are most at risk.
D. Common drug-resistant infections: Vancomycin-resistant enterococci (VRE), methicillin-resistant *Staphylococcus aureus* (MRSA), multidrug-resistant tuberculosis, carbapenem-resistant *Enterobacteriaceae* (CRE)
E. Illness and some medications such as immunosuppressants impair the normal defense mechanisms.

F. The hospital environment provides exposure to a variety of virulent organisms that the client has not been exposed to in the past; therefore, the client has not developed resistance to these organisms.

G. Infections can be transmitted by health care personnel who fail to practice proper standard precautions (i.e., hand-washing procedures or failing to change gloves between client contacts).

H. At many health care agencies, dispensers containing an alcohol-based solution for hand sanitization are mounted at the entrance to each client's room; it is important to note that alcohol-based sanitizers are not effective against some infectious agents such as *Clostridium difficile* spores; therefore, handwashing is necessary.

III. Standard Precautions

A. Description

1. Nurses must practice standard precautions with all clients in any setting, regardless of the diagnosis or presumed infectiveness.
2. Standard precautions include hand washing and the use of gloves, as well as washing hands after gloves are removed. Additionally, standard precautions include the use of masks, eye protection, and gowns, when appropriate, for client contact.
3. These precautions apply to blood, all body fluids (whether or not they contain blood), secretions and excretions, nonintact skin, and mucous membranes.

B. Interventions

1. Wash hands between client contacts; after contact with blood, body fluids, secretions or excretions, nonintact skin, or mucous membranes; after contact with equipment or contaminated articles; and immediately after removing gloves.
2. Wear gloves when touching blood, body fluids, secretions, excretions, nonintact skin, mucous membranes, or contaminated items; remove gloves and wash hands between client care contacts.
3. For routine decontamination of hands, use alcohol-based hand rubs when hands are not visibly soiled. For more information on hand hygiene from the Centers for Disease Control and Prevention (CDC), see www.cdc.gov/handhygiene/
4. Wear masks and eye protection, or face shields, if client care activities may generate splashes or sprays of blood or body fluid.
5. Wear gowns if soiling of clothing is likely from blood or body fluid; wash hands after removing a gown.
6. Steps for donning and removing personal protective equipment (PPE) (Table 13-2)

TABLE 13-2 Steps for Donning and Removing Personal Protective Equipment (PPE)

Donning of PPE	Removal of PPE*
Gown Fully cover front of body from neck to knees and upper arms to end of wrist. Fasten in the back at neck and waist, wrap around the back.	**Gloves** Grasp outside of glove with opposite hand with glove still on and peel off. Hold on to removed glove in gloved hand. Slide fingers of ungloved hand under clean side of remaining glove at wrist and peel off.
Mask or Respirator Secure ties or elastic band at neck and middle of head. Fit snug to face and below chin. Fit to nose bridge. Respirator fit should be checked per agency policy.	**Goggles/Face Shield** Remove by touching clean band or inner part.
Goggles/Face Shield Adjust to fit according to agency policy.	**Gown** Unfasten at neck, then at waist. Remove using a peeling motion, pulling gown from each shoulder toward the hands. Allow gown to fall forward, and roll into a bundle to discard.
Gloves Select appropriate size and extend to cover wrists of gown.	**Mask or Respirator** Grasp bottom ties then top ties to remove.

*Note: All equipment is considered contaminated on the outside.

7. Clean and reprocess client care equipment properly and discard single-use items.
8. Place contaminated linens in leak-proof bags and limit handling to prevent skin and mucous membrane exposure. Dispose according to agency policy.
9. Use needleless devices or special needle safety devices whenever possible to reduce the risk of needle sticks and sharps injuries to health care workers.
10. Discard all sharp instruments and needles in a puncture-resistant container; dispose of needles uncapped or engage the safety mechanism on the needle if available.
11. Clean spills of blood or body fluids with a solution of bleach and water (diluted 1:10) or agency-approved disinfectant.

! Handle all blood and body fluids from all clients as if they were contaminated.

IV. Transmission-Based Precautions

A. Transmission-based precautions include airborne, droplet, and contact precautions.

B. Airborne precautions

1. Diseases
   a. Measles

b. Chickenpox (varicella)
c. Disseminated varicella zoster
d. Pulmonary or laryngeal tuberculosis

2. Barrier protection
   a. Used for clients known or suspected to be infected with pathogens transmitted by the airborne route.
   b. Single room is maintained under negative pressure; door remains closed except upon entering and exiting.
   c. Negative airflow pressure is used in the room, with a minimum of 6 to 12 air exchanges per hour via high-efficiency particulate air (HEPA) filtration mask or according to agency protocol.
   d. Ultraviolet germicide irradiation or HEPA filter is used in the room.
   e. Health care workers wear a respiratory mask (N95 or higher level). A surgical mask is placed on the client when the client needs to leave the room; the client leaves the room only if necessary.

C. Droplet precautions
1. Diseases
   a. Adenovirus
   b. Diphtheria (pharyngeal)
   c. Epiglottitis
   d. Influenza (flu)
   e. Meningitis
   f. Mumps
   g. Mycoplasmal pneumonia or meningococcal pneumonia
   h. Parvovirus B19
   i. Pertussis
   j. Pneumonia
   k. Rubella
   l. Scarlet fever
   m. Sepsis
   n. Streptococcal pharyngitis
2. Barrier protection
   a. Used for clients with known or suspected infection with pathogens transmitted by respiratory droplets, generated when coughing, sneezing, or talking.
   b. Private room or cohort client (a client whose body cultures contain the same organism)
   c. Wear a surgical mask when within 3 feet of a client; place a mask on the client when the client needs to leave the room.

D. Contact precautions
1. Diseases
   a. Colonization or infection with a multidrug-resistant organism
   b. Enteric infections, such as *Clostridium difficile*
   c. Respiratory infections, such as respiratory syncytial virus
   d. Influenza: Infection can occur by touching something with flu viruses on it and then touching the mouth or nose.
   e. Wound infections
   f. Skin infections, such as cutaneous diphtheria, herpes simplex, impetigo, pediculosis, scabies, staphylococci, and varicella zoster
   g. Eye infections, such as conjunctivitis
   h. Indirect contact transmission may occur when contaminated object or instrument, or hands, are encountered.
2. Barrier protection
   a. Private room or cohort client
   b. Use gloves and a gown whenever entering the client's room.

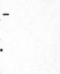

V. Emergency Response Plan and Disasters

A. Know the emergency response plan of the agency.
B. *Internal disasters* are those that occur within the health care facility.
C. *External disasters* occur in the community, and victims are brought to the health care facility for care.
D. When the health care facility is notified of a disaster, the nurse should follow the guidelines specified in the emergency response plan of the facility.
E. See Chapter 7 for additional information on disaster planning.

In the event of a disaster, the emergency response plan is activated immediately.

VI. Biological Warfare Agents

A. A warfare agent is a biological or chemical substance that can cause mass destruction or fatality.
B. Anthrax (Fig. 13-1)
1. The disease is caused by *Bacillus anthracis* and can be contracted through the digestive system, abrasions in the skin, or inhalation through the lungs.
2. Anthrax is transmitted by direct contact with bacteria and spores; spores are dormant encapsulated bacteria that become active when they enter a living host (no person-to-person spread) (Box 13-6).
3. The infection is carried to the lymph nodes and then spreads to the rest of the body by way of the blood and lymph systems; high levels of toxins lead to shock and death.

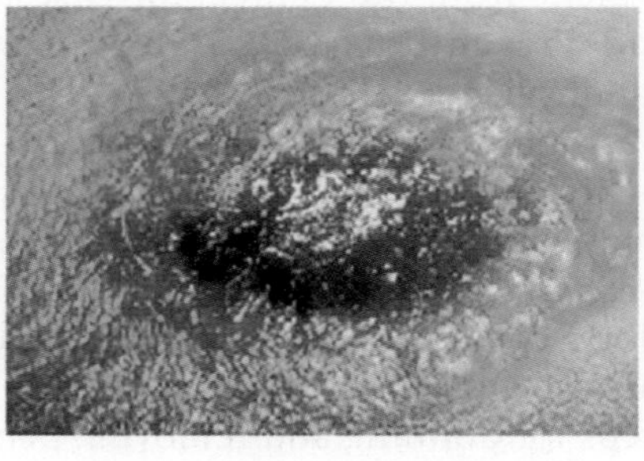

FIG. 13-1 Anthrax. (From Swartz, 2010.)

BOX 13-6 Anthrax: Transmission and Symptoms

Skin

Spores enter the skin through cuts and abrasions and are contracted by handling contaminated animal skin products.

Infection starts with an itchy bump like a mosquito bite that progresses to a small liquid-filled sac.

The sac becomes a painless ulcer with an area of black, dead tissue in the middle.

Toxins destroy surrounding tissue.

Gastrointestinal

Infection occurs following the ingestion of contaminated undercooked meat.

Symptoms begin with nausea, loss of appetite, and vomiting.

The disease progresses to severe abdominal pain, vomiting of blood, and severe diarrhea.

Inhalation

Infection is caused by the inhalation of bacterial spores, which multiply in the alveoli.

The disease begins with the same symptoms as the flu, including fever, muscle aches, and fatigue.

Symptoms suddenly become more severe with the development of breathing problems and shock.

Toxins cause hemorrhage and destruction of lung tissue.

4. In the lungs, anthrax can cause buildup of fluid, tissue decay, and death (fatal if untreated).
5. A blood test is available to detect anthrax (detects and amplifies *Bacillus anthracis* DNA if present in the blood sample).
6. Anthrax is usually treated with antibiotics such as ciprofloxacin, doxycycline, or penicillin.
7. The vaccine for anthrax has limited availability.

Anthrax is transmitted by direct contact with bacteria and spores and can be contracted through the digestive system, abrasions in the skin, or inhalation through the lungs.

C. Smallpox (Fig. 13-2)
1. Smallpox is transmitted in air droplets and by handling contaminated materials and is highly contagious.

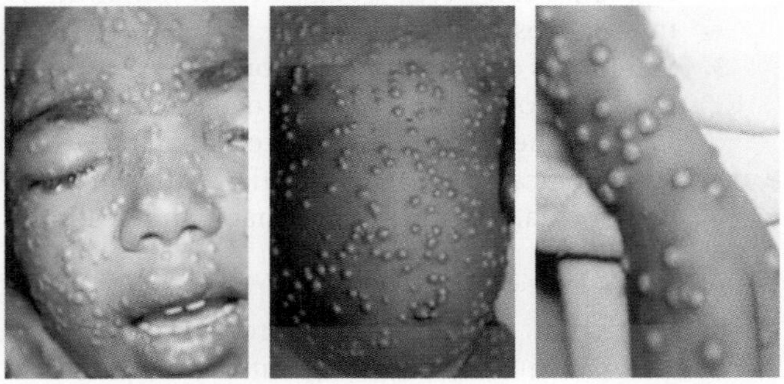

FIG. 13-2 Smallpox. (Courtesy Centers for Disease Control and Prevention [CDC]: *Evaluating patients for smallpox.* Atlanta, 2002, CDC.)

2. Symptoms begin 7 to 17 days after exposure and include fever, back pain, vomiting, malaise, and headache.
3. Papules develop 2 days after symptoms develop and progress to pustular vesicles that are abundant on the face and extremities initially.
4. A vaccine is available to those at risk for exposure to smallpox.

D. Botulism
1. Botulism is a serious paralytic illness caused by a nerve toxin produced by the bacterium *Clostridium botulinum* (death can occur within 24 hours).
2. Its spores are found in the soil and can spread through the air or food (improperly canned food) or via a contaminated wound.
3. Botulism cannot be spread from person to person.
4. Symptoms include abdominal cramps, diarrhea, nausea and vomiting, double vision, blurred vision, drooping eyelids, difficulty swallowing or speaking, dry mouth, and muscle weakness.
5. Neurological symptoms begin 12 to 36 hours after ingestion of food-borne botulism and 24 to 72 hours after inhalation and can progress to paralysis of the arms, legs, trunk, or respiratory muscles (mechanical ventilation is necessary).
6. If diagnosed early, food-borne and wound botulism can be treated with an antitoxin that blocks the action of toxin circulating in the blood.
7. For wound botulism, surgical removal of the source of the toxin-producing bacteria may be done; antibiotics may be prescribed.
8. No vaccine is available.

E. Plague
1. Plague is caused by *Yersinia pestis,* a bacteria found in rodents and fleas.
2. Plague is contracted by being bitten by a rodent or flea that is carrying the plague bacterium, by the ingestion of contaminated meat, or by handling an animal infected with the bacteria.
3. Transmission is by direct person-to-person spread.
4. Forms include bubonic (most common), pneumonic, and septicemic (most deadly).
5. Symptoms usually begin within 1 to 3 days and include fever, chest pain, lymph node swelling, and a productive cough (hemoptysis).
6. The disease rapidly progresses to dyspnea, stridor, and cyanosis; death occurs from respiratory failure, shock, and bleeding.
7. Antibiotics are effective only if administered immediately; the usual medications of choice include streptomycin or gentamicin.
8. A vaccine is available.

F. Tularemia
1. Tularemia (also called *deer fly fever* or *rabbit fever*) is an infectious disease of animals caused by the bacillus *Francisella tularensis.*

2. The disease is transmitted by ticks, deer flies, or contact with an infected animal.
3. Symptoms include fever, headache, and an ulcerated skin lesion with localized lymph node enlargement, eye infections, gastrointestinal ulcerations, or pneumonia.
4. Treatment is with antibiotics such as streptomycin, gentamicin, doxycycline, and ciprofloxacin.
5. Recovery produces lifelong immunity (a vaccine is available).

G. Hemorrhagic fever
1. Hemorrhagic fever is caused by several viruses, including Marburg, Lassa, Junin, and Ebola.
2. The virus is carried by rodents and mosquitoes.
3. The disease can be transmitted directly by person-to-person spread via body fluids.
4. Manifestations include fever, headache, malaise, conjunctivitis, nausea, vomiting, hypotension, hemorrhage of tissues and organs, and organ failure.
5. No known specific treatment is available; treatment is symptomatic.

H. Ebola Virus Disease (EVD)
1. Previously known as Ebola hemorrhagic fever
2. Caused by infection with a virus of the family *Filoviridae*, genus *Ebolavirus*
3. First discovered in 1976 in the Democratic Republic of the Congo. Outbreaks have appeared in Africa and in several other countries in the world.
4. The natural reservoir host of *Ebolavirus* remains unknown. It is believed that the virus is animal-borne and that bats are the most likely reservoir.
5. Spread of the virus is through contact with objects (such as clothes, bedding, needles, syringes/sharps, or medical equipment) that have been contaminated with the virus.
6. Symptoms similar to hemorrhagic fever may appear from 2 to 21 days after exposure.
7. Assessment: Ask the client if he or she traveled to an area with EVD such as Guinea, Nigeria, or Sierra Leone within the last 21 days or if he or she has had contact with someone with EVD and had any of the following symptoms:
   a. Fever at home or a current temperature of 38° C (100.4° F) or greater
   b. Severe headache
   c. Muscle pain
   d. Weakness
   e. Fatigue
   f. Diarrhea
   g. Vomiting
   h. Abdominal pain
   i. Unexplained bleeding or bruising
8. Interventions
   a. If the assessment indicates possible infection with EVD, the client needs to be isolated in a private room with a private bathroom or a covered bedside commode with the door closed.
   b. Health care workers need to wear the proper personal protective equipment (PPE) and follow updated procedures designated by the Centers for Disease Control and Prevention for donning (putting on) and removing PPE. Refer to the following Web site for updated information: http://www.cdc.gov/vhf/ebola/healthcare-us/ppe/guidance.html
   c. The number of health care workers entering the room should be limited, and a log of everyone who enters and leaves the room should be kept.
   d. Only necessary tests and procedures should be performed, and aerosol-generating procedures should be avoided.
   e. Refer to the CDC guidelines for cleaning, disinfecting, and managing waste (www.cdc.gov/vhf/ebola/healthcare-us/cleaning/hospitals.html).
   f. The agency's infection control program should be notified, as well as state and local public health authorities.

VII. Chemical Warfare Agents

A. Sarin
1. Sarin is a highly toxic nerve gas that can cause death within minutes of exposure.
2. It enters the body through the eyes and skin and acts by paralyzing the respiratory muscles.

B. Phosgene is a colorless gas normally used in chemical manufacturing that if inhaled at high concentrations for a long enough period will lead to severe respiratory distress, pulmonary edema, and death.

C. Mustard gas is yellow to brown and has a garlic-like odor that irritates the eyes and causes skin burns and blisters.

D. Nuclear warfare
1. Acute radiation exposure develops after a substantial exposure to radiation and is referred to as *nuclear warfare.*
2. Exposure can occur from external radiation or internal absorption.
3. Symptoms depend on the amount of exposure to the radiation and range from nausea and vomiting, diarrhea, fever, electrolyte imbalances, and neurological and cardiovascular impairment to leukopenia, purpura, hemorrhage, and death.

VIII. Nurse's Role in Exposure to Warfare Agents

A. Be aware that, initially, a bioterrorism attack may resemble a naturally occurring outbreak of an infectious disease.

B. Nurses and other health care workers must be prepared to assess and determine what type of event occurred, the number of clients who may be affected, and how and when clients will be expected to arrive at the health care agency.

C. It is essential to be aware that changes in the microorganism can occur that may increase its virulence or make it resistant to conventional antibiotics or vaccines.

D. See Chapter 7 for additional information on disasters and emergency response planning.

PRACTICE QUESTIONS

100. The nurse is preparing to initiate an intravenous (IV) line containing a high dose of potassium chloride using an IV infusion pump. While preparing to plug the pump cord into the wall, the nurse finds that no receptacle is available in the wall socket. The nurse should take which action?

1. Initiate the IV line without the use of a pump.
2. Contact the electrical maintenance department for assistance.
3. Plug in the pump cord in the available plug above the room sink.
4. Use an extension cord from the nurses' lounge for the pump plug.

101. The nurse obtains a prescription from a primary health care provider to restrain a client and instructs an assistive personnel (AP) to apply the safety device to the client. Which observation of unsafe application of the safety device would indicate that **further instruction is required** for the AP?

1. Placing a safety knot in the safety device straps
2. Safely securing the safety device straps to the side rails
3. Applying safety device straps that do not tighten when force is applied against them
4. Securing so that 2 fingers can slide easily between the safety device and the client's skin

102. The community health nurse is providing a teaching session about anthrax to members of the community and asks the participants about the methods of transmission. Which answers by the participants would indicate that teaching was **effective? Select all that apply.**

- ❑ 1. Bites from ticks or deer flies
- ❑ 2. Inhalation of bacterial spores
- ❑ 3. Through a cut or abrasion in the skin
- ❑ 4. Direct contact with an infected individual
- ❑ 5. Sexual contact with an infected individual
- ❑ 6. Ingestion of contaminated undercooked meat

103. The nurse is giving report to an assistive personnel (AP) who will be caring for a client in hand restraints (safety devices). How frequently should the nurse instruct the AP to check the tightness of the restrained hands?

1. Every 2 hours
2. Every 3 hours
3. Every 4 hours
4. Every 30 minutes

104. The nurse is reviewing a plan of care for a client with an internal radiation implant. Which intervention, if noted in the plan, **indicates the need for revision** of the plan?

1. Wearing gloves when emptying the client's bedpan
2. Keeping all linens in the room until the implant is removed
3. Wearing a lead apron when providing direct care to the client
4. Placing the client in a semiprivate room at the end of the hallway

105. Contact precautions are initiated for a client with a health care–associated (nosocomial) infection caused by methicillin-resistant *Staphylococcus aureus* (MRSA). The nurse prepares to provide colostomy care and should obtain which protective items to perform this procedure?

1. Gloves and gown
2. Gloves and goggles
3. Gloves, gown, and shoe protectors
4. Gloves, gown, goggles, and a mask or face shield

106. The nurse enters a client's room and finds that the wastebasket is on fire. The nurse immediately assists the client out of the room. What is the **next** nursing action?

1. Call for help.
2. Extinguish the fire.
3. Activate the fire alarm.
4. Confine the fire by closing the room door.

107. A mother calls a neighbor who is a nurse and tells the nurse that her 3-year-old child has just ingested liquid furniture polish. The nurse would direct the mother to take which **immediate** action?

1. Induce vomiting.
2. Call an ambulance.
3. Call the Poison Control Center.
4. Bring the child to the emergency department.

108. The emergency department (ED) nurse receives a telephone call and is informed that a tornado has hit a local residential area and that numerous casualties have occurred. The victims will be

brought to the ED. The nurse should take which **initial** action?
1. Prepare the triage rooms.
2. Activate the emergency response plan specific to the facility.
3. Obtain additional supplies from the central supply department.
4. Obtain additional nursing staff to assist in treating the casualties.

109. The nurse is caring for a client with meningitis and implements which transmission-based precaution for this client?
1. Private room or cohort client
2. Personal respiratory protection device
3. Private room with negative airflow pressure
4. Mask worn by staff when the client needs to leave the room

110. The nurse working in the emergency department (ED) is assessing a client who recently returned from Nigeria and presented complaining of a fever at home, fatigue, muscle pain, and abdominal pain. Which action should the nurse take **next**?
1. Check the client's temperature.
2. Isolate the client in a private room.
3. Check a complete set of vital signs.
4. Contact the primary health care provider.

ANSWERS

100. ***Answer:*** **2**
Rationale: Electrical equipment must be maintained in good working order and should be grounded; otherwise, it presents a physical hazard. An IV line that contains a dose of potassium chloride should be administered by an infusion pump. The nurse needs to use hospital resources for assistance. A regular extension cord should not be used because it poses a risk for fire. Use of electrical appliances near a sink also presents a hazard.
Test-Taking Strategy: Note the subject, electrical safety. Recalling safety issues will direct you to the correct option. Contacting the maintenance department is the only correct option, since the other options are not considered safe practice when implementing electrical actions. In addition, since potassium chloride is in the IV solution, a pump must be used.
Level of Cognitive Ability: Applying
Client Needs: Safe and Effective Care Environment
Integrated Process: Nursing Process—Implementation
Content Area: Foundations of Care: Safety
Health Problem: N/A
Priority Concepts: Clinical Judgment; Safety
Reference: Potter et al. (2017), pp. 389, 393.

101. ***Answer:*** **2**
Rationale: The safety device straps are secured to the bed frame and never to the side rails to avoid accidental injury in the event that the side rails are released. A half-bow or safety knot or device with a quick release buckle should be used to apply a safety device because it does not tighten when force is applied against it and it allows quick and easy removal of the safety device in case of an emergency. The safety device should be secure, and 1 or 2 fingers should slide easily between the safety device and the client's skin.
Test-Taking Strategy: Focus on the subject, the unsafe intervention. Also note the strategic words, *further instruction is required.* These words indicate a negative event query and the need to select the incorrect option. Read each option carefully. The words *securing the safety device straps to the side rails* in option 2 should direct your attention to this as an incorrect and unsafe action.
Level of Cognitive Ability: Evaluating
Client Needs: Safe and Effective Care Environment
Integrated Process: Teaching and Learning
Content Area: Foundations of Care: Safety
Health Problem: N/A
Priority Concepts: Health Care Quality; Safety
Reference: Potter et al. (2017), pp. 400-401.

102. ***Answer:*** **2, 3, 6**
Rationale: Anthrax is caused by *Bacillus anthracis* and can be contracted through the digestive system or abrasions in the skin, or inhaled through the lungs. It cannot be spread from person to person, and it is not contracted via bites from ticks or deer flies.
Test-Taking Strategy: Focus on the subject, routes of transmission of anthrax, and note the strategic word, *effective.* Knowledge regarding the methods of contracting anthrax is needed to answer this question. Remember that it is not spread by person-to-person contact or contracted via tick or deer fly bites.
Level of Cognitive Ability: Evaluating
Client Needs: Safe and Effective Care Environment
Integrated Process: Teaching and Learning
Content Area: Foundations of Care: Infection Control
Health Problem: Adult Health: Immune: Infections
Priority Concepts: Client Teaching; Infection
Reference: Ignatavicius, Workman, Rebar (2018), p. 429.

103. ***Answer:*** **4**
Rationale: The nurse should instruct the AP to check safety devices for tightness every 30 minutes. The neurovascular and circulatory status of the extremity should also be checked by the registered nurse every 30 minutes. In addition, the safety device should be removed at least every 2 hours to permit muscle exercise and to promote circulation. Agency guidelines regarding the use of safety devices should always be followed.
Test-Taking Strategy: Focus on the subject, checking the tightness of a safety devices. In this situation, selecting the option that identifies the most frequent time frame is best.
Level of Cognitive Ability: Applying
Client Needs: Safe and Effective Care Environment
Integrated Process: Teaching and Learning
Content Area: Leadership/Management: Delegating
Health Problem: N/A
Priority Concepts: Health Care Quality; Safety
Reference: Potter et al. (2017), p. 402.

104. *Answer:* 4

Rationale: A private room with a private bath is essential if a client has an internal radiation implant. This is necessary to prevent accidental exposure of other clients to radiation. The remaining options identify accurate interventions for a client with an internal radiation implant and protect the nurse from exposure.

Test-Taking Strategy: Note the strategic words, *indicates the need for revision*. These words indicate a negative event query and the need to select the incorrect nursing intervention. Remember that the client with an internal radiation implant needs to be placed in a private room.

Level of Cognitive Ability: Applying
Client Needs: Safe and Effective Care Environment
Integrated Process: Nursing Process—Planning
Content Area: Foundations of Care: Safety
Health Problem: N/A
Priority Concepts: Health Care Quality; Safety
Reference: Ignatavicius, Workman, Rebar (2018), p. 389.

105. *Answer:* 4

Rationale: Splashes of body secretions can occur when providing colostomy care. Goggles and a mask or face shield are worn to protect the face and mucous membranes of the eyes during interventions that may produce splashes of blood, body fluids, secretions, or excretions. In addition, contact precautions require the use of gloves, and a gown should be worn if direct client contact is anticipated. Shoe protectors are not necessary.

Test-Taking Strategy: Focus on the subject, protective items needed to perform colostomy care. Also, note the words *contact precautions*. Visualize care for this client to determine the necessary items required for self-protection. This will direct you to the correct option.

Level of Cognitive Ability: Applying
Client Needs: Safe and Effective Care Environment
Integrated Process: Nursing Process—Implementation
Content Area: Foundations of Care: Infection Control
Health Problem: Adult Health: Immune: Infections
Priority Concepts: Clinical Judgment; Safety
Reference: Ignatavicius, Workman, Rebar (2018), p. 419.

106. *Answer:* 3

Rationale: The order of priority in the event of a fire is to rescue the clients who are in immediate danger. The next step is to activate the fire alarm. The fire then is confined by closing all doors and, finally, the fire is extinguished.

Test-Taking Strategy: Note the strategic word, *next*. Remember the mnemonic *RACE* to prioritize in the event of a fire. *R* is rescue clients in immediate danger, *A* is alarm (sound the alarm), *C* is confine the fire by closing all doors, and *E* is extinguish or evacuate.

Level of Cognitive Ability: Applying
Client Needs: Safe and Effective Care Environment
Integrated Process: Nursing Process—Implementation
Content Area: Foundations of Care: Safety
Health Problem: N/A
Priority Concepts: Clinical Judgment; Safety
Reference: Potter et al. (2017), pp. 392-393.

107. *Answer:* 3

Rationale: If a poisoning occurs, the Poison Control Center should be contacted immediately. Vomiting should not be induced if the victim is unconscious or if the substance ingested is a strong corrosive or petroleum product. Bringing the child to the emergency department or calling an ambulance would not be the initial action because this would delay treatment. The Poison Control Center may advise the mother to bring the child to the emergency department; if this is the case, the mother should call an ambulance.

Test-Taking Strategy: Note the strategic word, *immediate*. Calling the Poison Control Center is the first action, since it will direct the mother on the next step to take based on the type of poisoning. The other options are unsafe or could cause a delay in treatment.

Level of Cognitive Ability: Applying
Client Needs: Safe and Effective Care Environment
Integrated Process: Nursing Process—Implementation
Content Area: Foundations of Care: Safety
Health Problem: Pediatric-Specific: Poisoning
Priority Concepts: Clinical Judgment; Safety
Reference: Potter et al. (2017), p. 375.

108. *Answer:* 2

Rationale: In an external disaster (a disaster that occurs outside of the institution or agency), many victims may be brought to the ED for treatment. The initial nursing action must be to activate the emergency response plan specific to the facility. Once the emergency response plan is activated, the actions in the other options will occur.

Test-Taking Strategy: Note the strategic word, *initial*, and determine the priority action. Note that the correct option is the umbrella option. The emergency response plan includes all of the other options.

Level of Cognitive Ability: Applying
Client Needs: Safe and Effective Care Environment
Integrated Process: Nursing Process—Implementation
Content Area: Foundations of Care: Safety
Health Problem: N/A
Priority Concepts: Clinical Judgment; Safety
Reference: Ignatavicius, Workman, Rebar (2018), pp. 153-154.

109. *Answer:* 1

Rationale: Meningitis is transmitted by droplet infection. Precautions for this disease include a private room or cohort client and use of a standard precaution mask. Private negative airflow pressure rooms and personal respiratory protection devices are required for clients with airborne disease such as tuberculosis. When appropriate, a mask must be worn by the client and not the staff when the client leaves the room.

Test-Taking Strategy: Focus on the subject, the correct precaution needs for a client with meningitis. Recalling that meningitis is transmitted by droplets will direct you to the correct option.

Level of Cognitive Ability: Applying
Client Needs: Safe and Effective Care Environment
Integrated Process: Nursing Process—Implementation
Content Area: Foundations of Care: Infection Control

Health Problem: Adult Health: Neurological: Inflammation/ Infections
Priority Concepts: Infection; Safety
Reference: Ignatavicius, Workman, Rebar (2018), p. 419-420.

110. *Answer:* 2
Rationale: The nurse should suspect the potential for Ebola virus disease (EVD) because of the client's recent travel to Nigeria. The nurse needs to consider the symptoms that the client is reporting, and clients who meet the exposure criteria should be isolated in a private room before other treatment measures are taken. Exposure criteria include a fever reported at home or in the ED of 38.0° C (100.4° F) *or* headache, fatigue, weakness, muscle pain, vomiting, diarrhea, abdominal pain, or signs of bleeding. This client is reporting a fever and is showing other signs of EVD, and therefore should be isolated. After isolating the client, it would be acceptable to then collect further data and notify the primary health care provider and other state and local authorities of the client's signs and symptoms.
Test-Taking Strategy: Note the **strategic word**, *next.* This indicates that some or all of the other options may be partially or totally correct, but the nurse needs to prioritize. Eliminate options 1 and 3 first because they are **comparable or alike.** Next note that the client recently traveled to Nigeria. Recall that isolation to prevent transmission of an infection is the immediate priority in the care of a client with suspected EVD.
Level of Cognitive Ability: Analyzing
Client Needs: Safe and Effective Care Environment
Integrated Process: Nursing Process—Implementation
Content Area: Foundations of Care: Infection Control
Health Problem: Adult Health: Immune: Infections
Priority Concepts: Clinical Judgment; Safety
Reference: Ignatavicius, Workman, Rebar (2018), p. 427.
www.cdc.gov/vhf/ebola/healthcare-us/emergency-services/emergency-departments.html

CHAPTER 14

Calculation of Medication and Intravenous Prescriptions

PRIORITY CONCEPTS **Clinical Judgment, Safety**

I. Medication Administration (Box 14-1)

In most clinical settings, an electronic infusion device is used to administer intravenous (IV) solutions and IV medications. However, the NCLEX-RN® examination is going to require that you correctly calculate an intravenous infusion rate via drops per minute, so be sure that you master this skill.

II. Medication Measurement Systems

A. Metric system (Box 14-2)
  1. The basic units of metric measures are the meter, liter, and gram.
  2. Meter measures length; liter measures volume; gram measures mass.

B. Apothecary and household systems
  1. The apothecary and household systems are the oldest of the medication measurement systems.
  2. Apothecary measures such as grain, dram, and minim are not commonly used in the clinical setting.
  3. Commonly used household measures include drop, teaspoon, tablespoon, ounce, pint, and cup.

⚠ The NCLEX will not present questions that require you to convert from the apothecary system of measurement to the metric system; however, this system is still important to know because, although it is not commonly used, you may encounter it in the clinical setting.

C. Additional common medication measures
  1. Milliequivalent
     a. Milliequivalent is abbreviated mEq.
     b. The milliequivalent is an expression of the number of grams of a medication contained in 1 mL of a solution.
     c. For example, the measure of serum potassium is given in milliequivalents.
  2. Unit
     a. Unit measures a medication in terms of its action, not its physical weight.
     b. For example, penicillin, heparin sodium, and insulin are measured in units.

III. Conversions

A. Conversion between metric units (Box 14-3)
  1. The metric system is a decimal system; therefore, conversions between the units in this system can be done by dividing or multiplying by 1000 or by moving the decimal point 3 places to the right or 3 places to the left.
  2. In the metric system, to convert larger to smaller, multiply by 1000 or move the decimal point 3 places to the right.
  3. In the metric system, to convert smaller to larger, divide by 1000 or move the decimal point 3 places to the left.

B. Conversion between household and metric systems
  1. Household and metric measures are equivalent and not equal measures.
  2. Conversion to equivalent measures between systems is necessary when a medication prescription is written in one system but the medication label is stated in another.
  3. Medications are not always prescribed and prepared in the same system of measurement; therefore, conversion of units from one system to another is necessary. However, the metric system is the most commonly used system in the clinical setting.
  4. Calculating equivalents between 2 systems may be done by using the method of ratio and proportion (Boxes 14-4 and 14-5).

⚠ Conversion is the first step in the calculation of dosages.

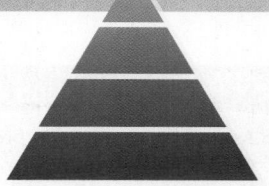

BOX 14-1 Medication Administration

- Assess the medication prescription.
- Compare the client's medication prescription with all medications that the client was previously taking (medication reconciliation).
- Ask the client about a history of allergies or use of herbal substances.
- Assess the client's current condition and the purpose for the medication or intravenous (IV) solution.
- Determine the client's understanding of the purpose of the prescribed medication or need for IV solution.
- Teach the client about the medication and about self-administration at home.
- Identify and address concerns (social, cultural, religious, spiritual) that the client may have about taking the medication.
- Assess the need for conversion when preparing a dose of medication for administration to the client.
- Assess the rights of medication administration such as: right prescription, right medication, right dose, right client, right route, right frequency/time, right reason, right education (medication name, purpose, action, and possible undesirable side or adverse effects), right assessment (performed by a qualified health care provider), right to refuse medication regardless of the consequences, right approach/technique, right evaluation/response, and right documentation.
- Inform the client of additional medication rights, which include not receiving unnecessary medication; being advised of the experimental nature of medication therapy and to give written consent for its use; being informed if prescribed medications are a part of a research study; and receiving appropriate supportive therapy in relation to medication therapy.
- Assess the vital signs, check significant laboratory results, and identify any potential interactions (food or medication interactions) before administering medication, when appropriate.
- Document the administration of the prescribed therapy and the client's response to the therapy.

BOX 14-2 Metric System

Abbreviations	Equivalents
meter: m	1 mcg = 0.000001 g
liter: L	1 mg = 1000 mcg or 0.001 g
milliliter: mL	1 g = 1000 mg
kilogram: kg	1 kg = 1000 g
gram: g	1 kg = 2.2 lb
milligram: mg	1 mL = 0.001 L
microgram: mcg	
milliequivalents: mEq	

IV. Medication Labels

A. A medication label always contains the **generic name** and may contain the **trade name** of the medication.

B. Always check expiration dates on medication labels.

BOX 14-3 Conversion Between Metric Units

Problem 1

Convert 2 g to milligrams.

Solution

Change a larger unit to a smaller unit:
2 g = 2000 mg (multiply by 1000 or move decimal point 3 places to the right)

Problem 2

Convert 250 mL to liters.

Solution

Change a smaller unit to a larger unit:
250 mL = 0.25 L (divide by 1000 or move decimal point 3 places to the left)

BOX 14-4 Ratio and Proportion

Ratio: The relationship between 2 numbers, separated by a colon; for example, 1:2 (1 to 2).

Proportion: The relationship between 2 ratios, separated by a double colon (::) or an equal sign (=).

Formula:

H(on hand) : V(vehicle) :: (=)(desired dose) : X(unknown)

To solve a ratio and proportion problem: The middle numbers (means) are multiplied and the end numbers (extremes) are multiplied.

Sample Problem

H = 1
V = 2
Desired dose = 3
X = unknown
Set up the formula: 1 : 2 :: 3 : X
Solve: Multiply means and extremes:
1X = 6
X = 6

The NCLEX tests you on generic names of medications. Trade names will not be presented on the exam for most medications, so be sure to learn medications by their generic names. However, you will likely still encounter the trade names in the clinical setting.

V. Medication Prescriptions (Box 14-6)

A. In a medication prescription, the name of the medication is written first, followed by the dosage, route, and frequency (depending on the frequency of the prescription, times of administration are usually established by the health care agency and written in an agency policy).

BOX 14-5 Calculating Equivalents Between Two Systems

Calculating equivalents between 2 systems may be done by using the method of ratio and proportion.

Problem

The primary health care provider prescribes nitroglycerin $\frac{1}{150}$ grain (gr).

The medication label reads 0.4 milligrams (mg) per tablet. The nurse prepares to administer how many tablets to the client?

If you knew that $\frac{1}{150}$ gr was equal to 0.4 mg, you would know that you need to administer 1 tablet. Otherwise, use the ratio and proportion formula.

Note that grain is a measure in the apothecary system but nitroglycerin is one medication that you may find prescribed in this unit of measure.

Ratio and Proportion Formula

$$H(\text{on hand}) : V(\text{vehicle}) :: (=)(\text{desired dose}) : X(\text{unknown})$$

$$1\,\text{gr} : 60\,\text{mg} :: \frac{1}{150}\,\text{gr} : X\,\text{mg}$$

$$60 \times \frac{1}{150} = X$$

$$X = 0.4\,\text{mg}\,(1\,\text{tablet})$$

BOX 14-6 Medication Prescriptions

- Name of client
- Date and time when prescription is written
- Name of medication to be given
- Dosage of medication
- Medication route
- Time and frequency of administration
- Signature of person writing the prescription

B. Medication prescriptions need to be written using accepted abbreviations, acronyms, and symbols approved by The Joint Commission; also follow agency guidelines.

If the nurse has any questions about or sees inconsistencies in the written prescription, the nurse must contact the person who wrote the prescription immediately and must verify the prescription.

VI. Oral Medications

A. Scored tablets contain an indented mark to be used for possible breakage into partial doses; when necessary, scored tablets (those marked for division) can be divided into halves or quarters according to agency policy.

B. Enteric-coated tablets and sustained-released capsules delay absorption until the medication reaches the small intestine; these medications should not be crushed.

C. Capsules contain a powdered or oily medication in a gelatin cover.

D. Orally administered liquids are supplied in solution form and contain a specific amount of medication in a given amount of solution, as stated on the label.

E. The medicine cup

1. The medicine cup has a capacity of 30 mL or 1 ounce (oz) and is used for orally administered liquids.
2. The medicine cup is calibrated to measure teaspoons, tablespoons, and ounces.
3. To pour accurately, place the medication cup on a level surface at eye level and then pour the liquid while reading the measuring markings

F. Volumes of less than 5 mL are measured using a syringe with the needle removed.

A calibrated syringe is used for giving medicine to children.

VII. Parenteral Medications

A. Parenteral means an injection route, and parenteral medications are administered by intravenous (IV), intramuscular, subcutaneous, or intradermal injection (see Fig. 14-1 for angles of injection).

B. Parenteral medications are packaged in single-use ampules, in single- and multiple-use rubber-stoppered vials, and in premeasured syringes and cartridges.

C. The standard 3-mL syringe is used to measure most injectable medications and is calibrated in tenths (0.1) of a milliliter.

D. The syringe is filled by drawing in solution until the top ring on the plunger (i.e., the ring closest to the needle), not the middle section or the bottom ring of the plunger, is aligned with the desired calibration (Fig. 14-2).

E. The nurse should not administer more than 3 mL per intramuscular injection site (2 mL for the deltoid) or 0.5 to 1.5 mL for an adult per subcutaneous injection site; larger volumes are difficult for an injection site to absorb and, if prescribed, need to be verified. Variations for pediatric clients are discussed in the pediatric sections of this text.

F. In an adult that is of normal size, a 25-gauge 5/8-inch needle at a 45-degree angle or a 1/2-inch needle at a 90-degree angle is used for subcutaneous injections.

G. For an intramuscular injection in an adult client, the client's weight, site for injection, and the amount of adipose tissue influences needle size. An obese person may require a needle 2 to 3 inches long, whereas a thin person requires only a 1/2- to 1-inch

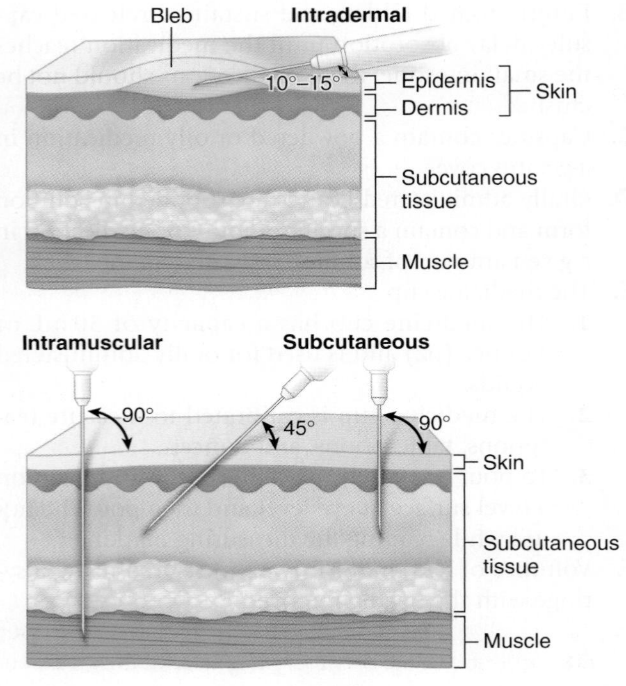

FIG. 14-1 Angles of injection.

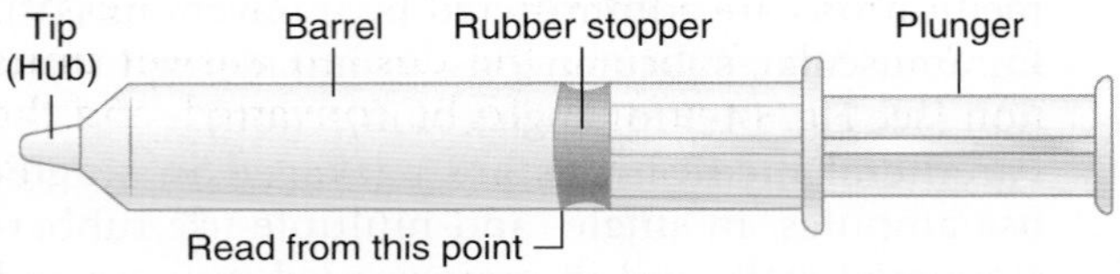

FIG. 14-2 Parts of a syringe.

needle; the gauge of the needle will depend on the viscosity of the solution being injected, with a larger gauge needed for more viscous solutions. If a Z-track method is used, a larger, deeper muscle such as the ventrogluteal muscle should be chosen as the site.

H. For an intradermal injection, a tuberculin or small syringe is used. The angle of insertion for an intradermal injection is 5 to 15 degrees.

⚠ Always question and verify excessively large or small volumes of medication.

I. Prefilled medication cartridge
1. The medication cartridge slips into the cartridge holder, which provides a plunger for injection of the medication.
2. The cartridge is designed to provide sufficient space to allow for the addition of a second medication when combined dosages are prescribed.
3. The prefilled medication cartridge is to be used once and discarded; if the nurse is to give less than the full single dose provided, the nurse needs to discard the extra amount before giving the client the injection, in accordance with agency policies and procedures.

J. In general, standard medication doses for adults are to be rounded to the nearest tenth (0.1 mL) of a milliliter and measured on the milliliter scale; for example, 1.28 mL is rounded to 1.3 mL (follow agency policy for rounding medication doses).

K. When volumes larger than 3 mL are required, the nurse may use a 5-mL syringe; these syringes are calibrated in fifths (0.2 mL) (Fig. 14-3).

L. Other syringe sizes may be available (10, 20, and 50 mL) and may be used for medication administration requiring dilution.

⚠ When performing a calculation, if rounding is necessary, perform the rounding at the end of the calculation. When taking the NCLEX, follow the instructions provided in the question regarding the need to round. For example, the NCLEX question may read: Record your answer using one decimal place.

M. Tuberculin syringe (Fig. 14-4)
1. The tuberculin syringe holds 1 mL and is used to measure small or critical amounts of medication, such as allergen extract, vaccine, or a child's medication.
2. The syringe is calibrated in hundredths (0.01) of a milliliter, with each one-tenth (0.1) marked on the metric scale.

N. Insulin syringe (Fig. 14-5)
1. The standard 100-unit insulin syringe is calibrated for 100 units of insulin (100 units = 1 mL); low-dose insulin syringes, such as a 30-unit insulin syringe or a 50-unit insulin syringe, are available for a more precise insulin draw for clients with low-dose insulin prescriptions.
2. Insulin should not be measured in any other type of syringe.

⚠ If the insulin prescription states to administer regular and NPH insulin, combine both types of insulin in the same syringe. Use the mnemonic *RN*: Draw *R*egular insulin into the insulin syringe first, and then draw the *N*PH insulin. Of note, with newer insulin types on the market, such as long-acting and rapid-acting insulin,

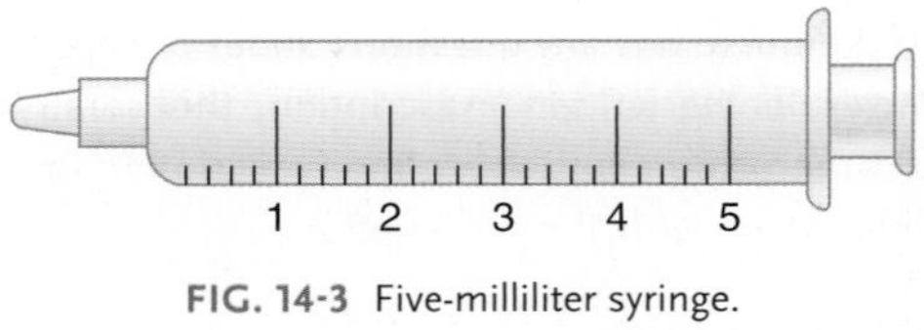

FIG. 14-3 Five-milliliter syringe.

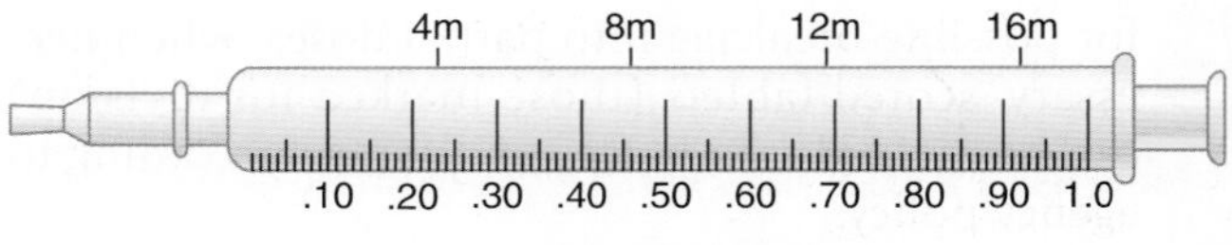

FIG. 14-4 Tuberculin syringe.

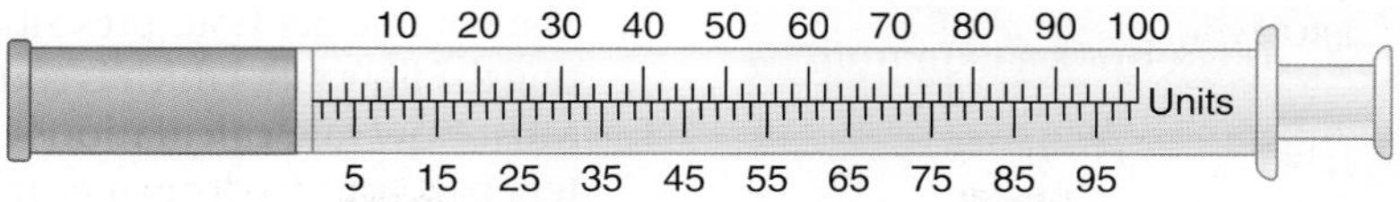

FIG. 14-5 A 100-unit insulin syringe.

Regular and NPH insulin are used less frequently because of safety and convenience factors.

O. Safety needles contain shielding devices that are attached to the needle and slipped over the needle to reduce the incidence of needlestick injuries.

VIII. Injectable Medications in Powder Form

A. Some medications become unstable when stored in solution form and are therefore packaged in powder form.

B. Powders must be dissolved with a sterile diluent before use; usually, sterile water or normal saline is used. The dissolving procedure is called reconstitution (Box 14-7).

IX. Calculating the Correct Dosage (see Box 14-8 for the standard formula)

A. When calculating dosages of oral medications, check the calculation and question the prescription if the calculation calls for more than 3 tablets.

B. When calculating dosages of parenteral medications, check the calculation and question the prescription if the amount to be given is too large a dose.

C. Be sure that all measures are in the same system and that all units are in the same size, converting when necessary; carefully consider what the reasonable amount of the medication that should be administered is.

D. Round standard injection doses to tenths and measure in a 3-mL syringe (follow agency policy).

E. Per agency policy, it may be acceptable to round down (avoid rounding up) small, critical amounts or children's doses to hundredths and measure in a 1-mL tuberculin syringe (example: 1.752 mL can be rounded to 1.75 mL).

BOX 14-7 Reconstitution

- In reconstituting a medication, locate the instructions on the label or in the vial package insert and read and follow the directions carefully.
- Instructions will state the volume of diluent to be used and the resulting volume of the reconstituted medication.
- Often, the powdered medication adds volume to the solution in addition to the amount of diluent added.
- The total volume of the prepared solution will exceed the volume of the diluent added.
- When reconstituting a multiple-dose vial, label the medication vial with the date and time of preparation, your initials, and the date of expiration.
- Indicating the strength per volume on the medication label also is important.

BOX 14-8 Standard Formula for Calculating a Medication Dosage

$$\frac{D}{A} \times Q = X$$

D (desired) is the dosage that the primary health care provider prescribed.
A (available) is the dosage strength as stated on the medication label.
Q (quantity) is the volume or form in which the dosage strength is available, such as tablets, capsules, or milliliters.

F. In addition to using the standard formula (see Box 14-8), calculations can be done using dimensional analysis, a method that uses conversion factors to move from one unit of measurement to another; the required elements of the equation include the desired answer units, conversion formula that includes the desired answer units and the units that need to be converted, and the original factors to convert, including quantity and units.

⚠ Regardless of the source or cause of a medication error, if the nurse gives an incorrect dose, the nurse is legally responsible for the action.

X. Percentage and Ratio Solutions

A. Percentage solutions
1. Express the number of grams (g) of the medication per 100 mL of solution.
2. For example, calcium gluconate 10% is 10 g of pure medication per 100 mL of solution.

B. Ratio solutions
1. Express the number of grams of the medication per total milliliters of solution.
2. For example, epinephrine 1:1000 is 1 g of pure medication per 1000 mL of solution.

XI. Intravenous Flow Rates (Box 14-9)

A. Monitor IV flow rate frequently even if the IV solution is being administered through an electronic infusion device (follow agency policy regarding frequency).

B. If an IV is running behind schedule, collaborate with the primary health care provider to determine the client's ability to tolerate an increased flow rate, particularly for older clients and those with cardiac, pulmonary, renal, or neurological conditions.

BOX 14-9 Formulas for Intravenous Calculations

Flow Rates

$$\frac{\text{Total volume} \times \text{Drop factor}}{\text{Time in minutes}} = \text{Drops per minute}$$

Infusion Time

$$\frac{\text{Total volume to infuse}}{\text{Milliliters per hour being infused}} = \text{Infusion time}$$

Number of Milliliters per Hour

$$\frac{\text{Total volume in milliliters}}{\text{Number of hours}} = \text{Number of milliliters per hour}$$

⚠ The nurse should never increase the rate of (i.e., speed up) an IV infusion to catch up if the infusion is running behind schedule. The nurse should include any IV fluid administered in the intake portion of the client's assessment.

C. Whenever a prescribed IV rate is increased, the nurse should assess the client for increased heart rate, increased respirations, and increased lung congestion, which could indicate fluid overload.
D. Intravenously administered fluids are prescribed most frequently based on milliliters per hour.
E. The volume per hour prescribed is administered by setting the flow rate, which is counted in drops per minute.
F. Most flow rate calculations involve changing milliliters per hour to drops per minute.
G. Intravenous tubing
   1. IV tubing sets are calibrated in drops per milliliter; this calibration is needed for calculating flow rates.
   2. A standard or macrodrip set is used for routine adult IV administrations; depending on the manufacturer and type of tubing, the set will require 10 to 20 drops (gtt) to equal 1 mL.
   3. A minidrip or microdrip set is used when more exact measurements are needed, such as in intensive care units and pediatric units.
   4. In a minidrip or microdrip set, 60 gtt is usually equal to 1 mL.
   5. The calibration, in drops per milliliter, is written on the IV tubing package.

XII. Calculation of Infusions Prescribed by Unit Dosage per Hour

A. The most common medications that will be prescribed by unit dosage per hour and run by continuous infusion are heparin sodium and regular insulin.
B. Calculation of these infusions can be done using a 2-step process (Box 14-10).

BOX 14-10 Infusions Prescribed by Unit Dosage per Hour

Calculation of these problems can be done using a 2-step process.
1. Determine the amount of medication per milliliter (mL).
2. Determine the infusion rate or milliliters per hour.

Problem 1

Prescription: Continuous heparin sodium by IV at 1000 units per hour

Available: IV bag of 500 mL D_5W with 20,000 units of heparin sodium

How many milliliters per hour are required to administer the correct dose?

Solution

Step 1: Calculate the amount of medication (units) per 1 mL.

$$\frac{\text{Known amount of medication in solution}}{\text{Total volume of diluent}} = \text{Amount of medication per milliliter}$$

$$\frac{20{,}000 \text{ units}}{500 \text{ mL}} = 40 \text{ units / 1 mL}$$

Step 2: Calculate milliliters per hour.

$$\frac{\text{Dose per hour desired}}{\text{Concentration per milliliter}} = \text{Infusion rate, or mL / hour}$$

$$\frac{1000 \text{ units}}{40 \text{ units}} = 25 \text{ mL / hour}$$

Problem 2

Prescription: Continuous regular insulin by IV at 10 units per hour

Available: IV bag of 100 mL NS with 50 units regular insulin

How many milliliters per hour are required to administer the correct dose?

Solution

Step 1: Calculate the amount of medication (units) per 1 mL.

$$\frac{\text{Known amount of medication in solution}}{\text{Total volume of diluent}} = \text{Amount of medication per milliliter}$$

$$\frac{50 \text{ units}}{100 \text{ mL}} = 0.5 \text{ units / 1 mL}$$

$$\frac{\text{Dose per hour desired}}{\text{Concentration per milliliter}} = \text{Infusion rate, or mL / hour}$$

$$\frac{10 \text{ units}}{0.5 \text{ units / mL}} = 20 \text{ mL / hour}$$

PRACTICE QUESTIONS

111. A prescription reads 1000 mL of normal saline (NS) to infuse over 12 hours. The drop factor is 15 drops (gtt)/1 mL. The nurse prepares to set the flow rate at how many drops per minute? **Fill in the blank. Record your answer to the nearest whole number.**
Answer: _______ drops per minute

112. A prescription reads to administer an intravenous (IV) dose of 400,000 units of penicillin G benzathine. The label on the 10-milliliters (mL) ampule sent from the pharmacy reads penicillin G benzathine, 300,000 units/mL. The nurse prepares how much medication to administer the correct dose? **Fill in the blank. Record your answer using 1 decimal place.**
Answer: _______ mL

113. A prescription reads potassium chloride 30 mEq to be added to 1000 mL normal saline (NS) and to be administered over a 10-hour period. The label on the medication bottle reads 40 mEq/20 mL. The nurse prepares how many milliliters (mL) of potassium chloride to administer the correct dose of medication? **Fill in the blank.**
Answer: _______ mL

114. A prescription reads clindamycin phosphate 0.3 g in 50 mL normal saline (NS) to be administered intravenously over 30 minutes. The medication label reads clindamycin phosphate 900 mg in 6 mL. The nurse prepares how many milliliters (mL) of the medication to administer the correct dose? **Fill in the blank.**
Answer: _______ mL

115. A prescription reads phenytoin 0.2 g orally twice daily. The medication label states that each capsule is 100 mg. The nurse prepares how many capsule(s) to administer 1 dose? **Fill in the blank.**
Answer: _______ capsule(s)

116. A prescription reads 1000 mL of normal saline 0.9% to infuse over 8 hours. The drop factor is 15 drops (gtt)/1 mL. The nurse sets the flow rate at how many drops per minute? **Fill in the blank. Record your answer to the nearest whole number.**
Answer: _______ drops per minute

117. A prescription reads heparin sodium, 1300 units/hr by continuous intravenous (IV) infusion. The pharmacy prepares the medication and delivers an IV bag labeled heparin sodium 20,000 units/250 mL D_5W. An infusion pump must be used to administer the medication. The nurse sets the infusion pump at how many milliliters (mL) per hour to deliver 1300 units/hour? **Fill in the blank. Record your answer to the nearest whole number.**
Answer: _______ mL/hr

118. A prescription reads 3000 mL of D_5W to be administered over a 24-hour period. The nurse determines that how many milliliters (mL) per hour will be administered to the client? **Fill in the blank.**
Answer: _______ mL/hr

119. Gentamicin sulfate, 80 mg in 100 mL normal saline (NS), is to be administered over 30 minutes. The drop factor is 10 drops (gtt)/1 mL. The nurse sets the flow rate at how many drops per minute? **Fill in the blank. Record your answer to the nearest whole number.**
Answer: _______ drops per minute

120. A prescription reads levothyroxine, 150 mcg orally daily. The medication label reads levothyroxine, 0.1 mg/tablet. The nurse administers how many tablet(s) to the client? **Fill in the blank.**
Answer: _______ tablet(s)

121. Cefuroxime sodium, 1 g in 50 mL normal saline (NS), is to be administered over 30 minutes. The drop factor is 15 drops (gtt)/1 mL. The nurse sets the flow rate at how many drops per minute? **Fill in the blank.**
Answer: _______ drops per minute

122. A prescription reads 1000 mL D_5W to infuse at a rate of 125 mL/hr. The nurse determines that it will take how many hours for 1 L to infuse? **Fill in the blank.**
Answer: _______ hour(s)

123. A prescription reads to infuse 1 unit of packed red blood cells over 4 hours. The unit of blood contains 250 mL. The drop factor is 10 drops (gtt)/1 mL. The nurse prepares to set the flow rate at how many drops per minute? **Fill in the blank. Record your answer to the nearest whole number.**
Answer: _______ drops per minute

124. A prescription reads morphine sulfate, 8 mg stat. The medication ampule reads morphine sulfate, 10 mg/mL. The nurse prepares how many milliliters (mL) to administer the correct dose? **Fill in the blank.**
Answer: _______ mL

125. A prescription reads regular insulin, 8 units/hr by continuous intravenous (IV) infusion. The pharmacy prepares the medication and then delivers an IV bag labeled 100 units of regular insulin in 100 mL normal saline (NS). An infusion pump must be used to administer the medication. The nurse sets the infusion pump at how many milliliters (mL) per hour to deliver 8 units/hr? **Fill in the blank.**
Answer: _______ mL/hr

ANSWERS

111. ***Answer:*** **21**
Rationale: Use the intravenous (IV) flow rate formula.
Formula:

$$\frac{\text{Total Volume} \times \text{Drop factor}}{\text{Time in minutes}} = \text{Drops per minute}$$

$$\frac{1000\text{ mL} \times 15\text{gtt}}{720\text{ minutes}} = \frac{15{,}000}{720} = 20.8\text{, or } 21\text{gtt/min}$$

Test-Taking Strategy: Focus on the subject, calculating an IV flow rate. Use the formula for calculating IV flow rates when answering the question. Once you have performed the calculation, verify your answer using a calculator and make sure that the answer makes sense. Remember to record the answer to the nearest whole number.
Level of Cognitive Ability: Applying
Client Needs: Physiological Integrity
Integrated Process: Nursing Process—Implementation
Content Area: Skills: Dosage Calculations
Health Problem: N/A
Priority Concepts: Clinical Judgment; Safety
Reference: Potter et al. (2017), pp. 978-979.

112. ***Answer:*** **1.3**
Rationale: Use the medication dose formula.
Formula:

$$\frac{\text{Desired} \times \text{mL}}{\text{Available}} = \text{Milliliters per dose}$$

$$\frac{400{,}000\text{ units} \times 1\text{mL}}{300{,}000\text{ units}} = \text{Milliliters per dose}$$

$$\frac{400{,}000}{300{,}000} = 1.33 = 1.3\text{mL}$$

Test-Taking Strategy: Focus on the subject, a dosage calculation. Follow the formula for the calculation of the correct medication dose. Once you have performed the calculation, verify your answer using a calculator and make sure that the answer makes sense. Remember to record your answer using 1 decimal place.
Level of Cognitive Ability: Applying
Client Needs: Physiological Integrity
Integrated Process: Nursing Process—Implementation
Content Area: Skills: Dosage Calculations
Health Problem: Adult Health: Immune: Infections
Priority Concepts: Clinical Judgment; Safety
Reference: Potter et al. (2017), pp. 618-620, 632.

113. ***Answer:*** **15**
Rationale: In most facilities, potassium chloride is premixed in the intravenous solution and the nurse will need to verify the correct dose before administration. In some cases the nurse will need to add the potassium chloride and will use the medication calculation formula to determine the mL to be added.
Formula:

$$\frac{\text{Desired} \times \text{mL}}{\text{Available}} = \text{Milliliters per dose}$$

$$\frac{30\text{mEq} \times 20\text{mL}}{40\text{mEq}} = 15\text{mL}$$

Test-Taking Strategy: Focus on the subject, a dosage calculation. Follow the formula for the calculation of the correct medication dose. Once you have performed the calculation, verify your answer using a calculator and make sure that the answer makes sense.
Level of Cognitive Ability: Applying
Client Needs: Physiological Integrity
Integrated Process: Nursing Process—Implementation
Content Area: Skills: Dosage Calculations
Health Problem: N/A
Priority Concepts: Clinical Judgment; Safety
Reference: Gahart, Nazareno, Ortega (2017), p. 1065; Potter et al. (2017), pp. 978-979.

114. ***Answer:*** **2**
Rationale: You must convert 0.3 g to milligrams. In the metric system, to convert larger to smaller, multiply by 1000 or move the decimal 3 places to the right. Therefore, 0.3 g = 300 mg. After conversion from grams to milligrams, use the formula to calculate the correct dose.
Formula:

$$\frac{\text{Desired} \times \text{mL}}{\text{Available}} = \text{Milliliters per dose}$$

$$\frac{300\text{mg} \times 6\text{mL}}{900\text{mg}} = \frac{1800}{900} = 2\text{mL}$$

Test-Taking Strategy: Focus on the subject, a dosage calculation. In this medication calculation problem, first you must convert grams to milligrams. Once you have performed the calculation, verify your answer using a calculator and make sure that the answer makes sense.
Level of Cognitive Ability: Applying
Client Needs: Physiological Integrity
Integrated Process: Nursing Process—Implementation
Content Area: Skills: Dosage Calculations
Health Problem: Adult Health: Immune: Infections
Priority Concepts: Clinical Judgment; Safety
Reference: Perry et al. (2018), pp. 514-515.

115. ***Answer:*** **2**
Rationale: You must convert 0.2 g to milligrams. In the metric system, to convert larger to smaller, multiply by 1000 or move the decimal point 3 places to the right. Therefore, 0.2 g equals 200 mg. After conversion from grams to milligrams, use the formula to calculate the correct dose.
Formula:

$$\frac{\text{Desired} \times \text{Capsule(s)}}{\text{Available}} = \text{Capsule(s) per dose}$$

$$\frac{200\text{mg} \times 1\text{Capsule}}{100\text{mg}} = 2\text{ Capsules}$$

Test-Taking Strategy: Focus on the subject, a dosage calculation. In this medication calculation problem, first you must convert grams to milligrams. Once you have done the conversion and reread the medication calculation problem, you will know that 2 capsules is the correct answer. Recheck your work using a calculator and make sure that the answer makes sense.

Level of Cognitive Ability: Applying
Client Needs: Physiological Integrity
Integrated Process: Nursing Process—Implementation
Content Area: Skills: Dosage Calculations
Health Problem: Adult Health: Neurological: Seizure disorder/epilepsy
Priority Concepts: Clinical Judgment; Safety
Reference: Potter et al. (2017), pp. 618-619.

116. ***Answer:*** **31**

Rationale: Use the intravenous (IV) flow rate formula.

Formula:

$$\frac{\text{Total volume} \times \text{Drop factor}}{\text{Time in Minutes}} = \text{Drop per minute}$$

$$\frac{1000\ \text{mL} \times 15\,\text{gtt}}{480\ \text{minutes}} = \frac{15{,}000}{480} = 31.2,\ \text{or}\ 31\,\text{gtt/min}$$

Test-Taking Strategy: Focus on the subject, an IV flow rate. Use the formula for calculating IV flow rates when answering the question. Once you have performed the calculation, verify your answer using a calculator and make sure that the answer makes sense. Remember to record the answer to the nearest whole number.

Level of Cognitive Ability: Applying
Client Needs: Physiological Integrity
Integrated Process: Nursing Process—Implementation
Content Area: Skills: Dosage Calculations
Health Problem: N/A
Priority Concepts: Clinical Judgment; Safety
Reference: Potter et al. (2017), pp. 978-979.

117. ***Answer:*** **16**

Rationale: Calculation of this problem can be done using a 2-step process. First, you need to determine the amount of heparin sodium in 1 mL. The next step is to determine the infusion rate, or milliliters per hour.

Formula:

Step 1:

$$\frac{\text{Known amount of medication in solution}}{\text{Total volume of diluent}}$$
$$= \text{Amount of medication per milliliter}$$

$$\frac{20{,}000\,\text{units}}{250\,\text{mL}} = 80\,\text{units/mL}$$

Step 2:

$$\frac{\text{Dose per hour desired}}{\text{Concentration per milliliter}} = \text{Infusion rate, or mL/hr}$$

$$\frac{1300\,\text{units}}{80\,\text{units / mL}} = 16.25,\ \text{or}\ 16\,\text{mL/hr}$$

Test-Taking Strategy: Focus on the subject, an IV flow rate. Read the question carefully, noting that 2 steps can be used to solve this medication problem. Follow the formula, verify your answer using a calculator, and make sure that the answer makes sense. Remember to record the answer to the nearest whole number.

Level of Cognitive Ability: Analyzing
Client Needs: Physiological Integrity
Integrated Process: Nursing Process—Implementation
Content Area: Skills: Dosage Calculations
Health Problem: Adult Health: Hematological: Bleeding/Clotting Disorders
Priority Concepts: Clinical Judgment; Safety
Reference: Potter et al. (2017), pp. 958, 978-979.

118. ***Answer:*** **125**

Rationale: Use the intravenous (IV) formula to determine milliliters per hour.

Formula:

$$\frac{\text{Total volume in milliliters}}{\text{Number of hours}} = \text{Milliliters per hour}$$

$$\frac{3000\ \text{mL}}{24\ \text{hours}} = 125\ \text{mL / hr}$$

Test-Taking Strategy: Focus on the subject, an IV infusion calculation of mL per hour. Read the question carefully, noting that the question is asking about milliliters per hour to be administered to the client. Use the formula for calculating milliliters per hour. Once you have performed the calculation, verify your answer using a calculator and make sure that the answer makes sense.

Level of Cognitive Ability: Applying
Client Needs: Physiological Integrity
Integrated Process: Nursing Process—Implementation
Content Area: Skills: Dosage Calculations
Health Problem: N/A
Priority Concepts: Clinical Judgment; Safety
Reference: Potter et al. (2017), pp. 978-979.

119. ***Answer:*** **33**

Rationale: Use the intravenous (IV) flow rate formula.

Formula:

$$\frac{\text{Total volume} \times \text{Drop factor}}{\text{Time in minutes}} = \text{Drops per minute}$$

$$\frac{100\ \text{mL} \times 10\,\text{gtt}}{30\ \text{minutes}} = \frac{1000}{30} = 33.3,\ \text{or}\ 33\,\text{gtt/min}$$

Test-Taking Strategy: Focus on the subject, an IV infusion calculation. Use the formula for calculating IV flow rates when answering the question. Once you have performed the calculation, verify your answer using a calculator and make sure that the answer makes sense. Remember to record the answer to the nearest whole number.

Level of Cognitive Ability: Applying
Client Needs: Physiological Integrity
Integrated Process: Nursing Process—Implementation
Content Area: Skills: Dosage Calculations
Health Problem: Adult Health: Immune: Infections
Priority Concepts: Clinical Judgment; Safety
Reference: Potter et al. (2017), pp. 978-979.

120. *Answer:* 1.5
Rationale: You must convert 150 mcg to milligrams. In the metric system, to convert smaller to larger, divide by 1000 or move the decimal 3 places to the left. Therefore, 150 mcg equals 0.15 mg. Next, use the formula to calculate the correct dose.
Formula:

$$\frac{\text{Desired}}{\text{Available}} \times \text{Tablet} = \text{Tablets per dose}$$

$$\frac{0.15\,\text{mg}}{0.1\,\text{mg}} \times 1\,\text{tablet} = 1.5\ \text{tablets}$$

Test-Taking Strategy: Focus on the **subject,** a dosage calculation. In this medication calculation problem, first you must convert micrograms to milligrams. Next, follow the formula for the calculation of the correct dose, verify your answer using a calculator, and make sure that the answer makes sense.
Level of Cognitive Ability: Applying
Client Needs: Physiological Integrity
Integrated Process: Nursing Process—Implementation
Content Area: Skills: Dosage Calculations
Health Problem: Adult Health: Endocrine: Thyroid Disorders
Priority Concepts: Clinical Judgment; Safety
Reference: Perry et al. (2018), pp. 514-515.

121. *Answer:* 25
Rationale: Use the intravenous (IV) flow rate formula.
Formula:

$$\frac{\text{Total volume} \times \text{Drop factor}}{\text{Time in minutes}} = \text{Drops per minute}$$

$$\frac{50\,\text{mL} \times 15\,\text{gtt}}{30\,\text{minutes}} = \frac{750}{30} = 25\,\text{gtt / min}$$

Test-Taking Strategy: Focus on the **subject,** an IV infusion calculation. Use the formula for calculating IV flow rates when answering the question. Once you have performed the calculation, verify your answer using a calculator and make sure that the answer makes sense.
Level of Cognitive Ability: Applying
Client Needs: Physiological Integrity
Integrated Process: Nursing Process—Implementation
Content Area: Skills: Dosage Calculations
Health Problem: Adult Health: Immune: Infections
Priority Concepts: Clinical Judgment; Safety
Reference: Potter et al. (2017), pp. 978-979.

122. *Answer:* 8
Rationale: You must determine that 1 L equals 1000 mL. Next, use the formula for determining infusion time in hours.
Formula:

$$\frac{\text{Total volume to infuse}}{\text{Milliliters per hour being infused}} = \text{Infusion time}$$

$$\frac{1000\,\text{mL}}{125\,\text{mL}} = 8\,\text{hours}$$

Test-Taking Strategy: Focus on the **subject,** an IV infusion time calculation. Read the question carefully, noting that the question is asking about infusion time in hours. First, convert 1 L to milliliters. Next, use the formula for determining infusion time in hours. Verify your answer using a calculator and make sure that the answer makes sense.
Level of Cognitive Ability: Applying
Client Needs: Physiological Integrity
Integrated Process: Nursing Process—Implementation
Content Area: Skills: Dosage Calculations
Health Problem: N/A
Priority Concepts: Clinical Judgment; Safety
Reference: Potter et al. (2017), p. 978.

123. *Answer:* 10
Rationale: Use the intravenous (IV) flow rate formula.
Formula:

$$\frac{\text{Total volume} \times \text{Drop factor}}{\text{Time in minute}} = \text{Drops per minute}$$

$$\frac{250\ \text{mL} \times 10\,\text{gtt}}{240\ \text{minutes}} = \frac{2500}{240} = 10.4, \text{or}\, 10\,\text{gtt/min}$$

Test-Taking Strategy: Focus on the **subject,** an IV infusion rate. Although an infusion pump would be used, use the formula to calculate drops per minute to answer the question. The formula for calculating IV flow rates when answering the question. Once you have performed the calculation, verify your answer using a calculator and make sure that the answer makes sense. Remember to record the answer to the nearest whole number.
Level of Cognitive Ability: Applying
Client Needs: Physiological Integrity
Integrated Process: Nursing Process—Implementation
Content Area: Skills: Dosage Calculations
Health Problem: N/A
Priority Concepts: Clinical Judgment; Safety
Reference: Potter et al. (2017), pp. 978-979.

124. *Answer:* 0.8
Rationale: Use the formula to calculate the correct dose.
Formula:

$$\frac{\text{Desired} \times \text{mL}}{\text{Available}} = \text{Milliliters per dose}$$

$$\frac{8\,\text{mg} \times 1\,\text{mL}}{10\,\text{mg}} = 0.8\,\text{mL}$$

Test-Taking Strategy: Focus on the **subject,** a dosage calculation. Follow the formula for the calculation of the correct dose. Once you have performed the calculation, verify your answer using a calculator and make sure that the answer makes sense.
Level of Cognitive Ability: Applying
Client Needs: Physiological Integrity
Integrated Process: Nursing Process—Implementation
Content Area: Skills: Dosage Calculations
Health Problem: Adult Health: Neurological: Pain
Priority Concepts: Clinical Judgment; Safety
Reference: Potter et al. (2017), pp. 618-620.

125. *Answer:* 8

Rationale: Calculation of this problem can be done using a 2-step process. First, you need to determine the amount of regular insulin in 1 mL. The next step is to determine the infusion rate, or milliliters per hour.

Formula:

Step 1:

$$\frac{\text{Known amount of medication in solution}}{\text{Total volume of diluent}} = \text{Amount of medication per milliliter}$$

$$\frac{100\,\text{units}}{100\,\text{mL}} = 1\,\text{unit} / \text{mL}$$

Step 2:

$$\frac{\text{Dose per hour desired}}{\text{Concentration per milliliter}} = \text{Infusion rate, or milliliters per hour}$$

$$\frac{8\,\text{units}}{1\,\text{unit} / \text{mL}} = 8\,\text{mL} / \text{hour}$$

Test-Taking Strategy: Focus on the **subject**, an IV flow rate. Read the question carefully, noting that 2 steps can be used to solve this medication problem. Once you have performed the calculation, verify your answer using a calculator and make sure that the answer makes sense. These steps can be used for similar medication problems related to the administration of heparin sodium or regular insulin by IV infusion.

Level of Cognitive Ability: Analyzing
Client Need: Physiological Integrity
Integrated Process: Nursing Process—Implementation
Content Area: Skills: Dosage Calculations
Health Problem: Adult Health: Endocrine: Diabetes Mellitus
Priority Concepts: Clinical Judgment; Safety
Reference: Potter et al. (2017), pp. 652, 978-979.

CHAPTER 15

Perioperative Nursing Care

PRIORITY CONCEPTS Infection; Safety

I. Preoperative Care

A client may return home shortly after having a surgical procedure because many surgical procedures are done through ambulatory care or 1-day stay surgical units. Perioperative care procedures apply even when the client returns home on the same day of the surgical procedure.

A. Obtaining informed consent
1. The surgeon is responsible for explaining the surgical procedure to the client and answering the client's questions. Often, the nurse is responsible for obtaining the client's signature on the consent form for surgery, which indicates the client's agreement to the procedure based on the surgeon's explanation.
2. The nurse may witness the client's signing of the consent form, but the nurse must be sure that the client has understood the surgeon's explanation of the surgery.
3. The nurse needs to document the witnessing of the signing of the consent form after the client acknowledges understanding the procedure.
4. Minors (clients younger than 18 years) may need a parent or legal guardian to sign the consent form.
5. Clients who are not alert or oriented may need power of attorney or legal guardian to sign the consent form.
6. Psychiatric clients have a right to refuse treatment until a court has legally determined that they are unable to make decisions for themselves.
7. No sedation should be administered to the client before the client signs the consent form.
8. Obtaining telephone consent from a legal guardian or power of attorney for health care is an acceptable practice if clients are unable to give consent themselves. The nurse must engage another nurse as a witness to the consent given over the telephone.

B. Nutrition
1. Review the surgeon's prescriptions regarding the NPO (nothing by mouth) status before surgery.
2. Withhold solid foods and liquids as prescribed to avoid aspiration, usually for 6 to 8 hours before general anesthesia and for approximately 3 hours before surgery with local anesthesia (as prescribed).
3. Insert an intravenous (IV) line and administer IV fluids, if prescribed; per agency policy, the IV catheter size should be large enough to administer blood products if they are required.

C. Elimination
1. If the client is to have intestinal or abdominal surgery, per surgeon's preference, an enema, laxative, or both may be prescribed for the day or night before surgery.
2. The client should void immediately before surgery.
3. Insert an indwelling urinary catheter, if prescribed; urinary catheter collection bags should be emptied immediately before surgery, and the nurse should document the amount and characteristics of the urine.

D. Surgical site
1. Clean the surgical site with a mild antiseptic or antibacterial soap on the night before surgery, as prescribed.
2. Shave the operative site, as prescribed; shaving may be done in the operative area.

Hair on the head or face (including the eyebrows) should be shaved only if prescribed.

E. Preoperative client teaching
1. Inform the client about what to expect postoperatively.
2. Inform the client to notify the nurse if the client experiences any pain postoperatively and that pain medication will be prescribed and given as the client requests. The client should be informed that some degree of pain should be expected and is normal.
3. Inform the client that requesting an opioid after surgery will not make the client a drug addict.

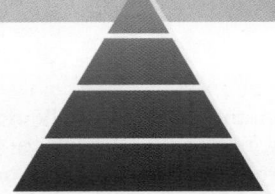

4. Demonstrate the use of a patient-controlled analgesia (PCA) pump if prescribed and explain that the client is the sole person who should push the button to administer medication.
5. Instruct the client how to use noninvasive pain relief techniques such as relaxation, distraction techniques, and guided imagery before the pain occurs and as soon as the pain is noticed.
6. The nurse should instruct the client not to smoke (for at least 24 hours before surgery); discuss smoking cessation treatments and programs.
7. Instruct the client in deep-breathing and coughing techniques, use of incentive spirometry, and the importance of performing the techniques postoperatively to prevent the development of pneumonia and atelectasis (Box 15-1).

BOX 15-1 Client Teaching

Deep-Breathing and Coughing Exercises

Instruct the client that a sitting position gives the best lung expansion for coughing and deep-breathing exercises.
Instruct the client to breathe deeply 3 times, inhaling through the nostrils and exhaling slowly through pursed lips.
Instruct the client that the third breath should be held for 3 seconds; then the client should cough deeply 3 times.
The client should perform this exercise every 1 to 2 hours.

Incentive Spirometry

Instruct the client to assume a sitting or upright position.
Instruct the client to place the mouth tightly around the mouthpiece.
Instruct the client to inhale slowly to raise and maintain the flow rate indicator, on the device as prescribed.
Instruct the client to hold the breath for 5 seconds and then to exhale through pursed lips.
Instruct the client to repeat this process 10 times every hour.

Leg and Foot Exercises

Gastrocnemius (calf) pumping: Instruct the client to move both ankles by pointing the toes up and then down.
Quadriceps (thigh) setting: Instruct the client to press the back of the knees against the bed and then to relax the knees; this contracts and relaxes the thigh and calf muscles to prevent thrombus formation.
Foot circles: Instruct the client to rotate each foot in a circle.
Hip and knee movements: Instruct the client to flex the knee and thigh and to straighten the leg, holding the position for 5 seconds before lowering (not performed if the client is having abdominal surgery or if the client has a back problem).

Splinting the Incision

If the surgical incision is abdominal or thoracic, instruct the client to place a pillow, or 1 hand with the other hand on top, over the incisional area.
During deep breathing and coughing, the client presses gently against the incisional area to splint or support it.

8. Instruct the client in leg and foot exercises and the purpose of sequential compression devices to prevent venous stasis of blood and to facilitate venous blood return (Fig. 15-1; see Box 15-1; see Fig. 15-3).
9. Instruct the client in how to splint an incision, turn, and reposition (Fig. 15-2; see Box 15-1).
10. Inform the client of any invasive devices that may be needed after surgery, such as a nasogastric tube, drain, urinary catheter, epidural catheter, or IV or subclavian lines.
11. Instruct the client not to pull on any of the invasive devices; they will be removed as soon as possible.

F. Psychosocial preparation
1. Be alert to the client's level of anxiety.
2. Answer any questions or concerns that the client may have regarding surgery.
3. Allow time for privacy for the client to prepare psychologically for surgery.
4. Provide support and assistance as needed.
5. Take cultural and spiritual aspects into consideration when providing care (Box 15-2).

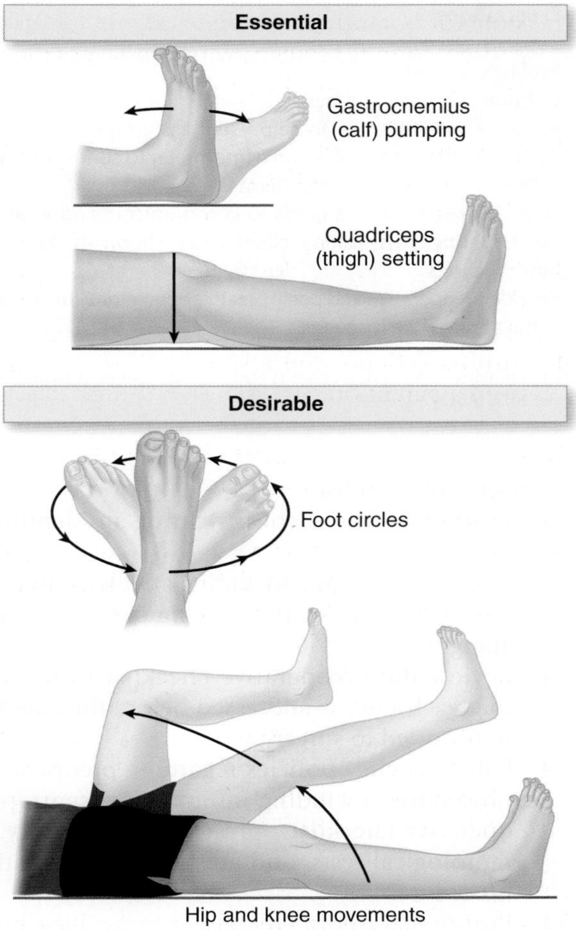

FIG. 15-1 Postoperative leg exercises.

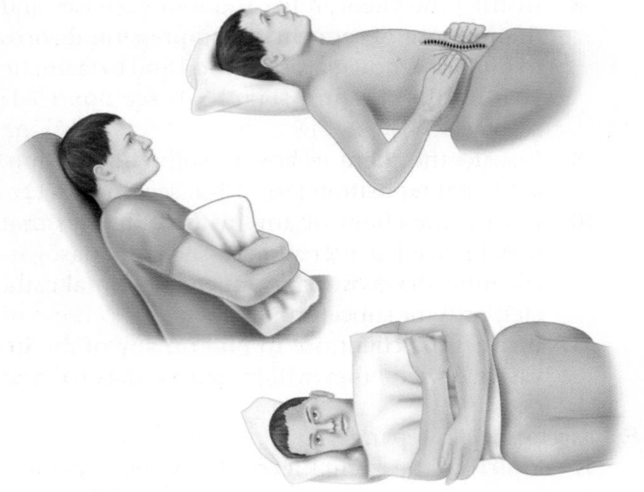

FIG. 15-2 Techniques for splinting a wound when coughing.

BOX 15-2 Cultural Aspects of Perioperative Nursing Care

- Primary language spoken
- Feelings related to surgery and pain
- Pain management
- Expectations
- Support systems
- Feelings toward self
- Cultural practices and beliefs
- Allow a family member to be present if appropriate.
- Secure the help of a professional interpreter to communicate with non–English-speaking clients.
- Use pictures or phrase cards to communicate and assess the non–English-speaking client's perception of pain or other feelings.
- Provide preoperative and postoperative educational materials in the appropriate language.

Adapted from Potter P, Perry A, Stockert P, Hall A: *Fundamentals of nursing*, ed 8, St. Louis, 2013, Mosby

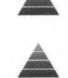

G. Preoperative checklist
1. Ensure that the client is wearing an identification bracelet.
2. Assess for allergies, including an allergy to latex (see Chapter 62 for information on latex allergy).
3. Review the preoperative checklist to be sure that each item is addressed before the client is transported to surgery.
4. Follow agency policies regarding preoperative procedures, including informed consents, preoperative checklists, prescribed laboratory or radiological tests, and any other preoperative procedure.
5. Ensure that informed consent forms have been signed for the operative procedure, any blood transfusions, disposal of a limb, or surgical sterilization procedures.
6. Ensure that a history and physical examination have been completed and documented in the client's record (Box 15-3).
7. Ensure that consultation requests have been completed and documented in the client's record.
8. Ensure that prescribed laboratory results are documented in the client's record.
9. Ensure that electrocardiogram and chest radiography reports are documented in the client's record.
10. Ensure that a blood type, screen, and crossmatch are performed and documented in the client's record within the established time frame per agency policy.
11. Remove jewelry, makeup, dentures, hairpins, nail polish (depending on agency procedures), glasses, and prostheses.
12. Document that valuables have been given to the client's family members or locked in the hospital safe.
13. Document the last time that the client ate or drank.
14. Document that the client voided before surgery.
15. Document that the prescribed preoperative medications were given (Box 15-4).
16. Monitor and document the client's vital signs.

H. Preoperative medications
1. Prepare to administer preoperative medications as prescribed before surgery.
2. Instruct the client about the desired effects of the preoperative medication.

After administering the preoperative medications, keep the client in bed with the side rails up (per agency policy). Place the call bell next to the client; instruct the client not to get out of bed and to call for assistance if needed.

BOX 15-3 Medical Problems That Increase Risk During Surgery

- Bleeding disorders such as thrombocytopenia or hemophilia
- Diabetes mellitus
- Chronic pain
- Heart disease, such as a recent myocardial infarction, dysrhythmia, heart failure, or peripheral vascular disease
- Obstructive sleep apnea
- Upper respiratory infection
- Liver disease
- Fever
- Chronic respiratory disease, such as emphysema, bronchitis, or asthma
- Immunological disorders, such as leukemia, infection with human immunodeficiency virus, acquired immunodeficiency syndrome, bone marrow depression, or use of chemotherapy or immunosuppressive agents
- Abuse of street drugs

Adapted from Potter P, Perry A, Stockert P, Hall A: *Fundamentals of nursing*, ed 8, St. Louis, 2013, Mosby.

BOX 15-4 Substances That Can Affect the Client in Surgery

Antibiotics

Antibiotics potentiate the action of anesthetic agents.

Anticholinergics

Medications with anticholinergic effects increase the potential for confusion, tachycardia, and intestinal hypotonicity and hypomotility.

Anticoagulants, Antiplatelets, and Thrombolytics

These medications alter normal clotting factors and increase the risk of hemorrhaging.

Acetylsalicylic acid (aspirin), clopidogrel, and nonsteroidal antiinflammatory drugs are commonly used medications that can alter platelet aggregation.

These medications should be discontinued at least 48 hours before surgery or as specified by the surgeon; clopidogrel usually has to be discontinued 5 days before surgery.

Anticonvulsants

Long-term use of certain anticonvulsants can alter the metabolism of anesthetic agents.

Antidepressants

Antidepressants may lower the blood pressure during anesthesia.

Antidysrhythmics

Antidysrhythmic medications reduce cardiac contractility and impair cardiac conduction during anesthesia.

Antihypertensives

Antihypertensive medications can interact with anesthetic agents and cause bradycardia, hypotension, and impaired circulation.

Corticosteroids

Corticosteroids cause adrenal atrophy and reduce the ability of the body to withstand stress.

Before and during surgery, dosages may be increased temporarily.

Diuretics

Diuretics potentiate electrolyte imbalances after surgery.

Herbal Substances

Herbal substances can interact with anesthesia and cause a variety of adverse effects. These substances may need to be stopped at a specific time before surgery. During the preoperative period, the client needs to be asked if he or she is taking an herbal substance.

Insulin

The need for insulin after surgery in a diabetic may be reduced because the client's nutritional intake is decreased, or the need for insulin may be increased because of the stress response and intravenous administration of glucose solutions.

Adapted from Potter P, Perry A, Stockert P, Hall A: *Fundamentals of nursing*, ed 8, St. Louis, 2013, Mosby.

I. Arrival in the operating room
   1. Guidelines to prevent wrong site and wrong procedure surgery
      a. The surgeon meets with the client in the preoperative area and uses a surgical marking pen to mark the operative site.
      b. In the operating room, the nurse and surgeon ensure and reconfirm that the operative site has been appropriately marked.
      c. Just before starting the surgical procedure, a time-out is conducted with all members of the operative team present to identify the correct client and appropriate surgical site again.
   2. When the client arrives in the operating room, the operating room nurse will verify the identification bracelet with the client's verbal response and will review the client's chart.
   3. The client's record will be checked for completeness and reviewed for informed consent forms, history and physical examination, and allergic reaction information.
   4. The surgeon's prescriptions will be verified and implemented.
   5. The IV line may be initiated at this time (or in the preoperative area), if prescribed.
   6. The anesthesia team will administer the prescribed anesthesia.

Verification of the client and the surgical operative site is critical.

II. Postoperative Care

A. Description
   1. Postoperative care is the management of a client after surgery and includes care given during the immediate postoperative period as well as during the days after surgery.
   2. The goal of postoperative care is to prevent complications, to promote healing of the surgical incision, and to return the client to a healthy state.

B. Respiratory system

Assess breath sounds; stridor, wheezing, or a crowing sound can indicate partial obstruction, bronchospasm, or laryngospasm, while crackles or rhonchi may indicate ateletasis, pneumonia, or pulmonary edema.

   1. Monitor vital signs per agency policy.
   2. Monitor airway patency and ensure adequate ventilation (prolonged mechanical ventilation during anesthesia may affect postoperative lung function).
   3. Remember that extubated clients who are lethargic may not be able to maintain an airway.
   4. Monitor for secretions; if the client is unable to clear the airway by coughing, suction the secretions from the client's airway.

5. Observe chest movement for symmetry and the use of accessory muscles.
6. Monitor oxygen administration if prescribed.
7. Monitor pulse oximetry and end tidal carbon dioxide (CO_2) as prescribed.
8. Encourage deep-breathing and coughing exercises as soon as possible after surgery.
9. Note the rate, depth, and quality of respirations; the respiratory rate should be greater than 10 and less than 30 breaths per minute.
10. Monitor for signs of respiratory distress, atelectasis, or other respiratory complications.

C. Cardiovascular system
1. Monitor circulatory status, such as skin color, peripheral pulses, and capillary refill, and for the absence of edema, numbness, and tingling.
2. Monitor for bleeding.
3. Assess the pulse for rate and rhythm (a bounding pulse may indicate hypertension, fluid overload, or client anxiety).
4. Monitor for signs of hypertension and hypotension.
5. Monitor for cardiac dysrhythmias.
6. Monitor for signs of thrombophlebitis, particularly in clients who were in the lithotomy position during surgery.
7. Encourage the use of antiembolism stockings or sequential compression devices (Fig. 15-3), if prescribed, to promote venous return, strengthen muscle tone, and prevent pooling of blood in the extremities.

D. Musculoskeletal system
1. Assess the client for movement of the extremities.
2. Review the surgeon's prescriptions regarding client positioning or restrictions.
3. Encourage ambulation if prescribed; before ambulation, instruct the client to sit at the edge of the bed with his or her feet supported to assume balance.
4. Unless contraindicated, place the client in a low-Fowler's position after surgery to increase the size of the thorax for lung expansion.
5. Avoid positioning the postoperative client in a **supine** position until pharyngeal reflexes have returned; if the client is comatose or semicomatose, position on the side (in addition, an oral airway may be needed).
6. If the client is unable to get out of bed, turn the client every 1 to 2 hours unless contraindicated.

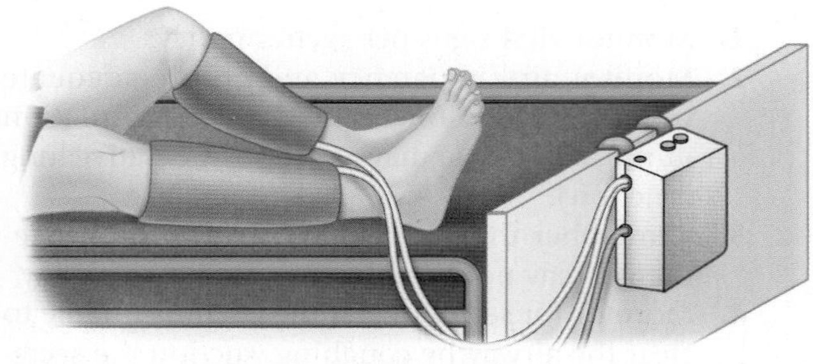

FIG. 15-3 Sequential compression device.

E. Neurological system
1. Assess level of consciousness.
2. Make frequent periodic attempts to awaken the client until the client fully awakens.
3. Orient the client to the environment.
4. Speak in a soft tone; filter out extraneous noises in the environment.
5. Maintain the client's body temperature and prevent heat loss by providing the client with warm blankets and raising the room temperature as necessary.

F. Temperature control
1. Monitor temperature.
2. Monitor for signs of hypothermia that may result from anesthesia, a cool operating room, or exposure of the skin and internal organs during surgery.
3. Apply warm blankets, continue oxygen, and administer medication as prescribed if the client experiences postoperative shivering.

G. Integumentary system
1. Assess the surgical site, drains, and wound dressings (serous drainage may occur from an incision, but notify the surgeon if excessive bleeding occurs from the site). Mark time and date for any drainage on surgical dressings and monitor for excessive drainage per agency policy.
2. Assess the skin for redness, abrasions, or breakdown that may have resulted from surgical positioning.
3. Monitor body temperature and wound for signs of infection.
4. Maintain a dry, intact dressing.
5. Change dressings as prescribed, noting the amount of bleeding or drainage, odor, and intactness of sutures or staples; commonly used dressings include 4 × 4 inch gauze, nonadherent pads, abdominal pads, gauze rolls, and split gauze that are commonly referred to as *drain sponges.*
6. Wound drains should be patent; prepare to assist with the removal of drains (as prescribed by the surgeon) when the drainage amount becomes insignificant. Empty drains as needed and document the output and drainage characteristics.
7. An abdominal binder may be prescribed for obese and debilitated individuals to prevent dehiscence of the incision.

H. Fluid and electrolyte balance
1. Monitor IV fluid administration as prescribed.
2. Record intake and output.
3. Monitor for signs of fluid or electrolyte imbalances.

I. Gastrointestinal system
1. Monitor intake and output and for nausea and vomiting.
2. Maintain patency of the nasogastric tube if present and monitor placement and drainage per agency procedure.
3. Monitor for abdominal distention.
4. Monitor for passage of flatus and return of bowel sounds.
5. Administer frequent oral care, at least every 2 hours.
6. Maintain the NPO status until the gag reflex and peristalsis return.
7. When oral fluids are permitted, start with ice chips and water.
8. Ensure that the client advances to clear liquids and then to a regular diet, as prescribed and as the client can tolerate.

To prevent aspiration, turn the client to a side-lying position if vomiting occurs; have suctioning equipment available and ready to use.

J. Renal system
1. Assess the bladder for distention.
2. Monitor urine output (urinary output should be at least 30 mL/hr).
3. If the client does not have a urinary catheter, the client is expected to void within 6 to 8 hours postoperatively depending on the type of anesthesia administered; ensure that the amount is at least 200 mL.

K. Pain management
1. Assess the type of anesthetic used and preoperative medication that the client received, and note whether the client received any pain medications in the postanesthesia period.
2. Assess for pain and inquire about the type and location of pain; ask the client to rate the degree of pain on a scale of 1 to 10, with 10 being the most severe.
3. If the client is unable to rate the pain using a numerical pain scale, use a descriptor scale that lists words that describe different levels of pain intensity, such as *no pain, mild pain, moderate pain,* and *severe pain,* or other available pain rating scales.
4. Monitor for objective data related to pain, such as facial expressions, body gestures, increased pulse rate, increased blood pressure, and increased respirations.
5. Inquire about the effectiveness of the last pain medication.
6. Assess respiratory rate, blood pressure, heart rate, oxygen saturation, and level of consciousness (LOC), and note if or when last medication was given prior to administering pain medication. Administer pain medication as prescribed.
7. Ensure that the client with a PCA pump understands how to use it.
8. If an opioid has been prescribed, after administration, assess the client every 30 minutes for respiratory rate and pain relief.
9. Use noninvasive measures to relieve postoperative pain, including provision of distraction, relaxation techniques, guided imagery, comfort measures, positioning, backrubs, heat or cold therapy, and a quiet and restful environment.
10. Document effectiveness of the pain medication and noninvasive pain relief measures.

Consider cultural and spiritual practices and beliefs when planning pain management.

III. Pneumonia and Atelectasis

A. Description (Box 15-5 and Fig. 15-4)
1. Pneumonia: An inflammation of the alveoli caused by an infectious process that may develop

BOX 15-5 Postoperative Complications

- Pneumonia and atelectasis
- Hypoxemia
- Pulmonary embolism
- Hemorrhage
- Shock
- Thrombophlebitis
- Urinary retention
- Constipation
- Paralytic ileus
- Wound infection
- Wound dehiscence
- Wound evisceration

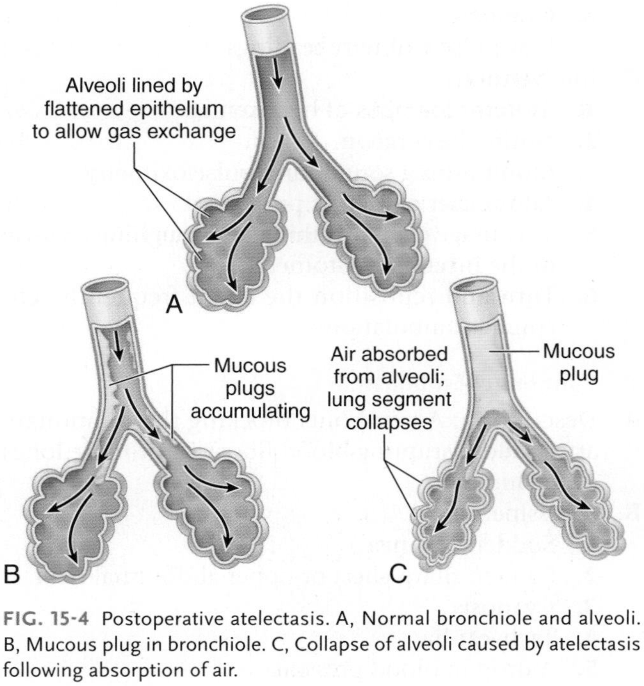

FIG. 15-4 Postoperative atelectasis. A, Normal bronchiole and alveoli. B, Mucous plug in bronchiole. C, Collapse of alveoli caused by atelectasis following absorption of air.

3 to 5 days postoperatively as a result of infection, aspiration, or immobility
2. Atelectasis: A collapsed or airless state of the lung that may be the result of airway obstruction caused by accumulated secretions or failure of the client to deep breathe or ambulate after surgery; a postoperative complication that usually occurs 1 to 2 days after surgery

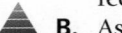

B. Assessment
1. Dyspnea and increased respiratory rate
2. Crackles over involved lung area
3. Elevated temperature
4. Productive cough and chest pain

C. Interventions
1. Assess lung sounds.
2. Reposition the client every 1 to 2 hours.
3. Encourage the client to deep breathe, cough, and use the incentive spirometer as prescribed.
4. Provide chest physiotherapy and postural drainage, as prescribed.
5. Encourage fluid intake and early ambulation.
6. Use suction to clear secretions if the client is unable to cough.

IV. Hypoxemia

A. Description: An inadequate concentration of oxygen in arterial blood; in the postoperative client, hypoxemia can be due to shallow breathing from the effects of anesthesia or medications.

B. Assessment
1. Restlessness
2. Dyspnea
3. Diaphoresis
4. Tachycardia
5. Hypertension
6. Cyanosis
7. Low pulse oximetry readings

C. Interventions
1. Monitor for signs of hypoxemia.
2. Notify the surgeon.
3. Monitor lung sounds and pulse oximetry.
4. Administer oxygen as prescribed.
5. Encourage deep breathing and coughing and use of the incentive spirometer.
6. Turn and reposition the client frequently; encourage ambulation.

V. Pulmonary Embolism

A. Description: An embolus blocking the pulmonary artery and disrupting blood flow to 1 or more lobes of the lung

B. Assessment
1. Sudden dyspnea
2. Sudden sharp chest or upper abdominal pain
3. Cyanosis
4. Tachycardia
5. A drop in blood pressure

C. Interventions
1. Notify the surgeon immediately, because pulmonary embolism may be life-threatening and requires emergency action.
2. Monitor vital signs.
3. Administer oxygen, medications, and treatments as prescribed.

VI. Hemorrhage

A. Description: The loss of a large amount of blood externally or internally in a short time period

B. Assessment
1. Restlessness
2. Weak and rapid pulse
3. Hypotension
4. Tachypnea
5. Cool, clammy skin
6. Reduced urine output

C. Interventions
1. Provide pressure to the site of bleeding.
2. Notify the surgeon.
3. Administer oxygen, as prescribed.
4. Administer IV fluids and blood, as prescribed.
5. Prepare the client for a surgical procedure, if necessary.

VII. Shock

A. Description: Loss of circulatory fluid volume, which usually is caused by hemorrhage

B. Assessment: Similar to assessment findings in hemorrhage

C. Interventions
1. If shock develops, elevate the legs.
2. Notify the surgeon.
3. Determine and treat the cause of shock.
4. Administer oxygen, as prescribed.
5. Monitor level of consciousness.
6. Monitor vital signs for increased pulse or decreased blood pressure.
7. Monitor intake and output.
8. Assess color, temperature, turgor, and moisture of the skin and mucous membranes.
9. Administer IV fluids, blood, and colloid solutions, as prescribed.

If the client had spinal anesthesia, do not elevate the legs any higher than placing them on the pillow; otherwise, the diaphragm muscles needed for effective breathing could be impaired.

VIII. Thrombophlebitis

A. Description
1. Thrombophlebitis is an inflammation of a vein, often accompanied by clot formation.
2. Veins in the legs are affected most commonly.

B. Assessment
1. Vein inflammation
2. Aching or cramping pain

3. Vein feels hard and cord-like and is tender to touch.
4. Elevated temperature

C. Interventions
1. Monitor legs for swelling, inflammation, pain, tenderness, venous distention, and cyanosis; notify the surgeon if any of these signs are present.
2. Elevate the extremity 30 degrees without allowing any pressure on the popliteal area.
3. Encourage the use of antiembolism stockings as prescribed; remove stockings twice a day to wash and inspect the legs.
4. Use a sequential compression device as prescribed (see Fig. 15-3).
5. Perform passive range-of-motion exercises every 2 hours if the client is confined to bed rest.
6. Encourage early ambulation, as prescribed.
7. Do not allow the client to dangle the legs.
8. Instruct the client not to sit in 1 position for an extended period of time.
9. Administer anticoagulants such as heparin sodium or enoxaparin, as prescribed.

IX. Urinary Retention

A. Description
1. Urinary retention is an involuntary accumulation of urine in the bladder as a result of loss of muscle tone.
2. It is caused by the effects of anesthetics or opioid analgesics and appears 6 to 8 hours after surgery.

B. Assessment
1. Inability to void
2. Restlessness and diaphoresis
3. Lower abdominal pain
4. Distended bladder
5. Hypertension
6. On percussion, the bladder sounds like a drum.

C. Interventions
1. Monitor for voiding.
2. Assess for a distended bladder by palpation and bladder scanning if indicated.
3. Encourage ambulation when prescribed.
4. Encourage fluid intake unless contraindicated.
5. Assist the client to void by helping the client stand.
6. Provide privacy.
7. Pour warm water over the perineum or allow the client to hear running water to promote voiding.
8. Contact the surgeon and catheterize the client as prescribed after all noninvasive techniques have been attempted.

X. Constipation

A. Description
1. Constipation is an abnormal infrequent passage of stool.
2. When the client resumes a solid diet postoperatively, failure to pass stool within 48 hours may indicate constipation.

B. Assessment
1. Absence of bowel movements
2. Abdominal distention
3. Anorexia, headache, and nausea

C. Interventions
1. Assess bowel sounds.
2. Encourage fluid intake up to 3000 mL/day unless contraindicated.
3. Encourage early ambulation.
4. Encourage consumption of fiber foods unless contraindicated.
5. Provide privacy and adequate time for bowel elimination.
6. Administer stool softeners and laxatives, as prescribed.

XI. Paralytic Ileus

A. Description
1. Paralytic ileus is failure of appropriate forward movement of bowel contents.
2. The condition may occur as a result of anesthetic medications or of manipulation of the bowel during the surgical procedure.

B. Assessment
1. Vomiting postoperatively
2. Abdominal distention
3. Absence of bowel sounds, bowel movement, or flatus

C. Interventions
1. Monitor intake and output.
2. Maintain NPO status until bowel sounds return.
3. Maintain patency of a nasogastric tube if in place; assess patency and drainage per agency procedure.
4. Encourage ambulation.
5. Administer IV fluids or parenteral nutrition, as prescribed.
6. Administer medications as prescribed to increase gastrointestinal motility and secretions.
7. If ileus occurs, it is treated first nonsurgically with bowel decompression by insertion of a nasogastric tube attached to intermittent or constant suction.

! Vomiting postoperatively, abdominal distention, and absence of bowel sounds may be signs of paralytic ileus.

XII. Wound Infection

A. Description
1. Wound infection may be caused by poor aseptic technique or a contaminated wound before surgical exploration; existing client conditions such as diabetes mellitus or immunocompromise may place the client at risk.

2. Infection usually occurs 3 to 6 days after surgery.
3. Purulent material may exit from the drains or separated wound edges.

B. Assessment
1. Fever and chills
2. Warm, tender, painful, and inflamed incision site
3. Edematous skin at the incision and tight skin sutures
4. Elevated white blood cell count

C. Interventions
1. Monitor temperature.
2. Monitor incision site for approximation of suture line, edema, or bleeding and signs of infection (*REEDA:* *r*edness, *e*rythema, *e*cchymosis, *d*rainage, *a*pproximation of the wound edges); notify the surgeon if signs of wound infection are present.
3. Maintain patency of drains, and assess drainage amount, color, and consistency.
4. Maintain asepsis, change the dressing, and perform wound irrigation, if prescribed (Box 15-6).
5. Anticipate prescriptions for wound culture and blood culture if infection is suspected.
6. Administer antibiotics, as prescribed.

XIII. Wound Dehiscence and Evisceration (Fig. 15-5)

A. Description
1. Wound dehiscence is separation of the wound edges at the suture line; it usually occurs 6 to 8 days after surgery.
2. Wound evisceration is protrusion of the internal organs through an incision; it usually occurs 6 to 8 days after surgery.
3. Dehiscence and evisceration is most common among obese clients, clients who have had abdominal surgery, or those who have poor wound-healing ability.
4. Wound evisceration is an emergency.

BOX 15-6 Procedure for Sterile Dressing Change and Wound Irrigation*

- Verify the prescription for the procedure in the medical record.
- Anticipate supplies that will be needed and gather supplies, including personal protective equipment (PPE) and additional equipment needed for protection (i.e., gown, face shield, clean and sterile gloves), a sterile dressing change kit if available, and any anticipated additional supplies such as gauze pads, drain sponges, cotton-tipped applicators, tape, an abdominal pad, a measuring tool, syringe for irrigation, irrigation basin, extra pair of sterile gloves, and underpad.
- Introduce self to client, identify the client with 2 accepted identifiers and compare against the medical record, provide privacy, and explain the procedure.
- Assess the client's pain level using an appropriate pain scale and medicate as necessary.
- Assess the client for allergies, particularly to tape or latex.
- Perform hand hygiene and don PPE.
- Position the client appropriately, apply clean gloves, and place the underpad underneath the client.
- Remove the soiled dressing, assess and characterize drainage noted on the dressing, and discard the removed dressing in the biohazard waste; note: if a moist-to-dry dressing adheres to the wound, gently free the dressing and warn the client of the discomfort; if a dry dressing adheres to the wound that is not to be debrided, moisten the dressing with normal saline and remove.
- Assess the wound and periwound for size (length, width, depth; measure using measuring tool), appearance, color, drainage, edema, approximation, granulation tissue, presence and condition of drains, and odor; and palpate edges for tenderness or pain.
- Cover the wound with sterile gauze by opening a sterile gauze pack and lightly placing the gauze on the wound without touching the dressing material; remove gloves and perform hand hygiene.
- Set up the sterile field: prepare sterile equipment using sterile technique on an overbed table. If irrigation is prescribed, pour any prescribed irrigation solution into a sterile basin and draw solution into the irrigating syringe. Gently irrigate the wound with the prescribed solution from the least contaminated area to the most contaminated area. Use an approved irrigation basin to collect solution from the irrigating procedure.
- Cleanse the wound with sterile gauze from the least contaminated area to the most contaminated area, using single-stroke motions. Discard the gauze from each stroke and use a new one for the next stroke. If drains are present, use cotton-tipped applicators to hold drains up and clean around drain sites using circular strokes, starting near the drain and moving outward from the insertion site using cotton-tipped applicators or sterile gauze. Dry sites in the same manner using sterile gauze.
- Apply any prescribed wound antiseptic with a cotton-tipped applicator or sterile gauze, using the same technique as when cleansing the wound.
- Dress the wound with the prescribed dressings using sterile technique and secure in place.
- Date/time/initial the dressing and discard supplies as indicated per agency procedures, and remove gloves.
- Assist the client to a comfortable position and ensure safety; assess pain level.
- Document the procedure, any related assessments, client response, and any additional procedural responses.

Adapted from Perry A, Potter P, Ostendorf W: *Clinical nursing skills and techniques*, ed 8, St. Louis, 2014, Mosby.

* *Note:* Adapt procedure if irrigation is not prescribed or if the client does not have drains or tubes in place. Always follow agency procedures for dressing changes and wound irrigations.

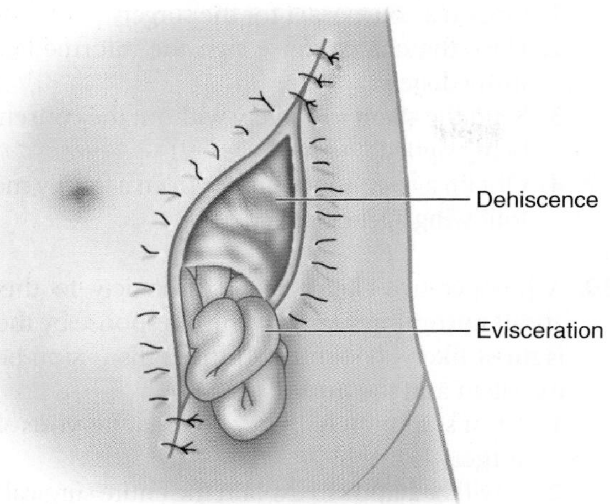

FIG. 15-5 Complications of wound healing.

B. Assessment: Dehiscence
1. Increased drainage
2. Opened wound edges
3. Appearance of underlying tissues through the wound

C. Assessment: Evisceration
1. Discharge of serosanguineous fluid from a previously dry wound
2. The appearance of loops of bowel or other abdominal contents through the wound
3. Client reports feeling a popping sensation after coughing or turning.

D. Interventions (see Priority Nursing Actions)

PRIORITY NURSING ACTIONS
Evisceration in a Wound

1. Call for help; ask that the surgeon be notified and that needed supplies be brought to the client's room.
2. Stay with the client.
3. While waiting for supplies to arrive, place the client in a low-Fowler's position with the knees bent.
4. Cover the wound with a sterile normal saline dressing and keep the dressing moist.
5. Take vital signs and monitor the client closely for signs of shock.
6. Prepare the client for surgery as necessary.
7. Document the occurrence, actions taken, and the client's response.

Reference
Ignatavicius. (2018). *Workman, Rebar,* 283.

XIV. Ambulatory Care or 1-Day Stay Surgical Units

A. General criteria for client discharge
1. Is alert and oriented.
2. Vital signs at baseline.
3. Laboratory values (if prescribed) within normal limits.
4. Has voided.
5. Has no respiratory distress.
6. Is able to ambulate, swallow, and cough.
7. Has minimal pain.
8. Is not vomiting.
9. Has minimal, if any, bleeding from the incision site with absence of purulent drainage.
10. Has a responsible adult available to drive the client home.
11. Discharge is appropriate and safe for client (i.e., to home or facility).
12. The surgeon has signed a release form.

B. Discharge teaching (Box 15-7)
1. Discharge teaching should be performed before the date of the scheduled procedure.
2. Provide written instructions to the client and family regarding the specifics of care.

BOX 15-7 Postoperative Discharge Teaching

- Assess the client's readiness to learn, educational level, and desire to change or modify lifestyle.
- Assess the need for resources needed for home care.
- Demonstrate care of the incision and how to change the dressing.
- Instruct the client to cover the incision with plastic if showering is allowed.
- Ensure that the client is provided with a 48-hour supply of dressings per agency procedure, for home use.
- Instruct the client on the importance of returning to the surgeon's office for follow-up.
- Instruct the client that sutures usually are removed in the surgeon's office 7 to 10 days after surgery.
- Inform the client that staples are removed 7 to 14 days after surgery and that the skin may become slightly reddened when staples are ready to be removed.
- Sterile adhesive strips (e.g., Steri-Strips®) may be applied to provide extra support after the sutures are removed.
- Instruct the client on the use of medications, their purpose, dosages, administration, and side effects or adverse effects.
- Instruct the client on diet and to drink 6 to 8 glasses of liquid a day unless contraindicated.
- Instruct the client about activity levels and to resume normal activities gradually.
- Instruct the client to avoid lifting for 6 weeks if a major surgical procedure was performed.
- Instruct the client with an abdominal incision not to lift anything weighing 10 pounds or more and not to engage in any activities that involve pushing or pulling.
- The client usually can return to work in 6 to 8 weeks depending on the procedure and as prescribed by the surgeon.
- Instruct the client about the signs and symptoms of complications and when to call the surgeon.

3. Instruct the client and family about postoperative complications that can occur.
4. Provide appropriate resources for home care support.
5. Instruct the client not to drive, make important decisions, or sign any legal documents for 24 hours after receiving general anesthesia.
6. Instruct the client to call the surgeon, ambulatory center, or emergency department if postoperative problems occur.
7. Instruct the client to keep follow-up appointments with the surgeon.

PRACTICE QUESTIONS

126. The nurse has just reassessed the condition of a postoperative client who was admitted 1 hour ago to the surgical unit. The nurse plans to monitor which parameter **most** carefully during the next hour?
1. Urinary output of 20 mL/hr
2. Temperature of 37.6° C (99.6° F)
3. Blood pressure of 100/70 mm Hg
4. Serous drainage on the surgical dressing

127. The nurse is teaching a client about coughing and deep-breathing techniques to prevent postoperative complications. Which statement is **most appropriate** for the nurse to make to the client at this time as it relates to these techniques?
1. "Use of an incentive spirometer will help prevent pneumonia."
2. "Close monitoring of your oxygen saturation will detect hypoxemia."
3. "Administration of intravenous fluids will prevent or treat fluid imbalance."
4. "Early ambulation and administration of blood thinners will prevent pulmonary embolism."

128. The nurse is creating a plan of care for a client scheduled for surgery. The nurse should include which activity in the nursing care plan for the client on the day of surgery?
1. Avoid oral hygiene and rinsing with mouthwash.
2. Verify that the client has not eaten for the last 24 hours.
3. Have the client void immediately before going into surgery.
4. Report immediately any slight increase in blood pressure or pulse.

129. A client with a gastric ulcer is scheduled for surgery. The client cannot sign the operative consent form because of sedation from opioid analgesics that have been administered. The nurse should take which **most appropriate** action in the care of this client?
1. Obtain a court order for the surgery.
2. Have the charge nurse sign the informed consent immediately.
3. Send the client to surgery without the consent form being signed.
4. Obtain a telephone consent from a family member, following agency policy.

130. A preoperative client expresses anxiety to the nurse about upcoming surgery. Which response by the nurse is **most likely** to stimulate further discussion between the client and the nurse?
1. "If it's any help, everyone is nervous before surgery."
2. "I will be happy to explain the entire surgical procedure to you."
3. "Can you share with me what you've been told about your surgery?"
4. "Let me tell you about the care you'll receive after surgery and the amount of pain you can anticipate."

131. The nurse is conducting preoperative teaching with a client about the use of an incentive spirometer. The nurse should include which piece of information in discussions with the client?
1. Inhale as rapidly as possible.
2. Keep a loose seal between the lips and the mouthpiece.
3. After maximum inspiration, hold the breath for 15 seconds and exhale.
4. The best results are achieved when sitting up or with the head of the bed elevated 45 to 90 degrees.

132. The nurse has conducted preoperative teaching for a client scheduled for surgery in 1 week. The client has a history of arthritis and has been taking acetylsalicylic acid. The nurse determines that the client **needs additional teaching** if the client makes which statement?
1. "Aspirin can cause bleeding after surgery."
2. "Aspirin can cause my ability to clot blood to be abnormal."
3. "I need to continue to take the aspirin until the day of surgery."
4. "I need to check with my doctor about the need to stop the aspirin before the scheduled surgery."

133. The nurse assesses a client's surgical incision for signs of infection. Which finding by the nurse would be interpreted as a normal finding at the surgical site?
1. Red, hard skin
2. Serous drainage
3. Purulent drainage
4. Warm, tender skin

134. The nurse is monitoring the status of a postoperative client in the immediate postoperative period. The nurse would become **most** concerned with which sign that could indicate an evolving complication?
1. Increasing restlessness
2. A pulse of 86 beats per minute
3. Blood pressure of 110/70 mm Hg
4. Hypoactive bowel sounds in all 4 quadrants

135. A client who has had abdominal surgery complains of feeling as though "something gave way" in the incisional site. The nurse removes the dressing and notes the presence of a loop of bowel protruding through the incision. Which interventions should the nurse take? **Select all that apply.**

- ❑ 1. Contact the surgeon.
- ❑ 2. Instruct the client to remain quiet.
- ❑ 3. Prepare the client for wound closure.
- ❑ 4. Document the findings and actions taken.
- ❑ 5. Place a sterile saline dressing and ice packs over the wound.
- ❑ 6. Place the client in a supine position without a pillow under the head.

136. A client who has undergone preadmission testing has had blood drawn for serum laboratory studies, including a complete blood count, coagulation studies, and electrolytes and creatinine levels. Which laboratory result should be reported to the surgeon's office by the nurse, knowing that it could cause surgery to be postponed?
1. Hemoglobin, 8.0 g/dL (80 mmol/L)
2. Sodium, 145 mEq/L (145 mmol/L)
3. Serum creatinine, 0.8 mg/dL (70.6 mcmol/L)
4. Platelets, 210,000 cells/mm^3 (210×10^9/L)

137. The nurse receives a telephone call from the postanesthesia care unit stating that a client is being transferred to the surgical unit. The nurse plans to take which action **first** on arrival of the client?
1. Assess the patency of the airway.
2. Check tubes or drains for patency.
3. Check the dressing to assess for bleeding.
4. Assess the vital signs to compare with preoperative measurements.

138. The nurse is reviewing a surgeon's prescription sheet for a preoperative client that states that the client must be nothing by mouth (NPO) after midnight. The nurse should call the surgeon to clarify that which medication should be given to the client and not withheld?
1. Prednisone
2. Ferrous sulfate
3. Cyclobenzaprine
4. Conjugated estrogen

ANSWERS

126. *Answer:* 1

Rationale: Urine output should be maintained at a minimum of 30 mL/hr for an adult. An output of less than 30 mL for 2 consecutive hours should be reported to the surgeon. A temperature higher than 37.7° C (100° F) or lower than 36.1° C (97° F) and a falling systolic blood pressure, lower than 90 mm Hg, are usually considered reportable immediately. The client's preoperative or baseline blood pressure is used to make informed postoperative comparisons. Moderate or light serous drainage from the surgical site is considered normal.

Test-Taking Strategy: Note the strategic word, *most.* Focus on the subject, expected postoperative assessment findings. To answer this question correctly, you must know the normal ranges for temperature, blood pressure, urinary output, and wound drainage. Note that the urinary output is the only observation that is not within the normal range.

Level of Cognitive Ability: Analyzing
Client Needs: Physiological Integrity
Integrated Process: Nursing Process—Planning
Content Area: Foundations of Care: Perioperative Care
Health Problem: N/A
Priority Concepts: Clinical Judgment; Perfusion
Reference: Ignatavicius, Workman, Rebar (2018), p. 276.

127. *Answer:* 1

Rationale: Postoperative respiratory problems are atelectasis, pneumonia, and pulmonary emboli. Pneumonia is the inflammation of lung tissue that causes productive cough, dyspnea, and lung crackles and can be caused by retained pulmonary secretions. Use of an incentive spirometer helps prevent pneumonia and atelectasis. Hypoxemia is an inadequate concentration of oxygen in arterial blood. While close monitoring of the oxygen saturation will help detect hypoxemia, monitoring is not directly related to coughing and deep-breathing techniques. Fluid imbalance can be a deficit or excess related to fluid loss or overload, and surgical clients are often given intravenous fluids to prevent a deficit; however, this is not related to coughing and deep breathing. Pulmonary embolus occurs as a result of a blockage of the pulmonary artery that disrupts blood flow to 1 or more lobes of the lung; this is usually due to clot formation. Early ambulation and administration of blood thinners helps prevent this complication; however, it is not related to coughing and deep-breathing techniques.

Test-Taking Strategy: Note the strategic words, *most appropriate.* Focus on the subject, client instructions related to coughing and deep-breathing techniques. Also, focus on the data in the question and note the relationship between the words *coughing* and *deep-breathing* in the question and *pneumonia* in the correct option.

Level of Cognitive Ability: Applying

Client Needs: Physiological Integrity
Integrated Process: Teaching and Learning
Content Area: Skills: Perioperative Care
Health Problem: N/A
Priority Concepts: Client Education; Gas Exchange
Reference: Ignatavicius, Workman, Rebar (2018), pp. 244, 281.

128. *Answer:* 3
Rationale: The nurse would assist the client to void immediately before surgery so that the bladder will be empty. Oral hygiene is allowed, but the client should not swallow any water. The client usually has a restriction of food and fluids for 6 to 8 hours (or longer as prescribed) before surgery instead of 24 hours. A slight increase in blood pressure and pulse is common during the preoperative period and is usually the result of anxiety.
Test-Taking Strategy: Focus on the subject, preoperative care measures. Think about the measures that may be helpful and promote comfort. Oral hygiene should be administered, since it may make the client feel more comfortable. A client should be nothing by mouth (NPO) for 6 to 8 hours before surgery rather than 24 hours. A slight increase in blood pressure or pulse is insignificant in this situation.
Level of Cognitive Ability: Creating
Client Needs: Physiological Integrity
Integrated Process: Nursing Process—Planning
Content Area: Foundations of Care: Perioperative Care
Health Problem: N/A
Priority Concepts: Clinical Judgment; Palliative Care
Reference: Lewis et al. (2017), p. 310.

129. *Answer:* 4
Rationale: Every effort should be made to obtain permission from a responsible family member to perform surgery if the client is unable to sign the consent form. A telephone consent must be witnessed by 2 persons who hear the family member's oral consent. The 2 witnesses then sign the consent with the name of the family member, noting that an oral consent was obtained. Consent is not informed if it is obtained from a client who is confused, unconscious, mentally incompetent, or under the influence of sedatives. In an emergency, a client may be unable to sign and family members may not be available. In this situation, a surgeon is permitted legally to perform surgery without consent, but the data in the question do not indicate an emergency. Options 1, 2, and 3 are not appropriate in this situation. Also, agency policies regarding informed consent should always be followed.
Test-Taking Strategy: Note the strategic words, *most appropriate.* Focus on the data in the question. Eliminate options 1 and 3 first. Option 1 will delay necessary surgery, and option 3 is inappropriate. Option 2 is not an acceptable and legal role of a charge nurse. Select option 4, since it is the only legally acceptable option: to obtain a telephone permission from a family member if it is witnessed by 2 persons.
Level of Cognitive Ability: Applying
Client Needs: Safe and Effective Care Environment
Integrated Process: Nursing Process—Implementation
Content Area: Foundations of Care: Perioperative Care
Health Problem: Adult Health: Gastrointestinal: Upper GI Disorders
Priority Concepts: Ethics; Health Care Law
Reference: Potter et al. (2017), p. 310.

130. *Answer:* 3
Rationale: Explanations should begin with the information that the client knows. By providing the client with individualized explanations of care and procedures, the nurse can assist the client in handling anxiety and fear for a smooth preoperative experience. Clients who are calm and emotionally prepared for surgery withstand anesthesia better and experience fewer postoperative complications. Option 1 does not focus on the client's anxiety. Explaining the entire surgical procedure may increase the client's anxiety. Option 4 avoids the client's anxiety and is focused on postoperative care.
Test-Taking Strategy: Note that the client expresses anxiety. Use therapeutic communication techniques. Note that the question contains strategic words, *most likely,* and also note the words *stimulate further discussion*. Also use the steps of the nursing process. The correct option addresses assessment and is the only therapeutic response.
Level of Cognitive Ability: Applying
Client Needs: Psychosocial Integrity
Integrated Process: Communication and Documentation
Content Area: Foundations of Care: Perioperative Care
Health Problem: Mental Health: Therapeutic Communication
Priority Concepts: Anxiety; Communication
Reference: Ignatavicius, Workman, Rebar (2018), pp. 237, 246.

131. *Answer:* 4
Rationale: For optimal lung expansion with the incentive spirometer, the client should assume the semi-Fowler's or high-Fowler's position. The mouthpiece should be covered completely and tightly while the client inhales slowly, with a constant flow through the unit. The breath should be held for 5 seconds before exhaling slowly.
Test-Taking Strategy: Focus on the subject, correct use of an incentive spirometer, and visualize the procedure. Note the words *rapidly, loose,* and *15 seconds* in the incorrect options. Options 1, 2, and 3 are incorrect steps regarding incentive spirometer use.
Level of Cognitive Ability: Applying
Client Needs: Physiological Integrity
Integrated Process: Teaching and Learning
Content Area: Skills: Perioperative Care
Health Problem: N/A
Priority Concepts: Client Education; Gas Exchange
Reference: Ignatavicius, Workman, Rebar (2018), pp. 243-244.

132. *Answer:* 3
Rationale: Antiplatelets alter normal clotting factors and increase the risk of bleeding after surgery. Aspirin has properties that can alter platelet aggregation and should be discontinued at least 48 hours before surgery. However, the client should always check with his or her surgeon regarding when to stop taking the aspirin when a surgical procedure is scheduled. Options 1, 2, and 4 are accurate client statements.
Test-Taking Strategy: Note the strategic words, *needs additional teaching*. These words indicate a negative event query and that you need to select the incorrect client statement. Eliminate options 1 and 2 first because they are comparable or alike. From the remaining options, recalling that aspirin has properties that can alter platelet aggregation will direct you to the correct option.
Level of Cognitive Ability: Evaluating

Client Needs: Physiological Integrity
Integrated Process: Teaching and Learning
Content Area: Foundations of Care: Perioperative Care
Health Problem: Adult Health: Musculoskeletal: Rheumatoid Arthritis and Osteoarthritis
Priority Concepts: Client Education; Clotting
Reference: Ignatavicius, Workman, Rebar (2018), pp. 241-242.

133. *Answer:* 2
Rationale: Serous drainage is an expected finding at a surgical site. The other options indicate signs of wound infection. Signs and symptoms of infection include warm, red, and tender skin around the incision. Wound infection usually appears 3 to 6 days after surgery. The client also may have a fever and chills. Purulent material may exit from drains or from separated wound edges. Infection may be caused by poor aseptic technique or a contaminated wound before surgical exploration; existing client conditions such as diabetes mellitus or immunocompromise may place the client at risk.
Test-Taking Strategy: Focus on the **subject,** normal findings in the postoperative period. Eliminate options 1, 3, and 4 because they are **comparable or alike** and are manifestations of infection.
Level of Cognitive Ability: Applying
Client Needs: Physiological Integrity
Integrated Process: Nursing Process—Assessment
Content Area: Foundations of Care: Perioperative Care
Health Problem: Adult Health: Integumentary: Wounds
Priority Concepts: Infection; Tissue Integrity
Reference: Ignatavicius, Workman, Rebar (2018), pp. 281-282.

134. *Answer:* 1
Rationale: Increasing restlessness is a sign that requires continuous and close monitoring because it could indicate a potential complication such as hemorrhage, shock, or pulmonary embolism. A blood pressure of 110/70 mm Hg with a pulse of 86 beats per minute is within normal limits. Hypoactive bowel sounds heard in all 4 quadrants are a normal occurrence in the immediate postoperative period.
Test-Taking Strategy: Note the **strategic word,** *most.* Focus on the **subject,** a manifestation of an evolving complication in the immediate postoperative period. Eliminate each of the incorrect options because they are **comparable or alike** and are normal expected findings, especially given the time frame noted in the question.
Level of Cognitive Ability: Analyzing
Client Needs: Physiological Integrity
Integrated Process: Nursing Process—Analysis
Content Area: Foundations of Care: Perioperative Care
Health Problem: N/A
Priority Concepts: Clinical Judgment; Safety
Reference: Lewis et al. (2017), p. 331.

135. *Answer:* 1, 2, 3, 4
Rationale: Wound dehiscence is the separation of the wound edges. Wound evisceration is protrusion of the internal organs through an incision. If wound dehiscence or evisceration occurs, the nurse should call for help, stay with the client, and ask another nurse to contact the surgeon and obtain needed supplies to care for the client. The nurse places the client in a low-Fowler's position, and the client is kept quiet and instructed not to cough. Protruding organs are covered with a sterile saline dressing. Ice is not applied because of its vasoconstrictive effect. The treatment for evisceration is usually immediate wound closure under local or general anesthesia. The nurse also documents the findings and actions taken.
Test-Taking Strategy: Focus on the **subject,** that the client is experiencing wound evisceration. Visualizing this occurrence will assist you in determining that the client would not be placed supine and that ice packs would not be placed on the incision.
Level of Cognitive Ability: Analyzing
Client Needs: Physiological Integrity
Integrated Process: Nursing Process—Implementation
Content Area: Skills: Perioperative Care
Health Problem: Adult Health: Integumentary: Wounds
Priority Concepts: Clinical Judgment; Tissue Integrity
Reference: Ignatavicius, Workman, Rebar (2018), p. 283.

136. *Answer:* 1
Rationale: Routine screening tests include a complete blood count, serum electrolyte analysis, coagulation studies, and a serum creatinine test. The complete blood count includes the hemoglobin analysis. All of these values are within normal range except for hemoglobin. If a client has a low hemoglobin level, the surgery likely could be postponed by the surgeon.
Test-Taking Strategy: Focus on the **subject,** an abnormal laboratory result that needs to be reported. Use knowledge of the normal reference intervals to assist in answering correctly. The hemoglobin value is the only abnormal laboratory finding.
Level of Cognitive Ability: Analyzing
Client Needs: Physiological Integrity
Integrated Process: Nursing Process—Implementation
Content Area: Foundations of Care: Perioperative Care
Health Problem: Adult Health: Hematological: Anemias
Priority Concepts: Clinical Judgment; Collaboration
Reference: Lewis et al. (2017), p. 600.

137. *Answer:* 1
Rationale: The first action of the nurse is to assess the patency of the airway and respiratory function. If the airway is not patent, the nurse must take immediate measures for the survival of the client. The nurse then takes vital signs followed by checking the dressing and the tubes or drains. The other nursing actions should be performed after a patent airway has been established.
Test-Taking Strategy: Note the **strategic word,** *first.* Use the principles of prioritization to answer this question. Use the **ABCs—airway, breathing, and circulation.** Ensuring airway patency is the first action to be taken, directing you to the correct option.
Level of Cognitive Ability: Analyzing
Client Needs: Physiological Integrity
Integrated Process: Nursing Process—Planning
Content Area: Foundations of Care: Perioperative Care
Health Problem: N/A
Priority Concepts: Care Coordination; Clinical Judgment
Reference: Lewis et al. (2017), p. 331.

138. *Answer:* 1

Rationale: Prednisone is a corticosteroid. With prolonged use, corticosteroids cause adrenal atrophy, which reduces the ability of the body to withstand stress. When stress is severe, corticosteroids are essential to life. Before and during surgery, dosages may be increased temporarily and may be given parenterally rather than orally. Ferrous sulfate is an oral iron preparation used to treat iron deficiency anemia. Cyclobenzaprine is a skeletal muscle relaxant. Conjugated estrogen is an estrogen used for hormone replacement therapy in postmenopausal women. These last 3 medications may be withheld before surgery without undue effects on the client.

Test-Taking Strategy: Focus on the **subject,** the medication that should be administered in the preoperative period. Use knowledge about medications that may have special implications for the surgical client. Prednisone is a corticosteroid. Recall that when stress is severe, such as with surgery, corticosteroids are essential to life.

Level of Cognitive Ability: Analyzing

Client Needs: Physiological Integrity

Integrated Process: Nursing Process—Analysis

Content Area: Foundations of Care: Perioperative Care

Health Problem: N/A

Priority Concepts: Clinical Judgment; Collaboration

Reference: Ignatavicius, Workman, Rebar (2018), p. 241.

CHAPTER 16

Positioning Clients

PRIORITY CONCEPTS **Mobility; Safety**

For reference throughout the chapter, please see Figure 16-1, 16-2, 16-3, and 16-4.

I. Guidelines for Positioning

A. Client safety and comfort
   1. Position client in a safe and appropriate manner to provide safety and comfort.
   2. Select a position that will prevent the development of complications related to an existing condition, prescribed treatment, or medical or surgical procedure.

B. Ergonomic principles related to body mechanics (Box 16-1)

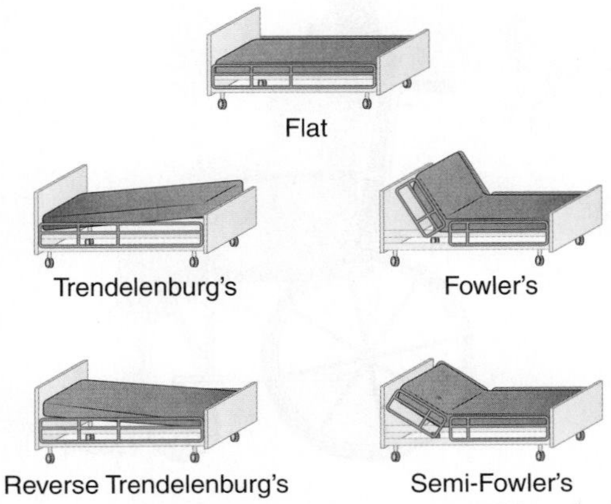

FIG. 16-1 Bed positions.

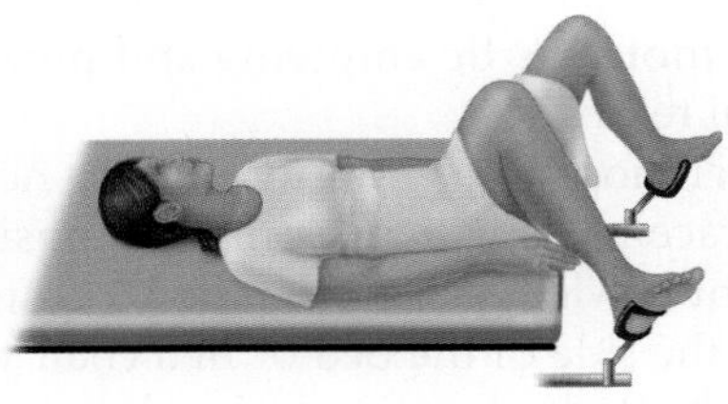

FIG. 16-2 Lithotomy position for examination.

Always review the primary health care provider's (PHCP's) or surgeon's prescription, especially after treatments or procedures, and take note of instructions regarding positioning and mobility.

II. Positions to Ensure Safety and Comfort

A. Integumentary system
   1. Autograft: After surgery, the site is immobilized usually for 3 to 7 days, or as prescribed, to provide the time needed for the graft to adhere and attach to the wound bed.
   2. Burns of the face and head: Elevate the head of the bed to prevent or reduce facial, head, and tracheal edema.
   3. Circumferential burns of the extremities: Elevate the extremities above the level of the heart to prevent or reduce dependent edema.
   4. Skin graft: Elevate and immobilize the graft site to prevent movement and shearing of the graft and disruption of tissue; avoid weight-bearing.

B. Reproductive system
   1. Mastectomy
      a. Position the client with the head of the bed elevated at least 30 degrees (semi-Fowler's position), with the affected arm elevated on a pillow to promote lymphatic fluid return after the removal of axillary lymph nodes.
      b. Turn the client only to the back and unaffected side.
   2. Perineal and vaginal procedures: Place the client in the lithotomy position.

C. Endocrine system
   1. Hypophysectomy: Elevate the head of the bed to prevent increased intracranial pressure.
   2. Thyroidectomy
      a. Place the client in the semi-Fowler's to Fowler's position to reduce swelling and edema in the neck area.
      b. Sandbags or pillows or other stabilization devices may be used to support the client's head or neck.

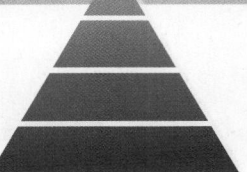

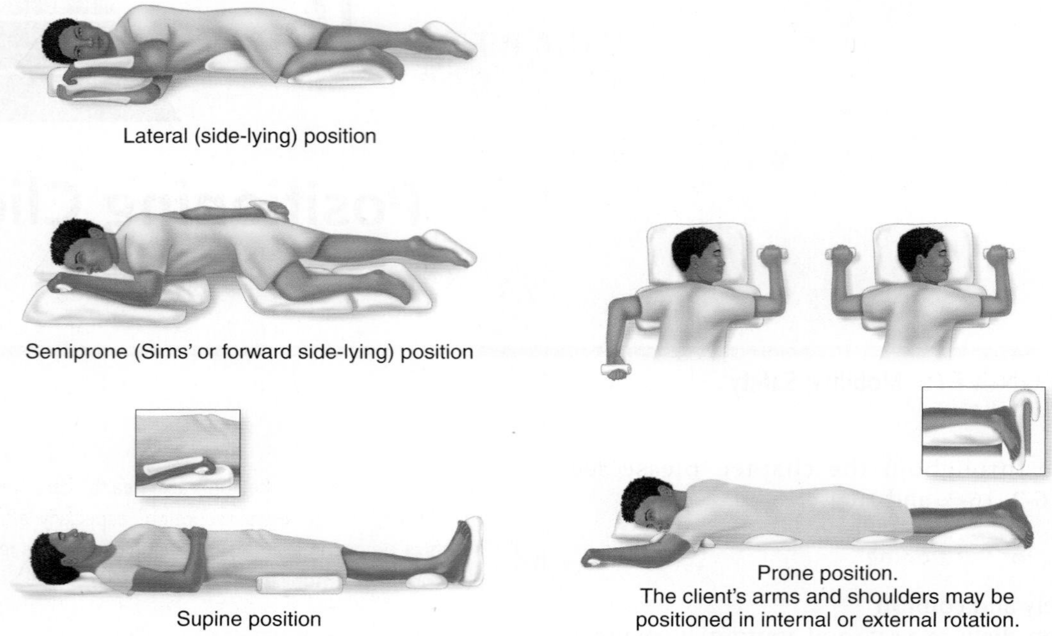

FIG. 16-3 Client positions.

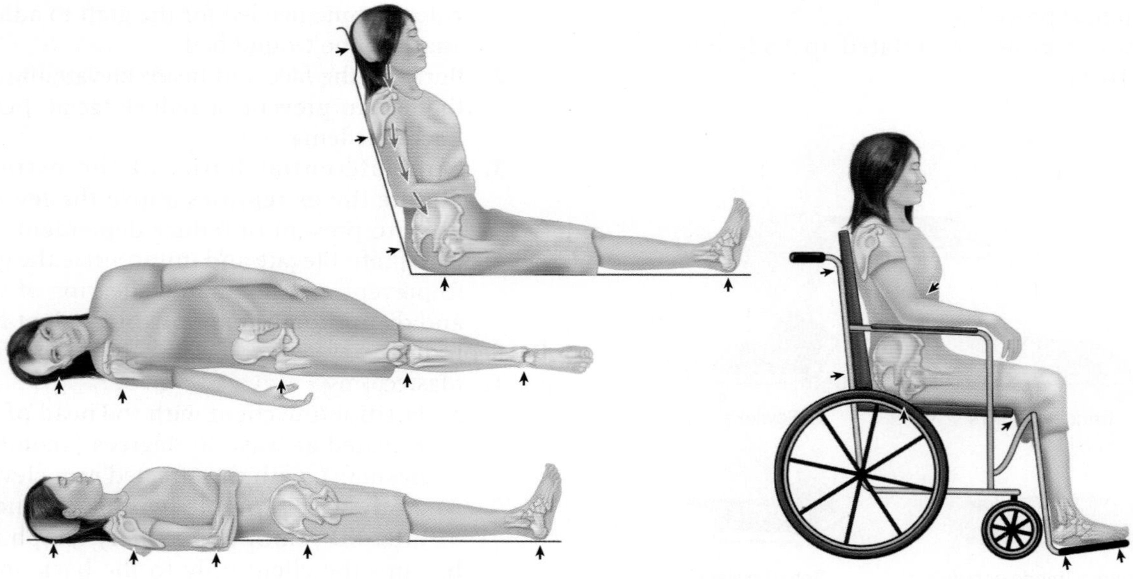

FIG. 16-4 Pressure points in lying and sitting positions.

c. Avoid neck extension to decrease tension on the suture line.

D. Gastrointestinal system

1. Hemorrhoidectomy: Assist the client to a **lateral (side-lying) position** to prevent pain and bleeding.
2. Gastroesophageal reflux disease: **Reverse Trendelenburg's position** may be prescribed to promote gastric emptying and prevent esophageal reflux.
3. Liver biopsy (see Priority Nursing Actions)
4. Paracentesis: Client is usually positioned in a semi-Fowler's position in bed, or sitting upright on the side of the bed or in a chair with the feet supported; client is assisted to a position of comfort after the procedure.

PRIORITY NURSING ACTIONS

Liver Biopsy

1. Explain the procedure to the client.
2. Ensure that informed consent has been obtained.
3. Position the client supine, with the right side of the upper abdomen exposed; the client's right arm is raised and extended behind the head and over the left shoulder.
4. Remain with the client during the procedure.
5. After the procedure, assist the client into a right lateral (side-lying) position and place a small pillow or folded towel under the puncture site.
6. Monitor vital signs closely after the procedure and monitor for signs of bleeding.
7. Document appropriate information about the procedure, client's tolerance, and postprocedure assessment findings.

Reference

Lewis et al. (2017), p. 850.

BOX 16-1 Body Mechanics (Ergonomic Principles) for Health Care Workers

- When planning to move a client, arrange for adequate help, including the use of mechanical aids. Use mechanical aids if help is unavailable.
- Encourage the client to assist as much as possible.
- Keep the back, neck and pelvis, and feet aligned. Avoid twisting.
- Flex knees and keep feet wide apart.
- Raise the client's bed so that the client's weight is at the level of the nurse's center of gravity.
- Position self close to the client (or object being lifted).
- Use arms and legs (not back).
- Slide client toward yourself, using a pull sheet. When transferring a client onto a stretcher, a slide board is more appropriate.
- Set (tighten) abdominal and gluteal muscles in preparation for the move.
- The person with the heaviest load coordinates efforts of the team involved by counting to 3.

Adapted from Potter P, Perry A, Stockert P, Hall A: *Fundamentals of nursing*, ed 8, St. Louis, 2013, Mosby. Perry, Potter, Ostendorf (2014), pp. 197-198. St. Louis: Mosby.

5. Nasogastric tube
   a. Insertion: Position the client in a **high-Fowler's position** with the head titled forward; this position will help close the trachea and open the esophagus.
   b. Irrigation and tube feedings: Elevate the head of the bed (semi-Fowler's to Fowler's position) to prevent aspiration; head elevation is maintained for 30 minutes to 1 hour (per agency procedure) after an intermittent feeding and should remain elevated for continuous feedings.

If the client receiving a continuous tube feeding needs to be placed in a supine position when providing care, such as when giving a bed bath or changing linens, shut off the feeding to prevent aspiration. Remember to turn the feeding back on and check the rate of flow when the client is placed back into the semi-Fowler's or Fowler's position.

6. Rectal enema and irrigations: Place the client in the left **Sims' position** to allow the solution to flow by gravity in the natural direction of the colon.
7. Sengstaken-Blakemore and Minnesota tubes
   a. Not commonly used because they are uncomfortable for the client and can cause complications, but their use may be necessary when other interventions are not feasible.
   b. If prescribed, maintain elevation of the head of the bed to enhance lung expansion and reduce portal blood flow, permitting effective esophagogastric balloon tamponade.

E. Respiratory system
   1. Chronic obstructive pulmonary disease: In advanced disease, place the client in a sitting position, leaning forward, with the client's arms over several pillows or an overbed table; this position will assist the client to breathe easier.
   2. Laryngectomy (radical neck dissection): Place the client in a semi-Fowler's or Fowler's position to maintain a patent airway and minimize edema.
   3. Bronchoscopy postprocedure: Place the client in a semi-Fowler's position to prevent choking or aspiration resulting from an impaired ability to swallow.
   4. Postural drainage: The lung segment to be drained should be in the uppermost position; **Trendelenburg's position** may be used.
   5. Thoracentesis
      a. During the procedure, to facilitate removal of fluid from the pleural space, position the client sitting on the edge of the bed or examining table and leaning over a bedside table with the feet supported on a stool, or lying on the unaffected side with the client in Fowler's position.
      b. After the procedure, assist the client to a position of comfort.

Always check the PHCP's prescription regarding positioning for the client who had a thoracotomy, lung wedge resection, lobectomy of the lung, or pneumonectomy.

F. Cardiovascular system
   1. Abdominal aneurysm resection
      a. After surgery, limit elevation of the head of the bed to 45 degrees to avoid flexion of the graft.
      b. The client may be turned from side to side.
   2. Amputation of the lower extremity
      a. During the first 24 hours after amputation, elevate the foot of the bed (the residual limb is supported with pillows but not elevated because of the risk of flexion contractures) to reduce edema.

b. Consult with the PHCP and, if prescribed, position the client in a prone position twice a day for a 20- to 30-minute period to stretch muscles and prevent flexion contractures of the hip.

3. Arterial vascular grafting of an extremity
   a. To promote graft patency after the procedure, bed rest usually is maintained for approximately 24 hours, and the affected extremity is kept straight.
   b. Limit movement and avoid flexion of the hip and knee.

4. Cardiac catheterization
   a. If the femoral vessel was accessed for the procedure, the client is maintained on bed rest for 4 to 6 hours (time for bed rest may vary depending on PHCP preference and if a vascular closure device was used); the client may turn from side to side.
   b. The affected extremity is kept straight and the head is elevated no more than 30 degrees (some PHCPs prefer a lower head position or the flat position) until hemostasis is adequately achieved.

5. Heart failure and pulmonary edema: Position the client upright, preferably with the legs dangling over the side of the bed, to decrease venous return and lung congestion.

⚠ Most often, clients with respiratory and cardiac disorders should be positioned with the head of the bed elevated.

6. Peripheral arterial disease
   a. Obtain the PHCP's prescription for positioning.
   b. Because swelling can prevent arterial blood flow, clients may be advised to elevate their feet at rest, but they should not raise their legs above the level of the heart, because extreme elevation slows arterial blood flow; some clients may be advised to maintain a slightly dependent position to promote perfusion.

7. Deep vein thrombosis
   a. If the extremity is red, edematous, and painful, traditional heparin sodium therapy may be initiated. Bed rest with leg elevation may also be prescribed for the client.
   b. Clients receiving low-molecular-weight heparin usually can be out of bed after 24 hours if pain level permits.

8. Varicose veins: Leg elevation above heart level usually is prescribed; the client also is advised to minimize prolonged sitting or standing during daily activities.

9. Venous insufficiency and leg ulcers: Leg elevation usually is prescribed.

G. Sensory system

1. Cataract surgery: Postoperatively, elevate the head of the bed (semi-Fowler's to Fowler's position) and position the client on the back or the nonoperative side to prevent the development of edema at the operative site.

2. Retinal detachment
   a. If the detachment is large, bed rest and bilateral eye patching may be prescribed to minimize eye movement and prevent extension of the detachment.
   b. Restrictions in activity and positioning after repair of the detachment depends on the PHCP's preference and the surgical procedure performed.

H. Neurological system

1. Autonomic dysreflexia: Elevate the head of the bed to a high-Fowler's position to assist with adequate ventilation and assist in the prevention of hypertensive stroke.

⚠ If autonomic dysreflexia occurs, immediately place the client in a high-Fowler's position.

2. Cerebral aneurysm: Bed rest is maintained with the head of the bed elevated 30 to 45 degrees to prevent pressure on the aneurysm site.

3. Cerebral angiography
   a. Maintain bed rest for the length of time as prescribed.
   b. The extremity into which the contrast medium was injected is kept straight and immobilized for about 6 to 8 hours.

4. Stroke (brain attack)
   a. In clients with hemorrhagic strokes, the head of the bed is usually elevated to 30 degrees to reduce intracranial pressure and to facilitate venous drainage.
   b. For clients with ischemic strokes, the head of the bed is usually kept flat.
   c. Maintain the head in a midline, neutral position to facilitate venous drainage from the head.
   d. Avoid extreme hip and neck flexion; extreme hip flexion may increase intrathoracic pressure, whereas extreme neck flexion prohibits venous drainage from the brain.

5. Craniotomy
   a. The client should not be positioned on the site that was operated on, especially if the bone flap has been removed, because the brain has no bony covering on the affected site.
   b. Elevate the head of the bed 30 to 45 degrees and maintain the head in a midline, neutral position to facilitate venous drainage from the head.
   c. Avoid extreme hip and neck flexion.

6. Laminectomy and other vertebral surgery
   a. Clients are often out of bed postoperatively with a back brace if prescribed.
   b. When the client is out of bed, the client's back is kept straight (the client is placed in

a straight-backed chair) with the feet resting comfortably on the floor.

7. Increased intracranial pressure
   - **a.** Elevate the head of the bed 30 to 45 degrees and maintain the head in a midline, neutral position to facilitate venous drainage from the head.
   - **b.** Avoid extreme hip and neck flexion.

Do not place a client with a head injury in a flat or Trendelenburg's position because of the risk of increased intracranial pressure.

8. Lumbar puncture
   - **a.** During the procedure, assist the client to the lateral (side-lying) position, with the back bowed at the edge of the examining table, the knees flexed up to the abdomen, and the neck flexed so that the chin is resting on the chest.
   - **b.** After the procedure, place the client in the **supine position** for 4 to 12 hours, as prescribed.
9. Spinal cord injury
   - **a.** Immobilize the client on a spinal backboard, with the head in a neutral position, to prevent incomplete injury from becoming complete.
   - **b.** Prevent head flexion, rotation, or extension; the head is immobilized with a firm, padded cervical collar.
   - **c.** Logroll the client; no part of the body should be twisted or turned, nor should the client be allowed to assume a sitting position.

I. Musculoskeletal system
1. Total hip replacement
   - **a.** Positioning depends on the surgical techniques used (anterior or posterior approach), the method of implantation, the prosthesis, and surgeon's preference.
   - **b.** Avoid extreme internal and external rotation.
   - **c.** Avoid adduction; in most cases side-lying is permitted as long as an abduction pillow is in place; some surgeons allow turning to only 1 side.
   - **d.** Maintain abduction when the client is in a supine position or positioned on the nonoperative side.
   - **e.** Place a wedge (abduction) pillow between the client's legs to maintain abduction; instruct the client not to cross the legs
   - **f.** Check the PHCP's prescriptions regarding elevation of the head of the bed and hip flexion.
2. Devices used to promote proper positioning (Box 16-2)

BOX 16-2 Devices Used for Proper Positioning

Bed Boards
These plywood boards are placed under the entire surface area of the mattress and are useful for increasing back support and body alignment. Many of the beds used in health care facilities have the capability of being adjusted to a softness or hardness desired for the mattress to meet the client's needs.

Foot Boots
Foot boots are made of rigid plastic or heavy foam and keep the foot flexed at the proper angle. They should be removed 2 or 3 times a day to assess skin integrity and joint mobility by providing range of motion.

Hand Rolls
Hand rolls maintain the fingers in a slightly flexed and functional position and keep the thumb slightly adducted in opposition to the fingers.

Hand-Wrist Splints
These splints are individually molded for the client to maintain proper alignment of the thumb in slight adduction and the wrist in slight dorsiflexion.

Pillows
Pillows provide support, elevate body parts, splint incisional areas, and reduce postoperative pain during activity, coughing, or deep breathing. They should be of the appropriate size for the body part to be positioned.

Sandbags
Sandbags are soft devices filled with a substance that can be shaped to body contours to provide support. They immobilize extremities and maintain specific body alignment.

Side Rails
These bars, positioned along the sides of the length of the bed, ensure client safety and are useful for increasing mobility. They also provide assistance in rolling from side to side or sitting up in bed. Laws regarding the use of side rails vary state to state, and these laws must be followed; some states view side rails as a form of restraint, and therefore, laws and agency policies must be followed.

Trapeze Bar
This bar descends from a securely fastened overhead bar attached to the bed frame. It allows the client to use the upper extremities to raise the trunk off the bed, assists in transfer from the bed to a wheelchair, and helps the client to perform upper arm–strengthening exercises.

Trochanter Rolls
These rolls prevent external rotation of the legs when the client is in the supine position. To form a roll, use a cotton bath blanket or a sheet folded lengthwise to a width extending from the greater trochanter of the femur to the lower border of the popliteal space.

Wedge Pillow
This triangular pillow is made of heavy foam and is used to maintain the legs in abduction after total hip replacement surgery.

Adapted from Potter P, Perry A, Stockert P, Hall A: *Fundamentals of nursing*, ed 8, St. Louis, 2013, Mosby.

PRACTICE QUESTIONS

139. A client is being prepared for a thoracentesis. The nurse should assist the client to which position for the procedure?
1. Lying in bed on the affected side
2. Lying in bed on the unaffected side
3. Sims' position with the head of the bed flat
4. Prone with the head turned to the side and supported by a pillow

140. The nurse is caring for a client following a craniotomy, in which a large cancerous tumor was removed from the left side. In which position can the nurse safely place the client? **Refer to the figures in options 1 to 4.**

1. 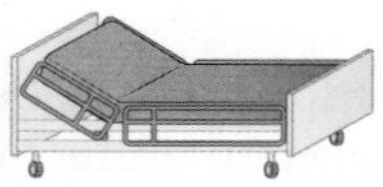

2. 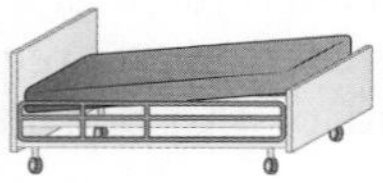

3. 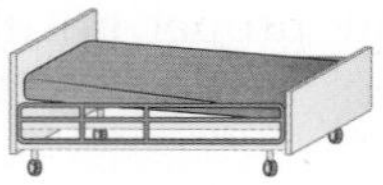

4. 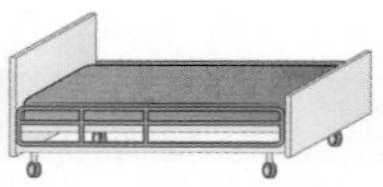

141. The nurse creates a plan of care for a client with deep vein thrombosis. Which client position or activity in the plan should be included?
1. Out-of-bed activities as desired
2. Bed rest with the affected extremity kept flat
3. Bed rest with elevation of the affected extremity
4. Bed rest with the affected extremity in a dependent position

142. The nurse is caring for a client who is 1 day postoperative for a total hip replacement. Which is the **best** position in which the nurse should place the client?
1. Head elevated lying on the operative side
2. On the nonoperative side with the legs abducted
3. Side-lying with the affected leg internally rotated
4. Side-lying with the affected leg externally rotated

143. The nurse is providing instructions to a client and the family regarding home care after right eye cataract removal. Which statement by the client would indicate an understanding of the instructions?
1. "I should sleep on my left side."
2. "I should sleep on my right side."
3. "I should sleep with my head flat."
4. "I should not wear my glasses at any time."

144. The nurse is administering a cleansing enema to a client with a fecal impaction. Before administering the enema, the nurse should place the client in which position?
1. Left Sims' position
2. Right Sims' position
3. On the left side of the body, with the head of the bed elevated 45 degrees
4. On the right side of the body, with the head of the bed elevated 45 degrees

145. A client has just returned to a nursing unit after an above-knee amputation of the right leg. The nurse should place the client in which position?
1. Prone
2. Reverse Trendelenburg's
3. Supine, with the residual limb flat on the bed
4. Supine, with the residual limb supported with pillows

146. The nurse is caring for a client with a severe burn who is scheduled for an autograft to be placed on the lower extremity. The nurse creates a postoperative plan of care for the client and should include which intervention in the plan?
1. Maintain the client in a prone position.
2. Elevate and immobilize the grafted extremity.
3. Maintain the grafted extremity in a flat position.
4. Keep the grafted extremity covered with a blanket.

147. The nurse is preparing to care for a client who has returned to the nursing unit after cardiac catheterization performed through the femoral vessel. The nurse checks the primary health care provider's (PHCP's) prescription and plans to allow which client position or activity after the procedure?
1. Bed rest in high-Fowler's position
2. Bed rest with bathroom privileges only
3. Bed rest with head elevation at 60 degrees
4. Bed rest with head elevation no greater than 30 degrees

148. The nurse is preparing to insert a nasogastric tube into a client. The nurse should place the client in which position for insertion?
1. Right side
2. Low-Fowler's
3. High-Fowler's
4. Supine with the head flat

ANSWERS

139. *Answer:* 2
Rationale: To facilitate removal of fluid from the chest, the client is positioned sitting at the edge of the bed leaning over the bedside table, with the feet supported on a stool; or lying in bed on the unaffected side with the head of the bed elevated 30 to 45 degrees. The prone and Sims' positions are inappropriate positions for this procedure.
Test-Taking Strategy: Focus on the subject, positioning for thoracentesis. To perform a thoracentesis safely, the site must be visible to the primary health care provider (PHCP) performing the procedure. The client should be placed in a position where he or she is as comfortable as possible with access to the affected side. A prone position would not give the PHCP access to the chest. Lying on the affected side would prevent access to the site.
Level of Cognitive Ability: Applying
Client Needs: Physiological Integrity
Integrated Process: Nursing Process—Implementation
Content Area: Foundations of Care: Diagnostic Tests
Health Problem: N/A
Priority Concepts: Clinical Judgment; Safety
Reference: Lewis et al. (2017), p. 471.

140. *Answer:* 1
Rationale: Clients who have undergone craniotomy should have the head of the bed elevated 30 to 45 degrees to promote venous drainage from the head. The client is positioned to avoid extreme hip or neck flexion and the head is maintained in a midline neutral position. The client should not be positioned on the site that was operated on, especially if the bone flap was removed, because the brain has no bony covering on the affected site. A flat position or Trendelenburg's position would increase intracranial pressure. A reverse Trendelenburg's position would not be helpful and may be uncomfortable for the client.
Test-Taking Strategy: Focus on the subject, positioning after craniotomy. Remember that a primary concern is the risk for increased intracranial pressure. Therefore, use concepts related to gravity and preventing edema and increased intracranial pressure to answer this question.
Level of Cognitive Ability: Analyzing
Client Needs: Physiological Integrity
Integrated Process: Nursing Process—Implementation
Content Area: Foundations of Care: Safety
Health Problem: Adult Health: Cancer: Brain Tumors
Priority Concepts: Intracranial Regulation; Safety
Reference: Ignatavicius, Workman, Rebar (2018), p. 953.

141. *Answer:* 3
Rationale: For the client with deep vein thrombosis, elevation of the affected leg facilitates blood flow by the force of gravity and also decreases venous pressure, which in turn relieves edema and pain. A flat or dependent position of the leg would not achieve this goal. Bed rest is indicated to prevent emboli and to prevent pressure fluctuations in the venous system that occur with walking.
Test-Taking Strategy: Focus on the subject, the safe position or activity for the client with deep vein thrombosis. Think about the pathophysiology associated with this disorder and the principles related to gravity flow and edema to answer the question.
Level of Cognitive Ability: Creating
Client Needs: Physiological Integrity
Integrated Process: Nursing Process—Planning
Content Area: Foundations of Care: Safety
Health Problem: Adult Health: Cardiovascular: Vascular Disorders
Priority Concepts: Perfusion; Safety
Reference: Lewis et al. (2017), p. 823.

142. *Answer:* 2
Rationale: Positioning after a total hip replacement depends on the surgical techniques used, the method of implantation, the prosthesis, and the primary health care provider's (PHCP's) preference. Abduction is maintained when the client is in a supine position or positioned on the nonoperative side. Internal and external rotation, adduction, or lying on the operative side (unless specifically prescribed by the PHCP) is avoided to prevent displacement of the prosthesis.
Test-Taking Strategy: Focus on the strategic word, *best.* Use knowledge regarding care of clients after total hip replacement to answer this question. After a total hip replacement, the client should never have the extremity internally or externally rotated. Lying on the surgical side can cause damage to the surgical replacement site.
Level of Cognitive Ability: Applying
Client Needs: Physiological Integrity
Integrated Process: Implementation
Content Area: Foundations of Care: Safety
Health Problem: Adult Health: Musculoskeletal: Skeletal Injury
Priority Concepts: Mobility; Safety
Reference: Lewis et al. (2017), p. 1483.

143. *Answer:* 1
Rationale: After cataract surgery, the client should not sleep on the side of the body that was operated on to prevent edema formation and intraocular pressure. The client also should be placed in a semi-Fowler's position to assist in minimizing edema and intraocular pressure. During the day, the client may wear glasses or a protective shield; at night, the protective shield alone is sufficient.
Test-Taking Strategy: Focus on the subject, right cataract surgery. Use of the principles of gravity and edema formation will assist in answering this question. Remember to instruct the client to remain off the operative side and to rest with the head elevated to minimize edema formation. This will assist you when answering questions related to cataract surgery.
Level of Cognitive Ability: Evaluating
Client Needs: Physiological Integrity
Integrated Process: Nursing Process—Evaluation
Content Area: Foundations of Care: Safety
Health Problem: Adult Health: Eye: Cataracts
Priority Concepts: Client Teaching; Sensory Perception
Reference: Lewis et al. (2017), pp. 375-376.

144. *Answer:* 1
Rationale: For administering an enema, the client is placed in a left Sims' position so that the enema solution can flow by gravity in the natural direction of the colon. The head of the bed is not elevated in the Sims' position.

Test-Taking Strategy: Focus on the subject, positioning for enema administration. Use knowledge regarding the anatomy of the bowel to answer the question. The descending colon is located on the lower left side of the body. The head of the bed should be flat during enema administration.
Level of Cognitive Ability: Applying
Client Needs: Physiological Integrity
Integrated Process: Nursing Process—Implementation
Content Area: Skills: Elimination
Health Problem: Adult Health: Gastrointestinal: Lower GI Disorders
Priority Concepts: Elimination; Safety
Reference: Potter et al. (2017), p. 1171.

145. ***Answer:*** **4**
Rationale: The residual limb is usually supported on pillows for the first 24 hours after surgery to promote venous return and decrease edema. After the first 24 hours, the residual limb usually is placed flat on the bed to reduce hip contracture. Edema also is controlled by limb-wrapping techniques. In addition, it is important to check the primary health care provider's or surgeon's prescriptions regarding positioning after amputation, because there are often differences in preference in terms of positioning after the procedure related to risks associated with hip and knee contracture.
Test-Taking Strategy: Focus on the subject, positioning after amputation, and note that the client has just returned from surgery. Using basic principles related to immediate postoperative care and preventing edema will assist in directing you to the correct option.
Level of Cognitive Ability: Applying
Client Needs: Physiological Integrity
Integrated Process: Nursing Process—Implementation
Content Area: Foundations of Care: Perioperative Care
Health Problem: Adult Health: Musculoskeletal: Amputation
Priority Concepts: Perfusion; Tissue Integrity
Reference: Ignatavicius, Workman, Rebar (2018), p. 1054.

146. ***Answer:*** **2**
Rationale: Autografts placed over joints or on lower extremities are elevated and immobilized after surgery for 3 to 7 days, depending on the surgeon's preference. This period of immobilization allows the autograft time to adhere and attach to the wound bed, and the elevation minimizes edema. Keeping the client in a prone position and covering the extremity with a blanket can disrupt the graft site.
Test-Taking Strategy: Focus on the subject, positioning after autograft. Use general postoperative principles; elevating the graft site will decrease edema to the graft. The client should not be placed in a prone position or have it covered after surgery, because this can disrupt a graft easily.
Level of Cognitive Ability: Creating
Client Needs: Physiological Integrity
Integrated Process: Nursing Process—Planning
Content Area: Foundations of Care: Perioperative Care
Health Problem: Adult Health: Integumentary: Burns
Priority Concepts: Perfusion; Tissue Integrity
Reference: Ignatavicius, Workman, Rebar (2018), pp. 500-501.

147. ***Answer:*** **4**
Rationale: After cardiac catheterization, the extremity into which the catheter was inserted is kept straight for 4 to 6 hours. The client is maintained on bed rest for 4 to 6 hours (time for bed rest may vary depending on the primary health care provider's (PHCPs) preference and on whether a vascular closure device was used), and the client may turn from side to side. The head is elevated no more than 30 degrees (although some PHCPs prefer a lower position or the flat position) until hemostasis is adequately achieved.
Test-Taking Strategy: Focus on the subject, positioning after cardiac catheterization. Think about this diagnostic procedure and what it entails. Understanding that the head of the bed is never elevated more than 30 degrees and bathroom privileges are restricted in the immediate postcatheterization period will assist in answering this question.
Level of Cognitive Ability: Applying
Client Needs: Physiological Integrity
Integrated Process: Nursing Process—Planning
Content Area: Foundations of Care: Diagnostic Tests
Health Problem: N/A
Priority Concepts: Perfusion; Safety
Reference: Ignatavicius, Workman, Rebar (2018), p. 659.

148. ***Answer:*** **3**
Rationale: During insertion of a nasogastric tube, the client is placed in a sitting or high-Fowler's position to facilitate insertion of the tube and reduce the risk of pulmonary aspiration if the client should vomit. The right side and low-Fowler's and supine positions place the client at risk for aspiration; in addition, these positions do not facilitate insertion of the tube.
Test-Taking Strategy: Focus on the subject, insertion of a nasogastric tube. Visualize each position and think about how it may facilitate insertion of the tube. Also, recall that a concern with insertion of a nasogastric tube is pulmonary aspiration. Placing the client in a high-Fowler's position with his or her chin to the chest will decrease the risk of aspiration.
Level of Cognitive Ability: Applying
Client Needs: Physiological Integrity
Integrated Process: Nursing Process—Implementation
Content Area: Skills: Tube Care
Health Problem: N/A
Priority Concepts: Clinical Judgment; Safety
Reference: Potter et al. (2017), p. 1086.

UNIT IV

Growth and Development Across the Life Span

Pyramid to Success

Normal growth and development proceed in an orderly, systematic, and predictable pattern, which provides a basis for identifying and assessing an individual's abilities. Understanding the normal path of growth and development across the life span assists the nurse in identifying appropriate and expected human behavior. The Pyramid to Success focuses on Sigmund Freud's theory of psychosexual development, Jean Piaget's theory of cognitive development, Erik Erikson's psychosocial theory, and Lawrence Kohlberg's theory of moral development. Growth and development concepts also focus on the aging process and on physical characteristics, nutritional behaviors, skills, play, and specific safety measures relevant to a particular age group that will ensure a safe and hazard-free environment. When a question is presented on the NCLEX-RN® examination, if an age is identified in the question, note the age and think about the associated growth and developmental concepts to answer the question correctly.

Client Needs: Learning Objectives

Safe and Effective Care Environment

Acting as a client advocate
Communicating with the interprofessional health care team
Ensuring home safety and security plans
Ensuring that informed consent has been obtained for invasive treatments or procedures
Establishing priorities of care
Maintaining confidentiality
Preventing accidents and errors considering risks related to age
Providing care in accordance with ethical and legal standards
Providing care using a nonjudgmental approach
Respecting client and family needs, based on their preferences
Upholding the client's rights

Health Promotion and Maintenance

Discussing high-risk behaviors and lifestyle choices
Identifying changes that occur as a result of the aging process
Identifying developmental stages and transitions
Maintaining health and wellness and self-care measures
Monitoring growth and development
Performing the necessary health and physical assessment techniques based on age
Providing client and family education
Respecting health care beliefs and preferences

Psychosocial Integrity

Assessing for abuse and neglect
Considering grief and loss issues and end-of-life care
Identifying coping mechanisms
Identifying cultural, religious, and spiritual practices and beliefs of the client and appropriate support systems
Identifying loss of quantity and quality of relationships with the older client
Monitoring for adjustment to potential deterioration in physical and mental health and well-being in the older client
Monitoring for changes and adjustment in role function in the older client (threat to independent functioning)
Monitoring for sensory and perceptual alterations
Providing resources for the client and family

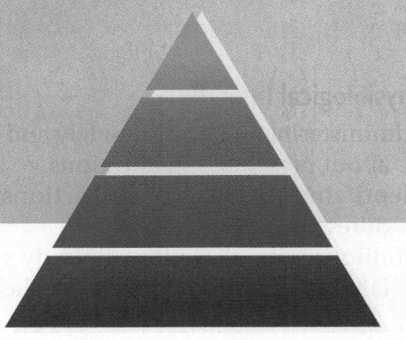

Physiological Integrity

Administering medication safely and teaching the client about prescribed medications

Identifying practices or restrictions related to procedures and treatments

Monitoring for alterations in body systems and the related risks associated with the client's age

Providing basic care and comfort needs

Providing interventions compatible with the client's age; cultural, spiritual, religious, and health care beliefs; education level; and language

CHAPTER 17

Theories of Growth and Development

PRIORITY CONCEPTS **Development, Health Promotion**

I. Psychosocial Development: Erik Erikson

A. The theory
   1. Erikson's theory of psychosocial development describes the human life cycle as a series of 8 developmental stages from birth to death.
   2. Each stage presents a psychosocial crisis in which the goal is to integrate physical, maturation, and societal demands.
   3. The result of 1 stage may not be permanent, but can be changed by experience(s) later in life.
   4. The theory focuses on psychosocial tasks that should be accomplished throughout the life cycle.

B. Psychosocial development: Occurs through a lifelong series of crises affected by social and cultural factors

According to Erikson's theory of psychosocial development, each psychosocial crisis must be resolved for the child or adult to progress emotionally. Unsuccessful resolution can leave the person emotionally disabled.

C. Stages of psychosocial development (Table 17-1)

D. Interventions to assist the client in achieving Erikson's stages of development (Box 17-1)

II. Cognitive Development: Jean Piaget

A. The theory
   1. Piaget's theory of cognitive development defines cognitive acts as ways in which the mind organizes and adapts to its environment (i.e., "mental mapping").
   2. *Schema* refers to an individual's cognitive structure or framework of thought.
   3. Schemata
      a. Schemata are categories that an individual forms in his or her mind to organize and understand the world.
      b. A young child has only a few schemata with which to understand the world, and gradually these are increased in number.
      c. Adults use a wide variety of schemata to understand the world.
   4. Assimilation
      a. Assimilation is the ability to incorporate new ideas, objects, and experiences into the framework of one's thoughts.
      b. The growing child will perceive and give meaning to new information according to what is already known and understood.
   5. Accommodation
      a. Accommodation is the ability to change a schema to introduce new ideas, objects, or experiences.
      b. Accommodation changes the mental structure so that new experiences can be added.

B. Stages of cognitive development
   1. Sensorimotor stage
      a. Birth to 2 years
      b. Development proceeds from reflex activity to imagining and solving problems through the senses and movement.
      c. The infant or toddler learns about reality and how it works.
      d. The infant or toddler does not recognize that objects continue to be in existence if they are out of the visual field.
   2. Preoperational stage
      a. 2 to 7 years
      b. The child learns to think in terms of past, present, and future.
      c. The child moves from knowing the world through sensation and movement to prelogical thinking and finding solutions to problems.
      d. The child is egocentric.
      e. The child is unable to conceptualize and requires concrete examples.
   3. Concrete operational
      a. 7 to 11 years
      b. The child is able to classify, order, and sort facts.
      c. The child moves from prelogical thought to solving concrete problems through logic.
      d. The child begins to develop abstract thinking.
      e. The child is less egocentric and thinks about how others may view a situation.

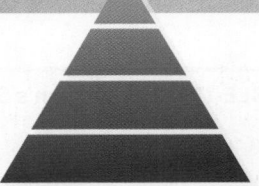

TABLE 17-1 Erik Erikson's Stages of Psychosocial Development

Age	Psychosocial Crisis	Task	Resolution of Crisis: Successful	Resolution of Crisis: Unsuccessful
Infancy (birth to 18 mo)	Trust versus mistrust	Attachment to the primary caregiver	Trust in persons; faith and hope about the environment and future	General difficulties relating to persons effectively; suspicion; trust-fear conflict, fear of the future
Early childhood (18 mo to 3 yr)	Autonomy versus shame and doubt	Gaining some basic control over self and environment	Sense of self-control and adequacy; willpower	Independence-fear conflict; severe feelings of self-doubt; lack self-control
Late childhood (3-6 yr)	Initiative versus guilt	Becoming purposeful and directive	Ability to initiate one's own activities; sense of purpose	Aggression-fear conflict; sense of inadequacy or guilt
School age (6-12 yr)	Industry versus inferiority	Developing social, physical, and learning skills	Competence; ability to learn and work	Sense of inferiority; difficulty learning and working
Adolescence (12-20 yr)	Identity versus role confusion	Developing sense of identity	Sense of personal identity	Unsure about one's identity; have a weak sense of self, experience role confusion, and are confused about the future
Early adulthood (20-35 yr)	Intimacy versus isolation	Establishing intimate bonds of love and friendship	Ability to love deeply and commit oneself	Emotional isolation, egocentricity
Middle adulthood (35-65 yr)	Generativity versus stagnation	Fulfilling life goals that involve family, career, and society	Ability to give and care for others	Self-absorption; inability to grow as a person
Later adulthood (65 yr to death)	Integrity versus despair	Looking back over one's life and accepting its meaning	Sense of integrity and fulfillment	Dissatisfaction with life

Adapted from Varcarolis E: *Foundations of psychiatric mental health nursing*, ed 6, St. Louis, 2010, Saunders.

BOX 17-1 Interventions to Assist the Client in Achieving Erikson's Stages of Development

Infancy
Hold the infant often.
Offer comfort after painful procedures.
Meet the infant's needs for food and hygiene.
Encourage parents to play an active role while the infant is hospitalized.

Early Childhood
Allow self-feeding opportunities.
Encourage child to remove and put on own clothes.
Allow for choice.

Late Childhood
Offer medical equipment for play.
Respect the child's choices and expressions of feelings.

School Age
Encourage the child to continue schoolwork while hospitalized.
Encourage the child to bring favorite pastimes to the hospital.

Adolescence
Take the health history and perform examinations without parents present.
Allow adolescent a choice in the plan of care.

Early Adulthood
Include support from client's partner or significant other.
Assist with rehabilitation and contacting support services as needed before return to work.

Middle Adulthood
Assist in choosing creative ways to foster social development.
Encourage volunteer activities.

Later Adulthood
Listen attentively to reminiscent stories about his or her life's accomplishments.
Assist with making changes to living arrangements.

4. Formal operational
   a. 11 years to adulthood
   b. The person is able to think abstractly and logically.
   c. Logical thinking is expanded to include solving abstract and concrete problems.

III. Moral Development: Lawrence Kohlberg

A. Moral development
   1. Moral development is a complicated process involving the acceptance of the values and rules of society in a way that shapes behavior.
   2. Moral development is classified in a series of levels and behaviors.
   3. Moral development is sequential.
   4. Stages or levels of moral development cannot be skipped.

B. Levels of moral development (Box 17-2)

IV. Psychosexual Development: Sigmund Freud

A. Components of the theory (Box 17-3)

B. Levels of awareness
   1. Unconscious level of awareness

BOX 17-2 Moral Development: Lawrence Kohlberg

Level One: Preconventional Morality

Stage 0 (Birth to 2 Years): Egocentric Judgment

The infant has no awareness of right or wrong.

Stage 1 (2 to 4 Years): Punishment-Obedience Orientation

At this stage, children cannot reason as mature members of society.

Children view the world in a selfish way, with no real understanding of right or wrong.

The child obeys rules and demonstrates acceptable behavior to avoid punishment and to avoid displeasing those who are in power, and because the child fears punishment from a superior force, such as a parent.

A toddler typically is at the first substage of the preconventional stage, involving punishment and obedience orientation, in which the toddler makes judgments based on avoiding punishment or obtaining a reward.

Physical punishment and withholding privileges tend to give the toddler a negative view of morals.

Withdrawing love and affection as punishment leads to feelings of guilt in the toddler.

Appropriate discipline includes providing simple explanations of why certain behaviors are unacceptable, praising appropriate behavior, and using distractions when the toddler is headed for an unsafe action.

Stage 2 (4 to 7 Years): Instrumental Relativist Orientation

The child conforms to rules to obtain rewards or have favors returned.

The child's moral standards are those of others, and the child observes them either to avoid punishment or obtain rewards.

A preschooler is in the preconventional stage of moral development.

In this stage, conscience emerges and the emphasis is on external control.

Level Two: Conventional Morality

The child conforms to rules to please others.

The child has increased awareness of others' feelings.

A concern for social order begins to emerge.

A child views good behavior as that which those in authority will approve.

If the behavior is not acceptable, the child feels guilty.

Stage 3 (7 to 10 Years): Good Boy or Nice Girl Orientation

Conformity occurs to avoid disapproval or dislike by others.

This stage involves living up to what is expected by individuals close to the child or what individuals generally expect of others in their roles such as daughter, son, brother, sister, and friend.

Being good is important and is interpreted as having good motives and showing concern about others.

Being good also means maintaining mutual relationships, such as trust, loyalty, respect, and gratitude.

Stage 4 (10 to 12 Years): Law and Order Orientation

The child considers society as a whole when making judgments.

Emphasis is on obeying laws to maintain social order.

Moral reasoning develops as the child shifts the focus of living to society.

The school-age child is at the conventional level of the conformity stage and has an increased desire to please others.

The child observes and to some extent internalizes the standards of others.

The child wants to be considered "good" by those individuals whose opinions matter to her or him.

Level Three: Postconventional Morality

The individual focuses on individual rights and principles of conscience.

The focus is on concerns regarding what is best for all.

Stage 5: Social Contract and Legalistic Orientation

The person is aware that others hold a variety of values and opinions and that most values and rules are relative to the group.

The adolescent in this stage gives and takes and does not expect to get something without paying for it.

At this stage, the person may disobey rules if they feel they are inconsistent with their personal values.

Stage 6: Universal Ethical Principles Orientation

Conformity is based on universal principles of justice and occurs to avoid self-condemnation.

This stage involves following self-chosen ethical principles.

The development of the postconventional level of morality occurs in the adolescent at about age 13 years, marked by the development of an individual conscience and a defined set of moral values.

The adolescent can now acknowledge a conflict between 2 socially accepted standards and try to decide between them.

Control of conduct is now internal in standards observed and in reasoning about right and wrong.

BOX 17-3 Components of Sigmund Freud's Psychosexual Development Theory

- Levels of awareness
- Agencies of the mind (id, ego, superego)
- Concept of anxiety and defense mechanisms
- Psychosexual stages of development

a. The unconscious is not logical and is governed by the Pleasure Principle, which refers to seeking immediate tension reduction.
b. Memories, feelings, thoughts, or wishes are repressed and are not available to the conscious mind.
c. These repressed memories, thoughts, or feelings, if made prematurely conscious, can cause anxiety

2. Preconscious level of awareness
   a. The preconscious is called the *subconscious*.
   b. The preconscious includes experiences, thoughts, feelings, or desires that might not be in immediate awareness but can be recalled to consciousness.
   c. The subconscious can help repress unpleasant thoughts or feelings and can examine and censor certain wishes and thinking.
3. Conscious level of awareness
   a. The conscious mind is logical and is regulated by the Reality Principle.
   b. Consciousness includes all experiences that are within an individual's awareness and that the individual is able to control and includes all information that is remembered easily and is immediately available to an individual.

C. Agencies of the mind: id, ego, and superego

! The id, ego, and superego are the 3 systems of personality. These psychological processes follow different operating principles. In a mature and well-adjusted personality, they work together as a team under the leadership of the ego.

1. The id
   a. Source of all drives, present at birth; operates according to the Pleasure Principle
   b. Does not tolerate uncomfortable states and seeks to discharge the tension and return to a more comfortable, constant level of energy
   c. Acts immediately in an impulsive, irrational way and pays no attention to the consequences of its actions; therefore, often behaves in ways harmful to self and others
   d. The primary process is a psychological activity in which the id attempts to reduce tension.
   e. The primary process by itself is not capable of reducing tension; therefore, a secondary psychological process must develop if the individual is to survive. When this occurs, the structure of the second system of the personality, the ego, begins to take form.
2. The ego
   a. Functions include reality testing and problem solving; follows the Reality Principle
   b. Begins its development during the fourth or fifth month of life
   c. Emerges out of the id and acts as an intermediary between the id and the external world
   d. Emerges because the needs, wishes, and demands of the id require appropriate exchanges with reality
   e. The ego distinguishes between things in the mind and things in the external world.
3. The superego
   a. Necessary part of socialization that develops during the phallic stage at 3 to 6 years of age
   b. Develops from interactions with the child's parents during the extended period of childhood dependency
   c. Includes internalization of the values, ideals, and moral standards of parents and society
   d. Superego consists of the conscience and the ego ideal.
   e. Conscience refers to capacity for self-evaluation and criticism; when moral codes are violated, the conscience punishes the individual by instilling guilt.

D. Anxiety and defense mechanisms
1. The ego develops defenses or defense mechanisms to fight off anxiety.
2. Defense mechanisms operate on an unconscious level, except for suppression, so the individual is not aware of their operation.
3. Defense mechanisms deny, falsify, or distort reality to make it less threatening.
4. An individual cannot survive without defense mechanisms; however, if the individual becomes too extreme in distorting reality, interference with healthy adjustment and personal growth may occur.

E. Psychosexual stages of development (Box 17-4)
1. Human development proceeds through a series of stages from infancy to adulthood.
2. Each stage is characterized by the inborn tendency of all individuals to reduce tension and seek pleasure.
3. Each stage is associated with a particular conflict that must be resolved before the child can move successfully to the next stage.
4. Experiences during the early stages determine an individual's adjustment patterns and the personality traits that the individual has as an adult.

BOX 17-4 Freud's Psychosexual Stages of Development

Oral Stage (Birth to 1 Year)

During this stage, the infant is concerned with self-gratification.

The infant is all id, operating on the Pleasure Principle and striving for immediate gratification of needs.

When the infant experiences gratification of basic needs, a sense of trust and security begins.

The ego begins to emerge as the infant begins to see self as separate from the caregiver; this marks the beginning of the development of a sense of self.

Anal Stage (1 to 3 Years)

Toilet training occurs during this period, and the child gains pleasure from learning to control his or her bodily needs. It provides a sense of accomplishment and independence.

The conflict of this stage is between those demands from society and the parents and the sensations of pleasure associated with the anus.

The child begins to gain a sense of control over instinctive drives and learns to delay immediate gratification to gain a future goal.

Phallic Stage (3 to 6 Years)

The child experiences pleasurable and conflicting feelings associated with the genital organs.

The pleasures of masturbation and the fantasy life of children set the stage for the Oedipus complex.

The child's unconscious sexual attraction to and wish to possess the parent of the opposite sex, the hostility and desire to remove the parent of the same sex, and the subsequent guilt about these wishes constitute the conflict the child faces.

The conflict is resolved when the child begins to identify with the parent of the same sex.

The emergence of the superego is the solution to and the result of these intense impulses.

Latency Stage (6 to 12 Years)

The latency stage is a tapering off of conscious biological and sexual urges.

The sexual impulses are channeled and elevated into a more culturally accepted level of activity such as intellectual pursuits and social communication.

Growth of ego functions and the ability to care about and relate to others outside the home is the task of this stage of development.

Genital Stage (12 Years and Beyond)

The genital stage emerges at adolescence with the onset of puberty, when the genital organs mature.

The individual gains gratification from his or her own body.

During this stage, the individual develops satisfying sexual and emotional relationships with members of the opposite sex.

The individual plans life goals and gains a strong sense of personal identity.

PRACTICE QUESTIONS

149. The clinic nurse is preparing to explain the concepts of Kohlberg's theory of moral development with a parent. The nurse should tell the parent that which factor motivates good and bad actions for the child at the preconventional level?

1. Peer pressure
2. Social pressure
3. Parents' behavior
4. Punishment and reward

150. The maternity nurse is providing instructions to a new mother regarding the psychosocial development of the newborn infant. Using Erikson's psychosocial development theory, the nurse instructs the mother to take which measure?

1. Allow the newborn infant to signal a need.
2. Anticipate all needs of the newborn infant.
3. Attend to the newborn infant immediately when crying.
4. Avoid the newborn infant during the first 10 minutes of crying.

151. The nurse notes that a 6-year-old child does not recognize that objects exist when the objects are outside of the visual field. Based on this observation, which action should the nurse take?

1. Report the observation to the pediatrician
2. Move the objects in the child's direct field of vision.
3. Teach the child how to visually scan the environment.
4. Provide additional lighting for the child during play activities.

152. A nursing student is presenting a clinical conference to peers regarding Freud's psychosexual stages of development, specifically the anal stage. The student explains to the group that which characteristic relates to the anal stage?

1. This stage is associated with toilet training.
2. This stage is characterized by the gratification of self.
3. This stage is characterized by a tapering off of conscious biological and sexual urges.
4. This stage is associated with pleasurable and conflicting feelings about the genital organs.

153. The nurse is describing Piaget's cognitive developmental theory to pediatric nursing staff. The nurse should tell that staff that which child behavior is characteristic of the formal operations stage?

1. The child has the ability to think abstractly.
2. The child begins to understand the environment.

3. The child is able to classify, order, and sort facts.
4. The child learns to think in terms of past, present, and future.

154. The mother of an 8-year-old child tells the clinic nurse that she is concerned about the child because the child seems to be more attentive to friends than anything else. Using Erikson's psychosocial development theory, the nurse should make which response?
1. "You need to be concerned."
2. "You need to monitor the child's behavior closely."
3. "At this age, the child is developing his own personality."
4. "You need to provide more praise to the child to stop this behavior."

155. The nurse educator is preparing to conduct a teaching session for the nursing staff regarding the theories of growth and development and plans to discuss Kohlberg's theory of moral development. What information should the nurse include in the session? **Select all that apply.**
- ☐ 1. Individuals move through all 6 stages in a sequential fashion.
- ☐ 2. Moral development progresses in relationship to cognitive development.
- ☐ 3. A person's ability to make moral judgments develops over a period of time.
- ☐ 4. The theory provides a framework for understanding how individuals determine a moral code to guide their behavior.
- ☐ 5. In stage 1 (punishment-obedience orientation), children are expected to reason as mature members of society.
- ☐ 6. In stage 2 (instrumental-relativist orientation), the child conforms to rules to obtain rewards or have favors returned.

156. A parent of a 3-year-old tells a clinic nurse that the child is rebelling constantly and having temper tantrums. Using Erikson's psychosocial development theory, which instructions should the nurse provide to the parent? **Select all that apply.**
- ☐ 1. Set limits on the child's behavior.
- ☐ 2. Ignore the child when this behavior occurs.
- ☐ 3. Allow the behavior, because this is normal at this age period.
- ☐ 4. Provide a simple explanation of why the behavior is unacceptable.
- ☐ 5. Punish the child every time the child says "no" to change the behavior.

ANSWERS

149. ***Answer:*** **4**
Rationale: In the preconventional stage, morals are thought to be motivated by punishment and reward. If the child is obedient and is not punished, then the child is being moral. The child sees actions as good or bad. If the child's actions are good, the child is praised. If the child's actions are bad, the child is punished. Options 1, 2, and 3 are not associated factors for this stage of moral development.
Test-Taking Strategy: Eliminate options 1 and 2; they are comparable or alike because peer pressure is the same as social pressure. To select from the remaining options, recalling that the preconventional stage occurs between birth and 7 years will assist in directing you to the correct option.
Level of Cognitive Ability: Applying
Client Needs: Health Promotion and Maintenance
Integrated Process: Teaching and Learning
Content Area: Developmental Stages: Toddler
Health Problem: N/A
Priority Concepts: Client Education; Development
Reference: McKinney et al. (2018), pp. 67, 70.

150. ***Answer:*** **1**
Rationale: According to Erikson, the caregiver should not try to anticipate the newborn infant's needs at all times but must allow the newborn infant to signal needs. If a newborn infant is not allowed to signal a need, the newborn will not learn how to control the environment. Erikson believed that a delayed or prolonged response to a newborn infant's signal would inhibit the development of trust and lead to mistrust of others.
Test-Taking Strategy: Eliminate options 2, 3, and 4 because of the closed-ended words "all," "immediately," and "avoid," in these options.
Level of Cognitive Ability: Applying
Client Needs: Health Promotion and Maintenance
Integrated Process: Teaching and Learning
Content Area: Developmental Stages: Infant
Priority Concepts: Client Education; Development
Reference: McKinney et al. (2018), pp. 67, 69.

151. ***Answer:*** **1**
Rationale: According to Jean Piaget's theory of cognitive development, it is normal for the infant or toddler not to recognize that objects continue to be in existence if out of the visual field; however, this is abnormal for the 6-year-old. If a 6-year-old child does not recognize that objects still exist even when outside the visual field, the child is not progressing normally through the developmental stages. The nurse should report this finding to the pediatrician. Options 2, 3, and 4 delay necessary follow-up and treatment.
Test-Taking Strategy: Focus on the data in the question. Also, note the age of the child and think about developmental concepts related to this age. Noting that the child is not able to recognize that objects continue to be in existence, even if out of the visual field, will direct you to the correct option. Also, note that options 2, 3, and 4 are comparable or alike and are interventions that will delay follow-up for an abnormal observation.

Level of Cognitive Ability: Applying
Client Needs: Physiological Integrity
Integrated Process: Nursing Process—Implementation
Content Area: Developmental Stages: Preschool and School Age
Health Problem: N/A
Priority Concepts: Clinical Judgment; Development
Reference: McKinney et al. (2018), pp. 67-69.

152. *Answer:* 1
Rationale: In general, toilet training occurs during the anal stage. According to Freud, the child gains pleasure from the elimination of feces and from their retention. Option 2 relates to the oral stage. Option 3 relates to the latency period. Option 4 relates to the phallic stage.
Test-Taking Strategy: Focus on the **subject,** the anal stage. Note the relationship between the words *anal* in the question and *toilet training* in the correct option.
Level of Cognitive Ability: Applying
Client Needs: Health Promotion and Maintenance
Integrated Process: Teaching and Learning
Content Area: Development Stages: Toddler
Health Problem: N/A
Priority Concepts: Development; Health Promotion
Reference: Hockenberry, Wilson, Rodgers (2017), p. 44.

153. *Answer:* 1
Rationale: In the formal operations stage, the child has the ability to think abstractly and logically. Option 2 identifies the sensorimotor stage. Option 3 identifies the concrete operational stage. Option 4 identifies the preoperational stage.
Test-Taking Strategy: Focus on the **subject,** the formal operational stage of Piaget's cognitive developmental theory, and note the relationship between the **subject** and the description in the correct option. Remember that in the formal operations stage, the child has the ability to think abstractly and logically.
Level of Cognitive Ability: Applying
Client Needs: Health Promotion and Maintenance
Integrated Process: Teaching and Learning
Content Area: Developmental Stages: Preschool and School Age
Health Problem: N/A
Priority Concepts: Client Education; Development
Reference: Hockenberry, Wilson, Rodgers (2017), pp. 45-46.

154. *Answer:* 3
Rationale: According to Erikson, during school-age years (6 to 12 years of age), the child begins to move toward peers and friends and away from the parents for support. The child also begins to develop special interests that reflect his or her own developing personality instead of the parents'. Therefore, options 1, 2, and 4 are incorrect responses.
Test-Taking Strategy: Use knowledge of Erikson's psychosocial development theory related to middle childhood. Options 1 and 2 can be eliminated first because they are **comparable or alike** and indicate that the mother should be concerned about the child. Eliminate option 4 next because although praising the child for accomplishments is important at this age, the behavior that the child is exhibiting is normal.
Level of Cognitive Ability: Applying
Client Needs: Health Promotion and Maintenance
Integrated Process: Nursing Process—Implementation
Content Area: Developmental Stages: Preschool and School Age
Health Problem: N/A
Priority Concepts: Development; Health Promotion
Reference: Hockenberry, Wilson, Rodgers (2017), pp. 430-431.

155. *Answer:* 2, 3, 4, 6
Rationale: Kohlberg's theory states that individuals move through stages of development in a sequential fashion but that not everyone reaches stages 5 and 6 in his or her development of personal morality. The theory provides a framework for understanding how individuals determine a moral code to guide their behavior. It states that moral development progresses in relationship to cognitive development and that a person's ability to make moral judgments develops over a period of time. In stage 1, ages 2 to 3 years (punishment-obedience orientation), children cannot reason as mature members of society. In stage 2, ages 4 to 7 years (instrumental-relativist orientation), the child conforms to rules to obtain rewards or have favors returned.
Test-Taking Strategy: Read each option carefully. Recalling that the theory provides a framework for understanding how individuals determine a moral code to guide their behavior and recalling the ages associated with each stage will assist in answering the question. Also noting the **closed-ended word** "all" in option 1 and the word *mature* in option 5 will assist in eliminating these options.
Level of Cognitive Ability: Applying
Client Needs: Health Promotion and Maintenance
Integrated Process: Teaching and Learning
Content Area: Developmental Stages: Infant
Health Problem: N/A
Priority Concepts: Client Education; Development
Reference: McKinney et al. (2018), pp. 67-68.

156. *Answer:* 1, 4
Rationale: According to Erikson, the child focuses on gaining some basic control over self and the environment and independence between ages 1 and 3 years. Gaining independence often means that the child has to rebel against the parents' wishes. Saying things like "no" or "mine" and having temper tantrums are common during this period of development. Being consistent and setting limits on the child's behavior are necessary elements. Providing a simple explanation of why certain behaviors are unacceptable is an appropriate action. Options 2 and 3 do not address the child's behavior. Option 5 is likely to produce a negative response during this normal developmental pattern.
Test-Taking Strategy: Options 2 and 3 can be eliminated first because they are **comparable or alike,** indicating that the mother should not address the child's behavior. Next, eliminate option 5, because this action is likely to produce a negative response during this normal developmental pattern. Also, note the **closed-ended word** "every" in option 5.
Level of Cognitive Ability: Applying
Client Needs: Health Promotion and Maintenance
Integrated Process: Teaching and Learning
Content Area: Developmental Stages: Toddler
Priority Concepts: Client Education; Development
Reference: Hockenberry, Wilson, Rodgers (2017), pp. 44-45.

CHAPTER 18

Growth, Development, and Stages of Life

PRIORITY CONCEPTS **Development, Family Dynamics**

I. The Hospitalized Infant and Toddler

A. Separation anxiety
1. Protest
a. Crying, screaming, searching for a parent; avoidance and rejection of contact with strangers
b. Verbal attacks on others
c. Physical fighting: Kicking, biting, hitting, pinching
2. Despair
a. Withdrawn, depressed, uninterested in the environment
b. Loss of newly learned skills
3. Detachment
a. Detachment is uncommon and occurs only after lengthy separations from the parent.
b. Superficially, the toddler appears to have adjusted to the loss.
c. During the detachment phase, the toddler again becomes more interested in the environment, plays with others, and seems to form new relationships; this behavior is a form of resignation and is not a sign of contentment.
d. The toddler detaches from the parent in an effort to escape the emotional pain of desiring the parent's presence.
e. During the detachment phase, the toddler copes by forming shallow relationships with others, becoming increasingly self-centered, and attaching primary importance to material objects.
f. Detachment is the most serious phase because reversal of the potential adverse effects is less likely to occur once detachment is established.
g. In most situations, the temporary separation imposed by hospitalization does not cause such prolonged parental absence that the toddler enters into detachment.

B. Fear of injury and pain: Affected by previous experiences, separation from parents, and preparation for the experience

C. Loss of control
1. Hospitalization, with its own set of rituals and routines, can severely disrupt the life of a toddler.
2. The lack of control often is exhibited in behaviors related to feeding, toileting, playing, and bedtime.
3. The toddler may demonstrate regression.

D. Interventions
1. Provide cuddling and touch and talk softly to the infant.
2. Provide opportunities for sucking and oral stimulation for the infant, using a pacifier if the infant is NPO (nothing by mouth).
3. Provide stimulation, if appropriate, for the infant, using objects of contrasting colors and textures.
4. Provide choices as much as possible to the toddler to enable him or her to have some control.
5. Approach the toddler with a positive attitude.
6. Allow the toddler to express feelings of protest.
7. Encourage the toddler to talk about parents or others in their lives.
8. Accept regressive behavior without ridiculing the toddler.
9. Provide the toddler with favorite and comforting objects.
10. Utilize play therapy for the toddler.
11. Allow the toddler as much mobility as possible.
12. Anticipate temper tantrums from the toddler and maintain a safe environment for physical acting out.
13. Employ pain reduction techniques, as appropriate.

For the hospitalized toddler, provide routines and rituals as close as possible to what he or she is used to at home.

II. The Hospitalized Preschooler

A. Separation anxiety
1. Separation anxiety is generally less obvious and less serious than in the toddler.

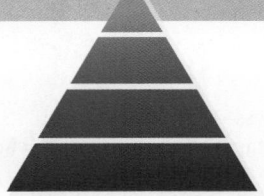

2. As stress increases, the preschooler's ability to separate from the parents decreases.
3. Protest
   a. Protest is less direct and aggressive than in the toddler.
   b. The preschooler may displace feelings onto others.
4. Despair
   a. The preschooler reacts in a manner similar to that of the toddler.
   b. The preschooler is quietly withdrawn, depressed, and uninterested in the environment.
   c. The child exhibits loss of newly learned skills.
   d. The preschooler becomes generally uncooperative, refusing to eat or take medication.
   e. The preschooler repeatedly asks when the parents will be visiting.
5. Detachment: Similar to the toddler

B. Fear of injury and pain
1. The preschooler has a general lack of understanding of body integrity.
2. The child fears invasive procedures and mutilation.
3. The child imagines things to be much worse than they are.
4. Preschoolers believe that they are ill because of something they did or thought.

C. Loss of control
1. The preschooler likes familiar routines and rituals and may show regression if not allowed to maintain some control.
2. Preschoolers' egocentric and magical thinking limits their ability to understand events, because they view all experiences from their own self-referenced (egocentric) perspective.
3. The child has attained a good deal of independence and self-care at home and may expect that to continue in the hospital.

D. Interventions
1. Provide a safe and secure environment.
2. Take time for communication.
3. Allow the preschooler to express anger.
4. Acknowledge fears and anxieties.
5. Accept regressive behavior; assist the preschooler in moving from regressive to appropriate behaviors according to age.
6. Encourage rooming-in or leaving a favorite toy.
7. Allow mobility and provide play and diversional activities.
8. Place the preschooler with other children of the same age if possible.
9. Encourage the preschooler to be independent.
10. Explain procedures simply, on the preschooler's level.
11. Avoid intrusive procedures when possible.
12. Allow the wearing of underpants.

III. The Hospitalized School-Age Child

A. Separation anxiety
1. The school-age child is accustomed to periods of separation from the parents, but as stressors are added, the separation becomes more difficult.
2. The child is more concerned with missing school and the fear that friends will forget her or him.
3. Usually, the stages of behavior of protest, despair, and detachment do not occur with school-age children.

B. Fear of injury and pain
1. The school-age child fears bodily injury and pain.
2. The child fears illness itself, disability, death, and intrusive procedures in genital areas.
3. The child is uncomfortable with any type of sexual examination.
4. The child groans or whines, holds rigidly still, and communicates about pain.

C. Loss of control
1. The child is usually highly social, independent, and involved with activities.
2. The child seeks information and asks relevant questions about tests and procedures and the illness.
3. The child associates his or her actions with the cause of the illness.
4. The child may feel helpless and dependent if physical limitations occur.

D. Interventions
1. Encourage rooming-in.
2. Focus on the school-age child's abilities and needs.
3. Encourage the school-age child to become involved with his or her own care.
4. Accept regression but encourage independence.
5. Provide choices to the school-age child.
6. Allow expression of feelings verbally and nonverbally.
7. Acknowledge fears and concerns and allow for discussion.
8. Explain all procedures, using body diagrams or outlines.
9. Provide privacy.
10. Avoid intrusive procedures if possible.
11. Allow the school-age child to wear underpants.
12. Involve the school-age child in activities appropriate to the developmental level and illness.
13. Encourage the school-age child to contact friends.
14. Provide for educational needs.
15. Use appropriate interventions to relieve pain.

IV. The Hospitalized Adolescent

A. Separation anxiety
1. Adolescents are not sure whether they want their parents with them when they are hospitalized.
2. Adolescents become upset if friends go on with their lives, excluding them.

For the hospitalized adolescent, separation from friends is a source of anxiety.

B. Fear of injury and pain
1. Adolescents fear being different from others and their peers.
2. Adolescents may give the impression that they are not afraid, even though they are terrified.
3. Adolescents become guarded when any areas related to sexual development are examined.

C. Loss of control
1. Behaviors exhibited include anger, withdrawal, and uncooperativeness.
2. Adolescents seek help and then reject it.

D. Interventions
1. Encourage questions about appearance and effects of the illness on the future.
2. Explore feelings about the hospital and the significance that the illness might have for relationships.
3. Encourage adolescents to wear their own clothes and carry out normal grooming activities.
4. Allow favorite foods to be brought into the hospital if possible.
5. Provide privacy.
6. Use body diagrams to prepare for procedures.
7. Introduce them to other adolescents in the nursing unit if appropriate and possible.
8. Encourage maintaining contact with peer groups.
9. Provide for educational needs.
10. Identify formation of future plans.
11. Help develop positive coping mechanisms.

V. Communication Approaches

A. General guidelines (Box 18-1)

B. Infant
1. Infants respond to nonverbal communication behaviors of adults, such as holding, rocking, patting, cuddling, and touching.
2. Use a slow approach and allow the infant to get to know the nurse.
3. Use a calm, soft, soothing voice.
4. Be responsive to cries.
5. Talk and read to infants.
6. Allow security objects such as blankets and pacifiers if the infant has them.

BOX 18-1 General Guidelines for Communication

Allow the child to feel comfortable with the nurse.
Communicate through the use of objects.
Allow the child to express fears and concerns.
Speak clearly and in a quiet, unhurried voice.
Offer choices when possible.
Be honest with the child.
Set limits with the child as appropriate.

C. Toddler
1. Approach the toddler cautiously.
2. Remember that toddlers accept the verbal communications of others literally.
3. Learn the toddler's words for common items and use them in conversations.
4. Use short, concrete terms.
5. Prepare the toddler for procedures immediately before the event.
6. Repeat explanations and descriptions.
7. Use play for demonstrations.
8. Use visual aids such as picture books, puppets, and dolls.
9. Allow the toddler to handle the equipment or instruments; explain what the equipment or instrument does and how it feels.
10. Encourage the use of comfort objects.

D. Preschooler
1. Seek opportunities to offer choices.
2. Speak in simple sentences.
3. Be concise and limit the length of explanations.
4. Allow asking questions.
5. Describe procedures as they are about to be performed.
6. Use play to explain procedures and activities.
7. Allow handling of equipment or instruments, which will ease fear and help to answer questions.

E. School-age child
1. Establish limits.
2. Provide reassurance to help in alleviating fears and anxieties.
3. Engage in conversations that encourage thinking.
4. Use medical play techniques.
5. Use photographs, books, dolls, and videos to explain procedures.
6. Explain in clear terms.
7. Allow time for composure and privacy.

F. Adolescent
1. Remember that the adolescent may be preoccupied with body image.
2. Encourage and support independence.
3. Provide privacy.
4. Use photographs, books, and videos to explain procedures.
5. Engage in conversations about the adolescent's interests.
6. Avoid becoming too abstract, too detailed, and too technical.
7. Avoid responding by prying, confronting, condescending, or expressing judgmental attitudes.

VI. Car Safety Seats and Guidelines

A. The safest place for all children to ride, regardless of age, is in the back seat of the car.

B. Lock the car doors; 4-door cars should be equipped with child safety locks on the back doors.

C. There are different types of car safety seats, and the manufacturer's guidelines need to be followed.

D. For specific information regarding car safety, refer to *Car seats: information for families* (copyright © 2018 American Academy of Pediatrics), found at https://www.healthychildren.org/English/safety-prevention/on-the-go/Pages/Car-Safety-Seats-Information-for-Families.aspx

VII. Preventive Pediatric Health Care

A. The American Academy of Pediatrics (AAP) and Bright Futures have developed guidelines regarding the recommended ages children should receive certain assessments and screenings. See Box 18-2 for more information regarding the recommended types of assessments and screenings and see Box 18-3 for the suggested timeline for preventive services, also known as well-child checks. For detailed information on these screenings and the timeline, access the following links:

https://brightfutures.aap.org/Pages/default.aspx
https://www.aap.org/en-us/Documents/periodicity_schedule.pdf

BOX 18-2 Preventive Services and Screenings: Infancy Through Adolescence

- History
- Measurements
  - Length/Height/Weight
  - Head Circumference
  - Body mass index (BMI)
  - Blood pressure
- Sensory Screening
  - Vision
  - Hearing
- Developmental/Behavioral Health
  - Developmental screening
  - Autism spectrum disorder screening
  - Developmental surveillance
  - Psychosocial/behavioral assessment
  - Depression screening
  - Maternal depression screening (as appropriate)
- Physical Examination
  - Procedures
    - Newborn blood
    - Newborn bilirubin
    - Critical congenital heart defect
    - Immunizations
    - Anemia
    - Lead
    - Tuberculosis
    - Dyslipidemia
    - Sexually transmitted infections
    - Human immunodeficiency virus
    - Cervical dysplasia
  - Oral Health
    - Fluoride varnish
    - Fluoride supplementation
  - Anticipatory Guidance

BOX 18-3 Preventive Services and Screenings: Well-Check Schedule

- Prenatal visit
- Newborn visit
- First week visit (3 to 5 days)
- 1 month visit
- 2 month visit
- 3 month visit
- 4 month visit
- 6 month visit
- 9 month visit
- 12 month visit
- 15 month visit
- 18 month visit
- 2 year visit
- 2½ year visit
- 3 year visit
- Annual visits from 4 years of age to 18 years of age; thereafter, the child should begin to visit a general practitioner

B. Well-checks are important in promoting health early in childhood and preventing diseases later in life. Childhood obesity, type 2 diabetes mellitus, and hyperlipidemia are noted to have an increased incidence in recent years. See Chapters 32 and 36 for more information on these problems.

VIII. Immunizations

A. Guidelines (see Priority Nursing Actions)

PRIORITY NURSING ACTIONS

Administering a Parenteral Vaccine

1. Verify the prescription for the vaccine.
2. Obtain an immunization history from the parents and assess for allergies.
3. Provide information to the parents about the vaccine.
4. Obtain parental consent.
5. Check the lot number and expiration date and prepare the injection.
6. Select the appropriate site for administration.
7. Administer the vaccine.
8. Document the administration and site of administration and lot number and expiration date of the vaccine.
9. Provide a vaccination record to the parents.

Reference

Hockenberry. (2017). Wilson, Rodgers, pp. 151–169.

1. Immunizations are an important aspect of health promotion during childhood.

2. In the United States, the recommended age for beginning primary immunizations of infants is at birth.
3. Children who began primary immunizations at the recommended age but failed to receive all required doses do not need to begin the series again; they need to receive only the missed doses.
4. If there is suspicion that the parent will not bring the child to the pediatrician or health care clinic for follow-up immunizations according to the optimal immunization schedule, any of the recommended vaccines can be administered simultaneously.

B. General contraindications and precautions
1. A vaccine is contraindicated if the child experienced an anaphylactic reaction to a previously administered vaccine or a component in the vaccine.
2. Live virus vaccines generally are not administered to individuals with severely deficient immune systems, individuals with a severe sensitivity to gelatin, or pregnant women.
3. A vaccine is administered with caution to an individual with a moderate or severe acute illness, with or without fever.
4. See Section IX, Recommended Childhood and Adolescent Immunizations, for specific information for each type of vaccine.

C. Guidelines for administration (Box 18-4)

⚠ Children born preterm should receive the full dose of each vaccine at the appropriate chronological age.

BOX 18-4 Guidelines for Administration of Vaccines

- Follow manufacturer's recommendations for route of administration, storage, and reconstitution of the vaccine.
- If refrigeration is necessary, store on a central shelf and not on the door; frequent temperature changes from opening the refrigerator door can alter the vaccine's potency.
- A vaccine information statement needs to be given to the parents or individual, and informed consent for administration needs to be obtained.
- Check the expiration date on the vaccine bottle.
- Parenteral vaccines are given in separate syringes in different injection sites.
- Vaccines administered intramuscularly are given in the vastus lateralis muscle (best site) or ventrogluteal muscle (the deltoid can be used for children 36 months of age and older).
- Vaccines administered subcutaneously are given in the fatty areas in the lateral upper arms and anterior thighs.
- Adequate needle length and gauge are as follows: intramuscular, 1 inch, 23-25 gauge; subcutaneous, {⅝} inch, 25 gauge (needle length may vary depending on the child's size).
- Mild side effects include fever, soreness, swelling, or redness at injection site.
- A topical anesthetic may be applied to injection site before the injection.
- For painful or red injection sites, advise the parent to apply cool compresses for the first 24 hours, and then use warm or cold compresses as long as needed.
- An age-appropriate dose of acetaminophen or ibuprofen, per health care provider's preference, may be administered every 4 to 6 hours for vaccine-associated discomfort.
- Maintain an immunization record—document day, month, year of administration; manufacturer and lot number of vaccine; name, address, and title of person administering the vaccine; and site and route of administration.
- A vaccine adverse event report needs to be filed and the health department needs to be notified if an adverse reaction to an immunization occurs.

IX. Recommended Childhood and Adolescent Immunizations (Box 18-5)

A. For the most up-to-date information, refer to Centers for Disease Control and Prevention (CDC) Web site: http://www.cdc.gov/vaccines/schedules/index.html.

B. Hepatitis B vaccine (HepB)
1. Administered by the intramuscular route
2. Contraindications: Severe allergic reaction to previous dose or vaccine component (components include aluminum hydroxide, yeast protein)
3. Precautions: An infant weighing less than 2000 g or an infant with moderate or severe acute illness with or without fever
4. HBsAg (hepatitis B surface antigen)-positive mothers
   a. Infant should receive HepB vaccine and hepatitis B immunoglobulin (HBIG) within 12 hours of birth.
   b. Infant should be tested for HBsAg and antibody to HBsAg after completion of HepB series (9 to 18 months of age).
5. Mother whose HBsAg status is unknown
   a. Infant should receive the first dose of hepatitis vaccine series within 12 hours of birth.
   b. Maternal blood should be drawn as soon as possible to determine the mother's HBsAg status.
   c. If the mother's HBsAg test result is positive, the infant should receive HBIG as soon as possible (no later than 1 week of age).

C. Rotavirus vaccine (RV)
1. Rotavirus is a cause of serious gastroenteritis and is a nosocomial (hospital-acquired) pathogen that is most severe in children 3 to 24 months of age; children younger than 3 months have some protection because of maternally acquired antibodies.
2. Vaccines are available and are administered by the oral route because the vaccine must replicate in the infant's gut.

BOX 18-5 Recommended Childhood and Adolescent Immunizations: 2018

Birth: Hepatitis B vaccine (HepB)
1 month: HepB
2 months: Inactivated poliovirus vaccine (IPV); diphtheria, tetanus, acellular pertussis (DTaP) vaccine; *Haemophilus influenzae* type b conjugate vaccine (Hib); pneumococcal conjugate vaccine (PCV), rotavirus (RV)
4 months: DTaP, Hib, IPV, PCV, RV
6 months: DTaP, Hib, HepB, IPV, PCV, RV (dose may be needed depending on type of vaccine used for first and second doses)
12-15 months: Hib; PCV; measles, mumps, rubella (MMR) vaccine; hepatitis A, first dose (second dose is given 6-18 months after the first dose); varicella vaccine
15-18 months: *DTaP*
18-33 months: Hepatitis A (second dose given 6-18 months after the first dose)
4-6 years: DTaP, IPV, MMR, varicella vaccine
11-12 years: MMR (if not administered at 4-6 years); diphtheria, tetanus, acellular pertussis adolescent preparation (Tdap); meningococcal vaccine (MCV4) with a booster at age 16 years; human papillomavirus (HPV) (first dose to girls at age 11 to 12 years, second dose 2 months after first dose, and third dose 6 months after first dose)

Updated yearly. See Centers for Disease Control and Prevention (CDC) Web site at http://www.cdc.gov/vaccines/schedules/index.html for current schedule.
Note: Influenza vaccine is recommended annually for children beginning at age 6 months.
From Centers for Disease Control and Prevention (CDC): *Immunization schedules*, Atlanta, 2018, CDC. Available at http://www.cdc.gov/vaccines/schedules/index.html.

3. Vaccine may be withheld if an infant is experiencing severe vomiting and diarrhea; it is administered as soon as the infant recovers.

D. Diphtheria, tetanus, acellular pertussis (DTaP); tetanus toxoid; reduced diphtheria toxoid and acellular pertussis vaccine (Tdap adolescent preparation)
   1. Administered by intramuscular route
   2. The Tdap (adolescent preparation) is recommended at 11 to 12 years of age for children who have completed the recommended childhood DTaP series but have not received a tetanus and diphtheria toxoid (Td) booster dose; children 13 to 18 years old who have not received Tdap should receive a dose.
   3. Td does not provide protection against pertussis; Td is used as a booster every 10 years after Tdap is administered at 11 to 18 years of age.
   4. Encephalopathy is a complication.
   5. Contraindications: Encephalopathy within 7 days of a previous dose or a severe allergic reaction to a previous dose or to a vaccine component

E. *Haemophilus influenzae* type b (Hib) conjugate vaccine (Hib)
   1. Protects against numerous serious infections caused by *H. influenzae* type b, such as bacterial meningitis, epiglottitis, bacterial pneumonia, septic arthritis, and sepsis
   2. Administered by the intramuscular route
   3. Contraindications: Severe allergic reaction to a previous dose or vaccine component

F. Influenza vaccine: Vaccine is recommended annually for children beginning at age 6 months.

G. Inactivated poliovirus vaccine (IPV)
   1. IPV is administered by the subcutaneous route (it may also be given by the intramuscular route).
   2. Contraindications: Severe allergic reaction to a previous dose or vaccine component; components may include formalin, neomycin, streptomycin, or polymyxin B

H. Measles, mumps, rubella (MMR) vaccine
   1. Vaccine is administered by the subcutaneous route.
   2. Contraindications: Severe allergic reaction to a previous dose or vaccine component (gelatin, neomycin, eggs), pregnancy, known immunodeficiency
   3. If the child received immunoglobulin, the MMR vaccine should be postponed for at least 3 to 6 months (immunoglobulin can inhibit the immune response to the MMR vaccine).

I. Varicella vaccine
   1. It is administered by the subcutaneous route.
   2. Children receiving the vaccine should avoid aspirin or aspirin-containing products because of the risk of Reye's syndrome.
   3. Contraindications: Severe allergic reaction to a previous dose or vaccine component (gelatin, bovine albumin, neomycin), significant suppression of cellular immunity, pregnancy

J. Pneumococcal conjugate vaccine (PCV)
   1. PCV prevents infection with *Streptococcus pneumoniae,* which may cause meningitis, pneumonia, septicemia, sinusitis, and otitis media.
   2. It is administered by the intramuscular route.
   3. Contraindications: Severe allergic reaction to a previous dose or vaccine component

K. Hepatitis A vaccine (HepA)
   1. It is administered by the intramuscular route.
   2. Contraindications: Severe allergic reaction to a previous dose or vaccine component

L. Meningococcal vaccine (MCV)
   1. Vaccine protects against *Neisseria meningitidis.*
   2. MCV4 is the preferred type of vaccine and is given intramuscularly.
   3. MCV4 should be administered to all children at age 11 to 12 years and to unvaccinated adolescents at high school entry (age 15 years); all college freshmen living in dormitories should be vaccinated.

4. Revaccination is recommended for children who remain at increased risk after 3 years (if the first dose was administered at age 2 to 6 years) or after 5 years (if the first dose was administered at age 7 years or older).
5. It is contraindicated in children with a history of Guillain-Barré syndrome.

M. Human papillomavirus vaccine (HPV)
1. Depending on the type of vaccine used (HPV2 or HPV4), the HPV vaccine guards against diseases that are caused by HPV types 6, 11, 16, and 18, such as cervical cancer, cervical abnormalities that can lead to cervical cancer, and genital warts.
2. The vaccine is most effective for boys and girls if administered before exposure to human papillomavirus through sexual contact.
3. The vaccine is administered as 3 injections over 6 months—first dose to girls at age 11 to 12 years, the second dose 2 months after the first dose, and the third dose 6 months after the first dose.
4. A 3-dose series may be administered to boys 9 to 18 years old to reduce their likelihood of acquiring genital warts.
5. The vaccine can cause pain, swelling, itching, and redness at the injection site; fever; nausea; and dizziness.
6. The vaccine is contraindicated in individuals with a reaction to a previous injection and in pregnant women.

X. Reactions to a Vaccine

A. Local reactions
1. Tenderness, erythema, swelling at injection site
2. Low-grade fever
3. Behavioral changes such as drowsiness, unusual crying, decreased appetite

B. Minimizing local reactions
1. Select a needle of adequate length to deposit vaccine deep into the muscle or subcutaneous mass.
2. Inject into the appropriate recommended site.

A. Anaphylactic reactions
1. Goals of treatment are to secure and protect the airway, restore adequate circulation, and prevent further exposure to the antigen.
2. For a mild reaction with no evidence of respiratory distress or cardiovascular compromise, a subcutaneous injection of an antihistamine, such as diphenhydramine, and epinephrine may be administered.
3. For moderate or severe distress, establish an airway; provide cardiopulmonary resuscitation if the child is not breathing; elevate the head; administer epinephrine, fluids, and vasopressors as prescribed; monitor vital signs; and monitor urine output.

B. Refer to Chapter 62 for additional information on allergic responses and anaphylactic reactions

XI. Developmental Characteristics

A. Infant
1. Physical
   a. Height increases by 1 inch per month in the first 6 months, and by 1 year the length has increased by 50%.
   b. Weight is doubled at 5 to 6 months and tripled at 12 months.
   c. At birth, head circumference is 33 to 35 cm (13.2 to 14 inches), approximately 2 to 3 cm more than chest circumference.
   d. By 1 to 2 years of age, head circumference and chest circumference are equal.
   e. Anterior fontanel (soft and flat in a normal infant) closes by 18 months of age.
   f. Posterior fontanel (soft and flat in a normal infant) closes by 4 months of age.
   g. The first primary teeth to erupt are the lower central incisors at approximately 6 to 10 months of age. Children at risk for development of dental caries should see a dentist 6 months after the first tooth erupts or by 1 year of age.
   h. Sleep patterns vary among infants; in general, by 3 to 4 months of age, most infants have developed a nocturnal pattern of sleep that lasts 9 to 11 hours.
2. Vital signs (Box 18-6)
3. Nutrition
   a. The infant may breast-feed or bottle-feed (with iron-fortified formula), depending on the mother's choice; however, breast milk is the preferred form of nutrition for all infants, especially during the first 6 months.
   b. Exclusively breast-fed infants and infants ingesting less than 1000 mL of vitamin D–fortified formula or milk per day should receive daily vitamin D supplementation (400 IU)

BOX 18-6 Vital Signs: Newborn and 1-Year-Old Infant

Newborn

Temperature: Axillary, 96.8° F to 99.0° F (36° C to 37.2° C)
Apical Heart Rate: 120-160 beats per minute
Respirations: 30-60 (average 40) breaths per minute
Blood Pressure: 80-90/40-50 mm Hg

1-Year-Old Infant

Temperature: Axillary, 97° F to 99° F (36.1° C to 37.2° C)
Apical Heart Rate: 90-130 beats per minute
Respirations: 20-40 breaths per minute
Blood Pressure: 90/56 mm Hg

starting in the first few days of life to prevent rickets and vitamin D deficiency.

c. Iron stores from birth are depleted by 4 months of age; if the infant is being breastfed only, iron supplementation, usually with a liquid iron supplement, is needed. Premature babies are at higher risk for iron deficiency due to smaller iron stores and often need additional supplementation. Infants should be screened at 12 months of age for iron deficiency.

d. Whole milk, low-fat milk, skim milk, other animal milk, or imitation milk should not be given to infants as a primary source of nutrition, because these food sources lack the necessary components needed for growth and have limited digestibility. If introduced, cow's milk should not be given to infants until 12 months of age.

e. Fluoride supplementation may be needed at about 6 months of age, depending on the infant's intake of fluoridated tap water.

f. Solid foods (strained, pureed, or finely mashed) are introduced at about 5 to 6 months of age; introduce solid foods one at a time, usually at intervals of 4 to 5 days, to identify food allergens.

g. Sequence of the introduction of solid foods varies depending on the pediatrician's preference and usually is as follows: iron-fortified rice cereal, fruits, vegetables, then meats.

h. At 12 months of age, eggs can be given (introduce egg whites in small quantities to detect an allergy); cheese may be used as a substitute for meat.

i. Avoid solid foods that place the infant at risk for choking, such as nuts, foods with seeds, raisins, popcorn, grapes, and hot dog pieces.

j. Avoid microwaving baby bottles and baby food because of the potential for uneven heating.

k. Never mix food or medications with formula.

l. Infants under 12 months should not be fed honey. Avoid adding honey to formula, water, or other fluid to prevent botulism.

m. Offer fruit juice from a cup (12 to 13 months or at a prescribed age) rather than a bottle to prevent nursing (bottle-mouth) caries; fruit juice is limited because of its high sugar content.

4. Skills (Box 18-7)

5. Play

a. Solitary

b. Birth to 3 months: Verbal, visual, and tactile stimuli

c. 4 to 6 months: Initiation of actions and recognition of new experiences

d. 6 to 12 months: Awareness of self, imitation, repetition of pleasurable actions

e. Enjoyment of soft stuffed animals, crib mobiles with contrasting colors, squeeze toys, rattles, musical toys, water toys during the bath, large picture books, and push toys after the infant begins to walk

6. Safety

a. Parents must baby-proof the home.

b. Guard the infant when on a bed or changing table.

c. Use gates to protect the infant from stairs.

BOX 18-7 Infant Skills

2 to 3 Months

- Smiles
- Turns head side to side
- Follows objects
- Holds head in midline

4 to 5 Months

- Grasps objects
- Switches objects from hands
- Rolls over for the first time
- Enjoys social interaction
- Begins to show memory
- Aware of unfamiliar surroundings

6 to 7 Months

- Creeps
- Sits with support
- Imitates
- Exhibits fear of strangers
- Holds arms out
- Frequent mood swings
- Waves "bye-bye"

8 to 9 Months

- Sits steadily unsupported
- Crawls
- May stand while holding on
- Begins to stand without help

10 to 11 Months

- Can change from prone to sitting position
- Walks while holding on to furniture
- Stands securely
- Entertains self for periods of time

12 to 13 Months

- Walks with 1 hand held
- Can take a few steps without falling
- Can drink from a cup

14 to 15 Months

- Walks alone
- Can crawl up stairs
- Shows emotions such as anger and affection
- Will explore away from mother in familiar surroundings

d. Be sure that bath water is not hot; do not leave the infant unattended in the bath.
e. Do not hold the infant while drinking or working near hot liquids or items such as a stove.
f. Cool vaporizers instead of steam should be used if needed, to prevent burn injuries.
g. Avoid offering food that is round and similar to the size of the airway to prevent choking.
h. Be sure that toys have no small pieces.
i. Toys or mobiles hanging over the crib should be well out of reach, to prevent strangulation.
j. Avoid placing large toys in the crib, because an older infant may use them as steps to climb.
k. Cribs should be positioned away from curtains and blind cords.
l. Cover electrical outlets.
m. Remove hazardous objects from low, reachable places.
n. Remove chemicals such as cleaning or other household products, medications, poisons, and plants from the infant's reach.
o. Keep the Poison Control Center number available.

⚠ Never shake an infant because of the risk of causing a closed head injury known as shaken baby syndrome, which is a life-threatening injury.

B. Toddler
1. Physical
   a. Height and weight increase in phases, reflecting growth spurts and lags.
   b. Head circumference increases about 1 inch (25.5 mm) between ages 1 and 2 years; thereafter head circumference increases about ½ inch (12.5 mm) per year until age 5 years.
   c. Anterior fontanel closes between ages 12 and 18 months.
   d. Weight gain is slower than in infancy; by age 2 years, the average weight is 22 to 27 pounds (10 to 12 kg).
   e. Normal height changes include a growth of about 3 inches (7.5 cm) per year; the average height of the toddler is 34 inches (86 cm) at age 2 years.
   f. Lordosis (pot belly) is noted.
   g. Regular dental care is essential, and the toddler will require assistance with brushing and flossing of teeth (fluoride supplements may be necessary if the water is not fluoridated).
   h. A toddler should never be allowed to fall asleep with a bottle containing milk, juice, soda pop, sweetened water, or any other sweet liquid because of the risk of nursing (bottle-mouth) caries.
   i. Typically, the toddler sleeps through the night and has 1 daytime nap; the daytime nap is normally discontinued at about age 3 years.
   j. A consistent bedtime ritual helps prepare the toddler for sleep.
   k. Security objects at bedtime may assist in sleep.
2. Vital signs (Box 18-8)
3. Nutrition
   a. The MyPlate food guide (see Fig. 11-1) provides dietary guidelines and applies to children as young as 2 years of age (see www.choosemyplate.gov).
   b. The toddler should average an intake of 2 to 3 servings of milk daily (24 to 30 oz [700 to 800 mL]) to ensure an adequate amount of calcium and phosphorus (low-fat milk may be given after 2 years of age).
   c. Trans-fatty acids and saturated fats need to be restricted; otherwise fat restriction is not appropriate for a toddler (mothers should be taught about the types of food that contain fat that should be selected).
   d. Iron-fortified cereal and a high-iron diet, adequate amounts of calcium and vitamin D, and vitamin C (4 to 6 oz [120 to 180 mL] of juice daily) are essential components for the toddler's diet.
   e. Most toddlers prefer to feed themselves.
   f. The toddler generally does best by eating several small nutritious meals each day rather than 3 large meals.
   g. Offer a limited number of foods at any one time.
   h. Offer finger foods and avoid concentrated sweets and empty calories.
   i. The toddler is at risk for aspiration of small foods that are not chewed easily, such as nuts, foods with seeds, raisins, popcorn, grapes, and hot dog pieces.
   j. Physiological anorexia may occur and is normal because of the alternating stages of fast and slow growth.
   k. Sit the toddler in a high chair at the family table for meals.
   l. Allow sufficient time to eat, but remove food when the toddler begins to play with it.
   m. The toddler drinks well from a cup held with both hands.
   n. Avoid using food as a reward or punishment.

BOX 18-8 The Toddler's Vital Signs

Temperature: Axillary, 97.5° F to 98.6° F (36.4° C to 37° C)
Apical Heart Rate: 80-120 beats per minute
Respirations: 20-30 breaths per minute
Blood Pressure: Average, 92/55 mm Hg

4. Skills
   a. The toddler begins to walk with 1 hand held by age 12 to 13 months.
   b. The toddler runs by age 2 years and walks backward and hops on 1 foot by age 3 years.
   c. The toddler usually cannot alternate feet when climbing stairs.
   d. The toddler begins to master fine motor skills for building, undressing, and drawing lines.
   e. The young toddler often uses "no" even when he or she means "yes" to assert independence.
   f. The toddler begins to use short sentences and has a vocabulary of about 300 words by age 2 years.
5. Bowel and bladder control
   a. Certain signs indicate that a toddler is ready for toilet training (Box 18-9).
   b. Bowel control develops before bladder control.
   c. By age 3 years, the toddler achieves fairly good bowel and bladder control.
   d. The toddler may stay dry during the day but may need a diaper at night until about age 4 years.
6. Play
   a. The major socializing mechanism is parallel play, and therapeutic play can begin at this age.
   b. The toddler has a short attention span, causing the toddler to change toys often.
   c. The toddler explores body parts of self and others.
   d. Typical toys include push-pull toys, blocks, sand, finger paints and bubbles, large balls, crayons, trucks and dolls, containers, Play-Doh, toy telephones, cloth books, and wooden puzzles.
7. Safety

⚠ Toddlers are eager to explore the world around them; they need to be supervised at play to ensure safety.

   a. Use back burners on the stove to prepare a meal; turn pot handles inward and toward the middle of the stove.
   b. Keep dangling cords from small appliances or other items away from the toddler.
   c. Place inaccessible locks on windows and doors, and keep furniture away from windows.
   d. Secure screens on all windows.
   e. Place safety gates at stairways.
   f. Do not allow the toddler to sleep or play in an upper bunk bed.
   g. Never leave the toddler alone near a bathtub, pail of water, swimming pool, or any other body of water.
   h. Keep toilet lids closed.
   i. Keep all medicines, poisons, household plants, and toxic products in high areas and locked out of reach.
   j. Keep the Poison Control Center number available.

C. Preschooler
1. Physical
   a. The preschooler grows 2.5 to 3 inches (6.5 to 7.5 cm) per year.
   b. Average height is 37 inches (94 cm) at age 3 years, 40.5 inches (103 cm) at age 4 years, and 43 inches (110 cm) at age 5 years.
   c. The preschooler gains approximately 5 pounds (2.25 kg) per year; average weight is 40 pounds (18 kg) at age 5 years.
   d. The preschooler requires about 12 hours of sleep each day.
   e. A security object and a nightlight help with sleeping.
   f. At the beginning of the preschool period, the eruption of the deciduous (primary) teeth is complete.
   g. Regular dental care is essential, and the preschooler may require assistance with brushing and flossing of teeth; fluoride supplements may be necessary if the water is not fluoridated.
2. Vital signs (Box 18-10)
3. Nutrition
   a. Nutritional needs are similar to those required for the toddler, although the daily amounts of minerals, vitamins, and protein may increase with age.
   b. The MyPlate food guide is appropriate for preschoolers (see www.choosemyplate.gov).

BOX 18-9 Signs of Readiness for Toilet Training

Child is able to stay dry for 2 hours.
Child is waking up dry from a nap.
Child is able to sit, squat, and walk.
Child is able to remove clothing.
Child recognizes the urge to defecate or urinate.
Child expresses willingness to please a parent.
Child is able to sit on the toilet for 5 to 10 minutes without fussing or getting off.

Data from Hockenberry M, Wilson D: *Nursing care of infants and children*, ed 9, St. Louis, 2011, Mosby.

BOX 18-10 The Preschooler's Vital Signs

Temperature: Axillary, 97.5° F to 98.6° F (36.4° C to 37° C)
Apical Heart Rate: 70-110 beats per minute
Respirations: 16-22 breaths per minute
Blood Pressure: Average, 95/57 mm Hg

c. The preschooler exhibits food fads and certain taste preferences and may exhibit finicky eating.
d. By 5 years old, the child tends to focus on social aspects of eating, table conversations, manners, and willingness to try new foods.

4. Skills
   a. The preschooler has good posture.
   b. The child develops fine motor coordination.
   c. The child can hop, skip, and run more smoothly.
   d. Athletic abilities begin to develop.
   e. The preschooler demonstrates increased skills in balancing.
   f. The child alternates feet when climbing stairs.
   g. The child can tie shoelaces by age 6 years.
   h. The child may talk continuously and ask many "why" questions.
   i. Vocabulary increases to about 900 words by age 3 years and to 2100 words by age 5 years.
   j. By age 3 years, the preschooler usually talks in 3- or 4-word sentences and speaks in short phrases.
   k. By age 4 years, the preschooler speaks 5- or 6-word sentences, and by age 5 years, speaks in longer sentences that contain all parts of speech.
   l. The child can be understood readily by others and can understand clearly what others are saying.
5. Bowel and bladder control
   a. By age 4 years, the preschooler has daytime control of bowel and bladder but may experience bed-wetting accidents at night.
   b. By age 5 years, the preschooler achieves bowel and bladder control, although accidents may occur in stressful situations.
6. Play
   a. The preschooler is cooperative.
   b. The preschooler has imaginary playmates.
   c. The child likes to build and create things, and play is simple and imaginative.
   d. The child understands sharing and is able to interact with peers.
   e. The child requires regular socialization with mates of similar age.
   f. Play activities include a large space for running and jumping.
   g. The preschooler likes dress-up clothes, paints, paper, and crayons for creative expression.
   h. Swimming and sports aid in growth development.
   i. Puzzles and toys aid with fine motor development.
7. Safety
   a. Preschoolers are active and inquisitive.
   b. Because of their magical thinking, they may believe that daring feats seen in cartoons are possible and may attempt them.
   c. The preschooler can learn simple safety practices because they can follow simple verbal directions and their attention span is longer.
   d. Teach the preschooler basic safety rules to ensure safety when playing in a playground such as near swings and ladders.
   e. Teach the preschooler never to play with matches or lighters.
   f. The preschooler should be taught what to do in the event of a fire or if clothes catch fire; fire drills should be practiced with the preschooler.
   g. Guns should be stored unloaded and secured under lock and key (ammunition should be locked in a separate place).
   h. Teach the preschooler his or her full name, address, parents' names, and telephone number.
   i. Teach the preschooler how to dial 911 in an emergency situation.
   j. Keep the Poison Control Center number available.

⚠ Teach a preschooler and school-age child to leave an area immediately if a gun is visible and to tell an adult. The preschooler should also be taught never to point a toy gun at another person.

D. School-age child
1. Physical
   a. Girls usually grow faster than boys.
   b. Growth is about 2 inches (5 cm) per year between ages 6 and 12 years.
   c. Height ranges from 45 inches (115 cm) at age 6 years to 59 inches (150 cm) at age 12 years.
   d. School-age children gain weight at a rate of about 4.5 to 6.5 pounds (2 to 3 kg) per year.
   e. Average weight is 46 pounds (21 kg) at age 6 years and 88 pounds (40 kg) at age 12 years.
   f. The first permanent (secondary) teeth erupt around age 6 years, and deciduous teeth are lost gradually.
   g. Regular dentist visits are necessary, and the school-age child needs to be
   h. Supervised with brushing and flossing teeth; fluoride supplements may be necessary if the water is not fluoridated.
   i. For school-age children with primary and permanent dentition, the best toothbrush is one with soft nylon bristles and an overall length of about 6 inches (15 cm).
   j. Sleep requirements range from 10 to 12 hours a night.
2. Vital signs (Box 18-11)
3. Nutrition

BOX 18-11 The School-Age Child's Vital Signs

Temperature: Oral, 97.5° F to 98.6° F (36.4° C to 37° C)
Apical Heart Rate: 60-100 beats per minute
Respirations: 18-20 breaths per minute
Blood Pressure: Average, 107/64 mm Hg

a. School-age children will have increased growth needs as they approach adolescence.
b. Children require a balanced diet from foods in the MyPlate food guide; healthy snacks should continue to be emphasized to prevent childhood obesity (see www.choosemyplate.gov).
c. Children still may be picky eaters but are usually willing to try new foods.

4. Skills
   a. School-age children exhibit refinement of fine motor skills.
   b. Development of gross motor skills continues.
   c. Strength and endurance increase.
5. Play
   a. Play is more competitive.
   b. Rules and rituals are important aspects of play and games.
   c. The school-age child enjoys drawing, collecting items, dolls, pets, guessing games, board games, listening to the radio, TV, reading, watching videos or DVDs, and computer games.
   d. The child participates in team sports.
   e. The child may participate in secret clubs, group peer activities, and scout organizations.
6. Safety
   a. The school-age child experiences less fear in play activities and frequently imitates real life by using tools and household items.
   b. Major causes of injuries include bicycles, skateboards, and team sports as the child increases in motor abilities and independence.
   c. Children should always wear a helmet when riding a bike or using in-line skates or skateboards.
   d. Teach the child water safety rules.
   e. Instruct the child to avoid teasing or playing roughly with animals.
   f. Teach the child never to play with matches or lighters.
   g. The child should be taught what to do in the event of a fire or if clothes catch fire; fire drills should be practiced with the child.
   h. Guns should be stored unloaded and secured under lock and key (ammunition should be locked in a separate place).
   i. Teach the child traffic safety rules.
   j. Teach the child how to dial 911 in an emergency situation.
   k. Keep the Poison Control Center number available.

! Teach the preschooler and school-age child that if another person touches his or her body in an inappropriate way, an adult should be told. Also teach the child to avoid speaking to strangers and never to accept a ride, toys, or gifts from a stranger.

E. Adolescent
1. Physical
   a. Puberty is the maturational, hormonal, and growth process that occurs when the reproductive organs begin to function and the secondary sex characteristics develop.
   b. Body mass increases to adult size.
   c. Sebaceous and sweat glands become active and fully functional.
   d. Body hair distribution occurs.
   e. Increases in height, weight, breast development, and pelvic girth occur in girls.
   f. Menstrual periods occur about 2.5 years after the onset of puberty.
   g. In boys, increases in height, weight, muscle mass, and penis and testicle size occur.
   h. The voice deepens in boys.
   i. Normal weight gain during puberty: Girls gain 15 to 55 pounds (7 to 25 kg); boys gain 15 to 65 pounds (7 to 30 kg).
   j. Careful brushing and care of the teeth are important, and many adolescents need to wear braces.
   k. Sleep patterns include a tendency to stay up late; therefore, in an attempt to catch up on missed sleep, adolescents sleep late whenever possible; an overall average of 8 hours per night is recommended.
2. Vital signs (Box 18-12)
3. Nutrition
   a. Teaching about the MyPlate food guide is important (see www.choosemyplate.gov).
   b. Adolescents typically eat whenever they have a break in activities.
   c. Calcium, zinc, iron, folic acid, and protein are especially important nutritional needs.
   d. Adolescents tend to snack on empty calories, and the importance of adequate and healthy nutrition needs to be stressed.
   e. Body image is important.

BOX 18-12 The Adolescent's Vital Signs

Temperature: Oral, 97.5° F to 98.6° F (36.4° C to 37° C)
Apical Heart Rate: 55-90 beats per minute
Respirations: 12-20 breaths per minute
Blood Pressure: Average, 121/70 mm Hg

4. Skills
   a. Gross and fine motor skills are well developed.
   b. Strength and endurance increase.
5. Play
   a. Games and athletic activities are the most common forms of play.
   b. Competition and strict rules are important.
   c. Adolescents enjoy activities such as sports, videos, movies, reading, parties, dancing, hobbies, computer games, music, communicating via the Internet, and experimenting, such as with makeup and hairstyles.
   d. Friends are important, and adolescents like to gather in small groups.
6. Safety
   a. Adolescents are risk takers.
   b. Adolescents have a natural urge to experiment and to be independent.
   c. Reinforce instructions about the dangers related to cigarette smoking, caffeine ingestion, alcohol, and drugs.
   d. Help adolescents to recognize that they have choices when difficult or potentially dangerous situations arise.
   e. Ensure that the adolescent uses a seat belt.
   f. Instruct adolescents in the consequences of injuries that motor vehicle accidents can cause.
   g. Instruct adolescents in water safety and emphasize that they should enter the water feet first as opposed to diving, especially when the depth of the water is unknown.
   h. Instruct adolescents about the dangers associated with guns, violence, and gangs.
   i. Instruct adolescents about the complications associated with body piercing, tattooing, and sun tanning.

! Discuss issues such as acquaintance rape, sexual relationships, and transmission of sexually transmitted infections with the adolescent. Also discuss the dangers of the Internet and social media related to communicating and setting up meetings (dates) with unknown persons.

F. Early adulthood
1. Description: Period between the late teens and mid to late 30s
2. Physical changes
   a. Person has completed physical growth by the age of 20 years.
   b. Person is active.
   c. Severe illnesses are less common than in older age groups.
   d. Person tends to ignore physical symptoms and postpone seeking health care.
   e. Lifestyle habits such as smoking, stress, lack of exercise, poor personal hygiene, and family history of disease increase the risk of future illness.
3. Cognitive changes
   a. Person has rational thinking habits.
   b. Conceptual, problem-solving, and motor skills increase.
   c. Person identifies preferred occupational areas.
4. Psychosocial changes
   a. Person separates from family of origin.
   b. Person gives much attention to occupational and social pursuits to improve socioeconomic status.
   c. Person makes decisions regarding career, marriage, and parenthood.
   d. Person is able to adapt to new situations.
5. Sexuality
   a. Person has the emotional maturity to develop mature sexual relationships.
   b. Person is at risk for sexually transmitted infections.

G. Middle adulthood
1. Description: Period between the mid- to late 30s and mid-60s
2. Physical changes
   a. Physical changes occur between 40 and 65 years of age.
   b. Individual becomes aware that changes in reproductive and physical abilities signify the beginning of another stage in life.
   c. Menopause occurs in women and climacteric occurs in men.
   d. Physiological changes often have an impact on self-concept and body image.
   e. Physiological concerns include stress, level of wellness, and the formation of positive health habits.
3. Cognitive changes
   a. Person may be interested in learning new skills.
   b. Person may become involved in educational or vocational programs for entering the job market or for changing careers.
4. Psychosocial changes
   a. Changes may include expected events, such as children moving away from home (postparental family stage), or unexpected events, such as the death of a close friend.
   b. Time and financial demands decrease as children move away from home, and couples face redefining their relationship.
   c. Adults may become grandparents.
   d. Adults are achieving generativity.
5. Sexuality
   a. Many couples renew their relationships and find increased marital and sexual satisfaction.

b. The onset of menopause and climacteric may affect sexual health.
c. Stress, health, and medications can affect sexuality.

H. Later adulthood (period between 65 years and death): Refer to Chapter 19.

XII. Gender Identity

A. Gender identity
1. Gender identity is one's personal sense of one's own gender.
2. It can be the same as the assigned sex at birth or it can be different.

B. Gender expression
1. Gender expression is how one expresses their gender to others.
2. Characteristics in personality, appearance, behavior, or the name one chooses to be called can relate to gender expression.

C. Sexual orientation
1. Sexual orientation refers to the gender to whom one is typically sexually attracted.
2. A person can be attracted to someone of the same gender and/or different gender(s).

D. Children
1. Children become aware of their physical difference from those of the opposite gender around age 2 and think of themselves as either a boy or a girl by age 3.
2. Children express their gender by their choices of toys, sports, preferred name, clothing, hairstyle, social behavior, and manner of behavior, such as through physical gestures.

E. Adolescents
1. Adolescents continue to develop their gender identity through their own personal sense of gender and from involvement with their social environment, such as family and friends.
2. Some adolescents are confident in their gender identity whereas others need time to develop their identity.
3. At puberty, some adolescents may realize that their gender identity is different from their assigned birth sex and sometimes they need to figure out who they are and their place in the world.

F. Family support interventions
1. Encourage the child to express themselves as to their sense of gender; avoid pressuring the child to change who they are.
2. Encourage love and unconditional support for the child and accept the child for who they are.
3. Suggest that the parents ask the school about how they support gender expression and what is taught about gender identity.
4. Support the child and prepare them for possible negative reactions or bullying from other children and the importance of sharing if these negative reactions or bullying surfaces against them.
5. Watch for signs of depression, anxiety, or other behaviors that affect the emotional health of the child.
6. Seek out medical professional assistance if concerned about the child's emotional health or if family members are having difficulty accepting the child's decision about one's own gender.
7. For additional information refer to: Rafferty, J. (2020). *Gender identity in children*. American Academy of Pediatrics at https://www.healthychildren.org/English/ages-stages/gradeschool/Pages/Gender-Identity-and-Gender-Confusion-In-Children.aspx

XIII. End-of-Life Care

A. Description: End-of-life care relates to death and dying.

B. Legal and ethical issues
1. Outcomes related to care during illness and the dying experience should be based on the client's wishes.
2. Issues for consideration may include organ and tissue donations, advance directives or other legal documents, withholding or withdrawing treatment, and cardiopulmonary resuscitation.

C. Cultural and religious considerations (Box 18-13)

BOX 18-13 Religion and End-of-Life Care

End-of-life care and practices may vary among members of each religious group. Therefore, culturally competent care requires that the nurse identify the specific preferences and needs of each individual. The nurse must ask the client and/or family what these preferences are and develop a plan of care that addresses these individualized preferences.

Buddhism

The decision to forego life-sustaining efforts is an individual matter that requires consultation with the person concerned and their family

Disposition of the body varies with the culture and denomination and the family needs to be consulted.

Beliefs on autopsy vary, therefore the individual or the individual's family must be consulted.

Guidelines for health care providers interacting with patients of the Buddhist religion and their families at: https://www.advocatehealth.com/assets/documents/faith/cgbuddhist.pdf

Catholic

Members look to a priest for prayers and support and comfort.

Sacraments before death include reconciliation and Holy Communion.

The Teachings of the Catholic Church: Caring for people at the end-of-life at: https://www.advocatehealth.com/assets/documents/faith/cgbuddhist.pdf

BOX 18-13 Religion and End-of-Life Care—cont'd

Church of Jesus Christ of Latter-Day Saints (Mormons)

Members look to church leaders for support and comfort.

Some may want to be blessed by the Mormon priesthood.

Caring for a Mormon Patient at: https://sites.google.com/site/culturalsensitivitytomormons/home/values-beliefs-norms/health-practices/caring-for-a-mormon-patient

Islam

A Muslim chaplain, a volunteer, or an Imam may be preferred to be present at the time of death and offer support to the family, read the Quran, and comfort the dying client.

Preference may be that the client face Mecca (west or southwest in the United States).

Ziyara, Muslim spiritual care: End-of-life care at: https://ziyara.org/programs/end-of-life-care/

Jehovah's Witnesses

Likely to refuse a blood transfusion whatever the possible consequences.

Congregational support is important.

Caring for the Jehovah Witness patient at: https://www.ashfordstpeters.info/images/other/PAS09.pdf

Judaism

A dying person should not be left alone (a rabbi's presence is desired).

If a client is mentally competent, Jewish tradition encourages them to reflect on their life, pass on wisdom, make amends if needed and say good-bye.

The culture connection: Judaism at end-of-life at: https://www.crossroadshospice.com/hospice-palliative-care-blog/2015/august/10/the-culture-connection-judaism-at-end-of-life/

Hinduism

Special prayers are said and often a relative must be present at the moment of death. A pandit (priest) may be called in to do a puja (prayer). Pujas may involve adorning the person's head with sandalwood paste, holy ash and red kum kum powder.

A red or yellow string may be tied around the wrist. After death, close family members will wash the body, close the eyes and straighten the legs. A death needs to be registered as soon as possible and the body cremated within 24 hour.

Caring for the Hindu patient: Cultural and clinical aspects at: http://www.pulsetoday.co.uk/caring-for-the-hindu-patient-cultural-and-clinical-aspects/10862719.article#:~:text=Caring%20for%20the%20Hindu%20patient%20is%20not%20complicated%2C%20but%20GPs,holistic%20and%20appropriate%20medical%20care.&text=Hinduism%20has%20no%20common%20roots,Judaism%2C%20Christianity%20and%20Islam).

Protestant

Some prefer specific rituals and practices at the time of one's dying and death.

Many prefer family members, friends and their own clergy to be present for comfort and prayers at this time. Consult with the family regarding their preference.

Guidelines for health care providers interacting with patients and their families who are members of Protestant religious groups at: https://www.advocatehealth.com/assets/documents/faith/cgprotestant.pdf

D. Palliative and hospice care
  1. Focuses on caring interventions and symptom management rather than cure for diseases or conditions that no longer respond to treatment and can be required at any age depending on the condition and prognosis.
  2. Pain and symptoms are controlled; the dying client should be as pain-free and as comfortable as possible.
  3. Provides support and care for clients of any age in the last phases of incurable diseases so that they might live as fully and as comfortably as possible; client and family needs are the focus of any intervention.

E. Near-death physiological manifestations
  1. As death approaches, metabolism is reduced, and the body gradually slows down until all functions end.
  2. Sensory: The client experiences blurred vision, decreased sense of taste and smell, decreased pain and touch perception, and loss of blink reflex and appears to stare (hearing is believed to be the last sense lost).
  3. Respirations
     a. Respirations may be rapid or slow, shallow, and irregular.
     b. Respirations may be noisy and wet sounding ("death rattle").
     c. Cheyne-Stokes respiration is alternating periods of apnea and deep, rapid breathing.
  4. Circulation
     a. Heart rate slows, and blood pressure falls progressively.
     b. Skin is cool to the touch, and the extremities become pale, mottled, and cyanotic.
     c. Skin is wax-like very near death.
  5. Urinary output decreases; incontinence may occur.
  6. Gastrointestinal motility and peristalsis diminish, leading to constipation, gas accumulation, and distention; incontinence may occur.
  7. Musculoskeletal system: The client gradually loses ability to move, has difficulty speaking and swallowing, and loses the gag reflex.

F. Death
  1. Death occurs when all vital organs and body systems cease to function.

2. In general, respirations cease first, and then the heartbeat stops a few minutes thereafter.
3. Brain death occurs when the cerebral cortex stops functioning or is irreversibly damaged.

G. Nursing care
1. Frequency of assessment depends on the client's stability (at least every 4 hours); as changes occur, assessment needs to be done more frequently.
2. Physical care (Box 18-14)
3. Psychosocial care
   a. Monitor for anxiety and depression.
   b. Monitor for fear (Box 18-15).
   c. Encourage the client and family to express feelings.
   d. Provide support and advocacy for the client and family.
   e. Provide privacy for the client and family.
   f. Provide a private room for the client.
4. See Chapter 67 for information on grief and loss.
5. Postmortem care (Box 18-16)
   a. Maintain respect and dignity for the client.
   b. Determine whether the client is an organ donor; if so, follow appropriate procedures related to the donation.
   c. Consider cultural and religious rituals, state laws, and agency procedures when performing postmortem care.
   d. Prepare the body for immediate viewing by the family.
   e. Provide privacy and time for the family to be with the deceased person.
   f. Medical examiner jurisdiction guidelines are determined by each state and usually include nonnatural, traumatic, or question of criminal involvement deaths; any forensic evidence is preserved and the body is not cleaned or prepared prior to transfer to the morgue.

BOX 18-15 Fear Associated With Dying

Fear of Pain

Fear of pain may occur, based on anxieties related to dying.

Do not delay or deny pain relief measures to a terminally ill client.

Fear of Loneliness and Abandonment

Allow family members to stay with the client.

Holding hands, touching (if culturally acceptable), and listening to the client are important.

Fear of Being Meaningless

Client may feel hopeless and powerless.

Encourage life reviews and focus on the positive aspects of the client's life.

Adapted from Lewis S, Dirksen S, Heitkemper M, Bucher L, Camera I: *Medical-surgical nursing: assessment and management of clinical problems*, ed 8, St. Louis, 2011, Mosby.

BOX 18-14 Physical Care of the Dying Client

Pain

Administer pain medication.

Do not delay or deny pain medication.

Dyspnea

Elevate the head of the bed or position the client on his or her side.

Administer supplemental oxygen for comfort.

Suction fluids from the airway as needed.

Administer medications as prescribed.

Skin

Assess color and temperature.

Assess for breakdown.

Implement measures to prevent breakdown.

Dehydration

Maintain regular oral care.

Encourage taking ice chips and sips of fluid.

Do not force the client to eat or drink.

Use moist cloths to provide moisture to the mouth.

Apply lubricant to the lips and oral mucous membranes.

Anorexia, Nausea, and Vomiting

Provide antiemetics before meals.

Have family members provide the client's favorite foods.

Provide frequent small portions of favorite foods.

Elimination

Monitor urinary and bowel elimination.

Place absorbent pads under the client and check frequently.

Weakness and Fatigue

Provide rest periods.

Assess tolerance for activities.

Provide assistance and support as needed for maintaining bed or chair positions.

Restlessness

Maintain a calm, soothing environment.

Do not restrain.

Limit the number of visitors at the client's bedside (consider cultural practices).

Allow a family member to stay with the client.

BOX 18-16 General Postmortem Procedures

Close the client's eyes.
Replace dentures.
Wash the body and change bed linens if needed.
Place pads under the perineum.
Remove tubes and dressings.
Straighten the body and place a pillow under the head in preparation for family viewing.

PRACTICE QUESTIONS

157. A 4-year-old child diagnosed with leukemia is hospitalized for chemotherapy. The child is fearful of the hospitalization. Which nursing intervention should be implemented to alleviate the child's fears?
1. Encourage the child's parents to stay with the child.
2. Encourage play with other children of the same age.
3. Advise the family to visit only during the scheduled visiting hours.
4. Provide a private room, allowing the child to bring favorite toys from home.

158. A 16-year-old client is admitted to the hospital for acute appendicitis and an appendectomy is performed. Which nursing intervention is **most appropriate** to facilitate normal growth and development postoperatively?
1. Encourage the client to rest and read.
2. Encourage the parents to room in with the client.
3. Allow the family to bring in the client's favorite computer games.
4. Allow the client to interact with others in his or her same age group.

159. Which car safety device should be used for a child who is 8 years old and 4 feet tall?
1. Seat belt
2. Booster seat
3. Rear-facing convertible seat
4. Front-facing convertible seat

160. The nurse assesses the vital signs of a 12-month-old infant with a respiratory infection and notes that the respiratory rate is 35 breaths per minute. On the basis of this finding, which action is **most appropriate**?
1. Administer oxygen.
2. Document the findings.
3. Notify the pediatrician.
4. Reassess the respiratory rate in 15 minutes.

161. The nurse is monitoring a 3-month-old infant for signs of increased intracranial pressure. On palpation of the fontanels, the nurse notes that the anterior fontanel is soft and flat. On the basis of this finding, which nursing action is **most appropriate**?
1. Increase oral fluids.
2. Document the finding.
3. Notify the pediatrician.
4. Elevate the head of the bed to 90 degrees.

162. The nurse is evaluating the developmental level of a 2-year-old. Which does the nurse expect to observe in this child?
1. Uses a fork to eat
2. Uses a cup to drink
3. Pours own milk into a cup
4. Uses a knife for cutting food

163. A 2-year-old child is treated in the emergency department for a burn to the chest and abdomen. The child sustained the burn by grabbing a cup of hot coffee that was left on the kitchen counter. The nurse reviews safety principles with the parents before discharge. Which statement by the parents indicates an understanding of measures to provide safety in the home?
1. "We will be sure not to leave hot liquids unattended."
2. "I guess our children need to understand what the word hot means."
3. "We will be sure that the children stay in their rooms when we work in the kitchen."
4. "We will install a safety gate as soon as we get home so the children cannot get into the kitchen."

164. A mother arrives at a clinic with her toddler and tells the nurse that she has a difficult time getting the child to go to bed at night. What measure is **most appropriate** for the nurse to suggest to the mother?
1. Allow the child to set bedtime limits.
2. Allow the child to have temper tantrums.
3. Avoid letting the child nap during the day.
4. Inform the child of bedtime a few minutes before it is time for bed.

165. The mother of a 3-year-old is concerned because her child still is insisting on a bottle at nap time and at bedtime. Which is the **most appropriate** suggestion to the mother?
1. Allow the bottle if it contains juice.
2. Allow the bottle if it contains water.
3. Do not allow the child to have the bottle.
4. Allow the bottle during naps but not at bedtime.

166. The nurse is preparing to care for a 5-year-old who has been placed in traction following a fracture of the femur. The nurse plans care, knowing that which is the **most appropriate** activity for this child?
1. A radio
2. A sports video
3. Large picture books
4. Crayons and a coloring book

167. The mother of a 3-year-old asks a clinic nurse about appropriate and safe toys for the child. The nurse should tell the mother that the **most appropriate** toy for a 3-year-old is which?
1. A wagon
2. A golf set
3. A farm set
4. A jack set with marbles

168. Which interventions are appropriate for the care of an infant? **Select all that apply.**
- ❑ 1. Provide swaddling.
- ❑ 2. Talk in a loud voice.
- ❑ 3. Provide the infant with a bottle of juice at nap time.
- ❑ 4. Hang mobiles with black and white contrast designs.
- ❑ 5. Caress the infant while bathing or during diaper changes.
- ❑ 6. Allow the infant to cry for at least 10 minutes before responding.

169. The nurse is preparing to care for a dying client, and several family members are at the client's bedside. Which therapeutic techniques should the nurse use when communicating with the family? **Select all that apply.**
- ❑ 1. Discourage reminiscing.
- ❑ 2. Make the decisions for the family.
- ❑ 3. Encourage expression of feelings, concerns, and fears.
- ❑ 4. Explain everything that is happening to all family members.
- ❑ 5. Touch and hold the client's or family member's hand if appropriate.
- ❑ 6. Be honest and let the client and family know they will not be abandoned by the nurse.

170. An infant receives a diphtheria, tetanus, and acellular pertussis (DTaP) immunization at a well-baby clinic. The parent returns home and calls the clinic to report that the infant has developed swelling and redness at the site of injection. Which intervention should the nurse suggest to the parent?
1. Monitor the infant for a fever.
2. Bring the infant back to the clinic.
3. Apply a hot pack to the injection site.
4. Apply a cold pack to the injection site.

171. A child is receiving a series of the hepatitis B vaccine and arrives at the clinic with his parent for the second dose. Before administering the vaccine, the nurse should ask the child and parent about a history of a severe allergy to which substance?
1. Eggs
2. Penicillin
3. Sulfonamides
4. A previous dose of hepatitis B vaccine or component

172. A parent brings her 4-month-old infant to a well-baby clinic for immunizations. The child is up to date with the immunization schedule. The nurse should prepare to administer which immunizations to this infant?
1. Varicella, hepatitis B vaccine (HepB)
2. Diphtheria, tetanus, acellular pertussis (DTaP); measles, mumps, rubella (MMR); inactivated poliovirus vaccine (IPV)
3. MMR, Haemophilus influenzae type b (Hib), DTaP
4. DTaP, Hib, IPV, pneumococcal vaccine (PCV), rotavirus vaccine (RV)

173. The clinic nurse is assessing a child who is scheduled to receive a live virus vaccine (immunization). What are the general contraindications associated with receiving a live virus vaccine? **Select all that apply.**
- ❑ 1. The child has symptoms of a cold.
- ❑ 2. The child had a previous anaphylactic reaction to the vaccine.
- ❑ 3. The mother reports that the child is having intermittent episodes of diarrhea.
- ❑ 4. The mother reports that the child has not had an appetite and has been fussy.
- ❑ 5. The child has a disorder that caused a severely deficient immune system.
- ❑ 6. The mother reports that the child has recently been exposed to an infectious disease.

ANSWERS

157. *Answer:* 1

Rationale: Although the preschooler already may be spending some time away from parents at a day care center or preschool, illness adds a stressor that makes separation more difficult. The child may ask repeatedly when parents will be coming for a visit or may constantly want to call the parents. Options 3 and 4 increase stress related to separation anxiety. Option 2 is unrelated to the subject of the question and, in addition, may not be appropriate for a child who may be immunocompromised and at risk for infection.

Test-Taking Strategy: Note that the **subject** relates to the child's fear. Options 3 and 4 will increase anxiety and fear further and should be eliminated. Bearing the **subject** of the question in mind and considering the child's diagnosis will assist you in eliminating option 2.

Level of Cognitive Ability: Applying
Client Needs: Health Promotion and Maintenance
Integrated Process: Caring
Content Area: Developmental Stages: Preschool and School Age
Health Problem: Pediatric-Specific: Cancers
Priority Concepts: Anxiety; Development
Reference: McKinney et al. (2018), pp. 787-788.

158. *Answer:* 4

Rationale: Adolescents often are not sure whether they want their parents with them when they are hospitalized. Because of the importance of their peer group, separation from friends is a source of anxiety. Ideally, the members of the peer group will support their ill friend. Options 1, 2, and 3 isolate the client from the peer group.

Test-Taking Strategy: Note the **strategic words,** *most appropriate.* Consider the psychosocial needs of the adolescent and remember that the peer group is very important. Options 1, 2, and 3 are **comparable or alike** in that they isolate the client from his or her own peer group.

Level of Cognitive Ability: Applying
Client Needs: Health Promotion and Maintenance
Integrated Process: Caring
Content Area: Developmental Stages: Adolescent
Health Problem: Pediatric-Specific: Appendicitis
Priority Concepts: Development; Health Promotion
Reference: McKinney et al. (2018), p. 791.

159. *Answer:* 2

Rationale: All children whose weight or height is above the forward-facing limit for their car safety seat should use a belt-positioning booster seat until the vehicle seat belt fits properly, typically when they have reached 4 feet, 9 inches in height (145 cm) and are between 8 and 12 years of age. Infants should ride in a car in a semireclined, rear-facing position in an infant-only seat or a convertible seat until they weigh at least 20 pounds (9 kg) and are at least 1 year of age. The transition point for switching to the forward-facing position is defined by the manufacturer of the convertible car safety seat but is generally at a body weight of 9 kilograms (20 pounds) and 1 year of age.

Test-Taking Strategy: Focus on the **subject,** car safety, and note the age and height of the child to identify the appropriate safety device. Remember that children should remain in a booster seat until they are 8 to 12 years old and at least 4 feet, 9 inches (145 cm) tall.

Level of Cognitive Ability: Applying
Client Needs: Safe and Effective Care Environment
Integrated Process: Nursing Process—Planning
Content Area: Foundations of Care: Safety
Health Problem: N/A
Priority Concepts: Clinical Judgment; Safety
References: Hockenberry, Wilson, Rodgers (2017), pp. 252-253. *https:*//www.healthychildren.org/English/safety-prevention/on-the-go/Pages/Car-Safety-Seats-Information-for-Families.aspx

160. *Answer:* 2

Rationale: The normal respiratory rate in a 12-month-old infant is 20 to 40 breaths per minute. The normal apical heart rate is 90 to 130 beats per minute, and the average blood pressure is 90/56 mm Hg. The nurse would document the findings.

Test-Taking Strategy: Focus on the **data in the question** and note the **strategic words,** *most appropriate.* Recalling the normal vital signs of an infant and noting that the respiratory rate identified in the question is within the normal range will direct you to the correct option.

Level of Cognitive Ability: Applying
Client Needs: Physiological Integrity
Integrated Process: Nursing Process—Implementation
Content Area: Developmental Stages: Infant
Health Problem: N/A
Priority Concepts: Clinical Judgment; Gas Exchange
Reference: Potter et al. (2017), pp. 499, 501.

161. *Answer:* 2

Rationale: The anterior fontanel is diamond-shaped and located on the top of the head. The fontanel should be soft and flat in a normal infant, and it normally closes by 12 to 18 months of age. The nurse would document the finding because it is normal. There is no useful reason to increase oral fluids, notify the pediatrician, or elevate the head of the bed to 90 degrees.

Test-Taking Strategy: Note the **strategic words,** *most appropriate,* and the words *soft* and *flat.* This should provide you with the clue that this is a normal finding. A bulging or tense fontanel may result from crying or increased intracranial pressure.

Level of Cognitive Ability: Applying
Client Needs: Physiological Integrity
Integrated Process: Nursing Process—Implementation
Content Area: Developmental Stages: Infant
Health Problem: N/A
Priority Concepts: Development; Intracranial Regulation
Reference: Hockenberry, Wilson, Rodgers (2017), pp. 198-199.

162. *Answer:* 2

Rationale: By age 2 years, the child can use a cup and spoon correctly but with some spilling. By age 3 to 4 years, the child begins to use a fork. By the end of the preschool period, the child should be able to pour milk into a cup and begin to use a knife for cutting.

Test-Taking Strategy: Focus on the **subject,** the developmental level of a 2-year-old. Option 4 can be eliminated first because of the word *knife.* Next, think about the fine motor skills

that need to be developed in selecting the correct option. With this in mind, eliminate options 1 and 3.
Level of Cognitive Ability: Applying
Client Needs: Health Promotion and Maintenance
Integrated Process: Nursing Process—Assessment
Content Area: Developmental Stages: Toddler
Health Problem: N/A
Priority Concepts: Clinical Judgment; Development
Reference: McKinney et al. (2018), p. 111.

163. *Answer:* 1
Rationale: Toddlers, with their increased mobility and development of motor skills, can reach hot water or hot objects placed on counters and stoves and can reach open fires or stove burners above their eye level. The nurse should encourage parents to remain in the kitchen when preparing a meal, use the back burners on the stove, and turn pot handles inward and toward the middle of the stove. Hot liquids should never be left unattended or within the child's reach, and the toddler should always be supervised. The statements in options 2, 3, and 4 do not indicate an understanding of the principles of safety.
Test-Taking Strategy: Note the words *indicates an understanding*. Option 2 can be eliminated because it is mandating that the toddler understand what is and is not safe. The toddler is not developmentally able to understand danger. Options 3 and 4 are comparable or alike in that they isolate the child from the environment. The correct option is the only one that reflects an understanding of safety principles by the parents.
Level of Cognitive Ability: Evaluating
Client Needs: Safe and Effective Care Environment
Integrated Process: Nursing Process—Evaluation
Content Area: Developmental Stages: Toddler
Health Problem: Pediatric-Specific: Burns
Priority Concepts: Development; Safety
Reference: McKinney et al. (2018), pp. 120-121.

164. *Answer:* 4
Rationale: Toddlers often resist going to bed. Bedtime protests may be reduced by establishing a consistent before-bedtime routine and enforcing consistent limits regarding the child's bedtime behavior. Informing the child of bedtime a few minutes before it is time for bed is the most appropriate option. Most toddlers take an afternoon nap and, until their second birthday, also may require a morning nap. Firm, consistent limits are needed for temper tantrums or when toddlers try stalling tactics.
Test-Taking Strategy: Note the strategic words, *most appropriate,* and focus on the subject, the toddler. Eliminate options 1, 2, and 3 by using concepts related to growth and development. Remember that preparing the toddler for an event will minimize resistive behavior.
Level of Cognitive Ability: Applying
Client Needs: Health Promotion and Maintenance
Integrated Process: Teaching and Learning
Content Area: Developmental Stages: Toddler
Health Problem: N/A
Priority Concepts: Client Education; Development
Reference: McKinney et al. (2018), p. 118.

165. *Answer:* 2
Rationale: A toddler should never be allowed to fall asleep with a bottle containing milk, juice, soda pop, sweetened water, or any other sweet liquid because of the risk of nursing (bottle-mouth) caries. If a bottle is allowed at nap time or bedtime, it should contain only water.
Test-Taking Strategy: Note the strategic words, *most appropriate*. Eliminate options 3 and 4 first because they are comparable or alike statements. From the remaining options, recalling that nursing (bottle-mouth) caries is a concern in a child will assist in directing you to the correct option.
Level of Cognitive Ability: Applying
Client Needs: Health Promotion and Maintenance
Integrated Process: Teaching and Learning
Content Area: Developmental Stages: Toddler
Health Problem: N/A
Priority Concepts: Development; Safety
Reference: McKinney et al. (2018), pp. 94-95.

166. *Answer:* 4
Rationale: In the preschooler, play is simple and imaginative and includes activities such as crayons and coloring books, puppets, felt and magnetic boards, and Play-Doh. A radio or a sports video is most appropriate for the adolescent. Large picture books are most appropriate for the infant.
Test-Taking Strategy: Note the strategic words, *most appropriate*. Note the age of the child, and think about the age-related activity that would be most appropriate. Eliminate options 1 and 2, knowing that they are most appropriate for the adolescent. From the remaining options, the word *large* in option 3 should provide you with the clue that this activity would be more appropriate for a child younger than age 5 years.
Level of Cognitive Ability: Applying
Client Needs: Health Promotion and Maintenance
Integrated Process: Nursing Process—Planning
Content Area: Developmental Stages: Preschool and School Age
Health Problem: Pediatric-Specific: Fractures
Priority Concepts: Coping; Development
Reference: Hockenberry, Wilson, Rodgers (2017), pp. 564-565.

167. *Answer:* 1
Rationale: Toys for the toddler must be strong, safe, and too large to swallow or place in the ear or nose. Toddlers need supervision at all times. Push-pull toys, large balls, large crayons, large trucks, and dolls are some of the appropriate toys. A farm set, a golf set, and jacks with marbles may contain items that the child could swallow.
Test-Taking Strategy: Note the strategic words, *most appropriate,* and focus on the subject, the appropriate toy for a 3-year-old. Options 2, 3, and 4 can be eliminated because they are comparable or alike and could contain items that the child could swallow. Remember that large and strong toys are safest for the toddler.
Level of Cognitive Ability: Applying
Client Needs: Safe and Effective Care Environment
Integrated Process: Teaching and Learning
Content Area: Developmental Stages: Toddler
Health Problem: N/A
Priority Concepts: Development; Safety
Reference: Hockenberry, Wilson, Rodgers (2017), pp. 359-360.

168. *Answer:* 1, 4, 5

Rationale: Holding, caressing, and swaddling provide warmth and tactile stimulation for the infant. To provide auditory stimulation, the nurse should talk to the infant in a soft voice and should instruct the mother to do so also. Additional interventions include playing a music box, radio, or television, or having a ticking clock or metronome nearby. Hanging a bright shiny object in midline within 20 to 25 cm of the infant's face and hanging mobiles with contrasting colors, such as black and white, provide visual stimulation. Crying is an infant's way of communicating; therefore, the nurse would respond to the infant's crying. The mother is taught to do so also. An infant or child should never be allowed to fall asleep with a bottle containing milk, juice, soda pop, sweetened water, or another sweet liquid because of the risk of nursing (bottle-mouth) caries.

Test-Taking Strategy: Focus on the subject, care of the infant. Noting the word *loud* and the words *at least 10 minutes before responding* will assist in eliminating these interventions. Also, recalling the concerns related to dental caries will assist in eliminating option 3.

Level of Cognitive Ability: Applying
Client Needs: Health Promotion and Maintenance
Integrated Process: Nursing Process—Implementation
Content Area: Developmental Stages: Infant
Health Problem: N/A
Priority Concepts: Development; Safety
Reference: Hockenberry, Wilson, Rodgers (2017), pp. 60-61.

169. *Answer:* 3, 5, 6

Rationale: The nurse must determine whether there is a spokesperson for the family and how much the client and family want to know. The nurse needs to allow the family and client the opportunity for informed choices and assist with the decision-making process if asked. The nurse should encourage expression of feelings, concerns, and fears and reminiscing. The nurse needs to be honest and let the client and family know they will not be abandoned. The nurse should touch and hold the client's or family member's hand, if appropriate.

Test-Taking Strategy: Use therapeutic communication techniques and recall client and family rights to assist in directing you to the correct options.

Level of Cognitive Ability: Analyzing
Client Needs: Psychosocial Integrity
Integrated Process: Caring
Content Area: Developmental Stages: End-of-Life Care
Health Problem: N/A
Priority Concepts: Family Dynamics; Palliation
Reference: Potter et al. (2017), pp. 761-762.

170. *Answer:* 4

Rationale: On occasion, tenderness, redness, or swelling may occur at the site of the DTaP injection. This can be relieved with cold packs for the first 24 hours, followed by warm or cold compresses if the inflammation persists. Bringing the infant back to the clinic is unnecessary. Option 1 may be an appropriate intervention but is not specific to the subject of the question, a localized reaction at the injection site. Hot packs are not applied and can be harmful by causing burning of the skin.

Test-Taking Strategy: Focus on the subject, a localized reaction at the injection site. Option 1 can be eliminated first because it does not relate specifically to the subject of the question. Eliminate option 2 next as an unnecessary intervention. From the remaining options, general principles related to the effects of heat and cold will direct you to the correct option. Also noting the word *hot* in option 3 will assist in eliminating this option.

Level of Cognitive Ability: Applying
Client Needs: Physiological Integrity
Integrated Process: Nursing Process—Implementation
Content Area: Pediatrics: Infectious/Communicable Diseases
Health Problem: Pediatric-Specific: Immunizations
Priority Concepts: Client Education; Health Promotion
References: Centers for Disease Control and Prevention (CDC), http://www.cdc.gov/vaccines/schedules/index.html; McKinney et al. (2018), p. 77.

171. *Answer:* 4

Rationale: A contraindication to receiving the hepatitis B vaccine is a previous anaphylactic reaction to a previous dose of hepatitis B vaccine or to a component (aluminum hydroxide or yeast protein) of the vaccine. An allergy to eggs, penicillin, and sulfonamides is unrelated to the contraindication to receiving this vaccine.

Test-Taking Strategy: Focus on the subject, a contraindication to receiving the hepatitis B vaccine. Note the relationship of the words *hepatitis B vaccine* in the question and the correct option.

Level of Cognitive Ability: Analyzing
Client Needs: Physiological Integrity
Integrated Process: Nursing Process—Assessment
Content Area: Pediatrics: Infectious/Communicable Diseases
Health Problem: Pediatric-Specific: Immunizations
Priority Concepts: Clinical Judgment; Safety
References: Centers for Disease Control and Prevention (CDC), http://www.cdc.gov/vaccines/schedules/index.html; McKinney et al. (2018), pp. 75, 77.

172. *Answer:* 4

Rationale: DTaP, Hib, IPV, PCV, and RV are administered at 4 months of age. DTaP is administered at 2, 4, and 6 months of age; at 15 to 18 months of age; and at 4 to 6 years of age. Hib is administered at 2, 4, and 6 months of age and at 12 to 15 months of age. IPV is administered at 2, 4, and 6 months of age and at 4 to 6 years of age. PCV is administered at 2, 4, and 6 months of age and at 12 to 15 months of age. The first dose of MMR vaccine is administered at 12 to 15 months of age; the second dose is administered at 4 to 6 years of age (if the second dose was not given by 4 to 6 years of age, it should be given at the next visit). The first dose of HepB is administered at birth, the second dose is administered at 1 month of age, and the third dose is administered at 6 months of age. Varicella-zoster vaccine is administered at 12 to 15 months of age and again at 4 to 6 years of age.

Test-Taking Strategy: Focus on the subject, immunization schedule for a 4-month-old infant, and use knowledge regarding the immunization schedule to answer this question. Noting the age of the infant will assist in directing you to the correct option.

Level of Cognitive Ability: Applying
Client Needs: Health Promotion and Maintenance
Integrated Process: Nursing Process—Implementation
Content Area: Pediatrics: Infectious/Communicable Diseases
Health Problem: Pediatric-Specific: Immunizations
Priority Concepts: Development; Health Promotion
References: Centers for Disease Control and Prevention (CDC), http://www.cdc.gov/vaccines/schedules/index.html; McKinney et al. (2018), p. 75.

173. ***Answer:*** **2, 5**
Rationale: The general contraindications for receiving live virus vaccines include a previous anaphylactic reaction to a vaccine or a component of a vaccine. In addition, live virus vaccines generally are not administered to individuals with a severely deficient immune system, individuals with a severe sensitivity to gelatin, or pregnant women. A vaccine is administered with caution to an individual with a moderate or severe acute illness, with or without fever. Options 1, 3, 4, and 6 are not contraindications to receiving a vaccine.
Test-Taking Strategy: Focus on the **subject**, contraindications for a live virus vaccine. This indicates that you need to select the situations in which a live virus vaccine cannot be given because doing so can cause harm to the child. Noting the word *anaphylactic* in option 2 and the words *severely deficient* in option 5 will direct you to these options.
Level of Cognitive Ability: Analyzing
Client Needs: Physiological Integrity
Integrated Process: Nursing Process—Assessment
Content Area: Pediatrics: Infectious/Communicable Diseases
Health Problem: Pediatric-Specific: Immunizations
Priority Concepts: Clinical Judgment; Safety
References: McKinney et al. (2018), p. 77; Centers for Disease Control and Prevention (CDC), http://www.cdc.gov/vaccines/schedules/index.html; Hockenberry, Wilson (2015), pp. 207-208.

CHAPTER 19

Care of the Older Client

PRIORITY CONCEPTS Development, Safety

I. Aging and Gerontology

A. Aging is the biopsychosocial process of change that occurs in a person between birth and death.

B. Gerontology is the study of the aging process.

II. Physiological Changes

A. Integumentary system
1. Loss of pigment in hair and skin
2. Wrinkling of the skin
3. Thinning of the epidermis and easy bruising and tearing of the skin
4. Decreased skin turgor, elasticity, and subcutaneous fat
5. Increased nail thickness and decreased nail growth
6. Decreased perspiration
7. Dry, itchy, scaly skin
8. Seborrheic dermatitis and keratosis formation (overgrowth and thickening of certain areas of the skin)

B. Neurological system
1. Slowed reflexes
2. Slight tremors and difficulty with fine motor movement
3. Loss of balance
4. Increased incidence of awakening after sleep onset
5. Increased susceptibility to hypothermia and hyperthermia
6. Short-term memory decline possible
7. Long-term memory usually maintained

C. Musculoskeletal system
1. Decreased muscle mass and strength and atrophy of muscles
2. Decreased mobility, range of motion, flexibility, coordination, and stability
3. Change of gait, with shortened step and wider base
4. Posture and stature changes causing a decrease in height, also known as kyphosis (Fig. 19-1)
5. Increased brittleness of the bones due to demineralization
6. Deterioration of joint capsule components

The older client is at risk for falls because of the changes that occur in the neurological and musculoskeletal systems.

D. Cardiovascular system
1. Diminished energy and endurance, with lowered tolerance to exercise
2. Decreased compliance of the heart muscle can be due to remodeling of the heart after myocardial infarction or long-standing hypertension, with heart valves becoming thicker and more rigid due to calcification
3. Decreased cardiac output and decreased efficiency of blood return to the heart
4. Decreased compensatory response, so less able to respond to increased demands on the cardiovascular system
5. Decreased resting heart rate, which may be medication-related
6. Peripheral pulses can be weak due to lower cardiac output
7. Increased blood pressure but susceptible to postural hypotension, especially with certain cardiac medications such as diuretics

E. Respiratory system
1. Decreased stretch and compliance of the chest wall
2. Decreased strength and function of respiratory muscles
3. Decreased size and number of alveoli
4. Respiratory rate usually unchanged
5. Decreased depth of respirations
6. Decreased ability to cough and expectorate sputum

F. Hematological system
1. Hemoglobin and hematocrit levels average toward the low end of normal

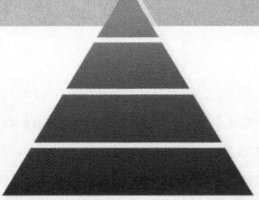

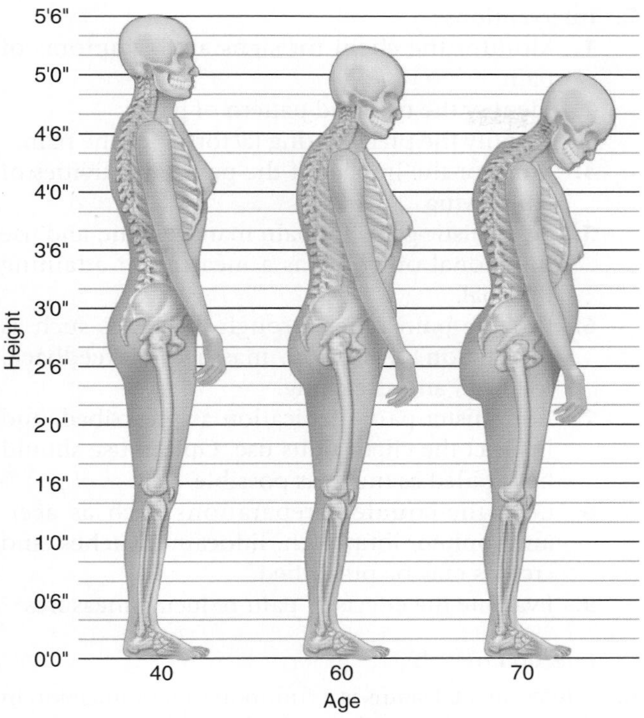

FIG. 19-1 A normal spine at 40 years of age and osteoporotic changes at 60 and 70 years of age. These changes can cause a loss of as much as 6 inches (15 cm) in height and can result in the so-called dowager's hump *(far right)* in the upper thoracic vertebrae.

2. Prone to increased blood clotting
3. Decreased protein available for protein-bound medications

G. Immune system
1. Tendency for lymphocyte counts to be low with altered immunoglobulin production
2. Decreased resistance to infection and disease

H. Gastrointestinal system
1. Decreased caloric needs because of lowered basal metabolic rate
2. Decreased appetite, thirst, and oral intake
3. Decreased lean body weight
4. Slowed gastric motility
5. Increased tendency toward constipation due to poor oral intake and slowed motility
6. Increased susceptibility for dehydration
7. Tooth loss
8. Difficulty in chewing and swallowing food

I. Endocrine system
1. Decreased secretion of hormones, with specific changes related to each hormone's function
2. Decreased metabolic rate
3. Decreased glucose tolerance, with resistance to insulin in peripheral tissues

J. Renal/urinary system
1. Decreased kidney size, function, and ability to concentrate urine
2. Decreased glomerular filtration rate
3. Decreased capacity of the bladder
4. Increased residual urine and increased incidence of infection and possibly incontinence
5. Impaired medication excretion

K. Reproductive system
1. Decreased testosterone production and decreased size of the testes
2. Changes in the prostate gland, leading to urinary problems such as retention, hesitancy, or stress incontinence, predisposing to urinary tract infections
3. Decreased secretion of hormones with the cessation of menses
4. Vaginal changes, including decreased muscle tone and lubrication
5. Impotence or sexual dysfunction for both sexes; sexual function varies and depends on general physical condition, mental health status, and medications

L. Special senses
1. Decreased visual acuity
2. Decreased accommodation in eyes, requiring increased adjustment time to changes in light
3. Decreased peripheral vision and increased sensitivity to glare
4. Presbyopia and cataract formation
5. Possible loss of hearing ability; low-pitched tones are heard more easily
6. Inability to discern taste of food
7. Decreased sense of smell
8. Changes in touch sensation
9. Decreased pain awareness

III. Psychosocial Concerns

A. Adjustment to deterioration in physical and mental health and well-being
B. Threat to independent functioning and fear of becoming a burden to loved ones
C. Adjustment to retirement and loss of income
D. Loss of skills and competencies developed early in life
E. Coping with changes in role function and social life
F. Diminished quantity and quality of relationships and coping with loss
G. Dependence on governmental and social systems
H. Access to social support systems
I. Costs of health care and medications
J. Loss of independence in living, driving, and other daily functions

IV. Mental Health Concerns

A. **Depression**: The increased dependency that older adults may experience can lead to hopelessness, helplessness, lowered sense of self-control, and decreased self-esteem and self-worth; these changes can interfere with daily functioning and lead to depression.

B. Grief: Client reacts to the perception of loss, including physical, psychological, social, and spiritual aspects.

C. Isolation: Client is alone and desires contact with others but is unable to make that contact.

D. Suicide: Depression can lead to thoughts of self-harm.

E. Depression differs from delirium and **dementia** (Table 19-1).

⚠ Any suicide threat made by an older client should be taken seriously.

V. Pain

A. Description

1. Pain can occur from numerous causes and most often occurs from degenerative changes in the musculoskeletal system.
2. The nurse needs to monitor the older client closely for signs of pain; failure to alleviate pain in the older client can lead to functional limitations affecting his or her ability to function independently.

B. Assessment

1. Restlessness
2. Verbal reporting of pain
3. Agitation
4. Moaning
5. Crying

C. Interventions

1. Monitor the client for signs and symptoms of pain.
2. Identify the type and pattern of pain.
3. Identify the precipitating factor(s) for the pain.
4. Monitor the impact of the pain on activities of daily living.
5. Set realistic goals for pain management, and use functional outcome as a measure of attaining the goal.
6. Provide pain relief through measures such as distraction, relaxation, massage, biofeedback, ice, heat, and stretching.
7. Administer pain medication as prescribed, and instruct the client in its use. Opioid use should be avoided as much as possible.
8. Over-the-counter preparations such as acetaminophen, ibuprofen, lidocaine patches, and creams may be prescribed.
9. Evaluate the effects of pain-reducing measures.

VI. Infection (Box 19-1)

A. Altered mental status is a common sign of infection in the older adult, especially infection of the urinary tract.

B. Carefully monitor the older adult with infection because of the diminished and altered immune response.

C. Nonspecific symptoms may indicate illness or infection (see Box 19-1).

TABLE 19-1 Differentiating Delirium, Depression, and Dementia

Characteristic	Delirium	Depression	Dementia
Onset	Sudden, abrupt	Recent, may relate to life change	Insidious, slow, over years and often unrecognized until deficits are obvious
Course over 24 hr	Fluctuating, often worse at night	Fairly stable, may be worse in the morning	Fairly stable, may see changes with stress; sundowning may occur
Consciousness	Reduced	Clear	Clear
Alertness	Increased, decreased, or variable	Normal	Generally normal
Psychomotor activity	Increased, decreased, or mixed	Variable; agitation or retardation	Normal; may have apraxia or agnosia; agitation can occur
Duration	Hours to weeks	Variable and may be chronic	Years
Attention	Disordered, fluctuates	Little impairment	Generally normal but may have trouble focusing; overwhelmed with multiple stimuli
Orientation	Usually impaired, fluctuates	Usually normal, may answer "I don't know" to questions or may not try to answer	Often impaired, may make up answers or answer close to the right thing, or may confabulate, but tries to answer
Speech	Often incoherent, slow or rapid, may call out repeatedly or repeat the same phrase	May be slow	Difficulty finding word, perseveration
Affect	Variable but may look disturbed, frightened	Flat	Slowed response, may be labile

Adapted from Sendelbach S, Guthrie PF, Schoenfelder DP: Acute confusion/delirium, *J Gerontol Nurse* 35(11):11–18, 2009.

BOX 19-1 Nonspecific Symptoms That Possibly Indicate Illness or Infection

- Anorexia
- Apathy
- Changes in functional status
- Altered mental status, including delirium
- Tachypnea
- Hyperglycemia
- Dyspnea
- Falling
- Fatigue
- Incontinence
- Self-neglect
- Shortness of breath
- Blood pressure below baseline

VII. Medications

A. Major problems with prescriptive medications include adverse effects, medication interactions, medication errors, nonadherence, polypharmacy, and cost. See Box 19-2 for information on medications to avoid in the older adult client. This information is based on Beers Criteria from the American Geriatrics Society. Information on this criteria and a full list of medications to avoid can be located at https://geriatricscareonline.org/ProductAbstract/american-geriatrics-society-updated-beers-criteria-for-potentially-inappropriate-medication-use-in-older-adults/CL001

B. Determine the use of over-the-counter medications.

C. Polypharmacy

1. Routinely monitor the number of prescription and nonprescription medications used and determine whether any can be eliminated or combined.
2. Keep the use of medications to a minimum.
3. Overprescribing medications leads to increased problems with more side and adverse effects, increased interaction between medications, duplication of medication treatment, diminished quality of life, and increased costs.

D. Medication dosages normally are prescribed at one-third to one-half of normal adult dosages.

E. Closely monitor the client for adverse effects and response to therapy because of the increased risk for medication toxicity (see Box 19-2).

F. Assess for medication interactions in the client taking multiple medications.

G. Advise the client to use one pharmacy and notify the consulting primary health care provider(s) of the medications taken.

A common sign of an adverse reaction to a medication in the older client is a sudden change in mental status.

H. Safety measures for medication administration (see Priority Nursing Actions box)

BOX 19-2 Medications to Avoid in the Older Client

Analgesics
- Indomethacin
- Ketorolac
- Nonsteroidal antiinflammatory drugs (NSAIDs)
- Meperidine

Antidepressants
- First-generation tricyclic antidepressants

Antihistamines
- First-generation antihistamines

Antihypertensives
- Alpha$_1$-blockers
- Centrally acting alpha$_2$-agonists

Urge Incontinence Medications
- Oxybutynin
- Tolterodine

Muscle Relaxants
- Carisoprodol
- Cyclobenzaprine
- Metaxalone
- Methocarbamol

Sedative-Hypnotics
- Barbiturates
- Benzodiazepines

Reference

Based on Beers Criteria from the American Geriatrics Society. Information on this criteria and a full list of medications to avoid can be located at https://geriatricscareonline.org/ProductAbstract/american-geriatrics-society-updated-beers-criteria-for-potentially-inappropriate-medication-use-in-older-adults/CL001

1. The client should be in a sitting position when taking medication.
2. The mouth is checked for dryness because medication may stick and dissolve in the mouth.
3. Liquid preparations can be used if the client has difficulty swallowing tablets.
4. Tablets can be crushed if necessary and given with textured food (nectar, applesauce) if not contraindicated.
5. Enteric-coated tablets are not crushed, and capsules are not opened.
6. If administering a suppository, avoid inserting the suppository immediately after removing it from the refrigerator; a suppository may take a while to dissolve because of decreased body core temperature.
7. When administering parenteral solution or medication, monitor the site because it may ooze or bleed because of decreased tissue

elasticity; an immobile limb is not used for administering parenteral medication.

8. Monitor client adherence with taking prescribed medications.
9. Monitor the client for safety in correctly taking medications, including an assessment of his or her ability to read the instructions and discriminate among the pills and their colors and shapes.
10. Use a medication cassette or checklists/schedules to facilitate proper administration of medication.
11. Encourage client to keep a complete and up-to-date list of medications with them at all times.
12. Educate the client on each medication, common side effects, and when to notify the primary health care provider.
13. Allow time for the client to ask questions, and use the teach-back method when appropriate. Include support persons in the teaching.

PRIORITY NURSING ACTIONS

Administering Oral Medications to a Client at Risk for Aspiration

1. Check the medication prescription and compare against the medical record. Clarify any incomplete prescriptions prior to administration. Check the rights of medication administration.
2. Review pertinent information related to the medication and any related nursing considerations, such as laboratory parameters.
3. Assess for any contraindications to the administration of oral medications, such as NPO (nothing by mouth) status or decreased level of consciousness.
4. Place the client in a sitting position. Assess aspiration risk using a screening tool or per agency policy. Check for an ability to swallow and cough on command. Check for the presence of a gag reflex. Following this assessment, if aspiration is a serious concern, the nurse would collaborate with the primary health care provider and speech therapist before administering the medication.
5. Prepare the medication in the form that is easiest to swallow, checking the rights of medication administration again. Mix medications whole or crush medications and mix with applesauce or pudding if indicated (use sugar-free and low carbohydrate products for clients with diabetes). Do not crush sustained-release tablets, and use liquid preparations when possible. Thicken liquids when indicated, and avoid the use of straws.
6. Check the rights of medication administration one more time, and administer the medications 1 at a time in the prepared form, ensuring that the client has effectively swallowed everything. Ensure that the client is comfortable and safe, and document the medications given using an electronic system or per agency policy.

Reference

Potter et al. (2017), pp. 634-635

VIII. Mistreatment of the Older Adult

A. Domestic mistreatment takes place in the home of the older adult and is usually carried out by a family member or significant other; this can include physical, psychological, financial, and sexual maltreatment, neglect, or abandonment.

B. Institutional mistreatment takes place when an older adult experiences abuse when hospitalized or living somewhere other than home (e.g., long-term care facility).

C. Self-neglect is the choice by a mentally competent individual to avoid medical care or other services that could improve optimal function, to not care for oneself, and to engage in actions that negatively affect his or her personal safety; unless declared legally incompetent, an individual has the right to refuse care.

⚠ Individuals at most risk for abuse include those who are dependent because of their immobility or altered mental status.

D. For additional information on abuse of the older client, see Chapter 67.

PRACTICE QUESTIONS

174. The nurse is providing medication instructions to an older client who is taking digoxin daily. The nurse explains to the client that decreased lean body mass and decreased glomerular filtration rate, which are age-related body changes, could place the client at risk for which complication with medication therapy?

1. Decreased absorption of digoxin
2. Increased risk for digoxin toxicity
3. Decreased therapeutic effect of digoxin
4. Increased risk for side effects related to digoxin

175. The nurse is caring for an older client in a long-term care facility. Which action contributes to encouraging autonomy in the client?

1. Planning meals
2. Decorating the room
3. Scheduling haircut appointments
4. Allowing the client to choose social activities

176. The home care nurse is visiting an older client whose spouse died 6 months ago. Which behaviors by the client indicates **effective** coping? **Select all that apply.**

- ☐ 1. Neglecting personal grooming
- ☐ 2. Looking at old snapshots of family
- ☐ 3. Participating in a senior citizens program
- ☐ 4. Visiting the spouse's grave once a month
- ☐ 5. Decorating a wall with the spouse's pictures and awards received

177. The nurse is providing instructions to the assistive personnel (AP) regarding care of an older client with hearing loss. What should the nurse tell the AP about older clients with hearing loss?

1. They are often distracted.
2. They have middle ear changes.
3. They respond to low-pitched tones.
4. They develop moist cerumen production.

178. The nurse is providing an educational session to new employees, and the topic is abuse of the older client. The nurse helps the employees identify which client as **most** typically a victim of abuse?

1. A man who has moderate hypertension
2. A man who has newly diagnosed cataracts
3. A woman who has advanced Parkinson's disease
4. A woman who has early diagnosed Lyme disease

179. The nurse is performing an assessment on an older client who is having difficulty sleeping at night. Which statement by the client indicates the **need for further teaching** regarding measures to improve sleep?

1. "I swim 3 times a week."
2. "I have stopped smoking cigars."
3. "I drink hot chocolate before bedtime."
4. "I read for 40 minutes before bedtime."

180. The visiting nurse observes that the older male client is confined by his daughter-in-law to his room. When the nurse suggests that he walk to the den and join the family, he says, "I'm in everyone's way; my daughter-in-law needs me to stay here." Which is the **most important** action for the nurse to take?

1. Say to the daughter-in-law, "Confining your father-in-law to his room is inhumane."
2. Suggest to the client and daughter-in-law that they consider a nursing home for the client.
3. Say nothing, because it is best for the nurse to remain neutral and wait to be asked for help.
4. Suggest appropriate resources to the client and daughter-in-law, such as respite care and a senior citizens center.

181. The nurse is performing an assessment on an older adult client. Which assessment data would indicate a potential complication associated with the skin?

1. Crusting
2. Wrinkling
3. Deepening of expression lines
4. Thinning and loss of elasticity in the skin

182. The home health nurse is visiting a client for the first time. While assessing the client's medication history, it is noted that there are 19 prescriptions and several over-the-counter medications that the client has been taking. Which intervention should the nurse take **first?**

1. Check for medication interactions.
2. Determine whether there are medication duplications.
3. Determine whether a family member supervises medication administration.
4. Call the prescribing primary health care provider (PHCP) and report polypharmacy.

183. The long-term care nurse is performing assessments on several of the residents. Which are normal age-related physiological changes the nurse should expect to note? **Select all that apply.**

- ❑ 1. Increased heart rate
- ❑ 2. Decline in visual acuity
- ❑ 3. Decreased respiratory rate
- ❑ 4. Decline in long-term memory
- ❑ 5. Increased susceptibility to urinary tract infections
- ❑ 6. Increased incidence of awakening after sleep onset

ANSWERS

174. ***Answer:* 2**

Rationale: The older client is at risk for medication toxicity because of decreased lean body mass and an age-associated decreased glomerular filtration rate. This age-related change is not specifically associated with decreased absorption, decreased therapeutic effect, or increased risk for side effects. Toxicity, or toxic effects, occurs as a result of excessive accumulation of the medication in the body.

Test-Taking Strategy: Focus on the subject, age-related body changes that could place the client at risk for medication toxicity. Recall that toxicity occurs as a result of medication accumulation in the body, which usually occurs as a result of decreased renal function. Note that the correct option is the only one that addresses renal excretion.

Level of Cognitive Ability: Applying
Client Needs: Physiological Integrity
Integrated Process: Teaching and Learning
Content Area: Developmental Stages: Early Adulthood to Later Adulthood
Health Problem: N/A
Priority Concepts: Client Education; Safety
Reference: Lewis et al. (2017), pp. 72-73.

175. ***Answer:* 4**

Rationale: Autonomy is the personal freedom to direct one's own life as long as it does not impinge on the rights of others. An autonomous person is capable of rational thought. This individual can identify problems, search for alternatives, and select solutions that allow continued personal freedom as long as others and their rights and property are not harmed. Loss of autonomy, and therefore independence, is a real fear of older clients. The correct option is the only one that allows the client to be a decision maker.

Test-Taking Strategy: Focus on the subject, encouraging autonomy. Recalling the definition of autonomy will direct you to the correct option. Remember that giving the client choices is essential to promote independence.
Level of Cognitive Ability: Applying
Client Needs: Safe and Effective Care Environment
Integrated Process: Caring
Content Area: Developmental Stages: Early Adulthood to Later Adulthood
Health Problem: N/A
Priority Concepts: Health Care Quality; Professionalism
Reference: Ignatavicius, Workman, Rebar (2018), p. 9.

176. *Answer:* 2, 3, 4, 5

Rationale: Coping mechanisms are behaviors used to decrease stress and anxiety. In response to a death, ineffective coping is manifested by an extreme behavior that in some cases may be harmful to the individual physically or psychologically. Neglecting personal grooming is indicative of a behavior that identifies ineffective coping in the grieving process. The remaining options identify appropriate and effective coping mechanisms.

Test-Taking Strategy: Note the strategic word, *effective,* and focus on the subject, effective coping behaviors. Note that options 2, 3, 4, and 5 are comparable or alike and are positive activities in which the individual is engaging to get on with his or her life.
Level of Cognitive Ability: Analyzing
Client Needs: Psychosocial Integrity
Integrated Process: Nursing Process—Assessment
Content Area: Mental Health
Health Problem: Mental Health: Coping
Priority Concepts: Coping; Family Dynamics
Reference: Potter et al. (2017), pp. 775, 777.

177. *Answer:* 3

Rationale: Presbycusis refers to the age-related irreversible degenerative changes of the inner ear that lead to decreased hearing ability. As a result of these changes, the older client has a decreased response to high-frequency sounds. Low-pitched voice tones are heard more easily and can be interpreted by the older client. Options 1, 2, and 4 are not accurate characteristics related to aging.

Test-Taking Strategy: Focus on the subject, age-related changes related to hearing. Think about the physiological changes associated with aging. Recalling that the client with a hearing loss responds to low-pitched tones will direct you to the correct option.
Level of Cognitive Ability: Applying
Client Needs: Physiological Integrity
Integrated Process: Teaching and Learning
Content Area: Developmental Stages: Early Adulthood to Later Adulthood
Health Problem: Adult Health: Ear: Hearing Loss
Priority Concepts: Development; Sensory Perception
Reference: Lewis et al. (2017), pp. 361, 391.

178. *Answer:* 3

Rationale: Elder abuse includes physical, sexual, or psychological abuse; misuse of property; and violation of rights. The typical abuse victim is a woman of advanced age with few social contacts and at least 1 physical or mental impairment that limits her ability to perform activities of daily living. In addition, the client usually lives alone or with the abuser and depends on the abuser for care.

Test-Taking Strategy: Focus on the subject, elder abuse. Note the strategic word, *most.* Read each option carefully and identify the client who is most defenseless as the result of the disease process. This will direct you to the correct option.
Level of Cognitive Ability: Analyzing
Client Needs: Safe and Effective Care Environment
Integrated Process: Nursing Process—Assessment
Content Area: Developmental Stages: Early Adulthood to Later Adulthood
Health Problem: Mental Health: Abusive Behaviors
Priority Concepts: Interpersonal Violence; Safety
Reference: Lewis et al. (2017), pp. 66-67.

179. *Answer:* 3

Rationale: Many nonpharmacological sleep aids can be used to influence sleep. However, the client should avoid caffeinated beverages and stimulants such as tea, cola, and chocolate. The client should exercise regularly, because exercise promotes sleep by burning off tension that accumulates during the day. A 20- to 30-minute walk, swim, or bicycle ride 3 times a week is helpful. Smoking and alcohol should be avoided. Reading is also a helpful measure and is relaxing.

Test-Taking Strategy: Note the strategic words, *need for further teaching.* These words indicate a negative event query and ask you to select an option that is an incorrect statement. Options 1, 2, and 4 are positive statements indicating that the client understands the methods of improving sleep. Remember that chocolate contains caffeine.
Level of Cognitive Ability: Evaluating
Client Needs: Physiological Integrity
Integrated Process: Teaching and Learning
Content Area: Developmental Stages: Early Adulthood to Later Adulthood
Health Problem: N/A
Priority Concepts: Client Education; Palliation
Reference: Potter et al. (2017), p. 1006.

180. *Answer:* 4

Rationale: Assisting clients and families to become aware of available community support systems is a role and responsibility of the nurse. Observing that the client has begun to be confined to his room makes it necessary for the nurse to intervene legally and ethically, so option 3 is not appropriate and is passive in terms of advocacy. Option 2 suggests committing the client to a nursing home and is a premature action on the nurse's part. Although the data provided tell the nurse that this client requires nursing care, the nurse does not know the extent of the nursing care required. Option 1 is incorrect and judgmental.

Test-Taking Strategy: Note the strategic words, *most important.* Using principles related to the ethical and legal responsibility of the nurse and knowledge of the nurse's role will direct you to the correct option. Option 1 is a nontherapeutic statement, option 2 is a premature action, and option 3 avoids the situation.
Level of Cognitive Ability: Applying
Client Needs: Safe and Effective Care Environment

Integrated Process: Nursing Process—Implementation
Content Area: Developmental Stages: Early Adulthood to Later Adulthood
Health Problem: Mental Health: Abusive Behaviors
Priority Concepts: Ethics; Health Care Law
Reference: Lewis et al. (2017), 69.

181. *Answer:* 1
Rationale: The normal physiological changes that occur in the skin of older adults include thinning of the skin, loss of elasticity, deepening of expression lines, and wrinkling. Crusting noted on the skin would indicate a potential complication.
Test-Taking Strategy: Note the subject, a potential complication. Think about the normal physiological changes that occur in the aging process in the integumentary system to direct you to the correct option.
Level of Cognitive Ability: Analyzing
Client Needs: Health Promotion and Maintenance
Integrated Process: Nursing Process—Assessment
Content Area: Developmental Stages: Early Adulthood to Later Adulthood
Health Problem: N/A
Priority Concepts: Clinical Judgment; Tissue Integrity
Reference: Lewis et al. (2017), p. 397.

182. *Answer:* 2
Rationale: Polypharmacy is a concern in the older client. Duplication of medications needs to be identified before medication interactions can be determined, because the nurse needs to know what the client is taking. Asking about medication administration supervision may be part of the assessment but is not a first action. The phone call to the PHCP is the intervention after all other information has been collected.
Test-Taking Strategy: Note the strategic word, *first.* Also note that the nurse is visiting the client for the first time. Options 1, 3, and 4 should be done after possible medication duplication has been identified.
Level of Cognitive Ability: Applying
Client Needs: Safe and Effective Care Environment
Integrated Process: Nursing Process—Implementation
Content Area: Foundations of Care: Safety
Health Problem: N/A
Priority Concepts: Clinical Judgment; Safety
Reference: Potter et al. (2017), pp. 187-188.

183. *Answer:* 2, 5, 6
Rationale: Anatomical changes to the eye affect the individual's visual ability, leading to potential problems with activities of daily living. Light adaptation and visual fields are reduced. Although lung function may decrease, the respiratory rate usually remains unchanged. Heart rate decreases and heart valves thicken. Age-related changes that affect the urinary tract increase an older client's susceptibility to urinary tract infections. Short-term memory may decline with age, but long-term memory usually is maintained. Change in sleep patterns is a consistent, age-related change. Older persons experience an increased incidence of awakening after sleep onset.
Test-Taking Strategy: Focus on the subject, normal age-related changes. Read each characteristic carefully and think about the physiological changes that occur with aging to select the correct items.
Level of Cognitive Ability: Analyzing
Client Needs: Health Promotion and Maintenance
Integrated Process: Nursing Process—Assessment
Content Area: Developmental Stages: Early Adulthood to Later Adulthood
Health Problem: N/A
Priority Concepts: Development; Safety
Reference: Potter et al. (2017), p. 36.

UNIT V

Maternity Nursing

Pyramid to Success

The Pyramid to Success focuses on the physiological and psychosocial aspects related to the experience of pregnancy, birth, and the postpartum period. Pyramid Points begin with the assessment and knowledge of expected findings of the pregnant client and fetus during the antepartum period. Instructing the pregnant client in measures that promote a healthy environment for the mother and the fetus is included. The focus is on the importance of antepartum follow-up, nutrition, and interventions for common discomforts that occur during pregnancy. Knowledge of the purpose of the commonly prescribed diagnostic tests and procedures in the antepartum period is also part of the Pyramid to Success. The focus is on disorders that can occur during pregnancy, particularly gestational hypertension and diabetes. The labor and birth process and the immediate interventions for conditions in which the maternal or fetal status is compromised, such as prolapsed cord or altered fetal heart rate, are part of the Pyramid to Success. Review of the fetus/newborn of a mother with human immunodeficiency virus or acquired immunodeficiency syndrome or a substance-abusing mother is recommended. The Pyramid to Success also includes a focus on the normal expectations of the postpartum period and the complications that can occur during this time. The next Pyramid Point focuses on the normal physical assessment findings and early identification of disorders in the neonate. The last Pyramid Point in this unit focuses on maternity and newborn medications.

Client Needs: Learning Objectives

Safe and Effective Care Environment

Consulting with the interprofessional health care team
Ensuring that informed consent for diagnostic tests and procedures has been obtained
Establishing priorities of care
Handling hazardous and infectious materials safely
Maintaining confidentiality
Providing continuity of client care
Promoting a safe environment to protect the client from potential teratogenic threats
Upholding client's rights
Using surgical asepsis when providing care
Using standard and transmission-based precautions when providing care

Health Promotion and Maintenance

Assessing for growth and development
Discussing expected body image changes with the client
Discussing family planning and birthing and parenting issues
Identifying at-risk clients during pregnancy
Identifying health and wellness concepts and providing health care screening
Identifying lifestyle choices and high-risk behaviors
Performing techniques of physical assessment
Providing antepartum, intrapartum, postpartum, and newborn care
Teaching regarding antepartum, intrapartum, and postpartum care, and care to the newborn

Psychosocial Integrity

Considering cultural, religious, and spiritual influences regarding birth and motherhood
Discussing situational role changes in the family
Ensuring therapeutic interactions within the family
Identifying available support systems
Identifying coping mechanisms

Physiological Integrity

Instructing the client about prescribed diagnostic tests and procedures
Monitoring for expected outcomes and effects related to pharmacological and parenteral therapies
Monitoring for normal expectations during pregnancy
Monitoring for side effects and adverse effects related to prescribed pharmacological and parenteral therapies

- Monitoring the client during the labor and birth process
- Providing interventions for unexpected events during pregnancy
- Providing nonpharmacological comfort interventions and pharmacological pain management during labor
- Supporting families who are experiencing fertility issues
- Teaching the client about nutrition during pregnancy and in the postpartum period
- Teaching the client about the physiological changes that occur during pregnancy

CHAPTER 20

Reproductive System

PRIORITY CONCEPTS **Reproduction, Sexuality**

I. Female Reproductive Structures

A. Ovaries
  1. Form and expel ova
  2. Secrete estrogen and progesterone

B. Fallopian tubes
  1. Muscular tubes (oviducts) lying near the ovaries and connected to the uterus
  2. Tubes that propel the ova from the ovaries to the uterus

C. Uterus
  1. Muscular, pear-shaped cavity in which the fetus develops
  2. Cavity from which menstruation occurs

D. Cervix
  1. The internal os of the cervix opens into the body of the uterine cavity.
  2. The cervical canal is located between the internal os and the external os.
  3. The external cervical os opens into the vagina.

E. Vagina
  1. Muscular tube that extends from the cervix to the vaginal opening in the perineum
  2. Known as the *birth canal*
  3. Passageway for menstrual blood flow, for penis for intercourse, and for the fetus

II. Male Reproductive Structures

A. Penis
  1. Structures include the body or shaft, glans penis, and urethra.
  2. Primary functions include pathway for urination and the organ used for intercourse.

B. Scrotum
  1. Structures include the testes, epididymis, and vas deferens.
  2. Normal temperature is slightly cooler than body temperature.

C. Prostate gland
  1. Secretes a milky alkaline fluid
  2. Enhances sperm movement and neutralizes acidic vaginal secretions

III. Menstrual Cycle (Box 20-1)

A. Ovarian hormones
  1. Ovarian hormones, released by the anterior pituitary gland, include follicle-stimulating hormone (FSH) and luteinizing hormone (LH).
  2. The hormones produce changes in the ovaries and in the endometrium.
  3. The menstrual cycle, the regularly recurring physiological changes in the endometrium that culminate in its shedding, may vary in length, with the average length being about 28 days.

B. Ovarian and uterine phases (Box 20-1)

IV. Female Pelvis and Measurements

A. True pelvis
  1. Lies below the pelvic brim
  2. Consists of the pelvic inlet, midpelvis, and pelvic outlet

B. False pelvis
  1. The shallow portion above the pelvic brim
  2. Supports the abdominal viscera

C. Types of pelvis
  1. Gynecoid
     a. Normal female pelvis
     b. Transversely rounded or blunt

The gynecoid pelvis is most favorable for successful labor and birth. If cephalopelvic disproportion (CPD) exists, the normal labor process will be delayed and most likely result in a cesarean delivery.

  2. Anthropoid
     a. Oval shape
     b. Adequate outlet, with a narrow pubic arch
  3. Android
     a. Heart-shaped or angulated
     b. Resembles a male pelvis
     c. Not favorable for labor and vaginal birth
     d. Narrow pelvic planes can cause slow descent and midpelvic arrest.

BOX 20-1 Menstrual Cycle

Ovarian Changes

Preovulatory Phase

Hypothalamus releases gonadotropin-releasing hormone through the portal system to the anterior pituitary system.

Secretion of follicle-stimulating hormone (FSH) by the anterior lobe of the pituitary gland stimulates growth of follicles.

Most follicles die, leaving one to mature into a large graafian follicle.

Estrogen produced by the follicle stimulates increased secretions of luteinizing hormone (LH) by the anterior lobe of the pituitary gland.

The follicle ruptures and releases an ovum into the peritoneal cavity.

Luteal Phase

Begins with ovulation.

Body temperature decreases and then increases by 0.5° F to 1° F around the time of ovulation.

Corpus luteum is formed from follicle cells that remain in the ovary after ovulation.

Corpus luteum secretes estrogen and progesterone during the remaining 14 days of the cycle.

Corpus luteum degenerates if the ovum is not fertilized, and secretion of estrogen and progesterone declines.

Decline of estrogen and progesterone stimulates the anterior pituitary to secrete more FSH and LH, initiating a new reproductive cycle.

Uterine Changes

Menstrual Phase

Consists of 4 to 6 days of bleeding as the endometrium breaks down because of the decreased levels of estrogen and progesterone.

The level of FSH increases, enabling the beginning of a new cycle.

Proliferative Phase

Lasts about 9 days.

Estrogen stimulates proliferation and growth of the endometrium.

As estrogen increases, it suppresses secretion of FSH and increases secretion of LH.

Secretion of LH stimulates ovulation and the development of the corpus luteum.

Ovulation occurs between days 12 and 16.

Estrogen level is high, and progesterone level is low.

Secretory Phase

Lasts about 12 days and follows ovulation.

This phase is initiated in response to the increase in LH level.

The graafian follicle is replaced by the corpus luteum.

The corpus luteum secretes progesterone and estrogen.

Progesterone prepares the endometrium for pregnancy if a fertilized ovum is implanted.

4. Platypelloid
   a. Flat with an oval inlet
   b. Wide transverse diameter, but short anteroposterior diameter, making labor and vaginal birth difficult

D. Pelvic inlet diameters
   1. Anteroposterior diameters
      a. Diagonal conjugate: Distance from the lower margin of the symphysis pubis to the sacral promontory
      b. True conjugate or conjugate vera: Distance from the upper margin of the symphysis pubis to the sacral promontory
      c. Obstetric conjugate: Extends from the sacral promontory to the top of the symphysis pubis. It is the smallest front-to-back distance through which the fetal head must pass in moving through the pelvic inlet.
   2. Transverse diameter: The largest of the pelvic inlet diameters; located at right angles to the true conjugate
   3. Oblique (diagonal) diameter: Not clinically measurable
   4. Posterior sagittal diameter: Distance from the point where the anteroposterior and transverse diameters cross each other to the middle of the sacral promontory

E. Pelvic midplane diameters
   1. Transverse (interspinous diameter)
   2. Midplane normally is the largest plane and has the longest diameter.

F. Pelvic outlet diameters
   1. Transverse (intertuberous diameter)
   2. Outlet presents the smallest plane of the pelvic canal.

V. Fertilization and Implantation

A. Fertilization

1. Fertilization occurs in the ampulla of the fallopian (uterine) tube when sperm and ovum unite.
2. When fertilized, the membrane of the ovum undergoes changes that prevent entry of other sperm.
3. Each reproductive cell carries 23 chromosomes.
4. Sperm carry an X or a Y chromosome—XY, male; XX, female.

B. Implantation

1. The zygote is propelled toward the uterus and implants 6 to 8 days after ovulation.

2. The blastocyst secretes chorionic gonadotropin to ensure that the corpus luteum remains viable and secretes estrogen and progesterone for the first 2 to 3 months of gestation.

VI. Fetal Development (Box 20-2)

BOX 20-2 Fetal Development

Preembryonic Period
First 2 weeks after conception

Embryonic Period
Beginning day 15 through approximately week 8 after conception

Fetal Period
Week 9 after conception to birth

Week 1
Blastocyst is free-floating.

Weeks 2 to 3
Embryo is 1.5 to 2 mm in length.
Lung buds appear.
Blood circulation begins.
Heart is tubular and begins to beat.
Neural plate becomes brain and spinal cord.

Week 5
Embryo is 0.4 to 0.5 cm in length.
Embryo is 0.4 g.
Double heart chambers are visible.
Heart is beating.
Limb buds form.

Week 8
Embryo is 3 cm in length.
Embryo is 2 g.
Eyelids begin to fuse.
Circulatory system through umbilical cord is well established.
Every organ system is present.

Week 12
Fetus is 6 to 9 cm in length.
Fetus is 19 g.
Face is well formed.
Limbs are long and slender.
Kidneys begin to form urine.
Spontaneous movements occur.
Heartbeat is detected by Doppler transducer between 10 and 12 weeks.

Week 16
Fetus is 11.5 to 13.5 cm in length.
Fetus is 100 g.
Active movements are present.
Fetal skin is transparent.
Lanugo hair begins to develop.
Skeletal ossification occurs.
Sex of fetus is visually recognizable on ultrasound.

Week 20
Fetus is 16 to 18.5 cm in length.
Fetus is 300 g.
Lanugo covers the entire body.
Fetus has nails.
Muscles are developed.
Enamel and dentin are depositing.
Heartbeat is detected by regular (nonelectronic) fetoscope.

Week 24
Fetus is 23 cm in length.
Fetus is 600 g.
Hair on head is well formed.
Skin is reddish and wrinkled.
Reflex hand grasp functions are present.
Vernix caseosa covers entire body.
Fetus has ability to hear.

Week 28
Fetus is 27 cm in length.
Fetus is 1100 g.
Limbs are well flexed.
Brain is developing rapidly.
Eyelids open and close.
Lungs are developed sufficiently to provide gas exchange (lecithin forming).
If born, neonate can breathe at this time.

Week 32
Fetus is 31 cm in length.
Fetus is 1800 to 2100 g.
Bones are fully developed.
Subcutaneous fat has collected.
Lecithin-to-sphingomyelin (L/S) ratio is 1.2:1.

Week 36
Fetus is 35 cm in length.
Fetus is 2200 to 2900 g.
Skin is pink and body is rounded.
Skin is less wrinkled.
Lanugo is disappearing.
L/S ratio is greater than 2:1.

Week 40
Fetus is 40 cm in length.
Fetus is more than 3200 g.
Skin is pinkish and smooth.
Lanugo may be present on upper arms and shoulders.
Vernix caseosa decreases.
Fingernails extend beyond fingertips.
Sole (plantar) creases run down to the heel.
Testes are in the scrotum.
Labia majora are well developed.

VII. Fetal Environment

A. Amnion
1. Encloses the amniotic cavity
2. Is the inner membrane that forms about the second week of embryonic development

3. Forms a fluid-filled sac that surrounds the embryo and later the fetus

B. Chorion
1. Is the outer membrane enclosing the amniotic cavity
2. Becomes vascularized and forms the fetal part of the placenta

C. Amniotic fluid
1. Consists of 800 to 1200 mL by the end of pregnancy
2. Surrounds, cushions, and protects the fetus and allows for fetal movement
3. Maintains the body temperature of the fetus
4. Contains fetal urine and is a measure of fetal kidney function
5. The fetus modifies the amniotic fluid through the processes of swallowing, urinating, and movement of fluid through the respiratory tract.

D. Placenta
1. The placenta provides for exchange of nutrients and waste products between the fetus and mother.
2. The placenta begins to form at implantation; the structure is complete by week 12.
3. It produces hormones to maintain pregnancy and assumes full responsibility for the production of these hormones by the 12th week of gestation.
4. In the third trimester, transfer of maternal immunoglobulin provides the fetus with passive immunity to certain diseases for the first few months after birth.
5. By week 10 to 12, genetic testing can be done via chorionic villus sampling (CVS).

Large particles such as bacteria cannot pass through the placenta, but nutrients, medications, alcohol, antibodies, and viruses can pass through the placenta.

VIII. Fetal Circulation

A. Umbilical cord
1. It contains 2 arteries and 1 vein.
2. The arteries carry deoxygenated blood and waste products from the fetus.
3. The vein carries oxygenated blood and provides oxygen and nutrients to the fetus.

B. Fetal heart rate (FHR)
1. FHR depends on gestational age; FHR is 160 to 170 beats per minute in the first trimester but slows with fetal growth to 110 to 160 beats per minute.
2. FHR is about twice the maternal heart rate.

C. Fetal circulation bypass (Fig. 20-1)
1. Fetal circulation bypass is present because of nonfunctioning lungs.
2. Bypasses must close after birth to allow blood to flow through the lungs and the liver.
3. The ductus arteriosus connects the pulmonary artery to the aorta, bypassing the lungs.
4. The ductus venosus connects the umbilical vein and the inferior vena cava, bypassing the liver.
5. The foramen ovale is the opening between the right and left atria of the heart, bypassing the lungs.

IX. Family Planning

A. Description
1. Involves choosing when to have children
2. Includes contraception, prevention of pregnancy, and methods to achieve pregnancy

B. Birth control
1. The focus of counseling on contraception must meet the needs and feelings of the woman and her partner.
2. Several factors should be considered when choosing a method of birth control, including effectiveness, safety, and personal preference.
3. The woman's preferences are most important, and cultural practices and beliefs and religious or other personal beliefs may affect the choice of contraceptives.
4. Other factors that bear on selection of a contraceptive method include family planning goals, age, frequency of intercourse, and the individual's capacity for compliance.
5. If family planning goals have already been met, sterilization of either the male or the female partner may be desirable (it is important for the couple to understand that tubal reconstruction may be unsuccessful).
6. For women who frequently engage in coitus, oral contraceptives or a long-term method such as implants or an intrauterine device (IUD) may be considered.
7. When sexual activity is limited, use of spermicide, condoms, or a diaphragm may be most appropriate.
8. Because some methods have adverse effects, a signed informed consent form may be needed.
9. For additional information on the use of contraceptives, see Chapter 28.

C. Infertility
1. Infertility is the involuntary inability to conceive when desired.
2. Some factors contributing to infertility in men include abnormalities of the sperm, abnormal erections or ejaculations, or abnormalities of the seminal fluid.
3. Some factors that contribute to infertility in women include disorders of ovulation or abnormalities of the fallopian tubes or cervix.
4. Several diagnostic tests are available to determine the probable cause of infertility, and the therapy recommended may depend on the cause of the infertility.

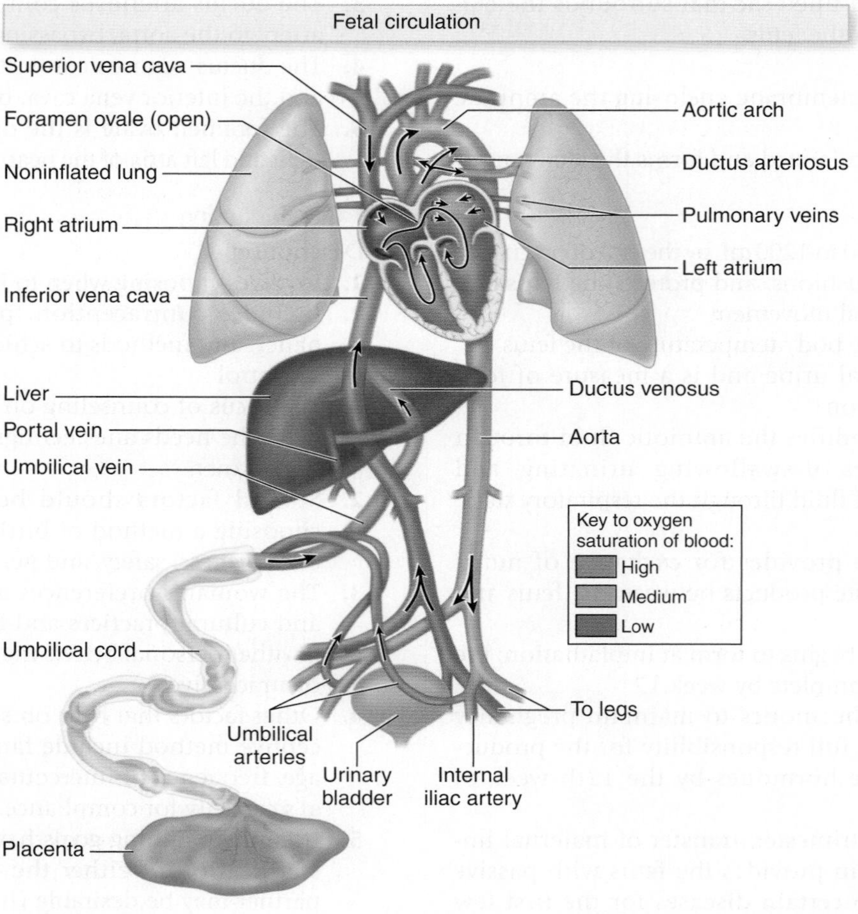

FIG. 20-1 Fetal circulation. Three shunts (ductus venosus, ductus arteriosus, and foramen ovale) allow most blood from the placenta to bypass the fetal lungs and liver.

5. Infertility options
   a. Options include medication, surgical procedures, and therapeutic insemination.
   b. Other therapies are available, such as in vitro fertilization, surrogate mothers, and embryo hosts.
   c. Adoption may also be an option.
6. The nurse needs to provide support to the couple in their decision-making process and during therapy.

PRACTICE QUESTIONS

184. The nurse is preparing to teach a prenatal class about fetal circulation. Which statements should be included in the teaching plan? **Select all that apply.**

❑ **1.** "The ductus arteriosus allows blood to bypass the fetal lungs."
❑ **2.** "One vein carries oxygenated blood from the placenta to the fetus."
❑ **3.** "The normal fetal heart beat range is 160 to 180 beats per minute in pregnancy."
❑ **4.** "Two arteries carry deoxygenated blood and waste products away from the fetus to the placenta."
❑ **5.** "Two veins carry blood that is high in carbon dioxide and other waste products away from the fetus to the placenta."

185. The nursing instructor asks the student to describe fetal circulation, specifically the ductus venosus. Which statement by the student indicates an understanding of the ductus venosus?

1. "It connects the pulmonary artery to the aorta."
2. "It is an opening between the right and left atria."
3. "It connects the umbilical vein to the inferior vena cava."
4. "It connects the umbilical artery to the inferior vena cava."

186. A pregnant client tells the clinic nurse that she wants to know the sex of her baby as soon as it can be determined. The nurse informs the client that

she should be able to find out the sex at 16 weeks' gestation because of which factor?
1. The appearance of the fetal external genitalia
2. The beginning of differentiation in the fetal groin
3. The fetal testes are descended into the scrotal sac
4. The internal differences in males and females become apparent

187. The nurse is performing an assessment on a client who is at 38 weeks' gestation and notes that the fetal heart rate (FHR) is 174 beats per minute. On the basis of this finding, what is the **priority** nursing action?
1. Document the finding.
2. Check the mother's heart rate.
3. Notify the obstetrician (OB).
4. Tell the client that the fetal heart rate is normal.

188. The nurse is conducting a prenatal class on the female reproductive system. When a client in the class asks why the fertilized ovum stays in the fallopian tube for 3 days, what is the nurse's **best** response?
1. "It promotes the fertilized ovum's chances of survival."
2. "It promotes the fertilized ovum's exposure to estrogen and progesterone."
3. "It promotes the fertilized ovum's normal implantation in the top portion of the uterus."
4. "It promotes the fertilized ovum's exposure to luteinizing hormone and follicle-stimulating hormone."

189. The nursing instructor asks a nursing student to explain the characteristics of the amniotic fluid. The student responds correctly by explaining which as characteristics of amniotic fluid? **Select all that apply.**
- ❑ 1. Allows for fetal movement
- ❑ 2. Surrounds, cushions, and protects the fetus
- ❑ 3. Maintains the body temperature of the fetus
- ❑ 4. Can be used to measure fetal kidney function
- ❑ 5. Prevents large particles such as bacteria from passing to the fetus
- ❑ 6. Provides an exchange of nutrients and waste products between the mother and the fetus

190. A couple comes to the family planning clinic and asks about sterilization procedures. Which question by the nurse should determine whether this method of family planning would be **most appropriate?**
1. "Have you ever had surgery?"
2. "Do you plan to have any other children?"
3. "Do either of you have diabetes mellitus?"
4. "Do either of you have problems with high blood pressure?"

191. The nurse should make which statement to a pregnant client found to have a gynecoid pelvis?
1. "Your type of pelvis has a narrow pubic arch."
2. "Your type of pelvis is the most favorable for labor and birth."
3. "Your type of pelvis is a wide pelvis, but it has a short diameter."
4. "You will need a cesarean section because this type of pelvis is not favorable for a vaginal delivery."

192. Which purposes of placental functioning should the nurse include in a prenatal class? **Select all that apply.**
- ❑ 1. It cushions and protects the baby.
- ❑ 2. It maintains the temperature of the baby.
- ❑ 3. It is the way the baby gets food and oxygen.
- ❑ 4. It prevents all antibodies and viruses from passing to the baby.
- ❑ 5. It provides an exchange of nutrients and waste products between the mother and developing fetus.

193. A 55-year-old male client confides in the nurse that he is concerned about his sexual function. What is the nurse's **best** response?
1. "How often do you have sexual relations?"
2. "Please share with me more about your concerns."
3. "You are still young and have nothing to be concerned about."
4. "You should not have a decline in testosterone until you are in your 80s."

ANSWERS

184. *Answer:* 1, 2, 4
Rationale: The ductus arteriosus is a unique fetal circulation structure that allows blood to bypass the nonfunctioning fetal lungs. Oxygenated blood is transported to the fetus by one umbilical vein. The normal fetal heart beat range is considered to be 110 to 160 beats per minute. Two arteries carry deoxygenated blood and waste products from the fetus, and one umbilical vein carries oxygenated blood and provides oxygen and nutrients to the fetus. Blood pumped by the embryo's heart leaves the embryo through two umbilical arteries.
Test-Taking Strategy: Focus on the subject, fetal circulation. Recall that three umbilical vessels are within the umbilical cord (two arteries and one vein) and that the vein carries oxygenated blood and the arteries carry deoxygenated blood. Also recalling the normal fetal heart beat will assist in answering correctly.
Level of Cognitive Ability: Applying
Client Needs: Physiological Integrity
Integrated Process: Teaching and Learning
Content Area: Maternity: Antepartum
Health Problem: N/A
Priority Concepts: Client Education; Perfusion
Reference: McKinney et al. (2018), pp. 210-211.

185. *Answer:* 3
Rationale: The ductus venosus connects the umbilical vein to the inferior vena cava. The foramen ovale is a temporary opening between the right and left atria. The ductus arteriosus joins the aorta and the pulmonary artery.
Test-Taking Strategy: Focus on the subject, the description of the ductus venosus. Note the relationship of the word *venosus* in the question and *vein* in the correct option.
Level of Cognitive Ability: Evaluating
Client Needs: Physiological Integrity
Integrated Process: Nursing Process/Evaluation
Content Area: Maternity: Antepartum
Health Problem: N/A
Priority Concepts: Perfusion; Reproduction
Reference: McKinney et al. (2018), pp. 210-211.

186. *Answer:* 1
Rationale: Between weeks 16 and 20, the external genitalia of the fetus have developed to such a degree that the sex of the fetus can be determined visually. Differentiation of the external genitalia occurs at the end of the ninth week. Testes begin to descend into the scrotal sac at the end of the 38th week. Internal differences in the male and female occur at the end of the seventh week.
Test-Taking Strategy: Focus on the subject, sex of the fetus. Remember that the sex of the fetus can be recognizable visually on ultrasound by the appearance of the external genitalia by gestational weeks 16 and 20.
Level of Cognitive Ability: Applying
Client Needs: Health Promotion and Maintenance
Integrated Process: Teaching and Learning
Content Area: Maternity: Antepartum
Health Problem: N/A
Priority Concepts: Development; Sexuality
Reference: Lowdermilk et al. (2016), p. 278.

187. *Answer:* 3
Rationale: The FHR depends on gestational age and ranges from 160 to 170 beats per minute in the first trimester but slows with fetal growth to 110 to 160 beats per minute. If the FHR is less than 110 beats per minute or more than 160 beats per minute with the uterus at rest, the fetus may be in distress. Because the FHR is increased from the reference range, the nurse should notify the OB. Options 2 and 4 are inappropriate actions based on the information in the question. Although the nurse documents the findings, based on the information in the question, the OB needs to be notified.
Test-Taking Strategy: Focus on the data in the question and note the strategic word, *priority*. Then, note if an abnormality exists. Also note the FHR and that the client is at 38 weeks of gestation. Remember that the normal FHR is 110 to 160 beats per minute.
Level of Cognitive Ability: Analyzing
Client Needs: Physiological Integrity
Integrated Process: Nursing Process—Implementation
Content Area: Maternity: Antepartum
Health Problem: Maternity: Fetal Distress/Demise
Priority Concepts: Clinical Judgment; Perfusion
Reference: McKinney et al. (2018), p. 339.

188. *Answer:* 3
Rationale: The tubal isthmus remains contracted until 3 days after conception to allow the fertilized ovum to develop within the tube. This initial growth of the fertilized ovum promotes its normal implantation in the fundal portion of the uterine corpus. Estrogen is a hormone produced by the ovarian follicles, corpus luteum, adrenal cortex, and placenta during pregnancy. Progesterone is a hormone secreted by the corpus luteum of the ovary, adrenal glands, and placenta during pregnancy. Luteinizing hormone and follicle-stimulating hormone are excreted by the anterior pituitary gland. The survival of the fertilized ovum does not depend on it staying in the fallopian tube for 3 days.
Test-Taking Strategy: Note the strategic word, *best*, and use knowledge of the anatomy and physiology of the female reproductive system. Remember that fertilization occurs in the fallopian tube and the fertilized ovum remains in the fallopian tube for about 3 days. This promotes its normal implantation.
Level of Cognitive Ability: Applying
Client Needs: Physiological Integrity
Integrated Process: Teaching and Learning
Content Area: Maternity: Antepartum
Health Problem: N/A
Priority Concepts: Development; Reproduction
Reference: McKinney et al. (2018), p. 198.

189. *Answer:* 1, 2, 3, 4
Rationale: The amniotic fluid surrounds, cushions, and protects the fetus. It allows the fetus to move freely and maintains the body temperature of the fetus. In addition, the amniotic fluid contains urine from the fetus and can be used to assess fetal kidney function. The placenta prevents large particles such as bacteria from passing to the fetus and provides an exchange of nutrients and waste products between the mother and the fetus.
Test-Taking Strategy: Focus on the subject, the characteristics of amniotic fluid. Visualizing the location of the amniotic

fluid will assist in answering this question.
Level of Cognitive Ability: Evaluating
Client Needs: Physiological Integrity
Integrated Process: Nursing Process/Evaluation
Content Area: Maternity: Antepartum
Health Problem: N/A
Priority Concepts: Client Education; Reproduction
Reference: McKinney et al. (2018), p. 209.

190. *Answer:* 2
Rationale: Sterilization is a method of contraception for couples who have completed their families. It should be considered a permanent end to fertility, because reversal surgery is not always successful. The nurse would ask the couple about their plans for having children in the future. Options 1, 3, and 4 are unrelated to this procedure.
Test-Taking Strategy: Note the strategic words, *most appropriate.* Focus on the subject, sterilization procedure. Note the relationship between the word *sterilization* and the words *plan to have any other children* in the correct option.
Level of Cognitive Ability: Applying
Client Needs: Health Promotion and Maintenance
Integrated Process: Nursing Process—Assessment
Content Area: Adult Health: Reproductive
Health Problem: N/A
Priority Concepts: Health Promotion; Reproduction
Reference: McKinney et al. (2018), p. 660.

191. *Answer:* 2
Rationale: A gynecoid pelvis is a normal female pelvis and is the most favorable for successful labor and birth. An android pelvis (resembling a male pelvis) would be unfavorable for labor because of the narrow pelvic planes. An anthropoid pelvis has an outlet that is adequate, with a normal or moderately narrow pubic arch. A platypelloid pelvis (flat pelvis) has a wide transverse diameter, but the anteroposterior diameter is short, making the outlet inadequate.
Test-Taking Strategy: Focus on the subject, female pelvis types. Recalling that the gynecoid pelvis is the normal female pelvis will direct you to the correct option.
Level of Cognitive Ability: Applying
Client Needs: Health Promotion and Maintenance
Integrated Process: Teaching and Learning
Content Area: Maternity: Antepartum
Health Problem: N/A
Priority Concepts: Health Promotion; Reproduction
Reference: McKinney et al. (2018), p. 578.

192. *Answer:* 3, 5
Rationale: The placenta provides an exchange of oxygen, nutrients, and waste products between the mother and the fetus. The amniotic fluid surrounds, cushions, and protects the fetus and maintains the body temperature of the fetus. Nutrients, medications, antibodies, and viruses can pass through the placenta.
Test-Taking Strategy: Focus on the subject, the purpose of the placenta. Remember that the placenta provides oxygen and nutrients.
Level of Cognitive Ability: Applying
Client Needs: Health Promotion and Maintenance
Integrated Process: Teaching and Learning
Content Area: Maternity: Antepartum
Health Problem: N/A
Priority Concepts: Development; Reproduction
Reference: McKinney et al. (2018), pp. 206-207, 209.

193. *Answer:* 2
Rationale: The nurse needs to establish trust when discussing sexual relationships with men. The nurse should open the conversation with broad statements to determine the true nature of the client's concerns. The frequency of intercourse is not a relevant first question to establish trust. Testosterone declines with the aging process.
Test-Taking Strategy: Note the strategic word, *best.* Determine whether further assessment or validation is needed. In this case, more information is needed to determine the nature of the client's concerns. Keeping these concepts in mind and using therapeutic communication techniques will assist in directing you to the correct option.
Level of Cognitive Ability: Applying
Client Needs: Psychosocial Integrity
Integrated Process: Caring
Content Area: Adult Health: Reproductive
Priority Concepts: Communication; Sexuality
Reference: Lewis et al. (2017), p. 1288.

Maternity

CHAPTER 21

Prenatal Period

PRIORITY CONCEPTS Development, Reproduction

I. Gestation

A. Time from fertilization of the ovum until the date of delivery
B. About 280 days
C. Näegele's rule for estimating the date of delivery, also known as date of birth (Box 21-1)
   1. Use of Näegele's rule requires that the woman have a regular 28-day menstrual cycle.
   2. Subtract 3 months and add 7 days to the first day of the last menstrual period; then add 1 year if appropriate. Alternatively, add 7 days to the first day of the last menstrual period and count forward 9 months.

II. Gravidity and Parity

A. Gravidity
   1. Gravida refers to a pregnant woman.
   2. *Gravidity* refers to the number of pregnancies.
   3. A nulligravida is a woman who has never been pregnant.
   4. A primigravida is a woman who is pregnant for the first time.
   5. A multigravida is a woman in at least her second pregnancy.
B. Parity
   1. Parity is the number of births (not the number of fetuses, e.g., twins) carried past 20 weeks of gestation, whether or not the fetus was born alive.
   2. A nullipara is a woman who has not had a birth at more than 20 weeks of gestation.
   3. A primipara is a woman who has had 1 birth that occurred after the 20th week of gestation.
   4. A multipara is a woman who has had 2 or more pregnancies to the stage of fetal viability.
C. Use of GTPAL: Pregnancy outcomes can be described with the acronym *GTPAL* (Box 21-2).
   1. *G* is gravidity, the number of pregnancies, including the present one.
   2. *T* is term births, the number born at term (longer than 37 weeks of gestation).
   3. *P* is preterm births, the number born before 37 weeks of gestation.
   4. *A* is abortions or miscarriages, the number of abortions or miscarriages (included in gravida if before 20 weeks of gestation)
   5. *L* is the number of current living children. This number can be greater than the P if multiples were delivered, or less than the P if a loss occurred.
   6. *Note:* Multiples count as a 1 for gravidity, as well as a 1 for term, preterm, or abortions, but are recorded as the actual number for living.

III. Pregnancy Signs

A. Presumptive signs
   1. Amenorrhea
   2. Nausea and vomiting
   3. Increased size and increased feeling of fullness in breasts
   4. Pronounced nipples
   5. Urinary frequency
   6. Quickening: The first perception of fetal movement by the mother may occur at the 16th to 20th week of gestation.
   7. Fatigue
   8. Discoloration of the vaginal mucosa
B. Probable signs
   1. Uterine enlargement
   2. Hegar's sign: Compressibility and softening of the lower uterine segment that occurs at about week 6
   3. Goodell's sign: Softening of the cervix that occurs at the beginning of the second month
   4. Chadwick's sign: Violet coloration of the mucous membranes of the cervix, vagina, and vulva that occurs at about week 6
   5. Ballottement: Rebounding of the fetus against the examiner's fingers on palpation
   6. Braxton Hicks contractions (irregular painless contractions that may occur intermittently throughout pregnancy)
   7. Positive pregnancy test for determination of the presence of human chorionic gonadotropin

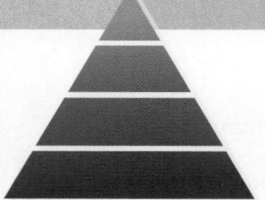

Box 21-1 Näegele's Rule for Estimating the Date of Delivery

First day of last menstrual period: September 12, 2021
Subtract 3 months: June 12, 2021
Add 7 days: June 19, 2021
Add 1 year: June 19, 2022
Estimated date of delivery: June 19, 2022

BOX 21-2 Describing Pregnancy Outcome with GTPAL

G = Gravidity
T = Term births
P = Preterm births
A = Abortions or miscarriages
L = Current living children

Example: A woman is pregnant for the fourth time. She had 1 elective abortion in the first trimester, a daughter who was born at 40 weeks of gestation, and a son who was born at 36 weeks of gestation. She is gravida (G), 4; term (T), 1 (the daughter born at 40 weeks); preterm (P), 1 (the son born at 36 weeks); abortion (A), 1 (the abortion is counted in the gravidity, but is not included in the parity because it occurred before 20 weeks); living children (L), 2. Parity is the number of births (not the number of fetuses) carried past 20 weeks of gestation, whether or not the fetus was born alive. Therefore, the parity for this woman is 2.

$$GTPAL = 4,1,1,1,2$$

C. Positive signs (diagnostic)
   1. Fetal heart rate detected by electronic device (Doppler transducer) at 10 to 12 weeks and by nonelectronic device (fetoscope) at 20 weeks of gestation
   2. Active fetal movements palpable by examiner
   3. Outline of fetus via radiography or ultrasonography

IV. Fundal Height (Box 21-3)

A. Fundal height is measured to evaluate the gestational age of the fetus.

B. During the second and third trimesters (weeks 18 to 30), fundal height in centimeters approximately equals fetal age in weeks ± 2 cm (Fig. 21-1).

BOX 21-3 Measuring Fundal Height

1. Place the client in the supine position.
2. Place the end of the tape measure at the level of the symphysis pubis.
3. Stretch the tape to the top of the uterine fundus.
4. Note and record the measurement.

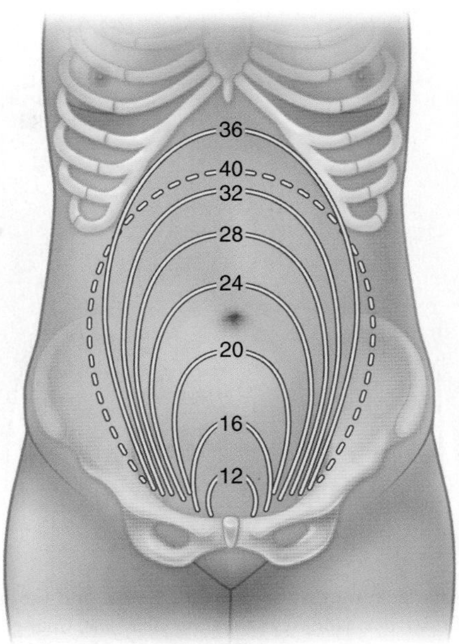

FIG. 21-1 Height of fundus by weeks of normal gestation with a single fetus. *Dashed line,* Height after lightening (descent of the fetus toward the pelvic inlet before labor).

C. At 16 weeks, the fundus can be found approximately halfway between the symphysis pubis and the umbilicus.

D. At 20 to 22 weeks, the fundus is approximately at the location of the umbilicus.

E. At 36 weeks, the fundus is at the xiphoid process.

⚠ When assessing fundal height, monitor the client closely for supine hypotension when placed in the supine position.

V. Physiological Maternal Changes

⚠ Culture often determines health beliefs, values, and family expectations. Therefore, it is important to assess cultural beliefs during care of the maternity client.

A. Cardiovascular system
   1. Circulating blood volume increases, plasma increases, and total red blood cell volume increases (total volume increases by approximately 40% to 50%).
   2. Physiological anemia occurs as the plasma increase exceeds the increase in production of red blood cells.
   3. Iron requirements are increased.
   4. Heart size increases, and the heart is elevated slightly upward and to the left because of displacement of the diaphragm as the uterus enlarges (Fig. 21-2).
   5. Retention of sodium and water may occur.

B. Respiratory system
   1. Oxygen consumption increases by approximately 15% to 20%.

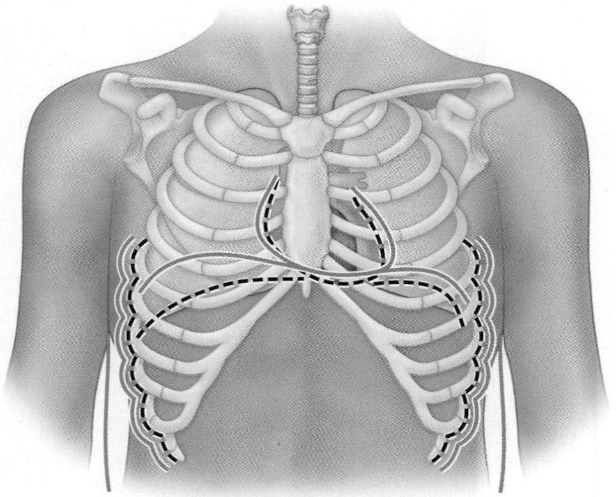

FIG. 21-2 Changes in position of heart, lungs, and thoracic cage in pregnancy. *Broken line,* Nonpregnant state. *Solid line,* Change that occurs in pregnancy.

2. Diaphragm is elevated because of the enlarged uterus (Fig. 21-2).
3. Shortness of breath may be experienced.

During pregnancy, a woman's pulse rate may increase about 10 to 15 beats per minute; the blood pressure slightly decreases in the second trimester, then increases in the third trimester, but not above the prepregnancy level; and the respiratory rate remains unchanged or slightly increases.

C. Gastrointestinal system
1. Nausea and vomiting may occur as a result of the secretion of human chorionic gonadotropin; it typically subsides by the third month.
2. Poor appetite may occur because of decreased gastric motility.
3. Alterations in taste and smell may occur.
4. Constipation may occur because of an increase in progesterone production or pressure of the uterus resulting in decreased gastrointestinal motility.
5. Flatulence and heartburn may occur because of decreased gastrointestinal motility and slowed emptying of the stomach caused by an increase in progesterone production.
6. Hemorrhoids may occur because of increased venous pressure.
7. Gum tissue may become swollen and easily bleed because of increasing levels of estrogen.
8. Ptyalism (excessive secretion of saliva) may occur because of increasing levels of estrogen.

D. Renal system
1. Frequency of urination increases in the first and third trimesters because of increased bladder sensitivity and pressure of the enlarging uterus on the bladder.
2. Decreased bladder tone may occur and is caused by an increase in progesterone and estrogen levels; bladder capacity increases in response to increasing levels of progesterone.
3. Renal threshold for glucose may be reduced.

E. Endocrine system
1. Basal metabolic rate increases and metabolic function increases.
2. The anterior lobe of the pituitary gland enlarges and produces serum prolactin needed for the lactation process.
3. The posterior lobe of the pituitary gland produces oxytocin, which stimulates uterine contractions.
4. The thyroid enlarges slightly, and thyroid activity increases.
5. The parathyroid increases in size.
6. Aldosterone levels gradually increase.
7. Body weight increases.
8. Water retention is increased, which can contribute to weight gain.

F. Reproductive system
1. Uterus
   a. Uterus enlarges, increasing in mass from approximately 60 to 1000 g as a result of hyperplasia (influence of estrogen) and hypertrophy.
   b. Size and number of blood vessels and lymphatics increase.
   c. Irregular contractions occur, typically beginning after 16 weeks of gestation.
2. Cervix
   a. Cervix becomes shorter, more elastic, and larger in diameter.
   b. Endocervical glands secrete a thick mucous plug, which is expelled from the canal when dilation begins.
   c. Increased vascularization and an increase in estrogen cause softening and a violet discoloration known as Chadwick's sign, which occurs at about 6 weeks of gestation.
3. Ovaries
   a. A major function of the ovaries is to secrete progesterone for the first 6 to 7 weeks of pregnancy.
   b. The maturation of new follicles is blocked.
   c. The ovaries cease ovum production.
4. Vagina
   a. Hypertrophy and thickening of the muscle occur.
   b. An increase in vaginal secretions is experienced; secretions are usually thick, white, and acidic.
5. Breasts: Breast changes occur because of the increasing effects of estrogen and progesterone.
   a. Breast size increases, and breasts may be tender.
   b. Nipples become more pronounced.

c. The areolae become darker in color.
d. Superficial veins become prominent.
e. Hypertrophy of Montgomery's follicles occurs.
f. Colostrum may leak from the breast.

G. Skin
1. Some changes occur because the levels of melanocyte-stimulating hormone increase as a result of an increase in estrogen and progesterone levels; these changes include the following:
a. Increased pigmentation
b. Dark streak down the midline of the abdomen (linea nigra)
c. Chloasma (mask of pregnancy)—a blotchy brownish hyperpigmentation over the forehead, cheeks, and nose
d. Reddish-purple stretch marks (striae gravidarum) on the abdomen, breasts, thighs, and upper arms
2. Vascular spider nevi may occur on the neck, chest, face, arms, and legs.
3. Rate of hair growth may increase.

H. Musculoskeletal system
1. Changes in the center of gravity begin in the second trimester and are caused by the hormones relaxin and progesterone.
2. The lumbosacral curve increases.
3. Aching, numbness, and weakness may result; walking becomes more difficult, and the woman develops a waddling gait and is at risk for falls.
4. Relaxation and increased mobility of pelvic joints occur, which permit enlargement of pelvic dimensions.
5. Abdominal wall stretches with loss of tone throughout pregnancy, regained postpartum.
6. Umbilicus flattens or protrudes.

! During pregnancy, postural changes occur as the increased weight of the uterus causes a forward pull of the bony pelvis. It is important for the nurse to encourage the client to implement measures that maintain safety and correct posture to prevent a backache.

VI. Psychological Maternal Changes

A. Ambivalence
1. Ambivalence may occur early in pregnancy, even when the pregnancy is planned.
2. The mother may experience a dependence–independence conflict and ambivalence related to role changes.
3. The partner may experience ambivalence related to the new role being assumed, increased financial responsibilities, and sharing the mother's attention with the child.

B. Acceptance: Factors that may be related to acceptance of the pregnancy are the woman's readiness for the experience and her identification with the motherhood role. Specific developmental tasks must be accomplished successfully for positive maternal role adaptation. These tasks include accepting the pregnancy, identifying with the mothering role, solidifying her relationship with her partner, establishing a relationship with her unborn infant, and preparing for her birth experience.

C. Emotional lability
1. Emotional lability may be manifested by frequent changes of emotional states or extremes in emotional states.
2. These emotional changes are common, but the mother may think that these changes are abnormal.

D. Body image changes
1. The changes in a woman's perception of her image during pregnancy occur gradually and may be positive or negative.
2. The physical changes and signs and symptoms that the woman experiences during pregnancy contribute to her body image.

E. Relationship with the fetus
1. The woman may daydream to prepare for motherhood and think about the maternal qualities that she would like to possess.
2. The woman first accepts the biological fact that she is pregnant.
3. The woman next accepts the growing fetus as distinct from herself and a person to nurture.
4. Finally, the woman prepares realistically for the birth and parenting of the child.

VII. Discomforts of Pregnancy

A. Nausea and vomiting
1. Occurs in the first trimester and usually subsides by the third month
2. Caused by elevated levels of human chorionic gonadotropin and other pregnancy hormones as well as changes in carbohydrate metabolism
3. Interventions
a. Eating dry crackers before arising
b. Avoiding brushing teeth immediately after arising
c. Eating small, frequent, low-fat meals during the day
d. Drinking liquids between meals rather than at meals
e. Avoiding fried foods and spicy foods
f. Asking the primary health care provider (PHCP) about acupressure (some types may require a prescription)
g. Asking the PHCP about the use of herbal remedies
h. Taking antiemetic medications as prescribed

B. Syncope
1. Usually occurs in the first trimester; supine hypotension occurs particularly in the second and third trimesters.

2. May be triggered hormonally or caused by the increased blood volume, anemia, fatigue, sudden position changes, or lying supine
3. Interventions
   a. Sitting with the feet elevated
   b. Risk for falls; teach to change positions slowly

! The nurse needs to instruct the pregnant woman to avoid lying in the supine position, particularly in the second and third trimesters. The supine position places the woman at risk for supine hypotension, which occurs as a result of pressure of the uterus on the inferior vena cava.

C. Urinary urgency and frequency
1. Usually occurs in the first and third trimesters
2. Caused by pressure of the uterus on the bladder
3. Interventions
   a. Drinking no less than 2000 mL of fluid during the day
   b. Limiting fluid intake in the evening
   c. Voiding at regular intervals
   d. Sleeping side-lying at night
   e. Wearing perineal pads, if necessary
   f. Performing Kegel exercises

D. Breast tenderness
1. Can occur in the first through the third trimesters
2. Caused by increased levels of estrogen and progesterone
3. Interventions
   a. Wearing a supportive bra
   b. Avoiding the use of soap on the nipples and areolar area to prevent drying of skin

E. Increased vaginal discharge
1. Can occur in the first through the third trimesters
2. Caused by hypertrophy and thickening of the vaginal mucosa and increased mucus production
3. Interventions
   a. Using proper cleansing and hygiene techniques
   b. Wearing cotton underwear
   c. Avoiding douching
   d. Consulting the PHCP if infection is suspected

F. Nasal stuffiness
1. Occurs in the first through third trimesters
2. Results from increased estrogen, which causes edema of the nasal tissues and dryness
3. Interventions
   a. Encouraging the use of a humidifier
   b. Avoiding the use of nasal sprays or antihistamines (the PHCP should be consulted about their use)

G. Fatigue
1. Occurs usually in the first and third trimesters
2. Usually results from hormonal changes
3. Interventions
   a. Arranging frequent rest periods throughout the day
   b. Using correct posture and body mechanics
   c. Obtaining regular exercise
   d. Performing muscle relaxation and strengthening exercises for the legs and hip joints
   e. Avoiding eating and drinking foods containing stimulants throughout the pregnancy

H. Heartburn
1. Occurs in the second and third trimesters
2. Results from increased progesterone levels, decreased gastrointestinal motility, esophageal reflux, and displacement of the stomach by the enlarging uterus
3. Interventions
   a. Eating small, frequent meals
   b. Sitting upright for 30 minutes after a meal
   c. Drinking milk between meals
   d. Avoiding fatty and spicy foods
   e. Performing tailor-sitting exercises
   f. Consulting with the PHCP about the use of antacids

I. Ankle edema
1. Usually occurs in the second and third trimesters
2. Results from vasodilation, venous stasis, and increased venous pressure below the uterus
3. Interventions
   a. Elevating the legs at least twice a day and when resting
   b. Sleeping in a side-lying position
   c. Wearing supportive stockings or support hose
   d. Avoiding sitting or standing in 1 position for long periods

J. Varicose veins
1. Usually occur in the second and third trimesters
2. Result from weakening walls of the veins or valves and venous congestion
3. Thrombophlebitis is rare, but it may occur.
4. Interventions
   a. Wearing supportive stockings or support hose
   b. Elevating the feet when sitting
   c. Lying with the feet and hips elevated
   d. Avoiding long periods of standing or sitting
   e. Moving about while standing to improve circulation
   f. Avoiding leg crossing
   g. Avoiding constricting articles of clothing such as knee-high stockings
   h. Teaching leg exercises
   i. Avoiding airline because of sitting position

K. Headaches
1. Usually considered benign in the first trimester. May need further investigation if occurring in the second and third trimesters
2. Result from changes in blood volume and vascular tone

3. Interventions
   a. Changing position slowly
   b. Applying a cool cloth to the forehead
   c. Eating a small snack
   d. Using acetaminophen only if prescribed by the PHCP

L. Hemorrhoids
1. Usually occur in the second and third trimesters
2. Result from increased venous pressure and constipation
3. Interventions
   a. Soaking in a warm sitz bath
   b. Sitting on a soft pillow
   c. Eating high-fiber foods and drinking sufficient fluids to avoid constipation
   d. Increasing exercise, such as walking
   e. Applying ointments, suppositories, or compresses as prescribed by the PHCP

M. Constipation
1. Usually occurs in the second and third trimesters
2. Results from an increase in progesterone production, decreased intestinal motility, displacement of the intestines, pressure of the uterus, and taking iron supplements
3. Interventions
   a. Eating high-fiber foods such as whole grains, fruits, and vegetables
   b. Drinking no less than 2000 mL per day
   c. Exercising regularly, such as a daily 20-minute walk
   d. Consulting with the PHCP about interventions such as the use of stool softeners, laxatives, or enemas

N. Backache
1. Usually occurs in the second and third trimesters
2. Caused by an exaggerated lumbosacral curve resulting from an enlarged uterus
3. Risk for falls; teach to move about slowly
4. Interventions
   a. Obtaining rest
   b. Using correct posture and body mechanics
   c. Wearing low-heeled, comfortable, and supportive shoes
   d. Performing pelvic tilt (rock) exercises and conscious relaxation exercises
   e. Sleeping on a firm mattress

O. Leg cramps
1. Usually occur in the second and third trimesters
2. Result from an altered calcium-phosphorus balance and pressure of the uterus on nerves or from fatigue
3. Interventions
   a. Getting regular exercise, especially walking
   b. Dorsiflexing the foot of the affected leg
   c. Increasing calcium intake

P. Shortness of breath
1. Can occur in the second and third trimesters
2. Results from pressure on the diaphragm from the enlarged uterus
3. Interventions
   a. Taking frequent rest periods
   b. Sitting and sleeping with the head elevated or on the side
   c. Avoiding overexertion

VIII. Maternal Risk Factors

A. Maternal age: Women younger than 20 years and older than 35 years are at risk for adverse perinatal outcomes.

B. Adolescent pregnancy
1. Factors that result in adolescent pregnancy include the early onset of menarche, sexual behaviors in this age group, problems with family relationships, poverty, and lack of knowledge of reproduction and birth control.
2. Major concerns related to adolescent pregnancy include poor nutritional status; emotional and behavioral difficulties; lack of support systems; increased risk of stillbirth; low-birth-weight infants; fetal mortality; cephalopelvic disproportion; and increased risk of maternal complications, such as hypertension, anemia, prolonged labor, and infections.
3. The role of the nurse in reducing risks and consequences of adolescent pregnancy is twofold: first, to encourage early and continued prenatal care; and second, to refer the adolescent, if necessary, for appropriate assistance, which can help counter the effects of a negative socioeconomic environment on the pregnancy.

C. Nutrition: Adequate nutrition is necessary for normal fetal growth and development. Nutrition needs are determined by the stage of pregnancy and nutrition should support recommended weight gain during the various stages.

⚠ Women of childbearing age should take folic acid supplements to prevent neural tube defects and orofacial clefts in the fetus.

D. Genetic considerations: Genetic abnormalities such as defective genes or transmissible inherited disorders can result in congenital anomalies; the nurse should perform a genetic risk assessment to determine an inheritable risk.

E. Health care: Failure to seek and obtain prenatal care, including dental care, increases the risk for preterm birth and low birth weight.

F. Abuse and violence: Physical abuse and violence can increase the risk for abruptio placentae, preterm birth, and infections from unwanted and forced sex.

G. Medical conditions: Concurrent medical conditions, such as, but not limited to, diabetes mellitus, hypertensive disorder, or cardiac disease, increase the risk of complications during pregnancy.

H. German measles (rubella): Maternal infection during the first 8 weeks of gestation carries the highest rate of fetal infection.

I. Sexually transmitted infections
   1. Syphilis
      a. Organism may cross the **placenta**.
      b. Infection usually leads to spontaneous abortions and increases the incidence of mental subnormality and physical deformities.
   2. Condyloma acuminatum (human papillomavirus)
      a. Transmission may occur during vaginal birth.
      b. Infection is associated with the development of epithelial tumors of the mucous membranes of the larynx in children.
   3. Gonorrhea
      a. Fetus is contaminated at the time of birth.
      b. Maternal infection may result in postpartum infection of the **neonate**.
      c. Risks to the neonate include ophthalmia neonatorum, pneumonia, and sepsis.
   4. Chlamydial infection
      a. Transmission may occur during vaginal birth and can result in neonatal conjunctivitis or pneumonitis.
      b. Infection can cause premature rupture of the membranes, premature labor, and postpartum endometritis.
   5. Trichomoniasis: Associated with premature rupture of the membranes and postpartum endometritis
   6. Genital herpes simplex virus
      a. Characterized by painful lesions, fever, chills, malaise, and severe dysuria and may last 2 to 3 weeks
      b. Assessment includes questioning all women about signs and symptoms and inspecting the vulvar, perineal, and vaginal areas for vesicles or areas of ulceration or crusting; this is done during pregnancy and at the onset of labor.
      c. Vaginal birth may be acceptable; cesarean birth is required if visible lesions are present.
      d. Infants who are born through an infected vagina should be observed carefully, and samples should be taken for culture.

J. Human immunodeficiency virus (HIV)
   1. HIV is transmitted through blood; blood products; and other bodily fluids such as urine, semen, and vaginal secretions; the virus is also transmitted through exposure to infected secretions during birth and through breast milk.
   2. Repeated exposure to the virus during pregnancy through unsafe sex practices or intravenous drug use can increase the risk of transmission to the fetus.
   3. Perinatal administration of zidovudine may be recommended to decrease the risk of transmission of HIV from mother to fetus.

K. Substance abuse
   1. Substance abuse threatens normal fetal growth and successful term completion of the pregnancy.
   2. Substance abuse places the pregnancy at risk for fetal growth restriction, abruptio placentae, and fetal bradycardia.
   3. Many substances cross the placenta and can be teratogenic (drugs, tobacco, alcohol, medications, certain foods such as raw fish); no over-the-counter medications should be taken unless prescribed by the PHCP.
   4. Smoking (tobacco) can result in low birth weight, a higher incidence of birth defects, and stillbirths.
   5. Physical signs of drug abuse may include dilated or contracted pupils, fatigue, track (needle) marks, skin abscesses, inflamed nasal mucosa, and inappropriate behavior by the mother.
   6. Consumption of alcohol during pregnancy may lead to fetal alcohol syndrome and can cause jitteriness, physical abnormalities, congenital anomalies, and growth deficits in the **newborn**.

L. Viral hepatitis (see Chapters 22, 33, and 48 for information regarding hepatitis B infection)

IX. Antepartum Diagnostic Testing

The usual schedule for antepartum health care visits is every 4 weeks for the first 28 to 32 weeks, every 2 weeks from 32 to 36 weeks, and every week from 36 to 40 weeks.

A. Blood type and Rh factor
   1. ABO typing is performed to determine the woman's blood type in the ABO antigen system.
   2. Rh typing is done to determine the woman's blood type in the rhesus antigen system. (*Rh positive* indicates the presence of the antigen; *Rh negative* indicates the absence of the antigen.)
   3. If the client is Rh negative and has a negative antibody screen, she will need repeat antibody screens and should receive $Rh_o(D)$ immune globulin (RhoGAM) at 28 weeks of gestation.

B. Rubella titer
   1. If the client has a negative titer (less than 1:8), indicating susceptibility to the rubella virus, she should receive the appropriate immunization postpartum.
   2. The client must be using effective birth control at the time of the immunization and must be counseled not to become pregnant for 1 to

3 months after immunization (as specified by the PHCP) and to avoid contact with anyone who is immunocompromised.

3. If the rubella vaccine is administered at the same time as $Rh_o(D)$ immune globulin, it may not be effective.
4. Rubella vaccine is administered postpartum (before discharge) via the subcutaneous route if the titer is less than 1:8; inquire about sensitivity to eggs.

Rubella vaccine is not given during pregnancy because the live attenuated virus may cross the placenta and present a risk to the developing fetus.

C. Hemoglobin and hematocrit levels
   1. Hemoglobin and hematocrit levels decline during gestation as a result of increased plasma volume.
   2. A decrease in the hemoglobin level to less than 10 g/dL (100 mmol/L) or in the hematocrit level to less than 30% indicates anemia.

D. Papanicolaou's smear may be done during the initial prenatal examination to screen for cervical neoplasia if the woman has not had a screening before or is beyond the recommended timeframe since her last screening.

E. Sexually transmitted infections (Table 21-1)

F. Sickle cell screening
   1. Screening is indicated for clients at risk for sickle cell disease.
   2. A positive test may indicate a need for further screening.

G. Tuberculin skin test
   1. The PHCP may prefer to perform this skin test after birth.
   2. A positive skin test indicates the need for a chest radiograph (using an abdominal lead shield) to rule out active disease; in a pregnant client, chest radiography would not be performed until after 20 weeks of gestation (after the fetal organs are formed).
   3. Converters to positive may be referred for treatment with medication after birth.

H. Hepatitis B surface antigens
   1. Testing for hepatitis antigens is recommended for all women because of the prevalence of the disease in the general population.
   2. Vaccination for hepatitis B antigen may be specifically indicated for the following:
      a. Health care workers
      b. Intravenous drug users
      c. Clients born in Asia, Africa, Haiti, or the Pacific islands
      d. Clients with previously undiagnosed jaundice or chronic liver disease
      e. Clients with tattoos
      f. Clients with histories of blood transfusions
      g. Clients with histories of multiple episodes of sexually transmitted infections
      h. Clients who have been rejected previously as blood donors
      i. Clients with histories of dialysis or renal transplantation
      j. Clients from households having members infected with hepatitis B or hemodialysis clients

TABLE 21-1 Monitoring for Sexually Transmitted Infections

Disease	Laboratory Test
Gonorrhea	Vaginal culture is done during initial prenatal examination to screen for gonorrhea. Culture may be repeated during third trimester in high-risk clients.
Syphilis	Culture of lesions (if present) is done during initial prenatal examination to screen for syphilis. Diagnosis depends on microscopic examination of primary and secondary lesion tissue and serology (Venereal Disease Research Laboratory [VDRL] or rapid plasma reagin [RPR] test) during latency and late infection. Culture may be repeated during the third trimester in high-risk clients.
Condyloma acuminatum (human papillomavirus)	Culture is indicated for clients with positive history or with active lesions. Test is performed to determine route of delivery. Weekly cultures may be done at week 35 or 36 of pregnancy until birth.
Chlamydia	Vaginal culture is indicated for all pregnant clients if client is in a high-risk group or if infants from previous pregnancies have developed neonatal conjunctivitis or pneumonia.
Trichomoniasis	Normal saline wet smear of vaginal secretions is checked for presence of protozoa. Associated with premature rupture of membranes and postpartum endometritis.
Genital herpes simplex virus (HSV-2)	Culture is done of lesions (if present) during initial prenatal examination to screen for HSV. Microscopic examination is done to determine presence of virus. Additional screening may be necessary as pregnancy progresses.
HIV	Testing may be done for a high-risk client. Common tests to determine the presence of antibodies include ELISA, Western blot, and immunofluorescence assay (IFA).

ELISA, Enzyme-linked immunosorbent assay; *HIV*, human immunodeficiency virus.

3. Hepatitis B vaccine is not contraindicated during pregnancy and may be recommended by the PHCP.
4. See Chapters 22, 33, and 48 for additional information about hepatitis.

I. Glucose challenge test (GCT)
1. Screening for gestational diabetes mellitus begins at the initial prenatal visit and is diagnosed by a fasting blood glucose greater than 126 mg/dL (7.0 mmol/L), A1C greater than 6.5%, or a random plasma glucose level greater than 200 mg/dL (11.1 mmol/L), then subsequently confirmed by an elevated fasting glucose level or A1C.
2. According to the American Congress of Obstetricians and Gynecologists (ACOG), a GCT using a two-step approach should be used in screening for gestational diabetes mellitus (GDM).
3. A 50-g oral glucose load without regard to time of day is given. After 1 hour a plasma or serum glucose level is drawn and is considered elevated if it is greater than 140 mg/dL (7.8 mmol/L) and a 3-hour GCT should be done.
4. If the 3-hour GCT is above 130 to 140 mg/dL (7.2 to 7.8 mmol/L), it is considered a positive result and may be indicative of GDM.
5. It is important to note that the GCT has 86% sensitivity, and some false positives may be noted.

J. Urinalysis and urine culture
1. A urine specimen for glucose and protein determinations should be obtained at every antepartum visit.
2. Glycosuria is a common result of decreased renal threshold that occurs during pregnancy.
3. If glycosuria persists, it may indicate diabetes.
4. White blood cells in the urine may indicate infection.
5. Ketonuria may result from insufficient food intake or vomiting.
6. Levels of 2 + to 4 + protein in the urine may indicate infection or preeclampsia.

K. Ultrasonography
1. Outlines and identifies fetal and maternal structures
2. Assists in confirming gestational age and estimated date of delivery and evaluating amniotic fluid volume (amniotic fluid index), which is done via special measurements
3. May be done abdominally or transvaginally during pregnancy
4. Can be used to determine the presence of premature dilation of the cervix (incompetent cervix). A transvaginal ultrasound is used during the first trimester to check the length of the cervix.
5. Interventions
   a. If an abdominal ultrasound is being performed, the woman may need to drink water to fill the bladder before the procedure to obtain a better image of the fetus.
   b. If a transvaginal ultrasound is being performed, a lubricated probe is inserted into the vagina.
   c. The client should be informed that the test presents no known risks to the client or the fetus.

L. Biophysical profile
1. Noninvasive assessment of the fetus that includes fetal breathing movements, fetal movements, fetal tone, amniotic fluid index, and fetal heart rate patterns via a nonstress test
2. Normal fetal biophysical activities indicate that the central nervous system is functional and that the fetus is not hypoxemic.

M. Doppler blood flow analysis: Noninvasive (ultrasonography) method of studying the blood flow in the fetus and placenta

N. Percutaneous umbilical blood sampling
1. Percutaneous umbilical blood sampling is performed if fetal blood sampling is necessary; it involves insertion of a needle directly into the fetal umbilical vessel under ultrasound guidance.
2. Fetal heart rate monitoring is necessary for 1 hour after the procedure, and a follow-up ultrasound to check for bleeding or hematoma formation is done 1 hour after the procedure.

O. α-Fetoprotein screening
1. Assesses the quantity of fetal serum proteins; abnormal protein levels are associated with open neural tube and abdominal wall defects
2. Assists in screening for spina bifida and Down syndrome
3. If abnormal, repeat test; false positive is common.
4. Interventions
   a. α-Fetoprotein level is determined by a maternal blood sample drawn between 16 and 18 weeks of gestation.
   b. If the level is abnormal and the gestation is less than 18 weeks, a second sample is drawn and screened.
   c. An ultrasound is performed for elevated levels to rule out fetal abnormalities or multiple gestation.

P. Deoxyribonucleic acid (DNA) genetic testing
1. Can be used to detect abnormalities related to an inherited condition
2. Assists in determining if the woman is at risk for having a fetus with Down syndrome (trisomy 21), Edwards syndrome (trisomy 18), or Patau syndrome (trisomy 13).
3. Interventions: This type of testing can be done as early as 7 weeks of gestation, and a blood sample is used.

Q. Chorionic villus sampling
1. Performed for the purpose of detecting genetic abnormalities; the PHCP aspirates a small sample of chorionic villus tissue at 10 to 13 weeks of gestation.
2. Interventions
a. Ensure informed consent was obtained.
b. The client may need to drink water to fill the bladder before the procedure to aid in the visualization of the uterus for catheter insertion.
c. Obtain baseline vital signs and fetal heart rate; monitor frequently after the procedure.
d. Rh-negative women may be given Rh_o(D) immune globulin, because chorionic villus sampling increases the risk of Rh sensitization.

R. Amniocentesis
1. Aspiration of amniotic fluid; best performed between 15 and 20 weeks of pregnancy because amniotic fluid volume is adequate and many viable fetal cells are present in the fluid by this time
2. Performed to determine genetic disorders, metabolic defects, and fetal lung maturity
3. Risks
a. Maternal hemorrhage
b. Infection
c. Rh isoimmunization
d. Abruptio placentae
e. Amniotic fluid emboli
f. Premature rupture of the membranes
4. Interventions
a. Ensure informed consent was obtained.
b. If less than 20 weeks of gestation, the client should have a full bladder to support the uterus; if performed after 20 weeks of gestation, the client should have an empty bladder to minimize the chance of puncture.
c. Prepare the client for ultrasonography, which is performed to locate the placenta and avoid puncture.
d. Obtain baseline vital signs and fetal heart rate; monitor every 15 minutes.
e. Position the client supine during the examination and on the left side after the procedure.

After chorionic villus sampling and amniocentesis, instruct the client that if chills, fever, bleeding, leakage of fluid at the needle insertion site, decreased fetal movement, uterine contractions, or cramping occurs, she must notify the PHCP.

S. Kick counts (fetal movement counting)
1. Beginning at 28 weeks' gestation, the client sits quietly or lies down on her side and counts fetal kicks as instructed.
2. Instruct the client to notify the PHCP if there are fewer than 10 kicks in 2 consecutive 2-hour periods or as instructed by the PHCP.

T. Fern test
1. The fern test is a microscopic slide test to determine the presence of amniotic fluid leakage.
2. Using sterile technique, a specimen is obtained from the external os of the cervix and vaginal pool and is examined on a slide under a microscope.
3. A fern-like pattern produced by the effects of salts of the amniotic fluid indicates the presence of amniotic fluid; may be done in conjunction with the Nitrazine test.
4. Interventions
a. Position the client in the dorsal lithotomy position.
b. Instruct the client to cough, which causes the amniotic fluid to leak from the uterus if the membranes are ruptured.

U. Nitrazine test
1. A nitrazine test strip is used to detect the presence of amniotic fluid in vaginal secretions.
2. Vaginal secretions have a pH of 4.5 to 5.5 and do not affect the nitrazine strip or swab.
3. Amniotic fluid has a pH of 7.0 to 7.5 and turns the nitrazine strip or swab blue.
4. Interventions
a. Position the client in the dorsal lithotomy position.
b. Touch the test tape to the fluid.
c. Assess the test tape for a blue-green, blue-gray, or deep blue color, which indicates that the membranes are ruptured, causing leakage of amniotic fluid.

V. Fibronectin test
1. Sampling of cervical and vaginal secretions for fetal fibronectin; done between week 22 and week 34 of pregnancy if the primary health care provider is concerned about preterm labor.
2. Positive results may indicate the onset of labor in 1 to 3 weeks; negative test results are more predictive that preterm labor will not begin.
3. Test used if at risk for preterm labor, before 37 weeks of gestation
4. Interventions
a. Client is placed in lithotomy position for sterile speculum exam.
b. Cervical secretions are obtained with cotton swab.
c. Laboratory tests are done for the presence of fibronectin.

W. Nonstress test (Box 21-4)

X. Contraction stress test (Box 21-5)

BOX 21-4 Nonstress Test

Description

Test is performed to assess placental function and oxygenation.
Test determines fetal well-being.
Test evaluates the fetal heart rate (FHR) response to fetal movement.

Interventions

An external ultrasound transducer and tocodynamometer are applied to the client, and a tracing of at least 20 minutes' duration is obtained so that the FHR and uterine activity can be observed.
Baseline blood pressure is obtained, and blood pressure is monitored frequently.
The client is placed in the lateral (side-lying) position to avoid vena cava compression.
The client may be asked to press a button every time she feels fetal movement; the monitor records a mark at each point of fetal movement, which is used as a reference point to assess the FHR response.

Results

Reactive Nonstress Test (Normal, Negative)
"Reactive" indicates a healthy fetus.
The result requires 2 or more FHR accelerations of at least 15 beats per minute, lasting at least 15 seconds from the beginning of the acceleration to the end, in association with fetal movement, during a 20-minute period.

Nonreactive Nonstress Test (Abnormal)
No accelerations or accelerations of less than 15 beats per minute or lasting less than 15 seconds in duration occur during a 40-minute observation.

Unsatisfactory
The result cannot be interpreted because of the poor quality of the FHR tracing.

BOX 21-5 Contraction Stress Test

Description

Test assesses placental oxygenation and function.
Test determines fetal ability to tolerate labor and determines fetal well-being.
Fetus is exposed to the stress of contractions to assess the adequacy of placental perfusion under simulated labor conditions.
Test is performed if nonstress test is abnormal.

Interventions

External fetal monitor is applied to the client, and a 20- to 30-minute baseline strip is recorded.
The uterus is stimulated to contract by the administration of a dilute dose of oxytocin or by having the client use nipple stimulation until 3 palpable contractions with a duration of 40 seconds or more in a 10-minute period have been achieved.
Frequent maternal blood pressure readings are done, and the mother is monitored closely while increasing doses of oxytocin are given.

Results

Negative Contraction Stress Test (Normal)
A negative result is represented by no late decelerations of the fetal heart rate (FHR).

Positive Contraction Stress Test (Abnormal)
A positive result is represented by late decelerations of the FHR, with 50% or more of the contractions in the absence of hyperstimulation of the uterus.

Equivocal
An equivocal result contains decelerations, but with less than 50% of the contractions, or uterine activity shows a hyperstimulated uterus.

Unsatisfactory
An unsatisfactory result means that adequate uterine contractions cannot be achieved, or the FHR tracing is of insufficient quality for adequate interpretation.

X. Nutrition

A. General guidelines
1. Guidelines for health and nutrition information for breast-feeding and pregnant women are located at the U.S. Department of Agriculture ChooseMyPlate website at https://www.myplate.gov/life-stages/pregnancy-and-breastfeeding. The woman should be assisted with accessing this site and preparing a nutritional plan.
2. The average expected weight gain during pregnancy is 25 to 35 lb (11 to 16 kg) for women with a normal prepregnancy weight.
3. An increase of about 300 calories/day is needed during pregnancy.
4. Calorie needs are greater in the last 2 trimesters than in the first.
5. An increase of about 500 calories/day is needed during lactation.
6. A diet high in folic acid or folic acid supplements is necessary for all women of childbearing age to prevent neural tube defects and orofacial clefts in the fetus.
7. At least 8 to 10 (8-oz) glasses of fluid are needed each day, of which 4 to 6 glasses should be water.
8. Sodium is not restricted unless specifically prescribed by the PHCP.

B. Vegan and Vegetarian Diets (see Chapter 11)
1. Ensure that the client eats a sufficient amount of varied foods to meet normal nutrient and energy needs.
2. Clients should be educated about consuming complementary proteins over the course of each day to ensure that all essential amino acids are provided.

3. Potential deficiencies in vegetarian diets include energy, protein, vitamin B_{12}, zinc, iron, calcium, omega-3 fatty acids, and vitamin D (if limited exposure to sunlight).
4. Protein consumption can be increased by consumption of a variety of vegetable protein sources based on whole grains, legumes, seeds, nuts, and vegetables combined to provide all essential amino acids.
5. To enhance absorption of iron, vegetarians should include a good source of iron and vitamin C with each meal.
6. Foods commonly eaten include tofu, tempeh, soy milk and soy products, meat analogs, legumes, nuts and seeds, sprouts, and a variety of fruits and vegetables.

C. Lactose intolerance
1. Lactose consumed by an individual with lactose intolerance can cause abdominal distention, discomfort, nausea, vomiting, cramps, and loose stools.
2. Clients with lactose intolerance need to incorporate sources of calcium other than dairy products into their dietary patterns regularly.
3. Milk may be tolerated in cooked form, such as in custards or fermented dairy products.
4. Cheese and yogurt sometimes are tolerated.
5. Lactase, an enzyme, may be prescribed and is taken before ingesting milk or milk products.
6. Lactase-treated milk or lactose-free products are also available commercially.

D. Pica
1. Pica refers to eating nonfood substances, such as dirt, clay, starch, and freezer frost.
2. The cause is unknown; cultural values, such as beliefs regarding the effect of a material on the mother or fetus, may make pica a common practice.
3. Iron deficiency anemia may occur as a result of pica.

PRACTICE QUESTIONS

194. The nurse is providing instructions to a pregnant client who is scheduled for an amniocentesis. What instruction should the nurse provide?
1. Strict bed rest is required after the procedure.
2. Hospitalization is necessary for 24 hours after the procedure.
3. An informed consent needs to be signed before the procedure.
4. A fever is expected after the procedure because of the trauma to the abdomen.

195. A pregnant client in the first trimester calls the nurse at a health care clinic and reports that she has noticed a thin, colorless vaginal drainage. The nurse should make which statement to the client?
1. "Come to the clinic immediately."
2. "The vaginal discharge may be bothersome, but is a normal occurrence."
3. "Report to the emergency department at the maternity center immediately."
4. "Use tampons if the discharge is bothersome, but be sure to change the tampons every 2 hours."

196. A nonstress test is performed on a client who is pregnant, and the results of the test indicate nonreactive findings. The primary health care provider prescribes a contraction stress test, and the results are documented as negative. How should the nurse document this finding?
1. A normal test result
2. An abnormal test result
3. A high risk for fetal demise
4. The need for a cesarean section

197. A rubella titer result of a 1-day postpartum client is less than 1:8, and a rubella virus vaccine is prescribed to be administered before discharge. The nurse provides which information to the client about the vaccine? **Select all that apply.**
- ❑ 1. Breast-feeding needs to be stopped for 3 months.
- ❑ 2. Pregnancy needs to be avoided for 1 to 3 months.
- ❑ 3. The vaccine is administered by the subcutaneous route.
- ❑ 4. Exposure to immunosuppressed individuals needs to be avoided.
- ❑ 5. A hypersensitivity reaction can occur if the client has an allergy to eggs.
- ❑ 6. The area of the injection needs to be covered with a sterile gauze for 1 week.

198. The nurse in a health care clinic is instructing a pregnant client how to perform "kick counts." Which statement by the client indicates a **need for further instruction**?
1. "I will record the number of movements or kicks."
2. "I need to lie flat on my back to perform the procedure."
3. "If I count fewer than 10 kicks in a 2-hour period, I should count the kicks again over the next 2 hours."
4. "I should place my hands on the largest part of my abdomen and concentrate on the fetal movements to count the kicks."

199. The nurse is performing an assessment of a pregnant client who is at 28 weeks of gestation. The nurse measures the fundal height in centimeters and notes that the fundal height is 30 cm. How should the nurse interpret this finding?

1. The client is measuring large for gestational age.
2. The client is measuring small for gestational age.
3. The client is measuring normal for gestational age.
4. More evidence is needed to determine size for gestational age.

200. The nurse is performing an assessment on a client who suspects that she is pregnant and is checking the client for probable signs of pregnancy. The nurse should assess for which probable signs of pregnancy? **Select all that apply.**

- ☐ 1. Ballottement
- ☐ 2. Chadwick's sign
- ☐ 3. Uterine enlargement
- ☐ 4. Positive pregnancy test
- ☐ 5. Fetal heart rate detected by a nonelectronic device
- ☐ 6. Outline of fetus via radiography or ultrasonography

201. A pregnant client is seen for a regular prenatal visit and tells the nurse that she is experiencing irregular contractions. The nurse determines that she is experiencing Braxton Hicks contractions. On the basis of this finding, which nursing action is appropriate?

1. Contact the primary health care provider.
2. Instruct the client to maintain bed rest for the remainder of the pregnancy.
3. Inform the client that these contractions are common and may occur throughout the pregnancy.
4. Call the maternity unit and inform them that the client will be admitted in a preterm labor condition.

202. A client arrives at the clinic for the first prenatal assessment. She tells the nurse that the first day of her last normal menstrual period was October 19, 2020. Using Näegele's rule, which expected date of delivery should the nurse document in the client's chart?

1. July 12, 2021
2. July 26, 2021
3. August 12, 2021
4. August 26, 2021

203. The nurse is collecting data during an admission assessment of a client who is pregnant with twins. The client has a healthy 5-year-old child who was delivered at 38 weeks and tells the nurse that she does not have a history of any type of abortion or fetal demise. Using GTPAL, what should the nurse document in the client's chart?

1. G = 3, T = 2, P = 0, A = 0, L = 1
2. G = 2, T = 1, P = 0, A = 0, L = 1
3. G = 1, T = 1, P = 1, A = 0, L = 1
4. G = 2, T = 0, P = 0, A = 0, L = 1

ANSWERS

194. *Answer:* 3

Rationale: Because amniocentesis is an invasive procedure, informed consent needs to be obtained before the procedure. After the procedure, the client is instructed to rest, but may resume light activity after the cramping subsides. The client is instructed to keep the puncture site clean and to report any complications, such as chills, fever, bleeding, leakage of fluid at the needle insertion site, decreased fetal movement, uterine contractions, or cramping. Amniocentesis is an outpatient procedure and may be done in the obstetrician's office or in a special prenatal testing unit. Hospitalization is not necessary after the procedure.

Test-Taking Strategy: Focus on the subject, nursing implications related to amniocentesis. Recalling that this procedure is invasive will direct you to the correct option.

Level of Cognitive Ability: Applying

Client Needs: Physiological Integrity

Integrated Process: Teaching and Learning

Content Area: Maternity: Antepartum

Health Problem: N/A

Priority Concepts: Client Education; Health Care Law

Reference: McKinney et al. (2018), pp. 17, 280.

195. *Answer:* 2

Rationale: Leukorrhea begins during the first trimester. Many clients notice a thin, colorless, or yellow vaginal discharge throughout pregnancy. Some clients become distressed about this condition, but it does not require that the client report to the health care clinic or emergency department immediately. If vaginal discharge is profuse, the client may use panty liners, but she should not wear tampons because of the risk of infection. If the client uses panty liners, she should change them frequently.

Test-Taking Strategy: Eliminate options 1 and 3 first because they are comparable or alike, indicating that the client requires medical attention. From the remaining options, recalling that this manifestation is a normal physiological occurrence or that tampons should be avoided will assist in directing you to the correct option.

Level of Cognitive Ability: Applying

Client Needs: Health Promotion and Maintenance

Integrated Process: Nursing Process—Implementation

Content Area: Maternity: Antepartum

Health Problem: N/A

Priority Concepts: Health Promotion; Reproduction

Reference: Lowdermilk et al. (2016), p. 289.

196. *Answer:* 1

Rationale: Contraction stress test results may be interpreted as negative (normal), positive (abnormal), or equivocal. A negative test result indicates that no late decelerations occurred in the fetal heart rate, although the fetus was stressed by 3 contractions of at least 40 seconds' duration in a 10-minute period. Options 2, 3, and 4 are incorrect interpretations.

Test-Taking Strategy: Note that options 2, 3, and 4 are comparable or alike in that they indicate an abnormal test result finding.

Level of Cognitive Ability: Applying

Client Needs: Physiological Integrity

Integrated Process: Nursing Process—Assessment

Content Area: Maternity: Antepartum

Health Problem: N/A

Priority Concepts: Perfusion; Reproduction

Reference: McKinney et al. (2018), pp. 283-284.

197. *Answer:* 2, 3, 4, 5

Rationale: Rubella vaccine is administered to women who have not had rubella or women who are not serologically immune. The vaccine may be administered in the immediate postpartum period to prevent the possibility of contracting rubella in future pregnancies. The live attenuated rubella virus is not communicable in breast milk; breast-feeding does not need to be stopped. The client is counseled not to become pregnant for 1 to 3 months after immunization or as specified by the obstetrician because of a possible risk to a fetus from the live virus vaccine; the client must be using effective birth control at the time of the immunization. The client should avoid contact with immunosuppressed individuals because of their low immunity toward live viruses and because the virus is shed in the urine and other body fluids. The vaccine is administered by the subcutaneous route. A hypersensitivity reaction can occur if the client has an allergy to eggs because the vaccine is made from duck eggs. There is no useful or necessary reason for covering the area of the injection with a sterile gauze.

Test-Taking Strategy: Focus on the subject, client instructions regarding the rubella vaccine. Recalling that the rubella vaccine is a live virus vaccine will assist in selecting options 2 and 5. Next, recalling the route of administration and the contraindications associated with its use will assist in selecting options 3 and 4.

Level of Cognitive Ability: Analyzing

Client Needs: Health Promotion and Maintenance

Integrated Process: Teaching and Learning

Content Area: Maternity: Postpartum

Health Problem: Maternity: Infections/Inflammations

Priority Concepts: Client Education; Immunity

Reference: McKinney et al. (2018), p. 401.

198. *Answer:* 2

Rationale: The client should sit or lie quietly on her side to perform kick counts. Lying flat on the back is not necessary to perform this procedure, can cause discomfort, and presents a risk of vena cava (supine hypotensive) syndrome. The client is instructed to place her hands on the largest part of the abdomen and concentrate on the fetal movements. The client records the number of movements felt during a specified time period. The client needs to notify the primary health care provider (PHCP) if she feels fewer than 10 kicks over two consecutive 2-hour intervals or as instructed by the PHCP.

Test-Taking Strategy: Note the strategic words, *need for further instruction*. These words indicate a negative event query and ask you to select an option that is an incorrect statement. If you are unfamiliar with this procedure, recalling that the risk of vena cava (supine hypotensive) syndrome exists when the client lies on her back will direct you to the correct option.

Level of Cognitive Ability: Evaluating

Client Needs: Health Promotion and Maintenance

Integrated Process: Teaching and Learning

Content Area: Maternity: Antepartum

Health Problem: N/A

Priority Concepts: Client Education; Perfusion

Reference: McKinney et al. (2018), p. 285.

199. *Answer:* 3

Rationale: During the second and third trimesters (weeks 18 to 30), fundal height in centimeters approximately equals the fetus's age in weeks ± 2 cm. Therefore, if the client is at 28 weeks' gestation, a fundal height of 30 cm would indicate that the client is measuring normal for gestational age. At 16 weeks, the fundus can be located halfway between the symphysis pubis and the umbilicus. At 20 to 22 weeks, the fundus is at the umbilicus. At 36 weeks, the fundus is at the xiphoid process.

Test-Taking Strategy: Focus on the subject, the location of fundal height. Remember that during the second and third trimesters (weeks 18 to 30), fundal height in centimeters approximately equals the fetus's age in weeks ± 2 cm.

Level of Cognitive Ability: Analyzing

Client Needs: Health Promotion and Maintenance

Integrated Process: Nursing Process—Assessment

Content Area: Maternity: Antepartum

Health Problem: N/A

Priority Concepts: Development; Reproduction

Reference: Lowdermilk et al. (2016), pp. 287, 315-316.

200. *Answer:* 1, 2, 3, 4

Rationale: The probable signs of pregnancy include uterine enlargement, Hegar's sign (compressibility and softening of the lower uterine segment that occurs at about week 6), Goodell's sign (softening of the cervix that occurs at the beginning of the second month), Chadwick's sign (violet coloration of the mucous membranes of the cervix, vagina, and vulva that occurs at about week 4), ballottement (rebounding of the fetus against the examiner's fingers on palpation), Braxton Hicks contractions, and a positive pregnancy test for the presence of human chorionic gonadotropin. Positive signs of pregnancy include fetal heart rate detected by electronic device (Doppler transducer) at 10 to 12 weeks and by nonelectronic device (fetoscope) at 20 weeks of gestation, active fetal movements palpable by the examiner, and an outline of the fetus by radiography or ultrasonography.

Test-Taking Strategy: Focusing on the subject, probable signs of pregnancy, will assist in answering this question. Remember that detection of the fetal heart rate and an outline of the fetus via radiography or ultrasonography are positive signs of pregnancy.

Level of Cognitive Ability: Analyzing

Client Needs: Health Promotion and Maintenance

Integrated Process: Nursing Process—Assessment

Content Area: Maternity: Antepartum

Health Problem: N/A
Priority Concepts: Development; Reproduction
Reference: Lowdermilk et al. (2016), pp. 286, 302.

201. *Answer:* 3
Rationale: Braxton Hicks contractions are irregular, painless contractions that may occur intermittently throughout pregnancy. Because Braxton Hicks contractions may occur and are normal in some pregnant women during pregnancy, there is no reason to notify the primary health care provider. This client is not in preterm labor and, therefore, does not need to be placed on bed rest or be admitted to the hospital to be monitored.
Test-Taking Strategy: Options 1 and 4 are comparable or alike and can be eliminated first. From the remaining options, knowing that Braxton Hicks contractions are common and normal and can occur throughout pregnancy will assist in directing you to the correct option.
Level of Cognitive Ability: Applying
Client Needs: Health Promotion and Maintenance
Integrated Process: Nursing Process—Implementation
Content Area: Maternity: Antepartum
Health Problem: N/A
Priority Concepts: Clinical Judgment; Reproduction
Reference: McKinney et al. (2018), pp. 214, 223-224.

202. *Answer:* 2
Rationale: Accurate use of Näegele's rule requires that the woman have a regular 28-day menstrual cycle. Subtract 3 months and add 7 days to the first day of the last menstrual period, and then add 1 year to that date: first day of the last menstrual period, October 19, 2020; subtract 3 months, July 19, 2020; add 7 days, July 26, 2020; add 1 year, July 26, 2021.
Test-Taking Strategy: Focus on the subject and use knowledge regarding Näegele's rule to answer this question. This rule requires addition and subtraction, so read all options carefully, noting the dates and years in the options, before selecting an answer.
Level of Cognitive Ability: Applying
Client Needs: Health Promotion and Maintenance
Integrated Process: Nursing Process—Assessment
Content Area: Maternity: Antepartum
Health Problem: N/A
Priority Concepts: Development; Reproduction
Reference: McKinney et al. (2018), p. 225.

203. *Answer:* 2
Rationale: Pregnancy outcomes can be described with the acronym *GTPAL*. *G* is gravidity, the number of pregnancies; *T* is term births, the number born at term (longer than 37 weeks); *P* is preterm births, the number born before 37 weeks of gestation; *A* is abortions or miscarriages, the number of abortions or miscarriages (included in gravida if before 20 weeks of gestation; included in parity [number of births] if past 20 weeks of gestation); and *L* is the number of current living children. A woman who is pregnant with twins and has a child has a gravida of 2. Because the child was delivered at 38 weeks, the number of term births is 1, and the number of preterm births is 0. The number of abortions is 0, and the number of living children is 1.
Test-Taking Strategy: Focus on the subject of the question. Recalling the meaning of the acronym *GTPAL* and focusing on the information in the question will direct you to the correct option.
Level of Cognitive Ability: Applying
Client Needs: Health Promotion and Maintenance
Integrated Process: Nursing Process—Assessment
Content Area: Maternity: Antepartum
Health Problem: N/A
Priority Concepts: Clinical Judgment; Reproduction
Reference: McKinney et al. (2018), p. 225.

CHAPTER 22

Risk Conditions Related to Pregnancy

PRIORITY CONCEPTS Reproduction, Safety

I. Bleeding During Pregnancy

A. Implantation bleeding: Bleeding that occurs 10 to 14 days after conception. Usually lasts 1 to 2 days and is lighter than the typical menstrual period. Often confused with a normal menstrual period. No treatment is necessary.

B. Other causes include abortion, malignancy, polyps, trauma, ectopic pregnancy, idiopathic, infection, molar pregnancy, subchorionic hemorrhage, vaginitis, urinary tract infection, cervicitis, cervical polyps, postcoital bleeding, placenta previa, and abruptio placentae.

II. Abortion

A. Description: A pregnancy that ends before 20 weeks' gestation, spontaneously or electively

B. Types (Box 22-1)

C. Risk factors

1. Advanced maternal age
2. Those who have experienced a previous miscarriage are at a higher risk
3. Previous elective abortion
4. Uterine abnormalities such as adhesions or fibroids
5. Prolonged time to achieve pregnancy
6. Low serum progesterone
7. Celiac disease
8. Polycystic ovarian syndrome
9. Thyroid dysfunction or Cushing's syndrome
10. Systemic lupus erythematosus
11. Infection, fever, trauma
12. Low body mass index (BMI), less than 18.5
13. Smoking, alcohol, cocaine use, certain medications, high caffeine intake

D. Assessment

1. Spontaneous vaginal bleeding
2. Low uterine cramping or contractions
3. Blood clots or tissue through the vagina
4. Hemorrhage and shock can result if bleeding is excessive.

E. Interventions

1. Maintain bed rest as prescribed.
2. Monitor vital signs.
3. Monitor for cramping and bleeding.
4. Count perineal pads to evaluate blood loss, and save expelled tissues and clots.
5. Maintain intravenous (IV) fluids as prescribed; monitor for signs of hemorrhage or shock.
6. Prepare the client for dilation and curettage as prescribed for incomplete abortion.
7. Administer $Rh_o(D)$ immune globulin, as prescribed, for an Rh-negative woman.
8. Provide psychological support.

III. Cardiac Disease

A. Description: A pregnant client with cardiac disease may be unable physiologically to cope with the added plasma volume and increased cardiac output that occur during pregnancy; blood volume peaks at weeks 32 to 34 and then declines slightly to week 40.

B. Maternal cardiac disease risk groups (Box 22-2)

C. Assessment

1. Signs and symptoms of cardiac decompensation
   a. Cough and respiratory congestion
   b. Dyspnea and fatigue
   c. Palpitations and tachycardia
   d. Peripheral edema
   e. Chest pain
2. Signs of respiratory infection
3. Signs of heart failure and pulmonary edema

D. Interventions

1. Monitor vital signs, fetal heart rate, and condition of the fetus.
2. Limit physical activities, and stress the need for sufficient rest.
3. Monitor for signs of cardiac stress and decompensation, such as cough, fatigue, dyspnea, chest pain, and tachycardia; also monitor for signs of heart failure and pulmonary edema.
4. Encourage adequate nutrition to prevent anemia, which would worsen the cardiac status; in addition, a low-sodium diet may be prescribed to prevent fluid retention and heart failure.

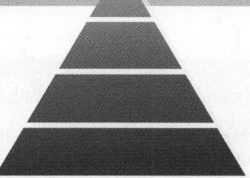

Maternity

BOX 22-1 Types of Abortions

Miscarriage: Pregnancy ends because of natural causes.
Induced: Therapeutic or elective reasons exist for terminating pregnancy.
Threatened: Spotting and cramping occur without cervical change.
Inevitable: Spotting and cramping occur and cervix begins to dilate and efface.
Incomplete: Loss of some of the products of conception occurs, with part of the products retained (most often placenta is retained).
Complete: Loss of all products of conception.
Missed: Products of conception are retained in utero after fetal death.
Habitual: Miscarriages occur in 3 or more successive pregnancies.

BOX 22-2 Maternal Cardiac Disease Risk Groups

Group I (Mortality Rate, 1%)

- Atrial septal defect
- Ventricular septal defect (uncomplicated)
- Patent ductus arteriosus
- Pulmonic and tricuspid disease
- Biosynthetic valve prosthesis (porcine and human allograft)
- Tetralogy of Fallot (corrected)
- Mitral stenosis (New York Heart Association [NYHA] class I and II) see http://www.heart.org/HEARTORG/Conditions/HeartFailure/AboutHeartFailure/Classes-of-Heart-Failure_UCM_306328_Article.jsp#.WyvejiAnY2w

Group II (Mortality Rate, 5% to 15%)

- Mitral stenosis NYHA class III and IV or with atrial fibrillation
- Aortic stenosis
- Coarctation of aorta (uncomplicated)
- Uncorrected tetralogy of Fallot
- Previous myocardial infarction
- Marfan syndrome with normal aorta
- Artificial heart valve

Group III (Mortality Rate, 25% to 50%)

- Pulmonary hypertension
- Coarctation of the aorta (complicated)
- Endocarditis
- Marfan syndrome with aortic involvement
- Eisenmenger syndrome

From Perry S, Hockenberry M, Lowdermilk D, Wilson D, *Maternal child nursing care,* ed 5, St. Louis, 2014, Mosby. Original source: Data from Gaddipati S, Troiano NH: Cardiac disorders in pregnancy. In Troiano NH, Harvey CJ, Chez BF, editors: *AWHONN's high risk and critical care obstetrics*, ed 3, Philadelphia, 2013, Lippincott Williams and Wilkins.

5. Avoid excessive weight gain.
6. During labor, prepare to do the following:
  a. Monitor vital signs frequently.
  b. Place the client on a cardiac monitor and on an external fetal monitor.
  c. Maintain bed rest, with the client lying on her side with her head and shoulders elevated.
  d. Administer oxygen as prescribed.
  e. Manage pain early in labor. Cardiology clearance may be required for epidural, spinal, or general anesthetic agents.
  f. Use controlled pushing efforts to decrease cardiac stress.

▲ Excessive weight gain places stress on the heart. In addition, obesity places the client at increased risk for complications during pregnancy.

IV. Chorioamnionitis

A. Description
  1. Bacterial infection of the amniotic cavity; can result from premature or prolonged rupture of the membranes, vaginitis, amniocentesis, or intrauterine procedures
  2. May result in the development of postpartum endometritis and neonatal sepsis
B. Assessment
  1. Uterine tenderness and contractions
  2. Elevated temperature
  3. Maternal or fetal tachycardia
  4. Foul odor to amniotic fluid
  5. Leukocytosis
C. Interventions
  1. Monitor maternal vital signs and fetal heart rate.
  2. Monitor for uterine tenderness, contractions, and fetal activity.
  3. Monitor results of blood cultures.
  4. Prepare for amniocentesis to obtain amniotic fluid for Gram stain and leukocyte count and other testing as prescribed.
  5. Administer antibiotics as prescribed after cultures are obtained.
  6. Administer oxytocic medications as prescribed to increase uterine tone.
  7. Prepare to obtain neonatal cultures after birth.

V. Diabetes Mellitus

A. Description
  1. Pregnancy places demands on carbohydrate metabolism and causes insulin requirements to change.
  2. Insulin resistance and hyperinsulinemia may predispose some women to diabetes.
  3. Maternal glucose crosses the placenta, but insulin does not.
  4. The fetus produces its own insulin and pulls glucose from the mother, which predisposes the mother to hypoglycemic reactions.
  5. The newborn of a diabetic mother may be large in size but has functions related to gestational age rather than size.
  6. The newborn of a diabetic mother is at risk for hypoglycemia, hyperbilirubinemia, respiratory distress syndrome, hypocalcemia, and congenital anomalies.

During the first trimester, maternal insulin needs decrease. During the second and third trimesters, increases in placental hormones cause an insulin-resistant state, requiring an increase in the client's insulin dose. After placental delivery, placental hormone levels abruptly decrease and insulin requirements decrease.

B. Gestational diabetes mellitus

1. Gestational diabetes occurs in pregnancy (during the second or third trimester) in clients not previously diagnosed as diabetic and occurs when the pancreas cannot respond to the demand for more insulin.
2. Women may be diagnosed with overt diabetes while pregnant as well, and as a result of personal risk factors such as being overweight or obese, there is an increased likelihood of overt, unrecognized diabetes. An HbA1C level may be helpful in making this determination.
3. There is an increased incidence of gestational diabetes when a woman also has polycystic ovarian syndrome.
4. Pregnant women should be screened for gestational diabetes between 24 and 28 weeks of gestation via the 1-hour glucose challenge test.
5. If the 1-hour glucose challenge test is abnormal, a 3-hour oral glucose tolerance test is performed to confirm gestational diabetes mellitus.
6. Gestational diabetes frequently can be treated by diet alone; however, some clients may need insulin (selected oral medications that are safe during pregnancy may be prescribed).
7. Most women with gestational diabetes return to a euglycemic state after birth; however, these individuals have an increased risk of developing diabetes mellitus in their lifetimes.
8. Early screening at an initial prenatal visit is done if the client has predisposing conditions as risk factors. See Chapter 21 for additional information on screening for gestational diabetes mellitus and interpreting glucose challenge test results.
9. The need for cesarean section is more likely, and neonatal hypoglycemia and macrosomia may be evident

C. Predisposing conditions/risk factors to gestational diabetes

1. Older than 35 years
2. Obesity—BMI greater than 30
3. Nonwhite race
4. Previous unexplained perinatal loss
5. Previous child born with congenital anomalies
6. Polycystic ovarian syndrome
7. Multiple gestation
8. First-degree relative with diabetes mellitus or gestational diabetes
9. Previous delivery of a fetus weighing greater than 9 lb
10. Maternal birth weight less than 6 lb or greater than 9 lb
11. Previous pregnancy with gestational diabetes
12. Glycosuria
13. Essential or pregnancy-related hypertension
14. Use of glucocorticoids

D. Assessment

1. Excessive thirst
2. Hunger
3. Weight loss
4. Frequent urination
5. Blurred vision
6. Recurrent urinary tract infections and vaginal yeast infections
7. Glycosuria and ketonuria
8. Signs of gestational hypertension and preeclampsia
9. Polyhydramnios
10. Large for gestational age fetus

E. Interventions

1. Employ diet, medications (if diet cannot control blood glucose levels), exercise, and blood glucose determinations 4 times daily (fasting and 1 to 2 hours after meals) to maintain blood glucose levels as follows: fasting less than 95 mg/dL (5.4 mmol/L), 1-hour post-prandial less than 130 to 140 mg/dL (7.4 to 8 mmol/L), 2-hour post-prandial less than 120 mg/dL (6.8 mmol/L).
2. Encourage moderate physical activity.
3. Facilitate referral to a diabetic educator and nutritionist.
4. Observe for signs of hyperglycemia, glycosuria and ketonuria, and hypoglycemia.
5. Monitor weight.
6. Maintain calorie intake as prescribed, with adequate oral medication or insulin therapy so that glucose moves into the cells.
7. Assess for signs of maternal complications such as preeclampsia, a serious blood pressure disorder that can affect all organs in the body (hypertension is characteristic of the condition).
8. Monitor for signs of infection.
9. Instruct the client to report burning and pain on urination, vaginal discharge or itching, or any other signs of infection to the primary health care provider (PHCP).
10. Assess fetal status and monitor for signs of fetal compromise.
11. Schedule visits every 2 weeks until 36 weeks, and then every week from 36 weeks and up.

F. Interventions during labor

1. Monitor fetal status continuously for signs of distress and, if noted, prepare the client for immediate cesarean section.

2. Carefully regulate insulin and provide glucose intravenously as prescribed because labor depletes glycogen.

G. Interventions during the postpartum period
1. Observe the mother closely for a hypoglycemic reaction because a precipitous decline in insulin requirements normally occurs (the mother may not require insulin for the first 24 hours).
2. Reregulate insulin needs as prescribed after the first day, according to blood glucose testing.
3. Assess dietary needs, based on blood glucose testing and insulin requirements.
4. Monitor for signs of infection or postpartum hemorrhage.

VI. Disseminated Intravascular Coagulation (DIC)

A. Description: DIC is a maternal condition in which the clotting cascade is activated, resulting in the formation of clots in the microcirculation (Fig. 22-1).

! The rapid and extensive formation of clots that occurs in DIC causes the platelets and clotting factors to be depleted; this results in bleeding and the potential vascular occlusion of organs from thromboembolus formation.

B. Predisposing conditions (Box 22-3)

C. Assessment
1. Uncontrolled bleeding
2. Bruising, purpura, petechiae, and ecchymosis
3. Presence of occult blood in excretions such as stool

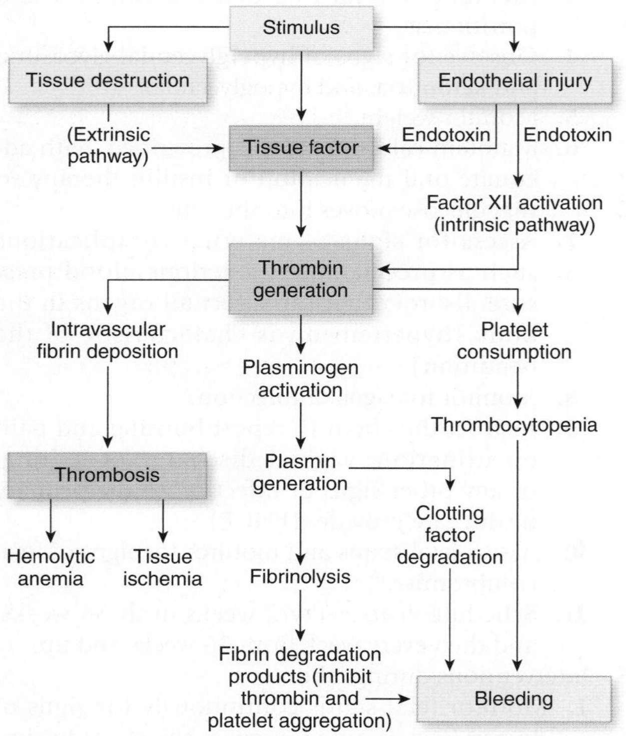

FIG. 22-1 Pathophysiology of disseminated intravascular coagulation.

BOX 22-3 Predisposing Conditions for Disseminated Intravascular Coagulation

- Abruptio placentae
- Amniotic fluid embolism
- Gestational hypertension
- HELLP syndrome
- Intrauterine fetal death
- Liver disease
- Sepsis
- Severe postpartum hemorrhage and blood loss

4. Hematuria, hematemesis, or vaginal bleeding
5. Signs of shock
6. Decreased fibrinogen level, platelet count, and hematocrit level
7. Increased prothrombin time and partial thromboplastin time, clotting time, and fibrin degradation products

D. Interventions
1. Remove underlying cause.
2. Monitor vital signs; assess for bleeding and signs of shock.
3. Prepare for oxygen therapy, volume replacement, blood component therapy, and possibly heparin therapy.
4. Monitor for complications associated with fluid and blood replacement and heparin therapy.
5. Monitor urine output and maintain at least 30 mL/hr (renal failure is a complication of DIC).

VII. Ectopic Pregnancy

A. Description
1. Implantation of the fertilized ovum outside of the uterine cavity
2. Most common location is the ampulla of the fallopian tube (Fig. 22-2).

B. Assessment
1. Missed menstrual period
2. Abdominal pain
3. Vaginal spotting to bleeding that is dark red or brown
4. Rupture: Increased pain, referred shoulder pain, signs of shock

C. Interventions
1. Obtain assessment data and vital signs.
2. Monitor bleeding and initiate measures to prevent rupture and shock.
3. Methotrexate, a folic acid antagonist, may be prescribed to inhibit cell division in the developing embryo.
4. Prepare the client for laparotomy and removal of the pregnancy and tube, if necessary, or repair of the tube.
5. Administer antibiotics; $Rh_o(D)$ immune globulin is prescribed for Rh-negative women.

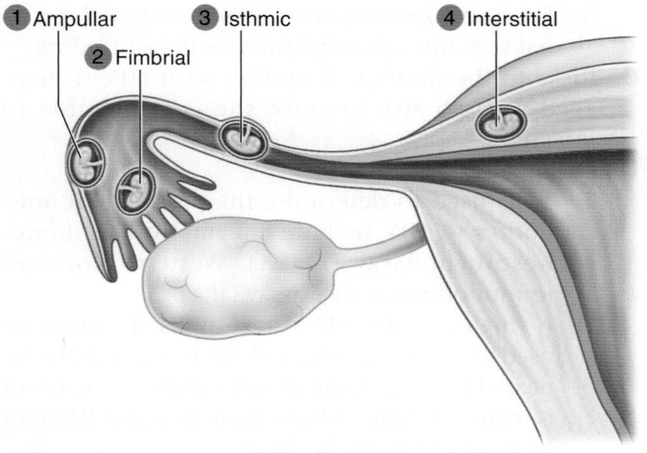

FIG. 22-2 Sites of tubal ectopic pregnancy. Numbers indicate the order of prevalence.

VIII. Fetal Death in Utero

A. Description
1. *Fetal death in utero* refers to the death of a fetus after the twentieth week of gestation and before birth.
2. The client can develop DIC if the dead fetus is retained in the uterus for 3 to 4 weeks or longer.

B. Assessment
1. Absence of fetal movement
2. Absence of fetal heart tones
3. Maternal weight loss
4. Lack of fetal growth or decrease in fundal height
5. No evidence of fetal cardiac activity
6. Other characteristics suggestive of fetal death noted on ultrasound

C. Interventions
1. Prepare for the birth of the fetus.
2. Support the client's decision about labor, birth, and the postpartum period.
3. Provide support and ask what can be helpful; provide assistance as appropriate and requested.
4. Accept behaviors such as sadness, anger, and hostility from the parents.
5. Refer the parents to an appropriate support group.

! Cultural, spiritual, and religious practices and beliefs are important to consider when caring for the parents of a fetus who has died. Be aware of these cultural, spiritual, and religious practices and beliefs and ensure that their beliefs are respected and implemented as appropriate.

IX. Hepatitis B

A. Description
1. The risks of prematurity, low birth weight, and neonatal death increase if the mother has hepatitis B infection.
2. Hepatitis is transmitted through blood, saliva, vaginal secretions, semen, and breast milk and across the placental barrier.

B. Interventions
1. Minimize the risk for intrapartum ascending infections (limit the number of vaginal examinations).
2. Remove maternal blood from the neonate immediately after birth.
3. Suction the fluids from the neonate immediately after birth.
4. Bathe the neonate before any invasive procedures including injections.
5. Clean and dry the face and eyes of the neonate before instilling eye prophylaxis.
6. Infection of the neonate can be prevented by the administration of hepatitis B immune globulin and hepatitis B vaccine soon after birth but after the newborn is bathed.
7. Discourage the mother from kissing the neonate until the neonate has received the vaccine.
8. Inform the mother that the hepatitis B vaccine will be administered to the neonate and that a second dose should be administered at 1 month after birth and a third dose at 6 months after birth.

! Support breast-feeding after neonatal treatment for hepatitis B; breast-feeding is not contraindicated if the neonate has been vaccinated.

X. Hematoma

A. Description
1. Hematoma occurs following the escape of blood into the maternal tissue after birth.
2. Predisposing conditions include operative delivery with forceps or injury to a blood vessel.

B. Assessment (Box 22-4)

C. Interventions
1. Monitor vital signs.
2. Monitor client for abnormal pain, especially when forceps delivery has been performed.
3. Apply ice to the hematoma site.
4. Administer analgesics as prescribed.
5. Monitor intake and output.

BOX 22-4 Hematoma: Assessment Findings

- Abnormal, severe pain
- Pressure in perineal area (client states that she feels like she has to have a bowel movement)
- Palpable, sensitive swelling in the perineal area, with discolored skin
- Inability to void
- Decreased hemoglobin and hematocrit levels
- Signs of shock, such as pallor, tachycardia, and hypotension, if significant blood loss has occurred

6. Encourage fluids and voiding; prepare for urinary catheterization if the client is unable to void.
7. Administer blood replacements as prescribed.
8. Monitor for signs of infection, such as increased temperature, pulse rate, and white blood cell count.
9. Administer antibiotics as prescribed; infection is common after hematoma formation.
10. Prepare for incision and evacuation of the hematoma if necessary.

XI. Human Immunodeficiency Virus (HIV) and Acquired Immunodeficiency Syndrome (AIDS)

A. Description
1. HIV is the causative agent of AIDS.
2. Women infected with HIV may first show signs and symptoms at the time of pregnancy or possibly develop life-threatening infections because normal pregnancy involves some suppression of the maternal immune system.
3. Repeated exposure to the virus during pregnancy through unsafe sex practices or intravenous (IV) drug use can increase the risk of transmission to the fetus.
4. Three-drug combination HAART (highly active antiretroviral therapy) treatment, which is monitored by an infectious disease specialist, is recommended to reduce mother-to-child transmission (MTCT). Zidovudine is recommended for the prevention of MTCT and is administered based on the following recommendations:
   a. Antepartum: Orally beginning after 12 weeks of gestation, maternal HAART is given to reduce the viral load to undetectable.
   b. Intrapartum: Intravenously during labor, zidovudine is given 1 hour before a vaginal birth and 3 hours before a cesarean section if the HIV RNA is greater than or equal to 400 copies/mL or unknown. Of note, this may not be required if the HIV RNA is less than 400 copies/mL but is given at the discretion of the provider. A vaginal birth is acceptable if the viral load is less than 1000 copies/mL; otherwise, a cesarean section is recommended.
   c. Postpartum: In the form of syrup to the newborn 2 hours after birth and every 12 hours for 6 weeks; depending on agency procedures, the newborn may need to be placed in the newborn intensive care unit (NICU) to begin initial therapy.

B. Transmission
1. Sexual exposure to genital secretions of an infected person
2. Parenteral exposure to infected blood and tissue
3. Perinatal exposure of an **infant** to infected maternal secretions through birth or breast-feeding

C. Risks to the mother: A mother with HIV is managed as high risk because she is vulnerable to infections.

D. Diagnosis
1. Tests used to determine the presence of antibodies to HIV include enzyme-linked immunosorbent assay (ELISA), Western blot, and immunofluorescence assay (IFA).
2. A single reactive ELISA test by itself cannot be used to diagnose HIV, and the test should be repeated with the same blood sample; if the result is again reactive, follow-up tests using Western blot or IFA should be done.
3. A positive Western blot or IFA is considered confirmatory for HIV.
4. A positive ELISA that fails to be confirmed by Western blot or IFA should not be considered negative, and repeat testing should be done in 3 to 6 months.

E. Assessment (see Chapter 62)

F. Interventions
1. Prenatal period
   a. Institute measures to prevent opportunistic infections.
   b. Avoid procedures that increase the risk of perinatal transmission, such as amniocentesis and fetal scalp sampling.
2. Intrapartum period
   a. If the fetus has not been exposed to HIV in utero, the highest risk exists during delivery through the birth canal.
   b. Avoid the use of internal scalp electrodes for monitoring of the fetus.
   c. Avoid episiotomy to decrease the amount of maternal blood in and around the birth canal.
   d. Avoid the administration of oxytocin, because contractions induced by oxytocin can be strong, causing vaginal tears or necessitating an episiotomy.
   e. Place heavy absorbent pads under the mother's hips to absorb amniotic fluid and maternal blood.
   f. Minimize the neonate's exposure to maternal blood and body fluids; promptly remove the neonate from the mother's blood after delivery.
   g. Suction fluids from the neonate promptly.
   h. Prepare to administer zidovudine as prescribed to the mother during labor and delivery.
3. Postpartum period
   a. Monitor for signs of infection.
   b. Place the mother in protective isolation if she is immunosuppressed.

c. Breast-feeding is likely to be restricted; follow PHCPs recommendations regarding breast-feeding.

d. Instruct the mother to monitor for signs of infection and report any signs if they occur.

e. The newborn can room with the mother; however, depending on agency procedures, the newborn may be placed in NICU for the first 24 hours of life to complete baseline laboratory studies and receive the initial treatment.

G. The newborn and HIV (refer to Chapter 27 for this information)

XII. Hydatidiform Mole

A. Description

1. Hydatidiform mole is a form of gestational trophoblastic disease that occurs when the trophoblasts, which are the peripheral cells that attach the fertilized ovum to the uterine wall, develop abnormally.
2. The mole manifests as an edematous grape-like cluster that may be nonmalignant or may develop into choriocarcinoma.

B. Assessment

1. Fetal heart rate not detectable
2. Vaginal bleeding, which may occur by the fourth week or not until the second trimester; may be bright red or dark brown in color and may be slight, profuse, or intermittent
3. Signs of preeclampsia (progressive blood pressure elevations) before the 20th week of gestation; note that preeclampsia usually occurs after 20 weeks of pregnancy, typically in the third trimester.
4. Fundal height greater than expected for gestational date
5. Elevated human chorionic gonadotropin levels
6. Characteristic snowstorm pattern shown on ultrasound

C. Interventions

1. Prepare the client for uterine evacuation (before evacuation, diagnostic tests are done to detect metastatic disease).
2. Evacuation of the mole is done by vacuum aspiration; oxytocin may be administered after evacuation to contract the uterus.
3. Monitor for postprocedure hemorrhage and infection.
4. Tissue is sent to the laboratory for evaluation, and follow-up is important to detect changes suggestive of malignancy.
5. Human chorionic gonadotropin levels are monitored every 1 to 2 weeks until normal prepregnancy levels are attained; levels are checked every 1 to 2 months for 1 year.
6. Instruct the client and her partner about birth control measures so that pregnancy can be prevented during the 1-year follow-up period.

XIII. Hyperemesis Gravidarum

A. Description: Intractable nausea and vomiting during the first trimester that causes disturbances in nutrition and fluid and electrolyte balance

B. Assessment

1. Nausea most pronounced on arising; may occur at other times during the day
2. Persistent vomiting
3. Weight loss
4. Signs of dehydration
5. Fluid and electrolyte imbalances

C. Interventions

1. Initiate measures to alleviate nausea, including medication therapy; if unsuccessful, and weight loss and fluid and electrolyte imbalances occur, intravenously administered fluid and electrolyte replacement or parenteral nutrition may be necessary.
2. Monitor vital signs, intake and output, weight, and calorie count.
3. Monitor laboratory data and for signs of dehydration and electrolyte imbalances.
4. Monitor urine for ketones.
5. Monitor fetal heart rate, activity, and growth.
6. Encourage intake of small portions of food (low-fat, easily digestible carbohydrates, such as cereals, rice, and pasta).
7. Encourage the intake of liquids between meals to avoid distending the stomach and triggering vomiting.
8. Encourage the client to sit upright after meals.

XIV. Hypertensive Disorders of Pregnancy

A. Description and types: Four major categories include preeclampsia, chronic/preexisting hypertension, chronic hypertension with superimposed preeclampsia, and gestational hypertension.

B. Blood pressure elevations can lead to preeclampsia and then eclampsia (seizures) (Table 22-1).

C. Women who have had preeclampsia, especially those who delivered preterm, have an increased risk later in life of cardiovascular disease and kidney disease, including heart attack, stroke, and high blood pressure.

D. Having preeclampsia once increases the risk of having it again in a future pregnancy.

E. Preeclampsia also can lead to eclampsia (seizures).

F. HELLP syndrome can result. HELLP stands for *hemolysis, elevated liver* enzymes, and *low platelet* count. In this condition, red blood cells are damaged or destroyed, blood clotting is impaired, and the liver can bleed internally, causing chest or abdominal pain. HELLP syndrome is a medical emergency; the woman can die from HELLP syndrome or have lifelong health problems as a result.

TABLE 22-1 Classification of Hypertensive Stages of Pregnancy

Type of Hypertension	Description
Normal	Less than 120/80 mm Hg
Elevated	Systolic between 120 and 129 and diastolic less than 80 mm Hg
Stage 1 hypertension	Systolic between 130 and 139 or diastolic between 80 and 89 mm Hg
Stage 2 hypertension	Systolic at least 140 or diastolic at least 90 mm Hg
Chronic hypertension	Hypertension that is present and observable before pregnancy or that occurs in the first half (before 20 weeks) of the pregnancy.
Gestational Hypertensive Disorders	
Gestational hypertension	Blood pressure elevation that first occurs in the second half (after 20 weeks) of pregnancy. Although gestational hypertension usually resolves after childbirth, it may increase the risk of developing hypertension in the future.
Preeclampsia	Usually occurs after 20 weeks of pregnancy, typically in the third trimester. When it occurs before 32 weeks of pregnancy, it is called early-onset preeclampsia. It also can occur in the postpartum period.
Eclampsia	Seizures occurring in pregnancy and linked to high blood pressure.

From The American College of Obstetricians and Gynecologists, May 2018 at: https://www.acog.org/Patients/FAQs/Preeclampsia-and-High-Blood-Pressure-During-Pregnancy

G. Assessment (Table 22-2)

Proteinuria is not a reliable indicator of preeclampsia. Evidence demonstrates that kidney or liver dysfunction can occur without signs of protein, and that the amount of protein in the urine does not predict how severely the disease will progress.

1. Persistent hypertension
2. Swelling of the face or hands
3. Headache
4. Changes in eyesight
5. Pain in the upper abdomen or shoulder
6. Nausea and vomiting (in the second half of pregnancy)
7. Sudden weight gain
8. Difficulty breathing

H. Risk factors

1. Previous preeclampsia or gestational hypertension, previous placental abruption, or fetal demise
2. Primigravida
3. Family history or first-degree relative with preeclampsia
4. Women who are 40 years or older
5. African American ethnicity
6. Women who are carrying more than one fetus
7. History of chronic hypertension, kidney disease, or both
8. Women who have medical conditions such as chronic hypertension, renal disease, connective tissue disease, diabetes mellitus, thrombophilia, or lupus erythematosus
9. BMI greater than 26
10. Metabolic syndrome
11. Multifetal pregnancy
12. Hydatidiform mole, hydrops fetalis, unexplained intrauterine growth retardation (IUGR)
13. Mother had IUGR as a newborn
14. Women who had in vitro **fertilization**

I. Complications of hypertension and gestational hypertension disorders

1. Abruptio placentae
2. Disseminated intravascular coagulopathy
3. Fetal growth restriction
4. Preeclampsia and eclampsia
5. Intracranial hemorrhage; maternal cerebral hemorrhage or infarction
6. Subcapsular hepatic hematoma
7. HELLP (*h*emolysis, *e*levated *l*iver enzyme levels, *l*ow *p*latelet count) syndrome
8. Oligohydramnios
9. Placental insufficiency
10. The need for preterm delivery or cesarean delivery
11. Maternal and/or fetal death

J. Interventions for hypertension and preeclampsia

1. Close blood pressure and weight monitoring throughout the pregnancy; the client may need to be taught how to take her blood pressure at home.
2. Weekly or twice weekly health care visits may be necessary; delivery may be recommended at 37 weeks of gestation (earlier if there is evidence of fetal distress).
3. Monitor fetal activity (teach the client how to perform Kick counts) and fetal growth (ultrasounds will be prescribed).
4. Encourage frequent rest periods, instructing the client to lie in the lateral position; for preeclampsia with severe features, the client may be hospitalized and bed rest may be prescribed (client should be placed in the lateral position).
5. Administer medications as prescribed to reduce blood pressure; blood pressure should not be reduced rapidly, because placental perfusion can be compromised.
6. Provide adequate fluids.
7. Monitor intake and output; a urinary output of 30 mL/hr indicates adequate renal perfusion.
8. Monitor neurological status, because changes can indicate cerebral hypoxia or impending seizure.
9. Monitor deep tendon reflexes and for the presence of hyperreflexia or clonus, because

TABLE 22-2 Assessment Findings in Preeclampsia

Parameter Evaluated	Preeclampsia	Preeclampsia with Severe Features
Blood pressure	Greater than or equal to 140 mm Hg systolic or greater than or equal to 90 mm Hg diastolic on two occasions at least 4 hours apart after 20 weeks of gestation in a woman with a previously normal blood pressure.	Persistent elevation and greater than or equal to 160 mm Hg systolic or greater than or equal to 110 mm Hg on 2 occasions at least 4 hours apart while on bedrest
Proteinuria Note: no longer used as a diagnostic measure	Less than or equal to 0.3 g in 24 hr, less than or equal to 1+ on dipstick, may be normal	Greater than or equal to 5 g in 24 hr, greater than or equal to 3+ on dipstick two times
Reflexes	May be normal	Hyperreflexia
Changes in mentation	Transient or absent	May be present
Placental perfusion	Somewhat reduced	Decreased with possible abnormal FHR
Creatinine, serum (renal function)	May be normal	Elevated (>1.0 mg/dL [>76.3 mcmol/L])
Protein/creatinine ratio	0.3 mg/dL (>22.89 mcmol/L)	>0.3 mg/dL (>22.89 mcmol/L)
Platelets	May be decreased	Decreased (<100,000 mm^3 [<100 × 10^9/L])
Liver enzymes (alanine aminotransferase or aspartate aminotransferase)	Normal or minimal increase in levels	Elevated levels (double or greater)
Uric acid	May be normal	>5.5 mg/dL (330 mcmol/L)
Urine output	Normal	Oliguria common, often <500 mL/day
Severe, unrelenting headache not attributable to other cause; mental confusion (cerebral edema)	Absent	Often present, persistent
Persistent right upper quadrant or epigastric pain or pain penetrating to back (distention of liver capsule); nausea and vomiting	Absent	May be present and often precedes seizure
Visual disturbances (spots or "sparkles"; temporary blindness; photophobia)	Absent to minimal	Common
Pulmonary edema; heart failure; cyanosis	Absent	May be present
Fetal growth restriction	Normal growth	Growth restriction; reduced amniotic fluid volume

Adapted from: The American College of Obstetricians and Gynecologists, May 2018 at: https://www.acog.org/Patients/FAQs/Preeclampsia-and-High-Blood-Pressure-During-Pregnancy
The American College of Obstetricians and Gynecologists, 2013, at: https://www.acog.org/topics/hypertension-and-preeclampsia-in-pregnancy
Preeclampsia Foundation, 2013.

hyperreflexia indicates increased central nervous system irritability (Box 22-5).

10. Monitor for HELLP syndrome.
11. Evaluate renal function through prescribed studies such as blood urea nitrogen, serum creatinine, and 24-hour urine levels for creatinine clearance and protein.
12. Magnesium sulfate (use a controlled infusion device) may be prescribed to prevent seizures; magnesium sulfate may be continued for 24 to 48 hours postpartum.
13. Monitor for signs of magnesium toxicity with the administration of magnesium sulfate, including flushing, sweating, hypotension, depressed deep tendon reflexes, decreased urine output, and central nervous system depression including respiratory depression; keep antidote (calcium gluconate) available for immediate use, if necessary.
14. Corticosteroids may be prescribed to promote fetal lung maturity.
15. Prepare the client for delivery as prescribed.

K. Eclampsia
1. Assessment: Characterized by generalized seizures (Box 22-6)
2. Interventions (see Priority Nursing Actions)

Maternity

BOX 22-5 Assessment of Reflexes

Biceps

Position thumb over client's biceps tendon, supporting client's elbow with the palm of the hand.
Strike a downward blow over the thumb with percussion hammer.
Normal response: Flexion of the arm at the elbow

Patellar

Position client with her legs dangling over the edge of the examining table or lying on her back with her legs slightly flexed.
Strike patellar tendon just below kneecap with percussion hammer.
Normal response: Extension or kicking out of the leg

Clonus

Position client with her legs dangling over the edge of examining table.
Support the leg with 1 hand and sharply dorsiflex client's foot with the other hand.
Maintain the dorsiflexed position for a few seconds and then release foot.
Normal response (negative clonus response):
Foot remains steady in dorsiflexed position.
No rhythmic oscillations or jerking of foot is felt.
When released, foot drops to plantar-flexed position with no oscillations.
Abnormal response (positive clonus response):
Rhythmic oscillations occur when foot is dorsiflexed.
Similar oscillations are noted when foot drops to plantar-flexed position.

Grading Response

0 Reflex absent
1 + Reflex present but hypoactive
2 + Normal reflex
3 + Hyperactive reflex
4 + Hyperactive reflex with clonus present

PRIORITY NURSING ACTIONS

Eclampsia Event

1. Remain with the client and call for help.
2. Ensure an open airway, turn the client on her side, and administer oxygen by face mask at 8 to 10 L/minute.
3. Monitor fetal heart rate patterns.
4. Administer medications to control the seizures as prescribed.
5. After the seizure has ended, insert an oral airway and suction the client's mouth as needed.
6. Prepare for delivery of the fetus after stabilization of the client, if warranted.
7. Document occurrence, client's response, and outcome.

Reference

Lowdermilk et al. (2016), p. 667

BOX 22-6 Eclampsia

1. Seizure typically begins with twitching around the mouth.
2. Body then becomes rigid in a state of tonic muscular contractions that last 15 to 20 seconds.
3. Facial muscles and then all body muscles alternately contract and relax in rapid succession (clonic phase may last about 1 minute).
4. Respiration ceases during seizure because diaphragm tends to remain fixed (breathing resumes shortly after the seizure).
5. Postictal sleep occurs.

XV. Incompetent Cervix

A. Description
1. *Incompetent cervix* refers to premature dilation of the cervix, which occurs most often in the fourth or fifth month of pregnancy and is associated with structural or functional defects of the cervix.
2. Treatment involves surgical placement of a cervical cerclage.

B. Assessment
1. Vaginal bleeding
2. Fetal membranes visible through the cervix

C. Interventions
1. Provide bed rest, hydration, and tocolysis, as prescribed, to inhibit uterine contractions.
2. Prepare for cervical cerclage (at 10 to 14 weeks of gestation as prescribed), in which a band of fascia or nonabsorbable ribbon is placed around the cervix beneath the mucosa to constrict the internal os.
3. After cervical cerclage, the client is told to refrain from intercourse and to avoid prolonged standing and heavy lifting.
4. The cervical cerclage is removed at 37 weeks of gestation or left in place and a cesarean birth is performed; if removed, cerclage needs to be repeated with each successive pregnancy.
5. After placement of the cervical cerclage, monitor for contractions, rupture of the membranes, and signs of infection.
6. Instruct the client to report to the PHCP immediately any postprocedure vaginal bleeding or increased uterine contractions.

XVI. Infections (TORCH Complex Acronym)

A. Toxoplasmosis ("T")
1. Caused by infection with the intracellular protozoan parasite *Toxoplasma gondii*
2. Produces a rash and symptoms of acute, flu-like infection in the mother
3. Transmitted to the mother through ingestion of raw meat or handling of cat litter of infected cats

4. Organism is transmitted to the fetus across the placenta
5. Can cause miscarriage in the first trimester
6. Client education regarding preventing infection is critical

B. Other Infections ("O," includes HIV—discussed earlier, syphilis—discussed under Sexually Transmitted Infections, parvovirus, hepatitis B virus [HBV], West Nile, etc.)

C. Rubella (German measles) ("R")
1. Teratogenic in the first trimester
2. Organism is transmitted to the fetus across the placenta.
3. Causes congenital defects of the eyes, heart, ears, and brain
4. Blood titer studies will be done. If not immune (titer less than 1:8), the client should be vaccinated in the postpartum period; the client must wait 1 to 3 months (as specified by the PHCP) before becoming pregnant.

D. Cytomegalovirus ("C")
1. Organism is transmitted through close personal contact; it is transmitted across the placenta to the fetus, or the fetus may be infected through the birth canal.
2. The mother may be asymptomatic; most infants are asymptomatic at birth.
3. Cytomegalovirus causes low birth weight, intrauterine growth restriction, enlarged liver and spleen, jaundice, blindness, hearing loss, and seizures.
4. Antiviral medications may need to be prescribed for severe infections in the mother, but these medications are toxic and may only temporarily suppress shedding of the virus; risk versus benefit will be considered by the PHCP.
5. Maintain contact precautions.

E. Herpes simplex virus ("H")
1. Herpes simplex virus affects the external genitalia, vagina, and cervix and causes draining, painful vesicles.
2. Acyclovir may be prescribed to treat recurrent outbreaks during pregnancy or used as suppressive therapy late in pregnancy to prevent an outbreak during labor and birth.
3. Virus usually is transmitted to the fetus during birth through the infected vagina or via an ascending infection after rupture of the membranes.
4. No vaginal examinations are done in the presence of active vaginal herpetic lesions.
5. Herpes can cause death or severe neurological impairment in the newborn.
6. Delivery of the fetus is usually by cesarean section if active lesions are present in the vagina; delivery may be performed vaginally if the lesions are in the anal, perineal, or inner thigh area (strict precautions are necessary to protect the fetus during delivery).
7. Maintain contact precautions.

F. Group B *Streptococcus* (GBS) (may be included as an "O" under TORCH complex)
1. GBS is a leading cause of life-threatening perinatal infections.
2. The gram-positive bacterium colonizes the rectum, vagina, cervix, and urethra of pregnant and nonpregnant women.
3. Meningitis, fasciitis, and intra-abdominal abscess can occur in the pregnant client if she is infected at the time of birth.
4. Transmission occurs during vaginal delivery.
5. Early-onset newborn GBS occurs within the first week after birth, usually within 48 hours, and can include infections such as sepsis, pneumonia, or meningitis; permanent neurological disability can result.
6. Diagnosis of the mother is done via vaginal and rectal cultures at 35 to 37 weeks of gestation.
7. Antibiotics may be prescribed for the mother during labor and birth; IV antibiotics may be prescribed for infected infants.
8. Maintain contact precautions.

XVII. Multiple Gestation

A. Description
1. Multiple gestation results from fertilization of 2 ova (fraternal or dizygotic) or a splitting of 1 fertilized ovum (identical or monozygotic).
2. Complications include miscarriage, anemia, congenital anomalies, hyperemesis gravidarum, intrauterine growth restriction, gestational hypertension, polyhydramnios, postpartum hemorrhage, premature rupture of membranes, and preterm labor and delivery.

B. Assessment
1. Excessive fetal activity
2. Uterus large for gestational age
3. Palpation of 3 or 4 large parts in the uterus
4. Auscultation of more than 1 fetal heart rate
5. Excessive weight gain

C. Interventions
1. Monitor vital signs.
2. Monitor fetal heart rates, activity, and growth.
3. Monitor for cervical changes.
4. Prepare the client for ultrasound as prescribed.
5. Monitor for anemia; administer supplemental vitamins as prescribed.
6. Monitor for preterm labor, and treat preterm labor promptly.
7. Prepare for cesarean delivery for abnormal presentations.
8. Prepare to administer oxytocic medications as prescribed after delivery to prevent postpartum hemorrhage from uterine overdistention.

XVIII. Placental Abnormalities

A. Description: Placenta accreta is an abnormally adherent placenta; placenta increta occurs when the placenta penetrates the uterine muscle itself; placenta percreta occurs when the placenta goes all the way through the uterus.

B. Assessment: May cause hemorrhage immediately after birth because the placenta does not separate easily

C. Intervention

1. Monitor for hemorrhage and shock.
2. Prepare the client for a hysterectomy if a large portion of the placenta is abnormally adherent.

XIX. Placenta Previa

A. Description

1. Placenta previa is an improperly implanted placenta in the lower uterine segment near or over the internal cervical os (Fig. 22-3).
2. Total (complete): The internal cervical os is covered entirely by the placenta when the cervix is dilated fully.
3. Partial: The lower border of the placenta is within 3 cm of the internal cervical os but does not fully cover it.
4. Marginal (low-lying): The placenta is implanted in the lower uterus, but its lower border is more than 3 cm from the internal cervical os.
5. Management depends on the classification of the placenta previa and gestational age of the fetus.

B. Assessment

1. Sudden onset of painless, bright red vaginal bleeding occurs in the last half of pregnancy.
2. Uterus is soft, relaxed, and nontender.
3. Fundal height may be more than expected for gestational age.

C. Interventions

1. Monitor maternal vital signs, fetal heart rate, and fetal activity.
2. Prepare for ultrasound to confirm the diagnosis.
3. Vaginal examinations or any other actions that would stimulate uterine activity are avoided.
4. Maintain bed rest in a side-lying position as prescribed.
5. Monitor amount of bleeding (treat signs of shock).
6. Administer intravenous (IV) fluids, blood products, or tocolytic medications as prescribed; Rh_o(D) immune globulin may be prescribed.
7. If bleeding is heavy, a cesarean delivery may be performed.

Vaginal exams are contraindicated if the client is suspected of having or has a known placenta previa.

XX. Abruptio Placentae

A. Description: Premature separation of the placenta from the uterine wall after the 20th week of gestation and before the fetus is delivered (Fig. 22-4)

B. Assessment

1. Dark red vaginal bleeding. If the bleeding is high in the uterus or is minimal, there can be an absence of visible blood.
2. Uterine pain or tenderness or both
3. Uterine rigidity
4. Severe abdominal pain
5. Signs of fetal distress
6. Signs of maternal shock if bleeding is excessive

C. Interventions

1. Monitor maternal vital signs and fetal heart rate.
2. Assess for excessive vaginal bleeding, abdominal pain, and an increase in fundal height.
3. Maintain bed rest; administer oxygen, IV fluids, and blood products as prescribed.

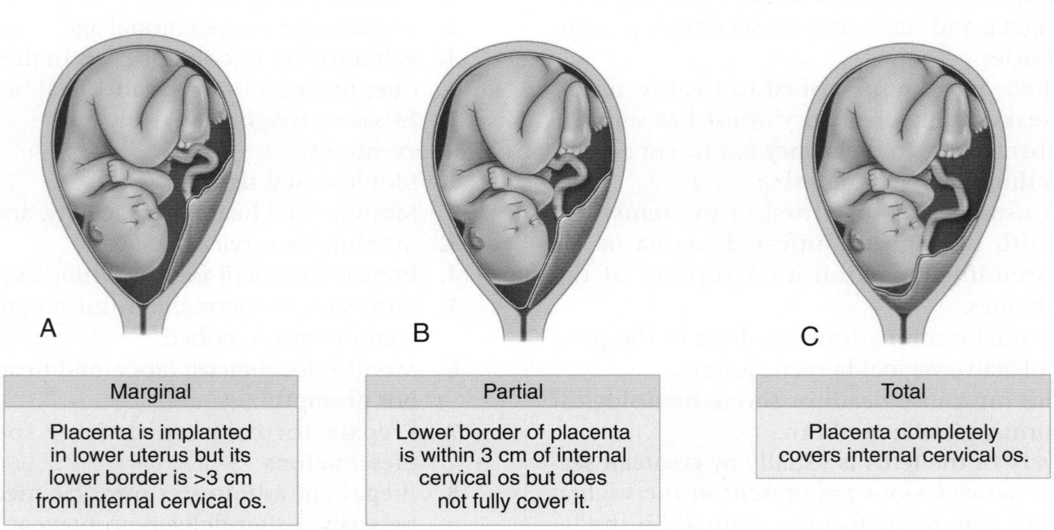
A
B
C
Marginal
Placenta is implanted in lower uterus but its lower border is >3 cm from internal cervical os.
Partial
Lower border of placenta is within 3 cm of internal cervical os but does not fully cover it.
Total
Placenta completely covers internal cervical os.

FIG. 22-3 Three classifications of placenta previa.

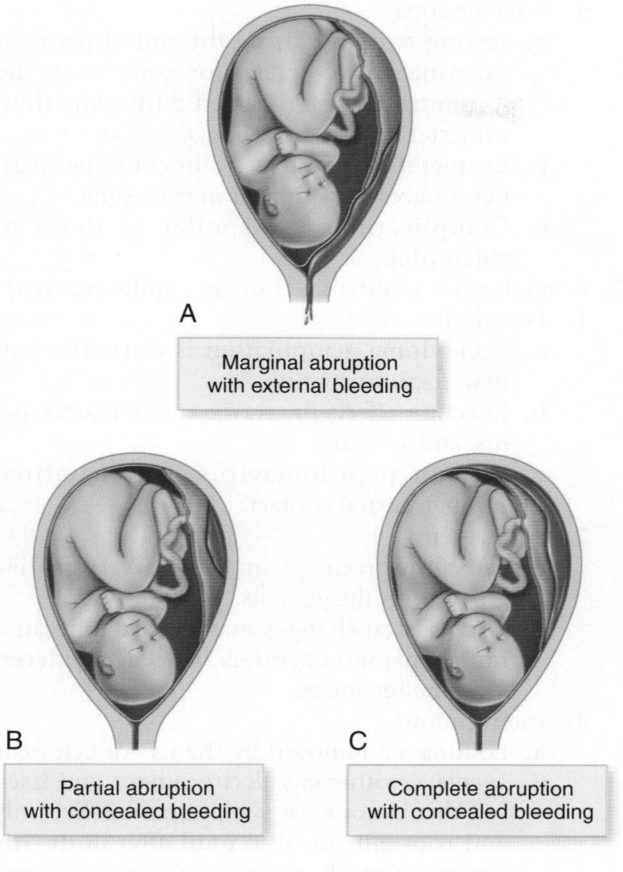

FIG. 22-4 Types of abruptio placentae.

4. Place the client in Trendelenburg's position if indicated to decrease the pressure of the fetus on the placenta, or place in the lateral position with the head of the bed flat if hypovolemic shock occurs.
5. Monitor and report any uterine activity.
6. Prepare for delivery of the fetus as quickly as possible, with vaginal delivery preferable if the fetus is healthy and stable and the presenting part is in the pelvis; emergency cesarean delivery is performed if the fetus is alive but shows signs of distress.
7. Monitor for signs of disseminated intravascular coagulation in the postpartum period.

! Know the differences between placenta previa and abruptio placentae. In placenta previa, there is painless, bright red vaginal bleeding, and the uterus is soft, relaxed, and nontender. In abruptio placentae, there is dark red vaginal bleeding, uterine pain or tenderness or both, and uterine rigidity.

XXI. Pyelonephritis

A. Description
1. Results from bacterial infections that extend upward from the bladder through the blood vessels and lymphatics (also see Section XXIV)
2. Frequently follows untreated urinary tract infections and is associated with increased incidence of anemia, low birth weight, gestational hypertension, premature labor and delivery, and premature rupture of the membranes

B. Assessment and Interventions (refer to Chapter 54)

XXII. Sexually Transmitted Infections

A. Chlamydia
1. Description
   a. Sexually transmitted pathogen associated with an increased risk for premature birth, stillbirth, neonatal conjunctivitis, and newborn chlamydial pneumonia
   b. Can cause salpingitis, pelvic abscesses, ectopic pregnancy, chronic pelvic pain, and infertility
   c. Diagnostic test is culture for *Chlamydia trachomatis.*
2. Assessment
   a. Usually asymptomatic—may have dysuria or dyspareunia
   b. Bleeding between periods or after coitus
   c. Mucoid or purulent cervical discharge
   d. Dysuria and pelvic pain
3. Interventions
   a. Screen the client to determine whether she is high risk; this is indicated for all pregnant clients if the client is in a high-risk group or if infants from previous pregnancies have developed neonatal conjunctivitis or pneumonia.
   b. Instruct the client in the importance of rescreening, because reinfection can occur as the client nears term.
   c. Ensure that the sexual partner is treated for the infection.
   d. Treatment for both gonorrhea and chlamydia should be done, which includes antibiotics.
   e. Complications in pregnancy may include septic spontaneous abortion or miscarriage, preterm delivery, premature rupture of the membranes (PROM), chorioamnionitis, disseminated gonococcal infection, ophthalmia neonatorum, postpartum metritis.

B. Syphilis
1. Description
   a. Syphilis is a chronic infectious disease caused by the organism *Treponema pallidum.*
   b. Transmission is by physical contact with syphilitic lesions, which usually are found on the skin, mucous membranes of the mouth, or genitals.
   c. The infection may cause abortion or premature labor and is passed to the fetus after the fourth month of pregnancy as congenital syphilis.
2. Assessment (Box 22-7)

BOX 22-7 Stages of Syphilis

Primary Stage
- Most infectious stage
- Appearance of ulcerative, painless lesions produced by spirochetes at point of entry into the body

Secondary Stage
- Highly infectious stage
- Appearance of lesions about 6 weeks to 6 months after primary stage; located anywhere on the skin and mucous membranes
- Generalized lymphadenopathy

Tertiary Stage
- Entrance of spirochetes into internal organs, causing permanent damage; symptoms occur 10 to 30 years after untreated primary lesion
- Invasion of central nervous system, causing meningitis, ataxia, general paresis, and progressive mental deterioration
- Deleterious effects on aortic valve and aorta

3. Interventions
  a. A serum test (Venereal Disease Research Laboratory or rapid plasma reagin) for syphilis is done on the first prenatal visit; prepare to repeat the test at 36 weeks of gestation because the disease may be acquired after the initial visit.
  b. If the test result is positive, treatment with an antibiotic may be necessary.
  c. Sonographic evaluation is necessary to assess for signs of placental syphilis.
  d. Instruct the client that treatment of her partner is necessary if infection is present, and intercourse should be avoided until treatment is instituted.
  e. Complications include transmission to fetus (100% in primary and secondary stages), congenital anomalies, deafness, neurological impairment (mortality rate is 50%).
  f. Those with syphilis should also be tested for HIV.

C. Gonorrhea
1. Description
  a. Gonorrhea is an infection caused by *Neisseria gonorrhoeae,* which causes inflammation of the mucous membranes of the genital and urinary tracts.
  b. Transmission of the organism is by sexual intercourse.
  c. Infection may be transmitted to the newborn's eyes during delivery, causing blindness (ophthalmia neonatorum).
2. Assessment: Usually asymptomatic; vaginal discharge, urinary frequency, and lower abdominal pain possible
3. Interventions
  a. Testing is done during the initial prenatal examination to screen for gonorrhea; the screening may be repeated during the third trimester in high-risk clients.
  b. Instruct the client that treatment of her partner is necessary if infection is present.
  c. Complications are similar to those of chlamydia.

D. Condyloma acuminatum (human papillomavirus)
1. Description
  a. Condyloma acuminatum is caused by human papillomavirus.
  b. Infection affects the cervix, urethra, anus, penis, and scrotum.
  c. Human papillomavirus is transmitted through sexual contact.
2. Assessment
  a. Infection produces small to large wart-like growths on the genitals.
  b. Cervical cell changes may be noted because human papillomavirus is associated with cervical malignancies.
3. Interventions
  a. Lesions are removed by the use of cytotoxic agents, cryotherapy, electrocautery, and laser, but this is done for symptomatic relief only and is usually delayed until after birth. The genital warts often regress after delivery, and treatment outcomes may be poor until after delivery.
  b. Encourage annual Papanicolaou test.
  c. Sexual contact should be avoided until lesions are healed (condoms reduce transmission).
  d. Cesarean delivery is indicated only if genital warts are obstructing the pelvic outlet or if vaginal delivery would result in excessive bleeding.

E. Trichomoniasis
1. Description
  a. Trichomoniasis is caused by *Trichomonas vaginalis* and is transmitted via sexual contact.
  b. A normal saline wet smear of vaginal secretions indicates the presence of protozoa.
  c. Infection is associated with premature rupture of the membranes and postpartum endometritis.
2. Assessment
  a. Yellowish to greenish, frothy, mucopurulent, copious, malodorous vaginal discharge
  b. Inflammation of vulva, vagina, or both may occur.
3. Interventions
  a. Metronidazole may be prescribed.
  b. Sexual partner may need to be treated.

F. Bacterial vaginosis

1. Description

a. Caused by *Haemophilus vaginalis (Gardnerella vaginalis)* and transmitted via sexual contact

b. Associated with premature labor and birth

2. Assessment

a. Client complains of "fishy odor" to vaginal secretions and increased odor after intercourse.

b. Microscopic examination of vaginal secretions identifies the infection.

3. Interventions

a. Metronidazole may be prescribed.

b. Sexual partner may need to be treated.

G. Vaginal candidiasis

1. Description

a. *Candida albicans* is the most common causative organism.

b. Predisposing factors include use of antibiotics, diabetes mellitus, and obesity.

c. Vaginal candidiasis is diagnosed by identifying spores of *Candida albicans.*

2. Assessment

a. Vulvar and vaginal pruritus

b. White, lumpy, cottage cheese–like discharge from vagina

3. Interventions

a. An antifungal vaginal preparation may be prescribed. Oral fluconazole should be avoided during pregnancy due to the risk of miscarriage.

b. For extensive irritation and swelling, sitz baths may be helpful.

c. Sexual partner may need to be treated.

XXIII. Tuberculosis

A. Description

1. Highly communicable disease caused by *Mycobacterium tuberculosis*

2. Transmitted by the airborne route

3. Multidrug-resistant strains of tuberculosis can result from improper compliance, noncompliance with treatment programs, or development of mutations in tubercle bacillus.

B. Transmission

1. Transplacental transmission is rare.

2. Transmission can occur during birth through aspiration of infected amniotic fluid.

3. The newborn can become infected from contact with infected individuals.

C. Risk to mother: Active disease during pregnancy has been associated with an increase in hypertensive disorders of pregnancy.

D. Diagnosis: If a chest radiograph is required for the mother, it is done only after 20 weeks of gestation, and a lead shield for the abdomen is required.

> ⚠ Tuberculin skin testing is safe during pregnancy; however, the PHCP may want to delay testing until after delivery.

E. Assessment

1. Mother

a. Possibly asymptomatic

b. Fever and chills

c. Night sweats

d. Weight loss

e. Fatigue

f. Cough with hemoptysis or green or yellow sputum

g. Dyspnea

h. Pleural pain

2. Newborn

a. Fever

b. Lethargy

c. Poor feeding

d. Failure to thrive

e. Respiratory distress

f. Hepatosplenomegaly

g. Meningitis

h. Disease may spread to all major organs

F. Interventions

1. Pregnant client

a. Administration of isoniazid, pyrazinamide, and rifampin daily for 9 months (as prescribed); ethambutol is added if medication resistance is likely.

b. Pyridoxine should be administered with isoniazid to the pregnant client to prevent fetal neurotoxicity caused by isoniazid.

c. Promote breast-feeding only if the client is noninfectious.

2. Newborn

a. Management focuses on preventing disease and treating early infection.

b. Skin testing is performed on the newborn at birth, and the newborn may be placed on isoniazid therapy; the skin test is repeated in 3 to 4 months, and isoniazid may be stopped if the skin test results remain negative.

c. If the skin test result is positive, the newborn should receive isoniazid for at least 6 months (as prescribed).

d. If the mother's sputum is free of organisms, the newborn does not need to be isolated from the mother while in the hospital.

XXIV. Urinary Tract Infection (Acute Cystitis and Acute Pyelonephritis)

A. Description: A urinary tract infection can occur during pregnancy (pregnancy is a predisposing factor). A urinary tract infection can be either lower urinary tract (cystitis) or upper urinary tract (pyelonephritis).

B. Women may also experience asymptomatic bacteriuria.

C. Predisposing conditions
   1. History of urinary tract infections
   2. Urinary tract anomalies
   3. Low socioeconomic status
   4. Sexual activity
   5. Young age
   6. Sickle cell trait
   7. Poor hygiene
   8. Anemia
   9. Diabetes mellitus
   10. Obesity
   11. Catheterization
D. Screening is done at the first prenatal visit or at 12 to 16 weeks' gestation. Rescreening is done based on risk factors.
E. Assessment and Interventions (refer to Chapter 54): It is important to differentiate between cystitis and the progression to pyelonephritis. If progressed to pyelonephritis, hospitalization may be required for antibiotic therapy and possible tocolysis.

XXV. Obesity in Pregnancy

A. Description: Obesity in every population, including adults and children, is a problem in the United States. Obesity in pregnancy places the client at risk for several complications during pregnancy, including gestational diabetes, gestational hypertension, preeclampsia, venous thromboembolism, and increased need for cesarean birth.
B. Delivery complications can result from difficulty obtaining IV access, epidural access, intubation, and decreased oxygen consumption with associated increased cardiac output, stressing the heart.
C. Obesity in pregnancy can have negative effects on the newborn, including stillbirth, premature birth, congenital anomalies, future obesity, heart disease, and difficulty with breast-feeding.
D. Obese women have lower prolactin response to suckling in the first week postpartum, contributing to high rates of breast-feeding failure in this population.
E. Potential postdelivery complications and associated interventions
   1. Thromboembolism formation is a concern; as prescribed, thromboembolism stockings, sequential compression devices (SCDs), and pharmacological venous thromboembolism prophylaxis may be necessary postdelivery.
   2. Postpartum hemorrhage is more common, as well as difficulty locating the fundus, predisposing further to this problem.
   3. Endometritis is common in this population.
   4. Early ambulation is encouraged to prevent venous thromboembolism formation.
   5. Frequent monitoring and cleaning of surgical incisions (episiotomy or cesarean incision) is needed to prevent infection or dehiscence due to excess abdominal fat

XXVI. Additional complications during pregnancy: See Table 22-3.

TABLE 22-3 Risk Factors and Management of Additional Complications During Pregnancy

Complication	Risk Factors	Prevention and Management
▪ Dental abscess ▪ Broken or missing teeth ▪ Pregnancy gingivitis ▪ Periodontal disease ▪ Pyogenic granuloma ▪ Oral cancer	▪ Tobacco use ▪ High sugar consumption ▪ Poor oral hygiene ▪ High stress level ▪ Substance use, particularly methamphetamine ▪ Diabetes ▪ HIV infection ▪ Immunosuppression ▪ Low income ▪ Poor nutrition ▪ Medications that reduce saliva ▪ Hormonal changes ▪ Genetic predisposition ▪ Poor access to oral health provider	▪ Adequate fluid intake ▪ Teeth brushing twice daily with fluoridated toothpaste ▪ Floss at least once daily ▪ Regular oral health checkups ▪ Avoid tobacco ▪ Avoid high-sugar drinks and sweet snacks ▪ Regular physical exercise ▪ Soft diet ▪ Warm towel or heating pad ▪ Analgesics ▪ Dental consult ▪ Antibiotics for abscess ▪ Surgical drainage as indicated
▪ Iron-deficiency anemia	▪ Low dietary intake of iron ▪ Adolescence ▪ Pregnancy and breastfeeding ▪ Low socioeconomic status ▪ African American, Hispanic, Native American, recent immigrant ▪ History of anemia before pregnancy ▪ Underweight before pregnancy ▪ Eating problems ▪ Multiparity	▪ Screening during pregnancy: complete blood cell count (CBC) at initial visit, at 24-28 weeks, and at 36 weeks ▪ Iron supplementation in addition to prenatal vitamins as prescribed ▪ Teach to take iron supplementation in between meals so that absorption of zinc is not affected ▪ Advise in foods high in iron ▪ Advise on medications inhibiting absorption of iron, such as antacids, proton pump inhibitors (PPIs), certain antibiotics ▪ Referral to dietitian ▪ May need blood transfusion or IV iron if severely anemic

TABLE 22-3 Risk Factors and Management of Additional Common Complications During Pregnancy—cont'd

Complication	Risk Factors	Prevention and Management
	▪ Short interval between pregnancies ▪ Pica ▪ Blood loss ▪ Menorrhagia before pregnancy ▪ Frequent blood donation ▪ Chronic infectious process ▪ Malabsorptive disorder ▪ Strict vegetarian diet ▪ Alcohol and substance abuse ▪ Tobacco use	
▪ Asthma	▪ Exposure to allergens, dust mites, animal dander, cockroaches, mold, pollen, grass, flowers, smoke, tobacco, air fresheners, chemical cleaners, sprays ▪ Upper respiratory infections ▪ Sinusitis ▪ Cold temperatures ▪ Physical activity ▪ Sulfites in food and drinks ▪ Gastroesophageal reflux disease (GERD) ▪ Weather changes	▪ Education on prevention or exacerbation ▪ Avoid triggers and exposures ▪ Asthma action plan education ▪ Asthma medications generally safe during pregnancy ▪ Short-acting beta-agonist (SABA), long-acting beta-agonist (LABA), and inhaled corticosteroid (ICS) use ▪ Instructions on use of inhalers and nebulizers ▪ Oral medications may be needed depending on severity ▪ Serial growth scans by ultrasound should be done starting at 32 weeks ▪ Frequent nonstress tests are advised depending on severity ▪ Daily fetal kick counts advised ▪ Influenza vaccine is important ▪ Smoking cessation
▪ Zika Virus	▪ Recent travel or history of residing in an area with local transmission within the past 6 months	▪ Treatment revolves around symptom relief ▪ Rest ▪ Fluids to prevent dehydration ▪ Acetaminophen for fever and pain ▪ Avoiding aspirin and nonsteroidal antiinflammatory drugs (NSAIDs) ▪ May need serial ultrasounds to monitor fetal well-being ▪ Newborn should be tested within 24 hours ▪ Microcephaly is possible ▪ Maternal-fetal specialist referral should be done

Adapted from: Cibulka NJ, Barron ML. *Guidelines for nurse practitioners in ambulatory obstetric settings*, ed 2, New York, 2017, Springer Publishing Company.

PRACTICE QUESTIONS

204. The nurse is providing instructions to a pregnant client with human immunodeficiency virus (HIV) infection regarding care to the newborn after delivery. The client asks the nurse about the feeding options that are available. Which response should the nurse make to the client?

1. "You will need to bottle-feed your newborn."
2. "You will need to feed your newborn by nasogastric tube feeding."
3. "You will be able to breast-feed for 6 months and then will need to switch to bottle-feeding."
4. "You will be able to breast-feed for 9 months and then will need to switch to bottle-feeding."

205. The home care nurse visits a pregnant client who has a diagnosis of preeclampsia. Which assessment finding indicates a worsening of the preeclampsia and the need to notify the primary health care provider (PHCP)?

1. Urinary output has increased.
2. Dependent edema has resolved.
3. Blood pressure reading is at the prenatal baseline.
4. The client complains of a headache and blurred vision.

206. A stillborn baby was delivered in the birthing suite a few hours ago. After the delivery, the family remained together, holding and touching the baby. Which statement by the nurse would assist the family in their period of grief?

1. "What can I do for you?"
2. "Now you have an angel in heaven."
3. "Don't worry, there is nothing you could have done to prevent this from happening."
4. "We will see to it that you have an early discharge so that you don't have to be reminded of this experience."

207. The nurse implements a teaching plan for a pregnant client who is newly diagnosed with gestational diabetes mellitus. Which statement made by the client indicates a **need for further teaching**?

1. "I should stay on the diabetic diet."
2. "I should perform glucose monitoring at home."
3. "I should avoid exercise because of the negative effects on insulin production."
4. "I should be aware of any infections and report signs of infection immediately to my obstetrician."

208. The nurse is performing an assessment on a pregnant client in the last trimester with a diagnosis of preeclampsia. The nurse reviews the assessment findings and determines that which finding is **most** closely associated with a complication of this diagnosis?
1. Enlargement of the breasts
2. Complaints of feeling hot when the room is cool
3. Periods of fetal movement followed by quiet periods
4. Evidence of bleeding, such as in the gums, petechiae, and purpura

209. The nurse in a maternity unit is reviewing the clients' records. Which clients should the nurse identify as being at the most risk for developing disseminated intravascular coagulation (DIC)? **Select all that apply.**
- ☐ 1. A primigravida with abruptio placenta
- ☐ 2. A primigravida who delivered a 10-lb infant 3 hours ago
- ☐ 3. A gravida 2 who has just been diagnosed with dead fetus syndrome
- ☐ 4. A gravida 4 who delivered 8 hours ago and has lost 500 mL of blood
- ☐ 5. A primigravida at 29 weeks of gestation who was recently diagnosed with gestational hypertension

210. The home care nurse is monitoring a pregnant client who is at risk for preeclampsia. At each home care visit, the nurse assesses the client for which sign of preeclampsia?
1. Hypertension
2. Low-grade fever
3. Generalized edema
4. Increased pulse rate

211. The nurse is assessing a pregnant client with type 1 diabetes mellitus about her understanding regarding changing insulin needs during pregnancy. The nurse determines that **further teaching is needed** if the client makes which statement?
1. "I will need to increase my insulin dosage during the first 3 months of pregnancy."
2. "My insulin dose will likely need to be increased during the second and third trimesters."
3. "Episodes of hypoglycemia are more likely to occur during the first 3 months of pregnancy."
4. "My insulin needs should return to prepregnant levels within 7 to 10 days after birth if I am bottle-feeding."

212. A pregnant client reports to a health care clinic, complaining of loss of appetite, weight loss, and fatigue. After assessment of the client, tuberculosis is suspected. A sputum culture is obtained and identifies *Mycobacterium tuberculosis.* Which instruction should the nurse include in the client's teaching plan?
1. Therapeutic abortion is required.
2. Isoniazid plus rifampin will be required for 9 months.
3. She will have to stay at home until treatment is completed.
4. Medication will not be started until after delivery of the fetus.

213. The nurse is providing instructions to a pregnant client with a history of cardiac disease regarding appropriate dietary measures. Which statement, if made by the client, indicates an understanding of the information provided by the nurse?
1. "I should increase my sodium intake during pregnancy."
2. "I should lower my blood volume by limiting my fluids."
3. "I should maintain a low-calorie diet to prevent any weight gain."
4. "I should drink adequate fluids and increase my intake of high-fiber foods."

214. The clinic nurse is performing a psychosocial assessment of a client who has been told that she is pregnant. Which assessment findings indicate to the nurse that the client is at risk for contracting human immunodeficiency virus (HIV)? **Select all that apply.**
- ☐ 1. The client has a history of intravenous drug use.
- ☐ 2. The client has a significant other who is heterosexual.
- ☐ 3. The client has a history of sexually transmitted infections.
- ☐ 4. The client has had one sexual partner for the past 10 years.
- ☐ 5. The client has a previous history of gestational diabetes mellitus.

215. The nurse in a maternity unit is providing emotional support to a client and her significant other who are preparing to be discharged from the hospital after the birth of a dead fetus. Which statement made by the client indicates a component of the normal grieving process?
1. "We want to attend a support group."
2. "We never want to try to have a baby again."

3. "We are going to try to adopt a child immediately."
4. "We are okay, and we are going to try to have another baby immediately."

216. The nurse evaluates the ability of a hepatitis B–positive mother to provide safe bottle-feeding to her newborn during postpartum hospitalization. Which maternal action **best** exemplifies the mother's knowledge of potential disease transmission to the newborn?
1. The mother requests that the window be closed before feeding.
2. The mother holds the newborn properly during feeding and burping.
3. The mother tests the temperature of the formula before initiating feeding.
4. The mother washes and dries her hands before and after self-care of the perineum and asks for a pair of gloves before feeding.

217. A client in the first trimester of pregnancy arrives at a health care clinic and reports that she has been experiencing vaginal bleeding. A threatened abortion is suspected, and the nurse instructs the client regarding management of care. Which statement made by the client indicates a **need for further instruction?**
1. "I will watch to see if I pass any tissue."
2. "I will maintain strict bed rest throughout the remainder of the pregnancy."
3. "I will count the number of perineal pads used on a daily basis and note the amount and color of blood on the pad."
4. "I will avoid sexual intercourse until the bleeding has stopped and for 2 weeks following the last episode of bleeding."

218. The nurse is planning to admit a pregnant client who is obese. In planning care for this client, which potential client needs should the nurse anticipate? **Select all that apply.**
- ❑ 1. Bed rest as a necessary preventive measure may be prescribed.
- ❑ 2. Administration of subcutaneous heparin postdelivery as prescribed.
- ❑ 3. An overbed lift may be necessary if the client requires a cesarean section.
- ❑ 4. Less frequent cleansing of a cesarean incision, if present, may be prescribed.
- ❑ 5. Thromboembolism stockings or sequential compression devices may be prescribed.

219. The nurse is assessing a pregnant client in the second trimester of pregnancy who was admitted to the maternity unit with a suspected diagnosis of abruptio placentae. Which assessment finding should the nurse expect to note if this condition is present?
1. Soft abdomen
2. Uterine tenderness
3. Absence of abdominal pain
4. Painless, bright red vaginal bleeding

220. The maternity nurse is preparing for the admission of a client in the third trimester of pregnancy who is experiencing vaginal bleeding and has a suspected diagnosis of placenta previa. The nurse reviews the primary health care provider's prescriptions and should question which prescription?
1. Prepare the client for an ultrasound.
2. Obtain equipment for a manual pelvic examination.
3. Prepare to draw a hemoglobin and hematocrit blood sample.
4. Obtain equipment for external electronic fetal heart rate monitoring.

221. An ultrasound is performed on a client at term gestation who is experiencing moderate vaginal bleeding. The results of the ultrasound indicate that abruptio placentae is present. On the basis of these findings, the nurse should prepare the client for which anticipated prescription?
1. Delivery of the fetus
2. Strict monitoring of intake and output
3. Complete bed rest for the remainder of the pregnancy
4. The need for weekly monitoring of coagulation studies until the time of delivery

222. The nurse in the postpartum unit is caring for a client who has just delivered a newborn infant following a pregnancy with placenta previa. The nurse reviews the plan of care and prepares to monitor the client for which risk associated with placenta previa?
1. Infection
2. Hemorrhage
3. Chronic hypertension
4. Disseminated intravascular coagulation

223. The nurse is performing an assessment on a client diagnosed with placenta previa. Which assessment findings should the nurse expect to note? **Select all that apply.**
- ❑ 1. Uterine rigidity
- ❑ 2. Uterine tenderness
- ❑ 3. Severe abdominal pain
- ❑ 4. Bright red vaginal bleeding
- ❑ 5. Soft, relaxed, nontender uterus
- ❑ 6. Fundal height may be greater than expected for gestational age

ANSWERS

204. *Answer:* 1

Rationale: Perinatal transmission of HIV can occur during the antepartum period, during labor and birth, or in the postpartum period if the mother is breast-feeding. Clients who have HIV will most likely be advised not to breast-feed; however, PHCPs recommendations regarding breast-feeding are always followed. There is no physiological reason why the newborn needs to be fed by nasogastric tube.

Test-Taking Strategy: Use knowledge regarding the transmission of HIV. Eliminate options 3 and 4 first because these options are comparable or alike in that they both address breast-feeding. From the remaining options, select the correct option, knowing that it is unnecessary to feed the newborn by nasogastric tube.

Level of Cognitive Ability: Applying
Client Needs: Safe and Effective Care Environment
Integrated Process: Teaching and Learning
Content Area: Maternity: Postpartum
Health Problem: Maternity: Infections/Inflammations
Priority Concepts: Client Education; Infection
Reference: McKinney et al. (2018), pp. 567-568.

205. *Answer:* 4

Rationale: If the client complains of a headache and blurred vision, the PHCP should be notified because these are signs of worsening preeclampsia. Options 1, 2, and 3 are normal findings.

Test-Taking Strategy: Note the word *worsening* in the question. Eliminate options 1, 2, and 3 because these options are comparable or alike and indicate normal findings.

Level of Cognitive Ability: Analyzing
Client Needs: Physiological Integrity
Integrated Process: Nursing Process—Assessment
Content Area: Maternity: Antepartum
Health Problem: Maternity: Gestational hypertension/preeclampsia and eclampsia
Priority Concepts: Clinical Judgment; Perfusion
Reference: Lowdermilk et al. (2016), pp. 654, 660.

206. *Answer:* 1

Rationale: When a loss or death occurs, the nurse should ensure that parents have been honestly told about the situation by their primary health care provider or others on the health care team. It is important for the nurse to be with the parents at this time and to use therapeutic communication techniques. The nurse must also consider cultural and religious/spiritual practices and beliefs. The correct option provides a supportive, giving, and caring response. Options 2, 3, and 4 are blocks to communication and devalue the parents' feelings.

Test-Taking Strategy: Use knowledge of therapeutic communication techniques to answer the question. The correct option is the only option that reflects use of therapeutic communication techniques.

Level of Cognitive Ability: Applying
Client Needs: Psychosocial Integrity
Integrated Process: Caring
Content Area: Maternity: Postpartum
Health Problem: Maternity: Fetal distress/demise
Priority Concepts: Communication; Coping
Reference: Lowdermilk et al. (2016), pp. 911, 918.

207. *Answer:* 3

Rationale: Exercise is safe for a client with gestational diabetes mellitus and is helpful in lowering the blood glucose level. Dietary modifications are the mainstay of treatment, and the client is placed on a standard diabetic diet. Many clients are taught to perform blood glucose monitoring. If the client is not performing the blood glucose monitoring at home, it is performed at the clinic or obstetrician's office. Signs of infection need to be reported to the obstetrician.

Test-Taking Strategy: Note the strategic words, *need for further teaching*. These words indicate a negative event query and the need to select an incorrect client statement. Also, noting the closed-ended word "avoid" in the correct option will assist in answering the question.

Level of Cognitive Ability: Evaluating
Client Needs: Physiological Integrity
Integrated Process: Teaching and Learning
Content Area: Maternity: Antepartum
Health Problem: Maternity: Diabetes
Priority Concepts: Client Education; Glucose Regulation
Reference: Lowdermilk et al. (2016), p. 703.

208. *Answer:* 4

Rationale: Severe preeclampsia can trigger disseminated intravascular coagulation (DIC) because of the widespread damage to vascular integrity. Bleeding is an early sign of DIC and should be reported to the primary health care provider if noted on assessment. Options 1, 2, and 3 are normal occurrences in the last trimester of pregnancy.

Test-Taking Strategy: Note the strategic word, *most*. Focus on the subject, a complication of preeclampsia. Eliminate options 1, 2, and 3 because they are comparable or alike and are normal occurrences in the last trimester of pregnancy.

Level of Cognitive Ability: Analyzing
Client Needs: Physiological Integrity
Integrated Process: Nursing Process—Assessment
Content Area: Maternity: Antepartum
Health Problem: Maternity: Gestational hypertension/preeclampsia and eclampsia
Priority Concepts: Clinical Judgment; Clotting
Reference: McKinney et al. (2018), p. 525.

209. *Answer:* 1, 3, 5

Rationale: In a pregnant client, DIC is a condition in which the clotting cascade is activated, resulting in the formation of clots in the microcirculation. Predisposing conditions include abruptio placentae, amniotic fluid embolism, gestational hypertension, HELLP syndrome, intrauterine fetal death, liver disease, sepsis, severe postpartum hemorrhage, and blood loss. Delivering a large newborn is not considered a risk factor for DIC. Hemorrhage is a risk factor for DIC; however, a loss of 500 mL is not considered hemorrhage.

Test-Taking Strategy: Note the strategic word, *most*. Focus on the subject, the client at most risk for DIC. Think about the pathophysiology associated with DIC and select the options that identify abnormal conditions. This will direct you to the correct options.

Level of Cognitive Ability: Analyzing
Client Needs: Physiological Integrity
Integrated Process: Nursing Process—Analysis

Content Area: Maternity: Intrapartum
Health Problem: Maternity: DIC
Priority Concepts: Clinical Judgment; Clotting
Reference: Lowdermilk et al. (2016), pp. 685-686.

210. *Answer:* 1

Rationale: A sign of preeclampsia is persistent hypertension. A low-grade fever or increased pulse rate is not associated with preeclampsia. Generalized edema may occur but is not a specific sign of preeclampsia because it can occur in many conditions.

Test-Taking Strategy: Focus on the subject, a sign of preeclampsia. Thinking about the pathophysiology associated with preeclampsia will direct you to the correct option. Remember that hypertension is associated with preeclampsia.

Level of Cognitive Ability: Analyzing
Client Needs: Physiological Integrity
Integrated Process: Nursing Process—Assessment
Content Area: Maternity: Antepartum
Health Problem: Maternity: Gestational hypertension/preeclampsia and eclampsia
Priority Concepts: Clinical Judgment; Perfusion
Reference: McKinney et al. (2018), pp. 537-538.

211. *Answer:* 1

Rationale: Insulin needs decrease in the first trimester of pregnancy because of increased insulin production by the pancreas and increased peripheral sensitivity to insulin. The statements in options 2, 3, and 4 are accurate and signify that the client understands control of her diabetes during pregnancy.

Test-Taking Strategy: Note the strategic words, *further teaching is needed*. These words indicate a negative event query and the need to select an incorrect client statement. Eliminate options 2, 3, and 4 because they are comparable or alike and are accurate statements. Remember that insulin needs decrease in the first trimester of pregnancy.

Level of Cognitive Ability: Evaluating
Client Needs: Physiological Integrity
Integrated Process: Teaching and Learning
Content Area: Maternity: Antepartum
Health Problem: Maternity: Diabetes
Priority Concepts: Client Education; Glucose Regulation
Reference: McKinney et al. (2018), p. 553.

212. *Answer:* 2

Rationale: More than one medication may be used to prevent the growth of resistant organisms in a pregnant client with tuberculosis. Treatment must continue for a prolonged period. The preferred treatment for the pregnant client is isoniazid plus rifampin daily for 9 months. Ethambutol is added initially if medication resistance is suspected. Pyridoxine (vitamin B_6) often is administered with isoniazid to prevent fetal neurotoxicity. The client does not need to stay at home during treatment, and therapeutic abortion is not required.

Test-Taking Strategy: Focus on the subject, therapeutic management for a client with tuberculosis. Recalling the pathophysiology associated with tuberculosis and its treatment will assist in eliminating options 1, 3, and 4.

Level of Cognitive Ability: Applying
Client Needs: Physiological Integrity
Integrated Process: Teaching and Learning
Content Area: Maternity: Antepartum
Health Problem: Maternity: Infections/Inflammations
Priority Concepts: Client Education; Infection
Reference: McKinney et al. (2018), pp. 569-570.

213. *Answer:* 4

Rationale: Constipation can cause the client to use the Valsalva maneuver. The Valsalva maneuver should be avoided in clients with cardiac disease because it can cause blood to rush to the heart and overload the cardiac system. Constipation can be prevented by the addition of fluids and a high-fiber diet. A low-calorie diet is not recommended during pregnancy and could be harmful to the fetus. Sodium should be restricted as prescribed by the primary health care provider, because excess sodium would cause an overload to the circulating blood volume and contribute to cardiac complications. Diets low in fluid can cause a decrease in blood volume, which could deprive the fetus of nutrients.

Test-Taking Strategy: Focus on the subject, the pregnant client with heart disease. Think about the physiology of the cardiac system, maternal and fetal needs, and the factors that increase the workload on the heart. This will direct you to the correct option.

Level of Cognitive Ability: Evaluating
Client Needs: Physiological Integrity
Integrated Process: Nursing Process—Evaluation
Content Area: Maternity: Antepartum
Health Problem: Maternity: Cardiac disease
Priority Concepts: Clinical Judgment; Perfusion
Reference: Lowdermilk et al. (2016), pp. 458, 719.

214. *Answer:* 1, 3

Rationale: HIV is transmitted by intimate sexual contact and the exchange of body fluids, exposure to infected blood, and passage from an infected woman to her fetus. Clients who fall into the high-risk category for HIV infection include individuals who have used intravenous drugs, individuals who experience persistent and recurrent sexually transmitted infections, and individuals who have a history of multiple sexual partners. Gestational diabetes mellitus does not predispose the client to HIV. A client with a heterosexual partner, particularly a client who has had only one sexual partner in 10 years, does not have a high risk for contracting HIV.

Test-Taking Strategy: Focus on the subject, risk factors for HIV. Recalling that exchange of blood and body fluids places the client at high risk for HIV infection will direct you to the correct options.

Level of Cognitive Ability: Analyzing
Client Needs: Safe and Effective Care Environment
Integrated Process: Nursing Process—Assessment
Content Area: Maternity: Antepartum
Health Problem: Maternity: Infections/Inflammations
Priority Concepts: Infection; Sexuality
Reference: Lowdermilk et al. (2016), p. 161.

215. *Answer:* 1

Rationale: A support group can help the parents work through their pain by nonjudgmental sharing of feelings. The correct option identifies a statement that indicates positive, normal

grieving. Although the other options may indicate reactions of the client and significant other, they are not specifically a part of the normal grieving process.
Test-Taking Strategy: Read all options carefully before selecting an answer and focus on the **subject,** the normal grieving process. Note that options 2, 3, and 4 are **comparable or alike** in that they relate to childbearing.
Level of Cognitive Ability: Applying
Client Needs: Psychosocial Integrity
Integrated Process: Caring
Content Area: Maternity: Postpartum
Health Problem: Maternity: Fetal distress/Demise
Priority Concepts: Coping; Family Dynamics
Reference: Lowdermilk et al. (2016), p. 918-919.

216. *Answer:* 4
Rationale: Hepatitis B virus is highly contagious and is transmitted by direct contact with blood and body fluids of infected persons. The rationale for identifying childbearing clients with this disease is to provide adequate protection of the fetus and the newborn, to minimize transmission to other individuals, and to reduce maternal complications. The correct option provides the best evaluation of maternal understanding of disease transmission. Option 1 will not affect disease transmission since hepatitis B does not spread through airborne transmission. Options 2 and 3 are appropriate feeding techniques for bottle-feeding but do not minimize disease transmission for hepatitis B.
Test-Taking Strategy: Note the **strategic word,** *best.* Focus on the **subject,** disease transmission to the newborn. This focus will direct you to the correct option.
Level of Cognitive Ability: Evaluating
Client Needs: Safe and Effective Care Environment
Integrated Process: Nursing Process—Evaluation
Content Area: Maternity: Postpartum
Health Problem: Maternity: Infections/Inflammations
Priority Concepts: Client Education; Infection
Reference: McKinney et al. (2018), p. 567.

217. *Answer:* 2
Rationale: Strict bed rest throughout the remainder of the pregnancy is not required for a threatened abortion. The client should watch for the evidence of the passage of tissue. The client is instructed to count the number of perineal pads used daily and to note the quantity and color of blood on the pad. The client is advised to curtail sexual activities until bleeding has ceased and for 2 weeks after the last evidence of bleeding or as recommended by the health care provider.
Test-Taking Strategy: Note the **strategic words,** *need for further instruction.* These words indicate a **negative event query** and the need to select an incorrect client statement. Noting the word *strict* in the correct option will assist in directing you to this option.
Level of Cognitive Ability: Evaluating
Client Needs: Physiological Integrity
Integrated Process: Teaching and Learning
Content Area: Maternity: Antepartum
Health Problem: Maternity: Abortions
Priority Concepts: Client Education; Reproduction
Reference: McKinney et al. (2018), pp. 525-526.

218. *Answer:* 2, 3, 5
Rationale: The obese pregnant client is at risk for complications such as venous thromboembolism and increased need for cesarean section. Additionally, the obese client requires special considerations pertaining to nursing care. To prevent venous thromboembolism, particularly in the client who required cesarean section, frequent and early ambulation (not bed rest), prior to and after surgery, is recommended. Routine administration of prophylactic pharmacological venous thromboembolism medications such as heparin is also commonly prescribed. An overbed lift may be needed to transfer a client from a bed to an operating table if cesarean section is necessary. Increased monitoring and cleansing of a cesarean incision, if present, is necessary due to the increased risk for infection secondary to increased abdominal fat. Thromboembolism stockings or sequential compression devices will likely be prescribed because of the client's increased risk of blood clots.
Test-Taking Strategy: Note the **subject,** planning care for the pregnant client who is obese. If you can recall the general complications associated with obesity, this will help you choose the correct options. Recall that preventive measures need to be taken to prevent blood clots and infection in clients at higher risk for these complications.
Level of Cognitive Ability: Applying
Client Needs: Safe and Effective Care Environment
Integrated Process: Nursing Process—Planning
Content Area: Maternity: Antepartum
Health Problem: Maternity: Infections/Inflammations
Priority Concepts: Infection; Perfusion
Reference: Lowdermilk et al. (2016), p. 778.

219. *Answer:* 2
Rationale: Abruptio placentae is the premature separation of the placenta from the uterine wall after the twentieth week of gestation and before the fetus is delivered. In abruptio placentae, acute abdominal pain is present. Uterine tenderness accompanies placental abruption, especially with a central abruption and trapped blood behind the placenta. The abdomen feels hard and board-like on palpation as the blood penetrates the myometrium and causes uterine irritability. A soft abdomen and painless, bright red vaginal bleeding in the second or third trimester of pregnancy are signs of placenta previa.
Test-Taking Strategy: Focus on the **subject,** assessment findings in abruptio placentae. Remember that the difference between placenta previa and abruptio placentae involves the presence of uterine pain and tenderness with abruptio placentae, as opposed to painless bleeding with placenta previa.
Level of Cognitive Ability: Analyzing
Client Needs: Physiological Integrity
Integrated Process: Nursing Process—Assessment
Content Area: Maternity: Intrapartum
Health Problem: Maternity: Abruptio placentae
Priority Concepts: Clinical Judgment; Perfusion
Reference: McKinney et al. (2018), pp. 531-532.

220. *Answer:* 2
Rationale: Placenta previa is an improperly implanted placenta in the lower uterine segment near or over the internal cervical os. Manual pelvic examinations are contraindicated when vaginal bleeding is apparent until a diagnosis is made

and placenta previa is ruled out. Digital examination of the cervix can lead to hemorrhage. A diagnosis of placenta previa is made by ultrasound. The hemoglobin and hematocrit levels are monitored, and external electronic fetal heart rate monitoring is initiated. Electronic fetal monitoring (external) is crucial in evaluating the status of the fetus, who is at risk for severe hypoxia.
Test-Taking Strategy: Focus on the subject, nursing care of the client with placenta previa. Use knowledge of the pathophysiology associated with placenta previa. Note the words *question which prescription* in the event query. Also, note that the correct option is the only procedure that is invasive to the pregnancy and endangers the physiological safety of the client and the fetus.
Level of Cognitive Ability: Analyzing
Client Needs: Physiological Integrity
Integrated Process: Nursing Process—Implementation
Content Area: Maternity: Intrapartum
Health Problem: Maternity: Placenta previa
Priority Concepts: Collaboration; Safety
Reference: McKinney et al. (2018), pp. 529-530.

221. *Answer:* 1
Rationale: Abruptio placentae is the premature separation of the placenta from the uterine wall after the 20th week of gestation and before the fetus is delivered. The goal of management in abruptio placentae is to control the hemorrhage and deliver the fetus as soon as possible. Delivery is the treatment of choice if the fetus is at term gestation or if the bleeding is moderate to severe and the client or fetus is in jeopardy. Because delivery of the fetus is necessary, options 2, 3, and 4 are incorrect regarding management of a client with abruptio placentae.
Test-Taking Strategy: Focus on the subject, management of abruptio placentae. Use knowledge regarding the pathophysiology and management of abruptio placentae to answer the question. Note the words *term gestation* and *moderate vaginal bleeding*. Knowing that the goal is to deliver the fetus will direct you easily to the correct option.
Level of Cognitive Ability: Analyzing
Client Needs: Physiological Integrity
Integrated Process: Nursing Process—Planning
Content Area: Complex Care: Emergency Situations/Management
Health Problem: Maternity: Abruptio placentae
Priority Concepts: Perfusion; Safety
Reference: Lowdermilk et al. (2016), p. 684.

222. *Answer:* 2
Rationale: In placenta previa, the placenta is implanted in the lower uterine segment. The lower uterine segment does not contain the same intertwining musculature as the fundus of the uterus, and this site is more prone to bleeding. Options 1, 3, and 4 are not risks that are related specifically to placenta previa.
Test-Taking Strategy: Focus on the subject, the risks associated with placenta previa. Thinking about the pathophysiology associated with this disorder and recalling that bleeding is a primary concern in this client will direct you easily to the correct option.
Level of Cognitive Ability: Analyzing
Client Needs: Physiological Integrity
Integrated Process: Nursing Process—Assessment
Content Area: Maternity: Postpartum
Health Problem: Maternity: Placenta previa
Priority Concepts: Clinical Judgment; Perfusion
Reference: Lowdermilk et al. (2016), p. 682.

223. *Answer:* 4, 5, 6
Rationale: Placenta previa is an improperly implanted placenta in the lower uterine segment near or over the internal cervical os. Painless, bright red vaginal bleeding in the second or third trimester of pregnancy is a sign of placenta previa. The client has a soft, relaxed, nontender uterus, and fundal height may be more than expected for gestational age. In abruptio placentae, severe abdominal pain is present. Uterine tenderness accompanies placental abruption. In addition, in abruptio placentae, the abdomen feels hard and board-like on palpation, as the blood penetrates the myometrium and causes uterine irritability.
Test-Taking Strategy: First, eliminate options 1 and 2 because they are comparable or alike. Next, remember that the difference between placenta previa and abruptio placentae involves the presence of uterine pain and tenderness with abruptio placentae, as opposed to painless bright red bleeding with placenta previa.
Level of Cognitive Ability: Analyzing
Client Needs: Physiological Integrity
Integrated Process: Nursing Process—Assessment
Content Area: Maternity: Intrapartum
Health Problem: Maternity: Placenta previa
Priority Concepts: Clinical Judgment; Perfusion
Reference: McKinney et al. (2018), pp. 529, 531.

CHAPTER 23

Labor and Birth

PRIORITY CONCEPTS Oxygenation, Perfusion

I. Process of Labor—4 Ps

A. Description
  1. Labor: Coordinated sequence of involuntary, intermittent uterine contractions
  2. Birth: Actual event of birth

B. Four major factors (4 Ps) interact during normal childbirth; the 4 Ps are interrelated and depend on each other for a safe birth and are Powers, Passageway, Passenger, and Psyche.

C. Powers: Uterine contractions
  1. Forces acting to expel the fetus
  2. Effacement: Shortening and thinning of the cervix during the first stage of labor
  3. Dilation: Enlargement of cervical os and cervical canal during the first stage of labor
  4. Pushing efforts of mother during the second stage

D. Passageway: The mother's rigid bony pelvis and the soft tissues of the cervix, pelvic floor, vagina, and introitus (external opening to the vagina)

E. Passenger: The fetus, membranes, and placenta

F. Psyche: A woman's emotional structure that can determine her entire response to labor and influence physiological and psychological functioning; the mother may experience anxiety or fear.

G. Attitude
  1. Attitude is the relationship of the fetal body parts to one another.
  2. Normal intrauterine attitude is flexion, in which the fetal back is rounded, the head is forward on the chest, and the arms and legs are folded in against the body. The other attitude, extension, tends to present larger fetal diameters.

H. Lie
  1. Relationship of the spine of the fetus to the spine of the mother
  2. Longitudinal or vertical (Fig. 23-1)
    a. Fetal spine is parallel to the mother's spine.
    b. Fetus is in cephalic or breech presentation.
  3. Transverse or horizontal (Fig. 23-1)
    a. Fetal spine is at a right angle, or perpendicular, to the mother's spine.
    b. Presenting part is the shoulder.
    c. Delivery by cesarean section is necessary.

I. Presentation
  1. Portion of the fetus that enters the pelvic inlet first
  2. Cephalic: Head first
    a. Cephalic is the most common presentation.
    b. Cephalic presentation has 4 variations: vertex, military, brow, and face.
  3. Breech: Buttocks present first.
    a. Delivery by cesarean section may be required, although vaginal birth is often possible.
    b. Breech presentation has 3 variations: frank, full (complete), and footling
  4. Shoulder
    a. Fetus is in a transverse lie, or the arm, back, abdomen, or side could present.
    b. If the fetus does not spontaneously rotate, or if it is impossible to turn the fetus manually, a cesarean section may need to be performed.

J. Presenting part: The specific fetal structure lying nearest to the cervix

K. Position: Relationship of assigned area of the presenting part or landmark to the maternal pelvis (Fig. 23-2 and Box 23-1)

L. Station
  1. The measurement of the progress of descent in centimeters above or below the midplane from the presenting part to the ischial spine
  2. Station 0: At ischial spine
  3. Minus station: Above ischial spine
  4. Plus station: Below ischial spine
  5. Engagement: When the widest diameter of the presenting part has passed the inlet; corresponds to a 0 station

II. Mechanisms of Labor (Box 23-2)

A. Assessment
  1. Lightening or dropping: Is also known as *engagement* and occurs when the fetus descends into the pelvis about 2 weeks before birth; lightening or dropping is most noticeable in first pregnancies.

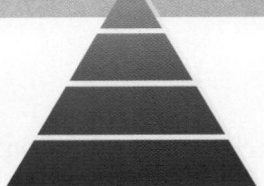

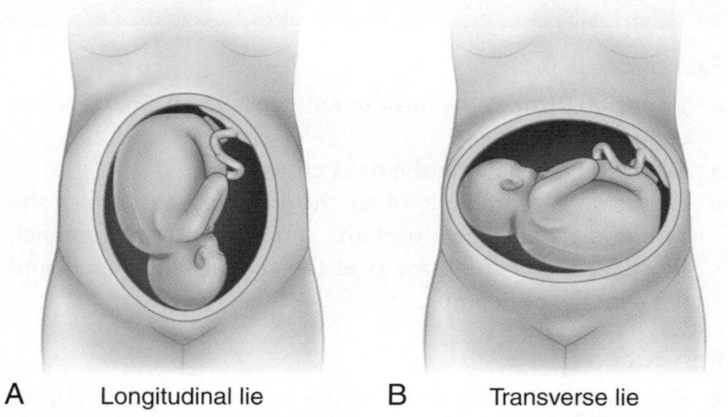

FIG. 23-1 Fetal lie. **A,** In a longitudinal lie, the long axis of the fetus is parallel to the long axis of the mother. **B,** In a transverse lie, the long axis of the fetus is at a right angle to the long axis of the mother. The mother's abdomen has a wide, short appearance.

BOX 23-1 Fetal Positions

Vertex Presentations

ROA: Right occipitoanterior
LOA: Left occipitoanterior
ROP: Right occipitoposterior
LOP: Left occipitoposterior
ROT: Right occipitotransverse
LOT: Left occipitotransverse

Face Presentations

RMA: Right mentoanterior
LMA: Left mentoanterior
RMP: Right mentoposterior

Breech Presentations

LSA: Left sacroanterior
LSP: Left sacroposterior

Other Presentations

Brow presentation
Shoulder presentation

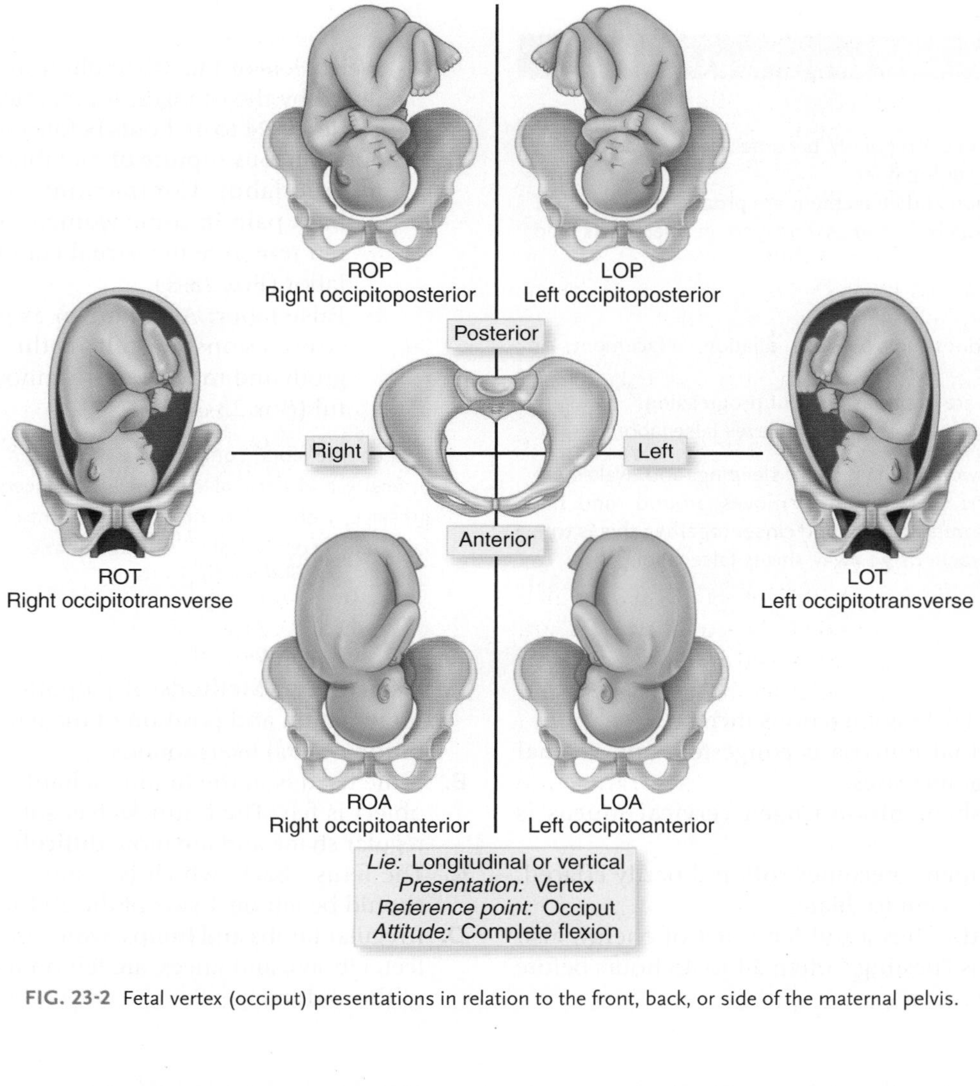

FIG. 23-2 Fetal vertex (occiput) presentations in relation to the front, back, or side of the maternal pelvis.

BOX 23-2 Mechanisms of Labor

Engagement
- Engagement is the mechanism whereby the fetus nestles into the pelvis.
- Engagement occurs when the presenting part reaches the level of the ischial spines.

Descent
- Descent is the process that the fetal head undergoes as it begins its journey through the pelvis.
- Descent is a continuous process from prior to engagement until birth and is assessed by the measurement called *station*.

Flexion
- Flexion is a process of nodding of the fetal head forward toward the fetal chest.

Internal Rotation
- Internal rotation of the fetus occurs most commonly from the occipitotransverse position, assumed at engagement into the pelvis, to the occipitoanterior position while continuously descending.

Extension
- Extension enables the head to emerge when the fetus is in a cephalic position.
- Extension begins after the head crowns.
- Extension is complete when the head passes under the symphysis pubis and occiput, and the anterior fontanel, brow, face, and chin pass over the sacrum and coccyx and are over the perineum.

Restitution
- Restitution is realignment of the fetal head with the body after the head emerges.

External Rotation
- The shoulders externally rotate after the head emerges and restitution occurs, so that the shoulders are in the anteroposterior diameter of the pelvis.

Expulsion
- Expulsion is the birth of the entire body.

BOX 23-3 True Labor Versus False Labor

True Labor
- Contractions occur regularly, become stronger, last longer, and occur closer together.
- Cervical dilation and effacement are progressive.
- The fetus usually becomes engaged in the pelvis and begins to descend.

False Labor
- False labor does not produce dilation, effacement, or descent.
- Contractions are irregular, without progression.
- Activity, such as walking, often relieves false labor.

Example: If a woman has been sleeping and wakes up with contractions, gets up, and moves around, and her contractions become stronger and closer together, this is true labor. If the contractions go away, this is false labor.

2. Braxton Hicks contractions increase.
3. The vaginal mucosa is congested, and vaginal discharge increases.
4. Brownish or blood-tinged cervical mucus is passed.
5. Cervix ripens, becomes soft and partly effaced, and may begin to dilate.
6. The mother has a sudden burst of energy, also known as "nesting," often 24 to 48 hours before onset of labor.
7. Weight loss of 1 to 3 lb results from fluid shifts produced by the changes in progesterone and estrogen levels 24 to 48 hours before the onset of labor.
8. Spontaneous rupture of membranes occurs.
   a. True labor: Contractions may manifest as back pain in some women; contractions often resemble menstrual cramps during early labor (Box 23-3).
   b. False labor: Also known as *prodromal labor,* contractions are felt in the abdomen and groin and may be more annoying than painful (Box 23-3).

⚠ In true labor, contractions increase in duration and intensity and cervical dilation and effacement are progressive, with engagement and descent of the fetus. In false labor, contractions are irregular and do not produce dilation, effacement, or descent.

III. Leopold's Maneuvers

A. Description: Methods of palpation to determine presentation and position of the fetus and aid in location of fetal heart sounds

B. If the head is in the fundus, a hard, round, movable object is felt. The buttocks feel soft and have an irregular shape and are more difficult to move.

C. The fetus's back, which is a smooth, hard surface, should be felt on 1 side of the abdomen.

D. Irregular knobs and lumps, which may be the hands, feet, elbows, and knees, are felt on the opposite side of the abdomen.

BOX 23-4 Breathing Techniques

First-Stage Breathing

Cleansing Breath

Each contraction begins and ends with a deep inspiration and expiration.

Slow-Paced Breathing

Slow-paced breathing promotes relaxation.

Slow-paced breathing is used for as long as possible during labor.

Modified-Paced Breathing

Modified-paced breathing is used when slow-paced breathing is no longer effective.

Breathing is shallow and fast.

Pattern-Paced Breathing

Pattern-paced breathing sometimes is referred to as *pant-blow*.

After a certain number of breaths (modified-paced breathing), the woman exhales with a slight blow and then begins modified-paced breathing again.

Breathing to Prevent Pushing

The woman blows repeatedly, using short puffs, when the urge to push is strong.

Second-Stage Breathing

Several variations of breathing can be used in the pushing stage of labor, and the woman may grunt, groan, sigh, or moan as she pushes. Prolonged breath holding while pushing with a closed glottis may result in a decrease in cardiac output. If breath holding while pushing is used, the open glottis method or limiting breath holding to less than 6 to 8 seconds should be done.

IV. Breathing Techniques (Box 23-4)

A. Provide a focus during contractions, interfering with pain sensory transmission

B. Promote relaxation and oxygenation

C. Begin with simple breathing patterns and progress to more complex ones as needed.

V. Fetal Monitoring

A. Description

1. The fetal monitor displays the fetal heart rate (FHR).
2. The device monitors uterine activity.
3. The monitor assesses frequency, duration, and intensity of contractions.
4. The monitor assesses FHR in relation to maternal contractions.
5. Baseline FHR is measured between contractions; the normal FHR at term is 110 to 160 beats per minute.

B. External fetal monitoring

1. External fetal monitoring is noninvasive and is performed with a tocotransducer or Doppler ultrasonic transducer.
2. Leopold's maneuvers are performed to determine on which side the fetal back is located, and the ultrasound transducer is placed over this area (fasten with a belt or stocking tubing).
3. The tocotransducer is placed over the fundus of the uterus, where contractions feel the strongest (fasten with a belt or stocking tubing).
4. The client is allowed to assume a comfortable position, avoiding vena cava compression (maternal supine hypotensive syndrome).
5. The preferred position is to have the client lie on her side to increase perfusion.

C. Internal fetal monitoring

1. Internal fetal monitoring is invasive and requires rupturing of the membranes and attaching an electrode to the presenting part of the fetus.
2. The client must be dilated 2 to 3 cm to perform internal monitoring.

D. Periodic patterns in FHR

1. Fetal bradycardia and tachycardia
   - **a.** Bradycardia: FHR is less than 110 beats per minute for 10 minutes or longer.
   - **b.** Tachycardia: FHR is more than 160 beats per minute for 10 minutes or longer.

⚠ If fetal bradycardia or tachycardia occurs, change the position of the mother, administer oxygen, and assess the mother's vital signs. Notify the primary health care provider (PHCP) as soon as possible.

2. Variability (Box 23-5)
   - **a.** Fluctuations in baseline FHR
   - **b.** Absent or undetected variability is considered nonreassuring.
   - **c.** Decreased variability can result from fetal hypoxemia, acidosis, or certain medications.
   - **d.** A temporary decrease in variability can occur when the fetus is in a sleep state (sleep states do not usually last longer than 30 minutes).
3. Accelerations
   - **a.** Brief, temporary increases in FHR of at least 15 beats per minute more than baseline and lasting at least 15 seconds

BOX 23-5 Variability in Fetal Heart Rate

Absent Variability: Undetected variability

Minimal Variability: Greater than undetected but not more than 5 beats per minute

Moderate Variability: Fetal heart rate fluctuations are 6 to 25 beats per minute

Marked Variability: Fetal heart rate fluctuations are greater than 25 beats per minute

b. Usually are a reassuring sign, reflecting a responsive, nonacidotic fetus
c. Usually occur with fetal movement
d. May be nonperiodic (having no relation to contractions) or periodic (with contractions)
e. May occur with uterine contractions, vaginal examinations, or mild cord compression, or when the fetus is in a breech presentation

4. Early decelerations (Fig. 23-3)
    a. Early decelerations are decreases in FHR below baseline; the rate at the lowest point of the deceleration usually remains greater than 100 beats per minute.
    b. Early decelerations occur during contractions as the fetal head is pressed against the mother's pelvis or soft tissues, such as the cervix, and return to baseline FHR by the end of the contraction.
    c. Tracing shows a uniform shape and mirror image of uterine contractions.
    d. Early decelerations are not associated with fetal compromise and require no intervention.

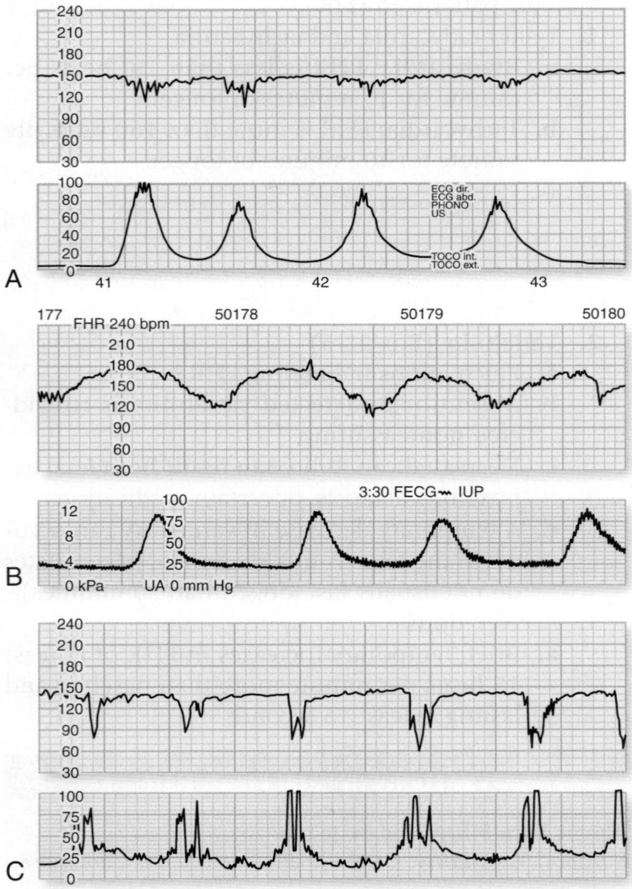

FIG. 23-3 Deceleration patterns. *Top graphs in each pair:* Fetal heart rate. *Bottom graphs in each pair:* Uterine contractions. **A,** Early decelerations caused by head compression. **B,** Late decelerations caused by uteroplacental insufficiency. **C,** Variable decelerations caused by cord compression.

5. Late decelerations (Fig. 23-3)
    a. Late decelerations are nonreassuring patterns that reflect impaired placental exchange or uteroplacental insufficiency.
    b. The patterns look similar to early decelerations but begin well after the contraction begins and return to baseline after the contraction ends.
    c. The degree of decline in FHR from baseline is not related to the amount of uteroplacental insufficiency.

Interventions for late decelerations include immediately improving placental blood flow and fetal oxygenation.

6. Variable decelerations (Fig. 23-3).
    a. Variable decelerations are caused by conditions that restrict flow through the umbilical cord.
    b. Variable decelerations do not have the uniform appearance of early and late decelerations.
    c. The shape, duration, and degree of decline below baseline FHR are variable; these fall and rise abruptly with the onset and relief of cord compression.
    d. Variable decelerations also may be nonperiodic, occurring at times unrelated to contractions.
    e. Baseline rate and variability are considered when evaluating variable decelerations.
    f. Variable decelerations are significant when FHR repeatedly declines to less than 70 beats per minute and persists at that level for at least 60 seconds before returning to baseline.

If variable decelerations occur, discontinue oxytocin if infusing, change the position of the mother, administer oxygen, and assess the mother's vital signs. Notify the PHCP. Assist with amnioinfusion (intrauterine instillation of warmed saline to decrease compression on the umbilical cord) if prescribed.

7. Hypertonic uterine activity
    a. Assessment of uterine activity includes frequency, duration, intensity of contractions, and uterine resting tone; assessment is performed either by palpating by hand or with an internal uterine pressure catheter (IUPC).
    b. The uterus should relax between contractions for 60 seconds or longer.
    c. Uterine contraction intensity is about 50 to 75 mm Hg (with an IUPC) during labor and may reach 110 mm Hg with pushing during the second stage.
    d. The average resting tone is 5 to 15 mm Hg.

BOX 23-6 Nonreassuring Fetal Heart Rate Patterns

- Bradycardia
- Tachycardia
- Late decelerations
- Prolonged decelerations
- Hypertonic uterine activity
- Decreased or absent variability
- Variable decelerations falling to less than 70 beats per minute for longer than 60 seconds

   e. In hypertonic uterine activity, the uterine resting tone between contractions is high, reducing uterine blood flow and decreasing fetal oxygen supply.

8. Nonreassuring FHR patterns (Box 23-6)
9. Interventions for nonreassuring patterns (see Priority Nursing Actions)

PRIORITY NURSING ACTIONS

Nonreassuring Fetal Heart Rate Pattern

1. Identify the cause.
2. Discontinue oxytocin infusion.
3. Change the mother's position.
4. Administer oxygen by face mask at 8 to 10 L/minute and infuse intravenous (IV) fluids as prescribed.
5. Prepare to initiate continuous electronic fetal monitoring with internal devices if not contraindicated.
6. Prepare for cesarean delivery if necessary.
7. Document the event, actions taken, and the mother's response.

Reference:
Lowdermilk et al. (2016), p. 423.

VI. Four Stages of Labor (Table 23-1)

A. Stage 1: Latent phase

1. Description: Stage 1 is the longest. A labor curve, such as the Friedman curve, may be used to identify whether a woman's cervical dilation is progressing at the expected rate (Fig. 23-4).
2. Assessment
   a. Cervical dilation is 1 to 4 cm.
   b. Uterine contractions occur every 15 to 30 minutes, are 15 to 30 seconds in duration, and are of mild intensity.
3. Interventions
   a. Encourage mother and partner to participate in care.
   b. Assist with comfort measures, changes of position, and ambulation.
   c. Keep mother and partner informed of progress.
   d. Offer fluids and ice chips.
   e. Encourage voiding every 1 to 2 hours.

B. Stage 1: Active phase

1. Assessment
   a. Cervical dilation is 4 to 7 cm.
   b. Uterine contractions occur every 3 to 5 minutes, are 30 to 60 seconds in duration, and are of moderate intensity.
2. Interventions
   a. Encourage maintenance of effective breathing patterns.
   b. Provide a quiet environment.
   c. Keep mother and partner informed of progress.
   d. Promote comfort with back rubs, sacral pressure, pillow support, and position changes.
   e. Instruct partner in effleurage (light stroking of abdomen).
   f. Offer fluids and ice chips and ointment for dry lips.
   g. Encourage voiding every 1 to 2 hours.

C. Stage 1: Transition phase

1. Assessment
   a. Cervical dilation is 8 to 10 cm.

TABLE 23-1 Four Stages of Labor

First Stage	Second Stage	Third Stage	Fourth Stage
Effacement and dilation of cervix	Expulsion of fetus	Separation of placenta	Physical recovery
Three stages—latent, active, and transition	Pushing stage Latent phase—known as "laboring down" Active phase—pushing	Expulsion of placenta	1-4 hr after expulsion of placenta
Mother is talkative and eager in latent phase, becoming tired, restless, and anxious as labor intensifies and contractions become stronger	Mother has intense concentration on pushing with contractions; may fall asleep between contractions	Mother is relieved after birth of newborn; mother is usually very tired	Mother is tired but is eager to become acquainted with her newborn

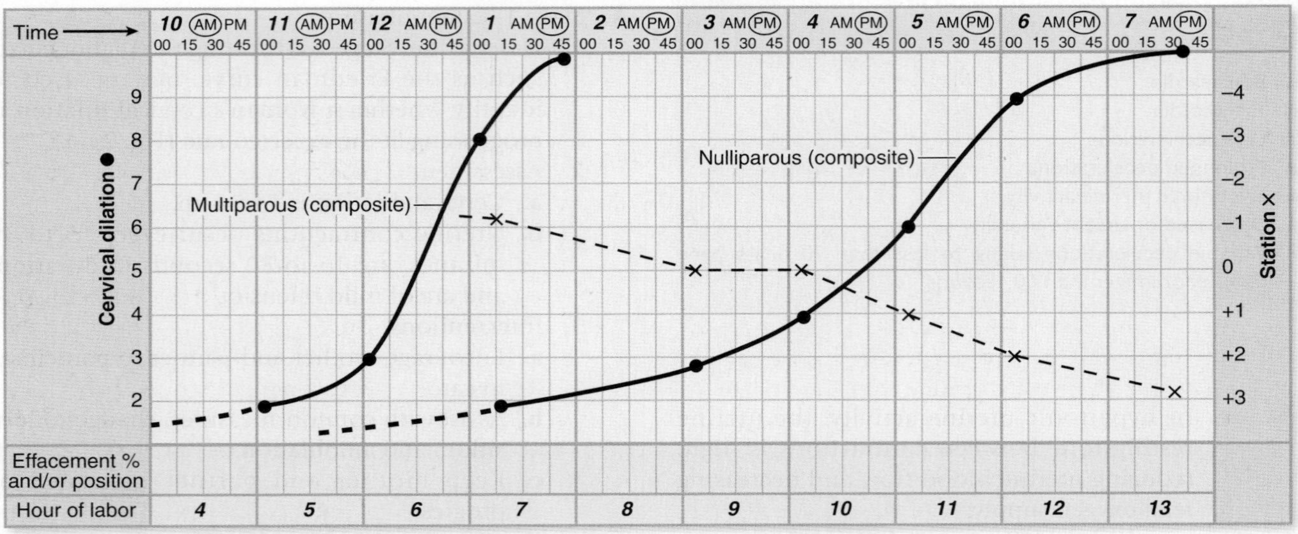

FIG. 23-4 A labor curve, often referred to as a partogram or *Friedman's curve*, may be used to identify whether a woman's cervical dilation and descent are progressing at the expected rate. The symbol for station (X), which represents descent, may be added to the labor curve. Typical labor curves for a multiparous woman and a nulliparous woman are illustrated for comparison of patterns.

b. Uterine contractions occur every 2 to 3 minutes, are 45 to 90 seconds in duration, and are of strong intensity.

2. Interventions
- **a.** Encourage rest between contractions.
- **b.** Wake mother at beginning of contraction so she can begin breathing pattern.
- **c.** Keep mother and partner informed of progress.
- **d.** Provide privacy.
- **e.** Offer fluids and ice chips and ointment for dry lips.
- **f.** Encourage voiding every 1 to 2 hours.

D. Interventions throughout stage 1
1. Monitor maternal vital signs.
2. Monitor FHR via ultrasound Doppler, fetoscope, or electronic fetal monitor.
3. Assess FHR before, during, and after a contraction, noting that the normal FHR is 110 to 160 beats per minute.
4. Monitor uterine contractions by palpation or tocodynamometer, determining frequency, duration, and intensity.
5. Assess status of cervical dilation and effacement.
6. Assess fetal station presentation and position by Leopold's maneuvers.
7. Assist with pelvic examination and prepare for a fern test.

⚠ If the membranes have ruptured, assess the FHR because of the risk of prolapsed umbilical cord, and assess the color of the amniotic fluid, because meconium-stained fluid can indicate fetal distress.

E. Stage 2

1. Assessment
- **a.** Cervical dilation is complete.
- **b.** Progress of labor is measured by descent of fetal head through the birth canal (change in fetal station).
- **c.** Uterine contractions occur every 2 to 3 minutes, lasting 60 to 75 seconds, and are of strong intensity.
- **d.** Increase in bloody show occurs.
- **e.** Mother feels urge to push (Ferguson reflex); assist mother in pushing efforts.

2. Interventions
- **a.** Perform assessments every 5 minutes.
- **b.** Monitor maternal vital signs.
- **c.** Monitor FHR via ultrasound Doppler, fetoscope, or electronic fetal monitor.
- **d.** Assess FHR before, during, and after a contraction, noting that the normal FHR is 110 to 160 beats per minute.
- **e.** Monitor uterine contractions by palpation or tocodynamometer, determining frequency, duration, and intensity.
- **f.** Provide mother with encouragement and praise and provide for rest between contractions.
- **g.** Keep mother and partner informed of progress.
- **h.** Maintain privacy.
- **i.** Provide ice chips and ointment for dry lips.
- **j.** Assist mother into a position that promotes comfort and facilitates pushing efforts, such as lithotomy, semisitting, kneeling, side-lying, or squatting.

k. Monitor for signs of approaching birth, such as perineal bulging or visualization of the fetal head.
l. Prepare for birth (expulsion of the fetus).

F. Stage 3
1. Assessment
a. Contractions occur until the placenta is expelled.
b. Placental separation and expulsion occur.
c. Expulsion of the placenta occurs 5 to 30 minutes after the birth of the infant.
d. Schultze mechanism: Center portion of the placenta separates first, and its shiny fetal surface emerges from the vagina.
e. Duncan mechanism: Margin of the placenta separates, and the dull, red, rough maternal surface emerges from the vagina first.
f. Method of placental presentation is of no clinical significance.
2. Interventions
a. Assess maternal vital signs.
b. Assess uterine status.
c. Provide parents with an explanation regarding expulsion of the placenta.
d. After expulsion of the placenta, uterine fundus remains firm and is located 2 fingerbreadths below the umbilicus.
e. Examine placenta for cotyledons and membranes to verify that it is intact.
f. Assess mother for shivering and provide warmth.
g. Promote parental-neonatal attachment.

G. Stage 4
1. Description: Period 1 to 4 hours after birth
2. Assessment
a. Blood pressure returns to prelabor level.
b. Pulse is slightly lower than during labor.
c. Fundus remains contracted, in the midline, 1 or 2 fingerbreadths below the umbilicus.

⚠ Monitor lochia discharge. Lochia may be moderate in amount and red in color in stage 4.

3. Interventions
a. Perform maternal assessments every 15 minutes for 1 hour, every 30 minutes for 1 hour, and hourly for 2 hours (or as per agency policy).
b. Provide warm blankets.
c. Apply ice packs to the perineum.
d. Massage the uterus if needed, and teach the mother to massage the uterus.
e. Provide breast-feeding support as needed.
f. See Chapter 27 for information on caring for the newborn.

VII. Anesthesia

A. Local anesthesia
1. Local anesthesia is used for blocking pain during episiotomy.
2. Local anesthesia is administered just before the birth of the infant.
3. The anesthetic has no effect on the fetus.

B. Lumbar epidural block
1. Injection site is in epidural space at L3 to L4.
2. The block is administered after labor is established or as partial anesthesia just before a scheduled cesarean birth.
3. The anesthetic relieves pain from contractions and numbs the vagina and perineum.
4. The block may cause hypotension, bladder distention, and a prolonged second stage.
5. The anesthetic does not cause a headache because the dura mater is not penetrated.
6. Assess maternal blood pressure and assess bladder frequently.
7. Maintain the mother in a side-lying position or place a rolled blanket beneath the right hip to displace the uterus from the vena cava.
8. Administer intravenous (IV) fluids as prescribed.
9. Increase fluids as prescribed if hypotension occurs.
10. Observe for any adverse effects from opioid epidurals, such as nausea and vomiting, pruritus, or respiratory depression.

C. Intrathecal opioid analgesics
1. The medication is injected into the subarachnoid space and has a rapid onset of action.
2. It may be used in combination with a lumbar epidural block.

D. Subarachnoid (spinal) block
1. Injection site is in the spinal subarachnoid space at L3 to L5.
2. The block is administered just before birth.
3. The anesthetic relieves uterine and perineal pain and numbs the vagina, perineum, and lower extremities.
4. The anesthetic may cause maternal hypotension.
5. The anesthetic may cause postpartum headache.
6. The mother must lie flat for 8 to 12 hours after spinal injection.
7. Administer IV fluids as prescribed.

E. General anesthesia
1. General anesthesia may be used for some surgical interventions.
2. The mother is not awake.

⚠ General anesthesia presents a maternal danger of respiratory depression, vomiting, and aspiration.

VIII. Obstetrical Procedures

A. Bishop score (Table 23-2)
1. The Bishop score is used to determine maternal readiness for labor and evaluates cervical status and fetal position.
2. The Bishop score is indicated before the induction of labor.
3. The 5 factors are assigned a score of 0 to 3, and the total score is calculated.
4. A score of 8 or greater indicates that the chance of a successful vaginal delivery is good and the cervix is favorable for induction.

B. Induction
1. Induction is a deliberate initiation of uterine contractions that stimulates labor.
2. Elective induction may be accomplished by oxytocin infusion.
3. Obtain a baseline tracing of uterine contractions and FHR.
4. Increase the IV dosage of oxytocin as prescribed only after assessing contractions, FHR, and maternal blood pressure and pulse.
5. Do not increase the rate of oxytocin when the desired contraction pattern is obtained (contraction frequency of 2 to 3 minutes and lasting 60 seconds).

! An oxytocin infusion is discontinued if uterine contraction frequency is less than 2 minutes or duration is longer than 90 seconds, or if fetal distress is noted.

C. Amniotomy
1. Artificial rupture of the membranes is performed by the obstetrician or nurse-midwife to stimulate labor.
2. Amniotomy is performed if the fetus is at 0 or a plus station.
3. Amniotomy increases the risk of prolapsed cord and infection.

TABLE 23-2 Factors of the Bishop Score

	Score			
	0	**1**	**2**	**3**
Dilation of cervix (cm)	0	1-2	3-4	>5
Effacement of cervix (%)	0-30	40-50	60-70	>80
Consistency of cervix	Firm	Medium	Soft	—
Position of cervix	Posterior	Midposition	Anterior	—
Station of presenting part	−3	−2	−1	+1, +2

4. Monitor FHR before and after amniotomy.
5. Record time of amniotomy, FHR, and characteristics of the fluid.
6. Meconium-stained amniotic fluid may be associated with fetal distress.
7. Bloody amniotic fluid may indicate abruptio placentae or fetal trauma.
8. An unpleasant odor to amniotic fluid is associated with infection.
9. Polyhydramnios is associated with maternal diabetes and certain congenital disorders.
10. Oligohydramnios is associated with intrauterine growth restriction and congenital disorders.
11. Expect more variable decelerations after rupture of the membranes as a result of possible cord compression during contractions.
12. Limit client activity if prescribed.

D. External version
1. External version is the manipulation of the fetus from an unfavorable presentation into a favorable presentation for birth.
2. External version is indicated for an abnormal presentation that exists after the 34th week.
3. Monitor vital signs.
4. If the mother is Rh-negative, ensure that Rho(D) immune globulin was given at 28 weeks of gestation.
5. Prepare for a nonstress test to evaluate fetal well-being.
6. IV fluids and tocolytic therapy may be administered to relax the uterus and permit easier manipulation of the fetus.
7. Ultrasound is used during the procedure to evaluate fetal position and placental placement and guide direction of the fetus.
8. The abdominal wall is manipulated to direct the fetus into a cephalic presentation if possible.
9. Monitor blood pressure to identify vena cava compression.
10. Monitor for unusual pain.
11. After the procedure, do the following:
   a. Perform a nonstress test to evaluate fetal well-being.
   b. Monitor for uterine activity, bleeding, ruptured membranes, and decreased fetal activity.
   c. With Rh-negative clients, perform Kleihauer-Betke test as prescribed to detect the presence and amount of fetal blood in the maternal circulation and to identify clients who need additional Rh_o(D) immune globulin.

E. Episiotomy
1. An episiotomy is an incision made into the perineum to enlarge the vaginal outlet and facilitate birth.

2. The use of this procedure has declined dramatically in recent years.
3. Check the episiotomy site.
4. Institute measures to relieve pain.
5. Provide ice packs during the first 24 hours.
6. Instruct the client in the use of an ice pack for the first 24 hours, and then sitz baths thereafter.
7. Apply analgesic spray or ointment as prescribed.
8. Provide perineal care, using clean technique.
9. Instruct the client in the proper care of the incision.
10. Instruct the client to dry the perineal area from front to back and to blot the area rather than wipe it.
11. Instruct the client to shower rather than bathe in a tub.
12. Apply a perineal pad without touching the inside surface of the pad.
13. Report any bleeding or discharge from the episiotomy site to the PHCP.

F. Forceps delivery
1. Two double-crossed, spoon-like articulated blades are used to assist in the delivery of the fetal head.
2. Reassure the mother and explain the need for forceps.
3. Monitor the mother and fetus during delivery.
4. Check the neonate and mother after delivery for any possible injury.
5. Assist with repair of any lacerations.

G. Vacuum extraction
1. A cap-like suction device is applied to the fetal head to facilitate extraction.
2. Suction is used to assist in delivery of the fetal head.
3. Traction is applied during uterine contractions until descent of the fetal head is achieved.
4. The suction device should not be kept in place any longer than 25 minutes.
5. Monitor FHR frequently; fetal monitoring should be used.
6. Assess infant at birth and throughout the postpartum period for signs of cerebral trauma.
7. Monitor for developing cephalhematoma.
8. Caput succedaneum is normal and resolves in 24 hours.

H. Cesarean delivery
1. Cesarean section is delivery of the fetus usually through a transabdominal, low-segment incision of the uterus.
2. Preoperative
   a. If planned, prepare the mother and partner.
   b. If an emergency, quickly explain the need and procedure to the mother and partner.
   c. Obtain informed consent.
   d. Ensure that the preoperative diagnostic tests are done, including Rh factor determination.
   e. Prepare to insert an IV line and an indwelling urinary catheter.
   f. Prepare the abdomen as prescribed.
   g. Monitor the mother and fetus continuously.
   h. Provide emotional support.
   i. Administer preoperative medications as prescribed.
3. Postoperative
   a. Monitor vital signs.
   b. Perform a fundal assessment; evaluate incision.
   c. Provide pain relief.
   d. Encourage turning, coughing, and deep breathing.
   e. Encourage ambulation.
   f. Encourage bonding and attachment with newborn.
   g. Provide psychological support.
   h. Monitor for signs of infection and bleeding.
   i. Burning and pain on urination may indicate a bladder infection.
   j. A tender uterus and foul-smelling lochia may indicate endometritis.
   k. A productive cough or chills may indicate pneumonia.
   l. Pain, redness, or edema of an extremity may indicate thrombophlebitis.

PRACTICE QUESTIONS

224. The nurse is caring for a client in labor. Which assessment findings indicate to the nurse that the client is beginning the second stage of labor? **Select all that apply.**

- ❑ 1. The contractions are regular.
- ❑ 2. The membranes have ruptured.
- ❑ 3. The cervix is dilated completely.
- ❑ 4. The client begins to expel clear vaginal fluid.
- ❑ 5. The Ferguson reflex is initiated from perineal pressure.

225. The nurse in the labor room is caring for a client in the active stage of the first phase of labor. The nurse is assessing the fetal patterns and notes a late deceleration on the monitor strip. What is the **most appropriate** nursing action?

1. Administer oxygen via face mask.
2. Place the mother in a supine position.
3. Increase the rate of the oxytocin intravenous infusion.
4. Document the findings and continue to monitor the fetal patterns.

226. The nurse is performing an assessment of a client who is scheduled for a cesarean delivery at 39 weeks of gestation. Which assessment finding indicates the need to contact the primary health care provider (PHCP)?
1. Hemoglobin of 11 g/dL (110 mmol/L)
2. Fetal heart rate of 180 beats per minute
3. Maternal pulse rate of 85 beats per minute
4. White blood cell count of 12.000/mm^3 (12× 10^9/L)

227. The nurse is reviewing the record of a client in the labor room and notes that the primary health care provider has documented that the fetal presenting part is at the +1 station. This documented finding indicates that the fetal presenting part is located at which area? **Refer to figure.**

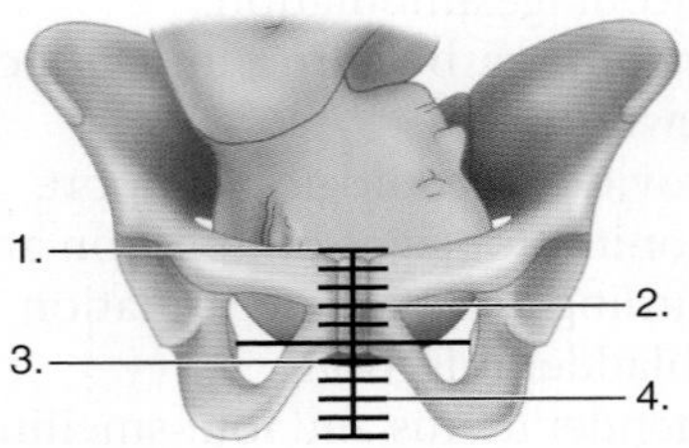

1. 1
2. 2
3. 3
4. 4

228. A client arrives at a birthing center in active labor. After examination, it is determined that her membranes are still intact and she is at a −2 station. The primary health care provider prepares to perform an amniotomy. What will the nurse relay to the client as the **most likely** outcomes of the amniotomy? **Select all that apply.**
- ☐ 1. Less pressure on her cervix
- ☐ 2. Decreased number of contractions
- ☐ 3. Increased efficiency of contractions
- ☐ 4. The need for increased maternal blood pressure monitoring
- ☐ 5. The need for frequent fetal heart rate monitoring to detect the presence of a prolapsed cord

229. The nurse is monitoring a client in labor. The nurse suspects umbilical cord compression if which is noted on the external monitor tracing during a contraction?
1. Variability
2. Accelerations
3. Early decelerations
4. Variable decelerations

230. A client in labor is transported to the delivery room and prepared for a cesarean delivery. After the client is transferred to the delivery room table, the nurse should place the client in which position?
1. Supine position with a wedge under the right hip
2. Trendelenburg's position with the legs in stirrups
3. Prone position with the legs separated and elevated
4. Semi-Fowler's position with a pillow under the knees

231. The nurse is monitoring a client in active labor and notes that the client is having contractions every 3 minutes that last 45 seconds. The nurse notes that the fetal heart rate between contractions is 100 beats per minute. Which nursing action is **most appropriate**?
1. Notify the primary health care provider (PHCP).
2. Continue monitoring the fetal heart rate.
3. Encourage the client to continue pushing with each contraction.
4. Instruct the client's coach to continue to encourage breathing techniques.

232. The nurse is caring for a client in labor and is monitoring the fetal heart rate patterns. The nurse notes the presence of episodic accelerations on the electronic fetal monitor tracing. Which action is **most appropriate**?
1. Notify the primary health care provider of the findings.
2. Reposition the mother and check the monitor for changes in the fetal tracing.
3. Take the mother's vital signs and tell the mother that bed rest is required to conserve oxygen.
4. Document the findings and tell the mother that the pattern on the monitor indicates fetal well-being.

233. The nurse is admitting a pregnant client to the labor room and attaches an external electronic fetal monitor to the client's abdomen. After attachment of the electronic fetal monitor, what is the **next** nursing action?
1. Identify the types of accelerations.
2. Assess the baseline fetal heart rate.
3. Determine the intensity of the contractions.
4. Determine the frequency of the contractions.

234. The nurse is reviewing true and false labor signs with a multiparous client. The nurse determines that the client understands the signs of true labor if she makes which statement?
1. "I won't be in labor until my baby drops."
2. "My contractions will be felt in my abdominal area."
3. "My contractions will not be as painful if I walk around."
4. "My contractions will increase in duration and intensity."

235. Which assessment finding after an amniotomy should be conducted **first?**
1. Cervical dilation
2. Bladder distention
3. Fetal heart rate pattern
4. Maternal blood pressure

236. The nurse has been working with a laboring client and notes that she has been pushing effectively for 1 hour. What is the client's **primary** physiological need at this time?
1. Ambulation
2. Rest between contractions
3. Change positions frequently
4. Consume oral food and fluids

237. The nurse is assisting a client undergoing induction of labor at 41 weeks of gestation. The client's contractions are moderate and occurring every 2 to 3 minutes, with a duration of 60 seconds. An internal fetal heart rate monitor is in place. The baseline fetal heart rate has been 120 to 122 beats per minute for the past hour. What is the **priority** nursing action?
1. Notify the health care provider.
2. Discontinue the infusion of oxytocin.
3. Place oxygen on at 8 to 10 L/minute via face mask.
4. Contact the client's primary support person(s) if not currently present.

ANSWERS

224. ***Answer:*** 3, 5
Rationale: The second stage of labor begins when the cervix is dilated completely and ends with birth of the neonate. The woman has a strong urge to push in stage 2 when the Ferguson reflex is activated. Options 1, 2, and 4 are not specific assessment findings of the second stage of labor and occur in stage 1.
Test-Taking Strategy: Eliminate options 2 and 4 first because they are comparable or alike. From the remaining options, recalling that regular contractions occur before the second stage of labor will direct you to the correct option.
Level of Cognitive Ability: Applying
Client Needs: Health Promotion and Maintenance
Integrated Process: Nursing Process—Assessment
Content Area: Maternity: Intrapartum
Health Problem: N/A
Priority Concepts: Clinical Judgment; Reproduction
Reference: McKinney et al. (2018), p. 299.

225. ***Answer:*** 1
Rationale: Late decelerations are due to uteroplacental insufficiency and occur because of decreased blood flow and oxygen to the fetus during the uterine contractions. Hypoxemia results; oxygen at 8 to 10 L/minute via face mask is necessary. The supine position is avoided because it decreases uterine blood flow to the fetus. The client should be turned onto her side to displace pressure of the gravid uterus on the inferior vena cava. An intravenous oxytocin infusion is discontinued when a late deceleration is noted. The oxytocin would cause further hypoxemia because of increased uteroplacental insufficiency resulting from stimulation of contractions by this medication. Although the nurse would document the occurrence, option 4 would delay necessary treatment.
Test-Taking Strategy: Note the strategic words, *most appropriate.* Use the ABCs—airway, breathing, and circulation—and knowledge related to the significance of a late deceleration to answer this question.
Level of Cognitive Ability: Analyzing
Client Needs: Physiological Integrity
Integrated Process: Nursing Process—Implementation
Content Area: Maternity: Intrapartum
Health Problem: Maternity: Fetal Distress/Demise
Priority Concepts: Clinical Judgment; Perfusion
Reference: McKinney et al. (2018), pp. 342, 344

226. ***Answer:*** 2
Rationale: A normal fetal heart rate is 110 to 160 beats per minute. A fetal heart rate of 180 beats per minute could indicate fetal distress and would warrant immediate notification of the PHCP. By full term, a normal maternal hemoglobin range is 11 to 13 g/dL (110 to 130 mmol/L) because of the hemodilution caused by an increase in plasma volume during pregnancy. The maternal pulse rate during pregnancy increases 10 to 15 beats per minute over prepregnancy readings to facilitate increased cardiac output, oxygen transport, and kidney filtration. White blood cell counts in a normal pregnancy begin to increase in the second trimester and peak in the third trimester, with a normal range of, 11,000–15,000/mm^3 (11–15 $\times$ 10^9/L) up to 18,000/mm^3 (18 $\times$ 10^9/L) During the immediate postpartum period, the white blood cell count may be 25,000–30,000/mm^3 (25–30 $\times$ 10^9/L) because of increased leukocytosis that occurs during delivery.
Test-Taking Strategy: Focus on the subject, normal assessment and laboratory findings and those that indicate the need to contact the PHCP. Knowledge regarding the normal and abnormal findings in a pregnant client and fetus will direct you to the correct option.
Level of Cognitive Ability: Analyzing
Client Needs: Physiological Integrity
Integrated Process: Nursing Process—Analysis
Content Area: Maternity: Intrapartum
Health Problem: Maternity: Fetal Distress/Demise
Priority Concepts: Collaboration; Perfusion
Reference: Lowdermilk et al. (2016), pp. 411, 788.

227. ***Answer:*** 3
Rationale: Station is the measurement of the progress of descent in centimeters above or below the midplane from the presenting part to the ischial spine. It is measured in centimeters and noted as a negative number above the line and as a positive number below the line. At the positive 1 (+1) station, the fetal presenting part is

1 cm below the ischial spine. Option 1 is at the negative 5 (−5) station and the fetal presenting part is 5 cm above the ischial spine. Option 2 is at the negative 2 (−2) station, and the fetal presenting part is 2 cm above the ischial spine. Option 4 is at the positive 3 (+3), and the fetal presenting part is 3 cm below the ischial spine.
Test-Taking Strategy: Recalling that station is measured in centimeters and uses the ischial spine as a reference point will assist in answering this question. Focus on the data in the question and note the location of the ischial spine and that the stations range from −5 cm to +5 cm above or below this reference point. Also, noting the location of the fetal head will assist in answering correctly.
Level of Cognitive Ability: Analyzing
Client Needs: Health Promotion and Maintenance
Integrated Process: Nursing Process—Assessment
Content Area: Maternity: Intrapartum
Health Problem: N/A
Priority Concepts: Clinical Judgment; Reproduction
Reference: McKinney et al. (2018), p. 300.

228. *Answer:* 3, 5
Rationale: Amniotomy (artificial rupture of the membranes) can be used to induce labor when the condition of the cervix is favorable (ripe) or to augment labor if the progress begins to slow. Rupturing of the membranes allows the fetal head to contact the cervix more directly and may increase the efficiency of contractions. Increased monitoring of maternal blood pressure is unnecessary after this procedure. The fetal heart rate needs to be monitored frequently, as there is an increased likelihood of a prolapsed cord with ruptured membranes and a high presenting part.
Test-Taking Strategy: Note the strategic words, *most likely.* Focus on the subject, an amniotomy. Recalling that amniotomy is performed to augment labor if the progress begins to slow will direct you to the correct option.
Level of Cognitive Ability: Applying
Client Needs: Physiological Integrity
Integrated Process: Nursing Process—Implementation
Content Area: Maternity: Intrapartum
Health Problem: N/A
Priority Concepts: Client Education; Reproduction
Reference: Lowdermilk et al. (2016), p. 783.

229. *Answer:* 4
Rationale: Variable decelerations occur if the umbilical cord becomes compressed, reducing blood flow between the placenta and the fetus. Variability refers to fluctuations in the baseline fetal heart rate. Accelerations are a reassuring sign and usually occur with fetal movement. Early decelerations result from pressure on the fetal head during a contraction.
Test-Taking Strategy: Focus on the subject, umbilical cord compression. Recalling that variable decelerations occur if the umbilical cord becomes compressed will direct you to the correct option.
Level of Cognitive Ability: Applying
Client Needs: Physiological Integrity
Integrated Process: Nursing Process—Assessment
Content Area: Maternity: Intrapartum
Health Problem: Maternity: Fetal Distress/Demise
Priority Concepts: Clinical Judgment; Perfusion
Reference: McKinney et al. (2018), p. 343.

230. *Answer:* 1
Rationale: Vena cava and descending aorta compression by the pregnant uterus impedes blood return from the lower trunk and extremities. This leads to decreasing cardiac return, cardiac output, and blood flow to the uterus and subsequently the fetus. The best position to prevent this would be side-lying, with the uterus displaced off the abdominal vessels. Positioning for abdominal surgery necessitates a supine position, however; a wedge placed under the right hip provides displacement of the uterus. Trendelenburg's position places pressure from the pregnant uterus on the diaphragm and lungs, decreasing respiratory capacity and oxygenation. A prone or semi-Fowler's position is not practical for this type of abdominal surgery.
Test-Taking Strategy: Focus on the subject, positioning the pregnant woman. Visualizing each of the positions identified in the options and considering the effect that the position may have on the mother and the fetus will direct you to the correct option.
Level of Cognitive Ability: Applying
Client Needs: Physiological Integrity
Integrated Process: Nursing Process—Implementation
Content Area: Maternity: Intrapartum
Health Problem: Maternity: Supine Hypotension
Priority Concepts: Clinical Judgment; Perfusion
Reference: McKinney et al. (2018), pp. 390-391.

231. *Answer:* 1
Rationale: A normal fetal heart rate is 110 to 160 beats per minute, and the fetal heart rate should be within this range between contractions. Fetal bradycardia between contractions may indicate the need for immediate medical management, and the PHCP or nurse-midwife needs to be notified. Options 2, 3, and 4 are inappropriate nursing actions in this situation and delay necessary intervention.
Test-Taking Strategy: Note the strategic words, *most appropriate.* Focus on the data in the question. Knowledge that the normal fetal heart rate is 110 to 160 beats per minute will assist you to recognize that fetal bradycardia is present.
Level of Cognitive Ability: Analyzing
Client Needs: Physiological Integrity
Integrated Process: Nursing Process—Implementation
Content Area: Maternity: Intrapartum
Health Problem: Maternity: Fetal Distress/Demise
Priority Concepts: Clinical Judgment; Perfusion
Reference: Lowdermilk et al. (2016), pp. 419-420.

232. *Answer:* 4
Rationale: Accelerations are transient increases in the fetal heart rate that often accompany contractions or are caused by fetal movement. Episodic accelerations are thought to be a sign of fetal well-being and adequate oxygen reserve. Options 1, 2, and 3 are inaccurate nursing actions and are unnecessary.
Test-Taking Strategy: Note the strategic words, *most appropriate.* Options 1, 2, and 3 are comparable or alike in that they indicate the need for further intervention. Also, knowing that accelerations indicate fetal well-being will direct you to the correct option.
Level of Cognitive Ability: Analyzing
Client Needs: Physiological Integrity
Integrated Process: Nursing Process—Implementation
Content Area: Maternity: Intrapartum

Health Problem: N/A
Priority Concepts: Clinical Judgment; Perfusion
Reference: Lowdermilk et al. (2016), p. 420.

233. *Answer:* 2
Rationale: Assessing the baseline fetal heart rate is important so that abnormal variations of the baseline rate can be identified if they occur. The intensity of contractions is assessed by an internal fetal monitor, not an external fetal monitor. Options 1 and 4 are important to assess, but not as the first priority. Fetal heart rate is evaluated by assessing baseline and periodic changes. Periodic changes occur in response to the intermittent stress of uterine contractions and the baseline beat-to-beat variability of the fetal heart rate.
Test-Taking Strategy: Note the **strategic word,** *next.* Use the **ABCs—airway, breathing, and circulation.** Fetal heart rate reflects the ABCs.
Level of Cognitive Ability: Applying
Client Needs: Physiological Integrity
Integrated Process: Nursing Process—Assessment
Content Area: Maternity: Intrapartum
Health Problem: N/A
Priority Concepts: Clinical Judgment; Perfusion
Reference: McKinney et al. (2018), pp. 338-339.

234. *Answer:* 4
Rationale: True labor is present when contractions increase in duration and intensity. Lightening or dropping leads to *engagement* (presenting part reaches the level of the ischial spine) and occurs when the fetus descends into the pelvis about 2 weeks before delivery. Contractions felt in the abdominal area and contractions that ease with walking are signs of false labor.
Test-Taking Strategy: Focus on the **subject,** the signs of true labor. Noting the word *true* in the question and its relationship to the words *increase in duration and intensity* in the correct option will direct you to this option.
Level of Cognitive Ability: Evaluating
Client Needs: Health Promotion and Maintenance
Integrated Process: Teaching and Learning
Content Area: Maternity: Intrapartum
Health Problem: N/A
Priority Concepts: Clinical Judgment; Reproduction
Reference: McKinney et al. (2018), pp. 298-299

235. *Answer:* 3
Rationale: Fetal heart rate is assessed immediately after amniotomy to detect any changes that may indicate cord compression or prolapse. When the membranes are ruptured, minimal vaginal examinations would be done because of the risk of infection. Bladder distention or maternal blood pressure would not be the first thing to check after an amniotomy.
Test-Taking Strategy: Note the **strategic word,** *first.* Because of the risk of a prolapsed cord after an amniotomy, the first action is to check the fetal heart rate for signs of nonreassuring fetal heart rate patterns.
Level of Cognitive Ability: Analyzing
Client Needs: Physiological Integrity
Integrated Process: Nursing Process—Assessment
Content Area: Maternity: Intrapartum
Health Problem: Maternity: Fetal Distress/Demise
Priority Concepts: Clinical Judgment; Perfusion
Reference: Lowdermilk et al. (2016), p. 783.

236. *Answer:* 2
Rationale: The birth process expends a great deal of energy, particularly during the transition stage. Encouraging rest between contractions conserves maternal energy, facilitating voluntary pushing efforts with contractions. Uteroplacental perfusion also is enhanced, which promotes fetal tolerance of the stress of labor. Ambulation is encouraged during early labor. Ice chips should be provided. Changing positions frequently is not the primary physiological need. Food and fluids are likely to be withheld at this time.
Test-Taking Strategy: Note the **strategic word,** *primary.* Also, noting the words *pushing effectively* will assist in directing you to the correct option.
Level of Cognitive Ability: Applying
Client Needs: Physiological Integrity
Integrated Process: Nursing Process—Implementation
Content Area: Maternity: Intrapartum
Health Problem: N/A
Priority Concepts: Clinical Judgment; Reproduction
Reference: McKinney et al. (2018), pp. 357, 370.

237. *Answer:* 2
Rationale: The priority nursing action is to stop the infusion of oxytocin. Oxytocin can cause forceful uterine contractions and decrease oxygenation to the placenta, resulting in decreased variability. After stopping the oxytocin, the nurse should reposition the laboring mother. Notifying the primary health care provider, applying oxygen, and increasing the rate of the intravenous (IV) fluid (the solution without the oxytocin) are also actions that are indicated in this situation, but not the priority action. Contacting the client's primary support person(s) is not the priority action at this time.
Test-Taking Strategy: Focus on the **strategic word,** *priority.* Focus on the **data in the question** and note the relationship of the words *undergoing induction* and the correct option. Also recall that physiological needs are prioritized over psychosocial needs.
Level of Cognitive Ability: Analyzing
Client Needs: Physiological Integrity
Integrated Process: Nursing Process—Implementation
Content Area: Maternity: Intrapartum
Health Problem: Maternity: Dystocia
Priority Concepts: Clinical Judgment; Perfusion
Reference: Lowdermilk et al. (2016), p. 784.

Maternity

CHAPTER 24

Problems with Labor and Birth

PRIORITY CONCEPTS **Reproduction, Safety**

I. Premature Rupture of the Membranes

A. Description
1. Premature rupture of the membranes refers to spontaneous rupture of the amniotic membranes before the onset of labor.
2. Gestational age usually determines the plan and intervention.
3. When the rupture of membranes is before term and birth will be delayed, infection becomes a risk.

B. Assessment
1. Presence of fluid pooling in vaginal vault; nitrazine test is positive.
2. Amount, color, consistency, and odor of fluid need to be assessed.
3. Vital signs are monitored; an elevated temperature may indicate infection.
4. Fetal monitoring is necessary; tachycardia in the fetus may indicate maternal infection.

C. Interventions
1. Assist with tests to assess gestational age.
2. Avoid vaginal examinations because of the risk of infection.
3. Monitor maternal and fetal status for signs of compromise or infection.
4. Administer antibiotics as prescribed.

II. Prolapsed Umbilical Cord

A. Description
1. The umbilical cord is displaced between the presenting part and the amnion or protruding through the cervix, causing compression of the cord and compromising fetal circulation (Fig. 24-1).

B. Assessment
1. The client has a feeling that something is coming through the vagina.
2. Umbilical cord is visible or palpable.
3. Fetal heart rate is irregular and slow.
4. Fetal heart monitor shows variable decelerations or bradycardia after rupture of the membranes.
5. If fetal hypoxia is severe, violent fetal activity may occur and then cease.

PRIORITY NURSING ACTIONS

Umbilical Cord Prolapse

1. Elevate the fetal presenting part that is lying on the cord by applying finger pressure with a gloved hand to relieve cord pressure.
2. Place the client into extreme Trendelenburg's or modified Sims' position or a knee-chest position.
3. Administer oxygen, 8 to 10 L/minute, by face mask to the client.
4. Monitor fetal heart rate and assess the fetus for hypoxia.
5. Prepare to start intravenous fluids or increase the rate of administration of an existing appropriate solution.
6. Prepare for immediate birth.
7. Document the event, actions taken, and the client's response.

Reference
McKinney et al. (2018), pp. 593-594.

C. Interventions (see Priority Nursing Actions)
1. The nurse stays with the client and asks another nurse to call the primary health care provider immediately.
2. The goal is to relieve cord pressure immediately so that the fetus receives adequate oxygenation.
3. The nurse never attempts to push the cord into the uterus.
4. If the umbilical cord is protruding from the vagina, the cord is wrapped loosely in a sterile towel saturated with warm sterile normal saline.
5. This situation is an emergency and delivery must occur, usually via a cesarean section.

III. Supine Hypotension (Vena Cava Syndrome)

A. Description
1. Supine hypotension (also known as vena cava syndrome) occurs when the venous return to the heart is impaired by the weight of the uterus on the vena cava.

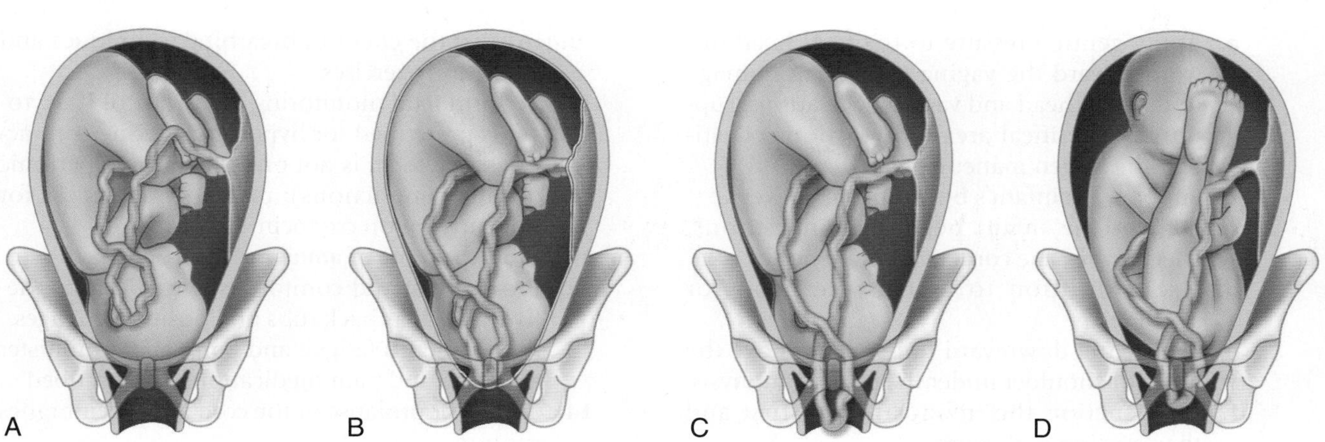

FIG. 24-1 Prolapse of umbilical cord. Note the pressure of the presenting part on the umbilical cord, which endangers fetal circulation. **A,** Occult (hidden) prolapse of cord. **B,** Complete prolapse of cord. Membranes are intact. **C,** Cord presenting in front of the fetal head may be seen in the vagina. **D,** Frank breech presentation with prolapsed cord.

2. The syndrome results in partial occlusion of the vena cava and aorta and in reduced cardiac return, cardiac output, and blood pressure.

B. Assessment
1. Pallor
2. Faintness, dizziness, breathlessness
3. Tachycardia, hypotension
4. Sweating, cool and damp skin
5. Fetal distress

C. Interventions
1. Position the client on her side to shift the weight of the fetus off the vena cava until the client's signs and symptoms subside and vital signs stabilize.
2. Monitor vital signs and fetal heart rate.

To prevent supine hypotension, avoid the supine position; position the client by placing a pillow or wedge under the client's hip to displace the gravid uterus off the vena cava.

IV. Preterm Labor

A. Description
1. Preterm labor occurs after the 20th week but before the 37th week of gestation.
2. Risk factors include a history of medical conditions; present and past obstetric problems; infection; and social and environmental factors, including substance abuse.
3. Additional risk factors include a multifetal pregnancy, which contributes to overdistention of the uterus; anemia, which decreases oxygen supply to the uterus; and age younger than 18 years or first pregnancy and age older than 40 years.

B. Assessment
1. Uterine contractions (painful or painless)
2. Abdominal cramping (may be accompanied by diarrhea)
3. Low back pain
4. Pelvic pressure or heaviness
5. Change in character and amount of usual discharge—may be thicker or thinner, bloody, brown or colorless, odorous
6. Rupture of amniotic membranes
7. Presence of fetal fibronectin in cervical canal
8. Shortening of cervical length

C. Interventions
1. Focus on stopping the labor: Identify and treat infection, restrict activity, and ensure hydration.
2. Maintain bed rest and a lateral position.
3. Monitor fetal status.
4. Administer fluids.
5. Administer medications as prescribed and monitor for side effects of tocolytics (see Table 28-1 for a description of medications used to treat preterm labor).
6. Use of 17 alpha-hydroxyprogesterone caproate known as 17P injection to decrease risk of preterm delivery.

V. Precipitous Labor and Delivery

A. Description: Labor lasting less than 3 hours

B. Interventions
1. Ensure that a precipitous delivery tray is available (hemostats, scissors, and cord clamp).
2. Stay with the client at all times.
3. Provide emotional support and keep the client calm.
4. Encourage the client to pant between contractions.
5. Prepare for rupturing membranes when the head crowns, if they are not already ruptured.
6. Do not try to prevent the fetus from being delivered.
7. If delivery is necessary before the arrival of the primary health care provider, do the following:

a. Apply gentle pressure to the fetal head upward toward the vagina to prevent damage to the fetal head and vaginal lacerations; support the perineal area. Both actions constitute the Ritgen maneuver.
b. Support the infant's body during delivery.
c. Deliver the infant between contractions, checking for the cord around the neck.
d. Use restitution to deliver the posterior shoulder.
e. Use gentle downward pressure to move the anterior shoulder under the pubic symphysis.
f. Bulb suction the infant's mouth first and then suction each naris.
g. Dry and cover the infant to keep the body warm.
h. Allow the placenta to separate naturally.
i. Place the infant on the mother's abdomen or breast to induce uterine contractions.

VI. Dystocia

A. Description
1. Dystocia is difficult labor that is prolonged or more painful.
2. Occurs because of problems caused by uterine contractions, the fetus, or the bones and tissues of the maternal pelvis.
3. The fetus may be excessively large, malpositioned, or in an abnormal presentation.
4. Contractions may be hypotonic or hypertonic.
5. Hypotonic contractions are short, irregular, and weak; amniotomy and oxytocin infusion may be treatment measures.
6. Hypertonic contractions are painful, occur frequently (6 or more in a 10-minute time period), and are uncoordinated; treatment depends on the cause and includes pain relief measures and rest.
7. Can result in maternal dehydration, infection, fetal injury, or death.

B. Assessment
1. Excessive abdominal pain
2. Abnormal contraction pattern
3. Fetal distress
4. Maternal or fetal tachycardia
5. Lack of progress in labor

C. Interventions
1. Assess fetal heart rate; monitor for fetal distress.
2. Monitor uterine contractions.
3. Monitor maternal temperature and heart rate.
4. Assist with pelvic examination, measurements, ultrasound, and other procedures.
5. Administer prophylactic antibiotics if prescribed to prevent infection.
6. Administer IV fluids as prescribed.
7. Monitor intake and output.
8. Maintain hydration.
9. Instruct the client in breathing techniques and relaxation exercises.
10. Perform fetal monitoring per protocol if oxytocin is prescribed for hypotonic uterine contractions (oxytocin is not prescribed for hypertonic uterine contractions); refer to Chapter 28 for information on oxytocin.
11. Monitor color of amniotic fluid.
12. Provide rest and comfort as with a normal delivery, such as back rubs and position changes.
13. Assess client's fatigue and pain, and administer sedatives and pain medications as prescribed.
14. Assess for prolapse of the cord after membranes rupture.

VII. Amniotic Fluid Embolism

A. Description
1. Amniotic fluid embolism is the escape of amniotic fluid into the maternal circulation.
2. The debris-containing amniotic fluid deposits in the pulmonary arterioles and is usually fatal to the mother.

B. Assessment
1. Abrupt onset of respiratory distress and chest pain
2. Cyanosis
3. Fetal bradycardia and distress if delivery has not occurred at the time of the embolism

C. Interventions
1. Institute emergency measures to maintain life.
2. Administer oxygen, 8 to 10 L/minute, by face mask or resuscitation bag delivering 100% oxygen.
3. Prepare for intubation and mechanical ventilation.
4. Position the client on her side.
5. Administer IV fluids, blood products, and medications as prescribed to correct coagulation failure.
6. Monitor fetal status.
7. Prepare for emergency delivery when the client is stabilized.
8. Provide emotional support to the client, partner, and family.

VIII. Fetal Distress

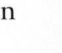

A. Assessment
1. Fetal heart rate less than 110 beats per minute or greater than 160 beats per minute
2. Meconium-stained amniotic fluid
3. Fetal hypoactivity or hyperactivity
4. Progressive decrease in baseline variability
5. Severe variable decelerations
6. Late decelerations

B. Interventions
1. Discontinue oxytocin if infusing.
2. Place the client in a lateral position.

3. Administer oxygen, 8 to 10 L/minute, via face mask.
4. Administer IV fluids (usually as a bolus)
5. Monitor maternal and fetal status.

In the event of fetal distress, prepare the client for emergency cesarean delivery.

IX. Intrauterine Fetal Demise

A. Assessment
1. Loss of fetal movement
2. Absence of fetal heart tones
3. Disseminated intravascular coagulation (DIC) screen (monitor for coagulation abnormalities because DIC is a complication related to intrauterine fetal demise)
4. Low hemoglobin and hematocrit; low platelet count; prolonged bleeding and clotting time
5. Bleeding from puncture sites (could indicate DIC)

B. Interventions
1. Encourage the client and her family to verbalize feelings; provide emotional support.
2. Incorporate religious, spiritual, and cultural health care beliefs and practices in the plan of care.
3. Allow the client choices relating to labor and delivery.
4. Administer IV fluids, medications, and blood and blood products as prescribed if DIC occurs.

X. Rupture of the Uterus

A. Description
1. Complete or incomplete separation of the uterine tissue as a result of a tear in the wall of the uterus from the stress of labor
2. Complete: Direct communication between the uterine and peritoneal cavities
3. Incomplete: Rupture into the peritoneum covering the uterus, but not into the peritoneal cavity
4. Manifestations vary with the degree of rupture.
5. Risk factors: Labor after previous cesarean section, overdistended uterus (e.g., multiple fetuses or hydramnios) after cesarean section, abdominal trauma

B. Assessment
1. Abdominal pain or tenderness
2. Chest pain
3. Contractions may stop or fail to progress
4. Rigid abdomen
5. Absent fetal heart rate
6. Signs of maternal shock
7. Fetus palpated outside the uterus (complete rupture)

C. Interventions
1. Monitor for and treat signs of shock (administer oxygen, IV fluids, and blood products).
2. Prepare the client for cesarean delivery (possible hysterectomy may be necessary).
3. Provide emotional support for the client and partner.

XI. Uterine Inversion

A. Description
1. Uterus completely or partly turns inside out.
2. This can occur during delivery or after delivery of the placenta.
3. Risk factors: Fundal implantation of the placenta, manual extraction of the placenta, short umbilical cord, uterine atony, leiomyomas, and abnormally adherent placental tissue

B. Assessment
1. A depression in the fundal area of the uterus is noted.
2. The interior of the uterus may be seen through the cervix or protruding through the vagina.
3. The client has severe pain.
4. Hemorrhage is evident.
5. The client shows signs of shock.

C. Interventions
1. Monitor for hemorrhage and signs of shock, and treat shock.
2. Prepare the client for a return of the uterus to the correct position via the vagina; if unsuccessful, laparotomy with replacement to the correct position is done.

PRACTICE QUESTIONS

238. The nurse is performing an assessment on a client who has just been told that a pregnancy test is positive. Which assessment finding indicates that the client is at risk for preterm labor?
1. The client is a 35-year-old primigravida.
2. The client has a history of cardiac disease.
3. The client's hemoglobin level is 13.5 g/dL (135 mmol/L).
4. The client is a 20-year-old primigravida of average weight and height.

239. The nurse is monitoring a client who is in the active stage of labor. The nurse documents that the client is experiencing labor dystocia. The nurse determines that which risk factors in the client's history placed her at risk for this complication? **Select all that apply.**
- ☐ 1. Age 54 years
- ☐ 2. Body mass index of 28
- ☐ 3. Previous difficulty with fertility
- ☐ 4. Administration of oxytocin for induction
- ☐ 5. Potassium level of 3.6 mEq/L (3.6 mmol/L)

240. The nurse in a birthing room is monitoring a client with dysfunctional labor for signs of fetal or maternal

compromise. Which assessment finding should alert the nurse to a compromise?
1. Maternal fatigue
2. Coordinated uterine contractions
3. Progressive changes in the cervix
4. Persistent nonreassuring fetal heart rate

241. The nurse in a labor room is preparing to care for a client with hypertonic uterine contractions. The nurse is told that the client is experiencing uncoordinated contractions that are erratic in their frequency, duration, and intensity. What is the **priority** nursing action?
1. Provide pain relief measures.
2. Prepare the client for an amniotomy.
3. Promote ambulation every 30 minutes.
4. Monitor the oxytocin infusion closely.

242. The nurse is reviewing the primary health care provider's (PHCP's) prescriptions for a client admitted for premature rupture of the membranes. Gestational age of the fetus is determined to be 37 weeks. Which prescription should the nurse question?
1. Monitor fetal heart rate continuously.
2. Monitor maternal vital signs frequently.
3. Perform a vaginal examination every shift.
4. Administer an antibiotic per prescription and per agency protocol.

243. The nurse has created a plan of care for a client experiencing dystocia and includes several nursing actions in the plan of care. What is the **priority** nursing action?
1. Providing comfort measures
2. Monitoring the fetal heart rate
3. Changing the client's position frequently
4. Keeping the significant other informed of the progress of the labor

244. Fetal distress is occurring with a laboring client. As the nurse prepares the client for a cesarean birth, what is the **most important** nursing action?
1. Slow the intravenous flow rate.
2. Continue the oxytocin drip if infusing.
3. Place the client in a high Fowler's position.
4. Administer oxygen, 8 to 10 L/minute, via face mask.

245. The nurse in a labor room is performing a vaginal assessment on a pregnant client in labor. The nurse notes the presence of the umbilical cord protruding from the vagina. What is the **first** nursing action with this finding?
1. Gently push the cord into the vagina.
2. Place the client in Trendelenburg's position.
3. Find the closest telephone and page the primary health care provider stat.
4. Call the delivery room to notify the staff that the client will be transported immediately.

ANSWERS

238. *Answer:* 2

Rationale: Preterm labor occurs after the 20th week but before the 37th week of gestation. Several factors are associated with preterm labor, including a history of medical conditions, present and past obstetric problems, social and environmental factors, and substance abuse. Other risk factors include a multifetal pregnancy, which contributes to overdistention of the uterus; anemia, which decreases oxygen supply to the uterus; and age younger than 18 years or first pregnancy at age older than 40 years.

Test-Taking Strategy: Options 1, 3, and 4 are comparable or alike and are average and normal findings. Also note that the correct option is the only option that identifies an abnormal condition.

Level of Cognitive Ability: Analyzing
Client Needs: Physiological Integrity
Integrated Process: Nursing Process—Assessment
Content Area: Maternity: Antepartum
Health Problem: Maternity: Preterm labor
Priority Concepts: Clinical Judgment; Perfusion
Reference: McKinney et al. (2018), p. 583.

239. *Answer:* 1, 2, 3

Rationale: Risk factors that increase a woman's risk for dysfunctional labor include the following: advanced maternal age, being overweight, electrolyte imbalances, previous difficulty with fertility, uterine overstimulation with oxytocin, short stature, prior version, masculine characteristics, uterine abnormalities, malpresentations and position of the fetus, cephalopelvic disproportion, maternal fatigue, dehydration, fear, administration of an analgesic early in labor, and use of epidural analgesia. Age 54 years is considered advanced maternal age, and a body mass index of 28 is considered overweight. Previous difficulty with fertility is another risk factor for labor dystocia. A potassium level of 3.6 mEq/L (3.6 mmol/L) is normal, and administration of oxytocin alone is not a risk factor; risk exists only if uterine hyperstimulation occurs.

Test-Taking Strategy: Focus on the subject, risk factors for labor dystocia. Additionally, focus on the data in the question, look at each option, and determine whether these are normal assessment findings.

Level of Cognitive Ability: Analyzing
Client Needs: Physiological Integrity
Integrated Process: Nursing Process: Assessment
Content Area: Maternity: Intrapartum
Health Problem: Maternity: Dystocia
Priority Concepts: Clinical Judgment; Perfusion
Reference: Lowdermilk et al. (2016), p. 773.

240. *Answer:* 4

Rationale: Signs of fetal or maternal compromise include a persistent, nonreassuring fetal heart rate, fetal acidosis, and

the passage of meconium. Maternal fatigue and infection can occur if the labor is prolonged but do not indicate fetal or maternal compromise. Coordinated uterine contractions and progressive changes in the cervix are a reassuring pattern in labor.
Test-Taking Strategy: Focus on the subject, signs of fetal or maternal compromise. Eliminate options 1, 2, and 3 because they are comparable or alike and are normal expectations during labor.
Level of Cognitive Ability: Analyzing
Client Needs: Physiological Integrity
Integrated Process: Nursing Process—Assessment
Content Area: Maternity: Intrapartum
Health Problem: Maternity: Dystocia
Priority Concepts: Clinical Judgment; Perfusion
Reference: McKinney et al. (2018), p. 315.

241. *Answer:* 1
Rationale: Hypertonic uterine contractions are painful, occur frequently, and are uncoordinated. Management of hypertonic labor depends on the cause. Relief of pain is the primary intervention to promote a normal labor pattern. An amniotomy and oxytocin infusion are not treatment measures for hypertonic contractions; however, these treatments may be used in clients with hypotonic dysfunction. A client with hypertonic uterine contractions would not be encouraged to ambulate every 30 minutes but would be encouraged to rest.
Test-Taking Strategy: Focus on the strategic word, *priority*. Also note that options 2, 3, and 4 are comparable or alike and are therapeutic measures for hypotonic dysfunction.
Level of Cognitive Ability: Analyzing
Client Needs: Physiological Integrity
Integrated Process: Nursing Process—Implementation
Content Area: Maternity: Intrapartum
Health Problem: Maternity: Dystocia
Priority Concepts: Clinical Judgment; Pain
Reference: McKinney et al. (2018), pp. 574-575.

242. *Answer:* 3
Rationale: Vaginal examinations should not be done routinely on a client with premature rupture of the membranes because of the risk of infection. The nurse would expect to monitor fetal heart rate, monitor maternal vital signs, and administer an antibiotic.
Test-Taking Strategy: Note the word *question*. This word indicates the activity that the nurse should not implement without clarification. Options 1, 2, and 4 are comparable or alike and are expected activities for the nurse to perform for a client with premature rupture of the membranes. Performing a vaginal examination every shift should not be done on a client with premature rupture of the membranes because of the risk of infection, so the nurse would question this prescription.
Level of Cognitive Ability: Analyzing
Client Needs: Physiological Integrity
Integrated Process: Nursing Process—Implementation
Content Area: Maternity: Intrapartum
Health Problem: Maternity: Premature rupture of the membranes
Priority Concepts: Collaboration; Safety
Reference: McKinney et al. (2018), pp. 580-581.

243. *Answer:* 2
Rationale: Dystocia is difficult labor that is prolonged or more painful than expected. The priority is to monitor the fetal heart rate. Although providing comfort measures, changing the client's position frequently, and keeping the significant other informed of the progress of the labor are components of the plan of care, the fetal status would be the priority.
Test-Taking Strategy: Note the strategic word, *priority*. Use Maslow's Hierarchy of Needs theory and the ABCs—airway, breathing, and circulation—to assist in answering the question. These strategies will direct you to the correct option.
Level of Cognitive Ability: Creating
Client Needs: Physiological Integrity
Integrated Process: Nursing Process—Planning
Content Area: Maternity: Intrapartum
Health Problem: Maternity: Dystocia
Priority Concepts: Clinical Judgment; Perfusion
Reference: Lowdermilk et al. (2016), pp. 773-774.

244. *Answer:* 4
Rationale: Oxygen is administered, 8 to 10 L/minute, via face mask to optimize oxygenation of the circulating blood. Option 1 is incorrect, because the intravenous infusion should be increased (per primary health care provider prescription) to increase the maternal blood volume. Option 2 is incorrect, because oxytocin stimulation of the uterus is discontinued if fetal heart rate patterns change for any reason. Option 3 is incorrect because the client is placed in the lateral position with her legs raised to increase maternal blood volume and improve fetal perfusion.
Test-Taking Strategy: Note the strategic words, *most important*. Use the ABCs—airway, breathing, and circulation. Oxygen is the only option that would improve cardiac output and improve perfusion to the fetus. The other options would not improve perfusion to the fetus.
Level of Cognitive Ability: Analyzing
Client Needs: Physiological Integrity
Integrated Process: Nursing Process—Implementation
Content Area: Complex Care: Emergency Situations/Management
Health Problem: Maternity: Fetal distress/Demise
Priority Concepts: Clinical Judgment; Perfusion
Reference: McKinney et al. (2018), p. 344.

245. *Answer:* 2
Rationale: When cord prolapse occurs, prompt actions are taken to relieve cord compression and increase fetal oxygenation. The client should be positioned with the hips higher than the head to shift the fetal presenting part toward the diaphragm. The nurse should push the call light to summon help, and other staff members should call the primary health care provider and notify the delivery room. If the cord is protruding from the vagina, no attempt should be made to replace it because to do so could traumatize it and reduce blood flow further. Also as a first action, the examiner should place a gloved hand into the vagina and hold the presenting part off the umbilical cord. Oxygen, 8 to 10 L/minute, by face mask is administered to the client to increase fetal oxygenation.
Test-Taking Strategy: Note the strategic word, *first*, and that the umbilical cord is protruding from the vagina. Options 3

and 4 can be eliminated first because these actions delay necessary and immediate treatment. Recalling that the goal is to relieve cord compression and to increase fetal oxygenation will direct you to the correct option. Also remember that the cord should not be pushed back into the vagina.
Level of Cognitive Ability: Analyzing
Client Needs: Physiological Integrity
Integrated Process: Nursing Process—Implementation
Content Area: Complex Care: Emergency Situations/Management
Health Problem: Maternity: Prolapsed umbilical cord
Priority Concepts: Clinical Judgment; Perfusion
Reference: McKinney et al. (2018), pp. 593-594.

CHAPTER 25

Postpartum Period

PRIORITY CONCEPTS Health Promotion, Reproduction

I. Postpartum

A. Description: Period when the reproductive tract returns to the normal, nonpregnant state

B. The postpartum period starts immediately after birth and is usually completed by week 6 following birth.

II. Physiological Maternal Changes

A. Involution

1. Description
   a. Involution is the rapid decrease in the size of the uterus as it returns to the nonpregnant state.
   b. Clients who breast-feed may experience a more rapid involution because of the release of oxytocin during breast-feeding.
2. Assessment
   a. The weight of the uterus decreases from approximately 2 lb (900 g) to 2 oz (57 g) in 6 weeks.
   b. The endometrium regenerates.
   c. The fundus steadily descends into the pelvis.
   d. Fundal height decreases about 1 cm/day (Fig. 25-1).
   e. By 10 days postpartum, the uterus cannot be palpated abdominally.
   f. A flaccid fundus indicates uterine atony, and it should be massaged until firm; a tender fundus indicates an infection.
   g. Afterpains decrease in frequency after the first few days.

B. Lochia

1. Description: Discharge from the uterus that consists of blood from the vessels of the placental site and debris from the decidua
2. Assessment (Box 25-1)
   a. Rubra is bright red discharge that occurs from day of birth to day 3.
   b. Serosa is brownish pink discharge that occurs from days 4 to 10.
   c. Alba is white discharge that occurs from days 11 to 14.
   d. Discharge should smell like normal menstrual flow.
   e. Discharge decreases daily in amount.
   f. Discharge may increase with ambulation.

C. Cervix: Cervical involution occurs, and the muscle begins to regenerate after 1 week.

D. Vagina: Vaginal distention decreases, although muscle tone is never restored completely to the pregravid state.

E. Ovarian function and menstruation

1. Ovarian function depends on the rapidity with which pituitary function is restored.
2. Menstrual flow resumes within 1 to 2 months in non–breast-feeding mothers.
3. Menstrual flow usually resumes within 3 to 6 months in breast-feeding mothers.
4. Breast-feeding mothers may experience amenorrhea during the entire period of lactation so long as they are exclusively breastfeeding.

! Women may ovulate without menstruating, so breast-feeding should not be considered a form of birth control.

F. Breasts

1. Breasts continue to secrete colostrum for the first 48 to 72 hours after birth.
2. A decrease in estrogen and progesterone levels after birth stimulates increased prolactin levels, which promote breast milk production.
3. Breasts become distended with milk on the third day.
4. Engorgement occurs on approximately day 4 in both breast-feeding and non–breast-feeding mothers. Box 25-2 summarizes care of breasts for non–breast-feeding mothers.
5. Breast-feeding relieves engorgement.

G. Urinary tract

1. The client may have urinary retention as a result of loss of elasticity and tone and loss of sensation in the bladder from trauma, medications, anesthesia, and lack of privacy.
2. Diuresis usually begins within the first 12 hours after birth.

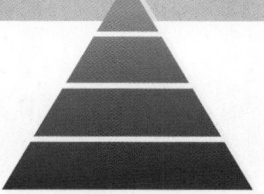

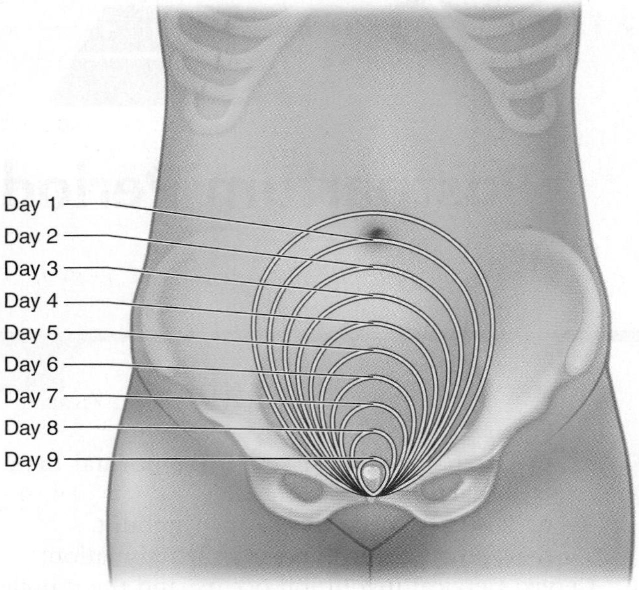

FIG. 25-1 Involution of the uterus. The height of the uterine fundus decreases by approximately 1 cm/day.

BOX 25-1 Amount of Lochia

Scant: Less than 2.5 cm (<1 inch) on menstrual pad in 1 hour
Light: Less than 10 cm (<4 inches) on menstrual pad in 1 hour
Moderate: Less than 15 cm (<6 inches) on menstrual pad in 1 hour
Heavy: Saturated menstrual pad in 1 hour
Excessive: Menstrual pad saturated in 15 minutes

From Murray S, McKinney E: *Foundations of maternal-newborn and women's health nursing*, ed 5, Philadelphia, 2010, Saunders.

BOX 25-2 Breast Care for Non–Breast-Feeding Mothers

- Avoid nipple stimulation.
- Apply a breast binder, wear a snug-fitting bra, apply ice packs, or take a mild analgesic for engorgement.
- Engorgement usually resolves within 24 to 36 hours after it begins.

H. Gastrointestinal tract
  1. Clients are usually hungry after birth.
  2. Constipation can occur, with bowel movement (soft, formed stool) by the second or third postpartum day.
  3. Hemorrhoids are common.

I. Vital signs (Table 25-1)

III. Postpartum Interventions

A. Assessment
  1. Monitor vital signs.
  2. Assess pain level.

TABLE 25-1 Normal Postpartum Vital Signs

Vital Sign	Description
Temperature	May increase to 100.4° F (38.0° C) during the first 24 hr postpartum because of dehydrating effects of labor. Any higher elevation may be caused by infection and must be reported.
Pulse	May decrease to 50 beats per minute (normal puerperal bradycardia). Pulse >100 beats per minute may indicate excessive blood loss or infection.
Blood pressure	Should be normal; suspect hypovolemia if it decreases.
Respirations	Rarely change; if respirations increase significantly, suspect pulmonary embolism, uterine atony, or hemorrhage.

  3. Assess height, consistency, and location of the fundus (have client empty the bladder before fundal assessment) (Fig. 25-2).
  4. Monitor color, amount, and odor of lochia.
  5. Assess breasts for engorgement.
  6. Monitor perineum for swelling or discoloration.
  7. Monitor for perineal lacerations or episiotomy for healing.
  8. Assess incisions or dressings of client who had a cesarean birth.
  9. Monitor bowel status.
  10. Monitor intake and output.
  11. Encourage frequent voiding.
  12. Encourage ambulation.
  13. Assess extremities for thrombophlebitis (redness, tenderness, or warmth of the leg).

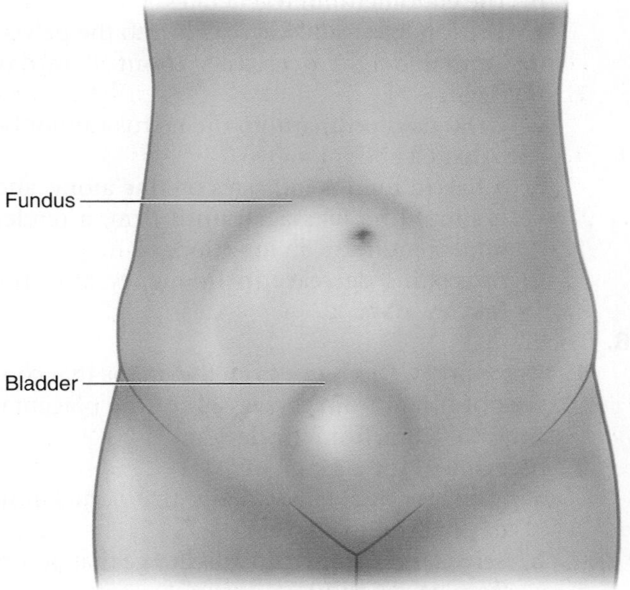

FIG. 25-2 A full bladder displaces and prevents contraction of the uterus.

14. Administer Rho(D) immune globulin if prescribed within 72 hours postpartum to Rh-negative client who has given birth to Rh-positive newborn.
15. Evaluate rubella immunity. If not immune, administer rubella immunization.
16. Assess bonding with the newborn.
17. Assess emotional status.

B. Client teaching
1. Demonstrate newborn care skills as necessary.
2. Provide the opportunity for the client to bathe the newborn.
3. Instruct in feeding technique.
4. Instruct the client to avoid heavy lifting for at least 3 weeks.
5. Instruct the client to plan at least 1 rest period per day.
6. Instruct the client that contraception should begin after birth or with the initiation of intercourse (intercourse should be postponed at least until lochia ceases). With rubella immunization, avoid conception for 1 to 3 months based on primary health care provider (PHCP) or obstetrician/gynecologist (OB/GYN) recommendation.
7. Instruct the client in the importance of follow-up, which should be scheduled at 4 to 6 weeks.
8. Instruct the client to report any signs of chills, fever, increased lochia, or depressed feelings to the PHCP immediately.

IV. Postpartum Discomforts

A. Afterbirth pains
1. Occur as a result of contractions of the uterus.
2. Are more common in multiparas, breast-feeding mothers, clients treated with oxytocin, and clients who had an overdistended uterus during pregnancy, such as with carrying twins.

B. Perineal discomfort
1. Apply ice packs to the perineum during the first 24 hours to reduce swelling.
2. After the first 24 hours, apply warmth by sitz baths.

C. Episiotomy
1. If done, instruct the client to administer perineal care after each voiding.
2. Encourage the use of an analgesic spray as prescribed.
3. Administer analgesics as prescribed if comfort measures are unsuccessful.

D. Perineal lacerations
1. Care as for an episiotomy; administer perineal care and use analgesic spray and analgesics for comfort.
2. Rectal suppositories and enemas may be contraindicated (to avoid injury to sutures).

E. Breast discomfort from engorgement
1. Encourage the client to wear a support bra at all times, even while she is sleeping.
2. Encourage the use of ice packs between feedings if the client is not breast-feeding. Use of ice packs could diminish milk supply in the breast-feeding mother.
3. Encourage the use of warm soaks or a warm shower before feeding for the breast-feeding mother.
4. Administer analgesics as prescribed if comfort measures are unsuccessful.

F. Constipation
1. Encourage adequate intake of fluids (2000 mL/day).
2. Encourage diet high in fiber.
3. Encourage ambulation.
4. Administer stool softener, laxative, enema, or suppository if needed and prescribed.

G. Postpartum emotional changes (Box 25-3)
1. Acknowledge the client's feelings and demonstrate a caring attitude.
2. Determine availability of family support and other support systems and resources as needed.
3. Encourage and assist the client to verbalize her feelings.
4. Monitor the newborn for appropriate growth and development expectations.
5. Assist the significant other and other appropriate family members to discuss feelings and identify ways to assist the client.

! All clients should be assessed for depression during pregnancy and in the postpartum period.

V. Nutritional Counseling

A. Discuss caloric intake with breast-feeding and non–breast-feeding mothers.

B. Nutritional needs depend on prepregnancy weight, ideal weight for height, and whether the client is breast-feeding.

C. If the client is breast-feeding, calorie needs increase by 200 to 500 calories/day, and the client may require increased fluids and the continuance of prenatal vitamins and minerals.

VI. Breast-Feeding

A. Interventions
1. Put the newborn to the mother's breast as soon as the mother's and newborn's conditions are stable (on delivery table, if possible).
2. Stay with the client each time she nurses until she feels secure and confident with the newborn and her feelings.
3. Assess *LATCH* (*l*atch achieved by newborn; *a*udible swallowing; *t*ype of nipple; *c*omfort of mother; *hold* or position of baby).
4. Uterine cramping may occur the first day after birth while the client is nursing, when oxytocin stimulation causes the uterus to contract.

BOX 25-3 Signs and Symptoms of Emotional Changes

Postpartum Blues
- Anger
- Anxiety
- Cries easily for no apparent reason
- Emotionally labile
- Expresses a let-down feeling
- Fatigue
- Headache
- Insomnia
- Restlessness
- Sadness

Postpartum Depression
- Anxiety
- Appetite changes
- Crying, sadness
- Difficulty concentrating or making decisions
- Fatigue, unable to sleep
- Feelings of guilt
- Irritability and agitation
- Lack of energy
- Less responsive to the infant
- Loss of pleasure in normal activities
- Suicidal thoughts

Postpartum Psychosis
- Break with reality
- Confusion
- Delirium
- Delusions
- Hallucinations
- Panic

Data from Lowdermilk D, Cashion MC, Perry S: *Maternity & women's health care*, ed 9, St. Louis, 2011, Mosby; Lowdermilk D, Perry S, Cashion MC, Alden K: *Maternity & women's health care*, ed 10, St. Louis, 2012, Mosby; and Perry S, Hockenberry M, Lowdermilk D, Wilson D: *Maternal-child nursing care*, ed 4, St. Louis, 2013, Mosby.

5. Instruct the client to use general hygiene and wash the breasts once daily.
6. If engorgement occurs, breast-feed frequently, apply warm packs before feeding, apply ice packs between feedings, and massage the breasts.
7. The client should not use soap on the breasts because it tends to remove natural oils, which increases the chance of cracked nipples.
8. If cracked nipples develop, the client should expose the nipples to air for 10 to 20 minutes after feeding, rotate the position of the baby for each feeding, and ensure that the baby is latched on to the areola, not just the nipple. Colostrum can also be expressed after the feeding as a moisturizer for the nipple to prevent cracked, dry skin.
9. The bra should be well fitted and supporting; avoid an underwire bra.
10. Breasts may leak between feedings or during coitus; place breast pad in bra.
11. Calories should be increased by 200 to 500 calories/day, and the diet should include additional fluids; prenatal vitamins should be taken as prescribed.
12. Newborn's stools are usually light yellow, seedy, watery, and frequent.
13. Medications, including over-the-counter medications, need to be avoided unless prescribed because they may be unsafe when breast-feeding.
14. Gas-producing foods and caffeine should be avoided.
15. Oral contraceptives containing estrogen are not recommended for breast-feeding mothers; progestin-only birth control pills are less likely to interfere with the milk supply.
16. The infant will develop her or his own feeding schedule.

B. Breast-feeding procedure for the mother (Box 25-4)

BOX 25-4 Breast-Feeding Procedure for the Mother

1. Wash hands and assume a comfortable position.
2. Start with the breast with which the last feeding ended.
3. Brush the newborn's lower lip with nipple.
4. Tickle the lips to have the newborn open the mouth wide.
5. Guide the nipple and surrounding areola into the newborn's mouth.
6. Encourage the newborn to nurse on each breast for 15 to 20 minutes.
7. After the newborn has nursed, release suction by depressing the newborn's chin or inserting a clean finger into the newborn's mouth.
8. Burp the newborn after the first breast.
9. Repeat the procedure on the second breast until the newborn stops nursing.
10. Burp the newborn again.
11. Listen for audible sucking and swallowing.

PRACTICE QUESTIONS

246. The postpartum nurse is taking the vital signs of a client who delivered a healthy newborn 4 hours ago. The nurse notes that the client's temperature is 100.2° F. What is the **priority** nursing action?
1. Document the findings.
2. Notify the obstetrician.
3. Retake the temperature in 15 minutes.
4. Increase hydration by encouraging oral fluids.

247. The nurse is assessing a client who is 6 hours postpartum after delivering a full-term healthy newborn. The client complains to the nurse of feelings of faintness and dizziness. Which nursing action is **most appropriate**?
1. Raise the head of the client's bed.
2. Obtain hemoglobin and hematocrit levels.
3. Instruct the client to request help when getting out of bed.
4. Inform the nursery room nurse to avoid bringing the newborn to the client until the client's symptoms have subsided.

248. The postpartum nurse is providing instructions to a client after birth of a healthy newborn. Which time frame should the nurse relay to the client regarding the return of bowel function?
1. 3 days postpartum
2. 7 days postpartum
3. On the day of birth
4. Within 2 weeks postpartum

249. The nurse is planning care for a postpartum client who had a vaginal delivery 2 hours ago. The client required an episiotomy and has several hemorrhoids. What is the **priority** nursing consideration for this client?
1. Client pain level
2. Inadequate urinary output
3. Client perception of body changes
4. Potential for imbalanced body fluid volume

250. The nurse is providing postpartum instructions to a client who will be breast-feeding her newborn. The nurse determines that the client has understood the instructions if she makes which statements? **Select all that apply.**
- ☐ 1. "I should wear a bra that provides support."
- ☐ 2. "Drinking alcohol can affect my milk supply."
- ☐ 3. "The use of caffeine can decrease my milk supply."
- ☐ 4. "I will start my estrogen birth control pills again as soon as I get home."
- ☐ 5. "I know if my breasts get engorged, I will limit my breast-feeding and supplement the baby."
- ☐ 6. "I plan on having bottled water available in the refrigerator so I can get additional fluids easily."

251. The nurse is teaching a postpartum client about breast-feeding. Which instruction should the nurse include?
1. The diet should include additional fluids.
2. Prenatal vitamins should be discontinued.
3. Soap should be used to cleanse the breasts.
4. Birth control measures are unnecessary while breast-feeding.

252. The nurse is preparing to assess the uterine fundus of a client in the immediate postpartum period. After locating the fundus, the nurse notes that the uterus feels soft and boggy. Which nursing intervention is appropriate?
1. Elevate the client's legs.
2. Massage the fundus until it is firm.
3. Ask the client to turn on her left side.
4. Push on the uterus to assist in expressing clots.

253. The nurse is caring for four 1-day postpartum clients. Which client assessment requires the **need for follow-up**?
1. The client with mild afterpains
2. The client with a pulse rate of 60 beats per minute
3. The client with colostrum discharge from both breasts
4. The client with lochia that is red and has a foul-smelling odor

254. When performing a postpartum assessment on a client, the nurse notes the presence of clots in the lochia. The nurse examines the clots and notes that they are larger than 1 cm. Which nursing action is **most appropriate**?
1. Document the findings.
2. Notify the obstetrician (OB).
3. Reassess the client in 2 hours.
4. Encourage increased oral intake of fluids.

255. The nurse is monitoring the amount of lochia drainage in a client who is 2 hours postpartum and notes that the client has saturated a perineal pad in 15 minutes. How should the nurse respond to this finding **initially**?
1. Document the finding.
2. Encourage the client to ambulate.
3. Encourage the client to increase fluid intake.
4. Contact the obstetrician (OB) and inform him or her of this finding.

256. The nurse has provided discharge instructions to a client who delivered a healthy newborn by cesarean delivery. Which statement made by the client indicates a **need for further instruction**?
1. "I will begin abdominal exercises immediately."
2. "I will notify my obstetrician if I develop a fever."

3. "I will turn on my side and push up with my arms to get out of bed."
4. "I will lift nothing heavier than my newborn baby for at least 2 weeks."

257. After a precipitous delivery, the nurse notes that the new mother is passive and touches her newborn infant only briefly with her fingertips. What should the nurse do to help the woman process the delivery?

1. Encourage the mother to breast-feed soon after birth.
2. Support the mother in her reaction to the newborn infant.
3. Tell the mother that it is important to hold the newborn infant.
4. Document a complete account of the mother's reaction on the birth record.

ANSWERS

246. *Answer:* 4
Rationale: The client's temperature should be taken every 4 hours while she is awake. Temperatures up to 100.4° F (38° C) in the first 24 hours after birth often are related to the dehydrating effects of labor. The appropriate action is to increase hydration by encouraging oral fluids, which should bring the temperature to a normal reading. Although the nurse also would document the findings, the appropriate action would be to increase hydration. Taking the temperature in another 15 minutes is an unnecessary action. Contacting the obstetrician is not necessary.
Test-Taking Strategy: Note the strategic word, *priority*, and use knowledge regarding the physiological findings in the immediate postpartum period to answer this question. Recalling that a temperature elevation often is related to the dehydrating effects of labor will direct you to the correct option. Also, increasing hydration relates to a physiological client need.
Level of Cognitive Ability: Applying
Client Needs: Physiological Integrity
Integrated Process: Nursing Process—Implementation
Content Area: Maternity: Postpartum
Health Problem: Maternity: Infections/Inflammation
Priority Concepts: Reproduction; Thermoregulation
Reference: Lowdermilk et al. (2016), p. 486.

247. *Answer:* 3
Rationale: Orthostatic hypotension may be evident during the first 8 hours after birth. Feelings of faintness or dizziness are signs that caution the nurse to focus interventions on the client's safety. The nurse should advise the client to get help the first few times she gets out of bed. Option 1 is not a helpful action in this situation and would not relieve the symptoms. Option 2 requires a prescription. Option 4 is unnecessary.
Test-Taking Strategy: Note the strategic words, *most appropriate.* Focus on the subject, client safety. Option 4 is unnecessary and should be eliminated first. Elevating the client's head is not a helpful intervention. To select from the remaining options, recall that safety is a primary issue.
Level of Cognitive Ability: Applying
Client Needs: Safe and Effective Care Environment
Integrated Process: Nursing Process—Implementation
Content Area: Maternity: Postpartum
Health Problem: N/A
Priority Concepts: Perfusion; Safety
Reference: McKinney et al. (2018), pp. 401, 408.

248. *Answer:* 1
Rationale: After birth, the nurse should auscultate the client's abdomen in all 4 quadrants to determine the return of bowel sounds. Normal bowel elimination usually returns 2 to 3 days postpartum. Surgery, anesthesia, and the use of opioids and pain control agents also contribute to the longer period of altered bowel functions. Options 2, 3, and 4 are incorrect.
Test-Taking Strategy: Focus on the subject and use general principles related to postpartum care. Eliminate options 2 and 4 first because of the length of time stated in these options. From the remaining options, eliminate option 3, because it would seem unreasonable that bowel function would return that quickly in the postpartum woman.
Level of Cognitive Ability: Applying
Client Needs: Physiological Integrity
Integrated Process: Teaching and Learning
Content Area: Maternity: Postpartum
Health Problem: N/A
Priority Concepts: Client Education; Elimination
Reference: McKinney et al. (2018), p. 398.

249. *Answer:* 1
Rationale: The priority nursing consideration for a client who delivered 2 hours ago and who has an episiotomy and hemorrhoids is client pain level. Most clients have some degree of discomfort during the immediate postpartum period. There are no data in the question that indicate inadequate urinary output, the presence of client perception of body changes, and potential for imbalanced body fluid volume.
Test-Taking Strategy: Note the strategic word, *priority*. Use Maslow's Hierarchy of Needs theory to eliminate option 3, because this is a psychosocial, not a physiological, need. To select from the remaining options, focus on the data in the question.
Level of Cognitive Ability: Analyzing
Client Needs: Physiological Integrity
Integrated Process: Nursing Process—Analysis
Content Area: Maternity: Postpartum
Health Problem: N/A
Priority Concepts: Pain; Reproduction
Reference: Lowdermilk et al. (2016), pp. 488-489.

250. *Answer:* 1, 2, 3, 6
Rationale: The postpartum client should wear a bra that is well fitted and supportive. Common causes of decreased milk supply include formula use; inadequate rest or diet; smoking

by the mother or others in the home; and use of caffeine, alcohol, or medications. Breast-feeding clients should increase their daily fluid intake; having bottled water available indicates that the postpartum client understands the importance of increasing fluids. If engorgement occurs, the client should not limit breast-feeding but should breast-feed frequently. Oral contraceptives containing estrogen are not recommended for breast-feeding mothers.
Test-Taking Strategy: Focus on the subject and note the words *understood the instructions*. Think about the physiology associated with milk production and the complications of breast-feeding to answer correctly.
Level of Cognitive Ability: Evaluating
Client Needs: Health Promotion and Maintenance
Integrated Process: Nursing Process—Evaluation
Content Area: Maternity: Postpartum
Health Problem: N/A
Priority Concepts: Health Promotion; Reproduction
Reference: Lowdermilk et al. (2016), pp. 620-621.

251. *Answer:* 1
Rationale: The diet for a breast-feeding client should include additional fluids. Prenatal vitamins should be taken as prescribed, and soap should not be used on the breasts because it tends to remove natural oils, which increases the chance of cracked nipples. Breast-feeding is not a method of contraception, so birth control measures should be resumed.
Test-Taking Strategy: Note the subject, teaching for the breast-feeding client. Remember that fluids and calories should be increased when the client is breast-feeding.
Level of Cognitive Ability: Applying
Client Needs: Physiological Integrity
Integrated Process: Teaching and Learning
Content Area: Maternity: Postpartum
Health Problem: N/A
Priority Concepts: Client Education; Nutrition
Reference: McKinney et al. (2018), pp. 268-269.

252. *Answer:* 2
Rationale: If the uterus is not contracted firmly, the initial intervention is to massage the fundus until it is firm and to express clots that may have accumulated in the uterus. Elevating the client's legs and positioning the client on the side would not assist in managing uterine atony. Pushing on an uncontracted uterus can invert the uterus and cause massive hemorrhage.
Test-Taking Strategy: Focus on the subject, a soft and boggy uterus. Visualize the situation and recall the therapeutic management for uterine atony. Remember that a full bladder displaces the uterus.
Level of Cognitive Ability: Applying
Client Needs: Health Promotion and Maintenance
Integrated Process: Nursing Process—Implementation
Content Area: Maternity: Postpartum
Health Problem: Maternity: Postpartum Uterine Problems
Priority Concepts: Health Promotion; Reproduction
Reference: McKinney et al. (2018), pp. 600-601.

253. *Answer:* 4
Rationale: Lochia, the discharge present after birth, is red for the first 1 to 3 days and gradually decreases in amount. Normal lochia has a fleshy odor or an odor similar to menstrual flow. Foul-smelling or purulent lochia usually indicates infection, and these findings are not normal. The other options are normal findings for a 1-day postpartum client.
Test-Taking Strategy: Note the strategic words, *need for follow-up*. These words indicate a negative event query and the need to select the abnormal assessment finding. Note the words *foul-smelling* in the correct option.
Level of Cognitive Ability: Analyzing
Client Needs: Physiological Integrity
Integrated Process: Nursing Process—Analysis
Content Area: Maternity: Postpartum
Health Problem: Maternity: Infection/Inflammations
Priority Concepts: Infection; Reproduction
Reference: McKinney et al. (2018), pp. 329, 396.

254. *Answer:* 2
Rationale: Normally, a few small clots may be noted in the lochia in the first 1 to 2 days after birth from pooling of blood in the vagina. Clots larger than 1 cm are considered abnormal. The cause of these clots, such as uterine atony or retained placental fragments, needs to be determined and treated to prevent further blood loss. Although the findings would be documented, the appropriate action is to notify the OB. Reassessing the client in 2 hours would delay necessary treatment. Increasing oral intake of fluids would not be a helpful action in this situation.
Test-Taking Strategy: Note the strategic words, *most appropriate*. Focus on the words *larger than 1 cm*. Think about the significance of lochial clots in the postpartum period to answer correctly.
Level of Cognitive Ability: Applying
Client Needs: Physiological Integrity
Integrated Process: Nursing Process—Implementation
Content Area: Maternity: Postpartum
Health Problem: Maternity: Postpartum Uterine Problems
Priority Concepts: Clinical Judgment; Clotting
Reference: McKinney et al. (2018), p. 329.

255. *Answer:* 4
Rationale: Lochia is the discharge from the uterus in the postpartum period; it consists of blood from the vessels of the placental site and debris from the decidua. The following can be used as a guide to determine the amount of flow: scant = less than 2.5 cm (<1 inch) on menstrual pad in 1 hour; light = less than 10 cm (<4 inches) on menstrual pad in 1 hour; moderate = less than 15 cm (<6 inches) on menstrual pad in 1 hour; heavy = saturated menstrual pad in 1 hour; and excessive = menstrual pad saturated in 15 minutes. If the client is experiencing excessive bleeding, the nurse should contact the OB in the event that postpartum hemorrhage is occurring. It may be appropriate to encourage increased fluid intake, but this is not the initial action. It is not appropriate to encourage ambulation at this time. Documentation should occur once the client has been stabilized.
Test-Taking Strategy: Note the strategic word, *initially*. Focus on the data in the question, a saturated perineal pad in 15 minutes. Next, determine if an abnormality exists. The data and the use of guidelines determine the amount of lochial flow will help you determine that this is abnormal and warrants notification of the OB.
Level of Cognitive Ability: Analyzing
Client Needs: Physiological Integrity

Integrated Process: Nursing Process—Implementation
Content Area: Complex Care: Emergency Situations/Management
Health Problem: Maternity: Postpartum Uterine Problems
Priority Concepts: Clotting; Reproduction
Reference: McKinney et al. (2018), p. 396.

256. *Answer:* 1
Rationale: A cesarean delivery requires an incision made through the abdominal wall and into the uterus. Abdominal exercises should not start immediately after abdominal surgery; the client should wait at least 3 to 4 weeks postoperatively to allow for healing of the incision. Options 2, 3, and 4 are appropriate instructions for the client after a cesarean delivery.
Test-Taking Strategy: Note the **strategic words,** *need for further instruction*. These words indicate a **negative event query** and ask you to select an option that is an incorrect statement. Keeping in mind that the client had a cesarean delivery and noting the word *immediately* in the correct option will assist in directing you to this option.
Level of Cognitive Ability: Evaluating
Client Needs: Health Promotion and Maintenance
Integrated Process: Teaching and Learning
Content Area: Maternity: Postpartum
Health Problem: N/A
Priority Concepts: Client Education; Reproduction
Reference: McKinney et al. (2018), pp. 405-406.

257. *Answer:* 2
Rationale: Precipitous labor is labor that lasts 3 hours or less. Women who have experienced precipitous labor often describe feelings of disbelief that their labor progressed so rapidly. To assist the client to process what has happened, the best option is to support the client in her reaction to the newborn infant. Options 1, 3, and 4 do not acknowledge the client's feelings.
Test-Taking Strategy: Use **therapeutic communication techniques**. The correct option is the only option that acknowledges the client's feelings.
Level of Cognitive Ability: Applying
Client Needs: Psychosocial Integrity
Integrated Process: Caring
Content Area: Maternity: Postpartum
Health Problem: Maternity: Precipitous Labor and Delivery
Priority Concepts: Caregiving; Reproduction
Reference: McKinney et al. (2018), pp. 27-28, 579.

CHAPTER 26

Postpartum Complications

PRIORITY CONCEPTS Caregiving, Reproduction

I. Cystitis

A. Description: Cystitis, an infection of the bladder, can occur in the postpartum period, and the postpartum woman should be encouraged to consume adequate fluids and void frequently to avoid bladder distention.

B. Assessment and interventions (refer to Chapter 54)

> If a urine specimen for culture and sensitivity is prescribed, obtain the specimen by straight catheterization (if prescribed) before initiating antibiotic therapy.

II. Hematoma

A. Description
1. A hematoma is a localized collection of blood in the tissues and can occur internally, involving the vaginal sulcus or other organs; vulvar hematomas are the most common (Fig. 26-1).
2. Predisposing conditions include operative delivery with forceps and injury to a blood vessel.
3. A hematoma can result in shock.

B. Assessment
1. Abnormal, severe pain not relieved with treatment or comfort measures
2. Pressure in the perineal area
3. Sensitive, bulging mass in the perineal area with discolored skin
4. Inability to void
5. Decreased hemoglobin and hematocrit levels
6. Restlessness; changes in vital signs indicating shock such as tachycardia and hypotension

C. Interventions
1. Monitor client for abnormal pain or perineal pressure, especially when forceps delivery has occurred.
2. Monitor vital signs and for signs of shock.
3. Place ice at the hematoma site.
4. Administer analgesics as prescribed.
5. Prepare for urinary catheterization if the client is unable to void.
6. Administer blood products as prescribed.
7. Monitor for signs of infection, such as increased temperature, pulse rate, and white blood cell count.
8. Administer antibiotics as prescribed because infection is common after hematoma formation.
9. Prepare for incision and evacuation of hematoma if necessary.

III. Uterine Atony

A. Description: A poorly contracted uterus that does not adequately compress large open vessels at the placental site; this can result in hemorrhage. This can involve the anterior, posterior, or both areas of the uterus.

B. Assessment: A soft (boggy) uterus noted on palpation of the uterine fundus

C. Interventions
1. Massage the uterus until firm (Fig. 26-2).
2. Empty the woman's bladder (by voiding or catheterization) if that is contributing to the uterine atony.
3. Notify the obstetrician (OB) if interventions do not resolve the atony, because this could be an indication of hemorrhage.

IV. Hemorrhage and Shock

A. Description
1. Bleeding of greater than 1000 mL or more after delivery or a 10% drop in hemoglobin and hematocrit from admission to postdelivery with signs and symptoms of hemorrhage.
2. Can occur early during the first 24 hours after delivery or later after the first 24 hours following delivery
3. Early postpartum hemorrhage is within the first 4 hours postpartum.
4. Late postpartum hemorrhage is anything beyond 4 hours postpartum.
5. While postpartum hemorrhage can occur any time during the postpartum period, the greatest risk is during the 4 hours immediately after delivery, and the second greatest risk is the first 24 hours following delivery.
6. Causes and predisposing factors (Box 26-1)

B. Assessment
1. Persistent significant bleeding: Perineal pad is soaked within 15 minutes.

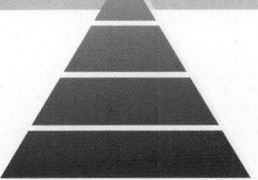

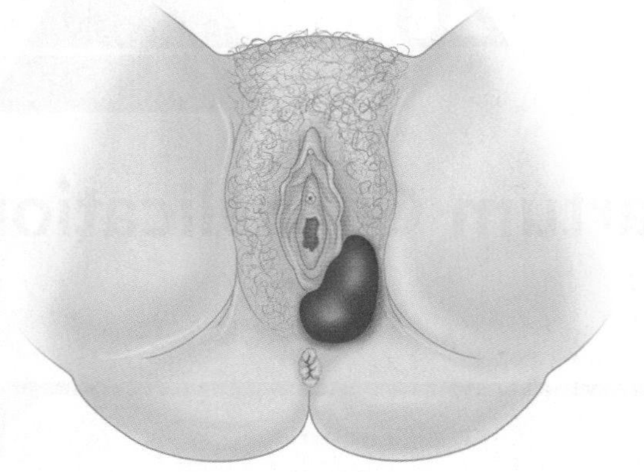

FIG. 26-1 A vulvar hematoma is caused by rapid bleeding into soft tissue. It causes severe pain and feelings of pressure.

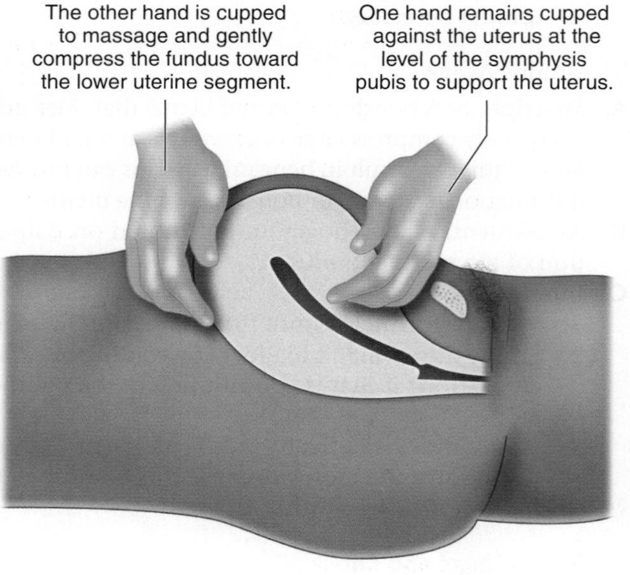
The other hand is cupped to massage and gently compress the fundus toward the lower uterine segment.
One hand remains cupped against the uterus at the level of the symphysis pubis to support the uterus.

FIG. 26-2 Technique for fundal massage.

BOX 26-1 Postpartum Hemorrhage

Causes

- Uterine atony
- Laceration of the cervix or vagina
- Hematoma development in the cervix, perineum, or labia
- Retained placental fragments

Predisposing Factors

- Previous history of postpartum hemorrhage
- Placenta previa
- Abruptio placentae
- Overdistention of the uterus—polyhydramnios, multiple gestation, large neonate
- Infection
- Multiparity
- Dystocia or labor that is prolonged
- Operative delivery—cesarean or forceps delivery, intrauterine manipulation

2. Restlessness and increased pulse rate (earlier signs), decrease in blood pressure, cool and clammy skin, ashen or grayish color
3. Complaints of weakness, lightheadedness, dyspnea

C. Interventions: See Priority Nursing Actions

PRIORITY NURSING ACTIONS

Hemorrhage and Shock in the Postpartum Client

1. Notify the obstetrician (OB); stay with the client and ask another nurse to contact the OB.
2. If uterus is atonic, massage firmly to cause it to contract.
3. Elevate her legs to at least a 30-degree angle.
4. Administer oxygen by nonrebreather face mask at 8 to 10 L/min.
5. Monitor vital signs and empty the bladder by catheterization if prescribed.
6. Administer uterotonic medications (e.g., oxytocin, prostaglandins) as prescribed to increase uterine tone.
7. Provide additional or maintain existing intravenous (IV) infusion of lactated Ringer's solution or normal saline solution to restore circulatory volume (woman should have 2 patent IV lines; insert the second IV line using 16- to 18-gauge IV catheter).
8. Administer blood or blood products as prescribed.
9. Insert an indwelling urinary catheter to monitor perfusion of kidneys.
10. Administer emergency medications as prescribed.
11. Prepare for possible surgery or other emergency treatments or procedures.
12. Record event, interventions instituted, and woman's response to interventions.

Reference

Lowdermilk et al. (2016), pp. 439, 486, 808-809.

V. Infection

A. Description: Any infection of the reproductive organs that occurs within 28 days of delivery or abortion; endometritis is inflammation/infection of the inner lining of the uterus.

B. Assessment
1. Fever
2. Chills
3. Anorexia
4. Pelvic discomfort or pain
5. Vaginal discharge that is malodorous; normal vaginal discharge has a fleshy odor or an odor similar to a menstrual period.
6. Elevated white blood cell count

A temperature up to 100.4° F (38° C) is normal during the first 24 hours postpartum because of dehydration; a temperature of 100.4° F (38° C) or greater after 24 hours postpartum indicates infection.

C. Interventions
1. Monitor vital signs and temperature every 2 to 4 hours.
2. Make the client as comfortable as possible; position the client to promote vaginal drainage.
3. Keep the client warm if chilled.
4. Isolate the newborn from the client only if the client can infect the newborn, such as with an airborne illness.
5. Provide a nutritious, high-calorie, high-protein diet.
6. Encourage fluids to 3000 to 4000 mL/day, if not contraindicated.
7. Encourage frequent voiding and monitor intake and output.
8. Monitor culture results if cultures were prescribed.
9. Administer antibiotics according to identified organism, as prescribed.

VI. Mastitis

A. Description
1. Mastitis is inflammation of the breast as a result of a blocked duct and infection.
2. Mastitis occurs primarily in breast-feeding mothers 2 to 3 weeks after delivery but may occur at any time during lactation.

B. Assessment (Fig. 26-3)
1. Localized heat and swelling
2. Pain; tender axillary lymph nodes
3. Elevated temperature
4. Complaints of flu-like symptoms

C. Interventions
1. Instruct the client in good hand-washing and breast hygiene techniques.
2. Promote comfort.
3. Apply heat to the site as prescribed.
4. Maintain lactation in breast-feeding mothers.
5. Encourage manual expression of breast milk or use of a breast pump every 3 to 4 hours.
6. Encourage the client to support the breasts by wearing a supportive bra; avoid wearing an underwire bra.
7. Administer analgesics as prescribed.
8. Administer antibiotics as prescribed.

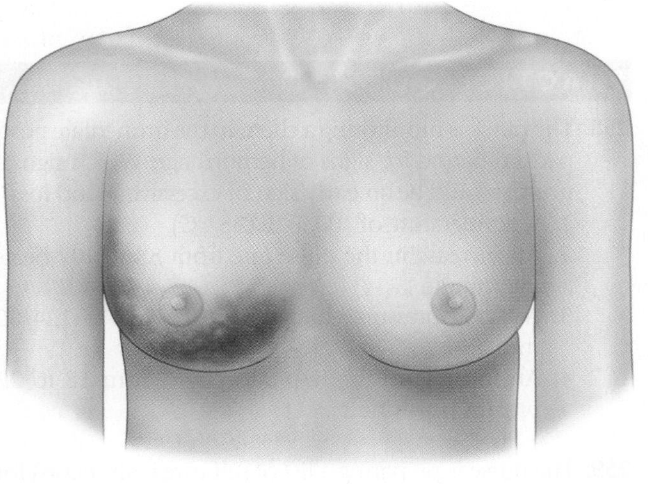

FIG. 26-3 Mastitis.

VII. Pulmonary Embolism

A. Description: Passage of a thrombus, often originating in a uterine or other pelvic vein, into the lungs, where it disrupts the circulation of the blood

B. Assessment
1. Sudden dyspnea and chest pain
2. Tachypnea and tachycardia
3. Cough and lung crackles
4. Hemoptysis
5. Feeling of impending doom

C. Interventions
1. Administer oxygen.
2. Position the client with the head of the bed elevated.
3. Monitor vital signs frequently, especially respiratory and heart rate and breath sounds.
4. Monitor for signs of respiratory distress and for signs of increasing hypoxemia.
5. Administer intravenous fluids as prescribed.
6. Administer anticoagulants as prescribed.
7. Prepare to assist the primary health care provider to administer medications to dissolve the clot, if prescribed.

VIII. Subinvolution

A. Description: Incomplete involution or failure of the uterus to return to its normal size and condition

B. Assessment
1. Uterine pain on palpation
2. Uterus larger than expected
3. More than normal vaginal bleeding

C. Interventions
1. Assess vital signs.
2. Assess uterus and fundus.
3. Monitor for uterine pain and vaginal bleeding.
4. Elevate legs to promote venous return.
5. Encourage frequent voiding.
6. Monitor hemoglobin and hematocrit.
7. Prepare to administer methylergonovine maleate, which provides sustained contraction of the uterus, as prescribed.

IX. Thrombophlebitis

A. Description
1. A clot forms in a vessel wall as a result of inflammation of the vessel wall.
2. A partial obstruction of the vessel can occur.
3. Increased blood-clotting factors in the postpartum period place the client at risk.
4. Early ambulation in the postoperative period after cesarean section is a preventive measure.

Maternity

B. Types
1. Superficial thrombophlebitis
2. Femoral thrombophlebitis
3. Pelvic thrombophlebitis

C. Assessment (Box 26-2)

D. Interventions
1. Specific therapies may depend on the location of thrombophlebitis.
2. Assess the lower extremities for edema, tenderness, varices, and increased skin temperature.
3. Maintain bed rest.
4. Elevate the affected leg.
5. Apply a bed cradle and keep bedclothes off the affected leg.
6. Never massage the leg.
7. Monitor for manifestations of pulmonary embolism.
8. Apply hot packs or moist heat to the affected site as prescribed to alleviate discomfort.
9. Apply elastic stockings (support hose) if prescribed.
10. Administer analgesics and antibiotics as prescribed.
11. Heparin sodium intravenously may be prescribed for femoral or pelvic thrombophlebitis to prevent further thrombus formation.

E. Client education (Box 26-3)

X. Perinatal Loss

A. Description
1. Perinatal loss is associated with miscarriage, neonatal death, stillbirth, and therapeutic abortion.
2. Loss and grief also may occur with the birth of a preterm baby, a **newborn** with complications of birth, or a newborn with congenital anomalies; it also may occur in a client who is giving up a child for adoption.

BOX 26-2 Assessment of Types of Thrombophlebitis

Superficial
- Palpable thrombus that feels bumpy and hard
- Tenderness and pain in affected lower extremity
- Warm and pinkish red color over the thrombus area

Femoral
- Malaise
- Chills and fever
- Diminished peripheral pulses
- Shiny white skin over affected area
- Pain, stiffness, and swelling of affected leg

Pelvic
- Severe chills
- Dramatic body temperature changes
- Pulmonary embolism may be the first sign

BOX 26-3 Client Education for Thrombophlebitis

- Never massage the leg.
- Avoid crossing the legs.
- Avoid prolonged sitting.
- Avoid constrictive clothing.
- Avoid pressure behind the knees.
- Know how to apply elastic stockings (support hose) if prescribed.
- Understand the importance of compliance with anticoagulant therapy if prescribed.
- Understand the importance of follow-up with the health care provider.

B. Interventions

Not all interventions are appropriate for every woman and her family who has experienced perinatal loss. It is crucial to consider religious, spiritual, and cultural health care practices and beliefs when planning care for a woman and family who have experienced perinatal loss.

1. Communicate therapeutically and actively listen, providing parents time to grieve.
2. Notify the hospital chaplain or other religious person as appropriate.
3. Discuss with the parents options such as seeing, holding, bathing, or dressing the deceased infant; visitation by other family members or friends; religious, spiritual, or cultural rituals; and funeral arrangements.
4. Prepare a special memories box with keepsakes such as footprints, handprints, locks of hair, and pictures, if appropriate.
5. Admit the mother to a private room; if possible, mark the door to the room with a special card (per agency procedure and maintaining confidentiality) that denotes to hospital staff that this family has experienced a loss.
6. See Chapter 24 for additional information on intrauterine fetal demise.

PRACTICE QUESTIONS

258. The nurse is monitoring a client in the immediate postpartum period for signs of hemorrhage. Which sign, if noted, would be an **early** sign of excessive blood loss?
1. A temperature of 100.4° F (38° C)
2. An increase in the pulse rate from 88 to 102 beats per minute
3. A blood pressure change from 130/88 to 124/80 mm Hg
4. An increase in the respiratory rate from 18 to 22 breaths per minute

259. The nurse is preparing a list of self-care instructions for a postpartum client who was diagnosed with mastitis.

Which instructions should be included on the list? **Select all that apply.**
- ☐ 1. Wear a supportive bra.
- ☐ 2. Rest during the acute phase.
- ☐ 3. Maintain a fluid intake of at least 3000 mL/day.
- ☐ 4. Continue to breast-feed if the breasts are not too sore.
- ☐ 5. Take the prescribed antibiotics until the soreness subsides.
- ☐ 6. Avoid decompression of the breasts by breast-feeding or breast pump.

260. The nurse is providing instructions about measures to prevent postpartum mastitis to a client who is breast-feeding her newborn. Which client statement would indicate a **need for further instruction?**
1. "I should breast-feed every 2 to 3 hours."
2. "I should change the breast pads frequently."
3. "I should wash my hands well before breast-feeding."
4. "I should wash my nipples daily with soap and water."

261. The postpartum nurse is assessing a client who delivered a healthy infant by cesarean section for signs and symptoms of superficial venous thrombosis. Which sign should the nurse note if superficial venous thrombosis were present?
1. Paleness of the calf area
2. Coolness of the calf area
3. Enlarged, hardened veins
4. Palpable dorsalis pedis pulses

262. A client in a postpartum unit complains of sudden sharp chest pain and dyspnea. The nurse notes that the client is tachycardic and the respiratory rate is elevated. The nurse suspects a pulmonary embolism. Which should be the **initial** nursing action?
1. Initiate an intravenous line.
2. Assess the client's blood pressure.
3. Prepare to administer morphine sulfate.
4. Administer oxygen, 8 to 10 L/minute, by face mask.

263. The nurse is assessing a client in the fourth stage of labor and notes that the fundus is firm, but that bleeding is excessive. Which should be the **initial** nursing action?
1. Record the findings.
2. Massage the fundus.
3. Notify the obstetrician (OB).
4. Place the client in Trendelenburg's position.

264. The nurse is preparing to care for four assigned clients. Which client is at **most** risk for hemorrhage?
1. A primiparous client who delivered 4 hours ago
2. A multiparous client who delivered 6 hours ago
3. A multiparous client who delivered a large baby after oxytocin induction
4. A primiparous client who delivered 6 hours ago and had epidural anesthesia

265. A postpartum client is diagnosed with cystitis. The nurse should plan for which **priority** action in the care of the client?
1. Providing sitz baths
2. Encouraging fluid intake
3. Placing ice on the perineum
4. Monitoring hemoglobin and hematocrit levels

266. The nurse is monitoring a postpartum client who received epidural anesthesia for delivery for the presence of a vulvar hematoma. Which assessment finding would **best** indicate the presence of a hematoma?
1. Changes in vital signs
2. Signs of heavy bruising
3. Complaints of intense pain
4. Complaints of a tearing sensation

267. The nurse is creating a plan of care for a postpartum client with a small vulvar hematoma. The nurse should include which specific action during the first 12 hours after delivery?
1. Encourage ambulation hourly.
2. Assess vital signs every 4 hours.
3. Measure fundal height every 4 hours.
4. Prepare an ice pack for application to the area.

268. On assessment of a postpartum client, the nurse notes that the uterus feels soft and boggy. The nurse should take which **initial** action?
1. Document the findings.
2. Elevate the client's legs.
3. Massage the fundus until it is firm.
4. Push on the uterus to assist in expressing clots.

ANSWERS

258. *Answer:* 2

Rationale: During the fourth stage of labor, the maternal blood pressure, pulse, and respiration should be checked every 15 minutes during the first hour. An increasing pulse is an early sign of excessive blood loss because the heart pumps faster to compensate for reduced blood volume. A slight increase in temperature is normal. The blood pressure decreases as the blood volume diminishes, but a decreased blood pressure would not be the earliest sign of hemorrhage. The respiratory rate is slightly increased from normal.

Test-Taking Strategy: Note the strategic word, *early*. Think about the physiological occurrences of hemorrhage and shock and the expected findings in the postpartum period. This should assist in directing you to the correct option.

Level of Cognitive Ability: Analyzing
Client Needs: Physiological Integrity
Integrated Process: Nursing Process—Assessment
Content Area: Maternity: Postpartum
Health Problem: Maternity: Postpartum Uterine Problems
Priority Concepts: Clotting; Perfusion
Reference: McKinney et al. (2018), p. 604.

259. *Answer:* 1, 2, 3, 4

Rationale: Mastitis is an inflammation of the lactating breast as a result of infection. Client instructions include resting during the acute phase, maintaining a fluid intake of at least 3000 mL/day (if not contraindicated), and taking analgesics to relieve discomfort. Antibiotics may be prescribed and are taken until the complete prescribed course is finished. They are not stopped when the soreness subsides. Additional supportive measures include the use of moist heat or ice packs and wearing a supportive bra. Continued decompression of the breast by breast-feeding or breast pump is important to empty the breast and prevent the formation of an abscess.

Test-Taking Strategy: Focus on the subject, treatment measures for mastitis. Think about the pathophysiology associated with mastitis to answer correctly. Recalling that supportive measures include rest, moist heat or ice packs, antibiotics, analgesics, increased fluid intake, breast support, and decompression of the breasts will assist in answering the question.

Level of Cognitive Ability: Applying
Client Needs: Physiological Integrity
Integrated Process: Teaching and Learning
Content Area: Maternity: Postpartum
Health Problem: Maternity: Infection/Inflammation
Priority Concepts: Client Education; Inflammation
Reference: McKinney et al. (2018), pp. 611-612.

260. *Answer:* 4

Rationale: Mastitis is inflammation of the breast as a result of infection. It generally is caused by an organism that enters through an injured area of the nipples, such as a crack or blister. Measures to prevent the development of mastitis include changing nursing pads when they are wet and avoiding continuous pressure on the breasts. Soap is drying and could lead to cracking of the nipples, and the client should be instructed to avoid using soap on the nipples. The mother is taught about the importance of hand washing and that she should breast-feed every 2 to 3 hours.

Test-Taking Strategy: Note the strategic words, *need for further instruction*. These words indicate a negative event query and the need to select the option that identifies the incorrect client statement. Recalling that the use of soap is drying to the skin and could cause cracking and provide an entry point for organisms will direct you easily to the correct option.

Level of Cognitive Ability: Evaluating
Client Needs: Health Promotion and Maintenance
Integrated Process: Teaching and Learning
Content Area: Maternity: Postpartum
Health Problem: Maternity: Infection/Inflammation
Priority Concepts: Client Education; Inflammation
Reference: Lowdermilk et al. (2016), pp. 625, 813.

261. *Answer:* 3

Rationale: Thrombosis of superficial veins usually is accompanied by signs and symptoms of inflammation, including swelling, redness, tenderness, and warmth of the involved extremity. It also may be possible to palpate the enlarged, hard vein. Clients sometimes experience pain when they walk. Palpable dorsalis pedis pulses is a normal finding.

Test-Taking Strategy: Eliminate option 4 first because this is a normal and expected finding. Next, eliminate options 1 and 2 because they are comparable or alike.

Level of Cognitive Ability: Analyzing
Client Needs: Physiological Integrity
Integrated Process: Nursing Process—Assessment
Content Area: Maternity: Postpartum
Health Problem: Maternity: Infection/Inflammation
Priority Concepts: Clotting; Perfusion
Reference: McKinney et al. (2018), p. 612.

262. *Answer:* 4

Rationale: If pulmonary embolism is suspected, oxygen should be administered, 8 to 10 L/minute, by face mask. Oxygen is used to decrease hypoxia. The client also is kept on bed rest with the head of the bed slightly elevated to reduce dyspnea. Morphine sulfate may be prescribed for the client, but this would not be the initial nursing action. An intravenous line also will be required, and vital signs need to be monitored, but these actions would follow the administration of oxygen.

Test-Taking Strategy: Note the strategic word, *initial*. Use the ABCs—airway, breathing, and circulation—to assist in directing you to the correct option.

Level of Cognitive Ability: Analyzing
Client Needs: Physiological Integrity
Integrated Process: Nursing Process—Implementation
Content Area: Complex Care: Emergency Situations/Management
Health Problem: Adult Health: Respiratory: Pulmonary Embolism
Priority Concepts: Gas Exchange; Perfusion
Reference: McKinney et al. (2018), pp. 608-609.

263. *Answer:* 3

Rationale: If bleeding is excessive, the cause may be laceration of the cervix or birth canal. Massaging the fundus if it is firm would not assist in controlling the bleeding. Trendelenburg's position should be avoided because it may interfere with cardiac and respiratory function. Although the nurse would record the findings, the initial nursing action would be to notify the OB.

Test-Taking Strategy: Note the strategic word, *initial.* Focus on the data in the question, noting the clinical manifestations identified in the question. Eliminate option 2 first because, if the uterus is firm, it would not be necessary to perform fundal massage. Knowing that Trendelenburg's position interferes with cardiac and respiratory function will assist in eliminating option 4. From the remaining options, noting the words *bleeding is excessive* will assist in directing you to the correct option.
Level of Cognitive Ability: Analyzing
Client Needs: Physiological Integrity
Integrated Process: Nursing Process—Implementation
Content Area: Complex Care: Emergency Situations/ Management
Health Problem: Maternity: Hematoma and Hemorrhage
Priority Concepts: Clinical Judgment; Clotting
Reference: McKinney et al. (2018), pp. 604-605.

264. *Answer:* 3
Rationale: The causes of postpartum hemorrhage include uterine atony; laceration of the vagina; hematoma development in the cervix, perineum, or labia; and retained placental fragments. Predisposing factors for hemorrhage include a previous history of postpartum hemorrhage, placenta previa, abruptio placentae, overdistention of the uterus from polyhydramnios, multiple gestation, a large neonate, infection, multiparity, dystocia or labor that is prolonged, operative delivery such as a cesarean or forceps delivery, and intrauterine manipulation. The multiparous client who delivered a large fetus after oxytocin induction has more risk factors associated with postpartum hemorrhage than do other clients. In addition, there are no specific data in the client descriptions in options 1, 2, and 4 that present the risk for hemorrhage.
Test-Taking Strategy: Note the strategic word, *most.* Focus on the subject, the client at most risk for hemorrhage. Read the client description in each option. Noting the words *large* and *oxytocin* in the correct option will direct you to this option.
Level of Cognitive Ability: Analyzing
Client Needs: Physiological Integrity
Integrated Process: Nursing Process—Assessment
Content Area: Maternity: Postpartum
Health Problem: Maternity: Hematoma and Hemorrhage
Priority Concepts: Clinical Judgment; Clotting
Reference: Lowdermilk et al. (2016), pp. 486, 810.

265. *Answer:* 2
Rationale: Cystitis is an infection of the bladder. The client should consume 3000 mL of fluids per day if not contraindicated. Sitz baths and ice would be appropriate interventions for perineal discomfort. Hemoglobin and hematocrit levels would be monitored with hemorrhage.
Test-Taking Strategy: Focus on the subject, measures to treat cystitis, and note the strategic word, *priority.* Remember that increased fluids are a priority intervention.
Level of Cognitive Ability: Applying
Client Needs: Physiological Integrity
Integrated Process: Nursing Process—Implementation
Content Area: Maternity: Postpartum
Health Problem: Maternity: Infection/Inflammation
Priority Concepts: Elimination; Infection
Reference: McKinney et al. (2018), p. 611.

266. *Answer:* 1
Rationale: Because the client has had epidural anesthesia and is anesthetized, she cannot feel pain, pressure, or a tearing sensation. Changes in vital signs indicate hypovolemia in an anesthetized postpartum client with vulvar hematoma. Option 2 (heavy bruising) may be seen, but vital sign changes indicate hematoma caused by blood collection in the perineal tissues.
Test-Taking Strategy: Note the strategic word, *best.* Also note that the client received epidural anesthesia. With this in mind, eliminate options 3 and 4. From the remaining options, use the ABCs—airway, breathing, and circulation—to direct you to the correct option.
Level of Cognitive Ability: Analyzing
Client Needs: Physiological Integrity
Integrated Process: Nursing Process—Assessment
Content Area: Maternity: Postpartum
Health Problem: Maternity: Hematoma and Hemorrhage
Priority Concepts: Clinical Judgment; Clotting
Reference: McKinney et al. (2018), p. 602.

267. *Answer:* 4
Rationale: A hematoma is a localized collection of blood in the tissues of the reproductive tissues after delivery. Vulvar hematoma is the most common. Application of ice reduces swelling caused by hematoma formation in the vulvar area. Options 1, 2, and 3 are not interventions that are specific to the plan of care for a client with a small vulvar hematoma. Ambulation hourly increases the risk for bleeding. Client assessment every 4 hours is too infrequent.
Test-Taking Strategy: Focus on the subject, a small vulvar hematoma. Think about the effect of each action in the options; this focus will assist in directing you to the correct option.
Level of Cognitive Ability: Creating
Client Needs: Physiological Integrity
Integrated Process: Nursing Process—Planning
Content Area: Maternity: Postpartum
Health Problem: Maternity: Hematoma and Hemorrhage
Priority Concepts: Clinical Judgment; Clotting
Reference: Lowdermilk et al. (2016), p. 804.

268. *Answer:* 3
Rationale: If the uterus is not contracted firmly (i.e., it is soft and boggy), the initial intervention is to massage the fundus until it is firm and to express clots that may have accumulated in the uterus. Elevating the client's legs would not assist in managing uterine atony. Documenting the findings is an appropriate action but is not the initial action. Pushing on an uncontracted uterus can invert the uterus and cause massive hemorrhage.
Test-Taking Strategy: Note the strategic word, *initial,* in the question. Focus on the subject, that the uterus is soft and boggy. Recalling the therapeutic management for uterine atony will assist in directing you to the correct option.
Level of Cognitive Ability: Applying
Client Needs: Physiological Integrity
Integrated Process: Nursing Process—Implementation
Content Area: Maternity: Postpartum
Health Problem: Maternity: Postpartum Uterine Problems
Priority Concepts: Clinical Judgment; Reproduction
Reference: McKinney et al. (2018), pp. 599-602.

CHAPTER 27

Care of the Newborn

PRIORITY CONCEPTS Development, Health Promotion

I. Initial Care of the Newborn

A. Assessment

1. Observe or assist with initiation of respirations.
2. Assess Apgar score.
3. Note characteristics of cry.
4. Monitor for nasal flaring, grunting, retractions, and abnormal respirations, such as a seesaw respiratory pattern (rise and fall of the chest and abdomen do not occur together).
5. Assess for central cyanosis and acrocyanosis.
6. Obtain vital signs.
7. Observe the newborn for signs of hypothermia or hyperthermia.
8. Assess for gross anomalies.

B. Interventions

1. Suction the mouth first and then the nares if needed with a bulb syringe.
2. Dry the newborn and stimulate crying by rubbing the back.
3. Maintain temperature stability; wrap the newborn in warm blankets and place a stockinette cap on the newborn's head.
4. Keep the newborn with the mother to facilitate bonding.
5. Place the newborn at the mother's breast if breast-feeding is planned, or place the newborn on the mother's chest for skin-to-skin.
6. Place the newborn in a radiant warmer.
7. Ensure the newborn's proper identification.
8. Footprint the newborn and fingerprint the mother on the identification sheet per agency policies and procedures; initiate other agency identification and safety procedures.
9. Place matching identification bracelets on the mother and the newborn.

C. Apgar scoring system

1. Assess each of 5 items to be scored and add the points to determine the newborn's total score.
2. Five vital indicators (Table 27-1)
3. Interventions: Apgar score (Table 27-2)

⚠ The newborn's Apgar score is routinely assessed and recorded at 1 minute and 5 minutes after birth, and may be repeated later if the score is and remains low.

II. Initial Physical Examination

A. General guidelines

1. Keep the newborn warm during the examination.
2. Begin with general observations, and then perform assessments that are least disturbing to the newborn first.
3. Initiate nursing interventions for abnormal findings and document findings.
4. The Ballard Scale may be used for gestational age assessment; in this scale, scores are assigned to physical and neurological criteria.

⚠ The phases of newborn instability occur during the first 6 to 8 hours after birth and are known as the transition period between intrauterine and extrauterine existence. These phases include the first period of reactivity, period of decreased responsiveness, and second period of reactivity.

B. Vital signs

1. Heart rate (resting): 110 to 160 beats per minute (apical), 90 to 110 beats per minute (if sleeping), up to 180 beats per minute (if crying); auscultate at the fourth intercostal space for 1 full minute to detect abnormalities.
2. Respirations: 30 to 60 breaths per minute; assess for 1 full minute.
3. Assess heart rate and respiratory rate first before assessing other vital signs while the newborn is resting or sleeping.
4. Axillary temperature: 97.7° F (36.5° C) to <100.3° F (37.9° C)
5. Blood pressure: Usually not done in term newborn unless a cardiac issue is suspected, 80 to 90/40 to 50 mm Hg

TABLE 27-1 Five Vital Indicators of Apgar Scoring

Indicator	0 Points	1 Point	2 Points
Heart rate	Absent	<100 beats per minute	≥100 beats per minute
Respiratory rate and effort	Absent	Slow, irregular breathing, weak cry	Good rate and effort, vigorous cry
Muscle tone	Flaccid, limp	Minimal flexion of extremities	Good flexion, active motion
Reflex irritability	No response	Minimal response (grimace) to suction or to gentle slap on soles	Responds promptly with a cry or active movement
Skin color	Pallor or cyanosis	Body skin color normal, extremities blue	Body and extremity skin color normal

TABLE 27-2 Apgar Score Interventions

Score	Intervention
8-10	No intervention required except to support newborn's spontaneous efforts
4-7	Stimulate; rub newborn's back; administer oxygen to newborn; rescore at specific intervals
0-3	Newborn requires full resuscitation; rescore at specific intervals

C. Body measurements (approximate)
1. Length: 18 to 22 inches (45 to 55 cm)
2. Weight: 2500 to 4000 g (5.5 to 8.75 lb)
3. Head circumference: 33 to 35 cm (13.2 to 14 inches)

D. Head
1. Head should be one-fourth of the body length (cephalocaudal development).
2. Bones of the skull are not fused.
3. Sutures (connective tissue between the skull bones) are palpable and may be overlapping because of head molding but should not be widened.
4. Fontanels are unossified membranous tissue at the junction of the sutures (Table 27-3).
5. Molding is asymmetry of the head resulting from pressure in the birth canal; molding disappears in about 72 hours (Fig. 27-1).

TABLE 27-3 Fontanels

Fontanel	Characteristics	Closure
Anterior	Soft, flat, diamond-shaped; 3-4 cm wide × 2-3 cm long	Between 12 and 18 mo of age
Posterior	Triangular; 0.5-1 cm wide Located between occipital and parietal bones	Between birth and 2-3 mo of age

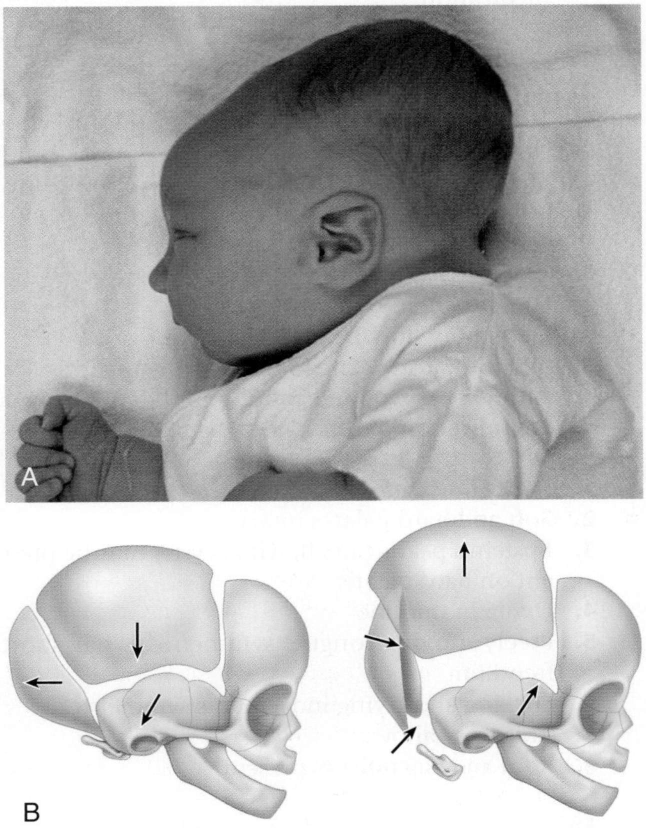

FIG. 27-1 Molding. **A**, Significant molding after vaginal birth. **B**, Schematic of bones of skull when molding is present. (**A**, From Perry et al, 2010. Courtesy Kim Molloy, Knoxville, Iowa.)

6. Masses from birth trauma
   a. Caput succedaneum is edema of the soft tissue over bone (crosses over suture line); it subsides within a few days.
   b. Cephalhematoma is swelling caused by bleeding into an area between the bone and its periosteum (does not cross over suture line); it usually is absorbed within 6 weeks with no treatment.
7. Head lag
   a. Common when pulling the newborn to a sitting position
   b. When prone, the newborn should be able to lift the head slightly and turn the head from side to side.

E. Eyes
1. Slate-gray (light skin), dark-blue, or brown-gray (dark skin)
2. Symmetrical and clear
3. Pupils equal, round, react to light and accommodation
4. Blink reflex present
5. Eyes cross because of weak extraocular muscles
6. Ability to track and fixate momentarily
7. Red reflex present
8. Eyelids often edematous as a result of pressure during the birth process and the effects of eye medication

F. Ears
1. Symmetrical
2. Firm cartilage with recoil
3. Top of pinna on or above line drawn from outer canthus of eye
4. Low-set ears associated with Down syndrome, renal anomalies, or other genetic or chromosomal syndromes

G. Nose
1. Flat, broad, in center of face
2. Obligatory nose breathing
3. Occasional sneezing to remove obstructions
4. Nares are patent and should not flare (flaring is an indication of respiratory distress).

H. Mouth
1. Pink, moist gums
2. Soft and hard palates intact
3. Epstein's pearls (small, white cysts) may be present on hard palate.
4. Uvula in midline
5. Freely moving tongue, symmetrical, has short frenulum
6. Sucking and crying movements symmetrical
7. Able to swallow
8. Root and gag reflexes present

When assessing the newborn's mouth, look for the presence of thrush (*Candida albicans*), which are white patchy areas on the tongue or gums that cannot be removed with a washcloth; these may be painful.

I. Neck
1. Short and thick
2. Head held in midline
3. Trachea midline
4. Good range of motion and ability to flex and extend
5. Assess for torticollis (head inclined to 1 side as a result of contraction of muscles on that side of the neck)

J. Chest
1. Circular appearance because anteroposterior and lateral diameters are about equal (approximately 30 to 33 cm [12 to 13.2 inches] at birth)
2. Diaphragmatic respirations—chest and abdomen should rise and fall in synchrony, not in a seesaw pattern
3. Bronchial sounds heard on auscultation
4. Nipples prominent and often edematous; milky secretion (witch's milk) common
5. Breast tissue present
6. Clavicles need to be palpated to assess for fractures.

K. Skin
1. Pinkish red (light-skinned newborn) to pinkish brown or pinkish yellow (dark-skinned newborn)
2. Vernix caseosa, a cheesy white substance, on entire body in preterm newborns, but is more prominent between folds closer to term; may be absent after 42 weeks of gestation
3. Lanugo, fine body hair, might be seen, especially on the back.
4. Milia, small white sebaceous glands, appear on the forehead, nose, and chin.
5. Dry, peeling skin, increased in postmature newborns
6. Dark-red color (plethoric) common in premature newborns
7. Cyanosis may be noted with hypothermia, infection, and hypoglycemia and with cardiac, respiratory, or neurological abnormalities.
8. Acrocyanosis (peripheral cyanosis of hands and feet) is normal in the first few hours after birth and may be noted intermittently for the next 7 to 10 days (Fig. 27-2).
9. Assess for ecchymosis and petechiae resulting from trauma of birth.
10. Assess skin turgor over the abdomen to determine hydration status.
11. Observe for forceps marks.
12. Harlequin sign
    a. Deep pink or red color develops over 1 side of newborn's body while the other side remains pale or of normal color.
    b. Harlequin sign may indicate shunting of blood that occurs with a cardiac problem or may indicate sepsis.
13. Birthmarks (Table 27-4)

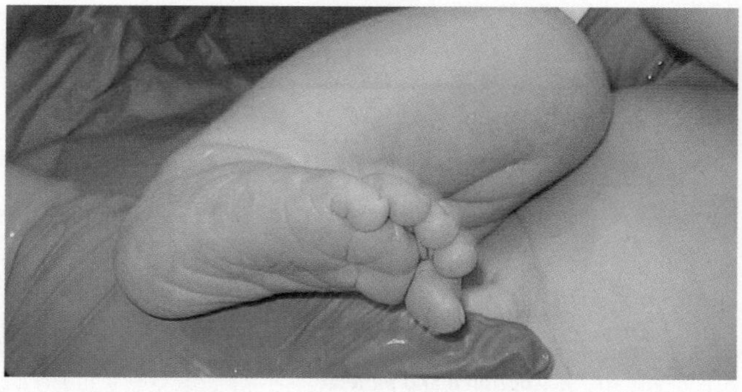

FIG. 27-2 Acrocyanosis. (From McKinney et al., 2013. Courtesy Todd Shiros, Santa Fe Springs, California.)

TABLE 27-4 Birthmarks

Birthmark	Characteristics
Telangiectatic nevi (stork bites)	Pale pink or red, flat, dilated capillaries On eyelids, nose, lower occipital bone, and nape of neck Blanch easily More noticeable during crying periods Disappear by age 2 yr
Nevus flammeus (port-wine stain)	Capillary angioma directly below epidermis Nonelevated, sharply demarcated, red to purple, dense areas of capillaries Commonly appear on face No fading with time May require future surgery
Nevus vasculosus (strawberry mark)	Capillary hemangioma Raised, clearly delineated, dark red, with rough surface Common in head region Disappears by age 7-9 yr
Mongolian spots	Bluish-black pigmentation On lumbar dorsal area and buttocks Gradually fade during first and second years of life Common in Asian and dark-skinned individuals

L. Abdomen
1. Umbilical cord
   a. Umbilical cord should have 3 vessels—2 arteries and 1 vein; if fewer than 3 vessels are noted, notify the primary health care provider (PHCP).
   b. While a 2-vessel cord (1 artery, 1 vein) may present no problems or concerns, there is a higher correlation to intrauterine growth restriction (IUGR) and genetic or chromosomal problems.
   c. Small, thin cord may be associated with poor fetal growth.
   d. Assess for intact cord and ensure that the cord clamp is secured.
   e. Cord should be clamped for at least the first 24 hours after birth; clamp can be removed when the cord is dried and occluded and is no longer bleeding.
   f. Note any bleeding or drainage from the cord.
   g. Cleansing of the cord needs to be done; hospital protocol and PHCP's preference determine the frequency, technique, and skin preparation used for cord care.
   h. If signs of infection, such as moistness, oozing, discharge, and a reddened base, occur, antibiotic treatment is prescribed.
2. Gastrointestinal
   a. Monitor cord for meconium staining.
   b. Assess for umbilical hernia.
   c. Assess for abdominal depression associated with diaphragmatic hernia.
   d. Assess for abdominal distention associated with obstruction, mass, or sepsis.
   e. Monitor bowel sounds (present within the first hour after birth).
3. Anus
   a. Ensure that the anal opening is present.
   b. First stool meconium should pass within first 24 hours.

M. Genitals
1. Female
   a. Labia may be swollen; clitoris may be enlarged.
   b. Smegma may be present (thick, white mucus discharge).
   c. Pseudomenstruation, caused by the withdrawal of the maternal hormone estrogen, is possible (blood-tinged mucus).
   d. Hymen tag may be visible.
   e. First voiding should occur within 24 hours.
2. Male
   a. Prepuce (foreskin) covers glans penis.
   b. Scrotum may be edematous.
   c. Verify meatus at tip of penis.
   d. Testes are descended but may retract with cold.
   e. Assess for hernia or hydrocele.
   f. First voiding should occur within 24 hours.

N. Spine
1. Straight
2. Posture flexed
3. Supportive of head momentarily when prone
4. Chin flexed on upper chest
5. Well-coordinated, sporadic movements
6. A degree of hypotonicity or hypertonicity may indicate central nervous system damage.
7. Assess for hair tufts and dimples along the spinal column (may be indicative of a possible opening).

O. Extremities
1. Flexed
2. Full range of motion; symmetrical movements
3. Fists clenched
4. Ten fingers and 10 toes, all separate
5. Legs bowed
6. Major gluteal folds even
7. Creases on soles of feet
8. Assess for fractures (especially clavicle) or dislocations (hip).
9. Assist PHCP to assess for developmental dysplasia of the hip; when thighs are rotated outward, no clicks should be heard (Ortolani's sign and Barlow's sign are the 2 assessment tools for developmental dysplasia of the hip).
10. Pulses palpable (radial, brachial, femoral)

Slight tremors noted in the newborn may be a common finding but could also be a sign of hypoglycemia, hypocalcemia, or drug withdrawal.

III. Body Systems Assessment and Interventions

A. Cardiovascular system
1. Keep the newborn warm.
2. Measure the apical heart rate for 1 full minute.
3. Listen for murmurs; assess oxygen saturation via pulse oximetry if a murmur is heard.
4. Palpate pulses.
5. Assess for cyanosis; blanch the skin on the trunk and extremities to assess circulation.
6. Observe for cardiac distress when the newborn is feeding.

B. Respiratory system
1. Suction the airway as necessary: Use a bulb syringe for upper airway suctioning (compress bulb before insertion) and a French catheter for deeper suctioning.
2. Observe for respiratory distress and hypoxemia.
   a. Nasal flaring
   b. Increasingly severe retractions
   c. Grunting
   d. Cyanosis
   e. Bradycardia and periods of apnea lasting longer than 15 seconds
3. Administer oxygen if necessary and as prescribed.

C. Hepatic system
1. Normal or physiological jaundice appears after the first 24 hours in full-term newborns and after the first 48 hours in premature newborns; jaundice occurring before this time (pathological jaundice) may indicate early hemolysis of red blood cells and must be reported to the PHCP.
2. Physiological jaundice peaks on about the fifth day of life (indirect bilirubin levels 6 to 7 mg/dL [90 to 105 mcmol/L).
3. Feed early to stimulate intestinal activity and to keep the bilirubin level low.
4. Prevent chilling because hypothermia can cause acidosis that interferes with bilirubin conjugation and excretion.
5. Liver stores the iron passed from the mother for 5 to 6 months.
6. Glycogen storage occurs in the liver.
7. The newborn is at risk for hemorrhagic disorders; coagulation factors synthesized in the liver depend on vitamin K, which is not synthesized until intestinal bacteria are present.
8. Handle the newborn carefully and monitor for any bruising or bleeding episodes.
9. Watch for meconium stool and subsequent stools.
10. Administer intramuscular dose of phytonadione to the newborn as prescribed to prevent hemorrhagic disorders (usually 0.5 to 1 mg is prescribed); administer in lateral aspect of the middle third of the vastus lateralis muscle (see Chapter 41).
11. Assess the newborn's hemoglobin and blood glucose levels.

D. Renal system
1. The immature kidneys are unable to concentrate urine.
2. A weight loss of 5% to 10% during the first week of life occurs as a result of water loss and limited intake; birth weight should be regained by 10 to 14 days after birth.
3. Weigh the newborn daily.
4. Monitor intake and output; weigh diapers if necessary (1 g of diaper weight equals 1 mL of urine).
5. If the diaper requires weighing, record the weight before putting it on the newborn; after the newborn voids, reweigh the diaper and subtract the prevoided weight.
6. Assess for signs of dehydration (dry mucous membranes, sunken eyeballs, poor skin turgor, sunken fontanels).

E. Immune system
1. Newborn receives passive immunity via the placenta (immunoglobulin G).
2. Newborn receives passive immunity from colostrum (immunoglobulin A).
3. Elevations in immunoglobulin M indicate infection in utero.
4. Use aseptic technique and standard precautions when caring for the newborn.
5. Ensure meticulous handwashing.
6. Ensure that an infection-free staff cares for the newborn.
7. Monitor the newborn's temperature.
8. Observe for any cracks or openings in the skin.
9. Administer eye medication within 1 hour after birth to prevent ophthalmia neonatorum (see Chapter 28).
10. Provide cord care.
    a. Umbilical clamp can be removed after 24 hours if cord is dried and occluded and is not bleeding.
    b. Teach the mother how to perform cord care.
    c. Keep the cord clean and dry; alcohol wipes may be prescribed for cleaning the cord only if it becomes soiled.
    d. Keep the diaper from covering the cord; fold the diaper below the cord.
    e. Assess the cord for odor, edema, or discharge.
    f. The newborn is typically washed via a sponge bath until the cord falls off (within 7 to 10 days). Follow alternate instructions if provided by PHCP.
11. Provide circumcision care.
    a. Apply petroleum jelly gauze to the penis except when a PlastiBell is used.

b. Remove petroleum jelly gauze, if applied, after the first voiding following circumcision.
c. Observe for edema, infection, or bleeding from the circumcision site.
d. Teach the mother how to care for the circumcision site.
e. Clean the penis after each voiding by squeezing warm water over the penis.
f. A milky covering over the glans penis is normal and should not be disrupted.
g. Monitor for urinary retention. Educate the parents and caregivers that the newborn needs to void within 24 hours after the circumcision.

F. Metabolic system and gastrointestinal system

1. Newborns are able to digest simple carbohydrates but are unable to digest fats because of the lack of lipase.
2. Proteins may be broken down only partially, so they may serve as antigens and provoke an allergic reaction.
3. The newborn has a small stomach capacity (less than 10 mL at birth, increasing to about 90 mL by day 10), with rapid intestinal peristalsis (bowel emptying time is 2.5 to 3 hours).
4. Breast-feeding usually can begin immediately after birth; based on PHCP preference and agency protocols, bottle-fed newborns may be initially offered no more than 30 mL of formula.
5. Observe feeding reflexes, such as rooting, sucking, and swallowing.
6. Assist the mother with breast-feeding or formula feeding; breast-feeding should be done every 2 to 3 hours, and formula feeding (minimum of 30 mL, or 1 oz by day 3) should be done every 3 to 4 hours (or per PHCP preference or agency protocols).
7. Burp the newborn during and after feeding.
8. Assess for regurgitation or vomiting.
9. Position the newborn on the right side after feeding; however, the side-lying position is not recommended for sleep because this position makes it easy for the newborn to roll to the prone position (prone position is contraindicated because it increases the risk of sudden infant death syndrome). Turning the head to the right is another option.
10. Observe for normal stool and the passage of meconium.
a. Meconium stool, which is greenish black with a thick, sticky, tar-like consistency, usually is passed within the first 24 hours of life.
b. Transitional stool, the second type of stool excreted by the newborn, is greenish brown and of looser consistency than meconium.
c. Seedy, yellow stools are usually noted in breast-fed newborns; pale yellow to light-brown stools are usually seen in formula-fed newborns.

11. Perform a newborn screening test (including the test for phenylketonuria [PKU]) as prescribed before discharge after sufficient protein intake occurs; the newborn should be on formula or breast milk for 24 hours before screening.

G. Neurological system

1. Newborn head size is proportionally larger than that of an adult because of cephalocaudal development.
2. Myelinization of nerve fibers is incomplete, so primitive reflexes are present.
3. Fontanels are open to allow for brain growth.
4. Assess for abnormal head size and a bulging or depressed anterior fontanel.
5. Measure and graph the head circumference in relation to chest circumference and length.
6. Assess the newborn's movements, noting symmetry, posture, and abnormal movements.
7. Observe for jitteriness, marked tremors, and seizures.
8. Test the newborn's reflexes.
9. Assess for lethargy.
10. Assess pitch of cry.

H. Thermal regulatory system

1. Prevent cold stress (Fig. 27-3).

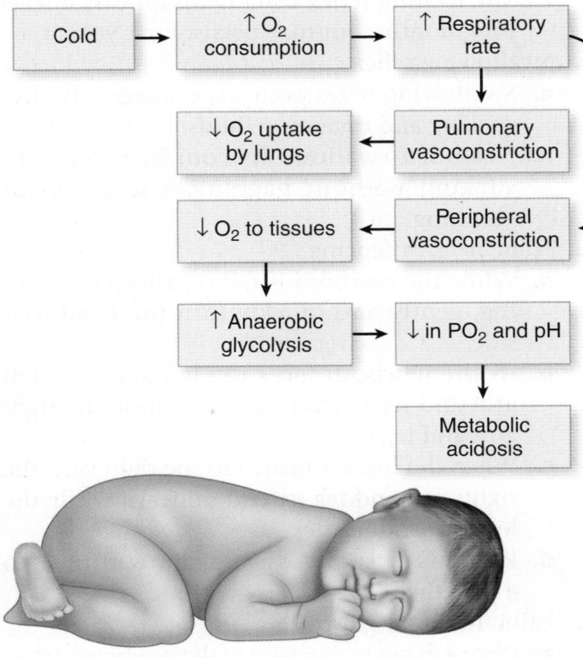

FIG. 27-3 Effects of cold stress. When a newborn is stressed by cold, oxygen (O_2) consumption increases and pulmonary and peripheral vasoconstriction occur, decreasing O_2 uptake by the lungs and O_2 delivery to the tissues; anaerobic glycolysis increases; and there is a decrease in partial pressure of oxygen (Po_2) and pH, leading to metabolic acidosis.

2. Newborns do not shiver to produce heat.
3. Newborns have brown fat deposits, which produce heat.
4. Prevent heat loss resulting from evaporation by keeping the newborn dry and well wrapped with a blanket.
5. Prevent heat loss resulting from radiation by keeping the newborn away from cold objects and outside walls.
6. Prevent heat loss resulting from convection by shielding the newborn from drafts.
7. Prevent heat loss resulting from conduction by performing all treatments on a warm, padded surface.
8. Keep the room temperature warm.
9. Take the newborn's axillary temperature every hour for the first 4 hours of life, every 4 hours for the remainder of the first 24 hours, and then every shift (as per agency protocol).

! Cold stress causes oxygen consumption and energy to be diverted from maintaining normal brain cell function and cardiac function, resulting in serious metabolic and physiological conditions.

I. Reflexes
1. Sucking and rooting
   a. Touch the newborn's lip, cheek, or corner of the mouth with a nipple.
   b. The newborn turns the head toward the nipple, opens the mouth, takes hold of the nipple, and sucks.
   c. The rooting reflex usually disappears after 3 to 4 months, but may persist for 1 year.
2. Swallowing reflex
   a. Swallowing reflex occurs spontaneously after sucking and obtaining fluids.
   b. Newborn swallows in coordination with sucking without gagging, coughing, or vomiting.
3. Tonic neck or fencing
   a. While the newborn is falling asleep or sleeping, gently and quickly turn the head to 1 side.
   b. As the newborn faces the left side, the left arm and leg extend outward while the right arm and leg flex.
   c. When the head is turned to the right side, the right arm and leg extend outward while the left arm and leg flex.
   d. Response usually disappears within 3 to 4 months.
4. Palmar-plantar grasp
   a. Place a finger in the palm of the newborn's hand and then place a finger at the base of the toes.
   b. The newborn's fingers curl around the examiner's fingers, and the newborn's toes curl downward.
   c. Palmar response lessens within 3 to 4 months.
   d. Plantar response lessens within 8 months.
5. Moro reflex
   a. Hold the newborn in a semisitting position and then allow the head and trunk to fall backward to at least a 30-degree angle.
   b. The newborn assumes sharp extension and abduction of the arms with the thumbs and forefingers in a "C" position; this is followed by flexion and adduction to an "embrace" position (legs follow a similar pattern).
   c. The Moro reflex is present at birth and is absent by 6 months of age if neurological maturation is not delayed.
   d. A body jerk motion may be the response between 8 and 18 weeks.
   e. A persistent response lasting more than 6 months may indicate a neurological abnormality.
6. Startle reflex (often considered the same as the Moro reflex but the response is different)
   a. The response is best elicited if the newborn is at least 24 hours old.
   b. The examiner makes a loud noise or claps hands to elicit the response.
   c. The newborn's arms adduct while the elbows flex.
   d. The hands stay clenched.
   e. The reflex should disappear within 4 months.
7. Pull-to-sit response
   a. Pull the newborn up by the wrist while the newborn is in the supine position.
   b. The head lags until the newborn is in an upright position, and then the head is level with the chest and shoulders momentarily before falling forward.
   c. The head then lifts for a few minutes.
   d. The response depends on the newborn's general muscle tone and condition and on maturity level.
8. Babinski's sign: Plantar reflex
   a. Beginning at the heel of the foot, use a finger to stroke gently upward along the lateral aspect of the sole, and then move the finger along the ball of the foot.
   b. The newborn's toes hyperextend while the big toe dorsiflexes.
   c. The reflex disappears after the newborn is 1 year old.
   d. Absence of this reflex indicates the need for a neurological examination.
9. Stepping or walking
   a. Hold the newborn in a vertical position, allowing 1 foot to touch a table surface.
   b. The newborn simulates walking, alternately flexing and extending the feet.

c. The reflex is usually present for 3 to 4 months.

10. Crawling
    a. Place the newborn on the abdomen.
    b. The newborn begins to make crawling movements with the arms and legs.
    c. The reflex usually disappears after about 6 weeks.

IV. Newborn Safety

A. Newborn identification
1. Information bracelets are applied to the mother and newborn immediately after birth and before the mother and newborn are separated; in addition, identification pictures of the newborn and footprints from the newborn may be obtained before the newborn leaves the mother's side in the delivery room.
2. The bracelets include name, sex, date, time of birth, and identification numbers.
3. Some agencies use identification bracelets that have radiofrequency transmitters that set off alarms if the newborn is removed from a certain area.
4. Agencies also conduct unit and hospital-wide drills to prevent newborn abductions.

B. Newborn abduction
1. The mother is taught to check the identification of any person who comes to remove the infant from her room and is taught other precautions to prevent newborn abduction (nurses must be wearing photo identification or some other security badge) (Box 27-1).
2. Closed-circuit televisions, code-alert bands, computer monitoring systems, or other monitoring systems may be used in some agencies.
3. The newborn is wheeled in a bassinette, not carried in a staff member's arms.

BOX 27-1 Precautions to Prevent Infant Abduction

- All personnel must wear identification that is easily visible at all times.
- Teach parents to allow only hospital staff with proper identification to take their infants from them.
- Question anyone with a newborn near an exit or in an unusual part of the facility.
- Never leave a newborn unattended.
- Teach the parents that the newborn must be observed at all times.
- When the newborn is in the mother's room, position the crib away from the doorway.
- Teach the parents home safety precautions; suggest that the parents not place announcements in the paper or signs in their yard that might alert an abductor that a new infant is in the home.

V. Parent Teaching

A. Formula feeding
1. Teach sterilization techniques if the water supply is located in areas where the purification process of the water is questionable.
2. Remind the mother not to heat the bottle of formula in a microwave oven.
3. Inform the mother that formula is a sufficient diet for the first 4 to 6 months.
4. Assess the mother's ability to burp the newborn.

B. Breast-feeding
1. Assess the newborn's ability to attach to the mother's breast and suck (Fig. 27-4).
2. Teach the mother how to pump her breasts and how to store breast milk properly.
3. Inform the mother that breast milk is a sufficient diet for the first 4 to 6 months.
4. Give the mother the phone numbers of local organizations that offer support to breast-feeding mothers.

C. Bathing
1. Bathe the newborn in a warm room before feeding.
2. Have all equipment for bathing available.
3. Use a mild soap (not on the face).
4. Proceed from the cleanest area to the dirtiest.
5. Clean eyes from the inner canthus outward.
6. Special care should be taken to clean under the folds of the neck, underarms, groin, and genitals.
7. Make bath time enjoyable for the newborn and the mother.

D. Clothing
1. Assess diaper and clothing needs for the newborn with the mother.
2. Instruct the mother that the newborn's head should be covered in cold weather to prevent heat loss.

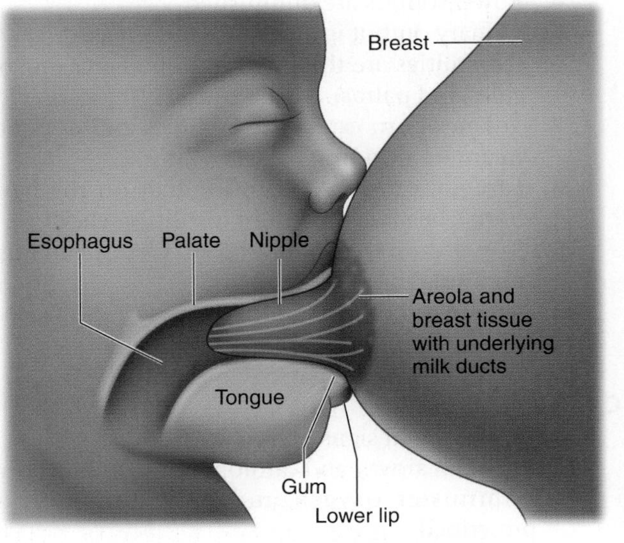

FIG. 27-4 Correct attachment (latch-on) of a newborn at breast.

3. Instruct the mother to layer the newborn's clothing in cooler weather.
4. To be comfortable, the newborn should be dressed in 1 more layer of clothing than what the parents are wearing.

E. Cord care: See earlier for cord care, "Body Systems Assessment and Interventions."

F. Circumcision: See earlier for circumcision care, "Body Systems Assessment and Interventions."

G. Uncircumcised newborn
1. Inform the mother that the foreskin and glans are 2 similar layers of cells that separate from each other and that the separation process normally is complete by 3 years of age, although the layers can remain adhered until puberty.
2. Instruct the mother not to pull back the foreskin, but to allow natural separation to occur.
3. Inform the mother that as the process of separation occurs, sloughed cells build up between the layers of the foreskin and the glans, and that when retraction occurs, daily gentle washing of the glans with soap and water is sufficient to maintain adequate cleanliness.

H. Stimulation: Providing stimulation to the newborn such as touching, cuddling, or talking is an important intervention.

VI. Preterm Newborn

A. Description
1. An infant born before 37 weeks of gestation but greater than 20 weeks of gestation.
2. Primary concern relates to immaturity of all body systems

B. Assessment
1. Respirations are irregular with periods of apnea.
2. Body temperature is below normal.
3. The newborn has poor suck and swallow reflexes.
4. Bowel sounds are diminished.
5. Urinary output is increased or decreased.
6. Extremities are thin, with minimal creasing on soles and palms.
7. The newborn extends extremities and does not maintain flexion.
8. Lanugo, on skin and in the hair on the newborn's head, is present in woolly patches.
9. Skin is thin, with visible blood vessels and minimal subcutaneous fat pads.
10. Skin may appear jaundiced.
11. Testes are undescended in boys.
12. Labia majora are narrow in girls.

C. Interventions
1. Monitor vital signs every 2 to 4 hours.
2. Maintain airway and cardiopulmonary functions.
3. Administer oxygen and humidification as prescribed.
4. Monitor intake and output and electrolyte balance.
5. Monitor daily weight.
6. Maintain the newborn in a warming device.
7. Avoid exposure to infections.

VII. Postterm Newborn

A. Description: Infant born after 42 weeks of gestation

B. Assessment
1. Hypoglycemia
2. Parchment-like skin (dry and cracked) without lanugo
3. Long fingernails, extended over ends of fingers
4. Profuse scalp hair
5. Long and thin body
6. Wasting of fat and muscle in extremities
7. Meconium staining possibly present on nails and umbilical cord

C. Interventions
1. Provide normal newborn care.
2. Monitor for hypoglycemia.
3. Maintain newborn's temperature.
4. Monitor for meconium aspiration.

VIII. Small for Gestational Age

A. Description: Newborn who is plotted at or below the 10th percentile on the intrauterine growth curve

B. Assessment
1. Fetal distress
2. Decreased or elevated body temperature
3. Physical abnormalities
4. Hypoglycemia
5. Signs of polycythemia
   a. Ruddy appearance
   b. Cyanosis
   c. Jaundice
6. Signs of infection
7. Signs of aspiration of meconium

C. Interventions
1. Maintain airway and cardiopulmonary function.
2. Maintain body temperature.
3. Observe for signs of respiratory distress.
4. Monitor for infection and initiate measures to prevent sepsis.
5. Monitor for hypoglycemia.
6. Initiate early feedings and monitor for signs of aspiration.

IX. Large for Gestational Age

A. Description: Newborn who is plotted at or above the 90th percentile on the intrauterine growth curve

B. Assessment
1. Birth trauma or injury
2. Respiratory distress
3. Hypoglycemia

C. Interventions
1. Monitor vital signs and for respiratory distress.
2. Monitor for hypoglycemia.

3. Initiate early feedings.
4. Monitor for infection and initiate measures to prevent sepsis.

X. Respiratory Distress Syndrome

A. Description: Serious lung disorder caused by immaturity and inability to produce surfactant, resulting in hypoxia and acidosis

B. Assessment
1. Respiratory distress; can include tachypnea, nasal flaring, expiratory grunting, retractions, seesaw respirations, decreased breath sounds, and apnea
2. Pallor and cyanosis
3. Hypothermia
4. Poor muscle tone

C. Interventions
1. Monitor color, respiratory rate, and degree of effort in breathing.
2. Maintain airway and cardiopulmonary function and support respirations as prescribed.
3. Monitor arterial blood gases and oxygen saturation levels as prescribed (arterial blood gases from umbilical artery); ensure that oxygen administered to the newborn is at the lowest possible concentration necessary to maintain adequate arterial oxygenation.
4. Any premature newborn who required oxygen support should be scheduled for an eye examination before discharge to assess for retinal damage.
5. Position the newborn on the side or back, with the neck slightly extended.
6. Administer respiratory therapy (percussion and vibration) as prescribed; use padded small plastic cup or small oxygen mask for percussion; use padded electric toothbrush for vibration.
7. Provide nutrition.
8. Support bonding.
9. Prepare parents for short-term to long-term period of oxygen dependency if necessary.
10. Encourage the mother to pump the breasts for future breast-feeding of her newborn if she desires.
11. Encourage as much parental participation in the newborn's care as the condition allows.

Prepare to administer surfactant replacement therapy (instilled into the endotracheal tube) to a newborn with respiratory distress syndrome.

XI. Meconium Aspiration Syndrome

A. Description
1. Occurs in term or postterm newborns
2. Exact etiology is unknown, but the release of meconium into the amniotic fluid is thought to be related to a stressful fetal event initiating a biochemical chain of events.
3. Aspiration can occur in utero or with the first breath.

B. Assessment
1. Respiratory distress is present at birth; tachypnea, cyanosis, retractions, nasal flaring, grunting, crackles, and rhonchi may be present.
2. The newborn's nails, skin, and umbilical cord may be stained a yellow-green color.

C. Interventions
1. If the newborn is delivered in an active, crying state with no evidence of respiratory distress, no intervention is necessary.
2. If the newborn is delivered and exhibits inactivity and lack of cry, endotracheal suctioning is performed. If the newborn also exhibits lack of respiratory effort and a low heart rate, additional interventions will be needed.
3. Newborns with severe meconium aspiration syndrome may benefit from extracorporeal membrane oxygenation; this therapy uses a modified heart-lung machine and provides oxygen to the circulation, allowing the lungs to rest and decreasing pulmonary hypertension and hypoxemia.

XII. Bronchopulmonary Dysplasia

A. Description
1. This chronic pulmonary condition affects newborns who have experienced respiratory failure or have been oxygen-dependent for more than 28 days.
2. X-ray findings are abnormal, indicating areas of overinflation and atelectasis.

B. Assessment
1. Tachypnea
2. Tachycardia
3. Retractions
4. Nasal flaring
5. Labored breathing
6. Crackles and decreased air movement
7. Occasional expiratory wheezing

C. Interventions
1. Monitor airway and cardiopulmonary function; provide oxygen therapy.
2. Fluid restriction may be prescribed.
3. Medications include surfactant at birth, bronchodilators, and possibly diuretics and corticosteroids.

XIII. Transient Tachypnea of the Newborn

A. Description
1. Respiratory condition that results from incomplete reabsorption of fetal lung fluid in full-term newborns
2. Usually disappears within 24 to 48 hours

B. Assessment
1. Tachypnea
2. Expiratory grunting
3. Retractions
4. Nasal flaring
5. Fluid breath sounds per auscultation
6. Cyanosis

C. Interventions
1. Supportive care
2. Oxygen administration

XIV. Intraventricular Hemorrhage

A. Description
1. Bleeding within the ventricles of the brain
2. Risk factors include prematurity, respiratory distress syndrome, trauma, and asphyxia.

B. Assessment: Diminished or absent Moro reflex, lethargy, apnea, poor feeding, high-pitched shrill cry, seizure activity

C. Interventions: Supportive treatment

XV. Retinopathy of Prematurity

A. Description
1. Vascular disorder involving gradual replacement of retina by fibrous tissue and blood vessels
2. Primarily caused by prematurity and use of supplemental oxygen (>30 days)

B. Assessment: Leukocoria (white tissue on the retrolental space), vitreous hemorrhage, strabismus, cataracts (check for red reflex)

C. Interventions: Laser photocoagulation surgery

XVI. Necrotizing Enterocolitis (NEC)

A. Description
1. Acute inflammatory disease of the gastrointestinal tract
2. Usually occurs 4 to 10 days after birth, and is most frequently seen in preterm newborns

B. Assessment: Increased abdominal girth, decreased or absent bowel sounds, bowel loop distention, vomiting, bile-stained emesis, abdominal tenderness, occult blood in stool

C. Prevention
1. Withhold feedings for 24 to 48 hours from infants believed to have suffered birth asphyxia. Breast milk is the preferred nutrient after this time period.
2. The use of probiotics with enteral feedings and breast milk has shown evidence of prevention of NEC.
3. Administration of corticosteroids to the mother prior to birth to promote early gut closure and maturation of the gut mucosa

D. Interventions
1. Hold oral feedings.
2. Insert oral gastric tube to decompress the abdomen.
3. Intravenous antibiotics
4. Intravenous fluids to correct fluid, electrolyte, and acid-base imbalances
5. Surgery if indicated

XVII. Hyperbilirubinemia

A. Description
1. Elevated serum bilirubin level
2. Evaluation is indicated when serum levels are greater than 12 mg/dL (180 mcmol/L) in a term newborn.
3. Therapy is aimed at preventing kernicterus, which results in permanent neurological damage resulting from the deposition of bilirubin in the brain cells.

B. Assessment
1. Jaundice
2. Elevated serum bilirubin levels
3. Enlarged liver
4. Poor muscle tone
5. Lethargy
6. Poor sucking reflex

C. Interventions
1. Monitor for the presence of jaundice; assess skin and sclera for jaundice.
   a. Examine the newborn's skin color in natural light.
   b. Press a finger over a bony prominence or tip of the newborn's nose to press out capillary blood from the tissues.
   c. Note that jaundice starts at the head first and spreads to the chest, abdomen, arms and legs, and hands and feet, which are the last to be jaundiced.
2. Keep the newborn well hydrated to maintain blood volume.
3. Facilitate early, frequent feeding to hasten passage of meconium and encourage excretion of bilirubin.
4. Report to the PHCP any signs of jaundice in the first 24 hours of life and any abnormal signs and symptoms.
5. Prepare for phototherapy (bili-light or bili-blanket), and monitor the newborn closely during the treatment.

At any serum bilirubin level, the appearance of jaundice during the first day of life indicates a pathological process.

D. Phototherapy
1. Description
   a. Phototherapy is use of light to reduce serum bilirubin levels in the newborn.
   b. Adverse effects from treatment, such as eye damage, dehydration, or sensory deprivation, can occur.

2. Interventions
   a. Follow specific instructions for phototherapy and biliblanket care.
   b. Expose as much of the newborn's skin as possible.
   c. Cover the genital area, and monitor the genital area for skin irritation or breakdown.
   d. Cover the newborn's eyes with eye shields or patches; ensure that the eyelids are closed when shields or patches are applied.
   e. Remove the shields or patches at least once per shift (during a feeding time) to inspect the eyes for infection or irritation and to allow for eye contact and bonding with the parents.
   f. Measure the lamp energy output to ensure efficacy of the treatment (done with a special device known as a *photometer*).
   g. Monitor skin temperature closely.
   h. Increase fluids to compensate for water loss.
   i. Expect loose green stools.
   j. Monitor the newborn's skin color with the fluorescent light turned off, every 4 to 8 hours.
   k. Monitor the skin for bronze baby syndrome, a grayish brown discoloration of the skin, a complication of phototherapy.
   l. Reposition the newborn every 2 hours; monitor the newborn closely.
   m. Provide stimulation.
   n. If treatment is done at home, teach the parents about care and indications of the need to notify the PHCP.
   o. After treatment, continue monitoring for signs of hyperbilirubinemia, because rebound elevations can occur after therapy is discontinued.
   p. Turn off the phototherapy lights before drawing a blood specimen for serum bilirubin levels, and do not leave the blood specimen uncovered under fluorescent lights (to prevent the breakdown of bilirubin in the blood specimen).

XVIII. Erythroblastosis Fetalis

A. Description
   1. Erythroblastosis fetalis is the destruction of red blood cells that results from an antigen-antibody reaction.
   2. The disorder is characterized by hemolytic anemia or hyperbilirubinemia.
   3. Exchange of fetal and maternal blood occurs primarily when the placenta separates at birth (Fig. 27-5).
   4. Antibodies are harmless to the mother but attach to the erythrocytes in the fetus and cause hemolysis.
   5. Sensitization is rare with the first pregnancy and ABO incompatibility is usually less severe.

B. Assessment
   1. Anemia
   2. Jaundice that develops rapidly after birth and before 24 hours
   3. Edema

C. Interventions
   1. Administer $Rh_0(D)$ immune globulin to the mother during the first 72 hours after birth if the Rh-negative mother delivers an Rh-positive fetus but remains unsensitized.
   2. Assist with exchange transfusion after birth or intrauterine transfusion as prescribed.
   3. The newborn's blood is replaced with Rh-negative blood to stop the destruction of the newborn's red blood cells; the Rh-negative blood is replaced with the newborn's own blood gradually.
   4. Provide support to the parents.

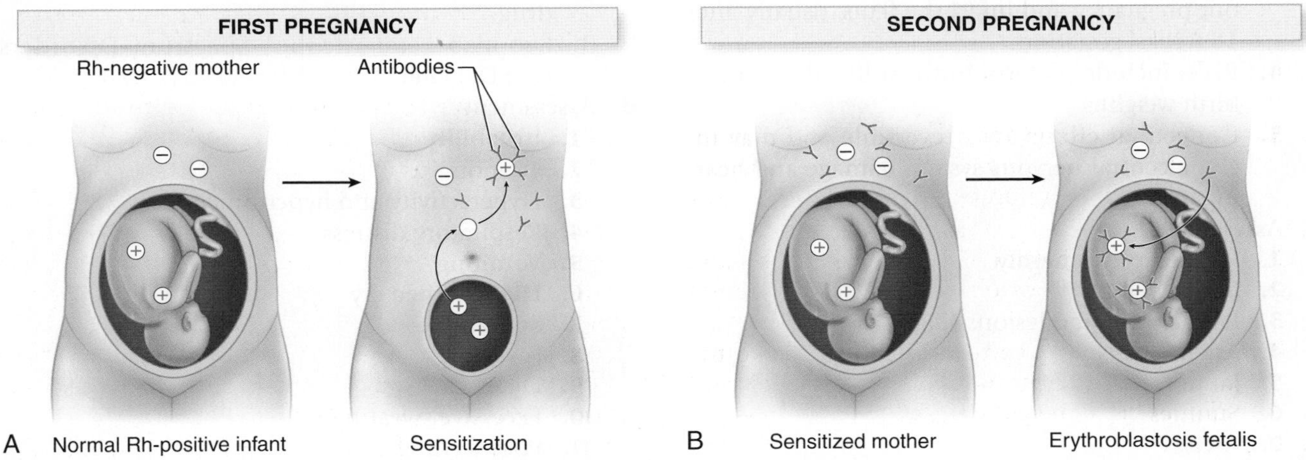

FIG. 27-5 Development of maternal sensitization to Rh antigens. **A,** Fetal Rh-positive erythrocytes enter the maternal system. Maternal anti-Rh antibodies are formed. **B,** Anti-Rh antibodies cross the placenta and attack fetal erythrocytes.

XIX. Sepsis

A. Description: Generalized infection resulting from the presence of bacteria in the blood, such as Group B streptococcal infection

B. Assessment
1. Pallor
2. Tachypnea, tachycardia
3. Poor feeding
4. Abdominal distention
5. Temperature instability

C. Interventions
1. Assess for periods of apnea or irregular respirations.
2. If apnea is present, stimulate by gently rubbing the chest or foot.
3. Administer oxygen as prescribed.
4. Monitor vital signs; assess for fever.
5. Maintain warmth in a radiant warmer.
6. Provide isolation as necessary.
7. Monitor intake and output, and obtain daily weight.
8. Monitor for diarrhea.
9. Assess feeding and sucking reflex, which may be poor.
10. Assess for jaundice.
11. Assess for irritability and lethargy.
12. Prepare for blood cultures and administer antibiotics as prescribed, and observe carefully for toxicity because a newborn's liver and kidneys are immature.

XX. TORCH Infections (see Chapter 22)

XXI. Syphilis

A. Description
1. Syphilis is a sexually transmitted infection.
2. Congenital syphilis can result in premature birth, skin lesions, and abnormal skeletal development.
3. The causative organism, *Treponema pallidum*, a spirochete, is able to cross the placenta throughout pregnancy and infect the fetus, usually after 18 weeks' gestation.
4. Risks include preterm birth, stillbirth, and low birth weight.
5. Congenital effects are irreversible and may include central nervous system damage and hearing loss.

B. Assessment
1. Hepatosplenomegaly
2. Joint swelling
3. Palmar rash and lesions (Fig. 27-6)
4. Anemia
5. Jaundice
6. Snuffles
7. Ascites
8. Pneumonitis
9. Cerebrospinal fluid changes

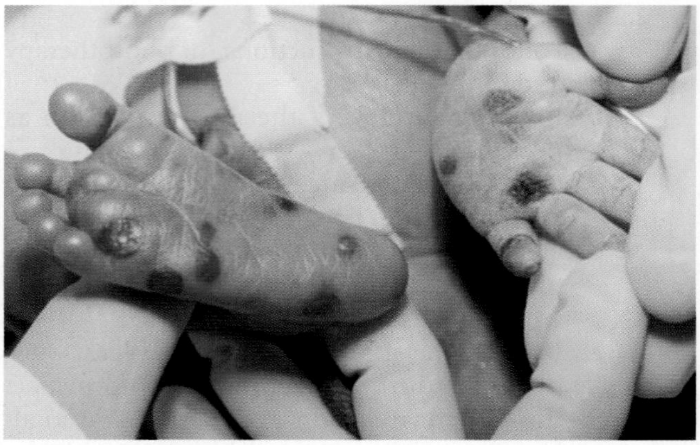

FIG. 27-6 Neonatal syphilitic lesions on hands and feet. (From Lowdermilk et al., 2012. Courtesy Mahesh Kotwal, MD, Phoenix, Arizona.)

C. Interventions
1. Monitor the newborn for signs of syphilis.
2. Prepare the newborn for serological testing if prescribed.
3. Administer antibiotic therapy as prescribed.
4. Use standard precautions and drainage and secretion (contact) precautions with suspected congenital syphilis.
5. Wear gloves when handling the newborn until antibiotic therapy has been administered for 24 hours.
6. Provide psychological support to the mother, and provide instructions regarding follow-up care to the newborn.

XXII. Addicted Newborn

A. Description
1. A newborn can become passively addicted to drugs that have passed through the placenta.
2. Assessment findings and withdrawal times may vary depending on the specific addicting drug.
3. See also Fetal Alcohol Spectrum Disorders (FASDs) later.

B. Assessment
1. Irritability
2. Tremors
3. Hyperactivity and hypertonicity
4. Respiratory distress
5. Vomiting
6. High-pitched cry
7. Sneezing
8. Fever
9. Diarrhea
10. Excessive sweating
11. Poor feeding
12. Extreme sucking of fists
13. Seizures

C. Interventions
1. Monitor respiratory and cardiac status frequently.
2. Monitor temperature and vital signs.
3. Hold newborn firmly and close to the body during feeding and when giving care.
4. Initiate seizure precautions (pad sides of the crib).
5. Provide small frequent feedings and allow a longer period for feeding.
6. Monitor intake and output.
7. Administer intravenous hydration if prescribed.
8. Protect the newborn's skin from injury that can be caused by the constant rubbing from hyperactive jitters.
9. Swaddle the newborn.
10. Place the newborn in a quiet room and reduce stimulation.
11. Allow the mother to express feelings such as anxiety and guilt.
12. Refer the mother for treatment of the substance abuse problem.

XXIII. Fetal Alcohol Spectrum Disorders (FASDs)

A. Description
1. FASDs are a group of conditions caused by maternal alcohol use during pregnancy.
2. The disorders are a result of teratogenesis.
3. FASDs cause cognitive and physical delays.
4. Fetal alcohol syndrome is the most severe of the FASDs. The other disorders included in this category are alcohol-related neurodevelopmental disorder (ARND) and alcohol-related birth defects (ARBDs).

B. Assessment
1. Facial changes (Fig. 27-7)
   a. Short palpebral fissures
   b. Hypoplastic philtrum
   c. Short, upturned nose
   d. Flat midface
   e. Thin upper lip
   f. Low nasal bridge
2. Abnormal palmar creases
3. Respiratory distress (apnea, cyanosis)
4. Congenital heart disorders
5. Irritability and hypersensitivity to stimuli
6. Tremors
7. Poor feeding
8. Seizures

C. Interventions
1. Monitor for respiratory distress.
2. Position the newborn on the side to facilitate drainage of secretions; initiate seizure precautions.
3. Keep resuscitation equipment at the bedside.
4. Monitor for hypoglycemia.
5. Assess suck and swallow reflex.
6. Administer small feedings and burp well.
7. Suction as necessary.

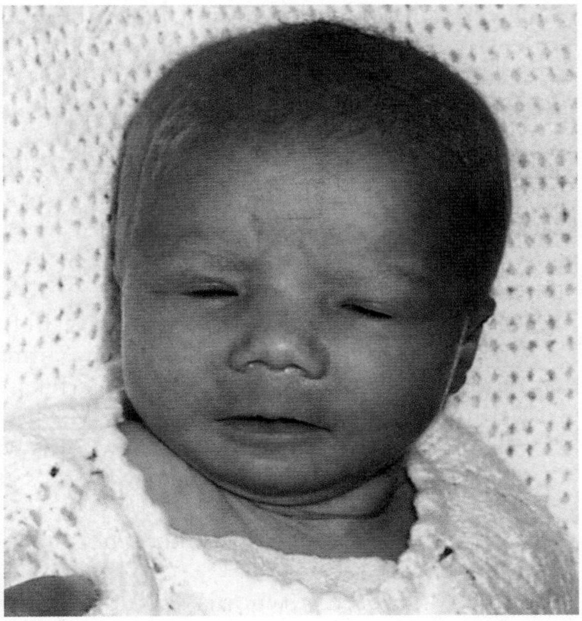

FIG. 27-7 Infant with fetal alcohol syndrome. (From Markiewicz, Abrahamson, 1999.)

8. Monitor intake and output.
9. Monitor weight and head circumference.
10. Decrease environmental stimuli.
11. Make referral to local early intervention system.

XXIV. Newborn of a Mother With Human Immunodeficiency Virus (HIV)

A. Description
1. The fetus of a mother who is positive for HIV antibody should be monitored closely throughout the pregnancy.
2. Serial ultrasound screenings should be done during pregnancy to identify IUGR.
3. Weekly nonstress testing after 32 weeks of gestation and biophysical profiles may be necessary during pregnancy.
4. Newborns born to HIV-positive mothers may test positive because the mother's antibodies may persist in the newborn for 18 months after birth.
5. The use of antiviral medication, the reduction of newborn exposure to maternal blood and body fluids, and the early identification of HIV in pregnancy reduce the risk of transmission to the newborn.
6. All newborns born to HIV-positive mothers acquire maternal antibody to HIV infection, but not all acquire the infection.
7. The newborn may be asymptomatic for the first several months to years of life.

B. Transmission
1. Across placental barrier
2. During labor and birth

3. Breast milk (breast-feeding not done if the mother is HIV-positive; follow PHCP prescription)

C. Assessment
1. Possibly no outward signs at birth
2. Signs of immunodeficiency
3. Hepatomegaly
4. Splenomegaly
5. Lymphadenopathy
6. Impairment in growth and development

D. Interventions
1. Clean the newborn's skin carefully before any invasive procedure, such as the administration of phytonadione, heel sticks, or venipunctures.
2. Circumcisions are not done on newborns with HIV-positive mothers until the newborn's status is determined.
3. Newborn can room with mother if hospital policies allow.
4. All HIV-exposed newborns should be treated with medication to prevent infection by *Pneumocystis jiroveci*.
5. Antiretroviral medications may be administered as prescribed for the first 6 weeks of life or longer if prescribed.
6. Monitor for early signs of immunodeficiency, such as enlarged spleen or liver, lymphadenopathy, and impairment in growth and development.
7. Newborns at risk for HIV infection should be seen by the PHCP at birth and at 1 week, 2 weeks, 1 month, and 2 months of age.
8. Inform the mother that HIV culture is recommended at 1 month and after 4 months of age.

E. Immunizations
1. Immunizations with live vaccines, such as measles-mumps-rubella and varicella, should not be done until the newborn's, infant's, or child's status is confirmed.
2. If infected, live vaccine will not be given.

Newborns at risk for HIV infection need to receive all recommended immunizations at the regular schedule; live vaccines are not administered until HIV status is determined.

XXV. Newborn of a Diabetic Mother

A. Description
1. Infant born to mother with type 1 or type 2 diabetes or gestational diabetes
2. Hypoglycemia, hyperbilirubinemia, respiratory distress syndrome, hypocalcemia, birth trauma, and congenital anomalies may be present.

B. Assessment
1. Excessive size and weight as a result of excess fat and glycogen in the tissues
2. Edema or puffiness in the face and cheeks
3. Signs of hypoglycemia, such as twitching, apnea, difficulty in feeding, lethargy, seizures, and cyanosis
4. Hyperbilirubinemia
5. Signs of respiratory distress, such as tachypnea, cyanosis, retractions, grunting, and nasal flaring

C. Interventions
1. Monitor for signs of respiratory distress, birth trauma, and congenital anomalies.
2. Monitor bilirubin and blood glucose levels.
3. Monitor weight.
4. Feed the newborn soon after birth with breast milk or formula as prescribed.
5. Administer glucose intravenously to treat hypoglycemia if necessary and as prescribed.
6. Monitor for edema.
7. Monitor for respiratory distress, tremors, or seizures.

XXVI. Hypoglycemia

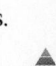

A. Description
1. Hypoglycemia is an abnormally low level of glucose in the blood (<45 mg/dL [<2.5 mmol/L]).
2. Normal blood glucose reference interval is 45 to 60 mg/dL (2.5 to 3.4 mmol/L) in a 1-day-old newborn and 50 to 90 mg/dL (2.9 to 5.1 mmol/L) in a newborn older than 1 day (institutional values for normal newborn blood glucose levels vary).

B. Assessment
1. Increased respiratory rate
2. Twitching, nervousness, or tremors
3. Unstable temperature
4. Lethargy, apnea, seizures, cyanosis

C. Interventions
1. Prevent low blood glucose level through early feedings.
2. Administer formula orally or glucose intravenously as prescribed.
3. Monitor blood glucose levels as prescribed.
4. Monitor for feeding problems.
5. Monitor for apneic periods.
6. Assess for shrill or intermittent cries.
7. Evaluate lethargy and poor muscle tone.

XXVII. Hypothyroidism

A. Description: Hypothyroidism is a decrease in the production of thyroid hormone.

B. Assessment
1. Protruding or thick tongue
2. Dull look; swollen face
3. Decreased muscle tone
4. Laboratory results reveal low thyroid production

C. Interventions: Focus on thyroid replacement

Maternity

PRIORITY NURSING ACTIONS

Choking Infant

1. Sit or kneel with the infant in your lap.
2. Remove clothing from the infant's chest if easily removed.
3. Hold the infant face down with the head lower than the chest while resting on your forearm. The infant's head and jaw should be supported with the hand. The forearm is rested on the thigh to support the infant (Fig. 27-8).

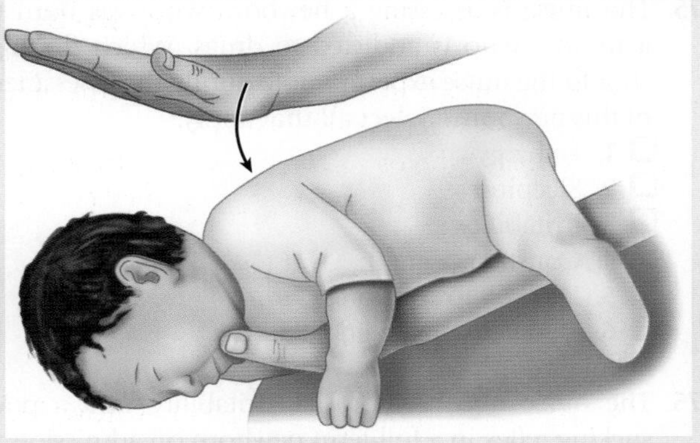

FIG. 27-8 Relief of choking in the newborn infant.

4. Deliver 5 back slaps between the infant's shoulder blades using the heel of the other hand with sufficient force. Place free hand on infant's back while supporting the back of the infant's head with the palm of the hand. Cradle the infant between the 2 forearms. Turn the infant as a unit while supporting the head and neck.
5. Rest the forearm on the thigh while holding the infant face up. Deliver 5 chest thrusts in the middle of the chest over the lower half of the sternum at a rate of 1 per second with enough force to dislodge the foreign body.
6. Repeat the sequence until the object is removed or the infant becomes unresponsive.
7. If the infant becomes unresponsive, call for help and activate the emergency response system.
8. Begin cardiopulmonary resuscitation (CPR) while checking for a foreign body each time the airway is opened. Do not perform blind finger sweeps.

Reference

American American Heart Association (2018). 2017 American Heart Association Focused Update on Pediatric Basic Life Support and Cardiopulmonary Resuscitation Quality: An Update to the American Heart Association Guidelines for Cardiopulmonary Resuscitation and Emergency Cardiovascular Care. *Circulation*, 137(1), e1–e6.

XXVIII. Relief of Choking in an Infant

A. Description: Choking is also known as foreign body airway obstruction (FBAO).

B. Assessment

1. Signs of mild airway obstruction include good air exchange, ability to cough forcefully, and wheezing between coughs.
2. Signs of severe airway obstruction include poor or no air exchange, weak or ineffective cough or no cough, a high-pitched noise while inhaling or no noise, increased respiratory difficulty, cyanosis, and inability to cry.

C. Interventions

1. For mild obstruction, do not interfere with the infant's own attempts to expel the object. Stay with them and continue to monitor. If the obstruction persists, activate the emergency response system and relieve the obstruction.
2. Severe obstruction must be relieved as soon as possible (see Priority Nursing Actions).

XXIX. Cardiopulmonary Resuscitation (CPR) Guidelines for Infants

A. Description: Infants include individuals who are 1 year of age or less. The basic life support (BLS) sequence for infants is very similar to that used for child and adult CPR. The main differences include the following:

1. Location of the pulse check is the brachial artery in infants.
2. Compression technique is to use 2 fingers for a single rescuer and to use a 2-thumb–encircling technique for 2 rescuers.
3. Compression depth should be one-third of the chest depth, which is approximately 1.5 inches or 4 cm.
4. The compression to ventilation ratio for 1 rescuer is 30:2; 2 rescuers is 15:2.
5. The emergency response system should be activated if the arrest is not witnessed and the rescuer is alone after providing 2 minutes of CPR; after 2 minutes the single rescuer can activate the emergency response system and get an automated external defibrillator.
6. The emergency response system should be activated and the automated external defibrillator should be retrieved before beginning CPR if the arrest is sudden and witnessed.

B. Refer to Chapter 52 for detailed information on the American Heart Association's recommendations for the CPR sequence.

PRACTICE QUESTIONS

269. The nurse assisted with the birth of a newborn. Which nursing action is **most effective** in preventing heat loss by evaporation?
1. Warming the crib pad
2. Closing the doors to the room
3. Drying the infant with a warm blanket
4. Turning on the overhead radiant warmer

270. The mother of a newborn calls the clinic and reports that when cleaning the umbilical cord, she noticed that the cord was moist and that discharge was present. What is the **most appropriate** nursing instruction for this mother?
1. Bring the infant to the clinic.
2. This is a normal occurrence and no further action is needed.
3. Increase the number of times that the cord is cleaned per day.
4. Monitor the cord for another 24 to 48 hours and call the clinic if the discharge continues.

271. The nurse in a neonatal intensive care unit (NICU) receives a telephone call to prepare for the admission of a 43-week gestation newborn with Apgar scores of 1 and 4. In planning for admission of this newborn, what is the nurse's **highest priority**?
1. Turn on the apnea and cardiorespiratory monitors.
2. Connect the resuscitation bag to the oxygen outlet.
3. Set up the intravenous line with 5% dextrose in water.
4. Set the radiant warmer control temperature at 36.5° C (97.6° F).

272. The nurse is assessing a newborn after circumcision and notes that the circumcised area is red with a small amount of bloody drainage. Which nursing action is **most appropriate**?
1. Apply gentle pressure.
2. Reinforce the dressing.
3. Document the findings.
4. Contact the primary health care provider (PHCP).

273. The nurse in a newborn nursery is monitoring a preterm newborn for respiratory distress syndrome. Which assessment findings should alert the nurse to the possibility of this syndrome? **Select all that apply.**
- ☐ 1. Cyanosis
- ☐ 2. Tachypnea
- ☐ 3. Hypotension
- ☐ 4. Retractions
- ☐ 5. Audible grunts
- ☐ 6. Presence of a barrel chest

274. The postpartum nurse is providing instructions to the mother of a newborn with hyperbilirubinemia who is being breast-fed. The nurse should provide which instruction to the mother?
1. Feed the newborn less frequently.
2. Continue to breast-feed every 2 to 4 hours.
3. Switch to bottle-feeding the infant for 2 weeks.
4. Stop breast-feeding and switch to bottle-feeding permanently.

275. The nurse is assessing a newborn who was born to a mother who is addicted to drugs. Which findings should the nurse expect to note during the assessment of this newborn? **Select all that apply.**
- ☐ 1. Lethargy
- ☐ 2. Sleepiness
- ☐ 3. Irritability
- ☐ 4. Constant crying
- ☐ 5. Difficult to comfort
- ☐ 6. Cuddles when being held

276. The nurse notes hypotonia, irritability, and a poor sucking reflex in a full-term newborn on admission to the nursery. The nurse suspects fetal alcohol syndrome and is aware that which additional sign would be consistent with this syndrome?
1. Length of 19 inches
2. Abnormal palmar creases
3. Birth weight of 6 lb, 14 oz (3120 g)
4. Head circumference appropriate for gestational age

277. The nurse is creating a plan of care for a newborn diagnosed with fetal alcohol syndrome. The nurse should include which **priority** intervention in the plan of care?
1. Allow the newborn to establish own sleep-rest pattern.
2. Maintain the newborn in a brightly lighted area of the nursery.
3. Encourage frequent handling of the newborn by staff and parents.
4. Monitor the newborn's response to feedings and weight gain pattern.

278. The nurse administers erythromycin ointment (0.5%) to the eyes of a newborn and the mother asks the nurse why this is performed. Which explanation is **best** for the nurse to provide about neonatal eye prophylaxis?
1. Protects the newborn's eyes from possible infections acquired while hospitalized.
2. Prevents cataracts in the newborn born to a woman who is susceptible to rubella.

3. Minimizes the spread of microorganisms to the newborn from invasive procedures during labor.
4. Prevents an infection called *ophthalmia neonatorum* from occurring after birth in a newborn born to a woman with an untreated gonococcal infection.

279. The nurse is preparing to care for a newborn receiving phototherapy. Which interventions should be included in the plan of care? **Select all that apply.**

- ☐ 1. Avoid stimulation.
- ☐ 2. Decrease fluid intake.
- ☐ 3. Expose all of the newborn's skin.
- ☐ 4. Monitor skin temperature closely.
- ☐ 5. Reposition the newborn every 2 hours.
- ☐ 6. Cover the newborn's eyes with eye shields or patches.

280. The nurse creates a plan of care for a woman with human immunodeficiency virus (HIV) infection and her newborn. The nurse should include which intervention in the plan of care?

1. Monitoring the newborn's vital signs routinely
2. Maintaining standard precautions at all times while caring for the newborn
3. Initiating referral to evaluate for blindness, deafness, learning problems, or behavioral problems
4. Instructing the breast-feeding mother regarding the treatment of the nipples with nystatin ointment

281. The nurse is planning care for a newborn of a mother with diabetes mellitus. What is the **priority** nursing consideration for this newborn?

1. Developmental delays because of excessive size
2. Maintaining safety because of low blood glucose levels
3. Choking because of impaired suck and swallow reflexes
4. Elevated body temperature because of excess fat and glycogen

282. Which statement reflects a new mother's understanding of the teaching about the prevention of newborn abduction?

1. "I will place my baby's crib close to the door."
2. "Some health care personnel won't have name badges."
3. "I will ask the nurse to attend to my infant if I am napping and my husband is not here."
4. "It's okay to allow the nurse assistant to carry my newborn to the nursery."

283. The nurse prepares to administer a phytonadione (vitamin K) injection to a newborn, and the mother asks the nurse why her infant needs the injection. What **best** response should the nurse provide?

1. "Your newborn needs the medicine to develop immunity."
2. "The medicine will protect your newborn from being jaundiced."
3. "Newborns have sterile bowels, and the medicine promotes the growth of bacteria in the bowel."
4. "Newborns are deficient in vitamin K, and this injection prevents your newborn from bleeding."

ANSWERS

269. *Answer:* 3

Rationale: Evaporation of moisture from a wet body dissipates heat along with the moisture. Keeping the newborn dry by drying the wet newborn at birth prevents hypothermia via evaporation. Hypothermia caused by conduction occurs when the newborn is on a cold surface, such as a cold pad or mattress, and heat from the newborn's body is transferred to the colder object (direct contact). Warming the crib pad assists in preventing hypothermia by conduction. Convection occurs as air moves across the newborn's skin from an open door and heat is transferred to the air. Radiation occurs when heat from the newborn radiates to a colder surface (indirect contact).
Test-Taking Strategy: Note the strategic words, *most effective*. Recalling that evaporation of moisture from a wet body dissipates heat along with the moisture will assist in directing you to the correct option.
Level of Cognitive Ability: Applying
Client Needs: Physiological Integrity
Integrated Process: Nursing Process—Implementation
Content Area: Maternity: Newborn
Health Problem: Newborn: Thermoregulation
Priority Concepts: Caregiving; Thermoregulation
Reference: Hockenberry, Wilson, Rodgers (2017), pp. 210, 239-240.

270. *Answer:* 1

Rationale: Signs of umbilical cord infection are moistness, oozing, discharge, and a reddened base around the cord. If signs of infection occur, the client should be instructed to notify the primary health care provider (PHCP). If these symptoms occur, antibiotics may be necessary. Options 2, 3, and 4 are not the most appropriate nursing interventions for an umbilical cord infection as described in the question.
Test-Taking Strategy: Note the strategic words, *most appropriate.* Focus on the clinical manifestations provided in the question to assist in answering. Noting the word *discharge* in the question will assist in directing you to the option that indicates that the newborn needs to be seen by the PHCP.
Level of Cognitive Ability: Applying
Client Needs: Physiological Integrity
Integrated Process: Nursing Process—Implementation
Content Area: Maternity: Newborn
Health Problem: Newborn: Infections
Priority Concepts: Clinical Judgment; Infection
Reference: McKinney et al. (2018), pp. 468, 473-474.

271. *Answer:* 2
Rationale: The highest priority on admission to the nursery for a newborn with a low Apgar score is the airway, which would involve preparing respiratory resuscitation equipment and oxygen. The remaining options are also important, although they are of lower priority. The newborn would be placed on an apnea and cardiorespiratory monitor. Setting up an intravenous line with 5% dextrose in water would provide circulatory support. The radiant warmer would provide an external heat source, which is necessary to prevent further respiratory distress.
Test-Taking Strategy: Note the strategic words, *highest priority*. This question asks you to prioritize care on the basis of information about a newborn's condition. Use the ABCs—airway, breathing, and circulation. A method of planning for airway support is to have the resuscitation bag connected to an oxygen source.
Level of Cognitive Ability: Analyzing
Client Needs: Physiological Integrity
Integrated Process: Nursing Process—Planning
Content Area: Complex Care: Emergency Situations/Management
Health Problem: Newborn: Respiratory Problems
Priority Concepts: Clinical Judgment; Gas Exchange
Reference: McKinney et al. (2018), p. 326.

272. *Answer:* 3
Rationale: The penis is normally red during the healing process after circumcision. A yellow exudate may be noted in 24 hours, and this is part of normal healing. The nurse would expect that the area would be red with a small amount of bloody drainage. Only if the bleeding were excessive would the nurse apply gentle pressure with a sterile gauze. If bleeding cannot be controlled, the blood vessel may need to be ligated, and the nurse would notify the PHCP. Because the findings identified in the question are normal, the nurse would document the assessment findings.
Test-Taking Strategy: Note the strategic words, *most appropriate*, and focus on the assessment findings in the question. This should assist in directing you to the correct option, because this is a normal occurrence after circumcision.
Level of Cognitive Ability: Applying
Client Needs: Physiological Integrity
Integrated Process: Nursing Process—Implementation
Content Area: Maternity: Newborn
Health Problem: Newborn: Circumcision
Priority Concepts: Clinical Judgment; Development
Reference: McKinney et al. (2018), pp. 471-472.

273. *Answer:* 1, 2, 4, 5
Rationale: A newborn infant with respiratory distress syndrome may present with clinical signs of cyanosis, tachypnea or apnea, nasal flaring, chest wall retractions, or audible grunts. Hypotension and a barrel chest are not clinical manifestations associated with respiratory distress syndrome.
Test-Taking Strategy: Focus on the subject, signs of respiratory distress syndrome. Eliminate hypotension, as this is not a finding associated with respiratory distress syndrome. Also, respiratory distress syndrome is an acute occurrence, and a barrel chest develops with a chronic condition. In addition, note the relationship between the diagnosis and the signs noted in the correct options.
Level of Cognitive Ability: Analyzing
Client Needs: Physiological Integrity
Integrated Process: Nursing Process—Assessment
Content Area: Maternity: Newborn
Health Problem: Newborn: Respiratory Problems
Priority Concepts: Gas Exchange; Perfusion
Reference: McKinney et al. (2018), p. 1053.

274. *Answer:* 2
Rationale: Hyperbilirubinemia is an elevated serum bilirubin level. At any serum bilirubin level, the appearance of jaundice during the first day of life indicates a pathological process. Early and frequent feeding hastens the excretion of bilirubin. Breast-feeding should be initiated within 2 hours after birth and every 2 to 4 hours thereafter. The infant should not be fed less frequently. Switching to bottle-feeding for 2 weeks or stopping breast-feeding permanently is unnecessary.
Test-Taking Strategy: Eliminate options 3 and 4 because they are comparable or alike. These options discourage the continuation of breast-feeding and should be eliminated. From the remaining options, recalling the pathophysiology associated with hyperbilirubinemia will assist you in eliminating option 1.
Level of Cognitive Ability: Applying
Client Needs: Physiological Integrity
Integrated Process: Teaching and Learning
Content Area: Maternity: Newborn
Health Problem: Newborn: Hyperbilirubinemia
Priority Concepts: Cellular Regulation; Client Education
Reference: McKinney et al. (2018), pp. 465, 467.

275. *Answer:* 3, 4, 5
Rationale: A newborn of a woman who uses drugs is irritable. The infant is overloaded easily by sensory stimulation. The infant may cry incessantly and be difficult to console. The infant would hyperextend and posture rather than cuddle when being held. This infant is not lethargic or sleepy.
Test-Taking Strategy: Lethargy and sleepiness are comparable or alike in that they indicate hypoactivity of the newborn, and therefore can be eliminated. From the remaining options, recalling the pathophysiology associated with an infant born to a drug-addicted mother and that the newborn is irritable will assist you in eliminating that this infant will be easily comforted and cuddle when held.
Level of Cognitive Ability: Analyzing
Client Needs: Physiological Integrity
Integrated Process: Nursing Process—Assessment
Content Area: Maternity: Newborn
Health Problem: Newborn: Addicted Newborn
Priority Concepts: Addiction; Clinical Judgment
Reference: Hockenberry, Wilson, Rodgers (2017), pp. 284-285.

276. *Answer:* 2
Rationale: Fetal alcohol syndrome, a diagnostic category of fetal alcohol spectrum disorders (FASDs), is caused by maternal alcohol use during pregnancy. Features of newborns diagnosed with fetal alcohol syndrome include craniofacial abnormalities, intrauterine growth restriction, cardiac abnormalities, abnormal palmar creases, and respiratory distress. Options 1, 3, and 4 are normal assessment findings in the full-term newborn infant.

Test-Taking Strategy: Use knowledge regarding normal assessment findings in the full-term newborn infant to answer this question. Length, birth weight, and head circumference are comparable or alike in that all are physical measurements assessed on a newborn and represent normal findings in a full-term newborn.
Level of Cognitive Ability: Analyzing
Client Needs: Physiological Integrity
Integrated Process: Nursing Process—Assessment
Content Area: Maternity: Newborn
Health Problem: Newborn: Addicted Newborn
Priority Concepts: Addiction; Clinical Judgment
Reference: Hockenberry, Wilson, Rodgers (2017), p. 290.

277. *Answer:* 4
Rationale: Fetal alcohol syndrome, a diagnostic category delineated under fetal alcohol spectrum disorders (FASDs), is caused by maternal alcohol use during pregnancy. A primary nursing goal for the newborn diagnosed with fetal alcohol syndrome is to establish nutritional balance after birth. These newborns may exhibit hyperirritability, vomiting, diarrhea, or an uncoordinated sucking and swallowing ability. A quiet environment with minimal stimuli and handling would help establish appropriate sleep-rest cycles in the newborn as well. Options 1, 2, and 3 are inappropriate interventions.
Test-Taking Strategy: Note the strategic word, *priority*. Think about the pathophysiology that occurs in a newborn with this condition. Also, use Maslow's Hierarchy of Needs theory to direct you to the correct option. Remember that nutrition is a priority.
Level of Cognitive Ability: Creating
Client Needs: Physiological Integrity
Integrated Process: Nursing Process—Planning
Content Area: Maternity: Newborn
Health Problem: Newborn: Addicted Newborn
Priority Concepts: Addiction; Clinical Judgment
Reference: McKinney et al. (2018), pp. 1348-1349.

278. *Answer:* 4
Rationale: Erythromycin ophthalmic ointment 0.5% is used as a prophylactic treatment for ophthalmia neonatorum, which is caused by the bacterium *Neisseria gonorrhoeae*. Preventive treatment of gonorrhea is required by law. Options 1, 2, and 3 are not the purposes for administering this medication to a newborn infant.
Test-Taking Strategy: Note the strategic word, *best*. Use knowledge of the purpose of administering erythromycin ophthalmic ointment to a newborn infant. Remember that this is done to prevent ophthalmia neonatorum.
Level of Cognitive Ability: Applying
Client Needs: Health Promotion and Maintenance
Integrated Process: Teaching and Learning
Content Area: Maternity: Newborn
Health Problem: Newborn: Infections
Priority Concepts: Health Promotion; Infection
Reference: McKinney et al. (2018), pp. 462-463.

279. *Answer:* 4, 5, 6
Rationale: Phototherapy (bili-light or bili-blanket) is the use of intense fluorescent light to reduce serum bilirubin levels in the newborn. Adverse effects from treatment, such as eye damage, dehydration, or sensory deprivation, can occur. Interventions include exposing as much of the newborn's skin as possible; however, the genital area is covered. The newborn's eyes are also covered with eye shields or patches, ensuring that the eyelids are closed when shields or patches are applied. The shields or patches are removed at least once per shift to inspect the eyes for infection or irritation and to allow eye contact. The nurse measures the lamp energy output to ensure efficacy of the treatment (done with a special device known as a *photometer*), monitors skin temperature closely, and increases fluids to compensate for water loss. The newborn may have loose green stools and green-colored urine. The newborn's skin color is monitored with the fluorescent light turned off every 4 to 8 hours and is monitored for bronze baby syndrome, a grayish brown discoloration of the skin. The newborn is repositioned every 2 hours, and stimulation is provided. After treatment, the newborn is monitored for signs of hyperbilirubinemia because rebound elevations can occur after therapy is discontinued.
Test-Taking Strategy: Focus on the subject, phototherapy. Recalling that adverse effects from treatment, such as eye damage, dehydration, or sensory deprivation, can occur will assist in determining the correct interventions.
Level of Cognitive Ability: Analyzing
Client Needs: Safe and Effective Care Environment
Integrated Process: Nursing Process—Implementation
Content Area: Maternity: Newborn
Health Problem: Newborn: Hyperbilirubinemia
Priority Concepts: Cellular Regulation; Safety
Reference: McKinney et al. (2018), pp. 647-648.

280. *Answer:* 2
Rationale: An infant born to a mother infected with HIV must be cared for with strict attention to standard precautions. This prevents the transmission of HIV from the newborn, if infected, to others and prevents transmission of other infectious agents to the possibly immunocompromised newborn. Options 1 and 3 are not associated specifically with the care of a potentially HIV-infected newborn. Mothers infected with HIV should not breast-feed.
Test-Taking Strategy: Eliminate options 1 and 3 first because they are comparable or alike and are not associated specifically with the care of a potentially HIV-infected newborn. Recalling that HIV-infected mothers should not breast-feed will direct you to the correct option.
Level of Cognitive Ability: Creating
Client Needs: Safe and Effective Care Environment
Integrated Process: Nursing Process—Planning
Content Area: Maternity: Newborn
Health Problem: Newborn: Newborn of a Mother with HIV/AIDS
Priority Concepts: Infection; Safety
Reference: McKinney et al. (2018), pp. 940-941.

281. *Answer:* 2
Rationale: The newborn of a diabetic mother is at risk for hypoglycemia, so maintaining safety because of low blood glucose levels would be a priority. The newborn would also be at risk for hyperbilirubinemia, respiratory distress, hypocalcemia, and congenital anomalies. Developmental delays, choking, and an elevated body temperature are not expected problems.

Test-Taking Strategy: Note the **strategic word,** *priority*. Read each option thoroughly and eliminate options 1, 3, and 4 because they are **comparable or alike** in that newborns of diabetic mothers are not at risk for these problems. Also, note the relationship of the words *diabetes mellitus* in the question and the word *glucose* in the correct option.
Level of Cognitive Ability: Analyzing
Client Needs: Physiological Integrity
Integrated Process: Nursing Process—Planning
Content Area: Maternity: Newborn
Health Problem: Newborn: Newborn of a Diabetic Mother
Priority Concepts: Clinical Judgment; Glucose Regulation
Reference: McKinney et al. (2018), pp. 652-653.

282. *Answer:* 3
Rationale: Precautions to prevent infant abduction include placing a newborn's crib away from the door, transporting a newborn only in the crib and never carrying the newborn, expecting health care personnel to wear identification that is easily visible at all times, and asking the nurse to attend to the newborn if the mother is napping and no family member is available to watch the newborn (the newborn is never left unattended). If the mother states that she will ask the nurse to watch the newborn while she is sleeping, she has understood the teaching. Options 1, 2, and 4 are incorrect and indicate that the mother needs further teaching.
Test-Taking Strategy: Focus on the **subject,** that the client understands precautions to prevent infant abduction. Read each option carefully and select the option that provides protection to the infant. This will direct you to the correct option.
Level of Cognitive Ability: Evaluating
Client Needs: Safe and Effective Care Environment
Integrated Process: Teaching and Learning
Content Area: Maternity: Newborn
Health Problem: N/A
Priority Concepts: Client Education; Safety
Reference: McKinney et al. (2018), pp. 469-470.

283. *Answer:* 4
Rationale: Phytonadione is necessary for the body to synthesize coagulation factors. It is administered to the newborn to prevent bleeding disorders. It also promotes liver formation of the clotting factors II, VII, IX, and X. Newborns are vitamin K–deficient because the bowel does not have the bacteria necessary to synthesize fat-soluble vitamin K. The normal flora in the intestinal tract produces vitamin K. The newborn's bowel does not support the normal production of vitamin K until bacteria adequately colonize it. The bowel becomes colonized by bacteria as food is ingested. Vitamin K does not promote the development of immunity or prevent the infant from becoming jaundiced.
Test-Taking Strategy: Note the **strategic word,** *best*. Because immunity and jaundice are not related to the action of vitamin K, eliminate options 1 and 2. From the remaining options, recall the action of vitamin K to direct you to the correct option. Remember that vitamin K does not promote the growth of bacteria but is administered to prevent bleeding.
Level of Cognitive Ability: Applying
Client Needs: Physiological Integrity
Integrated Process: Teaching and Learning
Content Area: Maternity: Newborn
Health Problem: N/A
Priority Concepts: Client Education; Clotting
Reference: McKinney et al. (2018), p. 463.

CHAPTER 28

Maternity and Newborn Medications

PRIORITY CONCEPTS Health Promotion, Safety

The Food and Drug Administration has initiated the Pregnancy and Lactation Labeling Rule (PLLR). This is a revision to the previous system that used Category A, B, C, D, and X. The PLLR provides more information on the risks and benefits of using medications during pregnancy. The PLLR also provides more information to assist the provider and pregnant mother to make informed decisions together, so as to not deter medication use during pregnancy when it is necessary.

I. Tocolytics

A. Description: Tocolytics are medications that produce uterine relaxation and suppress uterine activity (Table 28-1).

B. Uses: To halt uterine contractions and prevent preterm birth; dihydropyridine calcium channel blockers such as nifedipine and magnesium sulfate may be prescribed to achieve this goal. Terbutaline is another medication used for this effect.

C. Adverse effects and contraindications

1. See Table 28-1 for a description of adverse effects.
2. Maternal contraindications include severe preeclampsia and eclampsia, active vaginal bleeding, intrauterine infection, cardiac disease, placental abruption, or poorly controlled diabetes.
3. Fetal contraindications include estimated gestational age greater than 37 weeks, cervical dilation greater than 4 cm, fetal demise, lethal fetal anomaly, chorioamnionitis, acute fetal distress, and chronic intrauterine growth restriction.

D. Interventions for the client receiving tocolytic therapy

1. Position the client on her side to enhance placental perfusion and reduce pressure on the cervix.
2. Monitor maternal vital signs, fetal status, and labor status frequently according to agency protocol.
3. Monitor for signs of adverse effects to the medication.
4. Monitor daily weight and input and output status, and provide fluid intake as prescribed.
5. Offer comfort measures and provide psychosocial support to the client and family.
6. See Table 28-1 for interventions specific to each tocolytic medication.

II. Magnesium Sulfate

A. Description (Table 28-1)

1. Magnesium sulfate is a central nervous system depressant and antiseizure medication.
2. The medication causes smooth muscle relaxation.
3. The antidote is calcium gluconate.

B. Uses

1. Stopping preterm labor to prevent preterm birth, although it is less commonly used for this effect in practice
2. Preventing and controlling seizures in preeclamptic and eclamptic clients

C. Adverse effects and contraindications

1. Magnesium sulfate can cause respiratory depression, depressed reflexes, flushing, hypotension, extreme muscle weakness, decreased urine output, pulmonary edema, and elevated serum magnesium levels.
2. Continuous intravenous (IV) infusion increases the risk of magnesium toxicity in the newborn.
3. Magnesium sulfate is stopped for delivery only if the mother is having a C-section.
4. Magnesium sulfate may be prescribed for the first 12 to 24 hours postpartum if it is used for preeclampsia.
5. High doses can cause loss of deep tendon reflexes, heart block, respiratory paralysis, and cardiac arrest.
6. The medication is contraindicated in clients with heart block, myocardial damage, or kidney failure.
7. The medication is used with caution in clients with kidney impairment.

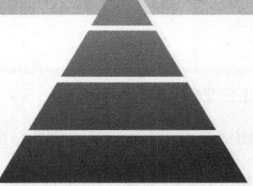

TABLE 28-1 Tocolytics

Medication, Classification, and Actions	Adverse Effects	Nursing Interventions
Terbutaline—selective $beta_2$ agonist that suppresses preterm labor by activating $beta_2$ receptors in the uterus—decreases both frequency and intensity of contractions; primarily used to delay birth for several hours to allow the fetus to mature more before being born	*Maternal*—Pulmonary edema, hypotension, hyperglycemia, and tachycardia	Administered by injection under the skin
	Fetus—Tachycardia	Dosing should stop after 48 hours and should be interrupted if the maternal heart rate exceeds 120 beats per minute
Magnesium sulfate—central nervous system depressant; relaxes smooth muscle, including the uterus; used to halt preterm labor contractions; used for preeclamptic clients to prevent seizures	*Maternal*—depressed respirations, depressed DTRs, hypotension, extreme muscle weakness, flushing, decreased urine output, pulmonary edema, serum magnesium levels >7.5 mEq/L (3.75 mmol/L)	Always use intravenous controller device for administration
	Fetus—hypotonia and sleepiness	Follow agency protocol for administration
		Discontinue infusion and notify OB if adverse effects occur
		Monitor for respirations <12/min, urine output <100 mL/4 hr (25-30 mL/hr)
		Monitor DTRs
		Monitor magnesium levels and report values outside therapeutic range of 4 to 7.5 mEq/L (2 to 3.75 mmol/L)
		Keep calcium gluconate readily accessible (antidote)
Nifedipine-calcium channel blocker; relaxes smooth muscles, including the uterus, by blocking calcium entry; in some health care agencies, this may be the first-line agent to halt preterm labor contractions	*Maternal*—tachycardia, hypotension, dizziness, headache, nervousness, facial flushing, fatigue, nausea *Fetus*—May cause vascular dilation	Follow agency protocol for administration Use with magnesium sulfate is avoided because severe hypotension can occur Monitor for adverse effects

DTRs, Deep tendon reflexes; *OB*, obstetrician.

D. Interventions

1. Monitor maternal vital signs, especially respirations, every 30 to 60 minutes.
2. Assess renal function and electrocardiogram for cardiac function.
3. Monitor magnesium levels every 6 hours or if signs and symptoms of toxicity are noted—the target range when used as a tocolytic agent is 4 to 7.5 mEq/L (2 to 3.75 mmol/L); if the magnesium level increases, notify the obstetrician (OB).
4. Always administer by IV infusion via an infusion monitoring device; carefully monitor the dose being administered, and follow agency protocol for administration.
5. Keep calcium gluconate readily accessible in case of a magnesium sulfate overdose, because calcium gluconate antagonizes the effect of magnesium sulfate.
6. Monitor deep tendon reflexes hourly for signs of developing toxicity.
7. Test the patellar reflex or knee jerk reflex before administering a repeat parenteral dose (used as an indicator of central nervous system depression; suppressed reflex may be a sign of impending respiratory arrest) (Table 28-2).
8. Patellar reflex must be present and respiratory rate must be greater than 12 breaths per minute (or as designated by agency protocol) before each parenteral dose.
9. Monitor intake and output hourly; output should be maintained at 25 to 30 mL/hr because the medication is eliminated through the kidneys.

Monitor a client receiving magnesium sulfate intravenously closely for signs of toxicity. Call the OB if respirations are less than 12 breaths per minute, indicating respiratory depression, or if any other adverse effects occur.

TABLE 28-2 Assessing Deep Tendon Reflexes

Grade	Deep Tendon Reflex Response
0	No response
1	Sluggish or diminished
2	Active or expected response
3	More brisk than expected, slightly hyperactive
4	Brisk, hyperactive, with intermittent or transient clonus

Data from Seidel H, Ball J, Dains J, Flynn J, Solomon B, Stewart R: *Mosby's guide to physical examination*, ed 6, St. Louis, 2011, Mosby.

III. Betamethasone and Dexamethasone

A. Description: Corticosteroids that increase the production of **surfactant** to accelerate fetal lung maturity and reduce the incidence or severity of respiratory distress syndrome

B. Use: For a client in preterm labor between 28 and 32 weeks' gestation whose labor can be inhibited for 48 hours without jeopardizing the mother or fetus

C. Adverse effects and contraindications
1. May decrease the mother's resistance to infection
2. Pulmonary edema secondary to sodium and fluid retention can occur.
3. Elevated blood glucose levels can occur in a client with diabetes mellitus.

D. Interventions
1. Monitor maternal vital signs and lung sounds, and for edema.
2. Monitor mother for signs of infection.
3. Monitor white blood cell count.
4. Monitor blood glucose levels.
5. Administer by deep intramuscular injection.

IV. Opioid Analgesics

A. Description
1. Used to relieve moderate to severe pain associated with **labor**
2. Administered by intramuscular or IV route
3. Regular use of opioids during pregnancy may produce withdrawal symptoms in the newborn (irritability, excessive crying, tremors, hyperactive reflexes, fever, vomiting, diarrhea, yawning, sneezing, and seizures).
4. Antidotes for opioids
   a. Naloxone is usually the treatment of choice because it rapidly reverses opioid toxicity; the dose may need to be repeated every few hours until opioid concentrations have decreased to nontoxic levels.
   b. These medications can cause withdrawal in opioid-dependent clients.

B. Hydromorphone hydrochloride
1. Can cause dizziness, nausea, vomiting, sedation, decreased blood pressure, decreased respirations, diaphoresis, flushed face, and urinary retention
2. May be prescribed to be administered with an antiemetic such as promethazine to prevent nausea
3. High dosages may result in respiratory depression, skeletal muscle flaccidity, cold clammy skin, cyanosis, and extreme somnolence progressing to seizures, stupor, and coma.
4. Used cautiously in clients delivering preterm newborns
5. Not administered in advanced labor (typically once transition phase during stage 1 of labor has been reached); if the medication is not adequately removed from the fetal circulation, respiratory depression can occur.

C. Fentanyl and sufentanil can cause respiratory depression, dizziness, drowsiness, hypotension, urinary retention, and fetal narcosis and distress; sufentanil is used less commonly than fentanyl.

D. Butorphanol tartrate and nalbuphine
1. May be prescribed depending on OB preference
2. Can cause confusion, sedation, sweating, nausea, vomiting, hypotension, and sinusoidal-like fetal heart rhythm
3. Use with caution in a client with preexisting opioid dependency, because these medications can precipitate withdrawal symptoms in the client and the newborn.

E. Interventions
1. Monitor vital signs, particularly respiratory status; if respirations are 12 breaths per minute or less, withhold the medication and contact the OB.
2. Monitor the fetal heart rate and characteristics of uterine contractions.
3. Monitor for blood pressure changes (hypotension); maintain the client in a recumbent position (elevate the hip with a wedge pillow or other device).
4. Record the level of pain relief.
5. Monitor the bladder for distention and retention.
6. Have the antidote naloxone readily accessible, especially if delivery is expected to occur during peak medication absorption time.

Obtain a medication history before the administration of an opioid analgesic. Some medications may be contraindicated if the client has a history of opioid dependency, because these medications can precipitate withdrawal symptoms in the client and newborn.

V. Prostaglandins (Box 28-1)

A. Description
1. Ripen the cervix, making it softer and causing it to begin to dilate and efface
2. Stimulate uterine contractions
3. Administered vaginally

BOX 28-1 Prostaglandins

Prostaglandin E_1: Misoprostol intravaginal tablet
Prostaglandin E_2: Dinoprostone vaginal gel, insert, or suppository

B. Uses
1. Preinduction cervical ripening (ripening of the cervix before the induction of labor when the Bishop score is ≤4)
2. Induction of labor
3. Induction of abortion (abortifacient agent)

C. Adverse effects and contraindications
1. Gastrointestinal effects, including diarrhea, nausea, vomiting, and stomach cramps
2. Fever, chills, flushing, headache, and hypotension
3. Uterine tachysystole (≥12 uterine contractions in 20 minutes without an alteration in the fetal heart rate pattern)
4. Hyperstimulation of the uterus
5. Fetal passage of meconium
6. Contraindications (Box 28-2)

D. Interventions
1. Monitor maternal vital signs, fetal heart rate pattern, and status of pregnancy, including indications for cervical ripening or the induction of labor, contraindications, adverse effects, signs of labor or impending labor, and the Bishop score (see Chapter 23, Table 23-2 for information about the Bishop score).
2. Have the client void before administration of medication and then have her maintain a supine with lateral tilt or side-lying position for 30 to 60 minutes (gel) up to 2 hours (insert) after administration, depending on the medication administered.
3. Treatment is discontinued when the Bishop score is 8 or more (cervix ripens) or an effective contraction pattern is established (3 or more contractions in a 10-minute period); in addition, signs of adverse effects indicate that the treatment needs to be discontinued.
4. Follow agency protocol for the induction of labor if cervical ripening has occurred and labor has not begun; oxytocin may be initiated if needed 6 to 12 hours after discontinuation of prostaglandin therapy.

BOX 28-2 Contraindications to the Use of Prostaglandins

- Active cardiac, hepatic, pulmonary, or kidney disease
- Acute pelvic inflammatory disease
- Clients in whom vaginal delivery is not indicated
- Fetal malpresentation
- History of cesarean section or major uterine surgery
- History of difficult labor or traumatic labor
- Hypersensitivity to prostaglandins
- Maternal fever or infection
- Nonreassuring fetal heart rate pattern
- Placenta previa or unexplained vaginal bleeding
- Regular progressive uterine contractions
- Significant cephalopelvic disproportion

VI. Uterine Stimulants (Oxytocics): Oxytocin

A. Description
1. Oxytocin stimulates the smooth muscle of the uterus and increases the force, frequency, and duration of uterine contractions.
2. Oxytocin also promotes milk letdown.
3. For induction of labor, oxytocin is administered by the IV route (other route of administration is intramuscular); if injecting intramuscularly, aspiration is necessary to avoid injection into a blood vessel.
4. Magnesium sulfate should be readily accessible in case relaxation of the myometrium is necessary.
5. Minimal cervical change usually is noted until the active phase of labor is achieved.

B. Uses
1. Induces or augments labor
2. Controls postpartum bleeding
3. Manages an incomplete abortion

C. Adverse effects and contraindications
1. Adverse effects include allergies, dysrhythmias, changes in blood pressure, uterine rupture, and water intoxication.
2. Oxytocin may produce uterine hypertonicity, resulting in fetal or maternal adverse effects.
3. High doses may cause hypotension, with rebound hypertension.
4. Postpartum hemorrhage can occur and should be monitored for, because the uterus may become atonic when the medication wears off.
5. Oxytocin should not be used in a client who cannot deliver vaginally or in a client with hypertonic uterine contractions; it is also contraindicated in a client with active genital herpes.

D. Interventions
1. Monitor maternal vital signs (every 15 minutes), especially the blood pressure and heart rate, weight, intake and output, level of consciousness, and lung sounds.
2. Monitor frequency, duration, and force of contractions and resting uterine tone every 15 minutes.
3. Monitor fetal heart rate every 15 minutes, and notify the OB if significant changes occur; use of an internal fetal scalp electrode may be prescribed.

4. Administered by IV infusion via an infusion monitoring device (most common route); prescribed additive solution is piggybacked at the port nearest the point of venous insertion (prescribed additive solution may be normal saline, lactated Ringer's, or 5% dextrose in water).
5. Carefully monitor the dose being administered; do not leave the client unattended while the oxytocin is infusing.
6. Administer oxygen if prescribed.
7. Monitor for hypertonic contractions or a nonreassuring fetal heart rate and notify the OB if these occur (see **Priority Nursing Actions**).
8. Stop the medication if uterine hyperstimulation or a nonreassuring fetal heart rate occurs; turn the client on her side, increase the IV rate of the prescribed additive solution, and administer oxygen via face mask.
9. Monitor for signs of water intoxication.
10. Have emergency equipment readily accessible.
11. Document the dose of the medication and the time the medication was started, increased, maintained, and discontinued; document the client's response.
12. Keep the client and family informed of the client's progress.
13. Calculating an oxytocin drip (Box 28-3)

PRIORITY NURSING ACTIONS

Hypertonic Contractions or a Nonreassuring Fetal Heart Rate during Oxytocin Infusion

1. Stop the oxytocin infusion.
2. Turn the client on her side, stay with the client, and ask another nurse to contact the obstetrician (OB).
3. Increase the flow rate of the intravenous (IV) solution that does not contain the oxytocin.
4. Administer oxygen, 8 to 10 L/minute, by snug face mask.
5. Assess maternal vital signs; fetal heart rate and patterns; and frequency, duration, and force of contractions.
6. Document the event, actions taken, and the response.

Reference
Lowdermilk et al. (2016), p. 784.

BOX 28-3 Calculating an Oxytocin Dose

Prescription: Oxytocin 2 milliunits (mU)/minute
Available: 20 units (U) in 1000 mL 5% dextrose in Water (D5W)

How many mL per hour?

Steps for calculating:
1. Do you need to convert? Yes, you need to change mU to U
2. What has been prescribed? Oxytocin 2 mU/minute
3. What do you have available? 1000 mL D5W containing 20 U oxytocin
4. Set up formula:

Convert:

$$1000\,mU : 1U = 2\,mU : X$$

How many mU are in 1 U? There are 1000 mU in 1 U.
If there are 1000 mU in 1 U, how many units in 2 mU?
Answer: 0.002 U in 2 mU
Now use the standard formula for calculation.

$$\text{Prescribed} / \text{Available} \times \text{Volume}$$

$$0.002\,U / 20\,U \times 1000\,mL = 0.1\,mL$$

Now, determine how many milliliters should be given in 1 hour if the prescription is for 0.1 mL/minute. 0.1 mL/minute × 60 minutes (1 hour) = 6 mL/hr

Note: Many electronic pumps allow for programming in units or milliunits per minute, eliminating the need to calculate the milliliters per hour, and this practice is recommended if available because medications are programmed in the pumps with dosage safeguards. If a dose that is too low or too high is programmed into the pump, the pump will flag or will not allow the nurse to proceed with administration.

Reference: Burcham & Rosenthal (2016), p. 782.

BOX 28-4 Medications Used to Manage Postpartum Hemorrhage

- Methylergonovine
- Oxytocin
- Prostaglandin $F_{2\alpha}$: Carboprost tromethamine

VII. Medications Used to Manage Postpartum Hemorrhage (Box 28-4)

A. Ergot alkaloid
1. Description
a. Methylergonovine maleate is an ergot alkaloid.
b. Directly stimulates uterine muscle, increases the force and frequency of contractions, and produces a firm tetanic contraction of the uterus
c. Can produce arterial vasoconstriction and vasospasm of the coronary arteries
d. An ergot alkaloid is administered postpartum and is not administered before the birth of the placenta.
2. Uses
a. Postpartum hemorrhage
b. Postabortal hemorrhage resulting from atony or involution
3. Adverse effects and contraindications
a. Can cause nausea, uterine cramping, bradycardia, dysrhythmias, myocardial infarction, and severe hypertension
b. High doses are associated with peripheral vasospasm or vasoconstriction, angina, miosis, confusion, respiratory depression, seizures, or unconsciousness; uterine tetany can occur.

c. Contraindicated during pregnancy and in clients with significant cardiovascular disease, peripheral vascular disease, or hypertension

4. Interventions
   a. Monitor maternal vital signs, weight, intake and output, level of consciousness, and lung sounds.
   b. Monitor the blood pressure closely; the medication produces vasoconstriction, and if an increase in blood pressure is noted, withhold the medication and notify the OB.
   c. Monitor uterine contractions (frequency, strength, and duration).
   d. Assess for chest pain, headache, shortness of breath, itching, pale or cold hands or feet, nausea, diarrhea, and dizziness.
   e. Assess the extremities for color, warmth, movement, and pain.
   f. Assess vaginal bleeding.
   g. Notify the OB if chest pain or other adverse effects occur.
   h. Administer analgesics as prescribed; they may be required because the medication produces painful uterine contractions.

⚠ Check the client's blood pressure before administering methylergonovine maleate. This medication can cause severe hypertension and is contraindicated in a client with hypertension.

B. Prostaglandin $F_{2\alpha}$: carboprost tromethamine
1. Description: Contracts the uterus
2. Uses: Postpartum hemorrhage
3. Adverse effects and contraindications
   a. Can cause headache, nausea, vomiting, diarrhea, fever, tachycardia, and hypertension
   b. Contraindicated if the client has asthma
4. Interventions
   a. Monitor vital signs.
   b. Monitor vaginal bleeding and uterine tone.

C. Oxytocin: See Section VI on uterine stimulants.

VIII. Rh_o(D) Immune Globulin

A. Description
1. Prevention of anti-Rh_o(D) antibody formation is most successful if the medication is administered twice, at 28 weeks' gestation and again within 72 hours after delivery.
2. Rh_o(D) immune globulin also should be administered within 72 hours after potential or actual exposure to Rh-positive blood and must be given with each subsequent exposure or potential exposure to Rh-positive blood.

B. Use: To prevent isoimmunization in Rh-negative clients who are negative for Rh antibodies and exposed or potentially exposed to Rh-positive red blood cells by amniocentesis, chorionic villus sampling, transfusion, termination of pregnancy, abdominal trauma, or bleeding during pregnancy or the birth process

C. Adverse effects and contraindications
1. Elevated temperature
2. Tenderness at the injection site
3. Contraindicated for Rh-positive clients
4. Contraindicated in clients with a history of systemic allergic reactions to preparations containing human immunoglobulins
5. Note: Not administered to a newborn

D. Interventions
1. Administer to the client by intramuscular injection at 28 weeks' gestation and within 72 hours after delivery.
2. Never administer by the IV route.
3. Monitor for temperature elevation.
4. Monitor injection site for tenderness.

⚠ Rh_o(D) immune globulin is of no benefit when the client has developed a positive antibody titer to the Rh antigen.

IX. Rubella Vaccine

A. Given subcutaneously before hospital discharge to a nonimmune postpartum client

B. Administered if the rubella titer is less than 1:8

C. Adverse effects: Transient rash, hypersensitivity

D. Contraindicated in a client with a hypersensitivity to eggs (check with the OB regarding administration)

E. Interventions
1. Assess for allergy to duck eggs and notify the OB before administration if an allergy exists.
2. Question administration if the client or other family members are immunocompromised.

⚠ The client should avoid pregnancy for 1 to 3 months (or as prescribed) after immunization with rubella vaccine. Inform the client about the need to use a contraception method during this time.

X. Lung Surfactants

A. Description
1. Replenish surfactant and restore surface activity to the lungs to prevent and treat respiratory distress syndrome.
2. Administered to the newborn by the intratracheal route.

B. Use: To prevent or treat respiratory distress syndrome in premature newborns

C. Adverse effects and contraindications
1. Adverse effects include transient bradycardia and oxygen desaturation; pulmonary hemorrhage, mucus plugging, and endotracheal tube reflux can also occur.
2. Surfactants are administered with caution in newborns at risk for circulatory overload.

D. Interventions
1. Instill surfactant through the catheter inserted into the newborn's endotracheal tube; avoid suctioning for at least 2 hours after administration.
2. Monitor for bradycardia and decreased oxygen saturation during administration.
3. Monitor respiratory status and lung sounds and for signs of adverse effects.

XI. Eye Prophylaxis for the Newborn

A. Description
1. Preventive eye treatment against ophthalmia neonatorum in the newborn is required by law in the United States.
2. Ophthalmic forms of erythromycin are prescribed because it is bacteriostatic and bactericidal and provides prophylaxis against *Neisseria gonorrhoeae* and *Chlamydia trachomatis*.

B. Use: As a prophylactic measure to protect against *N. gonorrhoeae* and *C. trachomatis*

C. Interventions
1. Clean the newborn's eyes before instilling the medication.
2. Do not flush the eyes after instillation.

Instillation of eye medication can be delayed for 1 hour after birth to facilitate eye contact and parent-newborn attachment and bonding.

XII. Phytonadione

A. Description
1. The newborn is at risk for hemorrhagic disorders; coagulation factors synthesized in the liver depend on phytonadione (also known as vitamin K), which is not synthesized until intestinal bacteria are present.
2. Newborns are deficient in phytonadione for the first 5 to 8 days of life because of the lack of intestinal bacteria.

B. Use: Prophylaxis and treatment of hemorrhagic disease of the newborn

C. Adverse effect: Can cause hyperbilirubinemia in the newborn (occurrence is rare)

D. Interventions
1. Protect the medication from light.
2. Administer during the early newborn period.
3. Administer by the intramuscular route in the lateral aspect of the middle third of the vastus lateralis muscle of the thigh.
4. Monitor for bruising at the injection site and for bleeding from the cord.
5. Monitor for jaundice and monitor the bilirubin level because, although rare, the medication can cause hyperbilirubinemia in the newborn.

XIII. Hepatitis B Vaccine, Recombinant

A. Description: Given intramuscularly to the newborn before discharge home

B. Use: Recommended for all newborns to prevent hepatitis B

C. Adverse effects: Rash, fever, erythema, and pain at injection site

D. Interventions
1. Parental consent must be obtained.
2. Administer intramuscularly in the lateral aspect of the middle third of the vastus lateralis muscle.
3. If the infant was born to a mother positive for hepatitis B surface antigen, hepatitis B immune globulin should be given within 12 hours of birth in addition to hepatitis B vaccine. Then follow the regularly scheduled hepatitis B vaccination schedule.
4. Document immunization administration on a vaccination card so that the parents have a record that the vaccine was administered.

XIV. Contraceptives

A. Description
1. These medications contain a combination of estrogen and a progestin or a progestin alone and come in several different forms, including oral and intramuscular preparations and implants.
2. Estrogen-progestin combinations suppress ovulation and change the cervical mucus, making it difficult for sperm to enter.
3. Medications that contain only progestins are less effective than the combined medications.
4. Contraceptives usually are taken for 21 consecutive days and stopped for 7 days; the administration cycle is then repeated.
5. Contraceptives provide reversible prevention of pregnancy.
6. Contraceptives are useful in controlling irregular or excessive menstrual cycles.
7. Risk factors associated with the development of complications related to the use of contraceptives include smoking, obesity, and hypertension.
8. Contraceptives are contraindicated in women with hypertension, thromboembolic disease, cerebrovascular or coronary artery disease, estrogen-dependent cancers, and pregnancy.
9. Contraceptives should be avoided with the use of hepatotoxic medications.
10. Contraceptives interfere with the activity of bromocriptine mesylate and anticoagulants and increase the toxicity of tricyclic antidepressants.
11. Contraceptives may alter blood glucose levels.

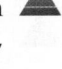

12. Antibiotics may decrease the absorption and effectiveness of oral contraceptives.

B. Side and adverse effects
1. Breakthrough bleeding
2. Excessive cervical mucus formation
3. Breast tenderness
4. Hypertension
5. Nausea, vomiting

C. Interventions
1. Monitor vital signs and weight.
2. Instruct the client in the administration of the medication (it may take up to 1 week for full contraceptive effect to occur when the medication is begun).
3. Instruct the client with diabetes mellitus to monitor blood glucose levels carefully.
4. Instruct the client to report signs of thromboembolic complications.
5. Instruct the client to notify the OB if vaginal bleeding or menstrual irregularities occur or if pregnancy is suspected.
6. Advise the client to use an alternative method of birth control when taking antibiotics because these may decrease absorption of the oral contraceptive.
7. Instruct the client to perform breast self-examination regularly and about the importance of annual physical examinations.
8. Contraceptive patches
   a. Designed to be worn for 3 weeks and removed for a 1-week period
   b. Applied on clean, dry, intact skin on the buttocks, abdomen, upper outer arm, or upper torso
   c. Instruct the client to peel away half of the backing on a patch, apply the sticky surface to the skin, remove the other half of the backing, and then press down on the patch with the palm for 10 seconds.
   d. Instruct the client to change the patch weekly, using a new location for each patch.
   e. If the patch falls off and remains off for less than 24 hours (such as when the client is sleeping or is unaware that it has fallen off), it can be reapplied if still sticky, or it can be replaced with a new patch.
   f. If the patch is off for more than 24 hours, a new 4-week cycle must be started immediately.
9. Vaginal ring
   a. Inserted into the vagina by the client, left in place for 3 weeks, and removed for 1 week
   b. The medication is absorbed through mucous membranes of the vagina.
   c. Removed rings should be wrapped in a foil pouch and discarded, not flushed down the toilet.
10. Implants and depot injections provide long-acting forms of birth control, from 3 months to 5 years in duration.

If the client decides to discontinue the contraceptive to become pregnant, recommend that the client use an alternative form of birth control for 2 months after discontinuation to ensure more complete excretion of hormonal agents before conception.

XV. Fertility Medications (Box 28-5)

A. Description
1. Fertility medications act to stimulate follicle development and ovulation in functioning ovaries and are combined with human chorionic gonadotropin to maintain the follicles once ovulation has occurred.
2. Fertility medications are contraindicated in the presence of primary ovarian dysfunction, thyroid or adrenal dysfunction, ovarian cysts, pregnancy, or idiopathic uterine bleeding.
3. Fertility medications should be used with caution in clients with thromboembolic or respiratory disease.

B. Side and adverse effects
1. Risk of multiple births and birth defects
2. Ovarian overstimulation (abdominal pain, distention, ascites, pleural effusion)
3. Headache, irritability
4. Fluid retention and bloating
5. Nausea, vomiting
6. Uterine bleeding
7. Ovarian enlargement
8. Gynecomastia
9. Rash
10. Orthostatic hypotension
11. Febrile reactions

C. Interventions
1. Instruct the client regarding administration of the medication.
2. Provide a calendar of treatment days and instructions on when intercourse should occur to increase therapeutic effectiveness of the medication.

BOX 28-5 Fertility Medications

- Chorionic gonadotropin
- Clomiphene citrate
- Follitropin alfa
- Follitropin beta
- Menotropins
- Urofollitropin
- Cetrorelix
- Ganirelix

3. Provide information about the risks and hazards of multiple births.
4. Instruct the client to notify the OB if signs of ovarian overstimulation occur.
5. Inform the client about the need for regular follow-up for evaluation.

PRACTICE QUESTIONS

284. The nurse is monitoring a client who is receiving oxytocin to induce labor. Which assessment findings should cause the nurse to **immediately** discontinue the oxytocin infusion? **Select all that apply.**
- ❑ 1. Fatigue
- ❑ 2. Drowsiness
- ❑ 3. Uterine hyperstimulation
- ❑ 4. Late decelerations of the fetal heart rate
- ❑ 5. Early decelerations of the fetal heart rate

285. A pregnant client is receiving magnesium sulfate for the management of preeclampsia. The nurse determines that the client is experiencing toxicity from the medication if which findings are noted on assessment? **Select all that apply.**
- ❑ 1. Proteinuria of 3+
- ❑ 2. Respirations of 10 breaths per minute
- ❑ 3. Presence of deep tendon reflexes
- ❑ 4. Urine output of 20 mL in an hour
- ❑ 5. Serum magnesium level of 4 mEq/L (2 mmol/L)

286. The nurse asks a nursing student to describe the procedure for administering erythromycin ointment to the eyes of a newborn. Which student statement indicates that **further teaching is needed** about administration of the eye medication?
1. "I will flush the eyes after instilling the ointment."
2. "I will clean the newborn's eyes before instilling ointment."
3. "I need to administer the eye ointment within 1 hour after delivery."
4. "I will instill the eye ointment into each of the newborn's conjunctival sacs."

287. A client in preterm labor (31 weeks) who is dilated to 4 cm has been started on magnesium sulfate and contractions have stopped. If the client's labor can be inhibited for the next 48 hours, the nurse anticipates a prescription for which medication?
1. Nalbuphine
2. Betamethasone
3. Rh_o(D) immune globulin
4. Dinoprostone vaginal insert

288. Methylergonovine is prescribed for a woman to treat postpartum hemorrhage. Before administration of methylergonovine, what is the **priority** assessment?
1. Uterine tone
2. Blood pressure
3. Amount of lochia
4. Deep tendon reflexes

289. The nurse is preparing to administer exogenous surfactant to a premature infant who has respiratory distress syndrome. The nurse prepares to administer the medication by which route?
1. Intradermal
2. Intratracheal
3. Subcutaneous
4. Intramuscular

290. An opioid analgesic is administered to a client in labor. The nurse assigned to care for the client ensures that which medication is readily accessible should respiratory depression occur?
1. Naloxone
2. Morphine sulfate
3. Betamethasone
4. Hydromorphone hydrochloride

291. Rh_o(D) immune globulin is prescribed for a client after delivery, and the nurse provides information to the client about the purpose of the medication. The nurse determines that the woman understands the purpose if the woman states that it will protect her next baby from which condition?
1. Having Rh-positive blood
2. Developing a rubella infection
3. Developing physiological jaundice
4. Being affected by Rh incompatibility

292. Methylergonovine is prescribed for a client with postpartum hemorrhage. Before administering the medication, the nurse should contact the obstetrician who prescribed the medication if which condition is documented in the client's medical history?
1. Hypotension
2. Hypothyroidism
3. Diabetes mellitus
4. Peripheral vascular disease

293. The nurse is monitoring a client in preterm labor who is receiving intravenous magnesium sulfate. The nurse should monitor for which adverse effects of this medication? **Select all that apply.**
- ❑ 1. Flushing
- ❑ 2. Hypertension
- ❑ 3. Increased urine output
- ❑ 4. Depressed respirations
- ❑ 5. Extreme muscle weakness
- ❑ 6. Hyperactive deep tendon reflexes

Maternity

ANSWERS

284. *Answer:* 3, 4

Rationale: Oxytocin stimulates uterine contractions and is a pharmacological method to induce labor. Late decelerations, a nonreassuring fetal heart rate pattern, is an ominous sign indicating fetal distress. Oxytocin infusion must be stopped when any signs of uterine hyperstimulation, late decelerations, or other adverse effects occur. Some obstetricians prescribe the administration of oxytocin in 10-minute pulsed infusions rather than as a continuous infusion. This pulsed method, which is more like endogenous secretion of oxytocin, is reported to be effective for labor induction and requires significantly less oxytocin use. Drowsiness and fatigue may be caused by the labor experience. Early decelerations of the fetal heart rate are a reassuring sign and do not indicate fetal distress.

Test-Taking Strategy: Note the strategic word, *immediately.* Focus on the subject, an adverse effect of oxytocin. Options 1 and 2 are comparable or alike and can be eliminated first. From the remaining options, recalling that early decelerations of the fetal heart rate are a reassuring sign will direct you to the correct options.

Level of Cognitive Ability: Analyzing

Client Needs: Physiological Integrity

Integrated Process: Nursing Process—Implementation

Content Area: Pharmacology: Maternity/Newborn: Uterine Stimulants

Health Problem: Maternity: Fetal Distress/Demise

Priority Concepts: Perfusion; Reproduction

References: Lowdermilk et al. (2016), p. 784.

285. *Answer:* 2, 4

Rationale: Magnesium toxicity can occur from magnesium sulfate therapy. Signs of magnesium sulfate toxicity relate to the central nervous system depressant effects of the medication and include respiratory depression, loss of deep tendon reflexes, and a sudden decline in fetal heart rate and maternal heart rate and blood pressure. Respiratory rate below 12 breaths per minute is a sign of toxicity. Urine output should be at least 25 to 30 mL per hour. Proteinuria of 3+ is an expected finding in a client with preeclampsia. Presence of deep tendon reflexes is a normal and expected finding. Therapeutic serum levels of magnesium are 4 to 7.5 mEq/L (2 to 3.75 mmol/L).

Test-Taking Strategy: Focus on the subject, magnesium toxicity. Eliminate option 3 first because it is a normal finding. Next, eliminate option 5, knowing that the therapeutic serum level of magnesium is 4 to 7.5 mEq/L (2 to 3.75 mmol/L). From the remaining options, recalling that proteinuria of 3+ would be noted and expected in a client with preeclampsia will direct you to the correct options.

Level of Cognitive Ability: Analyzing

Client Needs: Physiological Integrity

Integrated Process: Nursing Process—Assessment

Content Area: Pharmacology: Maternity/Newborn: Tocolytics

Health Problem: Maternity: Gestational hypertension/preeclampsia and eclampsia

Priority Concepts: Perfusion; Reproduction

Reference: McKinney et al. (2018), pp. 539, 544.

286. *Answer:* 1

Rationale: Eye prophylaxis protects the newborn against *Neisseria gonorrhoeae* and *Chlamydia trachomatis*. The eyes are not flushed after instillation of the medication because the flush would wash away the administered medication. Options 2, 3, and 4 are correct statements regarding the procedure for administering eye medication to the newborn.

Test-Taking Strategy: Note the strategic words, *further teaching is needed*. These words indicate a negative event query and ask you to select an option that is an incorrect statement. Eliminate options 3 and 4 first because they are comparable or alike and relate to instilling the eye medication. From the remaining options, visualize the effect of each. This will direct you to the correct option.

Level of Cognitive Ability: Evaluating

Client Needs: Health Promotion and Maintenance

Integrated Process: Teaching and Learning

Content Area: Pharmacology: Maternity/Newborn: Eye Prophylaxis for the newborn

Health Problem: Newborn: Infections

Priority Concepts: Health Promotion; Infection

Reference: McKinney et al. (2018), p. 463.

287. *Answer:* 2

Rationale: Betamethasone, a glucocorticoid, is given to increase the production of surfactant to stimulate fetal lung maturation. It is administered to clients in preterm labor at 28 to 32 weeks of gestation if the labor can be inhibited for 48 hours. Nalbuphine is an opioid analgesic. Rh_o(D) immune globulin is given to Rh-negative clients to prevent sensitization. Dinoprostone vaginal insert is a prostaglandin given to ripen and soften the cervix and to stimulate uterine contractions.

Test-Taking Strategy: Focus on the subject, a client at 31 weeks' gestation. Recall that the preterm infant is at risk for respiratory distress syndrome because of immaturity and the inability to produce surfactant. Next, recalling the actions of the medications in the options and that betamethasone is used to increase the production of surfactant will direct you to the correct option.

Level of Cognitive Ability: Analyzing

Client Needs: Physiological Integrity

Integrated Process: Nursing Process—Analysis

Content Area: Pharmacology: Maternity/Newborn: Lung Surfactant

Health Problem: Maternity: Preterm Labor

Priority Concepts: Gas Exchange; Perfusion

Reference: McKinney et al. (2018), p. 588.

288. *Answer:* 2

Rationale: Methylergonovine, an ergot alkaloid, is used to prevent or control postpartum hemorrhage by contracting the uterus. Methylergonovine causes continuous uterine contractions and may elevate the blood pressure. A priority assessment before the administration of the medication is to check the blood pressure. The obstetrician needs to be notified if hypertension is present. Although options 1, 3, and 4 may be components of the postpartum assessment, blood pressure is related specifically to the administration of this medication.

Test-Taking Strategy: Note the strategic word, *priority.* Eliminate options 1 and 3 first because they are comparable or alike and related to one another. To choose from the

remaining options, use the ABCs—airway, breathing, and circulation. Blood pressure is a method of assessing circulation.
Level of Cognitive Ability: Analyzing
Client Needs: Physiological Integrity
Integrated Process: Nursing Process—Assessment
Content Area: Pharmacology: Maternity/Newborn: Ergot alkaloids
Health Problem: Maternity: Postpartum uterine problems
Priority Concepts: Clotting; Reproduction
Reference: McKinney et al. (2018), p. 601.

289. *Answer:* 2
Rationale: Respiratory distress syndrome is a serious lung disorder caused by immaturity and the inability to produce surfactant, resulting in hypoxia and acidosis. It is common in premature infants and may be due to lung immaturity as a result of surfactant deficiency. The mainstay of treatment is the administration of exogenous surfactant, which is administered by the intratracheal route. Options 1, 3, and 4 are not routes of administration for this medication.
Test-Taking Strategy: Focus on the subject, route of administration for exogenous surfactant. Note the relationship between the diagnosis, *respiratory distress syndrome,* and the correct option, *intratracheal.*
Level of Cognitive Ability: Applying
Client Needs: Physiological Integrity
Integrated Process: Nursing Process—Planning
Content Area: Pharmacology: Maternity/Newborn: Lung Surfactant
Health Problem: Newborn: Respiratory Problems
Priority Concepts: Development; Gas Exchange
References: Lowdermilk et al. (2016), p. 826.

290. *Answer:* 1
Rationale: Opioid analgesics may be prescribed to relieve moderate to severe pain associated with labor. Opioid toxicity can occur and cause respiratory depression. Naloxone is an opioid antagonist, which reverses the effects of opioids and is given for respiratory depression. Morphine sulfate and hydromorphone hydrochloride are opioid analgesics. Betamethasone is a corticosteroid administered to enhance fetal lung maturity.
Test-Taking Strategy: Focus on the subject, the antidote for respiratory depression. Eliminate options 2 and 4 first because they are comparable or alike and are opioid analgesics. Next, eliminate option 3, knowing that this medication is a corticosteroid.
Level of Cognitive Ability: Applying
Client Needs: Physiological Integrity
Integrated Process: Nursing Process—Planning
Content Area: Pharmacology: Maternity/Newborn: Opioid analgesics
Health Problem: N/A
Priority Concepts: Gas Exchange; Safety
References: Lowdermilk et al. (2016), p. 395.

291. *Answer:* 4
Rationale: Rh incompatibility can occur when an Rh-negative mother becomes sensitized to the Rh antigen. Sensitization may develop when an Rh-negative woman becomes pregnant with a fetus who is Rh positive. During pregnancy and at delivery, some of the fetus's Rh-positive blood can enter the maternal circulation, causing the mother's immune system to form antibodies against Rh-positive blood. Administration of Rh_o(D) immune globulin prevents the mother from developing antibodies against Rh-positive blood by providing passive antibody protection against the Rh antigen.
Test-Taking Strategy: Note the subject, the purpose of Rh_o(D) immune globulin. Noting the relationship between the name of the medication, Rh_o(D) immune globulin, and the word *incompatibility* in the correct option will direct you to this option.
Level of Cognitive Ability: Evaluating
Client Needs: Physiological Integrity
Integrated Process: Nursing Process—Evaluation
Content Area: Pharmacology: Maternity/Newborn: Rho (D) Immune Globulin
Health Problem: Newborn: Erythroblastosis fetalis
Priority Concepts: Health Promotion; Reproduction
Reference: Lowdermilk et al. (2016), p. 494.

292. *Answer:* 4
Rationale: Methylergonovine is an ergot alkaloid used to treat postpartum hemorrhage. Ergot alkaloids are contraindicated in clients with significant cardiovascular disease, peripheral vascular disease, hypertension, preeclampsia, or eclampsia. These conditions are worsened by the vasoconstrictive effects of the ergot alkaloids. Options 1, 2, and 3 are not contraindications related to the use of ergot alkaloids.
Test-Taking Strategy: Focus on the subject, the purpose, action, and contraindications of methylergonovine. Recalling that ergot alkaloids produce vasoconstriction will direct you to the correct option.
Level of Cognitive Ability: Analyzing
Client Needs: Physiological Integrity
Integrated Process: Nursing Process—Implementation
Content Area: Pharmacology: Maternity/Newborn: Ergot alkaloids
Health Problem: Maternity: Postpartum uterine problems
Priority Concepts: Collaboration; Safety
Reference: McKinney et al. (2018), p. 601.

293. *Answer:* 1, 4, 5
Rationale: Magnesium sulfate is a central nervous system depressant and relaxes smooth muscle, including the uterus. It is used to halt preterm labor contractions and is used for preeclamptic clients to prevent seizures. Adverse effects include flushing, depressed respirations, depressed deep tendon reflexes, hypotension, extreme muscle weakness, decreased urine output, pulmonary edema, and elevated serum magnesium levels.
Test-Taking Strategy: Focus on the subject, adverse effects of magnesium sulfate. Recalling that this medication is a central nervous system depressant and relaxes smooth muscle will assist you in choosing the correct options.
Level of Cognitive Ability: Analyzing
Client Needs: Physiological Integrity
Integrated Process: Nursing Process—Assessment
Content Area: Pharmacology: Maternity/Newborn: Tocolytics
Health Problem: Maternity: Gestational hypertension/preeclampsia and eclampsia
Priority Concepts: Perfusion; Reproduction
References: Lowdermilk et al. (2016), pp. 663-664.

UNIT VI

Pediatric Nursing

Pyramid to Success

Pyramid Points focus on growth and development, safety, and age-appropriate measures to ensure a safe and hazard-free environment for the child; on protection of the child and the prevention of accidents; and on acute health problems that can occur in children. Preventive pediatric health care and well-check schedules are a focus along with nutrition, specific feeding techniques, positioning techniques, and interventions that will provide and maintain adequate airway, breathing, and circulation patterns in the child. In addition, neglect and/or abuse of the child is a focus. On the NCLEX-RN® examination, be alert to the age of the child if the age is presented in a question. If an age is presented in the question, think about the specific growth and development characteristics of the age group to answer the question correctly.

Client Needs: Learning Objectives

Safe and Effective Care Environment

Communicating with interprofessional health care team members
Considering issues related to informed consent regarding minors
Delegating care safely
Ensuring environmental safety, including home safety and personal safety, related to the developmental age of the child
Establishing priorities
Instituting measures related to the spread and control of infectious agents, particularly communicable diseases
Maintaining confidentiality
Preventing errors and accidents
Protecting the child and other contacts to prevent illness
Providing continuity of care
Providing protective measures
Upholding parent and child rights

Health Promotion and Maintenance

Ensuring that immunization schedules are up to date
Focusing on developmental stages when planning care
Performing physical assessment techniques specific to the pediatric client
Preventing disease in the pediatric population
Providing health promotion programs for the pediatric client such as preventive pediatric health care programs and well-check schedules
Providing instructions to the child and parents regarding care at home

Psychosocial Integrity

Assessing the child for neglect and/or abuse
Communicating with the pediatric client
Considering concepts of family dynamics when planning care
Considering cultural, religious, and spiritual beliefs when planning care
Considering end-of-life issues and grief and loss in the pediatric population
Identifying family and support systems for the child
Providing play therapies

Physiological Integrity

Following medication administration procedures
Following nutritional guidelines for the pediatric population
Identifying comfort measures appropriate for the child
Maintaining sensitivity for intrusive procedures needed for the pediatric client
Managing childhood health problems
Monitoring elimination patterns
Monitoring for age-appropriate normal body structure and function
Monitoring for infectious diseases of the pediatric client
Monitoring for responses to treatments
Providing for consistent rest and sleep patterns
Responding to medical emergencies

CHAPTER 29

Integumentary Problems

PRIORITY CONCEPTS Infection; Tissue Integrity

I. Eczema (Dermatitis)

A. Description
1. Superficial inflammatory process involving primarily the epidermis; there are many types, some of which include atopic dermatitis, contact dermatitis, and stasis dermatitis.
2. Associated with family history of the disorder, allergies, asthma, or allergic rhinitis
3. The major goals of management are to relieve pruritus, lubricate the skin, reduce inflammation, and prevent or control secondary infections.

B. Forms of eczema (Box 29-1)

C. Assessment
1. Redness
2. Scaliness
3. Itching
4. Minute papules (firm, elevated, circumscribed lesions <1 cm in diameter) and vesicles (similar to papules but fluid-filled)
5. Weeping, oozing, and crusting of lesions
6. Lesions can occur on scalp and face (infants), creases of elbows and knees, neck, wrists, ankles, or creases between the buttocks and legs.

D. Interventions
1. Baths and moisturizers are important; bathing water should be tepid and bath should be limited to 5 to 10 minutes, and the skin should be moisturized immediately after the bath; a thick cream or ointment should be used, such as petroleum jelly.
2. If topical medications are prescribed, they should be applied within 3 minutes after the bath.
3. Antihistamines and topical corticosteroids may be prescribed; corticosteroids are applied in a thin layer and are rubbed into the area thoroughly.
4. Antibiotics may be prescribed if secondary infections occur.
5. Avoid exposure to skin irritants such as irritating soaps, detergents, fabric softeners, diaper wipes, and powder.
6. Cool, wet compresses applied for short periods may help soothe the skin and alleviate itching; pat skin dry between cooling treatments.
7. Prevent or minimize scratching; keep nails short and clean, and place gloves or cotton socks over the hands.
8. Eliminate conditions that increase itching, such as wet diapers, excessive bathing, ambient heat, woolen clothes or blankets, and rough fabrics or furry stuffed animals; exposure to latex should also be avoided.
9. Instruct parents to wash clothing in a mild detergent and rinse thoroughly; putting the clothes through a second complete wash cycle without detergent minimizes the residue remaining on the fabric.
10. Instruct parents about measures to prevent skin infections.
11. Instruct parents to monitor lesions for signs of infection (honey-colored crusts with surrounding erythema) and to seek immediate medical intervention if such signs are noted.

BOX 29-1 Forms of Eczema

Infantile: Usually begins at 2 to 6 months of age and decreases in incidence with aging; spontaneous remission may occur by 3 years

Childhood: May follow the infantile form; occurs at 2 to 3 years of age

Preadolescent and Adolescent: Begins at about 12 years of age and may continue into the early adult years or indefinitely

! A child with an integumentary disorder needs to be monitored for signs of either a skin infection or a systemic infection.

II. Impetigo

A. Description
1. Impetigo is a contagious bacterial infection of the skin caused by β-hemolytic streptococci or staphylococci or both; it occurs most commonly during hot, humid months.

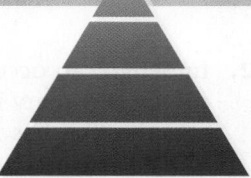

2. Impetigo can occur because of poor hygiene; it can be a primary infection or occur secondarily at a site that has been injured or sustained an insect bite, or at a site that was originally a rash, such as atopic dermatitis or poison ivy or poison oak.
3. The most common sites of infection are on the face and around the mouth, and then on the hands, neck, and extremities.
4. The lesions begin as vesicles or pustules surrounded by edema and redness (a pustule is similar to a vesicle except that its fluid content is purulent).
5. The lesions progress to an exudative and crusting stage; after the crusting of the lesions, the initially serous vesicular fluid becomes cloudy, and the vesicles rupture, leaving honey-colored crusts covering ulcerated bases.

B. Assessment (Fig. 29-1)

1. Blisters and crusts
2. Erythema
3. Pruritus
4. Burning
5. Secondary lymph node involvement can be present

C. Interventions

1. Institute contact isolation; also use standard precautions and implement agency-specific isolation procedures for the hospitalized child; strict hygiene practices are important, because impetigo is a highly contagious condition.
2. Apply topical antibiotic ointments with a clean/sterile cotton swab without touching the tube opening with fingers or skin, and instruct parents in the ointment and swab use; the infection is still communicable for 24 to 48 hours beyond initiation of antibiotic treatment.
3. Cover lesions with gauze bandages and tape to prevent the spread of infection.

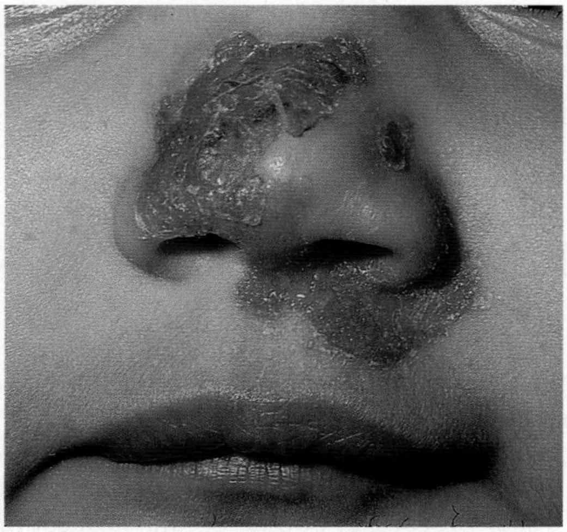

FIG. 29-1 Impetigo contagiosa. (From Weston, Lane, 2007.)

4. Assist the child with daily bathing with antibacterial soap, as prescribed.
5. Apply warm water compresses to the lesions 2 or 3 times daily, followed by mild soap and water rinse to soften crusts for removal and to promote healing.
6. Oral antibiotics may be prescribed if there is no response to topical antibiotic treatment; it is extremely important to comply with the prescribed antibiotic regimen, because secondary infections such as glomerulonephritis may result if the infectious agent is of a streptococcal type that can affect the nephrons.
7. To prevent skin cracking, apply emollients and instruct parents in the use of emollients.
8. Instruct parents in the methods to prevent the spread of the infection, especially careful hand-washing.
9. Inform parents that the child needs to use separate towels, linens, and eating utensils and dishes.
10. Inform parents that all linens and clothing used by the child should be washed with detergent in hot water separately from the linens and clothing of other household members.

III. Pediculosis capitis (Lice)

A. Description

1. *Pediculosis capitis* refers to an infestation of the hair and scalp with lice.
2. The most common sites of involvement are the occipital area, behind the ears at the nape of the neck, and occasionally the eyebrows and eyelashes.
3. The female louse lays her eggs (nits) on the hair shaft, close to the scalp; the incubation period is 7 to 10 days.
4. Lice can survive for 48 hours away from the host; nits shed in the environment can hatch in 7 to 10 days.
5. Head lice live and reproduce only on humans and are transmitted by direct and indirect contact, such as sharing of brushes, hats, towels, and bedding.
6. All contacts of the infested child, especially siblings, should be examined for lice infestation and referred for treatment as appropriate.

B. Assessment (Box 29-2)

C. Interventions

1. Use a pediculicide product as prescribed; follow package instructions for timing the application and for contraindications for use in children (most products used to treat pediculosis cannot be used on children younger than 6 months of age).
2. Daily removal of nits with an extra-fine-tooth metal nit comb should be done as a control

BOX 29-2 Assessment Findings: Pediculosis Capitis (Lice)

- Child scratches scalp excessively.
- Pruritus is caused by the crawling insect and insect saliva on the skin.
- Nits (white eggs) are observable on the hair shaft (it is important to differentiate nits from lint or dandruff, which flakes away easily).
- Adult lice are difficult to see and appear as small tan or grayish specks, which may crawl quickly.

measure after use of the pediculicide product (gloves should be worn for removal of nits); hairbrushes or combs should be discarded or soaked in boiling water for 10 minutes.

3. Instruct parents that siblings may also need treatment; grooming items should not be shared, and a single comb or brush should be used for each individual child.
4. Instruct parents that bedding and clothing used by the child for the previous 2 days before diagnosis should be laundered in hot water with detergent and dried in a hot dryer for 20 minutes; bedding and clothing needs to be changed daily and laundered.
5. Instruct parents that nonessential bedding and clothing can be stored in a tightly sealed plastic bag for 2 weeks and then washed.
6. Instruct parents to seal toys that cannot be washed or dry-cleaned in a plastic bag for 2 weeks.
7. Instruct parents that furniture and carpets need to be vacuumed frequently and that the dust bag from the vacuum should be discarded after vacuuming.
8. Teach the child not to share clothing, headwear, brushes, and combs.
9. Lice on the eyelashes or eyebrows may need to be removed manually.

IV. Scabies

A. Description

1. Scabies is a parasitic skin disorder caused by an infestation of *Sarcoptes scabiei* (itch mite).
2. Scabies is endemic among schoolchildren and institutionalized populations as a result of close personal contact.
3. Incubation period
   a. The female mite burrows into the epidermis, lays eggs, and dies in the burrow after 4 to 5 weeks.
   b. The eggs hatch in 3 to 5 days, and larvae mature and complete their life cycle.
4. Infectious period: During the entire course of the infestation

B. Assessment (Box 29-3 and Fig. 29-2)

⚠ Scabies is transmitted by close personal contact with an infected person. Household members and contacts of an infected child need to be treated simultaneously.

C. Interventions

1. Topical application of a scabicide is needed to kill the mites.
2. Various products are available, and a prescription is needed for the product.
3. One product known as lindane shampoo should not be used in children younger than 2 years because of the risk of neurotoxicity and seizures; all other products have contraindications regarding their use, and it is critical to know these contraindications.
4. Instruct parents in the application of the scabicide, because each product has different application methods; the scabicide is not applied to the face or head, only from the neck down.
5. When permethrin is prescribed, it is applied to cool dry skin at least 30 minutes after bathing; the cream is massaged thoroughly and gently into all skin surfaces (not just the areas that have the rash) from the head to the soles of the feet (avoid contact with the eyes), left on the skin for 8 to 14 hours, and then removed by bathing; a repeat treatment may be necessary.
6. Instruct the parents about the importance of frequent hand washing.
7. Instruct the parents that all clothing, bedding, and pillowcases used by the child need to be changed daily, washed in hot water with detergent, dried in a hot dryer, and ironed before reuse; this process should continue for at least 1 week.

BOX 29-3 Assessment Findings: Scabies

- Pruritic papular rash
- Burrows into the skin (fine grayish red lines that may be difficult to see)

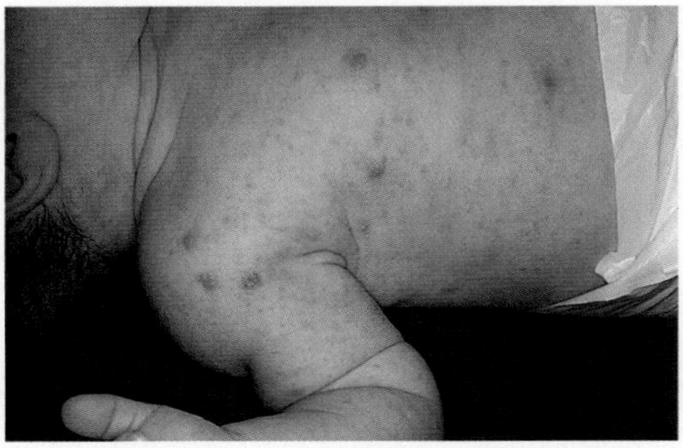

FIG. 29-2 Scabies rash on an infant.(From Calen et al., 1993. Courtesy Dr. Steve Estes.)

8. Instruct parents that nonwashable toys and other items should be sealed in plastic bags for at least 4 days.
9. Anti-itch topical treatment may be necessary, and antibiotics may be prescribed if a secondary infection develops.

V. Burn Injuries (see Priority Nursing Actions)

PRIORITY NURSING ACTIONS

A Major Burn Injury in the Child

1. Stop the burning process.
2. Assess for a patent airway.
3. Begin resuscitation measures if necessary using CAB—compressions, airway, and breathing.
4. Remove burned clothing and jewelry.
5. Cover the wound(s) with a clean cloth at the site of injury (sterile dressings on arrival to the health care facility).
6. Keep the child warm.
7. Transport the child to the emergency department.

Reference
Hockenberry, Wilson, Rodgers (2017), p. 402.

A. Pediatric considerations
   1. Very young children who have been burned severely have a higher mortality rate than older children and adults with comparable burns.
   2. Lower burn temperatures and shorter exposure to heat can cause a more severe burn in a child than in an adult, because a child's skin is thinner.
   3. The degree of pain experienced by the child and the ability to communicate it are different than in an adult with the same exposure.
   4. Severely burned children are at increased risk for fluid and heat loss, dehydration, and metabolic acidosis compared with adults.
   5. The higher proportion of body fluid to body mass in children increases the risk of cardiovascular problems.
   6. Burns involving more than 10% of the total body surface area require some form of fluid resuscitation.
   7. Infants and children are at increased risk for protein and calorie deficiency because they have smaller muscle mass and less body fat than adults.
   8. Scarring is more severe in a child; disturbed body image is a distinct issue for a child or adolescent, especially as growth continues.
   9. An immature immune system presents an increased risk of infection for infants and young children.
   10. A delay in growth may occur after a burn.

B. Extent of burn injury
   1. The rule of nines, used for adults with burn injuries, gives an inaccurate estimate in children because of the difference in body proportions between children and adults.
   2. In a pediatric client, the extent of the burn is expressed as a percentage of the total body surface area, using age-related charts (Fig. 29-3).

C. Fluid replacement therapy

! To determine adequacy of fluid resuscitation, vital signs (especially heart rate), urine output, adequacy of capillary filling, and sensorium status are assessed.

   1. Fluid replacement is necessary during the initial 24-hour period after burn injury because of the fluid shifts that occur as a result of the injury.
   2. Several formulas are available to calculate the child's fluid needs, and the formula used depends on the primary health care provider's preference.
   3. Crystalloid solutions are likely to be prescribed during the initial phase of therapy; colloid solutions such as albumin, Plasma-Lyte (combined electrolyte solution), or fresh-frozen plasma are useful in maintaining plasma volume.

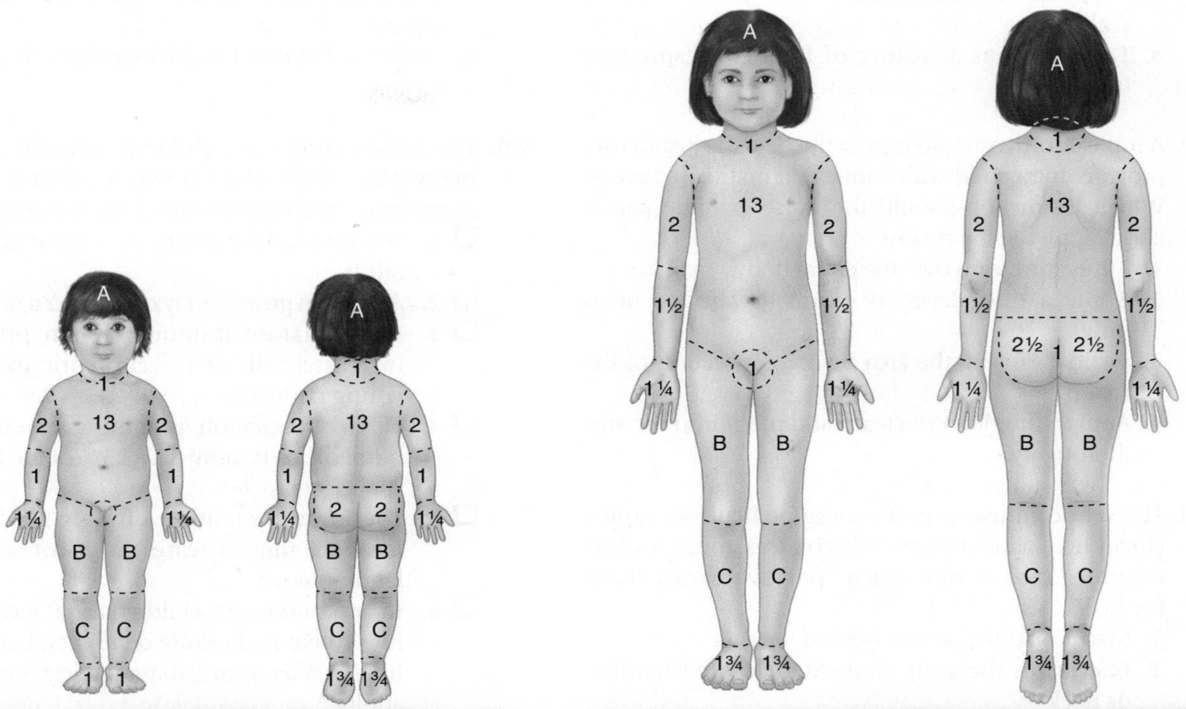

A

RELATIVE PERCENTAGES OF AREAS AFFECTED BY GROWTH			
AREA	BIRTH	AGE 1 YR	AGE 5 YR
A = ½ of head	9½	8½	6½
B = ½ of one thigh	2¾	3¼	4
C = ½ of one leg	2½	2½	2¾

B

RELATIVE PERCENTAGES OF AREAS AFFECTED BY GROWTH			
AREA	AGE 10 YR	AGE 15 YR	YOUNG ADULT
A = ½ of head	5½	4½	3½
B = ½ of one thigh	4½	4½	4¾
C = ½ of one leg	3	3¼	3½

FIG. 29-3 Estimation of distribution of burns in children. **A,** Children from birth to age 5 years. **B,** Older children.

PRACTICE QUESTIONS

294. The nurse is monitoring a child with burns during treatment. Which assessment provides the **most** accurate guide to determine the adequacy of fluid resuscitation?
1. Skin turgor
2. Level of edema at burn site
3. Adequacy of capillary filling
4. Amount of fluid tolerated in 24 hours

295. The mother of a 3-year-old child arrives at a clinic and tells the nurse that the child has been scratching the skin continuously and has developed a rash. The nurse assesses the child and suspects the presence of scabies. The nurse bases this suspicion on which finding noted on assessment of the child's skin?
1. Fine grayish red lines
2. Purple-colored lesions
3. Thick, honey-colored crusts
4. Clusters of fluid-filled vesicles

296. Permethrin is prescribed for a child with a diagnosis of scabies. The nurse should give which instruction to the parents regarding the use of this treatment?
1. Apply the lotion to areas of the rash only.
2. Apply the lotion and leave it on for 6 hours.
3. Avoid putting clothes on the child over the lotion.
4. Apply the lotion to cool, dry skin at least 30 minutes after bathing.

297. The school nurse has provided an instructional session about impetigo to parents of the children attending the school. Which statement, if made by a parent, indicates a **need for further instruction?**
1. "It is extremely contagious."
2. "It is most common in humid weather."
3. "Lesions most often are located on the arms and chest."
4. "It might show up in an area of broken skin, such as an insect bite."

298. The clinic nurse is reviewing the health care provider's prescription for a child who has been diagnosed with scabies. Lindane has been prescribed for the child. The nurse questions the prescription if which is noted in the child's record?
1. The child is 18 months old.
2. The child is being bottle-fed.

3. A sibling is using lindane for the treatment of scabies.
4. The child has a history of frequent respiratory infections.

299. A topical corticosteroid is prescribed by the health care provider for a child with contact dermatitis (eczema). Which instruction should the nurse give the parent about applying the cream?
1. Apply the cream over the entire body.
2. Apply a thick layer of cream to affected areas only.
3. Avoid cleansing the area before application of the cream.
4. Apply a thin layer of cream and rub it into the area thoroughly.

300. The school nurse is performing pediculosis capitis (head lice) assessments. Which assessment finding indicates that a child has a "positive" head check for lice?
1. Maculopapular lesions behind the ears
2. Lesions in the scalp that extend to the hairline or neck
3. White flaky particles throughout the entire scalp region
4. White sacs attached to the hair shafts in the occipital area

301. The nurse caring for a child who sustained a burn injury plans care based on which pediatric considerations associated with this injury? **Select all that apply.**
- ☐ 1. Scarring is less severe in a child than in an adult.
- ☐ 2. A delay in growth may occur after a burn injury.
- ☐ 3. An immature immune system presents an increased risk of infection for infants and young children.
- ☐ 4. Fluid resuscitation is unnecessary unless the burned area is more than 25% of the total body surface area.
- ☐ 5. The lower proportion of body fluid to body mass in a child increases the risk of cardiovascular problems.
- ☐ 6. Infants and young children are at increased risk for protein and calorie deficiency, because they have smaller muscle mass and less body fat than adults.

ANSWERS

294. *Answer:* 3

Rationale: Parameters such as vital signs (especially heart rate), urinary output volume, adequacy of capillary filling, and state of sensorium determine adequacy of fluid resuscitation. Although options 1, 2, and 4 may provide some information related to fluid volume, in a burn injury, and from the options provided, adequacy of capillary filling is most accurate.
Test-Taking Strategy: Note the strategic word, *most.* Use the ABCs—airway, breathing, and circulation—to assist in directing you to the correct option.
Level of Cognitive Ability: Evaluating
Client Needs: Physiological Integrity
Integrated Process: Nursing Process—Evaluation
Content Area: Pediatrics: Integumentary
Health Problem: Pediatric-Specific: Burns
Priority Concepts: Evidence; Fluids and Electrolytes
Reference: McKinney et al. (2018), p. 1202.

295. *Answer:* 1

Rationale: Scabies is a parasitic skin disorder caused by an infestation of *Sarcoptes scabiei* (itch mite). Scabies appears as burrows or fine, grayish red, thread-like lines. They may be difficult to see if they are obscured by excoriation and inflammation. Purple-colored lesions may indicate various disorders, including systemic conditions. Thick, honey-colored crusts are characteristic of impetigo or secondary infection in eczema. Clusters of fluid-filled vesicles are seen in herpesvirus infection.
Test-Taking Strategy: Focus on the subject, clinical manifestations of scabies. Think about the characteristic of this parasitic skin disorder. Recalling that scabies infestation produces burrows will assist in directing you to the correct option.
Level of Cognitive Ability: Analyzing
Client Needs: Physiological Integrity
Integrated Process: Nursing Process—Assessment
Content Area: Pediatrics: Integumentary
Health Problem: Pediatric-Specific: Skin Inflammation/Infection
Priority Concepts: Infection; Tissue Integrity
Reference: Hockenberry, Wilson, Rodgers (2017), pp. 180-182.

296. *Answer:* 4

Rationale: Permethrin is massaged thoroughly and gently into all skin surfaces (not just the areas that have the rash) from the head to the soles of the feet. Care should be taken to avoid contact with the eyes. The lotion should not be applied until at least 30 minutes after bathing and should be applied only to cool, dry skin. The lotion should be kept on for 8 to 14 hours, and then the child should be given a bath. The child should be clothed during the 8 to 14 hours of treatment contact time.
Test-Taking Strategy: Option 3 can be eliminated because the child should be clothed. Eliminate option 1 next because of the closed-ended word, "only," in this option. From the remaining options, recalling the procedure for the application of this lotion will direct you to the correct option.
Level of Cognitive Ability: Applying
Client Needs: Physiological Integrity

Integrated Process: Teaching and Learning
Content Area: Pediatrics: Integumentary
Health Problem: Pediatric-Specific: Skin Inflammation/Infection
Priority Concepts: Client Education; Tissue Integrity
References: Burchum, Rosenthal (2016) p. 1202.; McKinney et al. (2018), p. 1186.

297. *Answer:* 3
Rationale: Impetigo is a contagious bacterial infection of the skin caused by β-hemolytic streptococci or staphylococci, or both. Impetigo is most common during hot, humid summer months. Impetigo may begin in an area of broken skin, such as an insect bite or atopic dermatitis. Impetigo is extremely contagious. Lesions usually are located around the mouth and nose but may be present on the hands and extremities.
Test-Taking Strategy: Note the strategic words, *need for further instruction*. These words indicate a negative event query and ask you to select an option that is an incorrect statement. Think about the pathophysiology associated with impetigo. Knowledge regarding the cause and manifestations of impetigo will direct you to the correct option.
Level of Cognitive Ability: Evaluating
Client Needs: Safe and Effective Care Environment
Integrated Process: Teaching and Learning
Content Area: Pediatrics: Integumentary
Health Problem: Pediatric-Specific: Skin Inflammation/Infection
Priority Concepts: Client Education; Infection
Reference: McKinney et al. (2018), pp. 1178-1179.

298. *Answer:* 1
Rationale: Lindane is a pediculicide product that may be prescribed to treat scabies. It is contraindicated for children younger than 2 years because they have more permeable skin, and high systemic absorption may occur, placing the children at risk for central nervous system toxicity and seizures. Lindane also is used with caution in children between the ages of 2 and 10 years. Siblings and other household members should be treated simultaneously. Options 2 and 4 are unrelated to the use of lindane. Lindane is not recommended for use by a breast-feeding woman because the medication is secreted into breast milk.
Test-Taking Strategy: Focus on the subject, contraindications of lindane. Recall the concepts related to the body surface area of children and an 18-month-old, and medication administration. These concepts will direct you to the correct option.
Level of Cognitive Ability: Analyzing
Client Needs: Safe and Effective Care Environment
Integrated Process: Nursing Process—Analysis
Content Area: Pediatrics: Integumentary
Health Problem: Pediatric-Specific: Skin Inflammation/Infection
Priority Concepts: Clinical Judgment; Safety
Reference: McKinney et al. (2018), pp. 1186, 1188.

299. *Answer:* 4
Rationale: Contact dermatitis is a superficial inflammatory process involving primarily the epidermis. A topical corticosteroid may be prescribed and should be applied sparingly (thin layer) and rubbed into the area thoroughly. The affected area should be cleaned gently before application. A topical corticosteroid should not be applied over extensive areas. Systemic absorption is more likely to occur with extensive application.
Test-Taking Strategy: Focus on the subject, application of a topical corticosteroid. Eliminate option 3 first because it does not make sense not to clean an affected area. Eliminate option 1 because medicated cream should be applied only to areas that are affected. Eliminate option 2 because of the word *thick*.
Level of Cognitive Ability: Applying
Client Needs: Physiological Integrity
Integrated Process: Teaching and Learning
Content Area: Pediatrics: Integumentary
Health Problem: Pediatric-Specific: Skin Inflammation/Infection
Priority Concepts: Client Education; Tissue Integrity
Reference: McKinney et al. (2018), p. 1177.

300. *Answer:* 4
Rationale: Pediculosis capitis is an infestation of the hair and scalp with lice. The nits are visible and attached firmly to the hair shaft near the scalp. The occiput is an area in which nits can be seen. Maculopapular lesions behind the ears or lesions that extend to the hairline or neck are indicative of an infectious process, not pediculosis. White flaky particles are indicative of dandruff.
Test-Taking Strategy: Focus on the subject, the characteristics of pediculosis capitis. Option 3 can be eliminated first, because white flaky particles are indicative of dandruff. Recalling that in this infestation nit sacs attach to the hair shaft will direct you to the correct option.
Level of Cognitive Ability: Applying
Client Needs: Physiological Integrity
Integrated Process: Nursing Process—Assessment
Content Area: Pediatrics: Integumentary
Health Problem: Pediatric-Specific: Skin Inflammation/Infection
Priority Concepts: Clinical Judgment; Infection
Reference: McKinney et al. (2018), p. 1187.

301. *Answer:* 2, 3, 6
Rationale: Pediatric considerations in the care of a burn victim include the following: Scarring is more severe in a child than in an adult. A delay in growth may occur after a burn injury. An immature immune system presents an increased risk of infection for infants and young children. The higher proportion of body fluid to body mass in a child increases the risk of cardiovascular problems. Burns involving more than 10% of total body surface area require some form of fluid resuscitation. Infants and young children are at increased risk for protein and calorie deficiencies because they have smaller muscle mass and less body fat than adults.
Test-Taking Strategy: Focus on the subject, pediatric considerations in the care of a child who has sustained a burn injury. To answer correctly, read each option carefully and think about the physiology of a child related to body size.
Level of Cognitive Ability: Analyzing
Client Needs: Physiological Integrity
Integrated Process: Nursing Process—Planning
Content Area: Pediatrics: Integumentary
Health Problem: Pediatric-Specific: Burns
Priority Concepts: Development; Tissue Integrity
Reference: McKinney et al. (2018), p. 1194.

CHAPTER 30

Hematological Problems

PRIORITY CONCEPTS **Perfusion; Safety**

I. Sickle Cell Anemia

A. Description
1. Sickle cell anemia constitutes a group of diseases termed *hemoglobinopathies*, in which hemoglobin A is partly or completely replaced by abnormal sickle hemoglobin S.
2. It is caused by the inheritance of a gene for a structurally abnormal portion of the hemoglobin chain.
3. Risk factors include having parents heterozygous for hemoglobin S or being of African American descent.
4. For screening purposes, the sickle turbidity test (Sickledex) is frequently used because it can be performed on blood from a fingerstick and yields accurate results in 3 minutes. However, if the test result is positive, hemoglobin (Hgb) electrophoresis is necessary to distinguish between children with the trait and those with the disease.
5. Hemoglobin S is sensitive to changes in the oxygen content of the red blood cell.
6. Insufficient oxygen causes the cells to assume a sickle shape, and the cells become rigid and clumped together, obstructing capillary blood flow (Fig. 30-1).
7. The clinical manifestations occur primarily as a result of obstruction caused by sickled red blood cells and increased red blood cell destruction.
8. Situations that precipitate sickling include fever, dehydration, and emotional or physical stress; any condition that increases the need for oxygen or alters the transport of oxygen can result in sickle cell crisis (acute exacerbation).
9. Sickle cell crises are acute exacerbations of the disease, which vary considerably in severity and frequency; these include vaso-occlusive crisis, splenic sequestration, hyperhemolytic crisis, and aplastic crisis.
10. The sickling response is reversible under conditions of adequate oxygenation and hydration; after repeated sickling, the cell becomes permanently sickled.
11. An interprofessional approach to care is needed, and care focuses on the prevention (preventing exposure to infection and maintaining normal hydration) and treatment (hydration, oxygen, pain management, and bed rest) of the crisis.

B. Assessment of the crisis (Box 30-1)

C. Interventions
1. Maintain adequate hydration and blood flow through oral and intravenously (IV) administered fluids. Electrolyte replacement is also provided as needed; without adequate hydration, pain will not be controlled.
2. Administer oxygen and blood transfusions as prescribed to increase tissue perfusion; exchange transfusions, which reduce the number of circulating sickle cells and the risk of complications, may also be prescribed.
3. Administer analgesics as prescribed (around the clock).
4. Assist the child to assume a comfortable position so that the child keeps the extremities extended to promote venous return; elevate the head of the bed no more than 30 degrees, avoid putting strain on painful joints, and do not raise the knee gatch of the bed.
5. Encourage consumption of a high-calorie, high-protein diet, with folic acid supplementation.
6. Administer antibiotics as prescribed to prevent infection.
7. Monitor for signs of complications, including increasing anemia, decreased perfusion, and shock (mental status changes, pallor, vital sign changes).
8. Instruct the child and parents about the early signs and symptoms of crisis and the measures to prevent crisis.
9. Ensure that the child receives pneumococcal and meningococcal vaccines and an annual influenza vaccine, because of susceptibility to infection secondary to functional asplenia.

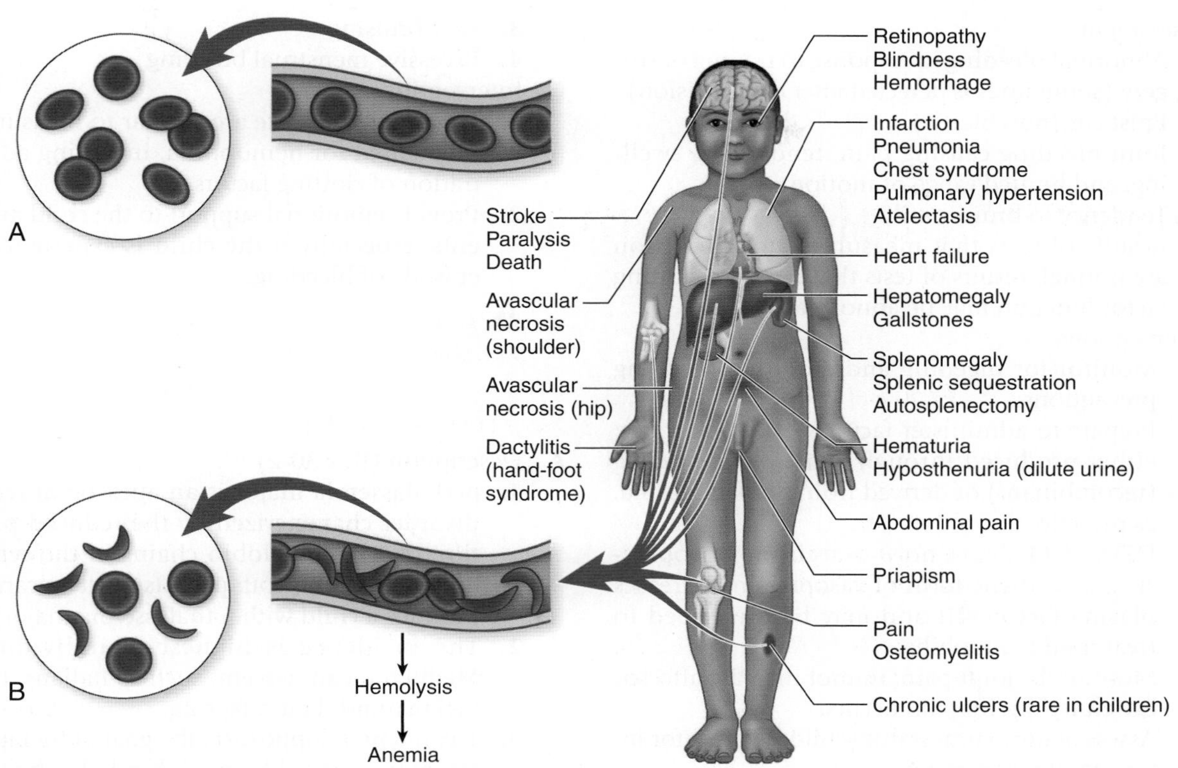

FIG. 30-1 Differences between effects of **(A)** normal red blood cells and **(B)** sickled red blood cells on circulation, with related complications.

10. A splenectomy may be necessary for clients who experience recurrent splenic sequestration.
11. Inform parents of the **hereditary** aspects of the disorder.

Administration of meperidine for pain is avoided because of the risk of normeperidine-induced seizures.

BOX 30-1 Sickle Cell Crisis

Vaso-Occlusive Crisis

Caused by stasis of blood with clumping of cells in the microcirculation, ischemia, and infarction

Manifestations: Fever; painful swelling of hands, feet, and joints; and abdominal pain

Splenic Sequestration

Caused by pooling and clumping of blood in the spleen (hypersplenism)

Manifestations: Profound anemia, hypovolemia, and shock

Hyperhemolytic Crisis

An accelerated rate of red blood cell destruction

Manifestations: Anemia, jaundice, and reticulocytosis

Aplastic Crisis

Caused by diminished production and increased destruction of red blood cells, triggered by viral infection or depletion of folic acid

Manifestations: Profound anemia and pallor

II. Hemophilia

A. Description

1. *Hemophilia* refers to a group of bleeding disorders resulting from a deficiency of specific coagulation proteins.
2. Identifying the specific coagulation deficiency is important so that definitive treatment with the specific replacement agent can be implemented; aggressive replacement therapy is initiated to prevent the chronic crippling effects from joint bleeding.
3. The most common types are factor VIII deficiency (hemophilia A or classic hemophilia) and factor IX deficiency (hemophilia B or Christmas disease).
4. Hemophilia is transmitted as an X-linked recessive disorder (it may also occur as a result of a gene mutation).
5. Carrier females pass on the defect to males; female offspring are rarely born with the disorder but may be if they inherit an affected gene from their mother and are offspring of a father with hemophilia.
6. The primary treatment is replacement of the missing clotting factor; additional medications, such as agents to relieve pain or corticosteroids, may be prescribed depending on the source of bleeding from the disorder.

B. Assessment
1. Abnormal bleeding in response to trauma or surgery (sometimes is detected after circumcision)
2. Epistaxis (nosebleeds)
3. Joint bleeding causing pain, tenderness, swelling, and limited range of motion
4. Tendency to bruise easily
5. Results of tests that measure platelet function are normal; results of tests that measure clotting factor function may be abnormal.

C. Interventions
1. Monitor for bleeding and maintain bleeding precautions.
2. Prepare to administer factor VIII concentrates, either produced through genetic engineering (recombinant) or derived from pooled plasma, as prescribed.
3. DDAVP (1-deamino-8-D-arginine vasopressin), a synthetic form of vasopressin, increases plasma factor VIII and may be prescribed to treat mild hemophilia.
4. Monitor for joint pain; immobilize the affected extremity if joint pain occurs.
5. Assess neurological status (child is at risk for intracranial hemorrhage).
6. Monitor urine for hematuria.
7. Control joint bleeding by immobilization, elevation, and application of ice; apply pressure (15 minutes) for superficial bleeding.
8. Instruct the child and parents about the signs of internal bleeding.
9. Instruct parents in how to control the bleeding.
10. Instruct parents regarding activities for the child, emphasizing the avoidance of contact sports and the need for protective devices while learning to walk; assist in developing an appropriate exercise plan.
11. Instruct the child to wear protective devices such as helmets and knee and elbow pads when participating in sports such as bicycling and skating.

III. von Willebrand's Disease

A. Description
1. von Willebrand's disease is a hereditary bleeding disorder that is characterized by a deficiency of or a defect in a protein termed *von Willebrand factor*.
2. The disorder causes platelets to adhere to damaged endothelium; the von Willebrand factor protein also serves as a carrier protein for factor VIII.
3. It is characterized by an increased tendency to bleed from mucous membranes.

B. Assessment
1. Epistaxis
2. Gum bleeding
3. Easy bruising
4. Excessive menstrual bleeding

C. Interventions
1. Treatment and care are similar to measures implemented for hemophilia, including administration of clotting factors.
2. Provide emotional support to the child and parents, especially if the child is experiencing an episode of bleeding.

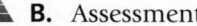

A child with a bleeding disorder needs to wear a MedicAlert bracelet.

IV. β-Thalassemia Major

A. Description (Box 30-2)
1. β-Thalassemia major is an autosomal recessive disorder characterized by the reduced production of 1 of the globin chains in the synthesis of hemoglobin (both parents must be carriers to produce a child with β-thalassemia major).
2. The incidence is highest in individuals of Mediterranean descent, such as Italians, Greeks, Syrians, and their offspring.
3. Treatment is supportive; the goal of therapy is to maintain normal hemoglobin levels by the administration of blood transfusions.
4. Bone marrow transplantation may be offered as an alternative therapy.
5. A splenectomy may be performed in a child with severe splenomegaly who requires repeated transfusions (assists in relieving abdominal pressure and may increase the life span of supplemental red blood cells).

B. Assessment
1. Frontal bossing
2. Maxillary prominence
3. Wide-set eyes with a flattened nose
4. Greenish yellow skin tone
5. Hepatosplenomegaly
6. Severe anemia
7. Microcytic, hypochromic red blood cells

C. Interventions
1. Administer blood transfusions as prescribed; monitor for transfusion reactions.
2. Monitor for iron overload; chelation therapy with deferasirox or deferoxamine may be prescribed to treat iron overload and to prevent

BOX 30-2 Types of β-Thalassemia

Thalassemia Minor: Asymptomatic silent carrier case
Thalassemia Trait: Produces mild microcytic anemia
Thalassemia Intermedia: Manifested as splenomegaly and moderate to severe anemia
Thalassemia Major: Results in severe anemia requiring transfusion support to sustain life (also known as Cooley's anemia)

organ damage from the elevated levels of iron caused by the multiple transfusion therapy.
3. If the child has had a splenectomy, instruct parents to report any signs of infection because of the risk of sepsis.
4. Ensure that parents understand the importance of the child receiving pneumococcal and meningococcal vaccines in addition to an annual influenza vaccine and the regularly scheduled vaccines.
5. Provide genetic counseling to parents.

V. Iron Deficiency Anemia

1. In iron deficiency anemia, iron stores are depleted, resulting in a decreased supply of iron for the manufacture of hemoglobin in red blood cells; red blood cells are microcytic and hypochromic.
2. Refer to Chapter 44 for additional information

VI. Aplastic anemia

1. A deficiency of circulating erythrocytes and all other formed elements of blood, resulting from the arrested development of cells within the bone marrow; pancytopenia, a deficiency of erythrocytes, leukocytes, and thrombocytes occurs.
2. Refer to Chapter 44 for additional information

⚠ Liquid iron preparation may be prescribed used to treat iron deficiency anemia. Teach the parents and child that liquid iron should be taken through a straw and that the teeth should be brushed after administration.

PRACTICE QUESTIONS

302. The nurse analyzes the laboratory results of a child with hemophilia. The nurse understands that which result will **most likely** be abnormal in this child?
1. Platelet count
2. Hematocrit level
3. Hemoglobin level
4. Partial thromboplastin time

303. The nurse is providing home care instructions to the parents of a 10-year-old child with hemophilia. Which sport activity should the nurse suggest for this child?
1. Soccer
2. Basketball
3. Swimming
4. Field hockey

304. The nursing student is presenting a clinical conference and discusses the cause of β-thalassemia. The nursing student informs the group that a child at greatest risk of developing this disorder is which of these?
1. A child of Mexican descent
2. A child of Mediterranean descent
3. A child whose intake of iron is extremely poor
4. A breast-fed child of a mother with chronic anemia

305. A child with β-thalassemia is receiving long-term blood transfusion therapy for the treatment of the disorder. Chelation therapy is prescribed as a result of too much iron from the transfusions. Which medication should the nurse anticipate being prescribed?
1. Fragmin
2. Meropenem
3. Metoprolol
4. Deferoxamine

306. The clinic nurse instructs parents of a child with sickle cell anemia about the precipitating factors related to sickle cell crisis. Which, if identified by the parents as a precipitating factor, indicates the **need for further instruction**?
1. Stress
2. Trauma
3. Infection
4. Fluid overload

307. A 10-year-old child with hemophilia A has slipped on the ice and bumped his knee. The nurse should prepare to administer which prescription?
1. Injection of factor X
2. Intravenous infusion of iron
3. Intravenous infusion of factor VIII
4. Intramuscular injection of iron using the Z-track method

308. The nurse is instructing the parents of a child with iron deficiency anemia regarding the administration of a liquid oral iron supplement. Which instruction should the nurse tell the parents?
1. Administer the iron at mealtimes.
2. Administer the iron through a straw.
3. Mix the iron with cereal to administer.
4. Add the iron to formula for easy administration.

309. Laboratory studies are performed for a child suspected to have iron deficiency anemia. The nurse reviews the laboratory results, knowing that which result indicates this type of anemia?
1. Elevated hemoglobin level
2. Decreased reticulocyte count
3. Elevated red blood cell count
4. Red blood cells that are microcytic and hypochromic

310. The nurse is reviewing a health care provider's prescriptions for a child with sickle cell anemia who was admitted to the hospital for the treatment of vaso-occlusive crisis. Which prescriptions documented in the child's record should the nurse question? **Select all that apply.**

- ☐ 1. Restrict fluid intake.
- ☐ 2. Position for comfort.
- ☐ 3. Avoid strain on painful joints.
- ☐ 4. Apply nasal oxygen at 2 L/minute.
- ☐ 5. Provide a high-calorie, high-protein diet.
- ☐ 6. Give meperidine, 25 mg intravenously, every 4 hours for pain.

311. The nurse is conducting staff in-service training on von Willebrand's disease. Which should the nurse include as characteristics of von Willebrand's disease? **Select all that apply.**

- ☐ 1. Easy bruising occurs.
- ☐ 2. Gum bleeding occurs.
- ☐ 3. It is a hereditary bleeding disorder.
- ☐ 4. Treatment and care are similar to that for hemophilia.
- ☐ 5. It is characterized by extremely high creatinine levels.
- ☐ 6. The disorder causes platelets to adhere to damaged endothelium.

ANSWERS

302. *Answer:* 4

Rationale: Hemophilia refers to a group of bleeding disorders resulting from a deficiency of specific coagulation proteins. Results of tests that measure platelet function are normal; results of tests that measure clotting factor function may be abnormal. Abnormal laboratory results in hemophilia indicate a prolonged partial thromboplastin time. The platelet count, hemoglobin level, and hematocrit level are normal in hemophilia.

Test-Taking Strategy: Focus on the subject, laboratory tests used to monitor hemophilia, and note the strategic words, *most likely*. Recalling the pathophysiology associated with this disorder and recalling that it results from a deficiency of specific coagulation proteins will direct you to the correct option.

Level of Cognitive Ability: Analyzing
Client Needs: Physiological Integrity
Integrated Process: Nursing Process—Assessment
Content Area: Pediatrics: Hematological
Health Problem: Pediatric-Specific: Bleeding Disorders
Priority Concepts: Clinical Judgment; Clotting
Reference: McKinney et al. (2018), p. 1130.

303. *Answer:* 3

Rationale: Hemophilia refers to a group of bleeding disorders resulting from a deficiency of specific coagulation proteins. Children with hemophilia need to avoid contact sports and to take precautions such as wearing elbow and knee pads and helmets with other sports. The safe activity for them is swimming.

Test-Taking Strategy: Focus on the subject, a safe activity. Recalling that bleeding is a major concern in this condition, eliminate options 1, 2, and 4, because these activities are comparable or alike in that they present the potential for injury.

Level of Cognitive Ability: Applying
Client Needs: Safe and Effective Care Environment
Integrated Process: Teaching and Learning
Content Area: Pediatrics: Hematological
Health Problem: Pediatric-Specific: Bleeding Disorder
Priority Concepts: Clotting; Safety
Reference: McKinney et al. (2018), p. 1133.

304. *Answer:* 2

Rationale: β-Thalassemia is an autosomal recessive disorder characterized by the reduced production of 1 of the globin chains in the synthesis of hemoglobin (both parents must be carriers to produce a child with β-thalassemia major). This disorder is found primarily in individuals of Mediterranean descent. Options 1, 3, and 4 are incorrect.

Test-Taking Strategy: Focus on the subject, the child at greatest risk for β-thalassemia major. Think about the pathophysiology of the disorder. Remember that this disorder occurs primarily in individuals of Mediterranean descent.

Level of Cognitive Ability: Applying
Client Needs: Physiological Integrity
Integrated Process: Teaching and Learning
Content Area: Pediatrics: Hematological
Health Problem: Pediatric-Specific: Anemias
Priority Concepts: Gas Exchange; Perfusion
Reference: McKinney et al. (2018), pp. 1128-1129.

305. *Answer:* 4

Rationale: β-Thalassemia is an autosomal recessive disorder characterized by the reduced production of 1 of the globin chains in the synthesis of hemoglobin (both parents must be carriers to produce a child with β-thalassemia major). The major complication of long-term transfusion therapy is hemosiderosis. To prevent organ damage from too much iron, chelation therapy with either deferasirox or deferoxamine may be prescribed. Deferoxamine is classified as an antidote for acute iron toxicity. Dalteparin is an anticoagulant used as prophylaxis for postoperative deep vein thrombosis. Meropenem is an antibiotic. Metoprolol is a beta blocker used to treat hypertension.

Test-Taking Strategy: Focus on the subject, chelation therapy. Specific knowledge regarding the antidote for iron toxicity is needed to answer this question. One way to remember this is to look at the prefix in the generic name of the medication used to treat iron overdose. Remember to associate *defer-* and removal of iron.

Level of Cognitive Ability: Analyzing
Client Needs: Physiological Integrity
Integrated Process: Nursing Process—Planning
Content Area: Pediatrics: Hematological
Health Problem: Pediatric-Specific: Anemias

Priority Concepts: Clinical Judgment; Gas Exchange
Reference: McKinney et al. (2018), pp. 1128-1129.

306. *Answer:* 4
Rationale: Sickle cell crises are acute exacerbations of the disease, which vary considerably in severity and frequency; these include vaso-occlusive crisis, splenic sequestration, hyperhemolytic crisis, and aplastic crisis. Sickle cell crisis may be precipitated by infection, dehydration, hypoxia, trauma, or physical or emotional stress. The mother of a child with sickle cell disease should encourage fluid intake of 1.5 to 2 times the daily requirement to prevent dehydration.
Test-Taking Strategy: Note the strategic words, *need for further instruction*. These words indicate a negative event query and ask you to select an option that is an incorrect statement. Recalling that fluids are a main component of treatment in sickle cell anemia to prevent crisis will direct you to the correct option. Remember that fluids are required to prevent dehydration.
Level of Cognitive Ability: Evaluating
Client Needs: Health Promotion and Maintenance
Integrated Process: Teaching and Learning
Content Area: Pediatrics: Hematological
Health Problem: Pediatric-Specific: Anemias
Priority Concepts: Client Education; Clotting
References: Hockenberry, Wilson, Rodgers (2017), pp. 791-792.

307. *Answer:* 3
Rationale: Hemophilia refers to a group of bleeding disorders resulting from a deficiency of specific coagulation proteins. The primary treatment is replacement of the missing clotting factor; additional medications, such as agents to relieve pain, may be prescribed depending on the source of bleeding from the disorder. A child with hemophilia A is at risk for joint bleeding after a fall. Factor VIII would be prescribed intravenously to replace the missing clotting factor and minimize the bleeding. Factor X and iron are not used to treat children with hemophilia A.
Test-Taking Strategy: Focus on the child's diagnosis. Eliminate options 2 and 4 because they are comparable or alike. Recalling that a child with hemophilia A is missing clotting factor VIII will direct you to the correct option from those remaining.
Level of Cognitive Ability: Analyzing
Client Needs: Physiological Integrity
Integrated Process: Nursing Process—Planning
Content Area: Pediatrics: Hematological
Health Problem: Pediatric-Specific: Bleeding Disorders
Priority Concepts: Clinical Judgment; Clotting
Reference: McKinney et al. (2018), pp. 1130, 1132.

308. *Answer:* 2
Rationale: In iron deficiency anemia, iron stores are depleted, resulting in a decreased supply of iron for the manufacture of hemoglobin in red blood cells. An oral iron supplement should be administered through a straw or medicine dropper placed at the back of the mouth, because the iron stains the teeth. The parents should be instructed to brush or wipe the child's teeth or have the child brush the teeth after administration. Iron is administered between meals because absorption is decreased if there is food in the stomach. Iron requires an acid environment to facilitate its absorption in the duodenum. Iron is not added to formula or mixed with cereal or other food items.
Test-Taking Strategy: Eliminate options 3 and 4 first because they are comparable or alike and because medication should not be added to formula and food. Next, note the word *liquid* in the question. This should assist you in recalling that iron in liquid form stains teeth.
Level of Cognitive Ability: Applying
Client Needs: Physiological Integrity
Integrated Process: Teaching and Learning
Content Area: Pediatrics: Hematological
Health Problem: Pediatric-Specific: Anemias
Priority Concepts: Client Education; Health Promotion
Reference: McKinney et al. (2018), p. 1121.

309. *Answer:* 4
Rationale: In iron deficiency anemia, iron stores are depleted, resulting in a decreased supply of iron for the manufacture of hemoglobin in red blood cells. The results of a complete blood cell count in children with iron deficiency anemia show decreased hemoglobin levels and microcytic and hypochromic red blood cells. The red blood cell count is decreased. The reticulocyte count is usually normal or slightly elevated.
Test-Taking Strategy: Focus on the subject, laboratory findings. Eliminate options 1 and 3 first, knowing that the hemoglobin and red blood cell counts would be decreased. From the remaining options, select the correct option over option 2 because of the relationship between anemia and red blood cells.
Level of Cognitive Ability: Analyzing
Client Needs: Physiological Integrity
Integrated Process: Nursing Process—Assessment
Content Area: Pediatrics: Hematological
Health Problem: Pediatric-Specific: Anemias
Priority Concepts: Cellular Regulation; Gas Exchange
Reference: McKinney et al. (2018), pp. 1120-1121.

310. *Answer:* 1, 6
Rationale: Sickle cell anemia is one of a group of diseases termed *hemoglobinopathies*, in which hemoglobin A is partly or completely replaced by abnormal sickle hemoglobin S. It is caused by the inheritance of a gene for a structurally abnormal portion of the hemoglobin chain. Hemoglobin S is sensitive to changes in the oxygen content of the red blood cell; insufficient oxygen causes the cells to assume a sickle shape, and the cells become rigid and clumped together, obstructing capillary blood flow. Oral and intravenous fluids are an important part of treatment. Meperidine is not recommended for a child with sickle cell disease because of the risk for normeperidine-induced seizures. Normeperidine, a metabolite of meperidine, is a central nervous system stimulant that produces anxiety, tremors, myoclonus, and generalized seizures when it accumulates with repetitive dosing. The nurse would question the prescription for restricted fluids and meperidine for pain control. Positioning for comfort, avoiding strain on painful joints, oxygen, and a high-calorie and high-protein diet are also important parts of the treatment plan.
Test-Taking Strategy: Focus on the subject, identifying the prescriptions that need to be questioned and on the pathophysiology

that occurs in sickle cell disease. Recalling that fluids are an important component of the treatment plan will assist in identifying that a fluid restriction prescription would need to be questioned. Also, recalling the effects of meperidine will assist in identifying that this prescription needs to be questioned.
Level of Cognitive Ability: Analyzing
Client Needs: Safe and Effective Care Environment
Integrated Process: Nursing Process—Implementation
Content Area: Pediatrics: Hematological
Health Problem: Pediatric-Specific: Anemias
Priority Concepts: Collaboration; Safety
Reference: McKinney et al. (2018), pp. 1125-1127.

311. ***Answer:*** **1, 2, 3, 4, 6**
Rationale: von Willebrand's disease is a hereditary bleeding disorder characterized by a deficiency of or a defect in a protein termed *von Willebrand factor*. The disorder causes platelets to adhere to damaged endothelium. It is characterized by an increased tendency to bleed from mucous membranes. Assessment findings include epistaxis, gum bleeding, easy bruising, and excessive menstrual bleeding. An elevated creatinine level is not associated with this disorder.
Test-Taking Strategy: Focus on the **subject,** assessment findings, and on the child's diagnosis. Recalling that this disorder is characterized by an increased tendency to bleed from mucous membranes will direct you to the correct options.
Level of Cognitive Ability: Analyzing
Client Needs: Physiological Integrity
Integrated Process: Nursing Process—Assessment
Content Area: Pediatrics: Hematological
Health Problem: Pediatric-Specific: Bleeding Disorders
Priority Concepts: Clinical Judgment; Clotting
Reference: McKinney et al. (2018), pp. 1132-1133.

CHAPTER 31

Oncological Problems

PRIORITY CONCEPTS Cellular Regulation; Safety

I. Leukemia

A. Description

1. Leukemia is a malignant increase in the number of leukocytes, usually at an immature stage, in the bone marrow.
2. In leukemia, proliferating immature white blood cells (WBCs) depress the bone marrow, causing anemia from decreased erythrocytes, infection from neutropenia, and bleeding from decreased platelet production (thrombocytopenia).
3. The cause is unknown; it seems to involve genetic damage of cells, leading to the transformation of cells from a normal state to a malignant state.
4. Risk factors include genetic, viral, immunological, and environmental factors and exposure to radiation, chemicals, and medications.
5. Acute lymphocytic leukemia is the most frequent type of cancer in children.
6. Leukemia is more common in boys than girls after 1 year of age.
7. Prognosis depends on various factors such as age at diagnosis, initial WBC count, type of cell involved, and sex of the child.
8. Treatment involves chemotherapy and possibly radiation and hematopoietic stem cell transplantation.
9. The phases of chemotherapy include induction, which achieves a complete remission or disappearance of leukemic cells; intensification or consolidation therapy, which decreases the tumor burden further; central nervous system prophylactic therapy, which prevents leukemic cells from invading the central nervous system; and maintenance, which serves to maintain the remission phase.

B. Assessment

1. Infiltration of the bone marrow by malignant cells causes fever, pallor, fatigue, anorexia, hemorrhage (usually petechiae), and bone and joint pain; pathological fractures can occur as a result of bone marrow invasion with leukemic cells.
2. Signs of infection occur as a result of neutropenia.
3. The child experiences hepatosplenomegaly and lymphadenopathy.
4. The child has a normal, elevated, or low WBC count, depending on the presence of infection or of immature versus mature WBCs.
5. The child has decreased hemoglobin and hematocrit levels.
6. The child has a decreased platelet count.
7. A positive bone marrow biopsy specimen identifies leukemic blast (immature)–phase cells.
8. Signs of increased intracranial pressure (ICP) occur as a result of central nervous system involvement (Box 31-1).
9. The child shows signs of cranial nerve (cranial nerve VII, or the facial nerve, is most commonly affected) or spinal nerve involvement; clinical manifestations relate to the area involved.
10. Clinical manifestations indicate the invasion of leukemic cells to the kidneys, testes, prostate, ovaries, gastrointestinal tract, and lungs.

C. Infection (Box 31-2)

1. Infection can occur through self-contamination or cross-contamination.
2. The most common sites for infection are the skin (any break in the skin is a potential site for infection), respiratory tract, and gastrointestinal tract.

D. Bleeding (Box 31-3)

1. Platelet transfusions are generally reserved for active bleeding episodes that do not respond to local treatment and that may occur during induction or relapse therapy.
2. Packed red blood cells may be prescribed for a child with severe blood loss.

E. Fatigue and nutrition

1. Assist the parents and child in selecting a well-balanced diet.
2. Provide small meals that require little chewing and are not irritating to the oral mucosa.
3. If the child cannot take oral feedings, parenteral nutrition or enteral feedings may be prescribed.
4. Assist the child in self-care and mobility activities.

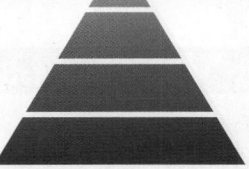

Pediatric

BOX 31-1 Manifestations of Increased Intracranial Pressure in Infants and Children

Infants

- Tense, bulging fontanel
- Separated cranial sutures
- Macewen's sign (cracked-pot sound on percussion)
- Irritability
- High-pitched cry
- Increased head circumference
- Distended scalp veins
- Poor feeding
- Crying when disturbed
- Setting sun sign (eyes appear downward, with the sclera seen over the iris, part of the lower pupil may be covered by the lower eyelid)

Children

- Headache
- Nausea
- Forceful vomiting
- Diplopia; blurred vision
- Seizures

Personality and Behavior Signs

- Irritability, restlessness
- Indifference, drowsiness
- Decline in school performance
- Diminished physical activity and motor performance
- Increased sleeping
- Inability to follow simple commands
- Lethargy

Late Signs

- Bradycardia
- Decreased motor response to command
- Decreased sensory response to painful stimuli
- Alterations in pupil size and reaction
- Decerebrate (extension) or decorticate (flexion) posturing
- Cheyne-Stokes respirations
- Papilledema
- Decreased consciousness
- Coma

From Perry S, Hockenberry M, Lowdermilk D, Wilson D: *Maternal-child nursing care*, ed 4, St. Louis, 2010, Mosby.

BOX 31-2 Protecting the Child from Infection

- Initiate protective isolation procedures.
- Maintain frequent and thorough hand washing.
- Maintain the child in a private room with high-efficiency particulate air filtration or laminar air flow system if possible.
- Ensure that the child's room is cleaned daily.
- Use strict aseptic technique for all nursing procedures.
- Limit the number of caregivers entering the child's room, and ensure that anyone entering the child's room wears a mask.
- Keep supplies for the child separate from supplies for other children.
- Reduce exposure to environmental organisms by eliminating raw fruits and vegetables from the diet, by not allowing fresh flowers in the child's room, and by not leaving standing water in the child's room.
- Assist the child with daily bathing, using antimicrobial soap.
- Assist the child to perform oral hygiene frequently.
- Assess for signs and symptoms of infection.
- Monitor temperature, pulse, and blood pressure.
- Change wound dressings daily, and inspect wounds for redness, swelling, or drainage.
- Assess urine for color and cloudiness.
- Assess the skin and oral mucous membranes for signs of infection.
- Auscultate lung sounds.
- Encourage the child to cough and deep-breathe.
- Monitor white blood cell and neutrophil counts.
- Notify the primary health care provider if signs of infection are present, and prepare to obtain specimens for culture of open lesions, urine, and sputum.
- Initiate a bowel program to prevent constipation and rectal trauma.
- Avoid invasive procedures such as injections, rectal temperatures, and urinary catheterization.
- Administer antibiotic, antifungal, and antiviral medications as prescribed.
- Administer granulocyte colony-stimulating factor as prescribed.
- Instruct parents to keep the child away from crowds and individuals with infections.
- Instruct parents that the child should not receive immunization with a live virus (measles, mumps, rubella, polio), because if the immune system is depressed, the attenuated virus can result in a life-threatening infection; also, the child should not receive the varicella vaccine.
- The Salk (inactivated) vaccine for poliomyelitis may be administered.
- Instruct parents to inform the teacher that they should be notified immediately if a case of a communicable disease occurs in another child at school.

5. Allow adequate rest periods during care.
6. Do not perform nursing care activities unless they are essential.

F. Chemotherapy

1. Monitor for severe bone marrow suppression; during the period of greatest bone marrow suppression (the nadir), blood cell counts are extremely low.
2. Monitor for infection and bleeding.
3. Protect the child from life-threatening infections.
4. Monitor for nausea, vomiting, and alteration in bowel function.
5. Administer stool softeners as prescribed and if needed to prevent straining if constipation occurs.

BOX 31-3 Protecting the Child from Bleeding

- Examine the child for signs and symptoms of bleeding.
- Handle the child gently.
- Measure abdominal girth; an increase can indicate internal hemorrhage.
- Instruct the child to use a soft toothbrush and avoid dental floss.
- Provide soft foods that are cool to warm in temperature.
- Avoid injections, if possible, to prevent trauma to the skin and bleeding.
- Apply firm and gentle pressure to a needle-stick site for at least 10 minutes.
- Pad side rails and sharp corners of the bed and furniture.
- Discourage the child from engaging in activities involving the use of objects that can cause injury.
- Instruct the child to avoid constrictive or tight clothing.
- Use caution when taking the blood pressure to prevent skin injury.
- Instruct the child to avoid blowing his or her nose.
- Avoid the use of rectal suppositories, enemas, and rectal thermometers.
- Examine all body fluids and excrement for the presence of blood.
- Count the number of pads or tampons used if the adolescent girl is menstruating.
- Instruct the child about the signs and symptoms of bleeding.
- Instruct parents to avoid administering nonsteroidal anti-inflammatory drugs and products that contain aspirin to the child.

6. Provide rectal hygiene gently as needed.
7. Administer antiemetics before beginning chemotherapy as prescribed.
8. Monitor for signs of dehydration.
9. Monitor for signs of hemorrhagic cystitis.
10. Monitor for signs of peripheral neuropathy.
11. Assess oral mucous membranes for mucositis; administer frequent mouth rinses per agency procedure and as prescribed to promote healing or prevent infection (local oral anesthetics may also be prescribed).
12. Instruct the parents and child in the signs and symptoms to watch for after chemotherapy and when to notify the primary health care provider (PHCP).
13. Inform the parents and child that hair loss may occur from chemotherapy (hair regrows in about 3 to 6 months and may be a slightly different color or texture).
14. Instruct the parents and child about the care of a central venous access device, as necessary (see Chapter 69).
15. Listen to the child and family, and encourage them to verbalize their feelings and express their concerns.
16. Introduce the family to other families of children with cancer, as appropriate
17. Consult social services and chaplains as necessary.

Monitor a child receiving chemotherapy closely for signs of infection. Infection is a major cause of death in the immunosuppressed child.

II. Hodgkin's Disease

A. Description

1. Hodgkin's disease (a type of lymphoma) is a malignancy of the lymph nodes that originates in a single lymph node or a single chain of nodes (Fig. 31-1).

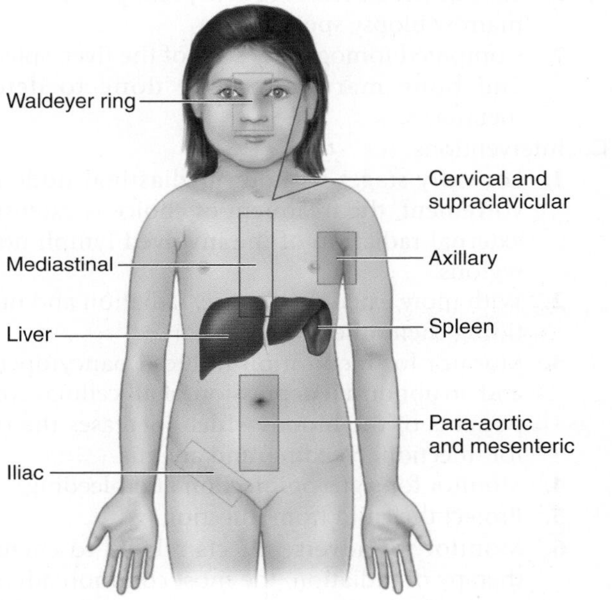

FIG. 31-1 Main areas of lymphadenopathy and organ involvement in Hodgkin's disease.

2. The disease predictably metastasizes to non-nodal or extralymphatic sites, especially the spleen, liver, bone marrow, lungs, and mediastinum.
3. Hodgkin's disease is characterized by the presence of Reed-Sternberg cells noted in a lymph node biopsy specimen.
4. Peak incidence is in mid-adolescence.
5. Possible causes include viral infections and previous exposure to alkylating chemical agents.
6. The prognosis is excellent, with long-term survival rates depending on the stage of the disease.
7. The primary treatment modalities are radiation and chemotherapy; each may be used alone or in combination, depending on the clinical stage of the disease.

B. Assessment
1. Painless enlargement of lymph nodes
2. Enlarged, firm, nontender, movable nodes in the supraclavicular area; in children, the "sentinel" node located near the left clavicle may be the first enlarged node
3. Nonproductive cough as a result of mediastinal lymphadenopathy
4. Abdominal pain as a result of enlarged retroperitoneal nodes
5. Advanced lymph node and extralymphatic involvement that may cause systemic symptoms, such as a low-grade or intermittent fever, anorexia, nausea, weight loss, night sweats, and pruritus
6. Positive biopsy specimen of a lymph node (presence of Reed-Sternberg cells) and positive bone marrow biopsy specimen
7. Computed tomography scan of the liver, spleen, and bone marrow may be done to detect metastasis.

C. Interventions
1. For early stages without mediastinal node involvement, the treatment of choice is extensive external radiation of the involved lymph node regions.
2. With more extensive disease, radiation and multidrug chemotherapy are used.
3. Monitor for medication-induced pancytopenia and an abnormal depression of all cellular components of the blood, which increases the risk for infection, bleeding, and anemia.
4. Monitor for signs of infection and bleeding.
5. Protect the child from infection.
6. Monitor for adverse effects related to chemotherapy or radiation; the most common adverse effect of extensive irradiation is malaise, which can be difficult for older children and adolescents to tolerate physically and psychologically (Table 31-1).
7. Monitor for nausea and vomiting, and administer antiemetics as prescribed.

TABLE 31-1 Adverse Effects of Radiation Therapy and Nursing Interventions

Body Area and Adverse Effects	Interventions
Gastrointestinal Tract	
Anorexia	Encourage fluids and foods as best tolerated
	Provide small, frequent meals
	Monitor for weight loss
Nausea, vomiting	Administer antiemetics around the clock
	Monitor for dehydration
Mucosal ulceration	Provide soothing oral hygiene and prescribed mouth rinses
	Topical anesthetic may be prescribed
Diarrhea	Administer antispasmodics and antidiarrheal preparations as prescribed
	Monitor for dehydration
Skin	
Alopecia (hair loss)	Introduce idea of a wig or head wraps to child
	Provide scalp hygiene
	Stress the need for head covering in cold weather
Dry or moist desquamation	Keep skin clean
	Wash skin daily, using a mild soap sparingly
	Do not remove skin markings for radiation
	Avoid exposure to the sun and other extreme temperature changes
	For dryness, apply lubricant as prescribed
Urinary Bladder	
Cystitis	Encourage fluid intake and frequent voiding
	Monitor for hematuria
Bone Marrow	
Myelosuppression	Monitor for fever
	Administer antibiotics as prescribed
	Avoid use of suppositories, enemas, and rectal temperatures
	Institute neutropenic or bleeding precautions as needed
	Monitor for signs of anemia

Adapted from Hockenberry M, Wilson D: *Wong's nursing care of infants and children*, ed 9, St. Louis, 2013, Mosby; and McKinney E, James S, Murray S, Ashwill J: *Maternal-child nursing*, ed 4, St. Louis, 2013, Saunders.

III. Nephroblastoma (Wilms' Tumor)

A. Description
1. Wilms' tumor is the most common intra-abdominal and kidney tumor of childhood; it may manifest unilaterally and localized or bilaterally, sometimes with metastasis to other organs.
2. The peak incidence is 3 years of age.
3. Occurrence is associated with a genetic inheritance and with several congenital anomalies.
4. Therapeutic management includes a combined treatment of surgery (partial to total nephrectomy) and chemotherapy with or without radiation, depending on the clinical stage and the histological pattern of the tumor.

B. Assessment
1. Swelling or mass within the abdomen (mass is characteristically firm, nontender, confined to 1 side, and deep within the flank)

2. Urinary retention or hematuria, or both
3. Anemia (caused by hemorrhage within the tumor)
4. Pallor, anorexia, and lethargy (resulting from anemia)
5. Hypertension (caused by secretion of excess amounts of renin by the tumor)
6. Weight loss and fever
7. Symptoms of lung involvement, such as dyspnea, shortness of breath, and pain in the chest, if metastasis has occurred

C. Preoperative interventions
1. Monitor vital signs, particularly blood pressure.
2. Avoid palpation of the abdomen; place a sign at bedside that reads, Do Not Palpate Abdomen.
3. Measure abdominal girth at least once daily.

D. Postoperative interventions
1. Monitor temperature and blood pressure closely.
2. Monitor for signs of hemorrhage and infection.
3. Monitor strict intake and urine output closely.
4. Monitor for abdominal distention; monitor bowel sounds and other signs of gastrointestinal activity because of the risk for intestinal obstruction.

Avoid palpation of the abdomen in a child with Wilms' tumor and be cautious when bathing, moving, or handling the child. It is important to keep the encapsulated tumor intact. Rupture of the tumor can cause the cancer cells to spread throughout the abdomen, lymph system, and bloodstream.

IV. Neuroblastoma

A. Description
1. Neuroblastoma is a tumor that originates from the embryonic neural crest cells that normally give rise to the adrenal medulla and the sympathetic ganglia.
2. Most tumors develop in the adrenal gland or the retroperitoneal sympathetic chain; other sites may be within the head, neck, chest, or pelvis.
3. Most children present with neuroblastoma before 10 years of age.
4. Most presenting signs are caused by the tumor compressing adjacent normal tissue and organs.
5. Diagnostic evaluation is aimed at locating the primary site of the tumor; analyzing the breakdown products excreted in the urine, namely vanillylmandelic acid, homovanillic acid, dopamine, and norepinephrine, permits detection of suspected tumor before and after medical-surgical intervention.
6. The prognosis is poor because of the frequency of invasiveness of the tumor and because, in most cases, a diagnosis is not made until after metastasis has occurred; the younger the child at diagnosis, the better the survival rate.
7. Therapeutic management
   a. Surgery is performed to remove as much of the tumor as possible and to obtain biopsy specimens; in the early stages, complete surgical removal of the tumor is the treatment of choice.
   b. Surgery usually is limited to biopsy in the later stages because of extensive metastasis.
   c. Radiation is used commonly with later-stage disease and provides palliation for metastatic lesions in bones, lungs, liver, and brain.
   d. Chemotherapy is used for extensive local or disseminated disease.

B. Assessment
1. Firm, nontender, irregular mass in the abdomen that crosses the midline
2. Urinary frequency or retention from compression of the kidney, ureter, or bladder
3. Lymphadenopathy, especially in the cervical and supraclavicular areas
4. Bone pain if skeletal involvement
5. Supraorbital ecchymosis, periorbital edema, and exophthalmos as a result of invasion of retrobulbar soft tissue
6. Pallor, weakness, irritability, anorexia, weight loss
7. Signs of respiratory impairment (thoracic lesion)
8. Signs of neurological impairment (intracranial lesion)
9. Paralysis from compression of the spinal cord

C. Preoperative interventions
1. Monitor for signs and symptoms related to the location of the tumor.
2. Provide emotional support to the child and parents.

D. Postoperative interventions
1. Monitor for postoperative complications related to the location (organ) of the surgery.
2. Monitor for complications related to chemotherapy or radiation if prescribed.
3. Provide support to the parents and encourage them to express their feelings; many parents feel guilt for not having recognized signs in the child earlier.
4. Refer parents to appropriate community services.

V. Osteosarcoma (Osteogenic Sarcoma)

A. Description
1. The most common bone cancer in children; it is also known as *osteogenic sarcoma*.
2. Cancer usually is found in the metaphysis of long bones, especially in the lower extremities, with most tumors occurring in the femur.
3. The peak age of incidence is between 10 and 25 years.
4. Symptoms in the earliest stage are almost always attributed to extremity injury or normal growing pains.

Pediatric

5. Treatment may include surgical resection (limb salvage procedure) to save a limb or remove affected tissue, or amputation.
6. Chemotherapy is used to treat the cancer and may be used before and after surgery.

B. Assessment
1. Localized pain at the affected site (may be severe or dull) that may be attributed to trauma or the vague complaint of "growing pains"; pain often is relieved by a flexed position.
2. Palpable mass
3. Limping if weight-bearing limb is affected
4. Progressive limited range of motion and the child's curtailing of physical activity
5. Child may be unable to hold heavy objects because of their weight and resultant pain in the affected extremity.
6. Pathological fractures occur at the tumor site.

C. Interventions
1. Prepare the child and family for prescribed treatment modalities, which may include surgical resection by limb salvage to remove affected tissue, amputation, and chemotherapy.
2. Communicate honestly with the child and family and provide support.
3. Prepare for prosthetic fitting as necessary.
4. Assist the child in dealing with problems of self-image.
5. Instruct the child and parents about the potential development of phantom limb pain that may occur after amputation, characterized by tingling, itching, and a painful sensation in the area where the limb was amputated.

VI. Brain Tumors

A. Description
1. An infratentorial (below the tentorium cerebelli) tumor, the most common brain tumor, is located in the posterior third of the brain (primarily in the cerebellum or brainstem) and accounts for the frequency of symptoms resulting from increased ICP.
2. A supratentorial tumor is located within the anterior two-thirds of the brain—mainly the cerebrum.
3. The signs and symptoms of a brain tumor depend on its anatomical location and size and, to some extent, on the age of the child; a number of tests may be used in the neurological evaluation, but the most common diagnostic procedure is magnetic resonance imaging (MRI), which determines the location and extent of the tumor.
4. Therapeutic management includes surgery, radiation, and chemotherapy; the treatment of choice is total removal of the tumor without residual neurological damage.

B. Assessment
1. Headache that is worse on awakening and improves during the day
2. Vomiting that is unrelated to feeding or eating
3. Ataxia
4. Seizures
5. Behavioral changes
6. Clumsiness; awkward gait or difficulty walking
7. Diplopia
8. Facial weakness

Monitor for signs of increased ICP in a child with a brain tumor and after a craniotomy. If signs of increased ICP occur, notify the PHCP immediately.

C. Preoperative interventions
1. Perform a neurological assessment at least every 4 hours.
2. Institute seizure precautions and safety measures.
3. Assess weight loss and nutritional status.
4. Shave the child's head as prescribed (provide a favorite cap or hat for the child); shaving the head may also be done in the surgical suite.
5. Prepare the child as much as possible; tell the child that he or she will wake up with a large head dressing.

D. Postoperative interventions
1. Assess neurological and motor function and level of consciousness.
2. Monitor temperature closely, which may be elevated because of hypothalamus or brainstem involvement during surgery; maintain a cooling blanket by the bedside.
3. Monitor for signs of respiratory infection.
4. Monitor for signs of meningitis (opisthotonos, Kernig's and Brudzinski's signs).
5. Monitor for signs of increased ICP (see Box 31-1; see also Chapter 38).
6. Monitor for hemorrhage, checking the back of the head dressing for posterior pooling of blood; mark drainage edges with marker, reinforce dressing if needed, and do not change dressing without a specific prescription.
7. Assess pupillary response; sluggish, dilated, or unequal pupils are reported immediately because they may indicate increased ICP and potential brainstem herniation.
8. Monitor for colorless drainage on the dressing or from the ears or nose, which indicates cerebrospinal fluid and should be reported immediately; assess for the presence of glucose in the drainage (dipstick).
9. Assess the surgeon's prescription for positioning, including the degree of neck flexion (Box 31-4).
10. Monitor intravenous fluids closely.

BOX 31-4 Positioning After Craniotomy

- Assess the surgeon's prescription for positioning, including the degree of neck flexion.
- If a large tumor has been removed, the child is not placed on the operative side, because the brain may shift suddenly to that cavity.
- In an infratentorial procedure, the child usually is positioned flat and on either side.
- In a supratentorial procedure, the head usually is elevated above the heart level to facilitate cerebrospinal fluid drainage and to decrease excessive blood flow to the brain to prevent hemorrhage.
- Never place the child in Trendelenburg's position because it increases intracranial pressure and the risk of hemorrhage.

11. Promote measures that prevent vomiting (vomiting increases ICP and the risk for incisional rupture).
12. Provide a quiet environment.
13. Administer analgesics as prescribed.
14. Provide emotional support to the child and parents, and promote optimal growth and development.

PRACTICE QUESTIONS

312. The nurse is monitoring a child for bleeding after surgery for removal of a brain tumor. The nurse checks the head dressing for the presence of blood and notes a colorless drainage on the back of the dressing. Which action should the nurse perform **immediately?**

1. Notify the surgeon.
2. Reinforce the dressing.
3. Document the findings and continue to monitor.
4. Circle the area of drainage and continue to monitor.

313. A child undergoes surgical removal of a brain tumor. During the postoperative period, the nurse notes that the child is restless, the pulse rate is elevated, and the blood pressure has decreased significantly from the baseline value. The nurse suspects that the child is in shock. Which is the **most appropriate** nursing action?

1. Place the child in a supine position.
2. Place the child in Trendelenburg's position.
3. Increase the flow rate of the intravenous fluids.
4. Notify the primary health care provider (PHCP).

314. The mother of a 4-year-old child tells the pediatric nurse that the child's abdomen seems to be swollen. During further assessment, the mother tells the nurse that the child is eating well and that the activity level of the child is unchanged. The nurse, suspecting the possibility of Wilms' tumor, should avoid which during the physical assessment?

1. Palpating the abdomen for a mass
2. Assessing the urine for the presence of hematuria
3. Monitoring the temperature for the presence of fever
4. Monitoring the blood pressure for the presence of hypertension

315. The nurse provides a teaching session to the nursing staff regarding osteosarcoma. Which statement by a member of the nursing staff indicates a **need for information**?

1. "The femur is the most common site of this sarcoma."
2. "The child does not experience pain at the primary tumor site."
3. "Limping, if a weight-bearing limb is affected, is a clinical manifestation."
4. "The symptoms of the disease in the early stage are almost always attributed to normal growing pains."

316. The nurse analyzes the laboratory values of a child with leukemia who is receiving chemotherapy. The nurse notes that the platelet count is 19,500 mm^3 (19.5 $\times 10^9/L$). On the basis of this laboratory result, which intervention should the nurse include in the plan of care?

1. Initiate bleeding precautions.
2. Monitor closely for signs of infection.
3. Monitor the temperature every 4 hours.
4. Initiate protective isolation precautions.

317. The nurse is monitoring a 3-year-old child for signs and symptoms of increased intracranial pressure (ICP) after a craniotomy. The nurse plans to monitor for which **early** sign or symptom of increased ICP?

1. Vomiting
2. Bulging anterior fontanel
3. Increasing head circumference
4. Complaints of a frontal headache

318. A 4-year-old child is admitted to the hospital for abdominal pain. The mother reports that the child has been pale and excessively tired and is bruising easily. On physical examination, lymphadenopathy and hepatosplenomegaly are noted. Diagnostic studies are being performed because acute lymphocytic leukemia is suspected. The nurse determines that which laboratory result confirms the diagnosis?

1. Lumbar puncture showing no blast cells
2. Bone marrow biopsy showing blast cells
3. Platelet count of 350,000 mm^3 ($350 \times 10^9/L$)
4. White blood cell count 4500 mm^3 ($4.5 \times 10^9/L$)

319. A 6-year-old child with leukemia is hospitalized and is receiving combination chemotherapy. Laboratory

results indicate that the child is neutropenic, and protective isolation procedures are initiated. The grandmother of the child visits and brings a fresh bouquet of flowers picked from her garden and asks the nurse for a vase for the flowers. Which response should the nurse provide to the grandmother?
1. "I have a vase in the utility room, and I will get it for you."
2. "I will get the vase and wash it well before you put the flowers in it."
3. "The flowers from your garden are beautiful, but should not be placed in the child's room at this time."
4. "When you bring the flowers into the room, place them on the bedside stand as far away from the child as possible."

320. A diagnosis of Hodgkin's disease is suspected in a 12-year-old child. Several diagnostic studies are performed to determine the presence of this disease. Which diagnostic test result will confirm the diagnosis of Hodgkin's disease?
1. Elevated vanillylmandelic acid urinary levels
2. The presence of blast cells in the bone marrow
3. The presence of Epstein-Barr virus in the blood
4. The presence of Reed-Sternberg cells in the lymph nodes

321. Which specific nursing interventions are implemented in the care of a child with leukemia who is at risk for infection? **Select all that apply.**
- ☐ 1. Maintain the child in a semiprivate room.
- ☐ 2. Reduce exposure to environmental organisms.
- ☐ 3. Use strict aseptic technique for all procedures.
- ☐ 4. Ensure that anyone entering the child's room wears a mask.
- ☐ 5. Apply firm pressure to a needle-stick area for at least 10 minutes.

322. The nurse is performing an assessment on a 10-year-old child suspected to have Hodgkin's disease. Which assessment findings are specifically characteristic of this disease? **Select all that apply.**
- ☐ 1. Abdominal pain
- ☐ 2. Fever and malaise
- ☐ 3. Anorexia and weight loss
- ☐ 4. Painful, enlarged inguinal lymph nodes
- ☐ 5. Painless, firm, and movable adenopathy in the cervical area

ANSWERS

312. *Answer:* 1
Rationale: Colorless drainage on the dressing in a child after craniotomy indicates the presence of cerebrospinal fluid and should be reported to the surgeon immediately. Options 2, 3, and 4 are not the immediate nursing action because they do not address the need for immediate intervention to prevent complications.
Test-Taking Strategy: Note the strategic word, *immediately*. Eliminate options 3 and 4 because they are comparable or alike and delay necessary intervention. Also, note the words *colorless drainage*. This should alert you quickly to the possibility of the presence of cerebrospinal fluid and direct you to the correct option.
Level of Cognitive Ability: Analyzing
Client Needs: Physiological Integrity
Integrated Process: Nursing Process—Implementation
Content Area: Pediatrics: Oncological
Health Problem: Complex Care: Emergency Situations/Management
Priority Concepts: Clinical Judgment; Intracranial Regulation
Reference: Hockenberry, Wilson, Rodgers (2017), p. 834.

313. *Answer:* 4
Rationale: In the event of shock, the PHCP is notified immediately before the nurse changes the child's position or increases intravenous fluids. After craniotomy, a child is never placed in the supine or Trendelenburg's position because it increases intracranial pressure (ICP) and the risk of bleeding. The head of the bed should be elevated. Increasing intravenous fluids can cause an increase in ICP.
Test-Taking Strategy: Focus on the subject, care for the child following craniotomy, and note the strategic words, *most appropriate*. Eliminate options 1 and 2 because these positions could increase ICP. Eliminate option 3 because increasing the flow rate could also increase ICP. In addition, the nurse should not increase intravenous fluids without a PHCP's prescription.
Level of Cognitive Ability: Synthesizing
Client Needs: Physiological Integrity
Integrated Process: Nursing Process—Implementation
Content Area: Complex Care: Emergency Situations/Management
Health Problem: Pediatric-Specific: Cancers
Priority Concepts: Clinical Judgment; Intracranial Regulation
Reference: Hockenberry, Wilson, Rodgers (2017), p. 834.

314. *Answer:* 1
Rationale: Wilms' tumor is the most common intra-abdominal and kidney tumor of childhood. If Wilms' tumor is suspected, the tumor mass should not be palpated by the nurse. Excessive manipulation can cause seeding of the tumor and spread of the cancerous cells. Hematuria, fever, and hypertension are clinical manifestations associated with Wilms' tumor.
Test-Taking Strategy: Focus on the subject, the action to avoid. Knowledge that this tumor is an intra-abdominal and kidney

tumor will assist in eliminating options 2 and 4 because of the relationship of these options to renal function. Next, thinking about the effect of palpating the tumor will direct you to the correct answer from the remaining options.
Level of Cognitive Ability: Applying
Client Needs: Physiological Integrity
Integrated Process: Nursing Process—Implementation
Content Area: Pediatrics: Oncological
Health Problem: Pediatric-Specific: Cancers
Priority Concepts: Cellular Regulation; Safety
Reference: McKinney et al. (2018), p. 1165.

315. *Answer:* 2
Rationale: Osteosarcoma is the most common bone cancer in children. Cancer usually is found in the metaphysis of long bones, especially in the lower extremities, with most tumors occurring in the femur. Osteosarcoma is manifested clinically by progressive, insidious, and intermittent pain at the tumor site. By the time these children receive medical attention, they may be in considerable pain from the tumor. Options 1, 3, and 4 are accurate regarding osteosarcoma.
Test-Taking Strategy: Note the strategic words, *need for information*. These words indicate a negative event query and ask you to select an option that is an incorrect statement. Knowledge that osteosarcoma is a malignant tumor of the bone will direct you to the correct option.
Level of Cognitive Ability: Evaluating
Client Needs: Physiological Integrity
Integrated Process: Teaching and Learning
Content Area: Pediatrics: Oncological
Health Problem: Pediatric-Specific: Cancers
Priority Concepts: Cellular Regulation; Clinical Judgment
Reference: McKinney et al. (2018), pp. 1162-1163.

316. *Answer:* 1
Rationale: Leukemia is a malignant increase in the number of leukocytes, usually at an immature stage, in the bone marrow. It affects the bone marrow, causing anemia from decreased erythrocytes, infection from neutropenia, and bleeding from decreased platelet production (thrombocytopenia). If a child is has a low platelet count usually less than 50,000 mm^3 ($50.0 \times 10^9/L$), bleeding precautions need to be initiated because of the increased risk of bleeding or hemorrhage. Precautions include limiting activity that could result in head injury, using soft toothbrushes, checking urine and stools for blood, and administering stool softeners to prevent straining with constipation. In addition, suppositories, enemas, and rectal temperatures are avoided. Options 2, 3, and 4 are related to the prevention of infection rather than bleeding.
Test-Taking Strategy: Note that the platelet count is low and recall that a low platelet count places the child at risk for bleeding. In addition, note that options 2, 3, and 4 are comparable or alike because they relate to prevention of and monitoring for infection.
Level of Cognitive Ability: Analyzing
Client Needs: Safe and Effective Care Environment
Integrated Process: Nursing Process—Planning
Content Area: Pediatrics: Oncological
Health Problem: Pediatric-Specific: Cancers
Priority Concepts: Cellular Regulation; Clotting
Reference: McKinney et al. (2018), pp. 1152-1153.

317. *Answer:* 1
Rationale: The brain, although well protected by the solid bony cranium, is highly susceptible to pressure that may accumulate within the enclosure. Volume and pressure must remain constant within the brain. A change in the size of the brain, such as occurs with edema or increased volume of intracranial blood or cerebrospinal fluid without a compensatory change, leads to an increase in ICP, which may be life-threatening. Vomiting, an early sign of increased ICP, can become excessive as pressure builds up and stimulates the medulla in the brainstem, which houses the vomiting center. Children with open fontanels (posterior fontanel closes at 2 to 3 months; anterior fontanel closes at 12 to 18 months) compensate for ICP changes by skull expansion and subsequent bulging fontanels. When the fontanels have closed, nausea, excessive vomiting, diplopia, and headaches become pronounced, with headaches becoming more prevalent in older children.
Test-Taking Strategy: Note the strategic word, *early;* focus on the age of the child, and use age as the key to principles of growth and development. Knowing when the fontanels close and focusing on the child's age as 3 years eliminates options 2 and 3. The subjective symptom of headache in option 4 is unreliable in a 3 year old, so eliminate this option.
Level of Cognitive Ability: Analyzing
Client Needs: Physiological Integrity
Integrated Process: Nursing Process—Assessment
Content Area: Pediatrics: Oncological
Health Problem: Pediatric-Specific: Cancers
Priority Concepts: Development; Intracranial Regulation
Reference: Hockenberry, Wilson, Rodgers (2017), p. 834.

318. *Answer:* 2
Rationale: Leukemia is a malignant increase in the number of leukocytes, usually at an immature stage, in the bone marrow. The confirmatory test for leukemia is microscopic examination of bone marrow obtained by bone marrow aspirate and biopsy, which is considered positive if blast cells are present. An altered platelet count occurs as a result of the disease but also may occur as a result of chemotherapy and does not confirm the diagnosis. The white blood cell count may be normal, high, or low in leukemia. A lumbar puncture may be done to look for blast cells in the spinal fluid that indicate central nervous system disease.
Test-Taking Strategy: Focus on the subject, bone marrow biopsy and leukemia, and note the word *confirms* in the question. This word and knowledge that the bone marrow is affected in leukemia will direct you to the correct option.
Level of Cognitive Ability: Analyzing
Client Needs: Physiological Integrity
Integrated Process: Nursing Process—Assessment
Content Area: Pediatrics: Oncological
Health Problem: Pediatric-Specific: Cancers
Priority Concepts: Cellular Regulation; Clinical Judgment
Reference: McKinney et al. (2018), p. 1149.

319. *Answer:* 3
Rationale: Leukemia is a malignant increase in the number of leukocytes, usually at an immature stage, in the bone marrow. It affects the bone marrow, causing anemia from decreased erythrocytes, infection from neutropenia, and bleeding from

decreased platelet production (thrombocytopenia). For a hospitalized neutropenic child, flowers or plants should not be kept in the room, because standing water and damp soil harbor *Aspergillus* and *Pseudomonas aeruginosa,* to which the child is susceptible. In addition, fresh fruits and vegetables harbor molds and should be avoided until the white blood cell count increases.
Test-Taking Strategy: Note that options 1 and 2 are comparable or alike and should be eliminated first; these options indicate that it is acceptable to place the flowers in the child's room. From the remaining options, select the correct option over option 4 because this response maintains the protective isolation procedures required.
Level of Cognitive Ability: Applying
Client Needs: Safe and Effective Care Environment
Integrated Process: Nursing Process—Implementation
Content Area: Pediatrics: Oncological
Health Problem: Pediatric-Specific: Cancers
Priority Concepts: Infection; Safety
Reference: McKinney et al. (2018), pp. 1151-1152.

320. *Answer:* 4
Rationale: Hodgkin's disease (a type of lymphoma) is a malignancy of the lymph nodes. The presence of giant, multinucleated cells (Reed-Sternberg cells) is the classic characteristic of this disease. Elevated levels of vanillylmandelic acid in the urine may be found in children with neuroblastoma. The presence of blast cells in the bone marrow indicates leukemia. Epstein-Barr virus is associated with infectious mononucleosis.
Test-Taking Strategy: Focus on the subject, confirmatory diagnostic tests for Hodgkin's disease. Think about the pathophysiology associated with Hodgkin's disease. Remember that the Reed-Sternberg cell is characteristic of Hodgkin's disease.
Level of Cognitive Ability: Analyzing
Client Needs: Physiological Integrity
Integrated Process: Nursing Process—Assessment
Content Area: Pediatrics: Oncological
Health Problem: Pediatric-Specific: Cancers
Priority Concepts: Cellular Regulation; Clinical Judgment
Reference: Hockenberry, Wilson, Rodgers (2017), pp. 829-830.

321. *Answer:* 2, 3, 4
Rationale: Leukemia is a malignant increase in the number of leukocytes, usually at an immature stage, in the bone marrow. It affects the bone marrow, causing anemia from decreased erythrocytes, infection from neutropenia, and bleeding from decreased platelet production (thrombocytopenia). A common complication of treatment for leukemia is overwhelming infection secondary to neutropenia. Measures to prevent infection include the use of a private room, strict aseptic technique, restriction of visitors and health care personnel with active infection, strict hand washing, ensuring that anyone entering the child's room wears a mask, and reducing exposure to environmental organisms by eliminating raw fruits and vegetables from the diet and fresh flowers from the child's room and by not leaving standing water in the child's room. Applying firm pressure to a needle-stick area for at least 10 minutes is a measure to prevent bleeding.
Test-Taking Strategy: Focus on the subject, preventing infection. Reading each intervention carefully and keeping this subject in mind will assist in answering the question. A semiprivate room places the child at risk for infection. Applying firm pressure to a needle-stick area is related to preventing bleeding.
Level of Cognitive Ability: Analyzing
Client Needs: Safe and Effective Care Environment
Integrated Process: Nursing Process—Implementation
Content Area: Pediatrics: Oncological
Health Problem: Pediatric-Specific: Cancers
Priority Concepts: Infection; Safety
Reference: McKinney et al. (2018), pp. 1151-1152.

322. *Answer:* 1, 5
Rationale: Hodgkin's disease (a type of lymphoma) is a malignancy of the lymph nodes. Specific clinical manifestations associated with Hodgkin's disease include painless, firm, and movable adenopathy in the cervical and supraclavicular areas and abdominal pain as a result of enlarged retroperitoneal nodes. Hepatosplenomegaly also is noted. Although fever, malaise, anorexia, and weight loss are associated with Hodgkin's disease, these manifestations are seen in many disorders.
Test-Taking Strategy: Note the words *specifically characteristic* in the question. Eliminate options 2 and 3 first because these symptoms are comparable or alike in that they are general and vague. Recalling that painless adenopathy is associated with Hodgkin's disease and abdominal pain will direct you to the correct options.
Level of Cognitive Ability: Analyzing
Client Needs: Physiological Integrity
Integrated Process: Nursing Process—Assessment
Content Area: Pediatrics: Oncological
Health Problem: Pediatric-Specific: Cancers
Priority Concepts: Cellular Regulation; Clinical Judgment
Reference: Hockenberry, Wilson, Rodgers (2017), pp. 829-830.

CHAPTER 32

Metabolic and Endocrine Problems

PRIORITY CONCEPTS Glucose Regulation; Thermoregulation

I. Fever

A. Description
1. Fever is an abnormal body temperature elevation.
2. A child's temperature can vary depending on activity, emotional stress, disease processes, medications, type of clothing the child is wearing, and temperature of the environment.
3. A fever in an infant less than 1 month old is considered an emergency, and the pediatric specialist should be contacted immediately if this occurs.
4. Assessment findings associated with the fever provide important indications of the seriousness of the fever.

B. Assessment
1. Temperature elevation: Normal temperature range for a child is 36.4° C to 37.0° C (97.5° F to 98.6° F); 38.0° C (100.4° F) is considered to be fever.
2. Flushed skin, warm to touch
3. Diaphoresis
4. Chills
5. Restlessness or lethargy

C. Interventions
1. Monitor vital signs; take the temperature via the electronic route or per agency procedures.
2. Remove excess clothing and blankets, reduce the room temperature, and increase the air circulation; use other cooling measures such as the application of a cool compress to the forehead if appropriate.
3. Administer a sponge bath with tepid water for 20 to 30 minutes and gently squeeze water from a facecloth over the back and chest. Recheck the temperature 30 minutes after the bath. Do not use alcohol because it can cause peripheral vasoconstriction.
4. Administer antipyretics such as ibuprofen as prescribed.
5. Aspirin should not be administered, unless specifically prescribed, because of the risk of Reye's syndrome.
6. Retake the temperature 30 to 60 minutes after the antipyretic is administered.
7. Provide adequate fluid intake as tolerated and as prescribed.
8. Monitor for signs and symptoms that indicate dehydration and electrolyte imbalances; monitor laboratory values.
9. Instruct the parents in how to take the temperature, how to medicate the child safely, and when it is necessary to call the primary health care provider (PHCP).

II. Dehydration

A. Description
1. Dehydration is a common fluid and electrolyte imbalance in infants and children.
2. In infants and children, the organs that conserve water are immature, placing them at risk for fluid volume deficit.
3. Causes can include decreased fluid intake, diaphoresis, vomiting, diarrhea, diabetic ketoacidosis, and extensive burns or other serious injuries.

> ! Infants and children are more vulnerable to fluid volume deficit because more of their body water is in the extracellular fluid compartment.

B. Assessment (Table 32-1)

C. Interventions
1. Treat and eliminate the cause of the dehydration.
2. Monitor vital signs.
3. Monitor weight and monitor for changes, including fluid gains and losses.
4. Monitor intake and output and urine for specific gravity.
5. Monitor level of consciousness.
6. Monitor skin turgor and mucous membranes for dryness.
7. For mild to moderate dehydration, provide oral rehydration therapy with Pedialyte or a similar rehydration solution as prescribed; avoid carbonated beverages because they are

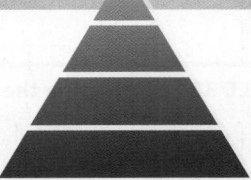

TABLE 32-1 Evaluating the Extent of Dehydration

	Level of Dehydration		
Clinical Signs	**Mild**	**Moderate**	**Severe**
Weight loss—infants	3%-5%	6%-9%	≥10%
Weight loss—children	3%-4%	6%-8%	10%
Pulse	Normal	Slightly increased	Very increased
Respiratory rate	Normal	Slight tachypnea (rapid)	Hyperpnea (deep and rapid)
Blood pressure	Normal	Normal to orthostatic (>10 mm Hg change)	Orthostatic to shock
Behavior	Normal	Irritable, more thirsty	Hyperirritable to lethargic
Thirst	Slight	Moderate	Intense
Mucous membranes*	Normal	Dry	Parched
Tears	Present	Decreased	Absent; sunken eyes
Anterior fontanel	Normal	Normal to sunken	Sunken
External jugular vein	Visible when supine	Not visible except with supraclavicular pressure	Not visible even with supraclavicular pressure
Skin*	Capillary refill 2 sec	Slowed capillary refill (2-4 sec [decreased turgor])	Very delayed capillary refill (>4 sec) and tenting; skin cool, acrocyanotic or mottled
Urine specific gravity	>1.020	>1.020; oliguria	Oliguria or anuria

* These signs are less prominent in the child who has hypernatremia.
Data from Jospe N, Forbes G: Fluids and electrolytes—clinical aspects, *Pediatr Rev* 17:395–403, 1996; and Steiner MJ, DeWalt DA, Byerley JS: Is this child dehydrated? *JAMA* 291:2746–2754, 2004. Table from Perry S, Hockenberry M, Lowdermilk D, Wilson D: *Maternal-child nursing care*, ed 4, St. Louis, 2010, Mosby.

gas-producing, and fluids that contain high amounts of sugar, such as apple juice.

8. For severe dehydration, maintain NPO (nothing by mouth) status to place the bowel at rest and provide fluid and electrolyte replacement by the intravenous (IV) route as prescribed; if potassium is prescribed for IV administration, ensure that the child has voided before administering and has adequate renal function.
9. Reintroduce a normal diet when rehydration is achieved.
10. Provide instructions to the parents about the types and amounts of fluid to encourage, signs of dehydration, and indications of the need to notify the PHCP.

III. Phenylketonuria

A. Description

1. Phenylketonuria is a genetic disorder (autosomal recessive disorder) that results in central nervous system damage from toxic levels of phenylalanine (an essential amino acid) in the blood.
2. It is characterized by blood phenylalanine levels greater than 20 mg/dL (1210 mcmol/L); normal level is 0 to 2 mg/dL (0 to 121 mcmol/L).
3. All 50 states require routine screening of all newborns for phenylketonuria.

B. Assessment

1. In all children
   a. Digestive problems and vomiting
   b. Seizures
   c. Musty odor of the urine
   d. Mental retardation
2. In older children
   a. Eczema
   b. Hypertonia
   c. Hypopigmentation of the hair, skin, and irises
   d. Hyperactive behavior

C. Interventions

1. Screening of newborn infants for phenylketonuria: The infant should have begun formula or breast milk feeding before specimen collection.
2. If initial screening is positive, a repeat test is performed, and further diagnostic evaluation is required to verify the diagnosis.
3. Rescreen newborns by 14 days of age if the initial screening was done before 48 hours of age.
4. If phenylketonuria is diagnosed, prepare to implement the following:
   a. Restrict phenylalanine intake; high-protein foods (meats and dairy products) and aspartame are avoided because they contain large amounts of phenylalanine.

b. Monitor physical, neurological, and intellectual development.
c. Stress the importance of follow-up treatment.
d. Encourage the parents to express their feelings about the diagnosis and discuss the risk of phenylketonuria in future children.
e. Educate the parents about the use of special preparation formulas and about the foods that contain phenylalanine.
f. Consult with social care services to assist the parents with the financial burdens of purchasing special prepared formulas.

IV. Childhood Obesity

A. Description
1. A condition where excess body fat negatively impacts the health and well-being of the child.
2. Body mass index (BMI) is a screening tool that can be used to measure obesity.
3. BMI is defined as a person's body weight in kilograms divided by the square of a person's height in meters.
4. As recommended by the Centers for Disease Control and Prevention (CDC), health professionals should use the BMI percentile when measuring children and adolescents aged 2 to 20 years.
5. Overweight is defined as being above the 85th percentile but less than the 95th percentile. Obesity is defined as having a BMI greater than the 95th percentile.

B. Effects of Obesity
1. Obesity can lead to problems later in life if diagnosed in childhood, such as physical, social, and emotional health problems.
2. Asthma, sleep apnea, bone and joint problems, type 2 diabetes, and risk factors leading to heart disease, such as hyperlipidemia, can occur.
3. A child who is obese is more likely to be obese as an adult, which results in the comorbidities associated with obesity later in life, such as type 2 diabetes, heart disease, metabolic syndrome, and cancer.

V. Diabetes Mellitus

A. Description (Fig. 32-1)
1. Type 1 diabetes mellitus is characterized by the destruction of the pancreatic beta cells, which produce insulin; this results in absolute insulin deficiency.
2. Type 2 diabetes mellitus usually arises because of insulin resistance, in which the body fails to use insulin properly, combined with relative (rather than absolute) insulin deficiency.
3. The rate of children and teens being diagnosed with prediabetes and type 2 diabetes is increasing. The number one risk factor for developing type 2 diabetes in childhood is being overweight. See Box 32-1 on prevention strategies for type 2 diabetes in childhood.

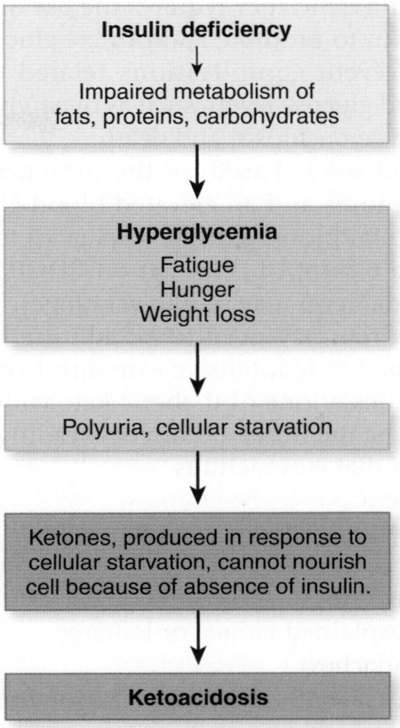

FIG. 32-1 Insulin deficiency leading to ketoacidosis.

BOX 32-1 Preventing Type 2 Diabetes Mellitus in Childhood

Eating Healthy to Lose Weight
- Drink water instead of sugared beverages, such as sodas, juices, and sports drinks.
- Eat more fruits and vegetables—fresh is the best, but frozen and canned in water (not syrup) is acceptable.
- Limit fast food.
- Make healthy snacks, such as grapes, carrots, or plain popcorn.

Increasing Physical Activity to Lose Weight
- Children and adolescents should have 60 minutes a day of physical activity.
- Dancing, walking, bike riding, taking the stairs, playing interactive video games.
- Limiting screen time (using computers, tablets, or phones) to 60 minutes per day.

Noticing Warning Signs
- Increased thirst
- Increased night-time urination
- Blurry vision
- Unusual fatigue

Adapted from American Diabetes Association. (2018). *Preventing type 2 in children.* Retrieved from http://www.diabetes.org/living-with-diabetes/parents-and-kids/children-and-type-2/preventing-type-2-in-children.html

4. Insulin deficiency requires the use of exogenous insulin to promote appropriate glucose use and to prevent complications related to elevated blood glucose levels, such as hyperglycemia, diabetic ketoacidosis, and death.
5. Diagnosis is based on the presence of classic symptoms and an elevated blood glucose level (normal blood glucose level is 70 to 99 mg/dL [4 to 6 mmol/L]); based on PHCP preference, normal level may be a lower range).
6. Children may need to be admitted directly to the pediatric intensive care unit because of the manifestations of diabetic ketoacidosis, which may be the initial occurrence leading to diagnosis of diabetes mellitus.

B. Assessment
1. Polyuria, polydipsia, polyphagia
2. Hyperglycemia
3. Weight loss
4. Unexplained fatigue or lethargy
5. Headaches
6. Occasional enuresis in a previously toilet-trained child
7. Vaginitis in adolescent girls (caused by *Candida*, which thrives in hyperglycemic tissues)
8. Fruity odor to breath
9. Dehydration
10. Blurred vision
11. Slow wound healing
12. Changes in level of consciousness

C. Long-term effects
1. Failure to grow at a normal rate
2. Delayed maturation
3. Recurrent infections
4. Neuropathy
5. Cardiovascular disease
6. Retinal microvascular disease
7. Renal microvascular disease

D. Complications
1. Hypoglycemia
2. Hyperglycemia
3. Diabetic ketoacidosis
4. Coma
5. Hypokalemia
6. Hyperkalemia
7. Microvascular changes
8. Cardiovascular changes

For a child with diabetes mellitus, plan to initiate a consultation with the diabetic specialist to plan the child's care.

E. Diet
1. Normal healthy nutrition is encouraged, and the total number of calories is individualized based on the child's age and **growth** expectations. For type 2 diabetes, the American Diabetes Association recommendations can be found at http://main.diabetes.org/dorg/PDFs/Type-2-Diabetes-in-Youth/Type-2-Diabetes-in-Youth_14-18.pdf.
2. As prescribed by the PHCP, children with diabetes need no special types of foods or supplements. They need sufficient calories to balance daily expenditure for energy and to satisfy the requirement for growth and development.
3. Dietary intake should include 3 well-balanced meals per day, eaten at regular intervals, plus a mid-afternoon snack and a bedtime snack; a consistent intake of the prescribed protein, fats, and carbohydrates at each meal and snack is needed (concentrated sweets are discouraged; fat is reduced to 30% or less of the total caloric requirement).
4. Instruct children and parents to carry a source of glucose, such as glucose tablets, with them at all times to treat hypoglycemia if it occurs.
5. Incorporate the diet into the individual child's needs, likes and dislikes, lifestyle, and cultural and socioeconomic patterns.
6. Allow the child to participate in making food choices to provide a sense of control.

F. Exercise
1. Instruct the child in dietary adjustments when exercising.
2. Extra food needs to be consumed for increased activity, usually 10 to 15 g of carbohydrates for every 30 to 45 minutes of activity.
3. Instruct the child to monitor the blood glucose level before exercising.
4. Plan an appropriate exercise regimen with the child, taking the developmental stage into account.

G. Insulin
1. Diluted insulin may be required for some infants to provide small enough doses to avoid hypoglycemia; diluted insulin should be labeled clearly to avoid dosage errors.
2. Laboratory evaluation of glycosylated hemoglobin (HgbA1c) should be performed every 3 months. Reference interval for HgbA1c is less than 6%.
3. Illness, infection, and stress increase the need for insulin, and insulin should not be withheld during illness, infection, or stress, because hyperglycemia and ketoacidosis can result.
4. When the child is not receiving anything by mouth for a special procedure, verify with the PHCP the need to withhold the morning insulin, and when food, fluids, and insulin are to be resumed.
5. Instruct the child and parents in the administration of insulin.
6. Instruct the child and parents to recognize symptoms of hypoglycemia and hyperglycemia.

7. Instruct the parents in the administration of glucagon intramuscularly or subcutaneously if the child has a hypoglycemic reaction and is unable to consume anything orally (if semiconscious or unconscious).
8. Instruct the child and parents always to have a spare bottle of insulin available.
9. Advise the parents to obtain a MedicAlert bracelet indicating the type and daily insulin dosage prescribed for the child.
10. See Chapter 47 for information on insulin types, administration sites, and administration procedure.

H. Blood glucose monitoring
1. Results provide information needed to maintain good glycemic control.
2. Blood glucose monitoring is more accurate than urine testing.
3. Monitoring requires that the child prick himself or herself several times a day as prescribed (Box 32-2).
4. Instruct the child and parents about the proper procedure for obtaining the blood glucose level.
5. Inform the child and parents that the procedure must be done precisely to obtain accurate results.
6. Stress the importance of hand washing before and after performing the procedure to prevent infection.
7. Stress the importance of following the manufacturer's instructions for the blood glucose monitoring device.
8. Instruct the child and parents to calibrate the monitor as instructed by the manufacturer.
9. Instruct the child and parents to check the expiration date on the test strips used for blood glucose monitoring.
10. Instruct the child and parents that if the blood glucose results do not seem reasonable, they should reread the instructions, reassess technique, check the expiration date of the test strips, and perform the procedure again to verify results.

I. Urine testing
1. Instruct the parents and child in the procedure for testing urine for ketones and glucose.
2. Teach the child that the second voided urine specimen is most accurate.
3. The presence of ketones may indicate impending ketoacidosis.

Urine glucose testing is an unreliable method of monitoring the glucose level; however, the urine should be tested for ketones when the child is ill or when the blood glucose level is consistently greater than 200 mg/dL (greater than 11.4 mmol/L) or as specified by the PHCP.

J. Hypoglycemia
1. Description
   a. Hypoglycemia is a blood glucose level less than 70 mg/dL (4 mmol/L) (or as specified by the PHCP).
   b. Hypoglycemia results from too much insulin, not enough food, or excessive activity.
2. Signs include headache, nausea, sweating, tremors, lethargy, hunger, confusion, slurred speech, tingling around the mouth, and anxiety.
3. Interventions (Boxes 32-3 and 32-4; see also Priority Nursing Actions)

K. Hyperglycemia
1. Description: Elevated blood glucose level (>200 mg/dL [11.4 mmol/L], or as specified by the PHCP)
2. Signs include polydipsia, polyuria, polyphagia, blurred vision, weakness, weight loss, and syncope.
3. Interventions (Box 32-5)
4. Sick day rules (Box 32-6)

BOX 32-2 Lessening the Pain of Blood Glucose Monitoring

Hold the finger under warm water for a few seconds before puncture (enhances blood flow to the finger).

Use the ring finger or thumb to obtain a blood sample, because blood flows more easily to these areas; puncture the finger just to the side of the finger pad, because there are more blood vessels in this area and fewer nerve endings.

Press the lancet device lightly against the skin to prevent a deep puncture.

Use glucose monitors that require very small blood samples for measurement.

Adapted from Perry S, Hockenberry M, Lowdermilk D, Wilson D: *Maternal-child nursing care*, ed 3, St. Louis, 2010, Mosby.

BOX 32-3 Interventions for Hypoglycemia

- If possible, confirm hypoglycemia with a blood glucose reading.
- Administer glucose immediately; rapid-releasing glucose is followed by a complex carbohydrate and protein, such as a slice of bread or a peanut butter cracker.
- Give an extra snack if the next meal is not planned for more than 30 minutes or if activity is planned.
- If the child becomes unconscious, squeeze cake frosting or glucose paste onto the gums and retest the blood glucose level in 15 minutes (monitor the child closely); if the reading remains low, administer additional glucose.
- If the child remains unconscious, the administration of glucagon may be necessary.
- In the hospital, prepare to administer dextrose intravenously if the child is unable to consume an oral glucose product.

Pediatric

BOX 32-4 Food Items to Treat Hypoglycemia

- ½ cup of orange juice or sugar-sweetened carbonated beverage
- 8 oz of milk
- 1 small box of raisins
- 3 or 4 hard candies
- 4 sugar cubes (1 Tbsp of sugar)
- 3 or 4 Life Savers candies
- 1 candy bar
- 1 tsp honey
- 2 or 3 glucose tablets

BOX 32-5 Interventions for Hyperglycemia

Instruct the parents to notify the primary health care provider when the following occur:

- Blood glucose results remain elevated (usually >200 mg/dL (>11.4 mmol/L)
- Moderate or high ketonuria is present
- Child is unable to take food or fluids
- Child vomits more than once
- Illness persists

BOX 32-6 Sick Day Rules for a Diabetic Child

- Always give insulin, even if the child does not have an appetite, or contact the primary health care provider (PHCP) for specific instructions.
- Test blood glucose levels at least every 4 hours.
- Test for urinary ketones with each voiding.
- Notify the PHCP if moderate or large amounts of urinary ketones are present.
- Follow the child's usual meal plan.
- Encourage liquids to aid in clearing ketones.
- Encourage rest, especially if urinary ketones are present.
- Notify the PHCP if vomiting, fruity odor to the breath, deep rapid respirations, decreasing level of consciousness, or persistent hyperglycemia occurs.

Adapted from Hockenberry M, Wilson D: *Nursing care of infants and children*, ed 9, St. Louis, 2011, Mosby.

L. Diabetic ketoacidosis

1. Description
   - **a.** Diabetic ketoacidosis is a complication of diabetes mellitus that develops when a severe insulin deficiency occurs.
   - **b.** Diabetic ketoacidosis is a life-threatening condition.
   - **c.** Hyperglycemia that progresses to metabolic acidosis occurs.
   - **d.** Diabetic ketoacidosis develops over several hours to days.
   - **e.** The blood glucose level is greater than 300 mg/dL (greater than 17.14 mmol/L), and urine and serum ketone tests are positive.

⚠ Manifestations of diabetic ketoacidosis include signs of hyperglycemia, Kussmaul's respirations, acetone (fruity) breath odor, increasing lethargy, and decreasing level of consciousness.

2. Interventions
   - **a.** Restore circulating blood volume, and protect against cerebral, coronary, or renal hypoperfusion.
   - **b.** Correct dehydration with IV infusions of 0.9% or 0.45% saline as prescribed.
   - **c.** Correct hyperglycemia with IV regular insulin administration as prescribed.
   - **d.** Monitor vital signs, urine output, and mental status closely.
   - **e.** Correct acidosis and electrolyte imbalances as prescribed.
   - **f.** Administer oxygen as prescribed.
   - **g.** Monitor blood glucose level frequently.
   - **h.** Monitor potassium level closely, because when the child receives insulin to reduce the blood glucose level, the serum potassium level changes; if the potassium level decreases, potassium replacement may be required.
   - **i.** The child should be voiding adequately before administering potassium; if the child does not have an adequate output, hyperkalemia may result.
   - **j.** Monitor the child closely for signs of fluid overload.
   - **k.** IV dextrose is added as prescribed when the blood glucose reaches an appropriate level.
   - **l.** Treat the cause of hyperglycemia.

PRIORITY NURSING ACTIONS

Hypoglycemia in a Hospitalized Child with Diabetes Mellitus

1. Check the child's blood glucose level.
2. Give the child ½ cup of fruit juice or other acceptable item.
3. Take the child's vital signs.
4. Retest the blood glucose level.
5. Give the child a small snack of carbohydrate and protein.
6. Document the child's signs and symptoms, actions taken, and outcome.

Reference

Hockenberry. (2017). *Wilson, Rodgers*, 292–294.

PRACTICE QUESTIONS

323. A school-age child with type 1 diabetes mellitus has soccer practice and the school nurse provides instructions regarding how to prevent hypoglycemia during practice. Which should the school nurse tell the child to do?
1. Eat twice the amount normally eaten at lunchtime.
2. Take half the amount of prescribed insulin on practice days.
3. Take the prescribed insulin at noontime rather than in the morning.
4. Eat a small box of raisins or drink a cup of orange juice before soccer practice.

324. The mother of a 6-year-old child who has type 1 diabetes mellitus calls a clinic nurse and tells the nurse that the child has been sick. The mother reports that she checked the child's urine and it was positive for ketones. The nurse should instruct the mother to take which action?
1. Hold the next dose of insulin.
2. Come to the clinic immediately.
3. Encourage the child to drink liquids.
4. Administer an additional dose of regular insulin.

325. A pediatrician prescribes an intravenous (IV) solution of 5% dextrose and half-normal saline (0.45%) with 40 mEq of potassium chloride for a child with hypotonic dehydration. The nurse performs which **priority** assessment before administering this IV prescription?
1. Obtains a weight
2. Takes the temperature
3. Takes the blood pressure
4. Checks the amount of urine output

326. An adolescent client with type 1 diabetes mellitus is admitted to the emergency department for treatment of diabetic ketoacidosis. Which assessment findings should the nurse expect to note?
1. Sweating and tremors
2. Hunger and hypertension
3. Cold, clammy skin and irritability
4. Fruity breath odor and decreasing level of consciousness

327. A mother brings her 2-week-old infant to a clinic for a phenylketonuria rescreening blood test. The test indicates a serum phenylalanine level of 1 mg/dL (60.5 mcmol/L). The nurse reviews this result and makes which interpretation?
1. It is positive.
2. It is negative.
3. It is inconclusive.
4. It requires rescreening at age 6 weeks.

328. A child with type 1 diabetes mellitus is brought to the emergency department by the mother, who states that the child has been complaining of abdominal pain and has been lethargic. Diabetic ketoacidosis is diagnosed. Anticipating the plan of care, the nurse prepares to administer which type of intravenous (IV) infusion?
1. Potassium infusion
2. NPH insulin infusion
3. 5% dextrose infusion
4. Normal saline infusion

329. The nurse has just administered ibuprofen to a child with a temperature of 102° F (38.8° C). The nurse should also take which action?
1. Withhold oral fluids for 8 hours.
2. Sponge the child with cold water.
3. Plan to administer salicylate in 4 hours.
4. Remove excess clothing and blankets from the child.

330. A child has fluid volume deficit. The nurse performs an assessment and determines that the child is improving and the deficit is resolving if which finding is noted?
1. The child has no tears.
2. Urine specific gravity is 1.035.
3. Capillary refill is less than 2 seconds.
4. Urine output is less than 1 mL/kg/hr.

331. The nurse should implement which interventions for a child older than 2 years with type 1 diabetes mellitus who has a blood glucose level of 60 mg/dL (3.4 mmol/L)? **Select all that apply.**
- ☐ 1. Administer regular insulin.
- ☐ 2. Encourage the child to ambulate.
- ☐ 3. Give the child a teaspoon of honey.
- ☐ 4. Provide electrolyte replacement therapy intravenously.
- ☐ 5. Wait 30 minutes and confirm the blood glucose reading.
- ☐ 6. Prepare to administer glucagon subcutaneously if unconsciousness occurs.

ANSWERS

323. *Answer:* 4

Rationale: Hypoglycemia is a blood glucose level less than 70 mg/dL (4 mmol/L) and results from too much insulin, not enough food, or excessive activity. An extra snack of 15 to 30 g of carbohydrates eaten before activities such as soccer practice would prevent hypoglycemia. A small box of raisins or a cup of orange juice provides 15 to 30 g of carbohydrates. The child or parents should not be instructed to adjust the amount or time of insulin administration. Meal amounts should not be doubled.

Test-Taking Strategy: Use general medication guidelines to eliminate options 2 and 3 first, noting that they are comparable or alike and indicate changing the amount of insulin or time of administration. From the remaining options, recalling the definition of hypoglycemia and its manifestations and associated treatment will direct you to the correct option.

Level of Cognitive Ability: Applying
Client Needs: Physiological Integrity
Integrated Process: Teaching and Learning
Content Area: Pediatrics: Metabolic/Endocrine
Health Problem: Pediatric-Specific: Diabetes mellitus
Priority Concepts: Glucose Regulation; Health Promotion
Reference: McKinney et al. (2018), p. 1267.

324. *Answer:* 3

Rationale: When the child is sick, the mother should test for urinary ketones with each voiding. If ketones are present, liquids are essential to aid in clearing the ketones. The child should be encouraged to drink liquids. Bringing the child to the clinic immediately is unnecessary. Insulin doses should not be adjusted or changed.

Test-Taking Strategy: Use general medication guidelines. Eliminate options 1 and 4, noting that they are comparable or alike. Recall that insulin doses should not be adjusted or changed. From the remaining options, note the words *positive for ketones* in the question. Recalling that liquids are essential to aid in clearing the ketones will direct you to the correct option.

Level of Cognitive Ability: Applying
Client Needs: Physiological Integrity
Integrated Process: Nursing Process—Implementation
Content Area: Pediatrics: Metabolic/Endocrine
Health Problem: Pediatric-Specific: Diabetes mellitus
Priority Concepts: Clinical Judgment; Glucose Regulation
Reference: McKinney et al. (2018), p. 1268.

325. *Answer:* 4

Rationale: In hypotonic dehydration, electrolyte loss exceeds water loss. The priority assessment before administering potassium chloride intravenously would be to assess the status of the urine output. Potassium chloride should never be administered in the presence of oliguria or anuria. If the urine output is less than 1 to 2 mL/kg/hr, potassium chloride should not be administered. Although options 1, 2, and 3 are appropriate assessments for a child with dehydration, these assessments are not related specifically to the IV administration of potassium chloride.

Test-Taking Strategy: Note the strategic word, *priority*. Focus on the IV prescription. Recalling that the kidneys play a key role in the excretion and reabsorption of potassium will direct you to the correct option.

Level of Cognitive Ability: Analyzing
Client Needs: Physiological Integrity
Integrated Process: Nursing Process—Assessment
Content Area: Pediatrics: Metabolic/Endocrine
Health Problem: Pediatric-Specific: Dehydration
Priority Concepts: Clinical Judgment; Fluids and Electrolytes
Reference: McKinney et al. (2018), p. 895.

326. *Answer:* 4

Rationale: Diabetic ketoacidosis is a complication of diabetes mellitus that develops when a severe insulin deficiency occurs. Hyperglycemia occurs with diabetic ketoacidosis. Signs of hyperglycemia include fruity breath odor and a decreasing level of consciousness. Hunger can be a sign of hypoglycemia or hyperglycemia, but hypertension is not a sign of diabetic ketoacidosis. Hypotension occurs because of a decrease in blood volume related to the dehydrated state that occurs during diabetic ketoacidosis. Cold clammy skin, irritability, sweating, and tremors all are signs of hypoglycemia.

Test-Taking Strategy: Focus on the subject, the signs of diabetic ketoacidosis, and recall that in this condition the blood glucose level is elevated. Eliminate options 1, 2, and 3 because these signs do not occur with hyperglycemia. Recall that fruity breath odor and a change in the level of consciousness can occur during diabetic ketoacidosis.

Level of Cognitive Ability: Analyzing
Client Needs: Physiological Integrity
Integrated Process: Nursing Process—Assessment
Content Area: Pediatrics: Metabolic/Endocrine
Health Problem: Pediatric-Specific: Diabetes mellitus
Priority Concepts: Clinical Judgment; Glucose Regulation
Reference: McKinney et al. (2018), pp. 1268, 1271-1272.

327. *Answer:* 2

Rationale: Phenylketonuria is a genetic (autosomal recessive) disorder that results in central nervous system damage from toxic levels of phenylalanine (an essential amino acid) in the blood. It is characterized by blood phenylalanine levels greater than 20 mg/dL (1210 mcmol/L); normal level is 0 to 2 mg/dL (0 to 121 mcmol/L). A result of 1 mg/dL is a negative test result.

Test-Taking Strategy: Eliminate options 3 and 4 first because they are comparable or alike, indicating no definitive finding. Note that the level identified in the question is a low level; this should assist in directing you to the correct option.

Level of Cognitive Ability: Applying
Client Needs: Physiological Integrity
Integrated Process: Nursing Process—Assessment
Content Area: Pediatrics: Metabolic/Endocrine
Health Problem: Pediatric-Specific: Phenylketonuria
Priority Concepts: Clinical Judgment; Health Promotion
Reference: Hockenberry, Wilson, Rodgers (2017), pp. 292-293.

328. *Answer:* 4

Rationale: Diabetic ketoacidosis is a complication of diabetes mellitus that develops when a severe insulin deficiency occurs. Hyperglycemia occurs with diabetic ketoacidosis. Rehydration is the initial step in resolving diabetic ketoacidosis. Normal

saline is the initial IV rehydration fluid. NPH insulin is never administered by the IV route. Dextrose solutions are added to the treatment when the blood glucose level decreases to an acceptable level. Intravenously administered potassium may be required, depending on the potassium level, but would not be part of the initial treatment.
Test-Taking Strategy: Focus on the subject, treatment for diabetic ketoacidosis. Eliminate option 3, knowing that dextrose would not be administered in a hyperglycemic state. Eliminate option 2 next, knowing that NPH insulin is not administered by the IV route. Recalling that hydration is the initial treatment in diabetic ketoacidosis will direct you to the correct option.
Level of Cognitive Ability: Analyzing
Client Needs: Physiological Integrity
Integrated Process: Nursing Process—Planning
Content Area: Pediatrics: Metabolic/Endocrine
Health Problem: Pediatric-Specific: Diabetes mellitus
Priority Concepts: Clinical Judgment; Glucose Regulation
Reference: McKinney et al. (2018), pp. 1271-1272.

329. *Answer:* 4
Rationale: After administering ibuprofen, excess clothing and blankets should be removed. The child can be sponged with tepid water but not cold water, because the cold water can cause shivering, which increases metabolic requirements above those already caused by the fever. Aspirin (a salicylate) is not administered to a child with fever because of the risk of Reye's syndrome. Fluids should be encouraged to prevent dehydration, so oral fluids should not be withheld.
Test-Taking Strategy: Focus on the subject, interventions for an elevated temperature. Remember that cooling measures such as removing excess clothing and blankets should be done when a child has a fever. Options 1, 2, and 3 are not interventions for a child with a fever.
Level of Cognitive Ability: Applying
Client Needs: Physiological Integrity
Integrated Process: Nursing Process—Implementation
Content Area: Pediatrics: Metabolic/Endocrine
Health Problem: Pediatric-Specific: Fever
Priority Concepts: Clinical Judgment; Thermoregulation
Reference: McKinney et al. (2018), p. 831.

330. *Answer:* 3
Rationale: Indicators that fluid volume deficit is resolving would be capillary refill less than 2 seconds, specific gravity of 1.003 to 1.030, urine output of at least 1 mL/kg/hr, and adequate tear production. A capillary refill time less than 2 seconds is the only indicator that the child is improving. Urine output of less than 1 mL/kg/hr, a specific gravity of 1.035, and no tears would indicate that the deficit is not resolving.
Test-Taking Strategy: Focus on the subject, assessment findings indicating that fluid volume deficit is resolving. Recall the parameters that indicate adequate hydration status. The only option that indicates an improving fluid balance is option 3. The other options indicate fluid imbalance.
Level of Cognitive Ability: Evaluating
Client Needs: Physiological Integrity
Integrated Process: Nursing Process—Evaluation
Content Area: Pediatrics: Metabolic/Endocrine
Health Problem: Pediatric-Specific: Dehydration
Priority Concepts: Evidence; Fluids and Electrolytes
Reference: McKinney et al. (2018), pp. 892, 894.

331. *Answer:* 3, 6
Rationale: Hypoglycemia is defined as a blood glucose level less than 70 mg/dL (4 mmol/L). Hypoglycemia occurs as a result of too much insulin, not enough food, or excessive activity. If possible, the nurse should confirm hypoglycemia with a blood glucose reading. Glucose is administered orally immediately; rapid-releasing glucose is followed by a complex carbohydrate and protein, such as a slice of bread or a peanut butter cracker. An extra snack is given if the next meal is not planned for more than 30 minutes or if activity is planned. If the child becomes unconscious, cake frosting or glucose paste is squeezed onto the gums, and the blood glucose level is retested in 15 minutes; if the reading remains low, additional glucose is administered. If the child remains unconscious, administration of glucagon may be necessary, and the nurse should be prepared for this intervention. Encouraging the child to ambulate and administering regular insulin would result in a lowered blood glucose level. Providing electrolyte replacement therapy intravenously is an intervention to treat diabetic ketoacidosis. Waiting 30 minutes to confirm the blood glucose level delays necessary intervention.
Test-Taking Strategy: Focus on the subject, a low blood glucose level, and on the information in the question. Think about the pathophysiology associated with hypoglycemia and how it is treated. Recalling that a blood glucose level of 60 mg/dL (3.4 mmol/L) indicates hypoglycemia will assist in determining the correct interventions.
Level of Cognitive Ability: Analyzing
Client Needs: Physiological Integrity
Integrated Process: Nursing Process—Implementation
Content Area: Pediatrics: Metabolic/Endocrine
Health Problem: Pediatric-Specific: Diabetes mellitus
Priority Concepts: Clinical Judgment; Glucose Regulation
Reference: Hockenberry, Wilson, Rodgers (2017), pp. 932, 936.

CHAPTER 33

Gastrointestinal Problems

PRIORITY CONCEPTS Elimination; Nutrition

I. Vomiting

A. Description
1. The major concerns when a child is vomiting are the risk of dehydration, the loss of fluid and electrolytes, and the development of metabolic alkalosis.
2. Additional concerns include aspiration and the development of atelectasis or pneumonia.
3. Causes of vomiting include acute infectious diseases, increased intracranial pressure, toxic ingestions, food intolerance, mechanical obstruction of the gastrointestinal tract, metabolic disorders, and psychogenic disorders.

B. Assessment
1. Character of vomitus
2. Signs of aspiration
3. Presence of pain and abdominal cramping
4. Signs of dehydration and fluid and electrolyte imbalances
5. Signs of metabolic alkalosis

C. Interventions
1. Maintain a patent airway.
2. Position the child on the side to prevent aspiration.
3. Monitor the character, amount, and frequency of vomiting.
4. Assess the force of the vomiting; projectile vomiting may indicate pyloric **stenosis** or increased intracranial pressure.
5. Monitor strict intake and output.
6. Monitor for signs and symptoms of dehydration, such as a sunken fontanel (age-appropriate), nonelastic skin turgor, dry mucous membranes, decreased tear production, vital sign changes, and oliguria.
7. Monitor electrolyte levels.
8. Provide oral rehydration therapy as tolerated and as prescribed; begin feeding slowly, with small amounts of fluid at frequent intervals.
9. Administer antiemetics as prescribed.
10. Assess for abdominal pain or diarrhea.
11. Advise the parents to inform the primary health care provider (PHCP) if signs of dehydration, blood in the vomitus, forceful vomiting, or abdominal pain are present.

II. Diarrhea

A. Description
1. Acute diarrhea is a cause of dehydration, particularly in children younger than 5 years.
2. Causes of acute diarrhea include acute infectious disorders of the gastrointestinal tract, antibiotic therapy, rotavirus, and parasitic infestation.
3. Causes of chronic diarrhea include malabsorption syndromes, inflammatory bowel disease, immunodeficiencies, food intolerances, and nonspecific factors.
4. Rotavirus is a cause of serious gastroenteritis and is a nosocomial (hospital-acquired) pathogen that is most severe in children 3 to 24 months old; children younger than 3 months have some protection because of maternally acquired antibodies.

! Many conditions can cause vomiting or diarrhea, such as but not limited to viral gastroenteritis, group B hemolytic streptococcal pharyngitis, food allergies, and food-borne illnesses.

B. Assessment
1. Character of stools
2. Presence of pain and abdominal cramping
3. Signs of dehydration and fluid and electrolyte imbalances
4. Signs of metabolic acidosis

C. Interventions
1. Monitor character, amount, and frequency of diarrhea.
2. Provide enteric isolation as required; instruct the parents in effective handwashing technique (children should be taught this technique also).
3. Monitor skin integrity.
4. Monitor strict intake and output.
5. Monitor electrolyte levels.

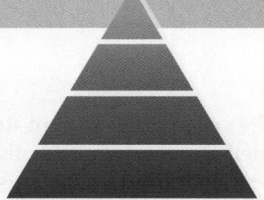

6. Monitor for signs and symptoms of dehydration.
7. For mild to moderate dehydration, provide oral rehydration therapy with Pedialyte or a similar rehydration solution as prescribed; avoid carbonated beverages because they are gas-producing, and fluids that contain high amounts of sugar, such as apple juice.
8. For severe dehydration, maintain NPO (nothing by mouth) status to place the bowel at rest and provide fluid and electrolyte replacement by the intravenous (IV) route as prescribed; if potassium is prescribed for IV administration, ensure that the child has voided before administering and has adequate renal function.
9. Reintroduce a normal diet when rehydration is achieved.

The major concerns when a child is having diarrhea are the risk of dehydration, the loss of fluid and electrolytes, and the development of metabolic acidosis. Orthostatic vital signs are helpful in assessing hydration status.

III. Cleft Lip and Cleft Palate

A. Description

1. Cleft lip and cleft palate are congenital anomalies that occur as a result of failure of soft tissue or bony structure to fuse during embryonic development.
2. The defects involve abnormal openings in the lip and palate that may occur unilaterally or bilaterally and are readily apparent at birth.
3. Causes include hereditary and environmental factors—exposure to radiation or rubella virus, chromosome abnormalities, family history, maternal smoking, and teratogenic factors such as medications taken during pregnancy.
4. Prenatal dietary supplementation of folic acid is important to decrease the risk of cleft lip and palate.
5. Closure of a cleft lip defect precedes closure of the cleft palate and is usually performed by age 3 to 6 months.
6. Cleft palate repair is usually performed around 1 year of age, following the successful repair of cleft lip if present, and to allow for the palatal changes that occur with normal growth; a cleft palate is closed as early as possible to facilitate speech development.
7. A child with cleft palate is at risk for developing frequent otitis media; this can result in hearing loss.
8. An interprofessional team approach, including audiologists, orthodontists, plastic surgeons, and occupational and speech therapists, is taken to address the many needs of the child.

B. Assessment (Fig. 33-1)

1. Cleft lip can range from a slight notch to a complete separation from the floor of the nose.

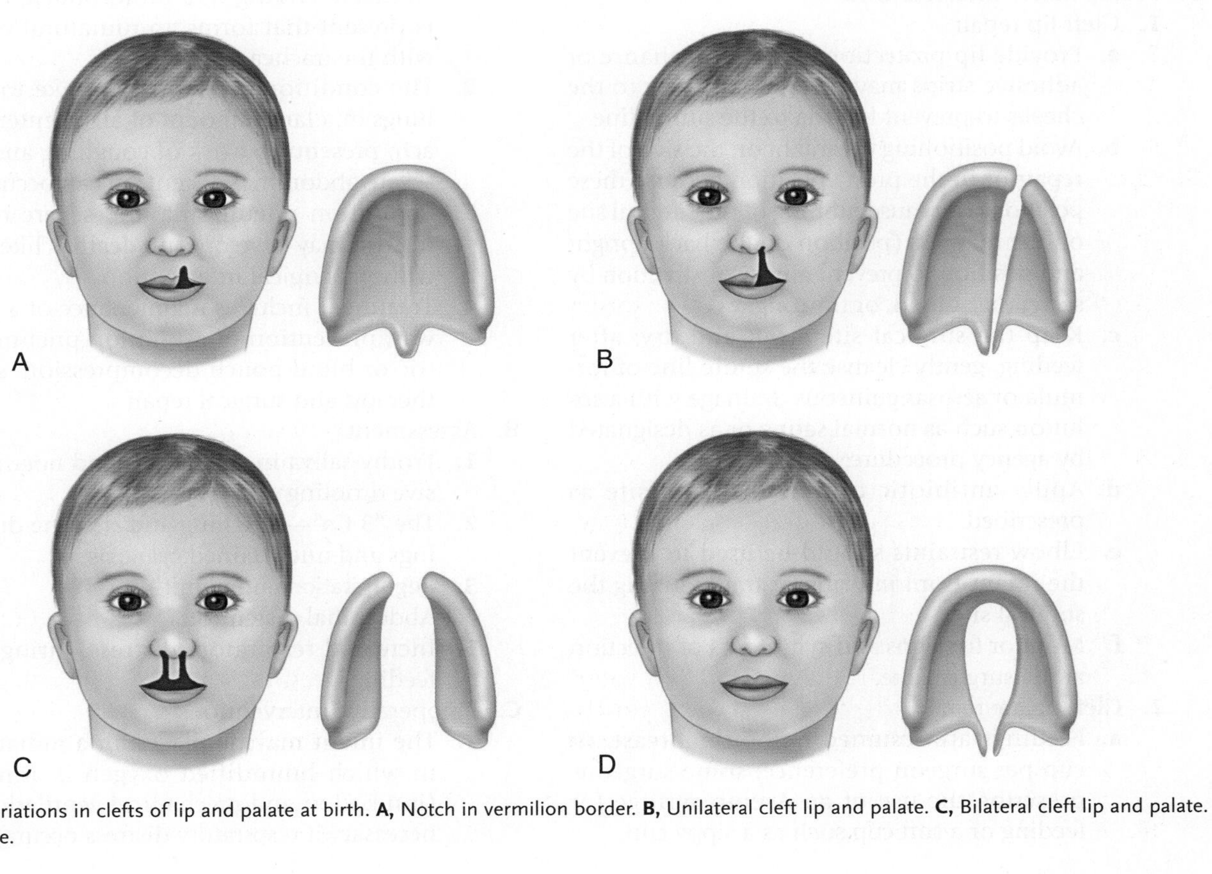

FIG. 33-1 Variations in clefts of lip and palate at birth. **A,** Notch in vermilion border. **B,** Unilateral cleft lip and palate. **C,** Bilateral cleft lip and palate. **D,** Cleft palate.

Pediatric

2. Cleft palate can include nasal distortion, midline or bilateral cleft, and variable extension from the uvula and soft and hard palate.

C. Interventions
1. Assess the ability to suck, swallow, handle normal secretions, and breathe without distress.
2. Assess fluid and calorie intake daily.
3. Monitor daily weight.
4. Modify feeding techniques; plan to use specialized feeding techniques, obturators, and special nipples and feeders.
5. Hold the infant in an upright position and direct the formula to the side and back of the mouth to prevent aspiration.
6. Feed small amounts gradually and burp frequently.
7. Keep suction equipment and a bulb syringe at the bedside.
8. Teach the parents special feeding or suctioning techniques.
9. Teach the parents the *ESSR* method of feeding—*e*nlarge the nipple, *s*timulate the sucking reflex, *s*wallow, *r*est to allow the infant to finish swallowing what has been placed in the mouth.
10. Encourage parents to express their feelings about the disorder.
11. Encourage parental bonding with the infant, including holding the infant and calling the infant by name.

D. Postoperative interventions
1. Cleft lip repair
   a. Provide lip protection; a metal appliance or adhesive strips may be taped securely to the cheeks to prevent trauma to the suture line.
   b. Avoid positioning the infant on the side of the repair or in the prone position because these positions can cause rubbing of the surgical site on the mattress (position on the back upright and position to prevent airway obstruction by secretions, blood, or the tongue).
   c. Keep the surgical site clean and dry; after feeding, gently cleanse the suture line of formula or serosanguineous drainage with a solution such as normal saline or as designated by agency procedure.
   d. Apply antibiotic ointment to the site as prescribed.
   e. Elbow restraints should be used to prevent the infant from injuring or traumatizing the surgical site.
   f. Monitor for signs and symptoms of infection at the surgical site.
2. Cleft palate repair
   a. Feedings are resumed by bottle, breast, or cup per surgeon preference; some surgeons prescribe the use of an Asepto syringe for feeding or a soft cup such as a sippy cup.
   b. Oral packing may be secured to the palate (usually removed in 2 to 3 days).
   c. Instruct the parents to avoid placing anything in the child's mouth that is harsh and could cause disruption of the surgical site.
3. Soft elbow or jacket restraints may be used (check agency policies and procedures) to keep the child from touching the repair site; remove restraints at least every 1 to 2 hours (or per agency procedure) to assess skin integrity and circulation and to allow for exercising the arms.
4. Avoid the use of oral suction or placing objects in the mouth such as a tongue depressor, thermometer, straws, spoons, forks, or pacifiers.
5. Provide analgesics for pain as prescribed.
6. Instruct the parents in feeding techniques and in the care of the surgical site.
7. Instruct the parents to monitor for signs of infection at the surgical site, such as redness, swelling, or drainage.
8. Encourage the parents to hold the child.
9. Initiate appropriate referrals such as a dental referral and speech therapy referral.

IV. Esophageal Atresia and Tracheoesophageal Fistula (Fig. 33-2)

A. Description
1. The esophagus terminates before it reaches the stomach, ending in a blind pouch, or a fistula is present that forms an unnatural connection with the trachea.
2. The condition causes oral intake to enter the lungs or a large amount of air to enter the stomach, presenting a risk of coughing and choking; severe abdominal distention can occur.
3. Aspiration pneumonia and severe respiratory distress may develop, and death is likely to occur without surgical intervention.
4. Treatment includes maintenance of a patent airway, prevention of aspiration pneumonia, gastric or blind pouch decompression, supportive therapy, and surgical repair.

B. Assessment
1. Frothy saliva in the mouth and nose and excessive drooling
2. The "3 Cs"—*c*oughing and *c*hoking during feedings and unexplained **cyanosis**
3. **Regurgitation** and vomiting
4. Abdominal distention
5. Increased respiratory distress during and after feeding

C. Preoperative interventions
1. The infant may be placed in a radiant warmer in which humidified oxygen is administered (intubation and mechanical ventilation may be necessary if respiratory distress occurs).

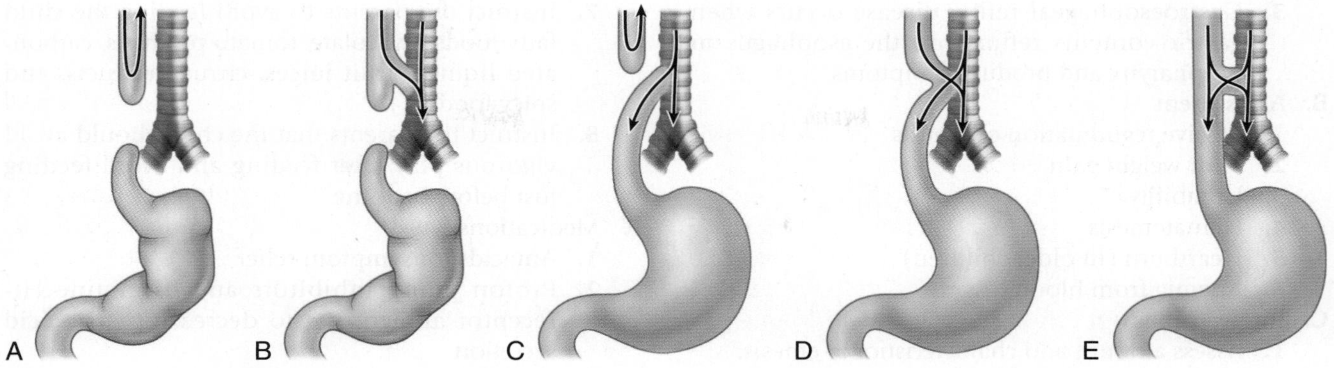

FIG. 33-2 Congenital atresia of esophagus and tracheoesophageal fistula. **A,** Upper and lower segments of esophagus end in blind sac (occurring in 5% to 8% of such infants). **B,** Upper segment of esophagus ends in atresia and connects to trachea by fistulous tract (occurring rarely). **C,** Upper segment of esophagus ends in blind pouch; lower segment connects with trachea by small fistulous tract (occurring in 80% to 95% of such infants). **D,** Both segments of esophagus connect by fistulous tracts to trachea (occurring in less than 1% of such infants). Infant may aspirate with first feeding. **E,** Esophagus is continuous but connects by fistulous tract to trachea (known as *H-type*).

2. Maintain NPO status.
3. Maintain IV fluids as prescribed.
4. Monitor respiratory status closely.
5. Suction accumulated secretions from the mouth and pharynx.
6. Maintain in a supine upright position (at least 30 degrees upright) to facilitate drainage and prevent aspiration of gastric secretions.
7. Keep the blind pouch empty of secretions by intermittent or continuous suction as prescribed; monitor its patency closely, because clogging from mucus can occur easily.
8. If a gastrostomy tube is inserted, it may be left open so that air entering the stomach through the fistula can escape, minimizing the risk of regurgitation of gastric contents into the trachea.
9. Broad-spectrum antibiotics may be prescribed because of the high risk for aspiration pneumonia.

D. Postoperative interventions
1. Monitor vital signs and respiratory status.
2. Maintain IV fluids, antibiotics, and parenteral nutrition as prescribed.
3. Monitor strict intake and output.
4. Monitor daily weight; assess for dehydration and possible fluid overload.
5. Assess for signs of pain.
6. Maintain chest tube if present.
7. Inspect the surgical site for signs and symptoms of infection.
8. Monitor for anastomotic leaks as evidenced by purulent drainage from the chest tube, increased temperature, and increased white blood cell count.
9. If a gastrostomy tube is present, it is usually attached to gravity drainage until the infant can tolerate feedings and the anastomosis is healed (usually postoperative day 5 to 7); then feedings are prescribed.
10. Before oral feedings and removal of the chest tube, prepare for an esophagogram as prescribed to check the integrity of the esophageal anastomosis.
11. Before feeding, elevate the gastrostomy tube and secure it above the level of the stomach to allow gastric secretions to pass to the duodenum and swallowed air to escape through the open gastrostomy tube.
12. Administer oral feedings with sterile water, followed by frequent small feedings of formula as prescribed.
13. Assess the cervical esophagostomy site, if present, for redness, breakdown, or exudate; remove accumulated drainage frequently, and apply protective ointment, barrier dressing, or a collection device as prescribed.
14. Provide nonnutritive sucking, using a pacifier for infants who remain NPO for extended periods (a pacifier should not be used if the infant is unable to handle secretions).
15. Instruct the parents in the techniques of suctioning, gastrostomy tube care and feedings, and skin site care as appropriate.
16. Instruct the parents to identify behaviors that indicate the need for suctioning, signs of respiratory distress, and signs of a constricted esophagus (e.g., poor feeding, dysphagia, drooling, coughing during feedings, regurgitated undigested food).

V. Gastroesophageal Reflux Disease

A. Description
1. Gastroesophageal reflux is backflow of gastric contents into the esophagus as a result of relaxation or incompetence of the lower esophageal or cardiac sphincter.
2. Most infants with gastroesophageal reflux have a mild problem that improves in about 1 year and requires medical therapy only.

3. Gastroesophageal reflux disease occurs when gastric contents reflux into the esophagus or oropharynx and produce symptoms.

B. Assessment
1. Passive regurgitation or emesis
2. Poor weight gain
3. Irritability
4. Hematemesis
5. Heartburn (in older children)
6. Anemia from blood loss

C. Interventions
1. Assess amount and characteristics of emesis.
2. Assess the relationship of vomiting to the times of feedings and infant activity.
3. Monitor breath sounds before and after feedings.
4. Assess for signs of aspiration, such as drooling, coughing, or dyspnea, after feeding.
5. Place suction equipment at the bedside.
6. Monitor intake and output.
7. Monitor for signs and symptoms of dehydration.
8. Maintain IV fluids as prescribed.

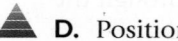

Complications of gastroesophageal reflux disease include esophagitis, esophageal strictures, aspiration of gastric contents, and aspiration pneumonia.

D. Positioning
1. The infant is placed in the supine position during sleep (to reduce the incidence of sudden infant death syndrome) unless the risk of death from aspiration or other serious complications of gastroesophageal reflux disease greatly outweighs the risks associated with the prone position (check the PHCP's prescription); otherwise, the prone position is acceptable only while the infant is awake and can be monitored.
2. In children older than 1 year, position with the head of the bed elevated.

E. Diet
1. Provide small, frequent feedings with predigested formula to decrease the amount of regurgitation.
2. Nutrition via nasogastric tube feedings may be prescribed if severe regurgitation and poor growth are present.
3. For infants, formula may be thickened by adding rice cereal to the formula (follow agency procedure); cross-cut the nipple.
4. Breast-feeding may continue, and the mother may provide more frequent feeding times or express milk for thickening with rice cereal.
5. Burp the infant frequently when feeding and handle the infant minimally after feedings; monitor for coughing during feeding and other signs of aspiration.
6. For toddlers, feed solids first, followed by liquids.
7. Instruct the parents to avoid feeding the child fatty foods, chocolate, tomato products, carbonated liquids, fruit juices, citrus products, and spicy foods.
8. Instruct the parents that the child should avoid vigorous play after feeding and avoid feeding just before bedtime.

F. Medications
1. Antacids for symptom relief
2. Proton pump inhibitors and histamine H_2-receptor antagonists to decrease gastric acid secretion

VI. Hypertrophic Pyloric Stenosis (Fig. 33-3)

A. Description
1. Hypertrophy of the circular muscles of the pylorus causes narrowing of the pyloric canal between the stomach and the duodenum.
2. The stenosis usually develops in the first few weeks of life, causing projectile vomiting, dehydration, metabolic alkalosis, and failure to thrive.

B. Assessment
1. Vomiting that progresses from mild regurgitation to forceful and projectile vomiting; it usually occurs after a feeding.

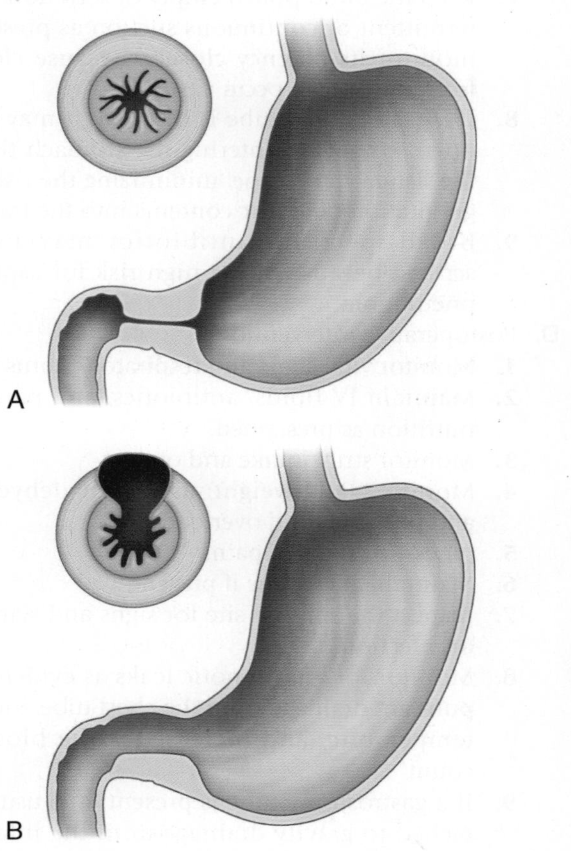

FIG. 33-3 Hypertrophic pyloric stenosis. **A,** Enlarged muscular area nearly obliterates pyloric channel. **B,** Longitudinal surgical division of muscle down to submucosa establishes adequate passageway.

2. Vomitus contains gastric contents such as milk or formula, may contain mucus, may be blood-tinged, and does not usually contain bile.
3. The child exhibits hunger and irritability.
4. Peristaltic waves are visible from left to right across the epigastrium during or immediately after a feeding.
5. An olive-shaped mass is in the epigastrium just right of the umbilicus.
6. Signs of dehydration and malnutrition
7. Signs of electrolyte imbalances
8. Metabolic alkalosis

C. Interventions
1. Monitor strict intake and output.
2. Monitor vomiting episodes and stools.
3. Obtain daily weights.
4. Monitor for signs of dehydration and electrolyte imbalances.
5. Prepare the child and parents for pyloromyotomy if prescribed.

D. Pyloromyotomy
1. Description: An incision through the muscle fibers of the pylorus; may be performed by laparoscopy
2. Preoperative interventions
   a. Monitor hydration status by daily weights, intake and output, and urine for specific gravity.
   b. Correct fluid and electrolyte imbalances; administer fluids intravenously as prescribed for rehydration.
   c. Maintain NPO status as prescribed.
   d. Monitor the number and character of stools.
   e. Maintain patency of the nasogastric tube placed for stomach decompression.
3. Postoperative interventions
   a. Monitor intake and output.
   b. Begin small, frequent feedings postoperatively as prescribed.
   c. Gradually increase amount and interval between feedings until a full feeding schedule has been reinstated.
   d. Feed the infant slowly, burping frequently, and handle the infant minimally after feedings.
   e. Monitor for abdominal distention.
   f. Monitor the surgical wound and for signs of infection.
   g. Instruct the parents about wound care and feeding.

VII. Lactose Intolerance

A. Description: Inability to tolerate lactose as a result of an absence or deficiency of lactase, an enzyme found in the secretions of the small intestine that is required for the digestion of lactose

B. Assessment
1. Symptoms occur after the ingestion of milk or other dairy products.
2. Abdominal distention
3. Crampy, abdominal pain; colic
4. Diarrhea and excessive flatus

C. Interventions
1. Eliminate the offending dairy product, or administer an enzyme tablet replacement.
2. Provide information to the parents about enzyme tablets that predigest the lactose in dairy products or supplement the body's own lactase.
3. Substitute soy-based formulas for cow's milk formula or human milk.
4. Allow milk consumption as tolerated.
5. Instruct the child and family that the child should drink milk with other foods rather than by itself.
6. Encourage consumption of hard cheese, cottage cheese, and yogurt, which contain the inactive lactase enzyme.
7. Encourage consumption of small amounts of dairy foods daily to help colonic bacteria adapt to ingested lactose.
8. Instruct the parents about the foods that contain lactose, including hidden sources.

A child with lactose intolerance can develop calcium and vitamin D deficiency. Instruct the parents about the importance of providing these supplements.

VIII. Celiac Disease

A. Description
1. Celiac disease is also known as gluten enteropathy or celiac sprue.
2. Intolerance to gluten, the protein component of wheat, barley, rye, and oats, is characteristic.
3. Celiac disease results in the accumulation of the amino acid glutamine, which is toxic to intestinal mucosal cells.
4. Intestinal villous atrophy occurs, which affects absorption of ingested nutrients.
5. Symptoms of the disorder occur most often between the ages of 1 and 5 years.
6. There is usually an interval of 3 to 6 months between the introduction of gluten in the diet and the onset of symptoms.
7. Strict dietary avoidance of gluten minimizes the risk of developing malignant lymphoma of the small intestine and other gastrointestinal malignancies.

B. Assessment
1. Acute or insidious diarrhea
2. Steatorrhea
3. Anorexia
4. Abdominal pain and distention
5. Muscle wasting, particularly in the buttocks and extremities

Pediatric

6. Vomiting
7. Anemia
8. Irritability

C. Celiac crisis
1. Precipitated by fasting, infection, or ingestion of gluten
2. Causes profuse watery diarrhea and vomiting
3. Can lead to rapid dehydration, electrolyte imbalance, and severe acidosis

D. Interventions
1. Maintain a gluten-free diet, substituting corn, rice, and millet as grain sources.
2. Instruct the parents and child about lifelong elimination of gluten sources such as wheat, rye, oats, and barley.
3. Administer mineral and vitamin supplements, including iron, folic acid, and fat-soluble vitamins A, D, E, and K.
4. Teach the child and parents about a gluten-free diet and about reading food labels carefully for hidden sources of gluten (Box 33-1).
5. Instruct the parents in measures to prevent celiac crisis.
6. Inform the parents about the Celiac Sprue Association.

IX. Appendicitis

A. Description
1. Inflammation of the appendix
2. When the appendix becomes inflamed or infected, perforation may occur within a matter of hours, leading to peritonitis, sepsis, septic shock, and potentially death.
3. Treatment is surgical removal of the appendix before perforation occurs.

B. Assessment
1. Pain in periumbilical area that descends to the right lower quadrant
2. Abdominal pain that is most intense at McBurney's point
3. Referred pain indicating the presence of peritoneal irritation
4. Rebound tenderness and abdominal rigidity
5. Elevated white blood cell count
6. Side-lying position with abdominal guarding (legs flexed) to relieve pain
7. Difficulty walking and pain in the right hip
8. Low-grade fever
9. Anorexia, nausea, and vomiting after pain develops
10. Diarrhea

C. Peritonitis
1. Description: Results from a perforated appendix
2. Assessment
a. Increased fever
b. Progressive abdominal distention
c. Tachycardia and tachypnea
d. Pallor
e. Chills
f. Restlessness and irritability

! An indication of a perforated appendix is the sudden relief of pain and then a subsequent increase in pain accompanied by right guarding of the abdomen.

D. Appendectomy
1. Description: Surgical removal of the appendix
2. Interventions preoperatively
a. Maintain NPO status.
b. Administer IV fluids and electrolytes as prescribed to prevent dehydration and correct electrolyte imbalances.
c. Monitor for changes in the level of pain.
d. Monitor for signs of a ruptured appendix and peritonitis.
e. Avoid the use of pain medications so as not to mask pain changes associated with perforation.
f. Administer antibiotics as prescribed.
g. Monitor bowel sounds.
h. Position in a right side-lying or low to semi-Fowler's position to promote comfort.
i. Apply ice packs to the abdomen for 20 to 30 minutes every hour if prescribed.
j. Avoid the application of heat to the abdomen.
k. Avoid laxatives or enemas.
3. Postoperative interventions
a. Monitor vital signs, particularly temperature.
b. Maintain NPO status until bowel function has returned, advancing the diet gradually as tolerated and as prescribed when bowel sounds return.
c. Assess the incision for signs of infection such as redness, swelling, drainage, and pain.
d. Monitor drainage from the drain, which may be inserted if perforation occurred.
e. Position the child in a right side-lying or low to semi-Fowler's position with the legs slightly flexed to facilitate drainage.

BOX 33-1 Basics of a Gluten-Free Diet

Foods Allowed

Meat such as beef, pork, poultry, and fish; eggs; milk and some dairy products; vegetables, fruits, rice, corn, gluten-free flour, puffed rice, cornflakes, cornmeal, and precooked gluten-free cereals are allowed.

Foods Prohibited

Commercially prepared ice cream; malted milk; prepared puddings; and grains, including anything made from wheat, rye, oats, or barley, such as breads, rolls, cookies, cakes, crackers, cereal, spaghetti, macaroni noodles, beer, and ale, are prohibited.

f. Change the dressing as prescribed, and record the type and amount of drainage.
g. Perform wound irrigations if prescribed.
h. Maintain nasogastric tube suction and patency of the tube if present.
i. Administer antibiotics and analgesics as prescribed.

X. Hirschsprung's Disease (Fig. 33-4)

A. Description
1. Hirschsprung's disease is a congenital anomaly also known as congenital aganglionosis or aganglionic megacolon.
2. The disease occurs as the result of an absence of ganglion cells in the rectum and other areas of the affected intestine.
3. Mechanical obstruction results because of inadequate motility in an intestinal segment.
4. The disease may be a familial congenital defect or may be associated with other anomalies, such as Down's syndrome and genitourinary abnormalities.
5. A rectal biopsy specimen shows histological evidence of the absence of ganglionic cells.
6. The most serious complication is enterocolitis; signs include fever, severe prostration, gastrointestinal bleeding, and explosive watery diarrhea.
7. Treatment for mild or moderate disease is based on relieving the chronic constipation with stool softeners and rectal irrigations; however, many children require surgery.
8. Treatment for moderate to severe disease involves a 2-step surgical procedure.
   a. Initially, in the neonatal period, a temporary colostomy is created to relieve obstruction and allow the normally innervated, dilated bowel to return to its normal size.
   b. When the bowel returns to its normal size, a complete surgical repair is performed via a pull-through procedure to excise portions of the bowel; at this time, the colostomy is closed.

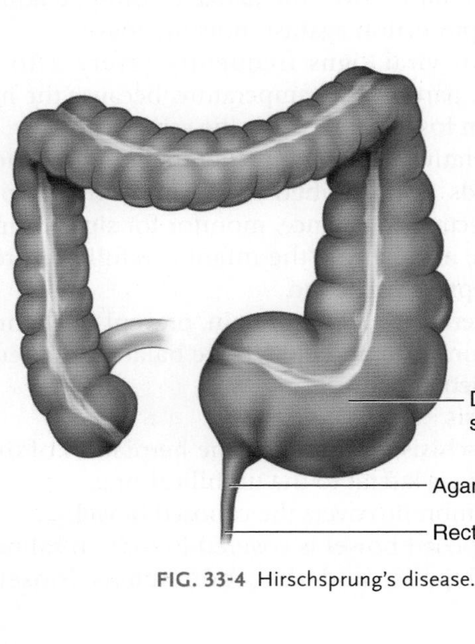

FIG. 33-4 Hirschsprung's disease.

B. Assessment
1. Newborns
   a. Failure to pass meconium stool
   b. Refusal to suck
   c. Abdominal distention
   d. Bile-stained vomitus
2. Children
   a. Failure to gain weight and delayed growth
   b. Abdominal distention
   c. Vomiting
   d. Constipation alternating with diarrhea
   e. Ribbon-like and foul-smelling stools

C. Interventions: Medical management
1. Maintain a low-fiber, high-calorie, high-protein diet; parenteral nutrition may be necessary in extreme situations.
2. Administer stool softeners as prescribed.
3. Administer daily rectal irrigations with normal saline to promote adequate elimination and prevent obstruction as prescribed.

D. Surgical management: Preoperative interventions
1. Assess bowel function.
2. Administer bowel preparation as prescribed.
3. Maintain NPO status.
4. Monitor hydration and fluid and electrolyte status; provide fluids intravenously as prescribed for hydration.
5. Administer antibiotics or colonic irrigations with an antibiotic solution as prescribed to clear the bowel of bacteria.
6. Monitor strict intake and output.
7. Obtain daily weight.
8. Measure abdominal girth daily.
9. Avoid taking the temperature rectally.
10. Monitor for respiratory distress associated with abdominal distention.

E. Surgical management: Postoperative interventions
1. Monitor vital signs, avoiding taking the temperature rectally.
2. Measure abdominal girth daily and PRN (as needed).
3. Assess the surgical site for redness, swelling, and drainage.
4. Assess the stoma if present for bleeding or skin breakdown (stoma should be red and moist).
5. Assess the anal area for the presence of stool, redness, or discharge.
6. Maintain NPO status as prescribed and until bowel sounds return or flatus is passed, usually within 48 to 72 hours.
7. Maintain nasogastric tube to allow intermittent suction until peristalsis returns.

8. Maintain IV fluids until the child tolerates appropriate oral intake, advancing the diet from clear liquids to regular as tolerated and as prescribed.
9. Assess for dehydration and fluid overload.
10. Monitor strict intake and output.
11. Obtain daily weight.
12. Assess for pain and provide comfort measures as required.
13. Provide the parents with instructions regarding colostomy care and skin care.
14. Teach the parents about the appropriate diet and the need for adequate fluid intake.

XI. Intussusception (Fig. 33-5)

A. Description
1. Telescoping of one portion of the bowel into another portion
2. The condition results in obstruction to the passage of intestinal contents.

B. Assessment
1. Colicky abdominal pain that causes the child to scream and draw the knees to the abdomen, similar to the fetal position
2. Vomiting of gastric contents
3. Bile-stained fecal emesis
4. Currant jelly–like stools containing blood and mucus
5. Hypoactive or hyperactive bowel sounds
6. Tender distended abdomen, possibly with a palpable sausage-shaped mass in the upper right quadrant

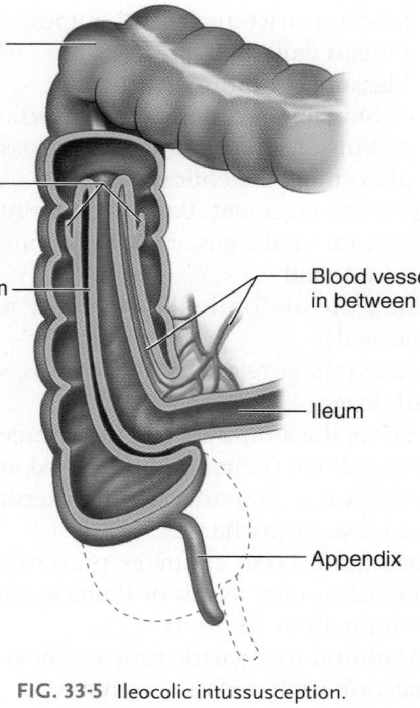

FIG. 33-5 Ileocolic intussusception.

C. Interventions
1. Monitor for signs of perforation and shock as evidenced by fever, increased heart rate, changes in level of consciousness or blood pressure, and respiratory distress, and report immediately.
2. Antibiotics, IV fluids, and decompression via nasogastric tube may be prescribed.
3. Monitor for the passage of normal, brown stool, which indicates that the intussusception has reduced itself.
4. Prepare for hydrostatic reduction as prescribed, if no signs of perforation or shock occur (in hydrostatic reduction, air or fluid is used to exert pressure on area involved to lessen, diminish, or resolve the prolapse).
5. Posthydrostatic reduction
   a. Monitor for the return of normal bowel sounds, for the passage of barium, and the characteristics of stool.
   b. Administer clear fluids, and advance the diet gradually as prescribed.
6. If surgery is required, postoperative care is similar to care after any abdominal surgery; procedure may be done via laparoscope.

XII. Abdominal Wall Defects

A. Omphalocele
1. *Omphalocele* refers to herniation of the abdominal contents through the umbilical ring, usually with an intact peritoneal sac.
2. The protrusion is covered by a translucent sac that may contain bowel or other abdominal organs.
3. Rupture of the sac results in evisceration of the abdominal contents.
4. Immediately after birth, the sac is covered with sterile gauze soaked in normal saline to prevent drying of abdominal contents; a layer of plastic wrap is placed over the gauze to provide additional protection against moisture loss.
5. Monitor vital signs frequently (every 2 to 4 hours), particularly temperature, because the infant can lose heat through the sac.
6. Preoperatively: Maintain NPO status, administer IV fluids as prescribed to maintain hydration and electrolyte balance, monitor for signs of infection, and handle the infant carefully to prevent rupture of the sac.
7. Postoperatively: Control pain, prevent infection, maintain fluid and electrolyte balance, and ensure adequate nutrition.

B. Gastroschisis
1. Gastroschisis occurs when the herniation of the intestine is lateral to the umbilical ring.
2. No membrane covers the exposed bowel.
3. The exposed bowel is covered loosely in saline-soaked pads, and the abdomen is loosely

wrapped in a plastic drape or or agency approved drape; wrapping directly around the exposed bowel is contraindicated, because if the exposed bowel expands, wrapping could cause pressure and necrosis.

4. Preoperatively: Care is similar to that for omphalocele; surgery is performed within several hours after birth because no membrane is covering the sac.
5. Postoperatively: Most infants develop prolonged ileus, require mechanical ventilation, and need parenteral nutrition; otherwise, care is similar to that for omphalocele.

XIII. Umbilical and Inguinal Hernia and Hydrocele

A. Description
1. An umbilical hernia is a protrusion of the bowel through an abnormal opening in the abdominal wall.
2. In children, hernias most commonly occur at the umbilicus and also through the inguinal canal.
3. A hydrocele is the presence of abdominal fluid in the scrotal sac.

B. Assessment
1. Umbilical hernia: Soft swelling or protrusion around the umbilicus that is usually reducible with a finger
2. Inguinal hernia
   a. Inguinal hernia refers to a painless inguinal swelling that is reducible.
   b. Swelling may disappear during periods of rest and is most noticeable when the infant cries or coughs.
3. Incarcerated hernia
   a. Incarcerated hernia occurs when the descended portion of the bowel becomes tightly caught in the hernial sac, compromising blood supply.
   b. This represents a medical emergency requiring surgical repair.
   c. Assessment findings include irritability, tenderness at site, anorexia, abdominal distention, and difficulty defecating.
   d. The protrusion cannot be reduced, and complete intestinal obstruction and gangrene may occur.
4. Noncommunicating hydrocele
   a. Noncommunicating hydrocele occurs when residual peritoneal fluid is trapped in the scrotum with no communication to the peritoneal cavity.
   b. Hydrocele usually disappears by age 1 year as the fluid is reabsorbed.
5. Communicating hydrocele
   a. Communicating hydrocele is associated with a hernia that remains open from the scrotum to the abdominal cavity.
   b. Assessment includes a bulge in the inguinal area or the scrotum that increases with crying or straining and decreases when the infant is at rest. Parents may also report the bulge is smaller in the morning but increases in size throughout the day.

C. Postoperative interventions (hernia)
1. Monitor vital signs.
2. Assess for wound infection.
3. Monitor for redness or drainage.
4. Monitor input and output and hydration status.
5. Advance the diet as tolerated.
6. Administer analgesics as prescribed.

D. Postoperative interventions (hydrocele)
1. Provide ice bags and a scrotal support to relieve pain and swelling.
2. Instruct the parents that tub bathing needs to be avoided until the incision heals.
3. Instruct the parents that strenuous physical activities need to be avoided.
4. Advise parent that the scrotum may not immediately return to normal size.

XIV. Constipation and Encopresis

A. Description
1. Constipation is the infrequent and difficult passage of dry, hard stools.
2. Encopresis is constipation with fecal incontinence; children often complain that soiling is involuntary and occurs without warning.
3. If the child does not have a neurological or anatomical disorder, encopresis is usually the result of fecal impaction and an enlarged rectum caused by chronic constipation.

B. Assessment
1. Constipation
   a. Abdominal pain and cramping without distention
   b. Palpable movable fecal masses
   c. Normal or decreased bowel sounds
   d. Malaise and headache
   e. Anorexia, nausea, and vomiting
2. Encopresis
   a. Evidence of soiling of clothing
   b. Scratching or rubbing of the anal area
   c. Fecal odor
   d. Social withdrawal

C. Interventions
1. Maintain a diet high in fiber and fluids to promote bowel elimination (Box 33-2).
2. Monitor treatment regimen for severe encopresis for 3 to 6 months.
3. Decrease sugar and milk intake.
4. Administer enemas as prescribed until impaction is cleared.
5. Monitor for hypernatremia or hyperphosphatemia when administering repeated enemas.

Pediatric

BOX 33-2 High-Fiber Foods

Bread and Grains

- Whole-grain bread or rolls
- Whole-grain cereals
- Bran
- Pancakes, waffles, and muffins with fruit or bran
- Unrefined (brown) rice

Vegetables

- Raw vegetables, especially broccoli, cabbage, carrots, cauliflower, celery, lettuce, and spinach
- Cooked vegetables, including those listed above and asparagus, beans, Brussels sprouts, corn, potatoes, rhubarb, squash, string beans, and turnips

Fruits

- Prunes, raisins, or other dried fruits
- Raw fruits, especially those with skins or seeds, other than ripe banana or avocado

Miscellaneous

- Legumes (beans), popcorn, nuts, and seeds
- High-fiber snack bars

Data from Perry S, Hockenberry M, Lowdermilk D, Wilson D: *Maternal-child nursing care*, ed 4, St. Louis, 2010, Mosby.

a. Signs of hypernatremia include increased thirst; dry, sticky mucous membranes; flushed skin; increased temperature; nausea and vomiting; oliguria; and lethargy.
b. Signs of hyperphosphatemia include tetany, muscle weakness, dysrhythmias, and hypotension.

6. Administer stool softeners or laxatives as prescribed.
7. Encourage the child to sit on the toilet for 5 to 10 minutes approximately 20 to 30 minutes after breakfast and dinner to assist with defecation.

XV. Irritable Bowel Syndrome

A. Description
1. Irritable bowel syndrome results from increased motility, which can lead to spasm and pain.
2. The diagnosis is based on the elimination of pathological conditions.
3. The syndrome is a self-limiting, intermittent problem with no definitive treatment.
4. Stress and emotional factors may contribute to its occurrence.

B. Assessment
1. Diffuse abdominal pain unrelated to meals or activity
2. Alternating constipation and diarrhea with the presence of undigested food and mucus in the stool

C. Interventions
1. Reassure the parents and child that the problem is self-limiting and intermittent and will resolve.
2. Anticholinergics may be prescribed (antidepressants may be needed in severe cases).
3. Encourage the maintenance of a healthy, well-balanced, moderate-fiber, and low-fat diet.
4. Encourage health promotion activities such as exercise and school activities.
5. Inform the parents of psychosocial resources if required.

XVI. Imperforate Anus

A. Description: Incomplete development or absence of the anus in its normal position in the perineum

B. Types
1. A membrane is noted over the anal opening, with a normal anus just above the membrane.
2. There is complete absence of the anus (anal agenesis) with a rectal pouch ending some distance above.
3. Rectum ends blindly or has a fistula connection to the perineum, urethra, bladder, or vagina.

C. Assessment (Box 33-3)

D. Preoperative interventions
1. Determine presence of an anal opening.
2. Monitor for the presence of stool in the urine and vagina (indicates a fistula) and report immediately.
3. Administer IV fluids as prescribed.
4. Prepare the child and parents for the surgical procedures, including the potential for colostomy.

E. Postoperative interventions
1. Monitor the skin for signs of infection.
2. The preferred position is a side-lying prone position with the hips elevated or a supine position with the legs suspended at a 90-degree angle to the trunk to reduce edema and pressure on the surgical site.
3. Keep the anal surgical incision clean and dry, and monitor for redness, swelling, or drainage.
4. Maintain NPO status and nasogastric tube if in place.
5. Maintain IV fluids until gastrointestinal motility returns.
6. Provide care for colostomy, if present, as prescribed.

BOX 33-3 Assessment Findings: Imperforate Anus

- Failure to pass meconium stool
- Absence or stenosis of the anal rectal canal
- Presence of an anal membrane
- External fistula to the perineum

7. A new colostomy stoma may be red and edematous, but the edema should decrease with time.
8. Instruct the parents to perform anal dilation if prescribed to achieve and maintain bowel patency.
9. Instruct the parents to use only anal dilators supplied by the PHCP and a water-soluble lubricant and to insert the dilator no more than 1 to 2 cm into the anus to prevent damage to the mucosa.

XVII. Hepatitis

A. This section contains specific information regarding hepatitis as it relates to infants and children; see also Chapters 22 and 48.

B. Description: An acute or chronic inflammation of the liver that may be caused by a virus, a medication reaction, or another disease process

C. Hepatitis A (HAV)
1. Highest incidence of HAV infection occurs among preschool or school-age children younger than 15 years.
2. Many infected children are asymptomatic, but mild nausea, vomiting, and diarrhea may occur.
3. Infected children who are asymptomatic still can spread HAV to others.

D. Hepatitis B (HBV)
1. Most HBV infection in children is acquired perinatally.
2. Newborns are at risk if the mother is infected with HBV or was a carrier of HBV during pregnancy.
3. Possible routes of maternal-fetal (newborn) transmission include leakage of the virus across the placenta late in pregnancy or during labor, ingestion of amniotic fluid or maternal blood, and breast-feeding, especially if the mother has cracked nipples.
4. The severity in the infant varies from no liver disease to fulminant (severe acute course) or chronic active disease.
5. In children and adolescents, HBV occurs in specific high-risk groups, including children with hemophilia or other disorders requiring multiple blood transfusions, children or adolescents involved in IV drug abuse, institutionalized children, preschool children in endemic areas, and children who have had heterosexual activity or sexual activity with homosexual men.
6. Infection with HBV can cause a carrier state and lead to eventual cirrhosis or hepatocellular carcinoma in adulthood.

E. Hepatitis C (HCV)
1. Transmission of HCV is primarily by the parenteral route.
2. Some children may be asymptomatic, but HCV often becomes a chronic condition and can cause cirrhosis and hepatocellular carcinoma.

F. Hepatitis D
1. Infection occurs in children already infected with HBV.
2. Acute and chronic forms tend to be more severe than HBV and can lead to cirrhosis.
3. Children with hemophilia are more likely to be infected, as are those who are IV drug users.

G. Hepatitis E
1. Infection is uncommon in children.
2. Infection is not a chronic condition, does not cause chronic liver disease, and has no carrier state.

H. Assessment (Box 33-4)

I. Laboratory diagnostic evaluation: See Chapters 10 and 48.

J. Prevention
1. Immunoglobulin provides **passive immunity** and may be effective for preexposure prophylaxis to prevent HAV infection.
2. Hepatitis B immunoglobulin provides passive immunity and may be effective in preventing infection after a 1-time exposure (should be given immediately after exposure), such as an accidental needle puncture or other contact of contaminated material with mucous membranes; immunoglobulin should also be given to newborns whose mothers are positive for hepatitis B surface antigen.
3. Hepatitis A **vaccine** and hepatitis B vaccine: See Chapters 18 and 40.

> ! Proper hand washing and standard precautions, as well as enteric precautions, can prevent the spread of viral hepatitis.

K. Interventions
1. Strict hand washing is required.
2. Hospitalization is required in the event of coagulopathy or fulminant hepatitis.
3. Standard precautions and enteric precautions are followed during hospitalization.

BOX 33-4 Assessment Findings: Hepatitis

Prodromal or Anicteric Phase
- Lasts 5 to 7 days
- Absence of jaundice
- Anorexia, malaise, lethargy, easy fatigability
- Fever (especially in adolescents)
- Nausea and vomiting
- Epigastric or right upper quadrant abdominal pain
- Arthralgia and rashes (more likely with hepatitis B virus)
- Hepatomegaly

Icteric Phase
- Jaundice, which is best assessed in the sclera, nail beds, and mucous membranes
- Dark urine and pale stools
- Pruritus

Pediatric

4. Provide enteric precautions for at least 1 week after the onset of jaundice with HAV.
5. The hospitalized child usually is not isolated in a separate room unless he or she is fecally incontinent and items are likely to become contaminated with feces.
6. Children are discouraged from sharing toys.
7. Instruct the child and parents in effective hand washing techniques.
8. Instruct the parents to disinfect diaper-changing surfaces thoroughly with a solution of ¼ cup (60 mL) bleach in 1 gallon (3.8 L) of water.
9. Maintain comfort and provide adequate rest and sleep.
10. Provide a low-fat, well-balanced diet.
11. Inform the parents that because HAV is not infectious 1 week after the onset of jaundice, the child may return to school at that time if he or she feels well enough.
12. Inform the parents that jaundice may appear worse before it resolves.
13. Caution the parents about administering any medications to the child; explain the role of the liver in detoxification and excretion of medications in understandable terms.
14. Instruct the parents about the signs of the child's condition worsening, such as changes in neurological status, bleeding, and fluid retention.

PRIORITY NURSING ACTIONS

Poisoning Treatment in the Emergency Department

1. Assess the child.
2. Terminate exposure to the poison.
3. Identify the poison.
4. Take measures to prevent absorption of the poison.
5. Document the occurrence, assessment findings, poison ingested, treatment measures, and the child's response.

Reference

Hockenberry. (2017). Wilson, Rodgers, 410.

XVIII. Ingestion of Poisons (see Priority Nursing Actions)

A. Lead poisoning
1. Description: Excessive accumulation of lead in the blood
2. Causes
   a. The pathway for exposure may be food, air, or water.
   b. Dust and soil contaminated with lead may be a source of exposure.
   c. Lead enters the child's body through ingestion or inhalation or through placental transmission to an unborn child when the mother is exposed; the most common route is hand to mouth lead-containing from contaminated objects, such as loose paint chips, pottery, or ceramic ware coupled with the inhalation of lead dust in the environment.
   d. When lead enters the body, it affects the erythrocytes, bones and teeth, and organs and tissues, including the brain and nervous system; the most serious consequences are the effects on the central nervous system.
3. Universal screening
   a. Screening is recommended for children 1 to 2 years old; children at high risk should be screened earlier.
   b. Any child between the ages of 3 and 6 years who has not been screened should be tested.
4. Targeted screening
   a. Targeted screening is acceptable in low-risk areas.
   b. A child at the age of 1 to 2 years (or a child between the ages of 3 and 6 years who has not been screened) may be targeted for screening if determined to be at risk.
5. Blood lead level test: Used for screening and diagnosis (Table 33-1)
6. Erythrocyte protoporphyrin test
   a. Indicator of anemia
   b. Normal value for a child: 35 mcg/100 mL of whole blood or lower
7. Chelation therapy
   a. Chelation therapy removes lead from the circulating blood and from some organs and tissues.
   b. Therapy does not counteract any effects of the lead.
   c. Medications include calcium disodium edetate, and succimer, an oral preparation; British anti-Lewisite is used in conjunction with ethylenediamine tetraacetic acid (EDTA).
   d. British anti-Lewisite is administered via the IV route or the deep intramuscular route and is contraindicated in children with an allergy to peanuts because the medication is prepared in a peanut oil solution; it is also contraindicated in children with glucose-6-phosphate dehydrogenase (G6PD) deficiency and should not be given with iron.
   e. The function of the renal, hepatic, and hematological systems must be monitored closely.
   f. Ensure adequate urinary output before administering the medication, and monitor the output and pH of the urine closely during and after therapy.

TABLE 33-1 Blood Lead Level Test Results and Interventions

Level (mcg/dL)	Intervention
<5	Reassess or rescreen in 1 yr or sooner if exposure status changes
5-14	Provide family lead education, follow-up testing, and social service referral for home assessment if necessary
15-19	Provide family education about lead, follow-up testing, and social service referral if necessary; on follow-up testing, initiate actions for blood lead level of 20-44 mcg/dL
20-44	Provide coordination of care and clinical management, including treatment, environmental investigation, and lead-hazard control
45-69	Provide coordination of care and clinical management within 48 hr, including treatment, environmental investigation, and lead-hazard control (the child must not remain in a lead-hazardous environment if resolution is necessary)
≥70	Medical treatment is provided immediately, including coordination of care, clinical management, environmental investigation, and lead-hazard control

Data from Perry S, Hockenberry M, Lowdermilk D, Wilson D: *Maternal-child nursing care*, ed 4, St. Louis, 2010, Mosby; and Centers for Disease Control and Prevention: *Blood lead levels in children* (website): https://www.cdc.gov/nceh/lead/default.htm.

g. Provide adequate hydration and monitor kidney function for nephrotoxicity when the medication is given, because the medication is excreted via the kidneys.
h. Follow-up of lead levels needs to be done to monitor progress.
i. Provide instructions to parents about safety from lead hazards, medication administration, and the need for follow-up.
j. Confirm that the child will be discharged to a home without lead hazards.

B. Acetaminophen
1. Description
a. Seriousness of ingestion is determined by the amount ingested and the length of time before intervention.
b. Toxic dose is 150 mg/kg or higher in children.
2. Assessment
a. First 2 to 4 hours: Malaise, nausea, vomiting, sweating, pallor, weakness
b. Latent period: 24 to 36 hours; child improves
c. Hepatic involvement: May last 7 days and may be permanent; right upper quadrant pain, jaundice, confusion, stupor, elevated liver enzyme and bilirubin levels, prolonged prothrombin time
3. Interventions
a. Administer antidote: *N*-Acetylcysteine.
b. Dilute antidote in juice or soda because of its offensive odor.
c. Loading dose is followed by maintenance doses.
d. In an unconscious child, prepare to administer gastric lavage with activated charcoal to decrease the absorption of acetaminophen.
e. If using activated charcoal with lavage, do not also use *N*-acetylcysteine because activated charcoal inactivates the antidote.

C. Acetylsalicylic acid (aspirin)
1. Description
a. Overdose may be caused by acute ingestion or chronic ingestion.
b. Acute: Severe toxicity with 300 to 500 mg/kg
c. Chronic: Ingestion of more than 100 mg/kg per day for 2 days or more, which can be more serious than acute ingestion
2. Assessment
a. Gastrointestinal effects: Nausea, vomiting, and thirst from dehydration
b. Central nervous system effects: Hyperpnea, confusion, tinnitus, seizures, coma, respiratory failure, circulatory collapse
c. Renal effects: Oliguria
d. Hematopoietic effects: Bleeding tendencies
e. Metabolic effects: Diaphoresis, fever, hyponatremia, hypokalemia, dehydration, hypoglycemia, metabolic acidosis
3. Interventions
a. Prepare to administer activated charcoal to decrease absorption of salicylate.
b. Emesis or cathartic measures may be prescribed.
c. Administer IV fluids; sodium bicarbonate may be prescribed to correct metabolic acidosis.
d. Other interventions include external cooling, anticonvulsants, vitamin K (if bleeding), and oxygen.
e. Prepare the child for dialysis as prescribed if the child is unresponsive to the therapy.

D. Corrosives
1. Description
a. Items that can cause poisoning include household cleaners, detergents, bleach, paint or paint thinners, and batteries.
b. Liquid corrosives can cause more damage to the victim than other types of corrosives, such as granular.

2. Assessment
   a. Severe burning in the mouth, throat, or stomach
   b. Edema of the mucous membranes, lips, tongue, and pharynx
   c. Vomiting
   d. Drooling and inability to clear secretions
3. Interventions
   a. Dilute corrosive with water or milk as prescribed (usually no more than 4 oz [120 mL])
   b. Inducing vomiting is contraindicated because vomiting redamages the mucous membranes.
   c. Neutralization of the ingested corrosive is not done because it can cause a reaction producing heat and burns.

Educate parents to call the Poison Control Center immediately in the event of poisoning. The parents need to post the Poison Control Center telephone number near each phone in the house and have it in their mobile phones.

XIX. Intestinal Parasites

A. Description: Common infections in children are giardiasis and pinworm infestation.
   1. Giardiasis is caused by protozoa and is prevalent among children in crowded environments, such as classrooms or day care centers.
   2. Pinworms (enterobiasis) are universally present in temperate climate zones and are easily transmitted in crowded environments.

B. Assessment
   1. Giardiasis
      a. Diarrhea and vomiting
      b. Anorexia
      c. Failure to thrive
      d. Abdominal cramps with intermittent loose stools and constipation
      e. Steatorrhea
      f. Stool specimens from 3 or more collections are used for diagnosis.
   2. Pinworms
      a. Intense perianal itching
      b. Irritability, restlessness
      c. Poor sleeping
      d. Bed wetting

C. Interventions
   1. Giardiasis
      a. Medications that kill the parasites may be prescribed; medications are not usually prescribed for children younger than 2 years.
      b. Caregivers should wash hands meticulously.
      c. Provide education to family and caregivers regarding sanitary practices.
   2. Pinworms
      a. Perform a visual inspection of the anus with a flashlight 2 to 3 hours after sleep.
      b. The tape test is the most common diagnostic test.
      c. Educate the family and caregivers regarding the tape test. A loop of transparent tape is placed firmly against the child's perianal area; it is removed in the morning and placed in a glass jar or plastic bag and transported to the laboratory for analysis.
      d. Medications that kill the parasites may be prescribed; medications are not usually prescribed for children younger than 2 years.
      e. The medication regimen may be repeated in 2 weeks to prevent reinfection.
      f. All members of the family are treated for the infection.
      g. Teach the family and caregivers about the importance of meticulous hand washing and about washing all clothes and bed linens in hot water.

PRACTICE QUESTIONS

332. The clinic nurse reviews the record of an infant and notes that the primary health care provider (PHCP) has documented a diagnosis of suspected Hirschsprung's disease. The nurse reviews the assessment findings documented in the record, knowing that which sign **most likely** led the mother to seek health care for the infant?
   1. Diarrhea
   2. Projectile vomiting
   3. Regurgitation of feedings
   4. Foul-smelling ribbon-like stools

333. An infant has just returned to the nursing unit after surgical repair of a cleft lip on the right side. The nurse should place the infant in which **best** position at this time?
   1. Prone position
   2. On the stomach
   3. Left lateral position
   4. Right lateral position

334. The nurse reviews the record of a newborn infant and notes that a diagnosis of esophageal atresia with tracheoesophageal fistula is suspected. The nurse expects to note which **most likely** sign of this condition documented in the record?
   1. Incessant crying
   2. Coughing at nighttime
   3. Choking with feedings
   4. Severe projectile vomiting

335. The nurse provides feeding instructions to a parent of an infant diagnosed with gastroesophageal reflux

disease. Which instruction should the nurse give to the parent to assist in reducing the episodes of emesis?
1. Provide less frequent, larger feedings.
2. Burp the infant less frequently during feedings.
3. Thin the feedings by adding water to the formula.
4. Thicken the feedings by adding rice cereal to the formula.

336. A child is hospitalized because of persistent vomiting. The nurse should monitor the child closely for which problem?
1. Diarrhea
2. Metabolic acidosis
3. Metabolic alkalosis
4. Hyperactive bowel sounds

337. The nurse is caring for a newborn with a suspected diagnosis of imperforate anus. The nurse monitors the infant, knowing that which is a clinical manifestation associated with this disorder?
1. Bile-stained fecal emesis
2. The passage of currant jelly–like stools
3. Failure to pass meconium stool in the first 24 hours after birth
4. Sausage-shaped mass palpated in the upper right abdominal quadrant

338. The nurse admits a child to the hospital with a diagnosis of pyloric stenosis. On assessment, which data would the nurse expect to obtain when asking the parent about the child's symptoms?
1. Watery diarrhea
2. Projectile vomiting
3. Increased urine output
4. Vomiting large amounts of bile

339. The nurse provides home care instructions to the parents of a child with celiac disease. The nurse should teach the parents to include which food item in the child's diet?
1. Rice
2. Oatmeal
3. Rye toast
4. Wheat bread

340. The nurse is preparing to care for a child with a diagnosis of intussusception. The nurse reviews the child's record and expects to note which sign of this disorder documented?
1. Watery diarrhea
2. Ribbon-like stools
3. Profuse projectile vomiting
4. Bright red blood and mucus in the stools

341. Which interventions should the nurse include when creating a care plan for a child with hepatitis? **Select all that apply.**
- ❑ 1. Providing a low-fat, well-balanced diet.
- ❑ 2. Teaching the child effective hand-washing techniques.
- ❑ 3. Scheduling playtime in the playroom with other children.
- ❑ 4. Notifying the primary health care provider (PHCP) if jaundice is present.
- ❑ 5. Instructing the parents to avoid administering medications unless prescribed.
- ❑ 6. Arranging for indefinite home schooling because the child will not be able to return to school.

ANSWERS

332. *Answer:* 4

Rationale: Hirschsprung's disease is a congenital anomaly also known as *congenital aganglionosis* or *aganglionic megacolon.* It occurs as the result of an absence of ganglion cells in the rectum and other areas of the affected intestine. Chronic constipation beginning in the first month of life and resulting in pellet-like or ribbon-like stools that are foul-smelling is a clinical manifestation of this disorder. Delayed passage or absence of meconium stool in the neonatal period is also a sign. Bowel obstruction, especially in the neonatal period; abdominal pain and distention; and failure to thrive are also clinical manifestations. Options 1, 2, and 3 are not associated specifically with this disorder.

Test-Taking Strategy: Note the strategic words, *most likely.* Use knowledge regarding the pathophysiology associated with Hirschsprung's disease to direct you to the correct option. Remember that chronic constipation beginning in the first month of life and resulting in pellet-like or ribbon-like, foul-smelling stools is a clinical manifestation of this disorder.

Level of Cognitive Ability: Analyzing
Client Needs: Physiological Integrity
Integrated Process: Nursing Process—Assessment
Content Area: Pediatrics: Gastrointestinal
Health Problem: Pediatric-Specific: Gastrointestinal and Rectal Problems
Priority Concepts: Clinical Judgment; Elimination
Reference: McKinney et al. (2018), pp. 988-989.

333. *Answer:* 3

Rationale: A cleft lip is a congenital anomaly that occurs as a result of failure of soft tissue or bony structure to fuse during embryonic development. After cleft lip repair, the nurse avoids positioning an infant on the side of the repair or in the prone position, because these positions can cause rubbing of the surgical site on the mattress. The nurse positions the infant on the side lateral to the repair or on the back upright and positions

the infant to prevent airway obstruction by secretions, blood, or the tongue. From the options provided, placing the infant on the left side immediately after surgery is best to prevent the risk of aspiration if the infant vomits.
Test-Taking Strategy: Note the strategic word, *best.* Eliminate options 1 and 2 because they are comparable or alike positions. Consider the anatomical location of the surgical site and note the words *right side* in the question to direct you to the correct option from those remaining.
Level of Cognitive Ability: Applying
Client Needs: Physiological Integrity
Integrated Process: Nursing Process—Implementation
Content Area: Pediatrics: Gastrointestinal
Health Problem: Pediatric-Specific: Disorders of Prenatal Development
Priority Concepts: Safety; Tissue Integrity
Reference: McKinney et al. (2018), pp. 963-965.

334. *Answer:* 3
Rationale: In esophageal atresia and tracheoesophageal fistula, the esophagus terminates before it reaches the stomach, ending in a blind pouch, and a fistula is present that forms an unnatural connection with the trachea. Any child who exhibits the "3 Cs"—coughing and choking with feedings and unexplained cyanosis—should be suspected to have tracheoesophageal fistula. Options 1, 2, and 4 are not specifically associated with tracheoesophageal fistula.
Test-Taking Strategy: Note the strategic words, *most likely.* Focus on the diagnosis and think about the pathophysiology of the disorder. Recalling the "3 Cs" associated with this disorder will assist in directing you to the correct option.
Level of Cognitive Ability: Analyzing
Client Needs: Physiological Integrity
Integrated Process: Nursing Process—Assessment
Content Area: Pediatrics: Gastrointestinal
Health Problem: Pediatric-Specific: Disorders of Prenatal Development
Priority Concepts: Clinical Judgment; Tissue Integrity
Reference: McKinney et al. (2018), pp. 965-966.

335. *Answer:* 4
Rationale: Gastroesophageal reflux is backflow of gastric contents into the esophagus as a result of relaxation or incompetence of the lower esophageal or cardiac sphincter. Small, more frequent feedings with frequent burping often are prescribed in the treatment of gastroesophageal reflux. Feedings thickened with rice cereal may reduce episodes of emesis. If thickened formula is used, cross-cutting of the nipple may be required.
Test-Taking Strategy: Note the subject, gastroesophageal reflux disease. Use basic principles related to feeding an infant to assist in eliminating options 1 and 2. Noting the words *reducing the episodes of emesis* in the question will assist in directing you to select the correct option over option 3.
Level of Cognitive Ability: Applying
Client Needs: Physiological Integrity
Integrated Process: Teaching and Learning
Content Area: Pediatrics: Gastrointestinal
Health Problem: Pediatric-Specific: Gastroesophageal Reflux Disease
Priority Concepts: Client Education; Nutrition
Reference: McKinney et al. (2018), pp. 971-972.

336. *Answer:* 3
Rationale: Vomiting causes the loss of hydrochloric acid and subsequent metabolic alkalosis. Metabolic acidosis would occur in a child experiencing diarrhea because of the loss of bicarbonate. Diarrhea might or might not accompany vomiting. Hyperactive bowel sounds are not associated with vomiting.
Test-Taking Strategy: Focus on the subject, complications related to vomiting. Recalling that gastric fluids are acidic and that the loss of these fluids leads to alkalosis will assist you in answering the question. No data in the question support options 1 and 4.
Level of Cognitive Ability: Analyzing
Client Needs: Physiological Integrity
Integrated Process: Nursing Process—Assessment
Content Area: Pediatrics: Gastrointestinal
Health Problem: Pediatric-Specific: Dehydration
Priority Concepts: Acid-Base Balance; Fluids and Electrolytes
Reference: McKinney et al. (2018), p. 891.

337. *Answer:* 3
Rationale: Imperforate anus is the incomplete development or absence of the anus in its normal position in the perineum. During the newborn assessment, this defect should be identified easily on sight. However, a rectal thermometer or tube may be necessary to determine patency if meconium is not passed in the first 24 hours after birth. Other assessment findings include absence or stenosis of the anal rectal canal, presence of an anal membrane, and an external fistula to the perineum. Options 1, 2, and 4 are findings noted in intussusception.
Test-Taking Strategy: Note the subject, manifestations of imperforate anus. Use the definition of the word *imperforate* to assist in answering this question. This should direct you to the correct option.
Level of Cognitive Ability: Analyzing
Client Needs: Physiological Integrity
Integrated Process: Nursing Process—Assessment
Content Area: Pediatrics: Gastrointestinal
Health Problem: Pediatric-Specific: Gastrointestinal and Rectal Problems
Priority Concepts: Clinical Judgment; Elimination
Reference: McKinney et al. (2018), pp. 968-969.

338. *Answer:* 2
Rationale: In pyloric stenosis, hypertrophy of the circular muscles of the pylorus causes narrowing of the pyloric canal between the stomach and the duodenum. Clinical manifestations of pyloric stenosis include projectile vomiting, irritability, hunger and crying, constipation, and signs of dehydration, including a decrease in urine output.
Test-Taking Strategy: Focus on the subject, the manifestations of pyloric stenosis. Considering the anatomical location of this disorder and its potential effects will assist in eliminating options 1 and 3. Thinking about the pathophysiology of the disorder and recalling that a major clinical manifestation is projectile vomiting will assist in directing you to the correct option from those remaining.

Level of Cognitive Ability: Analyzing
Client Needs: Physiological Integrity
Integrated Process: Nursing Process—Assessment
Content Area: Pediatrics: Gastrointestinal
Health Problem: Pediatric-Specific: Disorder of Prenatal Development
Priority Concepts: Clinical Judgment; Fluids and Electrolytes
Reference: Hockenberry, Wilson, Rodgers (2017), pp. 728-729.

339. *Answer:* 1
Rationale: Celiac disease also is known as *gluten enteropathy* or *celiac sprue* and refers to intolerance to gluten, the protein component of wheat, barley, rye, and oats. The important factor to remember is that all wheat, rye, barley, and oats should be eliminated from the diet and replaced with corn, rice, or millet. Vitamin supplements—especially the fat-soluble vitamins, iron, and folic acid—may be needed to correct deficiencies. Dietary restrictions are likely to be lifelong.
Test-Taking Strategy: Focus on the subject, home care instructions for the child with celiac disease. Recalling that corn, rice, and millet are substitute food replacements in this disease will direct you to the correct option.
Level of Cognitive Ability: Applying
Client Needs: Health Promotion and Maintenance
Integrated Process: Teaching and Learning
Content Area: Pediatrics: Gastrointestinal
Health Problem: Pediatric-Specific: Nutrition Problems
Priority Concepts: Client Education; Nutrition
Reference: Hockenberry, Wilson, Rodgers (2017), pp. 732-734.

340. *Answer:* 4
Rationale: Intussusception is a telescoping of 1 portion of the bowel into another. The condition results in an obstruction to the passage of intestinal contents. A child with intussusception typically has severe abdominal pain that is crampy and intermittent, causing the child to draw in the knees to the chest. Vomiting may be present, but is not projectile. Bright red blood and mucus are passed through the rectum and commonly are described as currant jelly–like stools. Watery diarrhea and ribbon-like stools are not manifestations of this disorder.
Test-Taking Strategy: Focus on the subject, the manifestations of intussusception. Think about the pathophysiology associated with this condition. Recalling that a classic manifestation is currant jelly–like stools will assist in directing you to the correct option.
Level of Cognitive Ability: Analyzing
Client Needs: Physiological Integrity
Integrated Process: Nursing Process—Assessment
Content Area: Pediatrics: Gastrointestinal
Health Problem: Pediatric-Specific: Gastrointestinal and Rectal Problems
Priority Concepts: Clinical Judgment; Elimination
Reference: Hockenberry, Wilson, Rodgers (2017), pp. 729-730.

341. *Answer:* 1, 2, 5
Rationale: Hepatitis is an acute or chronic inflammation of the liver that may be caused by a virus, a medication reaction, or another disease process. Because hepatitis can be viral, standard precautions should be instituted in the hospital. The child should be discouraged from sharing toys, so playtime in the playroom with other children is not part of the plan of care. The child will be allowed to return to school 1 week after the onset of jaundice, so indefinite home schooling would not need to be arranged. Jaundice is an expected finding with hepatitis and would not warrant notification of the PHCP. Provision of a low-fat, well-balanced diet is recommended. Parents are cautioned about administering any medication to the child, because normal doses of many medications may become dangerous owing to the liver's inability to detoxify and excrete them. Hand washing is the most effective measure for control of hepatitis in any setting, and effective hand washing can prevent the immunocompromised child from contracting an opportunistic type of infection.
Test-Taking Strategy: Focus on the subject, care for a child with hepatitis. Thinking about the pathophysiology associated with hepatitis and the method of transmission will assist you in answering the question. Because the infection can be transmitted to others, playing with other children in the playroom is not an appropriate intervention. Since jaundice is an expected finding, notifying the PHCP is unnecessary. Planning for an indefinite period of home schooling is not necessary.
Level of Cognitive Ability: Creating
Client Needs: Safe and Effective Care Environment
Integrated Process: Nursing Process—Planning
Content Area: Pediatrics: Gastrointestinal
Health Problem: Pediatric-Specific: Hepatitis
Priority Concepts: Clinical Judgment; Infection
Reference: McKinney et al. (2018), pp. 994-996.

Pediatric

CHAPTER 34

Eye, Ear, and Throat Problems

PRIORITY CONCEPTS **Safety; Sensory Perception**

I. Strabismus

A. Description
1. Called "squint" or "cross-eye"
2. Condition in which the eyes are not aligned because of lack of coordination of the extraocular muscles
3. Most often results from muscle imbalance or paralysis of extraocular muscles, but also may result from a congenital defect
4. Amblyopia (reduced visual acuity) may occur if not treated early, because the brain receives two messages as a result of the nonparallel visual axes.
5. Permanent loss of vision can occur if not treated early.
6. This condition, considered a normal finding in a young infant, should not be present after about age 4 months.
7. Treatment of the condition depends on the cause.

B. Assessment
1. Crossed eyes
2. Squinting; tilts the head or closes one eye to see
3. Loss of binocular vision
4. Impairment of depth perception
5. Frequent headaches
6. Diplopia; photophobia

C. Interventions
1. Corrective lenses may be indicated.
2. Instruct the parents regarding patching (occlusion therapy) of the "good" eye to strengthen the weak eye.
3. Prepare for surgery to realign the weak muscles as prescribed if nonsurgical interventions are unsuccessful.
4. Instruct the parents about the need for follow-up visits.

II. Conjunctivitis

A. Description
1. Also known as "pink eye"; an inflammation of the conjunctiva
2. Conjunctivitis usually is caused by allergy, infection, or trauma.
3. Types include viral, bacterial, or allergic; bacterial or viral conjunctivitis is extremely contagious.

B. Assessment
1. Itching, burning, or scratchy eyelids
2. Redness
3. Edema
4. Discharge

Chlamydial conjunctivitis is rare in older children; if diagnosed in a child who is not sexually active, the child should be assessed for possible sexual abuse.

C. Interventions
1. Viral conjunctivitis.
   a. The infection will usually resolve in 7 to 14 days; in some cases it can take 2 to 3 weeks or more to resolve.
   b. Antiviral medication may be prescribed to treat more serious forms of conjunctivitis, such as those caused by herpes simplex virus or varicella zoster virus; antibiotics are not effective against viruses.
2. Bacterial conjunctivitis
   a. Mild cases may improve without antibiotic treatment.
   b. An antibiotic, usually prescribed topically as eye drops or ointment, may be prescribed to shorten the length of infection, reduce complications, and reduce the spread to others.
3. Allergic conjunctivitis
   a. Removing the allergen from the environment often improves the condition.
   b. Allergy medications and eye drops such as topical antihistamine and vasoconstrictors may be prescribed.
4. General interventions
   a. The primary health care provider (PHCP) needs to be consulted regarding going to school and contact with others.
   b. Instruct the child and parents about the administration of the prescribed medications.

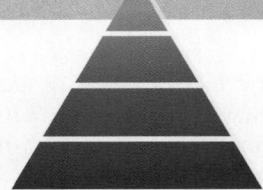

c. Instruct in infection control measures such as good hand washing and not sharing towels and washcloths.
d. Instruct the child to avoid rubbing the eye to prevent injury.
e. Instruct a child who is wearing contact lenses to discontinue wearing them and to obtain new lenses to eliminate the chance of reinfection that can occur from use of the old lenses.
f. Instruct an adolescent that eye makeup should be discarded and replaced.
g. For additional information, refer to Centers for Disease Control and prevention at https://www.cdc.gov/conjunctivitis/index.html.

III. Otitis Media

A. Description
1. An inflammatory disorder usually caused by an infection of the middle ear occurring as a result of a blocked eustachian tube, which prevents normal drainage; can be acute or chronic.
2. Otitis media is a common complication of an acute respiratory infection (most commonly from respiratory syncytial virus, influenza, or group A streptococcus).
3. Infants and children have eustachian tubes that are shorter, wider, and straighter, which makes them more prone to otitis media.

B. Prevention
1. Feed infants in an upright position, to prevent reflux.
2. Maintain routine immunizations.
3. Encourage breast-feeding for at least the first 6 months of life.
4. Avoid exposure to tobacco smoke and allergens.

C. Assessment
1. Fever
2. Acute onset of ear pain
3. Crying, irritability, lethargy
4. Loss of appetite
5. Rolling of head from side to side
6. Pulling on or rubbing the ear
7. Purulent ear drainage may be present
8. Red, opaque, bulging, immobile tympanic membrane on otoscopic examination
9. Signs of hearing loss (indicative of chronic otitis media)

D. Interventions
1. Encourage fluid intake (may be difficult if the child is in pain).
2. Instruct the child to avoid chewing as much as possible during the acute period, because chewing increases pain.
3. Provide local heat or cold as prescribed to relieve discomfort, and have the child lie with the affected ear down.
4. Instruct the parents in the appropriate procedure to clean drainage from the external ear canal with sterile swabs or gauze; frequent cleansing and the application of moisture barriers may be prescribed to prevent ear excoriation from the drainage.
5. Instruct the parents in the administration of analgesics or antipyretics such as acetaminophen or ibuprofen as prescribed to decrease fever and pain.
6. Instruct the parents in the administration of antibiotics if prescribed, emphasizing that the prescribed period of administration is necessary to eliminate infective organisms.
7. In healthy infants older than 6 months and children, careful use of antibiotics is recommended because of concerns about medication-resistant *Streptococcus pneumoniae;* usually, waiting up to 72 hours for spontaneous resolution is a safe and appropriate management of acute otitis media.
8. Instruct the parents that screening for hearing loss may be necessary.
9. Instruct the parents about the procedure for administering ear medications such as topical pain-relief drops, if prescribed.

E. Otitis Externa
1. Description: Inflammation of the external auditory canal, which can occur with or without infection; also known as "swimmer's ear."
2. Assessment
   a. Rapid onset of symptoms within 48 hours, symptoms include otalgia, pruritis, fullness, drainage, and impaired hearing.
   b. A low-grade fever may be present.
   c. Tenderness on manipulation of the pinna and tragus is noted on physical exam.
   d. May have regional lymphadenopathy.
3. Interventions: Treatment is indicated with topical antibiotics and may include neomycin with or without polymyxin B or a fluoroquinolone preparation.

To administer ear medications in a child younger than 3 years, pull the earlobe down and back. In a child older than 3 years, pull the pinna up and back.

F. Myringotomy
1. Description
   a. A surgical incision into the tympanic membrane to provide drainage of the purulent middle ear fluid; may be done by a laser-assisted procedure
   b. Tympanoplasty tubes, which are small cylinder-shaped tubes, may be inserted into the middle ear to allow continued drainage and to equalize pressure and allow ventilation of the middle ear.

2. Postoperative interventions
   a. Instruct the parents and child to keep the ears dry.
   b. The child should wear earplugs while bathing, shampooing, and swimming (diving and submerging under water are not allowed).
   c. Parents can administer an analgesic such as acetaminophen or ibuprofen to relieve discomfort after insertion of tympanoplasty tubes.
   d. Parents should be taught that the child should not blow her or his nose for 7 to 10 days after surgery.
   e. Instruct the parents that if the tubes fall out, it is not an emergency, but the PHCP should be notified; inform the parents of the appearance of the tubes (tiny, white, spool-shaped tubes).

IV. Tonsillitis and Adenoiditis

A. Description
1. *Tonsillitis* refers to inflammation and infection of the tonsils, which is lymphoid tissue located in the pharynx (Fig. 34-1).
2. *Adenoiditis* refers to inflammation and infection of the adenoids (pharyngeal tonsils), located on the posterior wall of the nasopharynx.
3. Enlarged tonsils and adenoids may lead to an obstructive sleep apnea in children, manifested by snoring and periods of sudden waking and fragmented sleep; a polysomnography and referral to ear, nose and throat specialist may be needed.
4. Can be the result of a viral, bacterial, or fungal infection. Group A streptococcus ("strep throat") is a common bacterial infection of the oropharynx, particularly in children, which can result in streptococcal toxic shock syndrome.

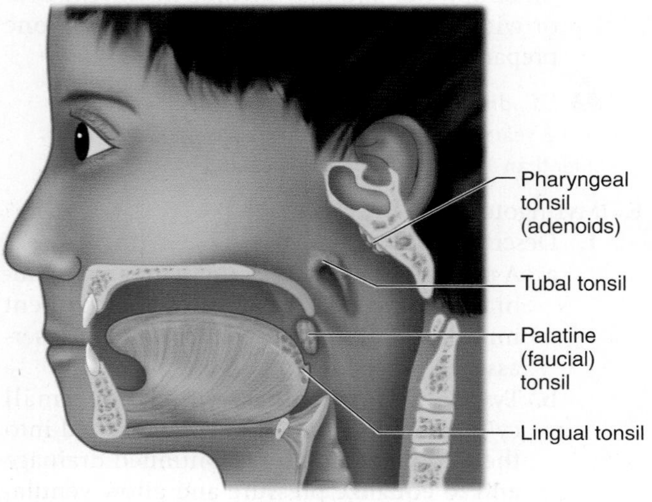

FIG. 34-1 Location of various tonsillar masses.

   Mononucleosis is another possible cause of tonsillitis and adenoiditis.
5. Tonsillectomy (surgical removal of the tonsils) and adenoidectomy (surgical removal of the adenoids) may be necessary depending on the number of infections per year as well as signs of obstructive respiratory disturbance.

B. Assessment
1. Persistent or recurrent sore throat
2. Enlarged, bright red tonsils that may be covered with white exudate
3. Difficulty in swallowing
4. Mouth breathing and an unpleasant mouth odor
5. Fever
6. Cough
7. Enlarged adenoids may cause nasal quality of speech, mouth breathing, hearing difficulty, snoring, or obstructive sleep apnea.

C. Preoperative interventions
1. Assess for signs of active infection.
2. Assess bleeding and clotting studies, because the throat is vascular.
3. Assess for any loose teeth to decrease the risk of aspiration during surgery.
4. Prepare the child for a sore throat postoperatively, and inform the child that she or he will need to drink liquids.

D. Interventions postoperatively
1. Position the child prone or side-lying to facilitate drainage.
2. Have suction equipment available but do not suction unless there is an airway obstruction.
3. Monitorforsignsofbleeding(frequentswallowing may indicate bleeding); if bleeding occurs, turn the child to the side and notify the PHCP.
4. Discourage coughing, clearing the throat, or nose blowing to prevent bleeding.
5. Provide an ice collar or analgesics (rectally or intravenously) for discomfort.
6. Administer antiemetics to prevent vomiting if prescribed.
7. Provide clear, cool, noncitrus and noncarbonated fluids (crushed ice, ice pops).
8. Avoid red, purple, or brown liquids, which simulate the appearance of blood if the child vomits.
9. Avoid milk products such as milk, ice cream, and pudding initially because they coat the throat, causing the child to cough to clear the throat.
10. Soft foods may be prescribed 1 to 2 days postoperatively.
11. Do not give the child any straws, forks, or sharp objects that can be put into the mouth.
12. Mouth odor, slight ear pain, and a low-grade fever may occur for a few days postoperatively,

but the parents should be instructed to notify the PHCP if bleeding, persistent earache, or fever occurs.

13. Instruct the parents to keep the child away from crowds until healing has occurred; usually the child is able to resume normal activities 1 to 2 weeks postoperatively.

V. Epistaxis (Nosebleed)

A. Description
   1. The nose, especially the septum, is a highly vascular structure, and bleeding usually results from direct trauma, foreign bodies, and nose picking or from mucosal inflammation.
   2. Recurrent epistaxis and severe bleeding may indicate an underlying disease.

B. Interventions
   1. See **Priority Nursing Actions**.
   2. If bleeding cannot be controlled, packing or cauterization of the bleeding vessel may be prescribed.

PRIORITY NURSING ACTIONS

Nosebleed in a Child

1. Remain calm and keep the child calm and quiet.
2. Have the child sit up and lean forward (not lie down).
3. Apply continuous pressure to the nose with the thumb and forefinger for at least 10 minutes.
4. Insert cotton or wadded tissue into each nostril, and apply ice or a cold cloth to the bridge of the nose if bleeding persists.

Reference
Hockenberry. (2017). Wilson, Rodgers, 805–806.

VI. Allergic Rhinitis

A. Description: a condition in which children are sensitized to environmental allergens

B. Assessment
   1. Itchy and watery eyes, runny nose, itchy throat
   2. May be a family history of atopic disease
   3. Dark circles under the eyes, cobblestoning of the conjunctiva, pale nasal mucosa, clear nasal drainage, nasal polyps, fluid in the middle ear, cobblestoning of the posterior pharynx, wheezes, rhonchi, eczema, hives, angioedema

A. Interventions
   1. Children with allergic rhinitis should be tested for environmental allergies, food allergies, atopic dermatitis, and asthma.
   2. Avoidance of triggers; administration of prescribed antihistamines, nasal corticosteroids, inhalers.

PRACTICE QUESTIONS

342. After a tonsillectomy, a child begins to vomit bright red blood. The nurse should take which **initial** action?
1. Turn the child to the side.
2. Administer the prescribed antiemetic.
3. Maintain NPO (nothing by mouth) status.
4. Notify the primary health care provider (PHCP).

343. The mother of a 6-year-old child arrives at a clinic because the child has been experiencing itchy, red, and swollen eyes. The nurse notes a discharge from the eyes and sends a culture to the laboratory for analysis. Chlamydial conjunctivitis is diagnosed. On the basis of this diagnosis, the nurse determines that which requires further investigation?
1. Possible trauma
2. Possible sexual abuse
3. Presence of an allergy
4. Presence of a respiratory infection

344. The nurse prepares a teaching plan for the mother of a child diagnosed with bacterial conjunctivitis. Which, if stated by the mother, indicates a **need for further teaching**?
1. "I need to wash my hands frequently."
2. "I need to clean the eye as prescribed."
3. "It is okay to share towels and washcloths."
4. "I need to give the eye drops as prescribed."

345. The nurse is reviewing the laboratory results for a child scheduled for a tonsillectomy. The nurse determines that which laboratory value is **most** significant to review?
1. Creatinine level
2. Prothrombin time
3. Sedimentation rate
4. Blood urea nitrogen level

346. The nurse is preparing to care for a child after a tonsillectomy. The nurse documents on the plan of care to place the child in which position?
1. Supine
2. Side-lying
3. High-Fowler's
4. Trendelenburg's

347. After a tonsillectomy, the nurse reviews the surgeon's postoperative prescriptions. Which prescription should the nurse question?
1. Monitor for bleeding.
2. Suction every 2 hours.
3. Give no milk or milk products.
4. Give clear, cool liquids when awake and alert.

348. The nurse is caring for a child after a tonsillectomy. The nurse monitors the child, knowing that which finding indicates the child is bleeding?

1. Frequent swallowing
2. A decreased pulse rate
3. Complaints of discomfort
4. An elevation in blood pressure

349. Antibiotics are prescribed for a child with otitis media who underwent a myringotomy with insertion of tympanostomy tubes. The nurse provides discharge instructions to the parents regarding the administration of the antibiotics. Which statement, if made by the parents, indicates understanding of the instructions provided?
1. "Administer the antibiotics until they are gone."
2. "Administer the antibiotics if the child has a fever."
3. "Administer the antibiotics until the child feels better."
4. "Begin to taper the antibiotics after 3 days of a full course."

350. The day care nurse is observing a 2-year-old child and suspects that the child may have strabismus. Which observation made by the nurse indicates the presence of this condition?
1. The child has difficulty hearing.
2. The child consistently tilts the head to see.
3. The child does not respond when spoken to.
4. The child consistently turns the head to hear.

351. A child has been diagnosed with acute otitis media of the right ear. Which interventions should the nurse include in the plan of care? **Select all that apply.**
- ❑ 1. Provide a soft diet.
- ❑ 2. Position the child on the left side.
- ❑ 3. Administer an antihistamine twice daily.
- ❑ 4. Irrigate the right ear with normal saline every 8 hours.
- ❑ 5. Administer ibuprofen for fever every 4 hours as prescribed and as needed.
- ❑ 6. Instruct the parents about the need to administer the prescribed antibiotics for the full course of therapy.

ANSWERS

342. *Answer:* 1
Rationale: After tonsillectomy, if bleeding occurs, the nurse immediately turns the child to the side to prevent aspiration and then notifies the PHCP. NPO status would be maintained, and an antiemetic may be prescribed; however, the initial nursing action would be to turn the child to the side.
Test-Taking Strategy: Note the strategic word, *initial*. Although all of the options may be appropriate to maintain physiological integrity, the initial action is to turn the child to the side to prevent aspiration.
Level of Cognitive Ability: Applying
Client Needs: Physiological Integrity
Integrated Process: Nursing Process—Implementation
Content Area: Pediatrics: Throat/Respiratory
Health Problem: Pediatric-Specific: Tonsillitis and Adenoiditis
Priority Concepts: Clinical Judgment; Safety
Reference: McKinney et al. (2018), pp. 1040-1041.

343. *Answer:* 2
Rationale: Conjunctivitis is an inflammation of the conjunctiva. A diagnosis of chlamydial conjunctivitis in a child who is not sexually active should signal the health care provider to assess the child for possible sexual abuse. Trauma, allergy, and infection can cause conjunctivitis, but the causative organism is not likely to be *Chlamydia*.
Test-Taking Strategy: Note the age of the child and the organism that is identified in the question. Also note that options 1, 3, and 4 are comparable or alike in that they can be recognized as the common causes of conjunctivitis and they relate to a physiological problem.
Level of Cognitive Ability: Analyzing
Client Needs: Psychosocial Integrity
Integrated Process: Nursing Process—Assessment
Content Area: Pediatrics: Infectious and Communicable Diseases
Health Problem: Pediatric-Specific: Conjunctivitis
Priority Concepts: Clinical Judgment; Infection
Reference: McKinney et al. (2018), pp. 926-927.

344. *Answer:* 3
Rationale: Conjunctivitis is an inflammation of the conjunctiva. Bacterial conjunctivitis is highly contagious, and the nurse should teach infection control measures. These include good hand washing and not sharing towels and washcloths. Options 1, 2, and 4 are correct treatment measures.
Test-Taking Strategy: Note the strategic words, *need for further teaching*. These words indicate a negative event query and ask you to select an option that is an incorrect statement. Options 1, 2, and 4 can be eliminated by recalling that bacterial conjunctivitis is highly contagious.
Level of Cognitive Ability: Evaluating
Client Needs: Safe and Effective Care Environment
Integrated Process: Teaching and Learning
Content Area: Pediatrics: Infectious and Communicable Diseases
Health Problem: Pediatric-Specific: Conjunctivitis
Priority Concepts: Client Education; Infection
Reference: Hockenberry, Wilson, Rodgers (2017), p. 171.

345. *Answer:* 2
Rationale: A tonsillectomy is the surgical removal of the tonsils. Because the tonsillar area is so vascular, postoperative bleeding is a concern. Prothrombin time, partial thromboplastin time, platelet count, hemoglobin and hematocrit, white blood cell count, and urinalysis are performed preoperatively. The prothrombin time results would identify a potential for bleeding. Creatinine level, sedimentation rate, and blood urea nitrogen would not determine the potential for bleeding.

Test-Taking Strategy: Note the strategic word, *most.* Focus on the surgical procedure and the subject of the question. The subject of the question relates to the potential for bleeding. Options 1 and 4 can be eliminated because they relate to kidney function. Option 3 can be eliminated because it is unrelated to the subject of the question.
Level of Cognitive Ability: Analyzing
Client Needs: Physiological Integrity
Integrated Process: Nursing Process—Assessment
Content Area: Pediatrics: Throat/Respiratory
Health Problem: Pediatric-Specific: Tonsillitis and Adenoiditis
Priority Concepts: Clinical Judgment; Clotting
References: McKinney et al. (2018), pp. 1040-1041; Pagana et al. (2015), p. 767.

346. *Answer:* 2
Rationale: A tonsillectomy is the surgical removal of the tonsils. The child should be placed in a prone or side-lying position after the surgical procedure to facilitate drainage. Options 1, 3, and 4 would not achieve this goal.
Test-Taking Strategy: Focus on the subject, positioning after tonsillectomy. Focus on the surgical procedure and visualize each of the positions described in the options. Keeping in mind that the goal is to facilitate drainage will direct you to the correct option.
Level of Cognitive Ability: Applying
Client Needs: Physiological Integrity
Integrated Process: Nursing Process—Planning
Content Area: Pediatrics: Throat/Respiratory
Health Problem: Pediatric-Specific: Tonsillitis and Adenoiditis
Priority Concepts: Caregiving; Safety
Reference: McKinney et al. (2018), p. 1041.

347. *Answer:* 2
Rationale: A tonsillectomy is the surgical removal of the tonsils. After tonsillectomy, suction equipment should be available, but suctioning is not performed unless there is an airway obstruction because of the risk of trauma to the surgical site. Monitoring for bleeding is an important nursing intervention after any type of surgery. Milk and milk products are avoided initially because they coat the throat, cause the child to clear the throat, and increase the risk of bleeding. Clear, cool liquids are encouraged.
Test-Taking Strategy: Focus on the subject, the prescription that the nurse questions. Option 1 can be eliminated first because this is a nursing action, not a medical prescription. From the remaining options, consider the anatomical location of the surgery. This should direct you to the correct option.
Level of Cognitive Ability: Analyzing
Client Needs: Safe and Effective Care Environment
Integrated Process: Nursing Process—Implementation
Content Area: Pediatrics: Throat/Respiratory
Health Problem: Pediatric-Specific: Tonsillitis and Adenoiditis
Priority Concepts: Collaboration; Safety
Reference: McKinney et al. (2018), p. 1041.

348. *Answer:* 1
Rationale: A tonsillectomy is the surgical removal of the tonsils. Frequent swallowing, restlessness, a fast and thready pulse, and vomiting bright red blood are signs of bleeding. An elevated blood pressure and complaints of discomfort are not indications of bleeding.
Test-Taking Strategy: Focus on the subject, a sign of bleeding, and use the concepts related to the signs of shock. These concepts should assist in eliminating options 2 and 4. From the remaining options, recalling that discomfort is expected and does not indicate bleeding will direct you to the correct option.
Level of Cognitive Ability: Analyzing
Client Needs: Physiological Integrity
Integrated Process: Nursing Process—Assessment
Content Area: Pediatrics: Throat/Respiratory
Health Problem: Pediatric-Specific: Tonsillitis and Adenoiditis
Priority Concepts: Clinical Judgment; Clotting
Reference: McKinney et al. (2018), p. 1041.

349. *Answer:* 1
Rationale: A myringotomy is the insertion of tympanoplasty tubes into the middle ear to promote drainage of purulent middle ear fluid, equalize pressure, and keep the ear aerated. The nurse must instruct parents regarding the administration of antibiotics. Antibiotics need to be taken as prescribed, and the full course needs to be completed. Options 2, 3, and 4 are incorrect. Antibiotics are not tapered but are administered for the full course of therapy.
Test-Taking Strategy: Focus on the subject, understanding of the instructions about antibiotics. Recall that antibiotics must be taken for the full course, regardless of whether the child is feeling better. This will assist in directing you to the correct option.
Level of Cognitive Ability: Evaluating
Client Needs: Physiological Integrity
Integrated Process: Nursing Process—Evaluation
Content Area: Pediatrics: Eye/Ear
Health Problem: Pediatric-Specific: Acute and Chronic Otitis
Priority Concepts: Client Education; Safety
Reference: Hockenberry, Wilson, Rodgers (2017), pp. 646-647.

350. *Answer:* 2
Rationale: Strabismus is a condition in which the eyes are not aligned because of lack of coordination of the extraocular muscles. The nurse may suspect strabismus in a child when the child complains of frequent headaches, squints, or tilts the head to see. Other manifestations include crossed eyes, closing one eye to see, diplopia, photophobia, loss of binocular vision, or impairment of depth perception. Options 1, 3, and 4 are not indicative of this condition.
Test-Taking Strategy: Eliminate options 1 and 4 first because they are comparable or alike and relate to hearing. To select from the remaining options, recall that this is a condition in which the eyes are not aligned because of lack of coordination of the extraocular muscles.
Level of Cognitive Ability: Analyzing
Client Needs: Physiological Integrity
Integrated Process: Nursing Process—Assessment
Content Area: Pediatrics: Eye/Ear
Health Problem: Pediatric-Specific: Eye Focus and Alignment Disorders
Priority Concepts: Clinical Judgment; Sensory Perception
Reference: Hockenberry, Wilson, Rodgers (2017), p. 543.

351. *Answer:* 1, 5, 6

Rationale: Acute otitis media is an inflammatory disorder caused by an infection of the middle ear. The child often has fever, pain, loss of appetite, and possible ear drainage. The child also is irritable and lethargic and may roll the head or pull on or rub the affected ear. Otoscopic examination may reveal a red, opaque, bulging, and immobile tympanic membrane. Hearing loss may be noted, particularly in chronic otitis media. The child's fever should be treated with ibuprofen. The child is positioned on her or his affected side to facilitate drainage. A soft diet is recommended during the acute stage to avoid pain that can occur with chewing. Antibiotics are prescribed to treat the bacterial infection and should be administered for the full prescribed course. The ear should not be irrigated with normal saline because it can exacerbate the inflammation further. Antihistamines are not usually recommended as a part of therapy.

Test-Taking Strategy: Focus on the subject, care for the child with acute otitis media, and on the child's diagnosis and note the words *acute* and *right ear.* Think about the pathophysiology associated with the disorder and the associated manifestations to select the correct options.

Level of Cognitive Ability: Analyzing

Client Needs: Physiological Integrity

Integrated Process: Nursing Process—Planning

Content Area: Pediatrics: Eye/Ear

Health Problem: Pediatric-Specific: Acute and Chronic Otitis

Priority Concepts: Clinical Judgment; Infection

Reference: McKinney et al. (2018), pp. 1038-1039.

CHAPTER 35

Respiratory Problems

PRIORITY CONCEPTS Gas Exchange; Health Promotion

I. Epiglottitis

A. Description
1. Bacterial form of croup
2. Inflammation of the epiglottis occurs, which may be caused by *Haemophilus influenzae* type b or *Streptococcus pneumoniae;* children immunized with *H. influenzae* type b (Hib vaccine) are at less risk for epiglottitis.
3. Occurs most frequently in children 2 to 8 years old, but can occur from infancy to adulthood
4. Onset is abrupt, and the condition occurs most often in winter.
5. Considered an emergency situation because it can progress rapidly to severe respiratory distress.

B. Assessment
1. High fever
2. Sore, red, and inflamed throat (large, cherry red, edematous epiglottis) and pain on swallowing (Fig. 35-1)
3. Absence of spontaneous cough
4. Dysphonia (muffled voice), dysphagia, dyspnea, and drooling
5. Agitation
6. Retractions as the child struggles to breathe
7. Inspiratory stridor aggravated by the supine position
8. Tachycardia
9. Tachypnea progressing to more severe respiratory distress (hypoxia, hypercapnia, respiratory acidosis, decreased level of consciousness)
10. Tripod positioning: While supporting the body with the hands, the child leans forward, thrusts the chin forward, and opens the mouth in an attempt to widen the airway.
11. A fiberoptic nasal laryngectomy may be necessary to assist in diagnosis.

C. Interventions
1. Maintain a patent airway.
2. Assess respiratory status and breath sounds, noting nasal flaring, the use of accessory muscles, retractions, and the presence of stridor (Fig. 35-2).
3. Do not measure the temperature by the oral route.
4. Monitor pulse oximetry.
5. Prepare the child for lateral neck films to confirm the diagnosis (accompany the child to the radiology department).
6. Do not leave the child unattended.
7. Avoid placing the child in a supine position, because this position would affect the respiratory status further.
8. Maintain NPO (nothing by mouth) status.
9. Do not restrain the child or take any other measure that may agitate the child.
10. Administer intravenous (IV) fluids as prescribed; insertion of an IV line may need to be delayed until an adequate airway is established because this procedure may agitate the child.
11. Administer IV antibiotics as prescribed; these are usually followed by oral antibiotics (blood cultures before initiation of antibiotics may be necessary to identify the organism).
12. Administer analgesics and antipyretics (acetaminophen or ibuprofen) to reduce fever and throat pain as prescribed.
13. Administer corticosteroids to decrease inflammation and reduce throat edema as prescribed.
14. Heliox (mixture of helium and oxygen) may be prescribed; this medication reduces the work of breathing, reduces airway turbulence, and helps relieve airway obstruction.
15. Provide cool mist oxygen therapy as prescribed; high humidification cools the airway and decreases swelling.
16. Have resuscitation equipment available, and prepare for endotracheal intubation or tracheotomy for severe respiratory distress.
17. Ensure that the child is up to date with immunizations, including Hib conjugate vaccine (see Chapter 18).

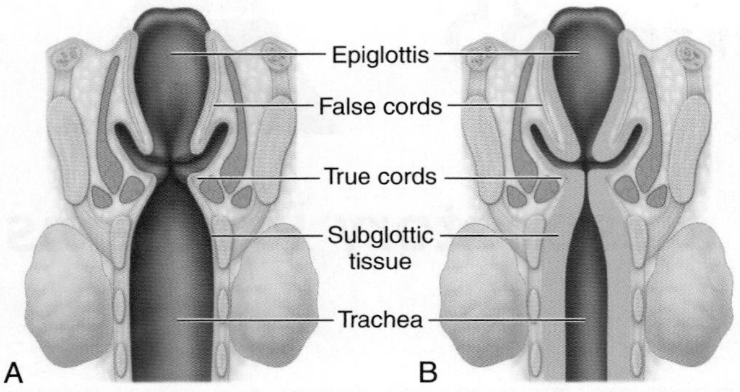

FIG. 35-1 **A,** Normal larynx. **B,** Obstruction and narrowing resulting from edema of croup.

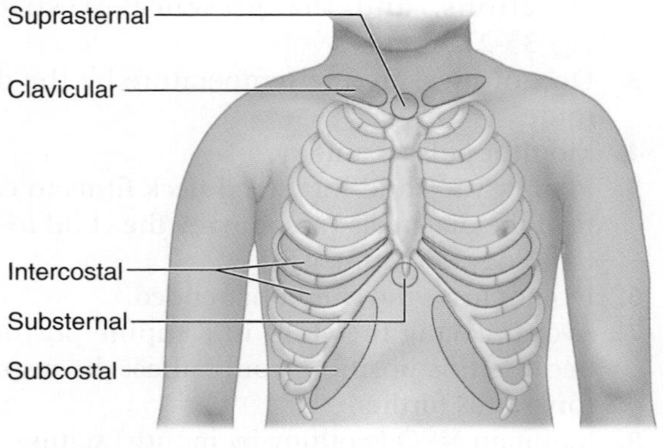

FIG. 35-2 Location of retractions.

⚠ If epiglottitis is suspected, no attempts should be made to visualize the posterior pharynx, obtain a throat culture, or take an oral temperature. Otherwise, spasm of the epiglottis can occur, leading to complete airway occlusion.

II. Laryngotracheobronchitis (Croup)

A. Description
1. Inflammation of the larynx, trachea, and bronchi.
2. Most common type of croup; may be viral or bacterial and most frequently occurs in children younger than 5 years.
3. Common causative organisms include parainfluenza virus types 2 and 3, respiratory syncytial virus (RSV), *Mycoplasma pneumoniae,* and influenza A and B.
4. Characterized by gradual onset that may be preceded by an upper respiratory infection.

B. Assessment (Box 35-1)

C. Interventions
1. Maintain a patent airway.
2. Assess respiratory status and monitor pulse oximetry; monitor for nasal flaring, sternal retraction, and inspiratory stridor (see Fig. 35-2).
3. Monitor for adequate respiratory exchange; monitor for pallor or **cyanosis**.
4. Elevate the head of the bed and provide rest.

BOX 35-1 Progression of Symptoms in Laryngotracheobronchitis

Stage I
- Low-grade fever
- Hoarseness
- Seal bark and brassy cough (croup cough)
- Inspiratory stridor
- Fear
- Irritability and restlessness

Stage II
- Continuous respiratory stridor
- Retractions
- Use of accessory muscles
- Crackles and wheezing
- Labored respirations

Stage III
- Continued restlessness
- Anxiety
- Pallor
- Diaphoresis
- Tachypnea
- Signs of anoxia and hypercapnia

Stage IV
- Intermittent cyanosis progressing to consistent cyanosis
- Apneic episodes progressing to cessation of breathing

Adapted from Perry S, Hockenberry M, Lowdermilk D, Wilson D: *Maternal-child nursing care,* ed 4, St. Louis, 2010, Mosby.

5. Provide humidified oxygen via a cool air or mist tent as prescribed for a hospitalized child (Table 35-1).
6. Instruct the parents to use a cool air vaporizer at home; other measures include having the child breathe in the cool night air or the air from an open freezer or taking the child to a cool basement or garage.
7. Provide and encourage fluid intake; IV fluids may be prescribed to maintain hydration status if the child is unable to take fluids orally.
8. Administer analgesics as prescribed to reduce fever.
9. Teach the parents to avoid administering cough syrups or cold medicines, which may dry and thicken secretions.
10. Administer corticosteroids if prescribed to reduce inflammation and edema.
11. Administer antibiotics as prescribed, noting that they are not indicated unless a bacterial infection is present.
12. Heliox (mixture of helium and oxygen) may be prescribed.
13. Have resuscitation equipment available.
14. Provide appropriate reassurance and education to the parents or caregivers.

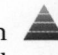

TABLE 35-1 Oxygen Delivery Systems: Advantages and Disadvantages

System	Advantages	Disadvantages
Oxygen mask	Various sizes available; delivers higher O_2 concentration than cannula Able to provide a predictable concentration of oxygen if Venturi mask is used, whether child breathes through nose or mouth	Skin irritation Fear of suffocation Accumulation of moisture on face Possibility of aspiration of vomitus Difficulty in controlling O_2 concentrations (except with Venturi mask)
Nasal cannula	Provides low-moderate O_2 concentration (22%-40%) Child is able to eat and talk while getting O_2 Possibility of more complete observation of child because nose and mouth remain unobstructed	Must have patent nasal passages May cause abdominal distention and discomfort or vomiting Difficulty controlling O_2 concentrations if child breathes through mouth Inability to provide mist if desired
Oxygen tent	Provides lower O_2 concentrations (FiO_2 up to 0.3-0.5) Child is able to receive desired inspired O_2 concentrations, even while eating	Necessity for tight fit around bed to prevent leakage of oxygen Cool and wet tent environment Poor access to child; inspired O_2 levels fall when tent is entered
Oxygen hood, face tent	Provides high O_2 concentrations (FiO_2 up to 1.00) Free access to child's chest for assessment	High-humidity environment Need to remove child for feeding and care

FiO_2, Fraction of inspired oxygen; *O_2*, oxygen.
Data from Hockenberry M, Wilson D: *Wong's nursing care of infants and children*, ed 9, St. Louis, 2011, Mosby.

Isolation precautions should be implemented for a hospitalized child with an upper respiratory infection until the cause of the infection is known.

III. Bronchitis

A. Description
1. Inflammation of the trachea and bronchi; may be referred to as *tracheobronchitis*
2. Usually occurs in association with an upper respiratory infection
3. Is usually a mild disorder; causative agent is most often viral

B. Assessment
1. Fever
2. Dry, hacking, and nonproductive cough that is worse at night and becomes productive in 2 to 3 days

C. Interventions
1. Treat symptoms as necessary.
2. Monitor for respiratory distress.
3. Provide cool, humidified air to the child.
4. Encourage increased fluid intake; child may drink beverages that he or she likes as long as the respiratory status is stable.
5. Administer antipyretics for fever as prescribed.
6. A cough suppressant may be prescribed to promote rest.

IV. Bronchiolitis and Respiratory Syncytial Virus (RSV)

A. Description
1. Bronchiolitis is an inflammation of the bronchioles that causes production of thick mucus that occludes bronchiole tubes and small bronchi.
2. RSV causes an acute viral infection and is a common cause of bronchiolitis (other organisms that cause bronchiolitis include adenoviruses, parainfluenza viruses, and human metapneumovirus).
3. RSV is highly communicable and is usually transferred via droplets or by direct contact with respiratory secretions.
4. RSV occurs primarily in the fall, winter, and spring.
5. RSV is rarer in children older than 2 years, with a peak incidence at approximately 6 months of age.
6. At-risk children include children who have a chronic or disabling condition and those who are immunocompromised.
7. Identification of the virus is done via testing of nasal or nasopharyngeal secretions.
8. Prevention measures include encouraging breast-feeding; avoiding tobacco smoke exposure; using good hand-washing techniques.
9. Administering palivizumab, a monoclonal antibody, to high-risk infants. See American Academy of Pediatrics for further information about palivizumab at http://www.aappublications.org/news/2017/10/19/RSV101917

B. Assessment (Box 35-2)

C. Interventions
1. For a child with bronchiolitis, interventions are aimed at treating symptoms and include airway maintenance, cool humidified air and oxygen, adequate fluid intake, and medications.

Pediatric

BOX 35-2 Assessment: Respiratory Syncytial Virus

Initial Manifestations
- Rhinorrhea
- Eye or ear drainage
- Pharyngitis
- Coughing
- Sneezing
- Wheezing
- Intermittent fever

Manifestations as Disease Progresses
- Increased coughing and wheezing
- Signs of air hunger
- Tachypnea and retractions
- Periods of cyanosis

Manifestations in Severe Illness
- Tachypnea more than 70 breaths per minute
- Decreased breath sounds and poor air exchange
- Listlessness
- Apneic episodes

Adapted from Perry S, Hockenberry M, Lowdermilk D, Wilson D: *Maternal-child nursing care*, ed 4, St. Louis, 2010, Mosby.

2. For a hospitalized child with RSV, place the child in a single room to prevent transmission of the virus.
3. Ensure that nurses caring for a child with RSV do not care for other high-risk children.
4. Use contact, droplet, and standard precautions during care; using good hand-washing techniques is necessary.
5. Monitor airway status and maintain a patent airway.
6. For most effective airway maintenance, position the child at a 30- to 40-degree angle with the neck slightly extended to maintain an open airway and decrease pressure on the diaphragm.
7. Provide cool, humidified oxygen as prescribed.
8. Monitor pulse oximetry levels.
9. Encourage fluids; fluids administered intravenously may be necessary until the acute stage has passed.
10. Periodic suctioning may be necessary if nasal secretions are copious; use of a bulb syringe for suctioning infants may be effective. Suctioning should be done before feeding to promote comfort and adequate intake.
11. Antiviral medication may be prescribed.

! Cough suppressants are administered with caution because they can interfere with the clearance of respiratory secretions.

V. Pneumonia

A. Description
1. Inflammation of the pulmonary parenchyma or alveoli or both, caused by a virus, mycoplasmal agents, bacteria, or aspiration of foreign substances.
2. The causative agent usually is introduced into the lungs through inhalation or from the bloodstream.
3. Viral pneumonia occurs more frequently than bacterial pneumonia, is seen in children of all ages, and often is associated with a viral upper respiratory infection.
4. Primary atypical pneumonia, usually caused by *Mycoplasma pneumoniae* or *Chlamydia pneumoniae*, occurs most often in the fall and winter months and is more common in crowded living conditions; it is most often seen in children 5 to 12 years old.
5. Bacterial pneumonia is often a serious infection requiring hospitalization when pleural effusion or empyema accompanies the disease; hospitalization is also necessary for children with staphylococcal pneumonia (*Streptococcus pneumoniae* is a common cause).
6. Aspiration pneumonia occurs when food, secretions, liquids, or other materials enter the lung and cause inflammation and a chemical pneumonitis. Classic symptoms include an increasing cough or fever with foul-smelling sputum, deteriorating results on chest x-rays, and other signs of airway involvement.
7. Prevention of viral and bacterial pneumonia includes immunization of infants and children with heptavalent pneumococcal conjugate vaccine (see Chapter 18).

B. Viral pneumonia
1. Assessment
   a. Acute or insidious onset
   b. Symptoms range from mild fever, slight cough, and malaise to high fever, severe cough, and diaphoresis.
   c. Nonproductive or productive cough of small amounts of whitish sputum
   d. Wheezes or fine **crackles**
2. Interventions
   a. Treatment is symptomatic.
   b. Administer oxygen with cool humidified air as prescribed.
   c. Increase fluid intake.
   d. Administer antipyretics for fever as prescribed.
   e. Administer chest physiotherapy and postural drainage as prescribed.

C. Primary atypical pneumonia
1. Assessment
   a. Acute or insidious onset
   b. Fever (lasting several days to 2 weeks), chills, anorexia, headache, malaise, and myalgia (muscle pain)

c. Rhinitis; sore throat; and dry, hacking cough
d. Nonproductive cough initially, progressing to production of seromucoid sputum that becomes mucopurulent or blood-streaked

2. Interventions
a. Treatment is symptomatic.
b. Recovery generally occurs in 7 to 10 days.

D. Bacterial pneumonia

1. Assessment
a. Acute onset
b. Infant: Irritability, lethargy, poor feeding; abrupt fever (may be accompanied by seizures); respiratory distress (air hunger, tachypnea, and circumoral cyanosis)
c. Older child: Headache, chills, abdominal pain, chest pain, meningeal symptoms (meningism)
d. Hacking, nonproductive cough
e. Diminished breath sounds or scattered crackles
f. With consolidation, decreased breath sounds are more pronounced.
g. As the infection resolves, the cough becomes productive and the child expectorates purulent sputum; coarse crackles and **wheezing** are noted.

2. Interventions
a. Blood cultures are taken and antibiotic therapy is initiated as soon as the diagnosis is suspected; in a hospitalized infant or child, IV antibiotics are usually prescribed.
b. Administer oxygen for respiratory distress as prescribed, and monitor oxygen saturation via pulse oximetry.
c. Place the child in a cool mist tent as prescribed; cool humidification moistens the airways and assists in temperature reduction.
d. Suction mucus from the infant, using a bulb syringe, to maintain a patent airway if the infant is unable to handle secretions.
e. Administer chest physiotherapy and postural drainage every 4 hours as prescribed.
f. Promote bed rest to conserve energy.
g. Encourage the child to lie on the affected side (if pneumonia is unilateral) to splint the chest and reduce the discomfort caused by pleural rubbing.
h. Encourage fluid intake (administer cautiously to prevent aspiration); intravenously administered fluids may be necessary.
i. Administer antipyretics for fever and bronchodilators as prescribed.
j. Monitor temperature frequently because of the risk for febrile seizures.
k. Institute isolation precautions with pneumococcal or staphylococcal pneumonia (according to agency policy).
l. Administer cough suppressant if prescribed before rest times and meals if the cough is disturbing (administered with caution because they can interfere with the clearance of respiratory secretions).
m. Continuous closed chest drainage may be necessary if purulent fluid is present (usually noted in *Staphylococcus* infections).
n. Fluid accumulation in the pleural cavity may be removed by thoracentesis; thoracentesis also provides a means for obtaining fluid for culture and for instilling antibiotics directly into the pleural cavity.

Children with a respiratory disorder should be monitored for weight loss and for signs of dehydration. Signs of dehydration include a sunken fontanel (infants), nonelastic skin turgor, decreased and concentrated urinary output, dry mucous membranes, and decreased tear production.

VI. Asthma

A. Description

1. Asthma is a chronic inflammatory disease of the airways (see Chapter 50).
2. Asthma is classified on the basis of disease severity; management includes medications, environmental control of allergens, and child and family education.
3. The allergic reaction in the airways caused by the precipitant can result in an immediate reaction with obstruction occurring, and it can result in a late bronchial obstructive reaction several hours after the initial exposure to the precipitant.
4. Mast cell release of histamine leads to a bronchoconstrictive process, bronchospasm, and obstruction.
5. Diagnosis is made on the basis of the child's symptoms, history and physical examination, chest radiograph, and laboratory tests (Box 35-3). See Table 35-2 for a classification system for asthma severity.
6. Precipitants may trigger an asthma attack (Box 35-4).
7. Status asthmaticus is the most severe form of an asthma attack that is unresponsive to repeated courses of beta-agonist therapy; this is a medical emergency that can result in respiratory failure and death if not recognized and vigorously treated.

B. Assessment

1. Child has episodes of dyspnea, wheezing, breathlessness, chest tightness, and cough, particularly at night or in the early morning or both.
2. Acute asthma attacks
a. Episodes include progressively worsening shortness of breath, cough, wheezing, chest tightness,

Pediatric

BOX 35-3 Laboratory Tests to Assist in Diagnosing Asthma

Pulmonary Function Tests: Spirometry testing assesses the presence and degree of disease and can determine the response to treatment.
Peak Expiratory Flow Rate Measurement: Measures maximum flow of air that can be forcefully exhaled in 1 second; child uses a peak expiratory flowmeter to determine a "personal best" value that can be used for comparison at other times, such as during and after an asthma attack.
Bronchoprovocation Testing: Testing that is done to identify inhaled allergens; mucous membranes are directly exposed to suspected allergen in increasing amounts.
Skin Testing: Done to identify specific allergens.
Exercise Challenges: Exercise is used to identify the occurrence of exercise-induced bronchospasm.
Radioallergosorbent Test: Blood test used to identify a specific allergen.
Chest Radiograph: May show hyperexpansion of the airways.

Note: Some tests place the child at risk for an asthma attack; testing should be done under close supervision.

decreases in expiratory airflow secondary to bronchospasm, mucosal edema, and mucus plugging; air is trapped behind occluded or narrow airways, and hypoxemia can occur.

b. The attack begins with irritability, restlessness, headache, feeling tired, or chest tightness; just before the attack, the child may present with itching localized at the front of the neck or over the upper part of the back.

c. Respiratory symptoms include a hacking, irritable, nonproductive cough caused by bronchial edema.

BOX 35-4 Examples of Precipitants Triggering an Asthma Attack

Allergens
Outdoor: Trees, shrubs, weeds, grasses, molds, pollen, air pollution, sand dust, spores
Indoor: Dust, dust mites, mold, cockroach antigen
Irritants: Tobacco smoke, wood smoke, odors, sprays
Exposure to Occupational Irritants
Exercise
Cold Air
Changes in Weather or Temperature
Environmental Change: Moving to a new home, starting a new school
Colds and Infections
Animals: Cats, dogs, rodents, horses
Medications: Aspirin, nonsteroidal antiinflammatory drugs, antibiotics, beta blockers
Strong Emotions: Fear, anger, laughing, crying
Conditions: Gastroesophageal reflux disease, tracheoesophageal fistula
Food Additives: Sulfite preservatives
Foods: Nuts, milk, other dairy products
Endocrine Factors: Menses, pregnancy, thyroid disease

Data from Perry S, Hockenberry M, Lowdermilk D, Wilson D: *Maternal-child nursing care*, ed 4, St. Louis, 2010, Mosby.

d. Accumulated secretions stimulate the cough; the cough becomes rattling, and there is production of frothy, clear, gelatinous sputum.

e. The child experiences retractions.

f. Hyperresonance on percussion of the chest is noted.

TABLE 35-2 Asthma Severity Classification System

Mild intermittent	Intermittent symptoms less than once per week Nighttime symptoms less than twice a month Asymptomatic and normal between exacerbations *FEV1 >80% predicted, *PFT >20% variability	Inhaled *SABA or cromolyn before exercise or allergen exposure No daily medications needed
Mild persistent	Symptoms more than 2 times/week but less than once/day May affect activity and sleep Nighttime symptoms more than twice a month FEV1 >80% predicted, PFT 20%-30% variability	One daily controlled medication, low-dose inhaled corticosteroid; cromolyn/nedocromil, leukotriene modifiers Inhaled SABA as needed
Moderate persistent	Daily symptoms, but not continual; nighttime symptoms more than once a week, but not every night Affect activity and sleep Daily use of SABA FEV1 60%-80% predicted, PFT >30%	Daily controller medications; combination inhaled medium-dose corticosteroid and LABA, especially for nighttime symptoms, cromolyn/nedocromil, leukotriene modifiers Inhaled SABA as needed
Severe persistent	Continuous daily symptoms Frequent nighttime symptoms Frequent exacerbations Physical activity limited by asthma FEV1 less than or equal to 60% predicted, PFT variability >30%	Inhaled SABA as needed Multiple daily controller meds, high-dose inhaled corticosteroid, *LABA, cromolyn/nedocromil, leukotriene modifiers, may need long-term corticosteroids

FEV1, Forced expiratory volume in 1 second; *LABA,* long-acting beta-adrenergic agonists; *PFT,* pulmonary function tests; *SABA,* short-acting beta-adrenergic agonists.
Adapted from Dunphy LM, Winland-Brown JE, Porter BO, Thomas DJ: *Primary care: the art and science of advanced practice nursing*, ed 4, Philadelphia, PA, 2015, FA Davis.

g. Breath sounds become coarse and loud, with crackles, coarse rhonchi, and inspiratory and expiratory wheezing; expiration is prolonged.
h. Child may be pale or flushed, and the lips may have a deep, dark-red color that may progress to cyanosis (also observed in the nail beds and skin, especially around the mouth).
i. Restlessness, apprehension, and diaphoresis occur.
j. Child speaks in short, broken phrases.
k. Younger children assume the tripod sitting position; older children sit upright, with the shoulders in a hunched-over position, the hands on the bed or a chair, and the arms braced to facilitate the use of the accessory muscles of breathing (child avoids a lying-down position).
l. Exercise-induced attack: Cough, shortness of breath, chest pain or tightness, wheezing, and endurance problems occur during exercise.
m. Severe spasm or obstruction: Breath sounds and wheezing cannot be heard (silent chest), and cough is ineffective (represents a lack of air movement).
n. Ventilatory failure and asphyxia: Shortness of breath, with air movement in the chest restricted to the point of absent breath sounds, is noted; this is accompanied by a sudden increase in the respiratory rate.

C. Interventions: Acute episode (see Priority Nursing Actions)

PRIORITY NURSING ACTIONS

Acute Asthma Attack

1. Assess airway patency and respiratory status.
2. Administer humidified oxygen by nasal cannula or face mask.
3. Administer quick-relief (rescue) medications.
4. Initiate an intravenous (IV) line.
5. Prepare the child for a chest radiograph and fiberoptic nasal laryngectomy if prescribed.
6. Prepare to obtain a blood sample for determining arterial blood gas levels if prescribed.

Reference
Hockenberry, Wilson, Rodgers (2017), p. 670.

D. Medications
1. Quick-relief medications (rescue medications): Used to treat symptoms and exacerbations (Box 35-5)
2. Long-term control medications (preventer medications): Used to achieve and maintain control of inflammation (Box 35-6)

BOX 35-5 Quick-Relief Medications (Rescue Medications)

- Short-acting β_2 agonists (for bronchodilation)
- Anticholinergics (for relief of acute bronchospasm)
- Systemic corticosteroids (for antiinflammatory action to treat reversible airflow obstruction)

BOX 35-6 Long-Term Control (Medications to Prevent Attacks)

- Inhaled corticosteroids (for antiinflammatory action)
- Antiallergy medications (to prevent an adverse response on exposure to an allergen)
- Nonsteroidal antiinflammatory drugs (for antiinflammatory action)
- Long-acting β_2 agonists (for long-acting bronchodilation)
- Leukotriene modifiers (to prevent bronchospasm and inflammatory cell infiltration)
- Monoclonal antibody (blocks binding of immunoglobulin E [IgE] to mast cells to inhibit inflammation)

⚠ Certain long-term control medications, such as long-acting beta-adrenergic agonists (LABAs), should not be given without an inhaled corticosteroid because of the risk for rebound bronchoconstriction.

3. Nebulizer, metered-dose inhaler (MDI): May be used to administer medications; if the child has difficulty using the MDI, medication can be administered by nebulization (medication is mixed with saline and then nebulized with compressed air by a machine).
4. If an MDI is used to administer a corticosteroid, a spacer should be used to prevent yeast infections in the child's mouth; the spacer prevents the medication being sprayed directly into the mouth, which can lead to irritation and possibly infection (thrush) in the mouth.
5. The child's growth patterns need to be monitored when corticosteroids are prescribed.

E. Chest physiotherapy
1. Includes breathing exercises and physical training.
2. Chest physiotherapy strengthens the respiratory musculature and produces more efficient breathing patterns.
3. Chest physiotherapy is not recommended during an acute exacerbation.

F. Allergen control
1. Testing may be done to identify allergens.
2. Teach the child and parents about measures to prevent and reduce exposure to allergens (see Box 35-4).

G. Home care measures
1. Instruct the family in measures to eliminate environmental allergens.
2. Avoid extremes of environmental temperature; in cold temperatures, instruct the child to breathe through the nose, not the mouth, and to cover the nose and mouth with a scarf.
3. Avoid exposure to individuals with a respiratory infection.
4. Instruct the child and family in how to recognize early symptoms of an asthma attack.
5. Teach the child and family about medications and how to use a nebulizer, MDI, or peak expiratory flowmeter (PEF).
6. The PEF measures how fast air comes out of the lungs after exhaling forcefully after inhaling fully.
7. Instruct the child and family about the importance of home monitoring of the peak expiratory flow rate; a decrease in the expiratory flow rate may indicate impending infection or exacerbation.
8. Instruct the child in the cleaning of devices used for inhaled medications (yeast infections can occur with the use of aerosolized corticosteroids).
9. Encourage adequate rest, sleep, and a well-balanced diet.
10. Instruct the child in the importance of adequate fluid intake to liquefy secretions.
11. Assist in developing an exercise program.
12. Instruct the child in the procedure for respiratory treatments and exercises as prescribed.
13. Encourage the child to cough effectively.
14. Encourage the parents to keep immunizations up to date; annual influenza vaccinations are recommended for children 6 months of age and older.
15. Inform other health care providers and school personnel of the asthma condition.
16. Allow the child to take control of self-care measures, based on age appropriateness.

VII. Cystic Fibrosis

A. Description (Fig. 35-3)
1. A chronic multisystem disorder (autosomal recessive trait disorder) characterized by exocrine gland dysfunction
2. The mucus produced by the exocrine glands is abnormally thick, tenacious, and copious, causing obstruction of the small passageways of the affected organs, particularly in the respiratory, gastrointestinal, and reproductive systems.
3. Common symptoms are associated with pancreatic enzyme deficiency and pancreatic fibrosis caused by duct blockage, progressive chronic lung disease as a result of infection, and sweat gland dysfunction resulting in increased sodium and chloride sweat concentrations.
4. An increase in sodium and chloride in sweat and saliva forms the basis for one diagnostic test, the sweat chloride test (Box 35-7).
5. Cystic fibrosis is a progressive and incurable disorder, and respiratory failure is a common cause of death; organ transplantations may be an option to increase survival rates.

B. Respiratory system
1. Symptoms are produced by the stagnation of mucus in the airway, leading to bacterial colonization and destruction of lung tissue.
2. Emphysema and atelectasis occur as the airways become increasingly obstructed.
3. Chronic hypoxemia causes contraction and hypertrophy of the muscle fibers in pulmonary arteries and arterioles, leading to pulmonary hypertension and eventual cor pulmonale.
4. Pneumothorax from ruptured bullae and hemoptysis from erosion of the bronchial wall occur as the disease progresses.
5. Other respiratory symptoms
   a. Wheezing and cough
   b. Dyspnea
   c. Cyanosis
   d. Clubbing of the fingers and toes
   e. Barrel chest
   f. Repeated episodes of bronchitis and pneumonia

C. Gastrointestinal system
1. Meconium ileus in the newborn is the earliest manifestation.
2. Intestinal obstruction (distal intestinal obstructive syndrome) caused by thick intestinal secretions can occur; signs include pain, abdominal distention, nausea, and vomiting.
3. Stools are frothy and foul-smelling.
4. Deficiency of the fat-soluble vitamins A, D, E, and K, which can result in easy bruising, bleeding, and anemia, occurs.
5. Malnutrition and failure to thrive is a concern.
6. Demonstration of hypoalbuminemia can occur from diminished absorption of protein, resulting in generalized edema.
7. Rectal prolapse can result from the large, bulky stools and increased intra-abdominal pressure.
8. Pancreatic fibrosis can occur and places the child at risk for diabetes mellitus.

D. Integumentary system
1. Abnormally high concentrations of sodium and chloride in sweat are noted.
2. Parents report that the infant tastes "salty" when kissed.
3. Dehydration and electrolyte imbalances can occur, especially during hyperthermic conditions.

E. Reproductive system
1. Cystic fibrosis can delay puberty in girls.

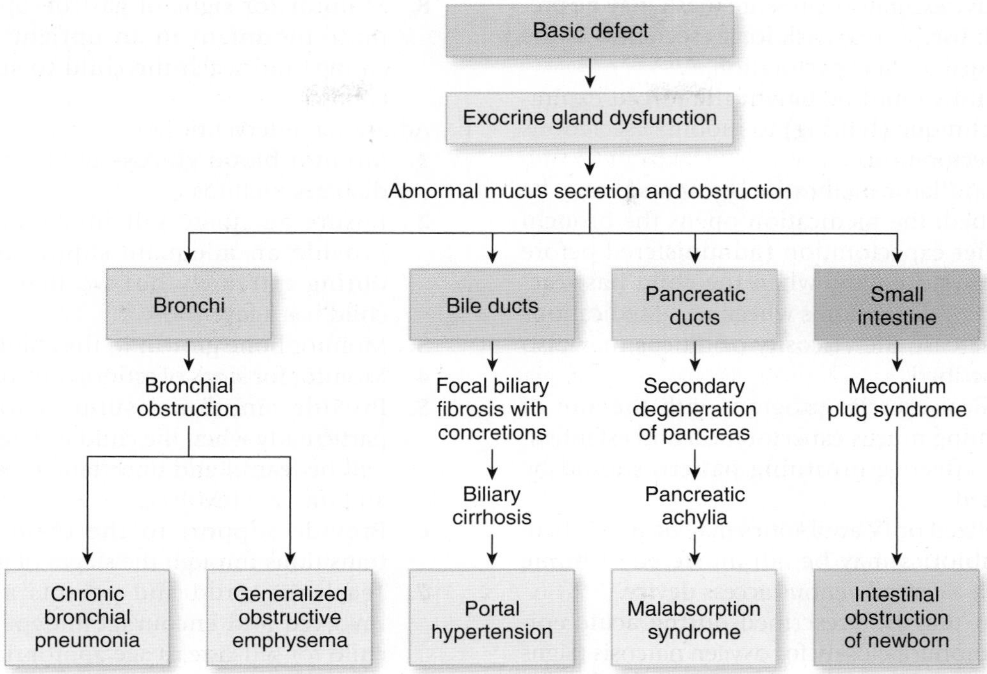

FIG. 35-3 Various effects of exocrine gland dysfunction in cystic fibrosis.

BOX 35-7 Quantitative Sweat Chloride Test

- Production of sweat is stimulated (pilocarpine iontophoresis), sweat is collected, and sweat electrolytes are measured (more than 75 mg of sweat is needed).
- Normally, the sweat chloride concentration is less than 40 mEq/L (40 mmol/L).
- Chloride concentration greater than 60 mEq/L (60 mmol/L) is a positive test result (higher than 40 mEq/L (40 mmol/L) is diagnostic in infants younger than 3 months of age.
- Chloride concentrations of 40 to 60 mEq/L (40 to 60 mmol/L) are highly suggestive of cystic fibrosis and require a repeat test.

2. Fertility can be inhibited by the highly viscous cervical secretions, which act as a plug and block sperm entry.
3. Males are usually sterile (but not impotent), caused by the blockage of the vas deferens by abnormal secretions or by failure of normal development of duct structures.

F. Diagnostic tests
1. Quantitative sweat chloride test is positive (see Box 35-7).
2. Newborn screening may be done in some states and may consist of immunoreactive trypsinogen analysis and direct DNA analysis for mutant genes.
3. Chest x-ray reveals atelectasis and obstructive emphysema.
4. Pulmonary function tests provide evidence of abnormal small airway function.
5. Stool, fat, enzyme analysis: A 72-hour stool sample is collected to check the fat or enzyme (trypsin) content, or both (food intake is recorded during the collection).

G. Interventions: Respiratory system
1. Goals of treatment include preventing and treating pulmonary infection by improving aeration, removing secretions, and administering antibiotic medications as prescribed.
2. Monitor respiratory status, including lung sounds and the presence and characteristics of a cough.
3. Chest physiotherapy (percussion and postural drainage) on awakening and in the evening (more frequently during pulmonary infection) needs to be done every day to maintain pulmonary hygiene; chest physiotherapy should not be performed before or immediately after a meal.
4. A Flutter mucus clearance device (a small, handheld plastic pipe with a stainless-steel ball on the inside) facilitates the removal of mucus and may be prescribed (store away from small children, because if the device separates, the steel ball poses a choking hazard).
5. Handheld percussors or a special vest device that provides high-frequency chest wall oscillation may be prescribed to help loosen secretions.

Pediatric

6. A positive expiratory pressure mask may be prescribed; use of this mask forces secretion to the upper airway for expectoration.
7. The child should be taught the forced expiratory technique (huffing) to mobilize secretions for expectoration.
8. Bronchodilator medication by aerosol may be prescribed; the medication opens the bronchi for easier expectoration (administered before chest physiotherapy when the child has reactive airway disease or is wheezing). Medications that decrease the viscosity of mucus may also be prescribed.
9. A physical exercise program with the aim of stimulating mucus expectoration and establishing an effective breathing pattern should be instituted.
10. Aerosolized or IV antibiotics may be prescribed; IV antibiotics may be administered at home through a central venous access device.
11. Oxygen may be prescribed during acute episodes; monitor closely for oxygen narcosis (signs include nausea and vomiting, malaise, fatigue, numbness and tingling of extremities, substernal distress), because a child with cystic fibrosis may have chronic carbon dioxide retention.
12. Lung transplantation may be an option.

H. Interventions: Gastrointestinal system
1. A child with cystic fibrosis requires a high-calorie, high-protein, and well-balanced diet to meet energy and growth needs; multivitamins and vitamins A, D, E, and K are also administered; for those with severe lung disease, energy requirements may be as high as 20% to 50% or more of the recommended daily allowance.
2. Monitor weight and for failure to thrive.
3. Monitor stool patterns and for signs of intestinal obstruction.
4. The goal of treatment for pancreatic insufficiency is to replace pancreatic enzymes; pancreatic enzymes are administered within 30 minutes of eating and administered with all meals and all snacks (enzymes should not be given if the child is NPO).
5. The amount of pancreatic enzymes administered depends on the primary health care provider's (PHCP's) preference and usually is adjusted to achieve normal growth and a decrease in the number of stools to 2 or 3 daily (additional enzymes are needed if the child is consuming high-fat foods).
6. Enteric-coated pancreatic enzymes should not be crushed or chewed; capsules can be taken apart, and the contents can be sprinkled on a small amount of food for administration.
7. Monitor for constipation, intestinal obstruction, and rectal prolapse.
8. Monitor for signs of gastroesophageal reflux; place the infant in an upright position after eating, and teach the child to sit upright after eating.

I. Additional interventions
1. Monitor blood glucose levels and for signs of diabetes mellitus.
2. Ensure adequate salt intake and fluids that provide an adequate supply of electrolytes during extremely hot weather and when the child has a fever.
3. Monitor bone growth in the child.
4. Monitor for signs of retinopathy or nephropathy.
5. Provide emotional support to the parents, particularly when the child is diagnosed; parents will be fearful and uncertain about the disorder and the care involved.
6. Provide support to the child as he or she transitions through the stages of growth.
7. Teach the child and parents about the care involved and encourage independence in the child for self-care as age appropriate.

J. Home care
1. Home care involves educating the parents and the child about all aspects of care for the disorder.
2. Inform the parents and child about the signs of complications and actions to take and that the importance of follow-up care is crucial.
3. Instruct the parents to ensure that the child receives the recommended immunizations on schedule; in addition, annual influenza vaccinations are recommended for children 6 months of age and older.
4. Inform the child and parents about the Cystic Fibrosis Foundation.

An alteration in respiratory status can be a frightening experience for the child and parents. A calm and reassuring nursing approach assists in reducing fear.

VIII. Sudden Infant Death Syndrome (SIDS)

A. Description
1. *SIDS* refers to unexpected death of an apparently healthy infant younger than 1 year for whom an investigation of the death and a thorough autopsy fail to show an adequate cause of death.
2. Several theories are proposed regarding the cause of SIDS, but the exact cause is unknown.
3. SIDS most frequently occurs during winter months.
4. Death usually occurs during sleep periods, but not necessarily at night.
5. SIDS most frequently affects infants 2 to 3 months of age.
6. Incidence is higher in boys.

7. Incidence is higher in Native Americans, African Americans, and Hispanics and in lower socioeconomic groups.
8. Incidence has been found to be lower in breast-fed infants and infants sleeping with a pacifier.
9. High-risk conditions for SIDS:
   a. Prone position
   b. Use of soft bedding, sleeping in a noninfant bed such as a sofa
   c. Overheating (thermal stress)
   d. Cosleeping
   e. Mother who smoked cigarettes or abused substances during pregnancy
   f. Exposure to tobacco smoke after birth

B. Assessment
1. Infant is apneic, blue, and lifeless.
2. Frothy blood-tinged fluid is in the nose and mouth.
3. Infant may be found in any position, but typically is found in a disheveled bed, with blankets over the head, and huddled in a corner.
4. Infants may appear to have been clutching bedding.
5. Diaper may be wet and full of stool.

C. Prevention and interventions
1. Infants should be placed in the supine position for sleep.
2. Mother needs to be taught about the risk factors: cigarette smoking and substance **abuse** during pregnancy; use of soft bedding, sleeping in a non-infant bed such as a sofa; overheating (thermal stress); cosleeping; exposure to tobacco smoke after birth. Stuffed animals or other toys should be removed from the crib while the infant is sleeping.
3. Teach the parents to monitor for positional plagiocephaly caused by the supine sleeping position; signs include flattened posterior occiput and development of a bald spot in the posterior occiput area.
4. To assist in preventing positional plagiocephaly, teach the parents to alter head position during sleep, avoid excessive time in infant seats and bouncers, and place the infant in a prone position while awake (monitor the infant when in the prone position).
5. If SIDS occurs, the parents need a great deal of support as they grieve and mourn, especially because the event was sudden, unexpected, and unexplained.

IX. Foreign Body Aspiration

A. Description (Fig. 35-4)
1. Swallowing and aspiration of a foreign body into the air passages
2. Most inhaled foreign bodies lodge in the main stem or lobar bronchus.
3. Most common offending foods are round in shape and include items such as hot dogs, candy, peanuts, popcorn, or grapes.

B. Assessment
1. Initially, choking, gagging, coughing, and retractions are general findings.
2. If the condition worsens, cyanosis may occur.
3. Laryngotracheal obstruction leads to dyspnea, stridor, cough, and hoarseness.
4. Bronchial obstruction produces paroxysmal cough, wheezing, asymmetrical breath sounds, and dyspnea.
5. If any obstruction progresses, unconsciousness and asphyxiation may occur.
6. Partial obstructions may occur without symptoms.
7. Distressed child cannot speak, becomes cyanotic, and collapses.

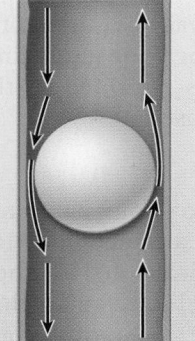

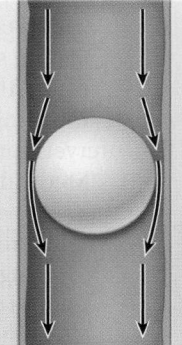

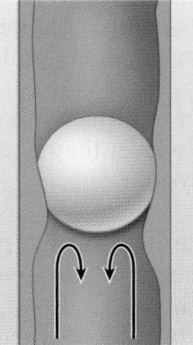

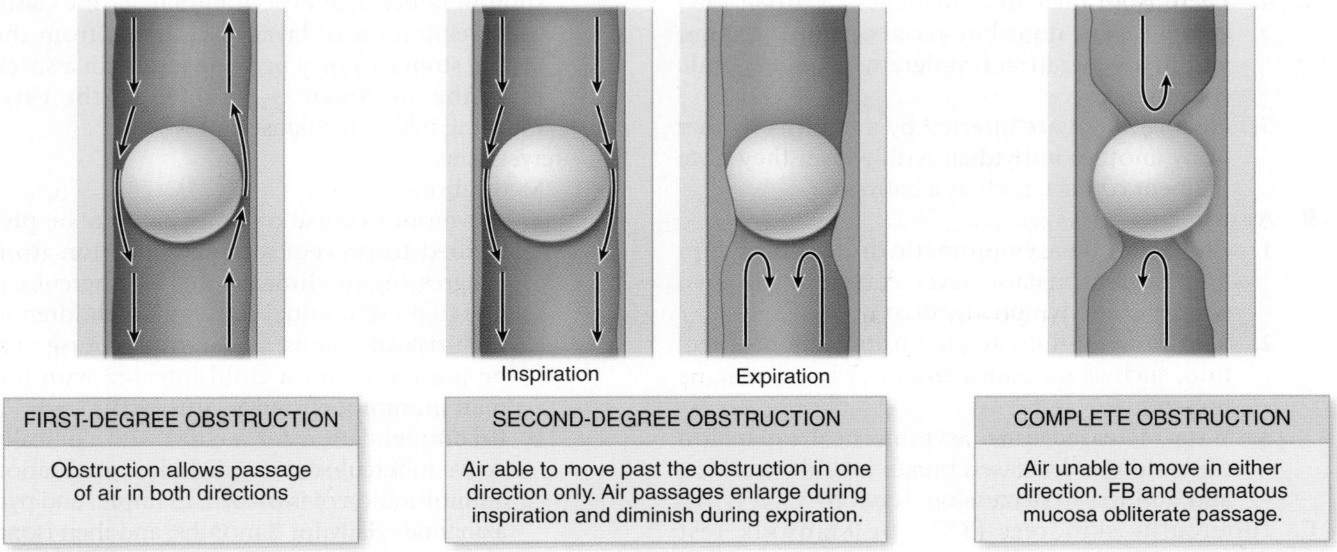

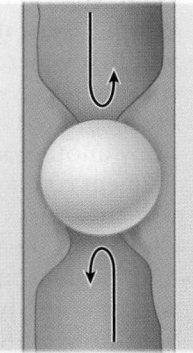

Inspiration
Expiration
FIRST-DEGREE OBSTRUCTION
Obstruction allows passage of air in both directions
SECOND-DEGREE OBSTRUCTION
Air able to move past the obstruction in one direction only. Air passages enlarge during inspiration and diminish during expiration.
COMPLETE OBSTRUCTION
Air unable to move in either direction. FB and edematous mucosa obliterate passage.

FIG. 35-4 Mechanisms of airway obstruction by a foreign body (FB).

C. Interventions: Abdominal thrust maneuver is used for the removal of a foreign body (or relief of choking) in a child; refer to the American Heart Association document at https://hinman.org/Clinicians/Handouts/2017/Th113-Th114-Fr141-Fr142.pdf.
1. Emergency care
2. After instituting emergency care measures, removal by endoscopy may be necessary.
   a. After endoscopy, the child receives high-humidity air.
   b. Observe for signs and symptoms of airway edema.
3. Prevention
   a. Keep small objects, including rubber balloons, out of reach of small children.
   b. Avoid giving small children small, round food items.
4. Parent, day care provider, and babysitter education
   a. Teach about the hazards of aspiration.
   b. Discuss potential situations in which small items may be aspirated.
   c. Teach about the symptoms of aspiration.
   d. Teach how to perform emergency care measures.

X. Tuberculosis

A. Description
1. Tuberculosis is a contagious disease caused by *Mycobacterium tuberculosis,* an acid-fast bacillus (see Chapter 50).
2. Multidrug-resistant strains of *M. tuberculosis* occur because of child or family noncompliance with therapeutic regimens.
3. The route of transmission of *M. tuberculosis* is through inhalation of droplets from an individual with active tuberculosis.
4. There is an increased incidence in urban low-income areas, nonwhite racial or ethnic groups, and first-generation immigrants from endemic countries.
5. Most children are infected by a family member or by another individual with whom they have frequent contact, such as a babysitter.

B. Assessment
1. Child may be asymptomatic or develop symptoms such as malaise, fever, cough, weight loss, anorexia, and lymphadenopathy.
2. Specific symptoms related to the site of infection, such as the lungs, brain, or bone, may be present.
3. With increased time, asymmetrical expansion of the lungs, decreased breath sounds, crackles, and dullness to percussion develop.

C. Tuberculin skin test (TST) or Mantoux test (Box 35-8)

BOX 35-8 Tuberculin Skin Test or Mantoux Test Interpretation

- Induration measuring 15 mm or more is considered to be a positive reaction in children 4 years or older who do not have any risk factors.
- Induration measuring 10 mm or more is considered to be a positive reaction in children younger than 4 years and in children with chronic illness or at high risk for exposure to tuberculosis.
- Induration measuring 5 mm or more is considered to be positive for the highest-risk groups, such as children with immunosuppressive conditions or human immunodeficiency virus (HIV) infection.

1. The test produces a positive reaction 2 to 10 weeks after the initial infection.
2. The test determines whether a child has been infected and has developed a sensitivity to the protein of the tubercle **bacillus**; a positive reaction does not confirm the presence of active disease (exposure versus presence).
3. After a child reacts positively, the child will always react positively; a positive reaction in a previously negative child indicates that the child has been infected since the last test.
4. Tuberculosis testing should not be done at the same time as measles immunization (viral interference from the measles vaccine may cause a false-negative result).

D. Sputum culture
1. A definitive diagnosis is made by showing the presence of mycobacteria in a culture.
2. Chest x-rays are supplemental to sputum cultures and are not definitive alone.
3. Because an infant or young child often swallows sputum rather than expectorates it, gastric washings (aspiration of lavaged contents from the fasting stomach) may be done to obtain a specimen; the specimen is obtained in the early morning before breakfast.

E. Interventions
1. Medications
   a. A 9-month course of isoniazid may be prescribed to prevent a latent infection from progressing to clinically active tuberculosis and to prevent initial infection in children in high-risk situations; a 12-month course may be prescribed for a child infected with human immunodeficiency virus (HIV).
   b. Recommendation for a child with clinically active tuberculosis may include combination administration of isoniazid, rifampin, and pyrazinamide daily for 2 months, and then isoniazid and rifampin twice weekly for 4 months.

c. Inform the parents and child that bodily fluids, including urine, may turn an orange-red color with some tuberculosis medications.
d. Directly observed therapy may be necessary for some children.

2. Place children with active disease who are contagious on respiratory isolation until medications have been initiated, sputum cultures show a diminished number of organisms, and cough is improving; this includes use of a personally fitted air-purifying N95 or N100 respirator (mask) by the nurse caring for the child.
3. Stress the importance of adequate rest and adequate diet.
4. Instruct the child and family about measures to prevent the transmission of tuberculosis.
5. Case finding and follow-up with known contacts is crucial to decrease the number of cases of individuals with active tuberculosis.

PRACTICE QUESTIONS

352. A 10-year-old child with asthma is treated for acute exacerbation in the emergency department. The nurse caring for the child should monitor for which sign, knowing that it indicates a worsening of the condition?
1. Warm, dry skin
2. Decreased wheezing
3. Pulse rate of 90 beats per minute
4. Respirations of 18 breaths per minute

353. The mother of an 8-year-old child being treated for right lower lobe pneumonia at home calls the clinic nurse. The mother tells the nurse that the child complains of discomfort on the right side and that ibuprofen is not effective. Which instruction should the nurse provide to the mother?
1. Increase the dose of ibuprofen.
2. Increase the frequency of ibuprofen.
3. Encourage the child to lie on the left side.
4. Encourage the child to lie on the right side.

354. A new parent expresses concern to the nurse regarding sudden infant death syndrome (SIDS). She asks the nurse how to position her new infant for sleep. In which position should the nurse tell the parent to place the infant?
1. Side or prone
2. Back or prone
3. Stomach with the face turned
4. Back rather than on the stomach

355. The clinic nurse is providing instructions to a parent of a child with cystic fibrosis regarding the immunization schedule for the child. Which statement should the nurse make to the parent?
1. "The immunization schedule will need to be altered."
2. "The child should not receive any hepatitis vaccines."
3. "The child will receive all of the immunizations except for the polio series."
4. "The child will receive the recommended basic series of immunizations along with a yearly influenza vaccination."

356. The emergency department nurse is caring for a child diagnosed with epiglottitis. In assessing the child, the nurse should monitor for which indication that the child may be experiencing airway obstruction?
1. The child exhibits nasal flaring and bradycardia.
2. The child is leaning forward, with the chin thrust out.
3. The child has a low-grade fever and complains of a sore throat.
4. The child is leaning backward, supporting herself or himself with the hands and arms.

357. A child with laryngotracheobronchitis (croup) is placed in a cool mist tent. The mother becomes concerned because the child is frightened, consistently crying, and trying to climb out of the tent. Which is the **most appropriate** nursing action?
1. Tell the mother that the child must stay in the tent.
2. Place a toy in the tent to make the child feel more comfortable.
3. Call the pediatrician and obtain a prescription for a mild sedative.
4. Let the mother hold the child and direct the cool mist over the child's face.

358. The clinic nurse reads the results of a tuberculin skin test (TST) on a 3-year-old child. The results indicate an area of induration measuring 10 mm. The nurse should interpret these results as which finding?
1. Positive
2. Negative
3. Inconclusive
4. Definitive and requiring a repeat test

359. The mother of a hospitalized 2-year-old child with viral laryngotracheobronchitis (croup) asks the nurse why the pediatrician did not prescribe antibiotics. Which response should the nurse make?
1. "The child may be allergic to antibiotics."
2. "The child is too young to receive antibiotics."
3. "Antibiotics are not indicated unless a bacterial infection is present."
4. "The child still has the maternal antibodies from birth and does not need antibiotics."

360. The nurse is caring for an infant with bronchiolitis, and diagnostic tests have confirmed respiratory syncytial virus (RSV). On the basis of this finding, which is the **most appropriate** nursing action?

1. Initiate strict enteric precautions.
2. Move the infant to a private room.
3. Leave the infant in the present room, because RSV is not contagious.
4. Inform the staff that using standard precautions is all that is necessary when caring for the child.

361. The nurse is preparing for the admission of an infant with a diagnosis of bronchiolitis caused by respiratory syncytial virus (RSV). Which interventions should the nurse include in the plan of care? **Select all that apply.**

- ☐ 1. Place the infant in a private room.
- ☐ 2. Ensure that the infant's head is in a flexed position.
- ☐ 3. Wear a mask, gown, and gloves when in contact with the infant.
- ☐ 4. Place the infant in a tent that delivers warm humidified air.
- ☐ 5. Position the infant on the side, with the head lower than the chest.
- ☐ 6. Ensure that nurses caring for the infant with RSV do not care for other high-risk children.

ANSWERS

352. ***Answer:*** 2

Rationale: Asthma is a chronic inflammatory disease of the airways. Decreased wheezing in a child with asthma may be interpreted incorrectly as a positive sign when it may actually signal an inability to move air. A "silent chest" is an ominous sign during an asthma episode. With treatment, increased wheezing actually may signal that the child's condition is improving. Warm, dry skin indicates an improvement in the child's condition, because the child is normally diaphoretic during exacerbation. The normal pulse rate in a 10-year-old is 70 to 110 beats per minute. The normal respiratory rate in a 10-year-old is 16 to 20 breaths per minute.

Test-Taking Strategy: Note the word *worsening* in the question. Options 3 and 4 can be eliminated because they are comparable or alike in that they are normal vital signs. From the remaining options, recall that a "silent chest" is an ominous sign during an asthma episode and indicates severe bronchial spasm or obstruction.

Level of Cognitive Ability: Analyzing

Client Needs: Physiological Integrity

Integrated Process: Nursing Process—Analysis

Content Area: Pediatrics: Throat/Respiratory

Health Problem: Pediatric-Specific: Asthma

Priority Concepts: Clinical Judgment; Gas Exchange

Reference: McKinney et al. (2018), p. 1057.

353. ***Answer:*** 4

Rationale: Pneumonia is an inflammation of the pulmonary parenchyma or alveoli, or both, caused by a virus, mycoplasmal agents, bacteria, or aspiration of foreign substances. Splinting of the affected side by lying on that side may decrease discomfort. It would be inappropriate to advise the mother to increase the dose or frequency of the ibuprofen. Lying on the left side would not be helpful in alleviating discomfort.

Test-Taking Strategy: Options 1 and 2 can be eliminated because they are comparable or alike. Recall that the nurse does not adjust the dose or frequency of medications. Recalling the principles related to splinting an incision in the postoperative client will assist in directing you to the correct option, because these principles can be applied in this situation.

Level of Cognitive Ability: Applying

Client Needs: Physiological Integrity

Integrated Process: Nursing Process—Implementation

Content Area: Pediatrics: Throat/Respiratory

Health Problem: Pediatric-Specific: Pneumonia

Priority Concepts: Client Education; Pain

Reference: McKinney et al. (2018), p. 1051.

354. ***Answer:*** 4

Rationale: SIDS is the unexpected death of an apparently healthy infant younger than 1 year for whom an investigation of the death and a thorough autopsy fail to show an adequate cause of death. Several theories are proposed regarding the cause, but the exact cause is unknown. Nurses should encourage parents to place the infant on the back (supine) for sleep. Infants in the prone position (on the stomach) may be unable to move their heads to the side, increasing the risk of suffocation. The infant may have the ability to turn to a prone position from the side-lying position.

Test-Taking Strategy: Eliminate options 1, 2, and 3 because they are comparable or alike. Remember that the infant needs to be placed on her or his back.

Level of Cognitive Ability: Applying

Client Needs: Safe and Effective Care Environment

Integrated Process: Teaching and Learning

Content Area: Pediatrics: Throat/Respiratory

Health Problem: Pediatric-Specific: Sudden infant death syndrome (SIDS)

Priority Concepts: Client Education; Safety

Reference: McKinney et al. (2018), p. 1056.

355. ***Answer:*** 4

Rationale: Cystic fibrosis is a chronic multisystem disorder (autosomal recessive trait disorder) characterized by exocrine gland dysfunction. The mucus produced by the exocrine glands is abnormally thick, tenacious, and copious, causing obstruction of the small passageways of the affected organs, particularly in the respiratory, gastrointestinal, and reproductive

systems. Adequately protecting children with cystic fibrosis from communicable diseases by immunization is essential. In addition to the basic series of immunizations, a yearly influenza immunization is recommended for children with cystic fibrosis. Options 1, 2, and 3 are incorrect.
Test-Taking Strategy: Eliminate options 1, 2, and 3 because they are comparable or alike, indicating that the immunization schedule will be adjusted in some way. Recalling the importance of protection from communicable diseases, particularly in children with a disorder such as cystic fibrosis, will assist in directing you to the correct option.
Level of Cognitive Ability: Applying
Client Needs: Health Promotion and Maintenance
Integrated Process: Teaching and Learning
Content Area: Pediatrics: Throat/Respiratory
Health Problem: Pediatric-Specific: Cystic fibrosis
Priority Concepts: Client Education; Health Promotion
Reference: McKinney et al. (2018), p. 1071.
https://www.cdc.gov/vaccines/schedules/hcp/child-adolescent.html

356. *Answer:* 2
Rationale: Epiglottitis is a bacterial form of croup. A primary concern is that it can progress to acute respiratory distress. Clinical manifestations suggestive of airway obstruction include tripod positioning (leaning forward while supported by arms, chin thrust out, mouth open), nasal flaring, the use of accessory muscles for breathing, and the presence of stridor. Option 4 is an incorrect position. Options 1 and 3 are incorrect because epiglottitis causes tachycardia and a high fever.
Test-Taking Strategy: Focus on the subject, manifestations of airway obstruction in a child with epiglottitis. Eliminate option 1 first, because tachycardia rather than bradycardia would occur in a child experiencing respiratory distress. Eliminate option 3 next, knowing that a high fever occurs with epiglottitis. From the remaining options, visualize the descriptions in each and determine which position would best assist a child experiencing respiratory distress.
Level of Cognitive Ability: Analyzing
Client Needs: Physiological Integrity
Integrated Process: Nursing Process—Assessment
Content Area: Pediatrics: Throat/Respiratory
Health Problem: Pediatric-Specific: Croup
Priority Concepts: Clinical Judgment; Gas Exchange
Reference: McKinney et al. (2018), pp. 1046-1047.

357. *Answer:* 4
Rationale: Laryngotracheobronchitis (croup) is the inflammation of the larynx, trachea, and bronchi and is the most common type of croup. Cool mist therapy may be prescribed to liquefy secretions and to assist in breathing. If the use of a tent or hood is causing distress, treatment may be more effective if the child is held by the parent and a cool mist is directed toward the child's face (blow-by). A mild sedative would not be administered to the child. Crying would increase hypoxia and aggravate laryngospasm, which may cause airway obstruction. Options 1 and 2 would not alleviate the child's fear.
Test-Taking Strategy: Note the strategic words, *most appropriate*. Focus on the subject, the child's fear. Options 1, 2, and 3 are comparable or alike in that they do not address the fear. The correct option is the one that addresses the subject of the question.
Level of Cognitive Ability: Applying
Client Needs: Psychosocial Integrity
Integrated Process: Caring
Content Area: Pediatrics: Throat/Respiratory
Health Problem: Pediatric-Specific: Croup
Priority Concepts: Caregiving; Clinical Judgment
Reference: Hockenberry, Wilson, Rodgers (2017), p. 650.

358. *Answer:* 1
Rationale: Induration measuring 10 mm or more is considered to be a positive result in children younger than 4 years of age and in children with chronic illness or at high risk for exposure to tuberculosis. A reaction of 5 mm or more is considered to be a positive result for the highest risk groups, such as a child with an immunosuppressive condition or a child with human immunodeficiency virus (HIV) infection. A reaction of 15 mm or more is positive in children 4 years or older without any risk factors.
Test-Taking Strategy: Options 3 and 4 are comparable or alike and can be eliminated first. From the remaining options, focus on the data in the question and note the child's age to assist in directing you to the correct option.
Level of Cognitive Ability: Analyzing
Client Needs: Physiological Integrity
Integrated Process: Nursing Process—Analysis
Content Area: Pediatrics: Throat/Respiratory
Health Problem: Pediatric-Specific: Tuberculosis
Priority Concepts: Evidence; Infection
Reference: Hockenberry, Wilson, Rodgers (2017), pp. 657-658.

359. *Answer:* 3
Rationale: Laryngotracheobronchitis (croup) is the inflammation of the larynx, trachea, and bronchi and is the most common type of croup. It can be viral or bacterial. Antibiotics are not indicated in the treatment of croup unless a bacterial infection is present. Options 1, 2, and 4 are incorrect. In addition, no supporting data in the question indicate that the child may be allergic to antibiotics.
Test-Taking Strategy: Focus on the subject, indications for the use of antibiotics. Eliminate option 1 because there are no supporting data in the question regarding the potential for allergies. Noting the word *viral* in the question and noting the age of the child will assist in eliminating options 2 and 4.
Level of Cognitive Ability: Applying
Client Needs: Physiological Integrity
Integrated Process: Teaching and Learning
Content Area: Pediatrics: Throat/Respiratory
Health Problem: Pediatric-Specific: Croup
Priority Concepts: Immunity; Inflammation
Reference: McKinney et al. (2018), p. 1043.

360. *Answer:* 2
Rationale: RSV is a highly communicable disorder and is transmitted via droplets and direct contact with respiratory secretions. Use of contact, droplet, and standard precautions during care is necessary. Using good hand-washing technique and wearing gloves, gown, and a mask should be done to prevent transmission. An infant with RSV should be placed in a private room to prevent transmission. Enteric precautions are unnecessary.

Test-Taking Strategy: Note the strategic words, *most appropriate.* Focus on the subject, the method of transmission of RSV. Remember that the virus is transmitted via droplets and direct contact with respiratory secretions. An infant with RSV is contagious and should be placed in a private room.
Level of Cognitive Ability: Applying
Client Needs: Safe and Effective Care Environment
Integrated Process: Nursing Process—Implementation
Content Area: Pediatrics: Throat/Respiratory
Health Problem: Pediatric-Specific: Bronchitis/bronchiolitis/respiratory syncytial virus
Priority Concepts: Infection; Safety
Reference: Hockenberry, Wilson, Rodgers (2017), pp. 652-653.

361. *Answer:* 1, 3, 6
Rationale: RSV is a highly communicable disorder and is transmitted via droplets or contact with respiratory secretions. Use of contact, droplet, and standard precautions during care (wearing gloves, mask, and a gown) reduces nosocomial transmission of RSV. In addition, it is important to ensure that nurses caring for a child with RSV do not care for other high-risk children to prevent the transmission of the infection. An infant with RSV should be placed in a private room. The infant should be positioned with the head and chest at a 30- to 40-degree angle and the neck slightly extended to maintain an open airway and decrease pressure on the diaphragm. Cool humidified oxygen is delivered to relieve dyspnea, hypoxemia, and insensible water loss from tachypnea.
Test-Taking Strategy: Focus on the subject, care of the child with bronchiolitis and RSV. Recalling the mode of transmission of RSV will assist in answering correctly. Remember that RSV is highly communicable and is transmitted via droplets or direct contact with respiratory secretions.
Level of Cognitive Ability: Analyzing
Client Needs: Safe and Effective Care Environment
Integrated Process: Nursing Process—Planning
Content Area: Pediatrics: Throat/Respiratory
Health Problem: Pediatric-Specific: Bronchitis/bronchiolitis/respiratory syncytial virus
Priority Concepts: Care Coordination; Safety
Reference: McKinney et al. (2018), pp. 1049-1050.

CHAPTER 36

Cardiovascular Problems

PRIORITY CONCEPTS Gas Exchange; Perfusion

I. Hyperlipidemia

A. Description

1. A condition in which there are high levels of lipids circulating in the blood, which can predispose a child to heart disease.

2. Laboratory values for lipids for individuals aged 2 to 19 years are as follows:

a. Total cholesterol: less than 170 mg/dL (4.25 mmol/L) is acceptable, 170 to 199 mg/dL (4.25 to 4.9 mmol/L) is borderline, 200 mg/dL (5 mmol/L) or greater is high.

b. Low-density lipoprotein cholesterol: less than 110 mg/dL (2.75 mmol/L) is acceptable, 110 to 129 mg/dL (2.75 to 3.22 mmol/L) is borderline, 130 mg/dL (3.25 mmol/L) or greater is high.

c. High-density lipoprotein cholesterol: greater than 45 mg/dL (1.12 mmol/L) is acceptable, 40 to 45 mg/dL (1.0 to 1.12 mmol/L) is borderline, less than 40 mg/dL (1.0 mmol/L) is low.

d. Triglycerides: less than 100 mg/dL (1.14 mmol/L) for 9 years and younger is acceptable; less than 130 mg/dL (1.48 mmol/L) for 10 years and older is acceptable.

e. Any person with hyperlipidemia as a child is likely to have the condition later in life, and it predisposes them to cardiac events.

f. Referral to a specialist (cardiology) should be made if there is an elevation in any of the above values.

g. Treatment focuses on lifestyle modifications and behavior changes. See Box 32-1 for recommended dietary and physical activity changes for preventing diabetes mellitus, which also applies with the treatment focus for hyperlipidemia.

II. Heart Failure (HF)

A. Description

1. HF (Box 36-1) is the inability of the heart to pump a sufficient amount of blood to meet the metabolic and oxygen needs of the body.

2. In infants and children, inadequate cardiac output most commonly is caused by congenital heart defects (**shunt**, obstruction, or a combination of both) that produce an excessive volume or pressure load on the myocardium.

3. In infants and children, a combination of left-sided and right-sided HF is usually present.

4. The goals of treatment are to improve cardiac function, remove accumulated fluid and sodium, decrease cardiac demands, improve tissue oxygenation, and decrease oxygen consumption; depending on the cause, surgery may be required.

B. Assessment of early signs

1. Tachycardia, especially during rest and slight exertion

2. Tachypnea

3. Profuse scalp diaphoresis, especially in infants

4. Fatigue and irritability

5. Sudden weight gain

6. Respiratory distress

C. Interventions

1. Monitor for early signs of HF.

2. Monitor for respiratory distress (count respirations for 1 minute).

3. Monitor apical pulse (count apical pulse for 1 minute), and monitor for dysrhythmias.

4. Monitor temperature for hyperthermia and for other signs of infection, particularly respiratory infection.

5. Monitor strict intake and output; weigh diapers as appropriate for most accurate output.

6. Monitor daily weight to assess for fluid retention; a weight gain of 0.5 kg (1 lb) in 1 day is caused by the accumulation of fluid.

7. Monitor for facial or peripheral dependent edema, auscultate lung sounds, and report abnormal findings indicating excessive fluid in the body.

8. Elevate the head of the bed in a semi-Fowler's position.

9. Maintain a neutral thermal environment to prevent cold stress in infants.

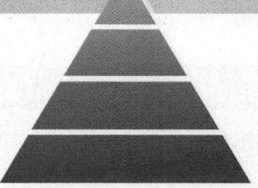

BOX 36-1 Signs and Symptoms of Heart Failure

Left-Sided Failure

- Crackles and wheezes
- Cough
- Dyspnea
- Grunting (infants)
- Head bobbing (infants)
- Nasal flaring
- Orthopnea
- Periods of cyanosis
- Retractions
- Tachypnea

Right-Sided Failure

- Ascites
- Hepatosplenomegaly
- Jugular vein distention
- Oliguria
- Peripheral edema, especially dependent edema, and periorbital edema
- Weight gain

10. Provide rest and decrease environmental stimuli.

11. Administer cool humidified oxygen as prescribed, using an oxygen hood for young infants and a nasal cannula or face mask for older infants and children.

12. Organize nursing activities to allow for uninterrupted sleep.

13. Maintain adequate nutritional status.

14. Feed when hungry and soon after awakening, conserving energy and oxygen supply.

15. Provide small, frequent feedings, conserving energy and oxygen supply.

16. Administer medications as prescribed, which may include digoxin, diuretics, and afterload reducers such as angiotensin-converting enzyme (ACE) inhibitors.

17. Administer digoxin as prescribed.

- **a.** Assess apical heart rate for 1 minute before administration.
- **b.** Withhold digoxin if the apical pulse is less than 90 to 110 beats per minute in infants and young children and less than 70 beats per minute in older children, as prescribed.
- **c.** Check the prescribed dose carefully to ensure it is a safe, age-appropriate dose; follow agency policy and question any unclear prescription.

18. Monitor digoxin levels and for signs of digoxin toxicity, including anorexia, poor feeding, nausea, vomiting, bradycardia, and dysrhythmias.

19. The optimal therapeutic digoxin level range is 0.8 to 2 ng/mL (1.02 to 2.55 nmol/L; toxicity is usually seen at >2 ng/mL (2.55 nmol/L) level.

20. Administer angiotensin-converting enzyme inhibitors as prescribed.

- **a.** Monitor for hypotension, renal dysfunction, and cough when ACE inhibitors are administered.
- **b.** Assess blood pressure; serum protein, albumin, blood urea nitrogen, and creatinine levels; white blood cell count; urine output; urinary specific gravity; and urinary protein level.

21. Administer diuretics such as furosemide as prescribed.

- **a.** Monitor for signs and symptoms of hypokalemia (serum potassium level <3.5 mEq/L [3.5 mmol/L]), including muscle weakness and cramping, confusion, irritability, restlessness, and inverted T waves or prominent U waves on the electrocardiogram.
- **b.** If signs and symptoms of hypokalemia are present and the child is also being administered digoxin, monitor closely for digoxin toxicity, because hypokalemia potentiates digoxin toxicity.

22. Administer potassium supplements and provide dietary sources of potassium as prescribed.

- **a.** Supplemental potassium should be given only if indicated by serum potassium levels and if adequate renal function is evident and is usually necessary when administering a potassium-losing diuretic such as furosemide.
- **b.** Encourage foods that the child will eat that are high in potassium, as appropriate, such as bananas, baked potato skins, and peanut butter.

23. Monitor serum electrolyte levels, particularly the potassium level (normal level is 3.5 to 5.0 mEq/L [3.5 to 5.0 mmol/L]).

24. Limit fluid intake as prescribed in the acute stage.

25. Monitor for signs and symptoms of dehydration, including sunken fontanel (infant), nonelastic skin turgor, dry mucous membranes, decreased tear production, decreased urine output, and concentrated urine.

26. Monitor sodium levels as prescribed.

- **a.** Normal level is 135 to 145 mEq/L (135 to 145 mmol/L).
- **b.** Many infant formulas have slightly more sodium than breast milk.

27. Instruct the parents regarding administration of digoxin (Box 36-2).

28. Instruct the parents in cardiopulmonary resuscitation (CPR). The guidelines for CPR for the child older than 1 year of age are the same as for an adult. For American Heart

BOX 36-2 Home Care Instructions for Administering Digoxin

- Administer as prescribed.
- Use an accurate measuring device as provided by the pharmacist.
- Administer 1 hour before or 2 hours after feedings.
- Use a calendar to mark off the dose administered.
- Do not mix medication with foods or fluid.
- If a dose is missed and more than 4 hours has elapsed, withhold the dose and give the next dose at the scheduled time; if less than 4 hours has elapsed, administer the missed dose.
- If the child vomits, do not administer a second dose. (Follow the pediatrician's prescription.)
- If more than 2 consecutive doses have been missed, notify the pediatrician; do not increase or double the dose for missed doses.
- If the child has teeth, give water after the medication; if possible, brush the teeth to prevent tooth decay from the sweetened liquid.
- Monitor for signs of toxicity, such as poor feeding or vomiting.
- If the child becomes ill, notify the pediatrician.
- Keep the medication in a locked cabinet.
- Call the Poison Control Center immediately if accidental overdose occurs.

Association current CPR guidelines, refer to https://cpr.heart.org/en/resuscitation-science/cpr-and-ecc-guidelines.

⚠ The parents should be provided with a medication guide for any medication prescribed for the infant or child. In addition, the nurse needs to review the instructions in the guide and provide an opportunity for the parents to demonstrate medication administration procedures.

III. Defects with Increased Pulmonary Blood Flow

A. Description
1. Intracardiac communication along the septum or an abnormal connection between the great arteries allows blood to flow from the high-pressure left side of the heart to the low-pressure right side of the heart.
2. The infant typically shows signs and symptoms of HF.

B. Atrial septal defect (ASD)
1. ASD is an abnormal opening between the atria that causes an increased flow of oxygenated blood into the right side of the heart.
2. Right atrial and ventricular enlargement occurs.
3. Infant may be asymptomatic or may develop HF.
4. Signs and symptoms of decreased cardiac output may be present (Box 36-3).

BOX 36-3 Signs and Symptoms of Decreased Cardiac Output

- Decreased peripheral pulses
- Activity intolerance
- Feeding difficulties
- Hypotension
- Irritability, restlessness, lethargy
- Oliguria
- Pale, cool extremities
- Tachycardia

5. Types
   a. ASD 1 (ostium primum): Opening is at the lower end of the septum.
   b. ASD 2 (ostium secundum): Opening is near the center of the septum.
   c. ASD 3 (sinus venosus defect): Opening is near the junction of the superior vena cava and the right atrium.
6. Management
   a. Defect may be closed during a cardiac catheterization.
   b. Open repair with cardiopulmonary bypass may be performed and usually is performed before school age.

C. Atrioventricular canal defect
1. The defect results from incomplete fusion of the endocardial cushions.
2. The defect is the most common cardiac defect in Down's syndrome.
3. A characteristic murmur is present.
4. The infant usually has mild to moderate HF, with **cyanosis** increasing with crying.
5. Signs and symptoms of decreased cardiac output may be present.
6. Management can include pulmonary artery banding for infants with severe symptoms (palliative) or complete repair via cardiopulmonary bypass.

D. Patent ductus arteriosus
1. Patent ductus arteriosus is failure of the fetal ductus arteriosus (shunt connecting the aorta and the pulmonary artery) to close within the first weeks of life.
2. A characteristic machinery-like murmur is present.
3. An infant may be asymptomatic or may show signs of HF.
4. A widened pulse pressure and bounding pulses are present.
5. Signs and symptoms of decreased cardiac output may be present.
6. Management
   a. Indomethacin, a prostaglandin inhibitor, may be administered to close a patent ductus in premature infants and some newborns.

b. The defect may be closed during cardiac catheterization, or the defect may require surgical management.

E. Ventricular septal defect (VSD)
1. VSD is an abnormal opening between the right and left ventricles.
2. Many VSDs close spontaneously during the first year of life in children with small or moderate defects.
3. A characteristic murmur is present.
4. Signs and symptoms of HF are commonly present.
5. Signs and symptoms of decreased cardiac output may be present.
6. Management
a. Closure during cardiac catheterization may be possible.
b. Open repair may be done with cardiopulmonary bypass.

IV. Obstructive Defects

A. Description
1. Blood exiting a portion of the heart meets an area of anatomical narrowing (**stenosis**), causing obstruction to blood flow.
2. The location of narrowing is usually near the valve of the obstructive defect.
3. Infants and children exhibit signs of HF.
4. Children with mild obstruction may be asymptomatic.

B. Aortic stenosis
1. Aortic stenosis is a narrowing or stricture of the aortic valve, causing resistance to blood flow from the left ventricle into the aorta, resulting in decreased cardiac output, left ventricular hypertrophy, and pulmonary vascular congestion.
2. Valvular stenosis is the most common type and usually is caused by malformed cusps, resulting in a bicuspid rather than a tricuspid valve, or fusion of the cusps.
3. A characteristic murmur is present.
4. Infants with severe defects show signs of decreased cardiac output.
5. Children show signs of activity intolerance, chest pain, and dizziness when standing for long periods.
6. Management
a. Dilation of the narrowed valve may be done during cardiac catheterization.
b. Surgical aortic valvotomy (palliative) may be done; a valve replacement may be required at a second procedure.

C. Coarctation of the aorta
1. Coarctation of the aorta is localized narrowing near the insertion of the ductus arteriosus.
2. Blood pressure is higher in the upper extremities than in the lower extremities; bounding pulses in the arms, weak or absent femoral pulses, and cool lower extremities may be present.
3. Signs of HF may occur in infants.
4. Signs and symptoms of decreased cardiac output may be present.
5. Children may experience headaches, dizziness, fainting, and epistaxis resulting from hypertension.
6. Management of the defect may be done via balloon angioplasty in children; restenosis can occur.
7. Surgical management
a. Mechanical ventilation and medications to improve cardiac output are often necessary before surgery.
b. Resection of the coarcted portion with end-to-end anastomosis of the aorta or enlargement of the constricted section, using a graft, may be required.
c. Because the defect is outside the heart, cardiopulmonary bypass is not required, and a thoracotomy incision is used.

! With coarctation of the aorta, the blood pressure is higher in the upper extremities than in the lower extremities. In addition, bounding pulses in the arms, weak or absent femoral pulses, and cool lower extremities may be present.

D. Pulmonary stenosis
1. Pulmonary stenosis is narrowing at the entrance to the pulmonary artery.
2. Resistance to blood flow causes right ventricular hypertrophy and decreased pulmonary blood flow; the right ventricle may be hypoplastic.
3. Pulmonary **atresia** is the extreme form of pulmonary stenosis in that there is total fusion of the commissures and no blood flow to the lungs.
4. A characteristic murmur is present.
5. Infants or children may be asymptomatic.
6. Newborns with severe narrowing are cyanotic.
7. If pulmonary stenosis is severe, HF occurs.
8. Signs and symptoms of decreased cardiac output may occur.
9. Management: Dilation of the narrowed valve may be done during cardiac catheterization.
10. Surgical management:
a. In infants: Transventricular (closed) valvotomy procedure
b. In children: Pulmonary valvotomy with cardiopulmonary bypass

V. Defects with Decreased Pulmonary Blood Flow

A. Description
1. Obstructed pulmonary blood flow and an anatomical defect (ASD or VSD) between the right and left sides of the heart are present.

2. Pressure on the right side of the heart increases, exceeding pressure on the left side, which allows desaturated blood to shunt right to left, causing desaturation in the left side of the heart and in the systemic circulation.
3. Typically hypoxemia and cyanosis appear.

B. Tetralogy of Fallot
1. Tetralogy of Fallot includes 4 defects—VSD, pulmonary stenosis, overriding aorta, and right ventricular hypertrophy.
2. If pulmonary vascular resistance is higher than systemic resistance, the shunt is from right to left; if systemic resistance is higher than pulmonary resistance, the shunt is from left to right.
3. Infants
   a. An infant may be acutely cyanotic at birth or may have mild cyanosis that progresses over the first year of life as the pulmonic stenosis worsens.
   b. A characteristic murmur is present.
   c. Acute episodes of cyanosis and hypoxia (hypercyanotic spells), called *blue spells* or *tet spells*, occur when the infant's oxygen requirements exceed the blood supply, such as during periods of crying, feeding, or defecating (see Priority Nursing Actions).

PRIORITY NURSING ACTIONS

Hypercyanotic Spell Occurring in an Infant

1. Place the infant in a knee-chest position.
2. Administer 100% oxygen.
3. Administer morphine sulfate.
4. Administer fluids intravenously.
5. Document occurrence, actions taken, and the infant's response.

Reference

McKinney et al. (2018), p. 1088.

4. Children: With increasing cyanosis, squatting, clubbing of the fingers, and poor growth may occur.
   a. Squatting is a compensatory mechanism to facilitate increased return of blood flow to the heart for oxygenation.
   b. Clubbing is an abnormal enlargement in the distal phalanges, seen in the fingers.
5. Surgical management: Palliative shunt
   a. The shunt increases pulmonary blood flow and increases oxygen saturation in infants who cannot undergo primary repair.
   b. The shunt provides blood flow to the pulmonary arteries from the left or right subclavian artery.
6. Surgical management: Complete repair
   a. Complete repair usually is performed in the first year of life.
   b. The repair requires a median sternotomy and cardiopulmonary bypass.

C. Tricuspid atresia
1. Tricuspid atresia is failure of the tricuspid valve to develop.
2. No communication exists from the right atrium to the right ventricle.
3. Blood flows through an ASD or a patent foramen ovale to the left side of the heart and through a VSD to the right ventricle and out to the lungs.
4. The defect often is associated with pulmonic stenosis and transposition of the great arteries.
5. The defect results in complete mixing of unoxygenated and oxygenated blood in the left side of the heart, resulting in systemic desaturation, pulmonary obstruction, and decreased pulmonary blood flow.
6. Cyanosis, tachycardia, and dyspnea are seen in the newborn.
7. Older children exhibit signs of chronic hypoxemia and clubbing.
8. Management: If the ASD is small, the defect may be closed during cardiac catheterization; otherwise, surgery is needed.

Clubbing is symptomatic of chronic hypoxia. Peripheral circulation is diminished, and oxygenation of vital organs and tissues is compromised.

VI. Mixed Defects

A. Description
1. Fully saturated systemic blood flow mixes with the desaturated blood flow, causing desaturation of the systemic blood flow.
2. Pulmonary congestion occurs and cardiac output decreases.
3. Signs of HF are present; symptoms vary with the degree of desaturation.

B. Hypoplastic left heart syndrome
1. Underdevelopment of the left side of the heart occurs, resulting in a hypoplastic left ventricle and aortic atresia.
2. Mild cyanosis and signs of HF occur until the ductus arteriosus closes; then progressive deterioration with cyanosis and decreased cardiac output are seen, leading to cardiovascular collapse.
3. The defect is fatal in the first few months of life without intervention.
4. Surgical treatment
   a. Surgical treatment is necessary; transplantation in the newborn period may be considered.

b. In the preoperative period, the newborn requires mechanical ventilation and a continuous infusion of prostaglandin E_1 to maintain ductal patency, ensuring adequate systemic blood flow.

C. Transposition of the great arteries or transposition of the great vessels
1. The pulmonary artery leaves the left ventricle, and the aorta exits from the right ventricle.
2. No communication exists between the systemic and pulmonary circulation.
3. Infants with minimal communication are severely cyanotic at birth.
4. Infants with large septal defects or a patent ductus arteriosus may be less severely cyanotic but may have symptoms of HF.
5. Cardiomegaly is evident a few weeks after birth.
6. Nonsurgical management
   a. Prostaglandin E_1 may be initiated to keep the ductus arteriosus open and to improve blood mixing temporarily.
   b. Balloon atrial septostomy during cardiac catheterization may be performed to increase mixing from both sides of the heart and to maintain cardiac output over a longer period.
7. Surgical management: The arterial switch procedure reestablishes normal circulation with the left ventricle acting as the systemic pump and creation of a new aorta.

D. Total anomalous pulmonary venous connection
1. The defect is a failure of the pulmonary veins to join the left atrium.
2. The defect results in mixed blood being returned to the right atrium and shunted from the right to the left through an ASD.
3. The right side of the heart hypertrophies, whereas the left side of the heart may remain small.
4. Signs and symptoms of HF develop.
5. Cyanosis worsens with pulmonary vein obstruction; when obstruction occurs, the infant's condition deteriorates rapidly.
6. Surgical management
   a. Corrective repair is performed in early infancy.
   b. The pulmonary vein is anastomosed to the left atrium, the ASD is closed, and the anomalous pulmonary venous connection is ligated.

E. Truncus arteriosus
1. Truncus arteriosus is failure of normal septation and division of the embryonic bulbar trunk into the pulmonary artery and the aorta, resulting in a single vessel that overrides both ventricles.
2. Blood from both ventricles mixes in the common great artery, causing desaturation and hypoxemia.
3. A characteristic murmur is present.
4. The infant exhibits moderate to severe HF and variable cyanosis, poor growth, and activity intolerance.
5. Surgical management: Corrective surgical repair is performed in the first few months of life.

VII. Interventions: Cardiovascular Defects (Box 36-4)

VIII. Cardiac Catheterization

A. Description
1. Invasive diagnostic procedure to determine cardiac defects.
2. Provides information about oxygen saturation of blood in great vessels and heart chambers.
3. May be done for diagnostic, interventional, or electrophysiological reasons.
4. May be carried out on an outpatient basis.
5. Risks include hemorrhage from the entry site, clot formation and subsequent blockage distally, and transient dysrhythmias.
6. General anesthesia is usually unnecessary.
7. See Chapter 52 for additional information about this procedure.

BOX 36-4 Interventions for Cardiovascular Defects

- Monitor for signs of a defect in the infant or child.
- Monitor vital signs closely.
- Monitor respiratory status for the presence of **nasal flaring**, use of accessory muscles, and for signs of impending respiratory distress, and notify the pediatrician if any changes occur.
- Auscultate breath sounds for crackles, rhonchi, or wheezes.
- If respiratory effort is increased, place the child in a reverse Trendelenburg's position, elevating the head and upper body, to decrease the work of breathing.
- Administer humidified oxygen as prescribed.
- Provide endotracheal tube and ventilator care if necessary as prescribed.
- Monitor for hypercyanotic spells and intervene immediately if they occur.
- Assess for signs of HF, such as periorbital edema or dependent edema in the hands and feet.
- Assess peripheral pulses.
- Maintain fluid restriction if prescribed.
- Monitor intake and output, and notify the pediatrician if a decrease in urine output occurs.
- Obtain daily weight.
- Provide adequate nutrition (high calorie requirements) as prescribed.
- Administer medications as prescribed.
- Plan interventions to allow maximal rest for the child; keep the child as stress-free as possible.
- Prepare the child and parents for cardiac catheterization, if appropriate.

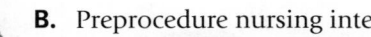

B. Preprocedure nursing interventions
1. Assess accurate height and weight, because this helps with the selection of the correct catheter size.
2. Obtain a history of the presence of allergic reactions to iodine.
3. Assess for symptoms of infection, including a diaper rash.
4. Assess and mark bilateral pulses, such as the dorsalis pedis and posterior tibial.
5. Assess baseline oxygen saturation.
6. Familiarize the parents and child with hospital procedures and equipment.
7. Educate the child, if age appropriate, and the parents about the procedure.
8. Allow the parents and child to verbalize feelings and concerns regarding the procedure and the disorder.

C. Postprocedure nursing interventions
1. Monitor findings on the cardiac monitor and oxygen saturation for 4 hours after procedure.
2. Assess pulses below the catheter site for presence, equality and symmetry.
3. Assess the temperature and color of the affected extremity and report coolness, which may indicate arterial obstruction.
4. Monitor vital signs frequently, usually every 15 minutes 4 times, every half-hour 4 times, and then every hour 4 times.
5. Assess the pressure dressing for intactness and signs of hemorrhage.
6. Check the bed sheets under the extremity for blood, which indicates bleeding from the entry site.
7. If bleeding is present, apply continuous, direct pressure at the cardiac catheter entry site and report it immediately.
8. Immobilize the affected extremity in a flat position for at least 4 to 6 hours for venous entry site and 6 to 8 hours for arterial entry site as prescribed.
9. Hydrate the child via the oral or intravenous route or both routes as prescribed.
10. Administer acetaminophen or ibuprofen for pain or discomfort as prescribed.
11. Prepare the parents and child, if appropriate, for surgery.

D. Discharge teaching for the child and parents
1. Remove the dressing on the day after the procedure and cover it with a bandage for 2 or 3 days as prescribed.
2. Keep the site clean and dry.
3. Avoid tub baths for 2 to 3 days.
4. Observe for redness, edema, drainage, bleeding, and fever, and report any of these signs immediately.
5. Avoid strenuous activity, if applicable.
6. The child may return to school, if appropriate.
7. Provide a diet as tolerated.
8. Administer acetaminophen or ibuprofen for pain, discomfort, or fever.
9. Keep follow-up appointment with the pediatrician.

IX. Cardiac Surgery

A. Postoperative interventions
1. Monitor vital signs frequently, especially temperature, and notify the surgeon if fever occurs.
2. Monitor for signs of sepsis such as fever, chills, diaphoresis, lethargy, and altered levels of consciousness.
3. Maintain strict aseptic technique.
4. Monitor lines, tubes, or catheters that are in place, and monitor for signs and symptoms of infection.
5. Assess for signs of discomfort such as irritability, restlessness, changes in heart rate, respiratory rate, and blood pressure.
6. Administer pain medications as prescribed.
7. Administer antibiotics and antipyretics as prescribed.
8. Promote rest and sleep periods.
9. Facilitate parent-child contact as soon as possible.

B. Postoperative home care (Box 36-5)

BOX 36-5 Home Care after Cardiac Surgery

- Omit play outside for several weeks as prescribed.
- Avoid activities in which the child could fall and be injured, such as bike riding, for 2 to 4 weeks.
- Avoid crowds for 2 weeks after discharge.
- Follow a no-added-salt diet, if prescribed.
- Do not add any new foods to the infant's diet (if an allergy exists to the new food, the manifestations may be interpreted as a postoperative complication).
- Do not place creams, lotions, or powders on the incision until completely healed.
- The child may return to school usually the third week after discharge, starting with half-days.
- The child should not participate in physical education for 2 months.
- Discipline the child normally.
- The 2-week follow-up is important.
- Avoid immunizations, invasive procedures, and dental visits for 2 months; following this time period, the immunization schedule and dental visits need to be resumed.
- The child should have a dental visit every 6 months after age 3 years and inform the dentist of the cardiac problem so that antibiotics can be prescribed if necessary.
- Call the pediatrician if coughing, tachypnea, cyanosis, vomiting, diarrhea, anorexia, pain, or fever occur, or any swelling, redness, or drainage occurs at the site of the incision.

Pediatric

X. Rheumatic Fever

A. Description

1. Rheumatic fever is an inflammatory autoimmune disease that affects the connective tissues of the heart, joints, skin (subcutaneous tissues), blood vessels, and central nervous system.
2. The most serious complication is rheumatic heart disease, which affects the cardiac valves, particularly the mitral valve.
3. Rheumatic fever manifests 2 to 6 weeks after an untreated or partially treated group A beta-hemolytic streptococcal infection of the upper respiratory tract.
4. Jones criteria are used to help determine the diagnosis (Box 36-6).

B. Assessment (Fig. 36-1)

1. Fever: Low-grade fever that spikes in the late afternoon
2. Elevated anti–streptolysin O titer
3. Elevated erythrocyte sedimentation rate
4. Elevated C-reactive protein level
5. Aschoff bodies (lesions): Found in the heart, blood vessels, brain, and serous surfaces of the joints and pleura

Assessment of a child with suspected rheumatic fever includes inquiring about a recent sore throat, because rheumatic fever manifests 2 to 6 weeks after an untreated or partially treated group A beta-hemolytic streptococcal infection of the upper respiratory tract.

C. Interventions

1. Assess vital signs.
2. Control joint pain and inflammation with massage and alternating hot and cold applications as prescribed.

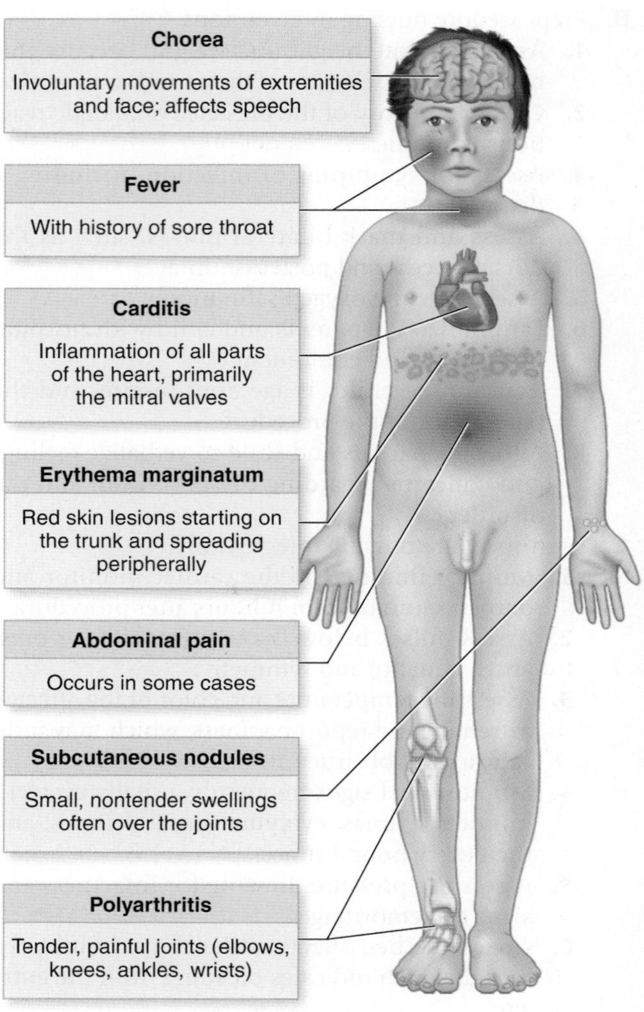

FIG. 36-1 Clinical manifestations of rheumatic fever.

3. Provide bed rest during the acute febrile phase.
4. Limit physical exercise in a child with carditis.
5. Administer antibiotics as prescribed.
6. Administer salicylates and antiinflammatory agents as prescribed; these medications should not be administered before the diagnosis is confirmed, because the medications mask the polyarthritis.
7. Initiate seizure precautions if the child is experiencing chorea.
8. Instruct the parents about the importance of follow-up and the need for antibiotic prophylaxis for dental work, infection, and invasive procedures.
9. Advise the child to inform the parents if anyone in school develops a streptococcal throat infection.

BOX 36-6 Jones Criteria for Diagnosis of Rheumatic Fever

Major Criteria

- Carditis
- Arthralgia
- Chorea
- Erythema marginatum
- Subcutaneous nodules

Minor Criteria

- Fever
- Arthralgia
- Elevated erythrocyte sedimentation rate or positive C-reactive protein level
- Prolonged PR interval on electrocardiogram

Note: For making a diagnosis, 2 major or 1 major and 2 minor manifestations must be accompanied by supporting evidence of a preceding streptococcal infection (positive throat culture for group A *Streptococcus* and an elevated or increasing anti–streptolysin O titer).

XI. Kawasaki Disease

A. Description

1. Kawasaki disease, also known as *mucocutaneous lymph node syndrome,* is an acute systemic inflammatory illness.

2. The cause is unknown, but may be associated with an infection from an organism or toxin.
3. Cardiac involvement is the most serious complication; aneurysms can develop.

B. Assessment
1. Acute stage
   a. Fever
   b. Conjunctival hyperemia
   c. Red throat
   d. Swollen hands, rash, and enlargement of cervical lymph nodes
2. Subacute stage
   a. Cracking lips and fissures
   b. Desquamation of the skin on the tips of the fingers and toes
   c. Joint pain
   d. Cardiac manifestations
   e. Thrombocytosis
3. Convalescent stage: Child appears normal, but signs of inflammation may be present.

C. Interventions
1. Monitor temperature frequently.
2. Assess heart sounds and heart rate and rhythm.
3. Assess extremities for edema, redness, and desquamation.
4. Examine eyes for conjunctivitis.
5. Monitor mucous membranes for inflammation.
6. Monitor strict intake and output.
7. Administer soft foods and liquids that are neither too hot nor too cold.
8. Weigh child daily.
9. Provide passive range-of-motion exercises to facilitate joint movement.
10. Administer acetylsalicylic acid as prescribed for its antipyretic and antiplatelet effects (additional anticoagulation may be necessary if aneurysms are present).
11. Administer immunoglobulin intravenously as prescribed to reduce the duration of the fever and the incidence of coronary artery lesions and aneurysms; intravenous immunoglobulin is a blood product, so blood precautions when administering it are warranted.
12. Parent education (Box 36-7)

BOX 36-7 Parent Education for Kawasaki Disease

- Follow-up care is essential to recovery.
- Signs and symptoms of Kawasaki disease include the following:
  - Irritability that may last for 2 months after the onset of symptoms
  - Peeling of the hands and feet
  - Pain in the joints that may persist for several weeks
  - Stiffness in the morning, after naps, and in cold temperatures
- Record the temperature (because fever is expected) until the child has been afebrile for several days.
- Notify the pediatrician if the temperature is 101° F (38.3° C) or higher.
- Salicylates such as acetylsalicylic acid (aspirin) may be prescribed.
- Signs of aspirin toxicity include tinnitus, headache, vertigo, and bruising; do not administer aspirin or aspirin-containing products if the child has been exposed to chickenpox or the flu.
- Signs and symptoms of bleeding include epistaxis (nosebleeds), hemoptysis (coughing up blood), hematemesis (vomiting up blood), hematuria (blood in urine), melena (blood in stool), and bruises on the body.
- Signs and symptoms of cardiac complications include chest pain or tightness (older children), cool and pale extremities, abdominal pain, nausea and vomiting, irritability, restlessness, and uncontrollable crying.
- The child should avoid contact sports, if age appropriate, if taking aspirin or anticoagulants.
- Avoid administration of measles, mumps, and rubella (MMR) or varicella vaccine to the child for 11 months after intravenous immunoglobulin therapy, if appropriate.

PRACTICE QUESTIONS

362. The nurse is monitoring an infant with congenital heart disease closely for signs of heart failure (HF). The nurse should assess the infant for which **early** sign of HF?
1. Pallor
2. Cough
3. Tachycardia
4. Slow and shallow breathing

363. The nurse reviews the laboratory results for a child with a suspected diagnosis of rheumatic fever, knowing that which laboratory study would assist in confirming the diagnosis?
1. Immunoglobulin
2. Red blood cell count
3. White blood cell count
4. Anti–streptolysin O titer

364. On assessment of a child admitted with a diagnosis of acute-stage Kawasaki disease, the nurse expects to note which clinical manifestation of the acute stage of the disease?
1. Cracked lips
2. Normal appearance
3. Conjunctival hyperemia
4. Desquamation of the skin

365. The nurse provides home care instructions to the parents of a child with heart failure regarding the procedure for administration of digoxin. Which statement made by the parent indicates the **need for further instruction**?

1. "I will not mix the medication with food."
2. "If more than 1 dose is missed, I will call the pediatrician."
3. "I will take my child's pulse before administering the medication."
4. "If my child vomits after medication administration, I will repeat the dose."

366. The nurse is closely monitoring the intake and output of an infant with heart failure who is receiving diuretic therapy. The nurse should use which **most appropriate** method to assess the urine output?
1. Weighing the diapers
2. Inserting a urinary catheter
3. Comparing intake with output
4. Measuring the amount of water added to formula

367. The clinic nurse reviews the record of a child just seen by the pediatrician and diagnosed with suspected aortic stenosis. The nurse expects to note documentation of which clinical manifestation specifically found in this disorder?
1. Pallor
2. Hyperactivity
3. Activity intolerance
4. Gastrointestinal disturbances

368. The nurse has provided home care instructions to the parents of a child who is being discharged after cardiac surgery. Which statement made by the parents indicates a **need for further instruction?**
1. "A balance of rest and activity is important."
2. "I can apply lotion or powder to the incision if it is itchy."
3. "Activities in which my child could fall need to be avoided for 2 to 4 weeks."
4. "Large crowds of people need to be avoided for at least 2 weeks after surgery."

369. A child with rheumatic fever will be arriving to the nursing unit for admission. On admission assessment, the nurse should ask the parents which question to elicit assessment information specific to the development of rheumatic fever?
1. "Has the child complained of back pain?"
2. "Has the child complained of headaches?"
3. "Has the child had any nausea or vomiting?"
4. "Did the child have a sore throat or fever within the last 2 months?"

370. A pediatrician has prescribed oxygen as needed for an infant with heart failure. In which situation should the nurse administer the oxygen to the infant?
1. During sleep
2. When changing the infant's diapers
3. When the mother is holding the infant
4. When drawing blood for electrolyte level testing

371. Assessment findings of an infant admitted to the hospital reveal a machinery-like murmur on auscultation of the heart and signs of heart failure. The nurse reviews congenital cardiac anomalies and identifies the infant's condition as which disorder? **Refer to figure** (the circled area) to determine the condition.

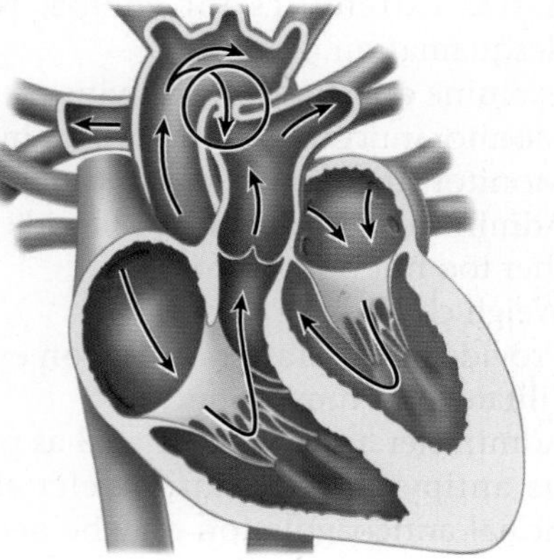

1. Aortic stenosis
2. Atrial septal defect
3. Patent ductus arteriosus
4. Ventricular septal defect

ANSWERS

362. *Answer:* 3

Rationale: HF is the inability of the heart to pump a sufficient amount of blood to meet the oxygen and metabolic needs of the body. The early signs of HF include tachycardia, tachypnea, profuse scalp sweating, fatigue and irritability, sudden weight gain, and respiratory distress. A cough may occur in HF as a result of mucosal swelling and irritation, but is not an early sign. Pallor may be noted in an infant with HF but is not an early sign.

Test-Taking Strategy: Note the strategic word, *early*. Think about the physiology and the effects on the heart when fluid overload occurs. These concepts will assist in directing you to the correct option.

Level of Cognitive Ability: Analyzing

Client Needs: Physiological Integrity

Integrated Process: Nursing Process—Assessment

Content Area: Pediatrics: Cardiovascular

Health Problem: Pediatric-Specific: Congestive Heart Failure

Priority Concepts: Clinical Judgment; Perfusion

Reference: Hockenberry, Wilson, Rodgers (2017), p. 753.

363. Answer: 4

Rationale: Rheumatic fever is an inflammatory autoimmune disease that affects the connective tissues of the heart, joints, skin (subcutaneous tissues), blood vessels, and central nervous system. A diagnosis of rheumatic fever is confirmed by the presence of 2 major manifestations or 1 major and 2 minor manifestations from the Jones criteria. In addition, evidence of a recent streptococcal infection is confirmed by a positive anti–streptolysin O titer, Streptozyme assay, or anti-DNase B assay. Options 1, 2, and 3 would not help confirm the diagnosis of rheumatic fever.

Test-Taking Strategy: Focus on the subject, definitive diagnosis of rheumatic fever. Recalling that rheumatic fever characteristically is associated with streptococcal infection will direct you to the correct option.

Level of Cognitive Ability: Analyzing
Client Needs: Physiological Integrity
Integrated Process: Nursing Process—Analysis
Content Area: Pediatrics: Cardiovascular
Health Problem: Pediatric-Specific: Rheumatic Fever
Priority Concepts: Clinical Judgment; Inflammation
Reference: Hockenberry, Wilson, Rodgers (2017), pp. 767-768.

364. Answer: 3

Rationale: Kawasaki disease, also known as *mucocutaneous lymph node syndrome*, is an acute systemic inflammatory illness. In the acute stage, the child has a fever, conjunctival hyperemia, red throat, swollen hands, rash, and enlargement of the cervical lymph nodes. In the subacute stage, cracking lips and fissures, desquamation of the skin on the tips of the fingers and toes, joint pain, cardiac manifestations, and thrombocytosis occur. In the convalescent stage, the child appears normal, but signs of inflammation may be present.

Test-Taking Strategy: Focus on the subject, the acute stage of Kawasaki disease. Option 2 can be eliminated first, because a normal appearance is not likely in the acute stage. From the remaining options, focusing on the words *acute stage* in the question will assist in directing you to the correct option.

Level of Cognitive Ability: Analyzing
Client Needs: Physiological Integrity
Integrated Process: Nursing Process—Assessment
Content Area: Pediatrics: Cardiovascular
Health Problem: Pediatric-Specific: Kawasaki Disease
Priority Concepts: Clinical Judgment; Inflammation
Reference: McKinney et al. (2018), p. 1111.

365. Answer: 4

Rationale: Digoxin is a cardiac glycoside. The parents need to be instructed that if the child vomits after digoxin is administered, they are not to repeat the dose. Options 1, 2, and 3 are accurate instructions regarding the administration of this medication. In addition, the parents should be instructed that if a dose is missed and is not identified until 4 hours later, the dose should not be administered.

Test-Taking Strategy: Note the strategic words, *need for further instruction*. These words indicate a negative event query and ask you to select an option that is an incorrect statement. General knowledge regarding digoxin administration will assist in eliminating option 2. Principles related to administering medications to children will assist in eliminating option 1. From the remaining options, select the correct option because if the child vomits, it would be difficult to determine whether the medication also was vomited or was absorbed by the body.

Level of Cognitive Ability: Evaluating
Client Needs: Physiological Integrity
Integrated Process: Teaching and Learning
Content Area: Pediatrics: Cardiovascular
Health Problem: Pediatric-Specific: Congestive Heart Failure
Priority Concepts: Client Education; Safety
Reference: McKinney et al. (2018), p. 1087.

366. Answer: 1

Rationale: Heart failure is the inability of the heart to pump a sufficient amount of blood to meet the oxygen and metabolic needs of the body. The most appropriate method for assessing urine output in an infant receiving diuretic therapy is to weigh the diapers. Comparing intake with output would not provide an accurate measure of urine output. Measuring the amount of water added to formula is unrelated to the amount of output. Although urinary catheter drainage is most accurate in determining output, it is not the most appropriate method in an infant and places the infant at risk for infection.

Test-Taking Strategy: Note the strategic words, *most appropriate*. Eliminate options 3 and 4 first because they are comparable or alike and will not provide an indication of urine output. Noting the strategic words will direct you to the correct option from the remaining options.

Level of Cognitive Ability: Applying
Client Needs: Physiological Integrity
Integrated Process: Nursing Process—Assessment
Content Area: Pediatrics: Cardiovascular
Health Problem: Pediatric-Specific: Congestive Heart Failure
Priority Concepts: Clinical Judgment; Perfusion
Reference: McKinney et al. (2018), p. 1084.

367. Answer: 3

Rationale: Aortic stenosis is a narrowing or stricture of the aortic valve, causing resistance to blood flow in the left ventricle, decreased cardiac output, left ventricular hypertrophy, and pulmonary vascular congestion. A child with aortic stenosis shows signs of activity intolerance, chest pain, and dizziness when standing for long periods. Pallor may be noted but is not specific to this type of disorder alone. Options 2 and 4 are not related to this disorder.

Test-Taking Strategy: Focus on the subject, the characteristics of aortic stenosis. Options 2 and 4 can be eliminated first, because they are not associated with a cardiac disorder. From the remaining options, noting the word *specifically* in the question will direct you to the correct option.

Level of Cognitive Ability: Analyzing
Client Needs: Physiological Integrity
Integrated Process: Nursing Process—Assessment
Content Area: Pediatrics: Cardiovascular
Health Problem: Pediatric-Specific: Congenital Cardiac Defects
Priority Concepts: Elimination; Perfusion
Reference: Hockenberry, Wilson, Rodgers (2017), p. 747.

368. Answer: 2

Rationale: The mother should be instructed that lotions and powders should not be applied to the incision site after cardiac

Pediatric

surgery. Lotions and powders can irritate the surrounding skin, which could lead to skin breakdown and subsequent infection of the incision site. Options 1, 3, and 4 are accurate instructions regarding home care after cardiac surgery.
Test-Taking Strategy: Note the strategic words, *need for further instruction*. These words indicate a negative event query and ask you to select an option that is an incorrect statement. Using general principles related to postoperative incisional site care will direct you to the correct option.
Level of Cognitive Ability: Evaluating
Client Needs: Physiological Integrity
Integrated Process: Teaching and Learning
Content Area: Pediatrics: Cardiovascular
Health Problem: Pediatric-Specific: Congenital Cardiac Defects
Priority Concepts: Client Education; Health Promotion
Reference: McKinney et al. (2018), p. 1104.

369. *Answer:* 4
Rationale: Rheumatic fever is an inflammatory autoimmune disease that affects the connective tissues of the heart, joints, skin (subcutaneous tissues), blood vessels, and central nervous system. Rheumatic fever characteristically manifests 2 to 6 weeks after an untreated or partially treated group A beta-hemolytic streptococcal infection of the upper respiratory tract. Initially, the nurse determines whether the child had a sore throat or an unexplained fever within the past 2 months. Options 1, 2, and 3 are unrelated to rheumatic fever.
Test-Taking Strategy: Focus on the subject, the pathophysiology and etiology associated with rheumatic fever. Also, note the similarity between the words *rheumatic fever* in the question and the word *fever* in the correct option.
Level of Cognitive Ability: Analyzing
Client Needs: Physiological Integrity
Integrated Process: Nursing Process—Assessment
Content Area: Pediatrics: Cardiovascular
Health Problem: Pediatric-Specific: Rheumatic Fever
Priority Concepts: Clinical Judgment; Inflammation
Reference: McKinney et al. (2018), pp. 1108-1109.

370. *Answer:* 4
Rationale: Heart failure (HF) is the inability of the heart to pump a sufficient amount of blood to meet the oxygen and metabolic needs of the body. Crying exhausts the limited energy supply, increases the workload of the heart, and increases the oxygen demands. Oxygen administration may be prescribed for stressful periods, especially during bouts of crying or invasive procedures. Options 1, 2, and 3 are not likely to produce crying in the infant.
Test-Taking Strategy: Focus on the subject, the need to administer oxygen to the infant with HF, and recall the situations that would place stress and an increased workload on the heart; this should direct you to the correct option. Drawing blood is an invasive procedure, which would likely cause the infant to cry.
Level of Cognitive Ability: Analyzing
Client Needs: Physiological Integrity
Integrated Process: Nursing Process—Implementation
Content Area: Pediatrics: Cardiovascular
Health Problem: Pediatric-Specific: Congestive Heart Failure
Priority Concepts: Clinical Judgment; Perfusion
Reference: McKinney et al. (2018), pp. 1084-1086.

371. *Answer:* 3
Rationale: A patent ductus arteriosus is failure of the fetal ductus arteriosus (artery connecting the aorta and the pulmonary artery) to close. A characteristic machinery-like murmur is present, and the infant may show signs of heart failure. Aortic stenosis is a narrowing or stricture of the aortic valve. Atrial septal defect is an abnormal opening between the atria. Ventricular septal defect is an abnormal opening between the right and left ventricles.
Test-Taking Strategy: Focus on the subject, the congenital cardiac anomaly and the location of the defect. Recalling the anatomical locations in the heart will direct you to the correct option.
Level of Cognitive Ability: Analyzing
Client Needs: Physiological Integrity
Integrated Process: Nursing Process—Assessment
Content Area: Pediatrics: Cardiovascular
Health Problem: Pediatric-Specific: Congenital Cardiac Defects
Priority Concepts: Clinical Judgment; Perfusion

CHAPTER 37

Renal and Genitourinary Problems

PRIORITY CONCEPTS Elimination; Inflammation

I. Urinary Tract Infection (UTI)

A. Bacterial invasion of the urinary tract from flora from the skin or gastrointestinal tract
B. Uncircumcised infants are more likely to develop a UTI than a circumcised infant; see: https://www.ncbi.nlm.nih.gov/pmc/articles/PMC1477524/
C. Hygiene (wiping from front to back) is important in children to prevent this problem
D. Children may experience asymptomatic bacteruria, so if there is a suspicion of infection in the urinary tract, they should be screened and treated accordingly.
E. See Chapter 54 for additional information.

II. Glomerulonephritis

A. Description
1. *Glomerulonephritis* refers to a group of kidney disorders characterized by inflammatory injury in the glomerulus, most of which are caused by an immunological reaction.
2. The disorder results in proliferative and inflammatory changes within the glomerular structure.
3. Destruction, inflammation, and sclerosis of the glomeruli of the kidneys occur.
4. Inflammation of the glomeruli results from an antigen-antibody reaction produced by an infection elsewhere in the body.
5. Loss of kidney function develops.

B. Causes
1. Immunological diseases
2. Autoimmune diseases
3. Antecedent group A β-hemolytic streptococcal infection of the pharynx or skin
4. History of pharyngitis or tonsillitis 2 to 3 weeks before symptoms

C. Types
1. Acute: Occurs 2 to 3 weeks after a streptococcal infection
2. Chronic: May occur after the acute phase or slowly over time

D. Complications
1. Kidney failure
2. Hypertensive encephalopathy
3. Pulmonary edema
4. Heart failure
5. Seizures

E. Assessment (Box 37-1)
F. Interventions (see Priority Nursing Actions)

PRIORITY NURSING ACTIONS

Fluid Volume Overload in a Child with Glomerulonephritis

1. Assess airway patency, vital signs, and weight.
2. Assess for dyspnea, bounding rapid pulse, dysrhythmias, and hypertension.
3. Assess for distended hand and neck veins.
4. Assess level of generalized edema (anasarca) and check amount of urinary output.
5. Notify the primary health care provider and carry out prescriptions, including water and sodium restriction and administration of diuretics.

Reference
McKinney et al. (2018), pp. 1016-1017.

1. Monitor vital signs, intake and output, and characteristics of urine.
2. Measure daily weights at the same time of day, using the same scale, and wearing the same clothing.
3. Limit activity; provide safety measures.
4. Diet restrictions of sodium depend on the stage and severity of the disease, especially the extent of the edema; in addition, potassium may be restricted during periods of oliguria.
5. Monitor for complications (e.g., kidney failure, hypertensive encephalopathy, seizures, pulmonary edema, heart failure).
6. Administer diuretics (if significant edema and fluid overload are present), antihypertensives (for hypertension), and antibiotics (to a child with evidence of persistent streptococcal infections) as prescribed.

Pediatric

BOX 37-1 Assessment Findings in Glomerulonephritis

- Periorbital and facial edema that is more prominent in the morning
- Anorexia
- Decreased urinary output
- Cloudy, smoky, brown-colored urine (hematuria)
- Pallor, irritability, lethargy
- In an older child: Headaches, abdominal or flank pain, dysuria
- Hypertension
- Proteinuria that produces a persistent and excessive foam in the urine
- Azotemia
- Increased blood urea nitrogen and creatinine levels
- Increased anti–streptolysin O titer (used to diagnose disorders caused by streptococcal infections)

7. Initiate seizure precautions and administer anticonvulsants as prescribed for seizures associated with hypertensive encephalopathy.
8. Instruct parents to report signs of bloody urine, headache, or edema.
9. Instruct parents that the child needs to obtain appropriate and immediate treatment for infections, specifically for sore throats, upper respiratory infections, and skin infections.

Measuring the daily weight and assessing for changes is the most useful and effective measure for determining fluid balance.

III. Nephrotic Syndrome

A. Description

1. Nephrotic syndrome is a kidney disorder characterized by massive proteinuria, hypoalbuminemia (hypoproteinemia), and edema (Fig. 37-1).
2. The primary objectives of therapeutic management are to reduce the excretion of urinary protein, maintain protein-free urine, reduce edema, prevent infection, and minimize complications.

B. Assessment (Box 37-2)

The classic manifestations of nephrotic syndrome are massive proteinuria, hypoalbuminemia, and edema.

C. Interventions

1. Monitor vital signs, intake and output, and daily weights.
2. Monitor urine for specific gravity and protein.
3. Monitor for edema.
4. Nutrition: A regular diet without added salt may be prescribed if the child is in remission; sodium is restricted during periods of massive edema (fluids may also be restricted).

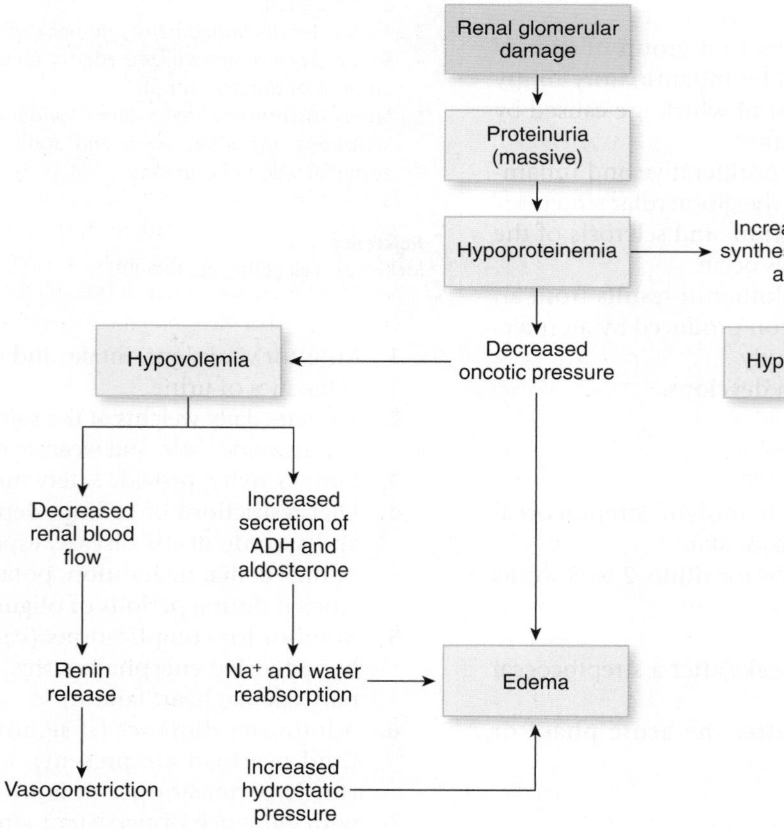

FIG. 37-1 Sequence of events in nephrotic syndrome. *ADH*, Antidiuretic hormone; *Na^+*, sodium.

BOX 37-2 Assessment Findings in Nephrotic Syndrome

- Child gains weight
- Periorbital and facial edema most prominent in the morning
- Leg, ankle, labial, or scrotal edema
- Urine output decreases; urine dark and frothy
- Ascites (fluid in abdominal cavity)
- Blood pressure normal or slightly decreased
- Lethargy, anorexia, and pallor
- Massive proteinuria
- Decreased serum protein (hypoproteinemia) and elevated serum lipid levels

5. Corticosteroid therapy is prescribed as soon as the diagnosis has been determined; monitor the child closely for signs of infection and other adverse effects of corticosteroids (see Chapter 47).
6. Immunosuppressant therapy may be prescribed to reduce the relapse rate and induce long-term remission, or, if the child is unresponsive to corticosteroid therapy, immunosuppressant therapy may be administered along with the corticosteroid.
7. Diuretics may be prescribed to reduce edema.
8. Plasma expanders such as salt-poor human albumin may be prescribed for a severely edematous child.
9. Instruct parents about testing the urine for protein, medication administration, side effects of medications, and general care of the child.
10. Instruct parents on the signs of infection and the need to avoid contact with other children who may be infectious.

IV. Hemolytic-Uremic Syndrome

A. Description
1. Hemolytic-uremic syndrome is thought to be associated with bacterial toxins, chemicals, and viruses that cause acute kidney injury in children.
2. It occurs primarily in infants and small children 6 months to 5 years old.
3. Clinical features include acquired hemolytic anemia, thrombocytopenia, kidney injury, and central nervous system symptoms.

B. Assessment
1. Triad of anemia, thrombocytopenia, and kidney failure (Box 37-3)
2. Proteinuria, hematuria, and presence of urinary casts
3. Blood urea nitrogen and serum creatinine levels elevated; hemoglobin and hematocrit levels decreased

BOX 37-3 Assessment Findings in Hemolytic-Uremic Syndrome

- Vomiting
- Irritability
- Lethargy
- Marked pallor
- Hemorrhagic manifestations: bruising, petechiae, jaundice, bloody diarrhea
- Oliguria or anuria
- Central nervous system involvement: seizures, stupor, coma

C. Interventions
1. Hemodialysis or peritoneal dialysis may be prescribed if a child is anuric (dialysate solution is prescribed to meet the child's electrolyte needs).
2. Strict monitoring of fluid balance is necessary; fluid restrictions may be prescribed if the child is anuric.
3. Institute measures to prevent infection.
4. Provide adequate nutrition.
5. Other treatments include medications to treat manifestations and the administration of blood products to treat severe anemia (administered with caution to prevent fluid overload).

V. Enuresis

A. Description
1. *Enuresis* refers to a condition in which a child is unable to control bladder function, even though the child has reached an age at which control of voiding is expected or the child has successfully completed a bladder control program.
2. A child does not have control over this condition.

B. Primary enuresis: Wetting that occurs in a child that has not fully mastered toilet training.

C. Nighttime (nocturnal) enuresis
1. Nighttime (nocturnal) enuresis is bedwetting in a child who has never been dry for extended periods.
2. The condition is common in children, and most children eventually outgrow bedwetting without therapeutic intervention.
3. The child is unable to sense a full bladder and does not awaken to void.
4. The child may have delayed maturation of the central nervous system.
5. The child should be evaluated for any pathological causes before the diagnosis of nighttime (nocturnal) enuresis is made.

D. Daytime (diurnal) enuresis: Wetting that occurs during the day.

E. Secondary enuresis
1. The onset of wetting occurs after a period of established urinary continence.

Pediatric

2. If the child complains of dysuria, urgency, or frequency the child should be assessed for urinary tract infections.

F. Assessment: A child older than 5 years wets their bed or their clothes 2 times a week or more, for at least 3 months.

G. Interventions
1. Perform urinalysis and urine culture as prescribed to rule out infection or an existing disorder.
2. Assist the family with identifying a treatment plan that best fits the needs of the child.
3. Limit fluid intake at night, and encourage the child to void just before going to bed.
4. Involve the child in caring for the wet sheets and changing the bed to assist the child to take ownership of the problem.
5. Provide reward systems as appropriate for the child.
6. Incorporate behavioral conditioning techniques.
7. Desmopressin may reduce urine production at night; anticholinergics may reduce bladder contractions and increase bladder capacity.
8. Encourage follow-up to determine the effectiveness of the treatment.

VI. Cryptorchidism

A. Description: Cryptorchidism is a condition in which one or both testes fail to descend through the inguinal canal into the scrotal sac.

B. Assessment: Testes are not palpable or easily guided into the scrotum.

C. Interventions
1. Monitor during the first 6 months of life to determine whether spontaneous descent occurs.
2. Surgical correction is commonly done at 6 months of age and before 12 months, depending on the pediatric surgeon's preference.
3. Monitor for bleeding and infection postoperatively.
4. Instruct parents in postoperative home care measures, including preventing infection, pain control, and activity restrictions.
5. Provide an opportunity for parental counseling if the parents are concerned about the future fertility of the child.

VII. Epispadias and Hypospadias (Fig. 37-2)

A. Description
1. Epispadias and hypospadias are congenital defects involving abnormal placement of the urethral orifice of the penis.
2. These anatomical defects can lead to the easy entry of bacteria into the urine.

B. Assessment
1. Epispadias: The urethral orifice is located on the dorsal surface of the penis; the condition often occurs with exstrophy of the bladder.

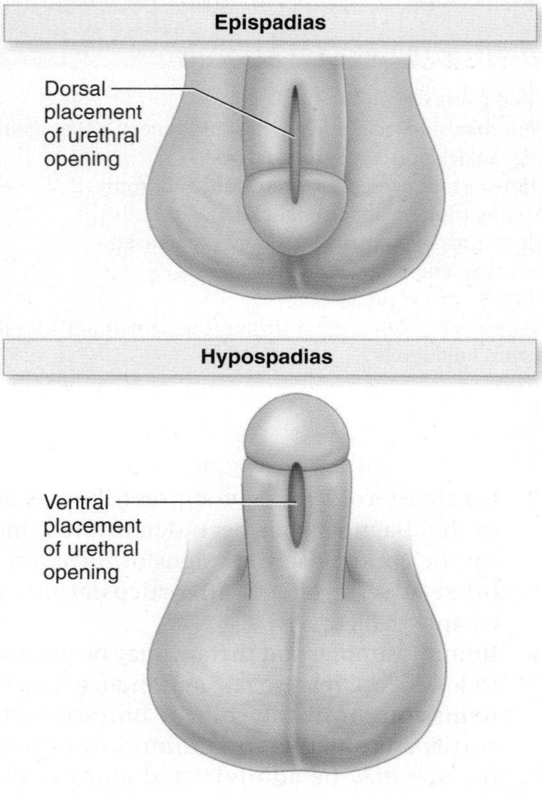

FIG. 37-2 Epispadias and hypospadias are genital anomalies in which the urethral opening is above or below its normal location on the glans of the penis.

2. Hypospadias: Urethral orifice is located below the glans penis along the ventral surface.

C. Surgical interventions: Surgery is done before the age of toilet training, between 6 and 12 months of age, depending on the pediatric surgeon's preference.

Circumcision may not be performed on a newborn with epispadias or hypospadias. Although there are other surgical techniques used to repair these defects, the pediatric surgeon may prefer using the foreskin for surgical reconstruction.

D. Postoperative interventions
1. The child has a pressure dressing and may have some type of urinary diversion or a urinary stent (used to maintain patency of the urethral opening) while the meatus is healing.
2. Monitor vital signs.
3. Encourage fluid intake to maintain adequate urine output and maintain patency of the stent if a stent was placed.
4. Monitor intake and output and the urine for cloudiness or a foul odor.
5. Notify the pediatric surgeon if there is no urinary output for 1 hour, because this may indicate kinks in the urinary diversion or stent or obstruction by sediment.

6. Provide pain medication or medication to relieve bladder spasms (anticholinergic) as prescribed.
7. Administer antibiotics as prescribed.
8. Instruct parents in the care of the child who has a urinary diversion or stent.
9. Instruct parents to avoid giving the child a tub bath until the stent, if present, is removed.
10. Instruct parents about fluid intake, medication administration, signs and symptoms of infection, and need for follow-up for dressing removal after surgery as prescribed.

VIII. Bladder Exstrophy

A. Description
1. Bladder exstrophy is a congenital anomaly characterized by extrusion of the urinary bladder to the outside of the body through a defect in the lower abdominal wall.
2. The cause is unknown; it is possibly a combination of genetic and environmental risk factors during pregnancy.
3. The condition can include specific defects of the abdominal wall, bladder, genitals, pelvic bones, rectum, and anus.
4. Children with bladder exstrophy will also experience vesicoureteral reflux, in which urine flows back up into the ureters to the kidneys; epispadias is also noted.
5. These defects are treated through surgical procedures that repair the affected organs, muscles, and bones.
6. Initial surgery for closure of the abdominal defect should occur within the first few days of life.
7. The goal of subsequent surgeries is to reconstruct the bladder and genitalia and enable the child to achieve urinary continence.

B. Assessment
1. Exposed bladder mucosa and epispadius in males
2. Defects of the abdominal wall
3. Vesicoureteral reflux
4. Defects of the rectum and anus

C. Interventions
1. Monitor urinary output.
2. Monitor for signs of urinary tract or wound infection.
3. Maintain the integrity of the exposed bladder mucosa.
4. Prevent the bladder tissue from drying, while allowing the drainage of urine, until surgical closure is performed. Immediately after birth, as prescribed, the exposed bladder is covered with a sterile, nonadherent dressing to protect it until closure can be performed.
5. Monitor laboratory values and urinalysis to assess renal function.
6. Administer antibiotics as prescribed.
7. Provide emotional support to the parents, and encourage verbalization of their fears and concerns.

Applying petroleum jelly to the bladder mucosa is avoided because it tends to dry out, adhere to the bladder mucosa, and damage the delicate tissues when the dressing is removed.

IX. Sexually Transmitted Infections (STIs)

A. Screening for certain STIs should be done for certain children and adolescents. See http://pediatrics.aappublications.org/content/early/2014/06/25/peds.2014-1024 for specific recommendations.

B. Refer to Chapters 21 and 22 for more detailed information on STIs.

PRACTICE QUESTIONS

372. The nurse reviews the record of a child who is suspected to have glomerulonephritis. Which statement by the child's parent should the nurse expect that is associated with this diagnosis?
1. "His pediatrician said his kidneys are working well."
2. "I noticed his urine was the color of cola lately."
3. "I'm so glad they didn't find any protein in his urine."
4. "The nurse who admitted my child said his blood pressure was low."

373. The nurse performing an admission assessment on a 2-year-old child who has been diagnosed with nephrotic syndrome notes that which **most** common characteristic is associated with this syndrome?
1. Hypertension
2. Generalized edema
3. Increased urinary output
4. Frank, bright red blood in the urine

374. The nurse is planning care for a child with hemolytic-uremic syndrome who has been anuric and will be receiving peritoneal dialysis treatment. The nurse should plan to implement which measure?
1. Restrict fluids as prescribed.
2. Care for the arteriovenous fistula.
3. Encourage foods high in potassium.
4. Administer analgesics as prescribed.

375. A 7-year-old child is seen in a clinic, and the pediatrician documents a diagnosis of nighttime (nocturnal) enuresis. The nurse should provide which information to the parents?
1. Nighttime (nocturnal) enuresis does not respond to treatment.
2. Nighttime (nocturnal) enuresis is caused by a psychiatric problem.

3. Nighttime (nocturnal) enuresis requires surgical intervention to improve the problem.
4. Nighttime (nocturnal) enuresis is usually outgrown without therapeutic intervention.

376. The nurse provided discharge instructions to the parents of a 2-year-old child who had an orchiopexy to correct cryptorchidism. Which statement by the parents indicates the **need for further instruction**?
1. "I'll check his temperature."
2. "I'll give him medication so he'll be comfortable."
3. "I'll check his voiding to be sure there's no problem."
4. "I'll let him decide when to return to his play activities."

377. The nurse is reviewing a treatment plan with the parents of a newborn with hypospadias. Which statement by the parents indicates their understanding of the plan?
1. "Caution should be used when straddling my infant on a hip."
2. "Vital signs should be taken daily to check for bladder infection."
3. "Catheterization will be necessary when my infant does not void."
4. "Circumcision has been delayed to save tissue for surgical repair."

378. The nurse is caring for an infant with a diagnosis of bladder exstrophy. To protect the exposed bladder tissue, the nurse should plan which intervention?
1. Cover the bladder with petroleum jelly gauze.
2. Cover the bladder with a nonadhering plastic wrap.
3. Apply sterile distilled water dressings over the bladder mucosa.
4. Keep the bladder tissue dry by covering it with dry sterile gauze.

379. Which question should the nurse ask the parents of a child suspected of having glomerulonephritis?
1. "Did your child fall off a bike onto the handlebars?"
2. "Has the child had persistent nausea and vomiting?"
3. "Has the child been itching or had a rash anytime in the last week?"
4. "Has the child had a sore throat or a throat infection in the last few weeks?"

380. The nurse collects a urine specimen preoperatively from a child with epispadias who is scheduled for surgical repair. When analyzing the results of the urinalysis, which should the nurse **most likely** expect to note?
1. Hematuria
2. Proteinuria
3. Bacteriuria
4. Glucosuria

381. The nurse is performing an assessment on a child admitted to the hospital with a probable diagnosis of nephrotic syndrome. Which assessment findings should the nurse expect to observe? **Select all that apply.**
- ☐ 1. Pallor
- ☐ 2. Edema
- ☐ 3. Anorexia
- ☐ 4. Proteinuria
- ☐ 5. Weight loss
- ☐ 6. Decreased serum lipids

ANSWERS

372. *Answer:* 2

Rationale: Glomerulonephritis refers to a group of kidney disorders characterized by inflammatory injury in the glomerulus. Gross hematuria, resulting in dark, smoky, cola-colored or brown-colored urine, is a classic symptom of glomerulonephritis. Blood urea nitrogen levels and serum creatinine levels may be elevated, indicating that kidney function is compromised. A mild to moderate elevation in protein in the urine is associated with glomerulonephritis. Hypertension is also common because of fluid volume overload secondary to the kidneys not working properly.

Test-Taking Strategy: Focus on the subject, the manifestations of glomerulonephritis. Eliminate options 1 and 3 first, because hypertension from fluid volume overload and proteinuria are most likely to occur in this kidney disorder. Recalling that this is a renal disorder and that blood urea nitrogen levels and serum creatinine levels increase in these type of disorders will assist in directing you to the correct option.

Level of Cognitive Ability: Analyzing
Client Needs: Physiological Integrity
Integrated Process: Nursing Process—Assessment
Content Area: Pediatrics: Renal and Urinary
Health Problem: Pediatric-Specific: Glomerulonephritis
Priority Concepts: Clinical Judgment; Elimination
Reference: Hockenberry, Wilson, Rodgers (2017), pp. 860-861.

373. *Answer:* 2

Rationale: Nephrotic syndrome is defined as massive proteinuria, hypoalbuminemia, hyperlipemia, and edema. Other manifestations include weight gain; periorbital and facial edema that is most prominent in the morning; leg, ankle, labial, or scrotal edema; decreased urine output and urine that is dark and frothy; abdominal swelling; and blood pressure that is normal or slightly decreased.

Test-Taking Strategy: Note the strategic word, *most.* Recall the pathophysiology associated with nephrotic syndrome. Associate edema with nephrotic syndrome. This will help you answer questions similar to this one.
Level of Cognitive Ability: Analyzing
Client Needs: Physiological Integrity
Integrated Process: Nursing Process—Assessment
Content Area: Pediatrics: Renal and Urinary
Health Problem: Pediatric-Specific: Nephrotic Syndrome
Priority Concepts: Clinical Judgment; Elimination
Reference: Hockenberry, Wilson, Rodgers (2017), pp. 858-859.

374. *Answer:* 1
Rationale: Hemolytic-uremic syndrome is thought to be associated with bacterial toxins, chemicals, and viruses that result in acute kidney injury in children. Clinical manifestations of the disease include acquired hemolytic anemia, thrombocytopenia, renal injury, and central nervous system symptoms. A child with hemolytic-uremic syndrome undergoing peritoneal dialysis because of anuria would be on fluid restriction. Pain is not associated with hemolytic-uremic syndrome, and potassium would be restricted, not encouraged, if the child is anuric. Peritoneal dialysis does not require an arteriovenous fistula (only hemodialysis).
Test-Taking Strategy: Note the subject, anuria. Focus on the child's diagnosis and recall knowledge about the care of a client with acute kidney injury. Also focus on the data in the question. Noting the word *peritoneal* will assist in eliminating option 2. From the remaining options, remember that because the child is anuric, fluids will be restricted.
Level of Cognitive Ability: Analyzing
Client Needs: Physiological Integrity
Integrated Process: Nursing Process—Planning
Content Area: Pediatrics: Renal and Urinary
Health Problem: Pediatric-Specific: Hemolytic Uremic Syndrome
Priority Concepts: Elimination; Fluids and Electrolytes
Reference: Hockenberry, Wilson, Rodgers (2017), p. 862.

375. *Answer:* 4
Rationale: Nighttime (nocturnal) enuresis occurs in a child who has never been dry at night for extended periods. The condition is common in children, and most children eventually outgrow bedwetting without therapeutic intervention. The child is unable to sense a full bladder and does not awaken to void. The child may have delayed maturation of the central nervous system. The condition is not caused by a psychiatric problem.
Test-Taking Strategy: Focus on the subject, the characteristics of nighttime (nocturnal) enuresis. Recall that the word *enuresis* refers to urinating, and the word *nocturnal* refers to nighttime.
Level of Cognitive Ability: Applying
Client Needs: Physiological Integrity
Integrated Process: Nursing Process—Implementation
Content Area: Pediatrics: Renal and Urinary
Health Problem: Pediatric-Specific: Enuresis
Priority Concepts: Development; Elimination
Reference: McKinney et al. (2018), pp. 1007-1008.

376. *Answer:* 4
Rationale: Cryptorchidism is a condition in which 1 or both testes fail to descend through the inguinal canal into the scrotal sac. Surgical correction may be necessary. All vigorous activities should be restricted for 2 weeks after surgery to promote healing and prevent injury. This prevents dislodging of the suture, which is internal. Normally, 2-year-olds want to be active; allowing the child to decide when to return to his play activities may prevent healing and cause injury. The parents should be taught to monitor the temperature, provide analgesics as needed, and monitor the urine output.
Test-Taking Strategy: Note the strategic words, *need for further instruction*. These words indicate a negative event query and ask you to select an option that is an incorrect statement. Option 1 is an important action to recognize signs of infection. Option 2 is appropriate to keep pain to a minimum. Option 3 monitors voiding pattern, which is also important after this type of surgery.
Level of Cognitive Ability: Evaluating
Client Needs: Physiological Integrity
Integrated Process: Teaching and Learning
Content Area: Pediatrics: Renal and Urinary
Health Problem: Pediatric-Specific: Urologic Structural Abnormalities
Priority Concepts: Client Education; Safety
Reference: Hockenberry, Wilson, Rodgers (2017), pp. 854-855.

377. *Answer:* 4
Rationale: Hypospadias is a congenital defect involving abnormal placement of the urethral orifice of the penis. In hypospadias, the urethral orifice is located below the glans penis along the ventral surface. The infant should not be circumcised, because the dorsal foreskin tissue will be used for surgical repair of the hypospadias. Options 1, 2, and 3 are unrelated to this disorder.
Test-Taking Strategy: Focus on the subject, treatment for hypospadias. Note the words *indicates their understanding*. Recalling that hypospadias is a congenital defect involving abnormal placement of the urethral orifice of the penis will direct you to the correct option.
Level of Cognitive Ability: Evaluating
Client Needs: Physiological Integrity
Integrated Process: Nursing Process—Evaluation
Content Area: Pediatrics: Renal and Urinary
Health Problem: Pediatric-Specific: Urologic Structural Abnormalities
Priority Concepts: Client Education; Elimination
Reference: Hockenberry, Wilson, Rodgers (2017), pp. 855-856.

378. *Answer:* 2
Rationale: In bladder exstrophy, the bladder is exposed and external to the body. In this disorder, one must take care to protect the exposed bladder tissue from drying, while allowing the drainage of urine. This is accomplished best by covering the bladder with a nonadhering plastic wrap. The use of petroleum jelly gauze should be avoided, because this type of dressing can dry out, adhere to the mucosa, and damage the delicate tissue when removed. Dry sterile dressings and dressings soaked in solutions (that can dry out) also damage the mucosa when removed.
Test-Taking Strategy: Focus on the subject, treatment for bladder exstrophy, and visualize this disorder. Noting the word *nonadhering* in the correct option will direct you to select this one.

Level of Cognitive Ability: Applying
Client Needs: Physiological Integrity
Integrated Process: Nursing Process—Planning
Content Area: Pediatrics: Renal and Urinary
Health Problem: Pediatric-Specific: Urologic Structural Abnormalities
Priority Concepts: Safety; Tissue Integrity
Reference: Hockenberry, Wilson, Rodgers (2017), pp. 856-857.

379. *Answer:* 4
Rationale: Glomerulonephritis refers to a group of kidney disorders characterized by inflammatory injury in the glomerulus. Group A β-hemolytic streptococcal infection is a cause of glomerulonephritis. Often, a child becomes ill with streptococcal infection of the upper respiratory tract and then develops symptoms of acute poststreptococcal glomerulonephritis after an interval of 1 to 2 weeks. The assessment data in options 1, 2, and 3 are unrelated to a diagnosis of glomerulonephritis.
Test-Taking Strategy: Note the **subject**, a question that will elicit information specific to the diagnosis of glomerulonephritis. Option 1 relates to a kidney injury, not an infectious process. From the remaining options, recalling that a streptococcal infection 1 to 2 weeks before the development of glomerulonephritis is the classic assessment finding will assist in directing you to the correct option.
Level of Cognitive Ability: Applying
Client Needs: Physiological Integrity
Integrated Process: Nursing Process—Assessment
Content Area: Pediatrics: Renal and Urinary
Health Problem: Pediatric-Specific: Glomerulonephritis
Priority Concepts: Clinical Judgment; Infection
Reference: McKinney et al. (2018), pp. 1015-1016.

380. *Answer:* 3
Rationale: Epispadias is a congenital defect involving abnormal placement of the urethral orifice of the penis. The urethral opening is located anywhere on the dorsum of the penis. This anatomical characteristic facilitates entry of bacteria into the urine. Options 1, 2, and 4 are not characteristically noted in this condition.
Test-Taking Strategy: Note the **strategic words**, *most likely.* Visualize the anatomical characteristics of epispadias to answer the question. Options 1, 2, and 4 do not relate to the potential for infection, which can be associated with epispadias.
Level of Cognitive Ability: Analyzing
Client Needs: Physiological Integrity
Integrated Process: Nursing Process—Assessment
Content Area: Pediatrics: Renal and Urinary
Health Problem: Pediatric-Specific: Urologic Structural Abnormalities
Priority Concepts: Clinical Judgment; Elimination
Reference: Hockenberry, Wilson, Rodgers (2017), pp. 856-857.

381. *Answer:* 1, 2, 3, 4
Rationale: Nephrotic syndrome is a kidney disorder characterized by massive proteinuria, hypoalbuminemia, edema, elevated serum lipids, anorexia, and pallor. The child gains weight.
Test-Taking Strategy: Focus on the **subject**, the characteristics of nephrotic syndrome. Thinking about the pathophysiology associated with this disorder and recalling the assessment findings for nephrotic syndrome will direct you to the correct options.
Level of Cognitive Ability: Analyzing
Client Needs: Physiological Integrity
Integrated Process: Nursing Process—Assessment
Content Area: Pediatrics: Renal and Urinary
Health Problem: Pediatric-Specific: Nephrotic Syndrome
Priority Concepts: Clinical Judgment; Elimination
Reference: McKinney et al. (2018), pp. 1018, 1021-1022.

CHAPTER 38

Neurological and Cognitive Problems

PRIORITY CONCEPTS Intracranial Regulation; Safety

I. Cerebral Palsy

A. Description
1. Disorder characterized by impaired movement and posture resulting from an abnormality in the extrapyramidal or pyramidal motor system
2. The most common clinical type is spastic cerebral palsy, which represents an upper motor neuron type of muscle weakness.
3. Less common types of cerebral palsy are athetoid, ataxic, and mixed.

B. Assessment
1. Extreme irritability and crying
2. Feeding difficulties
3. Abnormal motor performance
4. Alterations of muscle tone; stiff and rigid arms or legs
5. Delayed developmental milestones
6. Persistence of primitive infantile reflexes (Moro, tonic neck) after 6 months (most primitive reflexes disappear by 3 to 4 months of age)
7. Abnormal posturing, such as opisthotonos (exaggerated arching of the back) (Fig. 38-1)
8. Seizures may occur.

C. Interventions
1. The goal of management is early recognition and interventions to maximize the child's abilities.
2. An interprofessional team approach is implemented to meet the many needs of the child.
3. Therapeutic management includes physical therapy, occupational therapy, speech therapy, education, and recreation.
4. Assess the child's developmental level and intelligence.
5. Encourage early intervention and participation in school programs.
6. Prepare for using mobilizing devices to help prevent or reduce deformities.
7. Encourage communication and interaction with the child on her or his developmental level, rather than chronological age level.
8. Provide a safe environment by removing sharp objects, using a protective helmet if the child falls frequently, and implementing seizure precautions if necessary.
9. Provide safe, appropriate toys for the child's age and developmental level.
10. Position the child upright after meals.
11. Medications may be prescribed to relieve muscle spasms, which cause intense pain; antiseizure medications may also be prescribed.
12. Provide the parents with information about the disorder and treatment plan; encourage support groups for parents.

II. Head Injury

A. Description
1. Head injury is the pathological result of any mechanical force to the skull, scalp, meninges, or brain (Fig. 38-2).
   a. Open head injury occurs when there is a fracture of the skull or penetration of the skull by an object.
   b. Closed head injury is the result of blunt trauma (this is more serious than an open head injury because of the chance of increased intracranial pressure [ICP] in a "closed" vault); this type of injury can also be caused by shaken baby syndrome.
2. Manifestations depend on the type of injury and the subsequent amount of increased ICP.

B. Assessment: Increased ICP

> ⚠ The child's level of consciousness provides the earliest indication of an improvement or deterioration of the neurological condition.

1. Early signs
   a. Slight change in vital signs
   b. Slight change in level of consciousness
   c. Infant: Irritability, high-pitched cry, bulging fontanel, increased head circumference,

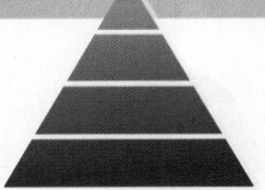

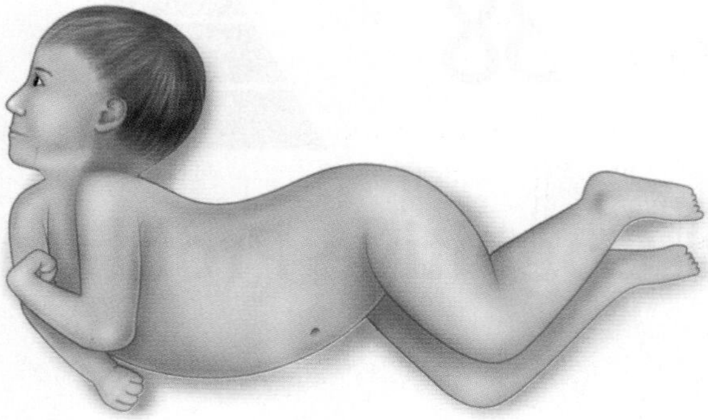

FIG. 38-1 Abnormal posturing: opisthotonos.

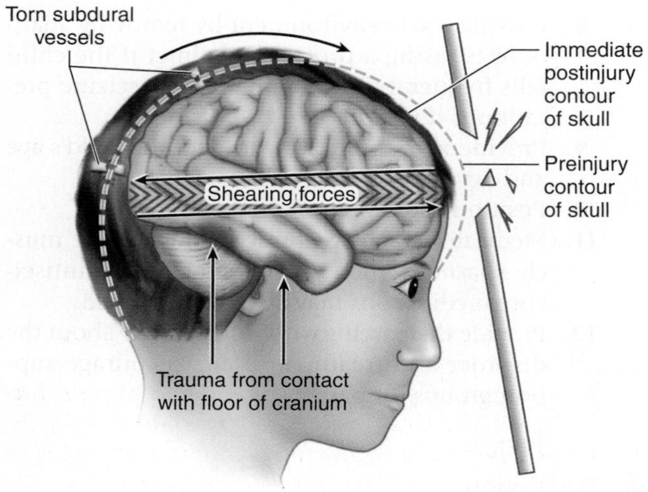

FIG. 38-2 Mechanical distortion of cranium during closed head injury.

dilated scalp veins, Macewen's sign (cracked-pot sound on percussion of the head), setting sun sign (sclera visible above the iris)

d. Child: Headache, nausea, vomiting, visual disturbances (diplopia), seizures

2. Late signs
   a. Significant decrease in level of consciousness
   b. Bradycardia
   c. Decreased motor and sensory responses
   d. Alteration in pupil size and reactivity
   e. Decorticate (flexion) posturing: Adduction of the arms at the shoulders; arms are flexed on the chest with the wrists flexed and the hands fisted, and the lower extremities are extended and adducted; seen with severe dysfunction of cerebral cortex (Fig. 38-3)
   f. Decerebrate (extension) posturing: Rigid extension and pronation of the arms and the legs; sign of dysfunction at the level of the midbrain (see Fig. 38-3)
   g. Cheyne-Stokes respirations
   h. Coma

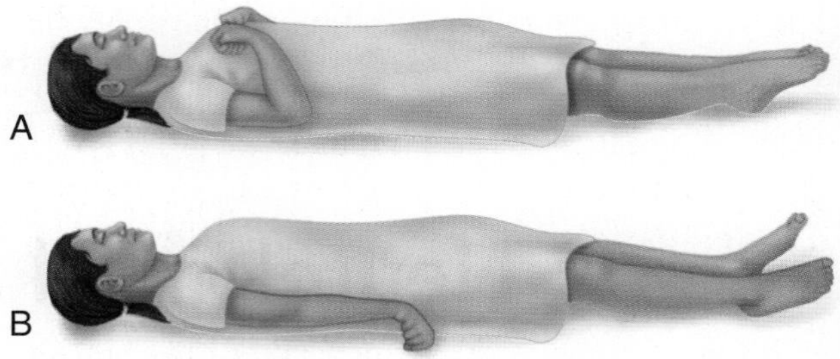

FIG. 38-3 **A,** Decorticate (flexion) posturing. **B,** Decerebrate (extension) posturing.

Immobilize the neck and spine after a head injury if a cervical or other spinal injury is suspected. When a spinal cord injury is ruled out, elevate the head of the bed 15 to 30 degrees, if not contraindicated and as prescribed, to facilitate venous drainage.

C. Interventions
1. Monitor the airway; administer oxygen as prescribed.
2. Assess injuries. (See Chapter 58 for information on spinal cord injuries.)
3. Position the client so that the head is maintained midline to avoid jugular vein compression, which can increase ICP.
4. Monitor vital signs and neurological function (assess level of consciousness closely).
5. Notify the primary health care provider (PHCP) if signs of increased ICP occur.
6. Keep stimuli to a minimum; attempt to minimize crying in an infant.
7. Withhold sedating medications during the acute phase of the injury so that changes in levels of consciousness can be assessed.
8. Initiate seizure precautions (Box 38-1).
9. Monitor for decreased responsiveness to pain (a significant sign of altered level of consciousness).
10. Maintain NPO (nothing by mouth) status or provide clear liquids, if prescribed, until it is determined that vomiting will not occur.

BOX 38-1 Seizure Precautions

- Raise side rails when child is sleeping or resting.
- Pad side rails and other hard objects.
- Place waterproof mattress or pad on bed or crib.
- Instruct child to wear or carry medical identification.
- Instruct child in precautions to take during potentially hazardous activities.
- Instruct child to swim with a companion.
- Instruct child to use a protective helmet and padding when engaged in bicycle riding, skateboarding, and in-line skating.
- Alert caregivers to need for any special precautions.

11. Monitor prescribed intravenous fluids carefully to avoid increasing any cerebral edema and to minimize the possibility of overhydration.
12. Monitor for a fluid or electrolyte alteration (could indicate injury to the hypothalamus or posterior pituitary).
13. Assess wounds and dressings for the presence of drainage, and monitor for nose or ear drainage, which could indicate leakage of cerebrospinal fluid (CSF).
14. Administer tepid sponge baths or place the child on a hypothermia blanket as prescribed if hyperthermia occurs.
15. Avoid suctioning through the nares because of the possibility of the catheter entering the brain through a fracture, which places the child at high risk for a secondary infection.
16. As prescribed, administer acetaminophen for headache, anticonvulsants for seizures, and antibiotics if a laceration is present; prepare to administer prophylactic tetanus toxoid.
17. A corticosteroid or osmotic diuretic may be prescribed to reduce cerebral edema.
18. Monitor for signs of brainstem involvement (Box 38-2).
19. Monitor for signs of epidural hematoma: Asymmetrical pupils (one dilated, nonreactive pupil) may indicate a neurosurgical emergency that requires evacuation of the hematoma.

⚠ Drainage from the nose or ear needs to be tested for the presence of glucose. Drainage that is positive for glucose (as tested with reagent strips) indicates leakage of CSF. The PHCP must be notified immediately if the drainage tests positive for glucose.

III. Hydrocephalus

A. Description
1. An imbalance of CSF absorption or production caused by malformations, tumors, hemorrhage, infections, or trauma
2. Results in head enlargement and increased ICP

B. Types
1. Communicating
   a. Hydrocephalus occurs as a result of impaired absorption within the subarachnoid space.
   b. Obstruction of the cerebrospinal fluid flow in the ventricular system does not occur.
2. Noncommunicating: Obstruction of cerebrospinal fluid flow in the ventricular system does occur.

C. Assessment
1. Infant
   a. Increased head circumference
   b. Thin, widely separated bones of the head that produce a cracked-pot sound (Macewen's sign) on percussion
   c. Anterior fontanel tense, bulging, and nonpulsating; sutures will separate prior to fontanel bulging
   d. Dilated scalp veins
   e. Frontal bossing
   f. "Setting sun" eyes
2. Child
   a. Behavior changes, such as irritability and lethargy
   b. Headache on awakening
   c. Nausea and vomiting
   d. Ataxia
   e. Nystagmus
3. Late signs: High, shrill cry and seizures

D. Surgical interventions
1. The goal of surgical treatment is to prevent further CSF accumulation by bypassing the blockage and draining the fluid from the ventricles to a location where it may be reabsorbed.
2. In a ventriculoperitoneal **shunt**, the CSF drains into the peritoneal cavity from the lateral ventricle (Fig. 38-4).
3. In a ventriculoatrial shunt, CSF drains into the right atrium of the heart from the lateral ventricle, bypassing the obstruction (used in older children and in children with pathological conditions of the abdomen).
4. Shunt revision may be necessary as the child grows.
5. An alternative to shunt placement is endoscopic third ventriculostomy, in which a small opening in the floor of the third ventricle is made that allows CSF to bypass the fourth ventricle and return to the circulation to be absorbed; this treatment may not be appropriate for some types of hydrocephalus.

E. Preoperative interventions
1. Monitor intake and output; give small, frequent feedings as tolerated until preoperative NPO status is prescribed.
2. Reposition the head frequently and use special devices such as an egg crate mattress under the head to prevent pressure sores.
3. Prepare the child and family for diagnostic procedures and surgery.

BOX 38-2 Signs of Brainstem Involvement

- Deep, rapid, or intermittent and gasping respirations
- Wide fluctuations or noticeable slowing of pulse
- Widening pulse pressure or extreme fluctuations in blood pressure
- Sluggish, dilated, or unequal pupils

Notify the primary health care provider immediately if these signs develop!

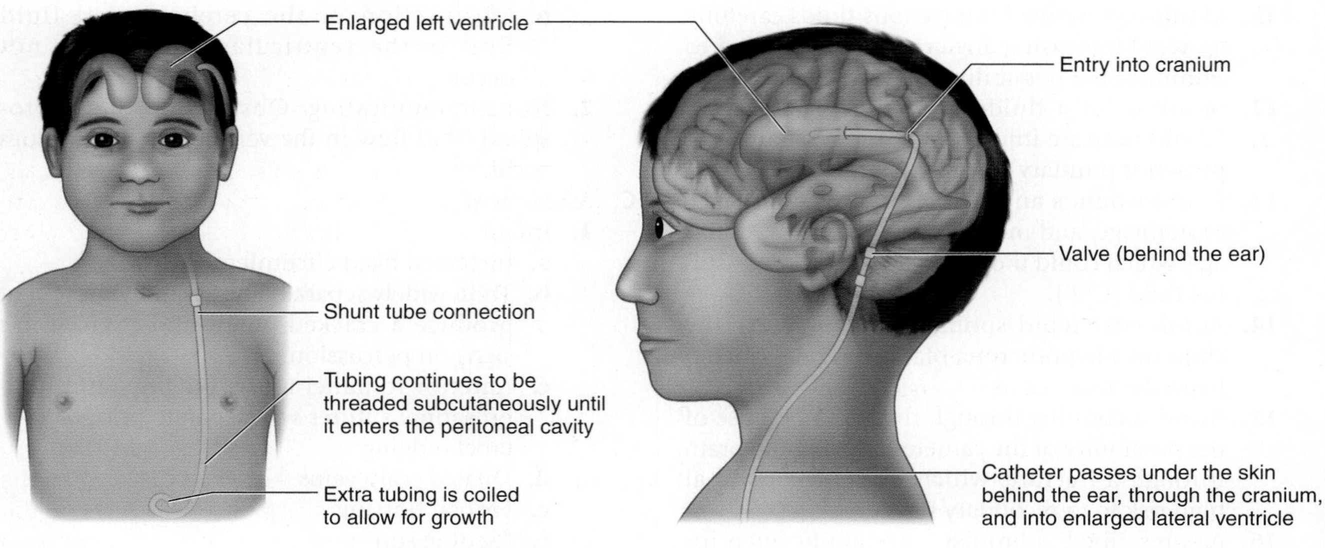

FIG. 38-4 Ventriculoperitoneal shunt.

F. Postoperative interventions
1. Monitor vital signs and neurological signs.
2. Position the child on the unoperated side to prevent pressure on the shunt valve.
3. Keep the child flat if prescribed to avoid rapid reduction of intracranial fluid.
4. Observe for increased ICP; if increased ICP occurs, elevate the head of the bed to 15 to 30 degrees to enhance gravity flow through the shunt.
5. Measure head circumference.
6. Monitor for signs of infection and assess dressings for drainage.
7. Monitor intake and output.
8. Provide comfort measures and administer medications as prescribed.
9. Instruct parents on how to recognize shunt infection or malfunction.
10. In an infant, irritability, a high, shrill cry, lethargy, and feeding poorly may indicate shunt malfunction or infection.
11. In a toddler, headache and a lack of appetite are the earliest common signs of shunt malfunction.
12. In older children, an indicator of shunt malfunction is an alteration in the child's level of consciousness.

A high, shrill cry in an infant can be a sign of increased ICP.

IV. Meningitis

A. Description
1. Meningitis is an infectious process of the central nervous system caused by bacteria or viruses that may be acquired as a primary disease or as a result of complications of neurosurgery, trauma, infection of the sinuses or ears, or systemic infections.
2. Diagnosis of bacterial meningitis is made by testing CSF obtained by lumbar puncture; the fluid is cloudy with increased pressure, increased white blood cell count, elevated protein, and decreased glucose levels.
3. Bacterial meningitis can be caused by various organisms, most commonly *Haemophilus influenzae* type b, *Streptococcus pneumoniae,* or *Neisseria meningitidis;* meningococcal meningitis occurs in epidemic form and can be transmitted by droplets from nasopharyngeal secretions.
4. Viral meningitis is associated with viruses such as mumps, paramyxovirus, herpesvirus, and enterovirus.

B. Assessment
1. Signs and symptoms vary, depending on the type, the age of the child, and the duration of the preceding illness.
2. Fever, chills, headache
3. Vomiting, diarrhea
4. Poor feeding or anorexia
5. Nuchal rigidity
6. Poor or high, shrill cry
7. Altered level of consciousness, such as lethargy or irritability
8. Bulging anterior fontanel in an infant
9. Positive Kernig's sign (inability to extend the leg when the thigh is flexed anteriorly at the hip) and Brudzinski's sign (neck flexion causes adduction and flexion movements of the lower extremities) in children and adolescents
10. Muscle or joint pain (meningococcal infection and *H. influenzae* infection)
11. Petechial or purpuric rashes (meningococcal infection)
12. Ear that chronically drains (pneumococcal meningitis)

C. Interventions
1. Provide respiratory isolation precautions and maintain it for at least 24 hours after antibiotics are initiated.
2. Administer antibiotics and antipyretics as prescribed (administer antibiotics as soon as they are prescribed after lumbar puncture); antiseizure medications may also be prescribed.
3. Perform neurological assessment and monitor for seizures; assess for the complication of inappropriate antidiuretic hormone secretion, causing fluid retention (cerebral edema) and dilutional hyponatremia.
4. Assess for changes in level of consciousness and irritability.
5. Monitor for a purpuric or petechial rash and for signs of thromboemboli.
6. Assess nutritional status; monitor intake and output.
7. Monitor for hearing loss.
8. Determine close contacts of the child with meningitis, because the contacts need prophylactic treatment.
9. Pneumococcal conjugate vaccine is recommended for all children beginning at age 2 months to protect against meningitis; streptococcal pneumococci can cause many bacterial infections, including meningitis (see Chapter 18 for information on vaccines).

V. Submersion Injury

A. Description
1. Survival of at least 24 hours after submersion in a fluid medium
2. Hypoxia/asphyxiation is the primary problem because it results in extensive cell damage; cerebral cells sustain irreversible damage after 4 to 6 minutes of submersion.
3. Additional problems include aspiration and hypothermia.
4. Outcome is predicted on the basis of the length of submersion in nonicy water; outcome may be good if submersion was for less than 5 minutes and the child exhibits neurological responsiveness, reactive pupils, and a normal cardiac rhythm.
5. A child who was submerged for more than 10 minutes and does not respond to cardiopulmonary life support measures within 25 minutes has an extremely poor prognosis (severe neurological impairment or death).

B. Interventions
1. Provide ventilatory and circulatory support; if the child has had a severe cerebral insult, endotracheal intubation and mechanical ventilation may be required.
2. Monitor respiratory status, because respiratory compromise and cerebral edema may occur 24 hours after the incident.
3. Monitor for aspiration pneumonia.
4. Monitor neurological status closely; if spontaneous purposeful movement and normal brainstem function are not apparent 24 hours after the event, the child most likely has sustained severe neurological deficits.
5. Teach parents to provide adequate supervision of infants and small children around water to prevent accidents.

VI. Reye's Syndrome

A. Description
1. Reye's syndrome is an acute encephalopathy that follows a viral illness and is characterized pathologically by cerebral edema and fatty changes in the liver; diagnosis is made by laboratory studies and liver biopsy.
2. The exact cause is unclear; it most commonly follows a viral illness such as influenza or varicella.
3. Administration of aspirin and aspirin-containing products is not recommended for children with a febrile illness or children with varicella or influenza because of its association with Reye's syndrome.
4. Acetaminophen or ibuprofen are considered the medications of choice.
5. Early diagnosis and aggressive treatment are important; the goal of treatment is to maintain effective cerebral perfusion and control increasing ICP.

B. Assessment
1. History of systemic viral illness 4 to 7 days before the onset of symptoms
2. Fever
3. Nausea and vomiting
4. Signs of altered hepatic function such as lethargy
5. Progressive neurological deterioration
6. Increased blood ammonia levels

C. Interventions
1. Provide rest and decrease stimulation in the environment.
2. Assess neurological status.
3. Monitor for altered level of consciousness and signs of increased ICP.
4. Monitor for signs of altered hepatic function and results of liver function studies.
5. Monitor intake and output.
6. Monitor for signs of bleeding and signs of impaired coagulation, such as a prolonged bleeding time.

VII. Seizure Disorders

A. Description (see Chapter 58 for additional information on seizures)

1. Excessive and unorganized neuronal discharges in the brain that activate associated motor and sensory organs
2. Classified as generalized, partial, or unclassified, depending on the area of the brain involved
3. Types of generalized seizures include tonic-clonic, absence, myoclonic, and atonic.
4. Partial seizures arise from a specific area in the brain and cause limited symptoms; types include simple partial and complex partial.

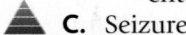

B. Assessment
1. Obtain information from the parents about the time of onset, precipitating events, and behavior before and after the seizure.
2. Determine the child's history related to seizures.
3. Ask the child about the presence of an aura (a warning sign of impending seizure).
4. Monitor for apnea and cyanosis.
5. Postseizure (postictal state): The child is disoriented and sleepy.

C. Seizure precautions (see Box 38-1)

D. Interventions (Box 38-3)

E. Antiseizure medications (see Chapter 59 for information on medications)

Never place anything, including an airway device, into the mouth of a child during a seizure.

VIII. Neural Tube Defects

A. Description
1. This central nervous system defect results from failure of the neural tube to close during embryonic development.
2. Folic acid is recommended during childbearing years and pregnancy to reduce the occurrence of these conditions.
3. Associated deficits include sensorimotor disturbance, dislocated hips, talipes equinovarus (clubfoot), and hydrocephalus.
4. Defect closure is performed soon after birth.

B. Types
1. Spina bifida occulta
   a. Posterior vertebral arches fail to close in the lumbosacral area.
   b. Spinal cord remains intact and usually is not visible.
   c. Meninges are not exposed on the skin surface.
   d. Neurological deficits are not usually present.
2. Closed neural tube defect
   a. This type consists of a diverse group of defects; the spinal cord is marked by malformations of fat, bone, or meninges.
   b. Usually there are few or no symptoms; in some situations the malformation causes incomplete paralysis with urinary and bowel dysfunction.
3. Meningocele
   a. Protrusion involves meninges and a sac-like cyst that contains CSF in the midline of the back, usually in the lumbosacral area.
   b. The spinal cord is not involved.
   c. Neurological deficits are usually not present.
4. Myelomeningocele
   a. Protrusion of the meninges, CSF, nerve roots, and a portion of the spinal cord occurs.
   b. The sac (defect) is covered by a thin membrane prone to leakage or rupture.
   c. Neurological deficits are evident.

C. Assessment
1. Depends on the spinal cord involvement
2. Visible spinal defect
3. Flaccid paralysis of the legs
4. Altered bladder and bowel function
5. Hip and joint deformities
6. Hydrocephalus

D. Interventions
1. Evaluate the sac and measure the lesion.
2. Perform neurological assessment.
3. Monitor for increased ICP, which might indicate developing hydrocephalus.
4. Measure head circumference; assess anterior fontanel for bulging.
5. Protect the sac; as prescribed, cover with a sterile, moist (normal saline), nonadherent dressing to maintain the moisture of the sac and contents.
6. Change the dressing covering the sac on a regular schedule or whenever it becomes soiled because of the risk of infection; diapering may be contraindicated until the defect has been repaired.

BOX 38-3 Interventions for Seizures

- Ensure airway patency.
- Have suction equipment and oxygen available.
- Time the seizure episode.
- If the child is standing or sitting, ease the child down to the floor and place the child in a side-lying position.
- Place a pillow or folded blanket under the child's head; if no bedding is available, place your own hands under the child's head or place the child's head in your own lap.
- Loosen restrictive clothing.
- Remove eyeglasses from the child if present.
- Clear the area of any hazards or hard objects.
- Allow the seizure to proceed and end without interference.
- If vomiting occurs, turn the child to one side as a unit.
- Do not restrain the child, place anything in the child's mouth, or give any food or liquids to the child.
- Prepare to administer medications as prescribed.
- Remain with the child until the child recovers fully.
- Observe for incontinence, which may have occurred during the seizure.
- Document the occurrence.

7. Use aseptic technique to prevent infection.
8. Assess the sac for redness, clear or purulent drainage, abrasions, irritation, and signs of infection.
9. Early signs of infection include elevated temperature (axillary), irritability, lethargy, and nuchal rigidity.
10. Place in a prone position to minimize tension on the sac and the risk of trauma; the head is turned to 1 side for feeding.
11. Assess for physical impairments such as hip and joint deformities.
12. Prepare the child and family for surgery.
13. Administer antibiotics preoperatively and postoperatively, as prescribed, to prevent infection.
14. Teach the parents and eventually the child about long-term home care.
    a. Positioning, feeding, skin care, and range-of-motion exercises
    b. Instituting a bladder elimination program and performing clean intermittent catheterization technique if necessary
    c. Administering antispasmodics (that act on the smooth muscle of the bladder) as prescribed to increase bladder capacity and improve continence
    d. Implement a bowel program, including a high-fiber diet, increased fluids, and suppositories as needed.
    e. The child is at high risk for allergy to latex and rubber products because of the frequent exposure to latex during implementation of care measures.

IX. Attention-Deficit Hyperactivity Disorder

A. Description
1. Behavior disorder characterized by developmentally inappropriate degrees of inattention, overactivity, and impulsivity
2. Childhood problems include lowered intellectual development, some minor physical abnormalities, sleeping disturbances, behavioral or emotional disorders, and difficulty in social relationships.
3. Early diagnosis is important to prevent impaired emotional and psychological development.
4. Diagnosis is established on the basis of self-reports, parent and teacher reports, and use of assessment tools.

B. Assessment
1. Fidgets with hands or feet or squirms in the seat
2. Easily distracted with external or internal stimuli
3. Difficulty with following through on instructions
4. Poor attention span
5. Shifts from 1 uncompleted activity to another
6. Talks excessively
7. Interrupts or intrudes on others
8. Engages in physically dangerous activities without considering the possible consequences

C. Interventions
1. Provide parents with information about the disorder and treatment plan; encourage support groups for parents.
2. Treatment includes behavioral therapy, medication, maintaining a consistent environment, and appropriate classroom placement.
3. Behavioral therapy focuses on preventing undesirable behavior.
4. Maintain a consistent home and classroom environment, and provide environmental and physical safety measures.
5. Promote self-esteem.
6. Stimulant medications may be prescribed; possible side effects include appetite suppression and weight loss, nervousness, tics, insomnia, and increased blood pressure.
7. Instruct the child and parents about medication administration and the need for regular follow-up.

X. Autism Spectrum Disorders

A. Description
1. Autism spectrum disorders (ASDs) are complex neurodevelopmental disorders of unknown etiology composed of qualitative alterations in social interaction and verbal impairment with repetitive, restricted, and stereotype behavioral patterns.
2. Autism spectrum disorder impairments range from mild to severe; types include autism, Asperger's syndrome, Rett's syndrome.
3. Symptoms are usually noticed by the parents by 3 years of age.
4. The cause of the disorder is not specifically known; however, it has been linked to a wide range of antepartum, intrapartum, and newborn conditions and exposure to hazardous chemicals; genetic predisposition is also linked to the disorder.
5. The disorder is accompanied by intellectual and social behavioral deficits, and the child exhibits peculiar and bizarre characteristics with social interactions, communication, and behaviors.
6. Despite their relatively moderate to severe disability, some children with autism (known as *savants*) excel in particular areas, such as art, music, memory, mathematics, or perceptual skills such as puzzle building.
7. Diagnosis is established on the basis of symptoms and the use of several screening tools.

B. Assessment
1. Social
    a. Abnormal or lack of comfort-seeking behaviors

b. Abnormal or lack of social play
c. Impairment in peer relationships
d. Lack of awareness of the existence or feelings of others
e. Abnormal imitation of others

2. Communication
a. Lack of, impaired, or abnormal speech, such as producing a monotone voice or echolalia
b. Abnormal nonverbal communication (does not use gestures to communicate)

3. Behavior
a. Lack of imaginative play
b. Persistent preoccupation or attachment to objects; range of interests restricted
c. Self-injurious behaviors
d. Must maintain routine; any environmental change produces marked distress
e. Produces repetitive body movements such as rocking or head banging

C. Interventions
1. Determine the child's routines, habits, and preferences and maintain consistency as much as possible.
2. Determine the specific ways in which the child communicates and use these methods.
3. Avoid placing demands on the child.
4. Implement safety precautions as necessary for self-injurious behaviors such as head banging.
5. Initiate referrals to special programs as required.
6. Provide support to parents.
7. The Modified Checklist for Autism in Toddlers—Revised (MCHAT-R) is used to screen toddlers for this disorder. For a copy of the tool, see https://www.autismspeaks.org/sites/default/files/docs/sciencedocs/m-chat/m-chat-r_f.pdf?v=1

Ensuring a safe environment for a child with autism is a priority.

XI. Intellectual Disability

A. Description
1. In intellectual disability, a child manifests subaverage intellectual functioning along with deficits in adaptive skills.
2. Down's syndrome is a congenital condition that results in moderate to severe intellectual disabilities and has been linked to an extra group G chromosome, chromosome 21 (trisomy 21).

B. Assessment
1. Deficits in cognitive skills and level of adaptive functioning
2. Delays in fine and gross motor skills
3. Speech delays
4. Decreased spontaneous activity
5. Nonresponsiveness
6. Irritability
7. Poor eye contact during feeding

C. Interventions
1. Medical strategies are focused on correcting structural deformities and treating associated behaviors.
2. Implement community and educational services, using a multidisciplinary approach.
3. Promote care skills as much as possible.
4. Assist with communication and socialization skills.
5. Facilitate appropriate play time.
6. Initiate safety precautions as necessary.
7. Assist the family with decisions regarding care.
8. Provide information regarding support services and community agencies.

PRACTICE QUESTIONS

382. The parents of a child recently diagnosed with cerebral palsy ask the nurse about the limitations of the disorder. The nurse responds by explaining that the limitations occur as a result of which pathophysiological process?
1. An infectious disease of the central nervous system
2. An inflammation of the brain as a result of a viral illness
3. A chronic disability characterized by impaired muscle movement and posture
4. A congenital condition that results in moderate to severe intellectual disabilities

383. The nurse notes documentation that a child is exhibiting an inability to flex the leg when the thigh is flexed anteriorly at the hip. Which condition does the nurse suspect?
1. Meningitis
2. Spinal cord injury
3. Intracranial bleeding
4. Decreased cerebral blood flow

384. A mother arrives at the emergency department with her 5-year-old child and states that the child fell off a bunk bed. A head injury is suspected. The nurse checks the child's airway status and assesses the child for early and late signs of increased intracranial pressure (ICP). Which is a **late** sign of increased ICP?
1. Nausea
2. Irritability
3. Headache
4. Bradycardia

385. The nurse is assigned to care for an 8-year-old child with a diagnosis of a basilar skull fracture. The nurse reviews the pediatrician's prescriptions and should contact the pediatrician to question which prescription?
1. Obtain daily weight.
2. Provide clear liquid intake.

3. Nasotracheal suction as needed.
4. Maintain a patent intravenous line.

386. The nurse is reviewing the record of a child with increased intracranial pressure and notes that the child has exhibited signs of decerebrate posturing. On assessment of the child, the nurse expects to note which characteristic of this type of posturing?
1. Flaccid paralysis of all extremities
2. Adduction of the arms at the shoulders
3. Rigid extension and pronation of the arms and legs
4. Abnormal flexion of the upper extremities and extension and adduction of the lower extremities

387. A child is diagnosed with Reye's syndrome. The nurse creates a nursing care plan for the child and should include which intervention in the plan?
1. Assessing hearing loss
2. Monitoring urine output
3. Changing body position every 2 hours
4. Providing a quiet atmosphere with dimmed lighting

388. The nurse creates a plan of care for a child at risk for tonic-clonic seizures. In the plan of care, the nurse identifies seizure precautions and documents that which item(s) need to be placed at the child's bedside?
1. Emergency cart
2. Tracheotomy set
3. Padded tongue blade
4. Suctioning equipment and oxygen

389. A lumbar puncture is performed on a child suspected to have bacterial meningitis, and cerebrospinal fluid (CSF) is obtained for analysis. The nurse reviews the results of the CSF analysis and determines that which results would verify the diagnosis?
1. Clear CSF, decreased pressure, and elevated protein level
2. Clear CSF, elevated protein, and decreased glucose levels
3. Cloudy CSF, elevated protein, and decreased glucose levels
4. Cloudy CSF, decreased protein, and decreased glucose levels

390. The nurse is planning care for a child with acute bacterial meningitis. Based on the mode of transmission of this infection, which precautionary intervention should be included in the plan of care?
1. Maintain enteric precautions.
2. Maintain neutropenic precautions.
3. No precautions are required as long as antibiotics have been started.
4. Maintain respiratory isolation precautions for at least 24 hours after the initiation of antibiotics.

391. An infant with a diagnosis of hydrocephalus is scheduled for surgery. Which is the **priority** nursing intervention in the preoperative period?
1. Test the urine for protein.
2. Reposition the infant frequently.
3. Provide a stimulating environment.
4. Assess blood pressure every 15 minutes.

392. The nurse is creating a plan of care for a child who is at risk for seizures. Which interventions apply if the child has a seizure? **Select all that apply.**
- ☐ 1. Time the seizure.
- ☐ 2. Restrain the child.
- ☐ 3. Stay with the child.
- ☐ 4. Place the child in a prone position.
- ☐ 5. Move furniture away from the child.
- ☐ 6. Insert a padded tongue blade in the child's mouth.

ANSWERS

382. *Answer:* 3

Rationale: Cerebral palsy is a chronic disability characterized by impaired movement and posture resulting from an abnormality in the extrapyramidal or pyramidal motor system. Meningitis is an infectious process of the central nervous system. Encephalitis is an inflammation of the brain that occurs as a result of viral illness or central nervous system infection. Down's syndrome is an example of a congenital condition that results in moderate to severe intellectual disabilities.

Test-Taking Strategy: Eliminate options 1 and 2 first, noting that they are comparable or alike. Next, note the relationship between the words *palsy* in the question and *impaired muscle movement* in the correct option.

Level of Cognitive Ability: Applying
Client Needs: Physiological Integrity
Integrated Process: Teaching and Learning
Content Area: Pediatrics: Neurological
Health Problem: Pediatric-Specific: Cerebral Palsy
Priority Concepts: Intracranial Regulation; Mobility
Reference: Hockenberry, Wilson, Rodgers (2017), pp. 979-980.

383. *Answer:* 1

Rationale: Meningitis is an infectious process of the central nervous system caused by bacteria and viruses. The inability to extend the leg when the thigh is flexed anteriorly at the hip is a positive Kernig's sign, noted in meningitis. Kernig's sign is not seen specifically with spinal cord injury, intracranial bleeding, or decreased cerebral blood flow.

Test-Taking Strategy: Note the data in the question and the subject, the characteristics of Kernig's sign. Knowledge regarding this sign is needed to answer correctly. Think about the neurological exam and physical assessment findings to answer correctly.
Level of Cognitive Ability: Applying
Client Needs: Physiological Integrity
Integrated Process: Nursing Process—Assessment
Content Area: Pediatrics: Neurological
Health Problem: Pediatric-Specific: Meningitis
Priority Concepts: Clinical Judgment; Intracranial Regulation
Reference: McKinney et al. (2018), p. 1302.

384. ***Answer:*** **4**
Rationale: Head injury is the pathological result of any mechanical force to the skull, scalp, meninges, or brain. A head injury can cause bleeding in the brain and result in increased ICP. In a child, early signs include a slight change in level of consciousness, headache, nausea, vomiting, visual disturbances (diplopia), and seizures. Late signs of increased ICP include a significant decrease in level of consciousness, bradycardia, decreased motor and sensory responses, alterations in pupil size and reactivity, posturing, Cheyne-Stokes respirations, and coma.
Test-Taking Strategy: Note the age of the child and the strategic word, *late*. Think about the pathophysiology that occurs when pressure increases in the cranial vault to assist in answering correctly.
Level of Cognitive Ability: Analyzing
Client Needs: Physiological Integrity
Integrated Process: Nursing Process—Assessment
Content Area: Pediatrics: Neurological
Health Problem: Pediatric-Specific: Head Injury
Priority Concepts: Clinical Judgment; Intracranial Regulation
Reference: Hockenberry, Wilson, Rodgers (2017), pp. 872-873.

385. ***Answer:*** **3**
Rationale: A basilar skull fracture is a type of head injury. Nasotracheal suctioning is contraindicated in a child with a basilar skull fracture. Because of the nature of the injury, there is a possibility that the catheter will enter the brain through the fracture, creating a high risk of secondary infection. Fluid balance is monitored closely by daily weight determination, intake and output measurement, and serum osmolality determination to detect early signs of water retention, excessive dehydration, and states of hypertonicity or hypotonicity. The child is maintained on NPO (nothing by mouth) status or restricted to clear liquids until it is determined that vomiting will not occur. An intravenous line is maintained to administer fluids or medications, if necessary.
Test-Taking Strategy: Note the words *question which prescription*. Eliminate options 1, 2, and 4 because they are comparable or alike in that they address the subject of fluids. Remember that nasotracheal suctioning is contraindicated in a child with a skull fracture because of the risk of infection.
Level of Cognitive Ability: Analyzing
Client Needs: Safe and Effective Care Environment
Integrated Process: Nursing Process—Implementation
Content Area: Pediatrics: Neurological
Health Problem: Pediatric-Specific: Head Injury
Priority Concepts: Collaboration; Intracranial Regulation
Reference: Hockenberry, Wilson, Rodgers (2017), p. 888.

386. ***Answer:*** **3**
Rationale: Decerebrate (extension) posturing is characterized by the rigid extension and pronation of the arms and legs. Option 1 is incorrect. Options 2 and 4 describe decorticate (flexion) posturing.
Test-Taking Strategy: Focus on the subject, characteristics of decerebrate (extension) posturing. Recalling the clinical manifestations associated with decerebrate posturing will direct you to the correct option. Remember that decerebrate posturing is characterized by the rigid extension and pronation of the arms and legs.
Level of Cognitive Ability: Analyzing
Client Needs: Physiological Integrity
Integrated Process: Nursing Process—Assessment
Content Area: Pediatrics: Neurological
Health Problem: Pediatric-Specific: Head Injury
Priority Concepts: Clinical Judgment; Intracranial Regulation
Reference: McKinney et al. (2018), p. 1283.

387. ***Answer:*** **4**
Rationale: Reye's syndrome is an acute encephalopathy that follows a viral illness and is characterized pathologically by cerebral edema and fatty changes in the liver. In Reye's syndrome, supportive care is directed toward monitoring and managing cerebral edema. Decreasing stimuli in the environment by providing a quiet environment with dimmed lighting would decrease the stress on the cerebral tissue and neuron responses. Hearing loss and urine output are not affected. Changing the body position every 2 hours would not affect the cerebral edema directly. The child should be positioned with the head elevated to decrease the progression of the cerebral edema and promote drainage of cerebrospinal fluid.
Test-Taking Strategy: Focus on the subject, nursing care for the child with Reye's syndrome. Think about the pathophysiology associated with Reye's syndrome. Recalling that cerebral edema is a concern for a child with Reye's syndrome will direct you to the correct option.
Level of Cognitive Ability: Creating
Client Needs: Physiological Integrity
Integrated Process: Nursing Process—Planning
Content Area: Pediatrics: Neurological
Health Problem: Pediatric-Specific: Reye Syndrome
Priority Concepts: Clinical Judgment; Intracranial Regulation
Reference: Hockenberry, Wilson, Rodgers (2017), pp. 895-896.

388. ***Answer:*** **4**
Rationale: A seizure results from the excessive and unorganized neuronal discharges in the brain that activate associated motor and sensory organs. A type of generalized seizure is a tonic-clonic seizure. This type of seizure causes rigidity of all body muscles, followed by intense jerking movements. Because increased oral secretions and apnea can occur during and after the seizure, oxygen and suctioning equipment are placed at the bedside. A tracheotomy is not performed during a seizure. No object, including a padded tongue blade, is placed into the child's mouth during a seizure. An emergency cart would not be left at the bedside but would be available in the treatment room or nearby on the nursing unit.
Test-Taking Strategy: Focus on the subject, seizure precautions. Note the words *need to be placed at the child's bedside.*

Eliminate option 2, knowing that a tracheotomy is not performed. Next, recalling that no object is placed into the mouth of a child experiencing a seizure assists in eliminating option 3. From the remaining options, focus on the primary concern during seizure activity. This will direct you to the correct option.
Level of Cognitive Ability: Creating
Client Needs: Physiological Integrity
Integrated Process: Nursing Process—Planning
Content Area: Pediatrics: Neurological
Health Problem: Pediatric-Specific: Seizures
Priority Concepts: Clinical Judgment; Intracranial Regulation
Reference: Hockenberry, Wilson, Rodgers (2017), p. 904.

389. *Answer:* 3
Rationale: Meningitis is an infectious process of the central nervous system caused by bacteria and viruses; it may be acquired as a primary disease or as a result of complications of neurosurgery, trauma, infection of the sinus or ears, or systemic infections. Meningitis is diagnosed by testing CSF obtained by lumbar puncture. In the case of bacterial meningitis, findings usually include an elevated pressure; turbid or cloudy CSF; and elevated leukocyte, elevated protein, and decreased glucose levels.
Test-Taking Strategy: Use knowledge regarding the diagnostic findings in meningitis. Eliminate options 1 and 2 first because they are comparable or alike; recall that clear CSF is not likely to be found in an infectious process such as meningitis. From this point, recall that an elevated protein level indicates a possible diagnosis of meningitis to direct you to the correct option.
Level of Cognitive Ability: Analyzing
Client Needs: Physiological Integrity
Integrated Process: Nursing Process—Analysis
Content Area: Pediatrics: Neurological
Health Problem: Pediatric-Specific: Meningitis
Priority Concepts: Infection; Intracranial Regulation
Reference: McKinney et al. (2018), pp. 1301-1302.

390. *Answer:* 4
Rationale: Meningitis is an infectious process of the central nervous system caused by bacteria and viruses; it may be acquired as a primary disease or as a result of complications of neurosurgery, trauma, infection of the sinus or ears, or systemic infections. A major priority of nursing care for a child suspected to have meningitis is to administer the prescribed antibiotic as soon as a culture is obtained. The child also is placed on respiratory isolation precautions for at least 24 hours while culture results are obtained and the antibiotic is having an effect. Enteric precautions and neutropenic precautions are not associated with the mode of transmission of meningitis. Enteric precautions are instituted when the mode of transmission is through the gastrointestinal tract. Neutropenic precautions are instituted when a child has a low neutrophil count.
Test-Taking Strategy: Focus on the subject, the mode of transmission of meningitis. Eliminate options 1 and 2 first because they are comparable or alike, and are unrelated to the mode of transmission. Recalling that it takes about 24 hours for antibiotics to reach a therapeutic blood level will assist in directing you to the correct option.
Level of Cognitive Ability: Applying
Client Needs: Safe and Effective Care Environment
Integrated Process: Nursing Process—Planning
Content Area: Pediatrics: Neurological
Health Problem: Pediatric-Specific: Meningitis
Priority Concepts: Infection; Safety
Reference: McKinney et al. (2018), pp. 1302-1303.

391. *Answer:* 2
Rationale: Hydrocephalus occurs as a result of an imbalance of cerebrospinal fluid absorption or production that is caused by malformations, tumors, hemorrhage, infections, or trauma. It results in head enlargement and increased intracranial pressure (ICP). In infants with hydrocephalus, the head grows at an abnormal rate, and if the infant is not repositioned frequently, pressure ulcers can occur on the back and side of the head. An egg crate mattress under the head is also a nursing intervention that can help prevent skin breakdown. Proteinuria is not specific to hydrocephalus. Stimulus should be kept at a minimum because of the increase in ICP. It is not necessary to check the blood pressure every 15 minutes.
Test-Taking Strategy: Note the strategic word, *priority.* Focus on the child's diagnosis. Eliminate option 4 because of the words *15 minutes*. From the remaining options, recall that because of the severe head enlargement, the nursing intervention that has priority is to reposition the infant frequently to prevent the development of pressure areas.
Level of Cognitive Ability: Applying
Client Needs: Physiological Integrity
Integrated Process: Nursing Process—Implementation
Content Area: Pediatrics: Neurological
Health Problem: Pediatric-Specific: Hydrocephalus
Priority Concepts: Intracranial Regulation; Tissue Integrity
Reference: Hockenberry, Wilson, Rodgers (2017), pp. 906-908.

392. *Answer:* 1, 3, 5
Rationale: A seizure is a disorder that occurs as a result of excessive and unorganized neuronal discharges in the brain that activate associated motor and sensory organs. During a seizure, the child is placed on her or his side in a lateral position. Positioning on the side prevents aspiration, because saliva drains out the corner of the child's mouth. The child is not restrained because this could cause injury to the child. The nurse would loosen clothing around the child's neck and ensure a patent airway. Nothing is placed into the child's mouth during a seizure, because this action may cause injury to the child's mouth, gums, or teeth. The nurse would stay with the child to reduce the risk of injury and allow for observation and timing of the seizure.
Test-Taking Strategy: Focus on the subject and visualize this clinical situation. Recalling that airway patency and safety is the priority will assist in determining the appropriate interventions.
Level of Cognitive Ability: Creating
Client Needs: Physiological Integrity
Integrated Process: Nursing Process—Implementation
Content Area: Pediatrics: Neurological
Health Problem: Pediatric-Specific: Seizures
Priority Concepts: Intracranial Regulation; Safety
Reference: Hockenberry, Wilson, Rodgers (2017), p. 904.

Pediatric

CHAPTER 39

Musculoskeletal Problems

PRIORITY CONCEPTS **Development; Mobility**

I. Developmental Dysplasia of the Hip

A. Description
1. Problems related to abnormal development of the hip that may develop during fetal life, infancy, or childhood; in these problems, the head of the femur is seated improperly in the acetabulum, or hip socket, of the pelvis.
2. Degrees of developmental dysplasia of the hip (Box 39-1)

B. Assessment (Fig. 39-1)
1. Neonate: Laxity of the ligaments around the hip
2. Infant
   a. Shortening of the limb on the affected side (Galeazzi sign, also known as *Allis sign*)
   b. Restricted abduction of the hip on the affected side when the infant is placed supine with knees and hips flexed (limited range of motion in the affected hip)
   c. Unequal gluteal folds when the infant is prone and legs are extended against the examining table
   d. Positive Ortolani's test: Ortolani's maneuver is a test to assess for hip instability. The examiner abducts the thigh and applies gentle pressure forward over the greater trochanter. A "clicking" sensation indicates a dislocated femoral head moving into the acetabulum.
   e. Positive Barlow's test: The examiner adducts the hips and applies gentle pressure down and back with the thumbs. In hip dysplasia, the examiner can feel the femoral head move out of the acetabulum.
3. Older infant and child
   a. Affected leg is shorter than the other.
   b. The head of the femur can be felt to move up and down in the buttock when the extended thigh is pushed first toward the child's head and then pulled distally.
   c. Positive Trendelenburg's sign: The child stands on one foot and then the other foot, holding on to a support and bearing weight on the affected hip; the pelvis tilts downward on the normal side instead of upward, as it would with normal stability.
   d. Greater trochanter is prominent.
   e. Marked lordosis or waddling gait is noted in bilateral dislocations.

C. Interventions
1. Birth to 6 months of age: Splinting of the hips with a Pavlik harness to maintain flexion and abduction and external rotation (worn continuously until hip is stable in about 3 to 6 months) (Fig. 39-2)
2. Age 6 to 18 months: Gradual reduction by traction followed by closed reduction or open reduction (if necessary) under general anesthesia; child is then placed in a hip spica cast for 2 to 4 months until the hip is stable, and then a flexion-abduction brace is applied for approximately 3 months
3. Older child: Operative reduction and reconstruction is usually required.

BOX 39-1 Degrees of Developmental Dysplasia of the Hip

Acetabular Dysplasia (Preluxation)
- Mildest form
- Neither subluxation nor dislocation
- Delay in acetabular development occurs
- Femoral head remains in acetabulum

Subluxation
- Incomplete dislocation of the hip
- Femoral head remains in acetabulum
- Stretched capsule and ligamentum teres causes head of the femur to be partially displaced

Dislocation
- Femoral head loses contact with acetabulum and is displaced posteriorly and superiorly over fibrocartilaginous rim
- Ligamentum teres is elongated and taut

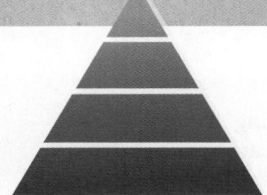

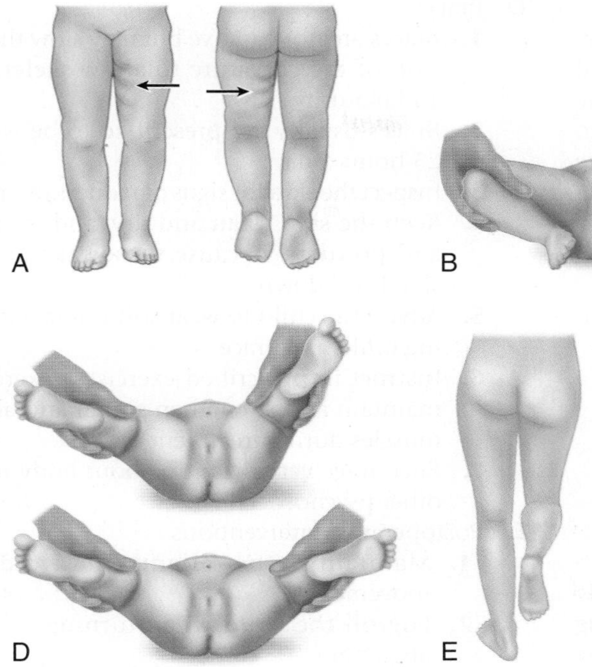

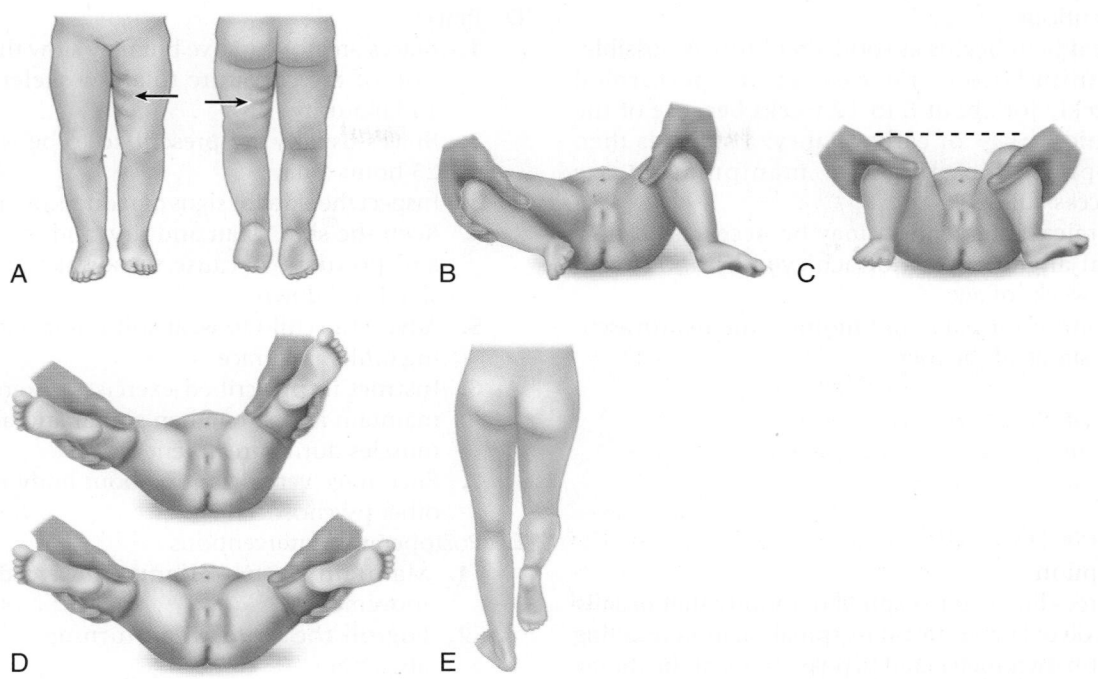

FIG. 39-1 Signs of developmental dysplasia of the hip. **A,** Asymmetry of gluteal and thigh folds. **B,** Limited hip abduction, as seen in flexion. **C,** Apparent shortening of the femur, as indicated by the level of the knees in flexion. **D,** Ortolani click (if infant is younger than 4 weeks old). **E,** Positive Trendelenburg's sign or gait (if child is weight-bearing).

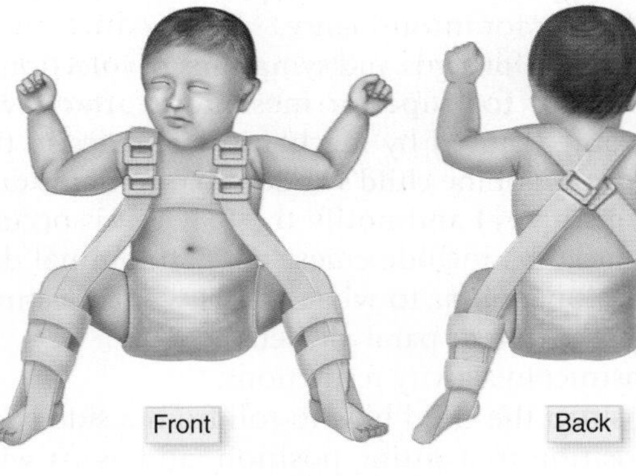

FIG. 39-2 Child in Pavlik harness.

4. Parents are instructed regarding proper care of a Pavlik harness, spica cast, or abduction brace.

II. Congenital Clubfoot

A. Description

1. Complex deformity of the ankle and foot that includes forefoot adduction, midfoot supination, hindfoot varus, and ankle equinus; defect may be unilateral or bilateral
2. The goal of treatment is to achieve a painless plantigrade (able to walk on the sole of the foot with the heel on the ground) and stable foot.
3. Long-term interval follow-up care is required until the child reaches skeletal maturity.

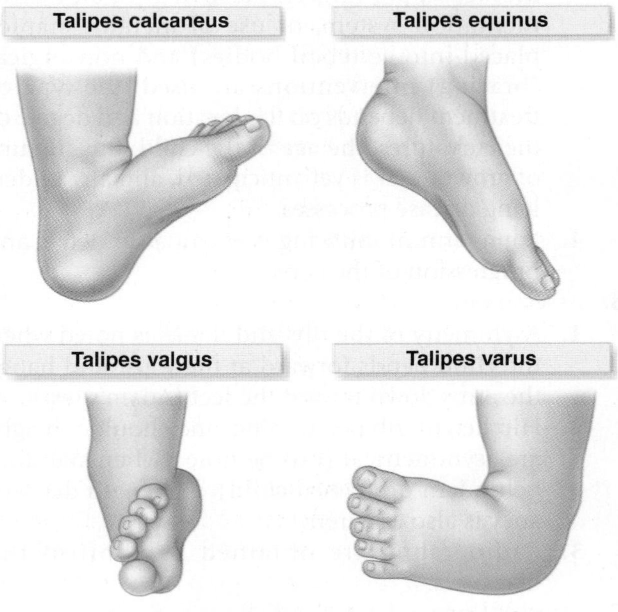

FIG. 39-3 Talipes clubfoot deformity positions.

B. Assessment: Deformities are described on the basis of the position of the ankle and foot (Fig. 39-3).

1. Talipes varus: Inversion or bending inward
2. Talipes valgus: Eversion or bending outward
3. Talipes equinus: Plantar flexion in which the toes are lower than the heel
4. Talipes calcaneus: Dorsiflexion in which the toes are higher than the heel

C. Interventions
1. Treatment begins as soon after birth as possible.
2. Manipulation and casting are performed weekly for about 8 to 12 weeks because of the rapid growth of early infancy; a splint is then applied if casting and manipulation are successful.
3. Surgical intervention may be necessary if normal alignment is not achieved by about 6 to 12 weeks of age.
4. Monitor for pain, and monitor the neurovascular status of the toes.

Contact the primary health care provider (PHCP) immediately if signs of neurovascular impairment are noted in a child with a cast or brace.

III. Idiopathic Scoliosis

A. Description
1. Three-dimensional spinal deformity that usually involves lateral curvature, spinal rotation resulting in rib asymmetry, and hypokyphosis of the thorax
2. Idiopathic scoliosis usually is diagnosed during the preadolescent growth spurt; screenings are important when growth spurts occur.
3. Surgical (spinal fusion, which may be done by thoracoscopic surgery, placement of an instrumentation system, or use of metallic staples placed into vertebral bodies) and nonsurgical (bracing) interventions are used; the type of treatment depends on the location and degree of the curvatures, the age of the child, the amount of growth that is yet anticipated, and any underlying disease processes.
4. Long-term monitoring is essential to detect any progression of the curve.

B. Assessment
1. Asymmetry of the ribs and flanks is noted when the child bends forward at the waist and hangs the arms down toward the feet (Adam's test).
2. Hip height, rib positioning, and shoulder height are asymmetrical (can be noted when standing behind an undressed child); leg length discrepancy is also apparent.
3. Radiographs are obtained to confirm the diagnosis.

C. Interventions
1. Monitor progression of the curvatures.
2. Prepare the child and parents for the use of a brace if prescribed.
3. Prepare the child and parents for surgery (spinal fusion, placement of internal instrumentation systems) if prescribed.

The potential for altered role performance, body image disturbance, fear, anger, and isolation exists for a child with a disabling condition and a condition that requires wearing a body brace.

D. Braces
1. Braces are not curative but may slow the progression of the curvature to allow skeletal growth and maturity.
2. Braces usually are prescribed to be worn 16 to 23 hours a day.
3. Inspect the skin for signs of redness or breakdown.
4. Keep the skin clean and dry, and avoid lotions and powders, because these cake and lead to skin breakdown.
5. Advise the child to wear soft nonirritating clothing under the brace.
6. Instruct in prescribed exercises (exercises help maintain and strengthen spinal and abdominal muscles during treatment).
7. Encourage verbalization about body image and other psychosocial issues.

E. Postoperative interventions
1. Maintain proper alignment; avoid twisting movements.
2. Logroll the child when turning to maintain alignment.
3. Assess extremities for adequate neurovascular status.
4. Encourage coughing and deep breathing and the use of incentive spirometry.
5. Assess pain and administer prescribed analgesics.
6. Monitor for incontinence.
7. Monitor for signs and symptoms of infection.
8. Monitor for superior mesenteric artery syndrome (caused by mechanical changes in the position of the child's abdominal contents during surgery) and notify the PHCP if it occurs; symptoms include emesis and abdominal distention similar to what occurs with intestinal obstruction or paralytic ileus.
9. Instruct in activity restrictions.
10. Instruct the child how to roll from a side-lying position to a sitting position, and assist with ambulation.
11. Address a potential body image disturbance when formulating a plan of nursing care.

IV. Juvenile Idiopathic Arthritis

A. Description
1. Autoimmune inflammatory disease affecting the joints and other tissues, such as articular cartilage; occurs most often in girls
2. Treatment is supportive (there is no cure) and directed toward preserving joint function, controlling inflammation, minimizing deformity, and reducing the impact that the disease may have on the development of the child.
3. Treatment includes medications, physical and occupational therapies, and child and family education.
4. A pediatric rheumatology team can manage the complex needs of the child and family most effectively. The team may consist of a pediatric

rheumatologist, physical and occupational therapist, social worker, and nurse specialist.
5. Surgical intervention may be implemented if the child has problems with joint contractures and unequal growth of extremities.

B. Assessment (Box 39-2)
1. There are no definitive tests to diagnose juvenile idiopathic arthritis.
2. Some laboratory tests, such as an elevated erythrocyte sedimentation rate or determination of the presence of leukocytosis, may support evidence of the disease.
3. Radiographs may show soft tissue swelling and joint space widening from increased synovial fluid in the joint.

C. Interventions
1. Facilitate social and emotional development.
2. Instruct parents and child in the administration of medications; medications may be given alone or in combination and are prescribed depending on the progression of the disease (Box 39-3).
3. Assist the child with range-of-motion exercises and instruct in prescribed exercises.
4. Encourage normal performance of activities of daily living.

BOX 39-2 Assessment Findings: Juvenile Idiopathic Arthritis

- Stiffness, swelling, and limited motion occur in affected joints.
- Affected joints are warm to touch, tender, and painful.
- Joint stiffness is present on arising in the morning and after inactivity.
- Uveitis (inflammation of structures in the uveal tract) can occur and cause blindness.

BOX 39-3 Medications Used in Juvenile Idiopathic Arthritis

Corticosteroid injections: Prescribed when only a few joints are involved. Usually do not have any significant side effects.

Oral corticosteroids: May be prescribed but only for as short a time and at the lowest dose possible. Long-term use is associated with side effects such as weight gain, poor growth, osteoporosis, cataracts, avascular necrosis, hypertension, and risk of infection.

Disease modifying antirheumatic drugs: Known as DMARDs are prescribed as a second-line treatment when many joints are involved or the child does not respond to corticosteroid joint injections. Biologics may also be prescribed, and these include antitumor necrosis factor agents. All of these medications cause side effects that need to be discussed with the child and/or parents.

Reference

American College of Rheumatology (2017), https://www.rheumatology.org/I-Am-A/Patient-Caregiver/Diseases-Conditions/Juvenile-Arthritis

5. Instruct parents and child in the use of hot or cold packs, splinting, and positioning the affected joint in a neutral position during painful episodes. Begin simple isometric exercises as soon as the child is able.
6. Encourage and support prescribed physical and occupational therapy.
7. Instruct in the importance of preventive eye care and reporting visual disturbances.
8. Assess the child's and family's perceptions regarding the chronic illness; plan to discuss the nature of a chronic illness and the associated life alterations that result from the chronic progression of the disorder.

V. Marfan's Syndrome

A. Description
1. Disorder of connective tissue that affects the skeletal system, cardiovascular system, eyes, and skin.
2. Marfan's syndrome is caused by defects in the fibrillin-1 gene, which serves as a building block for elastic tissue in the body; also, the disorder may be inherited.
3. There is no cure for the disorder.

B. Assessment
1. Tall and thin body structure: slender fingers, long arms and legs, curvature of the spine
2. Presence of visual problems
3. Presence of cardiac problems

C. Interventions
1. Monitor for vision problems and obtain visual examinations on a regular schedule.
2. Monitor for curvature of the spine, especially during adolescence.
3. Cardiac medications may be prescribed to slow the heart rate, to decrease stress on the aorta.
4. Instruct parents that the child should avoid participating in competitive athletics and contact sports to avoid injuring the heart.
5. Instruct parents to inform the dentist of the condition; antibiotics should be taken before dental procedures to prevent endocarditis.
6. Surgical replacement of the aortic root and valve may be necessary.

VI. Legg-Calve-Perthes Disease

A. Description
1. A condition affecting the hip where the femur and pelvis meet in the joint
2. Blood supply is temporarily interrupted to the head of the femur and the bone dies and stops growing.

B. Assessment
1. Limping
2. Pain or stiffness in the hip, groin, thigh, or knee
3. Limited range of motion in the affected joint

C. Interventions
1. Physical therapy, particularly stretching exercises
2. Use of crutches to avoid bearing weight on the affected hip
3. Bed rest and traction if pain is severe
4. Casting to keep the femoral head within its socket
5. Use of a nighttime brace
6. Hip replacement surgery

VII. Fractures

A. Description (see also Chapter 60)
1. A break in the continuity of the bone as a result of trauma, twisting, or bone decalcification
2. Fractures in children usually occur as a result of increased mobility and inadequate or immature motor and cognitive skills; they may result from trauma or bone diseases such as congenital bone disease or bone tumors.

Fractures in infancy are generally rare and warrant further investigation to rule out the possibility of child abuse and to identify bone structure defects.

B. Assessment
1. Pain or tenderness over the involved area
2. Obvious deformity
3. Edema
4. Ecchymosis
5. Muscle spasm
6. Loss of function
7. Crepitation

C. Initial care of a fracture (see Priority Nursing Actions)

PRIORITY NURSING ACTIONS

Extremity Fracture in a Child

1. Assess extent of injury and immobilize the affected extremity check neurovascular status of the extremity.
2. If a compound fracture exists, cover the wound with a sterile dressing (apply a clean dressing if a sterile dressing is unavailable).
3. Elevate the injured extremity if appropriate.
4. Apply cold to injured area.
5. Continue to monitor neurovascular status.
6. Transport to the nearest emergency department.

Reference
Hockenberry, Wilson, Rodgers (2017), p. 951.

D. Interventions
1. Reduction
a. Restoring the bone to proper alignment
b. Closed reduction: Accomplished by manual alignment of the fragments, followed by immobilization
c. Open reduction: Surgical insertion of internal fixation devices, such as rods, wires, or pins, that help maintain alignment while healing occurs
2. Retention: Application of traction or a cast to maintain alignment until healing occurs

E. Traction (see Chapter 60)
1. Russell skin traction
a. Used to stabilize a fractured femur before surgery
b. Similar to Buck's traction but provides a double pull using a knee sling that pulls at the knee and foot
2. Balanced suspension
a. Used with skin or skeletal traction to approximate fractures of the femur, tibia, or fibula
b. Balanced suspension is produced by a counterforce other than the child.
c. Provide pin care if pins are used with the skeletal traction.
3. 90-degree–90-degree traction
a. The lower leg is supported by a boot cast or a calf sling.
b. A skeletal Steinmann pin or Kirschner wire is placed in the distal fragment of the femur, allowing 90-degree flexion at the hip and the knee.
4. Interventions
a. Maintain correct amount of weight as prescribed.
b. Ensure that weights hang freely.
c. Check all ropes for fraying and all knots for tightness; be sure that the ropes are appropriately tracking in the grooves of the pulley wheels.
d. Monitor neurovascular status of the involved extremity.
e. Protect the skin from breakdown.
f. Monitor for signs and symptoms of complications of immobilization, such as constipation, skin breakdown, lung congestion, renal complications, and disuse syndrome of unaffected extremities.
g. Provide therapeutic and diversional play.

F. Casts (see Chapter 60)
1. Description
a. Made of plaster or fiberglass to provide immobilization of bone and joints after a fracture or injury
b. Fractures of the hip or knee may require a spica cast.
2. Interventions
a. Examine the cast for pressure areas.
b. Ensure that no rough casting material remains in contact with the skin; petal the cast edges with waterproof adhesive tape as necessary to ensure a smooth cast edge.

c. If a hip spica cast is placed, the cast edges around the perineum and buttocks may need to be taped with waterproof tape.
d. Monitor the extremity for circulatory impairment, such as pain greater than that expected for the type of injury, edema, rubor, pallor, numbness and tingling, coolness, decreased sensation or mobility, or diminished pulse.
e. Notify the PHCP if circulatory impairment occurs.
f. Prepare for bivalving or cutting the cast if circulatory impairment occurs; prepare for emergency fasciotomy if cast removal does not improve the neurocirculatory compromise.
g. Instruct parents and child not to stick objects down the cast.
h. Teach parents and child to keep the cast clean and dry.
i. Instruct parents and child in isometric exercises to prevent muscle atrophy.

PRACTICE QUESTIONS

393. A child has a right femur fracture caused by a motor vehicle crash and is placed in skin traction temporarily until surgery can be performed. During assessment, the nurse notes that the dorsalis pedis pulse is absent on the right foot. Which action should the nurse take?
1. Administer an analgesic.
2. Release the skin traction.
3. Apply ice to the extremity.
4. Notify the primary health care provider (PHCP).

394. A child is placed in skeletal traction for treatment of a fractured femur. The nurse creates a plan of care and should include which intervention?
1. Ensure that all ropes are outside the pulleys.
2. Ensure that the weights are resting lightly on the floor.
3. Restrict diversional and play activities until the child is out of traction.
4. Check the primary health care provider's (PHCP's) prescriptions for the amount of weight to be applied.

395. A 4-year-old child sustains a fall at home. After an x-ray examination, the child is determined to have a fractured arm and a plaster cast is applied. The nurse provides instructions to the parents regarding care for the child's cast. Which statement by the parents indicates a **need for further instruction**?
1. "The cast may feel warm as the cast dries."
2. "I can use lotion or powder around the cast edges to relieve itching."
3. "A small amount of white shoe polish can touch up a soiled white cast."
4. "If the cast becomes wet, a blow drier set on the cool setting may be used to dry the cast."

396. The parents of a child with juvenile idiopathic arthritis call the clinic nurse because the child is experiencing a painful exacerbation of the disease. The parents ask the nurse if the child can perform range-of-motion exercises at this time. The nurse should make which response?
1. "Avoid all exercise during painful periods."
2. "Range-of-motion exercises must be performed every day."
3. "Have the child perform simple isometric exercises during this time."
4. "Administer additional pain medication before performing range-of-motion exercises."

397. A child who has undergone spinal fusion for scoliosis complains of abdominal discomfort and begins to have episodes of vomiting. On further assessment, the nurse notes abdominal distention. On the basis of these findings, the nurse should take which action?
1. Administer an antiemetic.
2. Increase the intravenous fluids.
3. Place the child in a Sims' position.
4. Notify the primary health care provider (PHCP).

398. The nurse is providing instructions to the parents of a child with scoliosis regarding the use of a brace. Which statement by the parents indicates a **need for further instruction**?
1. "I will encourage my child to perform prescribed exercises."
2. "I will have my child wear soft fabric clothing under the brace."
3. "I should apply lotion under the brace to prevent skin breakdown."
4. "I should avoid the use of powder because it will cake under the brace."

399. The nurse is assisting a primary health care provider (PHCP) examine a 3-week-old infant with developmental dysplasia of the hip. What test or sign should the nurse expect the PHCP to assess?
1. Babinski's sign
2. The Moro reflex
3. Ortolani's maneuver
4. The palmar-plantar grasp

400. A 1-month-old infant is seen in a clinic and is diagnosed with developmental dysplasia of the hip. On assessment, the nurse understands that which finding should be noted in this condition?
1. Limited range of motion in the affected hip
2. An apparent lengthened femur on the affected side

3. Asymmetrical adduction of the affected hip when the infant is placed supine with the knees and hips flexed
4. Symmetry of the gluteal skinfolds when the infant is placed prone and the legs are extended against the examining table

401. Parents bring their 2-week-old infant to a clinic for treatment after a diagnosis of clubfoot made at birth. Which statement by the parents indicates a **need for further teaching** regarding this disorder?
1. "Treatment needs to be started as soon as possible."
2. "I realize my infant will require follow-up care until fully grown."
3. "I need to bring my infant back to the clinic in 1 month for a new cast."
4. "I need to come to the clinic every week with my infant for the casting."

402. The nurse prepares a list of home care instructions for the parents of a child who has a plaster cast applied to the left forearm. Which instructions should be included on the list? **Select all that apply.**
- ❑ 1. Use the fingertips to lift the cast while it is drying.
- ❑ 2. Keep small toys and sharp objects away from the cast.
- ❑ 3. Use a padded ruler or another padded object to scratch the skin under the cast if it itches.
- ❑ 4. Place a heating pad on the lower end of the cast and over the fingers if the fingers feel cold.
- ❑ 5. Elevate the extremity on pillows for the first 24 to 48 hours after casting to prevent swelling.
- ❑ 6. Contact the primary health care provider (PHCP) if the child complains of numbness or tingling in the extremity.

ANSWERS

393. *Answer:* 4
Rationale: An absent pulse to an extremity of the affected limb after a bone fracture could mean that the child is developing or experiencing compartment syndrome. This is an emergency situation, and the PHCP needs to be notified immediately. Administering analgesics would not improve circulation. The skin traction should not be released without a PHCP's prescription. Applying ice to an extremity with absent perfusion will worsen the problem. Ice may be prescribed when perfusion is adequate to decrease swelling.
Test-Taking Strategy: Use the ABCs—airway, breathing, and circulation. Focusing on the data in the question indicates that circulation is impaired. This should direct you to the correct option.
Level of Cognitive Ability: Applying
Client Needs: Physiological Integrity
Integrated Process: Nursing Process—Implementation
Content Area: Complex Care: Emergency Situations/ Management
Health Problem: Pediatric-Specific: Fractures
Priority Concepts: Clinical Judgment; Perfusion
Reference: McKinney et al. (2018), pp. 1213-1214.

394. *Answer:* 4
Rationale: When a child is in traction, the nurse would check the PHCP's prescription to verify the prescribed amount of traction weight. The nurse would maintain the correct amount of weight as prescribed, ensure that the weights hang freely, check the ropes for fraying and ensure that they are on the pulleys appropriately, monitor the neurovascular status of the involved extremity, and monitor for signs and symptoms of complications of immobilization. The nurse would provide therapeutic and diversional play activities for the child.
Test-Taking Strategy: Focus on the subject, care of the child in traction. Eliminate option 3 first because of the word *restrict.* Next recall the general principles related to traction, recalling that weights should hang freely and ropes should remain in the pulleys.
Level of Cognitive Ability: Creating
Client Needs: Physiological Integrity
Integrated Process: Nursing Process—Planning
Content Area: Pediatrics: Musculoskeletal
Health Problem: Pediatric-Specific: Fractures
Priority Concepts: Mobility; Safety
Reference: Hockenberry, Wilson, Rodgers (2017), p. 957.

395. *Answer:* 2
Rationale: Teaching about cast care is essential to prevent complications from the cast. The parents need to be instructed not to use lotion or powders on the skin around the cast edges or inside the cast. Lotions or powders can become sticky or caked and cause skin irritation. Options 1, 3, and 4 are appropriate statements and indicate the parents understand cast care.
Test-Taking Strategy: Note the strategic words, *need for further instruction.* These words indicate a negative event query and ask you to select an option that is an incorrect statement. Remember that lotions or powders can become sticky or caked and cause skin irritation.
Level of Cognitive Ability: Evaluating
Client Needs: Physiological Integrity
Integrated Process: Teaching and Learning
Content Area: Pediatrics: Musculoskeletal
Health Problem: Pediatric-Specific: Fractures
Priority Concepts: Client Education; Skin Integrity
Reference: McKinney et al. (2018), p. 1216.

396. *Answer:* 3
Rationale: Juvenile idiopathic arthritis is an autoimmune inflammatory disease affecting the joints and other tissues, such as articular cartilage. During painful episodes of juvenile

idiopathic arthritis, hot or cold packs and splinting and positioning the affected joint in a neutral position help reduce the pain. Although resting the extremity is appropriate, beginning simple isometric or tensing exercises as soon as the child is able is important. These exercises do not involve joint movement.
Test-Taking Strategy: Focus on the **subject,** exercise during an acute exacerbation of the disease. Eliminate options 1 and 2 because of the **closed-ended words** "all" and "must," and option 4 because of the word *additional*.
Level of Cognitive Ability: Applying
Client Needs: Physiological Integrity
Integrated Process: Teaching and Learning
Content Area: Pediatrics: Musculoskeletal
Health Problem: Pediatric-Specific: Juvenile Idiopathic Arthritis
Priority Concepts: Mobility; Pain
Reference: McKinney et al. (2018), pp. 1237-1238.

397. *Answer:* 4
Rationale: Scoliosis is a three-dimensional spinal deformity that usually involves lateral curvature, spinal rotation resulting in rib asymmetry, and hypokyphosis of the thorax. A complication after surgical treatment of scoliosis is superior mesenteric artery syndrome. This disorder is caused by mechanical changes in the position of the child's abdominal contents, resulting from lengthening of the child's body. The disorder results in a syndrome of emesis and abdominal distention similar to that which occurs with intestinal obstruction or paralytic ileus. Postoperative vomiting in children with body casts or children who have undergone spinal fusion warrants attention because of the possibility of superior mesenteric artery syndrome. Options 1, 2, and 3 are incorrect.
Test-Taking Strategy: Focus on the **subject,** complications after surgical treatment for scoliosis. Eliminate option 2 first because it should not be implemented unless prescribed by the PHCP. Eliminate option 3 next because this child requires logrolling, and Sims' position may cause injury after surgery. From the remaining options, note the assessment signs and symptoms in the question. These should alert you that notification of the PHCP is necessary.
Level of Cognitive Ability: Synthesizing
Client Needs: Physiological Integrity
Integrated Process: Nursing Process—Implementation
Content Area: Pediatrics: Musculoskeletal
Health Problem: Pediatric-Specific: Scoliosis
Priority Concepts: Clinical Judgment; Collaboration
Reference: Hockenberry, Wilson, Rodgers (2017), p. 970.

398. *Answer:* 3
Rationale: A brace may be prescribed to treat scoliosis. Braces are not curative but may slow the progression of the curvature to allow skeletal growth and maturity. The use of lotions or powders under a brace should be avoided because they can become sticky and cake under the brace, causing irritation. Options 1, 2, and 4 are appropriate interventions in the care of a child with a brace.
Test-Taking Strategy: Note the **strategic words,** *need for further instruction*. These words indicate a **negative event query** and ask you to select an option that is an incorrect statement. Careful reading of the options will assist in directing you to the correct option. Also, applying the principles associated with cast care will direct you to the correct option.
Level of Cognitive Ability: Evaluating
Client Needs: Physiological Integrity
Integrated Process: Teaching and Learning
Content Area: Pediatrics: Musculoskeletal
Health Problem: Pediatric-Specific: Scoliosis
Priority Concepts: Client Education; Mobility
Reference: McKinney et al. (2018), pp. 1224-1225.

399. *Answer:* 3
Rationale: In developmental dysplasia of the hip, the head of the femur is seated improperly in the acetabulum or hip socket of the pelvis. Ortolani's maneuver is a test to assess for hip instability and can be done only before 4 weeks of age. The examiner abducts the thigh and applies gentle pressure forward over the greater trochanter. A "clicking" sensation indicates a dislocated femoral head moving into the acetabulum. Babinski's sign is abnormal in anyone older than 2 years of age and indicates central nervous system abnormality. The Moro reflex is normally present at birth but is absent by 6 months; if still present at 6 months, there is an indication of neurological abnormality. The palmar-plantar grasp is present at birth and lessens within 8 months.
Test-Taking Strategy: Options 1 and 2 can be eliminated first because they are **comparable or alike** and are both tests of neurological function. To select from the remaining options, remember that Ortolani's maneuver is an assessment technique for hip dysplasia that must be done before 4 weeks of age. This will direct you to the correct option.
Level of Cognitive Ability: Applying
Client Needs: Physiological Integrity
Integrated Process: Nursing Process—Implementation
Content Area: Pediatrics: Musculoskeletal
Health Problem: Pediatric-Specific: Developmental Dysplasia of Hip
Priority Concepts: Clinical Judgment; Mobility
Reference: Hockenberry, Wilson, Rodgers (2017), pp. 960-961.

400. *Answer:* 1
Rationale: In developmental dysplasia of the hip, the head of the femur is seated improperly in the acetabulum or hip socket of the pelvis. Asymmetrical and restricted abduction of the affected hip, when the child is placed supine with the knees and hips flexed, would be an assessment finding in developmental dysplasia of the hip in infants beyond the newborn period. Other findings include an apparent short femur on the affected side, asymmetry of the gluteal skinfolds, and limited range of motion in the affected extremity.
Test-Taking Strategy: Note the **subject,** assessment findings in developmental dysplasia of the hip. Also, note the age of the infant and focus on the infant's diagnosis. Visualizing each of the assessment findings described in the options will direct you to the correct option.
Level of Cognitive Ability: Analyzing
Client Needs: Physiological Integrity
Integrated Process: Nursing Process—Assessment
Content Area: Pediatrics: Musculoskeletal
Health Problem: Pediatric-Specific: Developmental Dysplasia of Hip
Priority Concepts: Development; Mobility
Reference: McKinney et al. (2018), pp. 444, 743.

401. *Answer:* 3

Rationale: Clubfoot is a complex deformity of the ankle and foot that includes forefoot adduction, midfoot supination, hindfoot varus, and ankle equinus; the defect may be unilateral or bilateral. Treatment for clubfoot is started as soon as possible after birth. Serial manipulation and casting are performed at least weekly. If sufficient correction is not achieved in 3 to 6 months, surgery usually is indicated. Because clubfoot can recur, all children with clubfoot require long-term interval follow-up until they reach skeletal maturity to ensure an optimal outcome.

Test-Taking Strategy: Note the strategic words, *need for further teaching*. These words indicate a negative event query and ask you to select an option that is an incorrect statement. This will assist you in eliminating options 1 and 2. Recalling that serial manipulations and casting are required weekly will assist in directing you to the correct option.

Level of Cognitive Ability: Evaluating

Client Needs: Physiological Integrity

Integrated Process: Teaching and Learning

Content Area: Pediatrics: Musculoskeletal

Health Problem: Pediatric-Specific: Clubfoot

Priority Concepts: Client Education; Mobility

Reference: Hockenberry, Wilson, Rodgers (2017), p. 961.

402. *Answer:* 2, 5, 6

Rationale: While the cast is drying, the palms of the hands are used to lift the cast. If the fingertips are used, indentations in the cast could occur and cause constant pressure on the underlying skin. Small toys and sharp objects are kept away from the cast, and no objects (including padded objects) are placed inside the cast because of the risk of altered skin integrity. The extremity is elevated to prevent swelling, and the PHCP is notified immediately if any signs of neurovascular impairment develop. A heating pad is not applied to the cast or fingers. Cold fingers could indicate neurovascular impairment, and the PHCP should be notified.

Test-Taking Strategy: Use of the ABCs—airway, breathing, and circulation—and safety principles related to care of a child with a cast will assist in answering this question.

Level of Cognitive Ability: Applying

Client Needs: Physiological Integrity

Integrated Process: Teaching and Learning

Content Area: Pediatrics: Musculoskeletal

Health Problem: Pediatric-Specific: Fractures

Priority Concepts: Client Education; Safety

Reference: McKinney et al. (2018), p. 1216.

CHAPTER 40

Immune Problems and Infectious Diseases

PRIORITY CONCEPTS Infection; Safety

I. Immune Disorders: For information on the functions of the immune system, the immune response, immunodeficiency, and other immune disorders, hypersensitivity and allergies, and skin testing, see Chapter 62.

II. Human Immunodeficiency Virus Infection and Acquired Immunodeficiency Syndrome

A. Description
1. Acquired immunodeficiency syndrome (AIDS) is a disorder caused by human immunodeficiency virus (HIV) and characterized by generalized dysfunction of the immune system (Fig. 40-1).
2. The diagnosis of AIDS is associated with certain illnesses or conditions.
3. HIV infects CD4+ T cells; a gradual decrease in CD4+ T-cell count occurs, and this results in a progressive immunodeficiency; the risk for opportunistic infections is present (Box 40-1).
4. HIV is transmitted through blood, semen, vaginal secretions, and breast milk; the incubation period is months to years.
5. Horizontal transmission occurs through intimate sexual contact or parenteral exposure to blood or body fluids that contain the virus.
6. Vertical (perinatal) transmission occurs from an HIV-infected pregnant woman to her fetus (see Chapter 22).
7. The most common opportunistic infection that occurs in children infected with HIV is *Pneumocystis jiroveci* pneumonia; *P. jiroveci* pneumonia most frequently occurs between the ages of 3 and 6 months.

An infant or child infected with HIV is at risk for developing a life-threatening opportunistic infection. Monitor the infant or child closely for signs of infection and report these signs immediately if they occur.

B. Assessment (see Box 40-1 and Box 40-2)

C. Diagnostic tests: Before testing, counseling should be provided to parents; issues that should be addressed include the causes of HIV, reasons for testing, implications of positive test results, confidentiality issues, and beneficial effects of early intervention (Table 40-1).

III. Care of the Child with HIV Infection or AIDS

A. An interprofessional health care approach is taken; primary goals are to decelerate the replication of the virus, prevent opportunistic infections, provide nutritional support, treat symptoms, and treat opportunistic infections.

B. Prophylaxis (*P. jiroveci* pneumonia and other opportunistic infections)
1. Provide prophylaxis as prescribed against *P. jiroveci* pneumonia and other opportunistic infections, particularly during the first year of life of an infant born to an HIV-infected mother.
2. After 1 year of age, the need for prophylaxis is determined on the basis of the presence and severity of immunosuppression or a history of *P. jiroveci* pneumonia.
3. Continuing prophylaxis is based on the child's HIV status, history of opportunistic infections, and CD4+ counts.

C. Antiretroviral medications (refer to Chapter 63)

Before administering an antiretroviral medication, ensure that the medication is safe for pediatric administration. Also check the contraindications for use and the adverse effects.

1. The goal of antiretroviral medications is to suppress viral replication to slow the decline in the number of CD4+ cells, preserve immune function, reduce the incidence and severity of opportunistic infections, and delay disease progression.
2. The medications affect different stages of the HIV life cycle to prevent reproduction of new virus particles.
3. Combination therapy may be prescribed and includes the use of more than 1 antiretroviral medication.

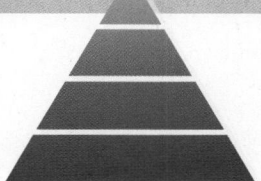

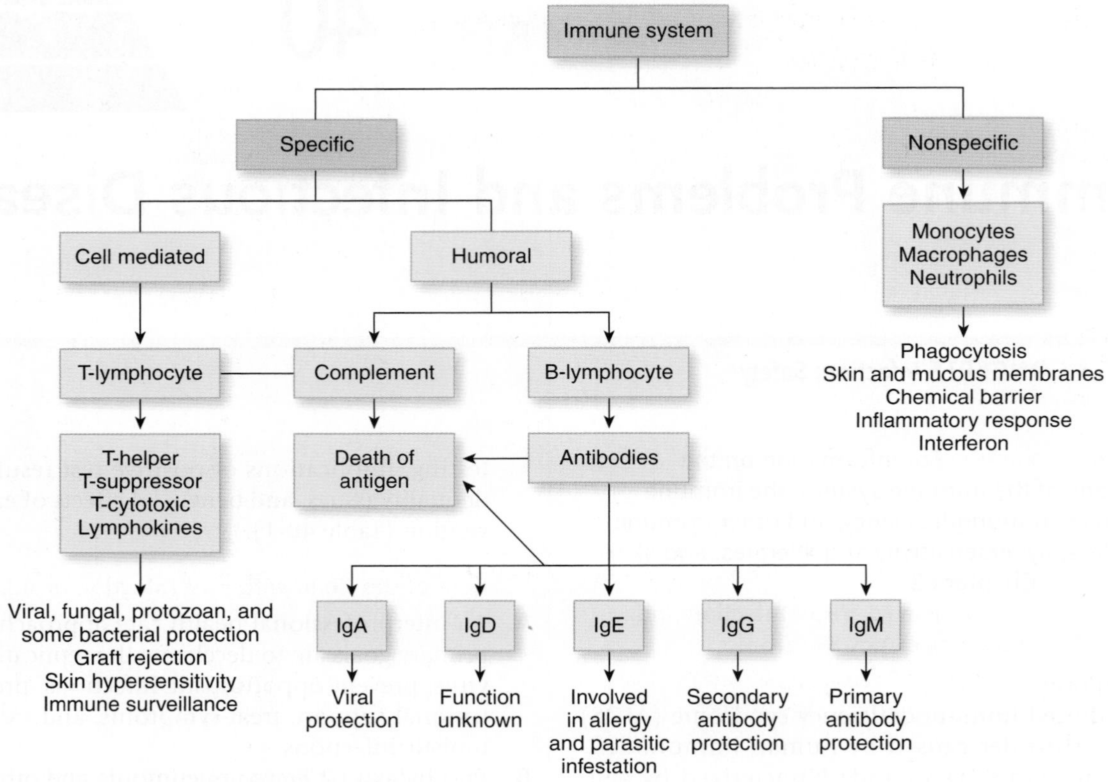

FIG. 40-1 Components of the immune system. *Ig,* Immunoglobulin.

BOX 40-1 Common Acquired Immunodeficiency Syndrome (AIDS)–Defining Conditions in Children

- Candidal esophagitis
- Cryptosporidiosis
- Cytomegalovirus disease
- Herpes simplex disease
- Human immunodeficiency virus encephalopathy
- Lymphoid interstitial pneumonitis
- *Mycobacterium avium-intracellulare* infection
- *Pneumocystis jiroveci* pneumonia
- Pulmonary candidiasis
- Recurrent bacterial infections
- Wasting syndrome

Data from Perry S, Hockenberry M, Lowdermilk D, Wilson D: *Maternal-child nursing care,* ed 4, St. Louis, 2010, Mosby.

BOX 40-2 Common Assessment Findings in Children with Human Immunodeficiency Virus (HIV) Infection

- Chronic cough
- Chronic or recurrent diarrhea
- Developmental delay or regression of developmental milestones
- Failure to thrive
- Hepatosplenomegaly
- Lymphadenopathy
- Malaise and fatigue
- Night sweats
- Oral candidiasis
- Parotitis
- Weight loss

Adapted from Perry S, Hockenberry M, Lowdermilk D, Wilson D: *Maternal-child nursing care,* ed 4, St. Louis, 2010, Mosby.

D. Immunizations (refer to Chapter 18 for specific information on childhood immunizations)

Immunization against childhood diseases is recommended for all children exposed to and infected with HIV.

1. If a child has symptomatic HIV infection or has severe immunosuppression, guidelines are as follows:
   - **a.** Only the inactivated influenza **vaccine** that is given intramuscularly should be used (influenza vaccine should be given yearly).
   - **b.** Measles vaccine should not be given; immunoglobulin may be prescribed after measles exposure.
   - **c.** Only the inactivated polio vaccine that is given intramuscularly should be used.
   - **d.** Rotavirus vaccine should not be given.

TABLE 40-1 Diagnostic Tests for Human Immunodeficiency Virus (HIV)

Test	Age-Appropriate Use	Test Determines	Special Considerations
Enzyme-linked immunosorbent assay	≥18 mo	Response of antibodies to HIV	If used and found to be positive in infants <18 mo, indicates only that mother is infected because maternal antibodies are transmitted transplacentally; use another diagnostic test
Western blot	≥18 mo	Presence of HIV antibodies	Same as above
Polymerase chain reaction	<18 mo	Presence of proviral DNA	Very accurate for diagnosing infants 1-4 mo of age
p24 antigen	<18 mo	HIV antigen specific	Very accurate for diagnosing infants 1-4 mo of age
$CD4^+$ lymphocyte count, T-lymphocyte count	Infant–13 yr	Immune system status related specifically to suppression	Age adjustment is essential, because normal counts are relatively high in infants and steadily decline until 6 yr of age. Severe suppression in all age groups is <15% total lymphocytes (<750 cells/L in infant <12 mo, <500 cells/L in child 1-5 yr, <200 cells/L in child 6-12 yr)

From Branson BM, Handsfield HH, Lampe MA, et al.: Centers for Disease Control and Prevention: Revised recommendations for HIV testing of adults, adolescents, and pregnant women in health-care settings. *MMWR Recomm Rep 2006*, 55(RR14):1–17. Available at http://www.cdc.gov/mmwr/preview/mmwrhtml/rr5514a1.htm.

e. Varicella-zoster virus vaccine should not be given; varicella-zoster immunoglobulin may be prescribed after chickenpox exposure.
f. Tetanus immunoglobulin may be prescribed for tetanus-prone wounds.

E. Caregiver instructions
1. Wash hands frequently.
2. Assess the child for fever, malaise, fatigue, weight loss, vomiting, diarrhea, altered activity level, and oral lesions; notify the pediatrician if any of these occur.
3. Assess the child for signs and symptoms of opportunistic infections, such as pneumonia.
4. Administer antiretroviral medications and other medications to the child as prescribed.
5. The child needs to be restricted from having contact with persons who have infections or other contagious or potentially contagious illnesses.
6. Keep the child's immunizations up to date.
7. Keep the child home when sick.
8. Avoid direct unprotected contact with the child's body fluids.
9. Monitor the child's weight.
10. Provide a high-calorie and high-protein diet to the child.
11. Administer appetite stimulants to the child as prescribed and as needed.
12. Do not share eating utensils with the child.
13. Wash all eating utensils in the dishwasher.
14. Cover any of the child's unused food and formula and refrigerate (discard unused refrigerated formula and food after 24 hours).
15. Do not allow the child to eat fresh fruits or vegetables or raw meat or fish (neutropenic diet if immunosuppressed).
16. Wear gloves when caring for the child, especially when in contact with body fluids and changing diapers.
17. Change the child's diapers frequently, away from food areas.
18. Fold the child's soiled disposable diapers inward, close with the tabs, and dispose in a tightly covered plastic-lined container.
19. Dispose of trash daily.
20. Clean up any of the child's body fluid spills with a bleach solution (10:1 ratio of water to bleach).

F. Education for an adolescent infected with HIV
1. Educate about high-risk behaviors and the importance of avoiding high-risk behaviors.
2. Identify the methods of transmission of HIV.
3. Emphasize the importance of abstinence from sexual contact, such as intercourse.
4. Emphasize the importance of using safe condoms if intercourse is planned.
5. Identify the resources available for support and other issues.

IV. Rubeola (Measles)

A. Description
1. Agent: Paramyxovirus
2. Incubation period: 10 to 20 days
3. Communicable period: From 4 days before to 5 days after rash appears, mainly during the **prodromal** stage (pertaining to early symptoms that may mark the onset of disease)
4. Source: Respiratory tract secretions, blood, or urine of infected person
5. Transmission: Airborne particles or direct contact with infectious droplets; transplacental

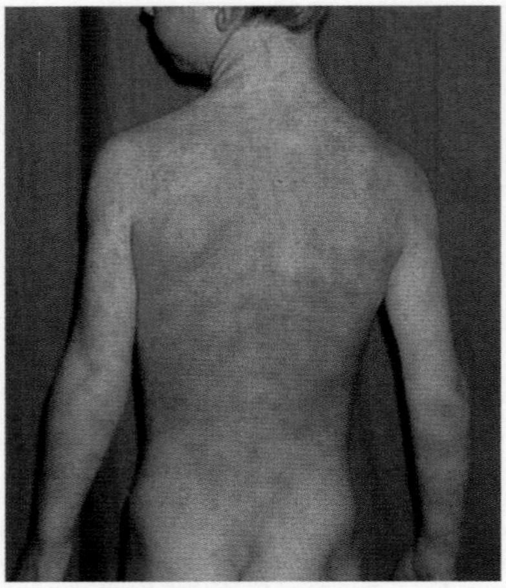

FIG. 40-2 Rubeola (measles). (From Hockenberry, Wilson, 2012.)

B. Assessment (Fig. 40-2)
1. Fever
2. Malaise
3. The 3 "Cs"—coryza, cough, conjunctivitis
4. Rash appears as red, erythematous maculopapular eruption starting on the face and spreading downward to the feet; blanches easily with pressure and gradually turns a brownish color (lasts 6 to 7 days); may have desquamation.
5. Koplik's spots: Small red spots with a bluish white center and a red base; located on the buccal mucosa and last 3 days

C. Interventions
1. Use airborne, droplet, and contact precautions if the child is hospitalized.
2. Restrict child to quiet activities and bed rest.
3. Use a cool mist vaporizer for cough and coryza.
4. Dim lights if photophobia is present.
5. Administer antipyretics for fever.
6. Administer vitamin A supplementation as prescribed.

V. Roseola (Exanthema Subitum)

A. Description
1. Agent: Human herpesvirus type 6
2. Incubation period: 5 to 15 days
3. Communicable period: Unknown, but thought to extend from the febrile stage to the time the rash first appears
4. Source: Unknown
5. Transmission: Unknown

B. Assessment (Fig. 40-3)
1. Sudden high (>38.8° C [>102° F]) fever of 3 to 5 days' duration in a child who appears well, followed by a rash (rose-pink macules that blanch with pressure); febrile seizures may occur
2. Rash appears several hours to 2 days after the fever subsides and lasts 1 to 2 days.

C. Interventions: Supportive

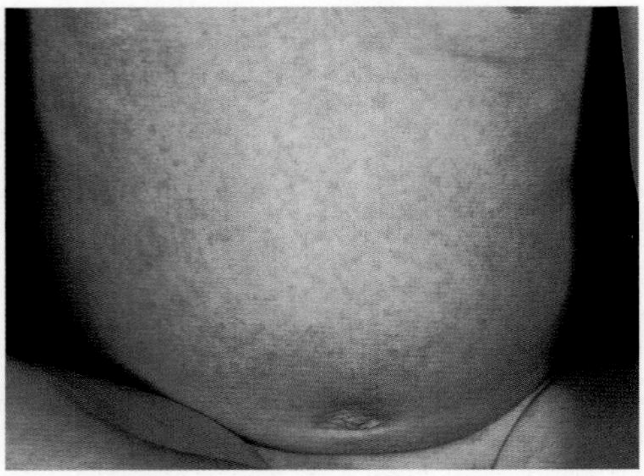

FIG. 40-3 Roseola (exanthema subitum). (From Habif, 2004.)

VI. Rubella (German Measles)

A. Description
1. Agent: Rubella virus
2. Incubation period: 14 to 21 days
3. Communicable period: From 7 days before to about 5 days after rash appears
4. Source: Nasopharyngeal secretions; virus is also present in blood, stool, and urine
5. Transmission
   a. Airborne or direct contact with infectious droplets
   b. Indirectly via articles freshly contaminated with nasopharyngeal secretions, feces, or urine
   c. Transplacental

B. Assessment (Fig. 40-4)
1. Low-grade fever
2. Malaise
3. Pinkish red maculopapular rash that begins on the face and spreads to the entire body within 1 to 3 days

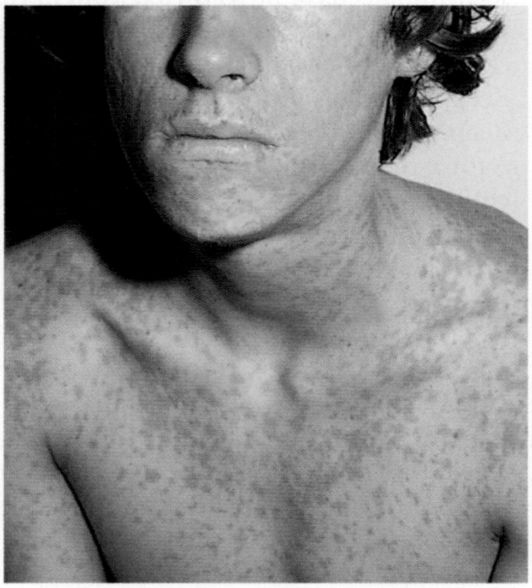

FIG. 40-4 Rubella (German measles). (From Zitelli, Davis, 2007. Courtesy Dr. Michael Sherlock, Lutherville, MD.)

4. Petechiae (red, pinpoint spots) may occur on the soft palate.

C. Interventions
   1. Use airborne, droplet, and contact precautions if the child is hospitalized; provide supportive treatment.
   2. Isolate the infected child from pregnant women.

VII. Mumps

A. Description
   1. Agent: Paramyxovirus
   2. Incubation period: 14 to 21 days
   3. Communicable period: Immediately before and after parotid gland swelling begins
   4. Source: Saliva of infected person and possibly urine
   5. Transmission: Direct contact or droplet spread from an infected person

B. Assessment
   1. Fever
   2. Headache and malaise
   3. Anorexia
   4. Jaw or ear pain aggravated by chewing, followed by parotid glandular swelling
   5. Orchitis or oophoritis may occur.
   6. Deafness may occur.
   7. Aseptic meningitis may occur.

C. Interventions
   1. Institute airborne, droplet, and contact precautions.
   2. Provide bed rest until the parotid gland swelling subsides.
   3. Avoid foods that require chewing.
   4. Apply hot or cold compresses as prescribed to the neck.
   5. Apply warmth and local support with snug-fitting underpants to relieve orchitis.
   6. Monitor for signs of aseptic meningitis (see Chapters 38 and 58 for information on meningitis).

VIII. Chickenpox (Varicella)

A. Description
   1. Agent: Varicella-zoster (VCZ) virus
   2. Incubation period: 13 to 17 days
   3. Communicable period: From 1 to 2 days before the onset of the rash to 6 days after the first crop of vesicles, when crusts have formed
   4. Source: Respiratory tract secretions of infected person; skin lesions
   5. Transmission: Direct contact, airborne, droplet spread, and contaminated objects

B. Assessment (Fig. 40-5)
   1. Slight fever, malaise, and anorexia are followed by a macular rash that first appears on the trunk and scalp and moves to the face and extremities.

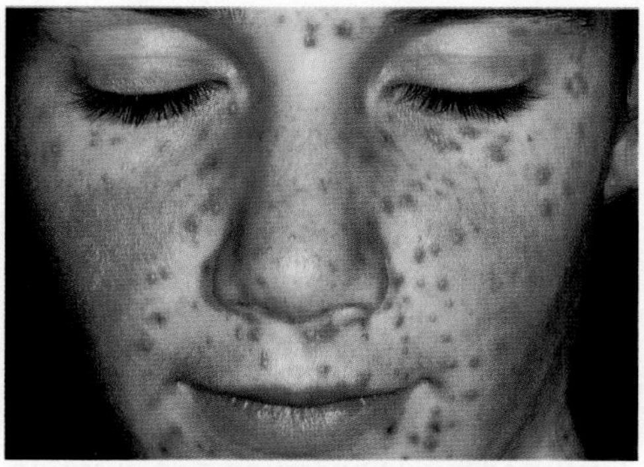

FIG. 40-5 Chickenpox (varicella). (From Habif, 2004.)

   2. Lesions become pustules, begin to dry, and develop a crust.
   3. Lesions may appear on the mucous membranes of the mouth, the genital area, and the rectal area.

C. Interventions
   1. In the hospital, ensure strict isolation (contact and, droplet, precautions).
   2. At home, isolate the infected child until the vesicles have dried.
   3. An antiviral agent may be used to treat varicella infections in susceptible immunocompromised persons to decrease the number of lesions; shorten the duration of fever; and decrease itching, lethargy, and anorexia.
   4. The use of varicella zoster (VCZ) immune globulin or intravenous immune globulin (IVIG) is recommended for children who are immunocompromised, who have no previous history of varicella, and who are likely to contract the disease and have complications as a result.
   5. Provide supportive care.

Isolate high-risk children, such as children who have immunosuppressive disorders, from a child with a communicable disease.

IX. Pertussis (Whooping Cough)

A. Description
   1. Agent: Bordetella pertussis
   2. Incubation period: 5 to 21 days (usually 10 days)
   3. Communicable period: Greatest during the catarrhal stage (when discharge from respiratory secretions occurs)
   4. Source: Discharge from the respiratory tract of the infected person
   5. Transmission: Direct contact or droplet spread from infected person; indirect contact with freshly contaminated articles

B. Assessment
   1. Symptoms of respiratory infection followed by increased severity of cough, with a loud whooping inspiration

2. May experience cyanosis, respiratory distress, and tongue protrusion
3. Listlessness, irritability, anorexia

C. Interventions
1. Isolate child during the catarrhal stage; if the child is hospitalized, institute airborne, droplet, and contact precautions.
2. Administer antimicrobial therapy as prescribed.
3. Reduce environmental factors that cause coughing spasms, such as dust, smoke, and sudden changes in temperature.
4. Ensure adequate hydration and nutrition.
5. Provide suction and humidified oxygen if needed.
6. Monitor cardiopulmonary status (via monitor as prescribed) and pulse oximetry.
7. Infants do not receive maternal immunity to pertussis; the tetanus–diphtheria–acellular pertussis (Tdap) vaccine should be administered to women in the postpartum period and those in close contact with the infant to prevent the spread of pertussis to infants.

X. Diphtheria

A. Description
1. Agent: Corynebacterium diphtheriae
2. Incubation period: 2 to 5 days
3. Communicable period: Variable, until virulent bacilli are no longer present (3 negative cultures of discharge from the nose and nasopharynx, skin, and other lesions); usually 2 weeks, but can be 4 weeks
4. Source: Discharge from the mucous membrane of the nose and nasopharynx, skin, and other lesions of the infected person
5. Transmission: Direct contact with infected person, carrier, or contaminated articles

B. Assessment
1. Low-grade fever, malaise, sore throat
2. Foul-smelling, mucopurulent nasal discharge
3. Dense pseudomembrane formation in the throat that may interfere with eating, drinking, and breathing
4. Lymphadenitis, neck edema, "bull neck"

C. Interventions
1. Ensure strict isolation for the hospitalized child.
2. Administer diphtheria antitoxin as prescribed (after a skin or conjunctival test to rule out sensitivity to horse serum).
3. Provide bed rest.
4. Administer antibiotics as prescribed.
5. Provide suction and humidified oxygen as needed.
6. Provide tracheostomy care if a tracheotomy is necessary.

XI. Poliomyelitis

A. Description
1. Agent: Enteroviruses
2. Incubation period: 7 to 14 days
3. Communicable period: Unknown; the virus is present in the throat and feces shortly after infection and persists for about 1 week in the throat and 4 to 6 weeks in the feces
4. Source: Oropharyngeal secretions and feces of the infected person
5. Transmission: Direct contact with infected person; fecal-oral and oropharyngeal routes

B. Assessment
1. Fever, malaise, anorexia, nausea, headache, sore throat
2. Abdominal pain followed by soreness and stiffness of the trunk, neck, and limbs that may progress to central nervous system paralysis

C. Interventions
1. Enteric and contact precautions
2. Supportive treatment
3. Bed rest
4. Monitoring for respiratory paralysis
5. Physical therapy

XII. Scarlet Fever

A. Description
1. Agent: Group A β-hemolytic streptococci
2. Incubation period: 1 to 7 days
3. Communicable period: About 10 days during the incubation period and clinical illness; during the first 2 weeks of the carrier stage, although may persist for months
4. Source: Nasopharyngeal secretions of infected person and carriers
5. Transmission: Direct contact with infected person or droplet spread; indirectly by contact with contaminated articles, ingestion of contaminated milk, or other foods

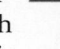

B. Assessment (Fig. 40-6)
1. Abrupt high fever, flushed cheeks, vomiting, headache, enlarged lymph nodes in the neck, malaise, abdominal pain
2. A red, fine sandpaper–like rash develops in the axilla, groin, and neck that spreads to cover the entire body except the face.
3. Rash blanches with pressure; pink or red lines of petechiae are noted in areas of deep creases and folds of the joints (Pastia's sign).
4. Desquamation, sheet-like sloughing of the skin on palms and soles, appears by weeks 1 to 3.
5. The tongue is initially coated with a white, furry covering with red projecting papillae (white strawberry tongue); by the third to fifth day, the white coat sloughs off, leaving a red swollen tongue (red strawberry tongue).

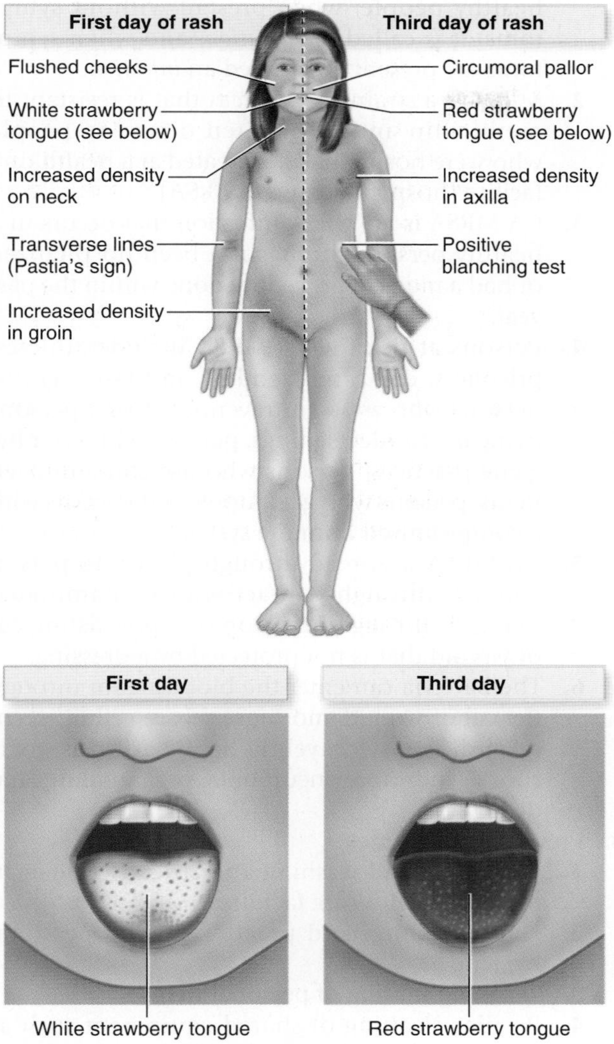

FIG. 40-6 Scarlet fever.

6. Tonsils are reddened, edematous, and covered with exudate.
7. Pharynx is edematous and beefy red.

C. Interventions
1. Institute contact and airborne (droplet) precautions until 24 hours after initiation of antibiotics.
2. Provide supportive therapy.
3. Provide bed rest.
4. Encourage fluid intake.

XIII. Erythema Infectiosum (Fifth Disease)

A. Description
1. Agent: Human parvovirus B19
2. Incubation period: 4 to 14 days; may be 20 days
3. Communicable period: Uncertain but before the onset of symptoms in most children
4. Source: Infected person
5. Transmission: Unknown; possibly respiratory secretions and blood

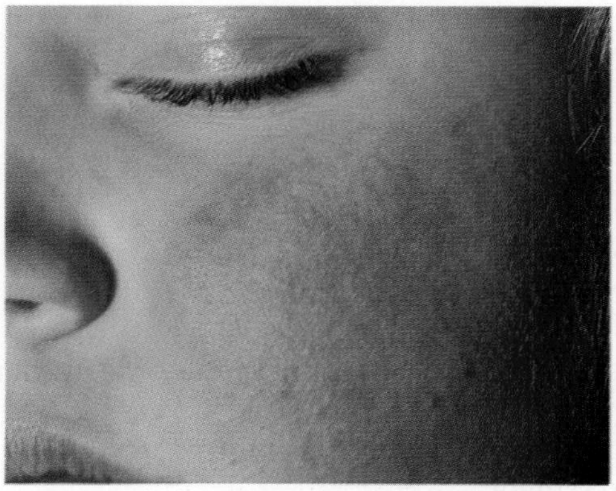

FIG. 40-7 Erythema infectiosum (fifth disease): Slapped-face appearance. (From Habif, 2004.)

B. Assessment
1. Before rash: Asymptomatic or mild fever, malaise, headache, runny nose
2. Stages of rash
   a. Erythema of the face (slapped-cheek appearance) develops and disappears by 1 to 4 days (Fig. 40-7).
   b. About 1 day after the rash appears on the face, maculopapular red spots appear, symmetrically distributed on the extremities; the rash progresses from proximal to distal surfaces and may last a week or more.
   c. The rash subsides but may reappear if the skin becomes irritated by the sun, heat, cold, exercise, or friction.

C. Interventions
1. Child is not usually hospitalized.
2. Pregnant women should avoid the infected individual.
3. Provide supportive care.
4. Administer antipyretics, analgesics, and anti-inflammatory medications as prescribed.

XIV. Infectious Mononucleosis

A. Description
1. Agent: Epstein-Barr virus
2. Incubation period: 4 to 6 weeks
3. Communicable period: Unknown
4. Source: Oral secretions
5. Transmission: Direct intimate contact

B. Assessment
1. Fever, malaise, headache, fatigue, nausea, abdominal pain, sore throat, enlarged red tonsils
2. Lymphadenopathy and hepatosplenomegaly
3. Discrete macular rash most prominent over the trunk may occur.

C. Interventions
1. Provide supportive care.
2. Monitor for signs of splenic rupture.

Teach the parents of a child with mononucleosis to monitor for signs of splenic rupture, which include abdominal pain, left upper quadrant pain, and left shoulder pain.

XV. Rocky Mountain Spotted Fever

A. Description
  1. Agent: *Rickettsia rickettsii*
  2. Incubation period: 2 to 14 days
  3. Source: Tick from a mammal, most often from wild rodents and dogs
  4. Transmission: Bite of infected tick

B. Assessment
  1. Fever, malaise, anorexia, vomiting, headache, myalgia
  2. Maculopapular or petechial rash primarily on the extremities (ankles and wrists), but may spread to other areas, characteristically on the palms and soles

C. Interventions
  1. Provide vigorous supportive care.
  2. Administer antibiotics as prescribed.
  3. Teach the child and parents about protection from tick bites (Box 40-3).

XVI. Community-Associated Methicillin-Resistant *Staphylococcus aureus* (CA-MRSA)

A. Description (also see Chapter 13)
  1. *Staphylococcus aureus* is a bacterium that is normally located on the skin or in the nose of healthy people; when present without symptoms, it is called *colonization,* and when symptoms are present, it is called an *infection.*
  2. MRSA is a strain of *S. aureus* that is resistant to methicillin and most often occurs in people who were hospitalized or treated at a health care facility (hospital-acquired MRSA).
  3. CA-MRSA is an MRSA infection that occurs in a healthy person who has not been hospitalized or had a medical procedure done within the past year.
  4. Persons at risk for CA-MRSA include athletes, prisoners, day care attendees, military recruits, persons who abuse intravenous drugs, persons living in crowded settings, persons with poor hygiene practices, persons who use contaminated items, persons who get tattoos, and persons with a compromised immune system.
  5. CA-MRSA is spread through person-to-person contact, through contact with contaminated items, or through infection of a preexisting cut or wound that is not protected by a dressing.
  6. The bacteria can enter the bloodstream through the cut or wound and cause sepsis, cellulitis, endocarditis, osteomyelitis, septic arthritis, toxic shock syndrome, pneumonia, organ failure, and death.

B. Prevention measures
  1. Frequent hand washing and strict aseptic technique in health care facilities
  2. Hand washing and practicing good personal hygiene
  3. Avoiding sharing of personal items
  4. Regular cleaning of shared equipment such as athletic equipment, whirlpools, or saunas
  5. Cleaning a cut or wound thoroughly
  6. Ensure tattoo or body piercing facilities adhere to strict guidelines regarding preventing infection

C. Assessment
  1. Appearance of a skin infection: Red, swollen area; warmth around the area; drainage of pus; pain at the site; fever
  2. Symptoms of a more serious infection: Chest pain, cough, fatigue, chills, fever, malaise, headache, muscle aches, shortness of breath, rash

D. Interventions
  1. Assess skin lesions.
  2. Prepare to drain an infected skin site and culture the wound and wound drainage.
  3. Prepare to obtain blood cultures, sputum cultures, and urine cultures.
  4. Prepare to administer antibiotics as prescribed.
  5. Educate the child and family about the causes and modes of transmission, signs and symptoms, and importance of treatment measures prescribed.

BOX 40-3 Measures to Protect Children from Tick Bites

- Wearing long-sleeved shirts, long pants tucked into long socks (socks should be pulled up over the pant legs), and a hat when walking in tick-infested areas
- Wearing light-colored clothing to make ticks more visible if they get onto the child
- Checking children for the presence of ticks after being in high-risk or tick-infested areas
- Following paths rather than walking in tall grass and shrub areas, because these are the places where most ticks are found
- Applying insect repellents containing diethyltoluamide (DEET) and permethrin before possible exposure to areas where ticks are found (use with caution in infants and small children)
- Keeping yards at home trimmed and free of accumulating leaves and other brush
- Applying tick repellent to dogs
- Saving the tick for later identification if it is removed from the child's body
- To remove the tick, grasp the tick at the point of closest contact to the skin with tweezers and pull straight up with steady, even pressure; remove any remaining parts with a sterile needle; if using bare hands, use a tissue during removal; wash hands with soap and water.

XVII. Influenza

A. Description

1. Various strains of influenza can occur.

2. It is a viral infection that affects the respiratory system and is highly contagious.

3. Children, pregnant women, persons with pre-existing health conditions, and persons with a compromised immune system are at high risk for developing complications.

4. It is caused by contact with an infected person or by touching something such as a toy or tissue that the infected person has touched.

B. Prevention

1. Flu vaccine

2. Wash the child's hands frequently and teach hand-washing techniques.

3. Avoid children who are ill.

4. Keep the child home from school or away from others until the child has been fever-free (without the use of antipyretics) for at least 24 hours.

5. For additional information, refer to Centers for Disease Control and Prevention (CDC) Web site: http://www.cdc.gov/vaccines/schedules/index.html.

The signs and symptoms of flu usually last a week. If they last longer, the presence of complications should be suspected.

C. Assessment

1. Fever that occurs suddenly and is high

2. Headache, body aches, fatigue, chills, cough, congestion, sore throat, loss of appetite, vomiting, diarrhea

D. Interventions

1. Antiviral medications if prescribed, fluids, rest, pain relievers such as acetaminophen or ibuprofen

2. Family and child teaching about prevention measures

PRACTICE QUESTIONS

403. An infant of a mother infected with human immunodeficiency virus (HIV) is seen in the clinic each month and is being monitored for symptoms indicative of HIV infection. With knowledge of the **most** common opportunistic infection of children infected with HIV, the nurse assesses the infant for which sign?

1. Cough
2. Liver failure
3. Watery stool
4. Nuchal rigidity

404. The nurse provides home care instructions to the parent of a child with acquired immunodeficiency syndrome (AIDS). Which statement by the parent indicates the **need for further teaching?**

1. "I will wash my hands frequently."
2. "I will keep my child's immunizations up to date."
3. "I will avoid direct unprotected contact with my child's body fluids."
4. "I can send my child to day care if he has a fever, as long as it is a low-grade fever."

405. The clinic nurse is instructing the parent of a child with human immunodeficiency virus (HIV) infection regarding immunizations. The nurse should provide which instruction to the parent?

1. The hepatitis B vaccine will not be given to the child.
2. The inactivated influenza vaccine will be given yearly.
3. The varicella vaccine will be given before 6 months of age.
4. A Western blot test needs to be performed and the results evaluated before immunizations.

406. A pediatrician prescribes laboratory studies for an infant of a woman positive for human immunodeficiency virus (HIV). The nurse anticipates that which laboratory study will be prescribed for the infant?

1. Chest x-ray
2. Western blot
3. $CD4^+$ cell count
4. p24 antigen assay

407. The mother with human immunodeficiency virus (HIV) infection brings her 10-month-old infant to the clinic for a routine checkup. The pediatrician has documented that the infant is asymptomatic for HIV infection. After the checkup, the mother tells the nurse that she is so pleased that the infant will not get HIV infection. The nurse should make which **most appropriate** response to the mother?

1. "I am so pleased also that everything has turned out fine."
2. "Because symptoms have not developed, it is unlikely that your infant will develop HIV infection."
3. "Everything looks great, but be sure to return with your infant next month for the scheduled visit."
4. "Most children infected with HIV develop symptoms within the first 9 months of life, and some become symptomatic sometime before they are 3 years old."

408. A 6-year-old child with human immunodeficiency virus (HIV) infection has been admitted to the hospital for pain management. The child asks the nurse if the pain will ever go away. The nurse should make which **best** response to the child?

1. "The pain will go away if you lie still and let the medicine work."
2. "Try not to think about it. The more you think it hurts, the more it will hurt."
3. "I know it must hurt, but if you tell me when it does, I will try to make it hurt a little less."
4. "Every time it hurts, press on the call button and I will give you something to make the pain go all away."

409. The home care nurse provides instructions regarding basic infection control to the parent of an infant with human immunodeficiency virus (HIV) infection. Which statement, if made by the parent, indicates the **need for further instruction**?
1. "I will clean up any spills from the diaper with diluted alcohol."
2. "I will wash baby bottles, nipples, and pacifiers in the dishwasher."
3. "I will be sure to prepare foods that are high in calories and high in protein."
4. "I will be sure to wash my hands carefully before and after caring for my infant."

410. Which home care instructions should the nurse provide to the parent of a child with acquired immunodeficiency syndrome (AIDS)? **Select all that apply.**
- ☐ 1. Monitor the child's weight.
- ☐ 2. Frequent hand washing is important.
- ☐ 3. The child should avoid exposure to other illnesses.
- ☐ 4. The child's immunization schedule will need revision.
- ☐ 5. Clean up body fluid spills with bleach solution (10:1 ratio of water to bleach).
- ☐ 6. Fever, malaise, fatigue, weight loss, vomiting, and diarrhea are expected to occur and do not require special intervention.

411. The nurse provides home care instructions to the parents of a child hospitalized with pertussis who is in the convalescent stage and is being prepared for discharge. Which statement by a parent indicates a **need for further instruction**?
1. "We need to encourage our child to drink fluids."
2. "Coughing spells may be triggered by dust or smoke."
3. "Vomiting may occur when our child has coughing episodes."
4. "We need to maintain droplet precautions and a quiet environment for at least 2 weeks."

412. The nurse caring for a child diagnosed with rubeola (measles) notes that the pediatrician has documented the presence of Koplik's spots. On the basis of this documentation, which observation is expected?
1. Pinpoint petechiae noted on both legs
2. Whitish vesicles located across the chest
3. Petechiae spots that are reddish and pinpoint on the soft palate
4. Small, blue-white spots with a red base found on the buccal mucosa

413. A mother of a child with mumps calls the health care clinic to tell the nurse that the child has been lethargic and vomiting. What instruction should the nurse give to the mother?
1. To continue to monitor the child
2. That lethargy and vomiting are normal with mumps
3. To bring the child to the clinic to be seen by the pediatrician
4. That, as long as there is no fever, there is nothing to be concerned about

414. The nurse is assessing a child admitted with a diagnosis of rheumatic fever. Which significant question should the nurse ask the child's parent during the assessment?
1. "Has your child had difficulty urinating?"
2. "Has your child been exposed to anyone with chickenpox?"
3. "Has any family member had a sore throat within the past few weeks?"
4. "Has any family member had a gastrointestinal disorder in the past few weeks?"

415. The nurse is caring for a child diagnosed with erythemia infectiosum (fifth disease). Which clinical manifestation should the nurse expect to note in the child?
1. An intense fiery red edematous rash on the cheeks
2. Pinkish-rose maculopapular rash on the face, neck, and scalp
3. Reddish and pinpoint petechiae spots found on the soft palate
4. Small bluish-white spots with a red base found on the buccal mucosa

ANSWERS

403. *Answer:* 1

Rationale: Acquired immunodeficiency syndrome (AIDS) is a disorder caused by HIV and characterized by generalized dysfunction of the immune system. The most common opportunistic infection of children infected with HIV is *Pneumocystis jiroveci* pneumonia, which occurs most frequently between the ages of 3 and 6 months, when HIV status may be indeterminate. Cough is a common sign of this opportunistic infection. Cytomegalovirus infection is also characteristic of HIV infection; however, it is not the most common opportunistic infection. Liver failure is a common sign of this complication. Although gastrointestinal disturbances and neurological abnormalities may occur in a child with HIV infection, options 3 and 4 are not specific opportunistic infections noted in the HIV-infected child. Watery stool is noted with gastroenteritis, and nuchal rigidity is seen in meningitis.

Test-Taking Strategy: Note the strategic word, *most*. This will direct you to the correct option. Remember that the most common opportunistic infection of children infected with HIV is *P. jiroveci* pneumonia, and that cough is a common sign with this complication.

Level of Cognitive Ability: Analyzing

Client Needs: Physiological Integrity

Integrated Process: Nursing Process—Assessment

Content Area: Pediatrics: Immune

Health Problem: Pediatric-Specific: Immunodeficiency disease

Priority Concepts: Clinical Judgment; Immunity

Reference: McKinney et al. (2018), pp. 938-939, 945.

404. *Answer:* 4

Rationale: AIDS is a disorder caused by human immunodeficiency virus (HIV) and characterized by generalized dysfunction of the immune system. A child with AIDS who is sick or has a fever should be kept home and not brought to a day care center. Options 1, 2, and 3 are correct statements and would be actions a caregiver should take when the child has AIDS.

Test-Taking Strategy: Note the strategic words, *need for further teaching*. These words indicate a negative event query and ask you to select an option that is an incorrect statement. Noting the word *fever* in the correct option will direct you to this option.

Level of Cognitive Ability: Evaluating

Client Needs: Safe and Effective Care Environment

Integrated Process: Teaching and Learning

Content Area: Pediatrics: Immune

Health Problem: Pediatric-Specific: Immunodeficiency disease

Priority Concepts: Client Education; Immunity

Reference: Hockenberry, Wilson, Rodgers (2017), p. 809.

405. *Answer:* 2

Rationale: Immunizations against common childhood illnesses are recommended for all children exposed to or infected with HIV. The inactivated influenza vaccine that is given intramuscularly will be administered (influenza vaccine should be given yearly). The hepatitis B vaccine is administered according to the recommended immunization schedule. Varicella-zoster virus vaccine should not be given, because it is a live virus vaccine; varicella-zoster immunoglobulin may be prescribed after chickenpox exposure. Option 4 is unnecessary and inaccurate.

Test-Taking Strategy: Focus on the subject, immunizations for the child with HIV. Option 4 can be eliminated first because the Western blot is a diagnostic test, not an evaluative test. From the remaining options, recalling that the child infected with HIV is at risk for opportunistic infections and that live virus vaccines are not administered to an immunodeficient child will assist in directing you to the correct option.

Level of Cognitive Ability: Applying

Client Needs: Health Promotion and Maintenance

Integrated Process: Teaching and Learning

Content Area: Pediatrics: Immune

Health Problem: Pediatric-Specific: Immunodeficiency disease

Priority Concepts: Client Education; Immunity

Reference: McKinney et al. (2018), p. 945.

406. *Answer:* 4

Rationale: Infants born to HIV-infected mothers need to be screened for the HIV antigen. The detection of HIV in infants is confirmed by a p24 antigen assay, virus culture of HIV, or polymerase chain reaction. A Western blot test confirms the presence of HIV antibodies. The $CD4^+$ cell count indicates how well the immune system is working. A chest x-ray evaluates the presence of other manifestations of HIV infection, such as pneumonia.

Test-Taking Strategy: Focus on the subject, laboratory study to determine the presence of HIV antigen, and note the word *infant*. Recall the laboratory tests used to determine the presence of HIV infection in the infant to answer this question.

Level of Cognitive Ability: Applying

Client Needs: Physiological Integrity

Integrated Process: Nursing Process—Assessment

Content Area: Pediatrics: Immune

Health Problem: Pediatric-Specific: Immunodeficiency disease

Priority Concepts: Clinical Judgment; Immunity

Reference: McKinney et al. (2018), pp. 939-940.

407. *Answer:* 4

Rationale: Acquired immunodeficiency syndrome (AIDS) is caused by HIV infection and characterized by generalized dysfunction of the immune system. Most children infected with HIV develop symptoms within the first 9 months of life. The remaining infected children become symptomatic sometime before age 3 years. With their immature immune systems, children have a much shorter incubation period than adults. Options 1, 2, and 3 are incorrect. Additionally, these options offer false reassurance.

Test-Taking Strategy: Note the strategic words, *most appropriate*. Eliminate options 1, 2, and 3 because they are comparable or alike in content. The correct option is the only one that provides specific and accurate data regarding HIV infection in an infant.

Level of Cognitive Ability: Applying

Client Needs: Psychosocial Integrity

Integrated Process: Nursing Process—Implementation

Content Area: Pediatrics: Immune

Health Problem: Pediatric-Specific: Immunodeficiency disease

Priority Concepts: Client Education; Immunity

Reference: Hockenberry, Wilson, Rodgers (2017), pp. 806-807.

408. *Answer:* 3

Rationale: The multiple complications associated with HIV are accompanied by a high level of pain. Aggressive pain management is essential for the child to have an acceptable quality of life. The nurse must acknowledge the child's pain and let the child know that everything will be done to decrease the pain. Telling the child that movement or lack thereof would eliminate the pain is inaccurate. Allowing a child to think that he or she can control the pain simply by thinking or not thinking about it oversimplifies the pain cycle associated with HIV. Giving false hope by telling the child that the pain will be taken "all away" is neither truthful nor realistic.

Test-Taking Strategy: Note the strategic word, *best.* Recall the general concept of pain and growth and development concepts of a 6-year-old child. Giving the child information about the pain in words that he or she can understand, but without providing false hope or not telling the truth, should guide you to the correct option. Options 1 and 2 provide inaccurate information about pain management. Option 4 provides false hope that the pain can be alleviated completely.

Level of Cognitive Ability: Applying
Client Needs: Physiological Integrity
Integrated Process: Nursing Process—Implementation
Content Area: Pediatrics: Immune
Health Problem: Pediatric-Specific: Immunodeficiency disease
Priority Concepts: Immunity; Pain
Reference: Hockenberry, Wilson, Rodgers (2017), pp. 808-809.

409. *Answer:* 1

Rationale: HIV is transmitted through blood, semen, vaginal secretions, and breast milk. The mother of an infant with HIV should be instructed to use a bleach solution for disinfecting contaminated objects or cleaning up spills from the child's diaper. Alcohol would not be effective in destroying the virus. Options 2, 3, and 4 are accurate instructions related to basic infection control.

Test-Taking Strategy: Note the strategic words, *need for further instruction.* These words indicate a negative event query and ask you to select an option that is an incorrect statement. Recalling basic infection control measures and the measures to prevent the spread of HIV will direct you to the correct option.

Level of Cognitive Ability: Evaluating
Client Needs: Safe and Effective Care Environment
Integrated Process: Teaching and Learning
Content Area: Pediatrics: Infectious and Communicable Diseases
Health Problem: Pediatric-Specific: Immunodeficiency disease
Priority Concepts: Client Education; Infection
Reference: McKinney et al. (2018), p. 945.

410. *Answer:* 1, 2, 3, 5

Rationale: AIDS is a disorder caused by human immunodeficiency virus (HIV) infection and is characterized by a generalized dysfunction of the immune system. Home care instructions include the following: frequent hand washing; monitoring for fever, malaise, fatigue, weight loss, vomiting, and diarrhea and notifying the pediatrician if these occur; monitoring for signs and symptoms of opportunistic infections; administering antiretroviral medications and other medications as prescribed; avoiding exposure to other illnesses; keeping immunizations up to date; monitoring weight and providing a high-calorie, high-protein diet; washing eating utensils in the dishwasher; and avoiding sharing eating utensils. Gloves are worn for care, especially when in contact with body fluids and changing diapers; diapers are changed frequently and away from food areas, and soiled disposable diapers are folded inward, closed with the tabs, and disposed of in a tightly covered plastic-lined container. Any body fluid spills are cleaned with a bleach solution (10:1 ratio of water to bleach).

Test-Taking Strategy: Focus on the subject, care of the child with AIDS. Recalling that AIDS is characterized by a generalized dysfunction of the immune system and recalling the modes of transmission of the virus will assist in selecting the correct home care instructions.

Level of Cognitive Ability: Analyzing
Client Needs: Safe and Effective Care Environment
Integrated Process: Teaching and Learning
Content Area: Pediatrics: Infectious and Communicable Diseases
Health Problem: Pediatric-Specific: Immunodeficiency disease
Priority Concepts: Client Education; Infection
Reference: McKinney et al. (2018), p. 945.

411. *Answer:* 4

Rationale: Pertussis is transmitted by direct contact or respiratory droplets from coughing. The communicable period occurs primarily during the catarrhal stage. Respiratory precautions are not required during the convalescent phase. Options 1, 2, and 3 are accurate components of home care instructions.

Test-Taking Strategy: Note the strategic words, *need for further instruction.* These words indicate a negative event query and ask you to select an option that is an incorrect statement. Also, note the word *convalescent* in the question. Options 1 and 3 can be eliminated because they are generally associated with convalescence. Knowing that 2 weeks of respiratory precautions is not required during the convalescent period will direct you to this option.

Level of Cognitive Ability: Evaluating
Client Needs: Health Promotion and Maintenance
Integrated Process: Teaching and Learning
Content Area: Pediatrics: Infectious and Communicable Diseases
Health Problem: Pediatric-Specific: Communicable Diseases
Priority Concepts: Client Education; Infection
Reference: Hockenberry, Wilson, Rodgers (2017), pp. 167, 656.

412. *Answer:* 4

Rationale: In rubeola (measles), Koplik's spots appear approximately 2 days before the appearance of the rash. These are small, blue-white spots with a red base that are found on the buccal mucosa. The spots last approximately 3 days, after which time they slough off. Based on this information, the remaining options are all incorrect.

Test-Taking Strategy: Eliminate options 1 and 3 that are comparable or alike and address petechiae spots. Focusing on the subject, Koplik's spots, will direct you to the correct option.

Level of Cognitive Ability: Applying
Client Needs: Physiological Integrity
Integrated Process: Nursing Process/Assessment

Content Area: Pediatrics: Infectious and Communicable Diseases
Health Problem: Pediatric-Specific: Communicable Diseases
Priority Concepts: Clinical Judgment; Infection
Reference: Hockenberry, Wilson, Rodgers (2017), p. 162.

413. *Answer:* 3
Rationale: Mumps generally affects the salivary glands, but it can also affect multiple organs. The most common complication is septic meningitis, with the virus being identified in the cerebrospinal fluid. Common signs include nuchal rigidity, lethargy, and vomiting. The child should be seen by the pediatrician.
Test-Taking Strategy: Focus on the **subject**, a child with mumps who has been lethargic and vomiting. Recalling that meningitis is a complication of mumps will direct you to the correct option.
Level of Cognitive Ability: Applying
Client Needs: Physiological Integrity
Integrated Process: Nursing Process/Implementation
Content Area: Pediatrics: Infectious and Communicable/ Diseases
Health Problem: Pediatric-Specific: Communicable Diseases
Priority Concepts: Clinical Judgment; Infection
Reference: Hockenberry, Wilson, Rodgers (2017), pp. 150; 167; 656.

414. *Answer:* 3
Rationale: Rheumatic fever characteristically presents 2 to 6 weeks after an untreated or partially treated group A beta-hemolytic streptococcal infection of the respiratory tract. Initially the nurse determines whether any family member has had a sore throat or unexplained fever within the past few weeks. The remaining options are unrelated to the assessment findings of rheumatic fever.
Test-Taking Strategy: Focus on the **subject**, rheumatic fever. Note the word *significant.* Recalling that rheumatic fever characteristically presents 2 to 6 weeks after a streptococcal infection of the respiratory tract will direct you to the correct option.
Level of Cognitive Ability: Analyzing
Client Needs: Physiological Integrity
Integrated Process: Nursing Process/Assessment
Content Area: Pediatrics: Infectious and Communicable Diseases
Health Problem: Pediatric-Specific: Rheumatic Fever
Priority Concepts: Clinical Judgment; Infection
Reference: Hockenberry, Wilson, Rodgers (2017), p. 641.

415. *Answer:* 1
Rationale: Fifth disease is characterized by the presence of an intense fiery red edematous rash on the cheeks, which gives an appearance that the child has been slapped. Options 2 and 3 are manifestations related to rubella (German measles). Koplik's spots (option 4) are found in rubeola (measles).
Test-Taking Strategy: Focus on the **subject**, erythema infectiosum (fifth disease). Recalling the "slapped cheek" appearance associated with fifth disease will direct you to the correct option.
Level of Cognitive Ability: Analyzing
Client Needs: Physiological Integrity
Integrated Process: Nursing Process/Assessment
Content Area: Pediatrics: Infectious and Communicable Diseases
Health Problem: Pediatric-Specific: Communicable Diseases
Priority Concepts: Clinical Judgment; Infection
Reference: Hockenberry, Wilson, Rodgers (2017), p. 162.

Pediatric

CHAPTER 41

Pediatric Medication Administration and Calculations

PRIORITY CONCEPTS Development; Safety

I. Oral Medications

A. Most oral pediatric medications are in liquid or suspension form or chewable tablet form, because children usually are unable to swallow a tablet or capsule.
B. Solutions may be measured by using an oral plastic syringe or other acceptable measurement or administration device; the device used depends on the developmental age of the child (Fig. 41-1).
C. Medications in suspension settle to the bottom of the bottle between uses, and thorough mixing is required before pouring the medication.
D. Suspensions must be administered immediately after measurement to prevent settling and resultant administration of an incomplete dose.
E. Administer oral medications with a child sitting in an upright position and with the head elevated to prevent aspiration if the child cries or resists.
F. Place a small child sideways on the lap; the child's closest arm should be placed under the adult's arm and behind the adult's back; cradle the child's head, hold the child's hand, and administer the medication slowly with a plastic spoon, small plastic cup, or syringe.
G. If a tablet or capsule has been administered, check the child's mouth to ensure that it has been swallowed; if swallowing is a problem, some tablets can be crushed and given in small amounts of puréed food or flavored syrup (enteric-coated tablets, timed-release tablets, and capsules should not be crushed).
H. Follow generally accepted medication administration guidelines for children (Box 41-1).

Newborns and infants have an immature liver and immature kidneys; therefore, metabolism and elimination of medications is delayed.

II. Parenteral Medications

A. Subcutaneously and intramuscularly administered medications
   1. Medications most often given via the subcutaneous route are insulin and some immunizations.
   2. Any site with sufficient subcutaneous tissue may be used for subcutaneous injections; common sites include the central third of the lateral aspect of the upper arm, the abdomen, and the central third of the anterior thigh.
   3. The safe use of injection sites is based on normal muscle development and the size of the child; the preferred site for intramuscular injections in infants is the vastus lateralis, but agency policies and procedures need to be followed (Table 41-1 and Fig. 41-2).
   4. The usual needle length and gauge for pediatric clients are 0.5 to 1 inch (1.25 to 2.5 cm) and 22 to 25 gauge; needle length also can be estimated by grasping the muscle between the thumb and forefinger—half the resulting distance would be the needle length.
   5. Pediatric dosages for subcutaneous and intramuscular administration are calculated to the nearest hundredth and measured by using a tuberculin syringe; always follow agency guidelines.
   6. Place a plain or decorated adhesive bandage over the puncture site to help the child view the experience in a pleasant way.
B. Intravenously administered medications
   1. Intravenous (IV) medications are diluted for administration.
   2. When an infant or child is receiving an IV medication, the IV site needs to be assessed for signs of inflammation and infiltration or extravasation immediately before, during, and after completion of each medication.
   3. IV medications may be prescribed in a manner that requires a continuous infusion through a primary infusion line.
   4. IV medications may be prescribed intermittently; several doses may be administered in a 24-hour period.
   5. Medications for IV administration are diluted according to the directions accompanying the medication and according to the pediatrician's prescriptions and agency procedures.

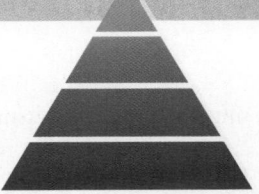

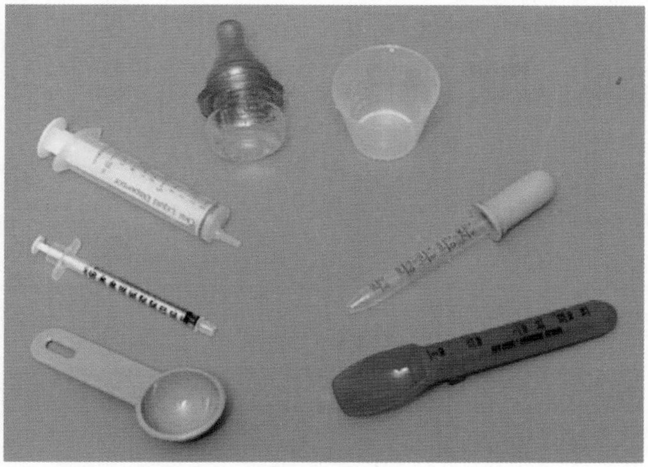

FIG. 41-1 Acceptable devices for measuring and administering oral medication to children *(clockwise from bottom left)*: Measuring spoon, plastic syringes, calibrated nipple, plastic medicine cup, calibrated dropper, hollow-handled medicine spoon. (From Hockenberry, Wilson, 2005.)

BOX 41-1 Medication Administration Guidelines for Children

- Two identifiers are required before medication administration—such as name, medical record number, and birth date. Bar code scanning systems are commonly used as an additional safeguard to ensure that medications are given to the correct client.
- Obtain information from parents about successful methods for administering medications to their children.
- Ask parents about any known allergies.
- To avoid aspiration, liquid forms of medication are safer to swallow than other forms.
- Straws often help older children to swallow pills.
- Avoid putting medications in foods such as milk, cereal, or baby food because it may cause an unpleasant taste to the food, and the child may refuse to accept the same food in the future. In addition, the child may not consume the entire serving and would not receive the required medication dosage.
- If the taste of the medication is unpleasant, it is acceptable to have the child pinch the nose and drink the medication through a straw.
- Offer juice, a soft drink, or a frozen juice bar after the child swallows a medication.
- Always read the pharmacological indications for administration. Some items such as fruit syrups can be acidic and should not be used with medications that react negatively in an acid medium.
- Record the most successful method of administering medications and pertinent nursing prescriptions on the child's care plan for other nursing staff to follow; this notation also saves the child frustration, fear, and anxiety.

Data from Potter P, Perry A, Stockert P, Hall A: *Fundamentals of nursing*, ed 8, St. Louis, 2013, Mosby; and Perry S, Hockenberry M, Lowdermilk D, Wilson D: *Maternal-child nursing care*, ed 4, St. Louis, 2010, Mosby.

6. Infusion time for IV medications is determined on the basis of the directions accompanying the medication, the pediatrician's prescription, and agency procedures.
7. Determine agency procedures related to the volume of flush (normal saline) for peripheral IV lines and for central lines.
8. The flush volume (3 to 20 mL) must be included in the child's intake; the flush is usually administered before administering an IV medication and after the IV medication is completed and is infused at the same rate as the medication.

C. Intermittent IV medication administration
1. Children receiving IV medications intermittently may or may not have a primary IV solution infusing.
2. If a primary IV solution is infusing, the medication may be administered by IV piggyback via a secondary line and via an infusion pump or infusion syringe device.
3. If a primary IV solution does not exist, an indwelling infusion catheter is used for medication administration, and the medication may be administered by push or piggyback; medication administration instructions must be checked for dilution and infusion time procedures.
4. All intermittent medication administrations are preceded and followed by a normal saline flush to ensure that the medication has cleared the IV tubing and that the total dose has been administered.
5. Electronic devices such as controllers or pumps are always used to regulate and administer IV fluids and intermittent IV medications.

D. Special IV administration sets
1. Special IV administration sets, such as a burette, may be used for medication preparation and administration via piggyback.
2. These special sets are all microdrip sets calibrated to deliver 60 drops (gtt)/mL.
3. The total capacity of these type of IV administration sets is 100 to 150 mL, calibrated in 1-mL increments so that exact measurements of small volumes are possible.
4. The medication is mixed with the appropriate amount of diluent, added to the IV administration set, and allowed to infuse at the prescribed rate.
5. The IV administration set needs to be labeled clearly to identify the medication and fluid dosage added.
6. During medication infusion time, a label (per agency guidelines) is attached that indicates that the medication is infusing.
7. During the flush infusion time, a label (per agency guidelines) is attached indicating that the flush is infusing.

TABLE 41-1 Intramuscular Injections: Amount of Medication (mL) by Muscle Group

Muscle	Neonate	Infant (1-12 mo old)	Toddler (1-2 yr old)	Preschool to Child (3-12 yr old)	Adolescent (12-18 yr old)
Vastus lateralis	0.5	0.5-1	0.5-2	2	2
Rectus femoris	Not safe	Not safe	0.5-1	2	2
Ventrogluteal	Not safe	Not safe	Not safe	0.5-3	2-3
Deltoid	Not safe	Not safe	0.5-1	0.5-1	1-1.5

Data from Kee J, Marshall S: *Clinical calculations: with applications to general and specialty areas*, ed 7, St. Louis, 2013, Saunders.

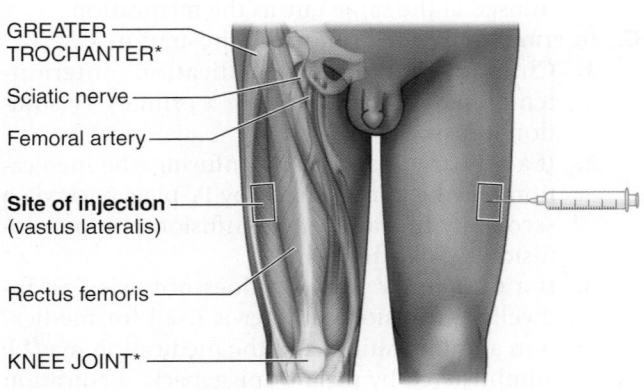

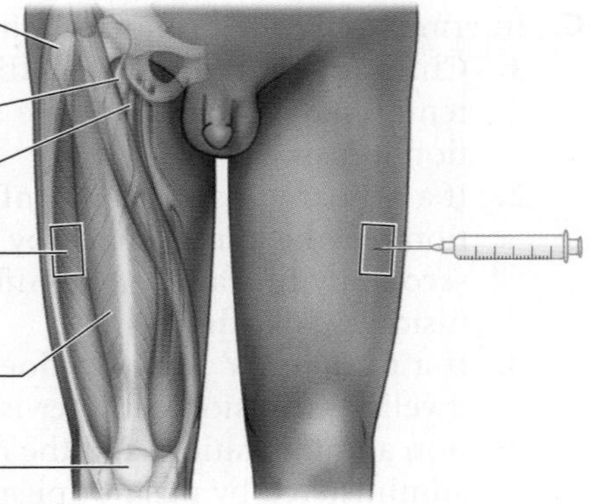

FIG. 41-2 Intramuscular injection site—vastus lateralis. Landmarks are indicated by asterisks.

E. Syringe pump for IV medication administration
1. A syringe containing the medication is fitted into a pump that is connected to the IV tubing through a Y connector.
2. The medication is administered over the prescribed time.

⚠ The 24-hour fluid intake must be monitored closely, and all IV fluid amounts including the amount of flush volume need to be documented accurately to prevent overhydration. For children, the maximum amount of IV fluid administered in a 24-hour period varies and is usually based on body weight and other factors. Check the prescription and agency guidelines for the procedures for the administration of IV fluids and medications.

III. Calculation of Medication Dosage by Body Weight

A. Conversion of body weight
1. There are many mobile application devices available to assist with calculating dosages, but it is important to know how to do these calculations without the use of a mobile device.
2. See Box 41-2 for body weight conversion.

B. Calculation of daily dosages based on weight
1. Abbreviations (Box 41-3)
2. Dosages are expressed in terms of milligrams per kilogram per day, milligrams per pound per day, or milligrams per kilogram per dose.
3. The total daily dosage usually is administered in divided (more than 1) doses per day as prescribed.
4. Express the child's body weight in kilograms or pounds to correlate with the dosage specifications.
5. Calculate the total daily dosage.
6. Divide the total daily dosage by the number of doses to be administered in 1 day.

BOX 41-2 Conversion of Body Weight

Measurements

1 lb = 16 oz

2.2 lb = 1 kg

Pounds to Kilograms

2.2 lb = 1 kg

When converting from pounds to kilograms, divide by 2.2. Kilograms are expressed to the nearest tenth.

Kilograms to Pounds

1 kg = 2.2 lb

When converting from kilograms to pounds, multiply by 2.2. Pounds are expressed to the nearest tenth.

BOX 41-3 Common Measurement Abbreviations

Abbreviation	Meaning
BSA	Body surface area
g	Gram(s)
gr	Grain(s)
kg	Kilogram(s)
lb	Pound(s)
m^2	Square meters
mcg	Microgram(s)
mg	Milligram(s)
mL	Milliliter(s)
SA	Surface area

IV. Calculation of Body Surface Area (BSA)

A. The BSA is determined by comparing body weight and height with averages or norms on a graph called a *nomogram*.

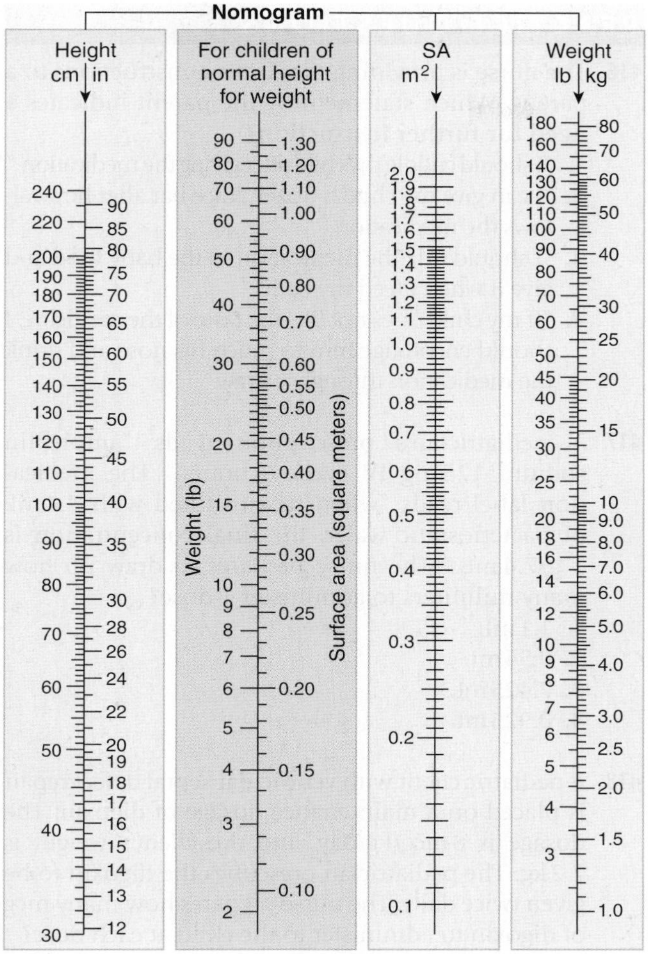

FIG. 41-3 West nomogram for estimation of surface areas in infants and children. First, find height; next, find weight; finally, draw a straight line connecting the height and weight. The body surface area (in square meters [m²]) is indicated where a straight line connecting the height and weight intersects the surface area (SA) column or, if the child is approximately of normal proportion, from weight alone *(darker blue area)*.

B. Not all children are the same size at the same age; the nomogram is used to determine the BSA of a child.

C. Look at the nomogram (Fig. 41-3) and note that the height is on the left-hand side of the chart and the weight is on the right-hand side of the chart.

D. Place a ruler across the chart.

E. Line up the left side of the ruler on the height and the right side of the ruler on the weight; read the BSA at the point where the straight edge of the ruler intersects the surface area (SA) column.

F. The estimated SA is given in square meters (m^2).

G. Box 41-4 gives a sample practice question using the nomogram.

V. Calculation Based on BSA

A. When dosage recommendations for children specify milligrams, micrograms, or units per square meter, calculating the dosage is simple multiplication (Box 41-5).

BOX 41-4 How to Use the Nomogram

Example: Use the nomogram (see Fig. 41-3) and calculate the body surface area (BSA) for a child whose height is 58 inches (147 cm) and weight is 12 kg.

1. Look at the nomogram chart and note that the height is on the left-hand side of the chart and the weight is on the right-hand side.
2. Place a ruler on the chart and line up the left side of the ruler on the height and the right side of the ruler on the weight; read the BSA at the point where the straight edge of the ruler intersects the surface area (SA) column.
3. The estimated SA is given in square meters.

Answer:

$$0.66\,m^2$$

BOX 41-5 Calculating Medication Dosage

When dosage recommendations for children specify milligrams, micrograms, or units per square meter, calculating the dosage is simple multiplication.

Example: The dosage recommendation is $4\,mg/m^2$. The child has a body surface area of $1.1\,m^2$. What is the dosage to be administered?

Answer:

$$1.1 \times 4\,mg = 4.4\,mg$$

BOX 41-6 Calculating a Child's Dosage from the Adult Dosage

When dosages are specified only for adults, a formula is used to calculate a child's dosage from the adult dosage. The adult dosage is based on a standardized body surface area (BSA) of $1.73\,m^2$.

Example: A pediatrician has prescribed an antibiotic for a child. The average adult dose is 250 mg. The child has a BSA of $0.41\,m^2$. What is the dose for the child?

Answer: 59.24 mg

Formula:

$$\frac{BSA\ of\ a\ child\left(m^2\right)}{1.73\,m^2} \times Adult\ dose = Child's\ dose$$

$$\frac{0.41}{1.73} \times 250\,mg = 59.24\,mg$$

B. When dosage recommendations are specified only for adults, a formula is used to calculate a child's dosage from the adult dosage (Box 41-6).

VI. Developmental Considerations for Administering Medications

A. When administering medications to children, developmental age must be taken into consideration to ensure safe and effective administration.

B. General interventions
1. Always be prepared for the procedure with all necessary equipment and assistance.
2. For a hospitalized child, ask the parent or child or both as appropriate if the parent should or should not remain for the procedure.
3. Determine appropriate preadministration and postadministration comfort measures.
4. Try to make the event as pleasant as possible.

C. Box 41-7 lists developmental considerations when giving medications.

BOX 41-7 Developmental Considerations for Administering Medications

Infants

Perform procedure quickly, allowing the infant to swallow; then offer comfort measures, such as holding, rocking, and cuddling.

Allow self-comforting measures, such as the use of a pacifier.

Toddlers

Offer a brief, concrete explanation of the procedure and then perform it.

Accept aggressive behavior, within reasonable limits, as a healthy response, and provide outlets for the toddler.

Provide comfort measures immediately after the procedure, such as touch, holding, cuddling, and providing a favorite toy.

Preschoolers

Offer a brief, concrete explanation of the procedure and then perform it.

Accept aggressive behavior, within reasonable limits, as a healthy response, and provide outlets for the child.

Provide comfort measures after the procedure, such as touch, holding, or providing a favorite toy.

School-Age Children

Explain the procedure, allowing for some control over the body and situation.

Explore feelings and concepts through therapeutic play, drawings of own body and self in the hospital, and the use of books and realistic hospital equipment.

Set appropriate behavior limits, such as it is all right to cry or scream, but not to bite.

Provide activities for releasing aggression and anger.

Use the opportunity to teach about how medication helps the disorder.

Adolescents

Explain the procedure, allowing for some control over body and situation.

Explore concepts of self, hospitalization, and illness, and correct any misconceptions.

Encourage self-expression, individuality, and self-care needs.

Encourage participation in the procedure.

Data from McKenry L, Salerno E: *Mosby's pharmacology in nursing*, St. Louis, 2003, Mosby.

PRACTICE QUESTIONS

416. The nurse is providing medication instructions to a parent. Which statement by the parent indicates a **need for further instruction?**
1. "I should cuddle my child after giving the medication."
2. "I can give my child a frozen juice bar after he swallows the medication."
3. "I should mix the medication in the baby food and give it when I feed my child."
4. "If my child does not like the taste of the medicine, I should encourage him to pinch his nose and drink the medication through a straw."

417. A pediatrician's prescription reads "ampicillin sodium 125 mg IV every 6 hours." The medication label reads "when reconstituted with 7.4 mL of bacteriostatic water, the final concentration is 1 g/7.4 mL." The nurse prepares to draw up how many milliliters to administer 1 dose?
1. 1.1 mL
2. 0.54 mL
3. 7.425 mL
4. 0.925 mL

418. A pediatric client with ventricular septal defect repair is placed on a maintenance dosage of digoxin. The dosage is 8 mcg/kg/day, and the client's weight is 7.2 kg. The pediatrician prescribes the digoxin to be given twice daily. The nurse prepares how many mcg of digoxin to administer to the child at each dose?
1. 12.6 mcg
2. 21.4 mcg
3. 28.8 mcg
4. 32.2 mcg

419. Sulfisoxazole, 1 g orally twice daily, is prescribed for an adolescent with a urinary tract infection. The medication label reads "500-mg tablets." The nurse has determined that the dosage prescribed is safe. The nurse administers how many tablets per dose to the adolescent?
1. ½ tablet
2. 1 tablet
3. 2 tablets
4. 3 tablets

420. Penicillin G procaine, 1,000,000 units IM (intramuscularly), is prescribed for an adolescent with an infection. The medication label reads "1,200,000 units per 2 mL." The nurse has determined that the dose prescribed is safe. The nurse administers how many milliliters per dose to the adolescent? **Round answer to the nearest tenth position.**
1. 0.8 mL
2. 1.2 mL
3. 1.4 mL
4. 1.7 mL

421. The nurse prepares to administer an intramuscular injection to a 4-month-old infant. The nurse selects which **best** site to administer the injection?

1. Ventrogluteal
2. Lateral deltoid
3. Rectus femoris
4. Vastus lateralis

422. Atropine sulfate, 0.6 mg intramuscularly, is prescribed for a child preoperatively. The nurse has determined that the dose prescribed is safe and prepares to administer how many milliliters to the child? **Fill in the blank (refer to figure).**

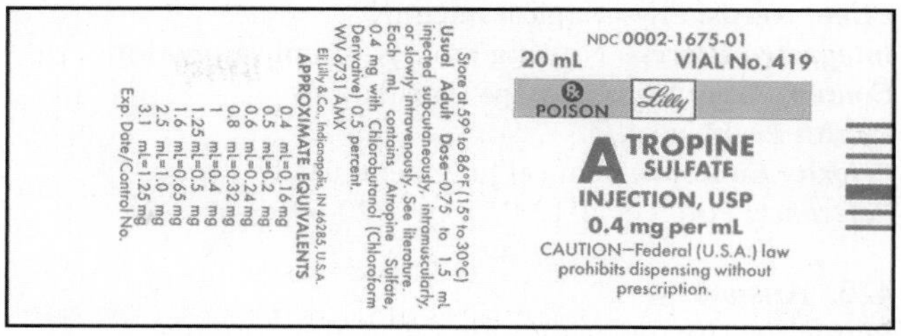

Answer: ________ mL

ANSWERS

416. ***Answer:*** **3**

Rationale: The nurse would teach the parent to avoid putting medications in foods because it may give an unpleasant taste to the food, and the child may refuse to accept the same food in the future. In addition, the child may not consume the entire serving and would not receive the required medication dosage. The mother should provide comfort measures immediately after medication administration, such as touching, holding, cuddling, and providing a favorite toy. The mother should offer juice, a soft drink, or a frozen juice bar to the child after the child swallows the medication. If the taste of the medication is unpleasant, the child should pinch the nose and drink the medication through a straw.

Test-Taking Strategy: Note the strategic words, *need for further instruction.* These words indicate a negative event query and the need to select the incorrect statement made by the mother. Read each statement carefully and think about the statement that may be unsafe and may not provide an accurate dose to the child. This will direct you to the correct option.

Level of Cognitive Ability: Evaluating
Client Needs: Physiological Integrity
Integrated Process: Teaching and Learning
Content Area: Skills: Client Teaching
Health Problem: N/A
Priority Concepts: Client Education; Safety
Reference: McKinney et al. (2018), pp. 855-856.

417. ***Answer:*** **4**

Rationale: Convert 1 g to milligrams. In the metric system, to convert larger to smaller, multiply by 1000 or move the decimal point 3 places to the right:

$$1\,g = 1000\,mg$$

Formula:

$$\frac{Desired}{Available} \times Volume = \frac{125\,mg}{1000\,mg} \times 7.4\,mL = 0.925\,mL\ per\ dose$$

Test-Taking Strategy: Focus on the subject, milliliters per dose. Convert grams to milligrams first. Next, use the formula to determine the correct dose, knowing that when reconstituted, 1000 mg = 7.4 mL. Verify the answer using a calculator.

Level of Cognitive Ability: Applying
Client Needs: Physiological Integrity
Integrated Process: Nursing Process—Implementation
Content Area: Skills: Dosage Calculations
Health Problem: N/A
Priority Concepts: Clinical Judgment; Safety
Reference: Potter et al. (2017), pp. 620-621.

418. ***Answer:*** **3**

Rationale: Calculate the daily dosage by weight first:

$$8\,mcg \times 7.2\,kg = 57.6\,mcg / day$$

The pediatrician prescribes digoxin twice daily; 2 doses in 24 hours will be administered:

$$\frac{57.6\,mcg / day}{2\,doses} = 28.8\,mcg\ for\ each\ dose$$

Test-Taking Strategy: Focus on the subject, mcg per dose, and note that the question states *twice daily* and *each dose*. Calculate the dosage per day by weight first, and then determine the micrograms per each dose by dividing the total daily dose by 2. Verify the answer using a calculator.

Level of Cognitive Ability: Applying
Client Needs: Physiological Integrity
Integrated Process: Nursing Process—Implementation
Content Area: Skills: Dosage Calculations
Health Problem: Pediatric-Specific: Congenital Cardiac Defects
Priority Concepts: Clinical Judgment; Safety
Reference: McKinney et al. (2018), p. 854.

419. ***Answer:*** **3**

Rationale: Change 1 g to milligrams, knowing that 1000 mg = 1 g. Also, when converting from grams to milligrams (larger to smaller), move the decimal point 3 places to the right:

$$1\,g = 1000\,mg$$

Next, use the formula to calculate the correct dose.

Formula:

$$\frac{Desired}{Available} \times Tablet = \frac{1000\,mg}{500\,mg} \times Tablet = 2\,tablets$$

Test-Taking Strategy: Focus on the subject, tablets per dose. Convert grams to milligrams first. Next, use the formula to determine the correct dose and verify the answer using a calculator.

Level of Cognitive Ability: Applying
Client Needs: Physiological Integrity
Integrated Process: Nursing Process—Implementation
Content Area: Skills: Dosage Calculations
Health Problem: N/A
Priority Concepts: Clinical Judgment; Safety
Reference: Potter et al. (2017), pp. 620-621.

420. *Answer:* 4
Rationale: Use the medication calculation formula.
Formula:

$$\frac{Desired}{Available} \times Volume = \frac{1,000,000}{1,200,000} \times 2\,mL$$
$$= 1.66 = 1.7\,mL\ per\ dose$$

Test-Taking Strategy: Focus on the **subject,** milliliters per dose. Use the formula to determine the correct dose, and verify the answer using a calculator.
Level of Cognitive Ability: Applying
Client Needs: Physiological Integrity
Integrated Process: Nursing Process—Implementation
Content Area: Skills: Dosage Calculations
Health Problem: N/A
Priority Concepts: Clinical Judgment; Safety
Reference: Potter et al. (2017), pp. 620-621.

421. *Answer:* 4
Rationale: Intramuscular injection sites are selected on the basis of the child's age and muscle development of the child. The vastus lateralis is the only safe muscle group to use for intramuscular injection in a 4-month-old infant. The sites identified in options 1, 2, and 3 are unsafe for a child of this age.
Test-Taking Strategy: Note the **strategic word,** *best,* and focus on the age of the child identified in the question. Thinking about the physiological development of the muscle groups in an infant at 4 months of age will assist in directing you to the correct option.
Level of Cognitive Ability: Applying
Client Needs: Physiological Integrity
Integrated Process: Nursing Process—Implementation
Content Area: Skills: Medication Administration
Health Problem: N/A
Priority Concepts: Clinical Judgment; Safety
Reference: Hockenberry, Wilson, Rodgers (2017), pp. 607-608.

422. *Answer:* 1.5
Rationale: Use the formula for calculating the medication dose.
Formula:

$$\frac{Desired}{Available} \times Volume = \frac{0.6\,mg}{0.4\,mg} \times 1\,mL = 1.5\,mL$$

Test-Taking Strategy: Focus on the **subject,** the milliliters to be administered. Note that the medication label indicates that there is 0.4 mg/mL. Use the formula to determine the correct dose, and verify the answer using a calculator.
Level of Cognitive Ability: Applying
Client Needs: Physiological Integrity
Integrated Process: Nursing Process—Implementation
Content Area: Skills: Dosage Calculations
Health Problem: N/A
Priority Concepts: Clinical Judgment; Safety
Reference: Potter et al. (2017), pp. 620-621.

UNIT VII

Integumentary Problems of the Adult Client

Pyramid to Success

The Pyramid to Success focuses on the concept that the integumentary system provides the first line of defense against infections. Focus is on the protective measures necessary to prevent infection, including infection from colonization with a multidrug-resistant organism, such as methicillin-resistant *Staphylococcus aureus* (MRSA). Pyramid Points address the risk factors related to the development of integumentary problems, and the preventive measures related to these problems, including skin cancer. Another important focus are the emergency measures related to bites and stings. Psychosocial issues related to the body image disturbances that can occur as the result of an integumentary problem and providing psychosocial support is a primary nursing consideration

Client Needs: Learning Objectives

Safe and Effective Care Environment

Consulting with interprofessional health care team members regarding treatments
Ensuring that informed consent has been obtained for treatments and procedures
Establishing priorities of care
Handling of hazardous and infectious materials
Instituting standard and other precautions
Maintaining confidentiality related to the skin problem
Making referrals to appropriate interprofessional health care team members
Practicing asepsis techniques and preventing infection

Health Promotion and Maintenance

Implementing disease prevention measures
Performing physical assessment techniques for the integumentary system
Promoting health screening and health promotion programs to prevent skin problems
Providing instructions to the client regarding prevention measures and care for an integumentary problem

Psychosocial Integrity

Addressing end-of-life issues
Discussing unexpected body image changes
Identifying coping mechanisms
Identifying situational role changes
Identifying support systems
Providing support to the client to assist in coping with the integumentary problem

Physiological Integrity

Assessing for alterations in body systems
Providing adequate nutrition for healing
Providing basic care and comfort
Providing emergency care for an integumentary injury such as a bite or sting
Monitoring for expected effects of treatments
Monitoring for fluid and electrolyte imbalances and other complications
Monitoring laboratory reference intervals

CHAPTER 42

Integumentary Problems

PRIORITY CONCEPTS Infection; Tissue Integrity

I. Anatomy and Physiology

A. The skin is the largest sensory organ of the body, with a surface area of 15 to 20 square feet (1.4 to 1.9 square meters) and a weight of about 9 lb (4 kg).

B. Functions
1. Acts as the first line of defense against infections
2. Protects underlying tissues and organs from injury
3. Receives stimuli from the external environment; detects touch, pressure, pain, and temperature stimuli; relays information to the nervous system
4. Regulates normal body temperature
5. Excretes salts, water, and organic wastes
6. Protects the body from excessive water loss
7. Synthesizes vitamin D_3, which converts to calcitriol, for normal calcium metabolism
8. Stores nutrients

C. Layers
1. Epidermis
2. Dermis
3. Hypodermis (subcutaneous fat)

D. Epidermal appendages
1. Nails
2. Hair
3. Glands
   a. Sebaceous
   b. Sweat

E. Normal bacterial flora
1. Types of normal bacterial flora include:
   a. Gram-positive and gram-negative staphylococci
   b. *Pseudomonas*
   c. *Streptococcus*
2. Organisms are shed with normal exfoliation.
3. A pH of 4.2 to 5.6 halts the growth of bacteria.

II. Risk Factors for Integumentary Problems

A. Exposure to chemical and environmental pollutants
B. Exposure to radiation
C. Race and age
D. Exposure to the sun or use of indoor tanning
E. Lack of personal hygiene habits
F. Use of harsh soaps or other harsh products
G. Some medications, such as long-term glucocorticoid use or herbal preparations
H. Nutritional deficiencies
I. Moderate to severe emotional stress
J. Infection, with injured areas as the potential entry points for infection
K. Repeated injury and irritation
L. Genetic predisposition
M. Systemic illnesses

III. Psychosocial Impact

A. Change in body image, decreased general well-being, and decreased self-esteem
B. Social isolation and fear of rejection (because of embarrassment about changes in skin appearance)
C. Restrictions in physical activity
D. Pain
E. Disruption or loss of employment
F. Cost of medications, hospitalizations, and follow-up care, including dressing supplies

IV. Phases of Wound Healing

A. Phases
1. Inflammatory: Begins at the time of injury and lasts 3 to 5 days; manifestations include local edema, pain, redness, and warmth.
2. Fibroblastic: Begins the fourth day after injury and lasts 2 to 4 weeks; scar tissue forms and granulation tissue forms in the tissue bed.
3. Maturation: Begins as early as 3 weeks after the injury and may last for 1 year; scar tissue becomes thinner and is firm and inelastic on palpation.

B. Healing by intention
1. First intention: Wound edges are approximated and held in place (i.e., with sutures) until healing occurs; wound is easily closed and dead space is eliminated.
2. Second intention: This type of healing occurs with injuries or wounds that have tissue loss and require gradual filling in of the dead space with connective tissue.

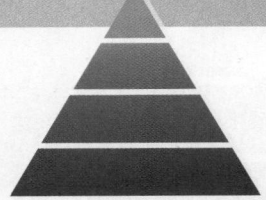

BOX 42-1 Types of Exudate from Wounds

Serous
- Clear or straw colored
- Occurs as a normal part of the healing process

Serosanguineous
- Pink colored due to the presence of a small amount of blood cells mixed with serous drainage
- Occurs as a normal part of the healing process

Sanguineous
- Red drainage from trauma to a blood vessel
- May occur with wound cleansing or other trauma to the wound bed
- Sanguineous drainage is abnormal in wounds

Hemorrhaging
- Frank blood from a leaking blood vessel
- May require emergency treatment to control bleeding
- Hemorrhage is an abnormal wound exudate

Purulent
- Yellow, gray, or green drainage due to infection in the wound

3. Third intention: This type of healing involves delayed primary closure and occurs with wounds that are intentionally left open for several days for irrigation or removal of debris and exudates; once debris has been removed and inflammation resolves, the wound is closed by first intention.

C. Types of wound drainage: Refer to Box 42-1.

V. Diagnostic Tests

A. Skin biopsy
1. Description
   a. Skin biopsy is the collection of a small piece of skin tissue for histopathological study.
   b. Methods include punch, excisional, and shave.
2. Preprocedure interventions
   a. Verify informed consent has been obtained.
   b. Cleanse site as prescribed.
3. Postprocedure interventions
   a. Place specimen in the appropriate container and send to pathology laboratory for analysis.
   b. Use surgically aseptic technique for biopsy site dressings.
   c. Assess the biopsy site for bleeding and infection.
   d. Instruct the client to keep dressing in place for at least 8 hours, and then clean daily and use antibiotic ointment as prescribed (sutures are usually removed in 7 to 10 days).
   e. Instruct the client to report signs of excessive drainage, redness, or other signs of infection.

B. Skin/wound cultures
1. A small skin culture sample is obtained with a sterile applicator and the appropriate type of culture tube (e.g., bacterial or viral). Methods include scraping, punch biopsy, and collecting fluid. Local anesthesia may be used.
2. A nasal swab is also commonly done to determine previous exposure to certain types of bacteria.
3. Postprocedure intervention
   a. Viral culture is placed immediately on ice.
   b. Sample is sent to the laboratory to identify an existing organism.

Obtain skin culture samples or any other type of culture specimens before instituting antibiotic therapy.

C. Wood's light examination
1. Description: Skin is viewed under ultraviolet light through a special glass (Wood's glass) to identify superficial infections of the skin.
2. Preprocedure intervention: Explain procedure to the client and reassure him or her that the light is not harmful to the skin or the eyes. Darken the room before the examination.
3. Postprocedure intervention: Assist the client during adjustment from the darkened room.

D. Diascopy
1. Technique allows clearer inspection of lesions by eliminating the erythema caused by increased blood flow to the area.
2. A glass slide is pressed over the lesion, causing blanching and revealing the lesion more clearly.

E. Skin assessment: See Chapter 12.

VI. *Candida albicans*

A. Description
1. A superficial fungal infection of the skin and mucous membranes
2. Also known as a *yeast infection* (oral candidiasis), or *thrush* when it occurs in the mouth
3. Risk factors include immunosuppression, long-term antibiotic therapy, diabetes mellitus, and obesity.
4. Common areas of occurrence include skin folds, perineum, vagina, axilla, and under the breasts.

B. Assessment
1. Skin: Red and irritated appearance that itches and stings
2. Mucous membranes of the mouth: Red and whitish patches

C. Interventions
1. Teach the client to keep skin fold areas clean and dry.
2. For the hospitalized client, inspect skin fold areas frequently, turn and reposition the client frequently, and keep the skin and bed linens clean and dry.
3. Provide frequent mouth care as prescribed and avoid irritating products.
4. Provide food and fluids that are tepid in temperature and nonirritating to mucous membranes.
5. Antifungal medications may be prescribed.

VII. Herpes Zoster (Shingles)

A. Description
1. With a history of chickenpox, shingles is caused by reactivation of the varicella zoster virus; shingles can occur during any immunocompromised state in a client with a history of chickenpox.
2. The dormant virus is located in the dorsal nerve root ganglia of the sensory cranial and spinal nerves.
3. Herpes zoster eruptions occur in a segmental distribution on the skin area along the infected nerve and show up after several days of discomfort in the area.
4. Diagnosis is determined by visual examination and by Tzanck smear to verify a herpes infection and viral culture to identify the organism.
5. Postherpetic neuralgia (severe pain) can remain after the lesions resolve.
6. Herpes zoster is contagious to individuals who never had chickenpox and who have not been vaccinated against the disease.
7. Herpes simplex virus is another type of virus; type 1 infection typically causes a cold sore (usually on the lip) and type 2 causes genital herpes typically below the waist (both types are contagious and may be present together).

B. Assessment
1. Unilaterally clustered skin vesicles along peripheral sensory nerves on the trunk, thorax, or face
2. Fever, malaise
3. Burning and pain
4. Paresthesia
5. Pruritus

C. Interventions
1. Isolate the client, because exudate from the lesions contains the virus (maintain standard and other precautions as appropriate, such as contact precautions, as long as vesicles are present).
2. Assess for signs and symptoms of infection, including skin infections and eye infections; skin necrosis can also occur.
3. Assess neurovascular status and seventh cranial nerve function; Bell's palsy is a complication.
4. Use an air mattress and bed cradle on the client's bed if hospitalized, and keep the environment cool; warmth and touch aggravate the pain.
5. Prevent the client from scratching and rubbing the affected area.
6. Instruct the client to wear lightweight, loose cotton clothing and to avoid wool and synthetic clothing.
7. Teach the client about the prescribed therapies; astringent compresses may be prescribed to relieve irritation and pain and to promote crust formation and healing.
8. Teach the client about measures to keep the skin clean to prevent infection.
9. Teach the client about topical treatment and antiviral medications; antiviral therapies begun within 3 days of rash reduce pain and lessen likelihood of postherpetic neuralgia.
10. The vaccination for shingles, is recommended for adults 50 years of age and older to reduce the risk of occurrence and the associated long-term pain.
11. Antiviral medications may be prescribed; refer to Chapter 63 for information on antiviral medications.

VIII. Methicillin-Resistant *Staphylococcus aureus* (MRSA)

A. Description
1. Skin or wound becomes infected with methicillin-resistant *Staphylococcus aureus* (MRSA). MRSA can be community acquired, such as through sports when skin-to-skin contact and sharing of equipment occurs. It can also be hospital acquired, such as in the case of a surgical site infection (SSI). See Chapter 13 for additional types of health care–associated infections.
2. An MRSA screening with a nasal swab may be done for clients who are having surgery, who have been previously hospitalized, or who live in group settings. Clients with positive cultures or with a history of a positive culture are isolated.
3. Infection can range from mild to severe and can present as folliculitis or furuncles.
4. Folliculitis is a superficial infection of the follicle caused by *Staphylococcus* and presents as a raised red rash and pustules; furuncles are also caused by *Staphylococcus* and occur deep in the follicle, presenting as very painful large, raised bumps that may or may not have a pustule.
5. If MRSA infects the blood, sepsis, organ damage, and death can occur.

⚠ MRSA is contagious and is spread to others by direct contact with infected skin or infected articles; for the client with MRSA, the infection can also be spread to many parts of the body.

B. Assessment: A culture and sensitivity test of the skin or wound confirms the presence of MRSA and leads to choice of appropriate antibiotic therapy.

C. Interventions
1. Maintain standard precautions and contact precautions as appropriate to prevent spread of infection to others.
2. Monitor the client closely for signs of further infection, which may result in systemic illness or organ damage.
3. Administer antibiotic therapy as prescribed.
4. For additional information on MRSA, refer to Chapters 13 and 40.

IX. Erysipelas and Cellulitis

A. Description
1. Erysipelas is an acute, superficial, rapidly spreading inflammation of the dermis and lymphatics caused by group A *Streptococcus*, which enters the tissue via an abrasion, bite, trauma, or wound.
2. Cellulitis is an infection of the dermis and underlying hypodermis; the causative organism is usually group A *Streptococcus* or *Staphylococcus aureus*.

B. Assessment
1. Pain and tenderness
2. Erythema and warmth
3. Edema
4. Fever

C. Interventions
1. Promote rest of the affected area.
2. Apply warm compresses as prescribed to promote circulation and to decrease discomfort, erythema, and edema.
3. Apply antibacterial dressings, ointments, or gels as prescribed.
4. Administer antibiotics as prescribed for an infection; obtain a culture of the area before initiating the antibiotics.

X. Poison Ivy, Poison Oak, and Poison Sumac

A. Description: A dermatitis that develops from contact with urushiol from poison ivy, oak, or sumac plants

B. Assessment
1. Papulovesicular lesions
2. Severe pruritus

C. Interventions
1. Cleanse the skin of the plant oils immediately.
2. Apply cool, wet compresses to relieve the itching.
3. Apply topical products to relieve the itching and discomfort.
4. Topical or oral glucocorticoids may be prescribed for severe reactions.

XI. Bites and Stings

A. Spider bites
1. Almost all types of spider bites are venomous and most are not harmful, but bites or stings from brown recluse spiders, black widow spiders, and tarantulas (as well as from scorpions, bees, and wasps) can produce toxic reactions in humans. Tetanus prophylaxis should be current because spider bites can be contaminated with tetanus spores.
2. Brown recluse spider
   a. Bite can cause a skin lesion, a necrotic wound, or systemic effects from the toxin (loxoscelism).
   b. Application of ice decreases enzyme activity of the venom and limits tissue necrosis; should be done immediately and intermittently for up to 4 days after the bite.
   c. Topical antiseptics and antibiotics may be necessary if the site becomes infected.
3. Black widow spider
   a. Bite causes a small red papule.
   b. Venom causes neurotoxicity.
   c. Ice is applied immediately to inhibit the action of the neurotoxin.
   d. Systemic toxicity can occur, and the victim may require supportive therapy in the hospital.
4. Tarantulas
   a. Bite causes swelling, redness, numbness, lymph inflammation, and pain at the bite site.
   b. The tarantula launches its barbed hairs, which can penetrate the skin and eyes of the victim, producing a severe inflammatory reaction.
   c. Tarantula hairs are removed as soon as possible, using sticky tape to pull hairs from the skin, and the skin is thoroughly irrigated; saline irrigations are done for eye exposure.
   d. The involved extremity is elevated and immobilized to reduce pain and swelling.
   e. Antihistamines and topical or systemic corticosteroids may be prescribed; tetanus prophylaxis is necessary.

B. Scorpion stings
1. Scorpions inject venom into the victim through a stinging apparatus on their tail.
2. Most stings cause local pain, inflammation, and mild systemic reactions that are treated with analgesics, wound care, and supportive treatment.

3. The bark scorpion can inflict a severe and potentially fatal systemic response, especially in children and the elderly; the venom is neurotoxic; the victim should be taken to the emergency department immediately (an antivenom is administered for bark scorpion bites).

C. Bees and wasps
1. Stings usually cause a wheal and flare reaction.
2. Emergency care involves quick removal of the stinger and application of an ice pack.
3. The stinger is removed by gently scraping or brushing it off with the edge of a needle or similar object; tweezers are not used because there is a risk of pinching the venom sac.
4. If the victim is allergic to the venom of a bee or wasp, a severe allergic response can occur (hives, pruritus, swelling of the lips and tongue) that can progress to life-threatening anaphylaxis; immediate emergency care is required.
5. Individuals who are allergic should carry an epinephrine autoinjector for self-administration of intramuscular epinephrine if a bee or wasp sting occurs. After use of the epinephrine autoinjector, the individual should seek emergency medical attention. Persons should have 2 injectors available and obtain a replacement as soon as possible.

D. Snake bites
1. Some snakes are venomous and can cause a serious systemic reaction in the victim.
2. The victim should be immediately moved to a safe area away from the snake and should rest to decrease venom circulation; the extremity is immobilized and kept below the level of the heart.
3. Constricting clothing and jewelry are removed before swelling occurs.
4. The victim is kept warm and is not allowed to consume caffeinated or alcoholic beverages, which may speed absorption of the venom.
5. If unable to seek emergency medical attention promptly, a constricting band may be applied proximal to the wound to slow the venom circulation; monitor the circulation frequently and loosen the band if edema occurs.
6. The wound is not incised or sucked to remove the venom; ice is not applied to the wound.
7. Emergency care in a hospital is required as soon as possible; an antivenom may be administered along with supportive care. The snake should not be transported with the victim for identification purposes unless it can be safely placed in a sealed container during transportation.

For spider bites, scorpion bites, or other stings or bites, the Poison Control Center should be contacted as soon as possible to determine the best initial management.

XII. Frostbite

A. Description
1. Frostbite is damage to tissues and blood vessels as a result of prolonged exposure to cold.
2. Fingers, toes, face, nose, and ears often are affected.

B. Assessment
1. First-degree: Involves white plaque surrounded by a ring of hyperemia and edema
2. Second-degree: Large, clear fluid–filled blisters with partial-thickness skin necrosis
3. Third-degree: Involves the formation of small hemorrhagic blisters, usually followed by eschar formation involving the hypodermis requiring debridement
4. Fourth-degree: No blisters or edema noted; full-thickness necrosis with visible tissue loss extending into muscle and bone, which may result in gangrene. Amputation may be required.

C. Interventions
1. Rewarm the affected part rapidly and continuously with a warm water bath or towels at 104.0° F to 107.6° F (40° C to 42° C) to thaw the frozen part.
2. Handle the affected area gently and immobilize.
3. Avoid using dry heat, and never rub or massage the part, which may result in further tissue damage.
4. The rewarming process may be painful; analgesics may be necessary.
5. Avoid compression of the injured tissues and apply only loose and nonadherent sterile dressings.
6. Monitor for signs of compartment syndrome.
7. Tetanus prophylaxis is necessary, and topical and systemic antibiotics may be prescribed.
8. Debridement of necrotic tissue may be needed; amputation may be necessary if gangrene develops.

XIII. Actinic Keratoses

A. Actinic keratoses are caused by chronic exposure to the sun and appear as rough, scaly, red, or brown lesions that are usually found on the face, scalp, arms, and backs of the hands.

B. Lesions are considered premalignant, and there is risk for slow progression to squamous cell carcinoma.

C. Treatment includes medications, excision, cryotherapy, curettage, and laser therapy.

D. See Chapter 43 for information on medications to treat this disorder.

XIV. Skin Cancer

A. Description
1. Skin cancer is a malignant lesion of the skin, which may or may not metastasize.
2. Overexposure to the sun is a primary cause; other causes and conditions that place the individual at risk include chronic skin damage

from repeated injury and irritation such as tanning and use of tanning beds, genetic predisposition, ionizing radiation, light-skinned race, age older than 60 years, an outdoor occupation, and exposure to chemical carcinogens.

3. Diagnosis is confirmed by skin biopsy.

B. Types

1. Basal cell: Basal cell cancer arises from the basal cells contained in the epidermis; metastasis is rare, but underlying tissue destruction can progress to organ tissue.
2. Squamous cell: Squamous cell cancer is a tumor of the epidermal keratinocytes and can infiltrate surrounding structures and metastasize to lymph nodes.
3. Melanoma: Melanoma may occur any place on the body, especially where birthmarks or new moles are apparent; it is highly metastatic to the brain, lungs, bone, and liver, with survival depending on early diagnosis and treatment.

C. Assessment (see Box 42-2)

1. Change in color, size, or shape of preexisting lesion
2. Pruritus
3. Local soreness

⚠ The client needs to be informed about the risks associated with overexposure to the sun and taught about the importance of performing monthly skin self-assessments.

D. Interventions

1. Instruct the client regarding the risk factors and preventive measures.
2. Instruct the client to perform monthly skin self-assessments and to monitor for lesions that do not heal or that change characteristics.
3. Advise the client to have moles or lesions that are subject to chronic irritation removed.
4. Advise the client to avoid contact with chemical irritants.
5. Instruct the client to wear layered clothing and use and reapply sunscreen lotions with an appropriate sun protection factor when outdoors.
6. Instruct the client to avoid sun exposure between 10 a.m. and 4 p.m.
7. Management may include surgical or nonsurgical interventions; if medication is prescribed, provide instructions about its use.
8. Assist with surgical management, which may include cryosurgery, curettage and electrodessication, or surgical excision of the lesion.

BOX 42-2 Appearance of Skin Cancer Lesions

Basal Cell Carcinoma

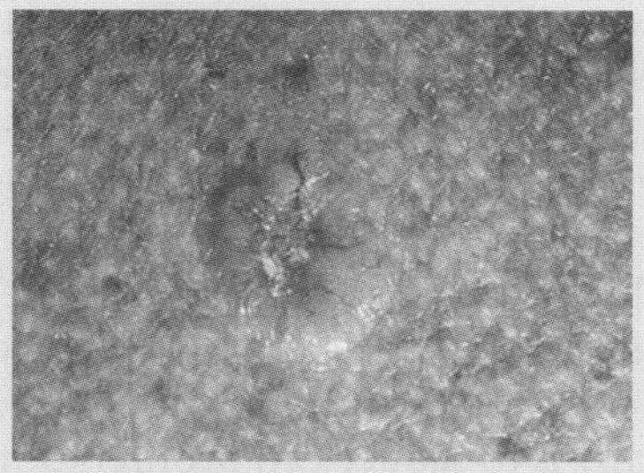

Waxy nodule with pearly borders
Papule, red, central crater
Metastasis is rare

Squamous Cell Carcinoma

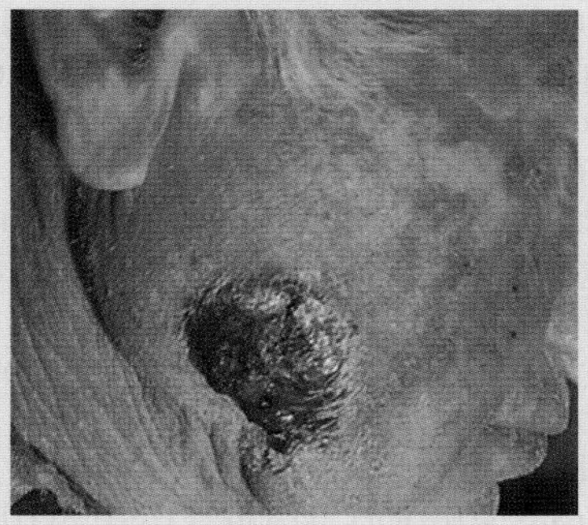

Oozing, bleeding, crusting lesion
Potentially metastatic
Larger tumors associated with a higher risk for metastasis

Melanoma

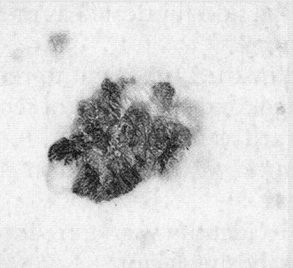

Irregular, circular, bordered lesion with hues of tan, black, or blue
Rapid infiltration into tissue, highly metastatic

Figures from Ignatavicius D, Workman ML: *Medical-surgical nursing: patient-centered collaborative care*, ed 8, Philadelphia, 2016, Saunders.

XV. Psoriasis

A. Description

1. Psoriasis is a chronic, noninfectious skin inflammation occurring with remissions and exacerbations involving keratin synthesis that results in psoriatic patches; it may lead to an infection in the affected area.
2. Various forms exist, with psoriasis vulgaris being the most common.
3. Possible causes of the disorder include stress, trauma, infection, hormonal changes, obesity,

an autoimmune reaction, and climate changes; a genetic predisposition may also be a cause.
4. The disorder may be exacerbated by the use of certain medications.
5. Koebner phenomenon is the development of psoriatic lesions at a site of injury, such as a scratched or sunburned area. Prompt cleansing of the area may prevent or lessen this phenomenon.
6. In some individuals with psoriasis, arthritis develops, which leads to joint changes similar to those seen in rheumatoid arthritis.
7. The goal of therapy is to reduce cell proliferation and inflammation, and the type of therapy prescribed depends on the extent of the disease and the client's response to treatment.

B. Assessment
1. Pruritus
2. Shedding: Silvery-white scales on a raised, reddened, round plaque that usually affects the scalp, knees, elbows, extensor surfaces of arms and legs, and sacral regions
3. Yellow discoloration, pitting, and thickening of the nails are noted if they are affected.
4. Joint inflammation with psoriatic arthritis

C. Pharmacological therapy: Refer to Chapter 43 for medications used to treat psoriasis.

D. Interventions and client education
1. Provide emotional support to the client with associated altered body image and decreased self-esteem.
2. Instruct the client in the use of prescribed therapies and to avoid over-the-counter medications.
3. Instruct the client not to scratch the affected areas and to keep the skin lubricated as prescribed to minimize itching.
4. Monitor for and instruct the client to recognize and report the signs and symptoms of secondary skin problems, such as infection.
5. Instruct the client to wear light cotton clothing over affected areas.
6. Assist the client to identify ways to reduce stress if stress is a predisposing factor.

XVI. Acne Vulgaris

A. Description
1. Acne is a chronic skin disorder that usually begins in puberty and is more common in males; lesions develop on the face, neck, chest, shoulders, and back.
2. Acne requires active treatment for control until it resolves.
3. The types of lesions include comedones (open and closed), pustules, papules, and nodules.
4. The exact cause is unknown but may include androgenic influence on sebaceous glands, increased sebum production, and proliferation of *Propionibacterium acnes*, the organism that converts sebum into irritant fatty acids.
5. Exacerbations coincide with the menstrual cycle in female clients because of hormonal activity; oily skin and a genetic predisposition may be contributing factors.

B. Assessment
1. Closed comedones are whiteheads and noninflamed lesions that develop as follicles enlarge, with the retention of horny cells.
2. Open comedones are blackheads that result from continuing accumulation of horny cells and sebum, which dilates the follicles.
3. Pustules and papules result as the inflammatory process progresses.
4. Nodules result from total disintegration of a comedone and subsequent collapse of the follicle.
5. Deep scarring can result from nodules.

C. Interventions
1. Instruct the client in prescribed skin-cleansing methods, with emphasis on not scrubbing the face and using only prescribed topical agents.
2. Instruct the client in the administration of topical or oral medications as prescribed.
3. Instruct the client not to squeeze, prick, or pick at lesions.
4. Instruct the client to use products labeled noncomedogenic and cosmetics that are water based and to avoid contact with products with an excessive oil base.
5. Instruct the client on the importance of follow-up treatment.
6. Refer to Chapter 43 for information on the medications used to treat acne.

XVII. Stevens-Johnson Syndrome

A. A medication-induced skin reaction that occurs through an immunological response; common medications causing the reaction include antibiotics (especially sulfonamides), antiseizure medications, and nonsteroidal antiinflammatory drugs (NSAIDs).

B. Similar to toxic epidermal necrolysis (TEN), another medication-induced skin reaction that results in diffuse erythema and large blister formation on the skin and mucous membranes

C. May be mild or severe, and may cause vesicles, erosions, and crusts on the skin; if severe, systemic reactions occur that involve the respiratory system, renal system, and eyes, resulting in blindness, and it can be fatal. Initial clinical manifestations include flu-like symptoms and erythema of the skin and mucous membranes. Serious systemic symptoms and complications occur when the ulcerations involve the larynx, bronchi, and esophagus.

D. Most commonly occurs in clients who have impaired immune systems

E. Treatment includes immediate discontinuation of the medication causing the syndrome; antibiotics, corticosteroids, and supportive therapy may be necessary.

XVIII. Pressure Injury

A. Description
1. A pressure injury is an impairment of skin integrity.
2. A pressure injury can occur anywhere on the body; tissue damage results when the skin and underlying tissue are compressed between a bony prominence and an external surface for an extended period.
3. The tissue compression restricts blood flow to the skin, which can result in tissue ischemia, inflammation, and necrosis; once a pressure injury forms, it is difficult to heal.
4. Prevention of skin breakdown in any part of the client's body is a major role for the nurse.

B. Risk factors
1. Skin pressure
2. Skin shearing and friction
3. Immobility
4. Malnutrition
5. Incontinence
6. Decreased sensory perception

C. Assessment and staging (Box 42-3)

D. Interventions

Avoid direct massage to a reddened skin area, because massage can damage the capillary beds and cause tissue necrosis.

1. Identify clients at risk for developing a pressure injury.
2. Institute measures to prevent pressure injury, such as appropriate positioning, using pressure relief devices, ensuring adequate nutrition, and developing a plan for skin cleansing and care.
3. Perform frequent skin assessments and monitor for an alteration in skin integrity (refer to Chapter 12 for more information on skin assessment).
4. Keep the client's skin dry and the sheets wrinkle-free; if the client is incontinent, check the client frequently and change pads or any items placed under the client immediately after they are soiled.
5. Use creams and lotions to lubricate the skin and a barrier protection ointment for the incontinent client.
6. Turn and reposition the immobile client every 2 hours or more frequently if necessary; provide active and passive range-of-motion exercises at least every 8 hours.
7. If a pressure injury is present, record the location and size of the wound (length, width, depth in centimeters), monitor and record the type and amount of exudates (a culture of the exudate may be prescribed), and assess for undermining and tunneling. Depending on agency policy, it may be required to have picture documentation on file of a pressure injury or other disruption in skin integrity that may include a client identifier, measuring device, and a label indicating wound laterality and location. If a wound or other skin problem is noted, it may be necessary to request a referral to a wound care and/or nutrition specialist.
8. Serosanguineous exudate (blood-tinged amber fluid) may be noted; purulent exudates indicate colonization of the wound with bacteria.
9. Use agency protocols for skin assessment and management of a wound.
10. Treatment may include wound dressings and debridement; skin grafting may be necessary (Tables 42-1 and 42-2).
11. Other treatments may include electrical stimulation to the wound area (increases blood vessel growth and stimulates granulation), vacuum-assisted wound closure (removes infectious material from the wound and promotes granulation), hyperbaric oxygen therapy (administration of oxygen under high pressure raises tissue oxygen concentration), and the use of topical growth factors (biologically active substances that stimulate cell growth).

BOX 42-3 Stages of Pressure Injuries

Stage I

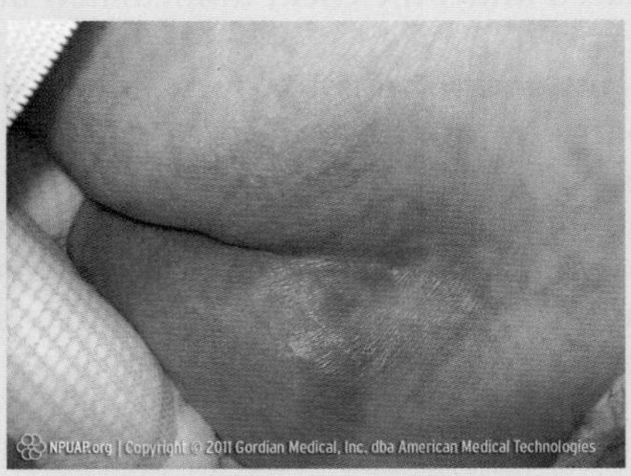

Skin is intact
Area is red and does not blanch with external pressure
Area may be painful, firm, soft, warmer, or cooler compared with adjacent tissue

Stage II

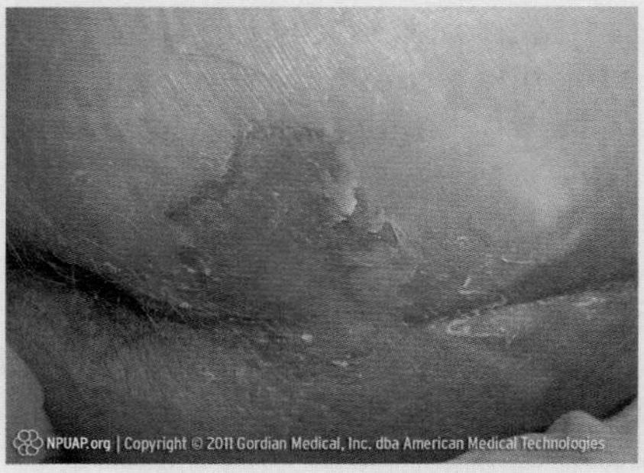

Skin is not intact
Partial-thickness skin loss of the dermis occurs
Presents as a shallow open ulceration with a red-pink wound bed or as intact or open/ruptured serum-filled blister

Stage III

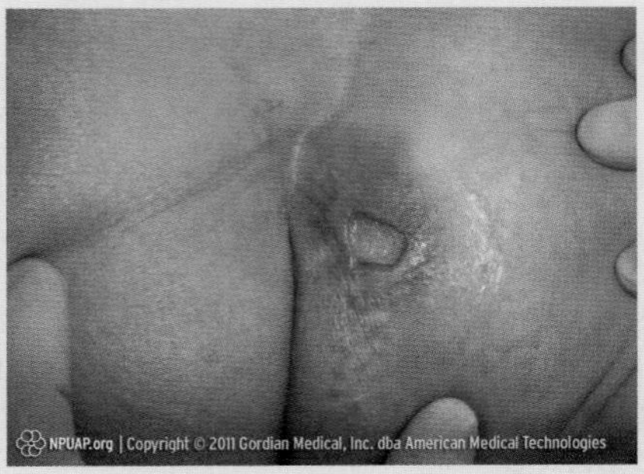

Full-thickness skin loss extends into the dermis and subcutaneous tissues, and slough may be present
Subcutaneous tissue may be visible
Undermining and tunneling may or may not be present

Stage IV

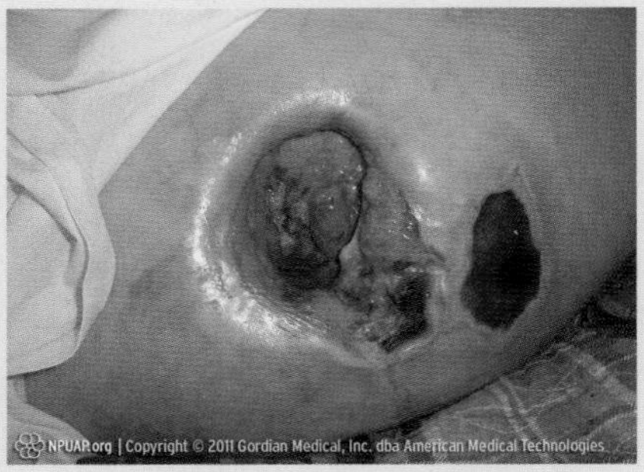

Full-thickness skin loss is present with exposed bone, tendon, or muscle
Slough or eschar may be present
Undermining and tunneling may develop

Suspected Deep-Tissue Injury

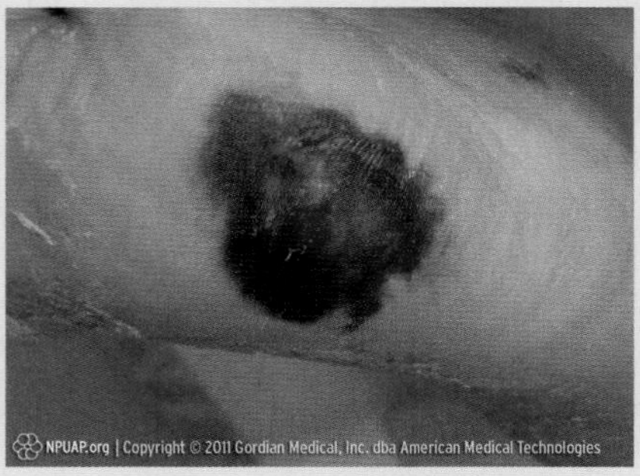

Ischemic subcutaneous tissue injury under intact skin
Appears purple or maroon colored
May be painful, firm, or boggy

Unstageable

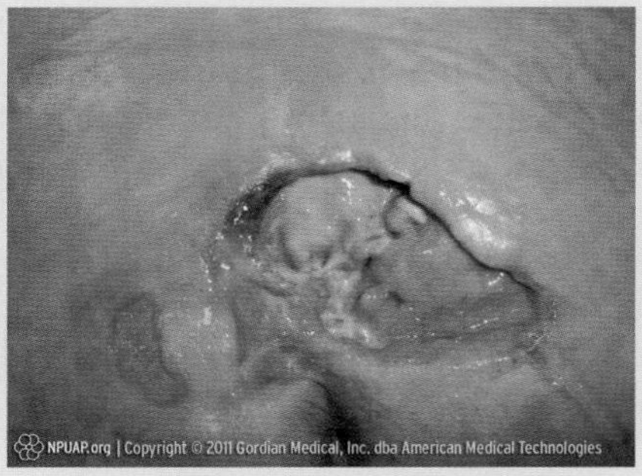

Full-thickness tissue loss in which the wound bed is covered by slough and/or eschar
The true depth, and therefore stage, of the wound cannot be determined until the slough and/or eschar is removed to visualize the wound bed

Adapted from Ignatavicius D, Workman ML: *Medical-surgical nursing: patient-centered collaborative care,* ed 8, Philadelphia, 2016, Saunders. Figures from National Pressure Ulcer Advisory Panel (NPUAP), copyright and used with permission.

TABLE 42-1 Types of Dressings and Mechanism of Action for Pressure Injuries

Pressure Injury Stage	Dressing Type	Mechanism of Action
I	None Transparent dressing Hydrocolloid dressing	Slow resolution within 7 to 10 days
II	Composite film Hydrocolloid dressing Hydrogel	Heals through reepithelialization
III	Hydrocolloid Hydrogel covered with foam dressing Gauze Growth factors	Heals through granulation and reepithelialization
IV	Hydrogel covered with foam dressing Calcium alginate Gauze	Heals through granulation, reepithelialization, and scar tissue development
Unstageable	Adherent film Gauze with a prescribed solution Enzymes None	Eschar loosens and lifts at edges as healing occurs; surgical debridement may be necessary

Data from Perry AG, Potter PA, Ostendorf W: *Clinical nursing skills & techniques*, ed 8, St. Louis, 2014, Mosby.

TABLE 42-2 Types of Dressing Materials

Type	Indications, Uses, and Considerations	Frequency of Dressing Changes
Alginate	Provides hemostasis, debridement, absorption, and protection Can be used as packing for deep wounds and for infected wounds Requires a secondary dressing for securing	When dressing is saturated (every 3 to 5 days) or more frequently
Biological	Provides protection and debridement after eschar removal May be used for dormant and nonhealing wounds that do not respond to other topical therapies May be used for burns or before pigskin and cadaver skin grafts Conforms to uneven wound surfaces; reduces pain Requires a secondary dressing for securing	Topical growth factors: changed daily Skin substitutes: the need for dressing change varies
Cotton gauze	Continuous dry dressing provides absorption and protection Continuous wet dressing provides protection, a means for the delivery of topical treatment, and debridement Wet to damp dressing provides atraumatic mechanical debridement May be painful on removal	Clean base: every 12 to 24 hr Necrotic base: every 4 to 6 hr
Foam	Provides absorption, protection, insulation, and debridement Conforms to uneven wound surfaces Requires a secondary dressing for securing	When dressing is saturated or more frequently; can remain for a maximum of 7 days
Hydrocolloidal	Provides absorption, protection, and debridement Is waterproof and painless on removal	Clean base: on leakage of exudates Necrotic base: every 24 hr
Hydrogel	Provides absorption, protection, and debridement Conducive to use with topical agents Conforms to uneven wound surfaces but allows only partial wound visualization Requires a secondary dressing for securing Can promote the growth of *Pseudomonas* and other microorganisms	Clean base: every 24 hr Necrotic base: every 6 to 8 hr
Adhesive transparent film	Provides protection for partial-thickness lesions and debridement and serves as a secondary (cover) dressing Provides good wound visualization Is waterproof and reduces pain Use is limited to superficial lesions Is nonabsorbent, adheres to normal and healing tissue Dressing may be difficult to apply	Clean base: on leakage of exudates Necrotic base: every 24 hr

From Ignatavicius D, Workman ML: *Medical-surgical nursing: patient-centered collaborative care*, ed 8, Philadelphia, 2016, Saunders.

PRACTICE QUESTIONS

423. The nurse is conducting a session about the principles of first aid and is discussing the interventions for a snakebite to an extremity. The nurse should inform those attending the session that the **first-priority** intervention in the event of this occurrence is which action?
1. Immobilize the affected extremity.
2. Remove jewelry and constricting clothing from the victim.
3. Place the extremity in a position so that it is below the level of the heart.
4. Move the victim to a safe area away from the snake and encourage the victim to rest.

424. A client calls the emergency department and tells the nurse that he came directly into contact with poison ivy shrubs. The client tells the nurse that he cannot see anything on the skin and asks the nurse what to do. The nurse should make which response?
1. "Come to the emergency department."
2. "Apply calamine lotion immediately to the exposed skin areas."
3. "Take a shower immediately, lathering and rinsing several times."
4. "It is not necessary to do anything if you cannot see anything on your skin."

425. A client is being admitted to the hospital for treatment of acute cellulitis of the lower left leg. During the admission assessment, the nurse expects to note which finding?
1. An inflammation of the epidermis only
2. A skin infection of the dermis and underlying hypodermis
3. An acute superficial infection of the dermis and lymphatics
4. An epidermal and lymphatic infection caused by *Staphylococcus*

426. The clinic nurse assesses the skin of a client with psoriasis after the client has used a new topical treatment for 2 months. The nurse identifies which characteristics as improvement in the manifestations of psoriasis? **Select all that apply.**
1. Presence of striae
2. Palpable radial pulses
3. Absence of any ecchymosis on the extremities
4. Thinner and decrease in number of reddish papules
5. Scarce amount of silvery-white scaly patches on the arms

427. The clinic nurse notes that the health care provider has documented a diagnosis of herpes zoster (shingles) in the client's chart. Based on an understanding of the cause of this disorder, the nurse determines that this definitive diagnosis was made by which diagnostic test?
1. Positive patch test
2. Positive culture results
3. Abnormal biopsy results
4. Wood's light examination indicative of infection

428. A client returns to the clinic for follow-up treatment after a skin biopsy of a suspicious lesion performed 1 week ago. The biopsy report indicates that the lesion is a melanoma. The nurse understands that melanoma has which characteristics? **Select all that apply.**
1. Lesion is painful to touch.
2. Lesion is highly metastatic.
3. Lesion is a nevus that has changes in color.
4. Skin under the lesion is reddened and warm to touch.
5. Lesion occurs in body areas exposed to outdoor sunlight.

429. When assessing a lesion diagnosed as basal cell carcinoma, the nurse **most likely** expects to note which findings? **Select all that apply.**
1. An irregularly shaped lesion
2. A small papule with a dry, rough scale
3. A firm, nodular lesion topped with crust
4. A pearly papule with a central crater and a waxy border
5. Location in the bald spot atop the head that is exposed to outdoor sunlight

430. A client arriving at the emergency department has experienced frostbite to the right hand. Which finding would the nurse note on assessment of the client's hand?
1. A pink, edematous hand
2. Fiery red skin with edema in the nailbeds
3. Black fingertips surrounded by an erythematous rash
4. A white color to the skin, which is insensitive to touch

431. The staff nurse reviews the nursing documentation in a client's chart and notes that the wound care nurse has documented that the client has a stage II pressure injury in the sacral area. Which finding would the nurse expect to note on assessment of the client's sacral area?
1. Intact skin
2. Full-thickness skin loss
3. Exposed bone, tendon, or muscle
4. Partial-thickness skin loss of the dermis

432. The nurse manager is planning the clinical assignments for the day. Which staff members cannot be assigned to care for a client with herpes zoster? **Select all that apply.**
1. The nurse who never had roseola
2. The nurse who never had mumps
3. The nurse who never had chickenpox
4. The nurse who never had German measles
5. The nurse who never received the varicella-zoster vaccine

ANSWERS

423. *Answer:* 4

Rationale: In the event of a snakebite, the first priority is to move the victim to a safe area away from the snake and encourage the victim to rest to decrease venom circulation. Next, jewelry and constricting clothing are removed before swelling occurs. Immobilizing the extremity and maintaining the extremity below heart level would be done next; these actions limit the spread of the venom. The victim is kept warm and calm. Stimulants such as alcohol or caffeinated beverages are not given to the victim because these products may speed the absorption of the venom. The victim should be transported to an emergency facility as soon as possible.

Test-Taking Strategy: Note the strategic words, *first priority*. Eliminate options 1 and 3 first because they are comparable or alike and relate to positioning of the affected extremity. For the remaining options, think about them and visualize each. Moving the victim to a safe area is the priority to prevent further injury from the snake.

Level of Cognitive Ability: Applying

Client Needs: Safe and Effective Care Environment

Integrated Process: Teaching and Learning

Content Area: Leadership/Management: Prioritizing

Health Problem: Adult Health: Integumentary: Bites and Stings

Priority Concepts: Clinical Judgment; Tissue Integrity

Reference: Ignatavicius, Workman, Rebar (2018), pp. 136, 138.

424. *Answer:* 3

Rationale: When an individual comes in contact with a poison ivy plant, the sap from the plant forms an invisible film on the human skin. The client should be instructed to cleanse the area by showering immediately and to lather the skin several times and rinse each time in running water. Removing the poison ivy sap will decrease the likelihood of irritation. Calamine lotion may be one product recommended for use if dermatitis develops. The client does not need to be seen in the emergency department at this time.

Test-Taking Strategy: Focus on the subject, contact with poison ivy. Recalling that dermatitis can develop from contact with an allergen and that contact with poison ivy results in an invisible film will assist in directing you to the correct option.

Level of Cognitive Ability: Applying

Client Needs: Physiological Integrity

Integrated Process: Nursing Process—Implementation

Content Area: Adult Health: Integumentary

Health Problem: Adult Health: Integumentary: Inflammations/Infections

Priority Concepts: Client Education; Tissue Integrity

Reference: Lewis et al. (2017), p. 1643.

425. *Answer:* 2

Rationale: Cellulitis is an infection of the dermis and underlying hypodermis that results in a deep red erythema without sharp borders and spreads widely throughout tissue spaces. The skin is erythematous, edematous, tender, and sometimes nodular. Erysipelas is an acute, superficial, rapidly spreading inflammation of the dermis and lymphatics. The infection is not superficial and extends deeper than the epidermis.

Test-Taking Strategy: Eliminate options 3 and 4 because they are comparable or alike and address the lymphatics. Eliminate option 1 because of the closed-ended word "only."

Level of Cognitive Ability: Applying

Client Needs: Physiological Integrity

Integrated Process: Nursing Process—Assessment

Content Area: Adult Health: Integumentary

Health Problem: Adult Health: Integumentary: Inflammations/Infections

Priority Concepts: Client Education; Tissue Integrity

Reference: Lewis et al. (2017), p. 414.

426. *Answer:* 4, 5

Rationale: Psoriasis skin lesions include thick reddened papules or plaques covered by silvery-white patches. A decrease in the severity of these skin lesions is noted as an improvement. The presence of striae (stretch marks), palpable pulses, or lack of ecchymosis is not related to psoriasis.

Test-Taking Strategy: Focus on the subject, manifestations of psoriasis. Use knowledge regarding the pathophysiology and signs and symptoms associated with psoriasis. This will direct you to the correct options detailing a decrease in the psoriatic signs.

Level of Cognitive Ability: Evaluating

Client Needs: Physiological Integrity

Integrated Process: Nursing Process—Evaluation

Content Area: Adult Health: Integumentary

Health Problem: Adult Health: Integumentary: Inflammations/Infections

Priority Concepts: Clinical Judgment; Tissue Integrity

Reference: Lewis et al. (2017), pp. 417, 419.

427. *Answer:* 2

Rationale: With the classic presentation of herpes zoster, the clinical examination is diagnostic. However, a viral culture of the lesion provides the definitive diagnosis. Herpes zoster (shingles) is caused by a reactivation of the varicella zoster virus, the virus that causes chickenpox. A patch test is a skin test that involves the administration of an allergen to the surface of the skin to identify specific allergies. A biopsy would provide a cytological examination of tissue. In a Wood's light examination, the skin is viewed under ultraviolet light to identify superficial infections of the skin.

Test-Taking Strategy: Focus on the subject, diagnosing herpes zoster. Recalling that herpes zoster is caused by a virus will assist in directing you to the correct option. Also remember that a biopsy will determine tissue type, whereas a culture will identify an organism.

Level of Cognitive Ability: Analyzing

Client Needs: Physiological Integrity

Integrated Process: Nursing Process—Assessment

Content Area: Adult Health: Integumentary

Health Problem: Adult Health: Integumentary: Inflammations/Infections

Priority Concepts: Clinical Judgment; Tissue Integrity

Reference: Ignatavicius, Workman, Rebar (2018), pp. 468-469.

428. *Answer:* 2, 3

Rationale: Melanomas are pigmented malignant lesions originating in the melanin-producing cells of the epidermis. Melanomas cause changes in a nevus (mole), including

color and borders. This skin cancer is highly metastatic, and a person's survival depends on early diagnosis and treatment. Melanomas are not painful or accompanied by sign of inflammation. Although sun exposure increases the risk of melanoma, lesions may occur any place on the body, especially where birthmarks or new moles are apparent.
Test-Taking Strategy: Focus on the subject, characteristics of melanoma skin cancer. It is necessary to know the normal characteristics associated with melanoma to answer this question correctly. Also, recalling that melanomas are highly metastatic will assist in directing you to the correct options.
Level of Cognitive Ability: Analyzing
Client Needs: Physiological Integrity
Integrated Process: Nursing Process—Assessment
Content Area: Adult Health: Integumentary
Health Problem: Adult Health: Cancer: Skin
Priority Concepts: Cellular Regulation; Tissue Integrity
Reference: Ignatavicius, Workman, Rebar (2018), pp. 475-476.

429. *Answer:* 4, 5
Rationale: Basal cell carcinoma appears as a pearly papule with a central crater and rolled waxy border. Exposure to ultraviolet sunlight is a major risk factor. A melanoma is an irregularly shaped pigmented papule or plaque with a red-, white-, or blue-toned color. Actinic keratosis, a premalignant lesion, appears as a small macule or papule with a dry, rough, adherent yellow or brown scale. Squamous cell carcinoma is a firm, nodular lesion topped with a crust or a central area of ulceration.
Test-Taking Strategy: Note the strategic words, *most likely*. Recall characteristics and etiology of basal cell cancer to direct you to the correct options.
Level of Cognitive Ability: Analyzing
Client Needs: Physiological Integrity
Integrated Process: Nursing Process—Assessment
Content Area: Adult Health: Integumentary
Health Problem: Adult Health: Cancer: Skin
Priority Concepts: Cellular Regulation; Tissue Integrity
Reference: Ignatavicius, Workman, Rebar (2018), pp. 475-476.

430. *Answer:* 4
Rationale: Assessment findings in frostbite include a white or blue color; the skin will be hard, cold, and insensitive to touch. As thawing occurs, flushing of the skin, the development of blisters or blebs, or tissue edema appears. Options 1, 2, and 3 are incorrect.
Test-Taking Strategy: Focus on the subject, assessment findings in frostbite. Noting the words *insensitive to touch* in the correct option should direct you to this option.
Level of Cognitive Ability: Analyzing
Client Needs: Physiological Integrity
Integrated Process: Nursing Process—Assessment
Content Area: Adult Health: Integumentary
Health Problem: Adult Health: Integumentary: Inflammations/Infections
Priority Concepts: Clinical Judgment; Tissue Integrity
Reference: Ignatavicius, Workman, Rebar (2018), pp. 144-145.

431. *Answer:* 4
Rationale: In a stage II pressure injury, the skin is not intact. Partial-thickness skin loss of the dermis has occurred. It presents as a shallow open ulceration with a red-pink wound bed, without slough. It may also present as an intact or open/ruptured serum-filled blister. The skin is intact in stage I. Full-thickness skin loss occurs in stage III. Exposed bone, tendon, or muscle is present in stage IV.
Test-Taking Strategy: Focus on the subject, assessment of a pressure injury. Focusing on the words *stage II* and visualizing the appearance of a stage II pressure injury will direct you to the correct option.
Level of Cognitive Ability: Applying
Client Needs: Physiological Integrity
Integrated Process: Nursing Process—Assessment
Content Area: Adult Health: Integumentary
Health Problem: Adult Health: Integumentary: Inflammations/Infections
Priority Concepts: Clinical Judgment; Tissue Integrity
Reference: Lewis et al. (2017), pp. 172-173.

432. *Answer:* 3, 5
Rationale: The nurses who have not had chickenpox or did not receive the varicella zoster vaccine are susceptible to the herpes zoster virus and should not be assigned to care for the client with herpes zoster. Nurses who have not contracted roseola, mumps, or rubella are not necessarily susceptible to herpes zoster. Herpes zoster (shingles) is caused by a reactivation of the varicella zoster virus, the causative virus of chickenpox. Individuals who have not been exposed to the varicella zoster virus or who did not receive the varicella zoster vaccine are susceptible to chickenpox. Health care workers who are unsure of their immune status should have varicella titers done before exposure to a person with herpes zoster.
Test-Taking Strategy: Focus on the subject, transmission of herpes zoster. Recalling that herpes zoster is caused by a reactivation of the varicella zoster virus, the causative virus of chickenpox, will direct you to the correct options.
Level of Cognitive Ability: Analyzing
Client Needs: Safe and Effective Care Environment
Integrated Process: Nursing Process—Planning
Content Area: Leadership/Management: Delegating
Health Problem: Adult Health: Integumentary: Inflammations/Infections
Priority Concepts: Infection; Safety
Reference: Ignatavicius, Workman, Rebar (2018), pp. 467-468.

CHAPTER 43

Integumentary Medications

PRIORITY CONCEPTS **Clinical Judgment; Safety**

I. Poison Ivy Treatment (Box 43-1)

A. Treatment of lesions includes calamine lotion and commercial products that soothe lesions, compresses and solutions that are astringent and antiseptic, and/or colloidal oatmeal baths to relieve discomfort.

B. Topical corticosteroids are effective to prevent or relieve inflammation, especially when used before blisters form.

C. Oral corticosteroids may be prescribed for severe reactions, and an antihistamine such as diphenhydramine may be prescribed.

II. Medications to Treat Dermatitis (Box 43-2)

A. Description
1. Superficial inflammatory process involving primarily the epidermis; there are many types, some of which include atopic dermatitis, contact dermatitis, and stasis dermatitis.
2. May be treated with moisturizer and topical glucocorticoids (preferred treatment); systemic immunosuppressants may need to be prescribed if topical treatment is ineffective.

B. Topical immunosuppressants
1. Tacrolimus and pimecrolimus creams
2. Side and adverse effects include redness, burning, and itching; causes sensitization of the skin to sunlight. Treated areas should be protected from direct sunlight.
3. Tacrolimus may increase the risk of contracting varicella zoster infection in children.
4. Tacrolimus may increase the risk of developing skin cancer and lymphoma.

BOX 43-1 Poison Ivy Treatment Products

- Bentoquatam—for preventive use
- Calamine lotion
- Hydrocortisone
- Zinc acetate; isopropanol
- Zinc acetate; isopropanol; benzyl alcohol

BOX 43-2 Medications to Treat Dermatitis

Systemic Immunosuppressants
- Azathioprine
- Cyclosporine
- Methotrexate
- Oral glucocorticoids

Topical Immunosuppressants
- Pimecrolimus 1% cream
- Tacrolimus

⚠ When administering any topical medication or topical patches, the nurse and family caregivers should always wear gloves to protect self from absorption of the medication. Caregivers should also be taught to wash hands thoroughly before and after administration.

III. Topical Glucocorticoids

A. Description
1. Antiinflammatory, antipruritic, and vasoconstrictive actions
2. Preparations vary in potency and depend on the concentration and type of preparation and method of application (occlusive dressings enhance absorption, increasing the effects).
3. Systemic effects are more likely to occur with prolonged therapy and when extensive skin surfaces are treated.

⚠ Topical glucocorticoids can be absorbed into the systemic circulation; absorption is greater in permeable skin areas (scalp, axilla, face and neck, eyelids, perineum) and less in areas where permeability is poor (palms, soles, back).

B. Contraindications
1. Clients demonstrating previous sensitivity to corticosteroids
2. Clients with current systemic fungal, viral, or bacterial infections
3. Clients with current complications related to glucocorticoid therapy

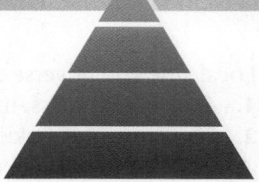

C. Local side and adverse effects
1. Burning, dryness, irritation, itching
2. Thinning of the skin, striae, purpura, telangiectasia (causes thread-like red lines on the skin)
3. Skin atrophy
4. Acneiform eruptions
5. Hypopigmentation
6. Overgrowth of bacteria, fungi, and viruses

D. Systemic adverse effects
1. Growth retardation in children
2. Adrenal suppression
3. Cushing's syndrome
4. Ocular effects (glaucoma and cataracts)

E. Interventions
1. Wear gloves; wash the area just before application to ensure cleanliness and to increase medication penetration.
2. Apply sparingly in a thin film, rubbing gently.
3. Avoid the use of a dry occlusive dressing unless specifically prescribed by the primary health care provider (PHCP).
4. Instruct the client to report signs of adverse effects to the PHCP.
5. Monitoring plasma cortisol levels may be prescribed if prolonged therapy is necessary.

⚠ In the adult, intact skin is generally impermeable to most topical medications. However, medications should not be applied to open areas unless prescribed, because undesired absorption and adverse effects can occur.

IV. Medications to Treat Actinic Keratosis (Box 43-3)

A. Description
1. Actinic keratoses are caused by prolonged exposure to the sun and appear as rough, scaly, red or brown lesions usually found on the face, scalp, arms, and back of the hands.
2. Lesions can progress to squamous cell carcinoma.
3. Treatment includes medications and therapies such as excision, cryotherapy, curettage, and laser therapy.

B. Medications (see Box 43-3)
1. Diclofenac sodium
   a. A nonsteroidal antiinflammatory topical medication; it may take up to 3 months to be effective.
   b. Side and adverse effects include dry skin, itching, redness, and rash.
2. Fluorouracil
   a. A topical medication that affects DNA and RNA synthesis and causes a sequence of responses that results in healing; results are usually seen in 2 to 6 weeks but may take 1 to 2 months longer for complete healing.
   b. Side and adverse effects include itching, burning, inflammation, rash, and increased sensitivity to sunlight.
3. Imiquimod 5% cream
   a. In addition to treating actinic keratoses, this topical medication has been used to treat venereal warts; it may take up to 4 months to be effective.
   b. Side and adverse effects include redness, skin swelling, itching, burning, sores, blisters, scabbing, and crusting of the skin.
4. Ingenol mebutate
   a. Indicated for the topical treatment of actinic keratosis; application recommendations need to be followed closely because of the risks of allergic reaction and development of herpes zoster.
   b. Side and adverse effects include skin reactions, erythema, flaking/scaling, crusting, swelling, postulation, and erosion/ulceration; allergic reactions; herpes zoster.

BOX 43-3 Medications to Treat Actinic Keratosis

- Diclofenac sodium 3% gel
- Fluorouracil
- Imiquimod 5% cream
- Ingenol mebutate

V. Sunscreens

A. Ultraviolet (UV) light can damage the skin and cause premalignant actinic keratoses and some types of skin cancer.

B. Sunscreens prevent the penetration of UV light and protect the skin.

C. Organic (chemical) sunscreens absorb UV light; inorganic (physical) sunscreens reflect and scatter UV light.

D. A sunscreen that protects against both UVB and UVA rays and one that has a sun protection factor (SPF) of at least 15 should be used.

E. Sunscreens are most effective when applied at least 30 minutes before exposure to the sun (sunscreens containing *para*-aminobenzoic acid or padimate O require application 2 hours before sun exposure).

F. Sunscreen should be reapplied every 2 to 3 hours and after swimming or sweating; otherwise, the duration of protection is reduced.

G. Products containing *para*-aminobenzoic acid need to be avoided by individuals allergic to benzocaine, sulfonamides, or thiazides.

H. Sunscreens can cause contact dermatitis and photosensitivity reactions.

⚠ The client should be informed that UV light is greatest between the hours of 10:00 a.m. and 4:00 p.m. and that sunglasses, protective clothing, and a hat should be worn to reduce the risk of skin damage from the sun.

VI. Medications to Treat Psoriasis (Box 43-4)

A. Description
  1. Psoriasis is a chronic inflammatory disorder that has varying degrees of severity.
  2. Treatment is based on the severity of symptoms and aims to suppress the proliferation of keratinocytes or suppress the activity of inflammatory cells.

B. Topical medications
  1. Glucocorticoids
    a. Used for mild psoriasis
    b. Should not be applied to the face, groin, axilla, or genitalia, because the medication is readily absorbable, making the skin vulnerable to glucocorticoid-induced atrophy
  2. Tazarotene
    a. Is a vitamin A derivative
    b. Local reactions include itching, burning, stinging, dry skin, and redness; other, less common effects include rash, desquamation, contact dermatitis, inflammation, fissuring, and bleeding.
    c. Sensitization to sunlight can occur, and the client should be instructed to use sunscreen and wear protective clothing.
    d. Medication is usually applied once daily in the evening to dry skin.

BOX 43-4 Medications and Treatments for Psoriasis

Topical Medications
- Calcipotriene
- Coal tar
- Glucocorticoids
- Keratolytics (topical salicylic acid; sulfur)
- Tazarotene

Systemic Medications
- Acitretin
- Cyclosporine
- Methotrexate

Systemic Biological Medications
- Adalimumab
- Brodalumab
- Etanercept
- Guselkumab
- Infliximab
- Ixekizumab
- Ustekinumab
- Secukinumab

Phototherapy
- Coal tar and ultraviolet B irradiation
- Photochemotherapy (psoralen and ultraviolet A therapy)

  3. Calcipotriene
    a. Is an analog of vitamin D
    b. May take up to 1 to 3 weeks to produce a desired effect
    c. Can cause local irritation; high-dose applications rarely have caused hypercalcemia.
  4. Coal tar
    a. Suppresses DNA synthesis, miotic activity, and cell proliferation
    b. Has an unpleasant odor and may cause irritation, burning, and stinging; can also stain the skin and hair and increase sensitivity to sun
    c. May increase risk for cancer development in high doses
  5. Keratolytics
    a. Soften scales and loosen the horny layer of the skin, resulting in minimal peeling to extensive desquamation
    b. Salicylic acid: Can be absorbed systemically and can cause salicylism, which is characterized by dizziness and tinnitus, hyperpnea, and psychological disturbances; salicylic acid is not applied to large surface areas or open wounds because of the risk of systemic effects.
    c. Sulfur: Promotes peeling and drying and is used to treat acne, dandruff, seborrheic dermatitis, and psoriasis

C. Systemic medications
  1. Methotrexate
    a. Reduces proliferation of epidermal cells
    b. Can be toxic; causes gastrointestinal effects such as diarrhea and ulcerative stomatitis and bone marrow depression leading to blood dyscrasias
    c. Can be hepatotoxic; hepatic function should be monitored during therapy
    d. This medication is teratogenic; women of child-bearing age should wait 3 months after discontinuation of the medication before becoming pregnant.
  2. Acitretin
    a. Inhibits keratinization, proliferation, and differentiation of cells; has antiinflammatory and immunomodulator actions; used for severe psoriasis and reserved for use in those who have not responded to safer medications
    b. Is embryotoxic and teratogenic: Medication is contraindicated during pregnancy; pregnancy must be ruled out, and 2 reliable forms of contraception need to be implemented before the medication is started (contraception must be implemented at least 1 month before treatment starts and be continued for at least 3 years after treatment is discontinued).
    c. If pregnancy occurs during treatment with the medication, the medication is discontinued

immediately and possible termination of the pregnancy is discussed.

d. Dermatological effects include hair loss, skin peeling, dry skin, rash, pruritus, and nail disorders; other effects include rhinitis from mucous membrane irritation, inflammation of the lips, dry mouth, dry eyes, nosebleed, gingivitis, stomatitis, bone and joint pain, and spinal disorders.
e. Can be hepatotoxic; can elevate triglyceride levels and reduce levels of high-density lipoprotein cholesterol
f. Should not be taken with alcohol, vitamin A supplementation, or tetracycline

3. Cyclosporine
   a. An immunosuppressant that inhibits proliferation of B and T cells
   b. Can be toxic and cause kidney damage
   c. Used for severe psoriasis and reserved for use in those who have not responded to safer medications

D. Systemic biological medications (clients should be tested for tuberculosis or other infections before initiation of medications)
1. These are injected into the skin or bloodstream; they block the altered immune system that is contributing to the psoriasis.
2. Some are tumor necrosis factor alpha-blockers, some bind to inflammation, causing proteins/interleukins; some are a human antibody that works against interleukins
3. Adverse effects, which are generally not severe, include upper respiratory infections, abdominal pain, headache, rash, injection site reactions, and urinary tract infections; may promote serious infections, including bacterial sepsis, invasive fungal infections, tuberculosis, and reactivation of hepatitis B; some medications increase the risk of developing lymphoma
4. Contraindicated for persons with history of certain cancers, severe or recurrent infections, heart failure, or demyelinating neurological diseases; given with caution to persons with numbness or tingling
5. The client should not receive any live virus vaccines, because the viruses used in some types of vaccines can cause infection in those with a weakened immune system; in addition, the PHCP needs to be informed if anyone in the household needs a vaccine.
6. The client should not receive the bacillus Calmette-Guérin (BCG) vaccine during the 1 year before taking or 1 year after taking the medication.
7. The client should inform the PHCP if he or she is receiving phototherapy, has any other medical condition, is pregnant or plans to become pregnant, or is breast-feeding or plans to breast-feed; safety with pregnancy has not been established with many of these medications.

E. Phototherapy
1. Coal tar and ultraviolet B (UVB) irradiation: Treatment that involves the application of coal tar for 8 to 10 hours; coal tar is washed off and the area is exposed to short-wave UV radiation (UVB).
2. Photochemotherapy (psoralen and ultraviolet A [UVA] therapy)
   a. Combines the use of long-wave radiation (UVA) with oral methoxsalen (used in very specific cases; photosensitive medication)
   b. Can cause pruritus, nausea, erythema; may accelerate the aging process of the skin; may increase the risk of skin cancer.

VII. Acne Products (Box 43-5; Fig. 43-1)

A. Description
1. Acne lesions that are mild may be treated with nonpharmacological measures such as gentle cleansing 2 or 3 times daily (oil-based moisturizing products need to be avoided), dermabrasion, or comedo extraction.
2. Mild acne is usually treated pharmacologically with topical agents (antimicrobials and retinoids).
3. Moderate acne is usually treated with oral antibiotics and comedolytics.
4. Severe acne is usually treated with isotretinoin.
5. Hormonal medications may be prescribed to treat acne in female clients.
6. A type of combination therapy may be prescribed to treat acne.

BOX 43-5 Acne Products

Topical Antibiotics
- Benzoyl peroxide
- Clindamycin and erythromycin
- Clindamycin/tretinoin combination gel
- Dapsone
- *Fixed dose combinations:* Clindamycin/benzoyl peroxide and erythromycin/benzoyl peroxide

Topical Retinoids
- Adapalene
- Azelaic acid
- Tazarotene
- Tretinoin

Oral Medications
- Doxycycline
- Erythromycin
- Isotretinoin
- Minocycline
- Tetracycline

Hormonal Medications
- Oral contraceptives
- Spironolactone

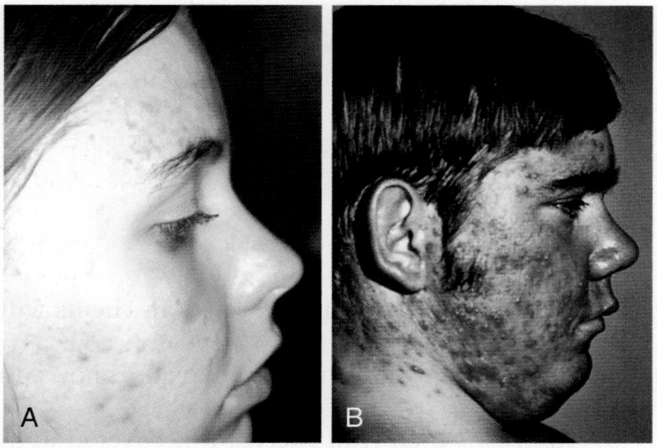

FIG. 43-1 Acne vulgaris. **A,** Comedones with a few inflammatory pustules. **B,** Papulopustular acne. (From Perry et al., 2010.)

7. Actions of the medications may include suppressing the growth of *Propionibacterium acnes*, reducing inflammation, promoting keratolysis, unplugging existing comedones and preventing their development, and normalizing hyperproliferation of epithelial cells within the hair follicles; some medications cause thinning of the skin, which facilitates penetration of other medications.
8. For topical applications: Site should be washed and allowed to dry completely before application; hands should be washed after application.
9. All topical products are kept away from the eyes, inside the nose, lips, mucous membranes, hair, and inflamed or denuded skin.

B. Topical antibiotic products
1. Benzoyl peroxide
   - **a.** Can produce drying and peeling
   - **b.** Severe local irritation (burning, blistering, scaling, swelling) may require reducing the frequency of applications.
   - **c.** Some products may contain sulfites; monitor for serious allergic reactions.
2. Salicylic acid and sulfur/sulfacetamide can be used as well.
3. Clindamycin and erythromycin
   - **a.** Both products are antibiotics that suppress the growth of *P. acnes.*
   - **b.** Combination therapy with benzoyl peroxide prevents the emergence of resistant bacteria; fixed-dose combinations include clindamycin/benzoyl peroxide and erythromycin/benzoyl peroxide.
4. Dapsone: Side and adverse effects include oiliness, peeling, dryness, and erythema of the skin (oral form of medication is used to treat leprosy).

C. Topical retinoids
1. Tretinoin
   - **a.** A derivative of vitamin A (vitamin A supplements should be discontinued during therapy)
   - **b.** In addition to treating acne, it may be prescribed to reduce fine wrinkles, skin roughness, and mottled hyperpigmentation, as with age spots.
   - **c.** Can cause localized side and adverse effects such as blistering, peeling, crusting, burning, and swelling of the skin
   - **d.** Abrasive products and keratolytic products are discontinued before using tretinoin to decrease localized adverse effects.
   - **e.** Instruct the client to apply a sunscreen with an SPF of 15 or greater and to wear protective clothing when outdoors due to sensitivity to UV light.
2. Adapalene: Similar to tretinoin and sensitizes the skin to UV light; adverse effects include burning and itching after application, redness, dryness, and scaling of the skin. Initially may worsen acne; benefits seen in 8 to 12 weeks.
3. Tazarotene
   - **a.** Is a derivative of vitamin A (vitamin A supplements should be discontinued during therapy)
   - **b.** In addition to acne, it is used to treat wrinkles and psoriasis.
   - **c.** Can cause itching, burning, and dry skin and sensitizes the skin to UV light
4. Azelaic acid can cause burning, itching, stinging, and redness of the skin; it can also cause hypopigmentation of the skin in clients with a dark complexion.

D. Oral antibiotics
1. Includes doxycycline, minocycline, tetracycline, erythromycin, trimethoprim-sulfamethoxazole, cephalosporins, penicillins
2. Improvement develops slowly with the use of oral antibiotics and may take 3 to 6 months for some improvement to be noted; after control of symptoms, the client is usually switched to a topical antibiotic.

E. Isotretinoin
1. Derivative of vitamin A (vitamin A supplements should be discontinued during therapy); in addition, the use of tetracyclines can increase the risk of adverse effects and should be discontinued before use of isotretinoin.
2. Used to treat severe cystic acne; reserved for persons who have not responded to other therapies, including systemic antibiotics
3. Side and adverse effects include nosebleeds; inflammation of the lips or eyes; dryness or itching of the skin, nose, or mouth; pain, tenderness, or stiffness in the joints, bones, or muscles; and back pain.

4. Less common side and adverse effects include rash, hair loss, peeling of the skin, headache, and reduction in night vision.
5. Causes sensitization of the skin to UV light
6. The medication elevates triglyceride levels, which should be measured before and during therapy; alcohol consumption should be eliminated during therapy because alcohol could potentiate elevation of serum triglyceride levels.
7. The medication may cause depression in some clients; if depression occurs, the medication should be discontinued.

⚠ Isotretinoin is highly teratogenic and can cause fetal abnormalities. If prescribed, the client needs to follow strict rules of the iPLEDGE program. It must not be used if the client is pregnant.

F. iPLEDGE program
1. A risk management program that ensures that no woman starting isotretinoin is pregnant and that no woman taking this medication becomes pregnant; refer to American Academy of Dermatology Association at https://www.aad.org/public/diseases/acne-and-rosacea/isotretinoin-treatment-for-severe-acne
2. Access to the medication is controlled through a central automated system.
3. Strict rules must be followed by the client, PHCP prescribing the medication, pharmacist dispensing the medication, and wholesaler of the medication to ensure safety and to ensure that no woman is pregnant on initiation of therapy or becomes pregnant while taking the medication.
4. Also see iPLEDGE® program at https://www.ipledgeprogram.com/iPledgeUI/home.u

G. Hormonal medications
1. Hormonal medications such as oral contraceptives and spironolactone may be prescribed to treat acne in female clients.
2. These medications decrease androgen activity, resulting in decreased production of sebum.
3. Spironolactone is teratogenic; therefore, contraception during its use is necessary.
4. Side and adverse effects of spironolactone include breast tenderness, menstrual irregularities, and hyperkalemia.

VIII. Burn Products: (Box 43-6) Refer to Chapter 69 for information on Caring for the Burn Client

A. Silver sulfadiazine
1. Has broad spectrum of activity against gram-negative bacteria, gram-positive bacteria, and yeast
2. Silver is released slowly from the cream, which is selectively toxic to bacteria.

BOX 43-6 Burn Products

- Mafenide acetate
- Silver sulfadiazine
- Bacitracin topical ointment (first-degree burns only)
- Povidone-iodine

3. Used primarily to prevent sepsis in clients with burns
4. Not a carbonic anhydrase inhibitor; does not cause acidosis
5. Apply 1/16-inch film (keep burn covered at all times with silver sulfadiazine).
6. Side and adverse effects include rash and itching, blue-green or gray skin discoloration, leukopenia, and interstitial nephritis.
7. Monitor complete blood cell count, particularly the white blood cells, frequently; if leukopenia develops, the PHCP is notified (medication is usually discontinued).

B. Mafenide acetate
1. Water-soluble cream that is bacteriostatic for gram-negative and gram-positive organisms
2. Used to treat burns to reduce the bacteria present in avascular tissues
3. Diffuses through the devascularized areas of the skin and may precipitate metabolic acidosis with the client displaying hyperventilation; monitor blood gases and electrolytes.
4. Apply 1/16-inch (1.5 mm) film directly to the burn.
5. Side effects can include local pain and rash; medicate for pain before application.
6. Adverse effects include bone marrow depression, hemolytic anemia, and metabolic acidosis.
7. Keep the burn covered with mafenide acetate at all times.
8. Notify the PHCP if hyperventilation occurs; if acidosis develops, mafenide acetate is washed off the skin and usually discontinued for 1 to 2 days.

PRACTICE QUESTIONS

433. Salicylic acid is prescribed for a client with a diagnosis of psoriasis. The nurse monitors the client, knowing that which finding indicates the presence of systemic toxicity from this medication?
1. Tinnitus
2. Diarrhea
3. Constipation
4. Decreased respirations

434. The health education nurse provides instructions to a group of clients regarding measures that will assist in preventing skin cancer. Which instructions should the nurse provide? **Select all that apply.**
1. Sunscreen should be applied every 8 hours.
2. Use sunscreen when participating in outdoor activities.
3. Wear a hat, opaque clothing, and sunglasses when in the sun.
4. Avoid sun exposure in the late afternoon and early evening hours.
5. Examine your body monthly for any lesions that may be suspicious.

435. Silver sulfadiazine is prescribed for a client with a burn injury. Which laboratory finding requires the **need for follow-up** by the nurse?
1. Glucose level of 99 mg/dL (5.65 mmol/L)
2. Platelet level of 300,000 mm^3 (300×10^9/L)
3. Magnesium level of 1.5 mEq/L (0.75 mmol/L)
4. White blood cell count of 3000 mm^3 (3.0×10^9/L)

436. A burn client is receiving treatments of topical mafenide acetate to the site of injury. The nurse monitors the client, knowing that which finding indicates that a systemic effect has occurred?
1. Hyperventilation
2. Elevated blood pressure
3. Local rash at the burn site
4. Local pain at the burn site

437. Isotretinoin is prescribed for a client with severe acne. Before the administration of this medication, the nurse anticipates that which laboratory test will be prescribed?
1. Potassium level
2. Triglyceride level
3. Hemoglobin A_1C
4. Total cholesterol level

438. A client with severe acne is seen in the clinic and the primary health care provider (PHCP) prescribes isotretinoin. The nurse reviews the client's medication record and would contact the PHCP if the client is also taking which medication?
1. Digoxin
2. Phenytoin
3. Vitamin A
4. Furosemide

439. The nurse is applying a topical corticosteroid to a client with eczema. The nurse understands that it is safe to apply the medication to which body areas? **Select all that apply.**
1. Back
2. Axilla
3. Eyelids
4. Soles of the feet
5. Palms of the hands

440. The clinic nurse is performing an admission assessment on a client and notes that the client is taking azelaic acid to treat acne. The nurse determines that which client complaint may be associated with use of this medication?
1. Itching
2. Euphoria
3. Drowsiness
4. Frequent urination

441. Silver sulfadiazine is prescribed for a client with a partial-thickness burn, and the nurse provides teaching about the medication. Which statement made by the client indicates a **need for further teaching** about the treatments?
1. "The medication is an antibacterial."
2. "The medication will help heal the burn."
3. "The medication should be applied directly to the wound."
4. "The medication is likely to cause stinging every time it is applied."

442. The camp nurse asks the children preparing to swim in the lake if they have applied sunscreen. The nurse reminds the children that chemical sunscreens are **most effective** when applied at which times?
1. Immediately before swimming
2. 5 minutes before exposure to the sun
3. Immediately before exposure to the sun
4. At least 30 minutes before exposure to the sun

ANSWERS

433. Answer: 1
Rationale: Salicylic acid is absorbed readily through the skin, and systemic toxicity (salicylism) can result. Symptoms include tinnitus, dizziness, hyperpnea, and psychological disturbances. Constipation and diarrhea are not associated with salicylism.
Test-Taking Strategy: Focus on the subject, systemic toxicity. Noting the name of the medication will assist in directing you to the correct option if you can recall the toxic effects that occur with acetylsalicylic acid (aspirin).
Level of Cognitive Ability: Analyzing
Client Needs: Physiological Integrity
Integrated Process: Nursing Process—Assessment
Content Area: Pharmacology: Integumentary: Antiinflammatory/Antiinfective
Health Problem: Adult Health: Integumentary: Inflammations/Infections
Priority Concepts: Clinical Judgment; Tissue Integrity
Reference: Burchum, Rosenthal (2016), p. 1279.

434. Answer: 2, 3, 5
Rationale: The client should be instructed to avoid sun exposure between the hours of brightest sunlight: 10 a.m. and 4 p.m. Sunscreen, a hat, opaque clothing, and sunglasses should be worn for outdoor activities. The client should be instructed to examine the body monthly for the appearance of any cancerous or precancerous lesions. Sunscreen should be applied 30 minutes to 1 hour before sun exposure, and reapplied every 2 to 3 hours, and after swimming or sweating; otherwise, the duration of protection is reduced.
Test-Taking Strategy: Focus on the subject, measures to prevent skin cancer. Read each option carefully. Noting the time frames in options 1 and 4 will assist in eliminating these options.
Level of Cognitive Ability: Analyzing
Client Needs: Health Promotion and Maintenance
Integrated Process: Teaching and Learning
Content Area: Pharmacology: Integumentary: Sunscreens
Health Problem: Adult Health: Integumentary: Burns
Priority Concepts: Client Education; Health Promotion
Reference: Ignatavicius, Workman, Rebar (2018), p. 476.

435. Answer: 4
Rationale: Silver sulfadiazine is used for the treatment of burn injuries. Adverse effects of this medication include rash and itching, blue-green or gray skin discoloration, leukopenia, and interstitial nephritis. The nurse should monitor a complete blood count, particularly the white blood cells, frequently for the client taking this medication. If leukopenia develops, the primary health care provider is notified and the medication is usually discontinued. The white blood cell count noted in option 4 is indicative of leukopenia. The other laboratory values are not specific to this medication and are also within normal limits.
Test-Taking Strategy: Note the strategic words, *need for follow-up.* Eliminate options 1, 2, and 3 because they are comparable or alike and are within normal limits. In addition, recall that leukopenia is an adverse effect requiring discontinuation of the medication.
Level of Cognitive Ability: Analyzing
Client Needs: Physiological Integrity
Integrated Process: Nursing Process—Implementation
Content Area: Pharmacology: Integumentary: Burn Products
Health Problem: Adult Health: Integumentary: Burns
Priority Concepts: Clinical Judgment; Tissue Integrity
Reference: Ignatavicius, Workman, Rebar (2018), p. 501.

436. Answer: 1
Rationale: Mafenide acetate is a carbonic anhydrase inhibitor and can suppress renal excretion of acid, thereby causing acidosis. Clients receiving this treatment should be monitored for signs of an acid-base imbalance (hyperventilation). If this occurs, the medication will probably be discontinued for 1 to 2 days. Options 3 and 4 describe local rather than systemic effects. An elevated blood pressure may be expected from the pain that occurs with a burn injury.
Test-Taking Strategy: Note the words *systemic effect.* Options 3 and 4 can be eliminated because they are comparable or alike and are local rather than systemic effects. From the remaining options, recall that the client in pain would likely have an elevated blood pressure. This should direct you to the correct option.
Level of Cognitive Ability: Analyzing
Client Needs: Physiological Integrity
Integrated Process: Nursing Process—Assessment
Content Area: Pharmacology: Integumentary: Burn Products
Health Problem: Adult Health: Integumentary: Burns
Priority Concepts: Gas Exchange; Tissue Integrity
Reference: Ignatavicius, Workman, Rebar (2018), p. 501.

437. Answer: 2
Rationale: Isotretinoin can elevate triglyceride levels. Blood triglyceride levels should be measured before treatment and periodically thereafter until the effect on the triglycerides has been evaluated. There is no indication that isotretinoin affects potassium, hemoglobin A_1C, or total cholesterol levels.
Test-Taking Strategy: Note the subject, laboratory values that should be monitored specifically for the client taking isotretinoin. Recall that the medication can affect triglyceride levels in the client.
Level of Cognitive Ability: Analyzing
Client Needs: Physiological Integrity
Integrated Process: Nursing Process—Assessment
Content Area: Pharmacology: Integumentary: Acne Products
Health Problem: Adult Health: Integumentary: Inflammations/Infections
Priority Concepts: Cellular Regulation; Tissue Integrity
Reference: Lewis et al. (2017), pp. 417, 419.

438. Answer: 3
Rationale: Isotretinoin is a metabolite of vitamin A and can produce generalized intensification of isotretinoin toxicity. Because of the potential for increased toxicity, vitamin A supplements should be discontinued before isotretinoin therapy. There are no contraindications associated with digoxin, phenytoin, or furosemide.
Test-Taking Strategy: Focus on the subject, the need to contact the PHCP to ensure client safety. Recall that isotretinoin is a metabolite of vitamin A. Vitamin A is a fat-soluble vitamin, and therefore it is possible to develop toxic levels. This will direct you to the correct option.

Level of Cognitive Ability: Analyzing
Client Needs: Safe and Effective Care Environment
Integrated Process: Nursing Process—Implementation
Content Area: Pharmacology: Integumentary: Acne Products
Health Problem: Adult Health: Integumentary: Inflammations/Infections
Priority Concepts: Collaboration; Safety
Reference: Burchum, Rosenthal (2016), p. 1283.

439. *Answer:* 1, 4, 5
Rationale: Topical corticosteroids can be absorbed into the systemic circulation. Absorption is higher from regions where the skin is especially permeable (scalp, axilla, face, eyelids, neck, perineum, genitalia), and lower from regions where permeability is poor (back, palms, soles). The nurse should avoid areas of higher absorption to prevent systemic absorption.
Test-Taking Strategy: Focus on the **subject**, permeability and the potential for increased systemic absorption. Eliminate options 2 and 3, because these body areas are **comparable or alike** in terms of skin substance. From the remaining options, think about permeability of the skin area. This should direct you to the correct options.
Level of Cognitive Ability: Applying
Client Needs: Physiological Integrity
Integrated Process: Nursing Process—Implementation
Content Area: Pharmacology: Integumentary: Antiinflammatory/Antiinfective
Health Problem: Adult Health: Integumentary: Inflammations/Infections
Priority Concepts: Safety; Tissue Integrity
Reference: Burchum, Rosenthal (2016), p. 1279.

440. *Answer:* 1
Rationale: Azelaic acid is a topical medication used to treat mild to moderate acne. Adverse effects include burning, itching, stinging, redness of the skin, and hypopigmentation of the skin in clients with a dark complexion. The effects noted in the other options are not specifically associated with this medication.
Test-Taking Strategy: Focus on the **subject**, an effect associated with the use of azelaic acid. Focusing on the name of the medication and recalling that acne medications commonly cause local irritation will direct you to the correct option.
Level of Cognitive Ability: Applying
Client Needs: Physiological Integrity
Integrated Process: Nursing Process—Assessment
Content Area: Pharmacology: Integumentary: Acne Products
Health Problem: Adult Health: Integumentary: Inflammations/Infections
Priority Concepts: Clinical Judgment; Tissue Integrity
Reference: Skidmore-Roth (2017), pp. 1286-1287.

441. *Answer:* 4
Rationale: Silver sulfadiazine is an antibacterial that has a broad spectrum of activity against gram-negative bacteria, gram-positive bacteria, and yeast. It is applied directly to the wound to assist in healing. It does not cause stinging when applied.
Test-Taking Strategy: Note the **strategic words**, *need for further teaching*. These words indicate a **negative event query** and ask you to select an option that is an incorrect statement. Recalling the characteristics of this medication will assist in answering correctly.
Level of Cognitive Ability: Evaluating
Client Needs: Physiological Integrity
Integrated Process: Teaching and Learning
Content Area: Pharmacology: Integumentary: Burn Products
Health Problem: Adult Health: Integumentary: Burns
Priority Concepts: Client Education; Tissue Integrity
Reference: Skidmore-Roth (2017), p. 1287.

442. *Answer:* 4
Rationale: Sunscreens are most effective when applied at least 30 minutes before exposure to the sun so that they can penetrate the skin. All sunscreens should be reapplied after swimming or sweating.
Test-Taking Strategy: Knowledge that sunscreens need to penetrate the skin will assist in eliminating options 2 and 3. Next, noting the **strategic words**, *most effective*, will assist in directing you to the correct option.
Level of Cognitive Ability: Applying
Client Needs: Safe and Effective Care Environment
Integrated Process: Teaching and Learning
Content Area: Pharmacology: Integumentary: Sunscreens
Health Problem: Adult Health: Integumentary: Burns
Priority Concepts: Client Education; Safety
Reference: Lewis et al. (2017), pp. 408-409.

UNIT VIII

Oncological and Hematological Problems of the Adult Client

Pyramid to Success

Pyramid Points focus on treatment modalities related to an oncological problem, such as pain management, internal and external radiation, and chemotherapy. In preparation for the NCLEX®, focus on the following oncological problems: skin cancer; leukemia; breast cancer; testicular cancer; stomach, bowel, and pancreatic cancers; bladder cancer; prostate cancer; and lung cancer. Particular attention is given to the nursing care related to these problems and treatment modalities, client adaptation to acceptance of diagnosis and associated lifestyle changes, and the impact of the treatment for the disorder on daily life. Also, concentrate on the complications related to chemotherapy, such as hematological problems, and the nursing measures required in monitoring for these complications and preventing life-threatening conditions, such as infection and bleeding.

Client Needs: Learning Objectives

Safe and Effective Care Environment

Discussing oncology-related consultations and referrals with the interprofessional health care team
Ensuring that advance directives are in the client's medical record
Ensuring advocacy related to the client's decisions
Ensuring that informed consent for treatments and procedures has been obtained
Establishing priorities
Handling hazardous and infectious materials related to radiation and chemotherapy safely
Implementing protective, standard, and other precautions
Maintaining medical and surgical asepsis and preventing infection
Providing confidentiality regarding diagnosis
Upholding client rights

Health Promotion and Maintenance

Discussing expected body image changes related to chemotherapy and treatments
Providing client and family instructions regarding home care
Providing instructions regarding regular breast or testicular self-examinations
Respecting the client's lifestyle choices
Teaching about health promotion programs regarding risks for cancer
Teaching about health screening measures for cancer

Psychosocial Integrity

Assessing the client's ability to cope, adapt, and/or solve problems during illness or stressful events
Assessing the concerns of the client who survived cancer
Assisting the client and family to cope with the alteration in body image
Discussing end-of-life and grief and loss issues related to death and the dying process
Mobilizing appropriate support and resource systems
Promoting a positive environment to maintain optimal quality of life
Respecting religious, spiritual, and cultural preferences

Physiological Integrity

Administering blood and blood products
Caring for central venous access devices and implanted ports
Caring for the client receiving chemotherapy or radiation therapy
Managing pain
Monitoring diagnostic tests and laboratory values, such as white blood cell and platelet counts
Monitoring for expected and unexpected responses to radiation and chemotherapy
Protecting the client from the life-threatening adverse effects of treatments
Providing basic care and comfort
Providing nutrition

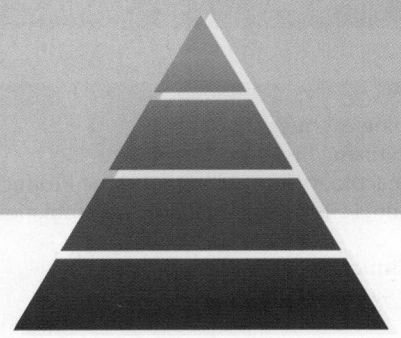

CHAPTER 44

Oncological and Hematological Problems

PRIORITY CONCEPTS Cellular Regulation; Safety

I. Cancer

A. Description
   1. Cancer is a malignant neoplastic disorder that can involve all body organs with manifestations that vary according to the body system affected and type of tumor cells.
   2. Cells lose their normal growth-controlling mechanism, and the growth of cells is uncontrolled.
   3. Cancer produces serious health problems such as impaired immune and hematopoietic (blood-producing) function, altered gastrointestinal tract structure and function, motor and sensory deficits, and decreased respiratory function.

B. Metastasis (Box 44-1)
   1. Cancer cells move from their original location to other sites.
   2. Routes of metastasis
      a. Local seeding: Distribution of shed cancer cells occurs in the local area of the primary tumor.
      b. Bloodborne metastasis: Tumor cells enter the blood, which is the most common cause of cancer spread.
      c. Lymphatic spread: Primary sites rich in lymphatics are more susceptible to early metastatic spread.

C. Cancer classification
   1. Solid tumors: Associated with the organs from which they develop, such as breast cancer or lung cancer
   2. Hematological cancers: Originate from blood cell–forming tissues, such as leukemias, lymphomas, and multiple myeloma

D. Grading and staging (Box 44-2)
   1. Grading and staging are methods used to describe the tumor.
   2. These methods describe the extent of the tumor, the extent to which malignancy has increased in size, the involvement of regional nodes, and metastatic development.

BOX 44-1 Common Sites of Metastasis

Bladder Cancer
- Lung
- Bone
- Liver
- Pelvic, retroperitoneal structures

Brain Tumors
- Central nervous system

Breast Cancer
- Bone
- Lung
- Brain
- Liver

Colorectal Cancer
- Liver

Lung Cancer
- Brain
- Liver

Prostate Cancer
- Bone
- Spine
- Lung
- Liver
- Kidneys

Testicular Cancer
- Lung
- Bone
- Liver
- Adrenal glands
- Retroperitoneal lymph nodes

   3. Grading a tumor classifies the cellular aspects of the cancer and is an indicator of tumor growth rate and spread.
   4. Staging classifies the severity and clinical aspects of the cancer and degree of metastasis at diagnosis.

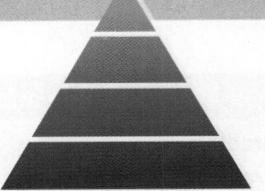

BOX 44-2 Grading and Staging

Grading

Grade I: Cells differ slightly from normal cells and are well differentiated (mild dysplasia).

Grade II: Cells are more abnormal and are moderately differentiated (moderate dysplasia).

Grade III: Cells are very abnormal and are poorly differentiated (severe dysplasia).

Grade IV: Cells are immature (anaplasia) and undifferentiated; cell of origin is difficult to determine.

Staging

Stage 0: Carcinoma in situ

Stage I: Tumor limited to the tissue of origin; localized tumor growth

Stage II: Limited local spread

Stage III: Extensive local and regional spread

Stage IV: Distant metastasis

E. Factors that influence cancer development
   1. Environmental factors
      a. Chemical carcinogen: Factors include industrial chemicals, medications, and tobacco.
      b. Physical carcinogen: Factors include ionizing radiation (diagnostic and therapeutic x-rays) and ultraviolet radiation (sun, tanning beds, and germicidal lights), chronic irritation, and tissue trauma.
      c. Viral carcinogen: Viruses capable of causing cancer are known as *oncoviruses,* such as Epstein-Barr virus, hepatitis B virus, and human papillomavirus.
      d. *Helicobacter pylori* infection is associated with an increased risk of gastric cancer.
   2. Obesity and dietary factors, including preservatives, contaminants, additives, alcohol, and nitrates
   3. Genetic predisposition: Factors include an inherited predisposition to specific cancers, inherited conditions associated with cancer, familial clustering, and chromosomal aberrations.
   4. Age: Advancing age is a significant risk factor for the development of cancer.
   5. Immune function: The incidence of cancer is higher in immunosuppressed individuals, such as those with acquired immunodeficiency syndrome and organ transplant recipients who are taking immunosuppressive medications.

F. Prevention: Avoidance of known or potential carcinogens and avoidance or modification of the factors associated with the development of cancer cells.

G. Early detection (Box 44-3)
   1. Mammography
   2. Papanicolaou (Pap) test
   3. Rectal exams and stools for occult blood
   4. Sigmoidoscopy, colonoscopy

BOX 44-3 Warning Signs of Cancer—CAUTION

- **C**hange in bowel or bladder habits
- **A**ny sore that does not heal
- **U**nusual bleeding or discharge
- **T**hickening or lump in breast or elsewhere
- **I**ndigestion
- **O**bvious change in wart or mole
- **N**agging cough or hoarseness

Data from WebMD: *Understanding cancer—symptoms.* www.webmd.com/cancer/understanding-cancer-symptoms; and Ignatavicius, Workman (2016), p. 367.

   5. Breast self-examination (BSE) and clinical breast examination
   6. Testicular self-examination
   7. Skin inspection

II. Diagnostic Tests

A. Diagnostic tests to be performed depend on the suspected primary or metastatic site of the cancer; invasive procedures require informed consent (Box 44-4).

B. Biopsy
   1. Description
      a. Biopsy is the definitive means of diagnosing cancer and provides histological proof of malignancy.
      b. Biopsy involves the surgical incision to obtain a small piece of tissue for microscopic examination.
   2. Types
      a. Needle: Aspiration of cells
      b. Incisional: Removal of a wedge of suspected tissue from a larger mass
      c. Excisional: Complete removal of the entire lesion
      d. Staging: Multiple needle or incisional biopsies in tissues where metastasis is suspected or likely (see Boxes 44-1 and 44-2)

BOX 44-4 Diagnostic Tests

- Biopsy
- Bone marrow examination (particularly if a hematolymphoid malignancy is suspected)
- Chest radiograph
- Complete blood count (CBC)
- Computed tomography (CT); positron emission tomography (PET)
- Cytological studies (Papanicolaou test)
- Evaluation of serum tumor markers (e.g., carcinoembryonic antigen and alpha-fetoprotein)
- Liver function studies
- Magnetic resonance imaging (MRI)
- Proctoscopic examination (including guaiac test for occult blood)
- Radiographic studies (mammography)
- Radioisotope scanning (liver, brain, bone, lung)
- Tumor markers

3. Tissue examination
   a. Following excision, a frozen section or a permanent paraffin section is prepared to examine the specimen.
   b. The advantage of the frozen section is the speed with which the section can be prepared and the diagnosis made, because only minutes are required for this test.
   c. Permanent paraffin section takes about 24 hours; however, it provides clearer details than the frozen section.
4. Interventions
   a. The procedure usually is performed in an outpatient surgical setting.
   b. Prepare the client for the diagnostic procedure and provide postprocedure instructions.
   c. Ensure that informed consent has been obtained.

III. Pain Control

A. Causes of pain
1. Bone destruction
2. Obstruction of an organ
3. Compression of peripheral nerves
4. Infiltration, distention of tissue
5. Inflammation, necrosis
6. Psychological factors, such as fear or anxiety; a distress screening tool may be used to assess emotional health (see http://www.cancer.org/treatment/treatmentsandsideeffects/emotional-sideeffects/distressinpeoplewithcancer/distress-in-people-with-cancer-tools-to-measure-distress).

B. Interventions
1. Collaborate with other members of the health care team to develop a pain management program.
2. Administer oral preparations if possible and if they provide adequate relief of pain; the transdermal or transmucosal route may also be prescribed.
3. Mild or moderate pain may be treated with salicylates, acetaminophen, and nonsteroidal anti-inflammatory drugs (NSAIDs).
4. Severe pain is treated with opioids, such as codeine sulfate, morphine sulfate, methadone, and hydromorphone hydrochloride. Neuropathic pain may be treated with a variety of anticonvulsants and antidepressants, as well as opioids.
5. Subcutaneous injections and continuous intravenous (IV) infusions of opioids provide rapid pain control; equianalgesic comparison charts should be used when switching routes of administration of opioids.
6. Monitor vital signs and for side effects of medications.
7. Monitor for effectiveness of medications and collaborate with the primary health care provider (PHCP) if mediation is ineffective.
8. Provide nonpharmacological techniques of pain control such as relaxation, guided imagery, biofeedback, massage, and heat-cold application.

⚠ Assess the client's pain; pain is what the client describes or says that it is. Do not undermedicate the client with cancer who is in pain.

IV. Surgery

A. Description: Surgery is indicated to diagnose, stage, and treat certain types of cancer.

B. Prophylactic surgery
1. Prophylactic surgery is performed in clients with an existing premalignant condition or a known family history or genetic mutation that strongly predisposes the person to the development of cancer.
2. An attempt is made to remove the tissue or organ at risk and thus prevent the development of cancer.

C. Curative surgery: All gross and microscopic tumor is removed or destroyed.

D. Control (cytoreductive or "debulking") surgery
1. Control surgery is a debulking procedure that consists of removing a large portion of a locally invasive tumor, such as advanced ovarian cancer.
2. Surgery decreases the number of cancer cells; therefore, it may increase the chance that other therapies will be successful.

E. Palliative surgery
1. Palliative surgery is performed to improve quality of life during the survival time.
2. Palliative surgery is performed to reduce pain, relieve airway obstruction, relieve obstructions in the gastrointestinal or urinary tract, relieve pressure on the brain or spinal cord, prevent hemorrhage, remove infected or ulcerated tumors, or drain abscesses.

F. Reconstructive or rehabilitative surgery is performed to improve quality of life by restoring maximal function and appearance, such as breast reconstruction after mastectomy.

G. Adverse effects of surgery
1. Loss or loss of function of a specific body part
2. Reduced function as a result of organ loss
3. Scarring or disfigurement
4. Grieving about altered body image or imposed change in lifestyle
5. Pain, infection, bleeding, thromboembolism

V. Chemotherapy

A. Description
1. Chemotherapy kills or inhibits the reproduction of neoplastic cells and kills normal cells.
2. The effects are systemic because chemotherapy is usually administered systemically.

3. Normal cells most profoundly affected include those of the skin, hair, and lining of the gastrointestinal tract; spermatocytes; and hematopoietic cells.
4. Usually, several chemotherapy and biotherapy agents are used in combination (combination therapy) to increase the therapeutic response.
5. Combination chemotherapy is planned by the PHCP so that medications with overlapping toxicities and **nadirs** (the time during which bone marrow activity and white blood cell counts are at their lowest) are not administered at or near the same time; this will minimize immunosuppression.
6. Chemotherapy may be combined with other treatments, such as surgery and radiation.

B. Common side effects include fatigue, alopecia, nausea and vomiting, mucositis, skin changes, and myelosuppression (neutropenia, anemia, and thrombocytopenia).

C. See Chapter 45 for information regarding care of the client receiving chemotherapy.

VI. Radiation Therapy

A. Description
1. Radiation therapy destroys cancer cells, with minimal exposure of normal cells to the damaging effects of radiation; the damaged cells die or become unable to divide.
2. Radiation therapy is effective on tissues directly within the path of the radiation beam.
3. Side effects include local skin changes and irritation, alopecia (hair loss), fatigue (most common side effect of radiation), and altered taste sensation; the effects vary according to the site of treatment.
4. External beam radiation (also called *teletherapy*) and internal radiation (also called *brachytherapy*) are the types of radiation therapy most commonly used to treat cancer.

B. External beam radiation (teletherapy): The actual radiation source is external to the client.
1. Instruct the client regarding self-care of the skin (Box 44-5).
2. The client does not emit radiation and does not pose a hazard to anyone else.

C. Brachytherapy
1. The radiation source comes into direct, continuous contact with tumor tissues for a specific time.
2. The radiation source is within the client; for a period of time, the client emits radiation and can pose a hazard to others.
3. Brachytherapy includes an unsealed source or a sealed source of radiation.
4. Unsealed radiation source
   a. Administration is via the oral or IV route or by instillation into body cavities.
   b. The source is not confined completely to one body area, and it enters body fluids and eventually is eliminated via various excreta, which are radioactive and harmful to others. Most of the source is eliminated from the body within 48 hours; then neither the client nor the excreta is radioactive or harmful.
5. Sealed radiation source (Priority Nursing Actions) (Box 44-6)
   a. A sealed, temporary or permanent radiation source (solid implant) is implanted within the tumor target tissues.

BOX 44-5 Client Education Guide: Radiation Therapy for Cancer

- Wash the irradiated area gently each day with warm water alone or with mild soap and water.
- Use the hand rather than a washcloth to wash the area.
- Rinse soap thoroughly from the skin.
- Take care not to remove the markings that indicate exactly where the beam of radiation is to be focused.
- Dry the irradiated area with patting motions rather than rubbing motions; use a clean, soft towel or cloth.
- Use no powders, ointments, lotions, or creams on the skin at the radiation site unless they are prescribed by the radiologist.
- Wear soft clothing over the skin at the radiation site.
- Avoid wearing belts, buckles, straps, or any type of clothing that binds or rubs the skin at the radiation site.
- Avoid exposure of the irradiated area to the sun.
- Avoid heat exposure.

BOX 44-6 Care of the Client with a Sealed Radiation Implant

- Place the client in a private room with a private bath.
- Place a radiation precaution sign on the client's door.
- Organize nursing tasks to minimize exposure to the radiation source.
- Nursing assignments to a client with a radiation implant should be rotated.
- Limit time to 30 minutes per care provider per shift.
- Wear a dosimeter film badge to measure radiation exposure.
- Lead shielding may be used to reduce exposure to radiation.
- The nurse should never care for more than 1 client with a radiation implant at 1 time.
- Do not allow a pregnant nurse to care for the client.
- Do not allow children younger than 16 years or a pregnant woman to visit the client.
- Limit visitors to 30 minutes per day; visitors should be at least 6 feet from the source.
- Save bed linens and dressings until the source is removed; then dispose of the linens and dressings in the usual manner.
- Other equipment can be removed from the room at any time.

b. The client emits radiation while the implant is in place, but the excreta are not radioactive.

6. Removal of sealed radiation sources
   a. The client is not radioactive after removal.
   b. Inform the client that cancer is not contagious.
   c. Inform the client to follow the PHCPs prescription regarding resumption of sexual intercourse if the implant was cervical or vaginal.
   d. Advise the client who had a cervical or vaginal implant to notify the PHCP if any of the following occurs: severe diarrhea, frequent urination, urethral burning for more than 24 hours, hematuria, heavy vaginal bleeding, extreme fatigue, abdominal pain, fever over 100° F (38° C), or other signs of infection.

PRIORITY NURSING ACTIONS

Sealed Radiation Implant that Dislodges

1. Encourage the client to lie still.
2. Use a long-handled forceps to retrieve the radioactive source.
3. Deposit the radioactive source in a lead container.
4. Contact the radiation oncologist.
5. Document the occurrence and the actions taken.

Reference

Ignatavicius, Workman, Rebar (2018), p. 389.

VII. Hematopoietic Stem Cell Transplantation

A. Description

1. Bone marrow transplantation (BMT) and peripheral blood stem cell transplantation (PBSCT) are procedures that replace stem cells that have been destroyed by high doses of chemotherapy and/or radiation therapy.
2. BMT and PBSCT are most commonly used in the treatment of leukemia and lymphoma but are also used to treat other cancers, such as neuroblastoma and multiple myeloma.
3. The goal of treatment is to rid the client of all leukemic or other **malignant** cells through treatment with high doses of chemotherapy and whole-body irradiation.
4. Because these treatments are damaging to bone marrow cells, without the replacement of blood-forming stem cell function through transplantation, the client would die of infection or hemorrhage.

B. Types of donor stem cells

1. Allogeneic: Stem cell donor is usually a sibling, a parent with a similar tissue type, or a person who is not related to the client (unrelated donor).
2. Syngeneic: Stem cells are from an identical twin.
3. Autologous
   a. Autologous donation is the most common type.
   b. The client receives his or her own stem cells.
   c. Stem cells are harvested during disease remission and are stored frozen to be reinfused later.

C. Procedure

1. Harvest
   a. The stem cells used in PBSCT come from the bloodstream in a 4- to 6-hour process called *apheresis* or *leukapheresis* (the blood is removed through a central venous catheter, and an apheresis machine removes the stem cells and returns the remainder of the blood to the donor).
   b. In BMT, marrow is harvested through multiple aspirations from the iliac crest to retrieve sufficient bone marrow for the transplant.
   c. Marrow from the client is filtered for residual cancer cells.
   d. Allogeneic marrow is transfused immediately; autologous marrow is frozen for later use (cryopreservation).
   e. Harvesting is done before the initiation of the conditioning regimen.
2. *Conditioning* refers to an immunosuppression therapy regimen used to eradicate all malignant cells, provide a state of immunosuppression, and create space in the bone marrow for the engraftment of the new marrow.
3. Transplantation
   a. Stem cells are administered through the client's central line in a manner similar to that for a blood transfusion.
   b. Stem cells may be administered by IV infusion or by IV push directly into the central line.
4. Engraftment
   a. The transfused stem cells move to the marrow-forming sites of the recipient's bones.
   b. Engraftment occurs when the white blood cell (WBC), erythrocyte, and platelet counts begin to rise.
   c. When successful, the engraftment process takes 2 to 5 weeks.

D. Posttransplantation period: Infection, bleeding, or neutropenia and thrombocytopenia are major concerns until engraftment occurs.

⚠ During the posttransplantation period, the client remains without any natural immunity until the donor stem cells begin to proliferate and engraftment occurs.

E. Complications

1. Failure to engraft: If the transplanted stem cells fail to engraft, the client will die unless another transplantation is attempted and is successful.

2. Graft-versus-host disease in allogeneic transplants
   a. Although the recipient cannot recognize the donated stem cells as foreign or nonself because of the total immunosuppression, the immune-competent cells of the donor recognize the recipient's cells as foreign and mount an immune offense against them.
   b. Graft-versus-host disease is managed cautiously with immunosuppressive agents to avoid suppressing the new immune system to such an extent that the client becomes more susceptible to infection, or the transplanted cells stop engrafting.
3. Hepatic veno-occlusive disease
   a. The disease involves occlusion of the hepatic venules by thrombosis or phlebitis.
   b. Signs include right upper quadrant abdominal pain, jaundice, ascites, weight gain, and hepatomegaly.
   c. Early detection is critical because there is no known way to open the hepatic vessels.
   d. The client will be treated with fluids and supportive therapy.

VIII. Skin Cancer (see Chapter 42)

IX. Leukemia (Box 44-7)

A. Description
1. Leukemias are a group of hematological malignancies involving abnormal overproduction of leukocytes, usually at an immature stage, in the bone marrow.
2. The 2 major types of leukemia are lymphocytic (involving abnormal cells from the lymphoid pathway) and myelocytic or myelogenous (involving abnormal cells from the myeloid pathways).

BOX 44-7 Classification of Leukemia

Acute Lymphocytic Leukemia
- Mostly lymphoblasts present in bone marrow
- Age of onset is younger than 15 years.

Acute Myelogenous Leukemia
- Mostly myeloblasts present in bone marrow
- Age of onset is between 15 and 39 years.

Chronic Myelogenous Leukemia
- Mostly granulocytes present in bone marrow
- Age of onset is in the fourth decade.

Chronic Lymphocytic Leukemia
- Mostly lymphocytes present in bone marrow
- Age of onset is after 50 years.

3. Leukemia may be acute, with a sudden onset, or chronic, with a slow onset and persistent symptoms over a period of years.
4. Leukemia affects the bone marrow, causing anemia, leukopenia, the production of immature cells, thrombocytopenia, and a decline in immunity.
5. The cause is unknown and appears to involve genetically damaged cells, leading to the transformation of cells from a normal state to a malignant state.
6. Risk factors include genetic, viral, immunological, and environmental factors and exposure to radiation, chemicals, and medications, such as previous chemotherapy.

B. Assessment
1. Anorexia, fatigue, weakness, weight loss
2. Anemia
3. Overt bleeding (nosebleeds, gum bleeding, rectal bleeding, hematuria, increased menstrual flow) and occult bleeding (e.g., as detected in a fecal occult blood test)
4. Ecchymoses, petechiae
5. Prolonged bleeding after minor abrasions or lacerations
6. Elevated temperature
7. Enlarged lymph nodes, spleen, liver
8. Palpitations, tachycardia, orthostatic hypotension
9. Pallor and dyspnea on exertion
10. Headache
11. Bone pain and joint swelling
12. Normal, elevated, or reduced WBC count
13. Decreased hemoglobin and hematocrit levels
14. Decreased platelet count
15. Positive bone marrow biopsy identifying leukemic blast–phase cells

C. Infection
1. Infection can occur through autocontamination or cross-contamination. The WBC count may be extremely low during the period of greatest bone marrow depression, known as the *nadir*.
2. Common sites of infection are the skin, respiratory tract, and gastrointestinal tract.
3. Initiate protective isolation procedures.
4. Ensure frequent and thorough hand washing by the client, family, and health care providers..
5. Staff and visitors with known infections or exposure to communicable diseases should avoid contact with the client.
6. Use strict aseptic technique for all procedures.
7. Keep supplies for the client separate from supplies for other clients; keep frequently used equipment in the room for the client's use only.
8. Limit the number of staff entering the client's room to reduce the risk of cross-infection.
9. Maintain the client in a private room with the door closed.

10. Place the client in a room with high-efficiency particulate air filtration or a laminar airflow system if possible.
11. Reduce exposure to environmental organisms by eliminating fresh or raw fruits and vegetables (low-bacteria diet) from the diet; eliminate fresh flowers and live plants from the client's room and avoid leaving standing water in the client's room.
12. Be sure that the client's room is cleaned daily.
13. Assist the client with daily bathing, using an antimicrobial soap.
14. Assist the client to perform oral hygiene frequently.
15. Initiate a bowel program to prevent constipation and prevent rectal trauma.
16. Avoid invasive procedures such as injections, insertion of rectal thermometers, and urinary catheterization.
17. Change wound dressings daily, and inspect the wounds for redness, swelling, or drainage.
18. Assess the urine for cloudiness and other characteristics of infection.
19. Assess skin and oral mucous membranes for signs of infection (Box 44-8).
20. Auscultate lung sounds, and encourage the client to cough and deep breathe.
21. Monitor temperature, pulse, respirations, blood pressure, and for pain.
22. Monitor WBC and neutrophil counts.
23. Notify the PHCP if signs of infection are present, and prepare to obtain specimens for culture of the blood, open lesions, urine, and sputum; chest radiograph may also be prescribed.
24. Administer prescribed antibiotic, antifungal, and antiviral medications.
25. Instruct the client to avoid crowds and those with infections.
26. Instruct the client about a low-bacteria diet.
27. Instruct the client to avoid activities that expose the client to infection, such as changing a pet's litter box or working with house plants or in the garden.
28. Instruct the client that neither they nor their household contacts should receive immunization with a live virus such as measles, mumps, rubella, polio, varicella, shingles, and some influenza, including the H1N1 vaccine.

⚠ Infection is a major cause of death in the immunosuppressed client.

BOX 44-8 Mouth Care for the Client with Mucositis

- Inspect the mouth daily.
- Offer complete mouth care before and after every meal and at bedtime.
- Brush the teeth and tongue with a soft-bristled toothbrush or sponges.
- Provide mouth rinses every 12 hours with the prescribed solution.
- Administer topical anesthetic agents to mouth sores as prescribed.
- Avoid the use of alcohol- or glycerin-based mouthwashes or swabs because they are irritating to the mucosa.
- Offer soft foods that are cool to warm in temperature rather than foods that are hard or spicy or cold or hot.

D. Bleeding

1. During the period of greatest bone marrow suppression (the nadir), the platelet count may be extremely low.
2. The client is at risk for bleeding when the platelet count falls below 50,000 mm^3 ($50 \times 10^9/L$), and spontaneous bleeding frequently occurs when the platelet count is lower than 20,000 mm^3 ($20 \times 10^9/L$).
3. Clients with platelet counts lower than 20,000 mm^3 ($20 \times 10^9/L$) may need a platelet transfusion.
4. For clients with anemia and fatigue, packed red blood cells may be prescribed.
5. Monitor laboratory values.
6. Examine the client for signs and symptoms of bleeding, such as petechiae; examine all body fluids and excrement for the presence of blood.
7. Handle the client gently; use caution when taking blood pressures to prevent skin injury.
8. Monitor for signs of internal hemorrhage (e.g., pain, rapid and weak pulse, increased abdominal girth, abdomen guarding, change in mental status).
9. Provide soft foods that are cool to warm to avoid oral mucosa damage.
10. Avoid injections, if possible, to prevent trauma to the skin and bleeding; apply firm and gentle pressure to a needle-stick site for at least 5 minutes, or longer if needed.
11. Pad side rails and sharp corners of the bed and furniture.
12. Avoid rectal suppositories, enemas, and thermometers.
13. If the female client is menstruating, count the number of pads or tampons used.
14. Administer blood products as prescribed.
15. Instruct the client to use a soft toothbrush and avoid dental floss.
16. Instruct the client to use only an electric razor for shaving.
17. Instruct the client to avoid blowing the nose.
18. Discourage the client from engaging in activities involving the use of sharp objects; contact sports also need to be avoided.
19. Instruct the client to avoid using NSAIDs and products that contain aspirin.

E. Fatigue and nutrition
1. Assist the client in selecting a well-balanced diet.
2. Provide small, frequent meals (high calorie, high protein, high carbohydrate) that require little chewing to reduce energy expenditure at mealtimes.
3. Assist the client in self-care and mobility activities.
4. Allow adequate rest periods during care.
5. Do not perform activities unless they are essential; assist the client in scheduling important or pleasurable activities during periods of highest energy.
6. Administer blood products for anemia as prescribed.

F. Additional interventions
1. Chemotherapy
   a. Induction therapy is aimed at achieving a rapid, complete remission of all manifestations of the disease.
   b. Consolidation therapy is administered early in remission with the aim of curing.
   c. Maintenance therapy may be prescribed for months or years after successful induction and consolidation therapy; the aim is to maintain remission.
2. Administer antibiotic, antibacterial, antiviral, and antifungal medications as prescribed.
3. Administer colony-stimulating factors as prescribed.
4. Administer blood replacements as prescribed.
5. Maintain infection and bleeding precautions.
6. Prepare the client for transplantation if indicated.
7. Instruct the client in appropriate home care measures.
8. Provide psychosocial support and support services for home care.

X. Lymphoma: Hodgkin's Disease

A. Description
1. Lymphomas, classified as Hodgkin's and non-Hodgkin's depending on the cell type, are characterized by abnormal proliferation of lymphocytes.
2. Hodgkin's disease is a malignancy of the lymph nodes that originates in a single lymph node or a chain of nodes.
3. Metastasis occurs to other, adjacent lymph structures and eventually invades nonlymphoid tissue.
4. The disease usually involves lymph nodes, tonsils, spleen, and bone marrow and is characterized by the presence of Reed-Sternberg cells in the nodes.
5. Possible causes include viral infections; clients treated with combination chemotherapy for Hodgkin's disease have a greater risk of developing acute leukemia and non–Hodgkin's lymphoma, among other secondary malignancies.
6. Prognosis depends on the stage of the disease.

B. Assessment
1. Fever
2. Malaise, fatigue, and weakness
3. Night sweats
4. Loss of appetite and significant weight loss
5. Anemia and thrombocytopenia
6. Enlarged lymph nodes, spleen, and liver
7. Positive biopsy of lymph nodes, with cervical nodes most often affected first
8. Presence of Reed-Sternberg cells in nodes
9. Positive computed tomography (CT) scan of the liver and spleen

C. Interventions
1. For earlier stages (stages I and II), without mediastinal node involvement, the treatment of choice is extensive external radiation of the involved lymph node regions.
2. With more extensive disease, radiation and multiagent chemotherapy are used.
3. Monitor for side effects related to chemotherapy or radiation therapy.
4. Monitor for signs of infection and bleeding.
5. Maintain infection and bleeding precautions.
6. Discuss the possibility of sterility with the client receiving chemotherapy and/or radiation, and inform the client of fertility options such as sperm banking.

XI. Multiple Myeloma

A. Description
1. A malignant proliferation of plasma cells within the bone
2. Excessive numbers of abnormal plasma cells invade the bone marrow and ultimately destroy bone; invasion of the lymph nodes, spleen, and liver occurs.
3. The abnormal plasma cells produce an abnormal antibody (myeloma protein or the Bence Jones protein) found in the blood and urine.
4. Multiple myeloma causes decreased production of immunoglobulin and antibodies and increased levels of uric acid and calcium, which can lead to kidney failure.
5. The disease typically develops slowly, and the cause is unknown.

B. Assessment
1. Bone (skeletal) pain, especially in the ribs, spine, and pelvis
2. Weakness and fatigue
3. Recurrent infections
4. Anemia
5. Urinalysis shows Bence Jones proteinuria and elevated total serum protein level.
6. Osteoporosis (bone loss and the development of pathological fractures)
7. Thrombocytopenia and leukopenia
8. Elevated calcium and uric acid levels

9. Kidney failure
10. Spinal cord compression and paraplegia
11. Bone marrow aspiration shows an abnormal number of immature plasma cells.

The client with multiple myeloma is at risk for pathological fractures. Therefore, provide skeletal support during moving, turning, and ambulating and provide a hazard-free environment.

C. Interventions
1. Administer chemotherapy as prescribed.
2. Provide supportive care to control symptoms and prevent complications, especially bone fractures, hypercalcemia, kidney failure, and infections.
3. Maintain neutropenic and bleeding precautions as necessary.
4. Monitor for signs of bleeding, infection, and skeletal fractures.
5. Encourage the consumption of at least 2 L of fluids per day to offset potential problems associated with hypercalcemia, hyperuricemia, and proteinuria, and encourage additional fluid as indicated and tolerated.
6. Monitor for signs of kidney failure. Collect 24-hour urine as prescribed.
7. Encourage ambulation to prevent renal problems and to slow down bone resorption.
8. Administer IV fluids and diuretics as prescribed to increase renal excretion of calcium.
9. Administer blood transfusions as prescribed for anemia.
10. Administer analgesics as prescribed and provide nonpharmacological therapies to control pain.
11. Administer antibiotics as prescribed for infection.
12. Prepare the client for local radiation therapy if prescribed.
13. Instruct the client in home care measures and the signs and symptoms of infection.
14. Administer bisphosphonate medications as prescribed to slow bone damage and reduce pain and risk of fractures.

XII. Testicular Cancer

A. Description
1. Testicular cancer arises from germinal epithelium from the sperm-producing germ cells or from nongerminal epithelium from other structures in the testicles.
2. Testicular cancer most often occurs between the ages of 15 and 40 years.
3. The cause of testicular cancer is unknown, but a history of undescended testicle (cryptorchidism) and genetic predisposition have been associated with testicular tumor development.
4. Metastasis occurs to the lung, liver, bone, and adrenal glands via the blood and to the retroperitoneal lymph nodes via lymphatic channels.

B. Early detection: Perform monthly testicular self-examination (Fig. 44-1).
1. Performing testicular self-examination: Perform monthly; a day of the month is selected and the examination is performed on the same day each month.
2. Client instructions (see Fig. 44-1)

C. Assessment
1. Painless testicular swelling occurs.
2. "Dragging" or "pulling" sensation is experienced in the scrotum.
3. Palpable lymphadenopathy, abdominal masses, and gynecomastia may indicate metastasis.
4. Late signs include back or bone pain and respiratory symptoms.

D. Interventions
1. Administer chemotherapy as prescribed.
2. Prepare the client for radiation therapy as prescribed.
3. Prepare the client for unilateral orchiectomy, if prescribed, for diagnosis and primary surgical management or radical orchiectomy (surgical removal of the affected testis, spermatic cord, and regional lymph nodes).
4. Prepare the client for retroperitoneal lymph node dissection, if prescribed, to stage the disease and reduce tumor volume so that chemotherapy and radiation therapy are more effective.

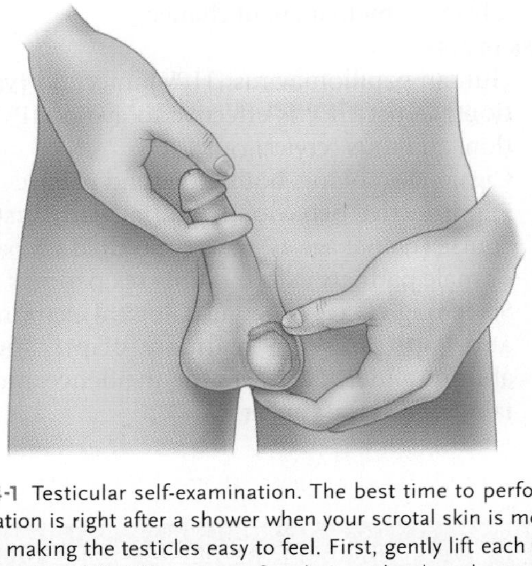

FIG. 44-1 Testicular self-examination. The best time to perform this examination is right after a shower when your scrotal skin is moist and relaxed, making the testicles easy to feel. First, gently lift each testicle. Each one should feel like an egg, firm but not hard, and smooth with no lumps. Then, using both hands, place your middle fingers on the underside of each testicle and your thumbs on top. Gently roll the testicle between the thumb and fingers to feel for any lumps, swelling, or mass. If you notice any changes from 1 month to the next, notify your primary health care provider.

5. Discuss reproduction, sexuality, and fertility information and options with the client.
6. Identify reproductive options such as sperm storage, donor insemination, and adoption.

E. Postoperative interventions
1. Monitor for signs of bleeding and wound infection; antibiotics may be administered to prevent wound infection.
2. Monitor intake and output.
3. Provide and explain pain management methods; to reduce swelling in the first 48 hours, apply an ice pack with an intervening protective layer of cloth.
4. Notify the PHCP if chills, fever, increasing pain or tenderness at the incision site, or drainage from the incision occurs.
5. After the orchiectomy, instruct the client to avoid heavy lifting and strenuous activity for the length of time prescribed by the PHCP.
6. Instruct the client to perform a monthly testicular self-examination on the remaining testicle (see Fig. 44-1).
7. Inform the client that sutures will be removed approximately 7 to 10 days after surgery.

XIII. Cervical Cancer

A. Description
1. Preinvasive cancer is limited to the cervix (Box 44-9).
2. Invasive cancer is in the cervix and other pelvic structures.
3. Metastasis usually is confined to the pelvis, but distant metastasis occurs through lymphatic spread.
4. Premalignant changes are described on a continuum from dysplasia, which is the earliest premalignancy change, to **carcinoma in situ**, the most advanced premalignant change.

B. Risk factors
1. Human papillomavirus (HPV) infection (vaccination against HPV is effective to avoid HPV infection, and thus cervical cancer)
2. Cigarette smoking, both active and passive
3. Reproductive behavior, including early first intercourse (before age 17 years), multiple sex partners, or male partners with multiple sex partners
4. Screening via regular gynecological examinations and Pap test, with treatment of precancerous abnormalities, decreases the incidence and mortality of cervical cancer.

C. Assessment
1. Painless vaginal postmenstrual and postcoital bleeding
2. Foul-smelling or serosanguineous vaginal discharge
3. Pelvic, lower back, leg, or groin pain
4. Anorexia and weight loss
5. Leakage of urine and feces from the vagina
6. Dysuria
7. Hematuria
8. Cytological changes on Pap test

D. Interventions (Box 44-10)

E. Laser therapy
1. Laser therapy is used when all boundaries of the lesion are visible during colposcopic examination.
2. Energy from the beam is absorbed by fluid in the tissues, causing them to vaporize.
3. Minimal bleeding is associated with the procedure.
4. Slight vaginal discharge is expected following the procedure, and healing occurs in 6 to 12 weeks.

F. Cryosurgery
1. Cryosurgery involves freezing of the tissues, using a probe, with subsequent necrosis and sloughing.
2. No anesthesia is required, although cramping may occur during the procedure.
3. A heavy watery discharge will occur for several weeks following the procedure.
4. Instruct the client to avoid intercourse and the use of tampons while the discharge is present.

G. Conization
1. A cone-shaped area of the cervix is removed.
2. Conization allows the woman to retain reproductive capacity.
3. Long-term follow-up care is needed, because new lesions can develop.
4. The risks of the procedure include hemorrhage, uterine perforation, incompetent cervix, cervical stenosis, and preterm labor in future pregnancies.

BOX 44-9 Premalignant Cancers: Stages of Cervical Intraepithelial Neoplasia

Stage I: Mild dysplasia
Stage II: Moderate dysplasia
Stage III: Severe dysplasia to carcinoma in situ

BOX 44-10 Treatment for Cervical Cancer

Nonsurgical
- Chemotherapy
- Cryosurgery
- External radiation
- Internal radiation implants (intracavitary)
- Laser therapy

Surgical
- Conization
- Hysterectomy
- Pelvic exenteration

Note: Internal radiation therapy is used for clients for whom surgery is not an option.

H. Hysterectomy
1. Description
a. Hysterectomy is performed for microinvasive cancer if childbearing is not desired.
b. A vaginal approach is most commonly used.
c. A radical hysterectomy and bilateral lymph node dissection may be performed for cancer that has spread beyond the cervix but not to the pelvic wall.
2. Postoperative interventions
a. Monitor vital signs
b. Assist with coughing and deep-breathing exercises.
c. Assist with range-of-motion exercises and provide early ambulation.
d. Apply antiembolism stockings or sequential compression devices as prescribed.
e. Monitor intake and output, urinary catheter drainage, and hydration status.
f. Monitor bowel sounds.
g. Assess incision site for signs of infection.
h. Administer pain medication as prescribed.
i. Instruct the client to limit stair climbing for 1 month as prescribed and to avoid tub baths and sitting for long periods.
j. Avoid strenuous activity or lifting anything weighing more than 20 pounds (9 kg).
k. Instruct the client to consume foods that promote tissue healing.
l. Instruct the client to avoid sexual intercourse for 3 to 6 weeks as prescribed.
m. Instruct the client in the signs associated with complications.

! Monitor vaginal bleeding following hysterectomy. More than 1 saturated pad per hour may indicate excessive bleeding.

I. Pelvic exenteration (Box 44-11)
1. Description
a. Pelvic exenteration, the removal of all pelvic contents, including bowel, vagina, and bladder, is a radical surgical procedure performed for recurrent cancer if no evidence of tumor outside the pelvis and no lymph node involvement exist.
b. When the bladder is removed, an ileal conduit is created and located on the right side of the abdomen to divert urine.
c. A colostomy may need to be created on the left side of the abdomen for the passage of feces.
2. Postoperative interventions
a. Similar to postoperative interventions following hysterectomy.
b. Monitor for signs of altered respiratory status.
c. Monitor incision site for infection.

BOX 44-11 Types of Pelvic Exenteration

Anterior
- Removal of the uterus, ovaries, fallopian tubes, vagina, bladder, urethra, and pelvic lymph nodes

Posterior
- Removal of the uterus, ovaries, fallopian tubes, descending colon, rectum, and anal canal

Total
- Combination of anterior and posterior

d. Monitor intake and output and for signs of dehydration.
e. Monitor for hemorrhage, shock, and deep vein thrombosis.
f. Apply antiembolism stockings or sequential compression devices as prescribed.
g. Administer prophylactic heparin as prescribed.
h. Administer perineal irrigations and sitz baths as prescribed.
i. Instruct the client to avoid strenuous activity for 6 months.
j. Instruct the client that the perineal opening, if present, may drain for several months.
k. Instruct the client in the care of the ileal conduit and colostomy, if created.
l. Provide sexual counseling, because vaginal intercourse is not possible after anterior and total pelvic exenteration.

XIV. Ovarian Cancer

A. Description
1. Ovarian cancer grows rapidly, spreads fast, and is often bilateral.
2. Metastasis occurs by direct spread to the organs in the pelvis, by distal spread through lymphatic drainage, or by peritoneal seeding.
3. In its early stages, ovarian cancer is often asymptomatic; because most women are diagnosed in advanced stages, ovarian cancer has a higher mortality rate than any other cancer of the female reproductive system, particularly among white women between 55 and 65 years of age of North American or European descent.
4. An exploratory laparotomy is performed to diagnose and stage the tumor.
5. A transvaginal ultrasound may also be done for screening purposes but will not provide a definitive diagnosis.

B. Assessment
1. Abdominal discomfort or swelling
2. Gastrointestinal disturbances
3. Dysfunctional vaginal bleeding
4. Abdominal mass
5. Elevated tumor marker (i.e., CA-125)

C. Interventions
1. External radiation may be used if the tumor has invaded other organs; intraperitoneal radioisotopes may be instilled for stage I disease.
2. Chemotherapy is used postoperatively for most stages of ovarian cancer.
3. Intraperitoneal chemotherapy involves the instillation of chemotherapy into the abdominal cavity.
4. Total abdominal hysterectomy and bilateral salpingo-oophorectomy with tumor debulking may be necessary.

XV. Endometrial (Uterine) Cancer

A. Description
1. Endometrial cancer is a slow-growing tumor arising from the endometrial mucosa of the uterus, associated with the menopausal years.
2. Metastasis occurs through the lymphatic system to the ovaries and pelvis; via the blood to the lungs, liver, and bone; or intra-abdominally to the peritoneal cavity.

B. Risk factors
1. Use of estrogen replacement therapy (ERT)
2. Nulliparity
3. Polycystic ovary disease
4. Increased age
5. Late menopause
6. Family history of uterine cancer or hereditary nonpolyposis colorectal cancer
7. Obesity
8. Hypertension
9. Diabetes mellitus

C. Assessment
1. Abnormal bleeding, especially in postmenopausal women
2. Vaginal discharge
3. Low back, pelvic, or abdominal pain (pain occurs late in the disease process)
4. Enlarged uterus (in advanced stages)

D. Nonsurgical interventions
1. External or internal radiation is used alone or in combination with surgery, depending on the stage of cancer.
2. Chemotherapy is used to treat advanced or recurrent disease.
3. Progesterone therapy with medication may be prescribed for estrogen-dependent tumors.
4. Antiestrogen medication may also be prescribed.

E. Surgical interventions: Total abdominal hysterectomy and bilateral salpingo-oophorectomy

XVI. Breast Cancer

A. Description
1. Breast cancer is classified as invasive when it penetrates the tissue surrounding the mammary duct and grows in an irregular pattern.
2. Metastasis occurs via lymph nodes.
3. Common sites of metastasis are the bone and lungs; metastasis may also occur to the brain and liver.
4. Diagnosis is made by breast biopsy through a needle aspiration or by surgical removal of the tumor with microscopic examination for malignant cells.

B. Risk factors
1. Age
2. Family history of breast cancer due to genetic predisposition
3. Early menarche and late menopause
4. Previous cancer of the breast, uterus, or ovaries
5. Nulliparity, late first birth
6. Obesity
7. High-dose radiation exposure to chest

C. Assessment
1. Mass felt during BSE (usually felt in the upper outer quadrant, beneath the nipple, or in axilla)
2. Presence of the lesion on mammography
3. A fixed, irregular nonencapsulated mass; typically painless except in the late stages
4. Asymmetry
5. Bloody or clear nipple discharge
6. Nipple retraction or elevation
7. Skin dimpling, retraction, or ulceration
8. Skin edema or peau d'orange skin
9. Axillary lymphadenopathy
10. Lymphedema of the affected arm
11. Symptoms of bone or lung metastasis in late stage

D. Early detection: Regular BSE
1. Performing BSE
   a. Perform regularly 7 to 10 days after menses.
   b. Postmenopausal clients or clients who have had a hysterectomy should perform BSE regularly as well.
2. Client instructions (Fig. 44-2)

E. Nonsurgical interventions
1. Chemotherapy
2. Radiation therapy
3. Hormonal manipulation via the use of medication in postmenopausal women or other medications for estrogen receptor–positive tumors
4. Monoclonal antibodies such as trastuzumab for human epidermal growth factor receptor 2–positive (HER-2 +) breast cancer

F. Surgical interventions: Surgical breast procedures, with possible breast reconstruction (Box 44-12)

G. Postoperative interventions
1. Monitor vital signs.
2. Position the client in a semi-Fowler's position; turn from the back to the unaffected side, with the affected arm elevated above the level of the heart to promote drainage and prevent lymphedema.

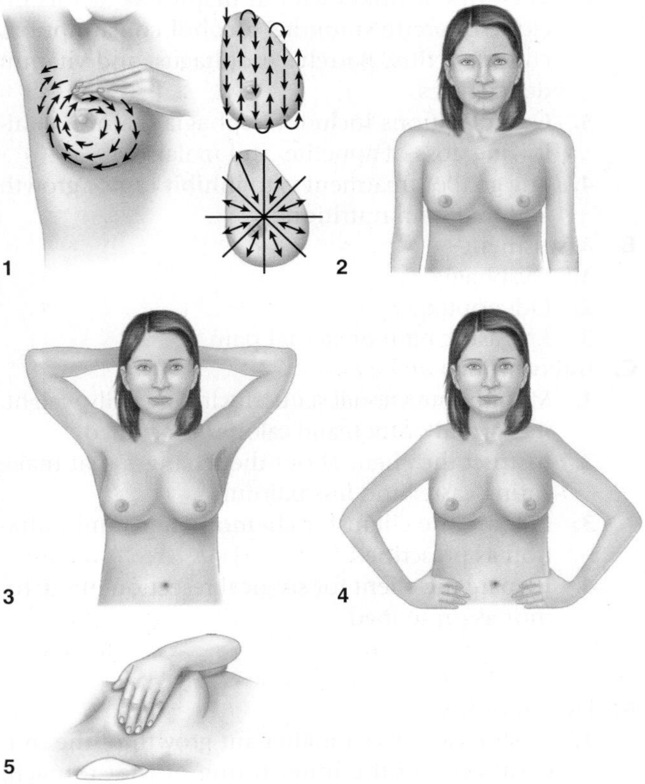

FIG. 44-2 Breast self-examination and client instructions. ***1,*** While in the shower or bath, when the skin is slippery with soap and water, examine your breasts. Use the pads of your second, third, and fourth fingers to press every part of the breast firmly. Use your right hand to examine your left breast, and use your left hand to examine your right breast. Using the pads of the fingers on your left hand, examine the entire right breast using small circular motions in a spiral or up-and-down motion so that the entire breast area is examined. Repeat the procedure using your right hand to examine your left breast. Repeat the pattern of palpation under the arm. Check for any lump, hard knot, or thickening of the tissue. ***2,*** Look at your breasts in a mirror. Stand with your arms at your side. ***3,*** Raise your arms overhead and check for any changes in the shape of your breasts, dimpling of the skin, or any changes in the nipple. ***4,*** Next, place your hands on your hips and press down firmly, tightening the pectoral muscles. Observe for asymmetry or changes, keeping in mind that your breasts probably do not match exactly. ***5,*** While lying down, feel your breasts as described in step *1*. When examining your right breast, place a folded towel under your right shoulder and put your right hand behind your head. Repeat the procedure while examining your left breast. Mark your calendar that you have completed your breast self-examination; note any changes or unique characteristics you want to check with your primary health care provider.

3. Encourage coughing and deep breathing.
4. If a drain (usually a Jackson-Pratt) is in place, maintain suction and record the amount of drainage and drainage characteristics; teach the client about home management of the drain (Fig. 44-3).
5. Assess operative site for infection, swelling, or the presence of fluid collection under the skin flaps or in the arm.

BOX 44-12 Surgical Breast Procedures

Lumpectomy
- Tumor is excised and removed.
- Lymph node dissection may also be performed.

Simple Mastectomy
- Breast tissue and the nipple are removed.
- Lymph nodes are usually left intact.

Modified Radical Mastectomy
- Breast tissue, nipple, and lymph nodes are removed.
- Muscles are left intact.

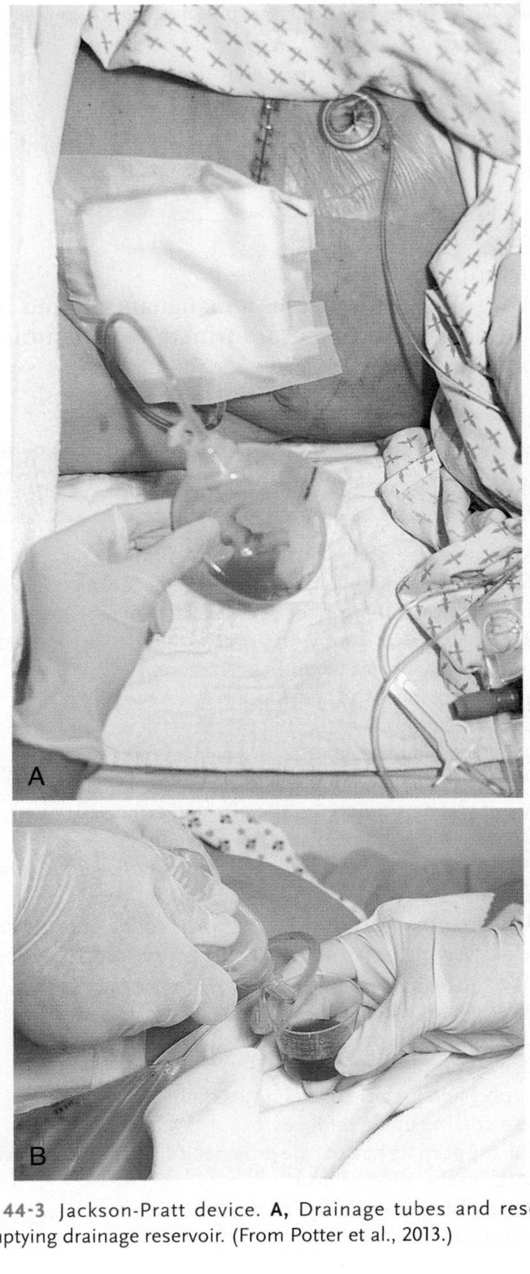

FIG. 44-3 Jackson-Pratt device. **A,** Drainage tubes and reservoir. **B,** Emptying drainage reservoir. (From Potter et al., 2013.)

6. Monitor incision site for restriction of dressing, impaired sensation, or color changes of the skin.
7. If breast reconstruction was performed, the client will return from surgery usually with a surgical brassiere and a prosthesis in place.
8. Provide the use of a pressure sleeve as prescribed if edema is severe.
9. Maintain fluid and electrolyte balance; administer diuretics and provide a low-salt diet as prescribed for severe lymphedema.
10. Consult with the PHCP and physical therapist regarding the appropriate exercise program, and assist the client with prescribed exercise.
11. Instruct the client about home care measures (Box 44-13).

No IVs, no injections, no blood pressure measurements, and no venipunctures should be done in the arm on the side of the mastectomy. The arm on the side of the mastectomy is protected, and any intervention that could traumatize the affected arm is avoided because of the risk for lymphedema on this side.

XVII. Esophageal Cancer

A. Description
1. Esophageal cancer is a malignancy found in the esophageal mucosa, formed by squamous cell carcinoma (SCC) or **adenocarcinoma**.

BOX 44-13 Client Instructions Following Mastectomy

- Avoid overuse of the arm during the first few months.
- To prevent lymphedema, keep the affected arm elevated; consultation with lymphedema specialist may be prescribed.
- Provide incision care with an emollient as prescribed, to soften and prevent wound contracture.
- Encourage use of support groups.
- Encourage the client to perform breast self-examination on the remaining breast and surgical site once healed.
- Protect the affected hand and arm.
- Avoid strong sunlight on the affected arm.
- Do not let the affected arm hang dependent.
- Do not carry a pocketbook or anything heavy over the affected arm.
- Avoid trauma, cuts, bruises, or burns to the affected side.
- Avoid wearing constricting clothing or jewelry on the affected side.
- Wear gloves when gardening.
- Use thick oven mitts when cooking.
- Use a thimble when sewing.
- Apply hand cream several times daily.
- Use cream cuticle remover.
- Call the primary health care provider if signs of inflammation occur in the affected arm.
- Wear a MedicAlert bracelet stating which arm is at risk for lymphedema.

2. The cause is unknown but major risk factors include cigarette smoking, alcohol consumption, chronic reflux, Barrett's esophagus, and vitamin deficiencies.
3. Complications include dysphagia, painful swallowing, loss of appetite, and malaise.
4. The goal of treatment is to inhibit tumor growth and maintain nutrition.

B. Assessment
1. Dysphagia
2. Odynophagia
3. Epigastric pain or sternal pain

C. Interventions
1. Monitor nutritional status, including daily weight, intake and output, and calories consumed.
2. Instruct the client about diet changes that make eating easier and less painful.
3. Prepare the client for chemotherapy and radiation as prescribed.
4. Prepare the client for surgical resection of the tumor as prescribed.

XVIII. Gastric Cancer

A. Description
1. Gastric cancer is a malignant growth of the mucosal cells in the inner lining of the stomach, with invasion to the muscle and beyond in advanced disease.
2. No single causative agent has been identified, but it is believed that *H. pylori* infection and a diet of smoked, highly salted, processed, or spiced foods have carcinogenic effects; other risk factors include smoking, alcohol and nitrate ingestion, and a history of gastric ulcers.
3. Complications include hemorrhage, obstruction, metastasis, and dumping syndrome.
4. The goal of treatment is to remove the tumor and provide a nutritional program.

B. Assessment
1. Early
   a. Indigestion
   b. Abdominal discomfort
   c. Full feeling
   d. Epigastric, back, or retrosternal pain
2. Late
   a. Weakness and fatigue
   b. Anorexia and weight loss
   c. Nausea and vomiting
   d. A sensation of pressure in the stomach
   e. Dysphagia and obstructive symptoms
   f. Iron deficiency anemia
   g. Ascites
   h. Palpable epigastric mass

C. Interventions
1. Monitor vital signs.
2. Monitor hemoglobin and hematocrit and administer blood transfusions as prescribed.

3. Monitor weight.
4. Assess nutritional status; encourage small, bland, easily digestible meals with vitamin and mineral supplements.
5. Administer pain medication as prescribed.
6. Prepare the client for chemotherapy or radiation therapy as prescribed.
7. Prepare the client for surgical resection of the tumor as prescribed (Box 44-14).

D. Postoperative interventions
1. Monitor vital signs.
2. Place in Fowler's position for comfort.
3. Administer analgesics and antiemetics, as prescribed.
4. Monitor intake and output; administer fluids and electrolyte replacement by IV as prescribed; administer parenteral nutrition as indicated.
5. Maintain NPO (nothing by mouth) status as prescribed for 1 to 3 days until peristalsis returns; assess for bowel sounds.
6. Monitor nasogastric suction. Following gastrectomy, drainage from the nasogastric tube is normally bloody for 24 hours postoperatively, changes to brown-tinged, and is then yellow or clear.
7. Do not irrigate or remove the nasogastric tube (follow agency procedures); assist the PHCP with irrigation or removal.
8. Advance the diet from NPO to sips of clear water to 6 small bland meals a day, as prescribed.
9. Monitor for complications such as hemorrhage, dumping syndrome, diarrhea, hypoglycemia, and vitamin B_{12} deficiency.

XIX. Pancreatic Cancer

A. Description
1. Most pancreatic tumors are highly malignant, rapidly growing adenocarcinomas originating from the epithelium of the ductal system.
2. Pancreatic cancer is associated with increased age, a history of diabetes mellitus, alcohol use, history of previous pancreatitis, smoking, ingestion of a high-fat diet, and exposure to environmental chemicals.
3. Symptoms usually do not occur until the tumor is large; therefore, the prognosis is poor.
4. Endoscopic retrograde cholangiopancreatography for visualization of the pancreatic duct and biliary system and collection of tissue and secretions may be done.

B. Assessment
1. Nausea and vomiting
2. Jaundice
3. Unexplained weight loss
4. Clay-colored stools
5. Glucose intolerance
6. Abdominal pain

C. Interventions
1. Radiation
2. Chemotherapy
3. Whipple procedure, which involves a pancreaticoduodenectomy with removal of the distal third of the stomach, pancreaticojejunostomy, gastrojejunostomy, and choledochojejunostomy (Fig. 44-4)
4. Postoperative care measures and complications are similar to those for the care of a client with pancreatitis and the client following gastric surgery; monitor blood glucose levels for transient hyperglycemia or hypoglycemia resulting from surgical manipulation of the pancreas.

XX. Intestinal Tumors

A. Description
1. Intestinal tumors are malignant lesions that develop in the cells lining the bowel wall or develop as adenomatous polyps in the colon or rectum.

BOX 44-14 Surgical Interventions for Gastric Cancer

Subtotal Gastrectomy

Billroth I
- Also called gastroduodenostomy
- Partial gastrectomy, with remaining segment anastomosed to the duodenum

Billroth II
- Also called gastrojejunostomy
- Partial gastrectomy, with remaining segment anastomosed to the jejunum

Total Gastrectomy
- Also called esophagojejunostomy
- Removal of the stomach, with attachment of the esophagus to the jejunum or duodenum

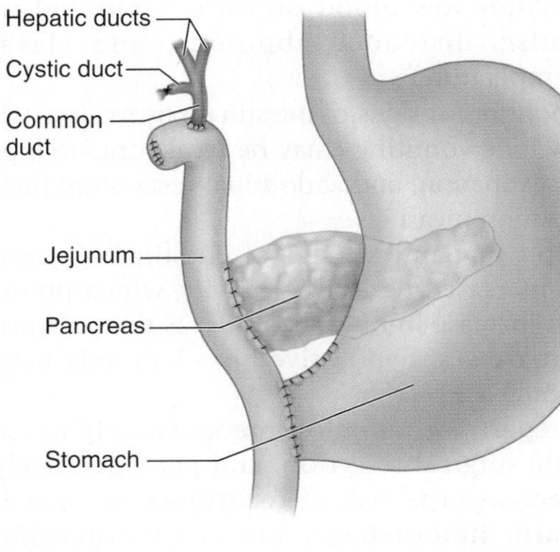

FIG. 44-4 Whipple procedure, or radical pancreaticoduodenectomy.

2. Tumor spread is by direct invasion and through the lymphatic and circulatory systems.
3. Complications include bowel perforation with peritonitis, abscess and fistula formation, hemorrhage, and complete intestinal obstruction.

B. Risk factors for colorectal cancer
1. Age older than 50 years
2. Familial polyposis, family history of colorectal cancer
3. Previous colorectal polyps, history of colorectal cancer
4. History of chronic inflammatory bowel disease
5. History of ovarian or breast, endometrial, and stomach cancers

C. Assessment
1. Blood in stool (most common manifestation) detected by fecal occult blood testing, sigmoidoscopy, and colonoscopy
2. Anorexia, vomiting, and weight loss
3. Anemia
4. Abnormal stools
   a. Ascending colon tumor: Diarrhea
   b. Descending colon tumor: Constipation or some diarrhea, or flat, ribbon-like stool caused by a partial obstruction
   c. Rectal tumor: Alternating constipation and diarrhea
5. Guarding or abdominal distention, abdominal mass (late sign)
6. Cachexia (late sign)
7. Masses noted on barium enema, colonoscopy, CT scan, sigmoidoscopy

D. General interventions
1. Monitor for signs of complications, which include bowel perforation with peritonitis, abscess or fistula formation (fever associated with pain), hemorrhage (signs of shock), and complete intestinal obstruction.
2. Monitor for signs of bowel perforation, which include low blood pressure, rapid and weak pulse, distended abdomen, and elevated temperature.
3. Monitor for signs of intestinal obstruction, which include vomiting (may be fecal contents), pain, constipation, and abdominal distention; provide comfort measures.
4. Note that an early sign of intestinal obstruction is increased peristaltic activity, which produces an increase in bowel sounds; as the obstruction progresses, hypoactive bowel sounds may be heard.
5. Prepare for radiation preoperatively to facilitate surgical resection, and postoperatively to decrease the risk of recurrence or to reduce pain, hemorrhage, bowel obstruction, or metastasis.

E. Nonsurgical interventions
1. Preoperative radiation for local control and postoperative radiation for palliation may be prescribed.
2. Postoperative chemotherapy to control symptoms and the spread of disease

F. Surgical interventions: Bowel resection, local lymph node resection, and creation of a colostomy or ileostomy

G. Colostomy, ileostomy
1. Preoperative interventions
   a. Consult with the enterostomal therapist to assist in identifying optimal placement of the ostomy.
   b. Instruct the client in prescribed preoperative diet; bowel preparation (laxatives and enemas) may be prescribed per surgeon preference.
   c. Intestinal antiseptics and antibiotics may be prescribed to decrease the bacterial content of the colon and to reduce the risk of infection from the surgical procedure.
2. Postoperative: Colostomy
   a. If a pouch system is not in place, apply a petroleum jelly gauze over the stoma to keep it moist, covered with a dry sterile dressing; place a pouch system on the stoma as soon as possible.
   b. Monitor the pouch system for proper fit and signs of leakage; empty the pouch when one-third full.
   c. Monitor the stoma for size, unusual bleeding, color changes, or necrotic tissue.
   d. Note that the normal stoma color is red or pink, indicating high vascularity.
   e. Note that a pale pink stoma indicates low hemoglobin and hematocrit levels.
   f. Assess the functioning of the colostomy.
   g. Expect that stool will be liquid postoperatively but will become more solid, depending on the area of the colostomy.
   h. Expect liquid stool from an ascending colon colostomy, loose to semiformed stool from a transverse colon colostomy, or close to normal stool from a descending colon colostomy.
   i. Fecal matter should not be allowed to remain on the skin.
   j. Administer analgesics and antibiotics as prescribed.
   k. Irrigate perineal wound if present and if prescribed, and monitor for signs of infection; provide comfort measures for perineal itching and pain.
   l. Instruct the client to avoid foods that cause excessive gas formation and odor.
   m. Instruct the client in stoma care and irrigations as prescribed.
   n. Instruct the client on when to resume normal activities, including work, travel, and sexual intercourse, as prescribed; provide psychosocial support.

3. Postoperative: Ileostomy
   a. Healthy stoma is red in color.
   b. Postoperative drainage will be dark green and progress to yellow as the client begins to eat.
   c. Stool is liquid.
   d. Risk for dehydration and electrolyte imbalance exists.

Monitor stoma color. A dark blue, purple, or black stoma indicates compromised circulation, requiring surgeon notification.

XXI. Lung Cancer

A. Description
   1. Lung cancer is a malignant tumor of the bronchi and peripheral lung tissue.
   2. The lungs are a common target for metastasis from other organs.
   3. Bronchogenic cancer (tumors originate in the epithelium of the bronchus) spreads through direct extension and lymphatic dissemination.
   4. Classified according to histological cell type; types include small cell lung cancer (SCLC) and non–small cell lung cancer (NSCLC); epidermal (squamous cell), adenocarcinoma, and large cell anaplastic carcinoma are classified as NSCLC because of their similar responses to treatment.
   5. Diagnosis is made by a chest x-ray study, CT and PET scan, or magnetic resonance imaging (MRI), which shows a lesion or mass, and by bronchoscopy and sputum studies, which demonstrate a positive cytological study for cancer cells.

B. Causes
   1. Cigarette smoking; also exposure to "passive" tobacco smoke
   2. Exposure to environmental and occupational pollutants

C. Assessment
   1. Cough
   2. Wheezing, dyspnea
   3. Hoarseness
   4. Hemoptysis, blood-tinged or purulent sputum
   5. Chest pain
   6. Anorexia and weight loss
   7. Weakness
   8. Diminished or absent breath sounds, respiratory changes

D. Interventions
   1. Monitor vital signs.
   2. Monitor breathing patterns and breath sounds and for signs of respiratory impairment; monitor for hemoptysis.
   3. Assess for tracheal deviation.
   4. Administer analgesics as prescribed for pain management.
   5. Place in a Fowler's position to help ease breathing.
   6. Administer oxygen as prescribed and humidification to moisten and loosen secretions.
   7. Monitor pulse oximetry.
   8. Provide respiratory treatments as prescribed.
   9. Administer bronchodilators and corticosteroids as prescribed to decrease bronchospasm, inflammation, and edema.
   10. Provide a high-calorie, high-protein, high-vitamin diet.
   11. Provide activity as tolerated, rest periods, and active and passive range-of-motion exercises.

E. Nonsurgical interventions
   1. Radiation therapy may be prescribed for localized intrathoracic lung cancer and for palliation of hemoptysis, obstructions, dysphagia, superior vena cava syndrome, and pain.
   2. Chemotherapy may be prescribed for treatment of nonresectable tumors or as adjuvant therapy.

F. Surgical interventions
   1. Laser therapy: To relieve endobronchial obstruction
   2. Thoracentesis and pleurodesis: To remove pleural fluid and relieve hypoxia
   3. Thoracotomy (opening into the thoracic cavity) with pneumonectomy: Surgical removal of 1 entire lung
   4. Thoracotomy with lobectomy: Surgical removal of 1 lobe of the lung for tumors confined to a single lobe
   5. Thoracotomy with segmental resection: Surgical removal of a lobe segment

G. Preoperative interventions
   1. Explain the potential postoperative need for chest tubes.
   2. Note that closed chest drainage usually is not used for a pneumonectomy, and the serous fluid that accumulates in the empty thoracic cavity eventually consolidates, preventing shifts of the mediastinum, heart, and remaining lung.

H. Postoperative interventions
   1. Monitor vital signs.
   2. Assess cardiac and respiratory status; monitor lung sounds.
   3. Maintain the chest tube drainage system, which drains air and blood that accumulates in the pleural space; monitor for excess bleeding. (See Chapter 69 for care of the client with a chest tube.)
   4. Administer oxygen as prescribed.
   5. Check the surgeon's prescriptions regarding client positioning; avoid complete lateral turning.
   6. Monitor pulse oximetry.
   7. Provide activity as tolerated.
   8. Encourage active range-of-motion exercises of the operative shoulder as prescribed.

The airway is the priority for a client with lung or laryngeal cancer.

XXII. Laryngeal Cancer

A. Description

1. Laryngeal cancer is a malignant tumor of the larynx (Fig. 44-5).
2. Laryngeal cancer presents as malignant ulcerations with underlying infiltration and is spread by local extension to adjacent structures in the throat and neck and by the lymphatic system.
3. Diagnosis is made by laryngoscopy and biopsy showing a positive cytological study for cancer cells.
4. Laryngoscopy allows for evaluation of the throat and biopsy of tissues; chest radiography, CT, and MRI are used for staging.

B. Risk factors

1. Cigarette smoking
2. Heavy alcohol use and the combined use of tobacco and alcohol
3. Exposure to environmental pollutants (e.g., asbestos, wood dust)
4. Exposure to radiation

C. Assessment

1. Persistent hoarseness or sore throat and ear pain
2. Painless neck mass
3. Feeling of a lump in the throat
4. Burning sensation in the throat
5. Dysphagia
6. Change in voice quality
7. Dyspnea
8. Weakness and weight loss
9. Hemoptysis
10. Foul breath odor

D. Interventions

1. Place in Fowler's position to promote optimal air exchange.
2. Monitor respiratory status.

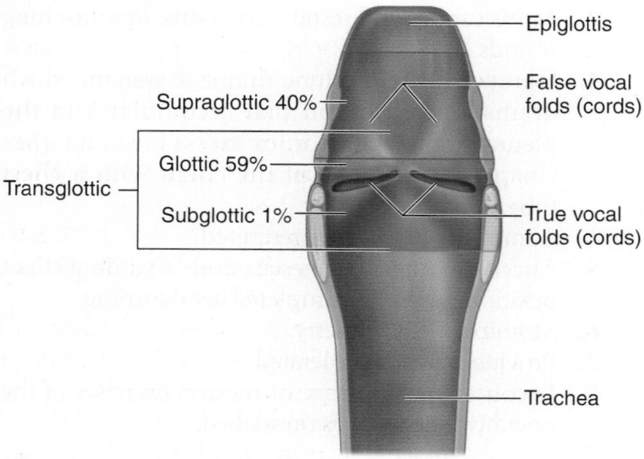

FIG. 44-5 Sites and incidence of primary laryngeal tumors.

3. Monitor for signs of aspiration of food and fluid.
4. Administer oxygen as prescribed.
5. Provide respiratory treatments as prescribed.
6. Provide activity as tolerated.
7. Provide a high-calorie and high-protein diet.
8. Provide nutritional support via parenteral nutrition, nasogastric tube feedings, or gastrostomy or jejunostomy tube, as prescribed.
9. Administer analgesics as prescribed for pain.
10. Encourage clients to stop smoking and drinking alcohol to increase effectiveness of treatments.

E. Nonsurgical interventions

1. Radiation therapy in specified situations
2. Chemotherapy, which may be given in combination with radiation and surgery

F. Surgical interventions

1. The goal is to remove the cancer while preserving as much normal function as possible.
2. Surgical intervention depends on the tumor size, location, and amount of tissue to be resected.
3. Types of resection include cordal stripping, cordectomy, partial laryngectomy, and total laryngectomy.
4. A tracheostomy is performed with a total laryngectomy; this airway opening is permanent and is referred to as a *laryngectomy stoma*.

G. Preoperative interventions

1. Discuss self-care of the airway, alternative methods of communication, suctioning, pain control methods, the critical care environment, and nutritional support.
2. Encourage the client to express feelings about changes in body image and loss of voice.
3. Describe the rehabilitation program and information about the tracheostomy and suctioning.

H. Postoperative interventions

1. Monitor vital signs.
2. Monitor respiratory status; monitor airway patency and provide frequent suctioning to remove bloody secretions.
3. Place the client in a high-Fowler's position.
4. Maintain mechanical ventilator support or a tracheostomy collar with humidification, as prescribed.
5. Monitor pulse oximetry.
6. Maintain surgical drains in the neck area if present.
7. Observe for hemorrhage and edema in the neck.
8. Monitor IV fluids or parenteral nutrition until nutrition is administered via a nasogastric, gastrostomy, or jejunostomy tube.
9. Provide oral hygiene.
10. Assess gag and cough reflexes and the ability to swallow.
11. Increase activity as tolerated.

12. Assess the color, amount, and consistency of sputum.
13. Provide stoma and laryngectomy care (Box 44-15).
14. Provide consultation with speech and language pathologist as prescribed.
15. Reinforce method of communication established preoperatively.
16. Prepare the client for rehabilitation and speech therapy (Box 44-16).

BOX 44-15 Stoma Care Following Laryngectomy

- Protect the neck from injury.
- Instruct the client in how to clean the incision and provide stoma care.
- Instruct the client to wear a stoma guard to shield the stoma.
- Demonstrate ways to prevent debris from entering the stoma.
- Advise the client to wear loose-fitting, high-collared clothing to cover the stoma.
- Avoid swimming, showering, and using aerosol sprays.
- Teach the client clean suctioning technique.
- Advise the client to increase humidity in the home.
- Increase fluid intake to 3000 mL/day as prescribed.
- Avoid exposure to persons with infections.
- Alternate rest periods with activity.
- Instruct the client in range-of-motion exercises for the arms, shoulders, and neck as prescribed.
- Advise the client to wear a MedicAlert bracelet.

BOX 44-16 Speech Rehabilitation Following Laryngectomy

Esophageal Speech

- The client produces esophageal speech by "burping" the air swallowed.
- The voice produced is monotone, cannot be raised or lowered, and carries no pitch.
- The client must have adequate hearing because his or her mouth shapes words as they are heard.

Mechanical Devices

- One device, the electrolarynx, is placed against the side of the neck; the air inside the neck and pharynx is vibrated, and the client articulates.
- Another device consists of a plastic tube that is placed inside the client's mouth and vibrates on articulation.

Tracheoesophageal Fistula

- A fistula is created surgically between the trachea and the esophagus, with eventual placement of a prosthesis to produce speech.
- The prosthesis provides the client with a means to divert air from the trachea into the esophagus, and out of the mouth.
- Lip and tongue movement produce the speech.

XXIII. Prostate Cancer

A. Description
1. Prostate cancer, a slow-growing malignancy of the prostate gland, is a common cancer in American men; most prostate tumors are adenocarcinomas arising from androgen-dependent epithelial cells.
2. The risk increases in men with each decade after the age of 50 years.
3. Prostate cancer can spread via direct invasion of surrounding tissues or by metastasis through the bloodstream and lymphatics, to the bony pelvis and spine.
4. Bone metastasis is a concern, as is spread to the lungs, liver, and kidneys.
5. The cause of prostate cancer is unclear, but advancing age, heavy metal exposure, smoking, and history of sexually transmitted infection are contributing factors; it is more common among men of African American descent.

B. Assessment
1. Asymptomatic in early stages
2. Hard, pea-sized nodule or irregularities palpated on rectal examination
3. Gross, painless hematuria
4. Late symptoms such as weight loss, urinary obstruction, and bone pain radiating from the lumbosacral area down the leg
5. The prostate-specific antigen level is elevated in various noncancerous conditions; therefore, it should not be used as a screening test without a digital rectal examination. It is routinely used to monitor response to therapy.
6. Diagnosis is made through biopsy of the prostate gland.

C. Nonsurgical interventions
1. Prepare the client for hormone manipulation therapy (androgen suppression therapy) as prescribed or active surveillance with prostate-specific antigen (PSA) and digital rectal examination (DRE).
2. Luteinizing hormone may be prescribed to slow the rate of growth of the tumor.
3. Medication adverse effects include reduced libido, hot flashes, breast tenderness, osteoporosis, loss of muscle mass, and weight gain. The client should be informed of these effects.
4. Pain medication, radiation therapy, corticosteroids, and bisphosphonates may be prescribed for palliation of advanced prostate cancer.
5. Prepare the client for external beam radiation or brachytherapy, which may be prescribed alone or with surgery, preoperatively or postoperatively, to reduce the lesion and limit metastasis.
6. Prepare the client for the administration of chemotherapy in cases of hormone treatment resistant tumors.

D. Surgical interventions
  1. Prepare the client for orchiectomy (palliative), if prescribed, which will limit the production of testosterone.
  2. Prepare the client for prostatectomy, if prescribed.
  3. The radical prostatectomy can be performed via a retropubic, perineal, or suprapubic approach.
  4. Cryosurgical ablation is a minimally invasive procedure that may be an alternative to radical prostatectomy; liquid nitrogen freezes the gland, and the dead cells are absorbed by the body.

E. Transurethral resection of the prostate (TURP) may be performed for palliation in prostate cancer clients.
  1. The procedure involves insertion of a scope into the urethra to excise prostatic tissue.
  2. Monitor for hemorrhage; bleeding is common following TURP.
  3. Postoperative continuous bladder irrigation (CBI) may be prescribed, which prevents catheter obstruction from clots.
  4. Assess for signs of transurethral resection syndrome, which include signs of cerebral edema and increased intracranial pressure, such as increased blood pressure, bradycardia, confusion, disorientation, muscle twitching, visual disturbances, and nausea and vomiting.
  5. Antispasmodics may be prescribed for bladder spasm.
  6. Instruct the client to monitor and report dribbling or incontinence postoperatively and teach perineal exercises.
  7. Sterility is possible following the surgical procedure.

F. Suprapubic prostatectomy
  1. Suprapubic prostatectomy is removal of the prostate gland by an abdominal incision with a bladder incision.
  2. The client will have an abdominal dressing that may drain copious amounts of urine, and the abdominal dressing will need to be changed frequently.
  3. Severe hemorrhage is possible, and monitoring for blood loss is an important nursing intervention.
  4. Antispasmodics may be prescribed for bladder spasms.
  5. CBI is prescribed and carried out to maintain pink-colored urine.
  6. Sterility occurs with this procedure.

G. Retropubic prostatectomy
  1. Retropubic prostatectomy is removal of the prostate gland by a low abdominal incision without opening the bladder.
  2. Less bleeding occurs with this procedure compared with the suprapubic procedure, and the client experiences fewer bladder spasms.
  3. Abdominal drainage is minimal.
  4. CBI may be used.
  5. Sterility occurs with this procedure.

H. Perineal prostatectomy
  1. The prostate gland is removed through an incision made between the scrotum and anus.
  2. Minimal bleeding occurs with this procedure.
  3. The client needs to be monitored closely for infection, because the risk of infection is increased with this type of prostatectomy.
  4. Urinary incontinence is common.
  5. The procedure causes sterility.
  6. Teach the client how to perform perineal exercises.

I. Postoperative interventions
  1. Monitor vital signs.
  2. Monitor urinary output and urine for hemorrhage or clots.
  3. Increase fluids to 2400 to 3000 mL/day, unless contraindicated.
  4. Monitor for arterial bleeding as evidenced by bright red urine with numerous clots; if it occurs, increase CBI and notify the surgeon immediately.
  5. Monitor for venous bleeding as evidenced by burgundy-colored urine output; if it occurs, inform the surgeon, who may apply traction on the catheter.
  6. Monitor hemoglobin and hematocrit levels.
  7. Expect red to light pink urine for 24 hours, turning to amber in 3 days.
  8. Ambulate the client as early as possible and as soon as urine begins to clear in color.
  9. Inform the client that a continuous feeling of an urge to void is normal.
  10. Instruct the client to avoid attempts to void around the catheter, because this will cause bladder spasms.
  11. Administer antibiotics, analgesics, stool softeners, and antispasmodics as prescribed.
  12. Monitor the 3-way urinary catheter, which usually has a 30- to 45-mL retention balloon.
  13. Maintain CBI with sterile bladder irrigation solution as prescribed to keep the catheter free of obstruction and keep the urine pink in color (Box 44-17).

Following TURP, monitor for transurethral resection syndrome or severe hyponatremia (water intoxication) caused by the excessive absorption of bladder irrigation during surgery. (Signs include altered mental status, bradycardia, increased blood pressure, and confusion.)

J. Postoperative interventions: Suprapubic prostatectomy
  1. Monitor suprapubic and urinary catheter drainage.
  2. Monitor CBI if prescribed.

BOX 44-17 Continuous Bladder Irrigation (CBI)

Description

- A 3-way (lumen) irrigation is used to decrease bleeding and to keep the bladder free from clots—1 lumen is for inflating the balloon (30 mL); 1 lumen is for instillation (inflow); 1 lumen is for outflow.

Interventions

- Maintain traction on the catheter, if applied and prescribed, to prevent bleeding by pulling the catheter taut and taping it to the abdomen or thigh.
- Instruct the client to keep the leg straight if traction is applied to the catheter and taped to the thigh.
- Catheter traction is not released without the surgeon's prescription; it usually is released after any bright red drainage has diminished.
- Use only sterile bladder irrigation solution or prescribed solution to prevent water intoxication.
- Run the solution at a rate, as prescribed, to keep the urine pink. Run the solution rapidly if bright red drainage or clots are present; monitor output closely. Run the solution at about 40 drops (gtt)/minute when the bright red drainage clears.
- If the urinary catheter becomes obstructed, turn off the CBI and irrigate the catheter with 30 to 50 mL of normal saline, if prescribed; notify the surgeon if obstruction does not resolve.
- Discontinue CBI and the urinary catheter as prescribed, usually 24 to 48 hours after surgery.
- Monitor for continence and urinary retention when the catheter is removed. Inform the client that some burning, frequency, and dribbling may occur following catheter removal.
- Inform the client that he should be voiding 150 to 200 mL of clear yellow urine every 3 to 4 hours by 3 days after surgery.
- Inform the client that he may pass small clots and tissue debris for several days.
- Teach the client to avoid heavy lifting, stressful exercise, driving, the Valsalva maneuver, and sexual intercourse for 2 to 6 weeks to prevent strain, and to call the surgeon if bleeding occurs or if there is a decrease in urinary stream.
- Instruct the client to drink 2400 to 3000 mL of fluid each day, preferably before 8 p.m., to avoid nocturia.
- Instruct the client to avoid alcohol, caffeinated beverages, and spicy foods and overstimulation of the bladder.
- Instruct the client that if the urine becomes bloody, to rest and increase fluid intake and, if the bleeding does not subside, to notify the surgeon.

3. Note that the urinary catheter will be removed 2 to 4 days postoperatively if the client has a suprapubic catheter.
4. If prescribed, clamp the suprapubic catheter after the urinary catheter is removed, and instruct the client to attempt to void; after the client has voided, assess the residual urine in the bladder by unclamping the suprapubic catheter and measuring the output.
5. Prepare for removal of the suprapubic catheter when the client consistently empties the bladder and residual urine is 75 mL or lessor as prescribed.
6. Monitor the suprapubic incision dressing, which may become saturated with urine, until the incision heals; dressing may need to be changed frequently.

K. Postoperative interventions: Retropubic prostatectomy
1. Note that because the bladder is not entered, there is no urinary drainage on the abdominal dressing; if urinary or purulent drainage is noted on the dressing, notify the surgeon.
2. Monitor for fever and increased pain, which may indicate an infection.

L. Postoperative interventions: Perineal prostatectomy
1. Note that the client will have an incision, which may or may not have a drain.
2. Avoid the use of rectal thermometers, rectal tubes, and enemas, because they may cause trauma and bleeding.

XXIV. Bladder Cancer

A. Description
1. Bladder cancer is a papillomatous growth in the bladder urothelium that undergoes malignant changes and that may infiltrate the bladder wall.
2. Predisposing factors include cigarette smoking, exposure to industrial chemicals, and exposure to radiation.
3. Common sites of metastasis include the liver, bones, and lungs.
4. As the tumor progresses, it can extend into the rectum, vagina, other pelvic soft tissues, and retroperitoneal structures.

B. Assessment
1. Gross or microscopic, painless hematuria (most common sign)
2. Frequency, urgency, dysuria
3. Clot-induced obstruction
4. Bladder wash specimens and biopsy confirm diagnosis

C. Radiation
1. Radiation therapy is indicated for advanced disease that cannot be eradicated by surgery; palliative radiation may be used to relieve pain and bowel obstruction and control potential hemorrhage and leg edema caused by venous or lymphatic obstruction.
2. Intracavitary radiation may be prescribed, which protects adjacent tissue.
3. External beam radiation combined with chemotherapy or surgery may be prescribed to improve survival.
4. Complications of radiation
   a. Abacterial cystitis
   b. Proctitis

c. Fistula formation
d. Ileitis or colitis
e. Bladder ulceration and hemorrhage

D. Chemotherapy
1. Intravesical instillation
a. An alkylating chemotherapeutic agent is instilled into the bladder.
b. This method provides a concentrated topical treatment with little systemic absorption.
c. The medication is injected into a urethral catheter and retained for 2 hours.
d. Following instillation, the client's position is rotated every 15 to 30 minutes, starting in the supine position, to avoid lying on a full bladder.
e. After 2 hours, the client voids in a sitting position and is instructed to increase fluids to flush the bladder.
f. Treat the urine as a biohazard and send to the radioisotope laboratory for monitoring.
g. For 6 hours following intravesical chemotherapy, disinfect the toilet with household bleach after the client has voided.
2. Systemic chemotherapy: Used to treat inoperable tumors or distant metastasis.
3. Complications of chemotherapy
a. Bladder irritation
b. Hemorrhagic cystitis

E. Surgical interventions
1. Transurethral resection of bladder tumor
a. Local resection and fulguration (destruction of tissue by electrical current through electrodes placed in direct contact with the tissue)
b. Performed for early tumors for cure or for inoperable tumors for palliation
2. Partial cystectomy
a. Partial cystectomy is the removal of up to half the bladder.
b. The procedure is done for early-stage tumors and for clients who cannot tolerate a radical cystectomy.
c. During the initial postoperative period, bladder capacity is reduced greatly to about 60 mL; however, as the bladder tissue expands, the capacity increases to 200 to 400 mL.
d. Maintenance of a continuous output of urine following surgery is critical to prevent bladder distention and stress on the suture line.
e. A urethral catheter and a suprapubic catheter may be in place, and the suprapubic catheter may be left in place for 2 weeks until healing occurs.
3. Cystectomy and urinary diversion (Fig. 44-6)
a. Various surgical procedures are performed to create alternative pathways for urine collection and excretion.
b. Urinary diversion may be performed with or without cystectomy (bladder removal).
c. The surgery may be performed in 2 stages if the tumor is extensive, with the creation of the urinary diversion first and the cystectomy several weeks later.
d. If a radical cystectomy is performed, lower extremity lymphedema may occur as a result of lymph node dissection, and male impotence may occur.
4. Ileal conduit
a. The ileal conduit is also called a *ureteroileostomy,* or Bricker's procedure.
b. Ureters are implanted into a segment of the ileum, with the formation of an abdominal stoma.
c. The urine flows into the conduit and is propelled continuously out through the stoma by peristalsis.
d. The client is required to wear an appliance over the stoma to collect the urine (Box 44-18).
e. Complications include obstruction, pyelonephritis, leakage at the anastomosis site, stenosis, hydronephrosis, calculi, skin irritation and ulceration, and stomal defects.
5. Kock pouch
a. The Kock pouch is a continent internal ileal reservoir created from a segment of the ileum and ascending colon.
b. The ureters are implanted into the side of the reservoir, and a special nipple valve is constructed to attach the reservoir to the skin.
c. Postoperatively, the client will have a urinary catheter in place to drain urine continuously until the pouch has healed.
d. The urinary catheter is irrigated gently with normal saline to prevent obstruction from mucus or clots.
e. Following removal of the urinary catheter, the client is instructed in how to self-catheterize and to drain the reservoir at 4- to 6-hour intervals (Box 44-19).
6. Indiana pouch
a. A continent reservoir is created from the ascending colon and terminal ileum, making a pouch larger than the Kock pouch (additional continent reservoirs include the Mainz and Florida pouch systems).
b. Postoperatively, care is similar to that for the Kock pouch.
7. Creation of a neobladder
a. Creation of a neobladder is similar to creation of an internal reservoir, with the difference being that instead of emptying through an abdominal stoma, the bladder empties through a pelvic outlet into the urethra.

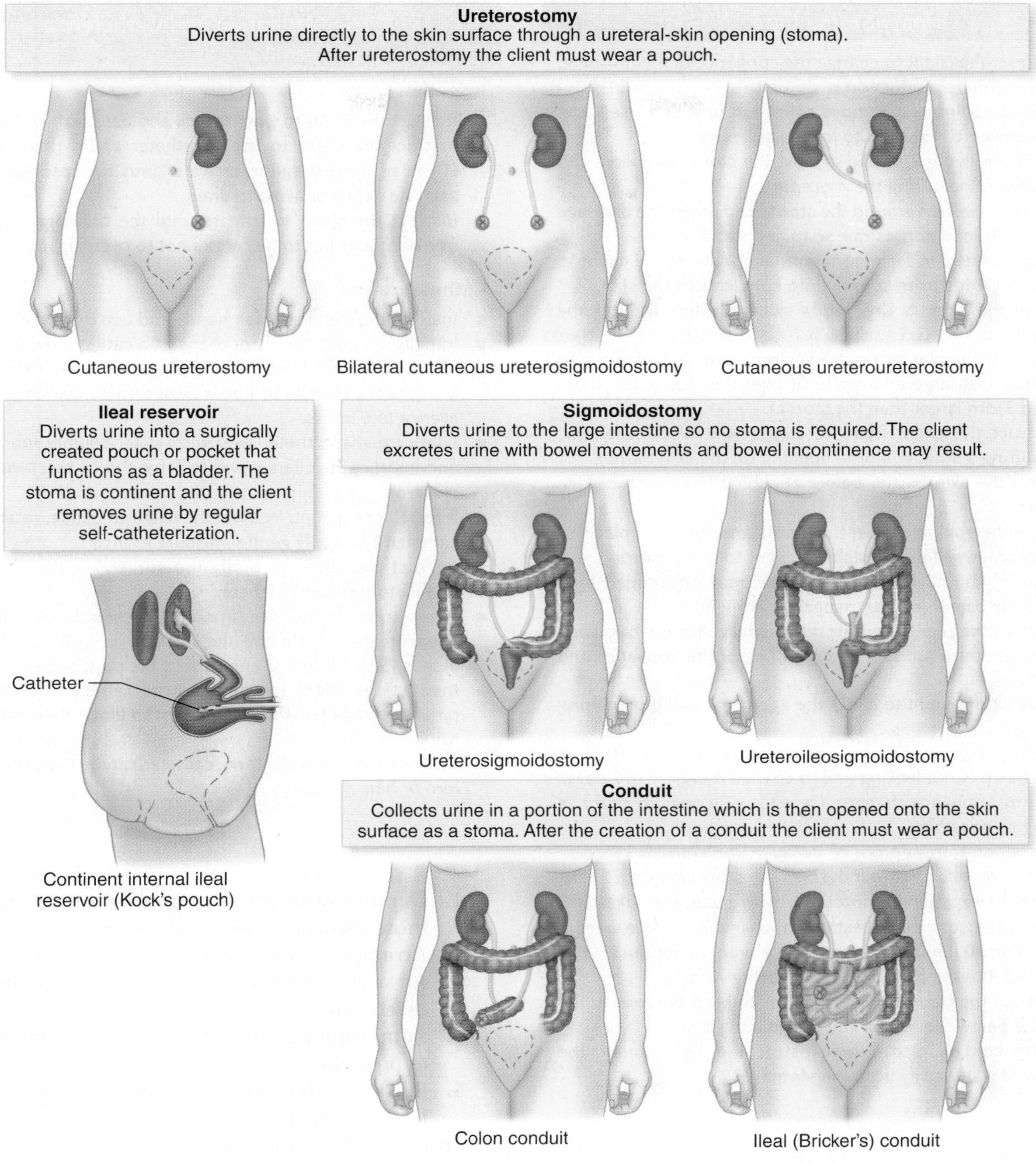
Ureterostomy
Diverts urine directly to the skin surface through a ureteral-skin opening (stoma). After ureterostomy the client must wear a pouch.
Cutaneous ureterostomy
Bilateral cutaneous ureterosigmoidostomy
Cutaneous ureteroureterostomy
Ileal reservoir
Diverts urine into a surgically created pouch or pocket that functions as a bladder. The stoma is continent and the client removes urine by regular self-catheterization.
Catheter
Continent internal ileal reservoir (Kock's pouch)
Sigmoidostomy
Diverts urine to the large intestine so no stoma is required. The client excretes urine with bowel movements and bowel incontinence may result.
Ureterosigmoidostomy
Ureteroileosigmoidostomy
Conduit
Collects urine in a portion of the intestine which is then opened onto the skin surface as a stoma. After the creation of a conduit the client must wear a pouch.
Colon conduit
Ileal (Bricker's) conduit

FIG. 44-6 Urinary diversion procedures used in the treatment of bladder cancer.

b. The client empties the neobladder by relaxing the external sphincter and creating abdominal pressure or by intermittent self-catheterization.

8. Percutaneous nephrostomy or pyelostomy

a. These procedures are used to prevent or treat obstruction.

b. The procedures involve a percutaneous or surgical insertion of a nephrostomy tube into the kidney for drainage.

c. Nursing interventions involve stabilizing the tube to prevent dislodgment and monitoring output.

9. Ureterostomy

a. Ureterostomy may be performed as a palliative procedure if the ureters are obstructed by the tumor.

b. The ureters are attached to the surface of the abdomen, where the urine flows directly into a drainage appliance without a conduit.

BOX 44-18 Urinary Stoma Care

- Instruct the client to change the appliance in the morning, when urinary production is slowest.
- Collect equipment, remove collection bag, and use water or commercial solvent to loosen adhesive.
- Hold a rolled gauze pad against the stoma to collect and absorb urine during the procedure.
- Cleanse the skin around the stoma and under the drainage bag with mild nonresidue soap and water.
- Inspect the skin for excoriation, and instruct the client to prevent urine from coming into contact with the skin.
- After the skin is dry, apply skin adhesive around the appliance.
- Instruct the client to cut the stoma opening of the skin barrier just large enough to fit over the stoma (no more than 3 mm larger than the stoma).
- Instruct the client that the stoma will begin to shrink, requiring a smaller stoma opening on the skin barrier.
- Apply the skin barrier before attaching the pouch or face plate.
- Place the appliance over the stoma and secure in place.
- Encourage self-care; teach the client to use a mirror.
- Instruct the client that the pouch may be drained by a bedside bag or leg bag, especially at night.
- Instruct the client to empty the urinary collection bag when it is one-third full to prevent pulling of the appliance and leakage.
- Instruct the client to check the appliance seal if perspiring occurs.
- Instruct the client to leave the urinary pouch in place as long as it is not leaking and to change it every 5 to 7 days.
- During appliance changes, leave the skin open to air for as long as possible.
- Use a non–karaya product, because urine erodes karaya.
- To control odor, instruct the client to drink adequate fluids, wash the appliance thoroughly with soap and lukewarm water, and soak the collection pouch in dilute white vinegar for 20 to 30 minutes; a special deodorant tablet can also be placed into the pouch while it is being worn.
- Instruct the client who takes baths to keep the level of the water below the stoma and to avoid oily soaps.
- If the client plans to shower, instruct the client to direct the flow of water away from the stoma.

c. Potential problems include infection, skin irritation, and obstruction to urinary flow as a result of strictures at the opening.

10. Vesicostomy
    a. The bladder is sutured to the abdomen, and a stoma is created in the bladder wall.
    b. The bladder empties through the stoma.

F. Preoperative interventions

1. Instruct the client in preoperative, operative, and postoperative management, including diet, medications, nasogastric tube placement, IV lines, NPO status, pain control, coughing and deep breathing, leg exercises, and postoperative activity.

BOX 44-19 Self-Irrigation and Catheterization of Stoma

Irrigation

- Instruct the client to wash hands and use clean technique.
- Instruct the client to use a catheter and syringe, instill 60 mL of normal saline or water into the reservoir, and aspirate gently or allow to drain.
- Instruct the client to irrigate until the drainage remains free of mucus but to be careful not to overirrigate.

Catheterization

- Instruct the client to wash hands and use clean technique.
- Initially, instruct the client to insert a catheter every 2 to 3 hours to drain the reservoir; during each week thereafter, increase the interval by 1 hour until catheterization is done every 4 to 6 hours.
- Lubricate the catheter well with water-soluble lubricant, and instruct the client never to force the catheter into the reservoir.
- If resistance is met, instruct the client to pause, rotate the catheter, and apply gentle pressure to insert.
- Instruct the client to notify the surgeon if the client is unable to insert the catheter.
- When urine has stopped, instruct the client to take several deep breaths and move the catheter in and out 2 to 3 inches (5 to 7.5 cm) to ensure that the pouch is empty.
- Instruct the client to withdraw the catheter slowly and pinch the catheter when withdrawn so that it does not leak urine.
- Instruct the client to carry catheterization supplies with him or her.

2. Demonstrate appliance application and use for those clients who will have a stoma.
3. Arrange an enterostomal nurse consult and for a visit with a person who has had urinary diversion.
4. Administer antimicrobials for bowel preparation as prescribed.
5. Encourage discussion of feelings, including the effects on sexual activities.

G. Postoperative interventions

Monitor urinary output closely following bladder surgery. Irrigate the ureteral catheter (if present and if prescribed) gently to prevent obstruction. Follow the surgeon's prescriptions and agency policy regarding irrigation.

1. Monitor vital signs.
2. Assess incision site.
3. Assess stoma (should be red and moist) every hour for the first 24 hours.
4. Monitor for edema in the stoma, which may be present in the immediate postoperative period.
5. Notify the surgeon if the stoma appears dark and dusky (indicates necrosis).
6. Monitor for prolapse or retraction of the stoma.

7. Assess bowel function; monitor for expected return of peristalsis in 3 to 4 days.
8. Maintain NPO status as prescribed until bowel sounds return.
9. Monitor for continuous urine flow (30 to 60 mL/hr).
10. Notify the surgeon if the urine output is less than 30 mL/hr or if no urine output occurs for more than 15 minutes.
11. Ureteral stents or catheters, if present, may be in place for 2 to 3 weeks or until healing occurs; maintain stability with catheters to prevent dislodgment.
12. Monitor for hematuria.
13. Monitor for signs of peritonitis.
14. Monitor for bladder distention following a partial cystectomy.
15. Monitor for shock, hemorrhage, thrombophlebitis, and lower extremity lymphedema after a radical cystectomy.
16. Monitor the urinary drainage pouch for leaks, and check skin integrity (see Box 44-18).
17. Monitor the pH of the urine (do not place the dipstick in the stoma), because highly alkaline or acidic urine can cause skin irritation and facilitate crystal formation.
18. Instruct the client regarding the potential for urinary tract infection or the development of calculi.
19. Instruct the client to assess the skin for irritation, monitor the urinary drainage pouch, and report any leakage.
20. Encourage the client to express feelings about changes in body image, embarrassment, and sexual dysfunction.

XXV. Oncological Emergencies

A. Sepsis and disseminated intravascular coagulation (DIC)
1. Description: The client with cancer is at increased risk for infection, particularly gram-negative organisms, in the bloodstream (sepsis or septicemia) and DIC, a life-threatening problem frequently associated with sepsis.
2. Interventions
   a. Prevent the complication through early identification of clients at high risk for sepsis and DIC.
   b. Maintain strict aseptic technique with the immunocompromised client and monitor closely for infection and signs of bleeding.
   c. Administer antibiotics intravenously as prescribed.
   d. Administer anticoagulants as prescribed during the early phase of DIC.
   e. Administer cryoprecipitated clotting factors, as prescribed, when DIC progresses and hemorrhage is the primary problem.

Notify the PHCP immediately if signs of an oncological emergency occur.

B. Syndrome of inappropriate antidiuretic hormone (SIADH)
1. Description
   a. Tumors can produce, secrete, or stimulate substances that mimic antidiuretic hormone.
   b. Mild symptoms include weakness, muscle cramps, loss of appetite, and fatigue; serum sodium levels range from 115 to 120 mEq/L (115 to 120 mmol/L).
   c. More serious signs and symptoms relate to water intoxication and include weight gain, personality changes, confusion, and extreme muscle weakness.
   d. As the serum sodium level approaches 110 mEq/L (110 mmol/L), seizures, coma, and eventually death will occur, unless the condition is treated rapidly.
2. Interventions
   a. Initiate fluid restriction and increased sodium intake as prescribed.
   b. As prescribed, administer an antagonist to antidiuretic hormone.
   c. Monitor serum sodium levels.
   d. Treat the underlying cause with chemotherapy or radiation to achieve tumor regression.

C. Spinal cord compression
1. Description
   a. Spinal cord compression occurs when a tumor directly enters the spinal cord or when the vertebral column collapses from tumor entry, impinging on the spinal cord.
   b. Spinal cord compression causes back pain, usually before neurological deficits occur.
   c. Neurological deficits relate to the spinal level of compression and include numbness; tingling; loss of urethral, vaginal, and rectal sensation; and muscle weakness.
2. Interventions
   a. Early recognition: Assess for back pain and neurological deficits.
   b. Administer high-dose corticosteroids to reduce swelling around the spinal cord and relieve symptoms.
   c. Prepare the client for immediate radiation and/or chemotherapy to reduce the size of the tumor and relieve compression.
   d. Surgery may need to be performed to remove the tumor and relieve the pressure on the spinal cord.
   e. Instruct the client in the use of neck or back braces if they are prescribed.

D. Hypercalcemia
1. Description

a. Hypercalcemia is a late manifestation of extensive malignancy that occurs most often with bone metastasis, when the bone releases calcium into the bloodstream.
b. Decreased physical mobility contributes to or worsens hypercalcemia.
c. Early signs include fatigue, anorexia, nausea, vomiting, constipation, and polyuria.
d. More serious signs and symptoms include severe muscle weakness, diminished deep tendon reflexes, paralytic ileus, dehydration, and changes in the electrocardiogram.

2. Interventions
a. Monitor serum calcium level and electrocardiographic changes.
b. Administer oral or parenteral fluids as prescribed.
c. Administer medications that lower the calcium level and control nausea and vomiting as prescribed.
d. Prepare the client for dialysis if the condition becomes life-threatening or is accompanied by renal impairment.
e. Encourage walking to prevent breakdown of bone.

E. Superior vena cava syndrome
1. Description
a. Superior vena cava (SVC) syndrome occurs when the SVC is compressed or obstructed by tumor growth (commonly associated with lung cancer and lymphoma).
b. Signs and symptoms result from blockage of blood flow in the venous system of the head, neck, and upper trunk.
c. Early signs and symptoms generally occur in the morning and include edema of the face, especially around the eyes, and tightness of the shirt or blouse collar (Stokes' sign).
d. As the condition worsens, edema in the arms and hands, dyspnea, erythema of the upper body, swelling of the veins in the chest and neck, and epistaxis occur.
e. Life-threatening signs and symptoms include airway obstruction, hemorrhage, cyanosis, mental status changes, decreased cardiac output, and hypotension.

2. Interventions
a. Assess for early signs and symptoms of SVC syndrome.
b. Place the client in semi-Fowler's position and administer corticosteroids and diuretics as prescribed.
c. Prepare the client for high-dose radiation therapy to the mediastinal area and possible surgery to insert a metal stent in the vena cava.

F. Tumor lysis syndrome
1. Description
a. Tumor lysis syndrome occurs when large quantities of tumor cells are destroyed rapidly and intracellular components such as potassium and uric acid are released into the bloodstream faster than the body can eliminate them.
b. Tumor lysis syndrome can indicate that cancer treatment is destroying tumor cells; however, if left untreated, it can cause severe tissue damage and death.
c. Hyperkalemia, hyperphosphatemia with resultant hypocalcemia, and hyperuricemia occur; hyperuricemia can lead to acute kidney injury.

2. Interventions
a. Encourage oral hydration; IV hydration may be prescribed; monitor renal function and intake and output, and ensure that the client is on a renal diet low in potassium and phosphorus.
b. Administer diuretics to increase the urine flow through the kidneys as prescribed.
c. Administer medications that increase the excretion of purines, such as allopurinol, as prescribed.
d. Prepare to administer IV infusion of glucose and insulin to treat hyperkalemia.
e. Prepare the client for dialysis if hyperkalemia and hyperuricemia persist despite treatment.

XXVI. Anemia

A. Description
1. Condition in which the blood lacks adequate healthy red blood cells or hemoglobin, with most common causes being acute blood loss, decreased or faulty red blood cell production, or the destruction of red blood cells.
2. There are several types of anemia, with the main types being anemia related to acute and chronic blood loss, anemia of chronic diseases (including cancers, immunodeficiency syndrome, renal disease, liver diseases, and autoimmune conditions), anemias caused by nutritional deficiencies (such as iron, folate, or vitamin B_{12} deficiency), and hereditary anemias (including sickle cell anemia and thalassemia).
3. Treatment of anemia focuses on treating the cause of the condition and varies based on the type of anemia.
4. Acute blood loss anemia is characterized by normal red blood cell size, shape, and color. Clients at risk include postoperative clients, clients with an active bleeding problem, or

immunocompromised clients with a reduction in blood components. Hemoglobin, hematocrit, or red blood cell levels can be low.

B. Assessment
1. Fatigue
2. Weakness
3. Pallor or slight jaundice if red blood cell destruction occurs
4. Shortness of breath
5. Dysrhythmias
6. Chest pain
7. Tachycardia
8. Cool extremities

C. Interventions
1. Administer blood products and hematopoietic medications as prescribed, which are used to treat anemia related to acute and chronic conditions.
2. Encourage a diet rich in the deficient nutrient if the anemia is caused by malnutrition, such as iron, folate, or vitamin B_{12} supplementation.
3. Control and address the source of bleeding if anemia is caused by acute blood loss and assess client for sources of frank and occult bleeding. Contact the PCHP and prepare for replacement therapy if acute blood loss occurs.

XXVII. Iron Deficiency Anemia

A. Description
1. Iron stores are depleted, resulting in a decreased iron supply for the manufacture of hemoglobin in red blood cells.
2. Commonly results from blood loss, increased metabolic demands, syndromes of gastrointestinal malabsorption, and dietary inadequacy.

B. Assessment
1. Pallor
2. Weakness and fatigue
3. Low hemoglobin, hematocrit, and mean cellular volume (MCV) levels
4. Red blood cells that are microcytic and hypochromic

C. Interventions
1. Increase oral intake of iron and instruct client in food choices that are high in iron (see Box 11-2 in Chapter 11 for iron-rich foods).
2. Administer iron supplements as prescribed.
3. Intramuscular injections of iron (using Z-track method) or IV administration of iron may be prescribed in severe cases of anemia.
4. Teach clients how to administer the iron supplements.
   - **a.** Take between meals for maximum absorption.
   - **b.** Take with a multivitamin or fruit juice, because vitamin C increases absorption.
   - **c.** Do not take with milk or antacids, because these items decrease absorption.
   - **d.** Instruct the client about the side effects of iron supplements (black stools, constipation, and foul aftertaste).
   - **e.** Liquid iron preparations stains the teeth. Teach the client that liquid iron should be taken through a straw and that the teeth should be brushed after administration.

XXVIII. Vitamin B_{12} Deficiency Anemia

A. Description
1. A macrocytic anemia that results from an inadequate intake of vitamin B_{12} or lack of absorption of ingested vitamin B_{12} from the intestinal tract.
2. Pernicious anemia results from a deficiency of intrinsic factor (normally secreted by the gastric mucosa), necessary for intestinal absorption of vitamin B_{12}; gastric disease or surgery can result in a lack of intrinsic factor.

B. Assessment
1. Severe pallor
2. Fatigue
3. Weight loss
4. Smooth, beefy red tongue
5. Slight jaundice
6. Paresthesias of the hands and feet
7. Disturbances with gait and balance

C. Interventions
1. Increase dietary intake of foods rich in vitamin B_{12} such as meats, poultry, fish, shellfish, eggs, dairy products, citrus fruits, dried beans, green leafy vegetables, liver, nuts, and brewer's yeast if the anemia is a result of a dietary deficiency.
2. Administer vitamin B_{12} injections as prescribed, weekly initially and then monthly for maintenance (lifelong) if the anemia is the result of a deficiency of intrinsic factor or disease or surgery of the ileum.

XXIX. Folate Deficiency Anemia

A. Description
1. A macrocytic anemia in which red blood cells are larger than normal and are oval-shaped rather than round-shaped due to the lack of inadequate intake of folate (vitamin B_9).
2. Folic acid is required for DNA synthesis required for red blood cell formation and maturation.
3. Common causes include dietary deficiency; malabsorption syndromes such as Celiac disease, Crohn's disease, or small bowel resection; medications (such as antiseizure medications) that decrease the absorption of folic acid, a condition (including pregnancy) that increases the requirement of folic acid; chronic alcoholism; and chronic hemodialysis.

B. Assessment
1. Dyspepsia
2. Smooth, beefy red tongue
3. Pallor, fatigue and weakness
4. Tinnitus
5. Tachycardia

C. Interventions
1. Encourage the client to eat foods rich in folic acid, such as green leafy vegetables, meat, liver, fish, legumes, peanuts, orange juice, and avocado.
2. Administer folic acid as prescribed.

XXX. Sickle Cell Anemia: See Chapter 30 for more information regarding sickle cell anemia

XXXI. Thalassemia: See Chapter 30 for more information regarding thalassemia

XXXII. Aplastic Anemia

A. Description
1. Aplastic anemia is a deficiency of circulating erythrocytes and all other formed elements of blood, resulting from the arrested development of cells within the bone marrow.
2. It can be primary (present at birth) or secondary (acquired).
3. Several possible causes exist, including chronic exposure to myelotoxic agents, viruses and infections such as hepatitis, Epstein-Barr virus, autoimmune disorders such as human immunodeficiency virus, and allergic states.
4. The definitive diagnosis is determined by bone marrow aspiration (shows conversion of red bone marrow to fatty bone marrow).
5. Therapeutic management focuses on restoring function to the bone marrow and involves immunosuppressive therapy and bone marrow transplantation (treatment of choice if a suitable donor exists).
6. If the cause is a myelotoxic medication that is being administered for another purpose, the medication may be discontinued to improve bone marrow function.

B. Assessment
1. Pancytopenia (deficiency of erythrocytes, leukocytes, and thrombocytes)
2. Petechiae, purpura, bleeding, pallor, weakness, tachycardia, and fatigue

C. Interventions
1. Prepare the client for bone marrow transplantation if planned.
2. Administer immunosuppressive medications as prescribed; antilymphocyte globulin or antithymocyte globulin may be prescribed to suppress the autoimmune response.
3. Colony-stimulating factors may be prescribed to enhance bone marrow production.
4. Corticosteroids and cyclosporine may be prescribed.
5. Administer blood transfusions if prescribed and monitor for transfusion reactions.

PRACTICE QUESTIONS

443. The nurse is reviewing the laboratory results of a client diagnosed with multiple myeloma. Which would the nurse expect to note specifically in this disorder?
1. Increased calcium level
2. Increased white blood cells
3. Decreased blood urea nitrogen level
4. Decreased number of plasma cells in the bone marrow

444. The nurse is creating a plan of care for the client with multiple myeloma and includes which **priority** intervention in the plan?
1. Encouraging fluids
2. Providing frequent oral care
3. Coughing and deep breathing
4. Monitoring the red blood cell count

445. When caring for a client with an internal radiation implant, the nurse should observe which principles? **Select all that apply.**
1. Limiting the time with the client to 1 hour per shift.
2. Keeping pregnant women out of the client's room.
3. Placing the client in a private room with a private bath.
4. Wearing a lead shield when providing direct client care.
5. Removing the dosimeter film badge when entering the client's room.
6. Allowing individuals younger than 16 years old in the room as long as they are 6 feet away from the client.

446. While giving care to a client with an internal cervical radiation implant, the nurse finds the implant in the bed. The nurse should take which **initial** action?
1. Call the primary health care provider (PHCP).
2. Reinsert the implant into the vagina.
3. Pick up the implant with gloved hands and flush it down the toilet.
4. Pick up the implant with long-handled forceps and place it in a lead container.

447. The nurse should plan to implement which intervention in the care of a client experiencing neutropenia as a result of chemotherapy?

1. Restrict all visitors.
2. Restrict fluid intake.
3. Teach the client and family about the need for hand hygiene.
4. Insert an indwelling urinary catheter to prevent skin breakdown.

448. The home health care nurse is caring for a client with cancer who is complaining of acute pain. The **most appropriate** determination of the client's pain should include which assessment?
1. The client's pain rating
2. Nonverbal cues from the client
3. The nurse's impression of the client's pain
4. Pain relief after appropriate nursing intervention

449. The nurse is caring for a client who is postoperative following a pelvic exenteration, and the surgeon changes the client's diet from NPO (nothing by mouth) status to clear liquids. The nurse should check which **priority** item before administering the diet?
1. Bowel sounds
2. Ability to ambulate
3. Incision appearance
4. Urine specific gravity

450. A client is admitted to the hospital with a suspected diagnosis of Hodgkin's disease. Which assessment finding would the nurse expect to note specifically in the client?
1. Fatigue
2. Weakness
3. Weight gain
4. Enlarged lymph nodes

451. During the admission assessment of a client with advanced ovarian cancer, the nurse recognizes which manifestation as typical of the disease?
1. Diarrhea
2. Hypermenorrhea
3. Abnormal bleeding
4. Abdominal distention

452. The nurse is caring for a client with lung cancer and bone metastasis. What signs and symptoms would the nurse recognize as indications of a possible oncological emergency? **Select all that apply.**
1. Facial edema in the morning
2. Weight loss of 20 lb (9 kg) in 1 month
3. Serum calcium level of 12 mg/dL (3.0 mmol/L)
4. Serum sodium level of 136 mg/dL (136 mmol/L)
5. Serum potassium level of 3.4 mg/dL (3.4 mmol/L)
6. Numbness and tingling of the lower extremities

453. A client who has been receiving radiation therapy for bladder cancer tells the nurse that it feels as if she is voiding through the vagina. The nurse interprets that the client may be experiencing which condition?
1. Rupture of the bladder
2. The development of a vesicovaginal fistula
3. Extreme stress caused by the diagnosis of cancer
4. Altered perineal sensation as a side effect of radiation therapy

454. The nurse is instructing a client to perform a testicular self-examination (TSE). The nurse should provide the client with which information about the procedure?
1. To examine the testicles while lying down
2. That the best time for the examination is after a shower
3. To gently feel the testicle with one finger to feel for a growth
4. That TSEs should be done at least every 6 months

455. The nurse is conducting a history and monitoring laboratory values on a client with multiple myeloma. What assessment findings should the nurse expect to note? **Select all that apply.**
- ☐ 1. Pathological fracture
- ☐ 2. Urinalysis positive for Bence Jones protein
- ☐ 3. Hemoglobin level of 15.5 g/dL (155 mmol/L)
- ☐ 4. Calcium level of 8.6 mg/dL (2.15 mmol/L)
- ☐ 5. Serum creatinine level of 2.0 mg/dL (176.6 mcmol/L)

456. A gastrectomy is performed on a client with gastric cancer. In the immediate postoperative period, the nurse notes bloody drainage from the nasogastric tube. The nurse should take which **most appropriate** action?
1. Measure abdominal girth.
2. Irrigate the nasogastric tube.
3. Continue to monitor the drainage.
4. Notify the primary health care provider (PHCP).

457. The nurse is teaching a client about the risk factors associated with colorectal cancer. The nurse determines that **further teaching is necessary** related to colorectal cancer if the client identifies which item as an associated risk factor?
1. Age younger than 50 years
2. History of colorectal polyps
3. Family history of colorectal cancer
4. Chronic inflammatory bowel disease

458. The nurse is assessing the perineal wound in a client who has returned from the operating room following an abdominal perineal resection and notes serosanguineous drainage from the wound. Which nursing intervention is **most appropriate**?

1. Clamp the surgical drain.
2. Change the dressing as prescribed.
3. Notify the surgeon.
4. Remove and replace the perineal packing.

459. The nurse is assessing the colostomy of a client who has had an abdominal perineal resection for a bowel tumor. Which assessment finding indicates that the colostomy is beginning to function?
1. The passage of flatus
2. Absent bowel sounds
3. The client's ability to tolerate food
4. Bloody drainage from the colostomy

460. The nurse is reviewing the history of a client with bladder cancer. The nurse expects to note documentation of which **most** common sign or symptom of this type of cancer?
1. Dysuria
2. Hematuria
3. Urgency on urination
4. Frequency of urination

461. The nurse is assessing a client who has a new ureterostomy. Which statement by the client indicates the **need for more education** about urinary stoma care?
1. "I change my pouch every week."
2. "I change the appliance in the morning."
3. "I empty the urinary collection bag when it is two-thirds full."
4. "When I'm in the shower I direct the flow of water away from my stoma."

462. A client with carcinoma of the lung develops syndrome of inappropriate antidiuretic hormone (SIADH) as a complication of the cancer. The nurse anticipates that the primary health care provider will request which prescriptions? **Select all that apply.**
1. Radiation
2. Chemotherapy
3. Increased fluid intake
4. Decreased oral sodium intake
5. Serum sodium level determination
6. Medication that is antagonistic to antidiuretic hormone

463. The nurse is monitoring a client for signs and symptoms related to superior vena cava syndrome. Which is an **early** sign of this oncological emergency?
1. Cyanosis
2. Arm edema
3. Periorbital edema
4. Mental status changes

464. The nurse manager is teaching the nursing staff about signs and symptoms related to hypercalcemia in a client with metastatic prostate cancer and tells the staff that which is a **late** sign or symptom of this oncological emergency?
1. Headache
2. Dysphagia
3. Constipation
4. Electrocardiographic changes

465. As part of chemotherapy education, the nurse teaches a female client about the risk for bleeding and self-care during the period of greatest bone marrow suppression (the nadir). The nurse understands that **further teaching is needed** if the client makes which statement?
1. "I should avoid blowing my nose."
2. "I may need a platelet transfusion if my platelet count is too low."
3. "I'm going to take aspirin for my headache as soon as I get home."
4. "I will count the number of pads and tampons I use when menstruating."

466. The community health nurse is instructing a group of young female clients about breast self-examination. The nurse should instruct the clients to perform the examination at which time?
1. At the onset of menstruation
2. Every month during ovulation
3. Weekly at the same time of day
4. One week after menstruation begins

467. A client is diagnosed as having a intestinal tumor. The nurse should monitor the client for which complications of this type of tumor? **Select all that apply.**
1. Flatulence
2. Peritonitis
3. Hemorrhage
4. Fistula formation
5. Bowel perforation
6. Lactose intolerance

468. The nurse is caring for a client following a mastectomy. Which nursing intervention would assist in preventing lymphedema of the affected arm?
1. Placing cool compresses on the affected arm
2. Elevating the affected arm on a pillow above heart level
3. Avoiding arm exercises in the immediate postoperative period
4. Maintaining an intravenous site below the antecubital area on the affected side

469. The nurse is providing dietary teaching for a client who underwent a partial gastrectomy to treat gastric cancer about foods high in vitamin B_{12}. The nurse would instruct the client to include which food items in the diet that are high in this vitamin? **Select all that apply.**

- ☐ 1. Milk
- ☐ 2. Fish
- ☐ 3. Beef
- ☐ 4. Apples
- ☐ 5. Turkey
- ☐ 6. Bananas

470. The nurse is instructing a client with iron deficiency anemia regarding the administration of a liquid oral iron supplement. Which instruction should the nurse tell the client?

1. Administer the iron at mealtimes.
2. Administer the iron through a straw.
3. Mix the iron with cereal to administer.
4. Add the iron to apple juice for easy administration.

471. Laboratory studies are performed for a client suspected to have iron deficiency anemia. The nurse reviews the laboratory results, knowing that which result indicates this type of anemia?

1. Elevated hemoglobin level
2. Decreased reticulocyte count
3. Elevated red blood cell count
4. Red blood cells that are microcytic and hypochromic

ANSWERS

443. *Answer:* 1
Rationale: Findings indicative of multiple myeloma are an increased number of plasma cells in the bone marrow, anemia, hypercalcemia caused by the release of calcium from the deteriorating bone tissue, and an elevated blood urea nitrogen level. An increased white blood cell count may or may not be present and is not related specifically to multiple myeloma.
Test-Taking Strategy: Focus on the subject, laboratory findings in multiple myeloma. Noting the name of the disorder and recalling the pathophysiology of the disease and that proliferation of plasma cells in the bone occurs will direct you to the correct option.
Level of Cognitive Ability: Analyzing
Client Needs: Physiological Integrity
Integrated Process: Nursing Process—Assessment
Content Area: Adult Health: Oncology
Health Problem: Adult Health: Cancer: Multiple Myeloma
Priority Concepts: Cellular Regulation; Clinical Judgment
Reference: Ignatavicius, Workman, Rebar (2018), pp. 829-830.

444. *Answer:* 1
Rationale: Hypercalcemia caused by bone destruction is a priority concern in the client with multiple myeloma. The nurse should administer fluids in adequate amounts to maintain a urine output of 1.5 to 2 L/day; this requires about 3 L of fluid intake per day. The fluid is needed not only to dilute the calcium overload but also to prevent protein from precipitating in the renal tubules. Options 2, 3, and 4 may be components of the plan of care but are not the priority in this client.
Test-Taking Strategy: Note the strategic word, *priority*. Recalling the pathophysiology of this disorder and that hypercalcemia can occur will direct you to the correct option.
Level of Cognitive Ability: Creating
Client Needs: Physiological Integrity
Integrated Process: Nursing Process—Planning
Content Area: Adult Health: Oncology
Health Problem: Adult Health: Cancer: Multiple Myeloma
Priority Concepts: Cellular Regulation; Clinical Judgment
Reference: Lewis et al. (2017), p. 646.

445. *Answer:* 2, 3, 4
Rationale: The time that the nurse spends in the room of a client with an internal radiation implant is 30 minutes per shift. The client must be placed in a private room with a private bath. Lead shielding can be used to reduce the transmission of radiation. The dosimeter film badge must be worn when in the client's room. Children younger than 16 years of age and pregnant women are not allowed in the client's room.
Test-Taking Strategy: Focus on the subject, radiation precautions. Recalling the time frame related to exposure to the client will assist in eliminating option 1. From the remaining options, select the correct options because of the possible risks associated with exposure to radiation.
Level of Cognitive Ability: Analyzing
Client Needs: Safe and Effective Care Environment
Integrated Process: Nursing Process—Implementation
Content Area: Foundations of Care: Safety
Health Problem: N/A
Priority Concepts: Cellular Regulation; Safety
Reference: Ignatavicius, Workman, Rebar (2018), p. 389.

446. *Answer:* 4
Rationale: In the event that a radiation source becomes dislodged, the nurse would first encourage the client to lie still until the radioactive source has been placed in a safe, closed container. The nurse would use long-handled forceps to place the source in the lead container that should be in the client's room. The nurse should then call the radiation oncologist and document the event and the actions taken. It is not within the scope of nursing practice to insert a radiation implant.
Test-Taking Strategy: Note the strategic word, *initial*. The initial action would be to prevent self-contamination from radiation exposure. This will direct you to the correct option.
Level of Cognitive Ability: Applying
Client Needs: Safe and Effective Care Environment
Integrated Process: Nursing Process—Implementation
Content Area: Foundations of Care: Safety
Health Problem: N/A
Priority Concepts: Cellular Regulation; Safety
Reference: Ignatavicius, Workman, Rebar (2018), p. 389.

447. Answer: 3
Rationale: In the neutropenic client, meticulous hand hygiene education is implemented for the client, family, visitors, and staff. Not all visitors are restricted, but the client is protected from persons with known infections. Fluids should be encouraged. Invasive measures such as an indwelling urinary catheter should be avoided to prevent infections.
Test-Taking Strategy: Eliminate option 1 because of the closed-ended word *all*. Next, eliminate option 2 because it is not reasonable to restrict fluids in a client receiving chemotherapy who is at risk for fluid and electrolyte imbalances. Eliminate option 4 because of the risk of infection that exists with this measure.
Level of Cognitive Ability: Applying
Client Needs: Safe and Effective Care Environment
Integrated Process: Nursing Process—Implementation
Content Area: Foundations of Care: Safety
Health Problem: N/A
Priority Concepts: Caregiving; Infection
Reference: Ignatavicius, Workman, Rebar (2018), p. 397.

448. Answer: 1
Rationale: The client's self-report is a critical component of pain assessment. The nurse should ask the client to describe the pain and listen carefully to the words the client uses to describe the pain. Nonverbal cues from the client are important but are not the most appropriate pain assessment measure. The nurse's impression of the client's pain is not appropriate in determining the client's level of pain. Assessing pain relief is an important measure, but this option is not related to the subject of the question.
Test-Taking Strategy: Note the strategic words, *most appropriate*. Eliminate option 3 because the nurse is not the client of the question. From the remaining options, the subjective data from the client will provide the most accurate description of the pain.
Level of Cognitive Ability: Analyzing
Client Needs: Physiological Integrity
Integrated Process: Caring
Content Area: Foundations of Care: Vital Signs
Health Problem: N/A
Priority Concepts: Caregiving; Pain
Reference: Lewis et al. (2017), pp. 107-108.

449. Answer: 1
Rationale: The client is kept NPO until peristalsis returns, usually in 4 to 6 days. When signs of bowel function return, clear fluids are given to the client. If no distention occurs, the diet is advanced as tolerated. The most important assessment is to assess bowel sounds before feeding the client. Options 2, 3, and 4 are unrelated to the data in the question.
Test-Taking Strategy: Note the strategic word, *priority*, and the words *NPO status to clear liquids* in the question. The correct option is the only one that relates to gastrointestinal function.
Level of Cognitive Ability: Analyzing
Client Needs: Physiological Integrity
Integrated Process: Nursing Process—Assessment
Content Area: Foundations of Care: Perioperative Care
Health Problem: N/A
Priority Concepts: Clinical Judgment; Nutrition
Reference: Lewis et al. (2017), pp. 342, 1261.

450. Answer: 4
Rationale: Hodgkin's disease is a chronic progressive neoplastic disorder of lymphoid tissue characterized by the painless enlargement of lymph nodes with progression to extralymphatic sites, such as the spleen and liver. Weight loss is most likely to be noted. Fatigue and weakness may occur but are not related significantly to the disease.
Test-Taking Strategy: Options 1 and 2 are comparable or alike and are rather vague symptoms that can occur in many disorders. Option 3 can be eliminated because, in such a disorder, weight loss is most likely to occur. Also, recalling that Hodgkin's disease affects the lymph nodes will direct you to the correct option.
Level of Cognitive Ability: Analyzing
Client Needs: Physiological Integrity
Integrated Process: Nursing Process—Assessment
Content Area: Adult Health: Oncology
Health Problem: Adult Health: Cancer: Lymphoma: Hodgkin's and non-Hodgkin's
Priority Concepts: Cellular Regulation; Clinical Judgment
Reference: Lewis et al. (2017), pp. 642-643.

451. Answer: 4
Rationale: Clinical manifestations of ovarian cancer include abdominal distention, urinary frequency and urgency, pleural effusion, malnutrition, pain from pressure caused by the growing tumor and the effects of urinary or bowel obstruction, constipation, ascites with dyspnea, and ultimately general severe pain. Abnormal bleeding, often resulting in hypermenorrhea, is associated with uterine cancer.
Test-Taking Strategy: Eliminate options 2 and 3 first because they are comparable or alike. From the remaining options, consider the anatomical location of the cancer. This will assist in directing you to the correct option.
Level of Cognitive Ability: Analyzing
Client Needs: Physiological Integrity
Integrated Process: Nursing Process—Assessment
Content Area: Adult Health: Oncology
Health Problem: Adult Health: Cancer: Cervical/Uterine/Ovarian
Priority Concepts: Cellular Regulation; Clinical Judgment
Reference: Lewis et al. (2017), pp. 1258-1259.

452. Answer: 1, 3, 6
Rationale: Oncological emergencies include sepsis, disseminated intravascular coagulation, syndrome of inappropriate antidiuretic hormone, spinal cord compression, hypercalcemia, superior vena cava syndrome, and tumor lysis syndrome. Blockage of blood flow to the venous system of the head resulting in facial edema is a sign of superior vena cava syndrome. A serum calcium level of 12 mg/dL (3.0 mmol/L) indicates hypercalcemia. Numbness and tingling of the lower extremities could be a sign of spinal cord compression. Mild hypokalemia and weight loss are not oncological emergencies. A sodium level of 136 mg/dL (136 mmol/L) is a normal level.
Test-Taking Strategy: Note the subject, an oncological emergency. Recalling the signs and symptoms of oncological emergencies will help you identify the correct options. Also, recalling the normal calcium, potassium, and sodium levels will direct you to the correct options.

Level of Cognitive Ability: Analyzing
Client Needs: Physiological Integrity
Integrated Process: Nursing Process—Assessment
Content Area: Adult Health: Oncology
Health Problem: Adult Health: Cancer: Laryngeal and Lung
Priority Concepts: Cellular Regulation; Clinical Judgment
Reference: Lewis et al. (2017), pp. 262-263.

453. *Answer:* 2
Rationale: A vesicovaginal fistula is a genital fistula that occurs between the bladder and vagina. The fistula is an abnormal opening between these two body parts, and if this occurs, the client may experience drainage of urine through the vagina. The client's complaint is not associated with options 1, 3, or 4.
Test-Taking Strategy: Focus on the **subject,** a complication of bladder cancer. Noting the words *voiding through the vagina* should direct you to the correct option.
Level of Cognitive Ability: Analyzing
Client Needs: Physiological Integrity
Integrated Process: Nursing Process—Analysis
Content Area: Adult Health: Oncology
Health Problem: Adult Health: Cancer: Bladder and Kidney
Priority Concepts: Cellular Regulation; Clinical Judgment
Reference: Lewis et al. (2017), p. 1263.

454. *Answer:* 2
Rationale: The TSE is recommended monthly after a warm bath or shower when the scrotal skin is relaxed. The client should stand to examine the testicles. Using both hands, with fingers under the scrotum and thumbs on top, the client should gently roll the testicles, feeling for any lumps.
Test-Taking Strategy: Focus on the **subject,** the procedure for performing TSE. Eliminate option 4 first because of the words *6 months*. Next, eliminate option 3 because of the word *one*. From the remaining options, eliminate option 1 by trying to visualize the process of the self-examination.
Level of Cognitive Ability: Applying
Client Needs: Health Promotion and Maintenance
Integrated Process: Teaching and Learning
Content Area: Health Assessment/Physical Exam: Testicles
Health Problem: Adult Health: Cancer: Testicular
Priority Concepts: Clinical Judgment; Health Promotion
Reference: Ignatavicius, Workman, Rebar (2018), p. 1486.

455. *Answer:* 1, 2, 5
Rationale: Multiple myeloma is a B cell neoplastic condition characterized by abnormal malignant proliferation of plasma cells and the accumulation of mature plasma cells in the bone marrow. The client with multiple myeloma may experience pathological fractures, hypercalcemia, anemia, recurrent infections, and renal failure. In addition, Bence Jones proteinuria is a finding. A serum calcium level of 8.6 mg/dL (2.15 mmol/L) and a hemoglobin level of 15.5 g/dL (155 mmol/L) are normal values. A serum creatinine level of 2.0 mg/dL (176.6 mcmol/L) is elevated indicating a renal problem.
Test-Taking Strategy: Focus on the **subject,** characteristics of multiple myeloma. Think about the pathophysiology of the disorder and analyze the values given to direct you to the correct option.
Level of Cognitive Ability: Analyzing
Client Needs: Physiological Integrity
Integrated Process: Teaching and Learning
Content Area: Adult Health: Oncology
Health Problem: Adult Health: Cancer: Multiple Myeloma
Priority Concepts: Cellular Regulation; Client Education
Reference: Ignatavicius, Workman, Rebar (2018), pp. 829-830.

456. *Answer:* 3
Rationale: Following gastrectomy, drainage from the nasogastric tube is normally bloody for 24 hours postoperatively, changes to brown-tinged, and is then yellow or clear. Because bloody drainage is expected in the immediate postoperative period, the nurse should continue to monitor the drainage. The nurse does not need to notify the PHCP (surgeon) at this time. Abdominal girth is measured to detect the development of distention. Following gastrectomy, a nasogastric tube should not be irrigated unless there are specific surgeon prescriptions to do so.
Test-Taking Strategy: Note the **strategic words,** *most appropriate*, and focus on the **subject,** the immediate postoperative period. This should direct you to the correct option. Remember that drainage from the nasogastric tube is normally bloody for 24 hours postoperatively, changes to brown-tinged, and then to yellow or clear.
Level of Cognitive Ability: Analyzing
Client Needs: Physiological Integrity
Integrated Process: Nursing Process—Implementation
Content Area: Foundations of Care: Perioperative Care
Health Problem: Adult Health: Cancer: Esophageal/Gastric/Intestinal
Priority Concepts: Cellular Regulation; Clinical Judgment
Reference: Ignatavicius, Workman, Rebar (2018), pp. 1207-1208.

457. *Answer:* 1
Rationale: Colorectal cancer risk factors include age older than 50 years, a family history of the disease, colorectal polyps, and chronic inflammatory bowel disease.
Test-Taking Strategy: Note the **strategic words,** *further teaching is necessary*. These words indicate a **negative event query** and ask you to select an option that is an incorrect statement. Noting the words *younger than* in option 1 will direct you to this option.
Level of Cognitive Ability: Evaluating
Client Needs: Health Promotion and Maintenance
Integrated Process: Teaching and Learning
Content Area: Adult Health: Oncology
Health Problem: Adult Health: Cancer: Esophageal/Gastric/Intestinal
Priority Concepts: Client Education; Health Promotion
Reference: Lewis et al. (2017), p. 954.

458. *Answer:* 2
Rationale: Immediately after surgery, profuse serosanguineous drainage from the perineal wound is expected. Therefore, the nurse should change the dressing as prescribed. A surgical drain should not be clamped, because this action will cause the accumulation of drainage within the tissue. The nurse does not need to notify the surgeon at this time. Drains and packing are removed gradually over a period of 5 to 7 days as prescribed. The nurse should not remove the perineal packing.
Test-Taking Strategy: Note the **strategic words,** *most appropriate*. Eliminate options 1 and 4, knowing that these are

inappropriate interventions. Recalling that serosanguineous drainage is expected following this type of surgery will assist in directing you to the correct option.
Level of Cognitive Ability: Applying
Client Needs: Physiological Integrity
Integrated Process: Nursing Process—Implementation
Content Area: Adult Health: Oncology
Health Problem: Adult Health: Cancer: Esophageal/Gastric/Intestinal
Priority Concepts: Clinical Judgment; Tissue Integrity
Reference: Lewis et al. (2017), pp. 343-344, 956.

459. *Answer:* 1
Rationale: Following abdominal perineal resection, the nurse would expect the colostomy to begin to function within 72 hours after surgery, although it may take up to 5 days. The nurse should assess for a return of peristalsis, listen for bowel sounds, and check for the passage of flatus. Absent bowel sounds would not indicate the return of peristalsis. The client would remain NPO (nothing by mouth) until bowel sounds return and the colostomy is functioning. Bloody drainage is not expected from a colostomy.
Test-Taking Strategy: Focus on the subject, the colostomy beginning to function. This should assist in eliminating option 2. Knowledge of general postoperative measures will assist in eliminating option 3. Focus on the subject to assist in eliminating option 4 as a correct option.
Level of Cognitive Ability: Analyzing
Client Needs: Physiological Integrity
Integrated Process: Nursing Process—Assessment
Content Area: Foundations of Care: Perioperative Care
Health Problem: Adult Health: Cancer: Esophageal/Gastric/Intestinal
Priority Concepts: Clinical Judgment; Elimination
Reference: Lewis et al. (2017), p. 956.

460. *Answer:* 2
Rationale: The most common sign in clients with cancer of the bladder is hematuria. The client also may experience irritative voiding symptoms such as frequency, urgency, and dysuria, and these symptoms often are associated with carcinoma in situ. Dysuria, urgency, and frequency of urination are also symptoms of a bladder infection.
Test-Taking Strategy: Focus on the subject, bladder cancer, and note the strategic word, *most*. Options 1, 3, and 4 are symptoms that are associated most often with bladder infection.
Level of Cognitive Ability: Analyzing
Client Needs: Physiological Integrity
Integrated Process: Nursing Process—Assessment
Content Area: Adult Health: Oncology
Health Problem: Adult Health: Cancer: Bladder and Kidney
Priority Concepts: Cellular Regulation; Elimination
Reference: Lewis et al. (2017), pp. 1053-1054.

461. *Answer:* 3
Rationale: The urinary collection bag should be changed when it is one-third full to prevent pulling of the appliance and leakage. The remaining options identify correct statements about the care of a urinary stoma.
Test-Taking Strategy: Note the strategic words, *need for more education*, and eliminate the options that indicate client understanding. Noting the words *two-thirds full* will assist in directing you to the correct option.
Level of Cognitive Ability: Evaluating
Client Needs: Physiological Integrity
Integrated Process: Teaching and Learning
Content Area: Adult Health: Oncology
Health Problem: Adult Health: Cancer: Bladder and Kidney
Priority Concepts: Client Education; Elimination
Reference: Perry et al. (2018), p. 939.

462. *Answer:* 1, 2, 5, 6
Rationale: Cancer is a common cause of SIADH. In SIADH, excessive amounts of water are reabsorbed by the kidney and put into the systemic circulation. The increased water causes hyponatremia (decreased serum sodium levels) and some degree of fluid retention. The syndrome is managed by treating the condition and cause and usually includes fluid restriction, increased sodium intake, and medication with a mechanism of action that is antagonistic to antidiuretic hormone. Sodium levels are monitored closely because hypernatremia can develop suddenly as a result of treatment. The immediate institution of appropriate cancer therapy, usually radiation or chemotherapy, can cause tumor regression so that antidiuretic hormone synthesis and release processes return to normal.
Test-Taking Strategy: Focus on the subject, treatment for SIADH, and recall that in SIADH excessive amounts of water are reabsorbed by the kidney and put into the systemic circulation. This will assist in answering this question.
Level of Cognitive Ability: Analyzing
Client Needs: Physiological Integrity
Integrated Process: Nursing Process—Analysis
Content Area: Adult Health: Oncology
Health Problem: Adult Health: Cancer: Laryngeal and Lung
Priority Concepts: Cellular Regulation; Clinical Judgment
Reference: Ignatavicius, Workman, Rebar (2018), pp. 954, 1251-1252.

463. *Answer:* 3
Rationale: Superior vena cava syndrome occurs when the superior vena cava is compressed or obstructed by tumor growth. Early signs and symptoms generally occur in the morning and include edema of the face, especially around the eyes, and client complaints of tightness of a shirt or blouse collar. As the compression worsens, the client experiences edema of the hands and arms. Cyanosis and mental status changes are late signs.
Test-Taking Strategy: Note the strategic word, *early*. Think about the pathophysiology associated with this disorder and focus on the strategic word to assist in eliminating options 1, 2, and 4.
Level of Cognitive Ability: Analyzing
Client Needs: Physiological Integrity
Integrated Process: Nursing Process—Assessment
Content Area: Adult Health: Oncology
Health Problem: N/A
Priority Concepts: Cellular Regulation; Clinical Judgment
Reference: Ignatavicius, Workman, Rebar (2018), pp. 408-409.

464. *Answer:* 4
Rationale: Hypercalcemia is a manifestation of bone metastasis in late-stage cancer. Headache and dysphagia are not

associated with hypercalcemia. Constipation may occur early in the process. Electrocardiogram changes include shortened ST segment and a widened T wave.
Test-Taking Strategy: Note the strategic word, *late*. Focus on the name of the oncological emergency, *hypercalcemia*, to direct you to the correct option. Eliminate options 1 and 2 because they are not signs of hypercalcemia. Eliminate option 3 because it is an early sign of hypercalcemia.
Level of Cognitive Ability: Applying
Client Needs: Physiological Integrity
Integrated Process: Teaching and Learning
Content Area: Adult Health: Oncology
Health Problem: Adult Health: Cancer: Prostate
Priority Concepts: Cellular Regulation; Fluids and Electrolytes
Reference: Ignatavicius, Workman, Rebar (2018), p. 408.

465. *Answer:* 3
Rationale: During the period of greatest bone marrow suppression (the nadir), the platelet count may be low, less than 20,000 cells mm^3 (20.0×10^9/L). The correct option describes an incorrect statement by the client. Aspirin and nonsteroidal antiinflammatory drugs and products that contain aspirin should be avoided because of their antiplatelet activity. Options 1, 2, and 4 are correct statements by the client to prevent and monitor bleeding.
Test-Taking Strategy: Note the strategic words, *further teaching is needed*. Recalling the effects of bone marrow suppression will direct you to the correct option.
Level of Cognitive Ability: Evaluating
Client Needs: Physiological Integrity
Integrated Process: Teaching and Learning
Content Area: Adult Health: Oncology
Health Problem: Adult Health: Hematological: Bleeding/Clotting Disorders
Priority Concepts: Cellular Regulation; Clinical Judgment
Reference: Lewis et al. (2017), pp. 250, 253.

466. *Answer:* 4
Rationale: The breast self-examination should be performed regularly, 7 days after the onset of the menstrual period. Performing the examination weekly is not recommended. At the onset of menstruation and during ovulation, hormonal changes occur that may alter breast tissue.
Test-Taking Strategy: Option 3 can be eliminated easily because of the word *weekly*. Eliminate options 1 and 2 next because they are comparable or alike in the similarity that exists regarding the hormonal changes that occur during these times.
Level of Cognitive Ability: Applying
Client Needs: Health Promotion and Maintenance
Integrated Process: Teaching and Learning
Content Area: Health Assessment/Physical Exam: Breasts
Health Problem: Adult Health: Cancer: Breast
Priority Concepts: Client Education; Health Promotion
Reference: Ignatavicius, Workman, Rebar (2018), pp. 1443-1444.

467. *Answer:* 2, 3, 4, 5
Rationale: Complications of intestinal tumors include bowel perforation, which can result in hemorrhage and peritonitis. Other complications include bowel obstruction and fistula formation. Flatulence can occur but is not a complication; lactose intolerance also is not a complication of intestinal tumor.
Test-Taking Strategy: Focus on the subject, complications of an intestinal tumor. Think about the location and pathophysiology associated with this type of tumor to answer correctly.
Level of Cognitive Ability: Analyzing
Client Needs: Physiological Integrity
Integrated Process: Nursing Process—Assessment
Content Area: Adult Health: Oncology
Health Problem: Adult Health: Cancer: Esophageal/Gastric/Intestinal
Priority Concepts: Cellular Regulation; Clinical Judgment
Reference: Lewis et al. (2017), p. 968.

468. *Answer:* 2
Rationale: Following mastectomy, the arm should be elevated above the level of the heart. Simple arm exercises should be encouraged. No blood pressure readings, injections, intravenous lines, or blood draws should be performed on the affected arm. Cool compresses are not a suggested measure to prevent lymphedema from occurring.
Test-Taking Strategy: Focus on the subject, preventing lymphedema. Note the relationship between the words *lymphedema* in the question and *elevating* in the correct option. Also, using general principles related to gravity will direct you to the correct option.
Level of Cognitive Ability: Applying
Client Needs: Physiological Integrity
Integrated Process: Nursing Process—Implementation
Content Area: Adult Health: Oncology
Health Problem: Adult Health: Cancer: Breast
Priority Concepts: Clinical Judgment; Tissue Integrity
Reference: Ignatavicius, Workman, Rebar (2018), p. 1454.

469. *Answer:* 1, 2, 3, 5
Rationale: Vitamin B_{12} aids in hemoglobin synthesis and energy metabolism, especially folic acid metabolism. It is also essential for normal functioning of all cells, especially the nervous system, bone marrow, and gastrointestinal tract. The client who had a partial gastrectomy is at risk for vitamin B_{12} deficiency because of loss of the intrinsic factor, which is produced in the lining of the stomach. Foods high in this vitamin include meat such as beef, organ meats such as liver, poultry such as chicken and turkey, fish, shellfish such as clams, eggs, and dairy products such as milk and eggs. Apples and bananas both contain vitamin C. Banana is also rich in potassium.
Test-Taking Strategy: Focus on the subject, foods high in vitamin B_{12}. Eliminate options 4 and 6 because they are comparable or alike and are fruits. For the remaining options it is necessary to recall that foods high in vitamin B_{12} include meat, organ meats, poultry, fish, shellfish, eggs, and dairy products.
Level of Cognitive Ability: Applying
Client Needs: Physiological Integrity
Integrated Process: Teaching and Learning
Content Area: Adult Health: Gastrointestinal
Health Problem: Adult Health: Cancer: Esophageal/Gastric/Intestinal
Priority Concepts: Client Education; Nutrition
References: Harding et al. (2020). *Lewis's Medical-surgical nursing: Assessment and management of clinical problems* (11th ed). p. 851; National Institutes of Health (NIH) (2020). *Vitamin B12*

fact Sheet for Health professionals at https://ods.od.nih.gov/factsheets/VitaminB12-HealthProfessional/#:~:text=of%20Vitamin%20B12-,Food,5%2C13%2D15%5D; Potter et al. (2021). *Fundamentals of nursing* (10th ed), St. Louis: Elsevier, p. 1104.

470. *Answer:* 2

Rationale: In iron deficiency anemia, iron stores are depleted, resulting in a decreased supply of iron for the manufacture of hemoglobin in red blood cells. An oral iron supplement should be administered through a straw or medicine dropper placed at the back of the mouth, because the iron stains the teeth. The client should be instructed to brush or wipe their teeth after administration. Iron is administered between meals, because absorption is decreased if there is food in the stomach. Iron requires an acid environment to facilitate its absorption in the duodenum. Iron is not mixed with cereal or other food items.

Test-Taking Strategy: Eliminate options 3 and 4 first because they are comparable or alike and because medication should not be added to formula and food. Next, note the word *liquid* in the question. This should assist you in recalling that iron in liquid form stains teeth.

Level of Cognitive Ability: Applying
Client Needs: Physiological Integrity
Integrated Process: Teaching and Learning
Content Area: Adult Health: Hematological
Health Problem: Adult Health: Hematological: Anemias
Priority Concepts: Client Education; Health Promotion
Reference: Burchum, Rosenthal (2016), pp. 652-653.

471. *Answer:* 4

Rationale: In iron deficiency anemia, iron stores are depleted, resulting in a decreased supply of iron for the manufacture of hemoglobin in red blood cells. The results of a complete blood cell count in clients with iron deficiency anemia show decreased hemoglobin levels and microcytic and hypochromic red blood cells. The red blood cell count is decreased. The reticulocyte count is usually normal or slightly elevated.

Test-Taking Strategy: Focus on the subject, laboratory findings. Eliminate options 1 and 3 first, knowing that the hemoglobin and red blood cell counts would be decreased. From the remaining options, select the correct option over option 2 because of the relationship between anemia and red blood cells.

Level of Cognitive Ability: Analyzing
Client Needs: Physiological Integrity
Integrated Process: Nursing Process—Assessment
Content Area: Adult Health: Hematological
Health Problem: Adult Health: Hematological: Anemias
Priority Concepts: Cellular Regulation; Gas Exchange
Reference: Ignatavicius, Workman, Rebar (2018), p. 803.

CHAPTER 45

Oncological and Hematological Medications

PRIORITY CONCEPTS **Cellular Regulation; Safety**

Note: Oncological medications are prescribed to treat cancer. Hematological medications are prescribed to treat conditions and diseases related to the blood and blood-forming organs. Blood components are affected when the client receives oncological medications. Hematological medications specific to treating the effects of oncological medications on the body are included in this chapter.

I. Antineoplastic Medications

A. Description
1. Antineoplastic medications kill or inhibit the reproduction of neoplastic cells.
2. Antineoplastic medications are used to cure, increase survival time, and decrease life-threatening complications.
3. The effect of antineoplastic medications may not be limited to neoplastic cells; normal cells also are affected by the medication.
4. Cell cycle phase–specific medications affect cells only during a certain phase of the reproductive cycle (Fig. 45-1).
5. Cell cycle phase–nonspecific medications affect cells in any phase of the reproductive cycle (Fig. 45-1).
6. Usually, several medications are used in combination to increase the therapeutic response.
7. Antineoplastic medications may be combined with other treatments, such as surgery and radiation.
8. Although the intravenous (IV) route is most common for administration, antineoplastic medication may be given by the oral, intra-arterial, isolated limb perfusion, or intracavitary route; dosing is usually based on the client's body surface area (BSA) and type of cancer.
9. Chemotherapy dosing is usually based on total BSA, which requires a current, accurate height and weight for BSA calculation (before each medication administration) to ensure that the client receives optimal doses of chemotherapy medications.

⚠ Side and adverse effects from chemotherapy result from the effects of the antineoplastic medication on normal cells.

B. Side and adverse effects
1. Mucositis
2. Alopecia
3. Anorexia, nausea, and vomiting
4. Diarrhea
5. Anemia
6. Low white blood cell count (neutropenia)
7. Thrombocytopenia
8. Infertility, sexual alterations
9. Neuropathy

C. General interventions
1. Physiological integrity
   a. Monitor complete blood cell count, white blood cell count, platelet count, uric acid level, and electrolytes.
   b. Initiate bleeding precautions if thrombocytopenia occurs.
   c. When the platelet count is less than 50,000 mm^3 ($50 \times 10^9/L$), minor trauma can lead to episodes of prolonged bleeding; when less than 20,000 mm^3 ($20 \times 10^9/L$), spontaneous and uncontrollable bleeding can occur; withhold the medication if the platelet count drops (according to agency policy) and notify the primary health care provider (PHCP). Bleeding precautions are initiated.
   d. Monitor for petechiae, ecchymoses, bleeding of the gums, and nosebleeds, because the decreased platelet count can precipitate bleeding tendencies.
   e. Avoid intramuscular injections and venipunctures as much as possible to prevent bleeding.
   f. Withhold the medication and initiate neutropenic precautions if the segmented neutrophil count decreases below 18% conventional units (0.18 SI units); notify the PHCP.
   g. Monitor for fever, sore throat, unusual bleeding, and signs and symptoms of infection.

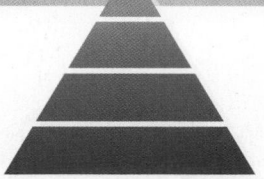

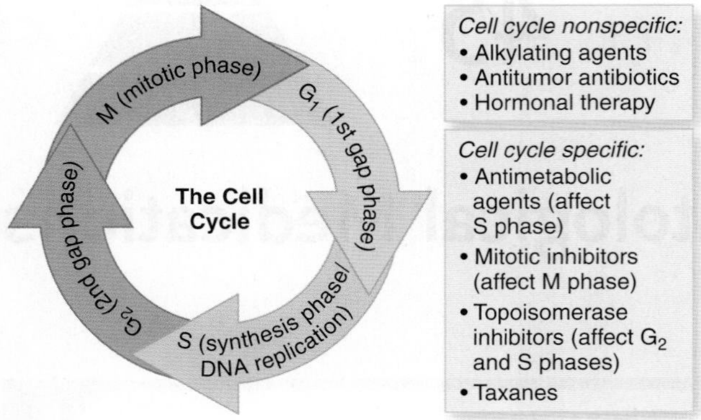

FIG. 45-1 The cell cycle. *G1*, the cell is preparing for division; *S* (synthesis phase/DNA replication), the cell doubles its DNA content through DNA synthesis; *G2*, the cell produces proteins to be used in cell division and in normal physiological function after cell division is complete; *M* (mitotic phase), the single cell splits apart into 2 cells.

   h. Inform the client that loss of appetite also may be the result of taste changes or a bitter taste in the mouth from the medications.
   i. Monitor for nausea and vomiting and provide a high-calorie diet with protein supplements.
   j. Administer antiemetics several hours before chemotherapy and for 12 to 48 hours after as prescribed, because antineoplastic medications stimulate the vomiting center in the brain.
   k. Encourage hydration; IV fluids are administered before and during therapy.
   l. Promote a fluid intake of at least 2000 mL/day to maintain adequate renal function.

⚠ Antineoplastic medication causes the rapid destruction of cells, resulting in the release of uric acid. Allopurinol may be prescribed to lower the serum uric acid level.

2. Safe and effective care environment
   a. Prepare IV chemotherapy in an air-vented space (biological safety cabinet).
   b. Wear appropriate personal protective equipment (PPE), including gloves, gown, eye protectors, and mask as indicated, to reduce exposure whenever there is a risk of hazardous medications being released into the environment.
   c. Nurses who are pregnant should avoid chemotherapy preparation or the administration of chemotherapy.
   d. Discard IV equipment in designated (biohazard) containers.
   e. Administer antineoplastic medication precisely as prescribed to maximize antineoplastic effects while allowing normal cells to recover.
   f. Monitor for phlebitis with IV administration, because these medications may irritate the veins.
   g. Vesicants should be administered through a central line when possible; if a peripheral line is used, blood return should be checked prior to administration.
   h. As prescribed, reduce IV site pain by altering IV rates or warming the injection site to distend the vein and increase blood flow.
   i. Monitor for extravasation (leakage of medication into surrounding skin and subcutaneous tissue, which causes tissue necrosis) and notify the PHCP if this occurs; heat or ice is applied depending on the medication, and an antidote may be injected into the site.

3. Psychosocial integrity
   a. Instruct the client about the possibility of hair loss and that varying degrees of hair loss may occur after the first or second treatment.
   b. Discuss the purchase of a wig before treatment starts and consider cutting hair short.
   c. Inform the client that new hair growth will occur several months after the final treatment.
   d. Instruct the client about the need for contraception, because these medications have teratogenic effects.
   e. Discuss the potential effect of infertility, which may be irreversible.
   f. Encourage pretreatment counseling and encourage sperm banking or preservation of eggs if the client is still of childbearing age.

4. Health promotion and maintenance
   a. Instruct the client, if diarrhea is a problem, to avoid spicy foods, high-fiber foods, and foods that are hot in temperature, which increase peristalsis.
   b. Instruct the client to inspect the oral mucosa frequently for erythema and ulcers, rinse the mouth after meals, and carry out good oral hygiene.
   c. Instruct the client to use mouth rinses as prescribed for mouth sores if necessary.
   d. Instruct the client in the use of antifungal agents for mouth sores, if prescribed, for the development of a fungal infection.
   e. Instruct the client to avoid crowds and persons with infections and to report signs of infection such as a low-grade fever, chills, or sore throat.
   f. Instruct individuals with colds or infections to wear a mask when visiting or to avoid visiting the client.
   g. Instruct the client to use a soft toothbrush and electric razor to minimize the risk of bleeding.
   h. Instruct the client to avoid aspirin-containing products to minimize the risk of bleeding.
   i. Instruct the client to consult the PHCP before receiving vaccinations (live vaccines should not be administered).

D. Anaphylactic reactions
 1. Precautions
  a. Obtain an allergy history.
  b. Administer a test dose when prescribed by the PHCP.
  c. Stay with the client during the administration of medication.
  d. Monitor vital signs.
  e. Have emergency equipment and medications readily available.
  f. Initiate IV access for the administration of emergency medications if needed.
 2. Signs of an anaphylactic reaction
  a. Dyspnea
  b. Chest tightness or pain
  c. Pruritus or urticaria
  d. Tachycardia
  e. Dizziness
  f. Anxiety or agitation
  g. Flushed appearance
  h. Hypotension
  i. Decreased sensorium
  j. Cyanosis
 3. Interventions for an anaphylactic reaction (see Priority Nursing Actions)

PRIORITY NURSING ACTIONS

Anaphylactic Reaction Occurring from Medication

1. Assess respiratory status.
2. Stop the medication.
3. Contact the primary health care provider (PHCP) and the Rapid Response Team if necessary.
4. Administer oxygen.
5. Maintain the intravenous (IV) access with normal saline.
6. Raise the client's feet and legs, if not contraindicated.
7. Administer prescribed emergency medications, such as epinephrine.
8. Monitor vital signs.
9. Document the event, actions taken, and the client's response.

Reference
Ignatavicius, Workman, Rebar (2018), p. 365.

II. Alkylating Medications (Box 45-1)

A. Description
 1. Break the DNA helix, thereby interfering with DNA replication
 2. Cell cycle phase–nonspecific medications
B. Side and adverse effects
 1. Anorexia, nausea, and vomiting may occur.
 2. Stomatitis may occur.
 3. Rash may occur.

BOX 45-1 Alkylating Medications

Nitrogen Mustards
- Bendamustine
- Chlorambucil
- Cyclophosphamide
- Ifosfamide
- Estramustine
- Mechlorethamine
- Melphalan

Nitrosoureas
- Carmustine
- Lomustine
- Streptozocin

Alkylating-Like Medications
- Altretamine
- Busulfan
- Carboplatin
- Cisplatin
- Dacarbazine
- Oxaliplatin
- Temozolomide
- Thiotepa

 4. Client may feel IV site pain during IV administration.
 5. Busulfan may cause hyperuricemia.
 6. Chlorambucil and mechlorethamine may cause gonadal suppression and hyperuricemia.
 7. Cisplatin, a platinum compound, may cause ototoxicity, tinnitus, hypokalemia, hypocalcemia, hypomagnesemia, and nephrotoxicity.
C. Interventions: Refer to Section I, C (Antineoplastic Medications—General Interventions).
 1. Cyclophosphamide may cause alopecia, gonadal suppression, hemorrhagic cystitis, and hematuria.
 2. Ifosfamide may cause hemorrhagic cystitis, and neurotoxicity.
 3. Assess results of pulmonary function tests.
 4. Assess results of chest radiography and renal and liver function studies.
 5. When administering cisplatin, assess the client for dizziness, tinnitus, hearing loss, incoordination, and numbness or tingling of extremities.
 6. Mesna may be administered with ifosfamide to reduce the potential for ifosfamide-induced cystitis.
 7. Instruct the client that cyclophosphamide, when prescribed orally, is administered without food.
 8. Instruct the client to follow a diet low in purines to alkalinize the urine and lower uric acid blood levels.
 9. Instruct the client about how to avoid infection.
 10. Instruct the client to report signs of infection or bleeding.
 11. Instruct the client about good oral hygiene and the use of a soft toothbrush.

Cyclophosphamide and ifosfamide are medications that can cause hemorrhagic cystitis. Encourage the client to drink increased fluids (2 to 3 L/day) during therapy, unless contraindicated.

BOX 45-2 Antitumor Antibiotic Medications

- Bleomycin sulfate
- Dactinomycin
- Daunorubicin
- Doxorubicin
- Epirubicin
- Idarubicin
- Mitomycin
- Mitoxantrone
- Valrubicin

III. Antitumor Antibiotic Medications (Box 45-2)

A. Description
  1. Interfere with DNA and RNA synthesis
  2. Cell cycle phase–nonspecific medications

B. Side and adverse effects
  1. Nausea and vomiting
  2. Fever
  3. Bone marrow depression
  4. Rash
  5. Alopecia
  6. Stomatitis
  7. Gonadal suppression
  8. Hyperuricemia
  9. Vesication (blistering of tissue at IV site)
  10. Daunorubicin may cause heart failure and dysrhythmias.
  11. Doxorubicin and idarubicin may cause cardiotoxicity, cardiomyopathy, and electrocardiographic changes (dexrazoxane, which is a cardioprotective agent, may be administered with doxorubicin to reduce cardiomyopathy).
  12. Pulmonary toxicity can occur with bleomycin.

C. Interventions: Refer to Section I, C (Antineoplastic Medications—General Interventions).
  1. Assess results of pulmonary function tests.
  2. Monitor for electrocardiographic changes.
  3. Assess lung sounds for crackles.
  4. Assess for signs of heart failure, including dyspnea, crackles, peripheral edema, and weight gain.
  5. Assess results of chest radiography and renal and liver function studies.
  6. Assess for myocardial toxicity, dyspnea, dysrhythmias, hypotension, and weight gain when administering doxorubicin or idarubicin.
  7. Monitor pulmonary status when administering bleomycin.

IV. Antimetabolite Medications (Box 45-3)

A. Description
  1. Antimetabolite medications halt the synthesis of cell protein; their presence impairs cell division.
  2. Antimetabolite medications are cell cycle phase–specific and affect the S phase.

B. Side and adverse effects
  1. Anorexia, nausea, and vomiting
  2. Diarrhea

BOX 45-3 Antimetabolite Medications

- Azacitidine
- Capecitabine
- Cladribine
- Clofarabine
- Cytarabine
- Decitabine
- Floxuridine
- Fludarabine
- Fluorouracil
- Gemcitabine
- Hydroxyurea
- Mercaptopurine
- Methotrexate
- Nelarabine
- Pemetrexed
- Pentostatin
- Pralatrexate
- Thioguanine
- Uracil

  3. Alopecia
  4. Stomatitis
  5. Depression of bone marrow
  6. Cytarabine may cause alopecia, stomatitis, hyperuricemia, and hepatotoxicity.
  7. Fluorouracil may cause alopecia, stomatitis, diarrhea, phototoxicity reactions, and cerebellar dysfunction.
  8. Mercaptopurine may cause hyperuricemia and hepatotoxicity.
  9. Methotrexate may cause alopecia; stomatitis; hyperuricemia; photosensitivity; hepatotoxicity; and hematological, gastrointestinal, and skin toxicity.

C. Interventions: Refer to Section I, C (Antineoplastic Medications—General Interventions).
  1. Monitor renal function studies.
  2. Monitor for cerebellar dysfunction.
  3. Assess for photosensitivity.
  4. When administering fluorouracil, assess for signs of cerebellar dysfunction, such as dizziness, weakness, and ataxia, and assess for stomatitis and diarrhea, which may necessitate medication discontinuation.
  5. When administering fluorouracil or methotrexate, instruct the client to use sunscreen and wear protective clothing to prevent photosensitivity reactions.

When administering methotrexate in large doses, prepare to administer leucovorin as prescribed to prevent toxicity. This is known as *leucovorin rescue.*

V. Mitotic Inhibitor Medications (*Vinca* Alkaloids) (Box 45-4)

A. Description
  1. Mitotic inhibitors prevent mitosis, causing cell death.
  2. Mitotic inhibitors are cell cycle phase–specific and act on the M phase.

B. Side and adverse effects
  1. Leukopenia

BOX 45-4 Mitotic Inhibitors

Vinca Alkaloids	Taxanes
Vinblastine sulfate	Docetaxel
Vincristine sulfate	Paclitaxel
Vinorelbine	

2. Neurotoxicity with vincristine, manifested as numbness and tingling in the fingers and toes; constipation, and paralytic ileus can also occur.
3. Ptosis
4. Hoarseness
5. Motor instability
6. Anorexia, nausea, and vomiting
7. Peripheral neuropathy
8. Alopecia
9. Stomatitis
10. Hyperuricemia
11. Phlebitis at IV site

C. Interventions: Refer to Section I, C (Antineoplastic Medications—General Interventions).
1. Monitor for hoarseness.
2. Assess eyes for ptosis.
3. Assess motor stability and initiate safety precautions as necessary.
4. Monitor for neurotoxicity with vincristine, manifested as numbness and tingling in the fingers and toes.
5. Monitor for constipation and paralytic ileus.

VI. Topoisomerase Inhibitors (Box 45-5)

A. Description
1. Block an enzyme needed for DNA synthesis and cell division
2. Cell cycle phase–specific; act on the G_2 and S phases

B. Side and adverse effects
1. Leukopenia, thrombocytopenia, and anemia
2. Anorexia, nausea, and vomiting
3. Diarrhea
4. Alopecia
5. Orthostatic hypotension
6. Hypersensitivity reaction

C. Interventions: Refer to Section I, C (Antineoplastic Medications—General Interventions).

VII. Hormonal Medications and Enzymes (Box 45-6)

A. Description

BOX 45-5 Topoisomerase Inhibitors

- Etoposide
- Irinotecan
- Teniposide
- Topotecan

BOX 45-6 Hormonal Medications and Enzymes

Estrogens
- Estramustine
- Ethinyl estradiol

Antiestrogens
- Anastrozole
- Exemestane
- Fulvestrant
- Letrozole
- Raloxifene
- Tamoxifen citrate
- Toremifene

Antiandrogens
- Bicalutamide
- Enzalutamide
- Flutamide
- Goserelin acetate
- Histrelin
- Nilutamide
- Triptorelin

Progestins
- Medroxyprogesterone
- Megestrol acetate

Other Hormonal Antagonists and Enzymes
- Asparaginase
- Leuprolide acetate
- Mitotane

1. Suppress the immune system and block normal hormones in hormone-sensitive tumors
2. Change the hormonal balance and slow the growth rates of certain tumors

B. Side and adverse effects
1. Anorexia, nausea, and vomiting
2. Leukopenia
3. Impaired pancreatic function with asparaginase
4. Sex characteristic alterations
   a. Masculinizing effect in women: Chest and facial hair, menses stops
   b. Feminine manifestations in men: Gynecomastia
5. Breast swelling
6. Hot flashes
7. Weight gain
8. Hemorrhagic cystitis, hypouricemia, and hypercholesterolemia, with mitotane
9. Hypertension
10. Thromboembolic disorders
11. Edema
12. Electrolyte imbalances
13. Tamoxifen citrate may cause edema, hypercalcemia, and elevated cholesterol and triglyceride levels.
14. Tamoxifen citrate decreases the effects of estrogen.

C. Interventions: Refer to Section I, C (Antineoplastic Medications—General Interventions).
1. Assess medications that the client is taking currently.
2. Monitor serum calcium levels with androgens.
3. Monitor for signs of alterations in sexual characteristics.
4. Monitor pancreatic function with asparaginase.
5. Monitor uric acid and cholesterol levels.
6. Monitor for signs of hemorrhagic cystitis.

VIII. Immunomodulator (Immunotherapy) Agents: Biological Response Modifiers (Box 45-7)

A. Description
  1. Immunomodulators stimulate the immune system to recognize cancer cells and take action to eliminate or destroy them.
  2. Interleukins help various immune system cells to recognize and destroy abnormal body cells.
  3. Interferons slow tumor cell division, stimulate proliferation, and cause cancer cells to differentiate into nonproliferative forms.

B. Colony-stimulating factors induce more rapid bone marrow recovery after suppression by chemotherapy (Box 45-8).

IX. Targeted Therapy

A. Description: (see Box 45-7)
  1. Medications used as targeted therapies are monoclonal antibodies and small molecule inhibitors that target a cellular element of the cancer cell or antisense medications that work at the gene level.
  2. Examples of monoclonal antibodies are rituximab, trastuzumab, alemtuzumab, bevacizumab, and cetuximab.

B. Adverse effects: Allergic reactions (monoclonal antibodies)

BOX 45-7 Immunomodulators and Targeted Therapies

Interleukins and Interferons
- Aldesleukin
- Interferon α-2a
- Interferon α-2b
- Interferon α-n3
- Recombinant interferon α-2a
- Recombinant interferon α-2b

Common Monoclonal Antibodies
- Bevacizumab
- Cetuximab
- Ibritumomab
- Infliximab
- Panitumumab
- Pembrolizumab
- Rituximab
- Trastuzumab

Small Molecule Inhibitors
- Bortezomib
- Dasatinib
- Erlotinib
- Gefitinib
- Imatinib
- Lapatinib
- Nilotinib
- Sorafenib
- Sunitinib
- Temsirolimus

BOX 45-8 Colony-Stimulating Factors

Granulocyte Macrophage Colony–Stimulating Factor
- Sargramostim

Granulocyte Colony–Stimulating Factor
- Filgrastim
- Pegfilgrastim

Erythropoietin
- Epoetin α
- Darbepoetin α

Thrombopoietic Growth Factor
- Oprelvekin

X. Other Antineoplastic Medications

A. Altretamine: Cytotoxic agent used to treat ovarian cancer

B. Denileukin diftitox: Recombinant DNA-derived medication used to treat cutaneous T-cell lymphoma

C. Pegaspargase: Used in combination chemotherapies for acute lymphoblastic leukemia in clients unable to take asparaginase

D. Bexarotene: Used to treat advanced-stage cutaneous T-cell lymphoma

XI. Medications to Treat Anemia (see Chapter 44 for more information)

A. Iron-deficiency anemia: Iron, oral or intravenous

B. Vitamin B_{12}-deficiency anemia: Vitamin B_{12}, oral or intramuscular

C. Folate-deficiency anemia: Folate, oral

D. Acute blood loss anemia: Blood transfusion, packed red blood cells, platelets, or fresh frozen plasma depending on cause

E. Anemia of chronic disease: Iron, oral or intravenous, erythropoietic growth factors, leukopoietic growth factors, and thrombopoietic growth factors (see Chapter 55 for more information).

PRACTICE QUESTIONS

472. Chemotherapy dosage is frequently based on total body surface area (BSA), so it is important for the nurse to perform which assessment before administering chemotherapy?
1. Measure the client's abdominal girth.
2. Calculate the client's body mass index.
3. Measure the client's current weight and height.
4. Ask the client about his or her weight and height.

473. A client with squamous cell carcinoma of the larynx is receiving bleomycin intravenously. The nurse caring for the client anticipates that which diagnostic study will be prescribed?
1. Echocardiography
2. Electrocardiography
3. Cervical radiography
4. Pulmonary function studies

474. A client with acute myelocytic leukemia is being treated with busulfan. Which laboratory value would

the nurse specifically monitor during treatment with this medication?
1. Clotting time
2. Uric acid level
3. Potassium level
4. Blood glucose level

475. A client with small cell lung cancer is being treated with etoposide. The nurse monitors the client during administration, knowing that which adverse effect is specifically associated with this medication?
1. Alopecia
2. Chest pain
3. Pulmonary fibrosis
4. Orthostatic hypotension

476. A clinic nurse prepares a teaching plan for a client receiving an antineoplastic medication. When implementing the plan, the nurse should make which statement to the client?
1. "You can take aspirin as needed for headache."
2. "You can drink beverages containing alcohol in moderate amounts each evening."
3. "You need to consult with the primary health care provider (PHCP) before receiving immunizations."
4. "It is fine to receive a flu vaccine at the local health fair without PHCP approval because the flu is so contagious."

477. A client with ovarian cancer is being treated with vincristine. The nurse monitors the client, knowing that which manifestation indicates an adverse effect specific to this medication?
1. Diarrhea
2. Hair loss
3. Chest pain
4. Peripheral neuropathy

478. The nurse is reviewing the history and physical examination of a client who will be receiving asparaginase, an antineoplastic agent. The nurse contacts the primary health care provider before administering the medication if which disorder is documented in the client's history?
1. Pancreatitis
2. Diabetes mellitus
3. Myocardial infarction
4. Chronic obstructive pulmonary disease

479. Tamoxifen citrate is prescribed for a client with metastatic breast carcinoma. The client asks the nurse if her family member with bladder cancer can also take this medication. The nurse **most appropriately** responds by making which statement?
1. "This medication can be used only to treat breast cancer."
2. "Yes, your family member can take this medication for bladder cancer as well."
3. "This medication can be taken to prevent and treat clients with breast cancer."
4. "This medication can be taken by anyone with cancer as long as their health care provider approves it."

480. A client with metastatic breast cancer is receiving tamoxifen. The nurse specifically monitors which laboratory value while the client is taking this medication?
1. Glucose level
2. Calcium level
3. Potassium level
4. Prothrombin time

481. Megestrol acetate, an antineoplastic medication, is prescribed for a client with metastatic endometrial carcinoma. The nurse reviews the client's history and should contact the primary health care provider if which diagnosis is documented in the client's history?
1. Gout
2. Asthma
3. Myocardial infarction
4. Venous thromboembolism

482. The nurse is monitoring the intravenous (IV) infusion of an antineoplastic medication. During the infusion, the client complains of pain at the insertion site. On inspection of the site, the nurse notes redness and swelling and that the infusion of the medication has slowed in rate. The nurse suspects extravasation and should take which actions? **Select all that apply.**
1. Stop the infusion.
2. Prepare to apply ice or heat to the site.
3. Restart the IV at a distal part of the same vein.
4. Notify the primary health care provider (PHCP).
5. Prepare to administer a prescribed antidote into the site.
6. Increase the flow rate of the solution to flush the skin and subcutaneous tissue.

483. The nurse is analyzing the laboratory results of a client with leukemia who has received a regimen of chemotherapy. Which laboratory value would the nurse specifically note as a result of the massive cell destruction that occurred from the chemotherapy?
1. Anemia
2. Decreased platelets
3. Increased uric acid level
4. Decreased leukocyte count

484. The nurse is providing medication instructions to a client with breast cancer who is receiving cyclophosphamide. The nurse should tell the client to take which action?
1. Take the medication with food.
2. Increase fluid intake to 2000 to 3000 mL daily.

3. Decrease sodium intake while taking the medication.
4. Increase potassium intake while taking the medication.

485. A client with non-Hodgkin's lymphoma is receiving daunorubicin. Which finding would indicate to the nurse that the client is experiencing an adverse effect related to the medication?
1. Fever
2. Sores in the mouth and throat
3. Complaints of nausea and vomiting
4. Crackles on auscultation of the lungs

486. The nurse is monitoring the laboratory results of a client receiving an antineoplastic medication by the intravenous route. The nurse plans to initiate bleeding precautions if which laboratory result is noted?
1. A clotting time of 10 minutes
2. An ammonia level of 10 mcg/dL (6 mcmol/L).
3. A platelet count of 50,000 mm^3 (50×10^9/L)
4. A white blood cell count of 5000 mm^3 (5.0×10^9/L)

ANSWERS

472. *Answer:* 3
Rationale: To ensure that the client receives optimal doses of chemotherapy, dosing is usually based on the total BSA, which requires a current accurate height and weight for BSA calculation (before each medication administration). Asking the client about his or her height and weight may lead to inaccuracies in determining a true BSA and dosage. Calculating body mass index and measuring abdominal girth will not provide the data needed.
Test-Taking Strategy: Recall the basis for dosing chemotherapy. Recalling that a current accurate height and weight need to be obtained for BSA calculation and chemotherapy dosing will direct you to the correct option. Eliminate option 4 because it is an unreliable way of obtaining the information. Next, eliminate options 1 and 2 because they are comparable or alike and do not relate to chemotherapy dosing.
Level of Cognitive Ability: Analyzing
Client Needs: Physiological Integrity
Integrated Process: Nursing Process—Assessment
Content Area: Adult Health: Oncology
Health Problem: N/A
Priority Concepts: Cellular Regulation; Clinical Judgment
Reference: Potter et al. (2017), p. 612.

473. *Answer:* 4
Rationale: Bleomycin is an antineoplastic medication that can cause interstitial pneumonitis, which can progress to pulmonary fibrosis. Pulmonary function studies along with hematological, hepatic, and renal function tests need to be monitored. The nurse needs to monitor lung sounds for dyspnea and crackles, which indicate pulmonary toxicity. The medication needs to be discontinued immediately if pulmonary toxicity occurs. Options 1, 2, and 3 are unrelated to the specific use of this medication.
Test-Taking Strategy: Eliminate options 1 and 2 first because they are cardiac related and are therefore comparable or alike. From the remaining options, use the ABCs—airway, breathing, and circulation—to direct you to the correct option.
Level of Cognitive Ability: Analyzing
Client Needs: Physiological Integrity
Integrated Process: Nursing Process—Analysis
Content Area: Pharmacology: Oncology Medications: Antitumor Antibiotics
Health Problem: Adult Health: Cancer: Laryngeal and Lung
Priority Concepts: Cellular Regulation; Clinical Judgment
Reference: Gahart, Nazareno, Ortega (2017), p. 183.

474. *Answer:* 2
Rationale: Busulfan can cause an increase in the uric acid level. Hyperuricemia can produce uric acid nephropathy, renal stones, and acute kidney injury. Options 1, 3, and 4 are not specifically related to this medication.
Test-Taking Strategy: Focus on the subject, a specific laboratory value. It is necessary to know the adverse effects associated with this medication. Recalling that busulfan increases the uric acid level will direct you to the correct option.
Level of Cognitive Ability: Analyzing
Client Needs: Physiological Integrity
Integrated Process: Nursing Process—Assessment
Content Area: Pharmacology: Oncology Medications: Alkylating
Health Problem: Adult Health: Cancer: Leukemia
Priority Concepts: Cellular Regulation; Clinical Judgment
Reference: Skidmore-Roth (2017), p. 178.

475. *Answer:* 4
Rationale: An adverse effect specific to etoposide is orthostatic hypotension. Etoposide should be administered slowly over 30 to 60 minutes to avoid hypotension. The client's blood pressure is monitored during the infusion. Hair loss occurs with nearly all antineoplastic medications. Chest pain and pulmonary fibrosis are unrelated to this medication.
Test-Taking Strategy: Eliminate option 1 first, because this adverse effect is associated with many of the antineoplastic agents. Eliminate options 2 and 3 next because they are comparable or alike and are unrelated to etoposide. Note that the question asks for the adverse effect *specific* to this medication. Correlate hypotension with etoposide.
Level of Cognitive Ability: Analyzing
Client Needs: Physiological Integrity
Integrated Process: Nursing Process—Assessment
Content Area: Pharmacology: Oncology Medications: Topoisomerase Inhibitors
Health Problem: Adult Health: Cancer: Laryngeal and Lung
Priority Concepts: Cellular Regulation; Clinical Judgment
Reference: Gahart, Nazareno, Ortega (2017), pp. 548-549.

476. Answer: 3

Rationale: Because antineoplastic medications lower the resistance of the body, clients must be informed not to receive immunizations without the PHCP's approval. Clients also need to avoid contact with individuals who have recently received a live virus vaccine. Clients need to avoid aspirin and aspirin-containing products to minimize the risk of bleeding, and they need to avoid alcohol to minimize the risk of toxicity and side/adverse effects.

Test-Taking Strategy: Focus on the **subject,** client teaching about an antineoplastic medication, and think about the side/adverse effects of antineoplastic medications. Recalling that antineoplastic medications lower the resistance of the body will direct you to the correct option.

Level of Cognitive Ability: Applying

Client Needs: Health Promotion and Maintenance

Integrated Process: Teaching and Learning

Content Area: Adult Health: Oncology

Health Problem: N/A

Priority Concepts: Cellular Regulation; Client Education

Reference: Lilley et al. (2017), p. 787; www.hrsa.gov/vaccinecompensation/index.html

477. Answer: 4

Rationale: An adverse effect specific to vincristine is peripheral neuropathy, which occurs in almost every client. Peripheral neuropathy can be manifested as numbness and tingling in the fingers and toes. Depression of the Achilles tendon reflex may be the first clinical sign indicating peripheral neuropathy. Constipation rather than diarrhea is most likely to occur with this medication, although diarrhea may occur occasionally. Hair loss occurs with nearly all antineoplastic medications. Chest pain is unrelated to this medication.

Test-Taking Strategy: Eliminate options 1 and 2 first because they are **comparable or alike** and are side/adverse effects associated with many of the antineoplastic agents. Note that the question asks for the adverse effect *specific* to this medication. Correlate peripheral neuropathy with vincristine.

Level of Cognitive Ability: Analyzing

Client Needs: Physiological Integrity

Integrated Process: Nursing Process—Assessment

Content Area: Pharmacology: Oncology Medications: Miotic Inhibitors

Health Problem: Adult Health: Cancer: Cervical/Uterine/Ovarian

Priority Concepts: Cellular Regulation; Clinical Judgment

Reference: Hodgson, Kizior (2018), p. 1227.

478. Answer: 1

Rationale: Asparaginase is contraindicated if hypersensitivity exists, in pancreatitis, or if the client has a history of pancreatitis. The medication impairs pancreatic function, and pancreatic function tests should be performed before therapy begins and when a week or more has elapsed between dose administrations. The client needs to be monitored for signs of pancreatitis, which include nausea, vomiting, and abdominal pain. The conditions noted in options 2, 3, and 4 are not contraindicated with this medication.

Test-Taking Strategy: Focus on the **subject,** a contraindication of asparaginase. It is necessary to know the contraindications associated with this medication. Recalling that this medication affects pancreatic function will direct you to the correct option.

Level of Cognitive Ability: Analyzing

Client Needs: Physiological Integrity

Integrated Process: Nursing Process—Assessment

Content Area: Pharmacology: Oncology Medications: Hormonal and Enzymes

Health Problem: N/A

Priority Concepts: Cellular Regulation; Clinical Judgment

Reference: Hodgson, Kizior (2018), p. 87.

479. Answer: 3

Rationale: Tamoxifen is an antineoplastic medication that competes with estradiol for binding to estrogen in tissues containing high concentrations of receptors. Tamoxifen is used to treat metastatic breast carcinoma in women and men. Tamoxifen is also effective in delaying the recurrence of cancer following mastectomy and for preventing breast cancer in those that are at high risk.

Test-Taking Strategy: Note the **strategic words,** *most appropriately.* Recalling that this medication is used for breast cancer will assist you in eliminating options 2 and 4. Note the **closed-ended word** "only" in option 1 to assist you in eliminating this option. Also, recall that this medication is used for both prevention and treatment of breast cancer.

Level of Cognitive Ability: Applying

Client Needs: Physiological Integrity

Integrated Process: Teaching and Learning

Content Area: Pharmacology: Oncology Medications: Selective Estrogen Receptor Modulators

Health Problem: Adult Health: Cancer: Breast

Priority Concepts: Cellular Regulation; Clinical Judgment

Reference: Lewis et al. (2017), 1217.

480. Answer: 2

Rationale: Tamoxifen may increase calcium, cholesterol, and triglyceride levels. Before the initiation of therapy, a complete blood count, platelet count, and serum calcium level should be assessed. These blood levels, along with cholesterol and triglyceride levels, should be monitored periodically during therapy. The nurse should assess for hypercalcemia while the client is taking this medication. Signs of hypercalcemia include increased urine volume, excessive thirst, nausea, vomiting, constipation, hypotonicity of muscles, and deep bone and flank pain.

Test-Taking Strategy: Focus on the **subject,** the laboratory value to monitor for tamoxifen. Think about the action of this medication. Recalling that this medication causes hypercalcemia will direct you to the correct option.

Level of Cognitive Ability: Analyzing

Client Needs: Physiological Integrity

Integrated Process: Nursing Process—Assessment

Content Area: Pharmacology: Oncology Medications: Selective Estrogen Receptor Modulators

Health Problem: Adult Health: Cancer: Breast

Priority Concepts: Cellular Regulation; Fluids and Electrolytes

Reference: Hodgson, Kizior (2018), p. 1115.

481. Answer: 4

Rationale: Megestrol acetate suppresses the release of luteinizing hormone from the anterior pituitary by inhibiting pituitary function and regressing tumor size. Megestrol is used with caution if the client has a history of venous thromboembolism. Options 1, 2, and 3 are not contraindications for this medication.

Test-Taking Strategy: Focus on the subject, a contraindication to megestrol acetate. It is necessary to know the adverse effects associated with this medication. Recalling that megestrol acetate is a hormonal antagonist enzyme and that an adverse effect is thrombotic disorders will direct you to the correct option.
Level of Cognitive Ability: Analyzing
Client Needs: Safe and Effective Care Environment
Integrated Process: Nursing Process—Implementation
Content Area: Pharmacology: Oncology Medications: Hormonal and Enzymes
Health Problem: Adult Health: Cancer: Cervical/Uterine/Ovarian
Priority Concepts: Clinical Judgment; Safety
Reference: Skidmore-Roth (2017), pp. 745-746.

482. *Answer:* 1, 2, 4, 5
Rationale: Redness and swelling and a slowed infusion indicate signs of extravasation. If the nurse suspects extravasation during the IV administration of an antineoplastic medication, the infusion is stopped and the PHCP is notified. Ice or heat may be prescribed for application to the site, and an antidote may be prescribed to be administered into the site. Increasing the flow rate can increase damage to the tissues. Restarting an IV in the same vein can increase damage to the site and vein.
Test-Taking Strategy: Focus on the assessment signs in the question and the words *suspects extravasation*. Visualize the situation to identify the nursing actions. Think about the actions that will cause further damage. Note that options 3 and 6 are comparable or alike and can cause further damage.
Level of Cognitive Ability: Analyzing
Client Needs: Physiological Integrity
Integrated Process: Nursing Process—Implementation
Content Area: Complex Care: Emergency Situations/Management
Health Problem: Adult Health: Integumentary: Inflammations/Infections
Priority Concepts: Clinical Judgment; Tissue Integrity
Reference: Ignatavicius, Workman, Rebar (2018), pp. 217, 392-393.

483. *Answer:* 3
Rationale: Hyperuricemia is especially common following treatment for leukemias and lymphomas, because chemotherapy results in massive cell kill. Although options 1, 2, and 4 also may be noted, an increased uric acid level is related specifically to cell destruction.
Test-Taking Strategy: Focus on the subject, the laboratory value that reflects massive cell destruction. Remember that uric acid is released when cells are destroyed. This will direct you to the correct option.
Level of Cognitive Ability: Analyzing
Client Needs: Physiological Integrity
Integrated Process: Nursing Process—Assessment
Content Area: Adult Health: Oncology
Health Problem: Adult Health: Cancer: Leukemia
Priority Concepts: Cellular Regulation; Clinical Judgment
Reference: Lewis et al. (2017), p. 252.

484. *Answer:* 2
Rationale: Hemorrhagic cystitis is an adverse effect that can occur with the use of cyclophosphamide. The client needs to be instructed to drink copious amounts of fluid during the administration of this medication. Clients also should monitor urine output for hematuria. The medication should be taken on an empty stomach, unless gastrointestinal upset occurs. Hyperkalemia can result from the use of the medication; therefore, the client would not be told to increase potassium intake. The client would not be instructed to alter sodium intake.
Test-Taking Strategy: Focus on the subject, client teaching about cyclophosphamide. Recalling that cyclophosphamide can cause hemorrhagic cystitis will direct you to the correct option.
Level of Cognitive Ability: Applying
Client Needs: Physiological Integrity
Integrated Process: Teaching and Learning
Content Area: Pharmacology: Oncology Medications: Alkylating
Health Problem: Adult Health: Cancer: Breast
Priority Concepts: Cellular Regulation; Client Education
Reference: Lewis et al. (2017), p. 1522.

485. *Answer:* 4
Rationale: Cardiotoxicity noted by abnormal electrocardiographic findings or cardiomyopathy manifested as heart failure (lung crackles) is an adverse effect of daunorubicin. Bone marrow depression is also an adverse effect. Fever is a frequent side effect, and sores in the mouth and throat can occur occasionally. Nausea and vomiting is a frequent side effect associated with the medication that begins a few hours after administration and lasts 24 to 48 hours. Options 1, 2, and 3 are not adverse effects.
Test-Taking Strategy: Keep in mind that the question is asking about an adverse effect. Use of the ABCs—airway, breathing, and circulation—will direct you to the correct option.
Level of Cognitive Ability: Analyzing
Client Needs: Physiological Integrity
Integrated Process: Nursing Process—Analysis
Content Area: Pharmacology: Oncology Medications: Antitumor Antibiotics
Health Problem: Adult Health: Cancer: Lymphoma: Hodgkin's and non-Hodgkins
Priority Concepts: Cellular Regulation; Clinical Judgment
Reference: Hodgson, Kizior (2018), p. 327.

486. *Answer:* 3
Rationale: Bleeding precautions need to be initiated when the platelet count decreases. The normal platelet count is 150,000 to 450,000 mm^3 (150 to 400 × 10^9/L). When the platelet count decreases, the client is at risk for bleeding. The normal white blood cell count is 5000 to 10,000 mm^3 (5.0 to 10.0× 10^9/L). When the white blood cell count drops, neutropenic precautions need to be implemented. The normal clotting time is 8 to 15 minutes. The normal ammonia value is 10 to 80 mcg/dL (6 to 47 mcmol/L).
Test-Taking Strategy: Use knowledge regarding normal laboratory values. Options 1, 2, and 4 are comparable or alike and identify normal laboratory values. Remember to correlate a low platelet count with the need for bleeding precautions and a low white blood cell count with the need for neutropenic precautions.
Level of Cognitive Ability: Synthesizing
Client Needs: Safe and Effective Care Environment
Integrated Process: Nursing Process—Planning
Content Area: Foundations of Care: Safety
Health Problem: Adult Health: Hematological: Bleeding/Clotting Disorders
Priority Concepts: Cellular Regulation; Safety
Reference: Ignatavicius, Workman, Rebar (2018), pp. 804-805.

UNIT IX

Endocrine Problems of the Adult Client

Pyramid to Success

The endocrine system is made up of organs or glands that secrete hormones and release them directly into the circulation. The endocrine system can be understood easily if you remember that basically 1 of 2 situations can occur—hypersecretion or hyposecretion of hormones from the organ or gland. When an excess of the hormone occurs, treatment is aimed at blocking the hormone release through medication or surgery. When a deficit of the hormone exists, treatment is aimed at replacement therapy. Pyramid Points focus on diabetes mellitus, including its prevention, the prevention and treatment of complications, insulin therapy, hypoglycemic and hyperglycemic reactions, and acute and chronic complications of diabetes; Addison's disease and addisonian crisis; Cushing's disease or Cushing's syndrome; thyroid problems and thyroid storm; and care of the client after thyroidectomy or adrenalectomy.

Client Needs: Learning Objectives

Safe and Effective Care Environment

Acting as a client advocate
Collaborating with the interprofessional team and appropriate care providers regarding treatment
Ensuring that informed consent for treatments and procedures has been obtained
Establishing priorities of care
Handling hazardous and infectious materials
Maintaining confidentiality related to the health problem
Preventing accidents and client injury
Using medical and surgical asepsis to prevent infection

Health Promotion and Maintenance

Discussing expected body image changes
Identifying lifestyle choices related to treatment
Performing physical assessment of the endocrine system
Preventing health problems
Providing health screening
Teaching about self-care measures

Psychosocial Integrity

Discussing grief and loss issues related to complications of the health problem
Discussing situational role changes related to the health problem
Discussing unexpected body image changes
Identifying coping mechanisms
Monitoring for sensory and perceptual alterations as a result of the health problem
Using support systems

Physiological Integrity

Monitoring for alterations in body systems as a result of the health problem
Monitoring for complications from surgical procedures and health alterations
Monitoring for complications of diagnostic tests, treatments, and procedures
Monitoring for expected outcomes and effects of pharmacological therapy
Monitoring for fluid and electrolyte imbalances that can occur
Monitoring for unexpected response to therapies
Monitoring laboratory values
Preparing the client for diagnostic tests
Providing emergency care to the client
Providing nonpharmacological comfort interventions
Providing nutrition and oral hydration measures

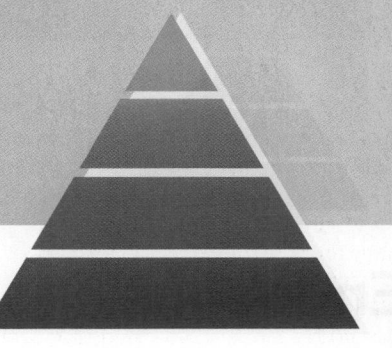

CHAPTER 46

Endocrine Problems

PRIORITY CONCEPTS Glucose Regulation; Hormonal Regulation

I. Anatomy and Physiology of Endocrine Glands (Box 46-1)

A. Functions
   1. Maintenance and regulation of vital functions
   2. Response to stress and injury
   3. Growth and development
   4. Energy metabolism
   5. Reproduction
   6. Fluid, electrolyte, and acid-base balance

B. Risk factors for endocrine problems (Box 46-2)

C. Hypothalamus (Box 46-3)
   1. Portion of the diencephalon of the brain, forming the floor and part of the lateral wall of the third ventricle
   2. Activates, controls, and integrates the peripheral autonomic nervous system, endocrine processes, and many somatic functions, such as body temperature, sleep, and appetite

D. Pituitary gland (Box 46-4; Fig. 46-1)
   1. The master gland; located at the base of the brain
   2. Influenced by the hypothalamus; directly affects the function of the other endocrine glands
   3. Promotes growth of body tissue, influences water absorption by the kidney, and controls sexual development and function

BOX 46-1 Endocrine Glands

- Adrenal
- Hypothalamus
- Ovaries
- Pancreas
- Parathyroid
- Pituitary
- Testes
- Thyroid

BOX 46-2 Risk Factors for Endocrine Problems

- Age
- Heredity
- Congenital factors
- Trauma
- Environmental factors
- Consequence of other health problems or surgery

BOX 46-3 Hypothalamus Hormones

- Corticotropin-releasing hormone (CRH)
- Gonadotropin-releasing hormone (GnRH)
- Growth hormone–inhibiting hormone (GHIH)
- Growth hormone–releasing hormone (GHRH)
- Melanocyte-inhibiting hormone (MIH)
- Prolactin-inhibiting hormone (PIH)
- Thyrotropin-releasing hormone (TRH)

BOX 46-4 Pituitary Gland Hormones

Anterior Lobe Production

- Adrenocorticotropic hormone (ACTH)
- Follicle-stimulating hormone (FSH)
- Growth hormone (GH)
- Luteinizing hormone (LH)
- Melanocyte-stimulating hormone (MSH)
- Prolactin (PRL)
- Somatotropic growth-stimulating hormone
- Thyroid-stimulating hormone (TSH)

Posterior Lobe

These hormones are produced by the hypothalamus, stored in the posterior lobe, and secreted into the blood when needed:

- Oxytocin
- Vasopressin, antidiuretic hormone (ADH)

E. Adrenal gland
   1. One adrenal gland is on top of each kidney.
   2. Regulates sodium and electrolyte balance; affects carbohydrate, fat, and protein metabolism; influences the development of sexual characteristics; and sustains the fight-or-flight response
   3. Adrenal cortex
      a. The cortex is the outer shell of the adrenal gland.
      b. The cortex synthesizes glucocorticoids and mineralocorticoids and secretes small amounts of sex hormones (androgens, estrogens; Box 46-5)

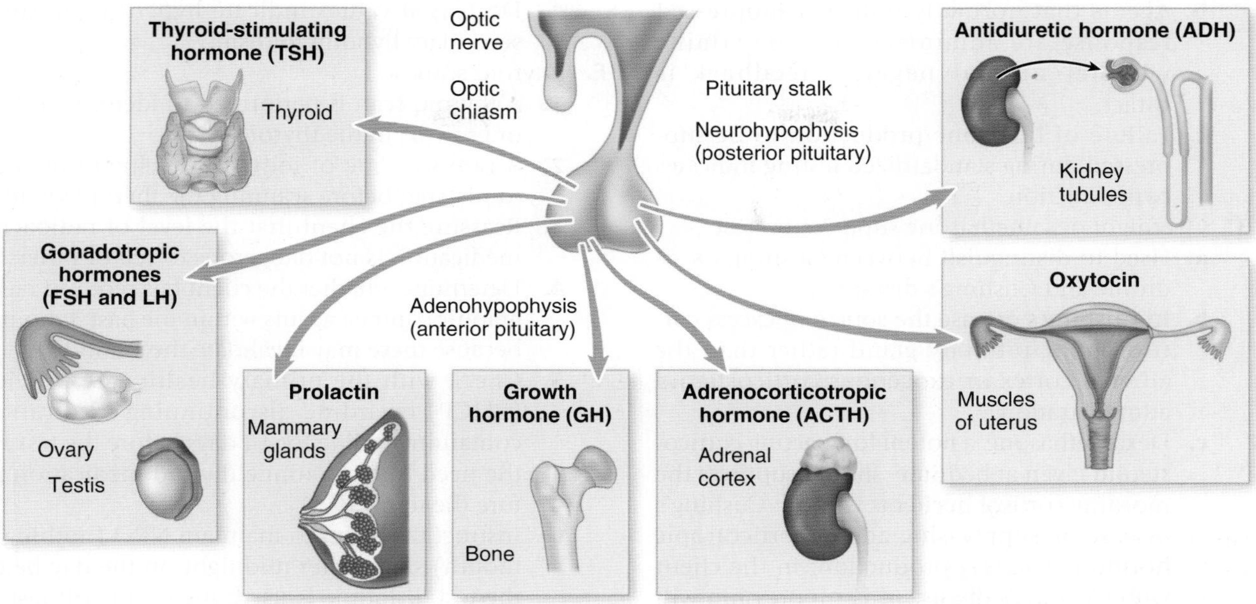

FIG. 46-1 Pituitary hormones. *FSH*, Follicle-stimulating hormone; *LH*, luteinizing hormone.

BOX 46-5 Adrenal Cortex

Glucocorticoids: Cortisol, Cortisone, Corticosterone

Responsible for glucose metabolism, protein metabolism, fluid and electrolyte balance, suppression of the inflammatory response to injury, protective immune response to invasion by infectious agents, and resistance to stress

Mineralocorticoids: Aldosterone

Regulation of electrolyte balance by promoting sodium retention and potassium excretion

4. Adrenal medulla
   a. The medulla is the inner core of the adrenal gland.
   b. The medulla works as part of the sympathetic nervous system and produces epinephrine and norepinephrine.

F. Thyroid gland
   1. Located in the anterior part of the neck
   2. Controls the rate of body metabolism and growth and produces thyroxine (T_4), triiodothyronine (T_3), and thyrocalcitonin

G. Parathyroid glands
   1. Located on the thyroid gland
   2. Controls calcium and phosphorus metabolism; produces parathyroid hormone

H. Pancreas
   1. Located posteriorly to the stomach
   2. Influences carbohydrate metabolism, indirectly influences fat and protein metabolism, and produces insulin and glucagon

I. Ovaries and testes
   1. The ovaries are located in the pelvic cavity and produce estrogen and progesterone.
   2. The testes are located in the scrotum, control the development of the secondary sex characteristics, and produce testosterone.

J. Negative-feedback loop
   1. Regulates hormone secretion by the hypothalamus and pituitary gland
   2. Increased amounts of target gland hormones in the bloodstream decrease secretion of the same hormone and other hormones that stimulate its release.

II. Diagnostic Tests

A. Stimulation and suppression tests
   1. Stimulation tests
      a. In the client with suspected underactivity of an endocrine gland, a stimulus may be provided to determine whether the gland is capable of normal hormone production.
      b. Measured amounts of selected hormones or substances are administered to stimulate the target gland to produce its hormone.
      c. Hormone levels produced by the target gland are measured.
      d. Failure of the hormone level to increase with stimulation indicates hypofunction.
   2. Suppression tests
      a. Suppression tests are used when hormone levels are high or in the upper range of normal.

b. Agents that normally induce a suppressed response are administered to determine whether normal negative feedback is intact.
c. Failure of hormone production to be suppressed during standardized testing indicates hyperfunction.
3. Overnight dexamethasone suppression test
a. Used to distinguish between Cushing's syndrome and Cushing's disease.
b. In Cushing's disease the source of excess cortisol is the pituitary gland rather than the adrenal cortex or exogenous corticosteroid administration.
c. Dexamethasone, a potent long-acting corticosteroid given at bedtime, should suppress the morning cortisol in clients without Cushing's disease by suppressing adrenocorticotropic hormone (ACTH) production; in the client with Cushing's disease, this suppression will not occur.

B. Radioactive iodine uptake
1. This thyroid function test measures the absorption of an iodine isotope to determine how the thyroid gland is functioning.
2. A small dose of radioactive iodine is given by mouth or intravenously; the amount of radioactivity is measured in 2 to 4 hours and again at 24 hours.
3. Normal values are approximately 3% to 10% at 2 to 4 hours, and 5% to 30% in 24 hours.
4. Elevated values indicate **hyperthyroidism**, decreased iodine intake, or increased iodine excretion.
5. Decreased values indicate a low T_4 level, the use of antithyroid medications, thyroiditis, myxedema, or **hypothyroidism**.
6. The test is contraindicated in pregnancy.

C. T_3 and T_4 resin uptake test
1. Blood tests are used to diagnose thyroid disorders.
2. T_3 and T_4 regulate thyroid-stimulating hormone.
3. Normal values (normal findings vary between laboratory settings)
a. Triiodothyronine, total T_3: 110.4 to 337.7 ng/dL (1.7 to 5.2 pmol/L)
b. Thyroxine, total T_4: 5 to 12 mcg/dL (64 to 154 nmol/L)
c. Thyroxine, free (FT_4): 0.8 to 2.8 ng/dL (10 to 36 pmol/L)
4. The T_4 level is elevated in hyperthyroidism and decreased in hypothyroidism.

D. Thyroid-stimulating hormone
1. Blood test is used to differentiate the diagnosis of primary hypothyroidism.
2. Normal value is 2 to 10 mcIU/mL (2 to 10 mIU/L).
3. Elevated values indicate primary hypothyroidism.
4. Decreased values indicate hyperthyroidism or secondary hypothyroidism.

E. Thyroid scan
1. A thyroid scan is performed to identify nodules or growths in the thyroid gland.
2. A radioisotope of iodine or technetium is administered before scanning the thyroid gland.
3. Reassure the client that the level of radioactive medication is not dangerous to self or others.
4. Determine whether the client has received radiographic contrast agents within the past 3 months, because these may invalidate the scan.
5. Check with the primary health care provider (PHCP) regarding discontinuing medications containing iodine for 14 days before the test and the need to discontinue thyroid medication before the test.
6. Instruct the client to maintain NPO (nothing by mouth) status after midnight on the day before the test; if iodine is used, the client will fast for an additional 45 minutes after ingestion of the oral isotope and the scan will be performed in 24 hours.
7. If technetium is used, it is administered by the intravenous (IV) route 30 minutes before the scan.
8. The test is contraindicated in pregnancy.

F. Needle aspiration of thyroid tissue
1. Aspiration of thyroid tissue is done for cytological examination.
2. No client preparation is necessary; NPO status may or may not be prescribed.
3. Light pressure is applied to the aspiration site after the procedure.

G. Glycosylated hemoglobin
1. HgbA1c is blood glucose bound to hemoglobin.
2. **Hemoglobin A1c** (glycosylated hemoglobin A; HbA1c) is a reflection of how well blood glucose levels have been controlled for the past 3 to 4 months.
3. **Hyperglycemia** in clients with diabetes is usually a cause of an increase in HbA1c.
4. Fasting is not required before the test.
5. Normal reference intervals: <6% (adult without diabetes)
6. HgbA1c and estimated average glucose (eAG) reference intervals: Refer to Table 10-4 for these reference intervals.

! Poor glycemic control in a client with diabetes mellitus is usually the cause of an increase in the HbA1c value.

H. 24-hour urine collection for vanillylmandelic acid (VMA)
1. Diagnostic tests for pheochromocytoma include a 24-hour urine collection for VMA, a product of catecholamine metabolism, metanephrine, and

catecholamines, all of which are elevated in the presence of pheochromocytoma.
2. The normal range of urinary catecholamines:
   a. Epinephrine: less than 20 mcg/day (less than 109 nmol/day)
   b. Norepinephrine: less than 100 mcg/day (less than 590 nmol/day)

III. Pituitary Gland Problems (Box 46-6)

A. Hypopituitarism
1. Description: Hyposecretion of 1 or more of the pituitary hormones caused by tumors, trauma, encephalitis, autoimmunity, or stroke
2. Hormones most often affected are growth hormone (GH) and gonadotropic hormones (luteinizing hormone, follicle-stimulating hormone), but thyroid-stimulating hormone (TSH), adrenocorticotropic hormone (ACTH), or antidiuretic hormone (ADH) may be involved.
3. Assessment
   a. Mild to moderate obesity (GH, TSH)
   b. Reduced cardiac output (GH, ADH)
   c. Infertility, sexual dysfunction (gonadotropins, ACTH)
   d. Fatigue, low blood pressure (TSH, ADH, ACTH, GH)
   e. Tumors of the pituitary also may cause headaches and visual defects (the pituitary is located near the optic nerve).
4. Interventions
   a. Client may need hormone replacement for the specific deficient hormones.
   b. Provide emotional support to the client and family.
   c. Encourage the client and family to express feelings related to disturbed body image or sexual dysfunction.
   d. Client education is needed regarding the signs and symptoms of hypofunction and hyperfunction related to insufficient or excess hormone replacement.

BOX 46-6 Pituitary Gland Problems

Anterior Pituitary
- Hyperpituitarism
- Hypopituitarism

Posterior Pituitary

These problems can be caused by damage to the posterior pituitary or hypothalamus:
- Diabetes insipidus
- Syndrome of inappropriate antidiuretic hormone secretion (SIADH)

B. Hyperpituitarism (acromegaly)
1. Description: Hypersecretion of growth hormone by the anterior pituitary gland in an adult; caused primarily by pituitary tumors
2. Assessment
   a. Large hands and feet
   b. Thickening and protrusion of the jaw
   c. Arthritic changes and joint pain, impingement syndromes
   d. Visual disturbances
   e. Diaphoresis
   f. Oily, rough skin
   g. Organomegaly
   h. Hypertension, atherosclerosis, cardiomegaly, heart failure
   i. Dysphagia
   j. Deepening of the voice
   k. Thickening of the tongue, narrowing of the airway, sleep apnea
   l. Hyperglycemia
   m. Colon polyps, increased colon cancer risk
3. Interventions
   a. Provide pharmacological interventions to suppress GH or to block the action of GH
   b. Prepare the client for radiation of the pituitary gland or for stereotactic radiosurgery if prescribed.
   c. Prepare the client for hypophysectomy if planned.
   d. Provide pharmacological and nonpharmacological interventions for joint pain.
   e. Provide emotional support to the client and family, and encourage the client and family to express feelings related to disturbed body image.

C. Hypophysectomy (pituitary adenectomy, sublabial transsphenoidal pituitary surgery)
1. Description
   a. Removal of a pituitary tumor via craniotomy or a sublabial transsphenoidal (endoscopic transnasal) approach (the latter approach is preferred because it is associated with fewer complications)
   b. Complications for craniotomy include increased intracranial pressure, bleeding, meningitis, and hypopituitarism.
   c. Complications for the sublabial transsphenoidal surgery include cerebrospinal fluid leak, infection, diabetes insipidus, and hypopituitarism.
   d. If the sublabial approach is used, an incision is made along the gum line of the inner upper lip.
2. Postoperative interventions
   a. Initial postoperative care is similar to craniotomy care (see Chapter 58).

b. Monitor vital signs, neurological status, and level of consciousness.
c. Elevate the head of the bed.
d. Monitor for increased intracranial pressure.
e. Instruct the client to avoid sneezing, coughing, and blowing the nose.
f. Monitor for bleeding.
g. Monitor for and report signs of temporary diabetes insipidus; monitor intake and output, and report excessive urinary output.
h. If the entire pituitary is removed, clients will require lifelong replacement of ADH, cortisol, and thyroid hormone.
i. Monitor for and report signs of infection and meningitis.
j. Administer antibiotics, analgesics, and antipyretics as prescribed.
k. Administer oral mouth rinses as prescribed. Clients may be instructed to avoid using a toothbrush or to brush teeth gently with an ultrasoft toothbrush for 10 days to 2 weeks after surgery.
l. Instruct the client in the administration of prescribed medications.

! Following transsphenoidal hypophysectomy, monitor for and report postnasal drip or clear nasal drainage, which might indicate a cerebrospinal fluid leak. Clear drainage should be checked for glucose.

D. Diabetes insipidus
1. Description
a. Hyposecretion of ADH by the posterior pituitary gland caused by stroke, trauma, or surgery, or it may be idiopathic
b. Kidney tubules fail to reabsorb water.
c. In central diabetes insipidus there is decreased ADH production.
d. In nephrogenic diabetes insipidus, ADH production is adequate, but the kidneys do not respond appropriately to the ADH.
2. Assessment
a. Excretion of large amounts of dilute urine
b. Polydipsia
c. Dehydration (decreased skin turgor and dry mucous membranes)
d. Inability to concentrate urine
e. Low urinary specific gravity; normal is 1.010 to 1.025 (1.005 to 1.030)
f. Fatigue
g. Muscle pain and weakness
h. Headache
i. Postural hypotension that may progress to vascular collapse without rehydration
j. Tachycardia
3. Interventions
a. Monitor vital signs and neurological and cardiovascular status.
b. Provide a safe environment, particularly for the client with postural hypotension.
c. Monitor electrolyte values and for signs of dehydration.
d. Maintain client intake of adequate fluids; IV hypotonic saline may be prescribed to replace urinary losses.
e. Monitor intake and output, weight, serum osmolality, and specific gravity of urine for excessive urinary output, weight loss, and low urinary specific gravity.
f. Instruct the client to avoid foods or liquids that produce diuresis.
g. Vasopressin or desmopressin acetate may be prescribed; these are used when the ADH deficiency is severe or chronic.
h. Instruct the client in the administration of medications as prescribed; desmopressin acetate may be administered by subcutaneous injection, intravenously, intranasally, or orally; watch for signs of water intoxication indicating overtreatment.
i. Instruct the client to wear a MedicAlert bracelet.

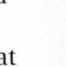

E. Syndrome of inappropriate antidiuretic hormone secretion (SIADH)
1. Description
a. Condition of hyperfunctioning of the posterior pituitary gland in which excess ADH is released, but not in response to the body's need for it
b. Causes include trauma, stroke, malignancies (often in the lungs or pancreas), medications, and stress.
c. The syndrome results in increased intravascular volume, water intoxication, and dilutional hyponatremia.
d. May cause cerebral edema, and the client is at risk for seizures.
2. Assessment
a. Signs of fluid volume overload
b. Changes in level of consciousness and mental status changes
c. Weight gain without edema
d. Hypertension
e. Tachycardia
f. Anorexia, nausea, and vomiting
g. Hyponatremia
h. Low urinary output and concentrated urine
3. Interventions
a. Monitor vital signs and cardiac and neurological status.
b. Provide a safe environment, particularly for the client with changes in level of consciousness or mental status.
c. Monitor for signs of increased intracranial pressure.

d. Implement seizure precautions.
e. Elevate the head of the bed a maximum of 10 degrees to promote venous return and decrease baroreceptor-induced ADH release.
f. Monitor intake and output and obtain weight daily.
g. Monitor fluid and electrolyte balance.
h. Monitor serum and urine osmolality.
i. Restrict fluid intake as prescribed.
j. Administer IV fluids (usually normal saline [NS] or hypertonic saline) as prescribed; monitor IV fluids carefully because of the risk for fluid volume overload.
k. Loop diuretics may be prescribed to promote diuresis, but only if serum sodium is at least 125 mEq/L (125 mmol/L); potassium replacement may be necessary if loop diuretics are prescribed.
l. Vasopressin antagonists may be prescribed to decrease the renal response to ADH.

IV. Adrenal Gland Problems (Box 46-7)

A. Adrenal cortex insufficiency (Addison's disease)
1. Primary adrenal insufficiency
a. Also known as **Addison's disease,** refers to hyposecretion of adrenal cortex hormones (glucocorticoids, mineralocorticoids, and androgen); autoimmune destruction is a common cause.
b. Requires lifelong replacement of glucocorticoids and possibly of mineralocorticoids if significant hyposecretion occurs; the condition is fatal if left untreated.
2. Secondary adrenal insufficiency is caused by hyposecretion of ACTH from the anterior pituitary gland; mineralocorticoid release is spared.
3. Loss of glucocorticoids in Addison's disease leads to decreased vascular tone, decreased vascular response to the catecholamines epinephrine and norepinephrine, and decreased gluconeogenesis.
4. In Addison's disease, loss of the mineralocorticoid aldosterone leads to dehydration, hypotension, hyponatremia, and hyperkalemia.
5. Assessment (Table 46-1)
6. Interventions

BOX 46-7 Adrenal Gland Problems

Adrenal Cortex
- Addison's disease
- Primary hyperaldosteronism (Conn's syndrome)
- Cushing's disease
- Cushing's syndrome

Adrenal Medulla
- Pheochromocytoma

TABLE 46-1 Assessment: Addison's Disease and Cushing's Disease and Cushing's Syndrome

Addison's Disease	Cushing's Disease and Cushing's Syndrome
Lethargy, fatigue, and muscle weakness	Generalized muscle wasting and weakness
Gastrointestinal disturbances	Moon face, buffalo hump
Weight loss	Truncal obesity with thin extremities, supraclavicular fat pads; weight gain
Menstrual changes in women; impotence in men	Hirsutism (masculine characteristics in females)
Hypoglycemia, hyponatremia	Hyperglycemia, hypernatremia
Hyperkalemia, hypercalcemia	Hypokalemia, hypocalcemia
Hypotension	Hypertension
Hyperpigmentation of skin (bronzed) with primary disease	Fragile skin that bruises easily Reddish-purple striae on the abdomen and upper thighs

a. Monitor vital signs (particularly for hypotension), for weight loss, and intake and output.
b. Monitor white blood cell (WBC) count; blood glucose; and potassium, sodium, and calcium levels.
c. Administer glucocorticoid and/or mineralocorticoid medications as prescribed.
d. Observe for **addisonian crisis** caused by stress, infection, trauma, or surgery.
7. Client education
a. Need for lifelong glucocorticoid replacement and possibly lifelong mineralocorticoid replacement.
b. Corticosteroid replacement will need to be increased during times of stress.
c. Avoid individuals with an infection.
d. Avoid strenuous exercise and stressful situations.
e. Avoid over-the-counter medications.
f. Diet should be high in protein and carbohydrates; clients taking glucocorticoids should be prescribed calcium and vitamin D supplements to maintain normal levels and to protect against corticosteroid-induced osteoporosis; some clients taking mineralocorticoids may be prescribed a diet high in sodium.
g. Wear a MedicAlert bracelet.
h. Report signs and symptoms of complications, such as underreplacement and overreplacement of corticosteroid hormones.

B. Addisonian crisis
1. Description (Box 46-8)
2. Assessment

BOX 46-8 Addisonian Crisis

- A life-threatening disorder caused by acute adrenal insufficiency
- Precipitated by stress, infection, trauma, surgery, or abrupt withdrawal of exogenous corticosteroid use
- Can cause hyponatremia, hyperkalemia, hypoglycemia, and shock

a. Severe headache
b. Severe abdominal, leg, and lower back pain
c. Generalized weakness
d. Irritability and confusion
e. Severe hypotension
f. Shock

3. Interventions
a. Prepare to administer glucocorticoids intravenously as prescribed.
b. Administer IV fluids as prescribed to replace fluids and restore electrolyte balance.
c. Following resolution of the crisis, administer glucocorticoid and mineralocorticoid orally as prescribed.
d. Monitor vital signs, particularly blood pressure.
e. Monitor neurological status, noting irritability and confusion.
f. Monitor intake and output.
g. Monitor laboratory values, particularly sodium, potassium, and blood glucose levels.
h. Protect the client from infection.
i. Maintain bed rest and provide a quiet environment.

⚠ Clients taking exogenous corticosteroids must establish a plan with their PHCPs or endocrinologist for increasing their corticosteroids during times of stress.

C. Cushing's syndrome and Cushing's disease (hypercortisolism)

1. **Cushing's syndrome**
a. A metabolic disorder resulting from the chronic and excessive production of cortisol by the adrenal cortex or from the administration of glucocorticoids in large doses for several weeks or longer (exogenous or iatrogenic).
b. ACTH secreting tumors (most often of the lung, pancreas, or gastrointestinal [GI] tract) can cause Cushing's syndrome.

2. **Cushing's disease** is a metabolic disorder characterized by abnormally increased secretion (endogenous) of cortisol, caused by increased amounts of ACTH secreted by the pituitary gland.

3. Assessment (Fig. 46-2; see Table 46-1)

4. Interventions
a. Monitor vital signs, particularly blood pressure.
b. Monitor intake and output and weight.
c. Monitor laboratory values, particularly WBC count and serum glucose, sodium, potassium, and calcium levels.
d. Prepare the client for radiation as prescribed if the condition results from a pituitary adenoma.
e. Administer chemotherapeutic agents as prescribed for inoperable adrenal tumors.
f. Prepare the client for removal of the pituitary tumor (hypophysectomy, sublabial transsphenoidal adenectomy) if the condition results from increased pituitary secretion of ACTH.
g. Prepare the client for **adrenalectomy** if the condition results from an adrenal adenoma; glucocorticoid replacement may be required following adrenalectomy.
h. Clients requiring lifelong glucocorticoid replacement following adrenalectomy should obtain instructions from their PHCPs about increasing their glucocorticoid during times of stress.
i. Assess for and protect against postoperative thrombus formation; Cushing's syndrome predisposes to thromboemboli.
j. Allow the client to discuss feelings related to body appearance.
k. Instruct the client about the need to wear a MedicAlert bracelet.

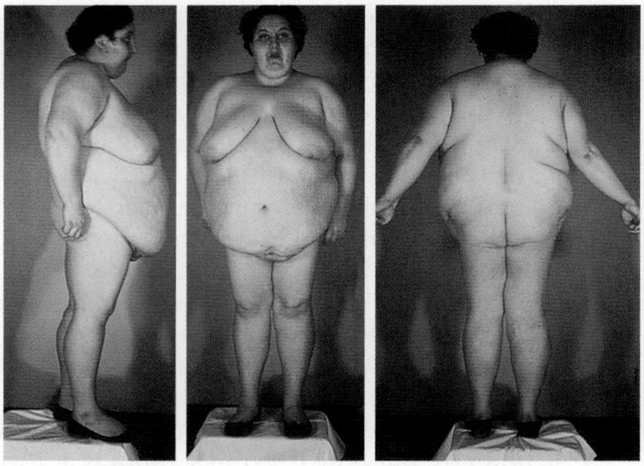

FIG. 46-2 Typical appearance of a client with Cushing's syndrome. Note truncal obesity, moon face, buffalo hump, thinner arms and legs, and abdominal striae. (From Wenig, Heffess, Adair, 1997.)

⚠ Addison's disease is characterized by the hyposecretion of adrenal cortex hormones, whereas Cushing's syndrome and Cushing's disease are characterized by a hypersecretion of glucocorticoids.

D. Primary hyperaldosteronism (Conn's syndrome)

1. Description
a. Hypersecretion of mineralocorticoids (aldosterone) from the adrenal cortex of the adrenal gland
b. Most commonly caused by an adenoma
c. Excess secretion of aldosterone causes sodium

and water retention and potassium excretion, leading to hypertension and hypokalemic alkalosis.

2. Assessment
   a. Symptoms related to hypokalemia, hypernatremia, and hypertension
   b. Headache, fatigue, muscle weakness
   c. Cardiac dysrhythmias
   d. Paresthesias, tetany
   e. Visual changes
   f. Glucose intolerance
   g. Elevated serum aldosterone levels
3. Interventions
   a. Monitor vital signs, particularly blood pressure.
   b. Monitor potassium and sodium levels.
   c. Monitor intake and output and urine for specific gravity.
   d. Monitor for hyperkalemia, particularly for clients with impaired renal function or excessive potassium intake, because potassium-retaining diuretics and aldosterone antagonists may be prescribed to promote fluid balance and control hypertension.
   e. Administer potassium supplements as prescribed to treat hypokalemia; clients taking potassium-retaining diuretics and potassium supplementation are at risk for hyperkalemia.
   f. Prepare the client for adrenalectomy.
   g. Maintain sodium restriction, if prescribed, preoperatively.
   h. Administer glucocorticoids preoperatively, as prescribed, to prevent adrenal hypofunction and prepare for stress of surgery.
   i. Monitor the client for adrenal insufficiency postoperatively.
   j. Instruct the client regarding the need for glucocorticoid therapy following adrenalectomy.
   k. Instruct the client about the need to wear a MedicAlert bracelet.

E. Pheochromocytoma

1. Description
   a. Catecholamine-producing tumor usually found in the adrenal medulla, but extraadrenal locations include the chest, bladder, abdomen, and brain; typically is a benign tumor but can be malignant
   b. Excessive amounts of epinephrine and norepinephrine are secreted.
   c. Diagnostic test includes a 24-hour urine collection for VMA.
   d. Surgical removal of the adrenal gland is the primary treatment.
   e. Symptomatic treatment is initiated if surgical removal is not possible.
   f. The complications associated with pheochromocytoma include hypertensive crisis; hypertensive retinopathy and nephropathy, cardiac enlargement, and dysrhythmias; heart failure; myocardial infarction; increased platelet aggregation; and stroke.
   g. Death can occur from shock, stroke, renal failure, dysrhythmias, or dissecting aortic aneurysm.
2. Assessment
   a. Paroxysmal or sustained hypertension
   b. Severe headaches
   c. Palpitations
   d. Flushing and profuse diaphoresis
   e. Pain in the chest or abdomen with nausea and vomiting
   f. Heat intolerance
   g. Weight loss
   h. Tremors
   i. Hyperglycemia
3. Interventions
   a. Monitor vital signs, particularly blood pressure and heart rate.
   b. Monitor for hypertensive crisis; monitor for complications that can occur with hypertensive crisis, such as stroke, cardiac dysrhythmias, and myocardial infarction.
   c. Instruct the client not to smoke, drink caffeine-containing beverages, or change position suddenly.
   d. Prepare to administer α-adrenergic blocking agents and β-adrenergic blocking agents as prescribed to control hypertension. α-Adrenergic blocking agents are started 7 to 10 days before β-adrenergic blocking agents.
   e. Monitor serum glucose level.
   f. Promote rest and a nonstressful environment.
   g. Provide a diet high in calories, vitamins, and minerals.
   h. Prepare the client for adrenalectomy.

For the client with pheochromocytoma, avoid stimuli that can precipitate a hypertensive crisis, such as increased abdominal pressure and vigorous abdominal palpation.

F. Adrenalectomy

1. Description (Box 46-9)
2. Preoperative interventions
   a. Monitor electrolyte levels and correct electrolyte imbalances.
   b. Assess for dysrhythmias.
   c. Monitor for hyperglycemia.
   d. Protect the client from infections.
   e. Administer glucocorticoids as prescribed.
3. Postoperative interventions
   a. Monitor vital signs.
   b. Monitor intake and output; if the urinary output is lower than 30 mL/hr, notify the PHCP or nephrologist, because this may result in acute kidney injury and indicate impending shock.

BOX 46-9 Adrenalectomy

- Surgical removal of an adrenal gland
- Lifelong glucocorticoid and mineralocorticoid replacement is necessary with bilateral adrenalectomy.
- Temporary glucocorticoid replacement, usually up to 2 years, is necessary after a unilateral adrenalectomy.
- Catecholamine levels drop as a result of surgery, which can result in cardiovascular collapse, hypotension, and shock, and the client needs to be monitored closely.
- Hemorrhage also can occur because of the high vascularity of the adrenal glands.

c. Monitor weight daily.
d. Monitor electrolyte and serum glucose levels.
e. Monitor for signs of hemorrhage and shock, particularly during the first 24 to 48 hours.
f. Monitor for manifestations of adrenal insufficiency (see Table 46-1).
g. Assess the dressing for drainage.
h. Monitor for paralytic ileus.
i. Administer IV fluids as prescribed to maintain blood volume.
j. Administer glucocorticoids and mineralocorticoids as prescribed.
k. Administer pain medication as prescribed.
l. Provide pulmonary interventions to prevent atelectasis (coughing and deep breathing, incentive spirometry, splinting of incision).
m. Instruct the client in the importance of hormone replacement therapy following surgery.
n. Instruct the client regarding signs and symptoms of complications such as underreplacement and overreplacement of hormones.
o. Instruct the client regarding the need to wear a MedicAlert bracelet.

V. Thyroid Gland Problems

A. Hypothyroidism

1. Description
   a. Hypothyroid state resulting from hyposecretion of thyroid hormones and characterized by a decreased rate of body metabolism
   b. The T_4 is low and the TSH is elevated.
   c. In primary hypothyroidism, the source of dysfunction is the thyroid gland, and the thyroid cannot produce the necessary amount of hormones. In secondary hypothyroidism, the thyroid is not being stimulated by the pituitary to produce hormones.
2. Assessment (Table 46-2)
3. Interventions
   a. Monitor vital signs, including heart rate and rhythm.
   b. Administer thyroid replacement; levothyroxine sodium is most commonly prescribed.

TABLE 46-2 Assessment: Hypothyroidism and Hyperthyroidism

Hypothyroidism	Hyperthyroidism
Lethargy and fatigue	Personality changes such as irritability, agitation, and mood swings
Weakness, muscle aches, paresthesias	Nervousness and fine tremors of the hands
	Weakness, muscle aches, paresthesias
Intolerance to cold	Heat intolerance
Weight gain	Weight loss
Dry skin and hair and loss of body hair	Smooth, soft skin and hair
Bradycardia	Palpitations, cardiac dysrhythmias, such as tachycardia or atrial fibrillation
Constipation	Diarrhea
Generalized puffiness and edema around the eyes and face (myxedema)	Protruding eyeballs (exophthalmos) may be present (see Fig. 46-3)
Forgetfulness and loss of memory	Diaphoresis
Menstrual disturbances	Hypertension
Goiter may or may not be present	Enlarged thyroid gland (goiter)
Cardiac enlargement, tendency to develop heart failure	

   c. Instruct the client about thyroid replacement therapy and about the clinical manifestations of both hypothyroidism and hyperthyroidism related to underreplacement or overreplacement of the hormone.
   d. Instruct the client in a low-calorie, low-cholesterol, low–saturated fat diet; discuss a daily exercise program such as walking.
   e. Assess the client for constipation; provide roughage and fluids to prevent constipation.
   f. Provide a warm environment for the client.
   g. Avoid sedatives and opioid analgesics because of increased sensitivity to these medications; may precipitate myxedema coma.
   h. Monitor for overdose of thyroid medications, characterized by tachycardia, chest pain, restlessness, nervousness, and insomnia.
   i. Instruct the client to report episodes of chest pain or other signs of overdose immediately.

B. Myxedema coma

1. Description (Box 46-10)
2. Assessment
   a. Hypotension

BOX 46-10 Myxedema Coma

- This rare but serious disorder results from persistently low thyroid production.
- Coma can be precipitated by acute illness, rapid withdrawal of thyroid medication, anesthesia and surgery, hypothermia, or the use of sedatives and opioid analgesics.

b. Bradycardia
c. Hypothermia
d. Hyponatremia
e. Hypoglycemia
f. Generalized edema
g. Respiratory failure
h. Coma

3. Interventions
 a. Maintain a patent airway.
 b. Institute aspiration precautions.
 c. Administer IV fluids (normal or hypertonic saline) as prescribed.
 d. Administer levothyroxine sodium intravenously as prescribed.
 e. Administer glucose intravenously as prescribed.
 f. Administer corticosteroids as prescribed.
 g. Assess the client's temperature hourly.
 h. Monitor blood pressure frequently.
 i. Keep the client warm.
 j. Monitor for changes in mental status.
 k. Monitor electrolyte and glucose levels.

C. Hyperthyroidism

1. Description
 a. Hyperthyroid state resulting from hypersecretion of thyroid hormones (T_3 and T_4)
 b. Characterized by an increased rate of body metabolism
 c. A common cause is Graves' disease, also known as toxic diffuse goiter.
 d. Clinical manifestations are referred to as *thyrotoxicosis*.
 e. The T_3 and T_4 are usually elevated and the TSH level is low.
2. Assessment (see Table 46-2; Fig. 46-3)
3. Interventions
 a. Provide adequate rest.
 b. Administer sedatives as prescribed.
 c. Provide a cool and quiet environment.
 d. Obtain weight daily.
 e. Provide a high-calorie diet.
 f. Avoid the administration of stimulants.
 g. Administer antithyroid medications, such as methimazole or propylthiouracil, that block thyroid synthesis as prescribed.
 h. Administer iodine preparations that inhibit the release of thyroid hormone as prescribed.

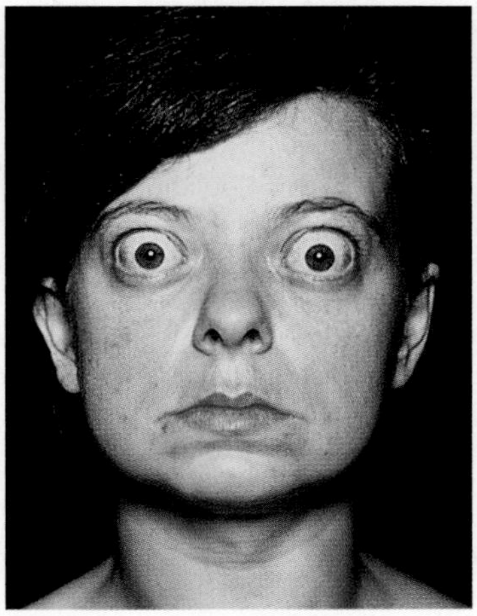

FIG. 46-3 Exophthalmos. (From Ignatavicius, Workman, 2016.)

 i. Administer propranolol for tachycardia as prescribed.
 j. Prepare the client for radioactive iodine therapy, as prescribed, to destroy thyroid cells.
 k. Prepare the client for subtotal thyroidectomy if prescribed.
 l. Elevate the head of the bed of a client experiencing exophthalmos; in addition, instruct on low-salt diet, administer artificial tears, encourage the use of dark glasses, and tape eyelids closed at night if necessary.
 m. Allow the client to express concerns about body image changes.

D. Thyroid storm

1. Description (Box 46-11)
2. Assessment
 a. Elevated temperature (fever)
 b. Tachycardia
 c. Systolic hypertension
 d. Nausea, vomiting, and diarrhea
 e. Agitation, tremors, anxiety
 f. Irritability, agitation, restlessness, confusion, and seizures as the condition progresses
 g. Delirium and coma
3. Interventions
 a. Maintain a patent airway and adequate ventilation.
 b. Administer antithyroid medications, iodides, propranolol, and glucocorticoids as prescribed.
 c. Monitor vital signs.
 d. Monitor continually for cardiac dysrhythmias.
 e. Administer nonsalicylate antipyretics as prescribed (salicylates increase free thyroid hormone levels).
 f. Use a cooling blanket to decrease temperature as prescribed.

BOX 46-11 Thyroid Storm

- This acute and life-threatening condition occurs in a client with uncontrollable hyperthyroidism.
- It can be caused by manipulation of the thyroid gland during surgery and the release of thyroid hormone into the bloodstream; it also can occur from severe infection and stress.
- Antithyroid medications, beta blockers, glucocorticoids, and iodides may be administered to the client before thyroid surgery to prevent its occurrence.

BOX 46-12 Signs of Tetany

- Cardiac dysrhythmias
- Carpopedal spasm
- Dysphagia
- Muscle and abdominal cramps
- Numbness and tingling of the face and extremities
- Positive Chvostek's sign
- Positive Trousseau's sign
- Visual disturbances (photophobia)
- Wheezing and dyspnea (bronchospasm, laryngospasm)
- Seizures

E. Thyroidectomy

1. Description
   a. Removal of the thyroid gland
   b. Performed when persistent hyperthyroidism exists
   c. Subtotal thyroidectomy, removal of a portion of the thyroid gland, is the preferred surgical intervention.
2. Preoperative interventions
   a. Obtain vital signs and weight.
   b. Assess electrolyte levels.
   c. Assess for hyperglycemia.
   d. Instruct the client in how to perform coughing and deep-breathing exercises and how to support the neck in the postoperative period when coughing and moving.
   e. Administer antithyroid medications, iodides, propranolol, and glucocorticoids as prescribed to prevent the occurrence of thyroid storm.
3. Postoperative interventions
   a. Monitor for respiratory distress.
   b. Have a tracheotomy set, oxygen, and suction at the bedside.
   c. Limit client talking, and assess level of hoarseness.
   d. Avoid neck flexion and stress on the suture line.
   e. Monitor for laryngeal nerve damage, as evidenced by airway obstruction, dysphonia, high-pitched voice, stridor, dysphagia, and restlessness.
   f. Monitor for signs of hypocalcemia and tetany, which can be caused by trauma to the parathyroid gland (Box 46-12).
   g. Prepare to administer calcium gluconate as prescribed for tetany.
   h. Monitor for thyroid storm.

Following thyroidectomy, maintain the client in a semi-Fowler's position. Monitor the surgical site for edema and for signs of bleeding and check the dressing anteriorly and at the back of the neck. Monitor for inflammation, which may block the airway. An emergency tracheostomy kit should be at the bedside.

VI. Parathyroid Gland Problems

A. Hypoparathyroidism

1. Description
   a. Condition caused by hyposecretion of parathyroid hormone by the parathyroid gland
   b. Can occur following thyroidectomy because of removal of parathyroid tissue
2. Assessment
   a. Hypocalcemia and hyperphosphatemia
   b. Numbness and tingling in the face
   c. Muscle cramps and cramps in the abdomen or in the extremities
   d. Positive Trousseau's sign or Chvostek's sign
   e. Signs of overt tetany, such as bronchospasm, laryngospasm, carpopedal spasm, dysphagia, photophobia, cardiac dysrhythmias, seizures
   f. Hypotension
   g. Anxiety, irritability, depression
3. Interventions
   a. Monitor vital signs.
   b. Monitor for signs of hypocalcemia and tetany.
   c. Initiate seizure precautions.
   d. Place a tracheotomy set, oxygen, and suctioning equipment at the bedside.
   e. Prepare to administer calcium gluconate intravenously for hypocalcemia.
   f. Provide a high-calcium, low-phosphorus diet.
   g. Instruct the client in the administration of calcium supplements as prescribed.
   h. Instruct the client in the administration of vitamin D supplements as prescribed; vitamin D enhances the absorption of calcium from the gastrointestinal (GI) tract.
   i. Instruct the client in the use of thiazide diuretics if prescribed, to protect the kidney if vitamin D is also taken.
   j. Instruct the client in the administration of phosphate binders as prescribed to promote the excretion of phosphate through the GI tract.
   k. Instruct the client to wear a MedicAlert bracelet.

B. Hyperparathyroidism

1. Description: Condition caused by hypersecretion of parathyroid hormone (PTH) by the parathyroid gland
2. Assessment
   a. Hypercalcemia and hypophosphatemia
   b. Fatigue and muscle weakness
   c. Skeletal pain and tenderness
   d. Bone deformities that result in pathological fractures
   e. Anorexia, nausea, vomiting, epigastric pain
   f. Weight loss
   g. Constipation
   h. Hypertension
   i. Cardiac dysrhythmias
   j. Renal stones
3. Interventions
   a. Monitor vital signs, particularly blood pressure.
   b. Monitor for cardiac dysrhythmias.
   c. Monitor intake and output and for signs of renal stones.
   d. Monitor for skeletal pain; move the client slowly and carefully.
   e. Encourage fluid intake.
   f. Administer furosemide as prescribed to lower calcium levels.
   g. Administer NS intravenously as prescribed to maintain hydration.
   h. Administer phosphates, which interfere with calcium reabsorption, as prescribed.
   i. Administer calcitonin as prescribed to decrease skeletal calcium release and increase renal excretion of calcium.
   j. Administer IV or oral bisphosphonates to inhibit bone resorption.
   k. Monitor calcium and phosphorus levels.
   l. Prepare the client for parathyroidectomy as prescribed.
   m. Encourage a high-fiber, moderate-calcium diet.
   n. Emphasize the importance of an exercise program and avoiding prolonged inactivity.

C. Parathyroidectomy

1. Description: Removal of 1 or more of the parathyroid glands
   a. Endoscopic radioguided parathyroidectomy with autotransplantation is a common procedure.
   b. Parathyroid tissue is transplanted in the forearm or near the sternocleidomastoid muscle, allowing PTH secretion to continue.
2. Preoperative interventions
   a. Monitor electrolytes, calcium, phosphate, and magnesium levels.
   b. Ensure that calcium levels are decreased to near-normal values.
   c. Inform the client that talking may be painful for the first day or two after surgery.
3. Postoperative interventions
   a. Monitor for respiratory distress.
   b. Place a tracheotomy set, oxygen, and suctioning equipment at the bedside.
   c. Monitor vital signs.
   d. Position the client in semi-Fowler's position.
   e. Assess neck dressing for bleeding.
   f. Monitor for hypocalcemic crisis, as evidenced by tingling and twitching in the extremities and face.
   g. Assess for positive Trousseau's sign or Chvostek's sign, which indicates tetany.
   h. Monitor for changes in voice pattern and hoarseness.
   i. Monitor for laryngeal nerve damage.
   j. Instruct the client in the administration of calcium and vitamin D supplements as prescribed.

VII. Problems of the Pancreas

A. Diabetes mellitus

1. Description
   a. Chronic disorder of impaired carbohydrate, protein, and lipid metabolism caused by a deficiency of insulin
   b. An absolute or relative deficiency of insulin results in hyperglycemia.
   c. Type 1 diabetes mellitus is a nearly absolute deficiency of insulin (primary beta cell destruction); if insulin is not given, fats are metabolized for energy, resulting in ketonemia (acidosis).
   d. Type 2 diabetes mellitus is a relative lack of insulin or resistance to the action of insulin; usually, insulin is sufficient to stabilize fat and protein metabolism but not carbohydrate metabolism.
   e. Metabolic syndrome is also known as syndrome X, and the individual has coexisting risk factors for developing type 2 diabetes mellitus; these risk factors include abdominal obesity, hyperglycemia, hypertension, high triglyceride level, and a lowered HDL (high-density lipoprotein) cholesterol level.
   f. Diabetes mellitus can lead to chronic health problems and early death as a result of complications that occur in the large and small blood vessels in tissues and organs.
   g. Macrovascular complications include coronary artery disease, cardiomyopathy, hypertension, cerebrovascular disease, and peripheral vascular disease. (Refer to Chapter 52 for information on cardiovascular problems.)
   h. Microvascular complications include retinopathy, nephropathy, and neuropathy.

i. Infection is also a concern because of reduced healing ability.
j. Male erectile dysfunction can also occur as a result of the disease.

Obesity is a major risk factor for diabetes mellitus.

2. Assessment
   a. Polyuria, polydipsia, polyphagia (more common in type 1 diabetes mellitus)
   b. Hyperglycemia
   c. Weight loss (common in type 1 diabetes mellitus, rare in type 2 diabetes mellitus)
   d. Blurred vision
   e. Slow wound healing
   f. Vaginal infections
   g. Weakness and paresthesias
   h. Signs of inadequate circulation to the feet
   i. Signs of accelerated atherosclerosis (renal, cerebral, cardiac, peripheral)
3. Diet
   a. The diabetic client's diet should take into account weight, medication, activity level, and other health problems.
   b. Day-to-day consistency in timing and amount of food intake helps control the blood glucose level.
   c. As prescribed by the PHCP or endocrinologist, the client may be advised to follow the recommendations of the American Diabetic Association diet or U.S. dietary guidelines (MyPlate; http://www.choosemyplate.gov/) issued by the U.S. Departments of Agriculture and Health and Human Services.
   d. Carbohydrate counting may be a simpler approach for some clients; it focuses on the total grams of carbohydrates eaten per meal. The client may be more compliant with carbohydrate counting, resulting in better glycemic control; it is usually necessary for clients undergoing intense insulin therapy.
   e. Incorporate the diet into individual client needs, lifestyle, and cultural and socioeconomic patterns.
4. Exercise
   a. Exercise lowers the blood glucose level, encourages weight loss, reduces cardiovascular risks, improves circulation and muscle tone, decreases total cholesterol and triglyceride levels, and decreases insulin resistance and glucose intolerance.
   b. Instruct the client in dietary adjustments when exercising; dietary adjustments are individualized.
   c. If the client requires extra food during exercise to prevent hypoglycemia, it need not be deducted from the regular meal plan.
   d. If the blood glucose level is higher than 250 mg/dL (13.9 mmol/L) and urinary ketones (type 1 diabetes mellitus) are present, the client is instructed not to exercise until the blood glucose level is closer to normal and urinary ketones are absent.
   e. The client should try to exercise at the same time each day and should exercise when glucose from the meal is peaking, not when insulin or glucose-lowering medications are peaking.
   f. Insulin should not be injected into an area of the body that will be exercised following injection, as exercise speeds absorption.

Instruct the client with diabetes mellitus to monitor the blood glucose level before, during, and after exercising.

5. Oral hypoglycemic medications: Oral medications are prescribed for clients with diabetes mellitus type 2 when diet and weight control therapy have failed to maintain satisfactory blood glucose levels (Chapter 47).
6. Insulin (refer to Chapter 47 for additional information on insulin)
   a. Insulin is used to treat type 1 diabetes mellitus and may be used to treat type 2 diabetes mellitus when diet, weight control therapy, and oral hypoglycemic agents have failed to maintain satisfactory blood glucose levels.
   b. Illness, infection, and stress increase the blood glucose level and the need for insulin; insulin should not be withheld during times of illness, infection, or stress because hyperglycemia and **diabetic ketoacidosis** can result.
   c. The peak action time of insulin is important to explain to the client because of the possibility of hypoglycemic reactions occurring during this time.

Regular insulin (U-100 strength) can be administered via IV injection (IV push). Regular insulin (U-100) and the short-duration insulins (lispro, aspart, and glulisine) can be administered via IV infusion.

B. Complications of insulin therapy
1. Local allergic reactions
   a. Redness, swelling, tenderness, and induration or a wheal at the site of injection may occur 1 to 2 hours after administration.
   b. Reactions usually occur during the early stages of insulin therapy.
   c. Instruct the client to cleanse the skin with alcohol before injection.
2. Insulin lipodystrophy
   a. The development of fibrous fatty masses at the injection site caused by repeated use of

an injection site; use of human insulin helps prevent this.

b. Instruct the client to avoid injecting insulin into affected sites.

c. Instruct the client about the importance of rotating insulin injection sites. Systematic rotation within 1 anatomical area is recommended to prevent lipodystrophy; the client should be instructed not to use the same site more than once in a 2- to 3-week period. Injections should be 1.5 inches (3.8 cm) apart within the anatomical area.

3. Dawn phenomenon

a. Dawn phenomenon is characterized by hyperglycemia upon morning awakening that results from excessive early morning release of GH and cortisol.

b. Treatment requires an increase in the client's insulin dose or a change in the time of insulin administration.

4. Somogyi phenomenon

a. Normal or elevated blood glucose levels are present at bedtime; hypoglycemia occurs at about 2 to 3 a.m., which causes an increase in the production of counterregulatory hormones.

b. By about 7 a.m., in response to the counterregulatory hormones, the blood glucose rebounds significantly to the hyperglycemic range.

c. Treatment includes a decrease in the client's insulin dose or increase in the bedtime snack, or both.

d. Clients experiencing the Somogyi phenomenon may complain of early morning headaches, night sweats, or nightmares caused by the early morning hypoglycemia.

C. Insulin administration

1. Subcutaneous injections and mixing insulin: See Chapter 47.

2. Insulin pumps

a. Continuous subcutaneous insulin infusion is administered by an externally worn device that contains a syringe and pump; different types of pumps are available and the one selected is based on the client's needs.

b. The client inserts the needle or Teflon catheter into the subcutaneous tissue (usually on the abdomen or upper arm) and secures it with tape or a transparent dressing; the needle or Teflon catheter is changed at least every 2 to 3 days.

c. A continuous basal rate of insulin infuses; in addition, on the basis of the blood glucose level, the anticipated food intake, and the activity level, the client delivers a bolus of insulin before each meal.

d. Both rapid-acting and regular short-acting insulin (buffered to prevent the precipitation of insulin crystals within the catheter) are appropriate for use in these pumps.

3. Insulin pump and skin sensor

a. A skin sensor device can be used that monitors the client's blood glucose continuously; the information is transmitted to the pump, which determines the need for insulin, and then the insulin is injected.

b. The pump holds up to a 3-day supply of insulin and can be disconnected easily if necessary for certain activities such as bathing.

4. Pancreas transplants

a. The goal of pancreatic transplantation is to halt or reverse the complications of diabetes mellitus.

b. Transplantations are performed on a limited number of clients (in general, these are clients who are undergoing kidney transplantation simultaneously).

c. Immunosuppressive therapy is prescribed to prevent and treat rejection.

D. Self-monitoring of blood glucose level

1. Self-monitoring provides the client with the current blood glucose level and information to maintain good glycemic control.

2. Monitoring requires a finger prick to obtain a drop of blood for testing.

3. Alternative site testing (obtaining blood from the forearm, upper arm, abdomen, thigh, or calf) is available, using specific measurement devices.

4. Tests must be used with caution in clients with diabetic neuropathy.

5. Client instructions (Box 46-13)

E. Urine testing

1. Urine testing for glucose is not a reliable indicator of the blood glucose level and is not used for monitoring purposes.

2. Instruct the client in the procedure for testing for urine ketones.

3. The presence of ketones may indicate impending ketoacidosis.

4. Urine ketone testing should be performed during illness and whenever the client with type 1 diabetes mellitus has persistently elevated blood glucose levels (higher than 250 mg/dL [13.9 mmol/L] or as prescribed for 2 consecutive testing periods).

VIII. Acute Complications of Diabetes Mellitus

A. Hypoglycemia

1. Description

a. Hypoglycemia occurs when the blood glucose level falls below 70 mg/dL (3.9 mmol/L), or when the blood glucose level drops rapidly from an elevated level.

BOX 46-13 Client Instructions: Self-Monitoring of Blood Glucose Level

- Use the proper procedure to obtain the sample for determining the blood glucose level.
- Perform the procedure precisely to obtain accurate results.
- Follow the manufacturer's instructions for the glucometer.
- Wash hands before and after performing the procedure to prevent infection.
- If needed, calibrate the monitor as instructed by the manufacturer.
- Check the expiration date on the test strips.
- If the blood glucose level results do not seem reasonable, reread the instructions, reassess technique, check the expiration date of the test strips, and perform the procedure again to verify results.

BOX 46-14 Simple Carbohydrates to Treat Hypoglycemia

- Commercially prepared glucose tablets or glucose gel
- 6 to 10 Life Savers or hard candy
- 4 tsp of sugar
- 4 sugar cubes
- 1 Tbsp of honey or syrup
- ½ cup of fruit juice or regular (nondiet) soft drink
- 8 oz (235 mL) of low-fat milk
- 6 saltine crackers
- 3 graham crackers

b. Hypoglycemia is caused by too much insulin or too large an amount of an oral hypoglycemic agent, too little food, or excessive activity.

c. The client needs to be instructed always to carry some form of fast-acting simple carbohydrate with him or her (Box 46-14).

d. If the client has a hypoglycemic reaction and does not have any of the recommended emergency foods available, any available food should be eaten; high-fat foods slow the absorption of glucose, and the hypoglycemic symptoms may not resolve quickly.

e. Clients who experience frequent episodes of hypoglycemia, older clients, and clients taking β-adrenergic blocking agents may not experience the warning signs of hypoglycemia until the blood glucose level is dangerously low; this phenomenon is termed *hypoglycemia unawareness.*

2. Assessment (Box 46-15)

a. Mild hypoglycemia: The client remains fully awake but displays adrenergic symptoms; the blood glucose level is lower than 70 mg/dL (3.9 mmol/L).

b. Moderate hypoglycemia: The client displays symptoms of worsening hypoglycemia; the blood glucose level is usually lower than 40 mg/dL (2.2 mmol/L).

c. Severe hypoglycemia: The client displays severe neuroglycopenic symptoms; the blood glucose level is usually lower than 20 mg/dL (1.1 mmol/L).

3. Interventions (see Priority Nursing Actions)

PRIORITY NURSING ACTIONS

Suspected Hypoglycemic Reaction (the 15/15 rule)

1. If a blood glucose monitor is readily available, check the client's blood glucose level. If the client is experiencing symptoms suggestive of hypoglycemia such as diaphoresis, hunger, pallor, and shakiness, and a blood glucose monitor is not readily available, assume hypoglycemia and treat accordingly.
2. For the client whose blood glucose is below 70 mg/dL (3.9 mmol/L), or for the client with an unknown blood glucose who is exhibiting signs of hypoglycemia, administer 15 g of a simple carbohydrate such as ½ cup of fruit juice or 15 g of glucose gel.
3. Recheck the blood glucose level in 15 minutes.
4. If the blood glucose remains below 70 mg/dL (3.9 mmol/L), administer another 15 g of a simple carbohydrate.
5. Recheck the blood glucose level in 15 minutes; if still below 70 mg/dL (3.9 mmol/L), treat with an additional 15 g of a simple carbohydrate.
6. Recheck the blood glucose level in 15 minutes; if still below 70 mg/dL (3.9 mmol/L), treat with 25 to 50 mL of 50% dextrose intravenously or, if no intravenous (IV) equipment is present, treat with 1 mg of glucagon subcutaneously or intramuscularly.
7. After the blood glucose level has recovered, have the client ingest a snack that includes a complex carbohydrate and a protein.
8. Document the client's complaints, actions taken, and outcome.
9. Explore the precipitating cause of the hypoglycemia with the client.
10. If the client is experiencing an altered level of consciousness, bypass oral treatment and start with injectable glucagon or 50% dextrose. If the client is at home and does not have access to injectable glucagon, the client should seek immediate medical care.

Reference

Lewis et al. (2017), pp. 1146-1147.
American Diabetes Association. *The 15/15 rule.* Retrieved from https://www.diabetes.org/

BOX 46-15 Assessment of Hypoglycemia

Mild
- Hunger
- Nervousness
- Palpitations
- Sweating
- Tachycardia
- Tremor

Moderate
- Confusion
- Double vision
- Drowsiness
- Emotional changes
- Headache
- Impaired coordination
- Inability to concentrate
- Irrational or combative behavior
- Lightheadedness
- Numbness of the lips and tongue
- Slurred speech

Severe
- Difficulty arousing
- Disoriented behavior
- Loss of consciousness
- Seizures

Do not attempt to administer oral food or fluids to the client experiencing a severe hypoglycemic reaction who is semiconscious or unconscious and is unable to swallow. This client is at risk for aspiration. For this client, an injection of glucagon is administered subcutaneously or intramuscularly. In the hospital or emergency department, the client may be treated with an IV injection of 25 to 50 mL (12.5 to 25 g) of 50% dextrose in water.

B. Diabetic ketoacidosis (DKA)

1. Description (Fig. 46-4)

a. Diabetic ketoacidosis is a life-threatening complication of type 1 diabetes mellitus that develops when a severe insulin deficiency occurs.

b. The main clinical manifestations include hyperglycemia, dehydration, ketosis, and acidosis.

2. Assessment (Table 46-3)

3. Interventions

a. Restore circulating blood volume and protect against cerebral, coronary, and renal hypoperfusion.

b. Treat dehydration with rapid IV infusions of 0.9% or 0.45% NS as prescribed; dextrose is added to IV fluids when the blood glucose level reaches 250 to 300 mg/dL (13.9 to 16.7 mmol/L). Too rapid administration of IV fluids; use of the incorrect types of IV fluids, particularly hypotonic solutions; and correcting the blood glucose level too rapidly can lead to cerebral edema.

c. Treat hyperglycemia with insulin administered intravenously as prescribed.

d. Correct electrolyte imbalances (potassium level may be elevated as a result of dehydration and acidosis).

e. Monitor potassium level closely, because when the client receives treatment for the dehydration and acidosis, the serum potassium level will decrease and potassium replacement may be required.

f. Cardiac monitoring should be in place for the client with DKA due to risks associated with abnormal serum potassium levels.

4. Insulin IV administration

a. Use short-duration insulin only.

b. An IV bolus dose of short-duration regular U-100 insulin (usually 5 to 10 units) may be prescribed before a continuous infusion is begun.

c. The prescribed IV dose of insulin for continuous infusion is prepared in 0.9% or 0.45% NS as prescribed.

d. Always place the insulin infusion on an IV infusion controller.

e. Insulin is infused continuously until subcutaneous administration resumes, to prevent a rebound of the blood glucose level.

f. Monitor vital signs.

g. Monitor urinary output and monitor for signs of fluid overload.

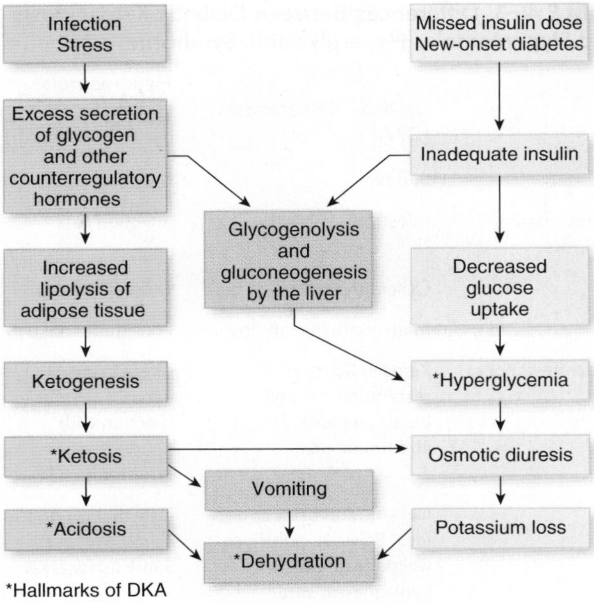

FIG. 46-4 Pathophysiology of diabetic ketoacidosis (DKA).

TABLE 46-3 Differences Between Diabetic Ketoacidosis and Hyperosmolar Hyperglycemic Syndrome

	Diabetic Ketoacidosis (DKA)	Hyperosmolar Hyperglycemic Syndrome (HHS)
Onset	Sudden	Gradual
Precipitating factors	Infection	Infection
	Other stressors	Other stressors
	Inadequate insulin dose	Poor fluid intake
Manifestations	Ketosis: Kussmaul's respiration, "fruity" breath, nausea, abdominal pain	Altered central nervous system function with neurological symptoms
	Dehydration or electrolyte loss: Polyuria, polydipsia, weight loss, dry skin, sunken eyes, soft eyeballs, lethargy, coma	Dehydration or electrolyte loss: Same as for DKA
Laboratory Findings		
Serum glucose	>300 mg/dL (>16.7 mmol/L)	>800 mg/dL (>44.5 mmol/L)
Osmolarity	Variable	>350 mOsm/kg (.350 mmol/kg)
Serum ketones	Positive at 1:2 dilution	Negative
Serum pH	<7.35	>7.4
Serum HCO_3	<15 mEq/L (15 mmol/L)	>20 mEq/L (>20 mmol/L)
Serum Na	Low, normal, or high	Normal or low
Serum K	Normal; elevated with acidosis, decreases following hydration	Normal or low
BUN	>20 mg/dL (>7.1 mmol/L); elevated because of dehydration	Elevated
Creatinine	>1.5 mg/dL (>132.5 mcmol/L); elevated because of dehydration	Elevated
Urine ketones	Positive	Negative

BUN, Blood urea nitrogen; *HCO_3*, bicarbonate; *K*, potassium; *Na*, sodium.

From Ignatavicius D, Workman M: *Medical-surgical nursing: patient-centered collaborative care*, ed 7, St. Louis, 2013, Saunders.

h. Monitor potassium and glucose levels and for signs of increased intracranial pressure.
i. The potassium level will fall rapidly within the first hour of treatment as the dehydration and the acidosis are treated.
j. Potassium is administered intravenously in a diluted solution as prescribed; ensure adequate renal function before administering potassium.

5. Client education (Box 46-16)

BOX 46-16 Client Education: Guidelines During Illness

- Take insulin or oral antidiabetic medications as prescribed.
- Determine the blood glucose level and test the urine for ketones every 3 to 4 hours.
- If the usual meal plan cannot be followed, substitute soft foods 6 to 8 times a day.
- If vomiting, diarrhea, or fever occurs, consume liquids every 30 to 60 minutes to prevent dehydration and to provide calories.
- Notify the primary health care provider if vomiting, diarrhea, or fever persists; if blood glucose levels are higher than 250 to 300 mg/dL (13.9 to 16.7 mmol/L); when ketonuria is present for more than 24 hours; when unable to take food or fluids for a period of 4 hours; or when illness persists for more than 2 days.

⚠ Monitor the client being treated for DKA closely for signs of increased intracranial pressure. If the blood glucose level falls too far or too fast before the brain has time to equilibrate, water is pulled from the blood to the cerebrospinal fluid and the brain, causing cerebral edema and increased intracranial pressure.

C. Hyperosmolar hyperglycemic syndrome (HHS)

1. Description
a. Extreme hyperglycemia occurs without ketosis or acidosis.
b. The syndrome occurs most often in individuals with type 2 diabetes mellitus.
c. The major difference between HHS and DKA is that ketosis and acidosis do not occur with HHS; enough insulin is present with HHS to prevent the breakdown of fats for energy, thus preventing ketosis.

2. Assessment (see Table 46-3)

3. Interventions
a. Treatment is similar to that for DKA.
b. Treatment includes fluid replacement, correction of electrolyte imbalances, and insulin administration.
c. Fluid replacement in the older client must be done very carefully because of the potential for heart failure.
d. Insulin plays a less critical role in the treatment of HHS than it does in the treatment of DKA because ketosis and acidosis do not occur; rehydration alone may decrease glucose levels.

IX. Chronic Complications of Diabetes Mellitus

A. Diabetic retinopathy

1. Description
a. Chronic and progressive impairment of the retinal circulation that eventually causes hemorrhage
b. Permanent vision changes and blindness can occur.

c. The client has difficulty with carrying out the daily tasks of blood glucose testing and insulin injections.

2. Assessment
   a. A change in vision is caused by the rupture of small microaneurysms in retinal blood vessels.
   b. Blurred vision results from macular edema.
   c. Sudden loss of vision results from retinal detachment.
   d. Cataracts result from lens opacity.
3. Interventions
   a. Maintain safety.
   b. Early prevention via the control of hypertension and blood glucose levels
   c. Photocoagulation (laser therapy) may be done to remove hemorrhagic tissue to decrease scarring and prevent progression of the disease process.
   d. Vitrectomy may be done to remove vitreous hemorrhages and thus decrease tension on the retina, preventing detachment.
   e. Cataract removal with lens implantation improves vision.

B. Diabetic nephropathy
1. Description: Progressive decrease in kidney function
2. Assessment
   a. Microalbuminuria
   b. Thirst
   c. Fatigue
   d. Anemia
   e. Weight loss
   f. Signs of malnutrition
   g. Frequent urinary tract infections
   h. Signs of a neurogenic bladder
3. Interventions
   a. Early prevention measures include the control of hypertension and blood glucose levels.
   b. Assess vital signs.
   c. Monitor intake and output.
   d. Monitor the blood urea nitrogen, creatinine, and urine albumin levels.
   e. Restrict dietary protein, sodium, and potassium intake as prescribed.
   f. Avoid nephrotoxic medications.
   g. Prepare the client for dialysis procedures if planned.
   h. Prepare the client for kidney transplant if planned.
   i. Prepare the client for pancreas transplant if planned.

C. Diabetic neuropathy
1. Description
   a. General deterioration of the nervous system throughout the body
   b. Complications include the development of nonhealing ulcers of the feet, gastric paresis, and erectile dysfunction.
2. Classifications
   a. Focal neuropathy or mononeuropathy: Involves a single nerve or group of nerves, most frequently cranial nerves III (oculomotor) and VI (abducens), resulting in diplopia
   b. Sensory or peripheral neuropathy: Affects distal portion of nerves, most frequently in the lower extremities
   c. Autonomic neuropathy: Symptoms vary according to the organ system involved.
   d. Cardiovascular: Cardiac denervation syndrome (heart rate does not respond to changes in oxygenation needs) and orthostatic hypotension occur.
   e. Pupillary: Pupil does not dilate in response to decreased light.
   f. Gastric: Decreased gastric emptying (gastroparesis)
   g. Urinary: Neurogenic bladder
   h. Skin: Decreased sweating
   i. Adrenal: Hypoglycemic unawareness
   j. Reproductive: Impotence (male), painful intercourse (female)
3. Assessment: Findings depend on the classification
   a. Paresthesias
   b. Decreased or absent reflexes
   c. Decreased sensation to vibration or light touch
   d. Pain, aching, and burning in the lower extremities
   e. Poor peripheral pulses
   f. Skin breakdown and signs of infection
   g. Weakness or loss of sensation in cranial nerves III (oculomotor), IV (trochlear), V (trigeminal), and VI (abducens)
   h. Dizziness and postural hypotension
   i. Nausea and vomiting
   j. Diarrhea or constipation
   k. Incontinence
   l. Dyspareunia
   m. Impotence
   n. Hypoglycemic unawareness
4. Interventions
   a. Early prevention measures include the control of hypertension and blood glucose levels.
   b. Careful foot care is required to prevent trauma (Box 46-17).
   c. Administer medications as prescribed for pain relief.
   d. Initiate bladder training programs.
   e. Instruct in the use of estrogen-containing lubricants for women with dyspareunia.

BOX 46-17 Preventive Foot Care Instructions

- Provide meticulous skin care and proper foot care.
- Inspect feet daily and monitor feet for redness, swelling, or break in skin integrity.
- Notify the primary health care provider if redness or a break in the skin occurs.
- Avoid thermal injuries from hot water, heating pads, and baths.
- Wash feet with warm (not hot) water and dry thoroughly (avoid foot soaks).
- Avoid treating corns, blisters, or ingrown toenails.
- Do not cross legs or wear tight garments that may constrict blood flow.
- Apply moisturizing lotion to the feet but not between the toes.
- Prevent moisture from accumulating between the toes.
- Wear loose socks and well-fitting (not tight) shoes; do not go barefoot.
- Wear clean cotton socks to keep the feet warm and change the socks daily.
- Avoid wearing the same pair of shoes 2 days in a row.
- Avoid wearing open-toed shoes or shoes with a strap that goes between the toes.
- Check shoes for cracks or tears in the lining and for foreign objects before putting them on.
- Break in new shoes gradually.
- Cut toenails straight across and smooth nails with an emery board.
- Avoid smoking.
- Follow-up with podiatry referral and recommendations as needed.

f. Prepare the male client with impotence for penile injections or other possible treatment options as prescribed.
g. Prepare for surgical decompression of compression lesions related to the cranial nerves as prescribed.

X. Care of the Diabetic Client Undergoing Surgery

A. Preoperative care
1. Check with PHCP regarding withholding oral hypoglycemic medications or insulin.
2. Some long-acting oral antidiabetic medications are discontinued 24 to 48 hours before surgery.
3. Metformin may need to be discontinued 48 hours before surgery and may not be restarted until renal function is normal postoperatively.
4. All other oral antidiabetic medications are usually withheld on the day of surgery.
5. Insulin dose may be adjusted or withheld if IV insulin administration during surgery is planned.
6. Monitor blood glucose level.
7. Administer IV fluids as prescribed.

B. Postoperative care
1. Administer IV glucose and insulin infusions as prescribed until the client can tolerate oral feedings.
2. Administer supplemental short-acting insulin as prescribed based on blood glucose results.
3. Monitor blood glucose levels frequently, especially if the client is receiving parenteral nutrition.
4. When the client is tolerating food, ensure that the client receives an adequate amount of carbohydrates daily to prevent hypoglycemia.
5. Client is at higher risk for cardiovascular and renal complications postoperatively.
6. Client is also at risk for impaired wound healing.

PRACTICE QUESTIONS

487. A client is brought to the emergency department in an unresponsive state, and a diagnosis of hyperosmolar hyperglycemic syndrome is made. The nurse would **immediately** prepare to initiate which anticipated primary health care provider's prescription?

1. Endotracheal intubation
2. 100 units of NPH insulin
3. Intravenous infusion of normal saline
4. Intravenous infusion of sodium bicarbonate

488. An external insulin pump is prescribed for a client with diabetes mellitus. When the client asks the nurse about the functioning of the pump, the nurse bases the response on which information about the pump?

1. It is timed to release programmed doses of either short-duration or NPH insulin into the bloodstream at specific intervals.
2. It continuously infuses small amounts of NPH insulin into the bloodstream while regularly monitoring blood glucose levels.
3. It is surgically attached to the pancreas and infuses regular insulin into the pancreas. This releases insulin into the bloodstream.
4. It administers a small continuous dose of short-duration insulin subcutaneously. The client can self-administer an additional bolus dose from the pump before each meal.

489. A client with a diagnosis of diabetic ketoacidosis (DKA) is being treated in the emergency department. Which findings support this diagnosis? **Select all that apply.**

- ☐ 1. Increase in pH
- ☐ 2. Comatose state
- ☐ 3. Deep, rapid breathing
- ☐ 4. Decreased urine output
- ☐ 5. Elevated blood glucose level

490. The nurse teaches a client with diabetes mellitus about differentiating between hypoglycemia and ketoacidosis. The client demonstrates an understanding of the teaching by stating that a form of glucose should be taken if which symptoms develop? **Select all that apply.**

- ☐ 1. Polyuria
- ☐ 2. Shakiness
- ☐ 3. Palpitations
- ☐ 4. Blurred vision
- ☐ 5. Lightheadedness
- ☐ 6. Fruity breath odor

491. A client with diabetes mellitus demonstrates acute anxiety when admitted to the hospital for the treatment of hyperglycemia. What is the appropriate intervention to decrease the client's anxiety?

1. Administer a sedative.
2. Convey empathy, trust, and respect toward the client.
3. Ignore the signs and symptoms of anxiety, anticipating that they will soon disappear.
4. Make sure that the client is familiar with the correct medical terms to promote understanding of what is happening.

492. The nurse provides instructions to a client newly diagnosed with type 1 diabetes mellitus. The nurse recognizes accurate understanding of measures to prevent diabetic ketoacidosis when the client makes which statement?

1. "I will stop taking my insulin if I'm too sick to eat."
2. "I will decrease my insulin dose during times of illness."
3. "I will adjust my insulin dose according to the level of glucose in my urine."
4. "I will notify my primary health care provider (PHCP) if my blood glucose level is higher than 250 mg/dL (13.9 mmol/L)."

493. A client is admitted to a hospital with a diagnosis of diabetic ketoacidosis (DKA). The initial blood glucose level is 950 mg/dL (52.9 mmol/L). A continuous intravenous (IV) infusion of short-acting insulin is initiated, along with IV rehydration with normal saline. The serum glucose level is now decreased to 240 mg/dL (13.3 mmol/L). The nurse would **next** prepare to administer which medication?

1. An ampule of 50% dextrose
2. NPH insulin subcutaneously
3. IV fluids containing dextrose
4. Phenytoin for the prevention of seizures

494. The nurse is monitoring a client newly diagnosed with diabetes mellitus for signs of complications. Which sign or symptom, if frequently exhibited in the client, indicates that the client is at risk for chronic complications of diabetes if the blood glucose is not adequately managed?

1. Polyuria
2. Diaphoresis
3. Pedal edema
4. Decreased respiratory rate

495. The nurse is preparing a plan of care for a client with diabetes mellitus who has hyperglycemia. The nurse places **priority** on which client problem?

1. Lack of knowledge
2. Inadequate fluid volume
3. Compromised family coping
4. Inadequate consumption of nutrients

496. The home health nurse visits a client with a diagnosis of type 1 diabetes mellitus. The client reports a history of vomiting and diarrhea and tells the nurse that no food has been consumed for the last 24 hours. Which additional statement by the client indicates a **need for further teaching**?

1. "I need to stop my insulin."
2. "I need to increase my fluid intake."
3. "I need to monitor my blood glucose every 3 to 4 hours."
4. "I need to call my primary health care provider (PHCP) because of these symptoms."

497. The nurse is caring for a client after hypophysectomy and notes clear nasal drainage from the client's nostril. The nurse should take which **initial** action?

1. Lower the head of the bed.
2. Test the drainage for glucose.
3. Obtain a culture of the drainage.
4. Continue to observe the drainage.

498. The nurse is admitting a client who is diagnosed with syndrome of inappropriate antidiuretic hormone secretion (SIADH) and has serum sodium of 118 mEq/L (118 mmol/L). Which primary health care provider prescriptions should the nurse anticipate receiving? **Select all that apply.**

- ☐ 1. Initiate an infusion of 3% NaCl.
- ☐ 2. Administer intravenous furosemide.
- ☐ 3. Restrict fluids to 800 mL over 24 hours.
- ☐ 4. Elevate the head of the bed to high-Fowler's.
- ☐ 5. Administer a vasopressin antagonist as prescribed.

499. A client is admitted to an emergency department, and a diagnosis of myxedema coma is made. Which action should the nurse prepare to carry out **initially**?

1. Warm the client.
2. Maintain a patent airway.
3. Administer thyroid hormone.
4. Administer fluid replacement.

500. The nurse is caring for a client admitted to the emergency department with diabetic ketoacidosis (DKA). In the acute phase, the nurse plans for which **priority** intervention?
1. Correct the acidosis.
2. Administer 5% dextrose intravenously.
3. Apply a monitor for an electrocardiogram.
4. Administer short-duration insulin intravenously.

501. A client with type 1 diabetes mellitus who takes NPH daily in the morning calls the nurse to report recurrent episodes of hypoglycemia with exercising. Which statement by the client indicates an adequate understanding of the peak action of NPH insulin and exercise?
1. "I should not exercise since I am taking insulin."
2. "The best time for me to exercise is after breakfast."
3. "The best time for me to exercise is mid- to late afternoon."
4. "NPH is a basal insulin, so I should exercise in the evening."

502. The nurse is completing an assessment on a client who is being admitted for a diagnostic workup for primary hyperparathyroidism. Which client complaints would be characteristic of this disorder? **Select all that apply.**
- ☐ 1. Polyuria
- ☐ 2. Headache
- ☐ 3. Bone pain
- ☐ 4. Nervousness
- ☐ 5. Weight gain

503. The nurse is teaching a client with hyperparathyroidism how to manage the condition at home. Which response by the client indicates the **need for additional teaching**?
1. "I should consume less than 1 liter of fluid per day."
2. "I should use my treadmill or go for walks daily."
3. "I should follow a moderate-calcium, high-fiber diet."
4. "My alendronate helps keep calcium from coming out of my bones."

504. A client with a diagnosis of addisonian crisis is being admitted to the intensive care unit. Which findings will the interprofessional health care team focus on? **Select all that apply.**
- ☐ 1. Hypotension
- ☐ 2. Leukocytosis
- ☐ 3. Hyperkalemia
- ☐ 4. Hypercalcemia
- ☐ 5. Hypernatremia

505. The nurse is monitoring a client who was diagnosed with type 1 diabetes mellitus and is being treated with NPH and regular insulin. Which manifestations would alert the nurse to the presence of a possible hypoglycemic reaction? **Select all that apply.**
- ☐ 1. Tremors
- ☐ 2. Anorexia
- ☐ 3. Irritability
- ☐ 4. Nervousness
- ☐ 5. Hot, dry skin
- ☐ 6. Muscle cramps

506. The nurse is performing an assessment on a client with pheochromocytoma. Which assessment data would indicate a potential complication associated with this disorder?
1. A urinary output of 50 mL/hr
2. A coagulation time of 5 minutes
3. A heart rate that is 90 beats per minute and irregular
4. A blood urea nitrogen level of 20 mg/dL (7.1 mmol/L)

507. The nurse is monitoring a client diagnosed with acromegaly who was treated with transsphenoidal hypophysectomy and is recovering in the intensive care unit. Which findings should alert the nurse to the presence of a possible postoperative complication? **Select all that apply.**
- ☐ 1. Anxiety
- ☐ 2. Leukocytosis
- ☐ 3. Chvostek's sign
- ☐ 4. Urinary output of 800 mL/hr
- ☐ 5. Clear drainage on nasal dripper pad

508. The nurse performs a physical assessment on a client with type 2 diabetes mellitus. Findings include a fasting blood glucose level of 70 mg/dL (3.9 mmol/L), temperature of 101° F (38.3° C), pulse of 82 beats per minute, respirations of 20 breaths per minute, and blood pressure of 118/68 mm Hg. Which finding would be the **priority** concern to the nurse?
1. Pulse
2. Respiration
3. Temperature
4. Blood pressure

509. The nurse is preparing a client with a new diagnosis of hypothyroidism for discharge. The nurse determines that the client understands discharge instructions if the client states that which signs and symptoms are associated with this diagnosis? **Select all that apply.**
- ☐ 1. Tremors
- ☐ 2. Weight loss
- ☐ 3. Feeling cold
- ☐ 4. Loss of body hair
- ☐ 5. Persistent lethargy
- ☐ 6. Puffiness of the face

510. A client has just been admitted to the nursing unit following thyroidectomy. Which assessment is the **priority** for this client?

1. Hoarseness
2. Hypocalcemia
3. Audible stridor
4. Edema at the surgical site

511. A client has been diagnosed with hyperthyroidism. The nurse monitors for which signs and symptoms indicating a complication of this disorder? **Select all that apply.**

- ☐ 1. Fever
- ☐ 2. Nausea
- ☐ 3. Lethargy
- ☐ 4. Tremors
- ☐ 5. Confusion
- ☐ 6. Bradycardia

ANSWERS

487. *Answer:* 3

Rationale: The primary goal of treatment in hyperosmolar hyperglycemic syndrome (HHS) is to rehydrate the client to restore fluid volume and to correct electrolyte deficiency. Intravenous (IV) fluid replacement is similar to that administered in diabetic ketoacidosis (DKA) and begins with IV infusion of normal saline. Regular insulin, not NPH insulin, would be administered. The use of sodium bicarbonate to correct acidosis is avoided because it can precipitate a further drop in serum potassium levels. Intubation and mechanical ventilation are not required to treat HHS.

Test-Taking Strategy: Focus on the subject, treatment of HHS, and note the strategic word, *immediately*. If you can recall the treatment for DKA, you will be able to answer this question easily. Treatment for HHS is similar to the treatment for DKA and begins with rehydration.

Level of Cognitive Ability: Analyzing

Client Needs: Physiological Integrity

Integrated Process: Nursing Process—Planning

Content Area: Adult Health: Endocrine

Health Problem: Adult Health: Endocrine: Diabetes Mellitus

Priority Concepts: Clinical Judgment; Glucose Regulation

Reference: Ignatavicius, Workman, Rebar (2018), pp. 1314-1316.

488. *Answer:* 4

Rationale: An insulin pump provides a small continuous dose of short-duration (rapid- or short-acting) insulin subcutaneously throughout the day and night. The client can self-administer an additional bolus dose from the pump before each meal as needed. Short-duration insulin is used in an insulin pump. An external pump is not attached surgically to the pancreas.

Test-Taking Strategy: Focus on the subject, use of an insulin pump. Recalling that short-duration insulin is used in an insulin pump will assist in eliminating options 1 and 2. Noting the word *external* in the question will assist in eliminating option 3.

Level of Cognitive Ability: Applying

Client Needs: Physiological Integrity

Integrated Process: Teaching and Learning

Content Area: Adult Health: Endocrine

Health Problem: Adult Health: Endocrine: Diabetes Mellitus

Priority Concepts: Client Education; Glucose Regulation

Reference: Lewis et al. (2017), pp. 1128-1129.

489. *Answer:* 2, 3, 5

Rationale: Because of the profound deficiency of insulin associated with DKA, glucose cannot be used for energy and the body breaks down fat as a secondary source of energy. Ketones, which are acid by-products of fat metabolism, build up, and the client experiences a metabolic ketoacidosis. High serum glucose contributes to an osmotic diuresis and the client becomes severely dehydrated. If untreated, the client will become comatose due to severe dehydration, acidosis, and electrolyte imbalance. Kussmaul's respirations, the deep rapid breathing associated with DKA, is a compensatory mechanism by the body. The body attempts to correct the acidotic state by blowing off carbon dioxide (CO_2), which is an acid. In the absence of insulin, the client will experience severe hyperglycemia. Option 1 is incorrect, because in acidosis the pH would be low. Option 4 is incorrect because a high serum glucose will result in an osmotic diuresis and the client will experience polyuria.

Test-Taking Strategy: Focus on the subject, findings associated with DKA. Recall that the pathophysiology of DKA is the breakdown of fats for energy. The breakdown of fats leads to a state of acidosis. The high serum glucose contributes to an osmotic diuresis. Knowing the pathophysiology of DKA will aid in identification of the correct answers.

Level of Cognitive Ability: Analyzing

Client Needs: Physiological Integrity

Integrated Process: Nursing Process—Assessment

Content Area: Adult Health: Endocrine

Health Problem: Adult Health: Endocrine: Diabetes Mellitus

Priority Concepts: Clinical Judgment; Glucose Regulation

Reference: Lewis et al. (2017), pp. 1143-1145.

490. *Answer:* 2, 3, 5

Rationale: Shakiness, palpitations, and lightheadedness are signs/symptoms of hypoglycemia and would indicate the need for food or glucose. Polyuria, blurred vision, and a fruity breath odor are manifestations of hyperglycemia.

Test-Taking Strategy: Focus on the subject, the treatment of hypoglycemia. Think about its pathophysiology and the manifestations that occur. Recalling the signs and symptoms of hypoglycemia will direct you to the correct option.

Level of Cognitive Ability: Evaluating

Client Needs: Physiological Integrity

Integrated Process: Nursing Process—Evaluation

Content Area: Adult Health: Endocrine

Health Problem: Adult Health: Endocrine: Diabetes Mellitus

Priority Concepts: Client Education; Glucose Regulation

Reference: Ignatavicius, Workman, Rebar (2018), p. 1309.

491. *Answer:* 2

Rationale: Anxiety is a subjective feeling of apprehension, uneasiness, or dread. The appropriate intervention is to address the client's feelings related to the anxiety. Administering a sedative is not the most appropriate intervention and does not address the source of the client's anxiety. The nurse should not ignore the client's anxious feelings. Anxiety needs to be managed before meaningful client education can occur.

Test-Taking Strategy: Use therapeutic communication techniques to answer the question. Remember that the client's feelings are the priority. Keeping this in mind will direct you easily to the correct option.

Level of Cognitive Ability: Applying
Client Needs: Psychosocial Integrity
Integrated Process: Caring
Content Area: Adult Health: Endocrine
Health Problem: Adult Health: Endocrine: Diabetes Mellitus
Priority Concepts: Anxiety; Caregiving
References: Lewis et al. (2017), pp. 302-303; Potter et al. (2017), pp. 327-329.

492. *Answer:* 4

Rationale: During illness, the client with type 1 diabetes mellitus is at increased risk of diabetic ketoacidosis, due to hyperglycemia associated with the stress response and due to a typically decreased caloric intake. As part of sick day management, the client with diabetes should monitor blood glucose levels and should notify the PHCP if the level is higher than 250 mg/dL (13.9 mmol/L). Insulin should never be stopped. In fact, insulin may need to be increased during times of illness. Doses should not be adjusted without the PHCP's advice and are usually adjusted on the basis of blood glucose levels, not urinary glucose readings.

Test-Taking Strategy: Use general medication guidelines to answer the question. Note that options 1, 2, and 3 are comparable or alike and all relate to adjustment of insulin doses.

Level of Cognitive Ability: Evaluating
Client Needs: Physiological Integrity
Integrated Process: Nursing Process—Evaluation
Content Area: Adult Health: Endocrine
Health Problem: Adult Health: Endocrine: Diabetes Mellitus
Priority Concepts: Client Education; Glucose Regulation
Reference: Ignatavicius, Workman, Rebar (2018), p. 1314.

493. *Answer:* 3

Rationale: Emergency management of DKA focuses on correcting fluid and electrolyte imbalances and normalizing the serum glucose level. If the corrections occur too quickly, serious consequences, including hypoglycemia and cerebral edema, can occur. During management of DKA, when the blood glucose level falls to 250 to 300 mg/dL (13.9 to 16.7 mmol/L), the IV infusion rate is reduced and a dextrose solution is added to maintain a blood glucose level of about 250 mg/dL (13.9 mmol/L), or until the client recovers from ketosis. Fifty percent dextrose is used to treat hypoglycemia. NPH insulin is not used to treat DKA. Phenytoin is not a usual treatment measure for DKA.

Test-Taking Strategy: Note the strategic word, *next.* Focus on the subject, management of DKA. Eliminate option 2 first, knowing that short-duration (rapid-acting) insulin is used in the management of DKA. Eliminate option 1 next, knowing that this is the treatment for hypoglycemia. Note the words *the serum glucose level is now decreased to 240 mg/dL (13.3 mmol/L).* This should indicate that the IV solution containing dextrose is the next step in the management of care.

Level of Cognitive Ability: Synthesizing
Client Needs: Physiological Integrity
Integrated Process: Nursing Process—Planning
Content Area: Adult Health: Endocrine
Health Problem: Adult Health: Endocrine: Diabetes Mellitus
Priority Concepts: Clinical Judgment; Glucose Regulation
Reference: Ignatavicius, Workman, Rebar (2018), pp. 1312-1313.

494. *Answer:* 1

Rationale: Chronic hyperglycemia, resulting from poor glycemic control, contributes to the microvascular and macrovascular complications of diabetes mellitus. Classic symptoms of hyperglycemia include polydipsia, polyuria, and polyphagia. Diaphoresis may occur in hypoglycemia. Hypoglycemia is an acute complication of diabetes mellitus; however, it does not predispose a client to the chronic complications of diabetes mellitus. Therefore, option 2 can be eliminated because this finding is characteristic of hypoglycemia. Options 3 and 4 are not associated with diabetes mellitus.

Test-Taking Strategy: Focus on the subject, chronic complications of diabetes mellitus. Recall that poor glycemic control contributes to development of the chronic complications of diabetes mellitus. Remember the 3 Ps associated with hyperglycemia—polyuria, polydipsia, and polyphagia.

Level of Cognitive Ability: Analyzing
Client Needs: Physiological Integrity
Integrated Process: Nursing Process—Analysis
Content Area: Adult Health: Endocrine
Health Problem: Adult Health: Endocrine: Diabetes Mellitus
Priority Concepts: Clinical Judgment; Glucose Regulation
Reference: Ignatavicius, Workman, Rebar (2018), pp. 1282-1283.

495. *Answer:* 2

Rationale: An increased blood glucose level will cause the kidneys to excrete the glucose in the urine. This glucose is accompanied by fluids and electrolytes, causing an osmotic diuresis leading to dehydration. This fluid loss must be replaced when it becomes severe. Options 1, 3, and 4 are not related specifically to the information in the question.

Test-Taking Strategy: Note the strategic word, *priority*, and focus on the information in the question. Use Maslow's Hierarchy of Needs theory. The correct option indicates a physiological need and is the priority. Options 1, 3, and 4 are problems that may need to be addressed after providing for the priority physiological needs.

Level of Cognitive Ability: Analyzing
Client Needs: Physiological Integrity
Integrated Process: Nursing Process—Planning
Content Area: Adult Health: Endocrine
Health Problem: Adult Health: Endocrine: Diabetes Mellitus
Priority Concepts: Clinical Judgment; Glucose Regulation
Reference: Lewis et al. (2017), p. 1143.

496. *Answer:* 1
Rationale: When a client with diabetes mellitus is unable to eat normally because of illness, the client still should take the prescribed insulin or oral medication. The client should consume additional fluids and should notify the PHCP. The client should monitor the blood glucose level every 3 to 4 hours. The client should also monitor the urine for ketones during illness.
Test-Taking Strategy: Note the strategic words, *need for further teaching*. These words indicate a negative event query and the need to select the incorrect statement. Remembering that the client needs to take insulin will direct you easily to the correct option.
Level of Cognitive Ability: Evaluating
Client Needs: Physiological Integrity
Integrated Process: Teaching and Learning
Content Area: Adult Health: Endocrine
Health Problem: Adult Health: Endocrine: Diabetes Mellitus
Priority Concepts: Client Education; Glucose Regulation
Reference: Ignatavicius, Workman, Rebar (2018), p. 1314.

497. *Answer:* 2
Rationale: After hypophysectomy, the client should be monitored for rhinorrhea, which could indicate a cerebrospinal fluid leak. If this occurs, the drainage should be collected and tested for the presence of cerebrospinal fluid. Cerebrospinal fluid contains glucose, and if positive, this would indicate that the drainage is cerebrospinal fluid. The head of the bed should remain elevated to prevent increased intracranial pressure. Clear nasal drainage would not indicate the need for a culture. Continuing to observe the drainage without taking action could result in a serious complication.
Test-Taking Strategy: Note the strategic word, *initial*, and determine whether an abnormality exists. This indicates that an action is required. Option 1 can be eliminated first by recalling that this action can increase intracranial pressure. Option 3 can be eliminated also, because the drainage is clear. Because an action is required, eliminate option 4.
Level of Cognitive Ability: Analyzing
Client Needs: Physiological Integrity
Integrated Process: Nursing Process—Implementation
Content Area: Adult Health: Endocrine
Health Problem: Adult Health: Endocrine: Pituitary Disorders
Priority Concepts: Clinical Judgment; Intracranial Regulation
Reference: Ignatavicius, Workman, Rebar (2018), p. 1249.

498. *Answer:* 1, 3, 5
Rationale: Clients with SIADH experience excess secretion of antidiuretic hormone (ADH), which leads to excess intravascular volume, a declining serum osmolarity, and dilutional hyponatremia. Management is directed at correcting the hyponatremia and preventing cerebral edema. Hypertonic saline is prescribed when the hyponatremia is severe, less than 120 mEq/L (120 mmol/L). An intravenous (IV) infusion of 3% saline is hypertonic. Hypertonic saline must be infused slowly as prescribed, and an infusion pump must be used. Fluid restriction is a useful strategy aimed at correcting dilutional hyponatremia. Vasopressin is an ADH; vasopressin antagonists are used to treat SIADH. Furosemide may be used to treat extravascular volume and dilutional hyponatremia in SIADH, but it is only safe to use if the serum sodium is at least 125 mEq/L (125 mmol/L). When furosemide is used, potassium supplementation should also occur and serum potassium levels should be monitored. To promote venous return, the head of the bed should not be raised more than 10 degrees for the client with SIADH. Maximizing venous return helps avoid stimulating stretch receptors in the heart that signal to the pituitary that more ADH is needed.
Test-Taking Strategy: Focus on the subject, treatment for SIADH. Think about the pathophysiology associated with SIADH. Remember that SIADH is associated with the increased secretion of ADH, or vasopressin. Excess vasopressin leads to increased intravascular fluid volume, decreased serum osmolality, and hyponatremia. When hyponatremia and decreased serum osmolality become severe, cerebral edema occurs.
Level of Cognitive Ability: Analyzing
Client Needs: Physiological Integrity
Integrated Process: Nursing Process—Planning
Content Area: Adult Health: Endocrine
Health Problem: Adult Health: Endocrine: Pituitary Disorders
Priority Concepts: Clinical Judgment; Fluids and Electrolytes
Reference: Ignatavicius, Workman, Rebar (2018), pp. 954, 1251-1253.

499. *Answer:* 2
Rationale: Myxedema coma is a rare but serious disorder that results from persistently low thyroid production. Coma can be precipitated by acute illness, rapid withdrawal of thyroid medication, anesthesia and surgery, hypothermia, and the use of sedatives and opioid analgesics. In myxedema coma, the initial nursing action is to maintain a patent airway. Oxygen should be administered, followed by fluid replacement, keeping the client warm, monitoring vital signs, and administering thyroid hormones by the intravenous route.
Test-Taking Strategy: Note the strategic word, *initially*. All the options are appropriate interventions, but use the ABCs—airway, breathing, and circulation—in selecting the correct option.
Level of Cognitive Ability: Applying
Client Needs: Physiological Integrity
Integrated Process: Nursing Process—Implementation
Content Area: Adult Health: Endocrine
Health Problem: Adult Health: Endocrine: Thyroid Disorders
Priority Concepts: Gas Exchange; Thermoregulation
Reference: Ignatavicius, Workman, Rebar (2018), p. 1271.

500. *Answer:* 4
Rationale: Lack of insulin (absolute or relative) is the primary cause of DKA. Treatment consists of insulin administration (short- or rapid-acting), intravenous fluid administration (normal saline initially, not 5% dextrose), and potassium replacement, followed by correcting acidosis. Cardiac monitoring is important due to alterations in potassium levels associated with DKA and its treatment, but applying an electrocardiogram monitor is not the priority action.
Test-Taking Strategy: Focus on the client's diagnosis. Note the strategic word, *priority*. Remember that in DKA, the initial treatment is short- or rapid-acting insulin. Normal saline is administered initially; therefore, option 2 is incorrect. Options 1 and 3 may be components of the treatment plan but are not the priority.

Level of Cognitive Ability: Analyzing
Client Needs: Physiological Integrity
Integrated Process: Nursing Process—Implementation
Content Area: Adult Health: Endocrine
Health Problem: Adult Health: Endocrine: Diabetes Mellitus
Priority Concepts: Clinical Judgment; Glucose Regulation
Reference: Lewis et al. (2017), p. 1144.

501. *Answer:* 2
Rationale: Exercise is an important part of diabetes management. It promotes weight loss, decreases insulin resistance, and helps control blood glucose levels. A hypoglycemic reaction may occur in response to increased exercise, so clients should exercise either an hour after mealtime or after consuming a 10- to 15-g carbohydrate snack, and they should check their blood glucose level before exercising. Option 1 is incorrect because clients with diabetes should exercise, though they should check with their primary health care provider before starting a new exercise program. Option 3 in incorrect; clients should avoid exercise during the peak time of insulin. NPH insulin peaks at 4 to 12 hours; therefore, afternoon exercise takes place during the peak of the medication. Option 4 is incorrect; NPH insulin is an intermediate-acting insulin, not a basal insulin.
Test-Taking Strategy: Focus on the subject, peak action of NPH insulin. Recalling that NPH insulin peaks at 4 to 12 hours and that exercise is beneficial for clients with diabetes will direct you to the correct option.
Level of Cognitive Ability: Evaluating
Client Needs: Physiological Integrity
Integrated Process: Nursing Process—Evaluation
Content Area: Adult Health: Endocrine
Health Problem: Adult Health: Endocrine: Diabetes Mellitus
Priority Concepts: Client Education; Glucose Regulation
Reference: Ignatavicius, Workman, Rebar (2018), pp. 1300-1301.

502. *Answer:* 1, 3
Rationale: The role of parathyroid hormone (PTH) in the body is to maintain serum calcium homeostasis. In hyperparathyroidism, PTH levels are high, which causes bone resorption (calcium is pulled from the bones). Hypercalcemia occurs with hyperparathyroidism. Elevated serum calcium levels produce osmotic diuresis and thus polyuria. This diuresis leads to dehydration (weight loss rather than weight gain). Loss of calcium from the bones causes bone pain. Options 2, 4, and 5 are not associated with hyperparathyroidism. Some gastrointestinal symptoms include anorexia, nausea, vomiting, and constipation.
Test-Taking Strategy: Focus on the subject, assessment findings in hyperparathyroidism. Think about the pathophysiology associated with hyperparathyroidism. Remember that hypercalcemia is associated with this disorder and that hypercalcemia leads to diuresis, and that calcium loss from bone leads to bone pain.
Level of Cognitive Ability: Analyzing
Client Needs: Physiological Integrity
Integrated Process: Nursing Process—Assessment
Content Area: Adult Health: Endocrine
Health Problem: Adult Health: Endocrine: Parathyroid Disorders
Priority Concepts: Clinical Judgment; Fluids and Electrolytes
Reference: Ignatavicius, Workman, Rebar (2018), pp. 1275-1276.

503. *Answer:* 1
Rationale: In hyperparathyroidism, clients experience excess parathyroid hormone (PTH) secretion. A role of PTH in the body is to maintain serum calcium homeostasis. When PTH levels are high, there is excess bone resorption (calcium is pulled from the bones). In clients with elevated serum calcium levels, there is a risk of nephrolithiasis. One to two liters of fluids daily should be encouraged to protect the kidneys and decrease the risk of nephrolithiasis. Moderate physical activity, particularly weight-bearing activity, minimizes bone resorption and helps protect against pathological fracture. Walking, as an exercise, should be encouraged in the client with hyperparathyroidism. Even though serum calcium is already high, clients should follow a moderate-calcium diet, because a low-calcium diet will surge PTH. Calcium causes constipation, so a diet high in fiber is recommended. Alendronate is a bisphosphate that inhibits bone resorption. In bone resorption, bone is broken down and calcium is deposited into the serum.
Test-Taking Strategy: Note the strategic words, *need for additional teaching*. These words indicate a negative event query and the need to select the incorrect statement. Consider the pathophysiology of hyperparathyroidism. Hyperparathyroidism leads to bone demineralization, which places the client at risk for pathological fracture, and high serum calcium, which places the client at risk for nephrolithiasis. Knowing that fluids should be encouraged rather than limited to help prevent nephrolithiasis should direct you to the correct option.
Level of Cognitive Ability: Evaluating
Client Needs: Physiological Integrity
Integrated Process: Teaching and Learning
Content Area: Adult Health: Endocrine
Health Problem: Adult Health: Endocrine: Parathyroid Disorders
Priority Concepts: Client Education; Fluids and Electrolytes
Reference: Lewis et al. (2017), pp. 1172-1173.

504. *Answer:* 1, 3
Rationale: In Addison's disease, also known as adrenal insufficiency, destruction of the adrenal gland leads to decreased production of adrenocortical hormones, including the glucocorticoid cortisol and the mineralocorticoid aldosterone. Addisonian crisis, also known as *acute adrenal insufficiency*, occurs when there is extreme physical or emotional stress and lack of sufficient adrenocortical hormones to manage the stressor. Addisonian crisis is a life-threatening emergency. One of the roles of endogenous cortisol is to enhance vascular tone and vascular response to the catecholamines epinephrine and norepinephrine. Hypotension occurs when vascular tone is decreased and blood vessels cannot respond to epinephrine and norepinephrine. The role of aldosterone in the body is to support the blood pressure by holding salt and water and excreting potassium. When there is insufficient aldosterone, salt and water are lost and potassium builds up; this leads to hypotension from decreased vascular volume, hyponatremia, and hyperkalemia. The remaining options are not associated with addisonian crisis.
Test-Taking Strategy: Focus on the subject, addisonian crisis. Think about the pathophysiology associated with Addison's disease. Recalling that in Addison's disease there is a decrease in the glucocorticoid cortisol and the mineralocorticoid aldosterone will assist in determining the correct answer.

Level of Cognitive Ability: Analyzing
Client Needs: Physiological Integrity
Integrated Process: Nursing Process—Planning
Content Area: Adult Health: Endocrine
Health Problem: Adult Health: Endocrine: Adrenal Disorders
Priority Concepts: Clinical Judgment; Fluids and Electrolytes
Reference: Ignatavicius, Workman, Rebar (2018), pp. 1253-1254.

505. *Answer:* 1, 3, 4
Rationale: Decreased blood glucose levels produce autonomic nervous system symptoms, which are manifested classically as nervousness, irritability, and tremors. Option 5 is more likely to occur with hyperglycemia. Options 2 and 6 are unrelated to the manifestations of hypoglycemia. In hypoglycemia, usually the client feels hunger.
Test-Taking Strategy: Focus on the subject, a hypoglycemic reaction. Think about the pathophysiology and manifestations that occur when the blood glucose is low. Recalling the signs of this type of reaction will direct you easily to the correct options.
Level of Cognitive Ability: Analyzing
Client Needs: Physiological Integrity
Integrated Process: Nursing Process—Assessment
Content Area: Adult Health: Endocrine
Health Problem: Adult Health: Endocrine: Diabetes Mellitus
Priority Concepts: Clinical Judgment; Glucose Regulation
Reference: Ignatavicius, Workman, Rebar (2018), p. 1309.

506. *Answer:* 3
Rationale: Pheochromocytoma is a catecholamine-producing tumor usually found in the adrenal medulla, but extra-adrenal locations include the chest, bladder, abdomen, and brain; it is typically a benign tumor but can be malignant. Excessive amounts of epinephrine and norepinephrine are secreted. The complications associated with pheochromocytoma include hypertensive retinopathy and nephropathy, myocarditis, increased platelet aggregation, and stroke. Death can occur from shock, stroke, kidney failure, dysrhythmias, or dissecting aortic aneurysm. An irregular heart rate indicates the presence of a dysrhythmia. A coagulation time of 5 minutes is normal. A urinary output of 50 mL/hr is an adequate output. A blood urea nitrogen level of 20 mg/dL (7.1 mmol/L) is a normal finding.
Test-Taking Strategy: Use the ABCs—airway, breathing, and circulation. An irregular heart rate is associated with circulation. In addition, knowing the normal hourly expectations associated with urinary output and the normal laboratory values for coagulation time and blood urea nitrogen level assists in selection of the correct option.
Level of Cognitive Ability: Analyzing
Client Needs: Physiological Integrity
Integrated Process: Nursing Process—Assessment
Content Area: Adult Health: Endocrine
Health Problem: Adult Health: Endocrine: Adrenal Disorders
Priority Concepts: Clinical Judgment; Perfusion
Reference: Ignatavicius, Workman, Rebar (2018), pp. 721, 1261-1262.

507. *Answer:* 2, 4, 5
Rationale: Acromegaly results from excess secretion of growth hormone, usually caused by a benign tumor on the anterior pituitary gland. Treatment is surgical removal of the tumor, usually with a sublingual transsphenoidal complete or partial hypophysectomy. The sublingual transsphenoidal approach is often through an incision in the inner upper lip at the gum line. Transsphenoidal surgery is a type of brain surgery, and infection is a primary concern. Leukocytosis, or an elevated white count, may indicate infection. Diabetes insipidus is a possible complication of transsphenoidal hypophysectomy. In diabetes insipidus there is decreased secretion of antidiuretic hormone, and clients excrete large amounts of dilute urine. Following transsphenoidal surgery, the nasal passages are packed and a dripper pad is secured under the nares. Clear drainage on the dripper pad is suggestive of a cerebrospinal fluid leak. The surgeon should be notified and the drainage should be tested for glucose. A cerebrospinal fluid leak increases the postoperative risk of meningitis. Anxiety is a nonspecific finding that is common to many disorders. Chvostek's sign is a test of nerve hyperexcitability associated with hypocalcemia and is seen as grimacing in response to tapping on the facial nerve. Chvostek's sign has no association with complications of sublingual transsphenoidal hypophysectomy.
Test-Taking Strategy: Focus on the subject, postoperative complications of sublingual transsphenoidal hypophysectomy. Knowing that infection, diabetes insipidus, and cerebrospinal fluid leak are possible complications will assist in determining the correct answer.
Level of Cognitive Ability: Analyzing
Client Needs: Physiological Integrity
Integrated Process: Nursing Process—Assessment
Content Area: Adult Health: Endocrine
Health Problem: Adult Health: Endocrine: Pituitary Disorders
Priority Concepts: Clinical Judgment; Intracranial Regulation
Reference: Ignatavicius, Workman, Rebar (2018), pp. 1247, 1249.

508. *Answer:* 3
Rationale: In the client with type 2 diabetes mellitus, an elevated temperature may indicate infection. Infection is a leading cause of hyperosmolar hyperglycemic syndrome in the client with type 2 diabetes mellitus. The other findings are within normal limits.
Test-Taking Strategy: Note the strategic word, *priority.* Use knowledge of the normal values of vital signs to direct you to the correct option. The client's temperature is the only abnormal value. Remember that an elevated temperature can indicate an infectious process that can lead to complications in the client with diabetes mellitus.
Level of Cognitive Ability: Analyzing
Client Needs: Physiological Integrity
Integrated Process: Nursing Process—Assessment
Content Area: Adult Health: Endocrine
Health Problem: Adult Health: Endocrine: Diabetes Mellitus
Priority Concepts: Glucose Regulation; Infection
Reference: Lewis et al. (2017), p. 1145.

509. *Answer:* 3, 4, 5, 6
Rationale: Feeling cold, hair loss, lethargy, and facial puffiness are signs of hypothyroidism. Tremors and weight loss are signs of hyperthyroidism.
Test-Taking Strategy: Focus on the subject, signs and symptoms associated with hypothyroidism. Options 1 and 2 can be eliminated if you remember that in *hypo*thyroidism there is

an *under*secretion of thyroid hormone that causes the metabolism to *slow* down.
Level of Cognitive Ability: Evaluating
Client Needs: Physiological Integrity
Integrated Process: Nursing Process—Evaluation
Content Area: Adult Health: Endocrine
Health Problem: Adult Health: Endocrine: Thyroid Disorders
Priority Concepts: Client Education; Clinical Judgment
Reference: Lewis et al. (2017), pp. 1168-1169.

510. *Answer:* 3
Rationale: Thyroidectomy is the removal of the thyroid gland, which is located in the anterior neck. It is very important to monitor airway status, as any swelling to the surgical site could cause respiratory distress. Although all of the options are important for the nurse to monitor, the priority nursing action is to monitor the airway.
Test-Taking Strategy: Note the **strategic word,** *priority*. Use the **ABCs—airway, breathing, and circulation,** to assist in directing you to the correct option.
Level of Cognitive Ability: Analyzing
Client Needs: Physiological Integrity
Integrated Process: Nursing Process—Assessment
Content Area: Adult Health: Endocrine
Health Problem: Adult Health: Endocrine: Thyroid Disorders
Priority Concepts: Clinical Judgment; Gas Exchange
Reference: Lewis et al. (2017), pp. 1167-1168.

511. *Answer:* 1, 2, 4, 5
Rationale: Thyroid storm is an acute and life-threatening complication that occurs in a client with uncontrollable hyperthyroidism. Signs and symptoms of thyroid storm include elevated temperature (fever), nausea, and tremors. In addition, as the condition progresses, the client becomes confused. The client is restless and anxious and experiences tachycardia.
Test-Taking Strategy: Focus on the **subject,** signs and symptoms indicating a complication of hyperthyroidism. Recall that thyroid storm is a complication of hyperthyroidism. Options 3 and 6 can be eliminated if you remember that thyroid storm is caused by the release of thyroid hormones into the bloodstream, causing uncontrollable *hyper*thyroidism. Lethargy and bradycardia (think: slow down) are signs of *hypo*thyroidism (slow metabolism).
Level of Cognitive Ability: Analyzing
Client Needs: Physiological Integrity
Integrated Process: Nursing Process—Assessment
Content Area: Adult Health: Endocrine
Health Problem: Adult Health: Endocrine: Thyroid Disorders
Priority Concepts: Clinical Judgment; Thermoregulation
Reference: Ignatavicius, Workman, Rebar (2018), p. 1270.

CHAPTER 47

Endocrine Medications

PRIORITY CONCEPTS Glucose Regulation; Hormonal Regulation

I. Pituitary Medications

A. Description
1. The anterior pituitary gland secretes growth hormone (GH), thyroid-stimulating hormone (TSH), adrenocorticotropic hormone (ACTH), prolactin, melanocyte-stimulating hormone (MSH), and gonadotropins (follicle-stimulating hormone [FSH] and luteinizing hormone [LH]).
2. The posterior pituitary gland secretes antidiuretic hormone (vasopressin) and oxytocin.

B. Growth hormones and related medications (Box 47-1)
1. Uses
   a. Growth hormones are used to treat pediatric or adult growth hormone deficiency.
   b. Growth hormone receptor antagonists are used to treat acromegaly.
   c. Growth hormone–releasing factor is used to evaluate anterior pituitary function.
2. Side and adverse effects
   a. May vary depending on the medication
   b. Development of antibodies to growth hormone
   c. Headache, muscle pain, weakness, vertigo
   d. Diarrhea, nausea, abdominal discomfort
   e. Mild **hyperglycemia**
   f. Hypertension
   g. Weight gain
   h. Allergic reaction (rash, swelling), pain at injection site
   i. Elevated aspartate aminotransferase (AST) and alanine aminotransferase (ALT)
3. Interventions
   a. Assess the child's physical growth and compare growth with standards.
   b. Recommend annual bone age determinations for children receiving growth hormones.
   c. Monitor vital signs, blood glucose levels, AST and ALT levels, and thyroid function tests.
   d. Teach the client and family about the clinical manifestations of hyperglycemia, other side and adverse effects of therapy, and the importance of follow-up regarding periodic blood tests.

II. Antidiuretic Hormones

A. Desmopressin acetate; vasopressin

B. Description
1. Antidiuretic hormones enhance reabsorption of water in the kidneys, promoting an antidiuretic effect and regulating fluid balance.
2. Antidiuretic hormones are used in **diabetes insipidus**.
3. Vasopressin is used less commonly than desmopressin acetate to treat diabetes insipidus; vasopressin is commonly used to treat septic shock.

C. Side and adverse effects
1. Flushing
2. Headache
3. Nausea and abdominal cramps
4. Water intoxication
5. Hypertension with water intoxication
6. Nasal congestion with nasal administration

D. Interventions
1. Monitor weight.
2. Monitor intake and output and urine osmolality.
3. Monitor electrolyte levels.
4. Monitor for signs of dehydration, indicating the need to increase the dosage.
5. Monitor for signs of water intoxication (drowsiness, listlessness, shortness of breath, and headache), indicating the need to decrease dosage.
6. Monitor blood pressure.
7. Instruct the client in how to use the intranasal medication.
8. Instruct the client to weigh herself or himself daily to identify weight gain.
9. Instruct the client to report signs of water intoxication or symptoms of headache or shortness of breath.

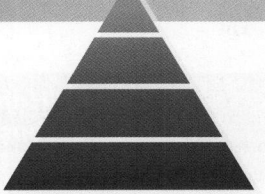

BOX 47-1 Growth Hormones and Related Medications

Growth Hormones
- Somatropin
- Norditropin
- Mecasermin

Growth Hormone Receptor Antagonists
- Octreotide acetate
- Lanreotide
- Pegvisomant

III. Thyroid Hormones (Box 47-2)

A. Description
1. Thyroid hormones control the metabolic rate of tissues and accelerate heat production and oxygen consumption.
2. Thyroid hormones are used to replace the thyroid hormone deficit in conditions such as **hypothyroidism** and **myxedema coma**.
3. Thyroid hormones enhance the action of oral anticoagulants, sympathomimetics, and antidepressants and decrease the action of insulin, oral hypoglycemics, and digitalis preparations; the action of thyroid hormones is decreased by phenytoin and carbamazepine.
4. Thyroid hormones should be given at least 4 hours apart from multivitamins, aluminum hydroxide and magnesium hydroxide, simethicone, calcium carbonate, phosphate binders, bile acid sequestrants, iron, and sucralfate, because these medications decrease the absorption of thyroid replacements.

B. Side and adverse effects
1. Nausea and decreased appetite
2. Abdominal cramps and diarrhea
3. Weight loss
4. Nervousness and tremors
5. Insomnia
6. Sweating
7. Heat intolerance
8. Tachycardia, dysrhythmias, palpitations, chest pain
9. Hypertension
10. Headache
11. Toxicity: **Hyperthyroidism**

C. Interventions
1. Assess the client for a history of medications currently being taken.
2. Monitor vital signs.
3. Monitor weight.
4. Monitor triiodothyronine (T3), thyroxine (T4) and TSH levels.
5. Instruct the client to take the medication at the same time each day, in the morning without food.
6. Instruct the client in how to monitor the pulse rate.
7. Inform the client that it is important to discuss which foods to specifically avoid that may inhibit thyroid secretion based on the client's individualized diet plan and medication regimen.
8. Advise the client to avoid over-the-counter medications.
9. Instruct the client to wear a MedicAlert bracelet.

BOX 47-2 Thyroid Hormones
- Levothyroxine sodium
- Liothyronine sodium
- Liotrix
- Thyroid, desiccated

Advise the client taking a thyroid hormone to report symptoms of hyperthyroidism, such as a fast heart beat (tachycardia), chest pain, palpitations, and excessive sweating. These indicate signs of toxicity.

IV. Antithyroid Medications (Box 47-3)

A. Description
1. Antithyroid medications inhibit the synthesis of thyroid hormone.
2. Antithyroid medications are used for hyperthyroidism, or Graves' disease.

B. Side and adverse effects
1. Nausea and vomiting
2. Diarrhea
3. Drowsiness, headache, fever
4. Hypersensitivity with rash
5. Agranulocytosis with leukopenia and thrombocytopenia
6. Alopecia and hyperpigmentation
7. Toxicity: Hypothyroidism
8. Iodism: Characterized by vomiting, abdominal pain, metallic or brassy taste in the mouth, rash, and sore gums and salivary glands.

Iodism is a concern for clients taking strong iodine solution, also known as Lugol's solution. Because of the risk of iodism, the use of strong iodine solution is limited to about 2 weeks, generally used for clients with hyperthyroidism in preparation for thyroid surgery.

BOX 47-3 Antithyroid Medications
- Methimazole
- Propylthiouracil
- Potassium iodide and strong iodine solution

C. Interventions
1. Monitor vital signs.
2. Monitor triiodothyronine, thyroxine, and TSH levels.
3. Monitor weight.
4. Instruct the client to take medication with meals to avoid gastrointestinal (GI) upset.
5. Instruct the client in how to monitor the pulse rate.
6. Inform the client of side and adverse effects and when to notify the primary health care provider (PHCP).
7. Instruct the client in the signs of hypothyroidism.
8. Instruct the client regarding the importance of medication compliance and that abruptly stopping the medication could cause **thyroid storm**.
9. Instruct the client to monitor for signs and symptoms of thyroid storm (fever, flushed skin, confusion and behavioral changes, tachycardia, dysrhythmias, and signs of heart failure).
10. Instruct the client to monitor for signs of iodism.
11. Advise the client to consult the PHCP before eating iodized salt and iodine-rich foods.
12. Instruct the client to avoid acetylsalicylic acid and medications containing iodine.

Methimazole causes agranulocytosis. Therefore, advise the client to contact the PHCP if a fever or sore throat develops.

V. Parathyroid Medications (Box 47-4)

A. Description
1. Parathyroid hormone regulates serum calcium levels.
2. Low serum levels of calcium stimulate parathyroid hormone release.
3. Hyperparathyroidism results in a high serum calcium level and bone demineralization; medication is used to lower the serum calcium level.
4. Hypoparathyroidism results in a low serum calcium level, which increases neuromuscular excitability; treatment includes calcium and vitamin D supplements.
5. Calcium salts administered with digoxin increase the risk of digoxin toxicity.
6. Oral calcium salts reduce the absorption of tetracycline hydrochloride.

B. Interventions
1. Monitor electrolyte and calcium levels.
2. Assess for signs and symptoms of hypocalcemia and hypercalcemia.
3. Assess for symptoms of tetany in the client with hypocalcemia.
4. Assess for renal calculi in the client with hypercalcemia.
5. Instruct the client in the signs and symptoms of hypercalcemia and hypocalcemia.

BOX 47-4 Medications to Treat Calcium Disorders

Oral Calcium Supplements
- Calcium acetate
- Calcium carbonate
- Calcium citrate
- Calcium glubionate
- Calcium gluconate
- Tribasic calcium phosphate

Vitamin D Supplements
- Cholecalciferol (vitamin D_3)
- Ergocalciferol (vitamin D_2)

Bisphosphonates and Calcium Regulators
- Alendronate sodium
- Calcitonin salmon
- Etidronate disodium
- Ibandronate
- Pamidronate disodium
- Risedronate sodium
- Zoledronic acid

Medications to Treat Hypercalcemia
- Cinacalcet hydrochloride
- Doxercalciferol
- Calcitonin
- Paricalcitol

6. Instruct the client to check over-the-counter medication labels for the possibility of calcium content.
7. Instruct the client receiving oral calcium supplements to maintain an adequate intake of vitamin D, because vitamin D enhances absorption of calcium.
8. Instruct the client receiving calcium regulators such as alendronate sodium to swallow the tablet whole with water at least 30 minutes before breakfast and not to lie down for at least 30 minutes.
9. Instruct the client using nasal spray of calcitonin to alternate nares.
10. Instruct the client using antihypercalcemic agents to avoid foods rich in calcium such as green, leafy vegetables; dairy products; shellfish; and soy.
11. Instruct the client not to take other medications within 1 hour of taking a calcium supplement.
12. Instruct the client to increase fluid and fiber in the diet to prevent constipation associated with calcium supplements.

VI. Corticosteroids: Mineralocorticoids

A. Fludrocortisone acetate
B. Description

1. Mineralocorticoids are steroid hormones that enhance the reabsorption of sodium and chloride and promote the excretion of potassium and hydrogen from the renal tubules, thereby helping maintain fluid and electrolyte balance.
2. Mineralocorticoids are used for replacement therapy in primary and secondary adrenal insufficiency in Addison's disease.

C. Side and adverse effects
1. Sodium and water retention, edema, hypertension
2. Hypokalemia
3. Hypocalcemia
4. Osteoporosis, compression fractures
5. Weight gain
6. Heart failure

D. Interventions
1. Monitor vital signs.
2. Monitor intake and output, weight, and for edema.
3. Monitor electrolyte and calcium levels.
4. Instruct the client to take medication with food or milk.
5. Instruct the client to consume a high-potassium diet.
6. Instruct the client to report signs of illness.
7. Instruct the client to notify the PHCP if low blood pressure, weakness, cramping, palpitations, or changes in mental status occur.
8. Instruct the client to wear a MedicAlert bracelet.

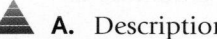

Instruct the client taking a corticosteroid not to stop the medication abruptly, because this could result in adrenal insufficiency.

VII. Corticosteroids: Glucocorticoids (Box 47-5)

A. Description
1. Glucocorticoids affect glucose, protein, and bone metabolism; alter the normal immune response and suppress inflammation; and produce anti-inflammatory, antiallergic, and antistress effects.
2. Glucocorticoids may be used as a replacement in adrenocortical insufficiency.
3. Glucocorticoids are used for their anti-inflammatory and immunosuppressant effects both short-term and long-term in the treatment of several nonendocrine disorders.

BOX 47-5 Corticosteroids: Glucocorticoids

- Betamethasone
- Cortisone acetate
- Dexamethasone
- Hydrocortisone
- Methylprednisolone
- Prednisolone
- Prednisone
- Triamcinolone

B. Side and adverse effects
1. Adrenal insufficiency
2. Hyperglycemia
3. Hypokalemia
4. Hypocalcemia, osteoporosis
5. Sodium and fluid retention
6. Weight gain and edema
7. Mood swings
8. Moon face, buffalo hump, truncal obesity
9. Increased susceptibility to infection and masking of the signs and symptoms of infection
10. Cataracts
11. Hirsutism, acne, fragile skin, bruising
12. Growth retardation in children
13. GI irritation, peptic ulcer, pancreatitis
14. Seizures
15. Psychosis (usually occurs with hydrocortisone and dexamethasone in clients receiving very high doses long-term and is most likely due to their effects on blood glucose)

C. Contraindications and cautions
1. Contraindicated in clients with hypersensitivity, psychosis, and fungal infections
2. Should be used with caution in clients with diabetes mellitus
3. Should be used with extreme caution in clients with infections because they mask the signs and symptoms of an infection
4. They can increase the potency of medications taken concurrently, such as aspirin and nonsteroidal antiinflammatory drugs, thus increasing the risk of GI bleeding and ulceration.
5. Use of potassium-losing diuretics increases potassium loss, resulting in hypokalemia.
6. Dexamethasone decreases the effects of orally administered anticoagulants and antidiabetic agents.
7. Barbiturates, phenytoin, and rifampin decrease the effect of prednisone.

D. Interventions
1. Monitor vital signs.
2. Monitor serum electrolyte and blood glucose levels.
3. Monitor for hypokalemia and hyperglycemia.
4. Monitor intake and output, weight, and for edema.
5. Monitor for hypertension.
6. Assess medical history for glaucoma, cataracts, peptic ulcer, mental health disorders, or diabetes mellitus.
7. Monitor the older client for signs and symptoms of increased osteoporosis.
8. Assess for changes in muscle strength.
9. Prepare a schedule as needed for the client, with information on short-term tapered doses.
10. Instruct the client that it is best to take medication in the early morning with food or milk.

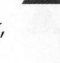

11. Advise the client to eat foods high in potassium.
12. Instruct the client to avoid individuals with infections.
13. Advise the client to inform all PHCPs of the medication regimen.
14. Instruct the client to report signs and symptoms of **Cushing's syndrome**, including a moon face, puffy eyelids, edema in the feet, increased bruising, dizziness, bleeding, and menstrual irregularities, which often results from the large doses of long-term glucocorticoids that may be used to treat nonendocrine conditions.
15. Note that the client may need additional doses during periods of stress, such as surgery.
16. Instruct the client not to stop the medication abruptly, because abrupt withdrawal can result in severe adrenal insufficiency.
17. Advise the client to consult with the PHCP before receiving vaccinations; live virus vaccines should not be administered to the client taking glucocorticoids.
18. Advise the client to wear a MedicAlert bracelet.

VIII. Androgens (Box 47-6)

A. Description
1. Used to replace deficient hormones or to treat hormone-sensitive disorders
2. Can cause bleeding if the client is taking oral anticoagulants (increase the effect of anticoagulants)
3. Can cause decreased serum glucose concentration, thereby reducing insulin requirements in the client with diabetes mellitus
4. Hepatotoxic medications are avoided with the use of androgens because of the risk of additive damage to the liver.
5. Androgens usually are avoided in men with known prostate or breast carcinoma, because androgens often stimulate growth of these tumors.

BOX 47-6 Androgens

- Methyltestosterone

Testosterone Preparations
- Testosterone, pellets
- Testosterone, transdermal
- Testosterone cypionate
- Testosterone enanthate
- Testosterone propionate
- Testosterone undecanoate
- Testosterone, buccal patch
- Testosterone, topical gel
- Testosterone, nasal gel

B. Side and adverse effects
1. Masculine secondary sexual characteristics (body hair growth, lowered voice, muscle growth)
2. Bladder irritation and urinary tract infections
3. Breast tenderness
4. Gynecomastia
5. Priapism
6. Menstrual irregularities
7. Virilism
8. Sodium and water retention with edema
9. Nausea, vomiting, or diarrhea
10. Acne
11. Changes in libido
12. Hepatotoxicity, jaundice
13. Hypercalcemia

C. Interventions
1. Monitor vital signs.
2. Monitor for edema, weight gain, and skin changes.
3. Assess mental status and neurological function.
4. Assess for signs of liver dysfunction, including right upper quadrant abdominal pain, malaise, fever, jaundice, and pruritus.
5. Assess for the development of secondary sexual characteristics.
6. Instruct the client to take medication with meals or a snack.
7. Instruct the client to notify the PHCP if priapism develops.
8. Instruct the client to notify the PHCP if fluid retention occurs.
9. Instruct women to use a nonhormonal contraceptive while on therapy.
10. For women, monitor for menstrual irregularities and decreased breast size.

IX. Estrogens and Progestins

A. Description
1. Estrogens are steroids that stimulate female reproductive tissue.
2. Progestins are steroids that specifically stimulate the uterine lining.
3. Estrogen and progestin preparations may be used to stimulate the endogenous hormones to restore hormonal balance or to treat hormone-sensitive tumors (suppress tumor growth) or for contraception (Boxes 47-7 and 47-8).

BOX 47-7 Estrogens

- Esterified estrogens
- Estradiol
- Estrogens, conjugated
- Ethinyl estradiol

BOX 47-8 Progestins

- Estradiol/drospirenone
- Estradiol/norgestimate
- Estradiol/levonorgestrel
- Estradiol/norethindrone
- Estradiol/etonogestrel
- Medroxyprogesterone acetate
- Medroxyprogesterone and conjugated estrogens
- Megestrol acetate
- Norethindrone acetate
- Levonorgestrel
- Progesterone

B. Contraindications and cautions
 1. Estrogens
  a. Estrogens are contraindicated in clients with breast cancer, endometrial hyperplasia, endometrial cancer, history of thromboembolism, known or suspected pregnancy, or lactation.
  b. Use estrogens with caution in clients with hypertension, gallbladder disease, or liver or kidney dysfunction.
  c. Estrogens increase the risk of toxicity when used with hepatotoxic medications.
  d. Barbiturates, phenytoin, and rifampin decrease the effectiveness of estrogen.
 2. Progestins are contraindicated in clients with thromboembolic disorders and should be avoided in clients with breast tumors or hepatic disease.
C. Side and adverse effects
 1. Breast tenderness, menstrual changes
 2. Nausea, vomiting, and diarrhea
 3. Malaise, depression, excessive irritability
 4. Weight gain
 5. Edema and fluid retention
 6. Atherosclerosis
 7. Hypertension, stroke, myocardial infarction
 8. Thromboembolism (estrogen)
 9. Migraine headaches and vomiting (estrogen)
D. Interventions
 1. Monitor vital signs.
 2. Monitor for hypertension.
 3. Assess for edema and weight gain.
 4. Advise the client not to smoke.
 5. Advise the client to undergo routine breast and pelvic examinations.

X. Medications for Diabetes Mellitus

A. Insulin and oral antidiabetic medications
 1. Description
  a. Insulin increases glucose transport into cells and promotes conversion of glucose to glycogen, decreasing serum glucose levels.
  b. Oral antidiabetic agents act in a number of ways: stimulate the pancreas to produce more insulin, increase the sensitivity of peripheral receptors to insulin, decrease hepatic glucose output, delay intestinal absorption of glucose, enhance the activity of incretins, and promote glucose loss through the kidney.
 2. Contraindications and concerns
  a. Oral antidiabetic agents, except the sodium-glucose cotransporter 2 (SGLT-2) inhibitors, are contraindicated in type 1 diabetes mellitus.
  b. β-Adrenergic blocking agents may mask signs and symptoms of hypoglycemia associated with hypoglycemia-producing medications.
  c. Anticoagulants, chloramphenicol, salicylates, propranolol, monoamine oxidase inhibitors, pentamidine, and sulfonamides may cause hypoglycemia.
  d. Corticosteroids, sympathomimetics, thiazide diuretics, phenytoin, thyroid preparations, oral contraceptives, and estrogen compounds may cause hyperglycemia.
  e. Side and adverse effects of the sulfonylureas include GI symptoms and dermatological reactions; hypoglycemia can occur when an excessive dose is administered or when meals are omitted or delayed, food intake is decreased, or activity is increased.

⚠ Sulfonylureas can cause a disulfiram type of reaction when alcohol is ingested.

B. Medications for type 2 diabetes mellitus (Table 47-1)
 1. Interventions
  a. Assess the client's knowledge of diabetes mellitus and the use of oral antidiabetic agents.
  b. Obtain a medication history regarding the medications that the client is taking currently.
  c. Assess vital signs and blood glucose levels.
  d. Instruct the client to recognize the signs and symptoms of hypoglycemia and hyperglycemia.
  e. Instruct the client to avoid over-the-counter medications unless prescribed by the PHCP.
  f. Instruct the client not to ingest alcohol with sulfonylureas.
  g. Inform the client that insulin may be needed during times of increased stress, surgery, or infection.
  h. Instruct the client on the necessity for compliance with prescribed medication.
  i. Instruct the client about how to take each specific medication, such as with the first bite of the meal for meglitinides and α-glucosidase inhibitors.
  j. Advise the client to wear a MedicAlert bracelet.

TABLE 47-1 Medications for Type 2 Diabetes

Class and Specific Agents	Actions	Major Adverse Effects
Oral Medications		
Biguanides		
Metformin	Decreases glucose production by the liver; increases tissue response to insulin	Gastrointestinal (GI) symptoms: decreased appetite, nausea, diarrhea
Second-Generation Sulfonylureas		
Glimepiride Glipizide Glyburide*	Promote insulin secretion by the pancreas; may also increase tissue response to insulin	Hypoglycemia Weight gain
Meglitinides (Glinides)		
Nateglinide Repaglinide	Promote insulin secretion by the pancreas	Hypoglycemia Weight gain
Thiazolidinediones (Glitazones)		
Pioglitazone Rosiglitazone	Decrease insulin resistance, and thereby increase glucose uptake by muscle and adipose tissue and decrease glucose production by the liver	Hypoglycemia, but only in the presence of excessive insulin Heart failure Bladder cancer Fractures (in women) Ovulation and thus possible unintended pregnancy
α-Glucosidase Inhibitors		
Acarbose Miglitol	Delay carbohydrate digestion and absorption, thereby decreasing the postprandial rise in blood glucose	GI symptoms: flatulence, cramps, abdominal distention, borborygmus
DPP-4 Inhibitors (Gliptins)		
Alogliptin Linagliptin Saxagliptin Sitagliptin	Enhance the activity of incretins (by inhibiting their breakdown by DPP-4), and thereby stimulate a decrease in blood glucose levels, increase insulin release, reduce glucagon release, and decrease hepatic glucose production	Pancreatitis Hypersensitivity reactions
Sodium-Glucose Cotransporter 2 (SGLT-2) Inhibitors		
Canagliflozin Dapagliflozin Empagliflozin Ertugliflozin (a combination with metformin is available)	Increase glucose excretion via the urine by inhibiting SGLT-2 in the kidney tubules, decreasing glucose levels and inducing weight loss via caloric loss through the urine	Genital mycotic infections Orthostatic hypotension
Dopamine Agonist		
Bromocriptine	Activates dopamine receptors in the central nervous system; how it improves glycemic control is unknown	Orthostatic hypotension Exacerbation of psychosis
Noninsulin Injectable Medications		
Incretin Mimetics		
Exenatide Exenatide extended-release Liraglutide Albiglutide Lixisenatide	Lower blood glucose by slowing gastric emptying, stimulating glucose-dependent insulin release, suppressing postprandial glucagon release, and reducing appetite	Hypoglycemia GI symptoms: nausea, vomiting, diarrhea Pancreatitis Renal insufficiency
Amylin Mimetics		
Pramlintide	Delays gastric emptying and suppresses glucagon secretion, decreasing the postprandial rise in glucose	Hypoglycemia Nausea Injection-site reactions

*Commonly known as *glibenclamide* outside the United States.
Adapted from Burchum JR, Rosenthal RD: *Lehne's pharmacology for nursing care*, ed 9, St. Louis, 2016, Saunders.

⚠ Metformin needs to be withheld temporarily before and for 48 hours after having any radiological study that involves the administration of intravenous contrast dye because of the risk of contrast-induced nephropathy and lactic acidosis. The PHCP needs to be consulted for specific prescriptions.

C. Insulin

1. Insulin acts primarily in the liver, muscle, and adipose tissue by attaching to receptors on cellular membranes and facilitating the passage of glucose, potassium, and magnesium.
2. Insulin is prescribed for clients with type 1 diabetes mellitus and for clients with type 2 diabetes mellitus whose blood glucose levels are not adequately controlled with oral antidiabetic agents.
3. The onset, peak, and duration of action depend on the insulin type (Tables 47-2 and 47-3).
4. Storing of insulin (Box 47-9)
5. Insulin injection sites
   a. The main areas for injections are the abdomen, arms (posterior surface), thighs (anterior surface), and hips (Fig. 47-1).
   b. Insulin injected into the abdomen may absorb more evenly and rapidly than at other sites.

TABLE 47-2 Types of Insulin: Time Course of Activity After Subcutaneous Injection

Generic Name	Time Course: Onset (min)	Peak (hr)	Duration (hr)
Short Duration: Rapid Onset			
Insulin lispro	15-30	0.5-2.5	3-6
Insulin aspart	10-20	1-3	3-5
Insulin glulisine	10-15	1-1.5	3-5
Short Duration: Slower Onset			
Regular insulin	30-60	1-5	6-10
Intermediate Duration			
NPH insulin	60-120	6-14	16-24
Long Duration			
Insulin glargine	70	None	18-24
Insulin detemir	60-120	12-24	Varies
Insulin degludec	60-120	None	>40 Hours

Adapted from Burchum JR, Rosenthal RD: *Lehne's pharmacology for nursing care*, ed 9, St. Louis, 2016, Saunders.

TABLE 47-3 Premixed Insulin Combinations*

Description	Time Course: Onset (min)	Peak (hr)	Duration (hr)
70% NPH insulin/30% regular insulin (Humulin)	30-60	1.5-16	10-16
70% NPH insulin/30% regular insulin (Novolin)	30-60	2-12	10-16
50% NPH insulin/50% regular insulin	30-60	2-12	10-16
70% insulin aspart protamine/30% insulin aspart	10-20	1-4	15-18
75% insulin lispro protamine/25% insulin lispro	15-30	1-6.5	10-16
50% insulin lispro protamine/50% insulin lispro	15-30	0.8-4.8	10-16

*Use only after the dosages and ratios of the components have been established as correct for the client.

Adapted from Burchum JR, Rosenthal RD: *Lehne's pharmacology for nursing care*, ed 9, St. Louis, 2016, Saunders.

BOX 47-9 Storing Insulin

- Avoid exposing insulin to extremes in temperature.
- Insulin should not be frozen or kept in direct sunlight or a hot car.
- Before injection, insulin should be at room temperature.
- If a vial of insulin will be used up in 1 month, it may be kept at room temperature; otherwise, the vial should be refrigerated.

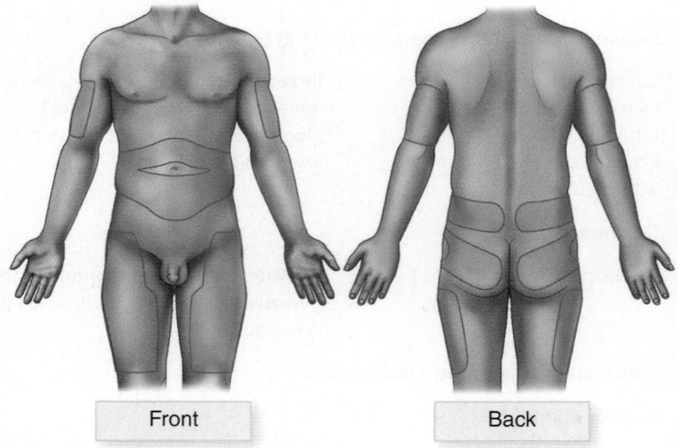

FIG. 47-1 Common insulin injection sites.

   c. Systematic rotation within 1 anatomical area is recommended to prevent lipodystrophy and to promote more even absorption; clients should be instructed not to use the same site more than once in a 2- to 3-week period.
   d. Injections should be 1 to 1.5 inches (2.5 to 3.8 cm) apart within the anatomical area.

e. Heat, massage, and exercise of the injected area can increase absorption rates and may result in hypoglycemia.
f. Injection into scar tissue may delay absorption of insulin.

6. Administering insulin (also see Chapter 46)

Insulin glargine cannot be mixed with any other types of insulin.

a. To prevent dosage errors, be certain that there is a match between the insulin concentration noted on the vial and the calibration of units on the insulin syringe; the usual concentration of insulin is U-100 (100 units/mL).
b. The Humulin R brand of regular insulin is the only insulin that is formulated in a U-500 strength. U-500 strength insulin is reserved for clients with severe insulin resistance who require large doses of insulin. A special syringe calibrated for use with U-500 insulin is required.
c. Prefilled syringes (pens) are commonly used; a new needle needs to be attached before each injection.
d. Most insulin syringes have a 27- to 29-gauge needle that is about 0.5-inch long (1.3 cm).
e. NPH insulin is an insulin suspension; the appearance is cloudy. All other insulin types are solutions; the appearance of all other insulin products is clear.
f. Before use, NPH insulins must be rotated, or rolled, between the palms to ensure that the insulin suspension is mixed well; otherwise, an inaccurate dose will be drawn; vigorously shaking the bottle will cause bubbles to form. It is not necessary to rotate or roll clear insulins before using.
g. Inject air into the insulin bottle (a vacuum makes it difficult to draw up the insulin).
h. When mixing insulins, draw up the shortest-acting insulin first.
i. Short-duration (i.e., regular, lispro, aspart, and glulisine) insulin may be mixed with NPH.
j. Administer a mixed dose of insulin within 5 to 15 minutes of preparation; after this time, the short-acting insulin binds with the NPH insulin and its action is reduced.
k. Aspiration after insertion of the needle generally is not recommended with self-injection of insulin.
l. Administer insulin at a 45- to 90-degree angle in clients with normal subcutaneous mass and at a 45- to 60-degree angle in thin persons or those with a decreased amount of subcutaneous mass.

Some rapid- and short-acting insulins can be administered intravenously.

D. Glucagon-like peptide (GLP-1) receptor agonists
1. Noninsulin injectable agents that are analogs of human GLP-1 and cause the same effects as the GLP-1 incretin hormone in the body, which are to stimulate the glucose level–dependent release of insulin, to suppress the postprandial release of glucagon, to slow gastric emptying, and to suppress appetite
2. Used for clients with type 2 diabetes mellitus (not recommended for clients taking insulin, nor should clients be taken off insulin and given a GLP-1 receptor agonist)
3. GLP-1 receptor agonists restore the first-phase insulin response (first 10 minutes after food ingestion), lower the production of glucagon after meals, slow gastric emptying (which limits the rise in blood glucose level after a meal), reduce fasting and postprandial blood glucose levels, and reduce caloric intake, resulting in weight loss
4. Packaged in premeasured doses (pens) that require refrigeration (cannot be frozen)
5. Administered as a subcutaneous injection in the thigh, abdomen, or upper arm. Exenatide is administered twice daily within 60 minutes before morning and evening meals (not taken after meals); if a dose is missed, the treatment regimen is resumed as prescribed with the next scheduled dose. Liraglutide is administered subcutaneously once daily without regard to meals. Albiglutide is injected subcutaneously once weekly.
6. Can cause mild to moderate nausea that abates with use.
7. Because delayed gastric emptying slows the absorption of other medications, other prescribed oral medications should be given an hour before injection of these medications.

E. Amylin Mimetic: Pramlintide
1. Synthetic form of amylin, a naturally occurring hormone secreted by the pancreas
2. Used for clients with types 1 and 2 diabetes mellitus who use insulin; administered subcutaneously before meals to lower blood glucose level after meals, leading to less fluctuation during the day and better long-term glucose control
3. Associated with an increased risk of insulin-induced severe hypoglycemia, particularly in clients with type 1 diabetes mellitus
4. GI effects, including nausea, can occur.
5. Unopened vials are refrigerated; opened vials can be refrigerated or kept at room temperature for up to 28 days.
6. Reduces postprandial hyperglycemia by delaying gastric emptying and suppressing postprandial glucagon release

7. Because pramlintide delays gastric emptying, other prescribed oral medications should be given 1 hour before or 2 hours after an injection of pramlintide.

F. Glucagon
1. Hormone secreted by the alpha cells of the islets of Langerhans in the pancreas
2. Increases blood glucose level by stimulating glycogenolysis in the liver
3. Can be administered subcutaneously, intramuscularly, or intravenously
4. Used to treat insulin-induced hypoglycemia when the client is semiconscious or unconscious and is unable to ingest liquids
5. The blood glucose level begins to increase within 5 to 20 minutes after administration.
6. Instruct the family in the procedure for administration.
7. See Chapter 46 for additional information regarding insulin and interventions for hypoglycemia.

PRACTICE QUESTIONS

512. The nurse is teaching a client with diabetes mellitus how to mix regular insulin and NPH insulin in the same syringe. Which action, if performed by the client, indicates the **need for further teaching?**
1. Withdraws the NPH insulin first
2. Withdraws the regular insulin first
3. Injects air into NPH insulin vial first
4. Injects an amount of air equal to the desired dose of insulin into each vial

513. The home care nurse visits a client recently diagnosed with diabetes mellitus who is taking Humulin NPH insulin daily. The client asks the nurse how to store the unopened vials of insulin. The nurse should tell the client to take which action?
1. Freeze the insulin.
2. Refrigerate the insulin.
3. Store the insulin in a dark, dry place.
4. Keep the insulin at room temperature.

514. Glimepiride is prescribed for a client with diabetes mellitus. The nurse instructs the client that which food items are **most** acceptable to consume while taking this medication? **Select all that apply.**
- ☐ 1. Alcohol
- ☐ 2. Red meats
- ☐ 3. Whole-grain cereals
- ☐ 4. Low-calorie desserts
- ☐ 5. Carbonated beverages

515. The nurse is providing discharge teaching for a client newly diagnosed with type 2 diabetes mellitus who has been prescribed metformin. Which client statement indicates the **need for further teaching**?
1. "It is okay if I skip meals once in a while."
2. "I need to let my doctor know if I get unusually tired."
3. "I need to constantly watch for signs of low blood sugar."
4. "I will be sure to not drink alcohol excessively while on this medication."

516. The primary health care provider (PHCP) prescribes exenatide for a client with type 1 diabetes mellitus who takes insulin. The nurse should plan to take which **most appropriate** intervention?
1. Withhold the medication and call the PHCP, questioning the prescription for the client.
2. Teach the client about the signs and symptoms of hypoglycemia and hyperglycemia.
3. Monitor the client for gastrointestinal side effects after administering the medication.
4. Withdraw the insulin from the prefilled pen into an insulin syringe to prepare for administration.

517. A client with diabetes mellitus is taking Humulin NPH insulin and regular insulin every morning. The nurse should provide which instructions to the client? **Select all that apply.**
1. Hypoglycemia may be experienced before dinnertime.
2. The insulin dose should be decreased if illness occurs.
3. The insulin should be administered at room temperature.
4. The insulin vial needs to be shaken vigorously to break up the precipitates.
5. The NPH insulin should be drawn into the syringe first, then the regular insulin.

518. The home health care nurse is visiting a client who was recently diagnosed with type 2 diabetes mellitus. The client is prescribed repaglinide and metformin. The nurse should provide which instructions to the client? **Select all that apply.**
- ☐ 1. Diarrhea may occur secondary to the metformin.
- ☐ 2. The repaglinide is not taken if a meal is skipped.
- ☐ 3. The repaglinide is taken 30 minutes before eating.
- ☐ 4. A simple sugar food item is carried and used to treat mild hypoglycemia episodes.
- ☐ 5. Muscle pain is an expected effect of metformin and may be treated with acetaminophen.
- ☐ 6. Metformin increases hepatic glucose production to prevent hypoglycemia associated with repaglinide.

519. The nurse is teaching the client about his prescribed prednisone. Which statement, if made by the client, indicates that **further teaching is necessary**?

1. "I can take aspirin or my antihistamine if I need it."
2. "I need to take the medication every day at the same time."
3. "I need to avoid coffee, tea, cola, and chocolate in my diet."
4. "If I gain 5 pounds or more a week, I will call my doctor."

520. A client with hyperthyroidism has been given methimazole. Which nursing considerations are associated with this medication? **Select all that apply.**

❑ 1. Administer methimazole with food.
❑ 2. Place the client on a low-calorie, low-protein diet.
❑ 3. Assess the client for unexplained bruising or bleeding.
❑ 4. Instruct the client to report side and adverse effects such as sore throat, fever, or headaches.
❑ 5. Use special radioactive precautions when handling the client's urine for the first 24 hours following initial administration.

521. The nurse is monitoring a client receiving levothyroxine sodium for hypothyroidism. Which findings indicate the presence of a side effect associated with this medication? **Select all that apply.**

❑ 1. Insomnia
❑ 2. Weight loss
❑ 3. Bradycardia
❑ 4. Constipation
❑ 5. Mild heat intolerance

522. The nurse provides instructions to a client who is taking levothyroxine. The nurse should tell the client to take the medication in which way?

1. With food
2. At lunchtime
3. On an empty stomach
4. At bedtime with a snack

523. The nurse should tell the client who is taking levothyroxine to notify the primary health care provider (PHCP) if which problem occurs?

1. Fatigue
2. Tremors
3. Cold intolerance
4. Excessively dry skin

524. The nurse is providing instructions to the client newly diagnosed with diabetes mellitus who has been prescribed pramlintide. Which instruction should the nurse include in the discharge teaching?

1. "Inject the pramlintide at the same time you take your other medications."
2. "Take your prescribed pills 1 hour before or 2 hours after the injection."
3. "Be sure to take the pramlintide with food so you don't upset your stomach."
4. "Make sure you take your pramlintide immediately after you eat so you don't experience a low blood sugar."

525. The nurse teaches the client who is newly diagnosed with diabetes insipidus about the prescribed intranasal desmopressin. Which statements by the client indicate understanding? **Select all that apply.**

❑ 1. "This medication will turn my urine orange."
❑ 2. "I should decrease my oral fluids when I start this medication."
❑ 3. "The amount of urine I make should increase if this medicine is working."
❑ 4. "I need to follow a low-fat diet to avoid pancreatitis when taking this medicine."
❑ 5. "I should report headache and drowsiness to my doctor since these symptoms could be related to my desmopressin."

526. A daily dose of prednisone is prescribed for a client. The nurse provides instructions to the client regarding administration of the medication and should instruct the client that which time is **best** to take this medication?

1. At noon
2. At bedtime
3. Early morning
4. Any time, at the same time, each day

527. The client with hyperparathyroidism is taking alendronate. Which statements by the client indicate understanding of the proper way to take this medication? **Select all that apply.**

❑ 1. "I should take this medication with food."
❑ 2. "I should take this medication at bedtime."
❑ 3. "I should sit up for at least 30 minutes after taking this medication."
❑ 4. "I should take this medication first thing in the morning on an empty stomach."
❑ 5. "I can pick a time to take this medication that best fits my lifestyle as long as I take it at the same time each day."

528. A client with diabetes mellitus visits a health care clinic. The client's diabetes mellitus previously had been well controlled with glyburide daily, but recently the fasting blood glucose level has been 180 to 200 mg/dL (10 to 11.1 mmol/L). Which medication, if added to the client's regimen, may have contributed to the hyperglycemia?

1. Atenolol
2. Prednisone
3. Phenelzine
4. Allopurinol

ANSWERS

512. *Answer:* 1

Rationale: When preparing a mixture of short-acting insulin, such as regular insulin, with another insulin preparation, the short-acting insulin is drawn into the syringe first. This sequence will avoid contaminating the vial of short-acting insulin with insulin of another type. Options 2, 3, and 4 identify correct actions for preparing NPH and short-acting insulin.

Test-Taking Strategy: Note the strategic words, *need for further teaching*. These words indicate a negative event query and ask you to select an option that is an incorrect action. Remember *RN*—draw up the *R*egular *(short-acting)* insulin before the *N*PH insulin.

Level of Cognitive Ability: Evaluating

Client Needs: Physiological Integrity

Integrated Process: Teaching and Learning

Content Area: Pharmacology: Endocrine Medications: Insulin

Health Problem: Adult Health: Endocrine: Diabetes mellitus

Priority Concepts: Client Education; Glucose Regulation

Reference: Lilley et al. (2017), pp. 504, 517.

513. *Answer:* 2

Rationale: Insulin in unopened vials should be stored under refrigeration until needed. Vials should not be frozen. When stored unopened under refrigeration, insulin can be used up to the expiration date on the vial. Options 1, 3, and 4 are incorrect.

Test-Taking Strategy: Note the subject, how to store unopened vials of insulin. Options 3 and 4 are comparable or alike regarding where to store the insulin and should be eliminated. Remembering that insulin should not be frozen will assist in eliminating option 1.

Level of Cognitive Ability: Applying

Client Needs: Physiological Integrity

Integrated Process: Teaching and Learning

Content Area: Pharmacology: Endocrine Medications: Insulin

Health Problem: Adult Health: Endocrine: Diabetes mellitus

Priority Concepts: Client Education; Safety

Reference: Lilley et al. (2017), p. 517.

514. *Answer:* 2, 3, 5

Rationale: When alcohol is combined with glimepiride, a disulfiram-like reaction may occur. This syndrome includes flushing, palpitations, and nausea. Alcohol can also potentiate the hypoglycemic effects of the medication. Clients need to be instructed to avoid alcohol consumption while taking this medication. Low-calorie desserts should also be avoided. Even though the calorie content may be low, carbohydrate content is most likely high and can affect the blood glucose. The items in options 2, 3, and 5 are acceptable to consume.

Test-Taking Strategy: Note the strategic word, *most*. Remembering that alcohol can affect the action of many medications will assist in eliminating option 1. Next, recalling that carbohydrates need to be controlled in a diabetic diet will assist in eliminating option 4.

Level of Cognitive Ability: Applying

Client Needs: Physiological Integrity

Integrated Process: Teaching and Learning

Content Area: Pharmacology: Endocrine Medications: Oral Hypoglycemic

Health Problem: Adult Health: Endocrine: Diabetes mellitus

Priority Concepts: Client Education; Glucose Regulation

Reference: Hodgson, Kizior (2018), p. 527.

515. *Answer:* 3

Rationale: Metformin is classified as a biguanide and is the most commonly used medication for type 2 diabetes mellitus initially. It is also often used as a preventive medication for those at high risk for developing diabetes mellitus. When used alone, metformin lowers the blood glucose after meal intake as well as fasting blood glucose levels. Metformin does not stimulate insulin release and therefore poses little risk for hypoglycemia. For this reason, metformin is well suited for clients who skip meals. Unusual somnolence as well as hyperventilation, myalgia, and malaise are early signs of lactic acidosis, a toxic effect associated with metformin. If any of these signs or symptoms occur, the client should inform the primary health care provider immediately. While it is best to avoid consumption of alcohol, it is not always realistic or feasible for clients to quit drinking altogether; for this reason, clients should be informed that excessive alcohol intake can cause an adverse reaction with metformin.

Test-Taking Strategy: Note the strategic words, *need for further teaching*. These words indicate a negative event query and the need to select the incorrect client statement as the answer. Recalling the adverse effects and drug interactions associated with this medication will assist you in eliminating options 2 and 4. Next, recalling the mechanism of action of this medication will help you determine that this medication is suited for clients who skip meals, thereby leading you to the correct option.

Level of Cognitive Ability: Evaluating

Client Needs: Physiological Integrity

Integrated Process: Teaching and Learning

Content Area: Pharmacology: Endocrine Medications: Oral Hypoglycemic

Health Problem: Adult Health: Endocrine: Diabetes mellitus

Priority Concepts: Client Education; Glucose Regulation

Reference: Lewis et al. (2017), pp. 1130-1131.

516. *Answer:* 1

Rationale: Exenatide is an incretin mimetic used for type 2 diabetes mellitus only. It is not recommended for clients taking insulin. Hence the nurse should withhold the medication and question the PHCP regarding this prescription. Although options 2 and 3 are correct statements about the medication, in this situation the medication should not be administered. The medication is packaged in prefilled pens ready for injection without the need for drawing it up into another syringe.

Test-Taking Strategy: Note the strategic words, *most appropriate*. Focus on the name of the medication, recalling that it is used for the treatment of type 2 diabetes mellitus. Eliminate option 4 because the medication is packaged in prefilled pens ready for injection. From the remaining options, focus on the data in the question. Although options 2 and 3 are appropriate when administering this medication, this client should not receive this medication.

Level of Cognitive Ability: Analyzing

Client Needs: Safe and Effective Care Environment

Integrated Process: Nursing Process—Planning

Content Area: Pharmacology: Endocrine Medications: Oral Hypoglycemic

Health Problem: Adult Health: Endocrine: Diabetes mellitus
Priority Concepts: Clinical Judgment; Glucose Regulation
Reference: Ignatavicius, Workman, Rebar (2018), p. 1292.

517. ***Answer:*** **1, 3**
Rationale: Humulin NPH is an intermediate-acting insulin. The onset of action is 60 to 120 minutes, it peaks in 6 to 14 hours, and its duration of action is 16 to 24 hours. Regular insulin is a short-acting insulin. Depending on the type, the onset of action is 30 to 60 minutes, it peaks in 1 to 5 hours, and its duration is 6 to 10 hours. Hypoglycemic reactions most likely occur during peak time. Insulin should be at room temperature when administered. Clients may need their insulin dosages increased during times of illness. Insulin vials should never be shaken vigorously. Regular insulin is always drawn up before NPH.
Test-Taking Strategy: Focus on the subject, client instructions regarding insulin. Eliminate option 4 because of the word *vigorously.* Use knowledge regarding the characteristics of insulin; procedures for administration; and the onset, peak, and duration of action for insulin and insulin administration to select from the remaining options. Remember that NPH insulin peaks in 6 to 14 hours and regular insulin peaks in 1 to 5 hours.
Level of Cognitive Ability: Applying
Client Needs: Physiological Integrity
Integrated Process: Teaching and Learning
Content Area: Pharmacology: Endocrine Medications: Insulin
Health Problem: Adult Health: Endocrine: Diabetes mellitus
Priority Concepts: Client Education; Glucose Regulation
Reference: Hodgson, Kizior (2018), p. 596.

518. ***Answer:*** **1, 2, 3, 4**
Rationale: Repaglinide, a rapid-acting oral hypoglycemic agent that stimulates pancreatic insulin secretion, should be taken before meals (approximately 30 minutes before meals) and should be withheld if the client does not eat. Hypoglycemia is a side effect of repaglinide and the client should always be prepared by carrying a simple sugar at all times. Metformin is an oral hypoglycemic given in combination with repaglinide and works by decreasing hepatic glucose production. A common side effect of metformin is diarrhea. Muscle pain may occur as an adverse effect from metformin, but it might signify a more serious condition that warrants primary health care provider notification, not the use of acetaminophen.
Test-Taking Strategy: Focus on the subject, oral medications to treat diabetes mellitus. Thinking about the pathophysiology of diabetes mellitus and recalling the actions and effects of these medications are needed to answer correctly.
Level of Cognitive Ability: Analyzing
Client Needs: Physiological Integrity
Integrated Process: Teaching and Learning
Content Area: Pharmacology: Endocrine Medications: Oral Hypoglycemic
Health Problem: Adult Health: Endocrine: Diabetes mellitus
Priority Concepts: Client Education; Glucose Regulation
Reference: Hodgson, Kizior (2018), pp. 732, 1017-1018.

519. ***Answer:*** **1**
Rationale: Aspirin and other over-the-counter medications should not be taken unless the client consults with the PHCP. The client needs to take the medication at the same time every day and should be instructed not to stop the medication. A slight weight gain as a result of an improved appetite is expected; however, after the dosage is stabilized, a weight gain of 5 pounds (2.25 kg) or more weekly should be reported to the PHCP. Caffeine-containing foods and fluids need to be avoided because they may contribute to steroid-ulcer development.
Test-Taking Strategy: Note the strategic words, *further teaching is necessary.* These words indicate a negative event query and ask you to select an option that is an incorrect statement. Remember that a client taking prednisone should not take other medications, especially over-the-counter medications, without first consulting with her or his PHCP.
Level of Cognitive Ability: Evaluating
Client Needs: Physiological Integrity
Integrated Process: Teaching and Learning
Content Area: Pharmacology: Endocrine Medications: Corticosteroids
Health Problem: N/A
Priority Concepts: Client Education; Safety
Reference: Skidmore-Roth (2017), pp. 966-967.

520. ***Answer:*** **1, 3, 4**
Rationale: Common side effects of methimazole include nausea, vomiting, and diarrhea. To address these side effects, this medication should be taken with food. Because of the increase in metabolism that occurs in hyperthyroidism, the client should consume a high-calorie diet. Antithyroid medications can cause agranulocytosis with leukopenia and thrombocytopenia. Sore throat, fever, headache, or bleeding may indicate agranulocytosis and the primary health care provider should be notified immediately. Methimazole is not radioactive and should not be stopped abruptly, due to the risk of thyroid storm.
Test-Taking Strategy: Focus on the subject, nursing considerations for administering methimazole. Focus on the client's diagnosis. Think about the pathophysiology associated with the diagnosis and the medication and the actions and effects of antithyroid medications to assist in answering correctly.
Level of Cognitive Ability: Analyzing
Client Needs: Physiological Integrity
Integrated Process: Nursing Process—Implementation
Content Area: Pharmacology: Endocrine Medications: Antithyroid Medications
Health Problem: Adult Health: Endocrine: Thyroid Disorders
Priority Concepts: Clinical Judgment; Safety
Reference: Skidmore-Roth (2017), pp. 761-762.

521. ***Answer:*** **1, 2, 5**
Rationale: Insomnia, weight loss, and mild heat intolerance are side effects of levothyroxine sodium. Bradycardia and constipation are not side effects associated with this medication, and rather are associated with hypothyroidism, which is the disorder that this medication is prescribed to treat.
Test-Taking Strategy: Focus on the subject, side effects of levothyroxine. Thinking about the pathophysiology of hypothyroidism and the action of the medication will assist you in determining that insomnia, weight loss, and mild heat intolerance are side effects of thyroid hormones.
Level of Cognitive Ability: Applying
Client Needs: Physiological Integrity
Integrated Process: Nursing Process—Assessment

Content Area: Pharmacology: Endocrine Medications: Thyroid Hormones
Health Problem: Adult Health: Endocrine: Thyroid Disorders
Priority Concepts: Clinical Judgment; Thermoregulation
Reference: Lewis et al. (2017), p. 1169.

522. *Answer:* 3
Rationale: Oral doses of levothyroxine should be taken on an empty stomach to enhance absorption. Dosing should be done in the morning before breakfast.
Test-Taking Strategy: Note that options 1, 2, and 4 are comparable or alike in that these options address administering the medication with food.
Level of Cognitive Ability: Applying
Client Needs: Physiological Integrity
Integrated Process: Teaching and Learning
Content Area: Pharmacology: Endocrine Medications: Thyroid Hormones
Health Problem: Adult Health: Endocrine: Thyroid Disorders
Priority Concepts: Client Education; Thermoregulation
Reference: Hodgson, Kizior (2018), p. 675.

523. *Answer:* 2
Rationale: Excessive doses of levothyroxine can produce signs and symptoms of hyperthyroidism. These include tachycardia, chest pain, tremors, nervousness, insomnia, hyperthermia, extreme heat intolerance, and sweating. The client should be instructed to notify the PHCP if these occur. Options 1, 3, and 4 are signs of hypothyroidism.
Test-Taking Strategy: Focus on the subject, the need to notify the PHCP. Recall the symptoms associated with hypothyroidism, the purpose of administering levothyroxine, and the effects of the medication. Options 1, 3, and 4 are symptoms related to hypothyroidism.
Level of Cognitive Ability: Applying
Client Needs: Physiological Integrity
Integrated Process: Teaching and Learning
Content Area: Pharmacology: Endocrine Medications: Thyroid Hormones
Health Problem: Adult Health: Endocrine: Thyroid Disorders
Priority Concepts: Client Education; Safety
Reference: Lewis et al. (2017), p. 1169.

524. *Answer:* 2
Rationale: Pramlintide is used for clients with types 1 and 2 diabetes mellitus who use insulin. It is administered subcutaneously before meals to lower blood glucose level after meals, leading to less fluctuation during the day and better long-term glucose control. Because pramlintide delays gastric emptying, any prescribed oral medications should be taken 1 hour before or 2 hours after an injection of pramlintide; therefore, instructing the client to take his or her pills 1 hour before or 2 hours after the injection is correct. Pramlintide should not be taken at the same time as other medications. Pramlintide is given immediately before the meal in order to control postprandial rise in blood glucose, not necessarily to prevent stomach upset. It is incorrect to instruct the client to take the medication after eating, as it will not achieve its full therapeutic effect.
Test-Taking Strategy: Focus on the subject, client instructions regarding pramlintide as it pertains to administration. Use knowledge regarding the action of the medication and treatment measures for diabetes mellitus to answer the question. Remember that this medication is used in conjunction with insulin to prevent postprandial rise in blood glucose, and that hypoglycemia is a potential adverse effect. Also remember that this medication causes delayed gastric emptying and should not be taken with other medications.
Level of Cognitive Ability: Applying
Client Needs: Physiological Integrity
Integrated Process: Teaching and Learning
Content Area: Pharmacology: Endocrine Medications: Oral Hypoglycemics
Health Problem: Adult Health: Endocrine: Diabetes mellitus
Priority Concepts: Client Education; Safety
Reference: Ignatavicius, Workman, Rebar (2018), p. 1293.

525. *Answer:* 2, 5
Rationale: In diabetes insipidus, there is a deficiency in antidiuretic hormone (ADH), resulting in large urinary losses. Desmopressin is an antidiuretic hormone that enhances reabsorption of water in the kidney. Clients with diabetes insipidus drink high volumes of fluid (polydipsia) as a compensatory mechanism to counteract urinary losses and maintain fluid balance. Once desmopressin is started, oral fluids should be decreased to prevent water intoxication. Therefore, clients with diabetes insipidus should decrease their oral fluid intake when they start desmopressin. Headache and drowsiness are signs of water intoxication in the client taking desmopressin and should be reported to the primary health care provider. Desmopressin does not turn urine orange. The amount of urine should decrease, not increase, when desmopressin is started. Desmopressin does not cause pancreatitis.
Test-Taking Strategy: Focus on the subject, understanding of desmopressin. Recall that in diabetes insipidus there is a deficiency of ADH and that desmopressin is an antidiuretic hormone. Recalling the pathophysiology of this disorder will assist you in answering correctly.
Level of Cognitive Ability: Evaluating
Client Needs: Physiological Integrity
Integrated Process: Nursing Process—Evaluation
Content Area: Pharmacology: Endocrine Medications: Antidiuretics
Health Problem: Adult Health: Endocrine: Pituitary disorders
Priority Concepts: Client Education; Fluids and Electrolytes
Reference: Skidmore-Roth (2017), pp. 343-344.

526. *Answer:* 3
Rationale: Corticosteroids (glucocorticoids) should be administered before 9 a.m. Administration at this time helps minimize adrenal insufficiency and mimics the burst of glucocorticoids released naturally by the adrenal glands each morning. Options 1, 2, and 4 are incorrect.
Test-Taking Strategy: Note the strategic word, *best.* Note the suffix *-sone* and recall that medication names that end with these letters are corticosteroids. Remember that a daily dose of a corticosteroid should be administered in the morning.
Level of Cognitive Ability: Applying
Client Needs: Physiological Integrity
Integrated Process: Teaching and Learning
Content Area: Pharmacology: Endocrine Medications: Corticosteroids
Health Problem: N/A

Priority Concepts: Client Education; Hormonal Regulation
Reference: Hodgson, Kizior (2018), pp. 967-968.

527. *Answer:* 3, 4
Rationale: Alendronate is a bisphosphonate used in hyperparathyroidism to inhibit bone loss and normalize serum calcium levels. Esophagitis is an adverse effect of primary concern in clients taking alendronate. For this reason the client is instructed to take alendronate first thing in the morning with a full glass of water on an empty stomach, not to eat or drink anything else for at least 30 minutes after taking the medication, and to remain sitting upright for at least 30 minutes after taking it.
Test-Taking Strategy: Focus on the subject, the correct method to take alendronate. Recall that the primary concern with alendronate is esophagitis. Eliminate options 1 and 2, since taking with food and taking at bedtime will each place the client at increased risk of reflux. Eliminate option 5 because alendronate should be taken first thing in the morning on an empty stomach.
Level of Cognitive Ability: Evaluating
Client Needs: Physiological Integrity
Integrated Process: Nursing Process—Evaluation
Content Area: Pharmacology: Endocrine Medications: Bisphosphonates and Calcium Regulators
Health Problem: Adult Health: Endocrine: Parathyroid Disorders
Priority Concepts: Client Education; Safety
Reference: Lewis et al. (2017), p. 1513.

528. *Answer:* 2
Rationale: Prednisone may decrease the effect of oral hypoglycemics, insulin, diuretics, and potassium supplements. Option 1, a beta blocker, and option 3, a monoamine oxidase inhibitor, have their own intrinsic hypoglycemic activity. Option 4 decreases urinary excretion of sulfonylurea agents, causing increased levels of the oral agents, which can lead to hypoglycemia.
Test-Taking Strategy: Focus on the subject, an increase in the blood glucose level. Recalling that prednisone is a corticosteroid and that corticosteroids decrease the effects of hypoglycemics will direct you to the correct option.
Level of Cognitive Ability: Analyzing
Client Needs: Physiological Integrity
Integrated Process: Nursing Process—Assessment
Content Area: Pharmacology: Endocrine Medications: Corticosteroids
Health Problem: Adult Health: Endocrine: Diabetes Mellitus
Priority Concepts: Clinical Judgment; Glucose Regulation
Reference: Skidmore-Roth (2017), pp. 571, 966-967.

UNIT X

Gastrointestinal Problems of the Adult Client

Pyramid to Success

Pyramid Points focus on diagnostic tests and nursing care related to the various gastric or intestinal tubes, gastric surgery, cirrhosis, hepatitis, pancreatitis, and colostomy care. Focus on preprocedure and postprocedure care of the client undergoing a gastrointestinal diagnostic test. Remember that an informed consent is required for any invasive procedure. Focus on diet restrictions before and after the diagnostic test and remember that the gag reflex or bowel sounds must return before allowing a client to consume food or fluids. Pyramid Points also include instructions to the client and family regarding the prevention of gastrointestinal problems and the complications associated with the problem. Focus on teaching the client and family about diet and nutrition specific to the problem, tube and wound care, preventing the transmission of infection such as with hepatitis, and care of a colostomy or ileostomy. Remember that body image disturbances can occur in clients with a gastrointestinal problem. Specific focus relates to the client with a diversion, such as an ileostomy or colostomy; the social isolation issues that can occur; and effective coping strategies.

Client Needs: Learning Objectives

Safe and Effective Care Environment

Consulting with the interprofessional team regarding the client's care and nutritional status
Ensuring that confidentiality issues related to the gastrointestinal problem are maintained
Ensuring that informed consent for treatments and surgical procedures has been obtained
Establishing priorities of care
Handling infectious drainage and secretions safely
Maintaining standard precautions and other precautions as appropriate
Obtaining referrals for home care and community services
Preventing disease transmission

Health Promotion and Maintenance

Performing physical assessment techniques of the gastrointestinal system
Preventing disease related to the gastrointestinal system
Providing health screening and health promotion programs related to gastrointestinal problems
Teaching related to colostomy or ileostomy care
Teaching related to prescribed dietary and other treatment measures
Teaching related to preventing the transmission of disease

Psychosocial Integrity

Assessing coping mechanisms
Considering end-of-life and grief and loss issues
Identifying available support systems
Monitoring for concerns related to body image changes

Physiological Integrity

Administering medications as prescribed specific to the gastrointestinal problem
Assessing for signs and symptoms of infectious diseases of the gastrointestinal tract
Assisting with personal hygiene
Monitoring elimination patterns
Monitoring for complications related to tests, procedures, and surgical interventions
Monitoring for fluid and electrolyte imbalances
Monitoring laboratory values related to gastrointestinal problems

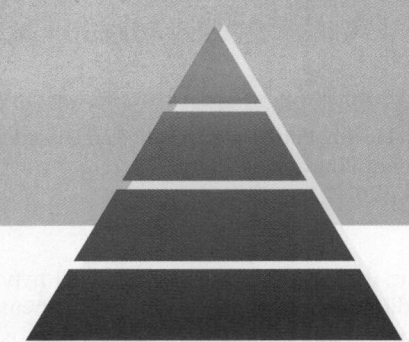

Monitoring parenterally administered fluids, including total parenteral nutrition (TPN)
Providing adequate nutrition and oral hydration
Providing care for gastrointestinal tubes
Providing nonpharmacological and pharmacological comfort measures
Providing preprocedure and postprocedure care for diagnostic tests related to the gastrointestinal system

CHAPTER 48

Gastrointestinal Problems

PRIORITY CONCEPTS **Elimination; Nutrition**

I. Anatomy and Physiology

A. Functions of the gastrointestinal (GI) system
1. Process food substances
2. Absorb the products of digestion into the blood
3. Excrete unabsorbed materials
4. Provide an environment for microorganisms to synthesize nutrients, such as vitamin K.
5. For risk factors associated with the GI system, see Box 48-1.

B. Mouth
1. Contains the lips, cheeks, palate, tongue, teeth, salivary glands, muscles, and maxillary bones
2. Saliva contains the enzyme amylase (ptyalin), which aids in digestion.

C. Esophagus
1. Collapsible muscular tube about 10 inches (25 cm) long
2. Carries food from the pharynx to the stomach

BOX 48-1 Risk Factors Associated with the Gastrointestinal System

- Allergic reactions to food or medications
- Cardiac, respiratory, and endocrine disorders that may lead to slowed gastrointestinal (GI) movement or constipation
- Chronic alcohol use
- Chronic high stress levels
- Chronic laxative use
- Chronic use of aspirin or nonsteroidal antiinflammatory drugs (NSAIDs)
- Diabetes mellitus, which may predispose to oral candidal infections or other GI disorders
- Family history of GI disorders
- Long-term GI conditions, such as ulcerative colitis, that may predispose to colorectal cancer
- Neurological disorders that can impair movement, particularly with chewing and swallowing
- Previous abdominal surgery or trauma, which may lead to adhesions
- Tobacco use

D. Stomach
1. Contains the cardia, fundus, body, and pylorus
2. Mucous glands are located in the mucosa and prevent autodigestion by providing an alkaline protective covering.
3. The lower esophageal (cardiac) sphincter prevents reflux of gastric contents into the esophagus.
4. The pyloric sphincter regulates the rate of stomach emptying into the small intestine.
5. Hydrochloric acid kills microorganisms, breaks food into small particles, and provides a chemical environment that facilitates gastric enzyme activation.
6. Pepsin is the chief coenzyme of gastric juice, which converts proteins into proteoses and peptones.
7. Intrinsic factor comes from parietal cells and is necessary for the absorption of vitamin B_{12}.
8. Gastrin controls gastric acidity.

E. Small intestine
1. The duodenum contains the openings of the bile and pancreatic ducts.
2. The jejunum is about 8 feet (2.4 meters) long.
3. The ileum is about 12 feet (3.7 meters) long.
4. The small intestine terminates in the cecum.

F. Pancreatic intestinal juice enzymes
1. Amylase digests starch to maltose.
2. Maltase reduces maltose to monosaccharide glucose.
3. Lactase splits lactose into galactose and glucose.
4. Sucrase reduces sucrose to fructose and glucose.
5. Nucleases split nucleic acids to nucleotides.
6. Enterokinase activates trypsinogen to trypsin.

G. Large intestine
1. About 5 feet (1.5 meters) long
2. Absorbs water and eliminates wastes
3. Intestinal bacteria play a vital role in the synthesis of some B vitamins and vitamin K.
4. Colon: Includes the ascending, transverse, descending, and sigmoid colons and rectum

5. The ileocecal valve prevents contents of the large intestine from entering the ileum.
6. The internal and external anal sphincters control the anal canal.

H. Peritoneum: Lines the abdominal cavity and forms the mesentery that supports the intestines and blood supply

I. Liver
1. The largest gland in the body, weighing 3 to 4 pounds (1.4 to 1.8 kg)
2. Contains Kupffer cells, which remove bacteria in the portal venous blood
3. Removes excess glucose and amino acids from the portal blood
4. Synthesizes glucose, amino acids, and fats
5. Aids in the digestion of fats, carbohydrates, and proteins
6. Stores and filters blood (200 to 400 mL of blood stored)
7. Stores vitamins A, D, and B and iron
8. The liver secretes bile to emulsify fats (500 to 1000 mL of bile/day).
9. Hepatic ducts
   a. Deliver bile to the gallbladder via the cystic duct and to the duodenum via the common bile duct
   b. The common bile duct opens into the duodenum, with the pancreatic duct at the ampulla of Vater.
   c. The sphincter prevents the reflux of intestinal contents into the common bile duct and pancreatic duct.

J. Gallbladder
1. Stores and concentrates bile and contracts to force bile into the duodenum during the digestion of fats
2. The cystic duct joins the hepatic duct to form the common bile duct.
3. The sphincter of Oddi is located at the entrance to the duodenum.
4. The presence of fatty materials in the duodenum stimulates the liberation of cholecystokinin, which causes contraction of the gallbladder and relaxation of the sphincter of Oddi.

K. Pancreas
1. Exocrine gland
   a. Secretes sodium bicarbonate to neutralize the acidity of the stomach contents that enter the duodenum
   b. Pancreatic juices contain enzymes for digesting carbohydrates, fats, and proteins.
2. Endocrine gland
   a. Secretes glucagon to raise blood glucose levels and secretes somatostatin to exert a hypoglycemic effect
   b. The islets of Langerhans secrete insulin.
   c. Insulin is secreted into the bloodstream and is important for carbohydrate metabolism.

II. Diagnostic Procedures (Box 48-2)

A. Upper GI tract study (barium swallow)
1. Description: Examination of the upper GI tract under fluoroscopy after the client drinks barium sulfate
2. Preprocedure: Withhold foods and fluids for 8 hours prior to the test.
3. Postprocedure
   a. A laxative may be prescribed.
   b. Instruct the client to increase oral fluid intake to help pass the barium.
   c. Monitor stools for the passage of barium (stools will appear chalky white for 24 to 72 hours postprocedure) because barium can cause a bowel obstruction.

B. Capsule endoscopy
1. Description: A procedure that uses a small wireless camera shaped like a medication capsule that the client swallows; the test will detect bleeding or changes in the lining of the small intestine.
2. The camera travels through the entire digestive tract and sends pictures to a small box that the client wears like a belt; the small box saves the pictures, which are then transferred to a computer for viewing once the test is complete.
3. The client visits the primary health care provider's (PHCP's) office in the morning and swallows the capsule, the recording belt is applied by the office staff, and then the client returns at the end of the day so that pictures can be transferred to the computer.
4. Preprocedure: A bowel preparation will be prescribed. The client will need to maintain a clear liquid diet on the evening before the exam;

BOX 48-2 Common Gastrointestinal System Diagnostic Studies

- Capsule endoscopy
- Endoscopic retrograde cholangiopancreatography (ERCP)
- Magnetic resonance cholangiopancreatogrraphy (MRCP)
- Endoscopic ultrasound
- Fiberoptic colonoscopy
- Gastric analysis
- Gastrointestinal motility studies
- Hydrogen and urea breath test
- Laparoscopy: Liver and pancreas laboratory studies
- Liver biopsy
- Paracentesis
- Stool specimens
- Upper gastrointestinal endoscopy or esophagogastroduodenoscopy
- Upper gastrointestinal tract study (barium swallow)
- Videofluoroscopic swallowing study
- Informed consent is obtained for a diagnostic study that is invasive.

additionally, NPO (nothing by mouth) status is maintained for 3 hours before and after swallowing the capsule (time for NPO status is prescribed by the PHCP but is usually 2 to 3 hours).

C. Gastric analysis
  1. Description
    a. Gastric analysis requires the passage of a nasogastric (NG) tube into the stomach to aspirate gastric contents for the analysis of acidity (pH), appearance, and volume; the entire gastric contents are aspirated, and then specimens are collected every 15 minutes for 1 hour.
    b. Medication, such as histamine or pentagastrin, may be administered subcutaneously to stimulate gastric secretions; some medications may produce a flushed feeling.
    c. Esophageal reflux of gastric acid may be diagnosed by ambulatory pH monitoring; a probe is placed just above the lower esophageal sphincter and connected to an external recording device. It provides a computer analysis and graphic display of results.
  2. Preprocedure
    a. Fasting for at least 12 hours is required before the test.
    b. Use of tobacco and chewing gum is avoided for 24 hours before the test.
    c. Medications that stimulate gastric secretions are withheld for 24 to 48 hours.
  3. Postprocedure
    a. Client may resume normal activities.
    b. Refrigerate gastric samples if not tested within 4 hours.

D. Upper GI endoscopy
  1. Description
    a. Also known as esophagogastroduodenoscopy
    b. Following sedation, an endoscope is passed down the esophagus to view the gastric wall, sphincters, and duodenum; tissue specimens can be obtained.
  2. Preprocedure
    a. The client must be NPO for 6 to 8 hours before the test.
    b. A local anesthetic (spray or gargle) is administered along with medication that provides moderate sedation just before the scope is inserted.
    c. Medication may be administered to reduce secretions, and medication may be administered to relax smooth muscle.
    d. The client is positioned on the left side to facilitate saliva drainage and to provide easy access of the endoscope.
    e. Airway patency is monitored during the test, and pulse oximetry is used to monitor oxygen saturation; emergency equipment should be readily available.
  3. Postprocedure
    a. Monitor vital signs.
    b. Client must be NPO until the gag reflex returns (1 to 2 hours).
    c. Monitor for signs of perforation (pain, bleeding, unusual difficulty in swallowing, elevated temperature).
    d. Maintain bed rest for the sedated client until alert.
    e. Lozenges, saline gargles, or oral analgesics can relieve a minor sore throat (not given to the client until the gag reflex returns).

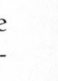

E. Fiberoptic colonoscopy
  1. Description
    a. Colonoscopy is a fiberoptic endoscopy study in which the lining of the large intestine is visually examined; biopsies and polypectomies can be performed.
    b. Cardiac and respiratory function is monitored continuously during the test.
    c. Colonoscopy is performed with the client lying on the left side with the knees drawn up to the chest; position may be changed during the test to facilitate passing of the scope.
  2. Preprocedure
    a. Adequate cleansing of the colon is necessary, as prescribed by the PHCP.
    b. A clear liquid diet is started on the day before the test. Red, orange, and purple (grape) liquids are to be avoided.
    c. Consult with the PHCP regarding medications that must be withheld before the test.
    d. Client is NPO for 4 to 6 hours prior to the test.
    e. Moderate sedation is administered intravenously.
    f. Medication may be administered to relax smooth muscle.
  3. Postprocedure
    a. Monitor vital signs.
    b. Provide bed rest until alert.
    c. Monitor for signs of bowel perforation and peritonitis (Box 48-3).
    d. Remind the client that passing flatus, abdominal fullness, and mild cramping are expected for several hours.
    e. Instruct the client to report any bleeding to the PHCP.

! The client receiving oral liquid bowel cleansing preparations or enemas is at risk for fluid and electrolyte imbalances.

F. Laparoscopy is performed with a fiberoptic laparoscope that allows direct visualization of organs and structures within the abdomen; biopsies may be obtained.

G. Endoscopic retrograde cholangiopancreatography (ERCP)

BOX 48-3 Signs of Bowel Perforation and Peritonitis

- Guarding of the abdomen
- Increased temperature and chills
- Pallor
- Progressive abdominal distention and abdominal pain
- Restlessness
- Tachycardia and tachypnea

1. Description
   a. Examination of the hepatobiliary system is performed via a flexible endoscope inserted into the esophagus to the descending duodenum; multiple positions are required during the procedure to pass the endoscope.
   b. If medication is administered before the procedure, the client is monitored closely for signs of respiratory and central nervous system depression, hypotension, oversedation, and vomiting.
2. Preprocedure
   a. Client is NPO for 6 to 8 hours.
   b. Inquire about previous exposure to contrast media and any sensitivities or allergies.
   c. Moderate sedation is administered.
3. Postprocedure
   a. Monitor vital signs.
   b. Monitor for the return of the gag reflex.
   c. Monitor for signs of perforation or peritonitis (see Box 48-3).

H. Magnetic resonance cholangiopancreatography (MRCP)
1. Description: Uses magnetic resonance to visualize the biliary and pancreatic ducts in a noninvasive way.
2. Preprocedure and postprocedure: see ERCP

I. Endoscopic ultrasonography
1. Description: Provides images of the GI wall and digestive organs.
2. Preprocedure and postprocedure: Care is similar to that implemented for endoscopy.

Following endoscopic procedures, monitor for the return of the gag reflex before giving the client any oral substance. If the gag reflex has not returned, the client could aspirate.

J. Computed tomography (CT) scan
1. Description
   a. Noninvasive cross-sectional view that can detect tissue densities in the abdomen, including in the liver, spleen, pancreas, and biliary tree.
   b. Can be performed with or without contrast medium.
2. Preprocedure
   a. Client is NPO for at least 4 hours.
   b. If contrast medium will be used, assess for previous sensitivities and allergies.
3. Postprocedure: No specific care is required.

K. Paracentesis
1. Description and preprocedure (see Priority Nursing Actions)

PRIORITY NURSING ACTIONS

Paracentesis

1. Ensure that the client understands the procedure and that informed consent has been obtained.
2. Obtain vital signs, including weight, and assist the client to void.
3. Position the client upright.
4. Assist the primary health care provider (PHCP), monitor vital signs, and provide comfort and support during the procedure.
5. Apply a dressing to the site of puncture.
6. Monitor vital signs, especially blood pressure and pulse, because these parameters provide information on rapid vasodilation postparacentesis; weigh the client postprocedure, and maintain the client on bed rest.
7. Measure the amount of fluid removed.
8. Label and send the fluid for laboratory analysis.
9. Document the event, client's response, and appearance and amount of fluid removed.

Reference: Ignatavicius, Workman, Rebar (2018), p. 1177.

2. Postprocedure
   a. Monitor vital signs.
   b. Measure fluid collected, describe, and record.
   c. Label fluid samples and send to the laboratory for analysis.
   d. Apply a dry sterile dressing to the insertion site; monitor the site for bleeding.
   e. Measure abdominal girth and weight.
   f. Monitor for hypovolemia, electrolyte loss, mental status changes, or encephalopathy.
   g. Monitor for hematuria caused by bladder trauma.
   h. Instruct the client to notify the PHCP if the urine becomes bloody, pink, or red.

The rapid removal of fluid from the abdominal cavity during paracentesis leads to decreased abdominal pressure, which can cause vasodilation and resultant shock; therefore, heart rate and blood pressure must be monitored closely.

L. Liver biopsy
1. Description: A needle is inserted through the abdominal wall to the liver to obtain a tissue sample for biopsy and microscopic examination.

2. Preprocedure
   a. Assess results of coagulation tests (prothrombin time, partial thromboplastin time, platelet count).
   b. Administer a sedative as prescribed.
   c. Note that the client is placed in the supine or left lateral position during the procedure to expose the right side of the upper abdomen.
3. Postprocedure
   a. Assess vital signs.
   b. Assess biopsy site for bleeding.
   c. Monitor for peritonitis (see Box 48-3).
   d. Maintain bed rest for several hours as prescribed.
   e. Place the client on the right side with a pillow under the costal margin for 2 hours to decrease the risk of bleeding, and instruct the client to avoid coughing and straining.
   f. Instruct the client to avoid heavy lifting and strenuous exercise for 1 week.

M. Stool specimens
1. Testing of stool specimens includes inspecting the specimen for consistency and color and testing for occult blood.
2. Tests for fecal urobilinogen, fat, nitrogen, parasites, pathogens, food substances, and other substances may be performed; these tests require that the specimen be sent to the laboratory.
3. Random specimens are sent promptly to the laboratory.
4. Quantitative 24- to 72-hour collections must be kept refrigerated until they are taken to the laboratory.
5. Some specimens require that a certain diet be followed or that certain medications be withheld; check agency guidelines regarding specific procedures.

N. Urea breath test
1. The urea breath test detects the presence of *Helicobacter pylori*, the bacteria that cause peptic ulcer disease.
2. The client consumes a capsule of carbon-labeled urea and provides a breath sample 10 to 20 minutes later.
3. Certain medications may need to be avoided before testing. These may include antibiotics or bismuth subsalicylate for 1 month before the test; sucralfate and omeprazole for 1 week before the test; and cimetidine, famotidine, ranitidine, and nizatidine for 24 hours before breath testing.
4. *H. pylori* can also be detected by assessing serum antibody levels.

O. Esophageal pH testing for gastroesophageal reflux disease
1. Used to diagnose or evaluate the treatment for heartburn or reflux disease
2. A probe is inserted into the nostril and is situated in the esophagus.
3. pH is tested over a period of 24 to 48 hours.

P. Liver and pancreas laboratory studies
1. Liver enzyme levels (alkaline phosphatase [ALP], aspartate aminotransferase [AST], and alanine aminotransferase [ALT]) are elevated with liver damage or biliary obstruction. Normal reference intervals: ALP, 38-126 U/L (0.65-2.14 μkat/L); AST, 0 to 35 U/L (0 to 35 U/L); ALT, 4 to 36 U/L (4 to 36 U/L).
2. Prothrombin time is prolonged with liver damage. Normal reference interval: 11 to 12.5 seconds.
3. The serum ammonia level assesses the ability of the liver to deaminate protein byproducts. Normal reference interval: 10 to 80 mcg/dL (6 to 47 mcmol/L).
4. An increase in cholesterol level indicates *pancreatitis* or biliary obstruction. Normal reference interval: less than 200 mg/dL (less than 5.0 mmol/L).
5. An increase in bilirubin level indicates liver damage or biliary obstruction. Normal reference intervals: total, 0.3 to 1.0 mg/dL (5.1 to 17 mcmol/L); indirect, 0.2 to 0.8 mg/dL (3.4 to 12 mcmol/L); direct, 0.1 to 0.3 mg/dL (1.7 to 5.1 mcmol/L).
6. Increased values for amylase and lipase levels indicate pancreatitis. Normal reference intervals: amylase, 60 to 120 Somogyi units/dL (100 to 300 U/L); lipase, 0 to 160 U/L (0 to 160 U/L).

III. Assessment: See Chapter 12 for abdominal assessment techniques.

IV. Gastrointestinal Tubes: See Chapter 69 for information regarding these tubes.

V. Gastroesophageal Reflux Disease

A. Description
1. The backflow of gastric and duodenal contents into the esophagus.
2. The reflux is caused by an incompetent lower esophageal sphincter (LES), pyloric stenosis, or motility disorder.

B. Assessment
1. Heartburn, epigastric pain
2. Dyspepsia
3. Nausea, regurgitation
4. Pain and difficulty with swallowing
5. Hypersalivation

C. Interventions
1. Instruct the client to avoid factors that decrease LES pressure or cause esophageal irritation, such as peppermint, chocolate, coffee, fried or fatty

foods, carbonated beverages, alcoholic beverages, and cigarette smoking.

2. Instruct the client to eat a low-fat, high-fiber diet and to avoid eating and drinking 2 hours before bedtime and wearing tight clothes; also, elevate the head of the bed on 6- to 8-inch (15 to 20 cm) blocks.
3. Avoid the use of anticholinergics, which delay stomach emptying; also, nonsteroidal anti-inflammatory medications (NSAIDs) and other medications that contain acetylsalicylic acid need to be avoided.
4. Instruct the client regarding prescribed medications, such as antacids, H_2-receptor antagonists, or proton pump inhibitors.
5. Instruct the client regarding the administration of prokinetic medications, if prescribed, which accelerate gastric emptying.
6. Surgery may be required in extreme cases when medical management is unsuccessful; this involves a fundoplication (wrapping a portion of the gastric fundus around the sphincter area of the esophagus); surgery may be performed by laparoscopy.

VI. Gastritis

A. Description

1. Inflammation of the stomach or gastric mucosa
2. Acute gastritis is caused by the ingestion of food contaminated with disease-causing microorganisms or food that is irritating or too highly seasoned, the overuse of aspirin or other NSAIDs, excessive alcohol intake, bile reflux, or radiation therapy.
3. Chronic gastritis is caused by benign or malignant ulcers or by the bacteria *H. pylori*, and also may be caused by autoimmune diseases, dietary factors, medications, alcohol, smoking, or reflux.

B. Assessment (Box 48-4)

C. Interventions

1. Acute gastritis: Food and fluids may be withheld until symptoms subside; afterward, and as prescribed, ice chips can be given, followed by clear liquids, and then solid food.
2. Monitor for signs of hemorrhagic gastritis such as hematemesis, tachycardia, and hypotension, and notify the PHCP if these signs occur.
3. Instruct the client to avoid irritating foods, fluids, and other substances, such as spicy and highly seasoned foods, caffeine, alcohol, and nicotine.
4. Instruct the client in the use of prescribed medications, such as antibiotics to treat *H. pylori*, and antacids.
5. Provide the client with information about the importance of vitamin B_{12} injections if a deficiency is present.

BOX 48-4 Assessment Findings in Acute and Chronic Gastritis

Acute

- Abdominal discomfort
- Anorexia, nausea, and vomiting
- Headache
- Hiccupping
- Reflux

Chronic

- Anorexia, nausea, and vomiting
- Belching
- Heartburn after eating
- Sour taste in the mouth
- Vitamin B_{12} deficiency

VII. Peptic Ulcer Disease

A. Description

1. A peptic ulcer is an ulceration in the mucosal wall of the stomach, pylorus, duodenum, or esophagus in portions accessible to gastric secretions; erosion may extend through the muscle.
2. The ulcer may be referred to as *gastric, duodenal,* or *esophageal,* depending on its location.
3. The most common peptic ulcers are gastric ulcers and duodenal ulcers.

B. Gastric ulcers

1. Description
   a. A gastric ulcer involves ulceration of the mucosal lining that extends to the submucosal layer of the stomach.
   b. Predisposing factors include stress, smoking, the use of corticosteroids, NSAIDs, alcohol, history of gastritis, family history of gastric ulcers, or infection with *H. pylori.*
   c. Complications include hemorrhage, perforation, and pyloric obstruction.
2. Assessment (Box 48-5)
3. Interventions
   a. Monitor vital signs and for signs of bleeding.
   b. Administer small, frequent bland feedings during the active phase.
   c. Administer H_2-receptor antagonists or proton pump inhibitors as prescribed to decrease the secretion of gastric acid.
   d. Administer antacids as prescribed to neutralize gastric secretions.
   e. Administer anticholinergics as prescribed to reduce gastric motility.
   f. Administer mucosal barrier protectants as prescribed 1 hour before each meal.
   g. Administer prostaglandins as prescribed for their protective and antisecretory actions.

BOX 48-5 Assessment: Gastric and Duodenal Ulcers

Gastric

- Gnawing, sharp pain in or to the left of the midepigastric region occurs 30 to 60 minutes after a meal (food ingestion accentuates the pain).
- Hematemesis is more common than melena.

Duodenal

- Burning pain occurs in the midepigastric area 1.5 to 3 hours after a meal and during the night (often awakens the client).
- Melena is more common than hematemesis.
- Pain is often relieved by the ingestion of food.

4. Client education
   a. Avoid consuming alcohol and substances that contain caffeine or chocolate.
   b. Avoid smoking.
   c. Avoid aspirin or NSAIDs.
   d. Obtain adequate rest and reduce stress.
5. Interventions during active bleeding
   a. Monitor vital signs closely.
   b. Assess for signs of dehydration, hypovolemic shock, sepsis, and respiratory insufficiency.
   c. Maintain NPO status and administer intravenous (IV) fluid replacement as prescribed; monitor intake and output.
   d. Monitor hemoglobin and hematocrit.
   e. Administer blood transfusions as prescribed.
   f. Prepare to assist with administering medications as prescribed to induce vasoconstriction and reduce bleeding.
6. Surgical interventions
   a. Total **gastrectomy**: Removal of the stomach with attachment of the esophagus to the jejunum or duodenum; also called *esophagojejunostomy* or *esophagoduodenostomy*
   b. **Vagotomy**: Surgical division of the vagus nerve to eliminate the vagal impulses that stimulate hydrochloric acid secretion in the stomach
   c. **Gastric resection**: Removal of the lower half of the stomach and usually includes a vagotomy; also called *antrectomy*
   d. Gastroduodenostomy: Partial gastrectomy, with the remaining segment anastomosed to the duodenum; also called **Billroth I** (Fig. 48-1)
   e. Gastrojejunostomy: Partial gastrectomy, with the remaining segment anastomosed to the jejunum; also called **Billroth II** (Fig. 48-2)
   f. **Pyloroplasty:** Enlargement of the pylorus to prevent or decrease pyloric obstruction, thereby enhancing gastric emptying

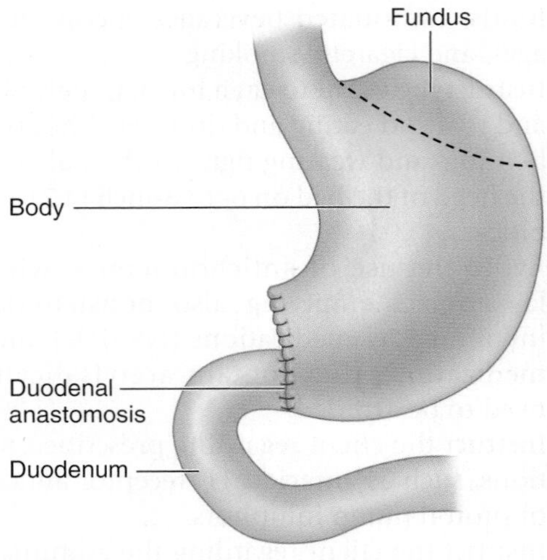

FIG. 48-1 The Billroth I procedure (gastroduodenostomy). The distal portion of the stomach is removed, and the remainder is anastomosed to the duodenum.

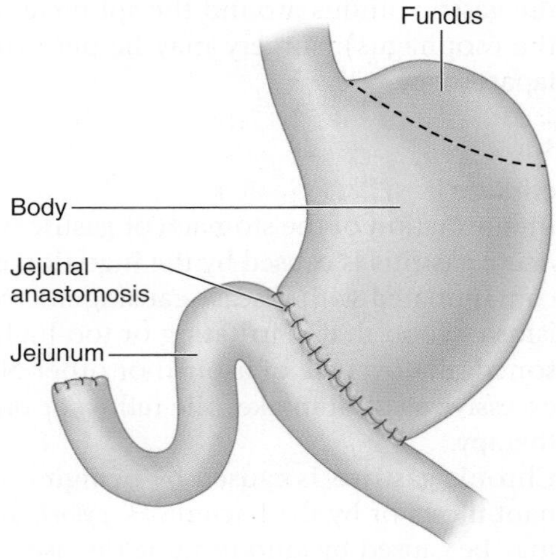

FIG. 48-2 The Billroth II procedure (gastrojejunostomy). The lower portion of the stomach is removed, and the remainder is anastomosed to the jejunum.

7. Postoperative interventions
   a. Monitor vital signs.
   b. Place in a Fowler's position for comfort and to promote drainage.
   c. Administer fluids and electrolyte replacements intravenously as prescribed; monitor intake and output.
   d. Assess bowel sounds.
   e. Monitor NG suction as prescribed.
   f. Maintain NPO status as prescribed for 1 to 3 days until peristalsis returns.
   g. Progress the diet from NPO to sips of clear water to 6 small bland meals a day, as prescribed when bowel sounds return.

h. Monitor for postoperative complications of hemorrhage, **dumping syndrome,** diarrhea, hypoglycemia, and vitamin B_{12} deficiency.

Following gastric surgery, do not irrigate or remove the NG tube unless specifically prescribed because of the risk for disruption of the gastric sutures. Monitor closely to ensure proper functioning of the NG tube to prevent strain on the anastomosis site. Contact the surgeon if the tube is not functioning properly.

C. Duodenal ulcers

1. Description

a. A duodenal ulcer is a break in the mucosa of the duodenum.

b. Risk factors and causes include infection with *H. pylori*; alcohol intake; smoking; stress; caffeine; and the use of aspirin, corticosteroids, and NSAIDs.

c. Complications include bleeding, perforation, gastric outlet obstruction, and intractable disease.

2. Assessment (see Box 48-5)

3. Interventions

a. Monitor vital signs.

b. Instruct the client about a bland diet, with small, frequent meals.

c. Provide for adequate rest.

d. Encourage the cessation of smoking.

e. Instruct the client to avoid alcohol intake; caffeine; and the use of aspirin, corticosteroids, and NSAIDs.

f. Administer medications to treat *H. pylori* and antacids to neutralize acid secretions as prescribed.

g. Administer H_2-receptor antagonists or proton pump inhibitors as prescribed to block the secretion of acid.

4. Surgical interventions: Surgery is performed only if the ulcer is unresponsive to medications or if hemorrhage, obstruction, or perforation occurs.

D. Dumping syndrome

1. Description: The rapid emptying of the gastric contents into the small intestine that occurs following gastric resection

2. Assessment

a. Symptoms occurring 30 minutes after eating

b. Nausea and vomiting

c. Feelings of abdominal fullness and abdominal cramping

d. Diarrhea

e. Palpitations and tachycardia

f. Perspiration

g. Weakness and dizziness

h. Borborygmi (loud gurgling sounds resulting from bowel hypermotility)

3. Client education (Box 48-6)

BOX 48-6 Client Education: Preventing Dumping Syndrome

- Avoid sugar, salt, and milk.
- Eat a high-protein, high-fat, low-carbohydrate diet.
- Eat small meals and avoid consuming fluids with meals.
- Lie down after meals.
- Take antispasmodic medications as prescribed to delay gastric emptying.

VIII. Vitamin B_{12} Deficiency: See Chapter 44 for more information.

IX. Bariatric Surgery

A. Description

1. Surgical reduction of gastric capacity or absorptive ability that may be performed on a client with morbid obesity to produce long-term weight loss

2. Surgery may be performed by laparoscopy; the decision is based on the client's weight, body build, history of abdominal surgery, and current medical disorders.

3. Obese clients are at increased postoperative risk for pulmonary and thromboembolic complications and death.

4. Surgery can prevent the complications of obesity, such as diabetes mellitus, hypertension and other cardiovascular disorders, or sleep apnea.

5. The client needs to agree to modify her or his lifestyle, lose weight and keep the weight off, and obtain support from available community resources such as the American Obesity Association, American Society of Bariatric Surgery, or Overeaters Anonymous.

B. Types (Fig. 48-3)

C. Postoperative interventions

1. Care is similar to that for the client undergoing laparoscopic or abdominal surgery.

2. As prescribed, if the client can tolerate water, clear liquids are introduced slowly in 1-ounce (30 mL) cups for each serving once bowel sounds have returned and the client passes flatus.

3. As prescribed, clear fluids are followed by puréed foods, juices, thin soups, and milk 24 to 48 hours after clear fluids are tolerated (the diet is usually limited to liquids or puréed foods for 6 weeks); then the diet is progressed to nutrient-dense regular food.

D. Client teaching points about diet (Box 48-7)

X. Gastric Cancer: See Chapter 44 for more information.

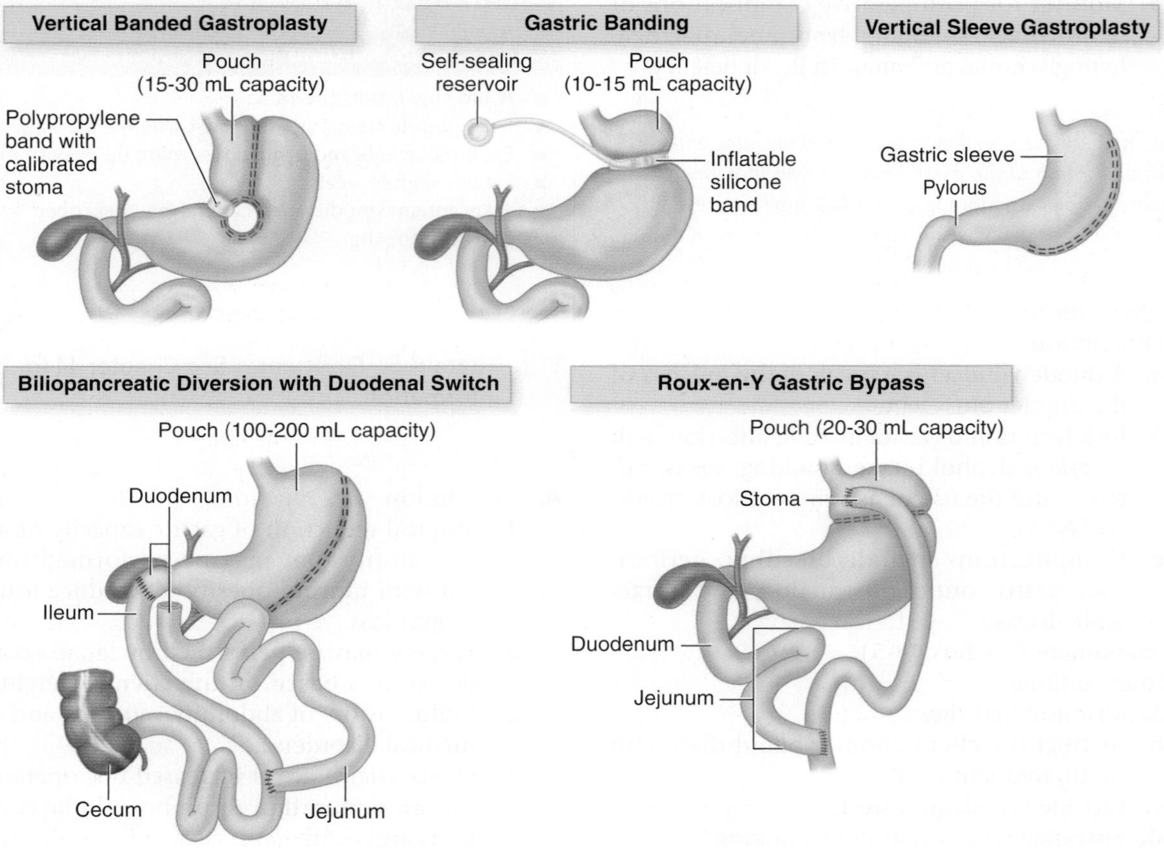

FIG. 48-3 Bariatric surgical procedures.

BOX 48-7 Dietary Measures for the Client Following Bariatric Surgery

- Avoid alcohol, high-protein foods, and foods high in sugar and fat.
- Eat slowly and chew food well.
- Progress food types and amounts as prescribed.
- Take nutritional supplements as prescribed, which may include calcium, iron, multivitamins, and vitamin B_{12}.
- Monitor and report signs and symptoms of complications, such as dehydration and gastric leak (persistent abdominal pain, nausea, vomiting).

XI. Hiatal Hernia

A. Description
1. A **hiatal hernia** is also known as *esophageal* or *diaphragmatic hernia.*
2. A portion of the stomach herniates through the diaphragm and into the thorax.
3. Herniation results from weakening of the muscles of the diaphragm and is aggravated by factors that increase abdominal pressure such as pregnancy, ascites, obesity, tumors, and heavy lifting.
4. Complications include ulceration, hemorrhage, regurgitation and aspiration of stomach contents, strangulation, and incarceration of the stomach in the chest with possible necrosis, peritonitis, and mediastinitis.

B. Assessment
1. Heartburn
2. Regurgitation or vomiting
3. Dysphagia
4. Feeling of fullness

C. Interventions
1. Medical and surgical management are similar to those for gastroesophageal reflux disease.
2. Provide small frequent meals and limit the amount of liquids taken with meals.
3. Advise the client not to recline for 1 hour after eating.
4. Avoid anticholinergics, which delay stomach emptying.

XII. Cholecystitis

A. Description
1. Inflammation of the gallbladder that may occur as an acute or chronic process
2. Acute inflammation is associated with gallstones (cholelithiasis).
3. Chronic **cholecystitis** results when inefficient bile emptying and gallbladder muscle wall disease cause a fibrotic and contracted gallbladder.

4. Acalculous cholecystitis occurs in the absence of gallstones and is caused by bacterial invasion via the lymphatic or vascular system.

B. Assessment
1. Nausea and vomiting
2. Indigestion
3. Belching
4. Flatulence
5. Epigastric pain that radiates to the right shoulder or scapula
6. Pain localized in the right upper quadrant and triggered by a high-fat or high-volume meal
7. Guarding, rigidity, and rebound tenderness
8. Mass palpated in the right upper quadrant
9. Murphy's sign (cannot take a deep breath when the examiner's fingers are passed below the hepatic margin because of pain)
10. Elevated temperature
11. Tachycardia
12. Signs of dehydration

C. Biliary obstruction (choledolithiasis)
1. Jaundice
2. Dark orange and foamy urine
3. Steatorrhea and clay-colored feces
4. Pruritus

D. Interventions
1. Maintain NPO status during nausea and vomiting episodes.
2. Maintain NG decompression as prescribed for severe vomiting.
3. Administer antiemetics as prescribed for nausea and vomiting.
4. Administer analgesics as prescribed to relieve pain and reduce spasm.
5. Administer antispasmodics (anticholinergics) as prescribed to relax smooth muscle.
6. Instruct the client with chronic cholecystitis to eat small, low-fat meals.
7. Instruct the client to avoid gas-forming foods.
8. Prepare the client for nonsurgical and surgical procedures as prescribed.

E. Surgical interventions
1. Cholecystectomy is the removal of the gallbladder.
2. Choledocholithotomy requires incision into the common bile duct to remove the stone.
3. Surgical procedures may be performed by laparoscopy.

F. Postoperative interventions
1. Monitor for respiratory complications caused by pain at the incisional site.
2. Encourage coughing and deep breathing.
3. Encourage early ambulation.
4. Instruct the client about splinting the abdomen to prevent discomfort during coughing.
5. Administer antiemetics as prescribed for nausea and vomiting.
6. Administer analgesics as prescribed for pain relief.
7. Maintain NPO status and NG tube suction as prescribed.
8. Advance diet from clear liquids to solids when prescribed and as tolerated by the client.
9. Maintain and monitor drainage from the T-tube, if present (Box 48-8).

XIII. Cirrhosis

A. Description
1. A chronic, progressive disease of the liver characterized by diffuse degeneration and destruction of hepatocytes
2. Repeated destruction of hepatic cells causes the formation of scar tissue.
3. Cirrhosis has many causes and is due to chronic damage and injury to liver cells; the most common are chronic hepatitis C, alcoholism, nonalcoholic fatty liver disease (NAFLD), and nonalcoholic steatohepatitis (NASH).

B. Complications
1. Portal hypertension: A persistent increase in pressure in the portal vein that develops as a result of obstruction to flow.
2. Ascites
   a. Accumulation of fluid in the peritoneal cavity that results from venous congestion of the hepatic capillaries
   b. Capillary congestion leads to plasma leaking directly from the liver surface and portal vein.

BOX 48-8 Care of a T-Tube

Purpose and Description

A T-tube is placed after surgical exploration of the common bile duct. The tube preserves the patency of the duct and ensures drainage of bile until edema resolves and bile is effectively draining into the duodenum. A gravity drainage bag is attached to the T-tube to collect the drainage.

Interventions

- Place the client in semi-Fowler's position to facilitate drainage.
- Monitor the output amount and the color, consistency, and odor of the drainage.
- Report sudden increases in bile output to the primary health care provider (PHCP).
- Monitor for inflammation and protect the skin from irritation.
- Keep the drainage system below the level of the gallbladder.
- Monitor for foul odor and purulent drainage and report its presence to the PHCP.
- Avoid irrigation, aspiration, or clamping of the T-tube without a PHCP's prescription.
- As prescribed, clamp the tube before a meal and observe for abdominal discomfort and distention, nausea, chills, or fever; unclamp the tube if nausea or vomiting occurs.

Adult—Gastrointestinal

3. Bleeding **esophageal varices**: Fragile, thin-walled, distended esophageal veins that become irritated and rupture
4. Coagulation defects
   a. Decreased synthesis of bile fats in the liver prevents the absorption of fat-soluble vitamins.
   b. Without vitamin K and clotting factors II, VII, IX, and X, the client is prone to bleeding.
5. Jaundice: Occurs because the liver is unable to metabolize bilirubin and because the edema, fibrosis, and scarring of the hepatic bile ducts interfere with normal bile and bilirubin secretion
6. Portal systemic encephalopathy: End-stage hepatic failure characterized by altered level of consciousness, neurological symptoms, impaired thinking, and neuromuscular disturbances; caused by failure of the diseased liver to detoxify neurotoxic agents such as ammonia
7. Hepatorenal syndrome
   a. Progressive renal failure associated with hepatic failure
   b. Characterized by a sudden decrease in urinary output, elevated blood urea nitrogen and creatinine levels, decreased urine sodium excretion, and increased urine osmolarity

C. Assessment (Fig. 48-4)

D. Interventions
1. Elevate the head of the bed to minimize shortness of breath.
2. If ascites and edema are absent and the client does not exhibit signs of impending coma, a high-protein diet supplemented with vitamins is prescribed.
3. Provide supplemental vitamins (B complex; vitamins A, C, and K; folic acid; and thiamine) as prescribed.
4. Restrict sodium intake and fluid intake as prescribed.
5. Initiate enteral feedings or parenteral nutrition as prescribed.
6. Administer diuretics as prescribed to treat ascites.
7. Monitor intake and output and electrolyte balance.
8. Weigh client and measure abdominal girth daily (Fig. 48-5).
9. Monitor level of consciousness; assess for precoma state (tremors, delirium).
10. Monitor for **asterixis**, a coarse tremor characterized by rapid, nonrhythmic extensions and flexions in the wrist and fingers (Fig. 48-6).
11. Monitor for **fetor hepaticus**, the fruity, musty breath odor of severe chronic liver disease.
12. Maintain gastric intubation to assess bleeding or esophagogastric balloon tamponade to control bleeding varices if prescribed.
13. Administer blood products as prescribed.
14. Monitor coagulation laboratory results; administer vitamin K if prescribed.
15. Administer antacids as prescribed.
16. Administer lactulose as prescribed, which decreases the pH of the bowel, decreases production of ammonia by bacteria in the bowel, and facilitates the excretion of ammonia.
17. Administer antibiotics as prescribed to inhibit protein synthesis in bacteria and decrease the production of ammonia.
18. Avoid medications such as opioids, sedatives, and barbiturates and any hepatotoxic medications or substances.
19. Instruct the client about the importance of abstinence of alcohol intake.
20. Prepare the client for paracentesis to remove abdominal fluid.
21. Prepare the client for surgical shunting procedures if prescribed to divert fluid from ascites into the venous system.

XIV. Esophageal Varices

A. Description
1. Dilated and tortuous veins in the submucosa of the esophagus
2. Caused by portal hypertension, often associated with liver **cirrhosis**; are at high risk for rupture if portal circulation pressure rises
3. Bleeding varices are an emergency.
4. The goal of treatment is to control bleeding, prevent complications, and prevent the recurrence of bleeding.

B. Assessment
1. Hematemesis
2. **Melena**
3. Ascites
4. Jaundice
5. Hepatomegaly and splenomegaly
6. Dilated abdominal veins
7. Signs of shock

Rupture and resultant hemorrhage of esophageal varices is the primary concern, because it is a life-threatening situation.

C. Interventions
1. Monitor vital signs.
2. Elevate the head of the bed.
3. Monitor for orthostatic hypotension.
4. Monitor lung sounds and for the presence of respiratory distress.
5. Administer oxygen as prescribed to prevent tissue hypoxia.
6. Monitor level of consciousness.
7. Maintain NPO status.
8. Administer fluids intravenously as prescribed to restore fluid volume and electrolyte imbalances; monitor intake and output.

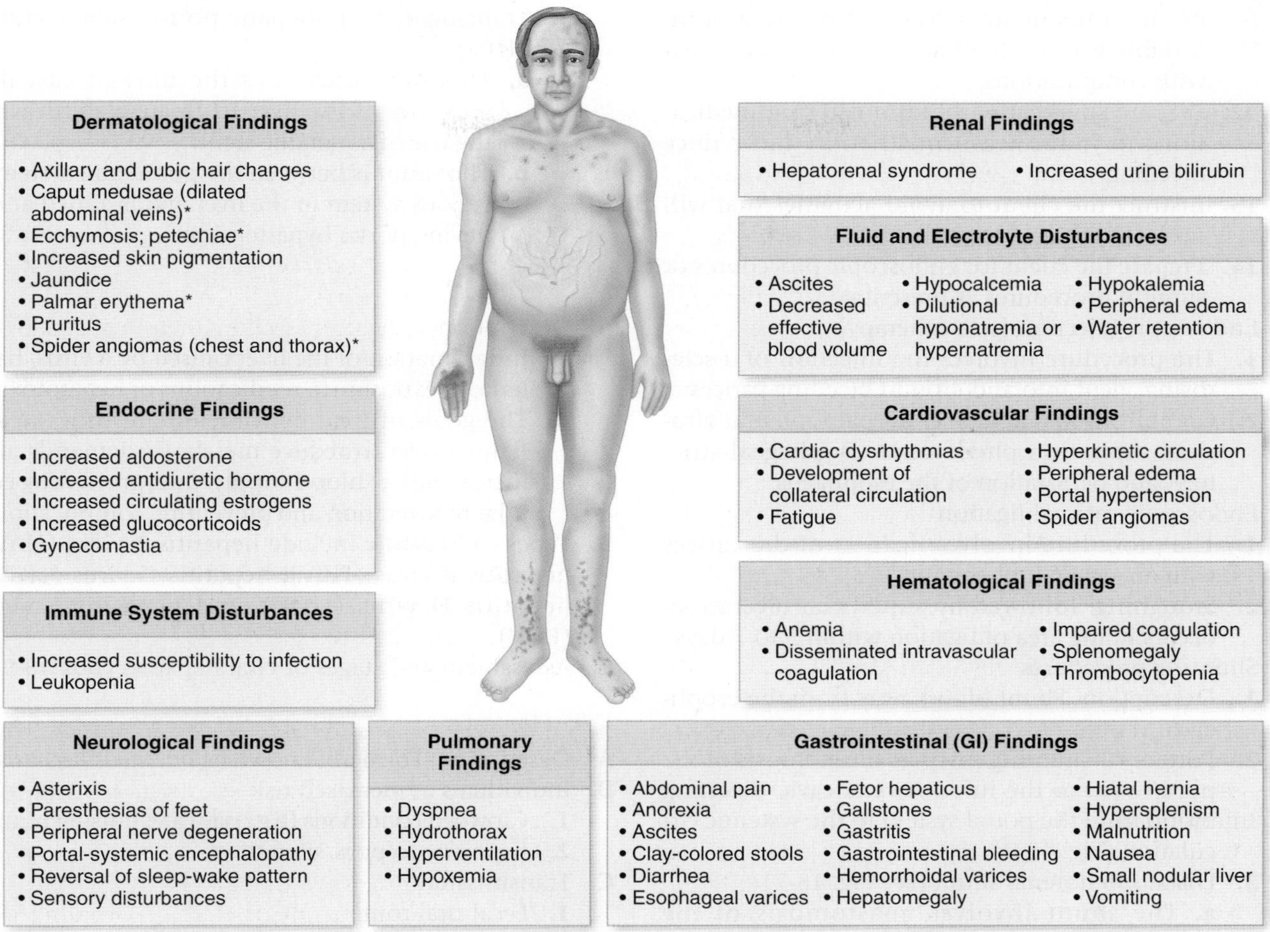

FIG. 48-4 Clinical picture of a client with liver dysfunction. Manifestations vary according to the progression of the disease. Some dermatological manifestations are noted in color (and marked with asterisks).

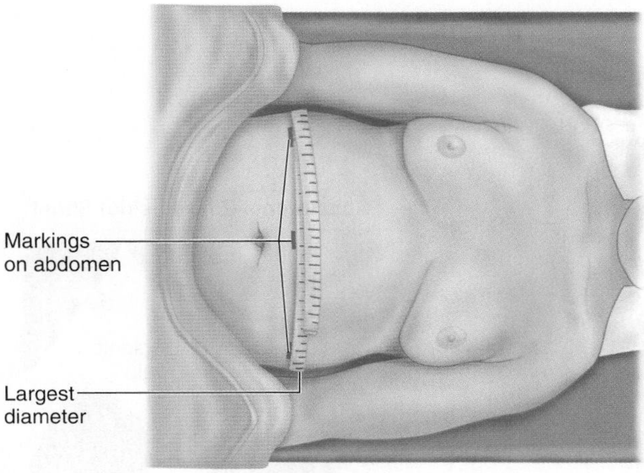

FIG. 48-5 How to measure abdominal girth. With the client supine, bring the tape measure around the client and take a measurement at the level of the umbilicus. Before removing the tape, mark the client's abdomen along the sides of tape on the client's flanks (sides) and midline to ensure that later measurements are taken at the same place.

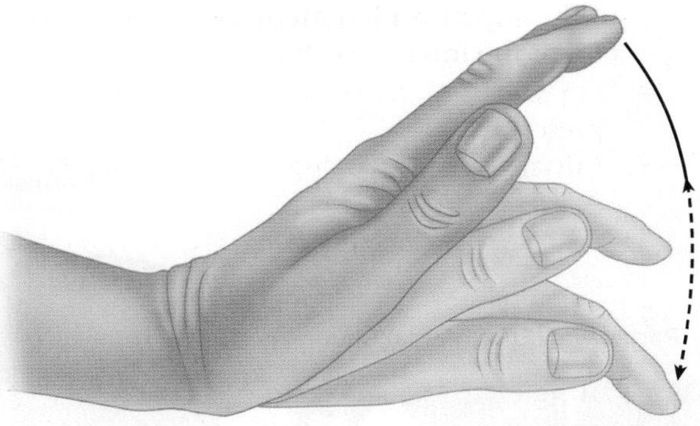

FIG. 48-6 Eliciting asterixis (flapping tremor). Have the client extend the arm, dorsiflex the wrist, and extend the fingers. Observe for rapid, nonrhythmic extensions and flexions.

9. Monitor hemoglobin and hematocrit values and coagulation factors.
10. Administer blood transfusions or clotting factors as prescribed.
11. Assist in inserting an NG tube or a balloon tamponade as prescribed; balloon tamponade is

not used frequently because it is very uncomfortable for the client and its use is associated with complications.

12. Prepare to assist with administering medications to induce vasoconstriction and reduce bleeding.
13. Instruct the client to avoid activities that will initiate vasovagal responses.
14. Prepare the client for endoscopic procedures or surgical procedures as prescribed.

D. Endoscopic injection (sclerotherapy)
1. The procedure involves the injection of a sclerosing agent into and around bleeding varices.
2. Complications include chest pain, pleural effusion, aspiration pneumonia, esophageal stricture, and perforation of the esophagus.

E. Endoscopic variceal ligation
1. The procedure involves ligation of the varices with an elastic rubber band.
2. Sloughing, followed by superficial ulceration, occurs in the area of ligation within 3 to 7 days.

F. Shunting procedures
1. Description: Shunt blood away from the esophageal varices
2. Portacaval shunting involves anastomosis of the portal vein to the inferior vena cava, diverting blood from the portal system to the systemic circulation (Fig. 48-7).
3. Distal splenorenal shunt (see Fig. 48-7)
   a. The shunt involves anastomosis of the splenic vein to the left renal vein.
   b. The spleen conducts blood from the high-pressure varices to the low-pressure renal vein.
4. Mesocaval shunting involves a side anastomosis of the superior mesenteric vein to the proximal end of the inferior vena cava.
5. Transjugular intrahepatic portosystemic shunt (TIPS)
   a. This procedure uses the normal vascular anatomy of the liver to create a shunt with the use of a metallic stent.
   b. The shunt is between the portal and systemic venous system in the liver and is aimed at relieving portal hypertension.

XV. Hepatitis

A. Description
1. Inflammation of the liver caused by a virus, bacteria, or exposure to medications or hepatotoxins
2. The goals of treatment include resting the inflamed liver to reduce metabolic demands and increasing the blood supply, thus promoting cellular regeneration and preventing complications.

B. Types of **hepatitis** include hepatitis A virus (HAV), hepatitis B virus (HBV), hepatitis C virus (HCV), hepatitis D virus (HDV), and hepatitis E virus (HEV).

C. Assessment and stages of viral hepatitis (Box 48-9)

XVI. Hepatitis A

A. Description: Formerly known as *infectious hepatitis*

B. Individuals at increased risk
1. Crowded conditions (e.g., day care, nursing home)
2. Exposure to poor sanitation

C. Transmission
1. Fecal-oral route
2. Person-to-person contact
3. Parenteral
4. Contaminated fruits or vegetables, or uncooked shellfish
5. Contaminated water or milk
6. Poorly washed utensils

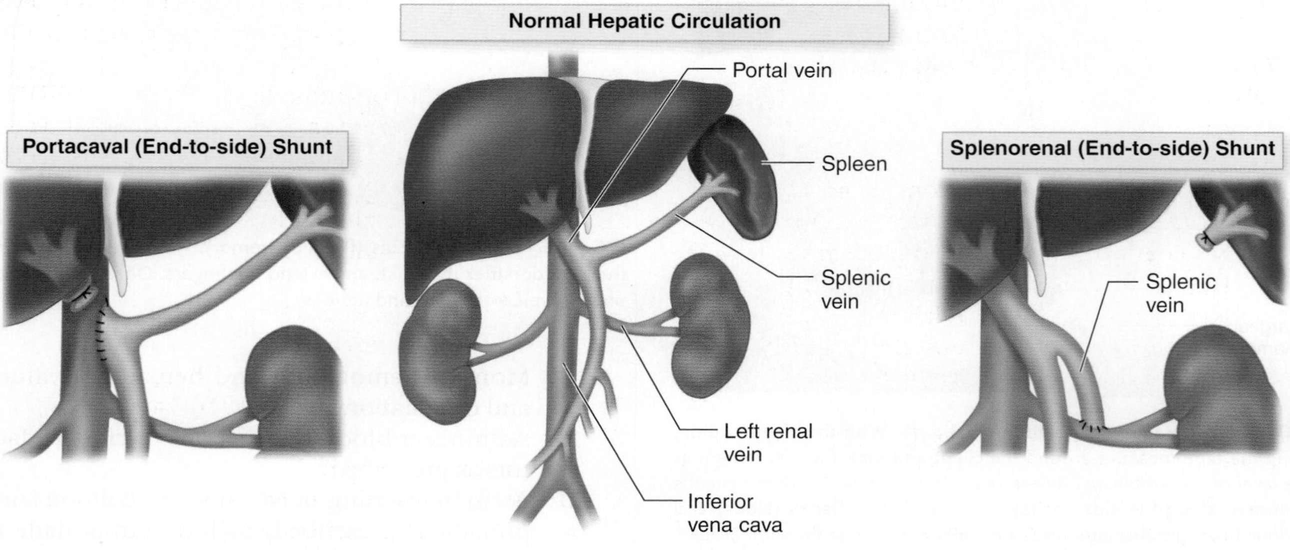

FIG. 48-7 Surgical shunting diverts portal venous blood flow from the liver to decrease portal and esophageal pressure.

BOX 48-9 Stages and Assessment of Viral Hepatitis

Preicteric Stage

The first stage of hepatitis, preceding the appearance of jaundice; includes flu-like symptoms—malaise, fatigue; anorexia, nausea, vomiting, diarrhea; pain—headache, muscle aches, polyarthritis; and elevated serum bilirubin and enzyme levels.

Icteric Stage

The second stage of hepatitis; includes the appearance of jaundice and associated symptoms such as elevated bilirubin levels, dark or tea-colored urine, and clay-colored stools; pruritus; and a decrease in preicteric-phase symptoms.

Posticteric Stage

The convalescent stage of hepatitis, in which the jaundice decreases and the color of the urine and stool returns to normal; energy increases, pain subsides, there is minimal to absent gastrointestinal symptoms, and bilirubin and enzyme levels return to normal.

D. Incubation and infectious period
 1. Incubation period is 2 to 6 weeks.
 2. Infectious period is 2 to 3 weeks before and 1 week after development of jaundice.

E. Testing
 1. Infection is established by the presence of HAV antibodies (anti-HAV) in the blood.
 2. Immunoglobulin M (IgM) and immunoglobulin G (IgG) are normally present in the blood, and increased levels indicate infection and inflammation.
 3. Ongoing inflammation of the liver is evidenced by the presence of elevated levels of IgM antibodies, which persist in the blood for 4 to 6 weeks.
 4. Previous infection is indicated by the presence of elevated levels of IgG antibodies.

F. Complication: Fulminant (severe acute and often fatal) hepatitis

G. Prevention
 1. Strict hand washing
 2. Stool and needle precautions
 3. Treatment of municipal water supplies
 4. Serological screening of food handlers
 5. Hepatitis A vaccine: Two doses are needed at least 6 months apart for lasting protection. For additional information, refer to http://www.cdc.gov/vaccines/hcp/vis/vis-statements/hep-a.html
 6. Immune globulin: For individuals exposed to HAV who have never received the hepatitis A vaccine; administer immune globulin during the period of incubation and within 2 weeks of exposure.
 7. Immune globulin and hepatitis A vaccine are recommended for household members and sexual contacts of individuals with hepatitis A.
 8. Preexposure prophylaxis with immune globulin is recommended to individuals traveling to countries with poor or uncertain sanitation conditions.

⚠ Strict and frequent hand washing is key to preventing the spread of all types of hepatitis.

XVII. Hepatitis B

A. Description
 1. Hepatitis B is nonseasonal.
 2. All age groups can be affected.

B. Individuals at increased risk
 1. IV drug users
 2. Clients undergoing long-term hemodialysis
 3. Health care personnel

C. Transmission
 1. Blood or body fluid contact
 2. Infected blood products
 3. Infected saliva or semen
 4. Contaminated needles
 5. Sexual contact
 6. Parenteral
 7. Perinatal period
 8. Blood or body fluid contact at birth

D. Incubation period: 6 to 24 weeks

E. Testing
 1. Infection is established by the presence of hepatitis B antigen–antibody systems in the blood.
 2. The presence of hepatitis B surface antigen (HBsAg) is the serological marker establishing the diagnosis of hepatitis B.
 3. The client is considered infectious if these antigens are present in the blood.
 4. If the serological marker (HBsAg) is present after 6 months, it indicates a carrier state or chronic hepatitis.
 5. Normally, the serological marker (HBsAg) level declines and disappears after the acute hepatitis B episode.
 6. The presence of antibodies to HBsAg (anti-HBs) indicates recovery and immunity to hepatitis B.
 7. Hepatitis B early antigen (HBeAg) is detected in the blood about 1 week after the appearance of HBsAg, and its presence determines the infective state of the client.

F. Complications
 1. Fulminant hepatitis
 2. Chronic liver disease
 3. Cirrhosis
 4. Primary hepatocellular carcinoma

G. Prevention
 1. Strict hand washing
 2. Screening blood donors
 3. Testing of all pregnant women
 4. Needle precautions

5. Avoiding intimate sexual contact and contact with body fluids if test for HBsAg is positive.
6. Hepatitis B vaccine: Adult and pediatric forms; there is also an adult vaccine that protects against hepatitis A and B.
7. Hepatitis B immune globulin is for individuals exposed to HBV through sexual contact or through the percutaneous or transmucosal routes who have never had hepatitis B and have never received hepatitis B vaccine.

XVIII. Hepatitis C

A. Description
1. HCV infection occurs year-round.
2. Infection can occur in any age group.
3. Infection with HCV is common among IV drug users and is the major cause of posttransfusion hepatitis.
4. Risk factors are similar to those for HBV, because hepatitis C is also transmitted parenterally.

B. Individuals at increased risk
1. Parenteral drug users
2. Clients receiving frequent transfusions
3. Health care personnel

C. Transmission: Same as for HBV, primarily through blood

D. Incubation period: 5 to 10 weeks

E. Testing: Anti-HCV is the antibody to HCV and is measured to detect chronic states of hepatitis C.

F. Complications
1. Chronic liver disease
2. Cirrhosis
3. Primary hepatocellular carcinoma

G. Prevention
1. Strict hand washing
2. Needle precautions
3. Screening of blood donors

XIX. Hepatitis D

A. Description
1. Hepatitis D is common in the Mediterranean and Middle Eastern areas.
2. Hepatitis D occurs with hepatitis B and causes infection only in the presence of active HBV infection.
3. Coinfection with the delta agent (HDV) intensifies the acute symptoms of hepatitis B.
4. Transmission and risk of infection are the same as for HBV, via contact with blood and blood products.
5. Prevention of HBV infection with vaccine also prevents HDV infection, because HDV depends on HBV for replication.

B. High-risk individuals
1. Drug users
2. Clients receiving hemodialysis
3. Clients receiving frequent blood transfusions

C. Transmission: Same as for HBV

D. Incubation period: 7 to 8 weeks

E. Testing: Serological HDV determination is made by detection of the hepatitis D antigen (HDAg) early in the course of the infection and by detection of anti-HDV antibody in the later disease stages.

F. Complications
1. Chronic liver disease
2. Fulminant hepatitis

G. Prevention: Because hepatitis D must coexist with hepatitis B, the precautions that help prevent hepatitis B are also useful in preventing delta hepatitis.

XX. Hepatitis E

A. Description
1. Hepatitis E is a waterborne virus.
2. Hepatitis E is prevalent in areas where sewage disposal is inadequate or where communal bathing in contaminated rivers is practiced.
3. Risk of infection is the same as for HAV.
4. Infection with HEV presents as a mild disease except in infected women in the third trimester of pregnancy, who have a high mortality rate.

B. Individuals with increased risk
1. Travelers to countries that have a high incidence of hepatitis E, such as India, Burma (Myanmar), Afghanistan, Algeria, and Mexico
2. Eating or drinking of food or water contaminated with the virus

C. Transmission: Same as for HAV

D. Incubation period: 2 to 9 weeks

E. Testing: Specific serological tests for HEV include detection of IgM and IgG antibodies to hepatitis E (anti-HEV).

F. Complications
1. High mortality rate in pregnant women
2. Fetal demise

G. Prevention
1. Strict hand washing
2. Treatment of water supplies and sanitation measures

XXI. Client and Family Home Care Instructions for Hepatitis: See Box 48-10

XXII. Pancreatitis

A. Description
1. Acute or chronic inflammation of the pancreas, with associated escape of pancreatic enzymes into surrounding tissue
2. Acute pancreatitis occurs suddenly as 1 attack or can be recurrent, with resolutions.
3. Chronic pancreatitis is a continual inflammation and destruction of the pancreas, with scar tissue replacing pancreatic tissue.

BOX 48-10 Home Care Instructions for the Client with Hepatitis

- Hand washing must be strict and frequent.
- Do not share bathrooms unless the client strictly adheres to personal hygiene measures.
- Individual washcloths, towels, drinking and eating utensils, and toothbrushes and razors must be labeled and used only by the client.
- The client must not prepare food for other family members.
- The client should avoid alcohol and over-the-counter medications, particularly acetaminophen and sedatives, because these medications are hepatotoxic.
- The client should increase activity gradually to prevent fatigue.
- The client should consume small, frequent meals consisting of high-carbohydrate, low-fat foods.
- The client is not to donate blood.
- The client may maintain normal contact with persons as long as proper personal hygiene is maintained.
- Close personal contact such as kissing and sexual activity should be discouraged with hepatitis B until surface antigen test results are negative.
- The client needs to carry a MedicAlert card noting the date of hepatitis onset.
- The client needs to inform other health professionals, such as medical or dental personnel, of the onset of hepatitis.
- The client needs to keep follow-up appointments with the primary health care provider.

4. Precipitating factors include trauma, the use of alcohol, biliary tract disease, viral or bacterial disease, hyperlipidemia, hypercalcemia, cholelithiasis, hyperparathyroidism, ischemic vascular disease, and peptic ulcer disease.

B. Acute pancreatitis
1. Assessment
   a. Abdominal pain, including a sudden onset at a midepigastric or left upper quadrant location with radiation to the back
   b. Pain aggravated by a fatty meal, alcohol, or lying in a recumbent position
   c. Abdominal tenderness and guarding
   d. Nausea and vomiting
   e. Weight loss
   f. Absent or decreased bowel sounds
   g. Elevated white blood cell count and elevated glucose, bilirubin, alkaline phosphatase, and urinary amylase levels
   h. Elevated serum lipase and amylase levels
   i. **Cullen's sign**
   j. **Turner's sign**

Cullen's sign is the discoloration of the abdomen and periumbilical area. Turner's sign is the bluish discoloration of the flanks. Both signs are indicative of pancreatitis.

2. Interventions
   a. Withhold food and fluid during the acute period and maintain hydration with IV fluids as prescribed.
   b. Administer parenteral nutrition for severe nutritional depletion.
   c. Administer supplemental preparations and vitamins and minerals to increase caloric intake if prescribed.
   d. An NG tube may be inserted if the client is vomiting or has biliary obstruction or paralytic ileus.
   e. Administer opiates as prescribed for pain.
   f. Administer H_2-receptor antagonists or proton pump inhibitors as prescribed to decrease hydrochloric acid production and prevent activation of pancreatic enzymes.
   g. Instruct the client in the importance of avoiding alcohol.
   h. Instruct the client in the importance of follow-up visits with the PHCP.
   i. Instruct the client to notify the PHCP if acute abdominal pain, jaundice, clay-colored stools, or dark-colored urine develops.

C. Chronic pancreatitis
1. Assessment
   a. Abdominal pain and tenderness
   b. Left upper quadrant mass
   c. Steatorrhea and foul-smelling stools that may increase in volume as pancreatic insufficiency increases
   d. Weight loss
   e. Muscle wasting
   f. Jaundice
   g. Signs and symptoms of diabetes mellitus
2. Interventions
   a. Instruct the client in the prescribed dietary measures (fat and protein intake may be limited).
   b. Instruct the client to avoid heavy meals.
   c. Instruct the client about the importance of avoiding alcohol.
   d. Provide supplemental preparations and vitamins and minerals to increase caloric intake.
   e. Administer pancreatic enzymes as prescribed to aid in the digestion and absorption of fat and protein.
   f. Administer insulin or oral hypoglycemic medications as prescribed to control diabetes mellitus, if present.
   g. Instruct the client in the use of pancreatic enzyme medications.
   h. Instruct the client in the treatment plan for glucose management.
   i. Instruct the client to notify the PHCP if increased steatorrhea, abdominal distention or cramping, or skin breakdown develops.

j. Instruct the client in the importance of follow-up visits.

XXIII. Pancreatic Tumors, Intestinal Tumors, and Bowel Obstructions: See Chapter 44 for more information.

XXIV. Irritable Bowel Syndrome (IBS)

A. Description
1. Functional disorder characterized by chronic or recurrent diarrhea, constipation, and/or abdominal pain and bloating
2. Cause is unclear but may be influenced by environmental, immunological, genetic, hormonal, and stress factors

B. Interventions
1. Increase dietary fiber.
2. Drink 8 to 10 cups of liquids per day.
3. Medication therapy: Depends on the predominant symptoms of IBS (antidiarrheals versus bulk-forming laxatives; lubiprostone or linaclotide for constipation-predominant IBS and alosetron for diarrhea-predominant IBS)

XXV. Ulcerative Colitis

A. Description
1. An ulcerative and inflammatory disease of the bowel that results in poor absorption of nutrients.
2. Commonly begins in the rectum and spreads upward toward the cecum
3. The colon becomes edematous and may develop bleeding lesions and ulcers; the ulcers may lead to perforation.
4. Scar tissue develops and causes loss of elasticity and loss of the ability to absorb nutrients.
5. Colitis is characterized by various periods of remissions and exacerbations.
6. Acute ulcerative colitis results in vascular congestion, hemorrhage, edema, and ulceration of the bowel mucosa.
7. Chronic ulcerative colitis causes muscular hypertrophy, fat deposits, and fibrous tissue, with bowel thickening, shortening, and narrowing.

B. Assessment
1. Anorexia
2. Weight loss
3. Malaise
4. Abdominal tenderness and cramping
5. Severe diarrhea that may contain blood and mucus
6. Malnutrition, dehydration, and electrolyte imbalances
7. Anemia
8. Vitamin K deficiency

C. Interventions
1. Acute phase: Maintain NPO status and administer fluids and electrolytes intravenously or via parenteral nutrition as prescribed.
2. Restrict the client's activity to reduce intestinal activity.
3. Monitor bowel sounds and for abdominal tenderness and cramping.
4. Monitor stools, noting color, consistency, and the presence or absence of blood.
5. Monitor for bowel perforation, peritonitis (see Box 48-3), and hemorrhage.
6. Following the acute phase, the diet progresses from clear liquids to a low-fiber diet as tolerated.
7. Instruct the client about diet. Usually a low-fiber diet is prescribed during an exacerbation episode; in addition, a high-protein diet with vitamins and iron supplements are prescribed.
8. Instruct the client to avoid gas-forming foods, milk products, and foods such as whole-wheat grains, nuts, raw fruits and vegetables, pepper, alcohol, and caffeine-containing products.
9. Instruct the client to avoid smoking.
10. Administer medications as prescribed, which may include a combination of medications such as salicylate compounds, corticosteroids, immunosuppressants, and antidiarrheals.

D. Surgical interventions
1. Performed in extreme cases if medical management is unsuccessful
2. Minimally invasive procedures are considered as a surgical option if the client is a candidate; clients who are obese, have had previous abdominal surgeries, or have adhesions may not be candidates.
3. Minimally invasive procedures can include laparoscopic procedures, robotic-assisted surgery, and natural orifice transluminal endoscopic surgery (NOTES).
4. Restorative proctocolectomy with ileal pouch–anal anastomosis (RPC-IPAA)
   a. Allows for bowel continence
   b. May be performed through laparoscopic procedure
   c. Involves a 2-stage procedure that includes removal of the colon and most of the rectum; the anus and anal sphincter remain intact.
   d. An internal pouch known as a reservoir (J-pouch, S-pouch, or pelvic pouch) is created using the small intestine and connected to the anus, followed by creation of a temporary ileostomy through the abdominal skin to allow healing of the internal pouch and all anastomosis sites.
   e. In the second surgical procedure (within 1 to 2 months), the ileostomy is closed.

5. Total proctocolectomy with permanent ileostomy
   a. Performed if the client is not a candidate for RPC-IPAA or if the client prefers this type of procedure.
   b. The procedure involves the removal of the entire colon (colon, rectum, and anus, with anal closure).
   c. The end of the terminal ileum forms the stoma or ostomy, which is located in the right lower quadrant.
6. Preoperative interventions
   a. Consult with the enterostomal therapist to help identify optimal placement of the ostomy.
   b. Instruct the client on dietary restrictions; the client may need to follow a low-fiber diet for 1 to 2 days before surgery.
   c. Parenteral antibiotics are administered 1 hour before the surgical opening.
   d. Address body image concerns and allow the client to express concerns; a visit from an ostomate may be helpful to the client.
7. Postoperative interventions
   a. A pouch system with a skin barrier is usually placed on the stoma postoperatively; if a pouch system is not covering the stoma, a petrolatum gauze dressing is placed over the stoma as prescribed to keep it moist, followed by a dry sterile dressing.
   b. Monitor the stoma for size, unusual bleeding, or necrotic tissue.
   c. Monitor for color changes in the stoma.
   d. Note that the normal stoma color is pink to bright red and shiny, indicating high vascularity.
   e. Note that a pale pink stoma indicates low hemoglobin and hematocrit levels and a purple-black stoma indicates compromised circulation, requiring PHCP notification.
   f. Assess the functioning of the ostomy.
   g. Expect that stool is liquid in the immediate postoperative period but becomes more solid depending on the area of creation—ascending colon, liquid; transverse colon, loose to semiformed; and descending colon, close to normal.
   h. Monitor the pouch system for proper fit and signs of leakage; the pouch is emptied when it is one-third full.
   i. Fecal matter should not be allowed to remain on the skin; skin assessment and care are a priority.
   j. Monitor for dehydration and electrolyte imbalance.
   k. Administer analgesics and antibiotics as prescribed.
   l. Instruct the client to avoid foods that cause excess gas formation and odor.
   m. Instruct the client about stoma care and irrigations if prescribed (Box 48-11).
   n. Instruct the client that normal activities may be resumed when approved by the PHCP.

⚠ A stoma that is purple-black in color indicates compromised circulation, requiring immediate PHCP notification.

XXVI. Crohn's Disease

A. Description
   1. An inflammatory disease that can occur anywhere in the gastrointestinal tract but most often affects the terminal ileum and leads to thickening and scarring, a narrowed lumen, fistulas, ulcerations, and abscesses
   2. Characterized by remissions and exacerbations
B. Assessment
   1. Fever
   2. Cramp-like and colicky pain after meals
   3. Diarrhea (semisolid), which may contain mucus and pus
   4. Abdominal distention
   5. Anorexia, nausea, and vomiting
   6. Weight loss
   7. Anemia
   8. Dehydration
   9. Electrolyte imbalances

BOX 48-11 Colostomy Irrigation

Purpose

An enema is given through the stoma to stimulate bowel emptying.

Description

Irrigation is performed by instilling 500 to 1000 mL of lukewarm tap water through the stoma and allowing the water and stool to drain into a collection bag.

Procedure

- If ambulatory, position the client sitting on the toilet.
- If on bed rest, position the client on her or his side.
- Hang the irrigation bag so that the bottom of the bag is at the level of the client's shoulder or slightly higher.
- Insert the irrigation tube carefully without force.
- Begin the flow of irrigation.
- Clamp the tubing if cramping occurs; release the tubing as cramping subsides.
- Avoid frequent irrigations, which can lead to loss of fluids and electrolytes.
- Perform irrigation at about the same time each day.
- Perform irrigation preferably 1 hour after a meal.
- To enhance effectiveness of the irrigation, massage the abdomen gently.

10. Malnutrition (may be worse than that seen in ulcerative colitis)

C. Interventions: Care is similar to that for the client with ulcerative colitis; however, surgery may be necessary but is avoided for as long as possible because recurrence of the disease process in the same region is likely to occur.

XXVII. Appendicitis

A. Description
1. Inflammation of the appendix
2. When the appendix becomes inflamed or infected, rupture may occur within a matter of hours, leading to peritonitis and sepsis.

B. Assessment
1. Pain in the periumbilical area that descends to the right lower quadrant
2. Abdominal pain that is most intense at McBurney's point
3. Rebound tenderness and abdominal rigidity
4. Low-grade fever
5. Elevated white blood cell count
6. Anorexia, nausea, and vomiting
7. Client in side-lying position, with abdominal guarding and legs flexed
8. Constipation or diarrhea

C. Peritonitis: Inflammation of the peritoneum (see Box 48-3)

D. Appendectomy: Surgical removal of the appendix
1. Preoperative interventions
   a. Maintain NPO status.
   b. Administer fluids intravenously to prevent dehydration.
   c. Monitor for changes in level of pain.
   d. Monitor for signs of ruptured appendix and peritonitis (see Box 48-3).
   e. Position the client in a right side–lying or low to semi-Fowler's position to promote comfort.
   f. Monitor bowel sounds.
   g. Apply ice packs to the abdomen for 20 to 30 minutes every hour if prescribed.
   h. Administer antibiotics as prescribed.
   i. Avoid laxatives or enemas.

! Avoid the application of heat to the abdomen of a client with appendicitis. Heat can cause rupture of the appendix leading to peritonitis, a life-threatening condition.

2. Postoperative interventions
   a. Monitor temperature for signs of infection.
   b. Assess incision for signs of infection such as redness, swelling, and pain.
   c. Maintain NPO status until bowel function has returned.
   d. Advance diet gradually as tolerated and as prescribed, when bowel sounds return.
   e. If rupture of the appendix occurred, expect a drain to be inserted, or the incision may be left open to heal from the inside out.
   f. Expect that drainage from the drain may be profuse for the first 12 hours.
   g. Position the client in a right side–lying or low to semi-Fowler's position, with legs flexed, to facilitate drainage.
   h. Change the dressing as prescribed and record the type and amount of drainage.
   i. Perform wound irrigations if prescribed.
   j. Maintain NG suction and patency of the NG tube if present.
   k. Administer antibiotics and analgesics as prescribed.

XXVIII. Diverticulosis and Diverticulitis

A. Description
1. Diverticulosis
   a. **Diverticulosis** is an outpouching or herniation of the intestinal mucosa.
   b. The disorder can occur in any part of the intestine but is most common in the sigmoid colon.
2. Diverticulitis
   a. **Diverticulitis** is the inflammation of 1 or more diverticula that occurs from penetration of fecal matter through the thin-walled diverticula; it can result in local abscess formation and perforation.
   b. A perforated diverticulum can progress to intra-abdominal perforation with generalized peritonitis.

B. Assessment
1. Left lower quadrant abdominal pain that increases with coughing, straining, or lifting
2. Elevated temperature
3. Nausea and vomiting
4. Flatulence
5. Cramp-like pain
6. Abdominal distention and tenderness
7. Palpable, tender rectal mass may be present.
8. Blood in the stools

C. Interventions
1. Provide bed rest during the acute phase.
2. Maintain NPO status or provide clear liquids during the acute phase as prescribed.
3. Introduce a fiber-containing diet gradually, when the inflammation has resolved.
4. Administer antibiotics, analgesics, and anticholinergics to reduce bowel spasms as prescribed.
5. Instruct the client to refrain from lifting, straining, coughing, or bending to avoid increased intra-abdominal pressure.
6. Monitor for perforation (see Box 48-3), hemorrhage, fistulas, and abscesses.
7. Instruct the client to increase fluid intake to 2500 to 3000 mL daily, unless contraindicated.

8. Instruct the client to eat soft high-fiber foods, such as whole grains; the client should avoid high-fiber foods when inflammation occurs, because these foods will irritate the mucosa further.
9. Instruct the client to avoid gas-forming foods or foods containing indigestible roughage, seeds, nuts, or popcorn, because these food substances become trapped in diverticula and cause inflammation.
10. Instruct the client to consume a small amount of bran daily and to take bulk-forming laxatives as prescribed to increase stool mass.

D. Surgical interventions
1. Colon resection with primary anastomosis may be an option.
2. Temporary or permanent colostomy may be required for increased bowel inflammation.

XXIX. Hemorrhoids

A. Description
1. Dilated varicose veins of the anal canal
2. May be internal, external, or prolapsed
3. Internal hemorrhoids lie above the anal sphincter and cannot be seen on inspection of the perianal area.
4. External hemorrhoids lie below the anal sphincter and can be seen on inspection.
5. Prolapsed hemorrhoids can become thrombosed or inflamed.
6. Hemorrhoids are caused from portal hypertension, straining, irritation, or increased venous or abdominal pressure.

B. Assessment
1. Bright red bleeding with defecation
2. Rectal pain
3. Rectal itching

C. Interventions
1. Apply cold packs to the anal-rectal area followed by sitz baths as prescribed.
2. Apply witch hazel soaks and topical anesthetics as prescribed.
3. Encourage a high-fiber diet and fluids to promote bowel movements without straining.
4. Administer stool softeners as prescribed.

D. Surgical interventions: May include ultrasound, sclerotherapy, circular stapling, band ligation, or simple resection of the hemorrhoids (hemorrhoidectomy)

E. Postoperative interventions following hemorrhoidectomy
1. Assist the client to a prone or side-lying position to prevent bleeding.
2. Maintain ice packs over the dressing as prescribed until the packing is removed by the PHCP.
3. Monitor for urinary retention.
4. Administer stool softeners as prescribed.
5. Instruct the client to increase fluids and high-fiber foods.
6. Instruct the client to limit sitting to short periods of time.
7. Instruct the client in the use of sitz baths three or four times a day as prescribed.

PRACTICE QUESTIONS

529. The nurse is monitoring a client admitted to the hospital with a diagnosis of appendicitis who is scheduled for surgery in 2 hours. The client begins to complain of increased abdominal pain and begins to vomit. On assessment, the nurse notes that the abdomen is distended and bowel sounds are diminished. Which is the **most appropriate** nursing intervention?
1. Administer the prescribed pain medication.
2. Notify the primary health care provider (PHCP).
3. Call and ask the operating room team to perform surgery as soon as possible.
4. Reposition the client and apply a heating pad on the warm setting to the client's abdomen.

530. A client admitted to the hospital with a suspected diagnosis of acute pancreatitis is being assessed by the nurse. Which assessment findings would be consistent with acute pancreatitis? **Select all that apply.**
- ☐ 1. Diarrhea
- ☐ 2. Black, tarry stools
- ☐ 3. Hyperactive bowel sounds
- ☐ 4. Gray-blue color at the flank
- ☐ 5. Abdominal guarding and tenderness
- ☐ 6. Left upper quadrant pain with radiation to the back

531. The nurse is assessing a client who is experiencing an acute episode of cholecystitis. Which of these clinical manifestations support this diagnosis? **Select all that apply.**
- ☐ 1. Fever
- ☐ 2. Positive Cullen's sign
- ☐ 3. Complaints of indigestion
- ☐ 4. Palpable mass in the left upper quadrant
- ☐ 5. Pain in the upper right quadrant after a fatty meal
- ☐ 6. Vague lower right quadrant abdominal discomfort

532. A client is diagnosed with viral hepatitis, complaining of "no appetite" and "losing my taste for food." What instruction should the nurse give the client to provide adequate nutrition?
1. Select foods high in fat.
2. Increase intake of fluids, including juices.
3. Eat a good supper when anorexia is not as severe.
4. Eat less often, preferably only 3 large meals daily.

533. A client has developed hepatitis A after eating contaminated oysters. The nurse assesses the client for which expected assessment finding?
1. Malaise
2. Dark stools
3. Weight gain
4. Left upper quadrant discomfort

534. A client has just had a hemorrhoidectomy. Which nursing interventions are appropriate for this client? **Select all that apply.**
- ☐ 1. Administer stool softeners as prescribed.
- ☐ 2. Instruct the client to limit fluid intake to avoid urinary retention.
- ☐ 3. Encourage a high-fiber diet to promote bowel movements without straining.
- ☐ 4. Apply cold packs to the anal-rectal area over the dressing until the packing is removed.
- ☐ 5. Help the client to a Fowler's position to place pressure on the rectal area and decrease bleeding.

535. The nurse is planning to teach a client with gastroesophageal reflux disease (GERD) about substances to avoid. Which items should the nurse include on this list? **Select all that apply.**
- ☐ 1. Coffee
- ☐ 2. Chocolate
- ☐ 3. Peppermint
- ☐ 4. Nonfat milk
- ☐ 5. Fried chicken
- ☐ 6. Scrambled eggs

536. A client has undergone esophagogastroduodenoscopy. The nurse should place **highest priority** on which item as part of the client's care plan?
1. Monitoring the temperature
2. Monitoring complaints of heartburn
3. Giving warm gargles for a sore throat
4. Assessing for the return of the gag reflex

537. The nurse has taught the client about an upcoming endoscopic retrograde cholangiopancreatography (ERCP) procedure. The nurse determines that the client **needs further information** if the client makes which statement?
1. "I know I must sign the consent form."
2. "I hope the throat spray keeps me from gagging."
3. "I'm glad I don't have to lie still for this procedure."
4. "I'm glad some intravenous medication will be given to relax me."

538. The primary health care provider has determined that a client has contracted hepatitis A based on flu-like symptoms and jaundice. Which statement made by the client supports this medical diagnosis?
1. "I have had unprotected sex with multiple partners."
2. "I ate shellfish about 2 weeks ago at a local restaurant."
3. "I was an intravenous drug abuser in the past and shared needles."
4. "I had a blood transfusion 30 years ago after major abdominal surgery."

539. The nurse is assessing a client 24 hours following a cholecystectomy. The nurse notes that the T-tube has drained 750 mL of green-brown drainage since the surgery. Which nursing intervention is **most appropriate**?
1. Clamp the T-tube.
2. Irrigate the T-tube.
3. Document the findings.
4. Notify the primary health care provider.

540. The nurse is monitoring a client with a diagnosis of peptic ulcer. Which assessment finding would **most likely** indicate perforation of the ulcer?
1. Bradycardia
2. Numbness in the legs
3. Nausea and vomiting
4. A rigid, board-like abdomen

541. The nurse is caring for a client following a gastrojejunostomy (Billroth II procedure). Which postoperative prescription should the nurse question and verify?
1. Leg exercises
2. Early ambulation
3. Irrigating the nasogastric tube
4. Coughing and deep-breathing exercises

542. The nurse is providing discharge instructions to a client following gastrectomy and should instruct the client to take which measure to assist in preventing dumping syndrome?
1. Ambulate following a meal.
2. Eat high-carbohydrate foods.
3. Limit the fluids taken with meals.
4. Sit in a high-Fowler's position during meals.

543. The nurse is reviewing the prescription for a client admitted to the hospital with a diagnosis of acute pancreatitis. Which interventions would the nurse expect to be prescribed for the client? **Select all that apply.**
- ☐ 1. Maintain NPO (nothing by mouth) status.
- ☐ 2. Encourage coughing and deep breathing.
- ☐ 3. Give small, frequent high-calorie feedings.
- ☐ 4. Maintain the client in a supine and flat position.
- ☐ 5. Give hydromorphone intravenously as prescribed for pain.
- ☐ 6. Maintain intravenous fluids at 10 mL/hr to keep the vein open.

544. The nurse is providing discharge teaching for a client with newly diagnosed Crohn's disease about dietary measures to implement during exacerbation episodes. Which statement made by the client indicates a **need for further instruction**?
1. "I should increase the fiber in my diet."
2. "I will need to avoid caffeinated beverages."
3. "I'm going to learn some stress reduction techniques."
4. "I can have exacerbations and remissions with Crohn's disease."

545. The nurse is reviewing the record of a client with a diagnosis of cirrhosis and notes that there is documentation of the presence of asterixis. How should the nurse assess for its presence?
1. Dorsiflex the client's foot.
2. Measure the abdominal girth.
3. Ask the client to extend the arms.
4. Instruct the client to lean forward.

546. The nurse is reviewing the laboratory results for a client with cirrhosis and notes that the ammonia level is 85 mcg/dL (51 mcmol/L). Which dietary selection does the nurse suggest to the client?
1. Roast pork
2. Cheese omelet
3. Pasta with sauce
4. Tuna fish sandwich

547. The nurse is doing an admission assessment on a client with a history of duodenal ulcer. To determine whether the problem is currently active, the nurse should assess the client for which manifestation of duodenal ulcer?
1. Weight loss
2. Nausea and vomiting
3. Pain relieved by food intake
4. Pain radiating down the right arm

548. A client with hiatal hernia chronically experiences heartburn following meals. The nurse should plan to teach the client to avoid which action because it is contraindicated with a hiatal hernia?
1. Lying recumbent following meals
2. Consuming small, frequent, bland meals
3. Taking H_2-receptor antagonist medication
4. Raising the head of the bed on 6-inch (15 cm) blocks

549. The nurse is providing care for a client with a recent transverse colostomy. Which observation requires **immediate** notification of the primary health care provider?
1. Stoma is beefy red and shiny
2. Purple discoloration of the stoma
3. Skin excoriation around the stoma
4. Semiformed stool noted in the ostomy pouch

550. A client had a new colostomy created 2 days earlier and is beginning to pass malodorous flatus from the stoma. What is the correct interpretation by the nurse?
1. This is a normal, expected event.
2. The client is experiencing early signs of ischemic bowel.
3. The client should not have the nasogastric tube removed.
4. This indicates inadequate preoperative bowel preparation.

551. A client has just had surgery to create an ileostomy. The nurse assesses the client in the immediate postoperative period for which **most** frequent complication of this type of surgery?
1. Folate deficiency
2. Malabsorption of fat
3. Intestinal obstruction
4. Fluid and electrolyte imbalance

552. The nurse provides instructions to a client about measures to treat inflammatory bowel syndrome (IBS). Which statement by the client indicates a **need for further teaching**?
1. "I need to limit my intake of dietary fiber."
2. "I need to drink plenty, at least 8 to 10 cups daily."
3. "I need to eat regular meals and chew my food well."
4. "I will take the prescribed medications because they will regulate my bowel patterns."

553. The nurse is monitoring a client for the **early** signs and symptoms of dumping syndrome. Which findings indicate this occurrence?
1. Sweating and pallor
2. Bradycardia and indigestion
3. Double vision and chest pain
4. Abdominal cramping and pain

ANSWERS

529. *Answer:* 2

Rationale: On the basis of the signs and symptoms presented in the question, the nurse should suspect peritonitis and notify the PHCP. Administering pain medication is not an appropriate intervention. Heat should never be applied to the abdomen of a client with suspected appendicitis because of the risk of rupture. Scheduling surgical time is not within the scope of nursing practice, although the PHCP probably would perform the surgery earlier than the prescheduled time.

Test-Taking Strategy: Note the strategic words, *most appropriate.* Determine if an abnormality exists, focus on the signs and symptoms in the question, and consider the complications that can occur with appendicitis. Noting that the signs presented in the question indicate a complication will assist in directing you to the correct option.

Level of Cognitive Ability: Analyzing

Client Needs: Physiological Integrity

Integrated Process: Nursing Process—Implementation

Content Area: Adult Health: Gastrointestinal

Health Problem: Adult Health: Gastrointestinal: GI Accessory Organs

Priority Concepts: Clinical Judgment; Inflammation

Reference: Ignatavicius, Workman, Rebar (2018), pp. 1147-1148.

530. *Answer:* 4, 5, 6

Rationale: Grayish-blue discoloration at the flank is known as Grey-Turner's sign and occurs as a result of pancreatic enzyme leakage to cutaneous tissue from the peritoneal cavity. The client may demonstrate abdominal guarding and may complain of tenderness with palpation. The pain associated with acute pancreatitis is often sudden in onset and is located in the epigastric region or left upper quadrant with radiation to the back. The other options are incorrect.

Test-Taking Strategy: Noting that options 1 and 3 are comparable or alike will assist you in eliminating these options first. Then recall that black, tarry stools occur when there is gastrointestinal bleeding, so this can also be eliminated. From the remaining options, recall the anatomical location of the pancreas, the pain characteristics, and the effect of enzymes leaking into the tissues to direct you to the correct options.

Level of Cognitive Ability: Analyzing

Client Needs: Physiological Integrity

Integrated Process: Nursing Process—Assessment

Content Area: Adult Health: Gastrointestinal

Health Problem: Adult Health: Gastrointestinal: GI Accessory Organs

Priority Concepts: Inflammation; Pain

Reference: Ignatavicius, Workman, Rebar (2018), p. 1199.

531. *Answer:* 1, 3, 5

Rationale: During an acute episode of cholecystitis, the client may complain of severe right upper quadrant pain that radiates to the right scapula or shoulder or experience epigastric pain after a fatty or high-volume meal. Fever and signs of dehydration would also be expected, as well as complaints of indigestion, belching, flatulence, nausea, and vomiting. Options 4 and 6 are incorrect because they are inconsistent with the anatomical location of the gallbladder. Option 2 (Cullen's sign) is associated with pancreatitis.

Test-Taking Strategy: Focus on the subject, the location and characteristics of pain associated with cholecystitis. Recalling the anatomical location of the gallbladder will also direct you to the correct option.

Level of Cognitive Ability: Analyzing

Client Needs: Physiological Integrity

Integrated Process: Nursing Process—Assessment

Content Area: Adult Health: Gastrointestinal

Health Problem: Adult Health: Gastrointestinal: GI Accessory Organs

Priority Concepts: Inflammation; Pain

Reference: Ignatavicius, Workman, Rebar (2018), p. 1193.

532. *Answer:* 2

Rationale: Although no special diet is required to treat viral hepatitis, it is generally recommended that clients consume a low-fat diet, as fat may be tolerated poorly because of decreased bile production. Small, frequent meals are preferable and may even prevent nausea. Frequently, appetite is better in the morning, so it is easier to eat a good breakfast. An adequate fluid intake of 2500 to 3000 mL/day that includes nutritional juices is also important.

Test-Taking Strategy: Focus on the subject, a diet for viral hepatitis. Think about the pathophysiology associated with hepatitis and focus on the client's complaints to direct you to the correct option.

Level of Cognitive Ability: Applying

Client Needs: Physiological Integrity

Integrated Process: Teaching and Learning

Content Area: Adult Health: Gastrointestinal

Health Problem: Adult Health: Gastrointestinal: GI Accessory Organs

Priority Concepts: Client Education; Infection

Reference: Ignatavicius, Workman, Rebar (2018), pp. 1184-1185.

533. *Answer:* 1

Rationale: Hepatitis causes gastrointestinal symptoms such as anorexia, nausea, right upper quadrant discomfort, and weight loss. Fatigue and malaise are common. Stools will be light- or clay-colored if conjugated bilirubin is unable to flow out of the liver because of inflammation or obstruction of the bile ducts.

Test-Taking Strategy: Focus on the subject, expected assessment findings. Recalling the function of the liver will direct you to the correct option. Remember that fatigue and malaise are common.

Level of Cognitive Ability: Analyzing

Client Needs: Physiological Integrity

Integrated Process: Nursing Process—Assessment

Content Area: Adult Health: Gastrointestinal

Health Problem: Adult Health: Gastrointestinal: GI Accessory Organs

Priority Concepts: Clinical Judgment; Infection

Reference: Ignatavicius, Workman, Rebar (2018), p. 1183.

534. *Answer:* 1, 3, 4

Rationale: Nursing interventions after a hemorrhoidectomy are aimed at management of pain and avoidance of bleeding and incision rupture. Stool softeners and a high-fiber diet will help the client avoid straining, thereby reducing the chances of rupturing the incision. An ice pack will increase comfort and decrease bleeding. Options 2 and 5 are incorrect interventions.

Test-Taking Strategy: Focus on the subject, postoperative hemorrhoidectomy care. Recall that decreasing fluid intake will cause difficulty with defecation because of hard stool. Recognize that Fowler's position will increase pressure in the rectal area, causing increased bleeding and increased pain.
Level of Cognitive Ability: Analyzing
Client Needs: Physiological Integrity
Integrated Process: Nursing Process—Implementation
Content Area: Adult Health: Gastrointestinal
Health Problem: Adult Health: Gastrointestinal: Lower GI Disorders
Priority Concepts: Elimination; Pain
Reference: Ignatavicius, Workman, Rebar (2018), p. 1140.

535. *Answer:* 1, 2, 3, 5
Rationale: Foods that decrease lower esophageal sphincter (LES) pressure and irritate the esophagus will increase reflux and exacerbate the symptoms of GERD and therefore should be avoided. Aggravating substances include coffee, chocolate, peppermint, fried or fatty foods, carbonated beverages, and alcohol. Options 4 and 6 do not promote this effect.
Test-Taking Strategy: Focus on the subject, food items to avoid. Use knowledge of the effect of various foods on LES pressure and GERD. However, if you are unsure, note that options 4 and 6 are the most healthful food items.
Level of Cognitive Ability: Analyzing
Client Needs: Physiological Integrity
Integrated Process: Teaching and Learning
Content Area: Adult Health: Gastrointestinal
Health Problem: Adult Health: Gastrointestinal: Upper GI Disorders
Priority Concepts: Client Education; Inflammation
Reference: Ignatavicius, Workman, Rebar (2018), pp. 1088, 1090.

536. *Answer:* 4
Rationale: The nurse places highest priority on assessing for return of the gag reflex. This assessment addresses the client's airway. The nurse also monitors the client's vital signs and for a sudden increase in temperature, which could indicate perforation of the gastrointestinal tract. This complication would be accompanied by other signs as well, such as pain. Monitoring for sore throat and heartburn are also important; however, the client's airway is the priority.
Test-Taking Strategy: Note the strategic words, *highest priority.* Use the ABCs—airway, breathing, and circulation. The correct option addresses the airway.
Level of Cognitive Ability: Analyzing
Client Needs: Safe and Effective Care Environment
Integrated Process: Nursing Process—Planning
Content Area: Foundations of Care: Diagnostic Tests
Health Problem: N/A
Priority Concepts: Clinical Judgment; Safety
Reference: Ignatavicius, Workman, Rebar (2018), p.1071.

537. *Answer:* 3
Rationale: The client does have to lie still for ERCP, which takes about 1 hour to perform. The client also has to sign a consent form. Intravenous sedation is given to relax the client, and an anesthetic spray is used to help keep the client from gagging as the endoscope is passed.
Test-Taking Strategy: Note the strategic words, *needs further information.* These words indicate a negative event query and ask you to select an option that is incorrect. Invasive procedures require consent, so option 1 can be eliminated. Noting the name of the procedure and considering the anatomical location will assist you in eliminating options 2 and 4.
Level of Cognitive Ability: Evaluating
Client Needs: Physiological Integrity
Integrated Process: Teaching and Learning
Content Area: Foundations of Care: Diagnostic Tests
Health Problem: N/A
Priority Concepts: Client Education; Safety
Reference: Lewis et al. (2017), p. 850.

538. *Answer:* 2
Rationale: Hepatitis A is transmitted by the fecal-oral route via contaminated water or food (improperly cooked shellfish), or infected food handlers. Hepatitis B, C, and D are transmitted most commonly via infected blood or body fluids, such as in the cases of intravenous drug abuse, history of blood transfusion, or unprotected sex with multiple partners.
Test-Taking Strategy: Focus on the subject, hepatitis A. Recalling the modes of transmission of the various types of hepatitis is required to answer this question. Remember that hepatitis A is transmitted by the fecal-oral route.
Level of Cognitive Ability: Analyzing
Client Needs: Safe and Effective Care Environment
Integrated Process: Nursing Process—Assessment
Content Area: Adult Health: Gastrointestinal
Health Problem: Adult Health: Gastrointestinal: GI Accessory Organs
Priority Concepts: Infection; Inflammation
Reference: Lewis et al. (2017), p. 975.

539. *Answer:* 3
Rationale: Following cholecystectomy, drainage from the T-tube is initially bloody and then turns a greenish-brown color. The drainage is measured as output. The amount of expected drainage will range from 500 to 1000 mL/day. The nurse would document the output.
Test-Taking Strategy: Note the strategic words, *most appropriate.* Options 1 and 2 can be eliminated because a T-tube is not irrigated and would not be clamped with this amount of drainage. From the remaining options, you must know normal expected findings following this surgical procedure.
Level of Cognitive Ability: Applying
Client Needs: Physiological Integrity
Integrated Process: Nursing Process—Implementation
Content Area: Adult Health: Gastrointestinal
Health Problem: Adult Health: Gastrointestinal: GI Accessory Organs
Priority Concepts: Clinical Judgment; Elimination
Reference: Lewis et al. (2017), pp. 344, 1009.

540. *Answer:* 4
Rationale: Perforation of an ulcer is a surgical emergency and is characterized by sudden, sharp, intolerable severe pain beginning in the midepigastric area and spreading over the abdomen, which becomes rigid and boardlike. Nausea and vomiting may occur. Tachycardia may occur as hypovolemic

shock develops. Numbness in the legs is not an associated finding.
Test-Taking Strategy: Focus on the subject, perforation. Option 2 can be eliminated easily because it is not related to perforation. Eliminate option 1 next because tachycardia rather than bradycardia would develop if perforation occurs. From the remaining options, note the strategic words, *most likely*, to help direct you to the correct option.
Level of Cognitive Ability: Analyzing
Client Needs: Physiological Integrity
Integrated Process: Nursing Process—Assessment
Content Area: Adult Health: Gastrointestinal
Health Problem: Adult Health: Gastrointestinal: Upper GI Disorders
Priority Concepts: Clinical Judgment; Safety
Reference: Lewis et al. (2017), p. 912-913.

541. *Answer:* 3
Rationale: In a gastrojejunostomy (Billroth II procedure), the proximal remnant of the stomach is anastomosed to the proximal jejunum. Patency of the nasogastric tube is critical for preventing the retention of gastric secretions. The nurse should never irrigate or reposition the gastric tube after gastric surgery, unless specifically prescribed by the primary health care provider. In this situation, the nurse should clarify the prescription. Options 1, 2, and 4 are appropriate postoperative interventions.
Test-Taking Strategy: Note the words *question and verify.* Eliminate options 1, 2, and 4 because they are comparable or alike and are general postoperative measures. Also, consider the anatomical location of the surgical procedure to assist in directing you to the correct option.
Level of Cognitive Ability: Analyzing
Client Needs: Physiological Integrity
Integrated Process: Nursing Process—Analysis
Content Area: Adult Health: Gastrointestinal
Health Problem: Adult Health: Gastrointestinal: Upper GI Disorders
Priority Concepts: Clinical Judgment; Safety
Reference: Ignatavicius, Workman, Rebar (2018), pp. 1208-1209.

542. *Answer:* 3
Rationale: *Dumping syndrome* is a term that refers to a constellation of vasomotor symptoms that occurs after eating, especially following a gastrojejunostomy (Billroth II procedure). Early manifestations usually occur within 30 minutes of eating and include vertigo, tachycardia, syncope, sweating, pallor, palpitations, and the desire to lie down. The nurse should instruct the client to decrease the amount of fluid taken at meals and to avoid high-carbohydrate foods, including fluids such as fruit nectars; to assume a low-Fowler's position during meals; to lie down for 30 minutes after eating to delay gastric emptying; and to take antispasmodics as prescribed.
Test-Taking Strategy: Eliminate options 1 and 4 first because these measures are comparable or alike and will promote gastric emptying. From the remaining options, select the measure that will delay gastric emptying.
Level of Cognitive Ability: Applying
Client Needs: Physiological Integrity
Integrated Process: Teaching and Learning
Content Area: Adult Health: Gastrointestinal
Health Problem: Adult Health: Gastrointestinal: Upper GI Disorders
Priority Concepts: Client Education; Nutrition
Reference: Lewis et al. (2017), pp. 917-918.

543. *Answer:* 1, 2, 5
Rationale: The client with acute pancreatitis normally is placed on NPO status to rest the pancreas and suppress gastrointestinal secretions, so adequate intravenous hydration is necessary. Because abdominal pain is a prominent symptom of pancreatitis, pain medications such as morphine or hydromorphone are prescribed. Meperidine is avoided, as it may cause seizures. Some clients experience lessened pain by assuming positions that flex the trunk, with the knees drawn up to the chest. A side-lying position with the head elevated 45 degrees decreases tension on the abdomen and may help ease the pain. The client is susceptible to respiratory infections because the retroperitoneal fluid raises the diaphragm, which causes the client to take shallow, guarded abdominal breaths. Therefore, measures such as turning, coughing, and deep breathing are instituted.
Test-Taking Strategy: Focus on the subject, care for the client with acute pancreatitis. Think about the pathophysiology associated with pancreatitis and note the word *acute*. This will assist in selecting the correct options.
Level of Cognitive Ability: Analyzing
Client Needs: Physiological Integrity
Integrated Process: Nursing Process—Analysis
Content Area: Adult Health: Gastrointestinal
Health Problem: Adult Health: Gastrointestinal: GI Accessory Organs
Priority Concepts: Pain; Inflammation
Reference: Lewis et al. (2017), pp. 1001-1002.

544. *Answer:* 1
Rationale: Crohn's disease is an inflammatory disease that can occur anywhere in the gastrointestinal tract but most often affects the terminal ileum and leads to thickening and scarring, a narrowed lumen, fistulas, ulcerations, and abscesses. It is characterized by exacerbations and remissions. If stress increases the symptoms of the disease, the client is taught stress management techniques and may require additional counseling. The client is taught to avoid gastrointestinal stimulants containing caffeine and to follow a high-calorie and high-protein diet. A low-fiber diet may be prescribed, especially during periods of exacerbation.
Test-Taking Strategy: Note the strategic words, *need for further instruction*. These words indicate a negative event query and ask you to select an option that is incorrect. Also, focus on the information in the question and that the question addresses exacerbation. Knowing that the client should consume a diet high in protein and calories and low in fiber will direct you to option 1. Options 2, 3, and 4 are correct statements.
Level of Cognitive Ability: Evaluating
Client Needs: Physiological Integrity
Integrated Process: Teaching and Learning
Content Area: Adult Health: Gastrointestinal
Health Problem: Adult Health: Gastrointestinal: Lower GI Disorders
Priority Concepts: Client Education; Elimination
Reference: Lewis et al. (2017), pp. 945-946.

545. *Answer:* 3

Rationale: Asterixis is irregular flapping movements of the fingers and wrists when the hands and arms are outstretched, with the palms down, wrists bent up, and fingers spread. Asterixis is the most common and reliable sign that hepatic encephalopathy is developing. Options 1, 2, and 4 are incorrect.

Test-Taking Strategy: Focus on the subject, the procedure for assessment of asterixis. Remember that asterixis is irregular flapping movements of the fingers and wrists. This will direct you to the correct option.

Level of Cognitive Ability: Applying

Client Needs: Health Promotion and Maintenance

Integrated Process: Nursing Process—Assessment

Content Area: Adult Health: Gastrointestinal

Health Problem: Adult Health: Gastrointestinal: GI Accessory Organs

Priority Concepts: Clinical Judgment; Inflammation

Reference: Ignatavicius, Workman, Rebar (2018), pp. 1173, 1378.

546. *Answer:* 3

Rationale: Cirrhosis is a chronic, progressive disease of the liver characterized by diffuse degeneration and destruction of hepatocytes. The serum ammonia level assesses the ability of the liver to deaminate protein byproducts. Normal reference interval is 10 to 80 mcg/dL (6 to 47 mcmol/L). Most of the ammonia in the body is found in the gastrointestinal tract. Protein provided by the diet is transported to the liver by the portal vein. The liver breaks down protein, which results in the formation of ammonia. Foods high in protein should be avoided since the client's ammonia level is elevated above the normal range; therefore, pasta with sauce would be the best selection.

Test-Taking Strategy: Focus on the subject, an ammonia level of 85 mcg/dL (51 mcmol/L). Realizing that this result is above the normal range will direct you away from selecting high-protein foods, such as pork, cheese, eggs, and fish.

Level of Cognitive Ability: Applying

Client Needs: Physiological Integrity

Integrated Process: Nursing Process—Planning

Content Area: Adult Health: Gastrointestinal

Health Problem: Adult Health: Gastrointestinal: GI Accessory Organs

Priority Concepts: Inflammation; Nutrition

Reference: Lewis et al. (2017), pp. 992-993, 995.

547. *Answer:* 3

Rationale: A frequent symptom of duodenal ulcer is pain that is relieved by food intake. These clients generally describe the pain as a burning, heavy, sharp, or "hungry" pain that often localizes in the midepigastric area. The client with duodenal ulcer usually does not experience weight loss or nausea and vomiting. These symptoms are more typical in the client with a gastric ulcer.

Test-Taking Strategy: Eliminate options 1 and 2 because they are comparable or alike; if the client is vomiting, weight loss will occur. Next, think about the symptoms of duodenal and gastric ulcer. Choose the correct option over option 4, knowing that the pain does not radiate down the right arm and that a pattern of pain-food-relief occurs with duodenal ulcer.

Level of Cognitive Ability: Analyzing

Client Needs: Physiological Integrity

Integrated Process: Nursing Process—Assessment

Content Area: Adult Health: Gastrointestinal

Health Problem: Adult Health: Gastrointestinal: Upper GI Disorders

Priority Concepts: Clinical Judgment; Inflammation

Reference: Heuther & McCance (2017), p. 916.

548. *Answer:* 1

Rationale: Hiatal hernia is caused by a protrusion of a portion of the stomach above the diaphragm where the esophagus usually is positioned. The client usually experiences pain from reflux caused by ingestion of irritating foods, lying flat following meals or at night, and eating large or fatty meals. Relief is obtained with the intake of small, frequent, and bland meals; use of H_2-receptor antagonists and antacids; and elevation of the thorax following meals and during sleep.

Test-Taking Strategy: Focus on the subject, the action contraindicated in hiatal hernia. Thinking about the pathophysiology that occurs in hiatal hernia will direct you to the correct option.

Level of Cognitive Ability: Analyzing

Client Needs: Physiological Integrity

Integrated Process: Teaching and Learning

Content Area: Adult Health: Gastrointestinal

Health Problem: Adult Health: Gastrointestinal: Upper GI Disorders

Priority Concepts: Client Education; Pain

Reference: Heuther & McCance (2017), pp. 911-912.

549. *Answer:* 2

Rationale: Ischemia of the stoma would be associated with a dusky or bluish or purple color. A beefy red and shiny stoma is normal and expected. Skin excoriation needs to be addressed and treated but does not require as immediate attention as purple discoloration of the stoma. Semiformed stool is a normal finding.

Test-Taking Strategy: Note the strategic word, *immediate,* and focus on the subject, the observation that requires primary health care provider notification. Note the words *purple discoloration* in option 2. Recall that purple indicates ischemia.

Level of Cognitive Ability: Analyzing

Client Needs: Physiological Integrity

Integrated Process: Nursing Process—Assessment

Content Area: Adult Health: Gastrointestinal

Health Problem: Adult Health: Gastrointestinal: Lower GI Disorders

Priority Concepts: Clinical Judgment; Tissue Integrity

Reference: Ignatavicius, Workman, Rebar (2018), p. 1132.

550. *Answer:* 1

Rationale: As peristalsis returns following creation of a colostomy, the client begins to pass malodorous flatus. This indicates returning bowel function and is an expected event. Within 72 hours of surgery, the client should begin passing stool via the colostomy. Options 2, 3, and 4 are incorrect interpretations.

Test-Taking Strategy: Focus on the subject, that the client is passing flatus from the stoma. Think about the normal functioning of the gastrointestinal tract and note the time frame in the question to assist in answering correctly.

Level of Cognitive Ability: Analyzing

Client Needs: Physiological Integrity

Integrated Process: Nursing Process—Assessment
Content Area: Adult Health: Gastrointestinal
Health Problem: Adult Health: Gastrointestinal: Lower GI Disorders
Priority Concepts: Clinical Judgment; Elimination
Reference: Lewis et al. (2017), p. 960.

551. *Answer:* 4
Rationale: A frequent complication that occurs following ileostomy is fluid and electrolyte imbalance. The client requires constant monitoring of intake and output to prevent this from occurring. Losses require replacement by intravenous infusion until the client can tolerate a diet orally. Intestinal obstruction is a less frequent complication. Fat malabsorption and folate deficiency are complications that could occur later in the postoperative period.
Test-Taking Strategy: Note the strategic word, *most.* Also note the subject, an ileostomy. Remember that ileostomy drainage is liquid, placing the client at risk for fluid and electrolyte imbalance.
Level of Cognitive Ability: Analyzing
Client Needs: Physiological Integrity
Integrated Process: Nursing Process—Assessment
Content Area: Adult Health: Gastrointestinal
Health Problem: Adult Health: Gastrointestinal: Lower GI Disorders
Priority Concepts: Clinical Judgment; Elimination
Reference: Lewis et al. (2017), p. 962.

552. *Answer:* 1
Rationale: IBS is a functional gastrointestinal disorder that causes chronic or recurrent diarrhea, constipation, and/or abdominal pain and bloating. Dietary fiber and bulk help produce bulky, soft stools and establish regular bowel elimination habits. Therefore, the client should consume a high-fiber diet. Eating regular meals, drinking 8 to 10 cups of liquid a day, and chewing food slowly help promote normal bowel function. Medication therapy depends on the main symptoms of IBS. Bulk-forming laxatives or antidiarrheal agents or other agents may be prescribed.
Test-Taking Strategy: Note the strategic words, *need for further teaching.* These words indicate a negative event query and the need to select the incorrect client statement. Think about the pathophysiology associated with IBS to answer correctly. Also, note the word *limit* in option 1. With IBS, dietary fiber and bulk is important to assist in controlling symptoms.
Level of Cognitive Ability: Evaluating
Client Needs: Physiological Integrity
Integrated Process: Teaching and Learning
Content Area: Adult Health: Gastrointestinal
Health Problem: Adult Health: Gastrointestinal: Lower GI Disorders
Priority Concepts: Client Education; Inflammation
Reference: Lewis et al. (2017), pp. 946, 949.

553. *Answer:* 1
Rationale: Early manifestations of dumping syndrome occur 5 to 30 minutes after eating. Symptoms include vertigo, tachycardia, syncope, sweating, pallor, palpitations, and the desire to lie down.
Test-Taking Strategy: Note the strategic word, *early.* Think about the pathophysiology associated with dumping syndrome and its etiology to answer correctly.
Level of Cognitive Ability: Analyzing
Client Needs: Physiological Integrity
Integrated Process: Nursing Process—Assessment
Content Area: Adult Health: Gastrointestinal
Health Problem: Adult Health: Gastrointestinal: Upper GI Disorders
Priority Concepts: Elimination; Nutrition
Reference: Ignatavicius, Workman, Rebar (2018), pp. 1117-1118.

CHAPTER 49

Gastrointestinal Medications

PRIORITY CONCEPTS Inflammation; Tissue Integrity

I. Antacids (Table 49-1; Fig. 49-1)

A. React with gastric acid to produce neutral salts or salts of low acidity
B. Inactivate pepsin and enhance mucosal protection but do not coat the ulcer crater
C. These medications are used for peptic ulcer disease and gastroesophageal reflux disease.
D. These medications should be taken on a regular schedule; some are prescribed to be taken 1 and 3 hours after each meal and at bedtime.
E. To provide maximum benefit, treatment should elevate the gastric pH above 5.
F. Antacid tablets should be chewed thoroughly and followed with a glass of water or milk.
G. Liquid preparations should be shaken before dispensing.

! To prevent interactions with other medications and interference with the action of other medications, allow 1 hour between antacid administration and the administration of other medications.

II. Gastric Protectants

A. Misoprostol
  1. An antisecretory medication that enhances mucosal defenses
  2. Suppresses secretion of gastric acid and maintains submucosal blood flow by promoting vasodilation
  3. Used to prevent gastric ulcers caused by nonsteroidal antiinflammatory drugs and aspirin
  4. Administered with meals
  5. Causes diarrhea and abdominal pain
  6. Contraindicated for use in pregnancy
B. Sucralfate
  1. Creates a protective barrier against acid and pepsin
  2. Administered orally; should be taken on an empty stomach
  3. May cause constipation
  4. May impede absorption of warfarin sodium, phenytoin, theophylline, digoxin, and some antibiotics; should be administered at least 2 hours apart from these medications

III. Histamine (H_2)-Receptor Antagonists

A. Description
  1. Suppress secretion of gastric acid
  2. Alleviate symptoms of heartburn and assist in preventing complications of peptic ulcer disease
  3. Prevent stress ulcers and reduce the recurrence of all ulcers
  4. Promote healing in gastroesophageal reflux disease
  5. Are contraindicated in hypersensitive clients
  6. Should be used with caution in clients with impaired renal or hepatic function
B. Cimetidine
  1. Can be administered orally, intramuscularly, or intravenously
  2. Food reduces the rate of absorption; if taken orally with meals, absorption will be slowed.
  3. Intravenous administration can cause hypotension and dysrhythmias.
  4. Antacids can decrease the absorption of oral cimetidine.
  5. Cimetidine and antacids should be administered at least 1 hour apart from each other.
  6. Cimetidine passes the blood–brain barrier, and central nervous system side and adverse effects can occur; it may cause mental confusion, agitation, psychosis, depression, anxiety, and disorientation.
  7. Dosage should be reduced in clients with renal impairment.
  8. Cimetidine inhibits hepatic drug-metabolizing enzymes and can cause many medication levels to rise; if administered with warfarin sodium, phenytoin, theophylline, or lidocaine, the dosages of these medications should be reduced.

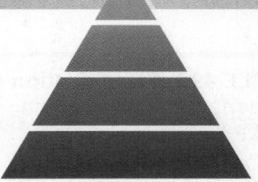

TABLE 49-1 Classification of Antacids and Considerations

Classification	Considerations
Aluminum compounds	Aluminum hydroxide is used to treat hyperphosphatemia; therefore, it can cause hypophosphatemia Aluminum hydroxide can reduce the effects of tetracyclines, warfarin sodium, and digoxin and can reduce phosphate absorption and thereby cause hypophosphatemia Aluminum compounds contain significant amounts of sodium; they should be used with caution in clients with hypertension and heart failure The most common side effect is constipation
Magnesium compounds	Magnesium hydroxide is also a saline laxative, and the most prominent side effect is diarrhea; it is usually administered in combination with aluminum hydroxide, an antacid that assists in preventing diarrhea. Magnesium compounds are contraindicated in clients with intestinal obstruction, appendicitis, or undiagnosed abdominal pain. In clients with renal impairment, magnesium can accumulate to high levels, causing signs of toxicity.
Calcium compounds	Calcium carbonate can cause acid rebound. Calcium compounds are rapid acting and release carbon dioxide in the stomach, causing belching and flatulence. A common side effect is constipation. Milk-alkali syndrome (headache, urinary frequency, anorexia, nausea/vomiting, fatigue) can occur (the client should avoid milk products and vitamin D supplements)
Sodium bicarbonate	Sodium bicarbonate has a rapid onset, liberates carbon dioxide, increases intra-abdominal pressure, and promotes flatulence. Sodium bicarbonate should be used with caution in clients with hypertension and heart failure. Sodium bicarbonate can cause systemic alkalosis in clients with renal impairment. Sodium bicarbonate is useful for treating acidosis and elevating urinary pH to promote excretion of acidic medications following overdose.

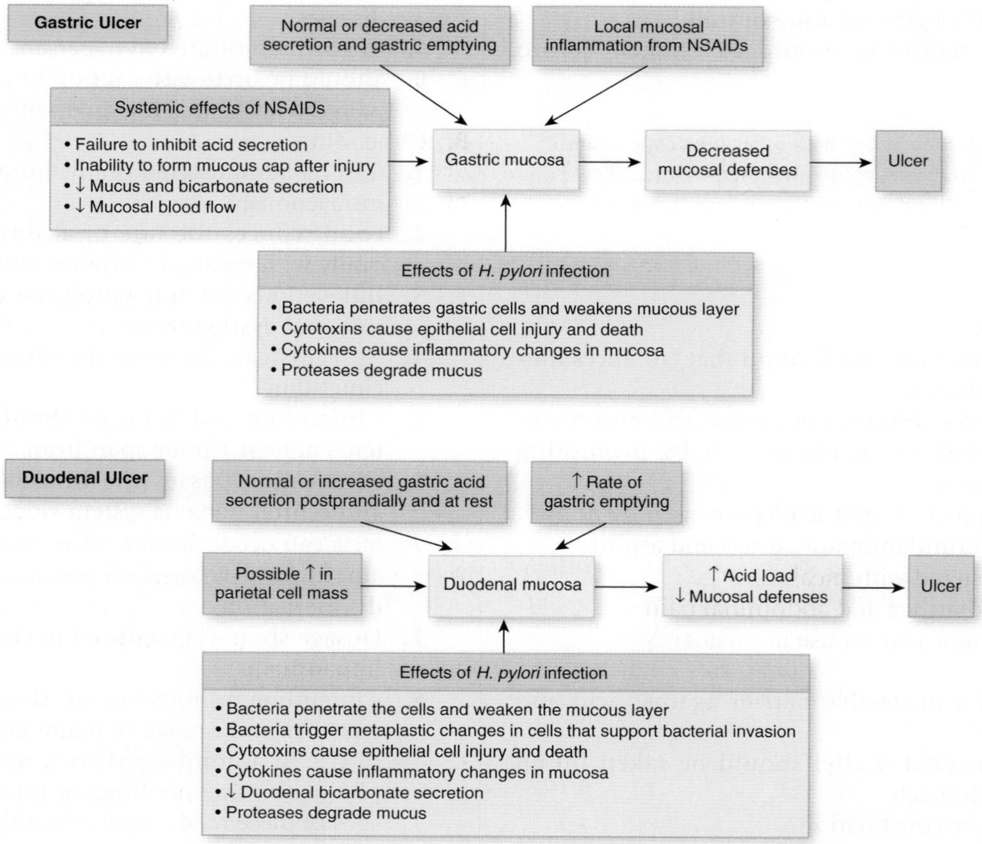

FIG. 49-1 Pathophysiological components of peptic ulcer. *H. pylori, Helicobacter pylori; NSAIDs,* nonsteroidal antiinflammatory drugs.

C. Ranitidine
   1. Can be administered orally, intramuscularly, or intravenously
   2. Side effects are uncommon, and it does not penetrate the blood–brain barrier as cimetidine does.
   3. Ranitidine is not affected by food.

D. Famotidine and nizatidine
   1. Famotidine and nizatidine are similar to ranitidine and cimetidine.
   2. These medications do not need to be administered with food.

IV. Proton Pump Inhibitors (Box 49-1)

A. Suppress gastric acid secretion
B. Used to treat active ulcer disease, erosive esophagitis, and pathological hypersecretory conditions
C. Contraindicated in hypersensitivity
D. Common side effects include headache, diarrhea, abdominal pain, and nausea.

V. Medication Regimens to Treat *Helicobacter pylori* Infections (Box 49-2)

A. An antibacterial agent alone is not effective for eradicating *H. pylori*, because the bacterium readily becomes resistant to the agent.
B. Triple or quadruple therapy with a variety of medication combinations is used (if triple therapy fails, quadruple therapy is recommended).

VI. Prokinetic Agent

A. Medication: Metoclopramide
B. Stimulates motility of the upper gastrointestinal tract and increases the rate of gastric emptying without stimulating gastric, biliary, or pancreatic secretions
C. Used to treat gastroesophageal reflux and paralytic ileus
D. May cause restlessness, drowsiness, extrapyramidal reactions, dizziness, insomnia, and headache
E. Usually administered 30 minutes before meals and at bedtime
F. Contraindicated in clients with sensitivity and in clients with mechanical obstruction, perforation, or gastrointestinal hemorrhage
G. Can precipitate hypertensive crisis in clients with pheochromocytoma
H. Safety in pregnancy has not been established
I. Metoclopramide can cause parkinsonian reactions; if this occurs, the medication will be discontinued by the health care provider.
J. Anticholinergics, such as atropine, and opioid analgesics, such as morphine, antagonize the effects of metoclopramide.
K. Alcohol, sedatives, cyclosporine, and tranquilizers produce an additive effect.

BOX 49-1 Proton Pump Inhibitors

- Esomeprazole
- Dexlansoprazole
- Lansoprazole
- Omeprazole
- Pantoprazole
- Rabeprazole

BOX 49-2 Medication Regimens to Treat *Helicobacter pylori* Infections

Triple Therapy
- Esomeprazole, amoxicillin, clarithromycin
- Lansoprazole, amoxicillin, clarithromycin
- Esomeprazole, metronidazole, clarithromycin

Quadruple Therapies
- Esomeprazole, metronidazole, tetracycline, bismuth subsalicylate

Note: Additional medications may be prescribed for each level of therapy.

VII. Bile Acid Sequestrants (Box 49-3)

A. Act by absorbing and combining with intestinal bile salts, which then are secreted in the feces, preventing intestinal reabsorption
B. Used to treat hypercholesterolemia in adults, biliary obstruction, and pruritus associated with biliary disease
C. With powdered forms, taste and palatability are often reasons for noncompliance and can be improved by the use of flavored products or mixing the medication with various juices.
D. Side and adverse effects include nausea, bloating, constipation, fecal impaction, and intestinal obstruction.
E. Stool softeners and other sources of fiber can be used to abate the gastrointestinal side effects.

Bile acid sequestrants should be used cautiously in clients with suspected bowel obstruction or severe constipation because they can worsen these conditions.

VIII. Treating Hepatic Encephalopathy

A. Medication: Lactulose
B. Used in the prevention and treatment of portal systemic encephalopathy, including hepatic precoma and coma; also used in the treatment of chronic constipation

BOX 49-3 Bile Acid Sequestrants

- Colesevelam
- Colestipol
- Cholestyramine

C. Promotes increased peristalsis and bowel evacuation, expelling ammonia from the colon and thus lowering the ammonia level (normal ammonia reference interval is 10 to 80 mcg/dL [6 to 47 mcmol/L])
D. Improves protein tolerance in clients with advanced hepatic cirrhosis
E. Administered orally in the form of a syrup or rectally

IX. Pancreatic Enzyme Replacements

A. Pancrelipase
B. Used to supplement or replace pancreatic enzymes and thus improve nutritional status and reduce the amount of fatty stools (a deficiency of pancreatic enzymes can compromise digestion, especially the digestion of fats)
C. Should be taken with all meals and snacks
D. Side and adverse effects include abdominal cramps or pain, nausea, vomiting, and diarrhea.
E. Products that contain calcium carbonate or magnesium hydroxide interfere with the action of these medications.

X. Treatment for Inflammatory Bowel Disease (Box 49-4)

A. Inflammatory bowel disease has 2 forms, Crohn's disease and ulcerative colitis.
B. Antimicrobials: May be prescribed to prevent or treat secondary infection (see Chapter 63 for information on antimicrobials)
C. 5-Aminosalicylates (5-ASAs): Decrease gastrointestinal inflammation; side and adverse effects include nausea, rash, arthralgia, and hematological disorders.
D. Corticosteroids: Act as an antiinflammatory to decrease gastrointestinal inflammation (see Chapter 47 for information on glucocorticoids and corticosteroids)
E. Immunomodulators: Monoclonal antibodies modulate the immune response to induce and maintain remission (see Box 49-4 for specific immunomodulators).

BOX 49-4 Medications to Treat Inflammatory Bowel Disease

Antimicrobials
- Ciprofloxacin
- Metronidazole
- Rifaximin
- Clarithromycin

5-Aminosalicylates
- Balsalazide
- Mesalamine
- Olsalazine
- Sulfasalazine

Corticosteroids
- Budesonide
- Prednisone
- Hydrocortisone

Immunosuppressants
- Azathioprine
- Cyclosporine
- Mercaptopurine
- Tacrolimus

Immunomodulators
- Adalimumab
- Certolizumab
- Infliximab
- Natalizumab

XI. Treatment for Irritable Bowel Syndrome (IBS)

A. Irritable bowel syndrome is a gastrointestinal disorder that is characterized by crampy abdominal pain accompanied by diarrhea, constipation, or both.
B. Pharmacological treatment depends on the main symptom, constipation or diarrhea.
C. Constipation-predominant IBS (IBS-C) treatment
   1. Bulk-forming laxatives, usually taken at mealtimes with a full glass of water.
   2. Lubiprostone: Chloride channel activator that increases fluid in the intestines to promote bowel elimination; needs to be taken with food and water.
   3. Linaclotide: Stimulates receptors in the intestines to promote bowel transit time; taken daily 30 minutes before breakfast.
   4. See Box 49-6 for a list of additional medications to treat constipation.
D. Diarrhea-predominant IBS (IBS-D) treatment
   1. Alosetron
      a. A selective serotonin receptor antagonist
      b. Can cause adverse effects such as constipation, impaction, bowel obstruction, perforation of the bowel, and ischemic colitis.
      c. A strict risk management procedure must be followed, including monitoring for serious adverse effects, reporting them, and immediate discontinuation of the medication if they arise.
   2. Antidiarrheal medications: See Box 49-7 for a list of additional medications to treat diarrhea.

XII. Antiemetics (Box 49-5)

A. Medications used to control vomiting and motion sickness
B. The choice of the antiemetic is determined by the cause of the nausea and vomiting.
C. Monitor vital signs and intake and output and for signs of dehydration and fluid and electrolyte imbalances.
D. Limit odors in the client's room when the client is nauseated or vomiting.
E. Limit oral intake to clear liquids when the client is nauseated or vomiting.

Antiemetics can cause drowsiness; therefore, a priority intervention is to protect the client from injury.

XIII. Laxatives (see Box 49-6)

A. Bulk-forming
   1. Description
      a. Absorb water into the feces and increase bulk to produce large and soft stools

BOX 49-5 Commonly Administered Antiemetics

Serotonin Antagonists
- Dolasetron
- Granisetron
- Ondansetron

Glucocorticoids
- Dexamethasone
- Methylprednisolone

Substance P/Neurokinin-1 Antagonists
- Aprepitant
- Fosaprepitant
- Rolapitant

Benzodiazepine
- Lorazepam

Dopamine Antagonists

Phenothiazines
- Chlorpromazine
- Perphenazine
- Prochlorperazine
- Promethazine

Butyrophenones
- Haloperidol
- Droperidol

Others
- Metoclopramide
- Trimethobenzamide

Cannabinoids
- Dronabinol
- Nabilone

Anticholinergics
- Scopolamine transdermal

Antihistamines
- Cyclizine
- Dimenhydrinate
- Diphenhydramine
- Hydroxyzine
- Meclizine hydrochloride

BOX 49-6 Laxatives

Bulk-Forming
- Methylcellulose
- Polycarbophil
- Psyllium

Stimulants
- Bisacodyl
- Senna

Emollient
- Docusate sodium

Osmotics
- Magnesium hydroxide
- Magnesium citrate
- Sodium phosphates
- Polyethylene glycol and electrolytes
- Lactulose

BOX 49-7 Medications to Control Diarrhea

Opioids and Related Medications
- Diphenoxylate with atropine sulfate
- Loperamide

Other Antidiarrheals
- Bismuth subsalicylate
- Bulk-forming medications
- Anticholinergic antispasmodics: dicyclomine, glycopyrrolate

b. Contraindicated in bowel obstruction
c. Dependency can occur with long-term use.

2. Side and adverse effects include gastrointestinal disturbances, dehydration, and electrolyte imbalances.

B. Stimulants: Stimulate motility of large intestine

C. Emollients
1. Inhibit absorption of water so fecal mass remains large and soft
2. Used to avoid straining

D. Osmotics: Attract water into the large intestine to produce bulk and stimulate peristalsis

⚠ The client receiving a laxative needs to increase fluid intake to prevent dehydration.

XIV. Medications to Control Diarrhea (see Box 49-7)

A. Identify and treat the underlying cause, treat dehydration, replace fluids and electrolytes, relieve abdominal discomfort and cramping, and reduce the passage of stool

B. Opioids
1. Opioids are effective antidiarrheal medications that decrease intestinal motility and peristalsis.
2. When poisons, infections, or bacterial toxins are the cause of the diarrhea, opioids worsen the condition by delaying the elimination of toxins.

PRACTICE QUESTIONS

554. A client with Crohn's disease is scheduled to receive an infusion of infliximab. What intervention by the nurse will determine the **effectiveness** of treatment?
1. Monitoring the leukocyte count for 2 days after the infusion
2. Checking the frequency and consistency of bowel movements
3. Checking serum liver enzyme levels before and after the infusion
4. Carrying out a Hematest on gastric fluids after the infusion is completed

555. A client has an as needed prescription for loperamide hydrochloride. For which condition should the nurse administer this medication?
1. Constipation
2. Abdominal pain
3. An episode of diarrhea
4. Hematest-positive nasogastric tube drainage

556. A client has an as-needed prescription for ondansetron. For which condition(s) should the nurse administer this medication?
1. Paralytic ileus
2. Incisional pain
3. Urinary retention
4. Nausea and vomiting

557. A client has begun medication therapy with pancrelipase. The nurse evaluates that the medication is having the optimal intended benefit if which effect is observed?
1. Weight loss
2. Relief of heartburn
3. Reduction of steatorrhea
4. Absence of abdominal pain

558. An older client recently has been taking cimetidine. The nurse monitors the client for which **most** frequent central nervous system side effect of this medication?
1. Tremors
2. Dizziness
3. Confusion
4. Hallucinations

559. A client with a gastric ulcer has a prescription for sucralfate 1 gram by mouth 4 times daily. The nurse should schedule the medication for which times?
1. With meals and at bedtime
2. Every 6 hours around the clock
3. One hour after meals and at bedtime
4. One hour before meals and at bedtime

560. A client who uses nonsteroidal antiinflammatory drugs (NSAIDs) has been taking misoprostol. The nurse determines that the misoprostol is having the intended therapeutic effect if which finding is noted?
1. Resolved diarrhea
2. Relief of epigastric pain
3. Decreased platelet count
4. Decreased white blood cell count

561. A client has been taking omeprazole for 4 weeks. The ambulatory care nurse evaluates that the client is receiving the optimal intended effect of the medication if the client reports the absence of which symptom?
1. Diarrhea
2. Heartburn
3. Flatulence
4. Constipation

562. A client with a peptic ulcer is diagnosed with a *Helicobacter pylori* infection. The nurse is teaching the client about the medications prescribed, including clarithromycin, esomeprazole, and amoxicillin. Which statement by the client indicates the **best** understanding of the medication regimen?
1. "My ulcer will heal because these medications will kill the bacteria."
2. "These medications are only taken when I have pain from my ulcer."
3. "The medications will kill the bacteria and stop the acid production."
4. "These medications will coat the ulcer and decrease the acid production in my stomach."

563. A client has a new prescription for metoclopramide. On review of the chart, the nurse identifies that this medication can be safely administered with which condition?
1. Intestinal obstruction
2. Peptic ulcer with melena
3. Diverticulitis with perforation
4. Vomiting following cancer chemotherapy

564. The nurse determines the client **needs further instruction** on cimetidine if which statements were made? **Select all that apply.**
- ☐ 1. "I will take the cimetidine with my meals."
- ☐ 2. "I'll know the medication is working if my diarrhea stops."
- ☐ 3. "My episodes of heartburn will decrease if the medication is effective."
- ☐ 4. "Taking the cimetidine with an antacid will increase its effectiveness."
- ☐ 5. "I will notify my primary health care provider if I become depressed or anxious."
- ☐ 6. "Some of my blood levels will need to be monitored closely since I also take warfarin for atrial fibrillation."

565. The nurse has given instructions to a client who has just been prescribed cholestyramine. Which statement by the client indicates a **need for further instruction**?
1. "I will continue taking vitamin supplements."
2. "This medication will help lower my cholesterol."
3. "This medication should only be taken with water."
4. "A high-fiber diet is important while taking this medication."

ANSWERS

554. *Answer:* 2

Rationale: The principal manifestations of Crohn's disease are diarrhea and abdominal pain. Infliximab is an immunomodulator that reduces the degree of inflammation in the colon, thereby reducing the diarrhea. Options 1, 3, and 4 are unrelated to this medication.

Test-Taking Strategy: Focus on the **subject**, treatment for Crohn's disease, and note the **strategic word**, *effectiveness*. Eliminate option 4, because gastric bleeding is not a characteristic of Crohn's disease. Monitoring the leukocyte count and liver enzyme levels is appropriate when infliximab is given but not to evaluate the effectiveness of treatment, eliminating options 1 and 3.

Level of Cognitive Ability: Evaluating
Client Needs: Physiological Integrity
Integrated Process: Nursing Process—Evaluation
Content Area: Pharmacology: Immune Medications: Immunosuppressants

Health Problem: Adult Health: Gastrointestinal: Lower GI disorders
Priority Concepts: Evidence; Immunity
Reference: Ignatavicius, Workman, Rebar (2018), pp. 1159-1160.

555. *Answer:* 3
Rationale: Loperamide is an antidiarrheal agent. It is used to manage acute and chronic diarrhea in conditions such as inflammatory bowel disease. Loperamide also can be used to reduce the volume of drainage from an ileostomy. It is not used for the conditions in options 1, 2, and 4.
Test-Taking Strategy: Focus on the subject, the action of loperamide. Recalling that this medication is an antidiarrheal agent will direct you to the correct option.
Level of Cognitive Ability: Applying
Client Needs: Physiological Integrity
Integrated Process: Nursing Process—Implementation
Content Area: Pharmacology: Gastrointestinal Medications: Antidiarrheals
Health Problem: Adult Health: Gastrointestinal: Lower GI disorders
Priority Concepts: Clinical Judgment; Elimination
Reference: Lewis et al. (2017), pp. 931-932.

556. *Answer:* 4
Rationale: Ondansetron is an antiemetic used to treat postoperative nausea and vomiting, as well as nausea and vomiting associated with chemotherapy. The other options are incorrect reasons for administering this medication.
Test-Taking Strategy: Focus on the subject, the action of ondansetron. Recalling that this medication is an antiemetic will direct you to the correct option.
Level of Cognitive Ability: Applying
Client Needs: Physiological Integrity
Integrated Process: Nursing Process—Implementation
Content Area: Pharmacology: Gastrointestinal Medications: Antiemetics
Health Problem: Adult Health: Gastrointestinal: Upper GI disorders
Priority Concepts: Clinical Judgment; Fluids and Electrolytes
Reference: Lewis et al. (2017), p. 895.

557. *Answer:* 3
Rationale: Pancrelipase is a pancreatic enzyme used in clients with pancreatitis as a digestive aid. The medication should reduce the amount of fatty stools (steatorrhea). Another intended effect could be improved nutritional status. It is not used to treat abdominal pain or heartburn. Its use could result in weight gain but should not result in weight loss if it is aiding in digestion.
Test-Taking Strategy: Focus on the subject, intended benefit of the medication and on the name of the medication. Use knowledge of physiology of the pancreas and the function of pancreatic enzymes to assist in directing you to the correct option.
Level of Cognitive Ability: Evaluating
Client Needs: Physiological Integrity
Integrated Process: Nursing Process—Evaluation
Content Area: Pharmacology: Gastrointestinal Medications: Pancreatic enzymes
Health Problem: Adult Health: Gastrointestinal: GI Accessory organs
Priority Concepts: Elimination; Inflammation
Reference: Hodgson, Kizior (2018), pp. 894-895.

558. *Answer:* 3
Rationale: Cimetidine is a histamine (H_2)-receptor antagonist. Older clients are especially susceptible to central nervous system side effects of cimetidine. The most frequent of these is confusion. Less common central nervous system side effects include headache, dizziness, drowsiness, and hallucinations.
Test-Taking Strategy: Note the strategic word, *most.* Use knowledge of the older client and medication effects to direct you to the correct option.
Level of Cognitive Ability: Analyzing
Client Needs: Physiological Integrity
Integrated Process: Nursing Process—Assessment
Content Area: Pharmacology: Gastrointestinal Medications: Histamine (H_2)-receptor antagonists
Health Problem: Adult Health: Gastrointestinal: Upper GI disorders
Priority Concepts: Clinical Judgment; Safety
Reference: Lewis et al. (2017), p. 903.

559. *Answer:* 4
Rationale: Sucralfate is a gastric protectant. The medication should be scheduled for administration 1 hour before meals and at bedtime. The medication is timed to allow it to form a protective coating over the ulcer before food intake stimulates gastric acid production and mechanical irritation. The other options are incorrect.
Test-Taking Strategy: Focus on the subject, times to administer sucralfate. Note the client's diagnosis and think about the pathophysiology associated with a gastric ulcer to assist in directing you to the correct option.
Level of Cognitive Ability: Applying
Client Needs: Physiological Integrity
Integrated Process: Nursing Process—Planning
Content Area: Pharmacology: Gastrointestinal Medications: Gastric protectants
Health Problem: Adult Health: Gastrointestinal: Upper GI disorders
Priority Concepts: Clinical Judgment; Tissue Integrity
Reference: Ignatavicius, Workman, Rebar (2018), p. 1112.

560. *Answer:* 2
Rationale: The client who uses NSAIDs is prone to gastric mucosal injury. Misoprostol is a gastric protectant and is given specifically to prevent this occurrence in clients taking NSAIDs frequently. Diarrhea can be a side effect of the medication but is not an intended effect. Options 3 and 4 are unrelated to the purpose of misoprostol.
Test-Taking Strategy: Focus on the subject, the intended therapeutic effect of misoprostol for a client who chronically uses NSAIDs. This indicates that the medication is being given to prevent the occurrence of specific symptoms. Recalling that NSAIDs can cause gastric mucosal injury will direct you to the correct option.
Level of Cognitive Ability: Evaluating
Client Needs: Physiological Integrity
Integrated Process: Nursing Process—Evaluation
Content Area: Pharmacology: Gastrointestinal Medications: Gastric protectants
Health Problem: Adult Health: Gastrointestinal: Upper GI disorders
Priority Concepts: Evidence; Tissue Integrity
Reference: Lewis et al. (2017), pp. 903, 914.

561. *Answer:* 2

Rationale: Omeprazole is a proton pump inhibitor classified as an antiulcer agent. The intended effect of the medication is relief of pain from gastric irritation, often called *heartburn* by clients. Omeprazole is not used to treat the conditions identified in options 1, 3, and 4.

Test-Taking Strategy: Focus on the **subject**, the optimal intended effect of omeprazole. Recalling that this medication is a proton pump inhibitor will direct you to the correct option.

Level of Cognitive Ability: Evaluating

Client Needs: Physiological Integrity

Integrated Process: Nursing Process—Evaluation

Content Area: Pharmacology: Gastrointestinal Medications: Proton pump inhibitors

Health Problem: Adult Health: Gastrointestinal: Upper GI disorders

Priority Concepts: Evidence; Tissue Integrity

Reference: Skidmore-Roth (2017), pp. 880-881.

562. *Answer:* 3

Rationale: Triple therapy for *H. pylori* infection usually includes 2 antibacterial medications and a proton pump inhibitor. Clarithromycin and amoxicillin are antibacterials. Esomeprazole is a proton pump inhibitor. These medications will kill the bacteria and decrease acid production.

Test-Taking Strategy: Focus on the **subject**, the medications and their actions, and note the **strategic word**, *best*. Eliminate option 1 because the medications do more than kill the bacteria. These medications are taken not only when there is pain but continually until gone, usually for 1 to 2 weeks. This will eliminate option 2. These medications do not coat the ulcer, eliminating option 4.

Level of Cognitive Ability: Evaluating

Client Needs: Physiological Integrity

Integrated Process: Nursing Process—Evaluation

Content Area: Pharmacology: Gastrointestinal Medications: Helicobacter pylori infection medications

Health Problem: Adult Health: Gastrointestinal: Upper GI disorders

Priority Concepts: Client Education; Infection

Reference: Lewis et al. (2017), pp. 911-912.

563. *Answer:* 4

Rationale: Metoclopramide is a gastrointestinal stimulant and antiemetic. Because it is a gastrointestinal stimulant, it is contraindicated with gastrointestinal obstruction, hemorrhage, or perforation. It is used in the treatment of vomiting after surgery, chemotherapy, or radiation.

Test-Taking Strategy: Focus on the **subject**, safe use of metoclopramide. Recalling the classification and action of this medication and that it is an antiemetic will direct you to the correct option.

Level of Cognitive Ability: Analyzing

Client Needs: Physiological Integrity

Integrated Process: Nursing Process—Implementation

Content Area: Pharmacology: Gastrointestinal Medications: Antiemetics

Health Problem: Adult Health—Gastrointestinal: Upper GI disorders

Priority Concepts: Clinical Judgment; Safety

Reference: Skidmore-Roth (2017), pp. 776-777.

564. *Answer:* 1, 2, 4

Rationale: Cimetidine, a histamine (H_2)-receptor antagonist, helps alleviate the symptom of heartburn, not diarrhea. Because cimetidine crosses the blood–brain barrier, central nervous system side and adverse effects, such as mental confusion, agitation, depression, and anxiety, can occur. Food reduces the rate of absorption, so if cimetidine is taken with meals, absorption will be slowed. Antacids decrease the absorption of cimetidine and should be taken at least 1 hour apart. If cimetidine is concomitantly administered with warfarin therapy, warfarin doses may need to be reduced, so prothrombin and international normalized ratio results must be followed.

Test-Taking Strategy: Note the **strategic words**, *needs further instruction*. These words indicate a **negative event query** and ask you to select the options that are incorrect statements. Think about the therapeutic effect, adverse effects, and potential medication interactions to direct you to the correct options.

Level of Cognitive Ability: Evaluating

Client Needs: Physiological Integrity

Integrated Process: Teaching and Learning

Content Area: Pharmacology: Gastrointestinal Medications: Histamine (H_2)-receptor antagonists

Health Problem: Adult Health: Gastrointestinal: Upper GI disorders

Priority Concepts: Client Education; Safety

Reference: Hodgson, Kizior (2018), pp. 244-245.

565. *Answer:* 3

Rationale: Cholestyramine is a bile acid sequestrant used to lower the cholesterol level, and client compliance is a problem because of its taste and palatability. The use of flavored products or fruit juices can improve the taste. Some side effects of bile acid sequestrants include constipation and decreased vitamin absorption.

Test-Taking Strategy: Note the **strategic words**, *need for further instruction*. These words indicate a **negative event query** and ask you to select an option that is an incorrect statement. Note the **closed-ended word** "only" in the correct option.

Level of Cognitive Ability: Evaluating

Client Needs: Physiological Integrity

Integrated Process: Teaching and Learning

Content Area: Pharmacology: Gastrointestinal Medications: Bile acid sequestrants

Health Problem: Adult Health: Gastrointestinal: GI Accessory organs

Priority Concepts: Client Education; Safety

Reference: Lewis et al. (2017), p. 711.

UNIT XI

Respiratory Problems of the Adult Client

Pyramid to Success

The Pyramid to Success focuses on infectious diseases, particularly tuberculosis, and respiratory care in relation to respiratory problems. Pyramid Points focus on the client with pneumonia, respiratory failure, chronic obstructive pulmonary disease, pneumothorax, influenza, and tuberculosis. The Pyramid to Success includes the care of the client with tuberculosis, especially regarding the importance of the medication regimen, providing adequate nutrition and adequate rest to promote the healing process, and prevention of transmission and progression of the disease. Focus on assisting the client to cope with the social isolation issues that exist during the period of illness and on teaching the client and family the critical measures of screening, preventing respiratory disease, and the transmission of infectious airborne disease. Another important area to consider is caring for a client with an acute pulmonary process such as pulmonary embolism.

Client Needs: Learning Objectives

Safe and Effective Care Environment

Collaborating with the interprofessional team in the management of the respiratory problem
Discussing consultations and referrals related to the respiratory problem
Ensuring that informed consent related to invasive procedures has been obtained
Establishing priorities
Handling infectious materials such as sputum or body fluids safely
Maintaining confidentiality related to the respiratory disorder
Maintaining respiratory precautions, standard precautions, and other precautions

Health Promotion and Maintenance

Educating the client about adequate fluid and nutritional intake
Educating the client about breathing exercises and respiratory therapy and care
Educating the client about medication administration
Educating the client about the need for follow-up care
Educating the client about the prevention of transmission of infection
Informing the client about health promotion programs
Performing respiratory assessment techniques
Preventing respiratory problems and infectious diseases
Providing health screening related to risks for respiratory problems

Psychosocial Integrity

Considering religious, cultural, and spiritual influences when providing care
Discussing body image changes related to respiratory problems
Discussing end-of-life and grief and loss issues
Discussing situational role changes
Identifying coping strategies
Identifying support systems and community resources

Physiological Integrity

Administering medications
Managing respiratory illnesses
Monitoring for acid-base imbalances
Monitoring for alterations in body systems
Monitoring for infectious diseases
Providing nutrition and oral hygiene
Providing personal hygiene and promoting rest and sleep
Providing comfort

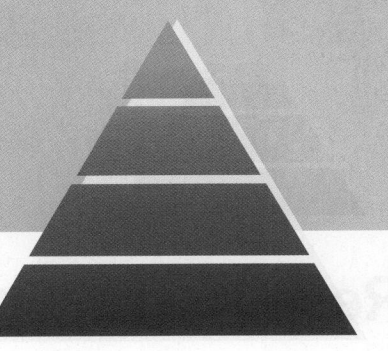

CHAPTER 50

Respiratory Problems

PRIORITY CONCEPTS **Gas Exchange; Perfusion**

I. Anatomy and Physiology

A. Primary functions of the respiratory system
   1. Provides oxygen for metabolism in the tissues
   2. Removes carbon dioxide, the waste product of metabolism

B. Secondary functions of the respiratory system
   1. Facilitates sense of smell
   2. Produces speech
   3. Maintains acid–base balance
   4. Maintains body water levels
   5. Maintains heat balance

C. Upper respiratory airway
   1. Nose: Humidifies, warms, and filters inspired air
   2. Sinuses: Air-filled cavities within the hollow bones that surround the nasal passages and provide resonance during speech
   3. Pharynx
      a. Passageway for the respiratory and digestive tracts located behind the oral and nasal cavities
      b. Divided into the nasopharynx, oropharynx, and laryngopharynx
   4. Larynx
      a. Located just below the pharynx at the root of the tongue; commonly called the *voice box*
      b. Contains 2 pairs of vocal cords, the false and true cords
      c. The opening between the true vocal cords is the glottis. The glottis plays an important role in coughing, which is the most fundamental defense mechanism of the lungs.
   5. Epiglottis
      a. Leaf-shaped elastic flap structure at the top of the larynx
      b. Prevents food from entering the tracheobronchial tree by closing over the glottis during swallowing

D. Lower respiratory airway
   1. Trachea: Located in front of the esophagus; branches into the right and left mainstem bronchi at the carina
   2. Mainstem bronchi
      a. Begin at the carina
      b. The right bronchus is slightly wider, shorter, and more vertical than the left bronchus.
      c. Divide into secondary or lobar bronchi that enter each of the 5 lobes of the lung
      d. The bronchi are lined with cilia, which propel mucus up and away from the lower airway to the trachea, where it can be expectorated or swallowed.
   3. Bronchioles
      a. Branch from the secondary bronchi and subdivide into the small terminal and respiratory bronchioles
      b. Contain no cartilage and depend on the elastic recoil of the lung for patency
      c. The terminal bronchioles contain no cilia and do not participate in gas exchange.
   4. Alveolar ducts and alveoli
      a. *Acinus* (plural, *acini*) is a term used to indicate all structures distal to the terminal bronchiole.
      b. Branch from the respiratory bronchioles
      c. Alveolar sacs, which arise from the ducts, contain clusters of alveoli, which are the basic units of gas exchange.
      d. Type 2 alveolar cells in the walls of the alveoli secrete surfactant, a phospholipid protein that reduces the surface tension in the alveoli; without surfactant, the alveoli would collapse.
   5. Lungs
      a. Located in the pleural cavity in the thorax
      b. Extend from just above the clavicles to the diaphragm, the major muscle of inspiration
      c. The right lung, which is larger than the left, is divided into 3 lobes: the upper, middle, and lower lobes.
      d. The left lung, which is narrower than the right lung to accommodate the heart, is divided into 2 lobes.

e. The respiratory structures are innervated by the phrenic nerve, the vagus nerve, and the thoracic nerves.
f. The parietal pleura lines the inside of the thoracic cavity, including the upper surface of the diaphragm.
g. The visceral pleura covers the pulmonary surfaces.
h. A thin fluid layer, which is produced by the cells lining the pleura, lubricates the visceral pleura and the parietal pleura, allowing them to glide smoothly and painlessly during respiration.
i. Blood flows throughout the lungs via the pulmonary circulation system.

6. Accessory muscles of respiration include the scalene muscles, which elevate the first 2 ribs; the sternocleidomastoid muscles, which raise the sternum; and the trapezius and pectoralis muscles, which fix the shoulders.
7. The respiratory process
a. The diaphragm descends into the abdominal cavity during inspiration, causing negative pressure in the lungs.
b. The negative pressure draws air from the area of greater pressure, the atmosphere, into the area of lesser pressure, the lungs.
c. In the lungs, air passes through the terminal bronchioles into the alveoli and diffuses into surrounding capillaries, then travels to the rest of the body to oxygenate the body tissues.
d. At the end of inspiration, the diaphragm and intercostal muscles relax and the lungs recoil.
e. As the lungs recoil, pressure within the lungs becomes higher than atmospheric pressure, causing the air, which now contains the cellular waste products carbon dioxide and water, to move from the alveoli in the lungs to the atmosphere.
f. Effective gas exchange depends on distribution of gas (ventilation) and blood (perfusion) in all portions of the lungs.

II. Diagnostic Tests

A. Risk factors for respiratory disorders (Box 50-1)

B. Chest x-ray film (radiograph)
1. Description: Provides information regarding the anatomical location and appearance of the lungs
2. Preprocedure
a. Remove all jewelry and other metal objects from the chest area.
b. Assess the client's ability to inhale and hold his or her breath.
3. Postprocedure: Help the client get dressed.

BOX 50-1 Risk Factors for Respiratory Disorders

- Environmental allergies
- Chest injury
- Crowded living conditions
- Exposure to chemicals and environmental pollutants
- Family history of infectious disease
- Frequent respiratory illnesses
- Geographical residence and travel to foreign countries
- Smoking
- Surgery
- Use of chewing tobacco
- Viral syndromes

! Question women regarding pregnancy or the possibility of pregnancy before performing radiography studies.

C. Sputum specimen
1. Description: Specimen obtained by expectoration or tracheal suctioning to assist in the identification of organisms or abnormal cells (see Priority Nursing Actions in Chapter 69)
2. Preprocedure
a. Determine the specific purpose of collection and check institutional policy for the appropriate method for collection.
b. Obtain an early morning sterile specimen by suctioning or expectoration after a respiratory treatment if a treatment is prescribed.
c. Instruct the client to rinse the mouth with water before collection.
d. Obtain 15 mL of sputum.
e. Instruct the client to take several deep breaths and then cough deeply to obtain sputum.
f. Collect the specimen before the client begins antibiotic therapy. If already started on antibiotic therapy, ensure the laboratory can utilize an antimicrobial removal device when analyzing the specimen.
3. Postprocedure
a. If a culture of sputum is prescribed, transport the specimen to the laboratory immediately.
b. Assist the client with mouth care.

! Ensure that an informed consent was obtained for any invasive procedure. Vital signs are measured before the procedure and monitored postprocedure to detect signs of complications.

D. Laryngoscopy and bronchoscopy
1. Description: Direct visual examination of the larynx, trachea, and bronchi with a fiberoptic bronchoscope
2. Preprocedure
a. Maintain NPO (nothing by mouth) status as prescribed.
b. Assess the results of coagulation studies.

c. Remove dentures and eyeglasses.
d. Establish an intravenous (IV) access as necessary and administer medication for sedation as prescribed.
e. Have emergency resuscitation supplies readily available.

3. Postprocedure
a. Maintain the client in a semi-Fowler's position.
b. Assess for the return of the gag reflex.
c. Maintain NPO status until the gag reflex returns.
d. Monitor for bloody sputum.
e. Monitor respiratory status, particularly if sedation has been administered.
f. Monitor for complications, such as bronchospasm or bronchial perforation, indicated by facial or neck crepitus, dysrhythmias, hemorrhage, hypoxemia, and pneumothorax.
g. Notify the primary health care provider (PHCP) if signs of complications occur.

E. Endobronchial ultrasound (EBUS)
1. Tissue samples are obtained from central lung masses and lymph nodes, using a bronchoscope with the help of ultrasound guidance.
2. Tissue samples are used for diagnosing and staging lung cancer, detecting infections, and identifying inflammatory diseases that affect the lungs, such as sarcoidosis.
3. Postprocedure, the client is monitored for signs of bleeding and respiratory distress.

F. Pulmonary angiography
1. Description
a. A fluoroscopic procedure in which a catheter is inserted through the antecubital or femoral vein into the pulmonary artery or 1 of its branches
b. Involves an injection of iodine or radiopaque contrast material

2. Preprocedure
a. Assess for allergies to iodine, seafood, or other radiopaque dyes.
b. Maintain NPO status as prescribed.
c. Assess results of coagulation studies.
d. Establish an IV access.
e. Administer sedation as prescribed.
f. Instruct the client to lie still during the procedure.
g. Instruct the client that he or she may feel an urge to cough, flushing, nausea, or a salty taste following injection of the dye.
h. Have emergency resuscitation equipment available.

3. Postprocedure
a. Avoid taking blood pressures for 24 hours in the extremity used for the injection.
b. Monitor peripheral neurovascular status of the affected extremity.
c. Assess insertion site for bleeding.
d. Monitor for reaction to the dye.

G. Thoracentesis
1. Description: Removal of fluid or air from the pleural space via transthoracic aspiration
2. Preprocedure
a. Prepare the client for ultrasound or chest radiograph, if prescribed, before the procedure.
b. Assess results of coagulation studies.
c. Note that the client is positioned sitting upright, with the arms and shoulders supported by a table at the bedside during the procedure (Fig. 50-1).
d. If the client cannot sit up, the client is placed lying in bed toward the unaffected side, with the head of the bed elevated.
e. Instruct the client not to cough, breathe deeply, or move during the procedure.

3. Postprocedure
a. Monitor respiratory status.
b. Apply a pressure dressing, and assess the puncture site for bleeding and crepitus.
c. Monitor for signs of pneumothorax, air embolism, and pulmonary edema.

H. Pulmonary function tests
1. Description: Tests used to evaluate lung mechanics, gas exchange, and acid–base disturbance through spirometric measurements, lung volumes, and arterial blood gas levels.
2. Preprocedure
a. Determine whether an analgesic that may depress the respiratory function is being administered.
b. Consult with the PHCP regarding withholding bronchodilators before testing, or alternatively if the testing will be done prior to and after administration of a bronchodilator.
c. Instruct the client to void before the procedure and to wear loose clothing.
d. Remove dentures.
e. Instruct the client to refrain from smoking or eating a heavy meal for 4 to 6 hours before the test.

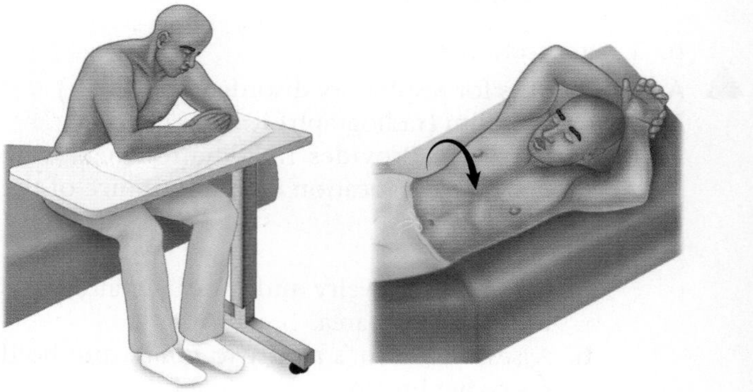

FIG. 50-1 Positions for thoracentesis.

3. Postprocedure: The client may resume a normal diet and any bronchodilators and respiratory treatments that were withheld before the procedure.

I. Lung biopsy
   1. Description
      a. A transbronchial biopsy and a transbronchial needle aspiration may be performed to obtain tissue for analysis by culture or cytological examination.
      b. An open lung biopsy is performed in the operating room.
   2. Preprocedure
      a. Maintain NPO status as prescribed.
      b. Inform the client that a local anesthetic will be used for a needle biopsy, but a sensation of pressure during needle insertion and aspiration may be felt.
      c. Administer analgesics and sedatives as prescribed.
   3. Postprocedure
      a. Apply a dressing to the biopsy site and monitor for drainage or bleeding.
      b. Monitor for signs of respiratory distress, and notify the PHCP if they occur.
      c. Monitor for signs of pneumothorax and air emboli, and notify the PHCP if they occur.
      d. Prepare the client for chest radiography if prescribed.

J. Spiral (helical) computed tomography (CT) scan
   1. Frequently used test to diagnose pulmonary embolism
   2. IV injection of contrast medium is used; if the client cannot have contrast medium, a ventilation-perfusion (V/Q) scan will be done.
   3. The scanner rotates around the body, allowing for a 3-dimensional picture of all regions of the lungs.

K. V/Q lung scan
   1. Description
      a. The perfusion scan evaluates blood flow to the lungs.
      b. The ventilation scan determines the patency of the pulmonary airways and detects abnormalities in ventilation.
      c. A radionuclide may be injected for the procedure.
   2. Preprocedure
      a. Assess the client for allergies to dye, iodine, or seafood.
      b. Remove jewelry around the chest area.
      c. Review breathing methods that may be required during testing.
      d. Establish an IV access.
      e. Administer sedation if prescribed.
      f. Have emergency resuscitation equipment available.
   3. Postprocedure
      a. Monitor the client for reaction to the radionuclide.
      b. Instruct the client that the radionuclide clears from the body in about 8 hours.
      c. Encourage increased fluid intake to clear the dye from the body if there is no fluid restriction.

L. Computed tomography pulmonary angiography
   1. Description
      a. The scan visualizes the pulmonary arteries and blood flow.
      b. Its main use is to diagnose pulmonary embolism and is the preferred method.
      c. A contrast dye is injected.
   2. Preprocedure: Similar to the V/Q lung scan; in addition, renal function should be adequate and dosing of the contrast should be done by a pharmacist.
   3. Postprocedure: Similar to the V/Q lung scan

M. Skin tests: A skin test uses an intradermal injection to help diagnose various infectious diseases (Box 50-2).

N. Arterial blood gases (ABGs)
   1. Description: Measurement of the dissolved oxygen and carbon dioxide in the arterial blood helps indicate the acid–base state and how well oxygen is being carried to the body.
   2. Preprocedure and postprocedure care, normal results, and analysis of results: See Chapter 9.

Avoid suctioning the client before drawing an ABG sample, because the suctioning procedure will deplete the client's oxygen, resulting in inaccurate ABG results.

O. Pulse oximetry: See Chapter 10.

BOX 50-2 Skin Test Procedure

1. Determine hypersensitivity or previous reactions to skin tests.
2. Use a skin site that is free of excessive body hair, dermatitis, and blemishes.
3. Apply the injection at the upper third of the inner surface of the left arm.
4. Circle and mark the injection test site.
5. Document the date, time, and test site.
6. Advise the client not to scratch the test site to prevent infection and possible abscess formation.
7. Instruct the client to avoid washing the test site.
8. Assess the reaction at the injection site 24 to 72 hours after administration of the test antigen.
9. Assess the test site for the amount of induration (hard swelling) in millimeters and for the presence of erythema and vesiculation (small blister-like elevations).

P. D-dimer

1. A blood test that measures clot formation and lysis that results from the degradation of fibrin
2. Helps diagnose (a positive test result) the presence of thrombus in conditions such as deep vein thrombosis, pulmonary embolism, or stroke; it is also used to diagnose disseminated intravascular coagulation (DIC) and to monitor the effectiveness of treatment.
3. The normal D-dimer level is less than 50 ng/mL (less than 3.0 mmol/L); normal fibrinogen is 60 to 100 mg/dL (2.0 to 5.0 g/L).

III. Respiratory Treatments (see Chapter 69)

IV. Chest Injuries

A. Rib fracture

1. Description
   a. Results from direct blunt chest trauma and causes a potential for intrathoracic injury, such as pneumothorax, hemothorax, or pulmonary contusion
   b. Pain with movement, deep breathing, and coughing results in impaired ventilation and inadequate clearance of secretions.
2. Assessment
   a. Pain and tenderness at the injury site that increases with inspiration
   b. Shallow respirations
   c. Client splints chest
   d. Fractures noted on chest x-ray
3. Interventions
   a. Note that the ribs usually reunite spontaneously.
   b. Open reduction and internal fixation of the ribs (rib plating) may be done.
   c. Place the client in a Fowler's position.
   d. Administer pain medication as prescribed to maintain adequate ventilatory status.
   e. Monitor for increased respiratory distress.
   f. Instruct the client to self-splint with the hands, arms, or a pillow.
   g. Prepare the client for an intercostal nerve block as prescribed if the pain is severe.

B. Flail chest

1. Description
   a. Occurs from blunt chest trauma associated with accidents, which may result in hemothorax and rib fractures.
   b. The loose segment of the chest wall becomes paradoxical to the expansion and contraction of the rest of the chest wall.
2. Assessment
   a. Paradoxical respirations (inward movement of a segment of the thorax during inspiration with outward movement during expiration)
   b. Severe pain in the chest
   c. Dyspnea
   d. Cyanosis
   e. Tachycardia
   f. Hypotension
   g. Tachypnea, shallow respirations
   h. Diminished breath sounds
3. Interventions
   a. Maintain the client in a Fowler's position.
   b. Administer oxygen as prescribed.
   c. Monitor for increased respiratory distress.
   d. Encourage coughing and deep breathing.
   e. Administer pain medication as prescribed.
   f. Maintain bed rest and limit activity to reduce oxygen demands.
   g. Open reduction and internal fixation of the ribs (rib plating) may be done.
   h. Prepare for intubation with **mechanical ventilation**, with positive end-expiratory pressure (PEEP) for severe flail chest associated with respiratory failure and shock (see Chapter 69).

C. Pulmonary contusion

1. Description
   a. Characterized by interstitial hemorrhage associated with intra-alveolar hemorrhage, resulting in decreased pulmonary compliance
   b. The major complication is acute respiratory distress syndrome.
2. Assessment
   a. Dyspnea
   b. Restlessness
   c. Increased bronchial secretions
   d. Hypoxemia
   e. Hemoptysis
   f. Decreased breath sounds
   g. Crackles and wheezes
3. Interventions
   a. Maintain a patent airway and adequate ventilation.
   b. Place the client in a Fowler's position.
   c. Administer oxygen as prescribed.
   d. Monitor for increased respiratory distress.
   e. Maintain bed rest and limit activity to reduce oxygen demands.
   f. Prepare for mechanical ventilation with PEEP if required.

D. **Pneumothorax** (Fig. 50-2)

1. Description
   a. Accumulation of atmospheric air in the pleural space, which results in a rise in intrathoracic pressure and reduced vital capacity, or the greatest amount of air expired from the lungs after taking a deep breath.
   b. The loss of negative intrapleural pressure results in collapse of the lung.

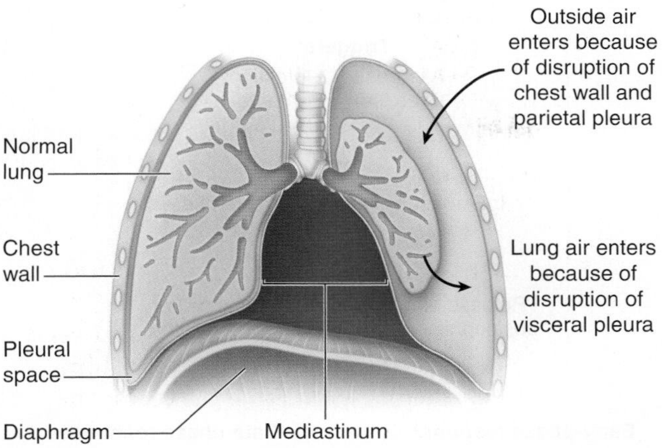

FIG. 50-2 Pneumothorax. Air in the pleural space causes the lungs to collapse around the hilus and may push the mediastinal contents (heart and great vessels) toward the other lung.

c. A spontaneous pneumothorax occurs with the rupture of a pulmonary bleb, or small air-containing spaces deep in the lung.
d. An open pneumothorax occurs when an opening through the chest wall allows the entrance of positive atmospheric air pressure into the pleural space.
e. A tension pneumothorax occurs from a blunt chest injury or from mechanical ventilation with PEEP when a buildup of positive pressure occurs in the pleural space.

2. Assessment (Box 50-3)
3. Interventions
   a. Diagnosis of pneumothorax is made by chest x-ray.
   b. Apply a nonporous dressing over an open chest wound.
   c. Administer oxygen as prescribed.
   d. Place the client in a Fowler's position.

BOX 50-3 Assessment Findings: Pneumothorax

- Absent or markedly decreased breath sounds on affected side
- Cyanosis
- Decreased chest expansion unilaterally
- Dyspnea
- Hypotension
- Sharp chest pain
- Subcutaneous emphysema as evidenced by crepitus on palpation
- Sucking sound with open chest wound
- Tachycardia
- Tachypnea
- Tracheal deviation to the unaffected side with tension pneumothorax

   e. Prepare for chest tube placement, which will remain in place until the lung has expanded fully.
   f. Monitor the chest tube drainage system.
   g. Monitor for subcutaneous emphysema.
   h. See Chapter 69 for information on caring for a client with chest tubes.

Clients with a respiratory disorder should be positioned with the head of the bed elevated.

V. Acute Respiratory Failure

A. Description
1. Occurs when insufficient oxygen is transported to the blood or inadequate carbon dioxide is removed from the lungs and the client's compensatory mechanisms fail
2. Causes include a mechanical abnormality of the lungs or chest wall, a defect in the respiratory control center in the brain, or an impairment in the function of the respiratory muscles.
3. In oxygenation failure, or hypoxemic respiratory failure, oxygen may reach the alveoli but cannot be absorbed or used properly, resulting in a PaO_2 lower than 60 mm Hg, arterial oxygen saturation (SaO_2) lower than 90%, or partial pressure of arterial carbon dioxide ($PaCo_2$) greater than 50 mm Hg occurring with acidemia.
4. Respiratory failure can be hypoxemic, hypercapnic, or both. Inadequate gas exchange is the mechanism behind failure. Arterial oxygen, carbon dioxide, or both are not kept at normal levels, resulting in failure.
5. Many clients experience both hypoxemic and hypercapnic respiratory failure and retained carbon dioxide in the alveoli displaces oxygen, contributing to the hypoxemia.
6. Manifestations of respiratory failure are related to the extent and rapidity of change in PaO_2 and $PaCo_2$.

B. Assessment
1. Dyspnea
2. Restlessness
3. Confusion
4. Tachycardia
5. Hypertension
6. Dysrhythmias
7. Decreased level of consciousness
8. Alterations in respirations and breath sounds
9. Headache (less common)

C. Interventions
1. Identify and treat the cause of the respiratory failure.
2. Administer oxygen to maintain the PaO_2 level higher than 60 to 70 mm Hg.
3. Place the client in a Fowler's position.
4. Encourage deep breathing.

5. Administer bronchodilators as prescribed.
6. Prepare the client for mechanical ventilation if supplemental oxygen cannot maintain acceptable PaO_2 and $PaCo_2$ levels.

VI. Acute Respiratory Distress Syndrome

A. Description
1. A form of acute respiratory failure that occurs as a complication caused by a diffuse lung injury or critical illness and leads to extravascular lung fluid.
2. The major site of injury is the alveolar capillary membrane.
3. The interstitial edema causes compression and obliteration of the terminal airways and leads to reduced lung volume and compliance.
4. The ABG levels identify respiratory acidosis and hypoxemia that do not respond to an increased percentage of oxygen.
5. The chest x-ray shows bilateral interstitial and alveolar infiltrates; interstitial edema may not be noted until there is a 30% increase in fluid content.
6. Causes include sepsis, fluid overload, shock, trauma, neurological injuries, burns, DIC, drug ingestion, aspiration, and inhalation of toxic substances.

B. Assessment
1. Tachypnea
2. Dyspnea
3. Decreased breath sounds
4. Deteriorating ABG levels
5. Hypoxemia despite high concentrations of delivered oxygen
6. Decreased pulmonary compliance
7. Pulmonary infiltrates

C. Interventions
1. Identify and treat the cause of the acute respiratory distress syndrome.
2. Administer oxygen as prescribed.
3. Place the client in a Fowler's position.
4. Restrict fluid intake as prescribed.
5. Provide respiratory treatments as prescribed.
6. Administer diuretics, anticoagulants, or corticosteroids as prescribed.
7. Prepare the client for intubation and mechanical ventilation using PEEP.

VII. Asthma (Fig. 50-3)

A. Description
1. Chronic inflammatory disorder of the airways that causes varying degrees of obstruction in the airways
2. Marked by airway inflammation and hyperresponsiveness to a variety of stimuli or triggers (Box 50-4).
3. Causes recurrent episodes of wheezing, breathlessness, chest tightness, and coughing associated with airflow obstruction that may resolve spontaneously; it is often reversible with treatment.
4. Severity is classified based on the clinical features before treatment (Box 50-5).
5. Status asthmaticus is a severe life-threatening **asthma** episode that is refractory to treatment and may result in pneumothorax, acute cor pulmonale, or respiratory arrest.

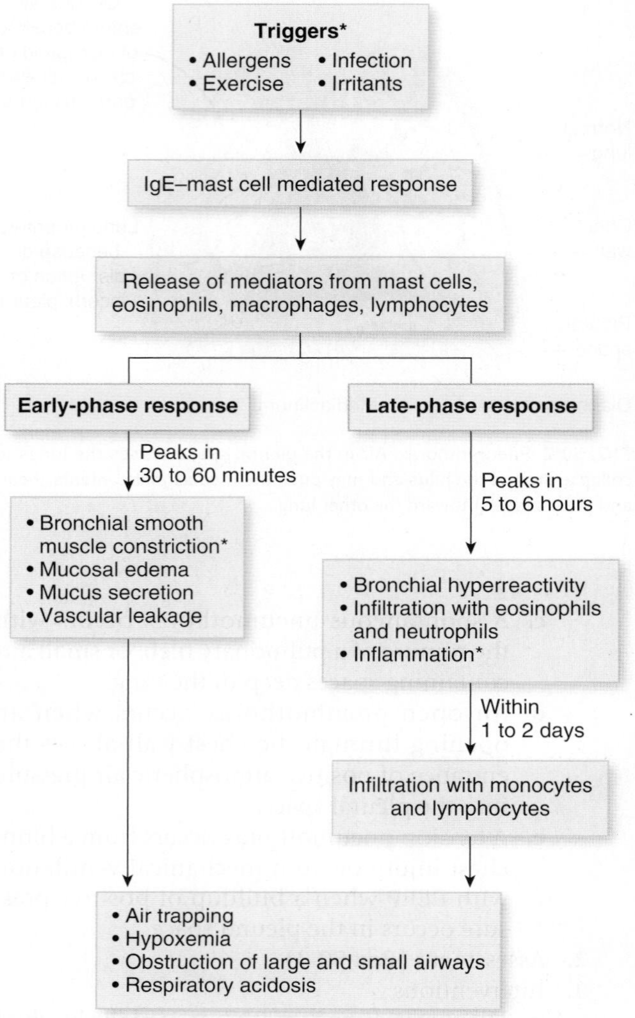

FIG. 50-3 Pathophysiology in asthma. Stems with asterisks are primary processes. *IgE*, Immunoglobulin E.

⚠ Silent breath sounds are associated with acute asthma exacerbation, may indicate impending respiratory failure due to diffuse bronchospasm, and is a life-threatening condition.

6. Refer to Chapter 35 for additional information on asthma.

B. Assessment
1. Restlessness
2. Wheezing or crackles
3. Absent or diminished lung sounds

BOX 50-4 Asthma Triggers

Environmental Factors
- Animal dander
- Cockroaches
- Dust
- Exhaust fumes
- Fireplaces
- Molds
- Perfumes or other products with aerosol sprays
- Pollen
- Smoke, including cigarette or cigar smoke
- Sudden weather changes

Physiological Factors
- Gastroesophageal reflux disease (GERD)
- Hormonal changes
- Sinusitis
- Stress
- Viral upper respiratory infection

Medications
- Acetylsalicylic acid (aspirin)
- β-Adrenergic blockers
- Nonsteroidal antiinflammatory drugs

Occupational Exposure Factors
- Metal salts
- Wood and vegetable dusts
- Industrial chemicals and plastics

Food Additives
- Sulfites (bisulfites and metabisulfites)
- Beer, wine, dried fruit, shrimp, processed potatoes
- Monosodium glutamate

From Lewis S, Dirksen S, Heitkemper M, Bucher L, Camera I: *Medical-surgical nursing: assessment and management of clinical problems*, ed 8, St. Louis, 2011, Mosby.

BOX 50-5 Classification of Asthma Severity

Severe Persistent
- Symptoms are continuous.
- Physical activity requires limitations.
- Frequent exacerbations occur.
- Nocturnal symptoms occur frequently.

Moderate Persistent
- Daily symptoms occur.
- Daily use of inhaled short-acting β-agonist is needed.
- Exacerbations affect activity.
- Exacerbations occur at least twice weekly and may last for days.
- Nocturnal symptoms occur more frequently than once weekly.

Mild Persistent
- Symptoms occur more frequently than twice weekly but less often than once daily.
- Exacerbations may affect activity.
- Nocturnal symptoms occur more frequently than twice a month.

Mild Intermittent
- Symptoms occur twice weekly or less.
- Client is asymptomatic between exacerbations.
- Exacerbations are brief (hours to days).
- Intensity of exacerbations varies.
- Nocturnal symptoms occur twice a month or less.

From Ignatavicius D, Workman M: *Medical-surgical nursing: patient-centered collaborative care*, ed 7, St. Louis, 2013, Saunders.

4. Hyperresonance
5. Use of accessory muscles for breathing
6. Tachypnea with hyperventilation
7. Prolonged exhalation
8. Tachycardia
9. Pulsus paradoxus
10. Diaphoresis
11. Cyanosis
12. Decreased oxygen saturation
13. Pulmonary function test results that demonstrate decreased airflow rates

C. Interventions
1. Monitor vital signs.
2. Monitor pulse oximetry.
3. Monitor peak flow.
4. During an acute asthma episode, provide interventions to assist with breathing (Box 50-6).

BOX 50-6 Nursing Interventions During an Acute Asthma Episode

- Position the client in a high-Fowler's position or sitting to aid in breathing.
- Administer oxygen as prescribed.
- Stay with the client to decrease anxiety.
- Administer bronchodilators as prescribed.
- Record the color, amount, and consistency of sputum, if any.
- Administer corticosteroids as prescribed.
- Administer magnesium sulfate as prescribed.
- Auscultate lung sounds before, during, and after treatments.

D. Client education
1. On the intermittent nature of symptoms and need for long-term management

2. To identify possible triggers and measures to prevent episodes
3. About the management of medication and proper administration
4. About the correct use of a peak flowmeter
5. About developing an asthma action plan with the PHCP and what to do if an asthma episode occurs

VIII. Chronic Obstructive Pulmonary Disease

A. Description
1. Also known as chronic obstructive lung disease and chronic airflow limitation
2. **Chronic obstructive pulmonary disease** is a disease state characterized by airflow obstruction.
3. Chronic bronchitis and emphysema are progressive lung diseases that fall under the general category of chronic obstructive pulmonary disease.
4. Chronic bronchitis is a condition in which the bronchial tubes become inflamed and excessive mucus production occurs as a result from irritants or injury.
5. Emphysema is a condition in which the air sacs in the lungs are damaged and enlarged, resulting in hyperinflation and breathlessness.
6. Progressive airflow limitation occurs, associated with an abnormal inflammatory response of the lungs that is not completely reversible.
7. Chronic obstructive pulmonary disease (COPD) leads to pulmonary insufficiency, pulmonary hypertension, and cor pulmonale.

B. Assessment
1. Cough
2. Exertional dyspnea
3. Wheezing and crackles
4. Sputum production
5. Weight loss
6. Barrel chest (emphysema) (Fig. 50-4)
7. Use of accessory muscles for breathing
8. Prolonged expiration
9. Orthopnea

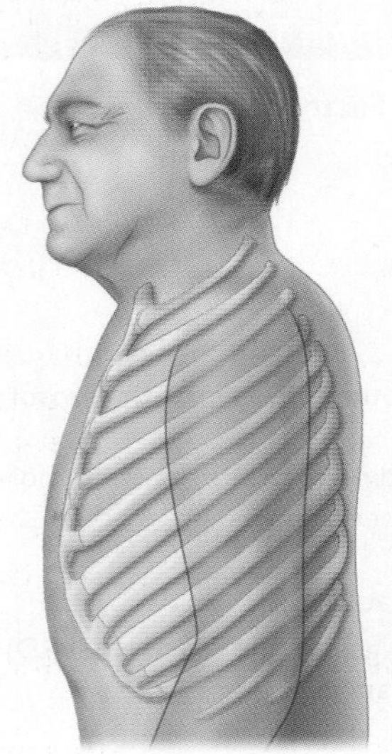

FIG. 50-4 Typical barrel chest in a client with chronic obstructive pulmonary disease.

10. Cardiac dysrhythmias
11. Congestion and hyperinflation seen on chest x-ray (Fig. 50-5)
12. ABG levels that indicate respiratory acidosis and hypoxemia
13. Pulmonary function tests that demonstrate decreased vital capacity

C. Interventions
1. Monitor vital signs.
2. Administer a concentration of oxygen based on ABG values and oxygen saturation by pulse oximetry as prescribed.
3. Monitor pulse oximetry.
4. Provide respiratory treatments and CPT.
5. Instruct the client in diaphragmatic or abdominal breathing techniques, tripod positioning, and pursed-lip breathing techniques, which

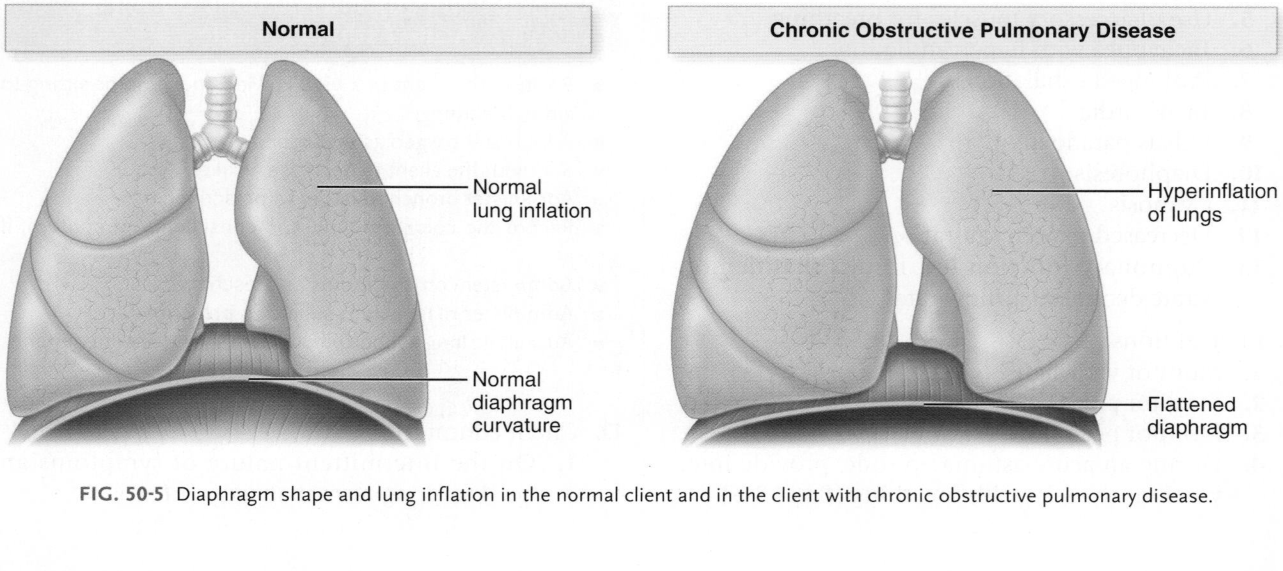

FIG. 50-5 Diaphragm shape and lung inflation in the normal client and in the client with chronic obstructive pulmonary disease.

increase airway pressure and keep air passages open, promoting maximal carbon dioxide expiration.
6. Record the color, amount, and consistency of sputum.
7. Suction the client's lungs, if necessary, to clear the airway and prevent infection.
8. Monitor weight.
9. Encourage small, frequent meals to maintain nutrition and prevent dyspnea.
10. Provide a high-calorie, high-protein diet with supplements.
11. Encourage fluid intake up to 3000 mL/day to keep secretions thin, unless contraindicated.
12. Place the client in a Fowler's position and leaning forward to aid in breathing (Fig. 50-6).
13. Allow activity as tolerated.
14. Administer bronchodilators as prescribed, and instruct the client in the use of oral and inhalant medications.
15. Administer corticosteroids as prescribed for exacerbations.
16. Administer mucolytics as prescribed to thin secretions.
17. Administer antibiotics for infection if prescribed.

D. Client education (Box 50-7)

BOX 50-7 Client Education: Chronic Obstructive Pulmonary Disease

- Adhere to activity limitations, alternating rest periods with activity.
- Avoid eating gas-producing foods, spicy foods, and extremely hot or cold foods.
- Avoid exposure to individuals with infections and avoid crowds.
- Avoid extremes in temperature.
- Avoid fireplaces, pets, feather pillows, and other environmental allergens.
- Avoid powerful odors.
- Meet nutritional requirements.
- Receive immunizations as recommended.
- Recognize the signs and symptoms of respiratory infection and hypoxia.
- Stop smoking.
- Use medications and inhalers as prescribed.
- Use oxygen therapy as prescribed.
- Use pursed-lip and diaphragmatic or abdominal breathing.
- When dusting, use a wet cloth.

IX. Pneumonia

A. Description
1. Infection of the pulmonary tissue, including the interstitial spaces, the alveoli, and the bronchioles
2. The edema associated with inflammation stiffens the lung, decreases lung compliance and vital capacity, and causes hypoxemia.
3. Pneumonia can be community-acquired or hospital-acquired.
4. The chest x-ray film shows lobar or segmental consolidation, pulmonary infiltrates, or pleural effusions.
5. A sputum culture identifies the organism.
6. The white blood cell count and the erythrocyte sedimentation rate are elevated.

B. Assessment
1. Chills
2. Elevated temperature
3. Pleuritic pain
4. Tachypnea
5. Rhonchi and wheezes
6. Use of accessory muscles for breathing
7. Mental status changes
8. Sputum production

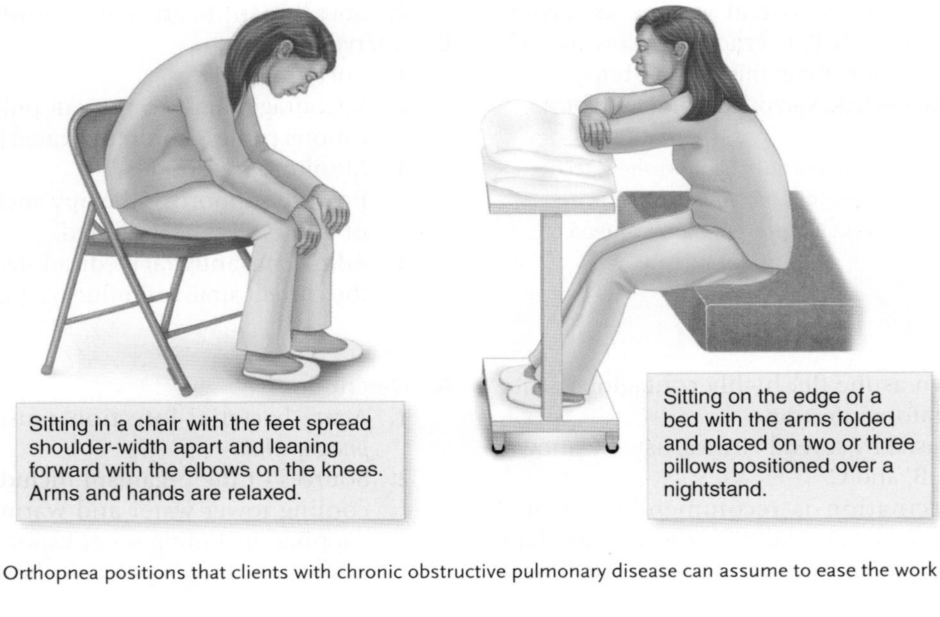
Sitting in a chair with the feet spread shoulder-width apart and leaning forward with the elbows on the knees. Arms and hands are relaxed.
Sitting on the edge of a bed with the arms folded and placed on two or three pillows positioned over a nightstand.

FIG. 50-6 Orthopnea positions that clients with chronic obstructive pulmonary disease can assume to ease the work of breathing.

C. Interventions
1. Administer oxygen as prescribed.
2. Monitor respiratory status.
3. Monitor for labored respirations, cyanosis, and cold and clammy skin.
4. Encourage coughing and deep breathing and use of the incentive spirometer.
5. Place the client in a semi-Fowler's position to facilitate breathing and lung expansion.
6. Change the client's position frequently and ambulate as tolerated to mobilize secretions.
7. Provide CPT (see Chapter 69).
8. Perform nasotracheal suctioning if the client is unable to clear secretions.
9. Monitor pulse oximetry.
10. Monitor and record color, consistency, and amount of sputum.
11. Provide a high-calorie, high-protein diet with small frequent meals.
12. Encourage fluids, up to 3 L/day, to thin secretions unless contraindicated.
13. Provide a balance of rest and activity, increasing activity gradually.
14. Administer antibiotics as prescribed.
15. Administer antipyretics, bronchodilators, cough suppressants, mucolytic agents, and expectorants as prescribed.
16. Prevent the spread of infection by hand washing and the proper disposal of secretions.

D. Client education
1. About the importance of rest, proper nutrition, and adequate fluid intake
2. To avoid chilling and exposure to individuals with respiratory infections or viruses
3. Regarding medications and the use of inhalants as prescribed
4. To notify the PHCP if chills, fever, dyspnea, hemoptysis, or increased fatigue occurs
5. To receive a pneumococcal vaccine as recommended by the PHCP; refer to the following Web site for information about this vaccine: http://www.cdc.gov/vaccines/vpd-vac/pneumo/default.htm.

Teach clients that using proper hand-washing techniques, disposing of respiratory secretions properly, and receiving vaccines will assist in preventing the spread of infection.

X. Influenza

A. Description
1. Also known as the flu; highly contagious acute viral respiratory infection
2. May be caused by several viruses, usually known as types A, B, and C
3. Yearly vaccination is recommended to prevent the disease, especially for those older than 50 years of age, individuals with chronic illness or who are immunocompromised, those living in institutions, and health care personnel providing direct care to clients (the vaccination is contraindicated in the individual with egg allergies).
4. Additional prevention measures include avoiding those who have developed influenza, frequent and proper hand washing, and cleaning and disinfecting surfaces that have become contaminated with secretions.
5. Avian influenza A (H5N1)
   a. Affects birds; does not usually affect humans; however, human cases have been reported in some countries.
   b. An H5N1 vaccine has been developed for use if a pandemic virus were to emerge.
   c. Reported symptoms are similar to those associated with influenza types A, B, and C.
   d. Prevention measures include thorough cooking of poultry products, avoiding contact with wild animals, frequent and proper hand washing, and cleaning and disinfecting surfaces that have become contaminated with secretions.
6. Swine (H1N1) influenza
   a. A strain of flu that consists of genetic materials from swine, avian, and human influenza viruses
   b. Signs and symptoms are similar to those that present with seasonal flu; in addition, vomiting and diarrhea commonly occur.
   c. Prevention measures and treatment are the same as for the seasonal flu.

B. Refer to Chapter 18 for information on vaccines.

C. Assessment
1. Acute onset of fever and muscle aches
2. Headache
3. Fatigue, weakness, anorexia
4. Sore throat, cough, and rhinorrhea

D. Interventions
1. Encourage rest.
2. Encourage fluids to prevent pulmonary complications (unless contraindicated).
3. Monitor lung sounds.
4. Provide supportive therapy such as antipyretics or antitussives as indicated.
5. Administer antiviral medications as prescribed for the current strain of influenza (see Chapter 51).

XI. Legionnaire's Disease

A. Description
1. Acute bacterial infection caused by *Legionella pneumophila*
2. Sources of the organism include contaminated cooling tower water and warm stagnant water supplies, including water vaporizers, water sonicators, whirlpool spas, and showers.

3. Person-to-person contact does not occur; the risk for infection is increased by the presence of other conditions.

B. Assessment: Influenza-like symptoms with a high fever, chills, muscle aches, and headache that may progress to dry cough, pleurisy, and sometimes diarrhea

C. Interventions: Treatment is supportive and antibiotics may be prescribed.

XII. Pleural Effusion

A. Description
1. Pleural effusion is the collection of fluid in the pleural space.
2. Any condition that interferes with secretion or drainage of this fluid will lead to pleural effusion.

B. Assessment
1. Pleuritic pain that is sharp and increases with inspiration
2. Progressive dyspnea with decreased movement of the chest wall on the affected side
3. Dry, nonproductive cough caused by bronchial irritation or mediastinal shift
4. Tachycardia
5. Elevated temperature
6. Decreased breath sounds over affected area
7. Chest x-ray film that shows pleural effusion and a mediastinal shift away from the fluid if the effusion is more than 250 mL

C. Interventions
1. Identify and treat the underlying cause.
2. Monitor breath sounds.
3. Place the client in a Fowler's position.
4. Encourage coughing and deep breathing.
5. Prepare the client for thoracentesis.
6. If pleural effusion is recurrent, prepare the client for pleurectomy or pleurodesis as prescribed.

D. Pleurectomy
1. Consists of surgically stripping the parietal pleura away from the visceral pleura
2. This produces an intense inflammatory reaction that promotes adhesion formation between the 2 layers during healing.

E. Pleurodesis
1. Involves the instillation of a sclerosing substance into the pleural space via a thoracotomy tube
2. The substance creates an inflammatory response that scleroses tissue together.

XIII. Empyema

A. Description
1. Collection of pus within the pleural cavity
2. The fluid is thick, opaque, and foul-smelling.
3. The most common cause is pulmonary infection and lung abscess caused by thoracic surgery or chest trauma, in which bacteria are introduced directly into the pleural space.
4. Treatment focuses on treating the infection, emptying the empyema cavity, re-expanding the lung, and controlling the infection.

B. Assessment
1. Recent febrile illness or trauma
2. Chest pain
3. Cough
4. Dyspnea
5. Anorexia and weight loss
6. Malaise
7. Elevated temperature and chills
8. Night sweats
9. Pleural exudate on chest x-ray

C. Interventions
1. Monitor breath sounds.
2. Place the client in a semi-Fowler's or high-Fowler's position.
3. Encourage coughing and deep breathing.
4. Administer antibiotics as prescribed.
5. Instruct the client to splint the chest as necessary.
6. Assist with thoracentesis or chest tube insertion to promote drainage and lung expansion.
7. If marked pleural thickening occurs, prepare the client for decortication, if prescribed; this surgical procedure involves removal of the restrictive mass of fibrin and inflammatory cells.

XIV. Pleurisy

A. Description
1. Inflammation of the visceral and parietal membranes; may be caused by pulmonary infarction or pneumonia.
2. The visceral and parietal membranes rub together during respiration and cause pain.
3. Pleurisy usually occurs on 1 side of the chest, usually in the lower lateral portions in the chest wall.

B. Assessment
1. Knife-like pain aggravated on deep breathing and coughing
2. Dyspnea
3. Pleural friction rub heard on auscultation

C. Interventions
1. Identify and treat the cause.
2. Monitor lung sounds.
3. Administer analgesics as prescribed.
4. Apply hot or cold applications as prescribed.
5. Encourage coughing and deep breathing.
6. Instruct the client to lie on the affected side to splint the chest.

XV. Pulmonary Embolism

A. Description
1. Occurs when a thrombus forms (most commonly in a deep vein), detaches, travels to the right side of the heart, and then lodges in a branch of the pulmonary artery

BOX 50-8 Assessment Findings: Pulmonary Embolism

- Apprehension and restlessness
- Blood-tinged sputum
- Chest pain
- Cough
- Crackles and wheezes on auscultation
- Cyanosis
- Distended neck veins
- Dyspnea accompanied by anginal and pleuritic pain, exacerbated by inspiration
- Feeling of impending doom
- Hypotension
- Petechiae over the chest and axilla
- Shallow respirations
- Tachypnea and tachycardia

2. Clients prone to pulmonary embolism are those at risk for deep vein thrombosis, including those with prolonged immobilization, surgery, obesity, pregnancy, heart failure, advanced age, or a history of thromboembolism.
3. Fat emboli can occur as a complication following fracture of a long bone and can cause pulmonary emboli.
4. Treatment is aimed at prevention through risk factor recognition and elimination.

B. Assessment (Box 50-8)
C. Interventions (see Priority Nursing Actions)

PRIORITY NURSING ACTIONS

Suspected Pulmonary Embolism

1. Notify the Rapid Response Team and primary health care provider (PHCP).
2. Reassure the client and elevate the head of the bed.
3. Prepare to administer the oxygen.
4. Obtain vital signs and check lung sounds.
5. Prepare to obtain an arterial blood gas.
6. Prepare for the administration of heparin therapy or other therapies.
7. Document the event, interventions taken, and the client's response to treatment.

Reference

Ignatavicius, Workman, Rebar, (2018) p. 619.

XVI. Lung Cancer and Laryngeal Cancer: See Chapter 44 for more information

XVII. Carbon Monoxide Poisoning: See Chapter 42 for more information

XVIII. Histoplasmosis

A. Description
1. Pulmonary fungal infection caused by spores of *Histoplasma capsulatum*
2. Transmission occurs by the inhalation of spores, which commonly are found in contaminated soil.
3. Spores also are usually found in bird droppings.

B. Assessment
1. Similar to pneumonia
2. Positive skin test for histoplasmosis
3. Positive agglutination test
4. Splenomegaly, hepatomegaly

C. Interventions
1. Administer oxygen as prescribed.
2. Monitor breath sounds.
3. Administer antiemetics, antihistamines, antipyretics, and corticosteroids as prescribed.
4. Administer fungicidal medications as prescribed.
5. Encourage coughing and deep breathing.
6. Place the client in a semi-Fowler's position.
7. Monitor vital signs.
8. Monitor for nephrotoxicity from fungicidal medications.
9. Instruct the client to wear a mask and spray the floor with water before sweeping barn and chicken coops.

XIX. Sarcoidosis

A. Description
1. Presence of epithelioid cell tubercles in the lung
2. The cause is unknown, but a high titer of Epstein-Barr virus may be noted.
3. Viral incidence is highest in African Americans and young adults.

B. Assessment
1. Night sweats
2. Fever
3. Weight loss
4. Cough and dyspnea
5. Skin nodules
6. Polyarthritis
7. Kveim test: Sarcoid node antigen is injected intradermally and causes a local nodular lesion in about 1 month.

C. Interventions
1. Administer corticosteroids to control symptoms.
2. Monitor temperature.
3. Increase fluid intake.
4. Provide frequent periods of rest.
5. Encourage small, frequent, nutritious meals.

XX. Occupational Lung Disease

A. Description
1. Caused by exposure to environmental or occupational fumes, dust, vapors, gases, bacterial or fungal antigens, and allergens; can result in

acute reversible effects or chronic lung disease
2. Common disease classifications include occupational asthma pneumoconiosis (silicosis or coal miner's [black lung] disease), diffuse interstitial fibrosis (asbestosis, talcosis, berylliosis), or extrinsic allergic alveolitis (farmer's lung, bird fancier's lung, or machine operator's lung).

B. Assessment: Manifestations depend on the type of disease and respiratory symptoms.

C. Interventions
1. Prevention through the use of respiratory protective devices
2. Treatment is based on the symptoms experienced by the client.

XXI. Tuberculosis

A. Description
1. Highly communicable disease caused by *Mycobacterium tuberculosis*
2. *M. tuberculosis* is a nonmotile, nonsporulating, acid-fast rod that secretes niacin; when the bacillus reaches a susceptible site, it multiplies freely.
3. Because *M. tuberculosis* is an aerobic bacterium, it primarily affects the pulmonary system, especially the upper lobes, where the oxygen content is highest, but it also can affect other areas of the body, such as the brain, intestines, peritoneum, kidney, joints, and liver.
4. An exudative response causes a nonspecific pneumonitis and the development of granulomas in the lung tissue.
5. Tuberculosis has an insidious onset, and many clients are not aware of symptoms until the disease is well advanced.
6. Improper or noncompliant use of treatment programs may cause the development of mutations in the tubercle bacilli, resulting in a **multidrug-resistant** strain of **tuberculosis** (MDR-TB).
7. The goal of treatment is to prevent transmission, control symptoms, and prevent progression of the disease.

B. Risk factors (Box 50-9)

C. Transmission
1. Via the airborne route by droplet infection
2. When an infected individual coughs, laughs, sneezes, or sings, droplet nuclei containing tuberculosis bacteria enter the air and may be inhaled by others.
3. Identification of those in close contact with the infected individual is important so that they can be tested and treated as necessary.
4. When contacts have been identified, these persons are assessed with a tuberculin skin test and chest x-rays to determine infection with tuberculosis.
5. After the infected individual has received tuberculosis medication for 2 to 3 weeks, the risk of transmission is reduced greatly.

BOX 50-9 Risk Factors for Tuberculosis

- Child younger than 5 years of age
- Drinking unpasteurized milk if the cow is infected with bovine tuberculosis
- Homeless individuals or those from a lower socioeconomic group, minority group, or refugee group
- Individuals in constant, frequent contact with an untreated or undiagnosed individual
- Individuals living in crowded areas, such as long-term care facilities, prisons, and mental health facilities
- Older client
- Individuals with malnutrition, infection, immune dysfunction, or human immunodeficiency virus infection; or immunosuppressed as a result of medication therapy
- Individuals who abuse alcohol or are intravenous drug users

D. Disease progression
1. Droplets enter the lungs, and the bacteria form a tubercle lesion.
2. The defense systems of the body encapsulate the tubercle, leaving a scar.
3. If encapsulation does not occur, bacteria may enter the lymph system, travel to the lymph nodes, and cause an inflammatory response termed *granulomatous inflammation*.
4. Primary lesions form; the primary lesions may become dormant but can be reactivated and become a secondary infection when re-exposed to the bacterium.
5. In an active phase, tuberculosis can cause necrosis and cavitation in the lesions, leading to rupture, the spread of necrotic tissue, and damage to various parts of the body.

E. Client history
1. Past exposure to tuberculosis
2. Client's country of origin and travel to foreign countries in which the incidence of tuberculosis is high
3. Recent history of influenza, pneumonia, febrile illness, cough, or foul-smelling sputum production
4. Previous tests for tuberculosis; results of the testing
5. Recent **bacillus Calmette-Guérin (BCG) vaccine** (a vaccine containing attenuated tubercle bacilli that may be given to persons in foreign countries or to persons traveling to foreign countries to produce increased resistance to tuberculosis)

⚠ An individual who has received a BCG vaccine will have a positive tuberculin skin test result and should be evaluated for tuberculosis with a chest x-ray.

F. Clinical manifestations
1. May be asymptomatic in primary infection
2. Fatigue

3. Lethargy
4. Anorexia
5. Weight loss
6. Low-grade fever
7. Chills
8. Night sweats
9. Persistent cough and the production of mucoid and mucopurulent sputum, which is occasionally streaked with blood
10. Chest tightness and a dull, aching chest pain may accompany the cough.

G. Chest assessment
1. A physical examination of the chest does not provide conclusive evidence of tuberculosis.
2. A chest x-ray is not definitive, but the presence of multinodular infiltrates with calcification in the upper lobes suggests tuberculosis.
3. If the disease is active, caseation and inflammation may be seen on the chest x-ray.
4. Advanced disease
   a. Dullness with percussion over involved parenchymal areas, bronchial breath sounds, rhonchi, and crackles indicate advanced disease.
   b. Partial obstruction of a bronchus caused by endobronchial disease or compression by lymph nodes may produce localized wheezing and dyspnea.

H. QuantiFERON-TB Gold test
1. A blood analysis test by an enzyme-linked immunosorbent assay
2. A sensitive and rapid test (results can be available in 24 hours) that assists in diagnosing the client

I. Sputum cultures
1. Sputum specimens are obtained for an acid-fast smear.
2. A sputum culture identifying *M. tuberculosis* confirms the diagnosis.
3. After medications are started, sputum samples are obtained again to determine the effectiveness of therapy.
4. Most clients have negative cultures after 3 months of treatment.

J. Tuberculin skin test (TST) (Table 50-1)
1. A positive reaction does not mean that active disease is present but indicates previous exposure to tuberculosis or the presence of inactive (dormant) disease.
2. Once the test result is positive, it will be positive in any future tests.
3. Skin test interpretation depends on 2 factors: measurement in millimeters of the induration and the person's risk of being infected with tuberculosis and progression to disease if infected.
4. Once an individual's skin test is positive, a chest x-ray is necessary to rule out active tuberculosis or to detect old healed lesions.

K. The hospitalized client
1. The client with active tuberculosis is placed under airborne isolation precautions in a negative-pressure room; to maintain negative pressure, the door of the room must be tightly closed.
2. The room should have at least 6 exchanges of fresh air per hour and should be ventilated to the outside environment, if possible.
3. The nurse wears a particulate respirator (a special individually fitted mask) when caring for the client and a gown when the possibility of clothing contamination exists.
4. Thorough hand washing is required before and after caring for the client.
5. If the client needs to leave the room for a test or procedure, the client is required to wear a surgical mask.

TABLE 50-1 Classification of the Tuberculin Skin Test Reaction

Induration ≥5 mm Considered Positive in:	Induration ≥10 mm Considered Positive in:	Induration ≥15 mm Considered Positive in:
HIV-infected persons	Recent immigrants from high-prevalence countries	Any person, including persons with no known risk factors for TB
Recent contact of a person with TB disease	Injection drug users	
Persons with fibrotic changes on chest x-ray consistent with prior TB	Residents and employees in high-risk congregate settings	
Clients with organ transplants	Mycobacteriology laboratory personnel	
Persons immunosuppressed for other reasons	Persons with clinical conditions that place them at high risk	
	Children <4 years of age	
	Infants, children, and adolescents exposed to adults in high-risk categories	

HIV, Human immunodeficiency virus; *TB*, tuberculosis.
From Centers for Disease Control and Prevention: *Tuberculosis (TB) fact sheets* (website): http://www.cdc.gov/tb/publications/factsheets/testing/skintesting.htm.

6. Respiratory isolation is discontinued when the client is no longer considered infectious.
7. After the infected individual has received tuberculosis medication for 2 to 3 weeks, the risk of transmission is reduced greatly.

L. Client education (Box 50-10)

BOX 50-10 Client Education: Tuberculosis

- Provide the client and family with information about tuberculosis and allay concerns about the contagious aspect of the infection.
- Instruct the client to follow the medication regimen exactly as prescribed and always to have a supply of the medication on hand.
- Advise the client that the medication regimen is continued up to 12 months depending on the situation.
- Advise the client of the side and adverse effects of the medication and ways of minimizing them to ensure compliance.
- Reassure the client that after 2 to 3 weeks of medication therapy, it is unlikely that the client will infect anyone.
- Advise the client to resume activities gradually.
- Instruct the client about the need for adequate nutrition and a well-balanced diet (foods rich in iron, protein, and vitamin C) to promote healing and to prevent recurrence of the infection.
- Inform the client and family that respiratory isolation is not necessary because family members already have been exposed.
- Instruct the client to cover the mouth and nose when coughing or sneezing and to put used tissues into plastic bags.
- Instruct the client and family about thorough hand washing.
- Inform the client that a sputum culture is needed every 2 to 4 weeks once medication therapy is initiated.
- Inform the client that when the results of 3 sputum cultures are negative, the client is no longer considered infectious and usually can return to former employment.
- Advise the client to avoid excessive exposure to silicone or dust because these substances can cause further lung damage.
- Instruct the client regarding the importance of compliance with treatment, follow-up care, and sputum cultures, as prescribed.

PRACTICE QUESTIONS

566. The emergency department nurse is assessing a client who has sustained a blunt injury to the chest wall. Which finding indicates the presence of a pneumothorax in this client?
1. A low respiratory rate
2. Diminished breath sounds
3. The presence of a barrel chest
4. A sucking sound at the site of injury

567. The nurse is caring for a client hospitalized with acute exacerbation of chronic obstructive pulmonary disease. Which findings would the nurse expect to note on assessment of this client? **Select all that apply.**
- ☐ 1. A low arterial PCo_2 level
- ☐ 2. A hyperinflated chest noted on the chest x-ray
- ☐ 3. Decreased oxygen saturation with mild exercise
- ☐ 4. A widened diaphragm noted on the chest x-ray
- ☐ 5. Pulmonary function tests that demonstrate increased vital capacity

568. The nurse is preparing a list of home care instructions for a client who has been hospitalized and treated for tuberculosis. Which instructions should the nurse include on the list? **Select all that apply.**
- ☐ 1. Activities should be resumed gradually.
- ☐ 2. Avoid contact with other individuals, except family members, for at least 6 months.
- ☐ 3. A sputum culture is needed every 2 to 4 weeks once medication therapy is initiated.
- ☐ 4. Respiratory isolation is not necessary, because family members already have been exposed.
- ☐ 5. Cover the mouth and nose when coughing or sneezing and put used tissues in plastic bags.
- ☐ 6. When 1 sputum culture is negative, the client is no longer considered infectious and usually can return to former employment.

569. The nurse is caring for a client after a bronchoscopy and biopsy. Which finding, if noted in the client, should be reported **immediately** to the primary health care provider?
1. Dry cough
2. Hematuria
3. Bronchospasm
4. Blood-streaked sputum

570. The nurse is assessing the respiratory status of a client who has suffered a fractured rib. The nurse should expect to note which finding?
1. Slow, deep respirations
2. Rapid, deep respirations
3. Paradoxical respirations
4. Pain, especially with inspiration

571. A client with a chest injury has suffered flail chest. The nurse assesses the client for which **most** distinctive sign of flail chest?
1. Cyanosis
2. Hypotension
3. Paradoxical chest movement
4. Dyspnea, especially on exhalation

572. The nurse is assessing a client with multiple trauma who is at risk for developing acute respiratory distress syndrome. The nurse should assess for which **earliest** sign of acute respiratory distress syndrome?
1. Bilateral wheezing
2. Inspiratory crackles

3. Intercostal retractions
4. Increased respiratory rate

573. The nurse has conducted discharge teaching with a client diagnosed with tuberculosis who has been receiving medication for 2 weeks. The nurse determines that the client has understood the information if the client makes which statement?
1. "I need to continue medication therapy for 1 month."
2. "I can't shop at the mall for the next 6 months."
3. "I can return to work if a sputum culture comes back negative."
4. "I should not be contagious after 2 to 3 weeks of medication therapy."

574. The nurse is preparing to give a bed bath to an immobilized client with tuberculosis. The nurse should wear which items when performing this care?
1. Surgical mask and gloves
2. Particulate respirator, gown, and gloves
3. Particulate respirator and protective eyewear
4. Surgical mask, gown, and protective eyewear

575. A client has experienced pulmonary embolism. The nurse should assess for which symptom, which is **most** commonly reported?
1. Hot, flushed feeling
2. Sudden chills and fever
3. Chest pain that occurs suddenly
4. Dyspnea when deep breaths are taken

576. A client who is human immunodeficiency virus (HIV)–positive has had a tuberculin skin test (TST). The nurse notes a 7-mm area of induration at the site of the skin test and interprets the result as which finding?
1. Positive
2. Negative
3. Inconclusive
4. Need for repeat testing

577. A client with acquired immunodeficiency syndrome (AIDS) has histoplasmosis. The nurse should assess the client for which expected finding?
1. Dyspnea
2. Headache
3. Weight gain
4. Hypothermia

578. The nurse provides discharge instructions to a client with pulmonary sarcoidosis. The nurse concludes that the client understands the information if the client indicates to report which **early** sign of exacerbation?
1. Fever
2. Fatigue
3. Weight loss
4. Shortness of breath

579. The nurse is taking the history of a client with occupational lung disease (silicosis). The nurse should assess whether the client wears which item during periods of exposure to silica particles?
1. Mask
2. Gown
3. Gloves
4. Eye protection

580. The nurse is instructing a hospitalized client with a diagnosis of emphysema about measures that will enhance the effectiveness of breathing during dyspneic periods. Which position should the nurse instruct the client to assume?
1. Sitting up in bed
2. Side-lying in bed
3. Sitting in a recliner chair
4. Sitting up and leaning on an overbed table

581. The community health nurse is conducting an educational session with community members regarding the signs and symptoms associated with tuberculosis. The nurse informs the participants that tuberculosis is considered as a diagnosis if which signs and symptoms are present? **Select all that apply.**
- ❑ 1. Dyspnea
- ❑ 2. Headache
- ❑ 3. Night sweats
- ❑ 4. A bloody, productive cough
- ❑ 5. A cough with the expectoration of mucoid sputum

582. The nurse performs an admission assessment on a client with a diagnosis of tuberculosis. The nurse should check the results of which diagnostic test that will confirm this diagnosis?
1. Chest x-ray
2. Bronchoscopy
3. Sputum culture
4. Tuberculin skin test

ANSWERS

566. *Answer:* 2

Rationale: This client has sustained a blunt or closed-chest injury. Basic symptoms of a closed pneumothorax are shortness of breath and chest pain. A larger pneumothorax may cause tachypnea, cyanosis, diminished breath sounds, and subcutaneous emphysema. Hyper-resonance also may occur on the affected side. A sucking sound at the site of injury would be noted with an open chest injury.

Test-Taking Strategy: Focus on the subject, a blunt chest injury. Noting the word *blunt* will assist in eliminating option 4, which describes a sucking chest wound injury. Knowing that in a respiratory injury increased respirations will occur will assist you in eliminating option 1. Option 3 can be eliminated because a barrel chest is a characteristic finding in a client with chronic obstructive pulmonary disease.

Level of Cognitive Ability: Analyzing

Client Needs: Physiological Integrity

Integrated Process: Nursing Process—Assessment

Content Area: Adult Health: Respiratory

Health Problem: Adult Health: Respiratory: Chest Injuries

Priority Concepts: Gas Exchange; Perfusion

Reference: Lewis et al. (2017), pp. 519-520.

567. *Answer:* 2, 3

Rationale: Clinical manifestations of chronic obstructive pulmonary disease (COPD) include hypoxemia, hypercapnia, dyspnea on exertion and at rest, oxygen desaturation with exercise, and the use of accessory muscles of respiration. Chest x-rays reveal a hyperinflated chest and a flattened diaphragm if the disease is advanced. Pulmonary function tests will demonstrate decreased vital capacity.

Test-Taking Strategy: Focus on the subject, manifestations of COPD. Think about the pathophysiology associated with this disorder. Remember that hypercapnia, a hyperinflated chest, a flat diaphragm, oxygen desaturation on exercise, and decreased vital capacity are manifestations.

Level of Cognitive Ability: Analyzing

Client Needs: Physiological Integrity

Integrated Process: Nursing Process—Assessment

Content Area: Adult Health: Respiratory

Health Problem: Adult Health: Respiratory: Obstructive Pulmonary Disease

Priority Concepts: Gas Exchange; Perfusion

Reference: Ignatavicius, Workman, Rebar (2018), p. 574.

568. *Answer:* 1, 3, 4, 5

Rationale: The nurse should provide the client and family with information about tuberculosis and allay concerns about the contagious aspect of the infection. The client needs to follow the medication regimen exactly as prescribed and always have a supply of the medication on hand. Side and adverse effects of the medication and ways of minimizing them to ensure compliance should be explained. After 2 to 3 weeks of medication therapy, it is unlikely that the client will infect anyone. Activities should be resumed gradually and a well-balanced diet that is rich in iron, protein, and vitamin C to promote healing and prevent recurrence of infection should be consumed. Respiratory isolation is not necessary, because family members already have been exposed. Instruct the client about thorough hand washing, to cover the mouth and nose when coughing or sneezing, and to put used tissues into plastic bags. A sputum culture is needed every 2 to 4 weeks once medication therapy is initiated. When the results of 3 sputum cultures are negative, the client is no longer considered infectious and can usually return to former employment.

Test-Taking Strategy: Focus on the subject, home care instructions for tuberculosis. Knowledge regarding the pathophysiology, transmission, and treatment of tuberculosis is needed to answer this question. Read each option carefully to answer correctly.

Level of Cognitive Ability: Analyzing

Client Needs: Safe and Effective Care Environment

Integrated Process: Teaching and Learning

Content Area: Adult Health: Respiratory

Health Problem: Adult Health: Respiratory: Tuberculosis

Priority Concepts: Client Education; Infection

Reference: Ignatavicius, Workman, Rebar (2018), p. 610.

569. *Answer:* 3

Rationale: If a biopsy was performed during a bronchoscopy, blood-streaked sputum is expected for several hours. Frank blood indicates hemorrhage. A dry cough may be expected. The client should be assessed for signs of complications, which would include cyanosis, dyspnea, stridor, bronchospasm, hemoptysis, hypotension, tachycardia, and dysrhythmias. Hematuria is unrelated to this procedure.

Test-Taking Strategy: Note the strategic word, *immediately*. Eliminate option 2 first because it is unrelated to the procedure. Next, eliminate option 1, because a dry cough may be expected. Noting that a biopsy has been performed will assist in eliminating option 4, because blood-streaked sputum would be expected. Note that the correct option relates to the airway.

Level of Cognitive Ability: Analyzing

Client Needs: Physiological Integrity

Integrated Process: Nursing Process—Implementation

Content Area: Complex Care: Emergency Situations/Management

Health Problem: N/A

Priority Concepts: Clinical Judgment; Gas Exchange

Reference: Ignatavicius, Workman, Rebar (2018), pp. 525-526.

570. *Answer:* 4

Rationale: Rib fractures result from a blunt injury or a fall. Typical signs and symptoms include pain and tenderness localized at the fracture site that is exacerbated by inspiration and palpation, shallow respirations, splinting or guarding the chest protectively to minimize chest movement, and possible bruising at the fracture site. Paradoxical respirations are seen with flail chest.

Test-Taking Strategy: Focus on the subject, findings associated with a rib fracture. Focusing on the anatomical location of the injury will direct you to the correct option.

Level of Cognitive Ability: Analyzing

Client Needs: Physiological Integrity

Integrated Process: Nursing Process—Assessment

Content Area: Adult Health: Respiratory

Health Problem: Adult Health: Respiratory: Chest Injuries

Priority Concepts: Gas Exchange; Pain

Reference: Lewis et al. (2017), p. 521.

571. Answer: 3

Rationale: Flail chest results from multiple rib fractures. This results in a "floating" section of ribs. Because this section is unattached to the rest of the bony rib cage, this segment results in paradoxical chest movement. This means that the force of inspiration pulls the fractured segment inward, while the rest of the chest expands. Similarly, during exhalation, the segment balloons outward while the rest of the chest moves inward. This is a characteristic sign of flail chest.

Test-Taking Strategy: Note the strategic word, *most.* Cyanosis and hypotension occur with many different disorders, so eliminate options 1 and 2 first. From the remaining options, choose paradoxical chest movement over dyspnea on exhalation by remembering that a flail chest has broken rib segments that move independently of the rest of the rib cage.

Level of Cognitive Ability: Analyzing

Client Needs: Physiological Integrity

Integrated Process: Nursing Process—Assessment

Content Area: Adult Health: Respiratory

Health Problem: Adult Health: Respiratory: Chest Injuries

Priority Concepts: Gas Exchange; Pain

Reference: Lewis et al. (2017), pp. 521-522.

572. Answer: 4

Rationale: The earliest detectable sign of acute respiratory distress syndrome is an increased respiratory rate, which can begin from 1 to 96 hours after the initial insult to the body. This is followed by increasing dyspnea, air hunger, retraction of accessory muscles, and cyanosis. Breath sounds may be clear or consist of fine inspiratory crackles or diffuse coarse crackles.

Test-Taking Strategy: Note the strategic word, *earliest.* Eliminate option 3 first, because intercostal retraction is a later sign of respiratory distress. Of the remaining options, recall that adventitious breath sounds (options 1 and 2) would occur later than an increased respiratory rate.

Level of Cognitive Ability: Analyzing

Client Needs: Physiological Integrity

Integrated Process: Nursing Process—Assessment

Content Area: Adult Health: Respiratory

Health Problem: Adult Health: Respiratory: Acute Respiratory Distress Syndrome/Failure

Priority Concepts: Gas Exchange; Perfusion

Reference: Lewis et al. (2017), pp. 1622-1623.

573. Answer: 4

Rationale: The client is continued on medication therapy for up to 12 months, depending on the situation. The client generally is considered noncontagious after 2 to 3 weeks of medication therapy. The client is instructed to wear a mask if there will be exposure to crowds until the medication is effective in preventing transmission. The client is allowed to return to work when the results of 3 sputum cultures are negative.

Test-Taking Strategy: Focus on the subject, client understanding of medication therapy. Knowing that the medication therapy lasts for up to 12 months helps you eliminate option 1 first. Knowing that 3 sputum cultures must be negative helps you eliminate option 3 next. From the remaining options, recalling that the client is not contagious after 2 to 3 weeks of therapy will direct you to the correct option.

Level of Cognitive Ability: Evaluating

Client Needs: Physiological Integrity

Integrated Process: Nursing Process—Evaluation

Content Area: Adult Health: Respiratory

Health Problem: Adult Health: Respiratory: Tuberculosis

Priority Concepts: Client Education; Infection

Reference: Ignatavicius, Workman, Rebar (2018), pp. 608-609.

574. Answer: 2

Rationale: The nurse who is in contact with a client with tuberculosis should wear an individually fitted particulate respirator. The nurse also would wear gloves as per standard precautions. The nurse wears a gown when the possibility exists that the clothing could become contaminated, such as when giving a bed bath.

Test-Taking Strategy: Focus on the subject, precautions when caring for the client with tuberculosis. Think about the nurse's task, a bed bath. Knowing that the nurse should wear a particulate respirator eliminates options 1 and 4. Knowledge of basic standard precautions directs you to the correct option.

Level of Cognitive Ability: Applying

Client Needs: Safe and Effective Care Environment

Integrated Process: Nursing Process—Implementation

Content Area: Foundations of Care: Infection Control

Health Problem: Adult Health: Respiratory: Tuberculosis

Priority Concepts: Infection; Safety

Reference: Potter et al. (2017), pp. 459-460.

575. Answer: 3

Rationale: The most common initial symptom in pulmonary embolism is chest pain that is sudden in onset. The next most commonly reported symptom is dyspnea, which is accompanied by an increased respiratory rate. Other typical symptoms of pulmonary embolism include apprehension and restlessness, tachycardia, cough, and cyanosis.

Test-Taking Strategy: Note the strategic word, *most.* Because pulmonary embolism does not result from an infectious process or an allergic reaction, eliminate options 1 and 2 first. To select between the correct option and option 4, look at them closely. Option 4 states dyspnea when deep breaths are taken. Although dyspnea commonly occurs with pulmonary embolism, dyspnea is not associated only with deep breathing. Therefore, eliminate option 4.

Level of Cognitive Ability: Analyzing

Client Needs: Physiological Integrity

Integrated Process: Nursing Process—Assessment

Content Area: Adult Health: Respiratory

Health Problem: Adult Health: Respiratory: Pulmonary Embolism

Priority Concepts: Gas Exchange; Perfusion

Reference: Ignatavicius, Workman, Rebar (2018), p. 618.

576. Answer: 1

Rationale: The client with HIV infection is considered to have positive results on tuberculin skin testing with an area of induration larger than 5 mm. The client without HIV is positive with an induration larger than 10 mm. The client with HIV is immunosuppressed, making a smaller area of induration positive for this type of client. It is possible for the client infected with HIV to have false-negative readings because of the immunosuppression factor. Options 2, 3, and 4 are incorrect interpretations.

Test-Taking Strategy: Eliminate options 3 and 4 first because they are comparable or alike. From the remaining options,

recalling that the client with HIV infection is immunosuppressed will assist in determining the interpretation of the area of induration.
Level of Cognitive Ability: Analyzing
Client Needs: Physiological Integrity
Integrated Process: Nursing Process—Analysis
Content Area: Adult Health: Respiratory
Health Problem: Adult Health: Respiratory: Tuberculosis
Priority Concepts: Evidence; Infection
Reference: Ignatavicius, Workman, Rebar (2018), p. 607.

577. *Answer:* 1
Rationale: Histoplasmosis is an opportunistic fungal infection that can occur in the client with AIDS. The infection begins as a respiratory infection and can progress to disseminated infection. Typical signs and symptoms include fever, dyspnea, cough, and weight loss. Enlargement of the client's lymph nodes, liver, and spleen may occur as well.
Test-Taking Strategy: Focus on the **subject,** manifestations of histoplasmosis. Recalling that histoplasmosis is an infectious process will help you eliminate option 4. Because the client has AIDS and another infection, weight gain is an unlikely symptom and can be eliminated next. Knowing that histoplasmosis begins as a respiratory infection helps you choose dyspnea over headache as the correct option.
Level of Cognitive Ability: Analyzing
Client Needs: Physiological Integrity
Integrated Process: Nursing Process—Assessment
Content Area: Adult Health: Respiratory
Health Problem: Adult Health: Respiratory: Viral, bacterial, fungal infections
Priority Concepts: Clinical Judgment; Infection
Reference: Ignatavicius, Workman, Rebar (2018), p. 347.

578. *Answer:* 4
Rationale: Dry cough and dyspnea are typical early manifestations of pulmonary sarcoidosis. Later manifestations include night sweats, fever, weight loss, and skin nodules.
Test-Taking Strategy: Note the **strategic word,** *early*. Because sarcoidosis is a pulmonary problem, eliminate options 1 and 3 first. Select the correct option over option 2 because the shortness of breath (and impaired ventilation) appears first and would cause the fatigue as a secondary symptom.
Level of Cognitive Ability: Evaluating
Client Needs: Physiological Integrity
Integrated Process: Nursing Process—Evaluation
Content Area: Adult Health: Respiratory
Health Problem: Adult Health: Respiratory: Environmental
Priority Concepts: Client Education; Gas Exchange
Reference: Lewis et al. (2017), pp. 528-529.

579. *Answer:* 1
Rationale: Silicosis results from chronic, excessive inhalation of particles of free crystalline silica dust. The client should wear a mask to limit inhalation of this substance, which can cause restrictive lung disease after years of exposure. Options 2, 3, and 4 are not necessary.
Test-Taking Strategy: Focus on the **subject,** prevention of silicosis. Recalling that exposure to silica dust causes the illness and that the dust is inhaled into the respiratory tract will direct you to the correct option.
Level of Cognitive Ability: Applying
Client Needs: Safe and Effective Care Environment
Integrated Process: Nursing Process—Assessment
Content Area: Adult Health: Respiratory
Health Problem: Adult Health: Respiratory: Environmental
Priority Concepts: Infection; Safety
Reference: Lewis et al. (2017), p. 513.

580. *Answer:* 4
Rationale: Positions that will assist the client with emphysema with breathing include sitting up and leaning on an overbed table, sitting up and resting the elbows on the knees, and standing and leaning against the wall.
Test-Taking Strategy: Eliminate options 1 and 3 first because they are **comparable or alike.** Next, eliminate option 2 because this position will not enhance breathing.
Level of Cognitive Ability: Applying
Client Needs: Physiological Integrity
Integrated Process: Teaching and Learning
Content Area: Adult Health: Respiratory
Health Problem: Adult Health: Respiratory: Obstructive Pulmonary Disease
Priority Concepts: Client Education; Gas Exchange
Reference: Ignatavicius, Workman, Rebar (2018), pp. 576, 578.

581. *Answer:* 1, 3, 4, 5
Rationale: Tuberculosis should be considered for any clients with a persistent cough, weight loss, anorexia, night sweats, hemoptysis, shortness of breath, fever, or chills. The client's previous exposure to tuberculosis should also be assessed and correlated with the clinical manifestations.
Test-Taking Strategy: Note the **subject,** clinical manifestations of tuberculosis. Note that headache is not specifically associated with tuberculosis, is not respiratory in nature, and is not associated with an infection to assist in eliminating this option.
Level of Cognitive Ability: Analyzing
Client Needs: Physiological Integrity
Integrated Process: Teaching and Learning
Content Area: Adult Health: Respiratory
Health Problem: Adult Health: Respiratory: Tuberculosis
Priority Concepts: Client Education; Infection
Reference: Lewis et al. (2017), pp. 507-508.

582. *Answer:* 3
Rationale: Tuberculosis is definitively diagnosed through culture and isolation of *Mycobacterium tuberculosis*. A presumptive diagnosis is made based on a tuberculin skin test, a sputum smear that is positive for acid-fast bacteria, a chest x-ray, and histological evidence of granulomatous disease on biopsy.
Test-Taking Strategy: Focus on the **subject,** confirming the diagnosis of tuberculosis. Confirmation is made by identifying the bacteria, *M. tuberculosis.*
Level of Cognitive Ability: Analyzing
Client Needs: Physiological Integrity
Integrated Process: Nursing Process—Assessment
Content Area: Adult Health: Respiratory
Health Problem: Adult Health: Respiratory: Tuberculosis
Priority Concepts: Evidence; Infection
Reference: Ignatavicius, Workman, Rebar (2018), pp. 605, 607.

CHAPTER 51

Respiratory Medications

PRIORITY CONCEPTS Gas Exchange; Infection

I. Medication Inhalation Devices

A. Metered-dose inhaler (MDI): Uses a chemical propellant to push the medication out of the inhaler (Fig. 51-1)

B. Dry powder inhaler (DPI): Delivers medication without using chemical propellants, but it requires strong and fast inhalation.

C. Nebulizer: Delivers fine liquid mists of medication through a tube or a mask that fits over the nose and mouth, or with a mouthpiece, using air or oxygen under pressure.

D. If 2 different inhaled medications are prescribed and 1 of the medications contains a glucocorticoid (corticosteroid), administer the bronchodilator first and the corticosteroid second.

⚠ If 2 different inhaled medications are prescribed, instruct the client to wait 5 minutes following administration of the first before inhaling the second. If a second dose of the same medication is needed, instruct the client to wait 1 to 2 minutes before taking the second dose.

II. Bronchodilators (Box 51-1)

A. Description
1. Sympathomimetic bronchodilators relax the smooth muscle of the bronchi and dilate the airways of the respiratory tree, making air exchange and respiration easier for the client. Examples include β_2-adrenergic agonists, such as albuterol.
2. Methylxanthine bronchodilators stimulate the central nervous system (CNS) and respiration, dilate coronary and pulmonary vessels, cause diuresis, and relax smooth muscle. An example is theophylline.
3. Used to treat acute bronchospasm, acute and chronic **asthma,** bronchitis, restrictive airway diseases, and reactive airway diseases
4. Contraindicated in individuals with hypersensitivity, peptic ulcer disease, severe cardiac disease and cardiac dysrhythmias, hyperthyroidism, or uncontrolled seizure disorders
5. Used with caution in clients with hypertension, diabetes mellitus, or narrow-angle glaucoma
6. Theophylline increases the risk of digoxin toxicity and decreases the effects of lithium and phenytoin. Theophylline should be a last-line medication.
7. If theophylline and a β_2-adrenergic agonist are administered together, cardiac dysrhythmias may result.
8. Beta blockers, cimetidine, and erythromycin increase the effects of theophylline.
9. Barbiturates and carbamazepine decrease the effects of theophylline.

B. Side and adverse effects
1. Palpitations and tachycardia
2. Dysrhythmias
3. Restlessness, nervousness, tremors
4. Anorexia, nausea, and vomiting
5. Headaches and dizziness
6. Hyperglycemia
7. Mouth dryness and throat irritation with inhalers
8. Tolerance and paradoxical bronchoconstriction with inhalers

C. Interventions
1. Assess lung sounds.
2. Monitor for cardiac dysrhythmias.
3. Assess for cough, wheezing, decreased breath sounds, and sputum production.
4. Monitor for restlessness and confusion.
5. Provide adequate hydration.
6. Administer the medication at regular intervals around the clock to maintain a sustained therapeutic level.
7. Administer oral medications with or after meals to decrease gastrointestinal irritation.
8. Monitor for a therapeutic serum theophylline level of 10 to 20 mcg/mL (55.5 to 111 mcmol/L).
9. Intravenously administered theophylline preparations should be administered slowly and always via an infusion pump.

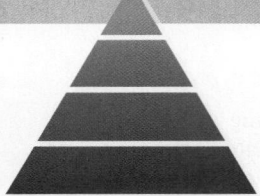

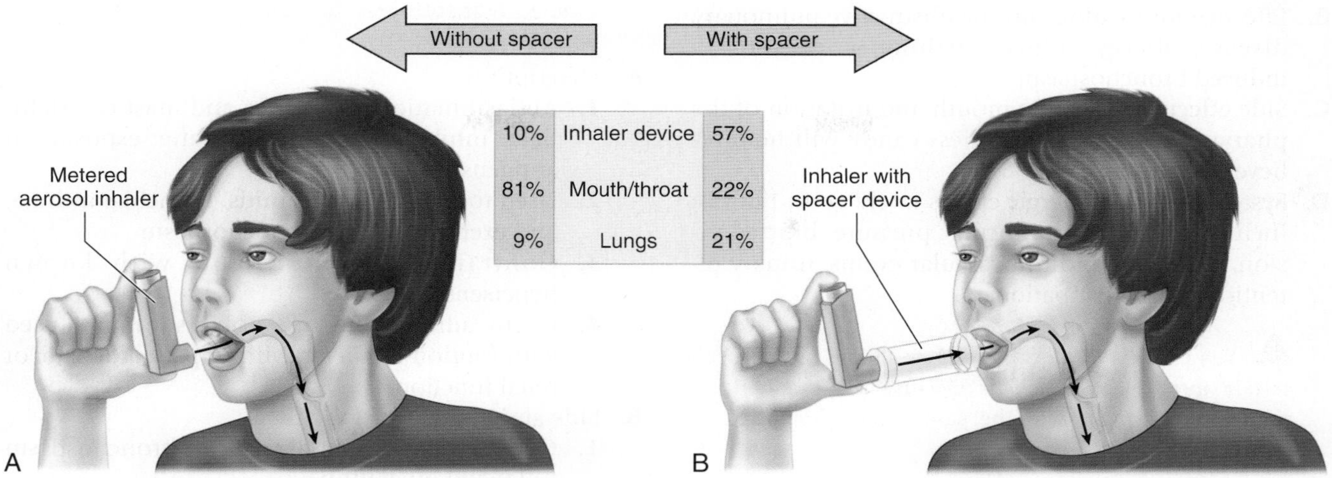

FIG. 51-1 Inhaled medications commonly used in asthma treatment include β-adrenergic bronchodilators, cromolyn sodium, and aerosol glucocorticoids. **A,** The metered-dose inhaler may be held about 2 fingerwidths (1.5 inches [4 cm]) in front of the mouth. **B,** Alternatively, an inhaler with a spacer device can be used. Clients should breathe deeply once before activating the inhaler and then continue breathing in for about 5 seconds. Clients then should hold their breath for 10 to 15 seconds before breathing out slowly. If a second dose is needed, clients should wait 1 to 2 minutes before taking the second dose.

BOX 51-1 Medications to Treat Restrictive Airway Problems

Bronchodilators

β_2-Adrenergic Agonists

Inhaled
- Albuterol
- Arformoterol
- Formoterol
- Levalbuterol
- Salmeterol

Oral
- Albuterol
- Terbutaline

Methylxanthines
- Theophylline, oral
- Aminophylline

Anticholinergics
- Ipratropium, inhaled
- Tiotropium, inhaled
- Aclidinium, inhaled
- Umeclidinium, inhaled

Glucocorticoids (Corticosteroids)

Inhaled
- Beclomethasone dipropionate
- Budesonide
- Ciclesonide
- Flunisolide
- Fluticasone propionate
- Mometasone furoate
- Triamcinolone acetonide

Oral
- Prednisone
- Prednisolone

Leukotriene Modifiers
- Montelukast, oral
- Zafirlukast, oral
- Zileuton, oral

Inhaled Nonsteroidal Antiallergy Agent
- Cromolyn sodium, inhaled

Monoclonal Antibody
- Omalizumab

Adapted from Burchum JR, Rosenthal LD: *Lehne's pharmacology for nursing care,* ed 9, St. Louis, 2016, Saunders.

10. Client education
  a. Not to crush enteric-coated or sustained-release tablets or capsules
  b. To avoid caffeine-containing products such as coffee, tea, cola, and chocolate, and over-the-counter medications
  c. About the side and adverse effects of bronchodilators
  d. How to monitor the pulse and to report any abnormalities to the primary health care provider (PHCP)
  e. How to use an inhaler, spacer (see Fig. 51-1), or nebulizer and how to monitor the amount of medication remaining in an inhaler canister
  f. The importance of smoking cessation and information regarding support resources
  g. To monitor blood glucose levels if diabetes mellitus is a coexisting condition
  h. To wear a MedicAlert bracelet, particularly if the client has asthma

Theophylline toxicity is likely to occur when the serum level is higher than 20 mcg/mL (111 mcmol/L). Early signs of toxicity include restlessness, nervousness, tremors, palpitations, and tachycardia.

III. Anticholinergics (see Box 51-1)

A. Inhaled medications that improve lung function by blocking muscarinic receptors in the bronchi, which prevents bronchoconstriction

B. Effective for treating chronic obstructive pulmonary disease, allergy-induced asthma, and exercise-induced bronchospasm
C. Side effects include dry mouth and irritation of the pharynx; sucking on sugarless candy will help relieve symptoms.
D. Systemic anticholinergic effects rarely occur but can include increased intraocular pressure, blurred vision, tachycardia, cardiovascular events, urinary retention, and constipation.

The client with a peanut allergy should not take certain ipratropium products because they contain soy lecithin, which is in the same plant family as peanuts.

IV. Glucocorticoids (Corticosteroids) (see Box 51-1)

A. Glucocorticoids act as antiinflammatory agents and reduce edema of the airways; they are used to treat asthma and other inflammatory respiratory conditions.
B. See Chapter 47 for information on glucocorticoids.

V. Leukotriene Modifiers (see Box 51-1)

A. Description
  1. Used in the prophylaxis and treatment of chronic bronchial asthma (not used for acute asthma episodes)
  2. Inhibit bronchoconstriction caused by specific antigens and reduce airway edema and smooth muscle constriction
  3. Contraindicated in clients with hypersensitivity and in breast-feeding mothers
  4. Should be used with caution in clients with impaired hepatic function
  5. Coadministration of inhaled glucocorticoids increases the risk of upper respiratory infection.
B. Side and adverse effects
  1. Headache
  2. Nausea and vomiting
  3. Dyspepsia
  4. Diarrhea
  5. Generalized pain, myalgia
  6. Fever
  7. Dizziness
C. Interventions
  1. Assess frequency of exacerbations.
  2. Assess changes in lung function.
  3. Assess liver function laboratory values.
  4. Monitor for cyanosis.
D. Client education
  1. To take medication 1 hour before or 2 hours after meals
  2. To increase fluid intake
  3. Not to discontinue the medication and to take it as prescribed, even during symptom-free periods

VI. Inhaled Nonsteroidal Antiallergy Agent (see Box 51-1)

A. Description
  1. Antiasthmatic, antiallergic, and mast cell stabilizers inhibit mast cell release after exposure to antigens.
  2. Used to treat allergic rhinitis, bronchial asthma, and exercise-induced bronchospasm
  3. Contraindicated in clients with known hypersensitivity
  4. Orally administered cromolyn sodium is used with caution in clients with impaired hepatic or renal function.
B. Side and adverse effects
  1. Cough, sneezing, nasal sting, or bronchospasm following inhalation
  2. Unpleasant taste in the mouth
C. Interventions: Monitor respirations and assess lung sounds for rhonchi or wheezing.
D. Client education
  1. To administer oral capsules at least 30 minutes before meals
  2. Not to discontinue the medication abruptly, because a rebound asthmatic attack can occur

Instruct the client taking inhaled medications to drink a few sips of water before and after inhalation to prevent a cough and an unpleasant taste in the mouth.

VII. Monoclonal Antibody (see Box 51-1)

A. Description
  1. Omalizumab is a recombinant DNA-derived humanized immunoglobulin G (IgG) murine monoclonal antibody that selectively binds to immunoglobulin E (IgE) to limit the release of mediators in the allergic response.
  2. Used to treat allergy-related asthma; administered subcutaneously every 2 to 4 weeks
  3. Dose is titrated on the basis of the serum IgE level and body weight.
  4. Contraindicated in those with hypersensitivity to the medication
B. Side and adverse effects
  1. Injection site reactions
  2. Viral infections
  3. Upper respiratory infections
  4. Sinusitis
  5. Headache
  6. Pharyngitis
  7. Anaphylaxis
  8. Malignancies
C. Interventions
  1. Assess respiratory rate, rhythm, and depth, and auscultate lung sounds.
  2. Assess for allergies and/or allergic reaction symptoms such as rash or urticaria.

3. Have medications for the treatment of severe hypersensitivity reactions available during initial administration in case anaphylaxis occurs.

D. Client education
1. That respiratory improvement will not be immediate
2. Not to stop taking or decrease the currently prescribed asthma medications unless instructed
3. To avoid receiving live virus vaccines for the duration of treatment

VIII. Antihistamines (Box 51-2)

A. Description
1. Called *histamine antagonists* or *H_1 blockers*; these medications compete with histamine for receptor sites, thus preventing a histamine response.
2. When the H_1 receptor is stimulated, the extravascular smooth muscles, including those lining the nasal cavity, are constricted.
3. Decrease nasopharyngeal, gastrointestinal, and bronchial secretions by blocking the H_1 receptor
4. Used for the common cold, rhinitis, nausea and vomiting, motion sickness, urticaria, and as a sleep aid
5. Can cause CNS depression if taken with alcohol, opioids, hypnotics, or barbiturates, particularly with first-generation antihistamines
6. Should be used with caution in clients with chronic obstructive pulmonary disease because of their drying effect
7. Diphenhydramine has an anticholinergic effect and should be avoided in clients with narrow-angle glaucoma.

B. Side and adverse effects
1. Drowsiness and fatigue
2. Dizziness
3. Urinary retention
4. Blurred vision
5. Wheezing
6. Constipation
7. Dry mouth
8. Gastrointestinal irritation
9. Hypotension
10. Hearing disturbances
11. Photosensitivity
12. Nervousness and irritability
13. Confusion
14. Nightmares

BOX 51-2 Antihistamines

■ Brompheniramine	■ Dimenhydrinate
■ Cetirizine	■ Diphenhydramine
■ Chlorpheniramine	■ Fexofenadine
■ Clemastine	■ Levocetirizine
■ Cyproheptadine	■ Loratadine
■ Desloratadine	■ Olopatadine

C. Interventions
1. Monitor for signs of urinary dysfunction.
2. Administer with food or milk.
3. Avoid subcutaneous injection, and administer by intramuscular injection in a large muscle if the intramuscular route is prescribed.

D. Client education
1. To avoid hazardous activities, alcohol, and other CNS depressants
2. If the medication is being taken for motion sickness, take it 30 minutes before the event and then before meals and at bedtime during the event as prescribed.
3. To suck on hard candy or ice chips for dry mouth

IX. Nasal Decongestants (Box 51-3)

A. Description
1. Nervousness
2. Restlessness, insomnia
3. Hypertension
4. Hyperglycemia

B. Side and adverse effects
1. Include adrenergic, anticholinergic, and corticosteroid medications
2. Shrink nasal mucosal membranes and reduce fluid secretion
3. Used for allergic rhinitis, hay fever, and acute coryza (profuse nasal discharge)
4. Contraindicated or used with extreme caution in clients with hypertension, cardiac disease, hyperthyroidism, or diabetes mellitus

C. Interventions
1. Monitor for cardiac dysrhythmias.
2. Monitor blood glucose levels.

D. Client education

Nasal decongestants can cause tolerance and rebound nasal congestion (vasodilation) caused by irritation of the nasal mucosa. Therefore, the client needs to be informed that these medications should not be used for longer than 48 hours.

1. To avoid consuming caffeine in large amounts because it can increase restlessness and palpitations

BOX 51-3 Nasal Decongestants

Nonglucocorticoids	Glucocorticoids
■ Oxymetazoline	■ Beclomethasone
■ Phenylephrine hydrochloride	■ Budesonide
■ Pseudoephedrine hydrochloride	■ Ciclesonide
	■ Flunisolide
	■ Fluticasone propionate
	■ Fluticasone furoate
	■ Mometasone
	■ Triamcinolone

2. About the importance of limiting the use of nasal sprays and drops to prevent rebound nasal congestion; consider weaning off one nare at a time to prevent this.

X. Expectorants and Mucolytic Agents (Box 51-4)

A. Description
   1. Expectorants loosen bronchial secretions so that they can be eliminated with coughing; they are used for a dry unproductive cough and to stimulate bronchial secretions.
   2. Mucolytic agents thin mucous secretions to help make the cough more productive.
   3. Mucolytic agents with dextromethorphan should not be used by clients with chronic obstructive pulmonary disease because they suppress the cough.
   4. Acetylcysteine can increase airway resistance and should not be used in clients with asthma. This medication can also be used to prevent liver damage in acetaminophen overdose, as well as to protect the kidneys in the event that diagnostic testing requiring contrast dye is done.

B. Side and adverse effects
   1. Gastrointestinal irritation
   2. Rash
   3. Oropharyngeal irritation

C. Interventions
   1. Acetylcysteine, administered by nebulization, should not be mixed with another medication.
   2. If acetylcysteine is administered with a bronchodilator, the bronchodilator should be administered 5 minutes before the acetylcysteine.
   3. Monitor for side effects of acetylcysteine such as nausea and vomiting, stomatitis, and runny nose.

D. Client education
   1. To take the medication with a full glass of water to loosen mucus
   2. To maintain adequate fluid intake
   3. To cough and deep breathe

XI. Antitussives (Box 51-5)

A. Description: Act on the cough control center in the medulla to suppress the cough reflex; used for a cough that is nonproductive and irritating

B. Side and adverse effects
   1. Dizziness, drowsiness, sedation
   2. Gastrointestinal irritation, nausea
   3. Dry mouth
   4. Constipation
   5. Respiratory depression

C. Interventions
   1. Encourage the client to take adequate fluids with the medication.
   2. Encourage the client to sleep with the head of the bed elevated.
   3. Note that medication dependency can occur.
   4. Avoid administration to the client with a head injury or a postoperative cranial surgery client.
   5. Avoid administration to the client using opioids, sedative-hypnotics, barbiturates, or select antidepressants, because CNS depression can occur.

D. Client education
   1. If the cough lasts longer than 1 week and a fever or rash occurs, to notify the PHCP
   2. To avoid hazardous activities
   3. To avoid the use of alcohol

XII. Opioid Antagonists (Box 51-6)

A. Description
   1. Reverses respiratory depression in opioid overdose
   2. Avoid its use for nonopioid respiratory depression.
   3. Reoccurrence of respiratory depression can occur if duration of opiate exceeds duration of opioid antagonist.
   4. This medication may be prescribed for clients at risk for opioid overdose.
   5. https://www.nsc.org/home-safety/safety-topics/opioids/prescription-nation?gclid=EAIaIQobChMIiJXd446a2wIViYizCh0-_ADOEAAYASAAEgKfc_D_BwE

B. Side and adverse effects
   1. Nausea, vomiting
   2. Tremors
   3. Sweating
   4. Increased blood pressure
   5. Tachycardia

BOX 51-4 Expectorants and Mucolytic Agents

Expectorant
- Guaifenesin

Mucolytic
- Acetylcysteine

BOX 51-5 Antitussives

Opioids
- Codeine phosphate, codeine sulfate
- Hydrocodone

Nonopioids
- Benzonatate
- Dextromethorphan
- Diphenhydramine hydrochloride

BOX 51-6 Opioid Antagonists

- Alvimopan
- Methylnaltrexone
- Naloxone
- Naltrexone

C. Interventions
1. Assess vital signs, especially respirations.
2. For intravenous administration, the dose is titrated every 2 to 5 minutes as prescribed.
3. Have oxygen and resuscitative equipment available during administration.

XIII. Tuberculosis Medications (Box 51-7)

A. Description
1. Offer the most effective method for treating the disease and preventing transmission
2. Treatment of identified lesions depends on whether the individual has active disease or has only been exposed to the disease.
3. Treatment is difficult because the bacterium has a waxy substance on the capsule that makes penetration and destruction difficult.
4. The use of a multidrug regimen destroys organisms as quickly as possible and minimizes the emergence of drug-resistant organisms.
5. Active tuberculosis is treated with a combination of medications to which the organism is susceptible.
6. Individuals with active tuberculosis are treated for 6 to 9 months; however, clients with immunosuppression (e.g., HIV) are treated for a longer period of time.
7. After the infected individual has received medication for 2 to 3 weeks, the risk of transmission is greatly reduced.
8. Most clients have negative sputum cultures after 3 months of compliance with medication therapy.
9. Individuals who have been exposed to active tuberculosis are treated with preventive isoniazid for 9 to 12 months.

B. First-line or second-line medications
1. First-line medications provide the most effective antituberculosis activity.
2. Second-line medications are used in combination with first-line medications but are more toxic.
3. Current infecting organisms are proving resistant to standard first-line medications; the resistant organisms develop because individuals with the disease fail to complete the course of treatment, so surviving bacteria adapt to the medication and become resistant.
4. Multidrug therapies are instituted because of the resistant organisms.

C. Multidrug-resistant strain of tuberculosis (MDR-TB)
1. Resistance occurs when a client receiving 2 medications (first-line and second-line medications) discontinues 1 of the medications.
2. The client briefly experiences some response from the single medication, but then large numbers of resistant organisms begin to grow.
3. The client, infectious again, transmits the drug-resistant organism to other individuals.
4. As this event is repeated, an organism develops that is resistant to many of the first-line tuberculosis medications.

D. General client education points for tuberculosis medications
1. Not to skip doses and to take medication for the full length of the prescribed therapy
2. Not to take any other medication without consulting with the PHCP
3. About the importance of follow-up PHCP visits and laboratory tests
4. To avoid alcohol
5. To take medication on an empty stomach with 8 oz of water 1 hour before or 2 hours after meals and to avoid taking antacids with the medication
6. About the adverse effects that require PHCP notification
7. Inform the client about direct observed therapy (DOT) to ensure adherence to the medication regimen.

BOX 51-7 First-Line and Second-Line Medications for Tuberculosis

First-Line Agents	Second-Line Agents
Isoniazid	Amikacin
Rifampin	Capreomycin sulfate
Ethambutol	Cycloserine
Pyrazinamide	Ethionamide
	Levofloxacin
	Moxifloxacin
	p-Aminosalicylic acid
	Rifabutin
	Rifapentine
	Streptomycin

XIV. First-Line Medications for Tuberculosis (see Box 51-7)

A. Isoniazid
1. Description
   a. Bactericidal
   b. Inhibits the synthesis of mycolic acids and acts to kill actively growing organisms in the extracellular environment
   c. Inhibits the growth of dormant organisms in the macrophages and caseating granulomas
   d. Is active only during cell division and is used in combination with other antitubercular medications

2. Contraindications and cautions
   a. Contraindicated in clients with hypersensitivity or with acute liver disease
   b. Use with caution in clients with chronic liver disease, alcoholism, or renal impairment.
   c. Use with caution in clients taking nicotinic acid.
   d. Use with caution in clients taking hepatotoxic medications because the risk for hepatotoxicity increases.
   e. Alcohol increases the risk of hepatotoxicity.
   f. May increase the risk of toxicity of carbamazepine and phenytoin
   g. May decrease ketoconazole concentrations
3. Side and adverse effects
   a. Hypersensitivity reactions
   b. Peripheral neuritis
   c. Neurotoxicity
   d. Hepatotoxicity and hepatitis; increased liver function test levels
   e. Pyridoxine deficiency
   f. Irritation at injection site with intramuscular administration
   g. Nausea and vomiting
   h. Dry mouth
   i. Dizziness
   j. Hyperglycemia
   k. Vision changes
4. Interventions
   a. Assess for hypersensitivity.
   b. Assess for hepatic dysfunction.
   c. Assess for sensitivity to nicotinic acid.
   d. Monitor liver function test results.
   e. Monitor for signs of hepatitis, such as anorexia, nausea, vomiting, weakness, fatigue, dark urine, or jaundice; if these symptoms occur, withhold the medication and notify the PHCP.
   f. Monitor for tingling, numbness, or burning of the extremities.
   g. Assess mental status.
   h. Monitor for visual changes, and notify the PHCP if they occur.
   i. Assess for dizziness and initiate safety precautions.
   j. Monitor complete blood count (CBC) and blood glucose levels.
   k. Administer isoniazid 1 hour before or 2 hours after a meal, because food may delay absorption.
   l. Administer isoniazid at least 1 hour before antacids.
   m. Administer pyridoxine as prescribed to reduce the risk of neurotoxicity.

! Many tuberculosis medications can cause toxic effects such as hepatotoxicity, nephrotoxicity, neurotoxicity, optic neuritis, or ototoxicity. Teach the client about the signs of toxicity and inform the client that the PHCP needs to be notified if any signs arise.

5. Client education
   a. To avoid tyramine-containing foods because they may cause a reaction such as red and itching skin, a pounding heartbeat, lightheadedness, a hot or clammy feeling, or a headache; if this occurs, the client should notify the PHCP.
   b. To recognize the signs of neurotoxicity, hepatitis, and hepatotoxicity
   c. To notify the PHCP if signs of neurotoxicity, hepatitis and hepatotoxicity, or visual changes occur.

B. Rifampin
1. Description
   a. Inhibits bacterial RNA synthesis
   b. Binds to DNA-dependent RNA polymerase and blocks RNA transcription
   c. Used with at least 1 other antitubercular medication
2. Contraindications and cautions
   a. Contraindicated in clients with hypersensitivity
   b. Used with caution in clients with hepatic dysfunction or alcoholism
   c. Use of alcohol or hepatotoxic medications may increase the risk of hepatotoxicity.
   d. Decreases the effects of several medications, including oral anticoagulants, oral hypoglycemics, chloramphenicol, digoxin, disopyramide phosphate, mexiletine, quinidine polygalacturonate, fluconazole, methadone hydrochloride, phenytoin, and verapamil hydrochloride
3. Side and adverse effects
   a. Hypersensitivity reaction, including fever, chills, shivering, headache, muscle and bone pain, and dyspnea
   b. Heartburn, nausea, vomiting, diarrhea
   c. Red-orange–colored body secretions
   d. Vision changes
   e. Hepatotoxicity and hepatitis
   f. Increased uric acid levels
   g. Blood dyscrasias
   h. Colitis
4. Interventions
   a. Assess for hypersensitivity.
   b. Evaluate CBC, uric acid, and liver function test results.
   c. Assess for signs of hepatitis; if they occur, withhold the medication and notify the PHCP.
   d. Monitor for signs of colitis.
   e. Assess for visual changes.
5. Client education
   a. That urine, feces, sweat, and tears will be red-orange and that soft contact lens can become permanently discolored
   b. To notify the PHCP if jaundice (yellow eyes or skin) develops or if weakness, fatigue,

nausea, vomiting, sore throat, fever, or unusual bleeding occurs

C. Ethambutol
1. Description
a. Bacteriostatic
b. Interferes with cell metabolism and multiplication by inhibiting 1 or more metabolites in susceptible organisms
c. Inhibits bacterial RNA synthesis and is active only during cell division
d. Slow-acting and must be used with other bactericidal agents
2. Contraindications and cautions
a. Contraindicated in clients with hypersensitivity or optic neuritis and in children younger than 13 years
b. Used with caution in clients with renal dysfunction, gout, ocular defects, diabetic retinopathy, cataracts, or ocular inflammatory conditions
c. Used with caution in clients taking neurotoxic medications because the risk for neurotoxicity increases
3. Side and adverse effects
a. Hypersensitivity reactions
b. Anorexia, nausea, vomiting
c. Dizziness
d. Malaise
e. Mental confusion
f. Joint pain
g. Dermatitis
h. Optic neuritis
i. Peripheral neuritis
j. Thrombocytopenia
k. Increased uric acid levels
l. Anaphylactoid reaction
4. Interventions
a. Assess the client for hypersensitivity.
b. Evaluate results of CBC, uric acid, and renal and liver function tests.
c. Monitor for visual changes such as altered color perception and decreased visual acuity; if changes occur, withhold the medication and notify the PHCP.
d. Administer once every 24 hours and administer with food to decrease gastrointestinal upset.
e. Monitor uric acid concentration and assess for painful or swollen joints or signs of gout.
f. Monitor intake and output and for adequate renal function.
g. Assess mental status.
h. Monitor for dizziness and initiate safety precautions.
i. Assess for peripheral neuritis (numbness, tingling, or burning of the extremities); if it occurs, notify the PHCP.
5. Client education
a. That nausea, related to the medication, can be prevented by taking the daily dose at bedtime or by taking the prescribed antinausea medications
b. To notify the PHCP immediately if any visual problems occur or if a rash; swelling and pain in the joints; or numbness, tingling, or burning in the hands or feet occurs

D. Pyrazinamide
1. Description
a. The exact mechanism of action is unknown.
b. May be bacteriostatic or bactericidal, depending on its concentration at the infection site and on the susceptibility of the infecting organism
c. Used with at least 1 other antitubercular medication if ineffectiveness of the primary medication(s) occurs
2. Contraindications and cautions
a. Contraindicated in clients with hypersensitivity
b. Used with caution in clients with diabetes mellitus, renal impairment, or gout and in children
c. May decrease the effects of allopurinol, colchicine, and probenecid
d. Cross-sensitivity is possible with isoniazid, ethionamide, or nicotinic acid.
3. Side and adverse effects
a. Increases liver function tests and uric acid levels
b. Arthralgia, myalgia
c. Photosensitivity
d. Hepatotoxicity
e. Thrombocytopenia
4. Interventions
a. Assess for hypersensitivity.
b. Evaluate CBC, liver function test results, and uric acid levels.
c. Observe for hepatotoxic effects; if they occur, withhold the medication and notify the PHCP.
d. Assess for painful or swollen joints.
e. Evaluate blood glucose level, because diabetes mellitus may be difficult to control while client is taking the medication.
5. Client education
a. To take the medication with food to reduce gastrointestinal distress
b. To avoid sunlight or ultraviolet light until photosensitivity is determined

Some tuberculosis medications can cause red-orange–colored body secretions. Inform the client that this is not a harmful effect but that the secretions can stain and permanently discolor items.

XV. Second-Line Medications for Tuberculosis (see Box 51-7)

A. Rifabutin
1. Description
   a. Inhibits mycobacterial DNA-dependent RNA polymerase and suppresses protein synthesis
   b. Used to prevent disseminated *Mycobacterium avium* complex (MAC) disease in clients with advanced HIV infection
   c. Used to treat active MAC disease and tuberculosis in clients with HIV infection
2. Cautions
   a. Can affect blood levels of some medications, including oral contraceptives and some medications used to treat HIV infection
   b. A nonhormonal method of birth control should be used instead of an oral contraceptive.
3. Side and adverse effects
   a. Rash
   b. Gastrointestinal disturbances
   c. Neutropenia
   d. Red-orange–colored body secretions
   e. Uveitis
   f. Myositis
   g. Arthralgia
   h. Hepatitis
   i. Chest pain with dyspnea
   j. Flu-like syndrome
4. Interventions
   a. Observe for hepatotoxic effects; if they occur, withhold the medication and notify the PHCP.
   b. Assess for painful or swollen joints.
   c. Assess for ocular pain or blurred vision.
5. Client education: That the medication can be taken without regard to food

B. Rifapentine
1. Description: Used only for pulmonary tuberculosis
2. Cautions: Can affect blood levels of some medications, including oral contraceptives and warfarin, and some medications used to treat HIV infection
3. Side and adverse effects
   a. Red-orange–colored body secretions
   b. Hepatotoxicity
4. Interventions
   a. Obtain baseline liver function studies and assess throughout therapy.
   b. Observe for hepatotoxic effects; if they occur, withhold the medication and notify the PHCP.
5. Client education
   a. That the medication can be taken without regard to food
   b. To avoid sunlight or ultraviolet light until photosensitivity is determined
   c. That red-orange–colored body secretions may occur

C. Capreomycin sulfate
1. Description
   a. Mechanism of action is unknown.
   b. Used to treat MDR-TB when significant resistance to other medications is expected
   c. Administered intramuscularly
2. Contraindications and cautions
   a. The risk of nephrotoxicity, ototoxicity, and neuromuscular blockade is increased with the use of aminoglycosides or loop diuretics.
   b. Used with caution in clients with renal insufficiency, acoustic nerve impairment, hepatic disorder, myasthenia gravis, or parkinsonism
   c. Not administered to clients receiving streptomycin
3. Side and adverse effects
   a. Nephrotoxicity
   b. Ototoxicity
   c. Neuromuscular blockade
4. Interventions
   a. Perform baseline audiometric testing.
   b. Assess renal, hepatic, and electrolyte levels before administration.
   c. Monitor intake and output.
   d. Reconstituted medication may be stored for 48 hours at room temperature.
   e. Administer intramuscularly, deep into a large muscle mass.
   f. Rotate injection sites.
   g. Observe injection site for redness, excessive bleeding, and inflammation.
5. Client education
   a. Not to perform tasks that require mental alertness
   b. To report any hearing loss, balance disturbances, respiratory difficulty, weakness, or signs of hypersensitivity reactions

D. Antibiotics
1. Description
   a. Aminoglycoside antibiotics or fluoroquinolones are given with at least 1 other antitubercular medication.
   b. Bactericidal because of receptor-binding action interfering with protein synthesis in susceptible microorganisms
   c. Gastrointestinal disturbances are the most common side effect.
   d. Fluoroquinolones are not recommended for use in children.
2. Contraindications and cautions
   a. Contraindicated in clients with hypersensitivity, neuromuscular disorders, or eighth cranial nerve damage

b. Used with caution in the older client, in neonates because of renal insufficiency and immaturity, and in young infants because it may cause CNS depression
c. The risk of toxicity increases if taken with other aminoglycosides or nephrotoxicity- or ototoxicity-producing medications.
3. Side and adverse effects
a. Hypersensitivity
b. Pain and irritation at the injection site
c. Nephrotoxicity is indicated by increased blood urea nitrogen and serum creatinine levels.
d. Ototoxicity is indicated by tinnitus, dizziness, ringing or roaring in the ears, and reduced hearing.
e. Neurotoxicity is indicated by headache, dizziness, lethargy, tremors, and visual disturbances.
f. Superinfections
4. Interventions
a. Assess for hypersensitivity.
b. Monitor for ototoxic, neurotoxic, and nephrotoxic reactions.
c. Monitor liver and renal function test results.
d. Obtain baseline audiometric test and repeat every 1 to 2 months, because the medication impairs the eighth cranial nerve.
e. Assess acuteness of hearing.
f. Monitor for visual changes.
g. Assess hydration status and maintain adequate hydration during therapy.
h. Monitor intake and output.
i. Assess urinalysis.
j. Monitor for superinfection.
5. Client education: To notify the PHCP if hearing loss, changes in vision, or urinary problems occur

E. Ethionamide
1. Description
a. Mechanism of action is unknown.
b. Used to treat MDR-TB when significant resistance to other medications is expected
2. Contraindications and cautions
a. Contraindicated in clients with hypersensitivity
b. Used with caution in clients with diabetes mellitus or renal dysfunction
3. Side and adverse effects
a. Anorexia, nausea, vomiting
b. Metallic taste in the mouth
c. Orthostatic hypotension
d. Jaundice
e. Mental changes
f. Peripheral neuritis
g. Rash
4. Interventions
a. Assess liver and renal function test results.
b. Monitor glucose levels in the client with diabetes mellitus.
c. Administer pyridoxine as prescribed to reduce the risk of neurotoxicity.
5. Client education
a. To take medication with food or meals to minimize gastrointestinal irritation
b. To change positions slowly
c. To report signs of a rash, which can progress to exfoliative dermatitis if the medication is not discontinued

F. Aminosalicylic acid
1. Description
a. Inhibits folic acid metabolism in mycobacteria
b. Used to treat MDR-TB when significant resistance to other medications is expected
2. Contraindications and cautions
a. Contraindicated with hypersensitivity to aminosalicylates, salicylates, or compounds containing the *para*-aminophenol group
b. Aminobenzoates block the absorption of aminosalicylate sodium.
3. Side and adverse effects
a. Hypersensitivity
b. Bitter taste in the mouth
c. Gastrointestinal tract irritation
d. Exfoliative dermatitis
e. Blood dyscrasias
f. Crystalluria
g. Changes in thyroid function
4. Interventions
a. Assess for hypersensitivity.
b. Offer water to rinse the mouth and chewing gum or hard candy to alleviate the bitter taste.
c. Encourage fluid intake to prevent crystalluria.
d. Monitor intake and output.
5. Client education
a. To discard the medication and obtain a new supply if a purplish-brown discoloration occurs
b. To take the medication with food
c. That urine may turn red on contact with hypochlorite bleach if bleach was used to clean a toilet
d. Not to take aspirin or over-the-counter medications without the PHCP's approval
e. To report signs of a blood dyscrasia, such as sore throat or mouth, malaise, fatigue, bruising, or bleeding

G. Cycloserine
1. Description
a. Interferes with cell wall biosynthesis
b. Used to treat MDR-TB when significant resistance to other medications is expected
2. Contraindications and cautions
a. Use of alcohol or ethionamide increases the risk of seizures

b. Used with caution in clients with a seizure disorder, depression, severe anxiety, psychosis, or renal insufficiency or in clients who use alcohol

3. Side and adverse effects
   a. Hypersensitivity
   b. CNS reactions
   c. Neurotoxicity
   d. Seizures
   e. Heart failure
   f. Headache
   g. Vertigo
   h. Altered level of consciousness
   i. Irritability, nervousness, anxiety
   j. Confusion
   k. Mood changes, depression, thoughts of suicide
4. Interventions
   a. Monitor level of consciousness.
   b. Monitor for changes in mental status and thought processes.
   c. Monitor renal and hepatic function tests.
   d. Monitor serum medication level to avoid the risk of neurotoxicity; the peak concentration, measured 2 hours after dosing, should be 25 to 35 mcg/mL (140 to 195 mcmol/L).
5. Client education
   a. To take the medication after meals to prevent gastrointestinal upset
   b. To report signs of a rash or signs of CNS toxicity
   c. To avoid driving or performing tasks that require alertness until the reaction to the medication has been determined
   d. About the need for monitoring serum medication levels weekly, as prescribed

H. Streptomycin
1. Description
   a. An aminoglycoside antibiotic used with at least 1 other antitubercular medication
   b. Bactericidal because of receptor-binding action that interferes with protein synthesis in susceptible organisms
2. Contraindications and cautions
   a. Contraindicated in clients with hypersensitivity, myasthenia gravis, parkinsonism, or eighth cranial nerve damage
   b. Used with caution in the older client, in neonates because of renal insufficiency and organ immaturity, and in young infants because the medication may cause CNS depression
   c. The risk of toxicity increases when taken with other aminoglycosides or nephrotoxicity- or ototoxicity-producing medications.
3. Side and adverse effects (Box 51-8)
4. Interventions
   a. Assess for hypersensitivity.
   b. Monitor liver and renal function test results.

BOX 51-8 Side and Adverse Effects of Streptomycin

Nephrotoxicity
- Changes in urine output
- Decreased appetite
- Increased thirst
- Nausea, vomiting

Neurotoxicity
- Muscle numbness
- Seizures
- Tingling
- Twitching

Vestibular Toxicity
- Clumsiness
- Dizziness
- Unsteadiness

Auditory Toxicity (Ototoxicity)
- A full feeling in the ears
- Ringing in the ears
- Loss of hearing

   c. Monitor for ototoxic, neurotoxic, and nephrotoxic reactions.
   d. Perform baseline audiometric testing and repeat every 1 to 2 months, because the medication impairs the eighth cranial nerve.
   e. Monitor for visual changes.
   f. Assess hydration status and maintain adequate hydration during therapy.
   g. Monitor intake and output.
   h. Assess urinalysis results.
   i. Monitor for signs of peripheral neuritis.
5. Client education: To notify the PHCP if hearing loss, changes in vision, or urinary problems occur

XVI. Influenza Medications

A. Vaccines
1. Description
2. Because the strain of influenza virus is different every year, annual vaccination is recommended (usually sometime during September to April); each time a flu vaccine is administered, the nurse should inform the client of any updated information regarding the vaccine.

! The trivalent influenza vaccine includes vaccination against H1N1 and H3N2 strains (influenza A strains) and an influenza B strain. Because the strain of influenza virus is different every year, vaccine components may change. The vaccine is recommended for all individuals unless a contraindication to receiving it exists.

   a. The nasal spray (live) vaccine, if available, is approved only for healthy people ages 2 through 49.
   b. The nasal spray vaccine is not approved for pregnant women.
   c. The flu shots (inactivated vaccine), depending on the manufacturer, are approved for children as young as 6 months of age and are safe for pregnant women.

d. The nasal spray contains a live flu virus that has been weakened to the point that it cannot cause the flu; its advantage is that it may elicit a stronger immune response than the flu shot in children who have never had the flu or a flu vaccine before.
e. The disadvantage of the nasal spray is that it may not be quite as protective as the flu shot for older people who have had the flu or flu vaccines before.
f. All individuals should receive an influenza vaccine. High-priority individuals include pregnant women; household contacts and caregivers of children younger than 6 months of age; people ages 6 months to 24 years; health care workers and emergency medical personnel; and adults ages 25 to 64 with a chronic medical condition, such as asthma, or a weakened immune system, which increases the risk of flu complications.

3. Contraindications and cautions
a. Contraindications of the inactivated vaccine include hypersensitivity, active infection, Guillain-Barré syndrome, active febrile illness, and children younger than 6 months.
b. Contraindications of the live attenuated vaccine include age younger than 2 years or adults 50 years or older; pregnant women; children or adolescents on long-term aspirin therapy; and those with severe nasal congestion or long-term conditions such as asthma; diabetes mellitus; anemia or blood disorders; or heart, kidney, or lung disease.

4. Side and adverse effects
a. Inactivated vaccine: Localized pain and swelling at the injection site, general body aches and pains, malaise, fever
b. Attenuated vaccine: Runny nose or nasal congestion, cough, headache, sore throat

5. Interventions
a. The intramuscular route is recommended for the inactivated vaccine; adults and older children should be vaccinated in the deltoid muscle.
b. Monitor for side and adverse effects of the vaccine.
c. Monitor for hypersensitivity reactions in clients receiving vaccination for the first time.

6. Client education
a. About the importance of an annual vaccination
b. That the inactivated vaccine contains noninfectious, killed viruses and cannot cause influenza
c. That any respiratory disease unrelated to influenza can occur after the vaccination
d. That if the attenuated vaccine is received, the virus may be shed in secretions up to 2 days after vaccination
e. That development of antibodies in adults takes approximately 2 weeks

7. Visit the Centers for Disease Control and Prevention for updates (http://www.cdc.gov/flu/protect/vaccine/index.htm).

C. Antiviral medications (Table 51-1)
1. Description
a. Use during outbreaks of influenza depends on the current strain of influenza
b. Diagnosis of influenza should include rapid diagnostic tests, because infection from other pathogens may cause symptoms similar to those of influenza infection.
c. May also be administered as prophylaxis against infection but should not replace vaccination
2. Contraindicated in hypersensitive clients
3. Side and adverse effects (see Table 51-1)
4. Interventions
a. Administer within 2 days of onset of symptoms and continue for the entire prescription.
b. Monitor for side and adverse effects of specific medications.
5. Client education
a. That the medication may not prevent the transmission of influenza to others

TABLE 51-1 Side and Adverse Effects of Antiviral Influenza Medications

Antiviral Medication	Side and Adverse Effects
Amantadine	Drowsiness, anxiety, psychosis, depression, hallucinations, tremors, confusion, insomnia, orthostatic hypotension, heart failure, blurred vision, constipation, dry mouth, urinary frequency and retention, leukopenia, photosensitivity, dermatitis
Oseltamivir	Insomnia, diarrhea, abdominal pain, cough
Rimantadine	Depression, hallucinations, tremors, seizures, insomnia, poor concentration, asthenia, gait abnormalities, anxiety, confusion, pallor, palpitations, hypotension, edema, tinnitus, eye pain, constipation, dry mouth, anorexia, abdominal pain, diarrhea, dyspepsia, rash
Zanamivir	Ear, nose, and throat infections; diarrhea; nasal symptoms; cough; sinusitis; bronchitis
Peramivir	Diarrhea, constipation, insomnia, high blood pressure

b. About the need to adjust activities if dizziness or fatigue occur
c. About management of side and adverse effects of various medications
d. To take medication exactly as prescribed and for the duration of prescription

XVII. Pneumococcal Conjugate Vaccine

A. Pneumococcal conjugate vaccine is used for the prevention of invasive pneumococcal disease in infants and children.
B. Pneumococcal polysaccharide vaccine is used for adults and high-risk children older than 2 years.
C. Side and adverse effects may include erythema, swelling, pain, and tenderness at the injection site; fever; irritability; drowsiness; and reduced appetite.
D. See Chapter 40 for additional information about vaccines for pneumonia.

PRACTICE QUESTIONS

583. A client has a prescription to take guaifenesin. The nurse determines that the client understands the proper administration of this medication if the client states that she or he will perform which action?
1. Take an extra dose if fever develops
2. Take the medication with meals only
3. Take the tablet with a full glass of water
4. Decrease the amount of daily fluid intake

584. The nurse is preparing to administer a dose of naloxone intravenously to a client with an opioid overdose. Which supportive medical equipment should the nurse plan to have at the client's bedside?
1. Nasogastric tube
2. Paracentesis tray
3. Resuscitation equipment
4. Central line insertion tray

585. The nurse teaches a client about the effects of diphenhydramine, which has been prescribed as a cough suppressant. The nurse determines that the client **needs further instruction** if the client makes which statement?
1. "I will take the medication on an empty stomach."
2. "I won't drink alcohol while taking this medication."
3. "I won't do activities that require mental alertness while taking this medication."
4. "I will use sugarless gum, candy, or oral rinses to decrease dryness in my mouth."

586. A cromolyn sodium inhaler is prescribed for a client with allergic asthma. The nurse provides instructions regarding the adverse effects of this medication and should tell the client that which undesirable effect is associated with this medication?
1. Insomnia
2. Constipation
3. Hypotension
4. Bronchospasm

587. Terbutaline is prescribed for a client with bronchitis. Which disorder in the client's medical history requires caution by the nurse?
1. Osteoarthritis
2. Hypothyroidism
3. Diabetes mellitus
4. Polycystic disease

588. Zafirlukast is prescribed for a client with bronchial asthma. Which laboratory test does the nurse expect to be prescribed before the administration of this medication?
1. Platelet count
2. Neutrophil count
3. Liver function tests
4. Complete blood count

589. A client has been taking isoniazid for 2 months. The client complains to the nurse about numbness, paresthesias, and tingling in the extremities. The nurse interprets that the client is experiencing which problem?
1. Hypercalcemia
2. Peripheral neuritis
3. Small blood vessel spasm
4. Impaired peripheral circulation

590. A client is to begin a 6-month course of therapy with isoniazid. The nurse should plan to teach the client to take which action?
1. Use alcohol in small amounts only.
2. Report yellow eyes or skin immediately.
3. Increase intake of Swiss or aged cheeses.
4. Avoid vitamin supplements during therapy.

591. A client has been started on long-term therapy with rifampin. The nurse should provide which information to the client about the medication?
1. Should always be taken with food or antacids
2. Should be double-dosed if 1 dose is forgotten
3. Causes orange discoloration of sweat, tears, urine, and feces
4. May be discontinued independently if symptoms are gone in 3 months

592. The nurse has given a client taking ethambutol information about the medication. The nurse determines that the client understands the instructions if the client states that they will **immediately** report which finding?
1. Impaired sense of hearing
2. Gastrointestinal side effects

3. Orange-red discoloration of body secretions
4. Difficulty in discriminating the color red from green

593. A client with tuberculosis is starting antituberculosis therapy with isoniazid. Before giving the client the first dose, the nurse should ensure that which baseline study has been completed?
1. Electrolyte levels
2. Coagulation times
3. Liver enzyme levels
4. Serum creatinine level

594. The nurse has a prescription to give a client salmeterol, 2 puffs, and beclomethasone dipropionate, 2 puffs, by metered-dose inhaler. The nurse should administer the medication using which procedure?
1. Beclomethasone first and then the salmeterol
2. Salmeterol first and then the beclomethasone
3. Alternating a single puff of each, beginning with the salmeterol
4. Alternating a single puff of each, beginning with the beclomethasone

595. Rifabutin is prescribed for a client with active *Mycobacterium avium* complex (MAC) disease and tuberculosis. The nurse should monitor for which side and adverse effects of rifabutin? **Select all that apply.**
- ☐ 1. Signs of hepatitis
- ☐ 2. Flu-like syndrome
- ☐ 3. Low neutrophil count
- ☐ 4. Vitamin B_6 deficiency
- ☐ 5. Ocular pain or blurred vision
- ☐ 6. Tingling and numbness of the fingers

596. A client begins therapy with theophylline. The nurse plans to teach the client to limit the intake of which items while taking this medication?
1. Coffee, cola, and chocolate
2. Oysters, lobster, and shrimp
3. Melons, oranges, and pineapple
4. Cottage cheese, cream cheese, and dairy creamers

597. The nurse has just administered the first dose of omalizumab to a client. Which statement by the client alerts the nurse of a life-threatening effect?
1. "I have a severe headache."
2. "My feet are quite swollen."
3. "I am nauseated and may vomit."
4. "My lips and tongue are swollen."

598. The nurse is teaching a client who is beginning antiviral therapy for influenza. Which statement by the client indicates an understanding of the instructions?
1. "I must take the medication exactly as prescribed."
2. "Once I start the medication, I will no longer be contagious."
3. "I will not get any colds or infections while taking this medication."
4. "This medication has minimal side effects and I can return to normal activities."

599. The nurse is caring for a client receiving an albuterol/ipratropium nebulized breathing treatment. Which report from the client should the nurse note as an expected side effect of this combination medication?
1. "I feel like my heart is racing."
2. "I feel more bloated than usual."
3. "My eyes have been watering lately."
4. "I haven't had a bowel movement in 4 days."

ANSWERS

583. *Answer:* 3

Rationale: Guaifenesin is an expectorant and should be taken with a full glass of water to decrease the viscosity of secretions. Extra doses should not be taken. The client should contact the primary health care provider if the cough lasts longer than 1 week or is accompanied by fever, rash, sore throat, or persistent headache. Fluids are needed to decrease the viscosity of secretions. The medication does not have to be taken with meals.

Test-Taking Strategy: Begin to answer this question by eliminating option 1 first, recalling that *extra doses* of medication should not be taken. Next, eliminate option 2 because of the closed-ended word "only." Next, knowing that increased fluid helps liquefy secretions for more effective coughing directs you to the correct option.

Level of Cognitive Ability: Evaluating
Client Needs: Physiological Integrity
Integrated Process: Nursing Process—Evaluation
Content Area: Pharmacology: Respiratory Medications: Expectorants and Mucolytic Agents
Health Problem: N/A
Priority Concepts: Client Education; Safety
Reference: Lilley et al. (2017), pp. 575-576.

584. *Answer:* 3

Rationale: The nurse administering naloxone for suspected opioid overdose should have resuscitation equipment readily

available to support naloxone therapy if it is needed. Other adjuncts that may be needed include oxygen, a mechanical ventilator, and vasopressors.
Test-Taking Strategy: Focus on the **subject**, supportive medical equipment. Note the words *opioid overdose*. Recalling the effects of these types of medications will direct you to the correct option. The correct option is also the **umbrella option**.
Level of Cognitive Ability: Applying
Client Needs: Physiological Integrity
Integrated Process: Nursing Process—Planning
Content Area: Pharmacology: Respiratory Medications: Opioid Antagonists
Health Problem: N/A
Priority Concepts: Clinical Judgment; Safety
Reference: Ignatavicius, Workman, Rebar (2018), p. 285.

585. *Answer:* 1
Rationale: Diphenhydramine has several uses, including as an antihistamine, antitussive, antidyskinetic, and sedative-hypnotic. Instructions for use include taking with food or milk to decrease gastrointestinal upset and using oral rinses, sugarless gum, or hard candy to minimize dry mouth. Because the medication causes drowsiness, the client should avoid use of alcohol or central nervous system depressants, operating a car, or engaging in other activities requiring mental awareness during use.
Test-Taking Strategy: Note the **strategic words**, *needs further instruction*. These words indicate a **negative event query** and ask you to select an option that is incorrect. Knowing that the medication has a sedative effect helps you eliminate options 2 and 3 first because they are **comparable or alike**. Recalling that the medication causes a dry mouth helps you choose the correct option as the answer, according to the way the question is stated.
Level of Cognitive Ability: Evaluating
Client Needs: Physiological Integrity
Integrated Process: Teaching and Learning
Content Area: Pharmacology: Respiratory Medications: Antitussives
Health Problem: N/A
Priority Concepts: Client Education; Safety
Reference: Lilley et al. (2017), p. 575.

586. *Answer:* 4
Rationale: Cromolyn sodium is an inhaled nonsteroidal antiallergy agent and a mast cell stabilizer. Undesirable effects associated with inhalation therapy of cromolyn sodium are bronchospasm, cough, nasal congestion, throat irritation, and wheezing. Clients receiving this medication orally may experience pruritus, nausea, diarrhea, and myalgia.
Test-Taking Strategy: Note the words *undesirable effect*. This should assist in directing you to the correct option. In addition, use the **ABCs—airway, breathing, and circulation**—to select the correct option. The correct option addresses the airway.
Level of Cognitive Ability: Applying
Client Needs: Physiological Integrity
Integrated Process: Teaching and Learning
Content Area: Pharmacology: Respiratory Medications: Restrictive Airway Disease Agents
Health Problem: Adult Health: Respiratory: Asthma
Priority Concepts: Client Education; Gas Exchange
Reference: Burchum, Rosenthal (2016), pp. 925, 937.

587. *Answer:* 3
Rationale: Terbutaline is a bronchodilator and is contraindicated in clients with hypersensitivity to sympathomimetics. It should be used with caution in clients with impaired cardiac function, diabetes mellitus, hypertension, hyperthyroidism, or a history of seizures. The medication may increase blood glucose levels.
Test-Taking Strategy: Focus on the **subject**, cautions for using terbutaline. Specific knowledge regarding the contraindications and cautions associated with the use of this medication is needed to answer this question. Remember that terbutaline is used with caution in the client with diabetes mellitus.
Level of Cognitive Ability: Analyzing
Client Needs: Physiological Integrity
Integrated Process: Nursing Process—Assessment
Content Area: Pharmacology: Respiratory Medications: Restrictive Airway Disease Agents
Health Problem: Adult Health: Respiratory: Upper Airway
Priority Concepts: Clinical Judgment; Safety
Reference: Burchum, Rosenthal (2016), pp. 936-937.

588. *Answer:* 3
Rationale: Zafirlukast is a leukotriene receptor antagonist used in the prophylaxis and long-term treatment of bronchial asthma. Zafirlukast is used with caution in clients with impaired hepatic function. Liver function laboratory tests should be performed to obtain a baseline, and the levels should be monitored during administration of the medication. It is not necessary to perform the other laboratory tests before administration of the medication.
Test-Taking Strategy: Eliminate options 2 and 4 first because they are **comparable or alike**, noting that a complete blood count would include a neutrophil count. From the remaining options, you would need to know that this medication affects hepatic function.
Level of Cognitive Ability: Analyzing
Client Needs: Physiological Integrity
Integrated Process: Nursing Process—Assessment
Content Area: Pharmacology: Respiratory Medications: Restrictive Airway Disease Agents
Health Problem: Adult Health: Respiratory: Asthma
Priority Concepts: Cellular Regulation; Gas Exchange
Reference: Hodgson, Kizior (2018), pp. 1246-1247.

589. *Answer:* 2
Rationale: Isoniazid is an antitubercular medication. A common side effect of isoniazid is peripheral neuritis, manifested by numbness, tingling, and paresthesias in the extremities. This can be minimized with pyridoxine (vitamin B_6) intake. Options 1, 3, and 4 are not associated with the information in the question.
Test-Taking Strategy: Focus on the **information in the question**, numbness, paresthesias, and tingling in the extremities. Options 3 and 4 would not cause the symptoms presented in the question but instead would cause pallor and coolness. From the remaining options, you should know that peripheral neuritis is an adverse effect of isoniazid, and that these signs and symptoms do not correlate with hypercalcemia.

Level of Cognitive Ability: Analyzing
Client Needs: Physiological Integrity
Integrated Process: Nursing Process—Analysis
Content Area: Pharmacology: Respiratory Medications: Tuberculosis Medications
Health Problem: Adult Health: Respiratory: Tuberculosis
Priority Concepts: Clinical Judgment; Perfusion
Reference: Burchum, Rosenthal (2016), p. 1084.

590. *Answer:* 2
Rationale: Isoniazid is hepatotoxic, and therefore the client is taught to report signs and symptoms of hepatitis immediately, which include yellow skin and sclera. For the same reason, alcohol should be avoided during therapy. The client should avoid intake of Swiss cheese, fish such as tuna, and foods containing tyramine, because they may cause a reaction characterized by redness and itching of the skin, flushing, sweating, tachycardia, headache, or lightheadedness. The client can avoid developing peripheral neuritis by increasing the intake of pyridoxine (vitamin B_6) during the course of isoniazid therapy.
Test-Taking Strategy: Focus on the subject, client teaching for isoniazid. Because alcohol intake is prohibited with the use of many medications, eliminate option 1 first. Because the client receiving this medication typically is given supplements of vitamin B_6, option 4 is incorrect and is eliminated next. Recalling that the medication is hepatotoxic will direct you to the correct option.
Level of Cognitive Ability: Applying
Client Needs: Physiological Integrity
Integrated Process: Teaching and Learning
Content Area: Pharmacology: Respiratory Medications: Tuberculosis Medications
Health Problem: Adult Health: Respiratory: Tuberculosis
Priority Concepts: Client Education; Safety
Reference: Skidmore-Roth (2017), pp. 658-659.

591. *Answer:* 3
Rationale: Rifampin causes orange-red discoloration of body secretions and will stain soft contact lenses permanently. Rifampin should be taken exactly as directed. Doses should not be doubled or skipped. The client should not stop therapy until directed to do so by a primary health care provider. It is best to administer the medication on an empty stomach unless it causes gastrointestinal upset, and then it may be taken with food. Antacids, if prescribed, should be taken at least 1 hour before the medication.
Test-Taking Strategy: Options 2 and 4 are comparable or alike and are inaccurate, based on general guidelines for medication administration; the client should not double-dose or discontinue medication independently. Eliminate option 1 next because of the closed-ended word "always."
Level of Cognitive Ability: Applying
Client Needs: Physiological Integrity
Integrated Process: Teaching and Learning
Content Area: Pharmacology: Respiratory Medications: Tuberculosis Medications
Health Problem: Adult Health: Respiratory: Tuberculosis
Priority Concepts: Client Education; Safety
Reference: Lewis et al. (2017), p. 509.

592. *Answer:* 4
Rationale: Ethambutol causes optic neuritis, which decreases visual acuity and the ability to discriminate between the colors red and green. This poses a potential safety hazard when a client is driving a motor vehicle. The client is taught to report this symptom immediately. The client also is taught to take the medication with food if gastrointestinal upset occurs. Impaired hearing results from antitubercular therapy with streptomycin. Orange-red discoloration of secretions occurs with rifampin.
Test-Taking Strategy: Note the strategic word, *immediately.* Option 2 is the least likely symptom to report; instead, it should be managed by taking the medication with food. To select among the other options, you must know that this medication causes optic neuritis, resulting in difficulty with red-green discrimination.
Level of Cognitive Ability: Evaluating
Client Needs: Physiological Integrity
Integrated Process: Nursing Process—Evaluation
Content Area: Pharmacology: Respiratory Medications: Tuberculosis Medications
Health Problem: Adult Health: Respiratory: Tuberculosis
Priority Concepts: Client Education; Safety
Reference: Lewis et al. (2017), p. 509.

593. *Answer:* 3
Rationale: Isoniazid therapy can cause an elevation of hepatic enzyme levels and hepatitis. Therefore, liver enzyme levels are monitored when therapy is initiated and during the first 3 months of therapy. They may be monitored longer in the client who is older than 50 years or abuses alcohol. The laboratory tests in options 1, 2, and 4 are not necessary.
Test-Taking Strategy: Focus on the subject, the laboratory value to monitor. Recalling that this medication can be toxic to the liver will direct you to the correct option.
Level of Cognitive Ability: Applying
Client Needs: Physiological Integrity
Integrated Process: Nursing Process—Implementation
Content Area: Pharmacology: Respiratory Medications: Tuberculosis Medications
Health Problem: Adult Health: Respiratory: Tuberculosis
Priority Concepts: Cellular Regulation; Safety
Reference: Hodgson, Kizior (2018), pp. 620-621.

594. *Answer:* 2
Rationale: Salmeterol is an adrenergic type of bronchodilator, and beclomethasone dipropionate is a glucocorticoid. Bronchodilators are always administered before glucocorticoids when both are to be given on the same time schedule. This allows for widening of the air passages by the bronchodilator, which then makes the glucocorticoid more effective.
Test-Taking Strategy: Focus on the subject, the procedure for administering inhaled medications. To answer this question correctly, you must know two different things. First, you must know that a bronchodilator is always given before a glucocorticoid. This would allow you to eliminate options 3 and 4, because you would not alternate the medications. To select between the remaining option and the correct option, you must know that salmeterol is a bronchodilator, whereas beclomethasone is a glucocorticoid.
Level of Cognitive Ability: Applying
Client Needs: Physiological Integrity

Integrated Process: Nursing Process—Implementation
Content Area: Pharmacology: Respiratory Medications: Restrictive Airway Disease Agents
Health Problem: N/A
Priority Concepts: Gas Exchange; Safety
Reference: Skidmore-Roth (2017), pp. 124-125.

595. *Answer:* 1, 2, 3, 5
Rationale: Rifabutin may be prescribed for a client with active MAC disease and tuberculosis. It inhibits mycobacterial DNA-dependent RNA polymerase and suppresses protein synthesis. Side and adverse effects include rash, gastrointestinal disturbances, neutropenia (low neutrophil count), red-orange–colored body secretions, uveitis (blurred vision and eye pain), myositis, arthralgia, hepatitis, chest pain with dyspnea, and flu-like syndrome. Vitamin B_6 deficiency and numbness and tingling in the extremities are associated with the use of isoniazid.
Test-Taking Strategy: Focus on the subject, side and adverse effects of rifabutin. Specific knowledge is needed to answer correctly. Remember that hepatitis, flu-like syndrome, neutropenia, and uveitis can occur.
Level of Cognitive Ability: Analyzing
Client Needs: Physiological Integrity
Integrated Process: Nursing Process—Assessment
Content Area: Pharmacology: Respiratory Medications: Tuberculosis Medications
Health Problem: Adult Health: Respiratory: Tuberculosis
Priority Concepts: Clinical Judgment; Safety
Reference: Ignatavicius, Workman, Rebar (2018), p. 608.

596. *Answer:* 1
Rationale: Theophylline is a methylxanthine bronchodilator. The nurse teaches the client to limit the intake of xanthine-containing foods while taking this medication. These foods include coffee, cola, and chocolate.
Test-Taking Strategy: Focus on the subject, food items that need to be limited. Recall that theophylline is a xanthine bronchodilator and that intake of excessive amounts of foods naturally high in xanthines needs to be limited. Also, recalling that these medications cause cardiac and central nervous system stimulation will direct you to the correct option.
Level of Cognitive Ability: Applying
Client Needs: Physiological Integrity
Integrated Process: Teaching and Learning
Content Area: Pharmacology: Respiratory Medications: Restrictive Airway Disease Agents
Health Problem: N/A
Priority Concepts: Client Education; Safety
Reference: Lilley et al. (2017), pp. 585, 590.

597. *Answer:* 4
Rationale: Omalizumab is an antiinflammatory and monoclonal antibody used for long-term control of asthma. Anaphylactic reactions can occur with the administration of omalizumab. The nurse administering the medication should monitor for adverse reactions of the medication. Swelling of the lips and tongue are an indication of an anaphylaxis. The client statements in options 1, 2, and 3 are not indicative of an adverse reaction.
Test-Taking Strategy: Focus on the subject, a life-threatening effect. Recall that anaphylactic reactions can occur with the administration of omalizumab. Knowing the signs of a reaction will direct you to the correct option.
Level of Cognitive Ability: Analyzing
Client Needs: Physiological Integrity
Integrated Process: Nursing Process—Assessment
Content Area: Pharmacology: Respiratory Medications: Restrictive Airway Disease Agents
Health Problem: Adult Health: Respiratory: Asthma
Priority Concepts: Clinical Judgment; Safety
Reference: Skidmore-Roth (2017), pp. 879-880.

598. *Answer:* 1
Rationale: Antiviral medications for influenza must be taken exactly as prescribed. These medications do not prevent the spread of influenza, and clients are usually contagious for up to 2 days after the initiation of antiviral medications. Secondary bacterial infections may occur despite antiviral treatment. Side effects occur with these medications and may necessitate a change in activities, especially when driving or operating machinery if dizziness occurs.
Test-Taking Strategy: Focus on the subject, client instructions for antiviral therapy, and note the words *indicates an understanding.* Using general medication guidelines will direct you to the correct option.
Level of Cognitive Ability: Evaluating
Client Needs: Physiological Integrity
Integrated Process: Nursing Process—Evaluation
Content Area: Pharmacology: Immune Medications: Antivirals
Health Problem: Adult Health: Respiratory: Viral, Bacterial, Fungal Infections
Priority Concepts: Client Education; Infection
Reference: Lilley et al. (2017), pp. 658.

599. *Answer:* 1
Rationale: Albuterol/ipratropium is a combination agent—one is a β_2-adrenergic agonist and the other is an anticholinergic medication, and in combination they produce an overall bronchodilation effect. Common side and adverse effects include headache, dizziness, dry mouth, tremors, nervousness, and tachycardia. Therefore, option 1 is correct. Options 2, 3, and 4 are not specifically associated with this medication.
Test-Taking Strategy: Begin to answer this question by eliminating options 2 and 4 first, noting they are **comparable or alike.** Next, eliminate option 3 because this medication causes anticholinergic effects such as dry eyes and dry mouth.
Level of Cognitive Ability: Evaluating
Client Needs: Physiological Integrity
Integrated Process: Nursing Process—Evaluation
Content Area: Pharmacology: Respiratory Medications: Reactive Airway Disease Agents
Health Problem: N/A
Priority Concepts: Client Education; Safety
Reference: Lilley et al. (2017), p. 940.

UNIT XII

Cardiovascular Problems of the Adult Client

Pyramid to Success

Pyramid Points focus on assessment data related to cardiovascular risks, health screening and promotion, complications of the various cardiovascular problems, emergency measures, and client education. Focus on the assessment findings and treatment in coronary artery disease, myocardial infarction, heart failure and pulmonary edema, pericarditis, aneurysms, hypertension, and arterial and venous problems. You must be able to identify the most common dysrhythmias and determine the appropriate interventions for these dysrhythmias, including the use of a pacemaker. Focus also on the care of the client following diagnostic treatments and surgical procedures. Note appropriate and therapeutic client positions, particularly with arterial and venous problems of the extremities. Focus on treatments and medications prescribed for the various cardiovascular problems and client teaching related to prescribed treatment plans. Be familiar with the components related to cardiac rehabilitation.

Client Needs: Learning Objectives

Safe and Effective Care Environment

Consulting with the interprofessional health care team
Establishing priorities
Maintaining asepsis
Maintaining standard and other precautions
Recognizing the need for consultations and referrals
Upholding client rights
Verifying that informed consent related to treatments and procedures has been obtained

Health Promotion and Maintenance

Discussing alterations in lifestyle
Mobilizing appropriate community resources
Performing cardiovascular assessment techniques
Preventing cardiovascular disease
Promoting cardiac rehabilitation
Providing health screening and health promotion programs
Teaching related to diet therapy, exercise, and medications

Psychosocial Integrity

Assisting the client to accept lifestyle changes
Considering religious, spiritual, and cultural influences on health
Discussing grief and loss and end-of-life issues
Discussing situational role changes
Discussing unexpected body image changes
Identifying coping mechanisms
Identifying fear, anxiety, and denial
Identifying support systems

Physiological Integrity

Administering intravenous medications
Discussing activity limitations and promoting rest and sleep
Monitoring for complications related to cardiovascular problems
Monitoring for therapeutic effects of medications
Monitoring hemodynamics
Monitoring of cardiac enzyme and troponin levels and other cardiovascular-related laboratory values
Providing interventions required in emergencies
Providing nonpharmacological and pharmacological comfort interventions
Responding to medical emergencies

CHAPTER 52

Cardiovascular Problems

PRIORITY CONCEPTS **Health Promotion; Perfusion**

I. Anatomy and Physiology

A. Heart and heart wall layers
 1. The heart is located in the left side of the mediastinum.
 2. The heart consists of 3 layers.
  a. The epicardium is the outermost layer of the heart.
  b. The myocardium is the middle layer and is the actual contracting muscle of the heart.
  c. The endocardium is the innermost layer and lines the inner chambers and heart valves.

B. Pericardial sac
 1. Encases and protects the heart from trauma and infection
 2. Has 2 layers
  a. The parietal pericardium is the tough, fibrous outer membrane that attaches anteriorly to the lower half of the sternum, posteriorly to the thoracic vertebrae, and inferiorly to the diaphragm.
  b. The visceral pericardium is the thin, inner layer that closely adheres to the heart.
 3. The pericardial space is between the parietal and visceral layers; it holds 5 to 20 mL of pericardial fluid, lubricates the pericardial surfaces, and cushions the heart.

C. There are 4 heart chambers.
 1. The right atrium receives deoxygenated blood from the body via the superior and inferior vena cava.
 2. The right ventricle receives blood from the right atrium and pumps it to the lungs via the pulmonary artery.
 3. The left atrium receives oxygenated blood from the lungs via 4 pulmonary veins.
 4. The left ventricle is the largest and most muscular chamber; it receives oxygenated blood from the lungs via the left atrium and pumps blood into the systemic circulation via the aorta.

D. There are 4 valves in the heart.
 1. There are 2 atrioventricular valves, the tricuspid and the mitral, which lie between the atria and ventricles.
  a. The tricuspid valve is located on the right side of the heart.
  b. The bicuspid (mitral) valve is located on the left side of the heart.
  c. The atrioventricular valves close at the beginning of ventricular contraction and prevent blood from flowing back into the atria from the ventricles; these valves open when the ventricles relax.
 2. There are 2 semilunar valves, the pulmonic and the aortic.
  a. The pulmonic semilunar valve lies between the right ventricle and the pulmonary artery.
  b. The aortic semilunar valve lies between the left ventricle and the aorta.
  c. The semilunar valves prevent blood from flowing back into the ventricles during relaxation; they open during ventricular contraction and close when the ventricles begin to relax.

E. Sinoatrial (SA) node
 1. The main pacemaker that initiates each heartbeat
 2. It is located at the junction of the superior vena cava and the right atrium.
 3. The SA node generates electrical impulses at 60 to 100 times per minute and is controlled by the sympathetic and parasympathetic nervous systems.

F. Atrioventricular (AV) node
 1. Located in the lower aspect of the atrial septum
 2. Receives electrical impulses from the SA node
 3. If the SA node fails, the AV node can initiate and sustain a heart rate of 40 to 60 beats per minute.

G. The bundle of His
 1. A continuation of the AV node; located at the interventricular septum

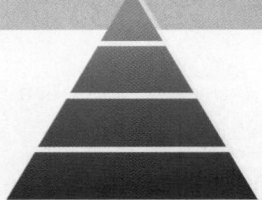

2. It branches into the right bundle branch, which extends down the right side of the interventricular septum; and the left bundle branch, which extends into the left ventricle.
3. The right and left bundle branches terminate in the Purkinje fibers.

H. Purkinje fibers
1. Purkinje fibers are a diffuse network of conducting strands located beneath the ventricular endocardium.
2. These fibers spread the wave of depolarization through the ventricles.
3. Purkinje fibers can act as the pacemaker with a rate between 20 and 40 beats per minute when higher pacemakers (such as the SA and AV nodes) fail.

I. Coronary arteries (Fig. 52-1)
1. The right main coronary artery supplies the right atrium and ventricle, the inferior portion of the left ventricle, the posterior septal wall, and the SA and AV nodes.
2. The left main coronary artery consists of 2 major branches, the left anterior descending (LAD) and the circumflex arteries.
3. The LAD artery supplies blood to the anterior wall of the left ventricle, the anterior ventricular septum, and the apex of the left ventricle.
4. The circumflex artery supplies blood to the left atrium and the lateral and posterior surfaces of the left ventricle.

The coronary arteries supply the capillaries of the myocardium with blood. If blockage occurs in these arteries, the client is at risk for myocardial infarction (MI).

J. Heart sounds
1. The first heart sound (S_1) is heard as the atrioventricular valves close and is heard loudest at the apex of the heart.

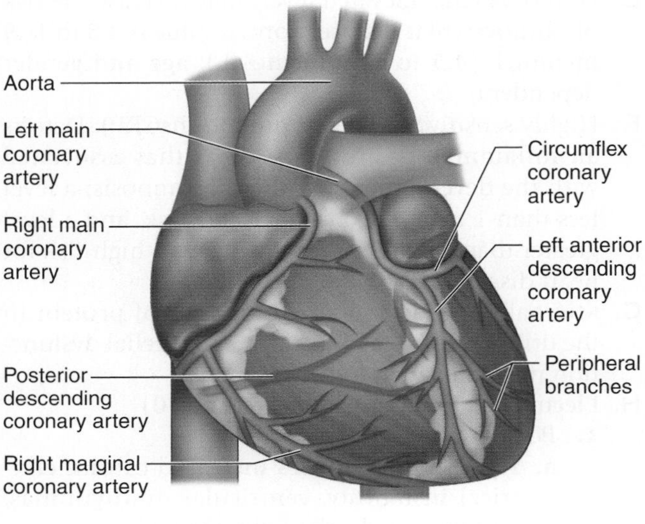

FIG. 52-1 Coronary arterial system.

2. The second heart sound (S_2) is heard when the semilunar valves close and is heard loudest at the base of the heart.
3. A third heart sound (S_3) may be heard if ventricular wall compliance is decreased and structures in the ventricular wall vibrate; this can occur in conditions such as heart failure or valvular regurgitation. However, a third heart sound may be normal in individuals younger than 30 years.
4. A fourth heart sound (S_4) may be heard on atrial systole if resistance to ventricular filling is present; this is an abnormal finding, and the causes include cardiac hypertrophy, disease, or injury to the ventricular wall.

K. Heart rate
1. The faster the heart rate, the less time the heart has for filling. At very fast rates the cardiac output decreases.
2. The normal sinus heart rate is 60 to 100 beats per minute.
3. Sinus tachycardia is a rate more than 100 beats per minute.
4. Sinus bradycardia is a rate less than 60 beats per minute.

L. Autonomic nervous system
1. Stimulation of sympathetic nerve fibers releases the neurotransmitter norepinephrine, producing an increased heart rate, increased conduction speed through the AV node, increased atrial and ventricular contractility, and peripheral vasoconstriction. Stimulation occurs when a decrease in pressure is detected.
2. Stimulation of the parasympathetic nerve fibers releases the neurotransmitter acetylcholine, which decreases the heart rate and lessens atrial and ventricular contractility and conductivity. Stimulation occurs when an increase in pressure is detected.

M. Blood pressure (BP) control
1. Baroreceptors (specialized nerve endings affected by changes in the arterial BP), also called *pressoreceptors*, are located in the walls of the aortic arch and carotid sinuses.
2. Increases in arterial pressure stimulate baroreceptors, and the heart rate and arterial pressure decrease.
3. Decreases in arterial pressure reduce stimulation of the baroreceptors and vasoconstriction occurs, as does an increase in heart rate.
4. Stretch receptors, located in the vena cava and the right atrium, respond to pressure changes that affect circulatory blood volume.
5. When the BP decreases as a result of hypovolemia, a sympathetic response occurs, causing an increased heart rate and blood vessel constriction; when the BP increases as a result of hypervolemia, an opposite effect occurs.

6. Antidiuretic hormone (vasopressin) influences BP indirectly by regulating vascular volume.
7. Increases in blood volume result in decreased antidiuretic hormone release, increasing diuresis, decreasing blood volume, and thus decreasing BP.
8. Decreases in blood volume result in increased antidiuretic hormone release; this promotes an increase in blood volume and therefore BP.
9. Renin, a potent vasoconstrictor, causes the BP to increase.
10. Renin converts angiotensinogen to angiotensin I; angiotensin I is then converted to angiotensin II in the lungs.
11. Angiotensin II stimulates the release of aldosterone, which promotes water and sodium retention by the kidneys; this action increases blood volume and BP.

N. The vascular system
1. Arteries are vessels through which the blood passes away from the heart to various parts of the body; they convey highly oxygenated blood from the left side of heart to the tissues.
2. Arterioles control the blood flow into the capillaries.
3. Capillaries allow the exchange of fluid and nutrients between the blood and the interstitial spaces.
4. Venules receive blood from the capillary bed and move blood into the veins.
5. Veins transport deoxygenated blood from the tissues back to the right heart and then to the lungs for oxygenation.
6. Valves help return blood to the heart against the force of gravity.
7. The lymphatics drain the tissues and return the tissue fluid to the blood.

II. Diagnostic Tests and Procedures (refer to Chapter 10 for further information on laboratory reference levels)

A. Cardiac markers
1. Troponin
   a. Troponin is composed of 3 proteins—troponin C, cardiac troponin I, and cardiac troponin T.
   b. Troponin I especially has a high affinity for myocardial injury; it rises within 3 hours and persists for up to 7 to 10 days.
   c. Normal values are low, with troponin I being less than 0.35 ng/mL (less than 0.35 mcg/L) and troponin T being less than 0.1 ng/mL (less than 0.1 mcg/L); thus, any rise can indicate myocardial cell damage.
2. CK-MB (creatine kinase, myocardial muscle)
   a. An elevation in value indicates myocardial damage.
   b. An elevation occurs within hours and peaks at 18 hours following an acute ischemic attack.
   c. Normal value for CK-MB (CK-2) is 2 to 6 ng/mL (2 to 6 mcg/L) for males and 2 to 5 ng/mL (2 to 5 mcg/L) for females.
3. Myoglobin
   a. Myoglobin is an oxygen-binding protein found in cardiac and skeletal muscle.
   b. The level rises within 2 hours after cell death, with a rapid decline in the level after 7 hours; however, it is not cardiac specific.

B. Complete blood count
1. The red blood cell count decreases in rheumatic heart disease and infective endocarditis and increases in conditions characterized by inadequate tissue oxygenation.
2. The white blood cell count increases in infectious and inflammatory diseases of the heart and after MI, because large numbers of white blood cells are needed to dispose of the necrotic tissue resulting from the infarction.
3. An elevated hematocrit level can result from vascular volume depletion.
4. Decreases in hemoglobin and hematocrit levels can indicate anemia.

C. Blood coagulation factors: An increase in coagulation factors can occur during and after MI, which places the client at greater risk for thrombophlebitis and formation of clots in the coronary arteries.

D. Serum lipids (refer to Chapter 10)
1. The lipid profile measures serum cholesterol, triglyceride, and lipoprotein levels.
2. The lipid profile is used to assess the risk of developing coronary artery disease.
3. Lipoprotein-*a* or *Lp(a)*, a modified form of low-density lipoprotein (LDL), increases atherosclerotic plaques and increases clots; value should be less than 30 mg/dL (300 mg/L).

E. Homocysteine: Elevated levels may increase the risk of cardiovascular disease; normal value is 4.5 to 11.9 mcmol/L (4.5 to 11.9 mcmol/L), age and gender dependent.

F. Highly sensitive C-reactive protein (hsCRP): Detects an inflammatory process such as that associated with the development of atherothrombosis; a level less than 1 mg/L is considered low risk, and a level greater than 3 mg/L places the client at high risk for heart disease.

G. Microalbuminuria: A small amount of protein in the urine has been a marker for endothelial dysfunction in cardiovascular disease.

H. Electrolytes (refer to Chapters 8 and 10)
1. Potassium
   a. Hypokalemia causes increased cardiac electrical instability, ventricular dysrhythmias, and increased risk of digoxin toxicity.

b. In hypokalemia, the electrocardiogram (ECG) shows flattening and inversion of the T wave, the appearance of a U wave, and ST depression.

c. Hyperkalemia causes asystole and ventricular dysrhythmias.

d. In hyperkalemia, the ECG may show tall, peaked T waves, widened QRS complexes, prolonged PR intervals, or flat P waves.

2. Sodium

a. The serum sodium level decreases with the use of diuretics.

b. The serum sodium level decreases in heart failure, indicating water excess.

I. Calcium

1. Hypocalcemia can cause ventricular dysrhythmias, prolonged ST and QT intervals, and cardiac arrest.

2. Hypercalcemia can cause a shortened ST segment and widened T wave, atrioventricular block, tachycardia or bradycardia, digitalis hypersensitivity, and cardiac arrest.

J. Phosphorus level: Phosphorus levels should be interpreted with calcium levels, because the kidneys retain or excrete one electrolyte in an inverse relationship to the other.

K. Magnesium

1. A low magnesium level can cause ventricular tachycardia and fibrillation.

2. Electrocardiographic changes that may be observed with hypomagnesemia include tall T waves and depressed ST segments.

3. A high magnesium level can cause muscle weakness, hypotension, and bradycardia.

4. Electrocardiographic changes that may be observed with hypermagnesemia include a prolonged PR interval and widened QRS complex.

▲ Electrolyte and mineral imbalances can cause cardiac electrical instability that can result in life-threatening dysrhythmias.

L. Blood urea nitrogen: The blood urea nitrogen level is elevated in heart disorders such as heart failure and cardiogenic shock that reduce renal circulation.

M. Blood glucose: An acute cardiac episode can elevate the blood glucose level.

▲ **N.** B-type natriuretic peptide (BNP)

1. BNP is released in response to atrial and ventricular stretch; it serves as a marker for heart failure.

2. BNP levels should be less than 100 ng/mL (less than 100 mcg/L); the higher the level, the more severe the heart failure.

O. Chest x-ray

1. Description: Radiography of the chest is done to determine anatomical changes such as the size, silhouette, and position of the heart.

2. Interventions

a. Prepare the client, explaining the purpose and procedure.

b. Remove jewelry.

c. Ensure that the client is not pregnant.

P. Electrocardiography (Box 52-1)

1. Description: This common noninvasive diagnostic test records the electrical activity of the heart and is useful for detecting cardiac dysrhythmias, location and extent of MI, and cardiac hypertrophy, and for evaluation of the effectiveness of cardiac medications.

BOX 52-1 Basics of Electrocardiography

- An electrocardiogram (ECG) reflects the electrical activity of cardiac cells and records electrical activity at a speed of 25 mm/second.
- An electrocardiographic strip consists of horizontal lines representing seconds and vertical lines representing voltage.
- Each small square represents 0.04 second.
- Each large square represents 0.20 second.
- The P wave represents atrial depolarization.
- The PR interval represents the time it takes an impulse to travel from the atria through the atrioventricular node, bundle of His, and bundle branches to the Purkinje fibers.
- Normal PR interval duration ranges from 0.12 to 0.2 second.
- The PR interval is measured from the beginning of the P wave to the end of the PR segment.
- The QRS complex represents ventricular depolarization.
- Normal QRS complex duration ranges from 0.04 to 0.1 second.
- The Q wave appears as the first negative deflection in the QRS complex and reflects initial ventricular septal depolarization.
- The R wave is the first positive deflection in the QRS complex.
- The S wave appears as the second negative deflection in the QRS complex.
- The J point marks the end of the QRS complex and the beginning of the ST segment.
- The QRS duration is measured from the end of the PR segment to the J point.
- The ST segment represents early ventricular repolarization.
- The T wave represents ventricular repolarization and ventricular diastole.
- The U wave may follow the T wave.
- A prominent U wave may indicate an electrolyte abnormality, such as hypokalemia.
- The QT interval represents ventricular refractory time or the total time required for ventricular depolarization and repolarization.
- The QT interval is measured from the beginning of the QRS complex to the end of the T wave.
- The QT interval normally lasts 0.32 to 0.4 second but varies with the client's heart rate, age, and gender.

2. Interventions
   a. Determine the client's ability to lie still; advise the client to lie still, breathe normally, and refrain from talking during the test.
   b. Reassure the client that an electrical shock will not occur.
   c. Document any cardiac medications the client is taking.

Q. Holter monitoring
1. Description
   a. A noninvasive test; the client wears a monitor and an electrocardiographic tracing is recorded continuously over a period of 24 hours or more while the client performs her or his activities of daily living.
   b. The monitor identifies dysrhythmias if they occur and evaluates the effectiveness of antidysrhythmics or pacemaker therapy.
2. Interventions
   a. Instruct the client to resume normal daily activities and to maintain a diary documenting activities and any symptoms that may develop for correlation with the electrocardiographic tracing.
   b. Instruct the client using a wired monitor to avoid tub baths, showers, or swimming, because they will interfere with the electrocardiographic recorder device.

R. Echocardiography
1. Description
   a. This noninvasive procedure is based on the principles of ultrasound and evaluates structural and functional changes in the heart.
   b. Used to detect valvular abnormalities, congenital heart defects, wall motion, ejection fraction, and cardiac function.
   c. Transesophageal echocardiography may be performed, in which the echocardiogram is done through the esophagus to view the posterior structures of the heart; this is an invasive exam and requires preparation and care similar to endoscopy procedures.
2. Interventions: Advise the client to lie still, breathe normally, and refrain from talking during the test.

S. Exercise electrocardiography testing (stress test)
1. Description
   a. This noninvasive test studies the heart during activity and detects and evaluates coronary artery disease.
   b. Treadmill testing is the most commonly used mode of stress testing.
   c. If the client is unable to tolerate exercise, an intravenous (IV) infusion of dipyridamole or dobutamine hydrochloride is given to dilate the coronary arteries and simulate the effect of exercise; the client may need to be NPO (nothing by mouth) for 3 to 6 hours preprocedure.
2. Preprocedure interventions
   a. Ensure that an informed consent is obtained if required.
   b. Encourage adequate rest the night before the procedure.
   c. Instruct the client having a noninvasive test to eat a light meal 1 to 2 hours before the procedure.
   d. Instruct the client to avoid smoking, alcohol, and caffeine before the procedure.
   e. Instruct the client to ask the primary health care provider (PHCP) or cardiologist about taking prescribed medication on the day of the procedure; theophylline products are usually withheld 12 hours before the test, and calcium channel blockers and beta blockers are usually withheld on the day of the test to allow the heart rate to increase during the stress portion of the test.
   f. Instruct the client to wear nonconstrictive, comfortable clothing and supportive rubber-soled shoes for the exercise stress test.
   g. Instruct the client to notify the PHCP if any chest pain, dizziness, or shortness of breath occurs during the procedure.
3. Postprocedure interventions: Instruct the client to avoid taking a hot bath or shower for at least 1 to 2 hours.

T. Myocardial nuclear perfusion imaging (MNPI)
1. Description
   a. Nuclear cardiology involves the use of radionuclide techniques and scanning for cardiovascular assessment.
   b. The most common tests include technetium pyrophosphate scanning, thallium imaging, and multigated cardiac blood pool imaging; these tests can evaluate cardiac motion and calculate the ejection fraction.
2. Preprocedure interventions
   a. Ensure that an informed consent is obtained.
   b. Inform the client that a small amount of radioisotope will be injected and that the radiation exposure and risks are minimal.
3. Postprocedure interventions
   a. Assess vital signs.
   b. Assess injection site for bleeding or discomfort.
   c. Inform the client that fatigue is possible.

U. Magnetic resonance imaging (MRI)
1. Description
   a. This is a noninvasive diagnostic test that produces an image of the heart or great vessels through the interaction of magnetic fields, radiowaves, and atomic nuclei.
   b. It provides information on chamber size and thickness, valve and ventricular function, and blood flow through the great vessels and coronary arteries.

2. Preprocedure interventions
   a. Evaluate the client for the presence of a pacemaker or other implanted items that present a contraindication to the test.
   b. Ensure that the client has removed all metallic objects such as a watch, jewelry, clothing with metal fasteners, and metal hair fasteners.
   c. Inform the client that she or he may experience claustrophobia while in the scanner.

V. Electrophysiological studies: An invasive procedure in which a programmed electrical stimulation of the heart is induced to cause dysrhythmias and conduction defects; assists in finding an accurate diagnosis and aids in determining treatment.

W. Electron-beam computed tomography (EBCT) scan: Determines whether calcifications are present in the arteries; a coronary artery calcium (CAC) score is provided (a score higher than 300 indicates high risk of myocardial infarction and requires intensive preventive treatment).

X. Cardiac catheterization (Fig. 52-2)
1. Description
   a. An invasive test involving insertion of a catheter into the heart and surrounding vessels

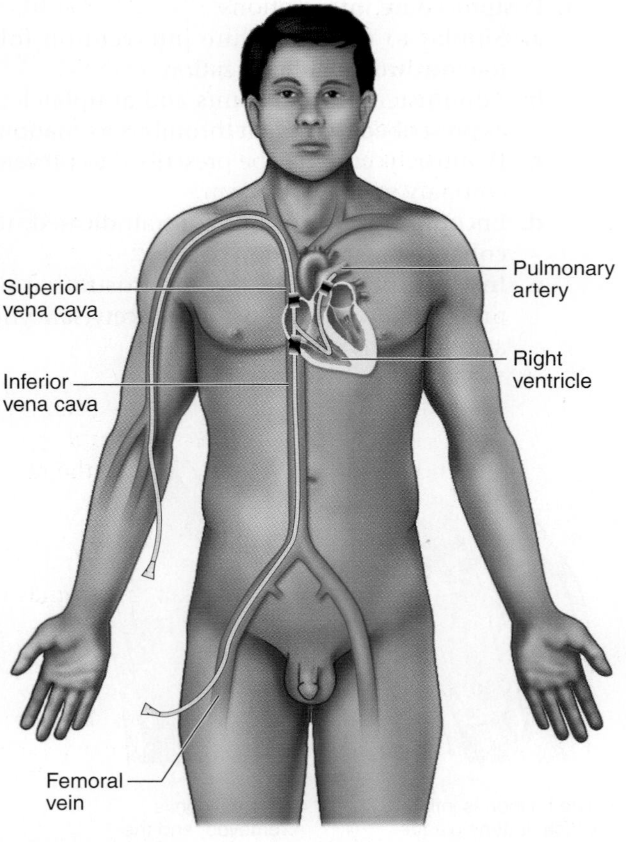

FIG. 52-2 Right-sided heart catheterization. The catheter is inserted into the femoral vein and advanced into the inferior vena cava (or, if into an antecubital or basilic vein, through the superior vena cava), right atrium, right ventricle, and pulmonary artery.

   b. Obtains information about the structure and performance of the heart chambers and valves and the coronary circulation
2. Preprocedure interventions
   a. Ensure that informed consent has been obtained.
   b. Assess for allergies to seafood, iodine, or radiopaque dyes; if allergic, the client may be premedicated with antihistamines and corticosteroids to prevent a reaction.
   c. Withhold solid food for 6 to 8 hours and liquids for 4 hours as prescribed to prevent vomiting and aspiration during the procedure.
   d. Document the client's height and weight, because these data will be needed to determine the amount of dye to be administered.
   e. Document baseline vital signs and note the quality and presence of peripheral pulses for postprocedure comparison.
   f. Inform the client that a local anesthetic will be administered before catheter insertion.
   g. Inform the client that she or he may feel a fluttery feeling as the catheter passes through the heart, a flushed and warm feeling when the dye is injected, a desire to cough, and palpitations caused by heart irritability.
   h. The insertion site is prepared by shaving or clipping the hair and cleaning with an antiseptic solution.
   i. Administer preprocedure medications such as sedatives if prescribed.
   j. Insert an IV line if prescribed.

If a client taking metformin is scheduled to undergo a procedure requiring the administration of iodine dye, the metformin is withheld for 24 hours prior to the procedure because of the risk of lactic acidosis. The medication is not resumed until prescribed by the PHCP (usually 48 hours after the procedure or after renal function studies are done and the results are evaluated).

3. Postprocedure interventions
   a. Monitor vital signs and cardiac rhythm for dysrhythmias at least every 30 minutes for 2 hours initially.
   b. Assess for chest pain and, if dysrhythmias or chest pain occurs, notify the PHCP.
   c. Monitor peripheral pulses and the color, warmth, and sensation of the extremity distal to the insertion site at least every 30 minutes for 2 hours initially.
   d. Notify the PHCP if the client reports numbness and tingling; if the extremity becomes cool, pale, or cyanotic; or if loss of the peripheral pulses occurs. This could indicate clot formation and is an emergency.

e. Apply a sandbag or compression device (if prescribed) to the insertion site to provide additional pressure if required.
f. Monitor for bleeding; if bleeding occurs, apply manual pressure immediately and notify the PHCP.
g. Monitor for hematoma; if a hematoma develops, notify the PHCP.
h. Keep the extremity extended for 4 to 6 hours, as prescribed, keeping the leg straight to prevent arterial occlusion.
i. Maintain strict bed rest for 6 to 12 hours, as prescribed; however, the client may turn from side to side. Do not elevate the head of the bed more than 15 degrees.
j. If the antecubital vessel was used, immobilize the arm with an armboard.
k. If the PHCP uses a vascular closure device to seal the arterial puncture site, there is no need for prolonged compression or bed rest, and clients may be out of bed in 1 to 2 hours.
l. Encourage fluid intake, if not contraindicated, to promote renal excretion of the dye and to replace fluid loss caused by the osmotic diuretic effect of the dye.
m. Monitor for nausea, vomiting, rash, or other signs of hypersensitivity to the dye.

Y. Intravascular ultrasonography (IVUS): A catheter with a transducer is used as an alternative to injecting a dye into the coronary arteries and detects plaque distribution and composition; it also detects arterial dissection and the degree of stenosis of an occluded artery.

III. Therapeutic Management

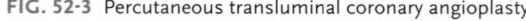

A. Percutaneous transluminal coronary angioplasty (PTCA)
1. Description (Fig. 52-3)
a. An invasive, nonsurgical technique in which 1 or more coronary arteries are dilated with a balloon catheter to open the vessel lumen and improve arterial blood flow
b. PTCA may be used for clients with an evolving MI, alone or in combination with medications, to achieve reperfusion.
c. The client can experience reocclusion after the procedure; thus, the procedure may need to be repeated.
d. Complications can include arterial dissection or rupture, embolization of plaque fragments, spasm, and acute MI.
e. Firm commitment is needed on the client's part to stop smoking, adhere to diet restrictions, lose weight, alter the exercise pattern, and stop any behaviors that lead to progressive artery occlusion.
2. Preprocedure interventions
a. Similar to preprocedure interventions for cardiac catheterization
b. The PHCP may prescribe preprocedure medications, including acetylsalicylic acid.
c. Instruct the client that chest pain may occur during balloon inflation and to report it if it does occur.
3. Postprocedure interventions
a. Similar to postprocedure intervention following cardiac catheterization
b. Administer anticoagulants and antiplatelets as prescribed to prevent thrombus formation.
c. IV nitroglycerin may be prescribed to prevent coronary artery vasospasm.
d. Encourage fluids, if not contraindicated, to enhance renal excretion of dye.
e. Instruct the client in the administration of prescribed medications; daily acetylsalicylic acid (aspirin) may be prescribed.

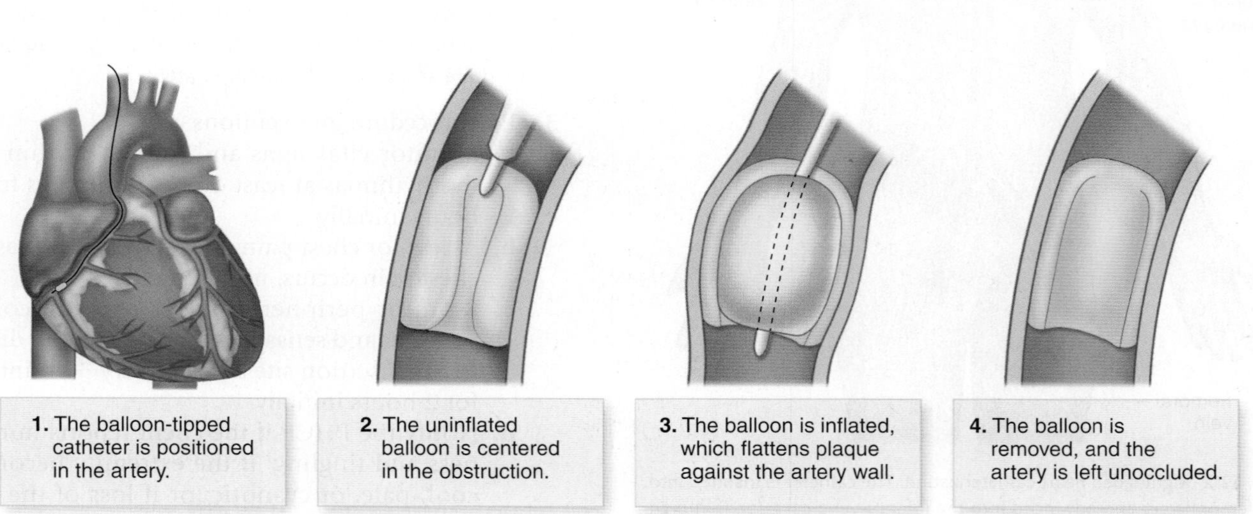

1. The balloon-tipped catheter is positioned in the artery.
2. The uninflated balloon is centered in the obstruction.
3. The balloon is inflated, which flattens plaque against the artery wall.
4. The balloon is removed, and the artery is left unoccluded.

FIG. 52-3 Percutaneous transluminal coronary angioplasty.

f. Assist the client with planning lifestyle modifications.

B. Laser-assisted angioplasty

1. Description
   a. A laser probe is advanced through a cannula similar to that used for PTCA.
   b. Used for clients with small occlusions in the coronary arteries, also the distal superficial femoral, proximal popliteal, and common iliac arteries.
   c. Heat from the laser vaporizes the plaque to open the occluded artery.
2. Preprocedure and postprocedure interventions
   a. Care is similar to that for PTCA.
   b. Monitor for complications of coronary dissection, acute occlusion, perforation, embolism, and MI.

C. Coronary artery stents

1. Description
   a. Coronary artery stents are used with PTCA to provide a supportive scaffold to eliminate the risk of acute coronary vessel closure and to improve long-term patency of the vessel.
   b. A balloon catheter bearing the stent is inserted into the coronary artery and positioned at the site of occlusion; balloon inflation deploys the stent.
   c. When placed in the coronary artery, the stent reopens the blocked artery.
2. Preprocedure and postprocedure interventions
   a. Care is similar to that for PTCA.
   b. Acute thrombosis is a major concern following the procedure; the client is placed on antiplatelet therapy such as clopidogrel and acetylsalicylic acid (aspirin) for several months following the procedure. Length of time of antiplatelet therapy is determined by the type of stent (metal or medication-coated) that has been deployed.
   c. Monitor for complications of the procedure such as stent migration or occlusion, coronary artery dissection, and bleeding resulting from anticoagulation.

D. Atherectomy

1. Description
   a. Atherectomy removes plaque from a coronary artery by the use of a cutting chamber on the inserted catheter or a rotating blade that pulverizes the plaque.
   b. Atherectomy is also used to improve blood flow to ischemic limbs in individuals with peripheral arterial disease.
2. Preprocedure and postprocedure interventions
   a. Care is similar to that for PTCA.
   b. Monitor for complications of perforation, embolus, and reocclusion.

E. Transmyocardial revascularization

1. May be used for clients with widespread atherosclerosis involving vessels that are too small and numerous for replacement or balloon catheterization; performed through a small chest incision
2. Transmyocardial revascularization uses a high-powered laser that creates 20 to 24 channels through the ventricular muscle of the left ventricle; blood enters these small channels, providing the affected region of the heart with oxygenated blood.
3. The opening on the surface of the heart heals; however, the main channels remain and perfuse the myocardium.

F. Coronary artery bypass grafting (Fig. 52-4)

1. Description
   a. The occluded coronary arteries are bypassed with the client's own venous or arterial blood vessels.
   b. The saphenous vein, internal mammary artery, or other arteries may be used to bypass lesions in the coronary arteries.

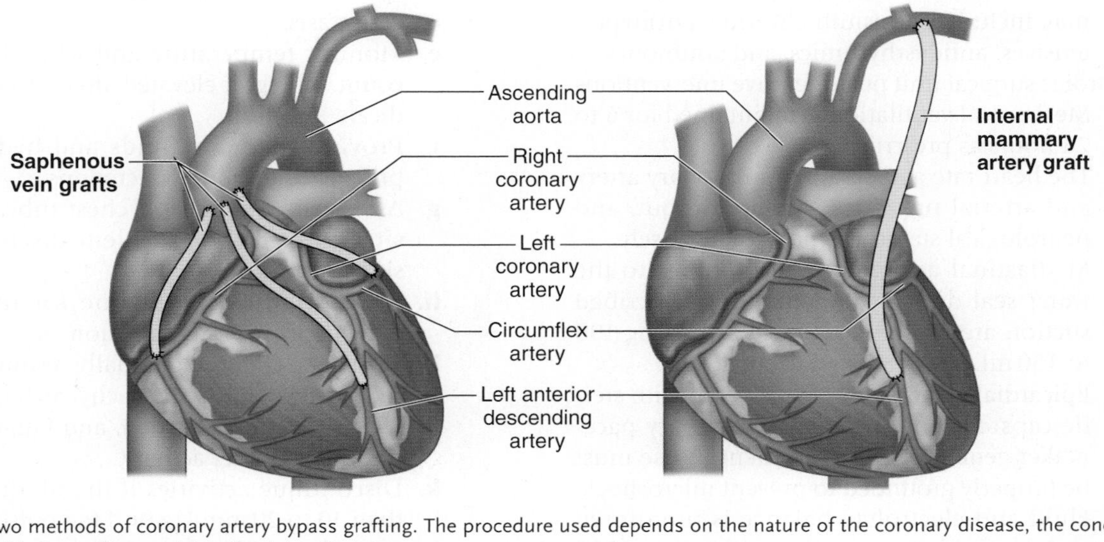

FIG. 52-4 Two methods of coronary artery bypass grafting. The procedure used depends on the nature of the coronary disease, the condition of the vessels available for grafting, and the client's health status.

c. Coronary artery bypass grafting is performed when the client does not respond to medical management of coronary artery disease or when vessels are severely occluded.
d. A minimally invasive direct coronary artery bypass (MIDCAB) may be an option for some clients who have a lesion in the LAD artery; a sternal incision is not required (usually a 2-inch [5-cm] left thoracotomy incision is done), and cardiopulmonary bypass is not required in this procedure.

2. Preoperative interventions
a. Familiarize the client and family with the cardiac surgical critical care unit.
b. Inform the client to expect a sternal incision, possible arm or leg incision(s), 1 or 2 chest tubes, a Foley catheter, and several IV fluid catheters.
c. Inform the client that an endotracheal tube will be in place for a short period of time and that she or he will be unable to speak.
d. Advise the client that she or he will be on mechanical ventilation and to breathe with the ventilator and not fight it.
e. Instruct the client that postoperative pain is expected and that pain medication will be available.
f. Instruct the client in how to splint the chest incision, cough and deep breathe, use the incentive spirometer, and perform arm and leg exercises.
g. Encourage the client and family to discuss anxieties and fears related to surgery.
h. Note that prescribed medications may be discontinued preoperatively (usually, diuretics 2 to 3 days before surgery, digoxin 12 hours before surgery, and aspirin and anticoagulants 1 week before surgery).
i. Administer medications as prescribed, which may include potassium chloride, antihypertensives, antidysrhythmics, and antibiotics.

3. Cardiac surgical unit postoperative interventions
a. Mechanical ventilation is maintained for 6 to 24 hours as prescribed.
b. The heart rate and rhythm, pulmonary artery and arterial pressures, urinary output, and neurological status are monitored closely.
c. Mediastinal and pleural chest tubes to the water seal drainage system with prescribed suction are present; drainage exceeding 100 to 150 mL/hr is reported to the PHCP.
d. Epicardial pacing wires are covered with sterile caps or connected to a temporary pacemaker generator; all equipment in use must be properly grounded to prevent microshock.
e. Fluid and electrolyte balance is monitored closely; fluids are usually restricted to 1500 to 2000 mL, because the client usually has edema.
f. The **blood pressure** is monitored closely, because hypotension can cause collapse of a vein graft; hypertension can cause increased pressure, promoting leakage from the suture line, causing bleeding.
g. Temperature is monitored and rewarming procedures are initiated using warm or thermal blankets if the temperature drops below 96.8° F (36.0° C); rewarm the client no faster than 1.8 degrees/hr to prevent shivering, and discontinue rewarming procedures when the temperature approaches 98.6° F (37.0° C).
h. Potassium is administered intravenously as prescribed to maintain the potassium level between 4 and 5 mEq/L (4 to 5 mmol/L) to prevent dysrhythmias.
i. The client is monitored for signs of cardiac tamponade, which will include sudden cessation of previously heavy mediastinal drainage, jugular vein distention with clear lung sounds, equalization of right atrial (RA) pressure and pulmonary artery wedge pressure, and pulsus paradoxus.
j. Pain is monitored, differentiating sternotomy pain from anginal pain, which would indicate graft failure.

4. Alarm safety and alarm fatigue: Refer to Chapter 69.

5. Transfer of the client from the cardiac surgical unit ▲
a. Monitor vital signs, level of consciousness, and peripheral perfusion.
b. Monitor for dysrhythmias.
c. Auscultate lungs and assess respiratory status.
d. Encourage the client to splint the incision, cough, deep breathe, and use the incentive spirometer to raise secretions and prevent atelectasis.
e. Monitor temperature and white blood cell count, which, if elevated after 3 to 4 days, indicate infection.
f. Provide adequate fluids and hydration as prescribed to liquefy secretions.
g. Assess suture line and chest tube insertion sites for redness, purulent discharge, and signs of infection.
h. Assess sternal suture line for instability, which may indicate infection.
i. Guide the client to gradually resume activity.
j. Assess the client for tachycardia, **postural (orthostatic) hypotension**, and fatigue before, during, and after activity.
k. Discontinue activities if the BP drops more than 10 to 20 mm Hg or if the pulse increases more than 10 beats per minute.

BOX 52-2 Home Care Instructions for the Client After Cardiac Surgery

- Progressive return to activities at home
- Limiting of pushing or pulling activities for 6 weeks following discharge
- Maintenance of incisional care and recording signs of redness, swelling, or drainage
- Sternotomy incision heals in about 6 to 8 weeks
- Avoidance of crossing legs; wearing elastic hose as prescribed until edema subsides, and elevating the surgical limb (if used to obtain the graft) when sitting in a chair
- Use of prescribed medications
- Dietary measures, including the avoidance of saturated fats and cholesterol and the use of salt
- Resumption of sexual intercourse on the advice of the primary health care provider or cardiologist after exercise tolerance is assessed (usually, if the client can walk 1 block or climb 2 flights of stairs without symptoms, she or he can resume sexual activity safely)

l. Monitor episodes of pain closely.
m. See Box 52-2 for home care instructions.

G. Heart transplantation
1. A donor heart from an individual with a comparable body weight and ABO compatibility is transplanted into a recipient within less than 6 hours of procurement.
2. The surgeon removes the diseased heart, leaving the posterior portion of the atria to serve as an anchor for the new heart.
3. Because a remnant of the client's atria remains, 2 unrelated P waves are noted on the ECG.
4. The transplanted heart is denervated and unresponsive to vagal stimulation; because the heart is denervated, clients do not experience angina.
5. Symptoms of heart rejection include hypotension, dysrhythmias, weakness, fatigue, and dizziness.
6. Endomyocardial biopsies are performed at regularly scheduled intervals and whenever rejection is suspected.
7. The client requires lifetime immunosuppressive therapy.
8. Strict aseptic technique and vigilant hand washing must be maintained when caring for the posttransplantation client because of increased risk for infection from immunosuppression.
9. The heart rate approximates 100 beats per minute and responds slowly to exercise or stress with regard to increases in heart rate, **contractility**, and **cardiac output**.

IV. Cardiac Dysrhythmias

A. Normal sinus rhythm (Fig. 52-5)
1. Rhythm originates from the SA node.
2. Description
   a. Atrial and ventricular rhythms are regular.
   b. Atrial and ventricular rates are 60 to 100 beats per minute (Fig. 52-6 and Box 52-3).
   c. PR interval and QRS width are within normal limits.

B. Sinus bradycardia
1. Description
   a. Atrial and ventricular rhythms are regular.
   b. Atrial and ventricular rates are less than 60 beats per minute.
   c. PR interval and QRS width are within normal limits.
   d. Treatment may be necessary if the client is symptomatic (signs of decreased cardiac output).
   e. A low heart rate may be normal for some individuals, such as athletes.
2. Interventions
   a. Attempt to determine the cause of sinus bradycardia; withhold medication suspected of causing the bradycardia and notify the PHCP.
   b. Administer oxygen as prescribed for the symptomatic client.
   c. Administer atropine sulfate as prescribed to increase the heart rate to 60 beats per minute.
   d. Be prepared to apply a noninvasive (transcutaneous) pacemaker initially if the atropine sulfate does not increase the heart rate sufficiently.
   e. Avoid additional doses of atropine sulfate, because this will induce tachycardia.

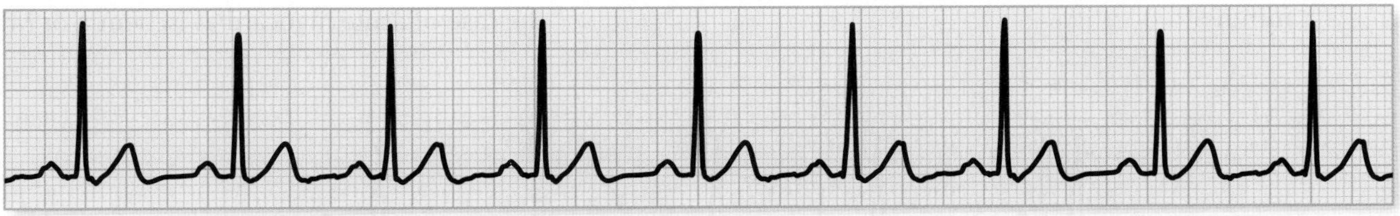

FIG. 52-5 Normal sinus rhythm. Both atrial and ventricular rhythms are essentially regular (a slight variation in rhythm is normal). Atrial and ventricular rates are both 83 beats per minute. There is one P wave before each QRS complex, and all P waves are of a consistent morphology, or shape. The PR interval measures 0.18 seconds and is constant; the QRS complex measures 0.06 seconds and is constant.

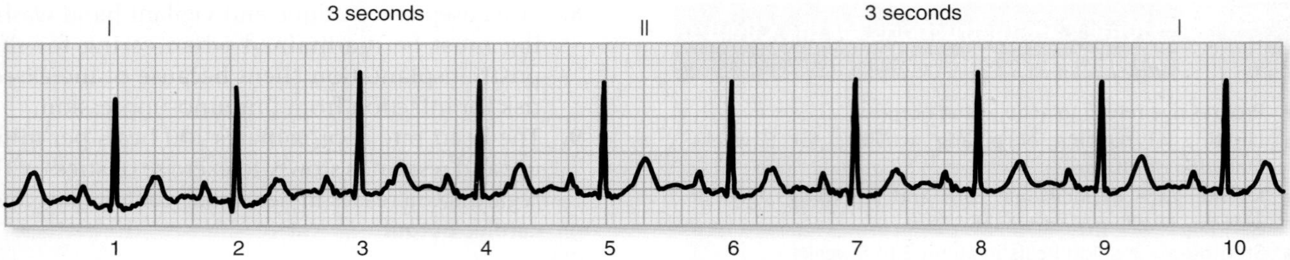

FIG. 52-6 Each segment between the dark lines (above the monitor strip) represents 3 seconds when the monitor is set at a speed of 25 mm/second. To estimate the ventricular rate, count the QRS complexes in a 6-second strip and then multiply that number by 10 to estimate the heart rate for 1 minute. In this example, there are 9 QRS complexes in 6 seconds. Therefore, the heart rate can be estimated as 90 beats per minute.

BOX 52-3 Determination of Heart Rate Using 6-Second Strip Method

- The method can be used to determine heart rate for regular and irregular rhythms.
- To determine atrial rate, count the number of P waves in 6 seconds and multiply by 10 to obtain a full minute rate.
- To determine ventricular rate, count the number of R waves or QRS complexes in 6 seconds and multiply by 10 to obtain a full minute rate.
- For accuracy, timing should begin on the P wave or the QRS complex and end exactly at 30 large blocks later.

f. Monitor for hypotension and administer fluids intravenously as prescribed.
g. Depending on the cause of the bradycardia, the client may need a permanent pacemaker.

C. Sinus tachycardia
1. Description
a. Atrial and ventricular rates are 100 to 180 beats per minute.
b. Atrial and ventricular rhythms are regular.
c. PR interval and QRS width are within normal limits.
2. Interventions
a. Identify the cause of the tachycardia.
b. Decrease the heart rate to normal by treating the underlying cause.

D. Atrial fibrillation (Fig. 52-7)
1. Description
a. Multiple rapid impulses from many foci depolarize in the atria in a totally disorganized manner at a rate of 350 to 600 times per minute.
b. The atria quiver, which can lead to the formation of thrombi.
c. Usually no definitive P wave can be observed, only fibrillatory waves before each QRS.
2. Interventions
a. Administer oxygen.
b. Administer anticoagulants as prescribed because of the risk of emboli.
c. Administer cardiac medications as prescribed to control the ventricular rhythm and assist in the maintenance of cardiac output.
d. Prepare the client for cardioversion as prescribed.
e. Instruct the client in the use of medications as prescribed to control the dysrhythmia.

E. Premature ventricular contractions (PVCs; Fig. 52-8 and Box 52-4)
1. Description
a. Early ventricular contractions result from increased irritability of the ventricles.
b. PVCs frequently occur in repetitive patterns such as bigeminy, trigeminy, and quadrigeminy.
c. The QRS complexes may be unifocal or multifocal.
2. Interventions
a. Identify the cause and treat on the basis of the cause.
b. Evaluate oxygen saturation to assess for hypoxemia, which can cause PVCs.
c. Evaluate electrolytes, particularly the potassium level, because hypokalemia can cause PVCs.
d. Oxygen and medication may be prescribed in the case of acute myocardial ischemia or MI.

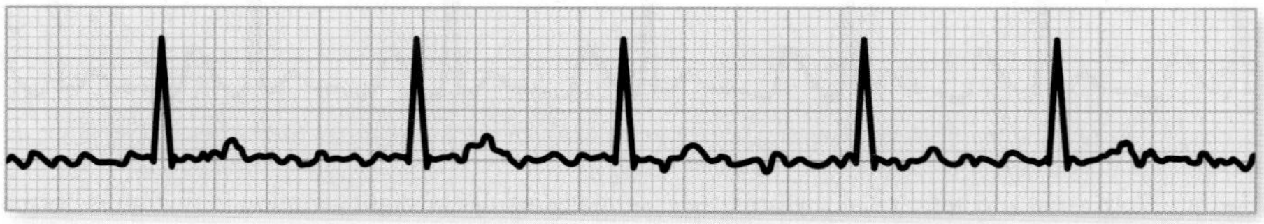

FIG. 52-7 Atrial dysrhythmias—atrial fibrillation.

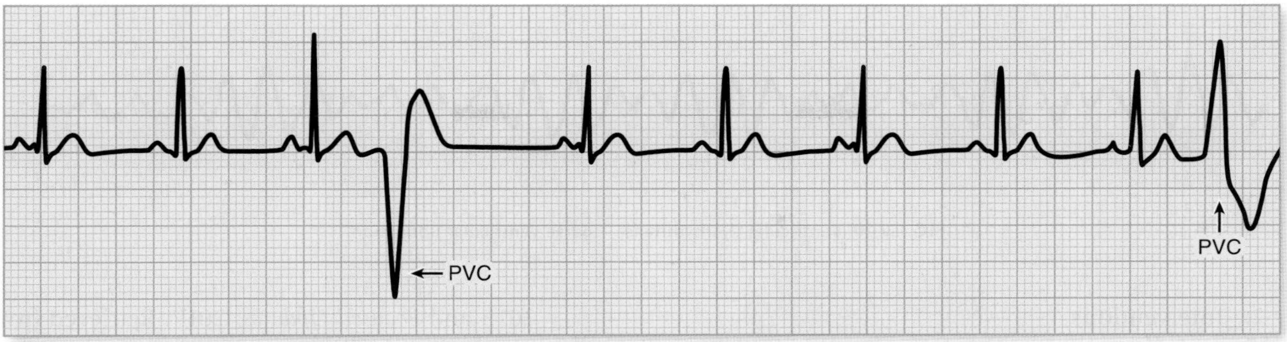

FIG. 52-8 Ventricular dysrhythmias—normal sinus rhythm with multifocal premature ventricular contractions (PVCs; one negative and the other positive).

BOX 52-4 Premature Ventricular Contractions

Bigeminy: Premature ventricular contraction (PVC) every other heartbeat
Trigeminy: PVC every third heartbeat
Quadrigeminy: PVC every fourth heartbeat
Couplet or pair: Two sequential PVCs
Unifocal: Uniform upward or downward deflection, arising from the same ectopic focus
Multifocal: Different shapes, with the impulse generation from different sites
R-on-T phenomenon: PVC falls on the T wave of the preceding beat; may precipitate ventricular fibrillation

! For the client experiencing PVCs, notify the PHCP or cardiologist if the client complains of chest pain or if the PVCs increase in frequency, are multifocal, occur on the T wave (R-on-T), or occur in runs of ventricular tachycardia.

F. Ventricular tachycardia (VT; Fig. 52-9)
  1. Description
    a. VT occurs because of a repetitive firing of an irritable ventricular ectopic focus at a rate of 140 to 250 beats per minute or more.
    b. VT may present as a paroxysm of 3 self-limiting beats or more, or may be a sustained rhythm.
    c. VT can lead to cardiac arrest.
  2. Stable client with sustained VT (with pulse and no signs or symptoms of decreased cardiac output)
    a. Administer oxygen as prescribed.
    b. Administer antidysrhythmics as prescribed.
  3. Unstable client with VT (with pulse and signs and symptoms of decreased cardiac output)
    a. Administer oxygen and antidysrhythmic therapy as prescribed.
    b. Prepare for synchronized cardioversion if the client is unstable.
    c. The PHCP may attempt cough cardiopulmonary resuscitation (CPR) by asking the client to cough hard every 1 to 3 seconds.
  4. Pulseless client with VT: Defibrillation and CPR

G. Ventricular fibrillation (VF; Fig. 52-10)
  1. Description
    a. Impulses from many irritable foci in the ventricles fire in a totally disorganized manner.
    b. VF is a chaotic rapid rhythm in which the ventricles quiver and there is no cardiac output.
    c. VF is fatal if not successfully resolved within 3 to 5 minutes.
    d. Client is unconscious with no pulse, BP, respirations, or heart sounds.

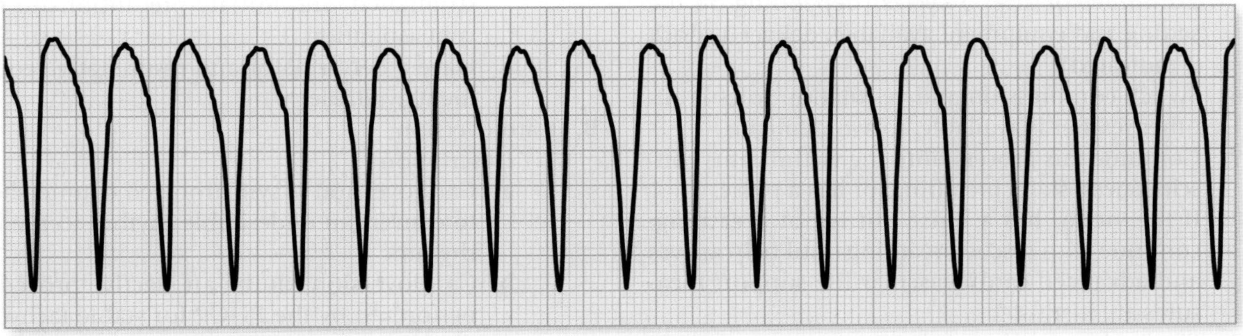

FIG. 52-9 Ventricular dysrhythmias—sustained ventricular tachycardia at a rate of 166 beats per minute.

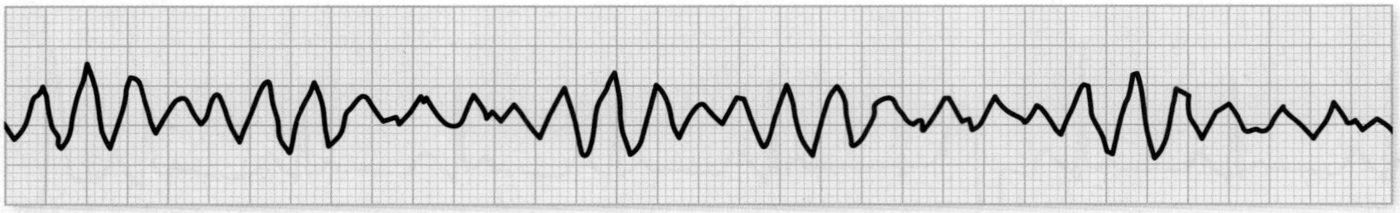

FIG. 52-10 Ventricular dysrhythmias—coarse ventricular fibrillation.

2. Interventions
   a. Initiate CPR until a defibrillator is available.
   b. The client is defibrillated immediately with 120 to 200 joules (biphasic defibrillator) or 360 joules (monophasic defibrillator); check the entire length of the client 3 times to make sure no one is touching the client or the bed; when clear, proceed with defibrillation.
   c. CPR is continued for 2 minutes, and the cardiac rhythm is reassessed to determine the need for further countershock.
   d. Administer oxygen as prescribed.
   e. Administer antidysrhythmic therapy as prescribed.

H. Guidelines for performing adult CPR
1. Follow CAB (compressions, airway, breathing) guidelines. If a victim is noted not breathing or only gasping, activate the emergency response system and obtain an automated external defibrillator (AED) or monophasic or biphasic defibrillator depending on the setting and equipment available.
2. Check the carotid pulse for a maximum of 10 seconds.
3. If no pulse is felt, begin chest compressions (100 to 120 per minute) at a depth of 2 inches (5 cm) for 2 minutes or 5 cycles of 30 compressions to 2 ventilations using a barrier device or bag valve mask.
4. To provide ventilations, the head-tilt chin-lift maneuver, or jaw thrust technique is used if neck injury is suspected.
5. Check rhythm and for presence of a pulse every 2 minutes or after 5 cycles (depending on the setting and equipment available, deliver a shock if indicated).
6. Switch compression and ventilation roles if another rescuer is available, to avoid fatigue.
7. Continue this process until the victim gains consciousness, starts breathing, or has a pulse.
8. If the victim has a pulse but is not breathing, continue with rescue breathing until help arrives and advanced cardiovascular life support measures are instituted.
9. For updated information, refer to American Heart Association: *Guidelines for CPR and ECC, 2015* and *Focused Updates*, 2017. Retrieved from https://eccguidelines.heart.org/index.php/circulation/cpr-ecc-guidelines-2/

V. Management of Dysrhythmias

A. Vagal maneuvers
1. Description: Vagal maneuvers induce vagal stimulation of the cardiac conduction system and are used to terminate supraventricular tachydysrhythmias.
2. Carotid sinus massage
   a. The PHCP instructs the client to turn the head away from the side to be massaged.
   b. The PHCP massages over 1 carotid artery for a few seconds to determine whether a change in cardiac rhythm occurs.
   c. The client must be on a cardiac monitor; an electrocardiographic rhythm strip before, during, and after the procedure should be documented on the chart.
   d. Have a defibrillator and resuscitative equipment available.
   e. Monitor vital signs, cardiac rhythm, and level of consciousness following the procedure.
3. Valsalva maneuver
   a. The PHCP instructs the client to bear down or induces a gag reflex in the client to stimulate a vagal response.
   b. Monitor the heart rate, rhythm, and BP.
   c. Observe the cardiac monitor for a change in rhythm.
   d. Record an electrocardiographic rhythm strip before, during, and after the procedure.
   e. Provide an emesis basin if the gag reflex is stimulated, and initiate precautions to prevent aspiration.
   f. Have a defibrillator and resuscitative equipment available.

B. Cardioversion
1. Description
   a. Cardioversion is synchronized countershock to convert an undesirable rhythm to a stable rhythm.
   b. Cardioversion can be an elective procedure performed by the PHCP for stable tachydysrhythmias resistant to medical therapies or an emergent procedure for hemodynamically

unstable ventricular or supraventricular tachydysrhythmias.

c. A lower amount of energy is used than with defibrillation.

d. The defibrillator is synchronized to the client's R wave to avoid discharging the shock during the vulnerable period (T wave).

e. If the defibrillator is not synchronized, it could discharge on the T wave and cause VF.

2. Preprocedure interventions

a. If an elective procedure, ensure that informed consent is obtained.

b. Administer sedation as prescribed.

c. If an elective procedure, hold digoxin for 48 hours preprocedure as prescribed to prevent postcardioversion ventricular irritability.

d. If an elective procedure for atrial fibrillation or atrial flutter, the client should receive anticoagulant therapy for 4 to 6 weeks preprocedure, and a transesophageal echocardiogram (TEE) should be performed to rule out clots in the atria prior to the procedure.

3. During the procedure

a. Ensure that the skin is clean and dry in the area where the electrode pads/hands-off pads will be placed.

b. Stop the oxygen during the procedure to avoid a fire hazard.

c. Be sure that no one is touching the bed or the client when delivering the countershock (check the entire length of the client 3 times).

4. Postprocedure interventions

a. Priority assessment includes ability of the client to maintain the airway and breathing.

b. Resume oxygen administration as prescribed.

c. Assess vital signs.

d. Assess level of consciousness.

e. Monitor cardiac rhythm.

f. Monitor for indications of successful response, such as conversion to sinus rhythm, strong peripheral pulses, an adequate BP, and adequate urine output.

g. Assess the skin on the chest for evidence of burns from the edges of the pads.

C. Defibrillation

1. Defibrillation is an asynchronous countershock used to terminate pulseless VT or VF.

2. The defibrillator is charged to 120 to 200 joules (biphasic) or 360 joules (monophasic) for 1 countershock from the defibrillator, and then CPR is resumed immediately and continued for 5 cycles or about 2 minutes.

3. Reassess the rhythm after 2 minutes, and if VF or pulseless VT continues, the defibrillator is charged to give a second shock at the same energy level previously used.

4. Resume CPR after the shock, and continue with the life support protocol.

⚠ Before defibrillating a client, be sure that the oxygen is shut off to avoid the hazard of fire and be sure that no one is touching the bed or the client.

D. Use of pad electrodes

1. One pad is placed at the third intercostal space to the right of the sternum; the other is placed at the fifth intercostal space on the left midaxillary line.

2. Apply firm pressure of at least 25 lb to each of the pads.

3. Be sure that no one is touching the bed or the client when delivering the countershock.

4. Pads for hands-off biphasic defibrillation may be applied in an anterior-posterior position or apex-posterior position, and placement directly over breast tissue should be avoided.

E. Automated external defibrillator (AED)

1. An AED is used by laypersons and emergency medical technicians for prehospital cardiac arrest.

2. Place the client on a firm, dry surface.

3. Turn on the AED and follow the voice prompts.

4. Place the electrode patches in the correct position on the client's chest.

5. Stop CPR.

6. Ensure that no one is touching the client to avoid motion artifact during rhythm analysis.

7. The machine will advise whether a shock is necessary.

8. Shocks are recommended for pulseless VT or VF only (usually 3 shocks are delivered).

9. If unsuccessful, CPR is continued for 1 minute and then another series of shocks is delivered.

F. Automated implantable cardioverter-defibrillator (AICD)

1. Description

a. An AICD monitors cardiac rhythm and detects and terminates episodes of VT and VF by delivering 25 to 30 joules up to 4 times, if necessary.

b. An AICD is used in clients with episodes of spontaneous sustained VT or VF unrelated to an MI or in clients whose medication therapy has been unsuccessful in controlling life-threatening dysrhythmias.

c. Transvenous electrode leads are placed in the right atrium and ventricle in contact with the endocardium; leads are used for sensing, pacing, and delivery of cardioversion or defibrillation.

d. The generator is most commonly implanted in the left pectoral region.

2. Client education
   a. Instruct the client in the basic functions of the AICD.
   b. Know the rate cutoff of the AICD and the number of consecutive shocks that it will deliver.
   c. Wear loose-fitting clothing over the AICD generator site.
   d. Instruct the client on activities to avoid, including contact sports, to prevent trauma to the AICD generator and lead wires.
   e. Report any fever, redness, swelling, or drainage from the insertion site.
   f. Report symptoms of fainting, nausea, weakness, blackouts, and rapid pulse rates to the PHCP.
   g. During shock discharge, the client may feel faint or short of breath.
   h. Instruct the client to sit or lie down if he or she feels a shock and to notify the PHCP.
   i. Advise the client to maintain a log of the date, time, and activity preceding the shock; the symptoms preceding the shock; and post-shock sensations.
   j. Instruct the client and family in how to access the emergency medical system.
   k. Encourage the family to learn CPR.
   l. Instruct the client to avoid electromagnetic fields directly over the AICD because they can inactivate the device.
   m. Instruct the client to move away from the magnetic field immediately if beeping tones are heard, and to notify the PHCP.
   n. Keep an AICD identification card in the wallet and obtain and wear a MedicAlert bracelet.
   o. Inform all PHCPs that an AICD has been inserted; certain diagnostic tests, such as MRI, and procedures using diathermy or electrocautery interfere with AICD function.

VI. Pacemakers

A. Description: Temporary or permanent device that provides electrical stimulation and maintains the heart rate when the client's intrinsic pacemaker fails to provide an adequate rate

B. Settings
   1. A synchronous (demand) pacemaker senses the client's rhythm and paces only if the client's intrinsic rate falls below the set pacemaker rate for stimulating depolarization.
   2. An asynchronous (fixed rate) pacemaker paces at a preset rate regardless of the client's intrinsic rhythm and is used when the client is asystolic or profoundly bradycardic.
   3. Overdrive pacing suppresses the underlying rhythm in tachydysrhythmias so that the sinus node will regain control of the heart.

C. Spikes
   1. When a pacing stimulus is delivered to the heart, a spike (straight vertical line) is seen on the monitor or ECG strip.
   2. Spikes precede the chamber being paced; a spike preceding a P wave indicates that the atrium is paced, and a spike preceding the QRS complex indicates that the ventricle is being paced.
   3. An atrial spike followed by a P wave indicates atrial depolarization, and a ventricular spike followed by a QRS complex represents ventricular depolarization; this is referred to as *capture*.

D. Temporary pacemakers
   1. Noninvasive transcutaneous pacing
      a. Noninvasive transcutaneous pacing is used as a temporary emergency measure in the profoundly bradycardic or asystolic client until invasive pacing can be initiated.
      b. Large electrode pads are placed on the client's chest and back and connected to an external pulse generator.
      c. Wash the skin with soap and water before applying electrodes.
      d. It is not necessary to shave the hair or apply alcohol or tinctures to the skin.
      e. Place the posterior electrode between the spine and left scapula behind the heart, avoiding placement over bone.
      f. Place the anterior electrode between V2 and V5 positions over the heart.
      g. Do not place the anterior electrode over female breast tissue; rather, displace breast tissue and place the electrode under the breast.
      h. Do not take the pulse or BP on the left side; the results will not be accurate because of the muscle twitching and electrical current.
      i. Ensure that electrodes are in good contact with the skin.
      j. Set pacing rate as prescribed; establish stimulation threshold to ensure capture.
      k. If loss of capture occurs, assess the skin contact of the electrodes and increase the current until capture is regained.
      l. Evaluate the client for discomfort from cutaneous and muscle stimulation; administer analgesics as needed.
   2. Invasive transvenous pacing
      a. Pacing lead wire is placed through the antecubital, femoral, jugular, or subclavian vein into the right atrium or right ventricle, so that it is in direct contact with the endocardium.
      b. Monitor the pacemaker insertion site.
      c. Restrict client movement to prevent lead wire displacement.
   3. Invasive epicardial pacing—applied by using a transthoracic approach; the lead wires are

threaded loosely on the epicardial surface of the heart after cardiac surgery.

4. Reducing the risk of microshock
   a. Use only inspected and approved equipment.
   b. Insulate the exposed portion of wires with plastic or rubber material (fingers of rubber gloves) when wires are not attached to the pulse generator; cover with nonconductive tape.
   c. Ground all electrical equipment, using a 3-pronged plug.
   d. Wear gloves when handling exposed wires.
   e. Keep dressings dry.

Vital signs are monitored and cardiac monitoring is done continuously for the client with a temporary pacemaker.

E. Permanent pacemakers
1. Pulse generator is internal and surgically implanted in a subcutaneous pocket below the clavicle.
2. The leads are passed transvenously via the cephalic or subclavian vein to the endocardium on the right side of the heart; postoperatively, limitation of arm movement on the operative side is required to prevent lead wire dislodgement.
3. Permanent pacemakers may be single-chambered, in which the lead wire is placed in the chamber to be paced; or dual-chambered, with lead wires placed in both the right atrium and the right ventricle.
4. Biventricular pacing of the ventricles allows for synchronized depolarization and is used for moderate to severe heart failure to improve cardiac output.
5. A permanent pacemaker is programmed when inserted and can be reprogrammed if necessary by noninvasive transmission from an external programmer to the implanted generator.
6. Pacemakers may be powered by a lithium battery with an average life span of 10 years, nuclear-powered with a life span of 20 years or longer, or designed to be recharged externally.
7. Pacemaker function can be checked in the PHCP's office or clinic by a pacemaker interrogator or programmer or from home, using a special telephone transmitter device.
8. The client may be provided with a device placed over the pacemaker battery generator with an attachment to the telephone; the heart rate then can be transmitted to the clinic.
9. Client teaching (Box 52-5).

BOX 52-5 Pacemakers: Client Education

- Instruct the client about the pacemaker, including the programmed rate.
- Instruct the client in the signs of battery failure and when to notify the primary health care provider (PHCP) or cardiologist.
- Instruct the client to report any fever, redness, swelling, or drainage from the insertion site.
- Report signs of dizziness, weakness or fatigue, swelling of the ankles or legs, chest pain, or shortness of breath.
- Keep a pacemaker identification card in the wallet and obtain and wear a MedicAlert bracelet.
- Instruct the client in how to take the pulse, to take the pulse daily, and to maintain a diary of pulse rates.
- Wear loose-fitting clothing over the pulse generator site.
- Avoid contact sports.
- Inform all PHCPs that a pacemaker has been inserted.
- Instruct the client to inform airport security that she or he has a pacemaker, because the pacemaker may set off the security detector.
- Instruct the client that most electrical appliances can be used without any interference with the functioning of the pacemaker; however, advise the client not to operate electrical appliances directly over the pacemaker site.
- Avoid transmitter towers and antitheft devices in stores.
- Instruct the client that if any unusual feelings occur when near any electrical devices, to move 5 to 10 feet away and check the pulse.
- Instruct the client about the methods of monitoring the function of the device.
- Emphasize the importance of follow-up with the PHCP.
- Use cellphones on the side opposite the pacemaker.

VII. Coronary Artery Disease

A. Description
1. Coronary artery disease is a narrowing or obstruction of 1 or more coronary arteries as a result of atherosclerosis, which is an accumulation of lipid-containing plaque in the arteries (Fig. 52-11).
2. The disease causes decreased perfusion of myocardial tissue and inadequate myocardial oxygen supply, leading to hypertension, angina, dysrhythmias, MI, heart failure, and death.
3. Collateral circulation, more than 1 artery supplying a muscle with blood, is normally present in the coronary arteries, especially in older persons.
4. The development of collateral circulation takes time and develops when chronic ischemia occurs to meet the metabolic demands; therefore, an occlusion of a coronary artery in a younger individual is more likely to be lethal than one in an older individual.
5. Symptoms occur when the coronary artery is occluded to the point that inadequate blood supply to the muscle occurs, causing ischemia.
6. Coronary artery narrowing is significant if the lumen diameter of the left main artery is reduced at least 50%, or if any major branch is reduced at least 75%.

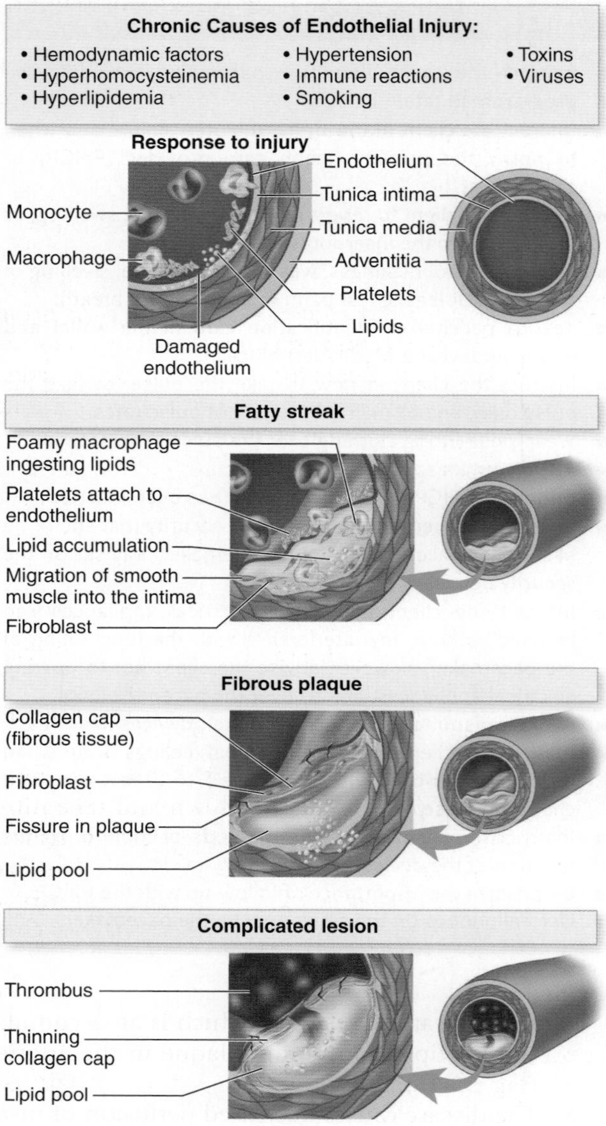

FIG. 52-11 Cross-sections of an atherosclerotic coronary artery.

7. The goal of treatment is to alter the atherosclerotic progression.

B. Assessment
1. Possibly normal findings during asymptomatic periods
2. Chest pain
3. Palpitations
4. Dyspnea
5. Syncope
6. Cough or hemoptysis
7. Excessive fatigue

C. Diagnostic studies
1. Electrocardiography
   a. When blood flow is reduced and ischemia occurs, ST-segment depression, T-wave inversion, or both is noted; the ST segment returns to normal when the blood flow returns.
   b. With infarction, cell injury results in ST-segment elevation, followed by T-wave inversion and an abnormal Q wave.
2. Cardiac catheterization: Cardiac catheterization shows the presence of atherosclerotic lesions.
3. Blood lipid levels
   a. Blood lipid levels may be elevated.
   b. Cholesterol-lowering medications may be prescribed to reduce the development of atherosclerotic plaques.

D. Interventions
1. Assist the client to identify risk factors that can be modified and to set goals to promote lifestyle changes to reduce the impact of risk factors.
2. Assist the client to identify barriers to adherence with the therapeutic plan and to identify methods to overcome barriers.
3. Instruct the client regarding a low-calorie, low-sodium, low-cholesterol, and low-fat diet, with an increase in dietary fiber.
4. Stress that dietary changes should be incorporated for the rest of the client's life; instruct the client regarding prescribed medications.
5. Provide community resources to the client regarding exercise, smoking cessation, and stress reduction as appropriate.

E. Surgical procedures
1. PTCA to compress the plaque against the walls of the artery and dilate the vessel
2. Laser angioplasty to vaporize the plaque
3. Atherectomy to remove the plaque from the artery
4. Vascular stent to prevent the artery from closing and to prevent restenosis
5. Coronary artery bypass grafting past the occluded artery to improve blood flow to the myocardial tissue at risk for ischemia or infarction

F. Medications
1. Nitrates to dilate the coronary arteries and decrease **preload** and **afterload**
2. Calcium channel blockers to dilate coronary arteries and reduce vasospasm
3. Cholesterol-lowering medications to reduce the development of atherosclerotic plaques
4. Beta blockers to reduce the BP in individuals who are hypertensive

VIII. Angina

A. Description
1. Angina is chest pain resulting from myocardial ischemia caused by inadequate myocardial blood and oxygen supply.
2. Angina is caused by an imbalance between oxygen supply and demand.
3. Causes include obstruction of coronary blood flow resulting from atherosclerosis, coronary artery spasm, or conditions increasing myocardial oxygen consumption.

The goal of treatment for angina is to provide relief from the acute attack, correct the imbalance between myocardial oxygen supply and demand, and prevent the progression of the disease and further attacks to reduce the risk of MI.

B. Patterns of angina
  1. Stable angina
    a. Also called exertional angina
    b. Occurs with activities that involve exertion or emotional stress; relieved with rest or nitroglycerin
    c. Usually has a stable pattern of onset, duration, severity, and relieving factors
  2. Unstable angina
    a. Also called preinfarction angina
    b. Associated with worsening cardiac ischemia
    c. Occurs with an unpredictable degree of exertion or emotion and increases in occurrence, duration, and severity over time
    d. Lasts longer than 15 minutes
    e. Pain may not be relieved with nitroglycerin.
  3. Variant angina
    a. Also called Prinzmetal's or vasospastic angina
    b. Results from coronary artery spasm
    c. May occur at rest
    d. Attacks may be associated with ST-segment elevation noted on the ECG.
  4. Intractable angina is a chronic, incapacitating angina unresponsive to interventions.

C. Assessment
  1. Pain
    a. Pain can develop slowly or quickly.
    b. Pain usually is described as mild or moderate.
    c. Substernal, crushing, squeezing pain may occur.
    d. Pain may radiate to the shoulders, arms, jaw, neck, or back.
    e. Pain intensity is unaffected by inspiration and expiration.
    f. Pain usually lasts less than 5 minutes; however, pain can last up to 15 to 20 minutes.
    g. Pain is relieved by nitroglycerin or rest.
  2. Dyspnea
  3. Pallor
  4. Sweating
  5. Palpitations and tachycardia
  6. Dizziness and syncope
  7. Hypertension
  8. Digestive disturbances

D. Diagnostic studies
  1. Electrocardiography: Readings are normal during rest, with ST depression or T-wave inversion during an episode of pain.
  2. Stress testing: Chest pain or changes in the ECG or vital signs during testing may indicate ischemia.
  3. Troponin and cardiac enzyme levels: Findings are normal in angina.
  4. Cardiac catheterization: Provides a definitive diagnosis by providing information about the patency of the coronary arteries.

E. Interventions
  1. Immediate management
    a. Assess pain; institute pain relief measures.
    b. Administer oxygen by nasal cannula as prescribed.
    c. Assess vital signs and provide continuous cardiac monitoring and nitroglycerin as prescribed to dilate the coronary arteries, reduce the oxygen requirements of the myocardium, and relieve the chest pain.
    d. Ensure that bed rest is maintained, place the client in semi-Fowler's position, and stay with the client.
    e. Obtain a 12-lead ECG.
    f. Establish an IV access route.
  2. Following the acute episode
    a. See section VII, D (Coronary Artery Disease, Interventions).
    b. Assist the client to identify angina-precipitating events.
    c. Instruct the client to stop activity and rest if chest pain occurs; sit down and take nitroglycerin as prescribed; the client is usually instructed to call emergency medical services if the nitroglycerin does not relieve the pain, and many PHCPs recommend that the client also chew an aspirin.

F. Surgical procedures: See section VII, E (Coronary Artery Disease, Surgical procedures).

G. Medications
  1. See section VII, F (Coronary Artery Disease, Medications).
  2. Antiplatelet therapy may be prescribed to inhibit platelet aggregation and reduce the risk of developing an acute MI.

IX. Myocardial Infarction

A. Description
  1. MI occurs when myocardial tissue is abruptly and severely deprived of oxygen.
  2. Ischemia can lead to necrosis of myocardial tissue if blood flow is not restored.
  3. Infarction does not occur instantly but evolves over several hours.
  4. Obvious physical changes do not occur in the heart until 6 hours after the infarction, when the infarcted area appears blue and swollen.
  5. After 48 hours, the infarct turns gray, with yellow streaks developing as neutrophils invade the tissue.
  6. By 8 to 10 days after infarction, granulation tissue forms.

7. Over 2 to 3 months, the necrotic area develops into a scar; scar tissue permanently changes the size and shape of the ventricle.
8. Not all clients experience the classic symptoms of an MI.
9. Women may experience atypical discomfort, shortness of breath, or fatigue and often present with non–ST-elevation myocardial infarction (NSTEMI) or T-wave inversion.
10. An older client may experience shortness of breath, pulmonary edema, dizziness, altered mental status, or a dysrhythmia.

B. Location of MI (see Fig. 52-1)
1. Obstruction of the LAD artery results in anterior wall or septal MI, or both.
2. Obstruction of the circumflex artery results in posterior wall MI or lateral wall MI.
3. Obstruction of the right coronary artery results in inferior wall MI.

C. Risk factors
1. Atherosclerosis
2. Coronary artery disease
3. Elevated cholesterol levels
4. Smoking
5. Hypertension
6. Obesity
7. Physical inactivity
8. Impaired glucose tolerance
9. Stress

D. Diagnostic studies
1. Troponin level: Level rises within 3 hours and remains elevated for up to 7 to 10 days.
2. Total CK level: Level rises within 6 hours after the onset of chest pain and peaks within 18 hours after damage and death of cardiac tissue.
3. CK-MB isoenzyme: Peak elevation occurs 18 hours after the onset of chest pain and returns to normal 48 to 72 hours later.
4. Myoglobin: Level rises within 2 hours after cell death, with a rapid decline in the level after 7 hours.
5. White blood cell count: An elevated white blood cell count appears on the second day following the MI and lasts up to 1 week.
6. Electrocardiogram
   a. ECG shows either ST segment elevation MI (STEMI), T-wave inversion, or NSTEMI; an abnormal Q wave may also present.
   b. Hours to days after the MI, ST- and T-wave changes will return to normal, but the Q-wave changes usually remain permanently.
7. Cardiac catheterization may be done emergently to determine the extent and location of obstructions of the coronary arteries; this allows for use of PTCA and restoration of bloodflow to the myocardium.
8. Diagnostic tests following the acute stage
   a. Exercise tolerance test or stress test to assess for electrocardiographic changes and ischemia and to evaluate for medical therapy or identify clients who may need invasive therapy.
   b. Thallium scans to assess for ischemia or necrotic muscle tissue.
   c. Multigated cardiac blood pool imaging scans may be used to evaluate left ventricular function.
   d. If not done urgently, cardiac catheterization to determine the coronary artery obstructions will be done after the client is stabilized.

E. Assessment
1. Pain
   a. Client may experience crushing substernal pain.
   b. Pain may radiate to the jaw, back, and left arm.
   c. Pain may occur without cause, primarily early in the morning.
   d. Pain is unrelieved by rest or nitroglycerin and is relieved only by opioids.
   e. Pain lasts 30 minutes or longer.
2. Nausea and vomiting
3. Diaphoresis
4. Dyspnea
5. Dysrhythmias
6. Feelings of fear and anxiety, impending doom
7. Pallor, cyanosis, coolness of extremities

F. Complications of MI (Box 52-6)

G. Interventions, acute stage

Pain relief increases oxygen supply to the myocardium; administer morphine as a priority in managing pain in the client having an MI.

1. Obtain a description of the chest discomfort.
2. Administer oxygen and institute pain relief measures (morphine, nitroglycerin as prescribed).
3. Assess vital signs and cardiovascular status and maintain cardiac monitoring.

BOX 52-6 Complications of Myocardial Infarction

- Dysrhythmias
- Heart failure
- Pulmonary edema
- Cardiogenic shock
- Thrombophlebitis
- Pericarditis
- Mitral valve insufficiency
- Postinfarction angina
- Ventricular rupture
- Dressler's syndrome (a combination of pericarditis, pericardial effusion, and pleural effusion, which can occur several weeks to months following a myocardial infarction)

4. Assess respiratory rate and breath sounds for signs of heart failure, as indicated by the presence of crackles or wheezes or dependent edema.
5. Ensure bed rest and place the client in a semi-Fowler's position to enhance comfort and tissue oxygenation; stay with the client.
6. Establish an IV access route.
7. Obtain a 12-lead ECG.
8. Monitor laboratory values.
9. Monitor for cardiac dysrhythmias, because tachycardia and PVCs frequently occur in the first few hours after MI; administer antidysrhythmics as prescribed.
10. Administer thrombolytic therapy, which may be prescribed within the first 6 hours of the coronary event if cardiac catheterization is not to be done emergently; monitor for signs of bleeding if the client is receiving thrombolytic therapy.
11. Assess distal peripheral pulses and skin temperature, because poor cardiac output may be identified by cool diaphoretic skin and diminished or absent pulses.
12. Monitor the BP closely after the administration of medications; if the **systolic pressure** is lower than 100 mm Hg or 25 mm Hg lower than the previous reading, lower the head of the bed and notify the PHCP.
13. Administer beta blockers as prescribed to slow the heart rate and increase myocardial perfusion while reducing the force of myocardial contraction.
14. Provide reassurance to the client and family.

H. Interventions following the acute episode
1. Maintain bed rest as prescribed.
2. Allow the client to stand to void or use a bedside commode if prescribed.
3. Provide range-of-motion exercises to prevent thrombus formation and maintain muscle strength.
4. Progress to dangling legs at the side of the bed or out of bed to the chair for 30 minutes 3 times a day as prescribed.
5. Progress to ambulation in the client's room and to the bathroom and then in the hallway 3 times a day.
6. Monitor for complications.
7. Administer angiotensin-converting enzyme (ACE) inhibitors, angiotensin-II receptor blockers (ARBs), calcium channel blockers, aspirin, thienopyridines (clopidogrel), and lipid-lowering agents as prescribed.
8. Encourage the client to verbalize feelings regarding the MI.

I. Cardiac rehabilitation: Process of actively assisting the client with cardiac disease to achieve and maintain a vital and productive life within the limitations of the heart disease; also refer to section VII, D (Coronary Artery Disease, Interventions).

X. Heart Failure

A. Description
1. Heart failure is the inability of the heart to maintain adequate cardiac output to meet the metabolic needs of the body because of impaired pumping ability.
2. Diminished cardiac output results in inadequate peripheral tissue perfusion.
3. Congestion of the lungs and periphery may occur; the client can develop acute pulmonary edema.

B. Classification
1. Acute heart failure occurs suddenly.
2. Chronic heart failure develops over time; however, a client with chronic heart failure can develop an acute episode.

C. Types of heart failure
1. Right ventricular failure, left ventricular failure
   a. Because the 2 ventricles of the heart represent 2 separate pumping systems, it is possible for 1 to fail alone for a short period.
   b. Most heart failure begins with left ventricular failure and progresses to failure of both ventricles.
   c. Acute pulmonary edema, a medical emergency, results from left ventricular failure.
   d. If pulmonary edema is not treated, death will occur from suffocation because the client literally drowns in her or his own fluids.
2. Forward failure, backward failure
   a. In forward failure, an inadequate output of the affected ventricle causes decreased perfusion to vital organs.
   b. In backward failure, blood backs up behind the affected ventricle, causing increased pressure in the atrium behind the affected ventricle.
3. Low output, high output
   a. In low-output failure, not enough cardiac output is available to meet the demands of the body.
   b. High-output failure occurs when a condition causes the heart to work harder to meet the demands of the body.
4. Systolic failure, diastolic failure
   a. Systolic failure, also known as heart failure with reduced ejection fraction (HFrEF), leads to problems with contraction and ejection of blood.
   b. Diastolic failure, also known as heart failure with preserved ejection fraction (HFpEF), leads to problems with the heart relaxing and filling with blood.

D. Compensatory mechanisms
1. Compensatory mechanisms act to restore cardiac output to near-normal levels.
2. Initially, these mechanisms increase cardiac output; however, they eventually have a damaging effect on pump action.

TABLE 52-1 Clinical Manifestations of Right-Sided and Left-Sided Heart Failure

Right-Sided Heart Failure	Left-Sided Heart Failure
Dependent edema (legs and sacrum)	Signs of pulmonary congestion
Jugular venous distention	Dyspnea
Abdominal distention	Tachypnea
Hepatomegaly	Crackles in the lungs
Splenomegaly	Dry, hacking cough
Anorexia and nausea	Paroxysmal nocturnal dyspnea
Weight gain	Increased BP (from fluid volume excess) or decreased BP (from pump failure)
Nocturnal diuresis	
Swelling of the fingers and hands	
Increased BP (from fluid volume excess) or decreased BP (from pump failure)	

BP, Blood pressure.

3. Compensatory mechanisms contribute to an increase in myocardial oxygen consumption; when this occurs, myocardial reserve is exhausted and clinical manifestations of heart failure develop.
4. Compensatory mechanisms include increased heart rate, improved **stroke volume**, arterial vasoconstriction, sodium and water retention, and myocardial hypertrophy.

E. Assessment (Table 52-1)
1. Right- and left-sided heart failure
2. Acute pulmonary edema
   a. Severe dyspnea
   b. Tachycardia, tachypnea
   c. Nasal flaring; use of accessory breathing muscles
   d. Wheezing and crackles on auscultation; gurgling respirations
   e. Expectoration of large amounts of blood-tinged, frothy sputum
   f. Acute anxiety, apprehension, restlessness
   g. Profuse sweating
   h. Cold, clammy skin
   i. Cyanosis

Signs of left ventricular failure are evident in the pulmonary system. Signs of right ventricular failure are evident in the systemic circulation.

F. Immediate management of acute episode (see Priority Nursing Actions)

PRIORITY NURSING ACTIONS

Pulmonary Edema

1. Place the client in a high-Fowler's position.
2. Administer oxygen.
3. Assess the client quickly, including assessing lung sounds.
4. Ensure that an intravenous (IV) access device is in place.
5. Prepare for the administration of a diuretic and morphine sulfate.
6. Insert a Foley catheter as prescribed.
7. Prepare for intubation and ventilator support, if required.
8. Document the event, actions taken, and the client's response.

G. Following the acute episode
1. Assist the client to identify precipitating risk factors of heart failure and methods of eliminating these risk factors.
2. Encourage the client to verbalize feelings about the lifestyle changes required as a result of the heart failure.
3. Instruct the client in the prescribed medication regimen, which may include digoxin, a diuretic, ACE inhibitors, low-dose beta blockers, and vasodilators.
4. Advise the client to notify the PHCP if side effects occur from the medications.
5. Advise the client to avoid over-the-counter medications.
6. Instruct the client to contact the PHCP if she or he is unable to take medications because of illness.
7. Instruct the client to avoid large amounts of caffeine, found in coffee, tea, cocoa, chocolate, and some carbonated beverages.
8. Instruct the client about the prescribed low-sodium, low-fat, and low-cholesterol diet.
9. Provide the client with a list of potassium-rich foods, because diuretics can cause hypokalemia (except for potassium-retaining diuretics).
10. Instruct the client regarding fluid restriction, if prescribed, advising the client to spread the fluid out during the day and to suck on hard candy to reduce thirst.
11. Instruct the client to balance periods of activity and rest.
12. Advise the client to avoid isometric activities, which increase pressure in the heart.
13. Instruct the client to monitor daily weight.
14. Instruct the client to report signs of fluid retention such as edema or weight gain.

XI. See Chapter 69 for a discussion on cardiogenic shock and associated invasive monitoring.

XII. Inflammatory Diseases of the Heart

A. Pericarditis
1. Description
a. Pericarditis is an acute or chronic inflammation of the pericardium.
b. Chronic pericarditis, a chronic inflammatory thickening of the pericardium, constricts the heart, causing compression.
c. The pericardial sac becomes inflamed.
d. Pericarditis can result in loss of pericardial elasticity or an accumulation of fluid within the sac.
e. Heart failure or cardiac tamponade may result.
2. Assessment
a. Pain in the anterior chest that radiates to the left side of the neck, shoulder, or back
b. Pain is grating and is aggravated by breathing (particularly inspiration), coughing, and swallowing
c. Pain is worse when in the supine position and may be relieved by leaning forward.
d. Pericardial friction rub (scratchy, high-pitched sound) is heard on auscultation and is produced by the rubbing of the inflamed pericardial layers.
e. Fever and chills
f. Fatigue and malaise
g. Elevated white blood cell count
h. Electrocardiographic changes with acute pericarditis; ST-segment elevation with the onset of inflammation; atrial fibrillation is common.
i. Signs of right ventricular failure in clients with chronic constrictive pericarditis
3. Interventions
a. Assess the nature of the pain.
b. Place the client in a high-Fowler's position, or upright and leaning forward.
c. Administer oxygen.
d. Administer analgesics, nonsteroidal anti-inflammatory drugs (NSAIDs), or corticosteroids for pain as prescribed.
e. Auscultate for a pericardial friction rub.
f. Check results of blood culture to identify the causative organism.
g. Administer antibiotics for bacterial infection as prescribed.
h. Administer diuretics and digoxin as prescribed to the client with chronic constrictive pericarditis; surgical incision of the pericardium (pericardial window) or pericardiectomy may be necessary.
i. Monitor for signs of cardiac tamponade.
j. Notify the PHCP if signs of cardiac tamponade occur.

B. Myocarditis
1. Description: Acute or chronic inflammation of the myocardium as a result of pericarditis, systemic infection, or allergic response
2. Assessment
a. Fever
b. Dyspnea
c. Tachycardia
d. Chest pain
e. Pericardial friction rub
f. Gallop rhythm
g. Murmur that sounds like fluid passing an obstruction
h. Pulsus alternans
i. Signs of heart failure
3. Interventions
a. Assist the client to a position of comfort, such as sitting up and leaning forward.
b. Administer oxygen as prescribed.
c. Administer analgesics, salicylates, and NSAIDs as prescribed to reduce fever and pain.
d. Administer digoxin as prescribed.
e. Administer antidysrhythmics as prescribed.
f. Administer antibiotics as prescribed to treat the causative organism.
g. Monitor for complications, which can include thrombus, heart failure, and cardiomyopathy.

C. Endocarditis
1. Description
a. Endocarditis is an inflammation of the inner lining of the heart and valves.
b. Occurs primarily in clients who are IV drug users, have had valve replacements or repair of valves with prosthetic materials, or have other structural cardiac defects
c. Ports of entry for the infecting organism include the oral cavity (especially if the client has had a dental procedure in the previous 3 to 6 months), infections (cutaneous, genitourinary, gastrointestinal, and systemic), and surgery or invasive procedures, including IV line placement.
2. Assessment
a. Fever
b. Anorexia, weight loss
c. Fatigue
d. Cardiac murmurs
e. Heart failure
f. Embolic complications from vegetation fragments traveling through the arterial circulation
g. Petechiae
h. Splinter hemorrhages in the nailbeds
i. Osler's nodes (reddish, tender lesions) on the pads of the fingers, hands, and toes
j. Janeway lesions (nontender hemorrhagic lesions) on the fingers, toes, nose, or earlobes

k. Splenomegaly
l. Clubbing of the fingers

3. Interventions
   a. Provide adequate rest balanced with activity to prevent thrombus formation.
   b. Monitor for signs of heart failure.
   c. Monitor for splenic emboli, as evidenced by sudden abdominal pain radiating to the left shoulder and the presence of rebound abdominal tenderness on palpation.
   d. Monitor for renal emboli, as evidenced by flank pain radiating to the groin, hematuria, and pyuria.
   e. Monitor for confusion, aphasia, or dysphasia, which may indicate central nervous system emboli.
   f. Monitor for pulmonary emboli as evidenced by pleuritic chest pain, dyspnea, and cough.
   g. Assess skin, mucous membranes, and conjunctiva for petechiae.
   h. Assess nailbeds for splinter hemorrhages.
   i. Assess for Osler's nodes on the pads of the fingers, hands, and toes.
   j. Assess for Janeway lesions on the fingers, toes, nose, or earlobes.
   k. Assess for clubbing of the fingers.
   l. Evaluate blood culture results.
   m. Administer antibiotics intravenously as prescribed.
   n. Plan and arrange for discharge, providing resources required for the continued administration of IV antibiotics.
4. Client education (Box 52-7)

BOX 52-7 Home Care Instructions for the Client with Infective Endocarditis

- Teach the client to maintain aseptic technique during setup and administration of intravenous (IV) antibiotics.
- Instruct the client to administer IV antibiotics at scheduled times to maintain the blood level.
- Instruct the client to monitor IV catheter sites for signs of infection and report this immediately to the primary health care provider (PHCP) or cardiologist.
- Instruct the client to record the temperature daily for up to 6 weeks and to report fever.
- Encourage oral hygiene at least twice a day with a soft toothbrush and rinse well with water after brushing.
- Client should avoid use of oral irrigation devices and flossing to avoid bacteremia.
- Teach the client to cleanse any skin lacerations thoroughly and apply an antibiotic ointment as prescribed.
- Client should inform all PHCPs of history of endocarditis and ask about the use of prophylactic antibiotics prior to invasive respiratory procedures and dentistry.
- Teach the client to observe for signs and symptoms of embolic conditions and heart failure.

XIII. Cardiac Tamponade

A. Description
1. A pericardial effusion occurs when the space between the parietal and visceral layers of the pericardium fills with fluid.
2. Pericardial effusion places the client at risk for cardiac tamponade, an accumulation of fluid in the pericardial cavity.
3. Tamponade restricts ventricular filling, and cardiac output drops.

⚠ Acute cardiac tamponade can occur when small volumes (20 to 50 mL) of fluid accumulate rapidly in the pericardium.

B. Assessment
1. Pulsus paradoxus
2. Increased CVP
3. Jugular venous distention with clear lungs
4. Distant, muffled heart sounds
5. Decreased cardiac output
6. Narrowing **pulse pressure**

C. Interventions
1. The client needs to be placed in a critical care unit for hemodynamic monitoring.
2. Administer fluids intravenously as prescribed to manage decreased cardiac output.
3. Prepare the client for chest x-ray or echocardiography.
4. Prepare the client for pericardiocentesis to withdraw pericardial fluid if prescribed.
5. Monitor for recurrence of tamponade following pericardiocentesis.
6. If the client experiences recurrent tamponade or recurrent effusions or develops adhesions from chronic pericarditis, a portion (pericardial window) or all of the pericardium (pericardiectomy) may be removed to allow adequate ventricular filling and contraction.

XIV. Valvular Heart Disease

A. Description
1. Valvular heart disease occurs when the heart valves cannot open fully (stenosis) or close completely (insufficiency or regurgitation).
2. Valvular heart disease prevents efficient blood flow through the heart.

B. Types
1. Mitral stenosis: Valvular tissue thickens and narrows the valve opening, preventing blood from flowing from the left atrium to the left ventricle.
2. Mitral insufficiency, regurgitation: Valve is incompetent, preventing complete valve closure during systole.
3. Mitral valve prolapse: Valve leaflets protrude into the left atrium during **systole**.

4. Aortic stenosis: Valvular tissue thickens and narrows the valve opening, preventing blood from flowing from the left ventricle into the aorta.
5. Aortic insufficiency: Valve is incompetent, preventing complete valve closure during diastole.
6. For aortic disorders, see Table 52-2.
7. For tricuspid disorders, see Table 52-3.
8. For pulmonary valve disorders, see Table 52-4.

TABLE 52-2 Aortic Valve Disorders

Aortic Stenosis	Aortic Insufficiency
Symptoms	
Dyspnea on exertion	Dyspnea
Angina	Angina
Syncope on exertion	Tachycardia
Fatigue	Fatigue
Orthopnea	Orthopnea
Paroxysmal nocturnal dyspnea	Paroxysmal nocturnal dyspnea
Harsh systolic crescendo-decrescendo murmur	Blowing decrescendo diastolic murmur
Interventions	
Refer to the section on repair procedures.	
Prepare the client for valve replacement as indicated.	

TABLE 52-3 Tricuspid Valve Disorders

Tricuspid Stenosis	Tricuspid Insufficiency
Symptoms	
Easily fatigued	Asymptomatic in mild situations
Effort intolerance	Signs of right ventricular failure, including ascites, hepatomegaly, peripheral edema
Reports fluttering sensations in the neck (obstructed venous flow)	Pleural effusion
Cyanosis	Systolic murmur heard at the left sternal border, fourth intercostal space
Signs of right ventricular failure, including ascites, hepatomegaly, peripheral edema, jugular vein distention with clear lung fields	
Symptoms of decreased cardiac output	
Rumbling diastolic murmur	
Interventions	
Refer to the section on repair procedures.	
Prepare the client for valve replacement as indicated.	

TABLE 52-4 Pulmonary Valve Disorders

Pulmonary Stenosis	Pulmonary Insufficiency
Symptoms	
Asymptomatic in a mild condition	Asymptomatic in mild condition
Dyspnea	Dyspnea
Fatigue	Fatigue
Syncope	Syncope
Signs of right ventricular failure, including ascites, hepatomegaly, peripheral edema	Signs of right ventricular failure, including ascites, hepatomegaly, peripheral edema
Systolic thrill heard at left sternal border	Systolic thrill heard at left sternal border
Interventions	
Refer to the section on repair procedures.	Refer to the section on repair procedures.
Prepare the client for pulmonary valve commissurotomy as indicated.	Prepare the client for pulmonary valve replacement as indicated.

C. Repair procedures
1. Percutaneous balloon valvuloplasty
   a. A balloon catheter is passed from the femoral vein through the atrial septum to the mitral valve or through the femoral artery to the aortic valve.
   b. The balloon is inflated to enlarge the orifice.
   c. Monitor for bleeding from the catheter insertion site.
   d. Institute precautions for arterial puncture if appropriate; site care and monitoring is similar to that after cardiac catheterization.
   e. Monitor for signs of systemic emboli.
   f. Monitor for signs of a regurgitant valve by monitoring cardiac rhythm, heart sounds, and cardiac output.
2. Mitral annuloplasty: Tightening and suturing the malfunctioning valve annulus to eliminate or greatly reduce regurgitation; percutaneous or open surgical approach.
3. Commissurotomy, valvotomy
   a. Thrombi are removed and calcium deposits are debrided; the valve is incised and widened.
   b. Percutaneous route or open heart surgical approach.

D. Valve replacement procedures
1. Mechanical prosthetic valves: These prosthetic valves are durable
2. Risk of clot formation is high as the body reacts to the artificial materials; anticoagulation is required.

⚠ Thromboembolism can be a problem following valve replacement with a mechanical prosthetic valve, and lifetime anticoagulant therapy is required.

3. Bioprosthetic valves
   a. Biological grafts are xenografts (valves from other species)—porcine valves (pig), bovine valves (cow), or homografts (human cadavers). These valves are less durable than mechanical prosthetic valves.
   b. The risk of clot formation is small; therefore, long-term anticoagulation may not be indicated.
4. Open heart surgical approach.
5. Preoperative interventions: Consult with the PHCP regarding discontinuing anticoagulants 72 hours before surgery.
6. Postoperative interventions
   a. Monitor closely for signs of bleeding.
   b. Monitor cardiac output and for signs of heart failure.
   c. Administer digoxin as prescribed to maintain cardiac output and prevent atrial fibrillation.
   d. Client education (Box 52-8).

XV. Cardiomyopathy (Table 52-5)

A. Description
   1. Cardiomyopathy is a subacute or chronic disorder of the heart muscle.
   2. Treatment is palliative, not curative, and the client needs to deal with numerous lifestyle changes and a shortened life span.

B. Types, signs and symptoms, and treatment (see Table 52-5)

XVI. Vascular Disorders

A. Venous thrombosis
   1. Description
      a. Thrombus can be associated with an inflammatory process.
      b. When a thrombus develops, inflammation occurs, thickening the vein wall and leading to embolization.
   2. Types
      a. Thrombophlebitis: Thrombus associated with vein inflammation
      b. Phlebothrombosis: Thrombus without vein inflammation
      c. Phlebitis: Vein inflammation associated with invasive procedures, such as IV lines
      d. Deep vein thrombophlebitis: More serious than a superficial thrombophlebitis because of the risk for pulmonary embolism
   3. Risk factors for thrombus formation
      a. Venous stasis from varicose veins, heart failure, immobility
      b. Hypercoagulability disorders
      c. Injury to the venous wall from IV injections; administration of vessel irritants (chemotherapy, hypertonic solutions)
      d. Following surgery, particularly orthopedic and abdominal surgery
      e. Pregnancy
      f. Ulcerative colitis
      g. Use of oral contraceptives
      h. Certain malignancies
      i. Fractures or other injuries of the pelvis or lower extremities

B. Phlebitis
   1. Assessment
      a. Red, warm area radiating up the vein and extremity
      b. Pain
      c. Swelling
   2. Interventions
      a. Apply warm, moist soaks as prescribed to dilate the vein and promote circulation (assess temperature of soak before applying).
      b. Assess for signs of complications such as tissue necrosis, infection, or pulmonary embolus.

C. Deep vein thrombophlebitis
   1. Assessment
      a. Calf or groin tenderness or pain with or without swelling

BOX 52-8 Client Instructions Following Valve Replacement

- Adequate rest is important, and fatigue is common.
- Anticoagulant therapy is necessary if a mechanical prosthetic valve has been inserted.
- Instruct the client concerning hazards related to anticoagulant therapy and to notify the primary health care provider (PHCP) or cardiologist if bleeding or excessive bruising occurs.
- Instruct the client concerning the importance of good oral hygiene to reduce the risk of infective endocarditis.
- Brush teeth twice daily with a soft toothbrush, followed by oral rinses.
- Avoid irrigation devices, electric toothbrushes, and flossing, because these activities can cause the gums to bleed, allowing bacteria to enter the mucous membranes and bloodstream.
- Monitor incision and report any drainage or redness.
- Avoid any dental procedures for 6 months.
- Heavy lifting (more than 10 lb [4.5 kg]) is to be avoided, and exercise caution when in an automobile to prevent injury to the sternal incision.
- If a prosthetic valve was inserted, a soft, audible, clicking sound may be heard.
- Instruct the client concerning the importance of prophylactic antibiotics before any invasive procedure and the importance of informing all PHCPs of history of valve replacement or repair.
- Obtain and wear a MedicAlert bracelet.

TABLE 52-5 Pathophysiology, Signs and Symptoms, and Treatment of Cardiomyopathies

	Hypertrophic Cardiomyopathy		
Dilated Cardiomyopathy	**Nonobstructed**	**Obstructed**	**Restrictive Cardiomyopathy**
Pathophysiology			
• Fibrosis of myocardium and endocardium • Dilated chambers • Mural wall thrombi prevalent	• Hypertrophy of the walls • Hypertrophied septum • Relatively small chamber size	• Same as for nonobstructed except for obstruction of left ventricular outflow tract associated with the hypertrophied septum and mitral valve incompetence	• Mimics constrictive pericarditis • Fibrosed walls cannot expandor contract • Chambers narrowed; emboli Common
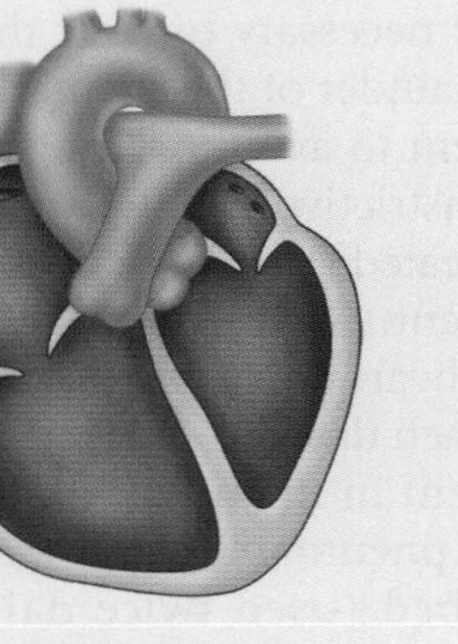	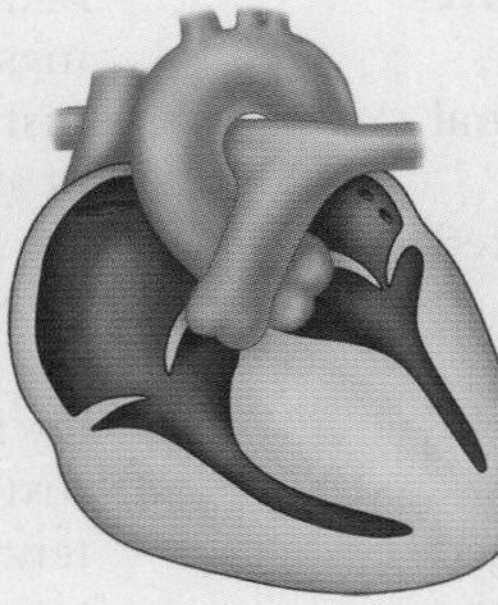		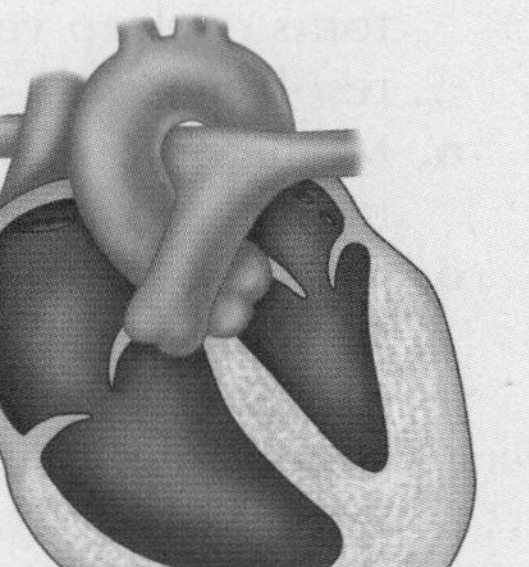
Signs and Symptoms			
• Fatigue and weakness • Heart failure (left side) • Dysrhythmias or heart block • Systemic or pulmonary emboli • S_3 and S_4 gallops • Moderate to severe cardiomegaly	• Dyspnea • Angina • Fatigue, syncope, palpitations • Mild cardiomegaly • S_4 gallop • Ventricular dysrhythmias • Sudden death common • Heart failure	• Same as for nonobstructed except with mitral regurgitation murmur • Atrial fibrillation	• Dyspnea and fatigue • Heart failure (right side) • Mild to moderate cardiomegaly • S_3 and S_4 gallops • Heart block • Emboli
Treatment			
• Symptomatic treatment of heart failure • Vasodilators • Control of dysrhythmias • Surgery: Heart transplant	For both nonobstructed and obstructed: • Symptomatic treatment • Beta blockers • Conversion of atrial fibrillation • Surgery: Ventriculomyotomy or muscle resection with mitralvalve replacement • Digoxin, nitrates, and other vasodilators contraindicated with the obstructed form		• Supportive treatment of symptoms • Treatment of hypertension • Conversion from dysrhythmias • Exercise restrictions • Emergency treatment of acute pulmonary edema

Adapted from Ignatavicius D, Workman ML: *Medical-surgical nursing: patient-centered collaborative care*, ed 7, Philadelphia, 2013, Saunders.

   b. Positive Homans' sign may be noted; however, false-positive results are common, so this is not a reliable assessment measure.
   c. Warm skin that is tender to touch

2. Interventions
   a. Provide bed rest as prescribed.
   b. Elevate the affected extremity above the level of the heart as prescribed.
   c. Avoid using the knee gatch or a pillow under the knees.
   d. Do not massage the extremity.
   e. Provide thigh-high or knee-high antiembolism stockings as prescribed to reduce venous stasis and assist in the venous return of blood to the heart; teach how to apply and remove stockings.
   f. Administer intermittent or continuous warm, moist compresses as prescribed.
   g. Palpate the site gently, monitoring for warmth and edema.
   h. Measure and record the circumferences of the thighs and calves.

i. Monitor for shortness of breath and chest pain, which can indicate pulmonary emboli.
j. Administer thrombolytic therapy (tissue plasminogen activator) if prescribed, which must be initiated within 5 days after the onset of symptoms.
k. Administer heparin therapy as prescribed to prevent enlargement of the existing clot and prevent the formation of new clots.
l. Monitor activated partial thromboplastin time during heparin therapy.
m. Administer warfarin as prescribed following heparin therapy when the symptoms of deep vein thrombophlebitis have resolved.
n. Monitor prothrombin time and international normalized ratio during warfarin therapy.
o. Monitor for the adverse effects associated with anticoagulant therapy.
p. Client education (Box 52-9)

D. Venous insufficiency
1. Description
a. Venous insufficiency results from prolonged venous hypertension, which stretches the veins and damages the valves.
b. The resultant edema and venous stasis cause venous stasis ulcers, swelling, and cellulitis.
c. Treatment focuses on decreasing edema and promoting venous return from the affected extremity.
d. Treatment for venous stasis ulcers focuses on healing the ulcer and preventing stasis and ulcer recurrence.
2. Assessment
a. Stasis dermatitis or brown discoloration along the ankles, extending up to the calf

BOX 52-9 Instructions for the Client with Deep Vein Thrombophlebitis

- Instruct the client concerning the hazards of anticoagulation therapy.
- Recognize the signs and symptoms of bleeding.
- Avoid prolonged sitting or standing, constrictive clothing, or crossing the legs when seated.
- Elevate the legs for 10 to 20 minutes every few hours each day.
- Plan a progressive walking program.
- Inspect the legs for edema, and measure the circumference of the legs.
- Wear antiembolism stockings as prescribed.
- Avoid smoking.
- Avoid any medications unless prescribed by the primary health care provider (PHCP) or cardiologist.
- Instruct the client concerning the importance of follow-up PHCP visits and laboratory studies.
- Obtain and wear a MedicAlert bracelet.

b. Edema
c. Ulcer formation: Edges are uneven, ulcer bed is pink, and granulation is present; usually located on the lateral malleolus.
3. Interventions

For venous insufficiency, leg elevation is usually prescribed to assist with the return of blood to the heart.

a. Instruct the client to wear elastic or compression stockings during the day and evening if prescribed (instruct the client to put on elastic stockings on awakening, before getting out of bed); it may be necessary to wear the stockings for the remainder of the client's life.
b. Instruct the client to avoid prolonged sitting or standing, constrictive clothing, or crossing the legs when seated.
c. Instruct the client to elevate the legs above the level of the heart for 10 to 20 minutes every few hours each day.
d. Instruct the client in the use of an intermittent sequential pneumatic compression system, if prescribed (used twice daily for 1 hour in the morning and evening).
e. Advise the client with an open ulcer that the compression system is applied over a dressing.
4. Wound care
a. Provide care to the wound as prescribed.
b. Assess the client's ability to care for the wound, and initiate home care resources as necessary.
c. If an Unna boot (dressing constructed of gauze moistened with zinc oxide) is prescribed, the PHCP will change it weekly.
d. The wound is cleansed with normal saline before application of the Unna boot; povidone-iodine and hydrogen peroxide are not used, because they destroy granulation tissue.
e. The Unna boot is covered with an elastic wrap that hardens to promote venous return and prevent stasis.
f. Monitor for signs of arterial occlusion from an Unna boot that may be too tight.
g. Keep tape off the client's skin.
h. Occlusive dressings such as polyethylene film or a hydrocolloid dressing may be used to cover the ulcer.
5. Medications
a. Apply topical agents to the wound as prescribed to debride the ulcer, eliminate necrotic tissue, and promote healing.
b. When applying topical debriding agents, apply an oil-based agent such as petroleum jelly on surrounding skin to protect healthy tissue.

c. Administer antibiotics as prescribed if infection or cellulitis occurs.

E. Varicose veins
1. Description
a. Distended, protruding veins that appear darkened and tortuous.
b. Vein walls weaken and dilate, and valves become incompetent.
2. Assessment
a. Pain in the legs with dull aching after standing
b. A feeling of fullness in the legs
c. Ankle edema
3. Trendelenburg's test
a. Place the client in a supine position with the legs elevated.
b. When the client sits up, if varicosities are present, veins fill from the proximal end; veins normally fill from the distal end.
4. Interventions
a. Emphasize the importance of antiembolism stockings as prescribed.
b. Instruct the client to elevate the legs as much as possible.
c. Instruct the client to avoid constrictive clothing and pressure on the legs.
d. Prepare the client for sclerotherapy or vein stripping as prescribed.
5. Sclerotherapy
a. A solution is injected into the vein, followed by the application of a pressure dressing.
b. Incision and drainage of the trapped blood in the sclerosed vein is performed 14 to 21 days after the injection, followed by the application of a pressure dressing for 12 to 18 hours.
6. Laser therapy: A laser fiber is used to heat and close the main vessel contributing to the varicosity.
7. Vein stripping: Varicose veins may be removed if they are larger than 4 mm in diameter or if they are in clusters; other treatments are usually tried before vein stripping.

XVII. Arterial Disorders

A. Peripheral arterial disease
1. Description
a. Chronic disorder in which partial or total arterial occlusion deprives the lower extremities of oxygen and nutrients
b. Tissue damage occurs below the level of the arterial occlusion.
c. Atherosclerosis is the most common cause of peripheral arterial disease.
2. Assessment
a. Intermittent claudication (pain in the muscles resulting from an inadequate blood supply)
b. Rest pain, characterized by numbness, burning, or aching in the distal portion of the lower extremities, which awakens the client at night and is relieved by placing the extremity in a dependent position
c. Lower back or buttock discomfort
d. Loss of hair and dry scaly skin on the lower extremities
e. Thickened toenails
f. Cold and gray-blue color of skin in the lower extremities
g. Elevational pallor and dependent rubor in the lower extremities
h. Decreased or absent peripheral pulses
i. Signs of arterial ulcer formation occurring on or between the toes or on the upper aspect of the foot that are characterized as painful
j. BP measurements at the thigh, calf, and ankle are lower than the brachial pressure (normally, BP readings in the thigh and calf are higher than those in the upper extremities).
3. Interventions

Because swelling in the extremities prevents arterial blood flow, the client with peripheral arterial disease is instructed to elevate the feet at rest but to refrain from elevating them above the level of the heart, because extreme elevation slows arterial blood flow to the feet. In severe cases of peripheral arterial disease, clients with edema may sleep with the affected limb hanging from the bed, or they may sit upright (without leg elevation) in a chair for comfort.

a. Assess pain.
b. Monitor the extremities for color, motion and sensation, and pulses.
c. Obtain BP measurements.
d. Assess for signs of ulcer formation or signs of gangrene.
e. Assist in developing an individualized exercise program, which is initiated gradually and increased slowly to improve arterial flow through the development of collateral circulation.
f. Instruct the client to walk to the point of claudication pain, stop and rest, and then walk a little farther.
g. Instruct the client with peripheral arterial disease to avoid crossing the legs, which interferes with blood flow.
h. Instruct the client to avoid exposure to cold (causes vasoconstriction) to the extremities and to wear socks or insulated shoes for warmth at all times.
i. Instruct the client never to apply direct heat to the limb, such as with a heating pad or hot water, because the decreased sensitivity in the limb can cause burning.

j. Instruct the client to inspect the skin on the extremities daily and to report any signs of skin breakdown.
k. Instruct the client to avoid tobacco and caffeine because of their vasoconstrictive effects.
l. Instruct the client in the use of hemorheological and antiplatelet medications as prescribed.

4. Procedures to improve arterial blood flow
a. Percutaneous transluminal angioplasty, with or without intravascular stent
b. Laser-assisted angioplasty
c. Atherectomy
d. Peripheral arterial bypass surgery: Graft material is sutured above and below the occlusion to facilitate blood flow around the occlusion. Inflow procedures bypass the occlusion above the superficial femoral arteries and include aortoiliac, aortofemoral, and axillofemoral bypasses; outflow procedures bypass the occlusion at or below the superficial femoral arteries and include femoropopliteal and femorotibial bypass (Fig. 52-12).

5. Preoperative interventions
a. Assess baseline vital signs and peripheral pulses.
b. Insert an IV line and urinary catheter as prescribed.
c. Maintain a central venous catheter and/or arterial line if inserted.

6. Postoperative interventions
a. Assess vital signs and notify the PHCP if changes occur.
b. Monitor for hypotension, which may indicate hypovolemia

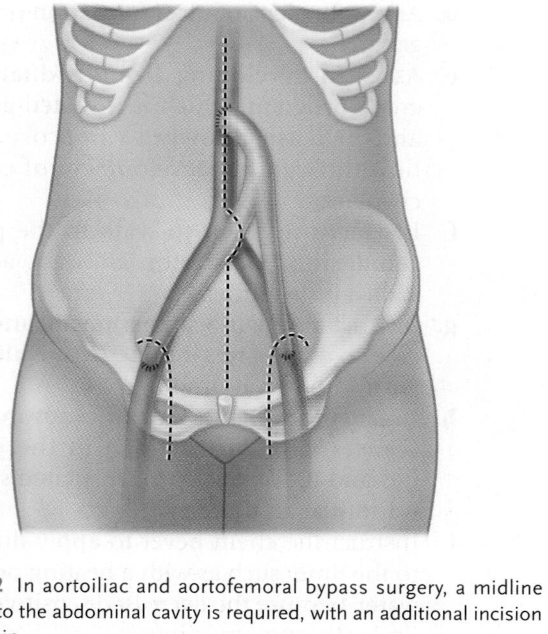

FIG. 52-12 In aortoiliac and aortofemoral bypass surgery, a midline incision into the abdominal cavity is required, with an additional incision in each groin.

c. Monitor for hypertension, which may place stress on the graft and cause clot formation.
d. Maintain bed rest for 24 hours as prescribed.
e. Instruct the client to keep the affected extremity straight, limit movement, and avoid bending the knee and hip.
f. Monitor for warmth, redness, and edema, which often are expected outcomes because of increased blood flow.
g. Monitor for vessel or graft occlusion, which often occurs within the first 24 hours.
h. Assess peripheral pulses and for adverse changes in color and temperature of the extremity.
i. Assess the incision for drainage, warmth, or swelling.
j. Monitor for excessive bleeding (a small amount of bloody drainage is expected).
k. Monitor the area over the graft for hardness, tenderness, and warmth, which may indicate infection; if this occurs, notify the PHCP immediately.
l. Instruct the client about proper foot care and measures to prevent ulcer formation.
m. Assist the client in modifying lifestyle to prevent further plaque formation.
n. Following arterial revascularization, monitor for a sharp increase in pain, because pain is frequently the first indicator of postoperative graft occlusion. If signs of graft occlusion occur, notify the PHCP immediately.

B. Raynaud's disease

1. Description
a. Raynaud's disease is vasospasm of the arterioles and arteries of the upper and lower extremities.
b. Vasospasm causes constriction of the cutaneous vessels.
c. Attacks occur with exposure to cold or stress.
d. Affects primarily fingers, toes, ears, and cheeks

2. Assessment
a. Blanching of the extremity, followed by cyanosis from vasoconstriction
b. Reddened tissue when the vasospasm is relieved
c. Numbness, tingling, swelling, and a cold temperature at the affected body part

3. Interventions
a. Monitor pulses.
b. Administer vasodilators as prescribed.
c. Instruct the client regarding medication therapy.
d. Assist the client to identify and avoid precipitating factors such as cold and stress.
e. Instruct the client to avoid smoking.

f. Instruct the client to wear warm clothing, socks, and gloves in cold weather.
g. Advise the client to avoid injuries to fingers and hands.

C. Buerger's disease (thromboangiitis obliterans)
1. Description
a. Buerger's disease is an occlusive disease of the median and small arteries and veins.
b. The distal upper and lower limbs are affected most commonly.
2. Assessment
a. Intermittent claudication
b. Ischemic pain occurring in the digits while at rest
c. Aching pain that is more severe at night
d. Cool, numb, or tingling sensation
e. Diminished pulses in the distal extremities
f. Extremities that are cool and red in the dependent position
g. Development of ulcerations in the extremities
3. Interventions: See Raynaud's disease

XVIII. Aortic Aneurysms

A. Description
1. An aortic aneurysm is an abnormal dilation of the arterial wall caused by localized weakness and stretching in the medial layer or wall of the aorta.
2. The aneurysm can be located anywhere along the abdominal aorta.
3. The goal of treatment is to limit the progression of the disease by modifying risk factors, controlling the BP to prevent strain on the aneurysm, recognizing symptoms early, and preventing rupture.

B. Types of aortic aneurysm
1. Fusiform: Diffuse dilation that involves the entire circumference of the arterial segment
2. Saccular: Distinct localized outpouching of the artery wall
3. Dissecting: Created when blood separates the layers of the artery wall, forming a cavity between them
4. False (pseudoaneurysm): Occurs when the clot and connective tissue are outside the arterial wall as a result of vessel injury or trauma to all 3 layers of the arterial wall.

C. Assessment
1. Thoracic aneurysm
a. Pain extending to neck, shoulders, lower back, or abdomen
b. Syncope
c. Dyspnea
d. Increased pulse
e. Cyanosis
f. Hoarseness, difficulty swallowing because of pressure from the aneurysm
2. Abdominal aneurysm
a. Prominent, pulsating mass in abdomen, at or above the umbilicus
b. Systolic bruit over the aorta
c. Tenderness on deep palpation
d. Abdominal or lower back pain
3. Rupturing aneurysm
a. Severe abdominal or back pain
b. Lumbar pain radiating to the flank and groin
c. Hypotension
d. Increased pulse rate
e. Signs of shock
f. Hematoma at flank area
4. Diagnostic tests
a. Diagnostic tests are done to confirm the presence, size, and location of the aneurysm.
b. Tests include abdominal ultrasound, computed tomography scan, and arteriography.
5. Interventions
a. Monitor vital signs.
b. Obtain information regarding back or abdominal pain.
c. Question the client regarding the sensation of pulsation in the abdomen.
d. Check peripheral circulation, including pulses, temperature, and color.
e. Observe for signs of rupture.
f. Note any tenderness over the abdomen.
g. Monitor for abdominal distention.
6. Nonsurgical interventions
a. Modify risk factors.
b. Instruct the client regarding the procedure for monitoring BP.
c. Instruct the client on the importance of regular PHCP visits to follow the size of the aneurysm.
d. Instruct the client that if severe back or abdominal pain or fullness, soreness over the umbilicus, sudden development of discoloration in the extremities, or a persistent elevation of BP occurs, to notify the PHCP immediately.

Instruct the client with an aortic aneurysm to report immediately the occurrence of chest or back pain, shortness of breath, difficulty swallowing, or hoarseness.

D. Pharmacological interventions
1. Administer antihypertensives to maintain the BP within normal limits and to prevent strain on the aneurysm.
2. Instruct the client about the purpose of the medications.
3. Instruct the client about the side effects and schedule of the medication.

E. Abdominal aortic aneurysm resection
1. Description: Surgical resection or excision of the aneurysm; the excised section is replaced with a graft that is sewn end to end (Fig. 52-13).

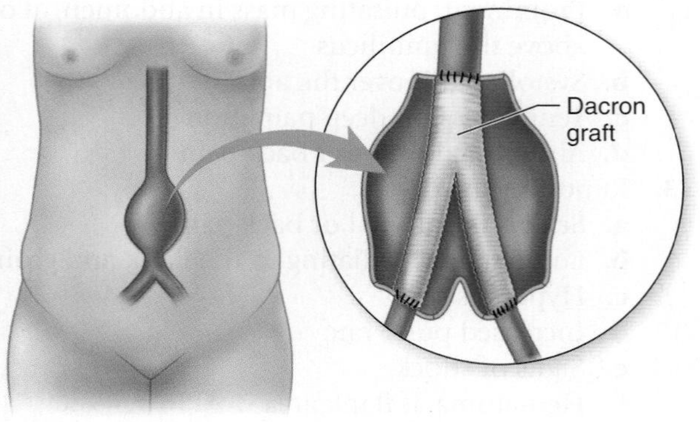

FIG. 52-13 Surgical repair of an abdominal aortic aneurysm with a woven Dacron graft.

2. Preoperative interventions
   a. Assess all peripheral pulses as a baseline for postoperative comparison.
   b. Instruct the client in coughing and deep-breathing exercises.
3. Postoperative interventions
   a. Monitor vital signs.
   b. Monitor peripheral pulses distal to the graft site.
   c. Monitor for signs of graft occlusion, including changes in pulses, cool to cold extremities below the graft, white or blue extremities or flanks, severe pain, or abdominal distention.
   d. Limit elevation of the head of the bed to 45 degrees to prevent flexion of the graft.
   e. Monitor for hypovolemia and kidney failure resulting from significant blood loss during surgery.
   f. Monitor urine output hourly, and notify the PHCP if it is lower than 30 to 50 mL/hr.
   g. Monitor serum creatinine and blood urea nitrogen levels daily.
   h. Monitor respiratory status and auscultate breath sounds to identify respiratory complications.
   i. Encourage turning, coughing and deep breathing, and splinting the incision.
   j. Ambulate as prescribed.
   k. Prepare the client for discharge by providing instructions regarding pain management, wound care, and activity restrictions.
   l. Instruct the client not to lift objects heavier than 15 to 20 lb for 6 to 12 weeks.
   m. Advise the client to avoid activities requiring pushing, pulling, or straining.
   n. Instruct the client not to drive a vehicle until approved by the PHCP.
   o. Endovascular aneurysm grafting involves insertion of a graft using a vascular catheter; it does not require an abdominal incision. The preoperative and postoperative care is similar to that of a surgical abdominal aneurysm repair.

F. Thoracic aneurysm repair
1. Description
   a. A thoracotomy or median sternotomy approach is used to enter the thoracic cavity.
   b. The aneurysm is exposed and excised, and a graft or prosthesis is sewn onto the aorta.
   c. Total cardiopulmonary bypass is necessary for excision of aneurysms in the ascending aorta.
   d. Partial cardiopulmonary bypass is used for clients with an aneurysm in the descending aorta.
2. Postoperative interventions
   a. Monitor vital signs and neurological and renal status.
   b. Monitor for signs of hemorrhage, such as a drop in BP and increased pulse rate and respirations, and report them to the PHCP immediately.
   c. Monitor chest tubes for an increase in chest drainage, which may indicate bleeding or separation at the graft site.
   d. Assess sensation and motion of all extremities and notify the PHCP if deficits are noted, which can occur because of a lack of blood supply to the spinal cord during surgery.
   e. Monitor respiratory status and auscultate breath sounds to identify respiratory complications.
   f. Encourage turning, coughing, and deep breathing while splinting the incision.
   g. Prepare the client for discharge by providing instructions regarding pain management, wound care, and activity restrictions.
   h. Instruct the client not to lift objects heavier than 15 to 20 lb for 6 to 12 weeks.
   i. Advise the client to avoid activities requiring pushing, pulling, or straining.
   j. Instruct the client not to drive a vehicle until approved by the PHCP.

XIX. Embolectomy

A. Description
1. Embolectomy is removal of an embolus from an artery, using a catheter.
2. A patch graft may be required to close the artery.

B. Preoperative interventions
1. Obtain a baseline vascular assessment.
2. Administer anticoagulants as prescribed.
3. Administer thrombolytics as prescribed.
4. Place a bed cradle on the bed to keep the weight of linens from causing pain and pressure.
5. Avoid bumping or jarring the bed.

6. Maintain the extremity in a slightly dependent position.

C. Postoperative interventions
1. Assess cardiac, respiratory, and neurological status.
2. Monitor affected extremity for color, temperature, and pulse.
3. Assess sensory and motor function of the affected extremity.
4. Monitor for signs and symptoms of new thrombi or emboli.
5. Administer oxygen as prescribed.
6. Monitor pulse oximetry.
7. Monitor for complications caused by reperfusion of the artery, such as spasms and swelling of the skeletal muscles.
8. Monitor for signs of swollen skeletal muscles such as edema, pain on passive movement, poor capillary refill, numbness, and muscle tenseness.
9. Maintain bed rest initially, with the client in a semi-Fowler's position.
10. Place a bed cradle on the bed.
11. Check the incision site for bleeding or hematoma.
12. Administer anticoagulants as prescribed.
13. Monitor laboratory values related to anticoagulant therapy.
14. Instruct the client to recognize the signs and symptoms of infection and edema.
15. Instruct the client to avoid prolonged sitting or crossing the legs when sitting.
16. Instruct the client to elevate the legs when sitting.
17. Instruct the client to wear antiembolism stockings as prescribed and how to remove and reapply the stockings.
18. Instruct the client to ambulate daily.
19. Instruct the client about anticoagulant therapy and the hazards associated with anticoagulants.

XX. Vena Cava Filter

A. Vena cava filter: Insertion of an intracaval filter (umbrella) that partially occludes the inferior vena cava and traps emboli to prevent pulmonary emboli (Fig. 52-14)

B. The filter is placed through a catheter placed in a large vein in the neck or groin and advanced to the inferior vena cava.

C. Preoperative interventions: If the client has been taking an anticoagulant, consult with the PHCP regarding discontinuation of the medication preoperatively to prevent hemorrhage.

D. Postoperative interventions: similar to care after embolectomy.

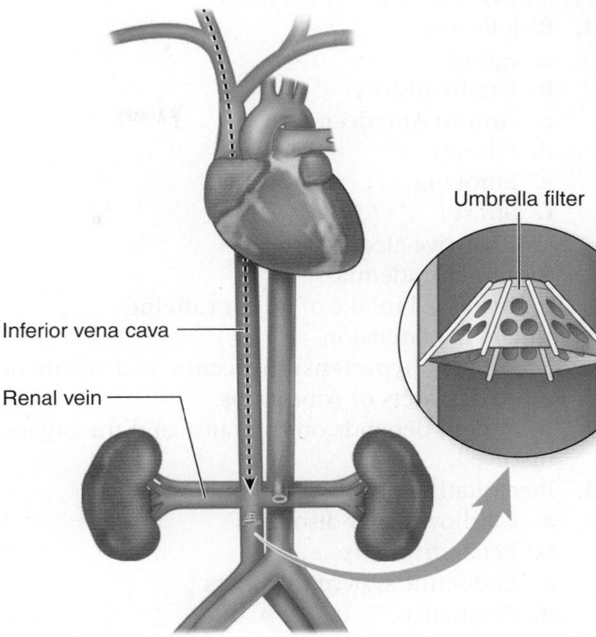

FIG. 52-14 An inferior vena cava filter.

XXI. Hypertension

A. Description
1. For an adult (ages 18 years and older), a normal BP is a systolic BP below 120 mm Hg and a diastolic pressure below 80 mm Hg.
2. Elevated blood pressure is defined as a systolic BP between 120 and 129 mm Hg and a diastolic BP below 80 mm Hg.
3. Hypertension (Stage 1) is defined as an SBP between 130 and 139 mm Hg or a diastolic BP between 80 and 89 mm Hg.
4. Hypertension (Stage 2) is defined as a SBP at least 140 mm Hg or a diastolic BP at least 90 mm Hg.
5. If either the SBP or DBP is outside of a range, the higher measurement will determine the classification.
6. Hypertension is a major risk factor for coronary, cerebral, renal, and peripheral vascular disease.
7. The disease is initially asymptomatic.
8. The goals of treatment include reduction of the BP and preventing or lessening the extent of organ damage.
9. Nonpharmacological approaches, such as lifestyle changes, may be prescribed initially; if the BP cannot be decreased after 1 to 3 months, the client may require pharmacological treatment.

B. Primary or essential hypertension
1. Risk factors
   a. Aging
   b. Family history
   c. African American race
   d. Obesity
   e. Smoking
   f. Stress
   g. Excessive alcohol
   h. Hyperlipidemia
   i. Increased intake of salt or caffeine

C. Secondary hypertension
1. Secondary hypertension occurs as a result of other disorders or conditions.
2. Treatment depends on the cause and the organs involved.
3. Precipitating disorders or conditions
   a. Cardiovascular disorders
   b. Renal disorders
   c. Endocrine system disorders
   d. Pregnancy
   e. Medications (e.g., estrogens, glucocorticoids, mineralocorticoids)

D. Assessment
1. May be asymptomatic
2. Headache
3. Visual disturbances
4. Dizziness
5. Chest pain
6. Tinnitus
7. Flushed face
8. Epistaxis

E. Interventions
1. Goals: To reduce the BP and to prevent or lessen the extent of organ damage
2. Question the client regarding the signs and symptoms of hypertension.
3. Obtain the BP 2 or more times on both arms, with the client supine and standing.
4. Compare the BP with prior documentation.
5. Determine family history of hypertension.
6. Identify current medication therapy.
7. Obtain weight.
8. Evaluate dietary patterns and sodium intake.
9. Assess for visual changes or retinal damage.
10. Assess for cardiovascular changes such as distended neck veins, increased heart rate, and dysrhythmias.
11. Evaluate chest x-ray for heart enlargement.
12. Assess the neurological system.
13. Evaluate renal function.
14. Evaluate results of diagnostic and laboratory studies.

F. Nonpharmacological interventions
1. Weight reduction, if necessary, or maintenance of ideal weight
2. Dietary sodium restriction to 2 g daily as prescribed
3. Moderate intake of alcohol and caffeine-containing products
4. Initiation of a regular exercise program
5. Avoidance of smoking
6. Relaxation techniques and biofeedback therapy
7. Elimination of unnecessary medications that may contribute to the hypertension

G. Pharmacological interventions
1. Medication therapy is individualized for each client, and the selection of the medication is based on such factors as the client's age, presence of coexisting conditions, severity of the hypertension, and client's preferences.
2. See Chapter 53 for medications to treat hypertension.

H. See Box 52-10 for client education.

BOX 52-10 Education for the Client with Hypertension

- Describe the importance of adherence with the treatment plan.
- Describe the disease process, explaining that symptoms usually do not develop until organs have suffered damage.
- Initiate and assist the client in planning a regular exercise program, avoiding heavy weight-lifting and isometric exercises.
- Emphasize the importance of beginning the exercise program gradually.
- Encourage the client to express feelings about daily stress.
- Assist the client to identify ways to reduce stress.
- Teach relaxation techniques.
- Instruct the client in how to incorporate relaxation techniques into the daily living pattern.
- Instruct the client and family in the technique for monitoring blood pressure (BP).
- Instruct the client to maintain a diary of BP readings.
- Emphasize the importance of lifelong medication.
- Instruct the client and family about dietary restrictions, which may include sodium, fat, calories, and cholesterol.
- Instruct the client in how to shop for and prepare low-sodium meals.
- Provide a list of products that contain sodium.
- Instruct the client to read labels of products to determine sodium content, focusing on substances listed as sodium, NaCl, or MSG (monosodium glutamate).
- Instruct the client to bake, roast, or boil foods; avoid salt in preparation of foods; and avoid using salt at the table.
- Instruct the client that fresh foods are best to consume, and to avoid canned foods.
- Instruct the client about the actions, side effects, and scheduling of medications.
- Advise the client that if uncomfortable side effects occur, to contact the primary health care provider or cardiologist and not to stop the medication.
- Instruct the client to avoid over-the-counter medications.
- Stress the importance of follow-up care.

XXII. Hypertensive Crisis

A. Description
1. A hypertensive crisis is an acute and life-threatening condition requiring immediate reduction in BP.
2. Emergency treatment is required, because target organ damage (brain, heart, kidneys, retina of the eye) can occur quickly.
3. Death can be caused by stroke, kidney failure, or cardiac disease.

B. Assessment
1. An extremely high BP; systolic over 180 mm Hg and/or diastolic over 120 mm Hg
2. Headache
3. Drowsiness and confusion
4. Blurred vision
5. Changes in neurological status
6. Tachycardia and tachypnea
7. Dyspnea
8. Cyanosis
9. Seizures

C. Interventions
1. Maintain a patent airway.
2. Administer antihypertensive medications intravenously as prescribed.
3. Monitor vital signs, assessing the BP every 5 minutes.
4. Monitor neurological status.
5. Maintain bed rest, with the head of the bed elevated at 45 degrees.
6. Assess for hypotension during the administration of antihypertensives; place the client in a supine position if hypotension occurs.
7. Have emergency medications and resuscitation equipment readily available.
8. Monitor IV therapy, assessing for fluid overload.
9. Insert a Foley catheter as prescribed.
10. Monitor intake and urinary output; if oliguria or anuria occurs, notify the PHCP.

PRACTICE QUESTIONS

600. A client is admitted to the emergency department with chest pain that is consistent with myocardial infarction based on elevated troponin levels. Heart sounds are normal. The nurse should alert the primary health care provider because the vital sign changes and client assessment are **most** consistent with which complication? **Refer to chart.**

Client's Chart

Time:	11:00 a.m.	11:15 a.m.	11:30 a.m.	11:45 a.m.
Pulse:	92 beats/min	96 beats/min	104 beats/min	118 beats/min
Respiratory rate:	24 breaths/min	26 breaths/min	28 breaths/min	32 breaths/min
Blood pressure:	140/88 mm Hg	128/82 mm Hg	104/68 mm Hg	88/58 mm Hg

1. Cardiogenic shock
2. Cardiac tamponade
3. Pulmonary embolism
4. Dissecting thoracic aortic aneurysm

601. A client with a history of type 2 diabetes is admitted to the hospital with chest pain. The client is scheduled for a cardiac catheterization. Which medication would need to be withheld for 24 hours before the procedure and for 48 hours after the procedure?
1. Glipizide
2. Metformin
3. Repaglinide
4. Regular insulin

602. A client in sinus bradycardia, with a heart rate of 45 beats per minute and blood pressure of 82/60 mm Hg, reports dizziness. Which intervention should the nurse anticipate will be prescribed?
1. Administer digoxin.
2. Defibrillate the client.
3. Continue to monitor the client.
4. Prepare for transcutaneous pacing.

603. The nurse in a medical unit is caring for a client with heart failure. The client suddenly develops extreme dyspnea, tachycardia, and lung crackles. The nurse immediately asks another nurse to contact the primary health care provider and prepares to implement which **priority** interventions? **Select all that apply.**
- ☐ 1. Administering oxygen
- ☐ 2. Inserting a Foley catheter
- ☐ 3. Administering furosemide
- ☐ 4. Administering morphine sulfate intravenously
- ☐ 5. Transporting the client to the coronary care unit
- ☐ 6. Placing the client in a low-Fowler's side-lying position

604. A client with myocardial infarction suddenly becomes tachycardic, shows signs of air hunger, and begins coughing frothy, pink-tinged sputum. Which finding would the nurse anticipate when auscultating the client's breath sounds?
1. Stridor
2. Crackles
3. Scattered rhonchi
4. Diminished breath sounds

605. A client with myocardial infarction is developing cardiogenic shock. What condition should the nurse carefully assess the client for?
1. Pulsus paradoxus
2. Ventricular dysrhythmias
3. Rising diastolic blood pressure
4. Falling central venous pressure

606. A client who had cardiac surgery 24 hours ago has had a urine output averaging 20 mL/hr for 2 hours. The client received a single bolus of 500 mL of intravenous fluid. Urine output for the subsequent hour was 25 mL. Daily laboratory results indicate that the blood urea nitrogen level is 45 mg/dL (16 mmol/L) and the serum creatinine level is 2.2 mg/dL (194 mcmol/L). On the basis of these findings, the nurse would anticipate that the client is at risk for which problem?
1. Hypovolemia
2. Acute kidney injury
3. Glomerulonephritis
4. Urinary tract infection

607. The nurse is reviewing an electrocardiogram rhythm strip. The P waves and QRS complexes are regular. The PR interval is 0.16 seconds, and QRS complexes measure 0.06 seconds. The overall heart rate is 64 beats per minute. Which action should the nurse take?
1. Check vital signs.
2. Check laboratory test results.
3. Monitor for any rhythm change.
4. Notify the primary health care provider.

608. A client is wearing a continuous cardiac monitor, which begins to sound its alarm. The nurse sees no electrocardiographic complexes on the screen. Which is the **priority** nursing action?
1. Call a code.
2. Check the client's status.
3. Call the health care provider.
4. Document the lack of complexes.

609. The nurse is watching the cardiac monitor and notices that a client's rhythm suddenly changes. There are no P waves, the QRS complexes are wide, and the ventricular rate is regular but more than 140 beats per minute. The nurse determines that the client is experiencing which dysrhythmia?
1. Sinus tachycardia
2. Ventricular fibrillation
3. Ventricular tachycardia
4. Premature ventricular contractions

610. A client has frequent bursts of ventricular tachycardia on the cardiac monitor. What should the nurse be **most** concerned about with this dysrhythmia?
1. It can develop into ventricular fibrillation at any time.
2. It is almost impossible to convert to a normal rhythm.
3. It is uncomfortable for the client, giving a sense of impending doom.
4. It produces a high cardiac output with cerebral and myocardial ischemia.

611. A client is having frequent premature ventricular contractions. The nurse should place **priority** on assessment of which item?
1. Causative factors, such as caffeine
2. Sensation of fluttering or palpitations
3. Blood pressure and oxygen saturation
4. Precipitating factors, such as infection

612. The client has developed atrial fibrillation, with a ventricular rate of 150 beats per minute. The nurse should assess the client for which associated signs and/or symptoms? **Select all that apply.**
- ☐ 1. Syncope
- ☐ 2. Dizziness
- ☐ 3. Palpitations
- ☐ 4. Hypertension
- ☐ 5. Flat neck veins

613. The nurse is watching the cardiac monitor, and a client's rhythm suddenly changes. There are no P waves; instead, there are fibrillatory waves before each QRS complex. How should the nurse interpret the client's heart rhythm?
1. Atrial fibrillation
2. Sinus tachycardia
3. Ventricular fibrillation
4. Ventricular tachycardia

614. The nurse is assisting to defibrillate a client in ventricular fibrillation. After placing the pads on the client's chest and before discharging the device, which intervention is a **priority**?
1. Ensure that the client has been intubated.
2. Set the defibrillator to the "synchronize" mode.
3. Administer an amiodarone bolus intravenously.
4. Confirm that the rhythm is ventricular fibrillation.

615. A client in ventricular fibrillation is about to be defibrillated. To convert this rhythm effectively, the monophasic defibrillator machine should be set at which energy level (in joules, J) for the first delivery?
1. 50 J
2. 120 J
3. 200 J
4. 360 J

616. The nurse should evaluate that defibrillation of a client was **most** successful if which observation was made?
1. Arousable, sinus rhythm, blood pressure (BP) 116/72 mm Hg
2. Nonarousable, sinus rhythm, BP 88/60 mm Hg
3. Arousable, marked bradycardia, BP 86/54 mm Hg
4. Nonarousable, supraventricular tachycardia, BP 122/60 mm Hg

617. The nurse is evaluating a client's response to cardioversion. Which assessment would be the **priority**?
1. Blood pressure
2. Airway patency
3. Oxygen flow rate
4. Level of consciousness

618. The nurse is caring for a client who has just had implantation of an automatic internal cardioverter-defibrillator. The nurse should assess which item based on **priority**?
1. Anxiety level of the client and family
2. Activation status and settings of the device
3. Presence of a MedicAlert card for the client to carry
4. Knowledge of restrictions on postdischarge physical activity

619. A client's electrocardiogram strip shows atrial and ventricular rates of 110 beats per minute. The PR interval is 0.14 seconds, the QRS complex measures 0.08 seconds, and the PP and RR intervals are regular. How should the nurse interpret this rhythm?
1. Sinus tachycardia
2. Sinus bradycardia
3. Sinus dysrhythmia
4. Normal sinus rhythm

620. The nurse is assessing the neurovascular status of a client who returned to the surgical nursing unit 4 hours ago after undergoing aortoiliac bypass graft. The affected leg is warm, and the nurse notes redness and edema. The pedal pulse is palpable. How should the nurse interpret the client's neurovascular status?
1. The neurovascular status is normal because of increased blood flow through the leg.
2. The neurovascular status is moderately impaired, and the surgeon should be called.
3. The neurovascular status is slightly deteriorating and should be monitored for another hour.
4. The neurovascular status shows adequate arterial flow, but venous complications are arising.

621. The nurse is evaluating the condition of a client after pericardiocentesis performed to treat cardiac tamponade. Which observation would indicate that the procedure was **effective**?
1. Muffled heart sounds
2. Client reports dyspnea
3. A rise in blood pressure
4. Jugular venous distention

622. The nurse is caring for a client who had a resection of an abdominal aortic aneurysm yesterday. The client has an intravenous (IV) infusion at a rate of 150 mL/hr, unchanged for the last 10 hours. The client's urine output for the last 3 hours has been 90, 50, and 28 mL (28 mL is most recent). The client's blood urea nitrogen level is 35 mg/dL (12.6 mmol/L), and the serum creatinine level is 1.8 mg/dL (159 mcmol/L), measured this morning. Which nursing action is the **priority?**
1. Check the serum albumin level.
2. Check the urine specific gravity.
3. Continue monitoring urine output.
4. Call the primary health care provider (PHCP).

623. A client with variant angina is scheduled to receive an oral calcium channel blocker twice daily. Which statement by the client indicates the **need for further teaching**?
1. "I should notify my cardiologist if my feet or legs start to swell."
2. "I am supposed to report to my cardiologist if my pulse rate decreases below 60."
3. "Avoiding grapefruit juice will definitely be a challenge for me, since I usually drink it every morning with breakfast."
4. "My spouse told me that since I have developed this problem, we are going to stop walking in the mall every morning."

624. The nurse notes that a client with sinus rhythm has a premature ventricular contraction that falls on the T wave of the preceding beat. The client's rhythm suddenly changes to one with no P waves, no definable QRS complexes, and coarse wavy lines of varying amplitude. How should the nurse interpret this rhythm?
1. Asystole
2. Atrial fibrillation
3. Ventricular fibrillation
4. Ventricular tachycardia

ANSWERS

600. *Answer:* 1

Rationale: Cardiogenic shock occurs with severe damage (more than 40%) to the left ventricle. Classic signs include hypotension; a rapid pulse that becomes weaker; decreased urine output; and cool, clammy skin. Respiratory rate increases as the body develops metabolic acidosis from shock. Cardiac tamponade is accompanied by distant, muffled heart sounds and prominent neck vessels. Pulmonary embolism presents suddenly with severe dyspnea accompanying the chest pain. Dissecting aortic aneurysms usually are accompanied by back pain.

Test-Taking Strategy: Note the strategic word, *most*. Recalling that the early serious complications of myocardial infarction include dysrhythmias, cardiogenic shock, and sudden death will direct you to the correct option. No information in the question is associated with the remaining options.

Level of Cognitive Ability: Synthesizing
Client Needs: Physiological Integrity
Integrated Process: Nursing Process—Analysis
Content Area: Complex Care: Shock
Health Problem: Adult Health: Cardiovascular: Shock
Priority Concepts: Clinical Judgment; Perfusion
Reference: Ignatavicius, Workman (2016), p. 741.

601. *Answer:* 2

Rationale: Metformin needs to be withheld 24 hours before and for 48 hours after cardiac catheterization because of the injection of contrast medium during the procedure. If the contrast medium affects kidney function, with metformin in the system the client would be at increased risk for lactic acidosis. The medications in the remaining options do not need to be withheld before and after cardiac catheterization.

Test-Taking Strategy: Eliminate glipizide and repaglinide first because they are comparable or alike. Although these medications may be withheld on the morning of the procedure because of the client's NPO (nothing by mouth) status, there is no indication for withholding the medication on the day prior to the procedure and postprocedure. Regular insulin may be administered if elevated blood glucose levels from infused intravenous solutions occur on the day of the procedure.

Level of Cognitive Ability: Analyzing
Client Needs: Physiological Integrity
Integrated Process: Nursing Process—Planning
Content Area: Pharmacology: Endocrine: Oral hypoglycemic
Health Problem: Adult Health: Cardiovascular: Coronary Artery Disease
Priority Concepts: Perfusion; Safety
Reference: Ignatavicius, Workman (2016), pp. 643, 1310.

602. *Answer:* 4

Rationale: Sinus bradycardia is noted with a heart rate less than 60 beats per minute. This rhythm becomes a concern when the client becomes symptomatic. Hypotension and dizziness are signs of decreased cardiac output. Transcutaneous pacing provides a temporary measure to increase the heart rate and thus perfusion in the symptomatic client. Defibrillation is used for treatment of pulseless ventricular tachycardia and ventricular fibrillation. Digoxin will further decrease the client's heart rate. Continuing to monitor the client delays necessary intervention.

Test-Taking Strategy: Focus on the subject, interventions for sinus bradycardia. Eliminate the option indicating to continue to monitor the client, because the client is symptomatic and requires intervention. Digoxin is eliminated because it will further decrease the client's heart rate. Defibrillation is used for treatment of pulseless ventricular tachycardia and ventricular fibrillation, so that option can be eliminated.

Level of Cognitive Ability: Applying
Client Needs: Physiological Integrity
Integrated Process: Nursing Process—Planning
Content Area: Complex Care: Emergency Situations/Management
Health Problem: Adult Health: Cardiovascular: Dysrhythmias
Priority Concepts: Gas Exchange; Perfusion
Reference: Ignatavicius, Workman (2016), p. 664.

603. *Answer:* 1, 2, 3, 4

Rationale: Extreme dyspnea, tachycardia, and lung crackles in a client with heart failure indicate pulmonary edema, a life-threatening event. In pulmonary edema, the left ventricle fails to eject sufficient blood, and pressure increases in the lungs because of the accumulated blood. Oxygen is always prescribed, and the client is placed in a high-Fowler's position to ease the work of breathing. Furosemide, a rapid-acting diuretic, will eliminate accumulated fluid. A Foley catheter is inserted to measure output accurately. Intravenously administered morphine sulfate reduces venous return (preload), decreases anxiety, and also reduces the work of breathing. Transporting the client to the coronary care unit is not a priority intervention. In fact, this may not be necessary at all if the client's response to treatment is successful.

Test-Taking Strategy: Note the strategic word, *priority*, and focus on the client's diagnosis. Recall the pathophysiology associated with pulmonary edema and use the ABCs—airway, breathing, and circulation—to help determine priority interventions.

Level of Cognitive Ability: Synthesizing
Client Needs: Physiological Integrity
Integrated Process: Nursing Process—Implementation
Content Area: Complex Care: Emergency Situations/Management
Health Problem: Adult Health: Cardiovascular: Heart Failure
Priority Concepts: Gas Exchange; Perfusion
Reference: Ignatavicius, Workman (2016), pp. 688-689.

604. *Answer:* 2

Rationale: Pulmonary edema is characterized by extreme breathlessness, dyspnea, air hunger, and the production of frothy, pink-tinged sputum. Auscultation of the lungs reveals crackles. Rhonchi and diminished breath sounds are not associated with pulmonary edema. Stridor is a crowing sound associated with laryngospasm or edema of the upper airway.

Test-Taking Strategy: Focus on the subject, breath sounds characteristic of pulmonary edema. Recalling that fluid produces sounds that are called *crackles* will assist you in eliminating the incorrect options.

Level of Cognitive Ability: Analyzing
Client Needs: Physiological Integrity
Integrated Process: Nursing Process—Assessment
Content Area: Complex Care: Emergency Situations/Management

Health Problem: Adult Health: Cardiovascular: Myocardial Infarction
Priority Concepts: Gas Exchange; Perfusion
Reference: Ignatavicius, Workman (2016), p. 699.

605. *Answer:* 2
Rationale: Dysrhythmias commonly occur as a result of decreased oxygenation and severe damage to greater than 40% of the myocardium. Classic signs of cardiogenic shock as they relate to myocardial ischemia include low blood pressure and tachycardia. The central venous pressure would rise as the backward effects of the severe left ventricular failure became apparent. Pulsus paradoxus is a finding associated with cardiac tamponade.
Test-Taking Strategy: Focus on the **subject**, cardiogenic shock, and note the words *myocardial ischemia*. Recall that ischemia makes the myocardium irritable, producing dysrhythmias. Also, knowledge of the classic signs of shock helps eliminate the incorrect options.
Level of Cognitive Ability: Analyzing
Client Needs: Physiological Integrity
Integrated Process: Nursing Process—Assessment
Content Area: Complex Care: Emergency Situations/Management
Health Problem: Adult Health: Cardiovascular: Shock
Priority Concepts: Clinical Judgment; Perfusion
Reference: Ignatavicius, Workman (2016), p. 759.

606. *Answer:* 2
Rationale: The client who undergoes cardiac surgery is at risk for renal injury from poor perfusion, hemolysis, low cardiac output, or vasopressor medication therapy. Renal injury is signaled by decreased urine output and increased blood urea nitrogen (BUN) and creatinine levels. Normal reference levels are BUN, 10 to 20 mg/dL (3.6 to 7.1 mmol/L), and creatinine 0.6 to 1.2 mg/dL (53 to 106 mcmol/L) for males and 0.5 to 1.1 mg/dL (44 to 97 mcmol/L) for females. The client may need medications to increase renal perfusion and possibly could need peritoneal dialysis or hemodialysis. No data in the question indicate the presence of hypovolemia, glomerulonephritis, or urinary tract infection.
Test-Taking Strategy: Eliminate glomerulonephritis and urinary tract infection first because they are **comparable or alike** in that there are no data indicating infection or inflammation. Noting that the creatinine level is elevated and the minimal urinary response to the fluid bolus will assist you in eliminating hypovolemia.
Level of Cognitive Ability: Synthesizing
Client Needs: Physiological Integrity
Integrated Process: Nursing Process—Analysis
Content Area: Adult Health: Renal and Urinary
Health Problem: Adult Health: Cardiovascular: Coronary Artery Disease
Priority Concepts: Clinical Judgment; Perfusion
References: Ignatavicius, Workman (2016), p. 777; Lewis et al. (2014), p. 1102.

607. *Answer:* 3
Rationale: Normal sinus rhythm is defined as a regular rhythm, with an overall rate of 60 to 100 beats per minute. The PR and QRS measurements are normal, measuring between 0.12 and 0.20 seconds and 0.04 and 0.10 seconds, respectively. There are no irregularities in this rhythm currently, so there is no immediate need to check vital signs or laboratory results, or to notify the primary health care provider. Therefore, the nurse would continue to monitor the client for any rhythm change.
Test-Taking Strategy: Focus on the **subject**, electrocardiogram rhythm strip measurements. A baseline knowledge of normal electrocardiographic measurements is needed to answer this question. Focusing on the **data in the question** and recalling the characteristics of normal sinus rhythm will help you prioritize your actions.
Level of Cognitive Ability: Analyzing
Client Needs: Physiological Integrity
Integrated Process: Nursing Process: Implementation
Content Area: Adult Health: Cardiovascular
Health Problem: Adult Health: Cardiovascular: Dysrhythmias
Priority Concepts: Clinical Judgment; Perfusion
Reference: Ignatavicius, Workman (2016), p. 656.

608. *Answer:* 2
Rationale: Sudden loss of electrocardiographic complexes indicates ventricular asystole or possibly electrode displacement. Accurate assessment of the client is necessary to determine the cause and identify the appropriate intervention. The remaining options are secondary to client assessment.
Test-Taking Strategy: Note the **strategic word**, *priority*. Use the **steps of the nursing process.** Always assess the client directly before taking any action related to equipment. The correct option is the only one that addresses assessment.
Level of Cognitive Ability: Applying
Client Needs: Physiological Integrity
Integrated Process: Nursing Process—Assessment
Content Area: Complex Care: Emergency Situations/Management
Health Problem: Adult Health: Cardiovascular: Dysrhythmias
Priority Concepts: Clinical Judgment; Perfusion
Reference: Lewis et al. (2014), p. 790.

609. *Answer:* 3
Rationale: Ventricular tachycardia is characterized by the absence of P waves, wide QRS complexes (longer than 0.12 seconds), and typically a rate between 140 and 180 impulses per minute. The rhythm is regular.
Test-Taking Strategy: Focus on the **subject**, the characteristics of an electrocardiogram pattern, and note the **data in the question**. Eliminate sinus tachycardia first, because there are no P waves. Premature ventricular contractions are isolated ectopic beats superimposed on an underlying rhythm, so that option is eliminated next. Recalling that there are no true QRS complexes with ventricular fibrillation will direct you to the correct option from those remaining.
Level of Cognitive Ability: Analyzing
Client Needs: Physiological Integrity
Integrated Process: Nursing Process—Assessment
Content Area: Complex Care: Emergency Situations/Management
Health Problem: Adult Health: Cardiovascular: Dysrhythmias
Priority Concepts: Clinical Judgment; Perfusion
Reference: Lewis et al. (2014), pp. 794, 799-800.

610. *Answer:* 1

Rationale: Ventricular tachycardia is a life-threatening dysrhythmia that results from an irritable ectopic focus that takes over as the pacemaker for the heart. Ventricular tachycardia can deteriorate into ventricular fibrillation at any time. Clients frequently experience a feeling of impending doom. The low cardiac output that results can lead quickly to cerebral and myocardial ischemia. Ventricular tachycardia is treated with antidysrhythmic medications, cardioversion (if the client is awake), or defibrillation (loss of consciousness).

Test-Taking Strategy: Note the strategic word, *most*. The option indicating that it is impossible to convert is incorrect and is eliminated first. From the remaining options, focusing on the strategic word will direct you to the correct option because this option identifies the life-threatening condition.

Level of Cognitive Ability: Analyzing
Client Needs: Physiological Integrity
Integrated Process: Nursing Process—Analysis
Content Area: Complex Care: Emergency Situations/Management
Health Problem: Adult Health: Cardiovascular: Dysrhythmias
Priority Concepts: Clinical Judgment; Perfusion
Reference: Ignatavicius, Workman (2016), p. 670.

611. *Answer:* 3

Rationale: Premature ventricular contractions can cause hemodynamic compromise. Therefore, the priority is to monitor the blood pressure and oxygen saturation. The shortened ventricular filling time can lead to decreased cardiac output. The client may be asymptomatic or may feel palpitations. Premature ventricular contractions can be caused by cardiac disorders; states of hypoxemia; any number of physiological stressors, such as infection, illness, surgery, or trauma; and intake of caffeine, nicotine, or alcohol.

Test-Taking Strategy: Note the strategic word, *priority*. Use the ABCs—airway, breathing, and circulation—to direct you to the correct option.

Level of Cognitive Ability: Analyzing
Client Needs: Physiological Integrity
Integrated Process: Nursing Process—Assessment
Content Area: Complex Care: Emergency Situations/Management
Health Problem: Adult Health: Cardiovascular: Dysrhythmias
Priority Concepts: Clinical Judgment; Perfusion
Reference: Lewis et al. (2014), p. 799.

612. *Answer:* 1, 2, 3

Rationale: The client with uncontrolled atrial fibrillation with a ventricular rate more than 100 beats per minute is at risk for low cardiac output because of loss of atrial kick. The nurse assesses the client for palpitations, chest pain or discomfort, hypotension, pulse deficit, fatigue, weakness, dizziness, syncope, shortness of breath, and distended neck veins. Hypertension and flat neck veins are not associated with the loss of cardiac output.

Test-Taking Strategy: Focus on the subject, signs and/or symptoms associated with atrial fibrillation. Flat neck veins are normal or indicate hypovolemia, so this option can be eliminated. From the remaining options, think of the consequences of a falling cardiac output to direct you to the correct option.

Level of Cognitive Ability: Analyzing
Client Needs: Physiological Integrity
Integrated Process: Nursing Process—Assessment
Content Area: Complex Care: Emergency Situations/Management
Health Problem: Adult Health: Cardiovascular: Dysrhythmias
Priority Concepts: Clinical Judgment; Perfusion
Reference: Lewis et al. (2014), p. 707.

613. *Answer:* 1

Rationale: Atrial fibrillation is characterized by a loss of P waves and fibrillatory waves before each QRS complex. The atria quiver, which can lead to thrombus formation.

Test-Taking Strategy: Focus on the subject, interpreting a heart rhythm. Note the data in the question. Noting the words *There are no P waves* should direct you to the correct option. Loss of P waves is characteristic of this dysrhythmia.

Level of Cognitive Ability: Analyzing
Client Needs: Physiological Integrity
Integrated Process: Nursing Process—Assessment
Content Area: Complex Care: Emergency Situations/Management
Health Problem: Adult Health: Cardiovascular: Dysrhythmias
Priority Concepts: Clinical Judgment; Perfusion
Reference: Ignatavicius, Workman (2016), pp. 666-667.

614. *Answer:* 4

Rationale: Until the defibrillator is attached and charged, the client is resuscitated by using cardiopulmonary resuscitation. Once the defibrillator has been attached, the electrocardiogram is checked to verify that the rhythm is ventricular fibrillation or pulseless ventricular tachycardia. Leads also are checked for any loose connections. A nitroglycerin patch, if present, is removed. The client does not have to be intubated to be defibrillated. The machine is not set to the synchronous mode because there is no underlying rhythm with which to synchronize.

Test-Taking Strategy: Note the strategic word, *priority*. Focus on the subject, ventricular fibrillation. Note that the correct option directly addresses this subject and also addresses assessment of the client.

Level of Cognitive Ability: Analyzing
Client Needs: Physiological Integrity
Integrated Process: Nursing Process—Assessment
Content Area: Complex Care: Basic Life Support/Cardiopulmonary Resuscitation/Cardiac Arrest
Health Problem: Adult Health: Cardiovascular: Dysrhythmias
Priority Concepts: Perfusion; Safety
Reference: Lewis et al. (2014), pp. 801-802.

615. *Answer:* 4

Rationale: The energy level used for all defibrillation attempts with a monophasic defibrillator is 360 joules.

Test-Taking Strategy: Focus on the subject, monophasic defibrillation. As a general rule, though, remember that lower levels of energy are used for cardioversion and biphasic defibrillation. Higher levels are used in monophasic defibrillation.

Level of Cognitive Ability: Analyzing
Client Needs: Physiological Integrity
Integrated Process: Nursing Process—Implementation

Content Area: Complex Care: Basic Life Support/Cardiopulmonary Resuscitation/Cardiac Arrest
Health Problem: Adult Health: Cardiovascular: Dysrhythmias
Priority Concepts: Perfusion; Safety
Reference: Lewis et al. (2014), p. 802.

616. *Answer:* 1
Rationale: After defibrillation, the client requires continuous monitoring of electrocardiographic rhythm, hemodynamic status, and neurological status. Respiratory and metabolic acidosis develop during ventricular fibrillation because of lack of respiration and cardiac output. These can cause cerebral and cardiopulmonary complications. Arousable status, adequate BP, and a sinus rhythm indicate successful response to defibrillation.
Test-Taking Strategy: Note the strategic word, *most*. Eliminate the options that contain the word *nonarousable*. From the remaining options, select the correct option, because a sinus rhythm is a more successful response compared with marked bradycardia.
Level of Cognitive Ability: Evaluating
Client Needs: Physiological Integrity
Integrated Process: Nursing Process—Evaluation
Content Area: Complex Care: Basic Life Support/Cardiopulmonary Resuscitation/Cardiac Arrest
Health Problem: Adult Health: Cardiovascular: Dysrhythmias
Priority Concepts: Evidence; Perfusion
Reference: Ignatavicius, Workman (2016), p. 672.

617. *Answer:* 2
Rationale: Nursing responsibilities after cardioversion include maintenance first of a patent airway, and then oxygen administration, assessment of vital signs and level of consciousness, and dysrhythmia detection.
Test-Taking Strategy: Note the strategic word, *priority*. Use the ABCs—airway, breathing, and circulation—to direct you to the correct option.
Level of Cognitive Ability: Analyzing
Client Needs: Physiological Integrity
Integrated Process: Nursing Process—Assessment
Content Area: Adult Health: Cardiovascular
Health Problem: Adult Health: Cardiovascular: Dysrhythmias
Priority Concepts: Clinical Judgment; Perfusion
Reference: Ignatavicius, Workman (2016), p. 668.

618. *Answer:* 2
Rationale: The nurse who is caring for the client after insertion of an automatic internal cardioverter-defibrillator needs to assess device settings, similar to after insertion of a permanent pacemaker. Specifically, the nurse needs to know whether the device is activated, the heart rate cutoff above which it will fire, and the number of shocks it is programmed to deliver. The remaining options are also nursing interventions but are not the priority.
Test-Taking Strategy: Note the strategic word, *priority*. Use Maslow's Hierarchy of Needs theory. The correct option is the one that identifies the physiological need.
Level of Cognitive Ability: Analyzing
Client Needs: Physiological Integrity
Integrated Process: Nursing Process—Assessment
Content Area: Adult Health: Cardiovascular
Health Problem: Adult Health: Cardiovascular: Dysrhythmias
Priority Concepts: Perfusion; Safety
Reference: Lewis et al. (2014), p. 803.

619. *Answer:* 1
Rationale: Sinus tachycardia has the characteristics of normal sinus rhythm, including a regular PP interval and normal-width PR and QRS intervals; however, the rate is the differentiating factor. In sinus tachycardia, the atrial and ventricular rates are greater than 100 beats per minute.
Test-Taking Strategy: Focus on the subject, interpreting a cardiac rhythm. Eliminate sinus bradycardia and normal sinus rhythm first, because the ventricular rate is 110 beats per minute. Next eliminate sinus dysrhythmia, because this is an irregular rhythm, with changing PP and RR intervals.
Level of Cognitive Ability: Analyzing
Client Needs: Physiological Integrity
Integrated Process: Nursing Process—Assessment
Content Area: Adult Health: Cardiovascular
Health Problem: Adult Health: Cardiovascular: Dysrhythmias
Priority Concepts: Clinical Judgment; Perfusion
Reference: Ignatavicius, Workman (2016), pp. 662-663.

620. *Answer:* 1
Rationale: An expected outcome of aortoiliac bypass graft surgery is warmth, redness, and edema in the surgical extremity because of increased blood flow. The remaining options are incorrect interpretations.
Test-Taking Strategy: Focus on the subject, expected outcomes following aortoiliac bypass graft surgery. Venous complications from immobilization resulting from surgery would not be apparent within 4 hours, so eliminate option 4. From the remaining options, note that the pedal pulse is unchanged from admission and think about the effects of sudden reperfusion in an ischemic limb. There would be redness from new blood flow and edema from the sudden change in pressure in the blood vessels.
Level of Cognitive Ability: Synthesizing
Client Needs: Physiological Integrity
Integrated Process: Nursing Process—Assessment
Content Area: Adult Health: Cardiovascular
Health Problem: Adult Health: Cardiovascular: Vascular disorders
Priority Concepts: Clinical Judgment; Perfusion
Reference: Lewis et al. (2014), p. 839.

621. *Answer:* 3
Rationale: Following pericardiocentesis, the client usually expresses immediate relief. Heart sounds are no longer muffled or distant and blood pressure increases. Distended neck veins are a sign of increased venous pressure, which occurs with cardiac tamponade.
Test-Taking Strategy: Focus on the subject, expected outcome following pericardiocentesis, and note the strategic word, *effective*. Successful therapy is measured by the disappearance of the original signs and symptoms of cardiac tamponade. This will direct you to the correct option.
Level of Cognitive Ability: Evaluating
Client Needs: Physiological Integrity
Integrated Process: Nursing Process—Evaluation
Content Area: Complex Care: Emergency Situations/Management

Health Problem: Adult Health: Cardiovascular: Cardiac Tamponade
Priority Concepts: Evidence; Perfusion
Reference: Lewis et al. (2014), pp. 815-816.

622. *Answer:* 4
Rationale: Following abdominal aortic aneurysm resection or repair, the nurse monitors the client for signs of acute kidney injury. Acute kidney injury can occur because often much blood is lost during the surgery and, depending on the aneurysm location, the renal arteries may be hypoperfused for a short period during surgery. Normal reference levels are BUN 10 to 20 mg/dL (3.6 to 7.1 mmol/L), and creatinine 0.6 to 1.2 mg/dL (53 to 106 mcmol/L) for males and 0.5 to 1.1 mg/dL (44 to 97 mcmol/L) for females. Continuing to monitor urine output or checking other parameters can wait. Urine output lower than 30 mL/hr is reported to the PHCP for urgent treatment
Test-Taking Strategy: Note the **strategic word**, *priority*. Focus on the **data in the question** and the abnormal assessment data. This question indicates elevations in blood urea nitrogen and creatinine levels and a significant drop in hourly urine output. These assessment findings should direct you to an option that includes active collaboration with the PHCP.
Level of Cognitive Ability: Synthesizing
Client Needs: Physiological Integrity
Integrated Process: Nursing Process—Implementation
Content Area: Complex Care—Emergency Situations/Management
Health Problem: Adult Health: Cardiovascular: Vascular Disorders
Priority Concepts: Clinical Judgment; Perfusion
Reference: Lewis et al. (2014), pp. 841-843.

623. *Answer:* 4
Rationale: Variant angina, or Prinzmetal's angina, is prolonged and severe and occurs at the same time each day, most often at rest. The pain is a result of coronary artery spasm. The treatment of choice is usually a calcium channel blocker, which relaxes and dilates the vascular smooth muscle, thus relieving the coronary artery spasm in variant angina. Adverse effects can include peripheral edema, hypotension, bradycardia, and heart failure. Grapefruit juice interacts with calcium channel blockers and should be avoided. If bradycardia occurs, the client should contact the primary health care provider or cardiologist. Clients should also be taught to change positions slowly to prevent orthostatic hypotension. Physical exertion does not cause this type of angina; therefore, the client should be able to continue morning walks with her or his spouse.
Test-Taking Strategy: Note the **strategic words**, *need for further teaching*, and focus on the **data in the question**. These words indicate a **negative event query** and the need to select the incorrect client statement. Recall that walking is a low-impact exercise and is usually recommended for clients with heart problems.
Level of Cognitive Ability: Evaluating
Client Needs: Physiological Integrity
Integrated Process: Teaching and Learning
Content Area: Adult Health: Cardiovascular
Health Problem: Adult Health: Cardiovascular: Coronary artery disease
Priority Concepts: Client Education; Safety
Reference: Ignatavicius, Workman (2016), pp. 759, 763.

624. *Answer:* 3
Rationale: Ventricular fibrillation is characterized by irregular chaotic undulations of varying amplitudes. Ventricular fibrillation has no measurable rate and no visible P waves or QRS complexes and results from electrical chaos in the ventricles.
Test-Taking Strategy: Focus on the **subject**, the characteristics of ventricular fibrillation. Note the words, *no definable QRS complexes*. The lack of visible QRS complexes eliminates atrial fibrillation and ventricular tachycardia. Recalling that asystole is lack of any electrical activity of the heart will direct you to the correct option.
Level of Cognitive Ability: Analyzing
Client Needs: Physiological Integrity
Integrated Process: Nursing Process—Assessment
Content Area: Complex Care: Emergency Situations/Management
Health Problem: Adult Health: Cardiovascular: Dysrhythmias
Priority Concepts: Clinical Judgment; Perfusion
Reference: Ignatavicius, Workman (2016), pp. 670-671.

CHAPTER 53

Cardiovascular Medications

PRIORITY CONCEPTS Clotting; Perfusion

I. Anticoagulants (Box 53-1)

A. Description

1. Anticoagulants prevent the extension and formation of clots by inhibiting factors in the clotting cascade and decreasing blood coagulability.

2. Anticoagulants are administered when there is evidence of or likelihood of clot formation—myocardial infarction, unstable angina, atrial fibrillation, deep vein thrombosis, pulmonary embolism, and the presence of mechanical heart valves.

3. Anticoagulants are contraindicated with active bleeding (except for disseminated intravascular coagulation), bleeding disorders or blood dyscrasias, ulcers, liver and kidney disease, and hemorrhagic brain injuries (Box 53-2).

B. Side and adverse effects

1. Hemorrhage
2. Hematuria
3. Epistaxis
4. Ecchymosis
5. Bleeding gums
6. Thrombocytopenia
7. Hypotension

C. Heparin sodium

1. Description

a. Heparin prevents thrombin from converting fibrinogen to fibrin.

b. Heparin prevents thromboembolism.

c. The therapeutic dose does not dissolve clots but prevents new thrombus formation.

2. Blood levels

a. The normal activated partial thromboplastin time (aPTT) is 30 to 40 seconds (conventional and SI units) in most laboratories (values depend on reagent and instrumentation used).

b. To maintain a therapeutic level of anticoagulation when the client is receiving a continuous infusion of heparin, the aPTT should be 1.5 to 2.5 times the normal value. Some agencies use 2 different protocols, a high-intensity protocol such as for acute coronary syndrome and a low-intensity protocol such as for venous thromboembolism prophylaxis, and the dosages and recommended aPTT ranges are slightly different for the two protocols.

c. Activated partial thromboplastin time therapy should be measured every 4 to 6 hours during initial continuous infusion therapy or until the client has been therapeutic for a specified time frame and then daily per agency policy.

d. If the aPTT is too long, per agency procedure, the dosage should be lowered.

e. If the aPTT is too short, per agency procedure, the dosage should be increased.

3. Interventions

a. Monitor aPTT.

b. Monitor platelet count.

c. Observe for bleeding gums, bruises, nosebleeds, hematuria, hematemesis, occult blood in the stool, and petechiae.

d. Instruct the client regarding measures to prevent bleeding.

e. The antidote to heparin is protamine sulfate.

f. When administering heparin subcutaneously, inject into the abdomen with a ⅝-inch (16-mm) needle (25 to 28 gauge) at a 90-degree angle and do not aspirate or rub the injection site.

g. Continuous IV infusions must be run on an infusion pump to ensure a precise rate of delivery.

D. Enoxaparin or Rivaroxaban—low-molecular-weight heparins

1. Description: Enoxaparin and rivaroxaban have the same mechanism of action and use as heparin but are not interchangeable with heparin; they have longer half-lives than heparin does.

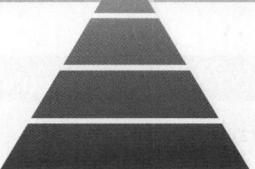

BOX 53-1 Anticoagulants

Oral
- Warfarin sodium
- Dabigatran etexilate mesylate
- Rivaroxaban
- Apixaban

Parenteral
- Argatroban
- Bivalirudin
- Dalteparin
- Desirudin
- Enoxaparin
- Fondaparinux
- Heparin sodium

BOX 53-2 Substances to Avoid with Anticoagulants

- Allopurinol
- Cimetidine
- Corticosteroids
- Green, leafy vegetables and other foods high in vitamin K
- Nonsteroidal antiinflammatory drugs
- Oral hypoglycemic agents
- Phenytoin
- Salicylates
- Sulfonamides
- Ginkgo and ginseng (herbs)

2. Interventions
   a. Administer enoxaparin only to the recumbent client by subcutaneous injection into the anterolateral or posterolateral abdominal wall; do not expel the air bubble from the prefilled syringe or aspirate during injection.
   b. Rivaroxaban is a taken orally, once daily.
   c. Monitor results of the Anti-Xa assay. The therapeutic range for anticoagulation is 0.5 to 1.2 IU/mL (conventional and SI units). Observe for bleeding.
   d. The antidote to low-molecular-weight heparins is protamine sulfate.

E. Warfarin sodium
1. Description
   a. Warfarin suppresses coagulation by acting as an antagonist of vitamin K by inhibiting 4 dependent clotting factors (X, IX, VII, and II).
   b. Warfarin prolongs clotting time and is monitored by the prothrombin time (PT) and the international normalized ratio (INR).
   c. It is used for long-term anticoagulation and is used mainly to prevent thromboembolic conditions such as thrombophlebitis, pulmonary embolism, and embolism formation caused by atrial fibrillation, thrombosis, myocardial infarction, or heart valve damage.
2. Blood levels
   a. The normal PT is 11 to 12.5 seconds (conventional and SI units).
   b. Warfarin sodium prolongs the PT; the therapeutic range is 1.5 to 2 times the control value.
3. INR
   a. The normal INR is 0.81 to 1.2 (0.81 to 1.2).
   b. The INR is determined by multiplying the observed PT ratio (the ratio of the client's PT to a control PT) by a correction factor specific to a particular thromboplastin preparation used in the testing.
   c. The treatment goal of warfarin sodium is to raise the INR to an appropriate value.
   d. An INR of 2 to 3 is appropriate for standard warfarin therapy; an INR of 3 to 4.5 is appropriate for high-dose warfarin therapy.
   e. If the PT value is longer than 30 seconds and the INR is greater than 3.0 in a client receiving standard warfarin therapy, initiate bleeding precautions.
   f. If the INR is below the recommended range, warfarin sodium should be increased.
   g. Clients may sometimes be prescribed "bridge therapy," whereby heparin sodium is used concurrently with warfarin sodium until the INR reaches the recommended range. Once this occurs, the heparin is discontinued.
4. Interventions
   a. Monitor PT and INR.
   b. Observe for bleeding gums, bruises, nosebleeds, hematuria, hematemesis, occult blood in the stool, and petechiae.
   c. Instruct the client regarding diet and measures to prevent bleeding.
   d. The antidote for warfarin is phytonadione.

F. Dabigatran etexilate
1. Description
   a. Dabigatran etexilate works through direct inhibition of thrombin, preventing the conversion of fibrinogen into fibrin and activation of factor XIII.
   b. Current approved use is for clot prevention associated with nonvalvular atrial fibrillation.
   c. It is administered in a fixed dose twice daily.
2. Blood levels: No blood testing is required.
3. Interventions: Same as for warfarin, except no routine monitoring is required.

II. Thrombolytic Medications (Box 53-3)

A. Description
1. Thrombolytic medications activate plasminogen; plasminogen generates plasmin (the enzyme that dissolves clots).

BOX 53-3 Thrombolytic Medications

- Alteplase
- Tenecteplase

2. Thrombolytic medications are used early in the course of myocardial infarction (within 4 to 6 hours of the onset of the infarct) to restore blood flow, limit myocardial damage, preserve left ventricular function, and prevent death.
3. Thrombolytics are also used in arterial thrombosis, deep vein thrombosis, occluded shunts or catheters, and pulmonary emboli.

B. Contraindications
1. Active internal bleeding
2. History of hemorrhagic stroke
3. Intracranial problems, including trauma
4. Intracranial or intraspinal surgery within the previous 2 months
5. Thoracic, pelvic, or abdominal surgery in the previous 10 days
6. History of hepatic or renal disease
7. Uncontrolled hypertension
8. Recent, prolonged cardiopulmonary resuscitation
9. Known allergy to the product or its preservatives

C. Side and adverse effects
1. Bleeding
2. Dysrhythmias
3. Allergic reactions

D. Interventions
1. Determine aPTT, PT, fibrinogen level, hematocrit, and platelet count.
2. Monitor vital signs.
3. Assess pulses.
4. Monitor for bleeding and check all excretions for occult blood.
5. Monitor for neurological changes such as slurred speech, lethargy, confusion, and hemiparesis.
6. Monitor for hypotension and tachycardia.
7. Avoid injections and venipunctures if possible.
8. Apply direct pressure over a puncture site for 20 to 30 minutes.
9. Handle the client gently and as little as possible when moving.
10. Instruct the client to use an electric razor for shaving and to brush teeth gently.
11. Withhold the medication if bleeding develops, and notify the primary health care provider (PHCP).
12. Antidote: Aminocaproic acid is the antidote.

Bleeding is the primary concern for a client taking an anticoagulant, thrombolytic, or antiplatelet medication.

III. Antiplatelet Medications (Box 53-4)

A. Description
1. Antiplatelet medications inhibit the aggregation of platelets in the clotting process, thereby prolonging the bleeding time.

BOX 53-4 Antiplatelet Medications

Oral	Parenteral
Acetylsalicylic acid	Abciximab
Anagrelide	Eptifibatide
Cilostazol	Tirofiban
Clopidogrel	
Dipyridamole	
Ticlopidine	
Ticagrelor	

2. Antiplatelet medications may be used with anticoagulants.
3. Used in the prophylaxis of long-term complications following myocardial infarction, coronary revascularization, stents, and stroke.
4. These medications are contraindicated in those with bleeding disorders and known sensitivity.

B. Side and adverse effects
1. Bruising
2. Hematuria
3. Gastrointestinal bleeding
4. Tarry stools

C. Interventions
1. A blood test may be prescribed to determine the client's sensitivity to the medication before beginning administration.
2. Monitor vital signs.
3. Instruct the client to take medication with food if gastrointestinal upset occurs.
4. Monitor bleeding time.
5. Instruct the client to monitor for side and adverse effects and in the measures to prevent bleeding.

IV. Positive Inotropic and Cardiotonic Medications (Box 53-5)

A. Description
1. These medications stimulate myocardial contractility and produce a positive inotropic effect.
2. These medications are used for short-term management of advanced heart failure; the increase in myocardial contractility improves cardiac, peripheral, and kidney function by increasing cardiac output, decreasing preload, improving blood flow to the periphery and kidneys, decreasing edema, and increasing fluid excretion. As a result, fluid retention in the lungs and extremities is decreased (Fig. 53-1).

B. Side and adverse effects
1. Dysrhythmias
2. Hypotension
3. Thrombocytopenia
4. Hepatotoxicity manifested by elevated liver enzyme levels

BOX 53-5 Positive Inotropic and Cardiotonic Medications

Dobutamine
- Used for short-term management of heart failure
- Increases myocardial contractility, thereby improving cardiac performance

Dopamine
- Used as a short-term rescue measure for clients with severe, acute heart failure
- Increases myocardial contractility, thereby improving cardiac performance
- Dilates renal blood vessels and increases renal blood flow and urine output

Milrinone Lactate
- Used for short-term management of heart failure; may be given before heart transplantation

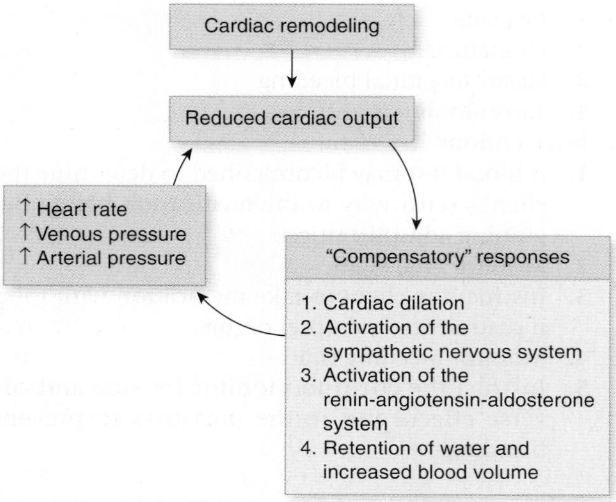

FIG. 53-1 The vicious cycle of maladaptive compensatory responses to a failing heart.

5. Hypersensitivity manifested by wheezing, shortness of breath, pruritus, urticaria, clammy skin, and flushing

C. Interventions
1. Positive inotropic and cardiotonic medications are used for intravenous (IV) administration.
   a. For continuous IV infusion, administer with an infusion pump.
   b. Stop the infusion if the client's blood pressure (BP) drops or dysrhythmias occur.
2. Monitor the apical pulse and BP.
3. Monitor for hypersensitivity.
4. Assess lung sounds for wheezing and crackles.
5. Monitor for edema.
6. Monitor for relief of heart failure as noted by reduction in edema and lessening of dyspnea, orthopnea, and fatigue.
7. Monitor electrolyte and liver enzyme levels, platelet count, and renal function studies; the medications may decrease potassium and increase liver enzyme levels; continuous electrocardiographic monitoring is done during administration.

V. Cardiac Glycosides

A. Digoxin
1. Description
   a. Cardiac glycosides inhibit the sodium-potassium pump, thus increasing intracellular calcium, which causes the heart muscle fibers to contract more efficiently.
   b. Cardiac glycosides produce a positive inotropic action, which increases the force of myocardial contractions.
   c. Cardiac glycosides produce a negative chronotropic action, which slows the heart rate.
   d. Cardiac glycosides produce a negative dromotropic action that slows conduction velocity through the atrioventricular (AV) node.
   e. The increase in myocardial contractility increases cardiac, peripheral, and kidney function by increasing cardiac output, decreasing preload, improving blood flow to the periphery and kidneys, decreasing edema, and increasing fluid excretion; as a result, fluid retention in the lungs and extremities is decreased.
   f. Cardiac glycosides are used second-line for heart failure (medications affecting the renin-angiotensin-aldosterone system are used more often) and cardiogenic shock, atrial tachycardia, atrial fibrillation, and atrial flutter; they are used less frequently for rate control in atrial dysrhythmias (beta blockers and calcium channel blockers are used more often).
   g. These medications are contraindicated in those with ventricular dysrhythmias and second- or third-degree heart block. They should be used with caution in clients with renal disease, hypothyroidism, and hypokalemia.
2. Side and adverse effects
   a. Anorexia, nausea, vomiting, diarrhea
   b. Bradycardia
   c. Visual disturbances: Diplopia, blurred vision, yellow vision, photophobia
   d. Headache
   e. Fatigue, weakness
   f. Drowsiness

Early signs of digoxin toxicity present as gastrointestinal manifestations (anorexia, nausea, vomiting, diarrhea); then, heart rate abnormalities and visual disturbances appear.

3. Interventions
   a. Monitor for toxicity as evidenced by anorexia, nausea, vomiting, visual disturbances (blurred or yellow vision), and dysrhythmias.
   b. Monitor serum digoxin level, electrolyte levels, and renal function test results.
   c. The optimal therapeutic range for digoxin is 0.5 to 2.0 ng/dL (0.63 to 2.56 nmol/L). However, a level on the low end of normal may be preferred to avoid toxicity.
   d. An increased risk of toxicity exists in clients with hypercalcemia, hypokalemia, hypomagnesemia, or hypothyroidism.
   e. Monitor the potassium level; if hypokalemia occurs (potassium lower than 3.5 mEq/L [3.5 mmol/L]), notify the PHCP.
   f. Instruct the client to avoid over-the-counter medications.
   g. Monitor the client taking a potassium-losing diuretic or corticosteroids closely for hypokalemia, because the hypokalemia can cause digoxin toxicity.
   h. Note that older clients are more sensitive to digoxin toxicity.
   i. Advise the client to eat foods high in potassium, such as fresh and dried fruits, fruit juices, vegetables, and potatoes.
   j. Monitor the apical pulse for 1 full minute; if the apical pulse rate is lower than 60 beats per minute, the medication should be withheld and the PHCP notified.
   k. Teach the client how to measure the pulse and to notify the PHCP if the pulse rate is lower than 60 or more than 100 beats per minute.
   l. Teach the client the signs and symptoms of toxicity.
   m. Antidote: Digoxin immune Fab is used in extreme toxicity.

VI. Antihypertensive Medications: Diuretics (Box 53-6)

A. Thiazide diuretics (Box 53-7)
1. Description
   a. Thiazide diuretics increase sodium and water excretion by inhibiting sodium reabsorption in the distal tubule of the kidney.
   b. Used for hypertension and peripheral edema

BOX 53-6 Classifications of Diuretics

- Loop diuretics
- Osmotic diuretics
- Potassium-retaining (sparing) diuretics
- Thiazide diuretics

BOX 53-7 Thiazide and Thiazide-Like Diuretics

- Chlorothiazide
- Chlorthalidone
- Hydrochlorothiazide
- Indapamide
- Metolazone

   c. Not effective for immediate diuresis
   d. Used in clients with normal renal function (contraindicated in clients with renal failure)
   e. Thiazide diuretics should be used with caution in the client taking lithium, because lithium toxicity can occur, and in the client taking digoxin, corticosteroids, or hypoglycemic medications.
2. Side and adverse effects
   a. Hypercalcemia, hyperglycemia, hyperuricemia
   b. Hypokalemia, hyponatremia
   c. Hypovolemia
   d. Hypotension
   e. Rashes
   f. Photosensitivity
   g. Dehydration
3. Interventions
   a. Monitor vital signs.
   b. Monitor weight.
   c. Monitor urine output.
   d. Monitor electrolytes, glucose, calcium, blood urea nitrogen (BUN), creatinine, and uric acid levels.
   e. Check peripheral extremities for edema.
   f. Monitor for signs of digoxin or lithium toxicity if the client is taking these medications.
   g. Instruct the client to take the medication in the morning to avoid nocturia and sleep interruption.
   h. Instruct the client in how to record the BP.
   i. Instruct the client to eat foods high in potassium.
   j. Instruct the client in how to take potassium supplements if prescribed.
   k. Instruct the client to take medication with food to avoid gastrointestinal upset.
   l. Instruct the client to change positions slowly to prevent **orthostatic hypotension.**
   m. Instruct the client to use sunscreen when in direct sunlight because of increased photosensitivity.
   n. Instruct the client with diabetes mellitus to have the blood glucose level checked periodically.

B. Loop diuretics (Box 53-8)
1. Description
   a. Loop diuretics inhibit sodium and chloride reabsorption from the loop of Henle and the distal tubule.
   b. Loop diuretics have little effect on the blood glucose level; however, they cause depletion

BOX 53-8 Loop Diuretics

- Bumetanide
- Ethacrynic acid
- Furosemide
- Torsemide

of water and electrolytes, increased uric acid levels, and the excretion of calcium.

c. Loop diuretics are more potent than thiazide diuretics, causing rapid diuresis, and thus decreasing vascular fluid volume, cardiac output, and BP.

d. Used for hypertension, pulmonary edema, edema associated with heart failure, hypercalcemia, and renal disease

e. Use loop diuretics with caution in the client taking digoxin or lithium and in the client taking aminoglycosides, anticoagulants, corticosteroids, or amphotericin B.

2. Side and adverse effects
- **a.** Hypokalemia, hyponatremia, hypocalcemia, hypomagnesemia
- **b.** Thrombocytopenia
- **c.** Hyperuricemia
- **d.** Orthostatic hypotension
- **e.** Rash
- **f.** Ototoxicity and deafness
- **g.** Thiamine deficiency
- **h.** Dehydration

3. Interventions: See section VI, A, 3 (Interventions for thiazide diuretics).
- **a.** Monitor electrolytes, calcium, magnesium, BUN, creatinine, and uric acid levels.
- **b.** Administer IV furosemide slowly over 1 to 2 minutes, because hearing loss can occur if injected rapidly.

C. Osmotic diuretics: See Chapter 59.

D. Potassium-retaining (sparing) diuretics (Box 53-9)

1. Description
- **a.** Potassium-retaining (sparing) diuretics act on the distal tubule to promote sodium and water excretion and potassium retention.
- **b.** Used for edema and hypertension, to increase urine output, and to treat fluid retention and overload associated with heart failure, ascites resulting from cirrhosis or nephrotic syndrome, and diuretic-induced hypokalemia.
- **c.** Potassium-retaining (sparing) diuretics are contraindicated in severe kidney or hepatic disease and in severe hyperkalemia.
- **d.** Potassium-retaining (sparing) diuretics should be used with caution in the client with diabetes mellitus, taking antihypertensives or lithium, or taking angiotensin-converting enzyme inhibitors or potassium supplements, because hyperkalemia can result.

⚠ The primary concern with administering potassium-retaining (sparing) diuretics is hyperkalemia.

2. Side and adverse effects
- **a.** Hyperkalemia
- **b.** Nausea, vomiting, diarrhea
- **c.** Rash
- **d.** Dizziness, weakness
- **e.** Headache
- **f.** Dry mouth
- **g.** Photosensitivity
- **h.** Anemia
- **i.** Thrombocytopenia

3. Interventions
- **a.** Monitor vital signs.
- **b.** Monitor urine output.
- **c.** Monitor for signs and symptoms of hyperkalemia such as nausea; diarrhea; abdominal cramps; tachycardia followed by bradycardia; tall, peaked T waves on the electrocardiogram; and oliguria.
- **d.** Monitor for a potassium level greater than 5.0 mEq/L (5.0 mmol/L), which indicates hyperkalemia.
- **e.** Instruct the client to avoid foods high in potassium.
- **f.** Instruct the client to avoid exposure to direct sunlight.
- **g.** Instruct the client to monitor for signs of hyperkalemia.
- **h.** Instruct the client to avoid salt substitutes because they contain potassium.
- **i.** Instruct the client to take the medication with or after meals to decrease gastrointestinal irritation.

VII. Peripherally Acting α-Adrenergic Blockers (Box 53-10)

A. Description

1. These medications decrease sympathetic vasoconstriction by reducing the effects of

BOX 53-9 Potassium-Retaining Diuretics

- Amiloride hydrochloride
- Eplerenone
- Spironolactone
- Triamterene

BOX 53-10 Peripherally Acting α-Adrenergic Blockers

- Doxazosin
- Prazosin
- Terazosin

norepinephrine at peripheral nerve endings, resulting in vasodilation and decreased BP.
2. These medications are used to maintain renal blood flow.
3. These medications are used to treat hypertension.

B. Side and adverse effects
1. Orthostatic hypotension
2. Reflex tachycardia
3. Sodium and water retention
4. Edema
5. Weight gain
6. Gastrointestinal disturbances
7. Drowsiness
8. Nasal congestion

C. Interventions
1. Monitor vital signs.
2. Monitor for fluid retention and edema.
3. Instruct the client to change positions slowly to prevent orthostatic hypotension.
4. Instruct the client in how to monitor the BP.
5. Instruct the client to monitor for edema.
6. Instruct the client to decrease salt intake.
7. Instruct the client to avoid over-the-counter medications.

VIII. Centrally Acting Sympatholytics (Adrenergic Blockers) (Box 53-11)

A. Description
1. Centrally acting sympatholytics stimulate α-receptors in the central nervous system to inhibit vasoconstriction, thus reducing peripheral resistance.
2. Used to treat hypertension
3. Contraindicated in impaired liver function

B. Side and adverse effects
1. Sodium and water retention
2. Edema
3. Drowsiness, dizziness
4. Dry mouth
5. Hypotension
6. Bradycardia
7. Impotence
8. Depression

C. Interventions
1. Monitor vital signs.
2. Instruct the client not to discontinue medication, because abrupt withdrawal can cause severe rebound hypertension.
3. Monitor liver function tests.

BOX 53-11 Centrally Acting Sympatholytics (Adrenergic Blockers)

- Clonidine
- Guanfacine
- Methyldopa

BOX 53-12 Angiotensin-Converting Enzyme Inhibitors and Angiotensin II Receptor Blockers

Angiotensin-Converting Enzyme Inhibitors	Angiotensin II Receptor Blockers
Benazepril	Candesartan
Captopril	Eprosartan
Fosinopril	Irbesartan
Enalapril	Losartan
Lisinopril	Olmesartan
Moexipril	Telmisartan
Perindopril	Valsartan
Quinapril	
Ramipril	
Trandolapril	

IX. Angiotensin-Converting Enzyme (ACE) Inhibitors and Angiotensin II Receptor Blockers (ARBs) (Box 53-12)

A. Description
1. ACE inhibitors prevent peripheral vasoconstriction by blocking conversion of angiotensin I to angiotensin II (AII).
2. ARBs prevent peripheral vasoconstriction and secretion of aldosterone and block the binding of AII to type 1 AII receptors.
3. These medications are used to treat hypertension and heart failure; also, ACE inhibitors are administered for their cardioprotective effect after myocardial infarction.
4. Avoid use with potassium supplements and potassium-retaining (sparing) diuretics.

B. Side and adverse effects
1. Nausea, vomiting, diarrhea
2. Persistent dry cough (ACE inhibitors)
3. Hypotension
4. Hyperkalemia
5. Tachycardia
6. Headache
7. Dizziness, fatigue
8. Insomnia
9. Hypoglycemic reaction in the client with diabetes mellitus
10. Bruising, petechiae, bleeding
11. Diminished taste (ACE inhibitors)

A persistent dry cough is a common complaint for those taking an ACE inhibitor, but this often subsides after a few weeks. Instruct the client to contact the PHCP if this occurs and persists.

C. Interventions
1. Monitor vital signs.
2. Monitor white blood cells, and protein, albumin, BUN, creatinine, and potassium levels.

3. Monitor for hypoglycemic reactions in the client with diabetes mellitus.
4. If captopril is prescribed, instruct the client to take the medication 20 to 60 minutes before a meal.
5. Monitor for bruising, petechiae, or bleeding with captopril.
6. Instruct the client not to discontinue medications, because rebound hypertension can occur.
7. Instruct the client not to take over-the-counter medications.
8. Instruct the client in how to take the BP.
9. Inform the client that the taste of food may be diminished during the first month of therapy.
10. Instruct the client to report adverse effects to the PHCP.

X. Antianginal Medications (Box 53-13)

A. Nitrates (see Priority Nursing Actions)

PRIORITY NURSING ACTIONS

Chest Pain in a Hospitalized Client with Cardiac Disease

1. Quickly assess the client, specifically characteristics of pain, heart rate and rhythm, and blood pressure (BP).
2. Administer a nitroglycerin tablet sublingually.
3. Stay with the client.
4. Reassess in 5 minutes.
5. Administer another nitroglycerin tablet sublingually if pain is not relieved and the BP is stable.
6. Reassess in 5 minutes.
7. Administer a third nitroglycerin tablet sublingually if pain is not relieved and the BP is stable.
8. Reassess in 5 minutes; contact the primary health care provider (PHCP) if the third nitroglycerin tablet does not relieve the pain.
9. Document the event, actions taken, and the client's response to treatment.

Reference

Burchum, Rosenthal (2016), pp. 604-605, 622.

1. Description
   a. Nitrates produce vasodilation, decrease preload and **afterload**, and reduce myocardial oxygen consumption.

BOX 53-13 Antianginal Medications (Organic Nitrates)

- Isosorbide dinitrate
- Isosorbide mononitrate
- Nitroglycerin, sublingual
- Nitroglycerin, translingual
- Nitroglycerin, transdermal patches
- Nitroglycerin ointment
- Intravenous nitroglycerin

   b. Contraindicated in the client with significant hypotension, increased intracranial pressure, or severe anemia and in those taking medication to treat erectile dysfunction
   c. Should be used with caution with severe renal or hepatic disease
   d. Avoid abrupt withdrawal of long-acting preparations to prevent the rebound effect of severe pain from myocardial ischemia.
2. Side and adverse effects
   a. Headache
   b. Orthostatic hypotension
   c. Dizziness, weakness
   d. Faintness
   e. Flushing or pallor
   f. Dry mouth
   g. Reflex tachycardia
3. Sublingual medications
   a. Monitor vital signs.
   b. Offer sips of water before giving, because dryness may inhibit medication absorption.
   c. Instruct the client to place under the tongue and leave until fully dissolved.
   d. Instruct the client not to swallow the medication.
   e. Instruct the at-home client to take 1 tablet for pain and to immediately contact emergency medical services if pain is not relieved; in the hospitalized client, 1 tablet is administered every 5 minutes for a total of 3 doses and the PHCP is notified immediately if pain is not relieved following the 3 doses (the BP is checked before each administration).
   f. Inform the client that a stinging or burning sensation may indicate that the tablet is fresh.
   g. Instruct the client to store medication in a dark, tightly closed bottle.
   h. Instruct the client to take acetaminophen for a headache.
4. Translingual medications (spray)
   a. Instruct the client to direct the spray against the oral mucosa.
   b. Instruct the client to avoid inhaling the spray.
5. Sustained-released medications: Instruct the client to swallow and not to chew or crush the medication.
6. Transdermal patch
   a. Instruct the client to apply the patch to a hairless area, using a new patch and different site each day.
   b. As prescribed, instruct the client to remove the patch after 12 to 14 hours, allowing 10 to 12 "patch-free" hours each day to prevent tolerance.
7. Topical ointments
   a. Instruct the client to remove the ointment on the skin from the previous dose.

b. Instruct the client to squeeze a ribbon of ointment of the prescribed length onto the applicator or dose-measuring paper.
c. Instruct the client to spread the ointment over a 2.5- by 3.5-inch (6.5 by 9 cm) area and cover with plastic wrap, using the chest, back, abdomen, upper arm, or anterior thigh (avoid hairy areas).
d. Instruct the client to rotate sites and to avoid touching the ointment when applying.

8. Patches and ointments
   a. Wear gloves when applying.
   b. Do not apply on the chest in the area of defibrillator-cardioverter pad placement, because skin burns can result if the pads need to be used.

Instruct the client using nitroglycerin tablets to check the expiration date on the medication bottle, because expiration may occur within 6 months of obtaining the medication. The tablets will not relieve chest pain if they have expired.

XI. β-Adrenergic Blockers (Box 53-14)

A. Description
1. β-Adrenergic blockers inhibit response to β-adrenergic stimulation, thus decreasing cardiac output.
2. They block the release of catecholamines, epinephrine, and norepinephrine, thus decreasing the heart rate and BP; they also decrease the workload of the heart and decrease oxygen demands.
3. Used for angina, dysrhythmias, hypertension, migraine headaches, prevention of myocardial infarction, and glaucoma
4. β-Adrenergic blockers are contraindicated in the client with asthma, bradycardia, heart failure (with exceptions), severe renal or hepatic disease, hyperthyroidism, or stroke; carvedilol, metoprolol, and bisoprolol have been approved for use in heart failure once the client has been stabilized by ACE inhibitor and diuretic therapy.
5. β-Adrenergic blockers should be used with caution in the client with diabetes mellitus, because the medication may mask symptoms of hypoglycemia.
6. β-Adrenergic blockers should be used with caution in the client taking antihypertensive medications.

B. Side and adverse effects
1. Bradycardia
2. Bronchospasm
3. Hypotension
4. Weakness, fatigue
5. Nausea, vomiting
6. Dizziness
7. Hyperglycemia
8. Agranulocytosis
9. Behavioral or psychotic response
10. Depression
11. Nightmares

C. Interventions
1. Monitor vital signs.
2. Withhold the medication if the pulse or BP is not within the prescribed parameters.
3. Monitor for signs of heart failure or worsening heart failure.
4. Assess for respiratory distress and for signs of wheezing and dyspnea.
5. Instruct the client to report dizziness, lightheadedness, or nasal congestion.
6. Instruct the client not to stop the medication, because rebound hypertension, rebound tachycardia, or an anginal attack can occur.
7. Advise the client taking insulin that the β-adrenergic blocker can mask early signs of hypoglycemia, such as tachycardia and nervousness.
8. Instruct the client taking insulin to monitor the blood glucose level.
9. Instruct the client in how to take pulse and BP.
10. Instruct the client to change positions slowly to prevent orthostatic hypotension.
11. Instruct the client to avoid over-the-counter medications, especially cold medications and nasal decongestants.

BOX 53-14 β-Adrenergic Blockers

Nonselective (Block β_1 and β_2)	Cardioselective (Block β_1)
Carvedilol	Acebutolol
Labetalol	Atenolol
Nadolol	Betaxolol
Pindolol	Bisoprolol
Propranolol	Esmolol
Sotalol	Metoprolol

XII. Calcium Channel Blockers (Box 53-15)

A. Description
1. Calcium channel blockers decrease cardiac contractility (negative inotropic effect by relaxing smooth muscle) and the workload of the heart, thus decreasing the need for oxygen.

BOX 53-15 Calcium Channel Blockers

Amlodipine	Nicardipine
Clevidipine	Nifedipine
Diltiazem	Nimodipine
Felodipine	Nisoldipine
Isradipine	Verapamil

2. Calcium channel blockers promote vasodilation of the coronary and peripheral vessels.
3. Used for angina, dysrhythmias, or hypertension
4. Should be used with caution in the client with heart failure, bradycardia, or atrioventricular block

B. Side and adverse effects
   1. Bradycardia
   2. Hypotension
   3. Reflex tachycardia as a result of hypotension
   4. Headache
   5. Dizziness, lightheadedness
   6. Fatigue
   7. Peripheral edema
   8. Constipation
   9. Flushing of the skin
   10. Changes in liver and kidney function

C. Interventions
   1. Monitor vital signs.
   2. Monitor for signs of heart failure.
   3. Monitor liver enzyme levels.
   4. Monitor kidney function tests.
   5. Instruct the client not to discontinue the medication.
   6. Instruct the client in how to take the pulse.
   7. Instruct the client to notify the PHCP if dizziness or fainting occurs.
   8. Instruct the client not to crush or chew sustained-release tablets.

XIII. Peripheral Vasodilators (Box 53-16)

A. Description
   1. Peripheral vasodilators decrease peripheral resistance by exerting a direct action on the arteries or on the arteries and the veins.
   2. These medications increase blood flow to the extremities and are used in peripheral vascular disorders of venous and arterial vessels.
   3. Peripheral vasodilators are most effective for disorders resulting from vasospasm (Raynaud's disease).

BOX 53-16 Peripheral Vasodilators

α-Adrenergic Blockers
- Doxazosin
- Prazosin
- Terazosin

Calcium Channel Blockers
- Diltiazem
- Nifedipine
- Nimodipine
- Verapamil

Hemorheological
- Pentoxifylline (increases microcirculation and tissue perfusion)

   4. These medications may decrease some symptoms of cerebral vascular insufficiency.

B. Side and adverse effects
   1. Lightheadedness, dizziness
   2. Orthostatic hypotension
   3. Tachycardia
   4. Palpitations
   5. Flushing
   6. Gastrointestinal distress

C. Interventions
   1. Monitor vital signs, especially the BP and the heart rate.
   2. Monitor for orthostatic hypotension and tachycardia.
   3. Monitor for signs of inadequate blood flow to the extremities, such as pallor, feeling cold, and pain.
   4. Instruct the client that it may take up to 3 months for a desired therapeutic response.
   5. Advise the client not to smoke, because smoking increases vasospasm.
   6. Instruct the client to avoid aspirin or aspirin-like compounds unless approved by the PHCP.
   7. Instruct the client to take the medication with meals if gastrointestinal disturbances occur.
   8. Instruct the client to avoid alcohol, because it may cause a hypotensive reaction.
   9. Encourage the client to change positions slowly to avoid orthostatic hypotension.

XIV. Direct-Acting Arteriolar Vasodilators (Box 53-17)

A. Description
   1. Direct-acting vasodilators relax the smooth muscles of the blood vessels, mainly the arteries, causing vasodilation; with vasodilation, the BP drops and sodium and water are retained, resulting in peripheral edema (diuretics may be given to decrease the edema).
   2. Direct-acting vasodilators promote an increase in blood flow to the brain and kidneys.
   3. These medications are used in the client with moderate to severe hypertension and for acute hypertensive emergencies.

B. Side and adverse effects
   1. Hypotension
   2. Reflex tachycardia caused by vasodilation and the drop in BP
   3. Palpitations
   4. Edema
   5. Dizziness

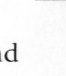

BOX 53-17 Direct-Acting Arteriolar Vasodilators

- Diazoxide
- Fenoldopam
- Hydralazine
- Nitroglycerin
- Sodium nitroprusside

6. Headaches
7. Nasal congestion
8. Gastrointestinal bleeding
9. Neurological symptoms
10. Confusion
11. With sodium nitroprusside, cyanide toxicity and thiocyanate toxicity can occur.

C. Interventions
1. Monitor vital signs, especially BP.
2. Sodium nitroprusside
   a. Monitor cyanide and thiocyanate levels.
   b. Protect from light because the medication decomposes.
   c. When administering, solution must be covered by a dark bag provided by the manufacturer and is stable for 24 hours.
   d. Discard if the medication is red, green, or blue.

Vasodilators cause orthostatic hypotension. Instruct the client about safety measures when taking these medications, such as when rising from a lying to a sitting or standing position slowly.

XV. Miscellaneous Vasodilator

A. Description
1. Nesiritide
   a. Recombinant version of human B-type natriuretic peptide that vasodilates arteries and veins
   b. Used for the treatment of decompensated heart failure
2. Side and adverse effects
   a. Hypotension
   b. Confusion
   c. Dizziness
   d. Dysrhythmias
3. Interventions
   a. Administer by continuous IV infusion via infusion device
   b. Monitor BP, cardiac rhythm, urine output, and body weight.
   c. Monitor for signs of resolving heart failure.

XVI. Antidysrhythmic Medications

A. Description: Antidysrhythmic medications suppress dysrhythmias by inhibiting abnormal pathways of electrical conduction through the heart.

B. Class I antidysrhythmics are sodium channel blockers, class II are beta blockers, class III are potassium channel blockers (medications that delay repolarization), and class IV are calcium channel blockers.

C. Class IA antidysrhythmics
1. Disopyramide
2. Procainamide
3. Quinidine sulfate

D. Class IB antidysrhythmics
1. Lidocaine
2. Mexiletine hydrochloride
3. Phenytoin

E. Class IC antidysrhythmics
1. Flecainide acetate
2. Propafenone hydrochloride
3. Side and adverse effects: Class I antidysrhythmics
   a. Hypotension
   b. Heart failure
   c. Worsened or new dysrhythmias
   d. Nausea, vomiting, or diarrhea

F. Class II antidysrhythmics
1. Acebutolol
2. Esmolol
3. Propranolol
4. Metoprolol
5. Nadolol
6. Atenolol
7. Side and adverse effects: Class II antidysrhythmics
   a. Dizziness
   b. Fatigue
   c. Hypotension
   d. Bradycardia
   e. Heart failure
   f. Dysrhythmias
   g. Heart block
   h. Bronchospasms
   i. Gastrointestinal distress

G. Class III antidysrhythmics
1. Amiodarone
2. Dofetilide
3. Ibutilide
4. Sotalol
5. Side and adverse effects: Class III antidysrhythmics
   a. Hypotension
   b. Bradycardia
   c. Nausea, vomiting
   d. Amiodarone hydrochloride may cause pulmonary fibrosis, photosensitivity, bluish skin discoloration, corneal deposits, peripheral neuropathy, tremor, poor coordination, abnormal gait, and hypothyroidism.
   e. The electrocardiogram should be monitored for clients receiving amiodarone or dofetilide, because they may prolong the QT interval, potentially leading to torsades de pointes.

H. Class IV antidysrhythmics
1. Verapamil
2. Diltiazem
3. Side and adverse effects: Class IV antidysrhythmics
   a. Dizziness
   b. Hypotension
   c. Bradycardia
   d. Edema
   e. Constipation

I. Other antidysrhythmics
1. Adenosine
2. Digoxin

J. Interventions for antidysrhythmics
1. Monitor heart rate, respiratory rate, and BP.
2. Monitor electrocardiogram.
3. Provide continuous cardiac monitoring.
4. Maintain therapeutic serum medication levels.
5. Before administering lidocaine, always check the vial label to prevent administering a form that contains epinephrine or preservatives, because these solutions are used for local anesthesia only.
6. Do not administer antidysrhythmics with food, because food may affect absorption.
7. Mexiletine may be administered with food or antacids to reduce gastrointestinal distress.
8. Always administer IV antidysrhythmics via an infusion pump.
9. Monitor for signs of fluid retention such as weight gain, peripheral edema, or shortness of breath.
10. Advise the client to limit fluid and salt intake to minimize fluid retention.
11. Monitor respiratory, thyroid, and neurological functions.
12. Instruct the client to change positions slowly to minimize orthostatic hypotension.
13. Instruct the client taking amiodarone to use sunscreen and protective clothing to prevent photosensitivity reactions.
14. Encourage the client to increase fiber intake to prevent constipation.

XVII. Adrenergic Agonists (Box 53-18)

A. Dobutamine
1. Increases myocardial force and cardiac output through stimulation of β-receptors
2. Used in clients with heart failure and for clients undergoing cardiopulmonary bypass surgery

B. Dopamine
1. Increases BP and cardiac output through positive inotropic action and increases renal blood flow through its action on α- and β-receptors
2. Used to treat mild kidney failure caused by low cardiac output

C. Epinephrine
1. Used for cardiac stimulation in cardiac arrest
2. Used for bronchodilation in asthma or allergic reactions
3. Produces mydriasis
4. Produces local vasoconstriction when combined with local anesthetics and prolongs anesthetic action by decreasing blood flow to the site

D. Norepinephrine
1. Stimulates the heart in cardiac arrest
2. Vasoconstricts and increases the BP in hypotension and shock

E. Side and adverse effects
1. Dysrhythmias
2. Tachycardia
3. Angina
4. Restlessness
5. Urgency or urinary incontinence

F. Interventions
1. Monitor vital signs.
2. Monitor lung sounds.
3. Monitor urinary output.
4. Monitor electrocardiogram.
5. Administer the medication through a large vein.

BOX 53-18 Adrenergic Agonists

- Dobutamine
- Dopamine
- Epinephrine
- Norepinephrine

XVIII. Antilipemic Medications

A. Description
1. Antilipemic medications reduce serum levels of cholesterol, triglycerides, or low-density lipoprotein.
2. When cholesterol, triglyceride, and low-density lipoprotein levels are elevated, the client is at increased risk for coronary artery disease.
3. In many cases, diet alone will not lower blood lipid levels; therefore, antilipemic medications will be prescribed.

B. Bile sequestrants (see Chapter 49)
1. Description
a. Bind with acids in the intestines, which prevents reabsorption of cholesterol
b. Should not be used as the only therapy in clients with elevated triglyceride levels because they may raise triglyceride levels
2. Side and adverse effects
a. Constipation
b. Gastrointestinal disturbances: Heartburn, nausea, belching, bloating
3. Interventions
a. Cholestyramine comes in a gritty powder that must be mixed thoroughly in juice or water before administration.
b. Monitor the client for early signs of peptic ulcer such as nausea and abdominal discomfort followed by abdominal pain and distention.
c. Instruct the client that the medication must be taken with and followed by sufficient fluids.

C. HMG-CoA reductase inhibitors (Box 53-19)
1. Description
a. Lovastatin is highly protein-bound and should not be administered with anticoagulants.

BOX 53-19 HMG-CoA Reductase Inhibitors

- Atorvastatin
- Fluvastatin
- Lovastatin
- Pitavastatin
- Pravastatin
- Rosuvastatin
- Simvastatin

b. Lovastatin should not be administered with gemfibrozil.
c. Administer lovastatin with caution to the client taking immunosuppressive medications.

2. Side and adverse effects
   a. Nausea
   b. Diarrhea or constipation
   c. Abdominal pain or cramps
   d. Flatulence
   e. Dizziness
   f. Headache
   g. Blurred vision
   h. Rash
   i. Pruritus
   j. Elevated liver enzyme levels
   k. Muscle cramps and fatigue
3. Interventions
   a. Monitor serum liver enzyme levels.
   b. Instruct the client to have an annual eye examination, because the medications can cause cataract formation.
   c. If lovastatin is not effective in lowering the lipid level after 3 months, it should be discontinued.

! Instruct the client who is taking an antilipemic medication to report any unexplained muscular pain to the PHCP immediately.

D. Other antilipemic medications (Box 53-20)
1. Description
   a. Gemfibrozil should not be taken with anticoagulants, because they compete for protein sites; if the client is taking an anticoagulant, the anticoagulant dose should be reduced during antilipemic therapy and the INR should be monitored closely.
   b. Do not administer gemfibrozil with HMG-CoA reductase inhibitors, because it increases the risk for myositis, myalgias, and rhabdomyolysis.

BOX 53-20 Other Antilipemic Medications

- Cholestyramine
- Colesevelam
- Colestipol
- Ezetimibe
- Lomitapide
- Fenofibrate
- Gemfibrozil
- Nicotinic acid

   c. Fish oil supplements have been associated with a decreased risk for cardiovascular heart disease; plant stanol and sterol esters and cholestin have been associated with reducing cholesterol levels.
2. Interventions
   a. Monitor vital signs.
   b. Monitor liver enzyme levels.
   c. Monitor serum cholesterol and triglyceride levels.
   d. Instruct the client that it will take several weeks before the lipid level declines.
   e. Instruct the client to restrict intake of fats, cholesterol, carbohydrates, and alcohol.
   f. Instruct the client to follow an exercise program.
   g. Instruct the client to have an annual eye examination and to report changes in vision.
   h. Instruct the client with diabetes mellitus who is taking gemfibrozil to monitor blood glucose levels regularly.
   i. Instruct the client to increase fluid intake.
   j. Nicotinic acid has numerous side and adverse effects, including gastrointestinal disturbances, flushing of the skin, elevated liver enzyme levels, hyperglycemia, and hyperuricemia.
   k. Instruct the client that taking aspirin or nonsteroidal antiinflammatory drugs 30 minutes before nicotinic acid may assist in reducing the side effect of cutaneous flushing.
   l. Instruct the client to take nicotinic acid with meals to reduce gastrointestinal discomfort.

PRACTICE QUESTIONS

625. A client with atrial fibrillation is receiving a continuous heparin infusion at 1000 units/hr. The nurse determines that the client is receiving the therapeutic effect based on which results?
1. Prothrombin time of 12.5 seconds
2. Activated partial thromboplastin time of 28 seconds
3. Activated partial thromboplastin time of 60 seconds
4. Activated partial thromboplastin time longer than 120 seconds

626. The nurse provides discharge instructions to a client with atrial fibrillation who is taking warfarin sodium. Which statement, by the client, reflects the **need for further teaching**?
1. "I will avoid alcohol consumption."
2. "I will take my pills every day at the same time."
3. "I have already called my family to pick up a MedicAlert bracelet."
4. "I will take coated aspirin for my headaches because it will coat my stomach."

627. A client who is receiving digoxin daily has a serum potassium level of 3 mEq/L (3 mmol/L) and reports anorexia. The health care provider prescribes a serum digoxin level to be done. The nurse checks the results and should recognize which level that is outside of the therapeutic range?

1. 0.5 ng/mL (0.63 nmol/L)
2. 0.8 ng/mL (1.02 nmol/L)
3. 0.9 ng/mL (1.14 nmol/L)
4. 2.2 ng/mL (2.8 nmol/L)

628. A client is being treated with procainamide for a cardiac dysrhythmia. Following intravenous administration of the medication, the client complains of dizziness. What intervention should the nurse take **first**?

1. Obtain a 12-lead electrocardiogram.
2. Check the client's fingerstick blood glucose level.
3. Auscultate the client's apical pulse and blood pressure.
4. Measure the QRS interval duration on the rhythm strip.

629. The nurse is monitoring a client with hypertension who is taking propranolol. Which assessment finding indicates a potential adverse complication associated with this medication?

1. Report of infrequent insomnia
2. Development of expiratory wheezes
3. A baseline blood pressure of 150/80 mm Hg followed by a blood pressure of 138/72 mm Hg after 2 doses of the medication
4. A baseline resting heart rate of 88 beats per minute followed by a resting heart rate of 72 beats per minute after 2 doses of the medication

630. A client with valvular heart disease who has a clot in the right atrium is receiving a heparin sodium infusion at 1000 units/hr and warfarin sodium 7.5 mg at 5:00 p.m. daily. The morning laboratory results are as follows: activated partial thromboplastin time (aPTT), 32 seconds; international normalized ratio (INR), 1.3. The nurse should take which action based on the client's laboratory results?

1. Collaborate with the primary health care provider (PHCP) to discontinue the heparin infusion and administer the warfarin sodium as prescribed.
2. Collaborate with the PHCP to obtain a prescription to increase the heparin infusion and continue the warfarin sodium as prescribed.
3. Collaborate with the PHCP to withhold the warfarin sodium since the client is receiving a heparin infusion and the aPTT is within the therapeutic range.
4. Collaborate with the PHCP to continue the heparin infusion at the same rate and to discuss use of dabigatran etexilate in place of warfarin sodium.

631. A client is diagnosed with an ST segment elevation myocardial infarction (STEMI) and is receiving a tissue plasminogen activator, alteplase. Which action is a **priority** nursing intervention?

1. Monitor for kidney failure.
2. Monitor psychosocial status.
3. Monitor for signs of bleeding.
4. Have heparin sodium available.

632. The nurse is monitoring a client for adverse effects of medications. Which findings are characteristic of adverse effects of hydrochlorothiazide? **Select all that apply.**

- ❑ 1. Sulfa allergy
- ❑ 2. Osteoporosis
- ❑ 3. Hypokalemia
- ❑ 4. Hypouricemia
- ❑ 5. Hyperglycemia
- ❑ 6. Hypercalcemia

633. The home health care nurse is visiting a client with coronary artery disease with elevated triglyceride levels and a serum cholesterol level of 398 mg/dL (10 mmol/L). The client is taking cholestyramine, and the nurse teaches the client about the medication. Which statement by the client indicates the **need for further teaching**?

1. "Constipation and bloating might be a problem."
2. "I'll continue to watch my diet and reduce my fats."
3. "Walking a mile each day will help the whole process."
4. "I'll continue my nicotinic acid from the health food store."

634. The nurse is monitoring a client with heart failure who is taking digoxin. Which findings are characteristic of digoxin toxicity? **Select all that apply.**

- ❑ 1. Tremors
- ❑ 2. Diarrhea
- ❑ 3. Irritability
- ❑ 4. Blurred vision
- ❑ 5. Nausea and vomiting

635. Prior to administering a client's daily dose of digoxin to treat heart failure, the nurse reviews the client's laboratory data and notes the following results: serum calcium, 9.8 mg/dL (2.45 mmol/L); serum magnesium, 1.0 mEq/L (0.4 mmol/L); serum potassium, 4.1 mEq/L (4.1 mmol/L); serum creatinine, 0.9 mg/dL (79.5 mcmol/L). Which result should alert the nurse that the client is at risk for digoxin toxicity?

1. Serum calcium level
2. Serum potassium level
3. Serum creatinine level
4. Serum magnesium level

636. The nurse administered intravenous bumetanide to a client being treated for heart failure. Which outcome indicates that the medication has achieved the expected effect?

1. Cough becomes productive of frothy pink sputum.
2. Urine output increases from 10 mL/hr to greater than 50 mL hourly.
3. The serum potassium level changes from 3.8 to 3.1 mEq/L (3.8 to 3.1 mmol/L).
4. B-type natriuretic peptide (BNP) factor increases from 200 to 262 ng/mL (200 to 262 mcg/L).

637. Intravenous heparin therapy is prescribed for a client with atrial fibrillation. While implementing this prescription, the nurse ensures that which medication is available on the nursing unit?

1. Vitamin K
2. Protamine sulfate
3. Potassium chloride
4. Aminocaproic acid

638. A client receiving thrombolytic therapy with a continuous infusion of alteplase suddenly becomes extremely anxious and reports itching. The nurse hears stridor and notes generalized urticaria and hypotension. Which interventions should the nurse anticipate? **Select all that apply.**

- ❑ 1. Stop the infusion.
- ❑ 2. Raise the head of the bed.
- ❑ 3. Administer protamine sulfate.
- ❑ 4. Administer diphenhydramine.
- ❑ 5. Call for the Rapid Response Team (RRT).

639. The nurse should report which assessment finding to the primary health care provider (PHCP) before initiating thrombolytic therapy in a client with pulmonary embolism?

1. Adventitious breath sounds
2. Temperature of 99.4° F (37.4° C) orally
3. Blood pressure of 198/110 mm Hg
4. Respiratory rate of 28 breaths per minute

640. The nurse provides instructions to the client about nicotinic acid prescribed for hyperlipidemia. Which statement by the client indicates understanding of the instructions?

1. "The medication should be taken with meals to decrease flushing."
2. "It is not necessary to avoid the use of alcohol when taking nicotinic acid."
3. "Clay-colored stools are a common side effect and should not be of concern."
4. "Ibuprofen taken 30 minutes before the nicotinic acid may decrease the flushing."

ANSWERS

625. *Answer:* 3

Rationale: Common laboratory ranges for activated partial thromboplastin time (aPTT) are 30 to 40 seconds. Because the aPTT should be 1.5 to 2.5 times the normal value, the client's aPTT would be considered therapeutic if it was 60 seconds. Prothrombin time assesses response to warfarin therapy.

Test-Taking Strategy: Focus on the **subject**, the therapeutic effect of heparin. Prothrombin time is eliminated because it assesses response to warfarin therapy. The aPTT of 28 seconds is eliminated because this result indicates that the client is receiving no therapeutic effect from the continuous heparin infusion. Finally, the aPTT greater than 120 seconds can be eliminated because this value is beyond the therapeutic range and the client is at risk for bleeding.

Level of Cognitive Ability: Evaluating

Client Needs: Physiological Integrity

Integrated Process: Nursing Process—Evaluation

Content Area: Pharmacology: Cardiovascular Medications: Anticoagulants

Health Problem: Adult Health: Cardiovascular: Dysrhythmias

Priority Concepts: Clotting; Safety

References: Gahart, Nazareno (2015), pp. 620-621, 624; Ignatavicius, Workman (2016), pp. 607-608.

626. *Answer:* 4

Rationale: Aspirin-containing products need to be avoided when a client is taking this medication. Alcohol consumption should be avoided by a client taking warfarin sodium. Taking the prescribed medication at the same time each day increases client compliance. The MedicAlert bracelet provides health care personnel with emergency information.

Test-Taking Strategy: Note the **strategic words**, *need for further teaching*. These words indicate a **negative event query** and ask you to select an option that is an incorrect statement. Recalling that warfarin is an anticoagulant and that coated aspirin is an aspirin-containing product will direct you to the correct option.

Level of Cognitive Ability: Evaluating

Client Needs: Physiological Integrity

Integrated Process: Teaching and Learning

Content Area: Pharmacology: Cardiovascular Medications: Anticoagulants

Health Problem: Adult Health: Cardiovascular: Dysrhythmias

Priority Concepts: Client Education; Safety

Reference: Hodgson, Kizior (2015), pp. 89, 1289-1290.

627. *Answer:* 4

Rationale: The optimal therapeutic range for digoxin is 0.5 to 2.0 ng/mL (0.63 to 2.56 nmol/L). If the client is experiencing symptoms such as anorexia and is experiencing hypokalemia as evidenced by a low potassium level, digoxin toxicity is a concern. Therefore, option 4 is correct because it is outside of the therapeutic level and elevated.

Test-Taking Strategy: Focus on the **subject**, a digoxin level outside of the therapeutic range. Additionally, **determine if an abnormality exists.** Note that the client is experiencing

anorexia and has a low serum potassium level. Therefore, it is best to select the option that identifies the highest level. Recall that in hypokalemia, the client is at greater risk for digoxin toxicity.
Level of Cognitive Ability: Analyzing
Client Needs: Physiological Integrity
Integrated Process: Nursing Process—Assessment
Content Area: Pharmacology: Cardiovascular Medications: Cardiac Glycosides
Health Problem: N/A
Priority Concepts: Clinical Judgment; Safety
Reference: Burchum, Rosenthal (2016), p. 527.

628. *Answer:* 3
Rationale: Signs of toxicity from procainamide include confusion, dizziness, drowsiness, decreased urination, nausea, vomiting, and tachydysrhythmias. If the client complains of dizziness, the nurse should assess the vital signs first. Although measuring the QRS duration on the rhythm strip and obtaining a 12-lead electrocardiogram may be interventions, these would be done after the vital signs are taken. Dizziness directly following the procainamide indicates that the medication was the likely cause and should be addressed before assessing for other possible causes such as hypoglycemia.
Test-Taking Strategy: Note the strategic word, *first.* Also use the steps of the nursing process to answer correctly. Remember to always assess the client first, not the monitoring devices. Therefore, auscultating the apical pulse and taking the blood pressure are the first actions.
Level of Cognitive Ability: Analyzing
Client Needs: Physiological Integrity
Integrated Process: Nursing Process—Implementation
Content Area: Pharmacology: Cardiovascular Medications: Antidysrhythmics
Health Problem: Adult Health: Cardiovascular: Dysrhythmias
Priority Concepts: Clinical Judgment; Perfusion
Reference: Gahart, Nazareno (2015), p. 1021.

629. *Answer:* 2
Rationale: Audible expiratory wheezes may indicate a serious adverse reaction, bronchospasm. Beta blockers may induce this reaction, particularly in clients with chronic obstructive pulmonary disease or asthma. Normal decreases in blood pressure and heart rate are expected. Insomnia is a frequent mild side effect and should be monitored.
Test-Taking Strategy: Focus on the subject, a potential adverse complication. Eliminate options indicating a decrease in blood pressure and a decrease in heart rate first, because these are expected effects from the medication. Next, focusing on the subject will direct you to the correct option.
Level of Cognitive Ability: Analyzing
Client Needs: Physiological Integrity
Integrated Process: Nursing Process—Assessment
Content Area: Pharmacology: Cardiovascular Medications: Beta blockers
Health Problem: Adult Health: Cardiovascular: Hypertension
Priority Concepts: Gas Exchange; Perfusion
Reference: Burchum, Rosenthal (2016), pp. 161, 163.

630. *Answer:* 2
Rationale: When a client is receiving warfarin for clot prevention due to atrial fibrillation, an INR of 2 to 3 is appropriate for most clients. Until the INR has achieved a therapeutic range, the client should be maintained on a continuous heparin infusion with the aPTT ranging between 60 and 80 seconds. Therefore, the nurse should collaborate with the HCP to obtain a prescription to increase the heparin infusion and to administer the warfarin as prescribed.
Test-Taking Strategy: Focus on the subject, laboratory result analysis related to these medications. First, eliminate the option that indicates to discuss use of dabigatran etexilate, recalling that it is contraindicated for use in atrial fibrillation associated with valvular heart disease. Next, recall that if the warfarin sodium has achieved the therapeutic range for the INR for clot prevention in atrial fibrillation, the heparin infusion is no longer necessary. This will help you eliminate the option that indicates to withhold the warfarin sodium because the INR is not therapeutic. Last, keep in mind that if both the aPTT and the INR are not within therapeutic range, the client is left unprotected from clot formation.
Level of Cognitive Ability: Synthesizing
Client Needs: Physiological Integrity
Integrated Process: Nursing Process—Implementation
Content Area: Pharmacology: Cardiovascular Medications: Anticoagulants
Health Problem: Adult Health: Cardiovascular: Dysrhythmias
Priority Concepts: Clotting; Collaboration
Reference: Burchum, Rosenthal (2016), pp. 621-623.

631. *Answer:* 3
Rationale: Tissue plasminogen activator is a thrombolytic. Hemorrhage is a complication of any type of thrombolytic medication. The client is monitored for bleeding. Monitoring for renal failure and monitoring the client's psychosocial status are important but are not the most critical interventions. Heparin may be administered after thrombolytic therapy, but the question is not asking about follow-up medications.
Test-Taking Strategy: Note the strategic word, *priority.* Remember that bleeding is a priority for thrombolytic medications.
Level of Cognitive Ability: Applying
Client Needs: Physiological Integrity
Integrated Process: Nursing Process—Implementation
Content Area: Pharmacology: Cardiovascular Medications: Thrombolytics
Health Problem: Adult Health: Cardiovascular: Myocardial infarction
Priority Concepts: Clotting; Safety
Reference: Burchum, Rosenthal (2016), pp. 617-618.

632. *Answer:* 1, 3, 5, 6
Rationale: Thiazide diuretics such as hydrochlorothiazide are sulfa-based medications, and a client with a sulfa allergy is at risk for an allergic reaction. Also, clients are at risk for hypokalemia, hyperglycemia, hypercalcemia, hyperlipidemia, and hyperuricemia.
Test-Taking Strategy: Focus on the subject, a concern related to administration of hydrochlorothiazide. Recall that thiazide diuretics chemical make-up carry a sulfa ring.

Level of Cognitive Ability: Analyzing
Client Needs: Physiological Integrity
Integrated Process: Nursing Process—Assessment
Content Area: Pharmacology: Cardiovascular Medications: Diuretics
Health Problem: Adult Health: Cardiovascular: Hypertension
Priority Concepts: Clinical Judgment; Safety
Reference: Burchum, Rosenthal (2016), pp. 452-453.

633. *Answer:* 4
Rationale: Nicotinic acid, even an over-the-counter form, should be avoided because it may lead to liver abnormalities. All lipid-lowering medications also can cause liver abnormalities, so a combination of nicotinic acid and cholestyramine resin needs to be avoided. Constipation and bloating are the 2 most common adverse effects. Walking and the reduction of fats in the diet are therapeutic measures to reduce cholesterol and triglyceride levels.
Test-Taking Strategy: Note the **strategic words**, *need for further teaching*. These words indicate a **negative event query** and ask you to select an option that is an incorrect statement. Remembering that over-the-counter medications should be avoided when a client is taking a prescription medication will direct you to the correct option.
Level of Cognitive Ability: Evaluating
Client Needs: Physiological Integrity
Integrated Process: Teaching and Learning
Content Area: Pharmacology: Cardiovascular Medications: Antilipemics
Health Problem: Adult Health: Cardiovascular: Coronary Artery Disease
Priority Concepts: Client Education; Safety
References: Hodgson, Kizior (2015), pp. 244-245; Burchum, Rosenthal (2016), p. 573.

634. *Answer:* 2, 4, 5
Rationale: Digoxin is a cardiac glycoside. The risk of toxicity can occur with the use of this medication. Toxicity can lead to life-threatening events and the nurse needs to monitor the client closely for signs of toxicity. Early signs of toxicity include gastrointestinal manifestations such as anorexia, nausea, vomiting, and diarrhea. Subsequent manifestations include headache; visual disturbances such as diplopia, blurred vision, yellow-green halos, and photophobia; drowsiness; fatigue; and weakness. Cardiac rhythm abnormalities can also occur. The nurse also monitors the digoxin level. The optimal therapeutic range for digoxin is 0.5 to 2.0 ng/mL (0.63 to 2.56 nmol/L).
Test-Taking Strategy: Focus on the **subject**, digoxin toxicity. Specific knowledge regarding the characteristics of digoxin toxicity is needed to answer this question. Recall that the early signs are gastrointestinal manifestations. Next, recall that visual disturbances can occur.
Level of Cognitive Ability: Analyzing
Client Needs: Physiological Integrity
Integrated Process: Nursing Process—Assessment
Content Area: Pharmacology: Cardiovascular Medications: Cardiac Glycosides
Health Problem: Adult Health: Cardiovascular: Heart Failure
Priority Concepts: Clinical Judgment; Safety
References: Hodgson, Kizior (2015), p. 363; Burchum, Rosenthal (2016), pp. 532-533.

635. *Answer:* 4
Rationale: An increased risk of toxicity exists in clients with hypercalcemia, hypokalemia, hypomagnesemia, hypothyroidism, and impaired renal function. The calcium, creatinine, and potassium levels are all within normal limits. The normal range for magnesium is 1.8–2.6 mEq/L (0.74–1.07 mmol/L), and the results in the correct option are reflective of hypomagnesemia.
Test-Taking Strategy: Focus on the **subject**, the laboratory result that places the client at risk for digoxin toxicity. Recalling the normal laboratory values for each electrolyte identified in the options will assist in answering correctly.
Level of Cognitive Ability: Analyzing
Client Needs: Physiological Integrity
Integrated Process: Nursing Process—Assessment
Content Area: Pharmacology: Cardiovascular Medications: Cardiac Glycosides
Health Problem: Adult Health: Cardiovascular: Heart Failure
Priority Concepts: Perfusion; Safety
Reference: Hodgson, Kizior (2015), p. 363.

636. *Answer:* 2
Rationale: Bumetanide is a diuretic and expected outcomes include increased urine output, decreased crackles, and decreased weight. Potassium loss is a side effect rather than an expected effect of the diuretic. Frothy pink sputum indicates progression to pulmonary edema. A BNP greater than 100 pg/mL (100 ng/L) is indicative of heart failure; thus, a rise from a previous level indicates worsening of the condition.
Test-Taking Strategy: Focus on the **subject**, assessment findings indicative of the expected effect of bumetanide. Keep in mind when answering this question that an expected effect of a medication refers to a positive outcome versus a side or adverse effect. This will help you eliminate the option that refers to the potassium loss.
Level of Cognitive Ability: Evaluating
Client Needs: Physiological Integrity
Integrated Process: Nursing Process—Evaluation
Content Area: Pharmacology: Cardiovascular Medications: Diuretics
Health Problem: Adult Health: Cardiovascular: Heart Failure
Priority Concepts: Evidence; Perfusion
Reference: Gahart, Nazareno (2015), pp. 191-192.

637. *Answer:* 2
Rationale: The antidote to heparin is protamine sulfate; it should be readily available for use if excessive bleeding or hemorrhage should occur. Vitamin K is an antidote for warfarin sodium. Potassium chloride is administered for a potassium deficit. Aminocaproic acid is the antidote for thrombolytic therapy.
Test-Taking Strategy: Focus on the **subject**, the antidote for heparin. Knowledge regarding the various antidotes is needed to answer this question. Remember that the antidote to heparin is protamine sulfate.
Level of Cognitive Ability: Applying
Client Needs: Physiological Integrity
Integrated Process: Nursing Process—Planning
Content Area: Pharmacology: Cardiovascular Medications: Anticoagulants
Health Problem: Adult Health: Cardiovascular: Dysrhythmias
Priority Concepts: Clotting; Safety
Reference: Gahart, Nazareno (2015), p. 626.

638. *Answer:* 1, 4, 5

Rationale: The client is experiencing an anaphylactic reaction. Therefore, the priority action is to stop the infusion and notify the RRT. The client may be treated with antihistamines. Raising the head of the bed would not be helpful, as that may exacerbate the hypotension. Protamine sulfate is the antidote for heparin, so it is not useful for a client receiving alteplase.

Test-Taking Strategy: Note the strategic word, *priority.* Recall that an allergic reaction and possible anaphylaxis are risks associated with alteplase therapy. Also, focusing on the signs and symptoms in the question will assist in answering correctly. When a severe allergic reaction occurs, the offending substance should be stopped, and lifesaving treatment should begin.

Level of Cognitive Ability: Analyzing

Client Needs: Physiological Integrity

Integrated Process: Nursing Process—Implementation

Content Area: Complex Care: Shock

Health Problem: Adult Health: Cardiovascular: Shock

Priority Concepts: Clinical Judgment; Gas Exchange

Reference: Ignatavicius, Workman (2016), pp. 352-353, 607, 939.

639. *Answer:* 3

Rationale: Thrombolytic therapy is contraindicated in severe uncontrolled hypertension because of the risk of cerebral hemorrhage. Therefore, the nurse would report the results of the blood pressure to the PHCP before initiating therapy.

Test-Taking Strategy: Focus on the subject, a contraindication for the use of thrombolytic therapy. Adventitious breath sounds, temperature of 99.4° F (37.4° C), and respiratory rate of 28 breaths per minute may be present in the client with pulmonary embolism but are not necessarily signs that warrant reporting before thrombolytic therapy is initiated.

Level of Cognitive Ability: Analyzing

Client Needs: Physiological Integrity

Integrated Process: Nursing Process—Assessment

Content Area: Pharmacology: Cardiovascular: Thrombolytics

Health Problem: Adult Health: Respiratory: Pulmonary Embolism

Priority Concepts: Clinical Judgment; Clotting

Reference: Ignatavicius, Workman (2016), pp. 731-732.

640. *Answer:* 4

Rationale: Flushing is an adverse effect of this medication. Aspirin or a nonsteroidal antiinflammatory drug, as prescribed, can be taken 30 minutes prior to taking the medication to decrease flushing. Alcohol consumption needs to be avoided because it will enhance this effect. The medication should be taken with meals to decrease gastrointestinal upset; however, taking the medication with meals has no effect on the flushing. Clay-colored stools are a sign of hepatic dysfunction and should be reported to the primary health care provider (PHCP) immediately.

Test-Taking Strategy: Focus on the subject, client understanding of the medication. Alcohol must be abstained from, so this option can be eliminated. Taking the medication with meals helps decrease the gastrointestinal symptoms rather than flushing. Clay-colored stools are a sign of hepatic dysfunction and should be reported to the PHCP immediately.

Level of Cognitive Ability: Evaluating

Client Needs: Physiological Integrity

Integrated Process: Nursing Process—Evaluation

Content Area: Pharmacology: Cardiovascular Medications: Antilipemics

Health Problem: Adult Health: Cardiovascular: Coronary Artery Disease

Priority Concepts: Client Education; Safety

Reference: Burchum, Rosenthal (2016), pp. 578-579.

UNIT XIII

Renal and Urinary Problems of the Adult Client

Pyramid to Success

Pyramid Points focus on acute kidney injury and chronic kidney disease, dialysis procedures, urinary diversions, and postoperative care following urinary or renal surgery. Be familiar with medical conditions and diagnostic tests that place the client at risk for acute kidney injury. Focus on the major problems associated with kidney failure and the rationale for the prescribed treatment modalities. Be familiar with the complications associated with hemodialysis and peritoneal dialysis, the specific assessment data related to complications, and the expected treatment. Focus on the care of a peritoneal catheter and hemodialysis access devices, the complications associated with these access devices, and the appropriate nursing interventions if a complication is suspected. Review assessment data indicating rejection following kidney transplantation. Be familiar with care for the client following prostatectomy and treatment measures for the client with urinary or renal calculi.

Client Needs: Learning Objectives

Safe and Effective Care Environment

Consulting with the interprofessional health care team
Establishing priorities
Identifying conditions and diagnostic procedures that increase the risk of developing renal problems
Identifying the guidelines related to kidney organ donation
Maintaining asepsis related to wound care and dialysis access devices
Maintaining confidentiality related to the renal disorder
Maintaining standard and other precautions related to care for the client
Preventing injury related to complications of the disorder
Upholding client rights
Verifying that informed consent related to diagnostic and surgical procedures has been obtained

Health Promotion and Maintenance

Performing urinary and renal physical assessment techniques
Providing client instructions regarding prescribed treatments related to the urinary or renal disorder
Providing client instructions regarding the prevention of the recurrence of a urinary or renal problem

Psychosocial Integrity

Assisting the client to use appropriate coping mechanisms
Discussing body image disturbances
Discussing the loss of renal function
Identifying cultural, religious, and spiritual influences on health
Identifying grief and loss and end-of-life issues
Identifying support systems and appropriate community resources

Physiological Integrity

Ensuring elimination measures
Informing the client about diagnostic tests and laboratory results
Monitoring for fluid and electrolyte imbalances and acid-base disorders
Obtaining assessment data indicating rejection of kidney transplant
Preventing complications arising as a result of dialysis
Providing adequate rest and sleep
Providing care related to hemodialysis and peritoneal dialysis and dialysis access devices
Providing care to the client following prostatectomy
Providing comfort interventions
Providing pharmacological therapy
Providing treatment measures for the client with renal or urinary calculi
Teaching the client about the prescribed nutrition and fluid measures

CHAPTER 54

Renal and Urinary Problems

PRIORITY CONCEPTS **Fluids and Electrolytes; Elimination**

I. Anatomy and Physiology

A. Kidney anatomy
1. Each person has 2 kidneys, which are located behind the peritoneum; attached at the level of the last thoracic and first 3 lumbar vertebrae, on the right and left sides.
2. The kidneys are enclosed in the renal capsule.
3. The renal cortex is the outer layer of the renal capsule, which contains blood-filtering mechanisms (glomeruli).
4. The renal medulla is the inner region, which contains the renal pyramids and renal tubules.
5. Together, the renal cortex, pyramids, and medulla constitute the parenchyma.
6. Nephrons
   a. Located within the parenchyma
   b. Composed of glomerulus and tubules
   c. Selectively secretes and reabsorbs ions and filtrates, including fluid, wastes, electrolytes, acids, and bases

! The nephrons are the functional units of the kidney.

7. Glomerulus
   a. Each nephron contains tufts of capillaries, which filter large plasma proteins and blood cells.
   b. Blood flows into the glomerular capillaries from the afferent arteriole and flows out of the glomerular capillaries into the efferent arteriole.
8. Bowman's capsule
   a. Thin double-walled capsule that surrounds the glomerulus
   b. Fluid and particles from the blood such as electrolytes, glucose, amino acids, and metabolic waste (glomerular filtrate) are filtered through the glomerular membrane into a fluid-filled space in Bowman's capsule (Bowman's space) and then enter the proximal convoluted tubule (PCT).
9. Tubules
   a. The tubules include the PCT, the loop of Henle, and the distal convoluted tubule (DCT).
   b. The PCT receives filtrate from the glomerular capsule and reabsorbs water and electrolytes through active and passive transport.
   c. The descending loop of Henle passively reabsorbs water from the filtrate.
   d. The ascending loop of Henle passively reabsorbs sodium and chloride from the filtrate and helps maintain osmolality.
   e. The DCT actively and passively removes sodium and water.
   f. The filtered fluid is converted to urine in the tubules, and then the urine moves to the pelvis of the kidney.
   g. The urine flows from the pelvis of the kidneys through the ureters and empties into the bladder.

B. Functions of kidneys
1. Maintain acid–base balance
2. Excrete end products of body metabolism
3. Control fluid and electrolyte balance
4. Excrete bacterial toxins, water-soluble medications, and medication metabolites
5. Secrete renin to regulate the blood pressure (BP) and erythropoietin to stimulate the bone marrow to produce red blood cells
6. Synthesize vitamin D for calcium absorption and regulation of the parathyroid hormones

C. Urine production
1. As fluid flows through the tubules, water, electrolytes, and solutes are reabsorbed, and other solutes such as creatinine, hydrogen ions, and potassium are secreted.
2. Water and solutes that are not reabsorbed become urine.
3. The process of selective reabsorption determines the amount of water and solutes to be secreted.

D. Homeostasis of water
1. Antidiuretic hormone (ADH) is primarily responsible for the reabsorption of water by the kidneys.
2. ADH is produced by the hypothalamus and secreted from the posterior lobe of the pituitary gland.

3. Secretion of ADH is stimulated by dehydration or high sodium intake and by a decrease in blood volume.
4. ADH makes the distal convoluted tubules and collecting duct permeable to water.
5. Water is drawn out of the tubules by osmosis and returns to the blood; concentrated urine remains in the tubule to be excreted.
6. When ADH is lacking, the client develops diabetes insipidus (DI).
7. Clients with DI produce large amounts of dilute urine; treatment is necessary because the client cannot drink sufficient water to survive.

E. Homeostasis of sodium
1. When the amount of sodium increases, extra water is retained to preserve osmotic pressure.
2. An increase in sodium and water produces an increase in blood volume and BP.
3. When the BP increases, glomerular filtration increases, and extra water and sodium are lost; blood volume is reduced, returning the BP to normal.
4. Reabsorption of sodium in the distal convoluted tubules is controlled by the renin-angiotensin system.
5. Renin, an enzyme, is released from the nephron when the BP or fluid concentration in the distal convoluted tubule is low.
6. Renin catalyzes the splitting of angiotensin I from angiotensinogen; angiotensin I converts to angiotensin II as blood flows through the lung.
7. Angiotensin II, a potent vasoconstrictor, stimulates the secretion of aldosterone.
8. Aldosterone stimulates the distal convoluted tubules to reabsorb sodium and secrete potassium.
9. The additional sodium increases water reabsorption and increases blood volume and BP, returning the BP to normal; the stimulus for the secretion of renin then is removed.

F. Homeostasis of potassium
1. Increases in the serum potassium level stimulate the secretion of aldosterone.
2. Aldosterone stimulates the distal convoluted tubules to secrete potassium; this action returns the serum potassium concentration to normal.

G. Homeostasis of acidity (pH)
1. Blood pH is controlled by maintaining the concentration of buffer systems.
2. Carbonic acid and sodium bicarbonate form the most important buffers for neutralizing acids in the plasma.
3. The concentration of carbonic acid is controlled by the respiratory system.
4. The concentration of sodium bicarbonate is controlled by the kidneys.
5. Normal arterial pH is 7.35 to 7.45, maintained by keeping the ratio of concentrations of sodium bicarbonate to carbon dioxide constant at 20:1.
6. Strong acids are neutralized by sodium bicarbonate to produce carbonic acid and the sodium salts of the strong acid; this process quickly restores the ratio and thus blood pH.
7. The carbonic acid dissociates into carbon dioxide and water; because the concentration of carbon dioxide is maintained at a constant level by the respiratory system, the excess carbonic acid is rapidly excreted.
8. Sodium combined with the strong acid is actively reabsorbed in the distal convoluted tubules in exchange for hydrogen or potassium ions. The strong acid is neutralized by ammonia and is excreted as ammonia or potassium salts.

H. Adrenal glands (see Chapter 46 for information about the adrenal glands)
1. One adrenal gland is on top of each kidney.
2. The adrenal glands influence BP and sodium and water retention.

I. Bladder
1. The bladder detrusor muscle, composed of smooth muscle, distends during bladder filling and contracts during bladder emptying.
2. The ureterovesical sphincter prevents reflux of urine from the bladder to the ureter.
3. The total bladder capacity is 1 L; normal adult urine output is 1500 mL/day.

J. Prostate gland
1. The prostate gland surrounds the male urethra.
2. The prostate gland contains a duct that opens into the prostatic portion of the urethra and secretes the alkaline portion of seminal fluid, which protects sperm.

K. Risk factors associated with renal disorders (Box 54-1)

II. Diagnostic Tests

A. See Chapter 10 and Box 54-2 for information regarding normal values for renal function studies.

BOX 54-1 Risk Factors Associated with Renal Problems

- Chemical or environmental toxin exposure
- Contact sports
- Diabetes mellitus
- Family history of renal disease
- Frequent urinary tract infections
- Heart failure
- High-sodium diet
- Hypertension
- Medications
- Polycystic kidney disease
- Trauma
- Urolithiasis or nephrolithiasis

BOX 54-2 Normal Renal Function Values

- Blood urea nitrogen (BUN) level, 10 to 20 mg/dL (3.6 to 7.1 mmol/L)
- Serum creatinine level, 0.6 to 1.2 mg/dL (53 to 106 mcmol/L) for males and 0.5 to 1.1 mg/dL (44 to 97 mcmol/L) for females
- BUN/creatinine ratio, 6 to 25

B. Determination of serum creatinine level
1. Description: A test that measures the amount of creatinine in the serum. Creatinine is an end product of protein and muscle metabolism.
2. Analysis
   a. Creatinine level reflects the glomerular filtration rate.
   b. Kidney disease is the only pathological condition that increases the serum creatinine level.
   c. Serum creatinine level increases only when at least 50% of renal function is lost.

C. Determination of blood urea nitrogen (BUN) level
1. Description: A serum test that measures the amount of nitrogenous urea, a byproduct of protein metabolism in the liver.
2. Analysis
   a. BUN levels indicate the extent of renal clearance of urea nitrogenous waste products.
   b. An elevation does not always mean that renal disease is present.
   c. Some factors that can elevate the BUN level include dehydration, poor renal perfusion, intake of a high-protein diet, infection, stress, corticosteroid use, gastrointestinal (GI) bleeding, and factors that cause muscle breakdown.

D. BUN/creatinine ratio
1. The BUN level is divided by the creatinine level to obtain the ratio.
2. When the BUN and serum creatinine levels increase at the same rate, the ratio of BUN to creatinine remains constant.
3. Elevated serum creatinine and BUN levels suggest renal dysfunction.
4. A decreased BUN/creatinine ratio occurs with fluid volume deficit, obstructive uropathy, catabolic state, and a high-protein diet.
5. An increased BUN/creatinine ratio occurs with fluid volume excess.

E. Urinalysis
1. Description: A urine test for evaluation of the renal system and renal disease (Table 54-1)
2. Interventions
   a. Wash perineal area and use a clean container for collection.
   b. Obtain 10 to 15 mL of the first morning voiding if possible.

TABLE 54-1 Normal Urinalysis Values

Color	Amber yellow
Odor	Specific aromatic odor, similar to ammonia
pH	4.0-8.0 (4.0-8.0)
Osmolality	300-1300 mOsm/kg (300-1300 mmol/kg)
Specific gravity	1.003-1.030
Glucose	Negative
Ketones	Negative
Protein	Negative
Bilirubin	Negative
Casts	Negative
Bacteria	None or <1000/mL
Hemoglobin	Negative
Myoglobin	Negative
Culture for organisms	Negative

   c. Refrigerating samples may alter the specific gravity.
   d. If the client is menstruating, note this on the laboratory requisition form.

F. A 24-hour urine collection
1. Check with the laboratory about specific instructions for the client to follow, such as dietary or medication restrictions.
2. Instruct the client about the urine collection.
3. At the start time, instruct the client to void and discard that sample.
4. Collect all urine for the prescribed time (24 hours).
5. Keep the urine specimen on ice or refrigerated and check with the laboratory regarding adding a preservative to the specimen during collection.
6. At the end of the prescribed time, instruct the client to empty the bladder and add that urine to the collection container.

G. Specific gravity determination
1. Description: A urine test that measures the ability of the kidneys to concentrate urine
2. Interventions
   a. Specific gravity can be measured by a multiple-test dipstick method (most common method), refractometer (an instrument used in the laboratory setting), or urinometer (least accurate method).
   b. Factors that interfere with an accurate reading include radiopaque contrast agents, glucose, and proteins.
   c. Cold specimens may produce a false high reading.
   d. Normal random reference interval is 1.003 to 1.030 (may vary depending on the laboratory).

e. An increase in specific gravity (more concentrated urine) occurs with insufficient fluid intake, decreased renal perfusion, or increased ADH.
f. A decrease in specific gravity (less concentrated urine) occurs with increased fluid intake or diabetes insipidus; it may also indicate renal disease or the kidneys' inability to concentrate urine.

H. Urine culture and sensitivity testing
1. Description: A urine test that identifies the presence of microorganisms (culture) and determines the specific antibiotics to treat the existing microorganism (sensitivity) appropriately
2. Interventions
a. Clean the perineal area and urinary meatus with a bacteriostatic solution.
b. Collect the midstream sample in a sterile container (clean catch specimen); if the client is unable to obtain a clean catch specimen, a specimen obtained by straight catheterization may be prescribed.
c. Send the collected specimen to the laboratory immediately.
d. Identify any sources of potential contaminants during the collection of the specimen, such as the hands, skin, clothing, hair, or vaginal or rectal secretions; if contamination occurs, the specimen is discarded and a new specimen needs to be collected. Urine from the client who drank a very large amount of fluids may be too dilute to provide a positive culture.

I. Creatinine clearance test
1. Description
a. The creatinine clearance test evaluates how well the kidneys remove creatinine from the blood, and is an estimate of glomerular filtration rate (GFR).
b. The test includes obtaining a blood sample and timed urine specimens.
c. Blood is drawn when the urine specimen collection is complete.
d. The urine specimen for the creatinine clearance is usually collected for 24 hours, but shorter periods such as 8 or 12 hours could be prescribed.

! The creatinine clearance test provides the best estimate of the GFR; the normal GFR is 125 mL per minute in a young adult. The GFR decreases with age (10% for each decade). By age 65 years the GFR approximately 65 mL per minute.

2. Interventions
a. Encourage fluids before and during the test.
b. Instruct the client to avoid caffeinated beverages during testing.
c. Check with the primary health care provider (PHCP) regarding the administration of any prescribed medications during testing.
d. Instruct the client about the urine collection.
e. At the start time, ask the client to void (or empty the tubing and drainage bag if the client has a urinary catheter) and discard the first sample.
f. Collect all urine for the prescribed time.
g. Keep the urine specimen on ice or refrigerated and check with the laboratory regarding adding a preservative to the specimen during collection.
h. At the end of the prescribed time, ask the client to empty the bladder (or empty the tubing and drainage bag if the client has a urinary catheter) and add that final urine to the collection container.
i. Send the labeled urine specimen to the laboratory.
j. Document specimen collection, time started and completed, and pertinent assessments.

J. KUB (kidneys, ureters, and bladder) radiography
1. Description: An x-ray of the urinary system and adjacent structures to detect urinary calculi.
2. Interventions: No specific preparation is necessary.

K. Bladder ultrasonography (bladder scanning)
1. Bladder ultrasonography is a noninvasive method for measuring the volume of urine in the bladder.
2. Bladder ultrasonography may be performed to evaluate urinary frequency, inability to urinate, or amount of residual urine (the amount of urine remaining in the bladder after voiding).

L. Intravenous urography
1. Description: An x-ray procedure in which an intravenous (IV) injection of a radiopaque dye is used to visualize and identify abnormalities in the renal system.
2. Preprocedure interventions
a. Verify that an informed consent was obtained.
b. Assess the client for allergies to iodine, seafood, and radiopaque dyes and contraindications for the test, including a positive pregnancy test; cautions include medical history of asthma, significant cardiac disease, and renal insufficiency.
c. Withhold food and fluids for the time prescribed.
d. Administer laxatives if prescribed.
e. Inform the client about possible throat irritation, flushing of the face, warmth, or a salty or metallic taste during the test.
3. Postprocedure interventions
a. Monitor vital signs.
b. Instruct the client to drink at least 1 L of fluid unless contraindicated.

c. Monitor urinary output.
d. Monitor for signs of a possible allergic reaction to the dye used during the test and instruct the client to notify the PHCP if any signs of an allergic reaction occur.
e. Contrast dye is potentially damaging to kidneys; the risk is greater in older clients and those experiencing dehydration.

! The dye (contrast media) used in IV urography may be nephrotoxic; therefore, encourage increased fluids unless contraindicated and monitor urinary output. It is essential that preprocedure BUN and creatinine levels are assessed on any client undergoing a procedure where dye might be injected. The PHCP may institute precautionary measures to prevent AKI or use smaller amounts of the dye.

M. Renography (kidney scan)
1. Description: An IV injection of a radioisotope for visual imaging of renal blood flow, glomerular filtration, tubular function, and excretion
2. Preprocedure interventions
a. Verify that an informed consent was obtained.
b. Assess for allergies.
c. Inform the client that the test requires no dietary or activity restrictions.
d. Instruct the client to remain motionless during the test and that imaging may be repeated at various intervals before the test is complete.
3. Postprocedure interventions
a. Encourage fluid intake unless contraindicated.
b. Assess the client for signs of an allergic reaction.
c. The radioisotope is eliminated in 24 hours; wear gloves for excretion precautions.
d. Follow standard precautions when caring for incontinent clients and double-bag client linens per agency policy.
e. If captopril was administered during the procedure, the client's BP should be checked frequently.

N. Cystoscopy and biopsy of the bladder
1. Description: The bladder mucosa is examined for inflammation, calculi, or tumors by means of a cystoscope; a sample for biopsy may be obtained.
2. Preprocedure interventions
a. Verify that an informed consent was obtained.
b. If a biopsy is planned, withhold food and fluids for the time prescribed.
c. If a cystoscopy alone is planned, no special preparation is necessary, and the procedure may be performed in the PHCP's office; postprocedure interventions include increasing fluid intake.
3. Postprocedure interventions following biopsy
a. Monitor vital signs.
b. Increase fluid intake as prescribed.
c. Monitor intake and output and assess urine characteristics.
d. Encourage deep-breathing exercises to relieve bladder spasms and administer analgesics as prescribed.
e. Administer sitz or tub baths for back and abdominal pain if prescribed.
f. Note that leg cramps are common because of the lithotomy position maintained during the procedure.
g. Inform the client that burning on urination, pink-tinged or tea-colored urine, and urinary frequency are common after cystoscopy and resolve in a few days.
h. Monitor for bright red urine or clots, and notify the PHCP if a fever occurs; an increase in white blood cell (WBC) count suggests infection.

O. Renal biopsy
1. Description: Insertion of a needle into the kidney to obtain a sample of tissue for examination; usually done percutaneously
2. Preprocedure interventions
a. Assess vital signs.
b. Assess baseline coagulation studies; notify the PHCP if abnormal results are noted.
c. Verify that an informed consent was obtained.
d. Withhold food and fluids as prescribed.
3. Intervention during the procedure: Position the client prone with a pillow under the abdomen and shoulders.
4. Postprocedure interventions
a. Monitor vital signs, especially for hypotension and tachycardia, which could indicate bleeding.
b. Provide pressure to the biopsy site for 30 minutes or as prescribed.
c. Monitor the hemoglobin and hematocrit levels for decreases, which could indicate bleeding.
d. Place the client on strict bed rest in the supine position with a back roll for additional support for 2 to 6 hours after the biopsy.
e. Check the biopsy site and under the client for bleeding.
f. Encourage fluid intake of 1500 to 2000 mL as prescribed.
g. Observe the urine for gross and microscopic bleeding.
h. Instruct the client to avoid heavy lifting and strenuous activity for 1 to 2 weeks.
i. Instruct the client to notify the PHCP if either a temperature greater than 100° F (37.8° C) or hematuria occurs after the first 24 hours postprocedure.

III. Acute Kidney Injury

A. Description

1. Acute kidney injury (AKI) is the rapid loss of kidney function from renal cell damage.
2. Occurs abruptly and can be reversible
3. AKI leads to cell hypoperfusion, cell death, and decompensation of renal function.
4. The prognosis depends on the cause and the condition of the client.
5. Near-normal or normal kidney function may resume gradually.

B. Causes

1. Prerenal: Outside the kidney; caused by intravascular volume depletion such as with blood loss associated with trauma or surgery, dehydration, decreased cardiac output (as with cardiogenic shock), decreased peripheral vascular resistance, decreased renovascular blood flow, and prerenal infection or obstruction.
2. Intrarenal: Within the parenchyma of the kidney; caused by tubular necrosis, prolonged prerenal ischemia, intrarenal infection or obstruction, and nephrotoxicity (Box 54-3)
3. Postrenal: Between the kidney and urethral meatus, such as bladder neck obstruction, bladder cancer, calculi, and postrenal infection

C. Phases of AKI and interventions (Box 54-4)

1. Onset: Begins with precipitating event
2. Oliguric phase
   - **a.** For some clients, oliguria does not occur and the urine output is normal; otherwise, the duration of oliguria is 8 to 15 days; the longer the duration, the less chance of recovery.
   - **b.** Sudden decrease in urine output; urine output is less than 400 mL/day.
   - **c.** Signs of excess fluid volume: Hypertension, edema, pleural and pericardial effusions, dysrhythmias, heart failure, and pulmonary edema
   - **d.** Signs of uremia: Anorexia, nausea, vomiting, and pruritus
   - **e.** Signs of metabolic acidosis: Kussmaul's respirations
   - **f.** Signs of neurological changes: Tingling of extremities, drowsiness progressing to disorientation, and then coma
   - **g.** Signs of pericarditis: Friction rub, chest pain with inspiration, and low-grade fever
   - **h.** Laboratory analysis (see Box 54-4)
   - **i.** With early recognition or potential for AKI, client may be treated with fluid challenges (IV boluses of 500 to 1000 mL over 1 hour).
   - **j.** Restrict fluid intake; if hypertension is present, daily fluid allowances may be 400 to 1000 mL plus the measured urinary output.
   - **k.** Administer medications, such as diuretics, as prescribed to increase renal blood flow and diuresis of retained fluid and electrolytes.

BOX 54-3 Potentially Nephrotoxic Substances

Medications

Antibiotics: Anti-infectives
- Amphotericin B
- Methicillin
- Polymyxin B
- Rifampin
- Sulfonamides
- Tetracycline hydrochloride
- Vancomycin

Aminoglycoside Antibiotics
- Gentamicin
- Kanamycin
- Neomycin
- Tobramycin

Antineoplastics
- Cisplatin
- Cyclophosphamide
- Methotrexate

Nonsteroidal Anti-inflammatory Drugs (NSAIDs)
- Celecoxib
- Flurbiprofen
- Ibuprofen
- Indomethacin
- Ketorolac
- Meclofenamate
- Meloxicam
- Nabumetone
- Naproxen
- Oxaprozin
- Rofecoxib
- Tolmetin

Other Medications
- Acetaminophen
- Captopril
- Cyclosporine
- Fluorinate anesthetics
- D-Penicillamine
- Phenazopyridine hydrochloride
- Quinine

Other Substances
- Organic solvents
- Carbon tetrachloride
- Ethylene glycol

Nonpharmacological Chemical Agents
- Radiographic contrast dye
- Pesticides
- Fungicides
- Myoglobin (from breakdown of skeletal muscle)

Heavy Metals and Ions
- Arsenic
- Bismuth
- Copper sulfate
- Gold salts
- Lead
- Mercuric chloride

Adapted from Ignatavicius D, Workman ML: *Medical-surgical nursing: patient-centered collaborative care*, ed 7, Philadelphia, 2013, Saunders.

3. Diuretic phase
   - **a.** Urine output rises slowly, followed by diuresis (4 to 5 L/day).
   - **b.** Excessive urine output indicates that damaged nephrons are recovering their ability to excrete wastes.
   - **c.** Dehydration, hypovolemia, hypotension, and tachycardia can occur.
   - **d.** Level of consciousness improves.
   - **e.** Laboratory analysis (see Box 54-4)
   - **f.** Administer IV fluids as prescribed, which may contain electrolytes to replace losses.
4. Recovery phase (convalescent)
   - **a.** Recovery is a slow process; complete recovery may take 1 to 2 years.
   - **b.** Urine volume returns to normal.
   - **c.** Memory improves.
   - **d.** Strength increases.
   - **e.** The older adult is less likely than a younger adult to regain full kidney function.

BOX 54-4 Acute Kidney Injury: Phases and Laboratory Findings

Onset
- Begins with precipitating event

Oliguric Phase
- Elevated blood urea nitrogen (BUN) and serum creatinine levels
- Decreased urine specific gravity (prerenal causes) or normal (intrarenal causes)
- Decreased glomerular filtration rate (GFR) and creatinine clearance
- Hyperkalemia
- Normal or decreased serum sodium level
- Hypervolemia
- Hypocalcemia
- Hyperphosphatemia

Diuretic Phase
- Gradual decline in BUN and serum creatinine levels, but still elevated
- Continued low creatinine clearance with improving GFR
- Hypokalemia
- Hyponatremia
- Hypovolemia

Recovery Phase (Convalescent)
- Increased GFR
- Stabilization or continual decline in BUN and serum creatinine levels toward normal
- Complete recovery (may take 1 to 2 years)

f. Laboratory analysis (see Box 54-4)
g. AKI can progress to **chronic kidney disease (CKD)**.

⚠ The signs and symptoms of AKI are primarily caused by the retention of nitrogenous wastes, the retention of fluids, and the inability of the kidneys to regulate electrolytes.

D. Assessment: Assess objective and subjective data noted in the phases of AKI (see Box 54-4).

E. Other interventions
1. Monitor vital signs, especially for signs of hypertension, tachycardia, tachypnea, and an irregular heart rate.
2. Monitor urine and intake and output hourly and urine color and characteristics.
3. Monitor daily weight (same scale, same clothes, same time of day), noting that an increase of 0.5 to 1 lb/day (0.25 to 0.5 kg/day) indicates fluid retention.
4. Monitor for changes in the BUN, serum creatinine, and serum electrolyte levels.
5. Monitor for acidosis (may need to be treated with sodium bicarbonate).
6. Monitor urinalysis for protein level, hematuria, casts, and specific gravity.
7. Monitor for altered level of consciousness caused by uremia.
8. Monitor for signs of infection because the client may not exhibit an elevated temperature or an increased WBC count.
9. Monitor the lungs for wheezes and rhonchi and monitor for edema, which can indicate fluid overload.
10. Administer the prescribed diet, which is usually a low- to moderate-protein (to decrease the workload on the kidneys) and high-carbohydrate diet; ill clients may require nutritional support with supplements, enteral feedings, or parenteral nutrition.
11. Restrict potassium and sodium intake as prescribed based on the electrolyte level.
12. Administer medications as prescribed; be alert to the mechanism for metabolism and excretion of all prescribed medications.
13. Be alert to nephrotoxic medications, which may be prescribed (see Box 54-3).
14. Be alert to the PHCP's adjustment of medication dosages for kidney injury.
15. Prepare the client for **dialysis** if prescribed; continuous renal replacement therapy may be used in AKI to treat fluid volume overload or rapidly developing **azotemia** and metabolic acidosis.
16. Provide emotional support by allowing opportunities for the client to express concerns and fears and by encouraging family interactions.
17. Promote consistency in caregivers.
18. Also refer to Section IV, E in this chapter (Special problems in kidney disease and interventions).

IV. Chronic Kidney Disease (CKD)

A. Description
1. CKD is a slow, progressive, irreversible loss in kidney function, with a GFR less than or equal to 60 mL per minute for 3 months or longer.
2. It occurs in stages (with loss of 75% of functioning nephrons, the client becomes symptomatic) and eventually results in uremia or end-stage kidney disease (with loss of 90% to 95% of functioning nephrons) (Table 54-2).
3. Hypervolemia can occur because of the kidneys' inability to excrete sodium and water; hypovolemia can occur because of the kidneys' inability to conserve sodium and water.

⚠ CKD affects all major body systems and may require dialysis or kidney transplantation to maintain life.

B. Primary causes
1. May follow AKI
2. Diabetes mellitus and other metabolic disorders
3. Hypertension

TABLE 54-2 Progression of Chronic Kidney Disease

Stage of CKD	Estimated GFR
At risk; normal kidney function (early kidney disease may or may not be present)	>90 mL/min
Mild CKD	60-89 mL/min
Moderate CKD	30-59 mL/min
Severe CKD	15-29 mL/min
ESRD	<15 mL/min

CKD, Chronic kidney disease; *ESRD*, end-stage renal disease; *GFR*, glomerular filtration rate.

Data from Ignatavicius D, Workman ML: *Medical-surgical nursing: patient-centered collaborative care*, ed 7, Philadelphia, 2013, Saunders.

4. Chronic urinary obstruction
5. Recurrent infections
6. Renal artery occlusion
7. Autoimmune disorders

C. Assessment
1. Assess body systems for the manifestations of CKD (Box 54-5).
2. Assess psychological changes, which could include emotional lability, withdrawal, depression, anxiety, denial, dependence–independence conflict, changes in body image, and suicidal behavior.

D. Interventions
1. Same as the interventions for AKI.
2. Administer a prescribed diet, which is usually a moderate-protein (to decrease the workload on the kidneys) and high-carbohydrate, low-potassium, and low-phosphorus diet.
3. Provide oral care to prevent stomatitis and reduce discomfort from mouth sores.
4. Provide skin care to prevent pruritus.
5. Teach the client about fluid and dietary restrictions and the importance of daily weights.
6. Provide support to promote acceptance of the chronic illness and prepare the client for long-term dialysis and transplantation, or explain to the client about her or his choice to decline dialysis or transplantation; with elderly clients, provide information that kidney function is declining and in time may reach end-stage renal disease and require dialysis; encourage healthy lifestyle and discuss choices.

E. Special problems in kidney disease and interventions (Box 54-6)
1. Activity intolerance and insomnia
   - **a.** Fatigue results from anemia and the buildup of wastes from the diseased kidneys.
   - **b.** Provide adequate rest periods.
   - **c.** Teach the client to plan activities to avoid fatigue.
   - **d.** Mild central nervous system (CNS) depressants may be prescribed to promote rest.

BOX 54-5 Key Features of Chronic Kidney Disease

Neurological Manifestations
- Asterixis
- Ataxia (alteration in gait)
- Inability to concentrate or decreased attention span
- Lethargy and daytime drowsiness
- Myoclonus
- Paresthesias
- Seizures
- Slurred speech
- Tremors, twitching, or jerky movements
- Coma

Cardiovascular Manifestations
- Hypertension
- Heart failure
- Peripheral edema
- Cardiomyopathy
- Pericardial effusion
- Pericardial friction rub
- Uremic pericarditis
- Cardiac tamponade

Respiratory Manifestations
- Crackles
- Deep sighing, yawning
- Depressed cough reflex
- Shortness of breath
- Tachypnea
- Kussmaul's respirations
- Pleural effusion
- Pulmonary edema
- Uremic halitosis
- Uremic pneumonia

Hematological Manifestations
- Abnormal bleeding and bruising
- Anemia

Gastrointestinal Manifestations
- Anorexia, nausea, vomiting
- Changes in taste acuity and sensation
- Constipation
- Diarrhea
- Metallic taste in the mouth
- Stomatitis
- Uremic colitis (diarrhea)
- Uremic fetor
- Uremic gastritis (possible gastrointestinal bleeding)

Urinary Manifestations
- Polyuria, nocturia (early)
- Proteinuria
- Diluted, straw-colored appearance
- Hematuria
- Oliguria, anuria (later)

Integumentary Manifestations
- Decreased skin turgor
- Dry skin
- Yellow-gray pallor
- Ecchymosis
- Pruritus
- Purpura
- Soft tissue calcifications
- Uremic frost (late, premorbid)

Musculoskeletal Manifestations
- Bone pain
- Muscle weakness and cramping
- Pathological fractures
- Renal osteodystrophy

Reproductive Manifestations
- Decreased fertility
- Decreased libido
- Impotence
- Infrequent or absent menses

From Ignatavicius D, Workman ML: *Medical-surgical nursing: patient-centered collaborative care*, ed 7, Philadelphia, 2013, Saunders.

2. Anemia
   - **a.** Anemia results from the decreased secretion of erythropoietin by damaged nephrons, resulting in decreased production of red blood cells.
   - **b.** Monitor for decreased hemoglobin and hematocrit levels.

BOX 54-6 Special Problems in Kidney Disease

- Activity intolerance and insomnia
- Anemia
- Gastrointestinal bleeding
- Hyperkalemia
- Hypermagnesemia
- Hyperphosphatemia
- Hypertension
- Hypervolemia
- Hypocalcemia
- Hypovolemia
- Infection
- Metabolic acidosis
- Muscle cramps
- Neurological changes
- Ocular irritation
- Potential for injury
- Pruritus
- Psychosocial problems

c. Administer hematopoietics such as epoetin alfa or darbepoetin alfa, as prescribed to promote maturity of the red blood cells.
d. Administer folic acid as prescribed.
e. Administer iron orally as prescribed, but not at the same time as phosphate binders.
f. Administer stool softeners as prescribed because of the constipating effects of iron.
g. Note that oral iron is not well absorbed by the GI tract in CKD and causes nausea and vomiting; parenteral iron may be used if iron deficiencies persist despite folic acid or oral iron administration.
h. Administer blood transfusions; prescribed only when necessary (acute blood loss, symptomatic anemia), because they decrease the stimulus to produce red blood cells.
i. Blood transfusions also cause the development of antibodies against human tissues, which can make matching for organ transplantation difficult.

3. Gastrointestinal bleeding
   a. Urea is broken down by the intestinal bacteria to ammonia; ammonia irritates the GI mucosa, causing ulceration and bleeding.
   b. Monitor for decreasing hemoglobin and hematocrit levels.
   c. Monitor stools for occult blood.
   d. Avoid the administration of acetylsalicylic acid, because it is excreted by the kidneys; if administered, aspirin toxicity can occur and prolong the bleeding time.

Place the client with kidney disease on continuous telemetry. The client can develop hyperkalemia, resulting in the risk for dysrhythmias.

4. Hyperkalemia
   a. Monitor vital signs for hypertension or hypotension and the apical heart rate; an irregular heart rate could indicate dysrhythmias.
   b. Monitor the serum potassium level; an elevated serum potassium level can cause decreased cardiac output, heart blocks, fibrillation, or asystole (Fig. 54-1).

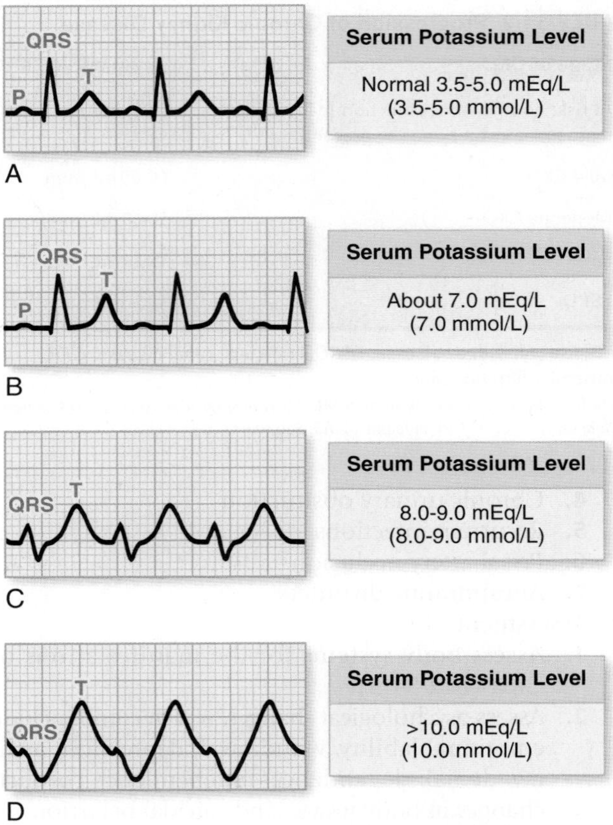

FIG. 54-1 Cardiac rhythm changes with hyperkalemia.

   c. Provide a low-potassium diet (see Chapter 11 for a list of foods that are high in potassium).
   d. Administer electrolyte-binding and electrolyte-excreting medications such as oral or rectal sodium polystyrene sulfonate as prescribed to lower the serum potassium level.
   e. Administer prescribed medications: 50% dextrose and regular insulin IV may be prescribed to shift potassium into the cells; calcium gluconate IV may be prescribed to reduce myocardial irritability from hyperkalemia; and sodium bicarbonate IV may be prescribed to correct acidosis.
   f. Administer prescribed loop diuretics to excrete potassium.
   g. Avoid potassium-retaining medications such as spironolactone and triamterene, because these medications will increase the potassium level
   h. Prepare the client for peritoneal dialysis (PD) or hemodialysis as prescribed.
5. Hypermagnesemia
   a. Results from decreased renal excretion of magnesium.
   b. Monitor for cardiac manifestations such as bradycardia, peripheral vasodilation, and hypotension.

c. Monitor CNS changes, such as drowsiness or lethargy.
d. Monitor neuromuscular manifestations, such as reduced or absent deep tendon reflexes or weak or absent voluntary skeletal muscle contractions.
e. Administer loop diuretics as prescribed to excrete magnesium.
f. Administer calcium as prescribed for resulting cardiac problems.
g. Avoid medications that contain magnesium, such as antacids; some laxatives and enemas may also contain magnesium.
h. During severe elevations, avoid foods that increase magnesium levels (see Chapter 11 for a list of foods that are high in magnesium).

6. Hyperphosphatemia
   a. As the phosphorus level rises, the calcium level drops; this leads to the stimulation of parathyroid hormone, causing bone demineralization.
   b. Treatment is aimed at lowering the serum phosphorus level.
   c. Administer phosphate binders as prescribed with meals to lower serum phosphate levels.
   d. Administer stool softeners and laxatives as prescribed, because phosphate binders are constipating.
   e. Teach the client about the need to limit the intake of foods high in phosphorus (see Chapter 11 for a list of foods that are high in phosphorus).
7. Hypertension
   a. Caused by failure of the kidneys to maintain BP homeostasis.
   b. Monitor vital signs for elevated BP.
   c. Maintain fluid and sodium restrictions as prescribed.
   d. Administer diuretics and antihypertensives as prescribed.
8. Hypervolemia
   a. Monitor vital signs for an elevated BP.
   b. Monitor intake and output and daily weight for indications of fluid retention.
   c. Monitor for periorbital, sacral, and peripheral edema.
   d. Monitor the serum electrolyte levels.
   e. Monitor for hypertension and notify the PHCP if there are sustained elevations.
   f. Monitor for signs of heart failure and pulmonary edema, such as restlessness, heightened anxiety, tachycardia, dyspnea, basilar lung crackles, and blood-tinged sputum; notify the PHCP immediately if signs occur.
   g. Maintain fluid restriction.
   h. Avoid the administration of large amounts of IV fluids.
   i. Administer diuretics as prescribed.
   j. Teach the client to maintain a low-sodium diet.
   k. Teach the client to avoid over-the-counter medications without checking with the PHCP.
9. Hypocalcemia
   a. Results from a high phosphorus level and the inability of the diseased kidney to activate vitamin D
   b. The absence of vitamin D causes poor calcium absorption from the intestinal tract.
   c. Monitor the serum calcium level.
   d. Administer calcium supplements as prescribed.
   e. Administer activated vitamin D as prescribed.
   f. See Chapter 11 for a list of foods that are high in calcium.
10. Hypovolemia
   a. Monitor the vital signs for hypotension and tachycardia.
   b. Monitor for decreasing intake and output and a reduction in the daily weight.
   c. Monitor for dehydration.
   d. Monitor electrolyte levels.
   e. Provide replacement therapy based on the serum electrolyte level values.
11. Infection
   a. The client is at risk for infection caused by a suppressed immune system, dialysis access site, and possible malnutrition.
   b. Monitor for signs of infection.
   c. Avoid urinary catheters when possible; if used, provide catheter care per protocol.
   d. Provide strict asepsis during urinary catheter insertion and other invasive procedures.
   e. Instruct the client to avoid fatigue and avoid persons with infections.
   f. Administer antibiotics as prescribed, monitoring for nephrotoxic effects.
12. Metabolic acidosis
   a. The kidneys are unable to excrete hydrogen ions or manufacture bicarbonate, resulting in acidosis.
   b. Administer alkalizers such as sodium bicarbonate as prescribed.
   c. Note that clients with CKD adjust to low bicarbonate levels and as a result do not become acutely ill.
13. Muscle cramps
   a. Occur from electrolyte imbalances and the effects of uremia on peripheral nerves
   b. Monitor serum electrolyte levels.
   c. Administer electrolyte replacements and medications to control muscle cramps as prescribed.
   d. Administer heat and massage as prescribed.

14. Neurological changes
    a. The buildup of active particles and fluids causes changes in the brain cells and leads to confusion and impairment in decision-making ability.
    b. Peripheral neuropathy results from the effects of uremia on peripheral nerves.
    c. Monitor the level of consciousness and for confusion.
    d. Monitor for restless leg syndrome, which is also common during dialysis treatments.
    e. Teach the client to examine areas of decreased sensation for signs of injury.
15. Ocular irritation
    a. Calcium deposits in the conjunctivae cause burning and watering of the eyes.
    b. Administer medications to control the calcium and phosphate levels as prescribed.
    c. Administer lubricating eye drops.
    d. Protect the client from injury.
16. Potential for injury
    a. The client is at risk for fractures caused by alterations in the absorption of calcium, excretion of phosphate, and vitamin D metabolism.
    b. Provide for a safe environment.
    c. Avoid injury; tissue breakdown causes increased serum potassium levels.
17. Pruritus
    a. To rid the body of excess wastes, urate crystals are excreted through the skin, causing pruritus.
    b. The deposit of urate crystals (uremic frost) occurs in advanced stages of kidney disease.
    c. Monitor for skin breakdown, rash, and uremic frost.
    d. Provide meticulous skin care and oral hygiene.
    e. Avoid the use of soaps.
    f. Administer antihistamines and antipruritics as prescribed to relieve itching.
    g. Teach the client to keep the nails trimmed to prevent local infection from scratching.
18. Psychosocial problems
    a. Listen to the client's concerns to determine how the client is handling the situation.
    b. Allow the client time to mourn the loss of kidney function.
    c. With client permission, include the family members in discussions of the client's concerns.
    d. Provide education about treatment options and support the client's decision; elderly clients with CKD may progress slowly toward end-stage kidney disease or require dialysis, and clients may decide on no treatment and opt for end-of-life care.
    e. Offer information about support groups.

V. Uremic Syndrome

A. Description: Systemic clinical and laboratory manifestations of severe and/or end-stage kidney disease due to accumulation of nitrogenous waste products in the blood caused by the kidneys' inability to filter out these waste products.

B. Assessment
1. Oliguria
2. Presence of protein, red blood cells, and casts in the urine
3. Elevated levels of urea, uric acid, potassium, and magnesium in the urine
4. Hypotension or hypertension
5. Alterations in the level of consciousness
6. Electrolyte imbalances
7. Stomatitis
8. Nausea or vomiting
9. Diarrhea or constipation

C. Interventions
1. Monitor vital signs for hypertension, tachycardia, and an irregular heart rate.
2. Monitor serum electrolyte levels.
3. Monitor intake and output and for oliguria.
4. Provide a limited but high-quality protein diet as prescribed.
5. Provide a limited sodium, nitrogen, potassium, and phosphate diet as prescribed.
6. Assist the client to cope with body image disturbances caused by uremic syndrome.

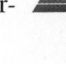

VI. Hemodialysis

A. Description
1. Hemodialysis is an intermittent renal replacement therapy involving the process of cleansing the client's blood.
2. It involves the diffusion of dissolved particles from 1 fluid compartment into another across a semipermeable membrane; the client's blood flows through 1 fluid compartment of a dialysis filter, and the dialysate is in another fluid compartment.

B. Functions of hemodialysis
1. Cleanses the blood of accumulated waste products
2. Removes the byproducts of protein metabolism such as urea, creatinine, and uric acid from the blood
3. Removes excess body fluids
4. Maintains or restores the buffer system of the body
5. Corrects electrolyte levels in the body

C. Principles of hemodialysis
1. The semipermeable membrane is made of a thin, porous cellophane.
2. The pore size of the membrane allows small particles to pass through, such as urea, creatinine, uric acid, and water molecules.

3. Proteins, bacteria, and some blood cells are too large to pass through the membrane.
4. The client's blood flows into the dialyzer; the movement of substances occurs from the blood to the dialysate by the principles of osmosis, diffusion, and ultrafiltration.
5. Osmosis is the movement of fluids across a semipermeable membrane from an area of lower concentration of particles to an area of higher concentration of particles.
6. Diffusion is the movement of particles from an area of higher concentration to one of lower concentration.
7. Ultrafiltration is the movement of fluid across a semipermeable membrane as a result of an artificially created pressure gradient.

D. Dialysate bath
1. A dialysate bath is composed of water and major electrolytes.
2. The dialysate need not be sterile because bacteria and viruses are too large to pass through the pores of the semipermeable membrane; however, the dialysate must meet specific standards, and water is treated to ensure a safe water supply.

E. Interventions
1. Monitor vital signs before, during, and after dialysis; the client's temperature may elevate because of slight warming of the blood from the dialysis machine (notify the PHCP about excessive temperature elevations because this could indicate sepsis, requiring blood cultures to be collected).
2. Monitor laboratory values, specifically the BUN, creatinine, and complete blood cell counts before, during, and after dialysis.
3. Assess the client for fluid overload before dialysis and fluid volume deficit following dialysis.
4. Weigh the client before and after dialysis to determine fluid loss. Note that the client will not urinate or will urinate small amounts (may be less than 30 mL/hr).
5. Assess the patency of the blood access device before, during, and after dialysis.
6. Monitor for bleeding; heparin is added to the dialysis bath to prevent clots from forming in the dialyzer or the blood tubing.
7. Monitor for hypovolemia during dialysis, which can occur from blood loss or excess fluid and electrolyte removal.
8. Provide adequate nutrition; the client may eat before or during dialysis.
9. Identify the client's reactions to the treatment and support coping mechanisms; encourage independence and involvement in care.

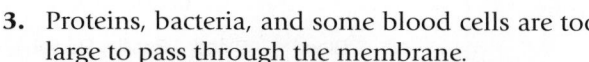

Withhold antihypertensives and other medications that can affect the BP or result in hypotension until after hemodialysis treatment. Also withhold medications that could be removed by dialysis, such as water-soluble vitamins, certain antibiotics, and digoxin.

VII. Access for Hemodialysis

A. Subclavian and femoral catheters
1. Description
   a. A subclavian (subclavian vein) or femoral (femoral vein) catheter may be inserted for short-term or temporary use in AKI.
   b. The catheter is used until a fistula or graft matures or develops, which is typically 6 weeks, or may be required when the client's fistula or graft access has failed because of infection or clotting.
2. Interventions
   a. Assess insertion site for hematoma, bleeding, catheter dislodgement, and infection.
   b. These catheters should only be used for dialysis treatments and accessed by dialysis personnel.
   c. Maintain an occlusive dressing over the catheter insertion site.
3. Subclavian vein catheter
   a. The catheter is usually filled with heparin and capped to maintain patency between dialysis treatments. Heparin is aspirated from the line before dialysis.
   b. The catheter should not be uncapped except for dialysis treatments.
   c. The catheter may be left in place for up to 6 weeks if no complications occur.
4. Femoral vein catheter
   a. Assess the extremity for circulation, temperature, and pulses.
   b. Prevent pulling or disconnecting of the catheter when giving care.
   c. Because the groin is not a clean site, meticulous perineal care is required.
   d. Use an IV infusion pump or controller with microdrip tubing if a heparin infusion through the catheter to maintain patency is prescribed.

The client with a femoral vein catheter should not sit up more than 45 degrees or lean forward, because the catheter may kink and occlude.

B. External arteriovenous shunt (Fig. 54-2)
1. Description
   a. Two Silastic cannulas are surgically inserted into an artery and vein in the forearm or leg to form an external blood path.

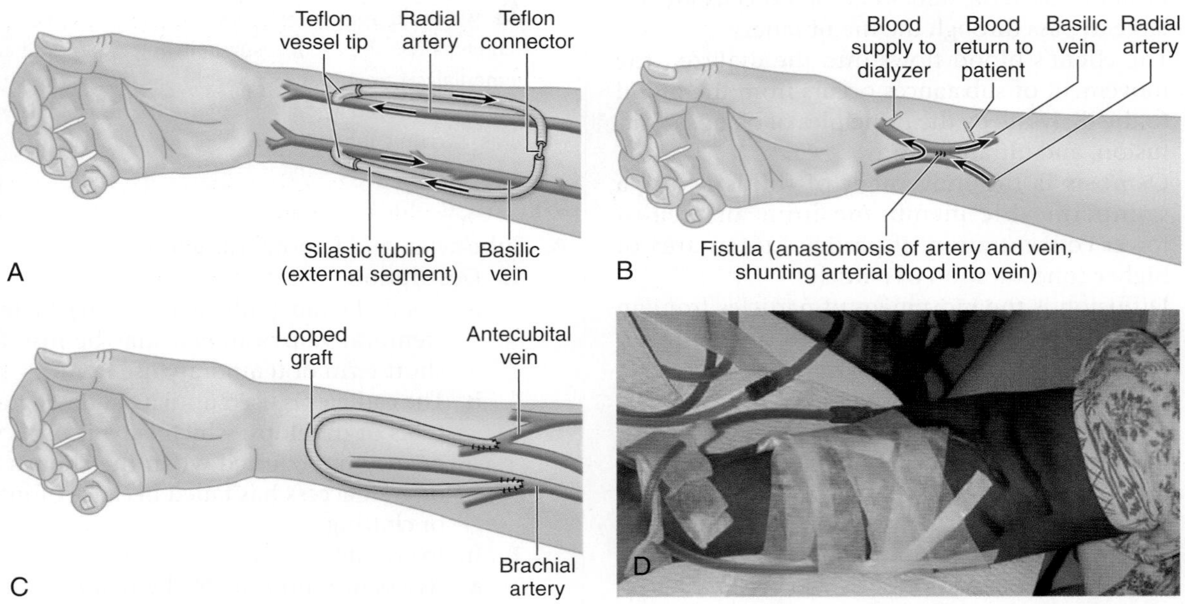

FIG. 54-2 Vascular access for hemodialysis. **A,** External shunt. **B,** Internal arteriovenous fistula. **C,** Internal arteriovenous graft. **D,** A hemodialysis graft while connected to a hemodialysis machine. (**D,** From Lewis et al., 2011.)

b. The cannulas are connected to form a U shape; blood flows from the client's artery through the shunt into the vein.
c. A tube leading to the membrane compartment of the dialyzer is connected to the arterial cannula.
d. Blood fills the membrane compartment, passes through the dialyzer, and is returned to the client through a tube connected to the venous cannula.
e. When dialysis is complete, the cannulas are clamped and reattached, reforming the U shape.

2. Advantages
a. The external arteriovenous shunt can be used immediately following its creation.
b. No venipuncture is necessary for dialysis.

3. Disadvantages
a. Disconnection or dislodgment of the external shunt
b. Risk of hemorrhage, infection, or clotting
c. Potential for skin erosion around the catheter site

4. Interventions
a. Avoid getting the shunt wet.
b. Wrap a dressing completely around the shunt and keep it dry and intact.
c. Keep cannula clamps at the client's bedside or attached to the arteriovenous dressing for use in case of accidental disconnection.
d. Teach the client that the shunt extremity should not be used for monitoring BP, drawing blood, placing IV lines, or administering injections.
e. Fold back the dressing to expose the shunt tubing and assess for signs of hemorrhage, infection, or clotting.
f. Monitor skin integrity around the insertion site.
g. Auscultate for a bruit and palpate for a thrill, although a bruit may not be heard with the shunt.
h. Notify the PHCP immediately if signs of clotting, hemorrhage, or infection occur.

5. Signs of clotting
a. Fibrin: White flecks in the tubing
b. Separation of serum and cells
c. Absence of a previously heard bruit; thrill absent on palpation
d. Coolness of the tubing or extremity
e. Tingling sensation at site or in extremity

C. Internal **arteriovenous fistula** (see Fig. 54-2)
1. Description
a. A permanent access of choice for the client with CKD requiring dialysis.
b. The fistula is created surgically by anastomosis of a large artery and large vein in the arm.
c. The flow of arterial blood into the venous system causes the vein to become engorged (matured or developed).
d. Maturity takes about 4 to 6 weeks, depending on the client's ability to do hand-flexing exercises such as ball squeezing, which help the fistula mature.

e. The fistula is required to be mature before it can be used, because the engorged vein is punctured with a large-bore needle for the dialysis procedure.
f. Subclavian or femoral catheters, PD, or an external arteriovenous shunt can be used for dialysis while the fistula is maturing or developing.
g. Avoid taking BP or performing venipuncture for intravenous access or lab draws to protect the integrity of the fistula.
h. Fistulas are dressed with pressure dressings after hemodialysis to prevent bleeding. Ensure the removal of the pressure dressing within the prescribed time frame or according to agency policy.

2. Advantages
a. Because the fistula is internal, the risk of clotting and bleeding is low.
b. The fistula can be used indefinitely.
c. The fistula has a decreased incidence of infection, because it is internal and is not exposed.
d. Once healing has occurred, no external dressing is required.
e. The fistula allows freedom of movement.

3. Disadvantages
a. The fistula cannot be used immediately after insertion, so planning ahead for an alternative access for dialysis is important.
b. Needle insertions through the skin and tissues to the fistula are required for dialysis.
c. Infiltration of the needles during dialysis can occur and cause hematomas.
d. An aneurysm can form in the fistula.
e. Heart failure can occur from the increased blood flow in the venous system.

Arterial steal syndrome can develop in a client with an internal arteriovenous fistula. In this complication, too much blood is diverted to the vein, and arterial perfusion to the hand is compromised.

D. Internal arteriovenous graft (see Fig. 54-2)
1. Description
a. The internal graft may be used for chronic dialysis clients who do not have adequate blood vessels for the creation of a fistula.
b. An artificial graft made of Gore-Tex or a bovine (cow) carotid artery is used to create an artificial vein for blood flow.
c. The procedure involves the anastomosis of an artery to a vein, using an artificial graft.
d. The graft can be used 2 weeks after insertion.
e. Complications of the graft include clotting, aneurysms, and infection.

2. Advantages and disadvantages: Same as for internal arteriovenous fistula

E. Interventions for an arteriovenous fistula and arteriovenous graft
1. Teach the client that the extremity should not be used for monitoring BP, drawing blood, placing IV lines, or administering injections, and that the client should inform all health care personnel of its presence.
2. Teach the client with an arteriovenous fistula to perform hand-flexing exercises such as ball squeezing (if prescribed) to promote graft maturity.
3. Note the temperature and capillary refill of the extremity.
4. Palpate pulses below the fistula or graft, and monitor for hand swelling as an indication of ischemia.
5. Monitor for clotting.
a. Complaints of tingling or discomfort in the extremity
b. Inability to palpate a thrill or auscultate a bruit over the fistula or graft
6. Monitor for **arterial steal syndrome**.
7. Monitor for infection.
8. Monitor lung and heart sounds for signs of heart failure.
9. Notify the PHCP immediately if signs of clotting, infection, or arterial steal syndrome occur.

To ensure patency, palpate for a thrill or auscultate for a bruit over the fistula or graft. Notify the PHCP if a thrill or bruit is absent.

VIII. Complications of Hemodialysis (Box 54-7)

A. If signs of complications occur, the dialysis is slowed or stopped, depending on the complication, and the PHCP is notified immediately.
B. The nurse stays with the client and monitors the client, including vital signs, while another nurse obtains initial prescriptions from the PHCP.
C. See Priority Nursing Actions for air embolism.

PRIORITY NURSING ACTIONS

Air Embolism in a Client Receiving Hemodialysis

1. Stop the hemodialysis.
2. Turn the client on the left side, with the head down (Trendelenburg's position).
3. Notify the primary health care provider (PHCP) and Rapid Response Team for the hospitalized client.
4. Administer oxygen.
5. Assess vital signs and pulse oximetry.
6. Document the event, actions taken, and the client's response.

Reference

Ignatavicius, Workman, Rebar (2018), p. 214.

BOX 54-7 Complications of Hemodialysis

- Air embolus
- Disequilibrium syndrome
- Electrolyte alterations
- Encephalopathy
- Hemorrhage
- Hepatitis
- Hypotension
- Sepsis
- Shock

IX. Peritoneal Dialysis

A. Description
  1. The peritoneum acts as the dialyzing membrane (semipermeable membrane) to achieve dialysis, and the membrane is accessed by insertion of a PD catheter through the abdomen.
  2. PD works on the principles of osmosis, diffusion, and ultrafiltration; PD occurs via the transfer of fluid and solute from the bloodstream through the peritoneum into the dialysate solution.
  3. The peritoneal membrane is large and porous, allowing solutes and fluid to move via osmosis from an area of higher concentration in the body to an area of lower concentration in the dialyzing fluid.
  4. The peritoneal cavity is rich in capillaries; therefore, it provides a ready access to the blood supply.

B. Contraindications to PD
  1. Peritonitis
  2. Recent abdominal surgery
  3. Abdominal adhesions
  4. Other GI problems such as diverticulosis

C. Access for PD (Fig. 54-3)
  1. A siliconized rubber catheter such as a Tenckhoff catheter is surgically inserted into the client's peritoneal cavity to allow infusion of dialysis fluid; the catheter site is covered by a sterile dressing that is changed daily and when soiled or wet.
  2. The preferred insertion site is 3 to 5 cm below the umbilicus; this area is relatively avascular and has less fascial resistance.
  3. The catheter is tunneled under the skin, through the fat and muscle tissue to the peritoneum; it is stabilized with inflatable Dacron cuffs in the muscle and under the skin.
  4. Over a period of 1 to 2 weeks following insertion, fibroblasts and blood vessels grow around the cuffs, fixing the catheter in place and providing an extra barrier against dialysate leakage and bacterial invasion.
  5. If the client is scheduled for transplant surgery, the PD catheter may be either removed or left in place if the need for dialysis is suspected post-transplantation.

D. Dialysate solution
  1. The solution is sterile.
  2. All dialysis solutions are prescribed by the PHCP; the solution contains electrolytes and minerals and has a specific osmolarity, specific glucose concentration, and other medication additives as prescribed.
  3. The higher the glucose concentration, the greater the hypertonicity and the amount of fluid removed during a PD exchange.
  4. Increasing the glucose concentration increases the concentration of active particles that cause osmosis, increases the rate of ultrafiltration, and increases the amount of fluid removed.
  5. If hyperkalemia is not a problem, potassium may be added to each bag of dialysate solution.

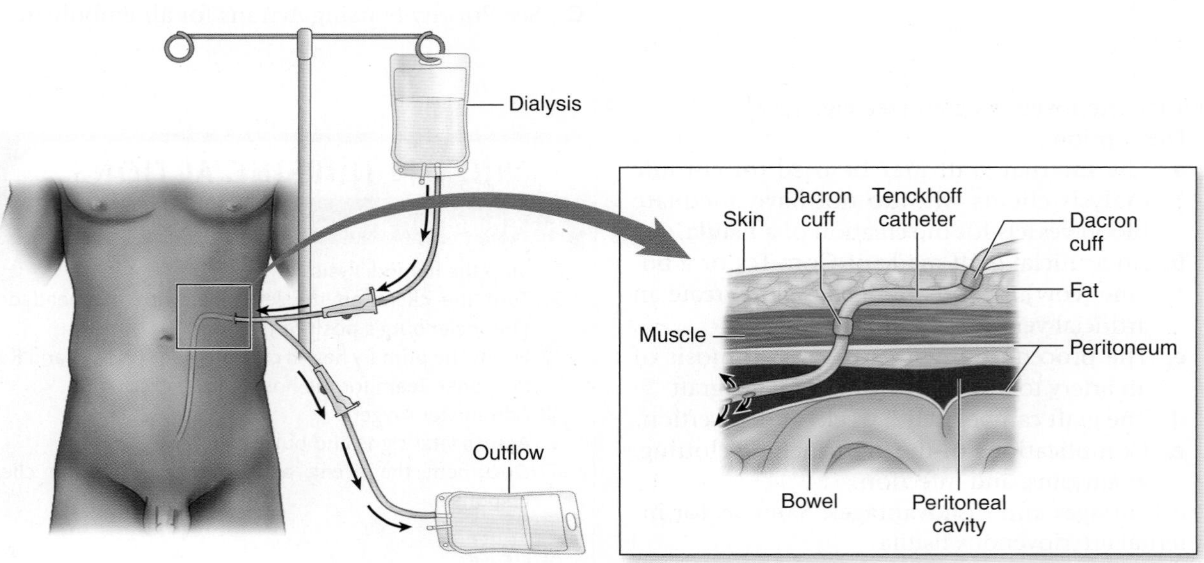

FIG. 54-3 Manual peritoneal dialysis via an implanted abdominal catheter (Tenckhoff catheter).

6. Heparin is added to the dialysate solution to prevent clotting of the catheter.
7. Prophylactic antibiotics may be added to the dialysate solution to prevent peritonitis.
8. Insulin may be added to the dialysate solution for the client with diabetes mellitus.

E. PD infusion
1. Description
   a. One infusion (fill), dwell, and drain is considered 1 exchange.
   b. Fill: 1 to 2 L of dialysate as prescribed is infused by gravity into the peritoneal space, which usually takes 10 to 20 minutes.
   c. Dwell time: The amount of time that the dialysate solution remains in the peritoneal cavity is prescribed by the PHCP and can last 20 to 30 minutes to 8 or more hours, depending on the type of dialysis used.
   d. Drain (outflow): Fluid drains out of body by gravity into the drainage bag.
2. Interventions before treatment
   a. Monitor vital signs.
   b. Monitor daily weight on the same scale.
   c. Have the client void, if possible.
   d. Assess electrolyte and glucose levels.
   e. Assess the peritoneal catheter dressing and site.
3. Interventions during treatment
   a. Monitor vital signs.
   b. Monitor for respiratory distress, pain, or discomfort.
   c. Monitor for signs of pulmonary edema.
   d. Monitor for hypotension and hypertension.
   e. Monitor for malaise, nausea, and vomiting.
   f. Assess the catheter site dressing for wetness or bleeding.
   g. Monitor dwell time as prescribed by the PHCP.
   h. Do not allow dwell time to extend beyond the PHCP's prescription, because this increases the risk for hyperglycemia.
   i. Initiate outflow; turn the client from side to side if the outflow is slow to start.
   j. Monitor outflow, which should be a continuous stream after the clamp is opened.
   k. Monitor outflow for color and clarity.
   l. Monitor intake and output accurately; if outflow is less than inflow, the difference is equal to the amount absorbed or retained by the client during dialysis and should be counted as intake.
   m. An outflow greater than inflow as well as the appearance of frank blood or cloudiness in the outflow should be reported to the PHCP.

F. Types of PD
1. Continuous ambulatory peritoneal dialysis (CAPD)
   a. Closely resembles renal function because it is a continuous process
   b. Does not require a machine for the procedure
   c. Promotes client independence
   d. The client performs self-dialysis 24 hours a day, 7 days a week.
   e. Four dialysis cycles are usually administered in a 24-hour period, including an overnight 8-hour dwell time.
   f. Dialysate, 1.5 to 2 L, is instilled into the abdomen 4 times daily and allowed to dwell as prescribed (bags are weighed to determine output); the catheter is clamped and the bag is rolled up during dwell time.
   g. After dwell, the bag is placed lower than the insertion site and the clamp is opened so that fluid drains out by gravity flow.
   h. After fluid is drained, the bag is changed, new dialysate is instilled into the abdomen, and the process continues.
   i. Between exchanges, the catheter is clamped.
2. Automated peritoneal dialysis (Box 54-8)
   a. Automated dialysis requires a peritoneal cycling machine.
   b. Automated dialysis can be done as intermittent peritoneal dialysis, continuous cycling peritoneal dialysis, or nightly peritoneal dialysis.
   c. The exchanges are automated instead of manual.

BOX 54-8 Types of Automated Peritoneal Dialysis

Continuous Cycling Peritoneal Dialysis
- Dialysis requires a peritoneal cycling machine.
- Dialysis usually consists of 3 cycles done at night and 1 cycle with an 8-hour dwell done in the morning.
- The sterile catheter system is opened only for the on-and-off procedures, which reduces the risk of infection.
- The client does not need to do exchanges during the day.

Intermittent Peritoneal Dialysis
- Dialysis requires a peritoneal cycling machine.
- Dialysis is not a continuous procedure.
- Dialysis is performed for 10 to 14 hours, 3 or 4 times a week.

Nightly Peritoneal Dialysis
- Dialysis requires a cycling machine.
- Dialysis is performed for 8 to 12 hours each night, with no daytime exchanges or dwells.

X. Complications of Peritoneal Dialysis

⚠ Infection is a concern with PD; sites of infection are either the catheter insertion site or the peritoneum, causing peritonitis.

A. Peritonitis
1. Monitor for signs and symptoms of peritonitis: Fever, cloudy outflow, rebound abdominal tenderness, abdominal pain, general malaise, nausea, and vomiting.
2. Cloudy or opaque outflow is an early sign of peritonitis.
3. If peritonitis is suspected, obtain a sample for culture and sensitivity of the outflow to determine the infective organism.
4. Antibiotics may be added to the dialysate.
5. Avoid infections by maintaining meticulous sterile technique when connecting and disconnecting PD solution bags and when caring for the catheter insertion site.
6. Prevent the catheter insertion site dressing from becoming wet during care of the client or the dialysis procedure; change the dressing if wet or soiled.
7. Follow institutional procedure for connecting and disconnecting PD solution bags, which may include scrubbing the connection sites with an antiseptic solution.

B. Abdominal pain
1. Peritoneal irritation during inflow commonly causes abdominal cramping and discomfort during the first few exchanges; the pain usually disappears after 1 to 2 weeks of dialysis treatments.
2. Warm the dialysate before administration, using a special dialysate warmer pad, because the cold temperature of the dialysate can cause discomfort.

C. Abnormal outflow characteristics indicative of complications
1. Bloody outflow after the first few exchanges indicates vascular complications (the outflow should be clear after the initial exchanges).
2. Brown outflow indicates bowel perforation.
3. Urine-colored outflow indicates bladder perforation.
4. Cloudy outflow indicates peritonitis.

D. Insufficient outflow
1. The main cause of insufficient outflow is a full colon; encourage a high-fiber diet, because constipation can cause inflow and outflow problems. Administer stool softeners as prescribed.
2. Insufficient outflow may also be caused by catheter migration out of the peritoneal area; if this occurs, an x-ray will be prescribed to evaluate catheter position.
3. Maintain the drainage bag below the client's abdomen.
4. Check for kinks in the tubing.
5. Change the client's outflow position by turning the client to a side-lying position or ambulating the client.
6. Check for fibrin clots in the tubing and milk the tubing to dislodge the clot as prescribed.

E. Leakage around the catheter site
1. Clear fluid that leaks from the catheter exit site will be noted.
2. It takes 1 to 2 weeks following insertion of the catheter before fibroblasts and blood vessels grow into the catheter cuffs, which fix it in place and provide an extra barrier against dialysate leakage and bacterial invasion.
3. Smaller amounts of dialysate need to be used; it may take up to 2 weeks for the client to tolerate a full 2-L exchange without leaking around the catheter site.

XI. Kidney Transplantation (Fig. 54-4)

A. Description
1. A human kidney from a compatible donor is implanted into a recipient.
2. Kidney transplantation is performed for irreversible kidney failure; specific criteria are established for eligibility for a transplant.
3. The recipient must take immunosuppressive medications for life.

B. Donors
1. Donors may be living donors (related or unrelated to the client), non-heart-beating donors (NHBDs), or cadaver donors.
2. The most desirable source of kidneys for transplantation is living related donors who closely match the client.
3. Non-heart-beating donors are those who have been declared dead by cardiopulmonary criteria and have organs harvested immediately after death; these persons have consented previously to organ donation.
4. Cadaver donors are those who have suffered irreversible brain injury; these persons are maintained with mechanical ventilation and must have adequate perfusion to the kidneys.
5. Physical criteria for donors include absence of systemic disease and infection, no history of cancer, no kidney disease or hypertension, and adequate kidney function.
6. Donors are screened for ABO blood group, tissue-specific antigen, human leukocyte antigen suitability, and mixed lymphocyte culture index (histocompatibility); donors are also screened for the presence of any communicable diseases

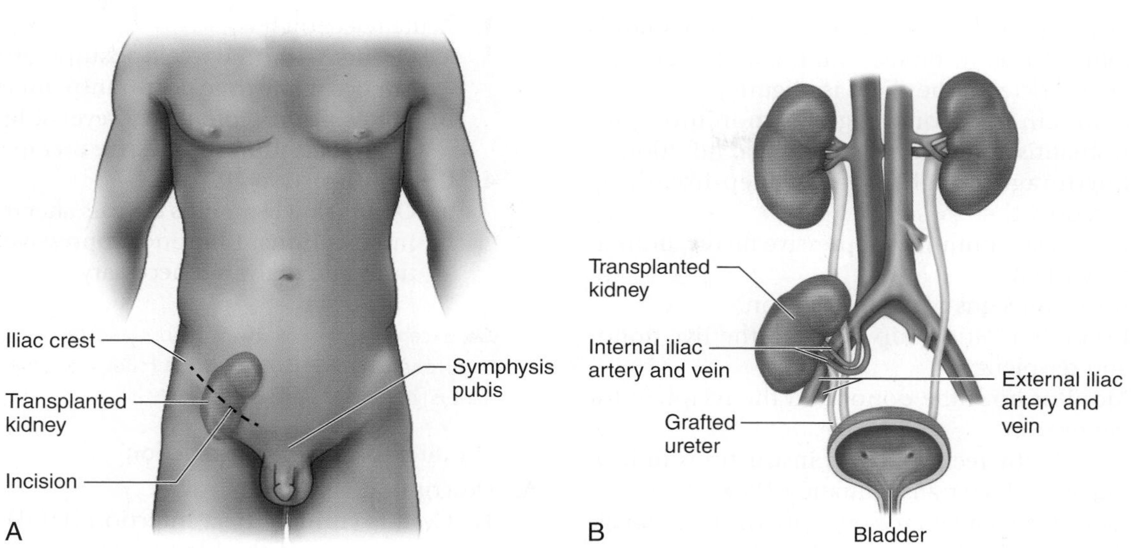

FIG. 54-4 **A,** Surgical incision for renal transplantation. **B,** Surgical placement of transplanted kidney.

and undergo a complete medical evaluation as well as a nephrology consultation.

7. The donor must be in excellent health, with 2 properly functioning kidneys.
8. The emotional well-being of the donor is determined.
9. Complete understanding of the donation process and outcome by the donor is necessary; usually kidney removal from the donor is done using a laparoscopic procedure.

C. Preoperative interventions
1. Verify histocompatibility tests of donor, which will be done by organ bank personnel.
2. Administer immunosuppressive medications to the recipient as prescribed.
3. Maintain strict aseptic technique.
4. Verify that hemodialysis of the recipient was completed 24 hours before transplantation.
5. Ensure that the recipient is free of any infections.
6. Assess renal function studies.
7. Encourage discussion of feelings of the live donor and the recipient.
8. Provide psychological support to the live donor, NHBD, or cadaver donor family and to the recipient.

D. Postoperative interventions for the recipient
1. The transplanted kidney is placed in the anterior iliac fossa; usually the recipient's diseased kidneys are left in place, except for those with polycystic kidney disease, in which the kidneys are often very enlarged and painful.
2. Urine output usually begins immediately if the donor was a living donor; it may be delayed for a few days or more with other donor types.
3. Hemodialysis may be performed until adequate kidney function is established.
4. Monitor vital signs and for signs of complications such as rejection, thrombosis, renal artery stenosis, or wound problems.
5. Monitor urine output hourly; immediately report an abrupt decrease in output.
6. Monitor IV fluids closely; for the first 12 to 24 hours, IV fluid replacement is based on hourly urine output.
7. Administer prescribed diuretics and osmotic agents.
8. Monitor daily weight to evaluate fluid status.
9. Monitor daily laboratory results to evaluate renal function, including hematocrit, BUN, and serum creatinine levels, and monitor urine for blood and specific gravity.
10. Position the client in a semi-Fowler's position to promote gas exchange, turning from the back to the nonoperative side.
11. Monitor urinary catheter patency; the urinary catheter usually remains in the bladder for 3 to 5 days to allow for anastomosis healing; it is removed as soon as possible to prevent infection.
12. Note that urine is pink and may be bloody initially but gradually returns to normal within several days to weeks.
13. Notify the PHCP if gross hematuria and clots are noted in the urine.
14. Monitor the 3-way bladder irrigation, if present, for clots; irrigate only if an PHCP's prescription is present.
15. Maintain aseptic technique and monitor for infection.
16. Maintain strict aseptic technique with wound care.
17. Monitor for bowel sounds and for the passage of flatus; initiate a specific diet and oral fluids

as prescribed when flatus and bowel sounds return (usually, fluids, sodium, and potassium are restricted if the client is oliguric).

18. Maintain good oral hygiene, monitoring for stomatitis and bacterial and fungal infections.

19. Encourage coughing and deep-breathing exercises.

20. Administer immunosuppressive medications as prescribed.

21. Assess for signs of organ rejection.

22. Promote relationship between the live donor and recipient.

23. Monitor both the donor and the recipient for depression.

24. Provide the recipient with instructions following the kidney transplantation (Box 54-9).

25. Assist the recipient to cope with the body image disturbances that occur from long-term use of immunosuppressants.

26. Advise the recipient of available support groups.

E. Graft rejection

1. Assessment (Box 54-10)

2. Hyperacute rejection

a. Hyperacute rejection occurs within 48 hours after the transplant.

b. Intervention: Removal of rejected kidney

3. Acute rejection

a. Occurs within 1 week postoperatively, but can occur any time post-transplantation.

b. Intervention: Potentially reversible with increased immunosuppressive therapy.

4. Chronic rejection

a. Occurs slowly months to years after transplant.

b. Interventions: Immunosuppressive medications and dialysis if necessary.

Except in identical twin donors and recipients, the major postoperative complication following renal transplant is graft rejection.

XII. Cystitis (Urinary Tract Infection)

A. Description

1. Cystitis (urinary tract infection [UTI]) is an inflammation of the bladder from an infection, obstruction of the urethra, or other irritants (Box 54-11).

2. The most common causative organisms are *Escherichia coli* and *Enterobacter, Pseudomonas,* and *Serratia* species.

3. Cystitis is more common in women, because women have a shorter urethra than men and the urethra in the woman is located close to the rectum.

4. Sexually active and pregnant women are most vulnerable to cystitis.

B. Assessment

1. Frequency and urgency

2. Burning on urination

3. Voiding in small amounts

4. Inability to void

5. Incomplete emptying of the bladder

6. Lower abdominal discomfort or back discomfort; bladder spasms

BOX 54-9 Client Instructions Following Kidney Transplantation

- Avoid prolonged periods of sitting.
- Monitor intake and output.
- Recognize the signs and symptoms of infection and rejection.
- Use medications as prescribed, and maintain immunosuppressive therapy for life.
- Avoid contact sports.
- Avoid exposure to persons with infections.
- Know the signs and symptoms that require the need to contact the primary health care provider or nephrologist.
- Ensure follow-up care.

BOX 54-10 Clinical Signs of Renal Transplant (Graft) Rejection

- Temperature higher than 100° F (37.8° C)
- Pain or tenderness over the grafted kidney
- 2- to 3-lb (0.9 to 1.4 kg) weight gain in 24 hours
- Edema
- Hypertension
- Malaise
- Elevated blood urea nitrogen and serum creatinine levels
- Decreased creatinine clearance
- Elevated white blood cell count
- Rejection indicated by ultrasound or biopsy

BOX 54-11 Causes of Cystitis

- Allergens or irritants, such as soaps, sprays, bubble bath, perfumed sanitary napkins
- Bladder distention
- Calculus
- Hormonal changes, influencing alterations in vaginal flora
- Indwelling urinary catheters
- Invasive urinary tract procedures
- Loss of bactericidal properties of prostatic secretions in the male
- Microorganisms
- Poor-fitting vaginal diaphragms
- Sexual intercourse
- Synthetic underwear and pantyhose
- Urinary stasis
- Use of spermicides
- Wet bathing suits

7. Cloudy, dark, foul-smelling urine
8. Hematuria
9. Malaise, chills, fever
10. WBC count greater than 11,000 mm^3 ($11.0 \times 10^9/L$) on urinalysis

⚠ Altered mentation is a sign of a UTI in older adults; frequency and urgency may not be specific symptoms of UTI because of urinary elimination changes that occur with aging.

C. Interventions
1. Before administering prescribed antibiotics, obtain a urine specimen for culture and sensitivity, if prescribed, to identify bacterial growth.
2. Encourage the client to increase fluids up to 3000 mL/day, especially if the client is taking a sulfonamide; sulfonamides can form crystals in concentrated urine.
3. Administer prescribed medications, which may include analgesics, antiseptics, antispasmodics, antibiotics, and antimicrobials.
4. Maintain an acid urine pH (5.5); instruct the client about foods to consume to maintain acidic urine.
5. Provide heat to the abdomen or sitz baths for complaints of discomfort.
6. Note that if the client is prescribed an aminoglycoside, sulfonamide, or nitrofurantoin, the actions of these medications are decreased by acidic urine.
7. Use sterile technique when inserting a urinary catheter.
8. Provide meticulous perineal care for the client with an indwelling catheter.
9. Discourage caffeine products such as coffee, tea, and cola.
10. Client education
    a. Avoid alcohol.
    b. Take medications as prescribed.
    c. Take antibiotics on schedule and complete the entire course of medications as prescribed, which may be 10 to 14 days.
    d. Repeat the urine culture following treatment.
    e. Prevent recurrence of cystitis (Box 54-12).

BOX 54-12 Client Instructions for Prevention of Cystitis

- Use good perineal care, wiping front to back.
- Avoid bubble baths, tub baths, and vaginal deodorants or sprays.
- Void every 2 to 3 hours.
- Wear cotton pants and avoid wearing tight clothes or pantyhose with slacks.
- Avoid sitting in a wet bathing suit for prolonged periods of time.
- If pregnant, void every 2 hours.
- If menopausal, use estrogen vaginal creams to restore pH.
- Use water-soluble lubricants for intercourse, especially after menopause.
- Void and drink a glass of water after intercourse.

XIII. Urethritis

A. Description
1. Inflammation of the urethra commonly associated with a sexually transmitted infection (STI); may occur with cystitis.
2. In men, urethritis most often is caused by gonorrhea or chlamydial infection.
3. In women, urethritis most often is caused by feminine hygiene sprays, perfumed toilet paper or sanitary napkins, spermicidal jelly, UTI, or changes in the vaginal mucosal lining.

B. Assessment
1. Pain or burning on urination
2. Frequency and urgency
3. Nocturia
4. Difficulty voiding
5. Males may have clear to mucopurulent discharge from the penis.
6. Females may have lower abdominal discomfort.

C. Interventions
1. Encourage fluid intake.
2. Prepare the client for testing to determine whether an STI is present.
3. Administer antibiotics as prescribed.
4. Instruct the client in the administration of sitz or tub baths.
5. If stricture occurs, prepare the client for dilation of the urethra and instillation of an antiseptic solution.
6. Instruct the female client to avoid the use of perfumed toilet paper or sanitary napkins and feminine hygiene sprays.
7. Instruct the client to avoid intercourse until the symptoms subside or treatment of the STI is complete.
8. Instruct the client about STIs if this is the cause.
    a. Prevent STIs by the use of latex condoms or abstinence.
    b. All sexual partners during the 30 days before diagnosis with chlamydial infection should be notified, examined, and treated if indicated.
    c. Chlamydial infection often coexists with gonorrhea; diagnostic testing is done for both STIs.
    d. Treatment for STIs includes antibiotics as prescribed to treat the causative organism.
    e. A serious primary complication of chlamydial infection is sterility.
    f. Follow-up culture may be requested in 4 to 7 days to evaluate the effectiveness of medications.

XIV. Ureteritis

A. Description: An inflammation of the ureter commonly associated with bacterial or viral infections and pyelonephritis

B. Assessment

C. Interventions

1. Dysuria
2. Frequent urination
3. Clear to mucopurulent penile discharge in males
4. Treatment includes identifying and treating the underlying cause and providing symptomatic relief.
5. Metronidazole or clotrimazole may be prescribed for treating *Trichomonas* infection.
6. Nystatin or fluconazole may be prescribed for treating yeast infections.
7. Doxycycline or azithromycin may be prescribed for treating chlamydial infections.

XV. Pyelonephritis

A. Description

1. An inflammation of the renal pelvis and the parenchyma, commonly caused by bacterial invasion
2. Acute pyelonephritis often occurs after bacterial contamination of the urethra or following an invasive procedure of the urinary tract.
3. Chronic pyelonephritis most commonly occurs following chronic urinary flow obstruction with reflux.
4. *E. coli* is the most common causative bacterial organism.

B. Acute pyelonephritis

1. Acute pyelonephritis occurs as a new infection or recurs as a relapse of a previous infection.
2. It can progress to bacteremia or chronic pyelonephritis.
3. Assessment
   - **a.** Fever and chills
   - **b.** Tachycardia and tachypnea
   - **c.** Nausea
   - **d.** Flank pain on the affected side
   - **e.** Costovertebral angle tenderness
   - **f.** Headache
   - **g.** Dysuria
   - **h.** Frequency and urgency
   - **i.** Cloudy, bloody, or foul-smelling urine
   - **j.** Increased WBCs in the urine

C. Chronic pyelonephritis

1. A slow, progressive disease usually associated with recurrent acute attacks
2. Causes contraction of the kidney and dysfunction of the nephrons, which are replaced by scar tissue
3. Causes the ureter to become fibrotic and narrowed by strictures
4. Can lead to AKI or CKD
5. Assessment
   - **a.** Frequently diagnosed incidentally when a client is being evaluated for hypertension
   - **b.** Inability to conserve sodium
   - **c.** Poor urine-concentrating ability
   - **d.** Pyuria
   - **e.** Azotemia
   - **f.** Proteinuria

D. Interventions

1. Monitor vital signs, especially for elevated temperature.
2. Encourage fluid intake up to 3000 mL/day to reduce fever and prevent dehydration.
3. Monitor intake and output (ensure that output is a minimum of 1500 mL in 24 hours).
4. Monitor weight.
5. Encourage adequate rest.
6. Instruct the client about a high-calorie, low-protein diet.
7. Provide warm, moist compresses to the flank area to help relieve pain.
8. Encourage the client to take warm baths for pain relief.
9. Administer analgesics, antipyretics, antibiotics, urinary antiseptics, and antiemetics as prescribed.
10. Monitor for signs of AKI or CKD.
11. Encourage follow-up urine culture.

XVI. Glomerulonephritis: Refer to Chapter 37

XVII. Nephrotic Syndrome: Refer to Chapter 37

XVIII. Polycystic Kidney Disease

A. Description

1. Cyst formation and hypertrophy of the kidneys, which leads to cystic rupture, infection, formation of scar tissue, and damaged nephrons
2. There is no specific treatment to arrest the progress of the destructive cysts.
3. The ultimate result of this disease is CKD.

B. Types

1. Infantile polycystic disease: An inherited autosomal recessive trait that results in the death of the infant within a few months after birth
2. Adult polycystic disease: An autosomal dominant trait that manifests between 30 and 40 years of age and results in end-stage kidney disease.

C. Assessment

1. Often asymptomatic until the age of 30 to 40 years
2. Flank, lumbar, or abdominal pain that worsens with activity and is relieved when lying down
3. Fever and chills
4. Recurrent UTIs
5. Hematuria, proteinuria, pyuria
6. Calculi

7. Hypertension
8. Palpable abdominal masses and enlarged kidneys
9. Increased abdominal girth

D. Interventions
1. Monitor for gross hematuria, which indicates cyst rupture.
2. Increase sodium and water intake because sodium loss rather than retention occurs.
3. Provide bed rest if ruptured cysts and bleeding occur.
4. Monitor pain, teach use of pain medications (avoid nonsteroidal antiinflammatory drugs [NSAIDs] and aspirin because of the risk for bleeding), and use dry heat to abdomen and flank areas for comfort when cysts are infected.
5. Prevent constipation from pressure of cysts on colon by adequate fiber in diet, stool softeners, adequate fluid intake, and exercise.
6. Prepare the client for percutaneous cyst puncture for relief of obstruction or for draining an abscess.
7. Administer antihypertensives as prescribed.
8. Prevent and/or treat UTIs.
9. Prepare the client for dialysis or renal transplantation.
10. Encourage the client to seek genetic counseling.
11. Provide psychological support to the client and family.
12. Provide psychosocial support and genetic counseling for family members without polycystic kidney disease who may want to donate a kidney.

XIX. Hydronephrosis

A. Description (Fig. 54-5)
1. Distention of the renal pelvis and calices caused by an obstruction of normal urine flow
2. The urine becomes trapped proximal to the obstruction.
3. The causes include calculus, tumors, scar tissue, ureter obstructions, and hypertrophy of the prostate.

B. Assessment
1. Hypertension
2. Headache
3. Colicky or dull flank pain that radiates to the groin

C. Interventions
1. Monitor vital signs frequently.
2. Monitor for fluid and electrolyte imbalances, including dehydration after the obstruction is relieved.
3. Monitor for diuresis, which can lead to fluid depletion.
4. Monitor weight daily.

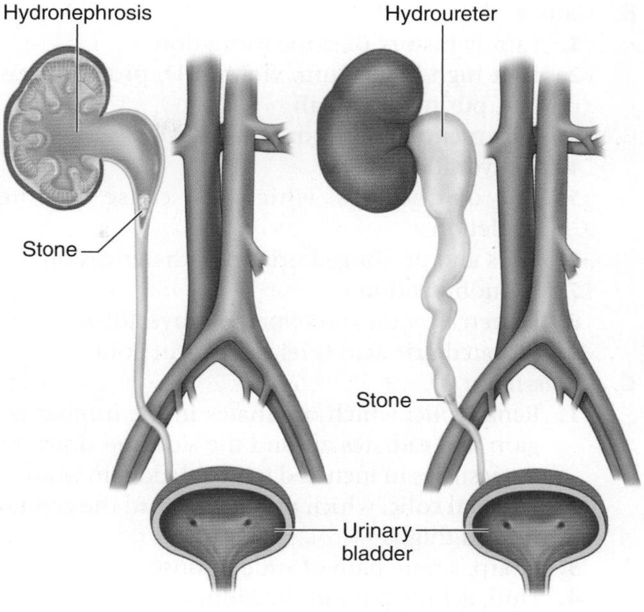

FIG. 54-5 Hydronephrosis and hydroureter.

5. Monitor urine for specific gravity and albumin and glucose levels.
6. Administer fluid replacement as prescribed.
7. Prepare the client for insertion of a nephrostomy tube or a surgical procedure to relieve the obstruction if prescribed.

XX. Renal Calculi

A. Description
1. Calculi are stones that can form anywhere in the urinary tract; however, the most frequent site is the kidneys.
2. Problems resulting from calculi are severe intermittent pain, obstruction, tissue trauma, secondary hemorrhage, and infection.
3. The stone can be located through radiography of the kidneys, ureters, and bladder; IV pyelography; computed tomography (CT) scanning; and renal ultrasonography.
4. A stone analysis is done after passage to determine the type of stone and assist in determining treatment.
5. **Urolithiasis** refers to the formation of urinary calculi; these form in the ureters.
6. **Nephrolithiasis** refers to the formation of kidney calculi; these form in the renal parenchyma.
7. When a calculus occludes the ureter and blocks the flow of urine, the ureter dilates, producing hydroureter (see Fig. 54-5).
8. If the obstruction is not removed, urinary stasis results in infection, impairment of renal function on the side of the blockage, hydronephrosis (see Fig. 54-5), and irreversible kidney damage.

B. Causes
1. Family history of stone formation
2. Diet high in calcium, vitamin D, protein, oxalate, purines, or alkali
3. Obstruction and urinary stasis
4. Dehydration
5. Use of diuretics, which can cause volume depletion
6. UTIs and prolonged urinary catheterization
7. Immobilization
8. Hypercalcemia and hyperparathyroidism
9. Elevated uric acid level, such as in gout

C. Assessment
1. Renal colic, which originates in the lumbar region and radiates around the side and down to the testicles in men and to the bladder in women
2. Ureteral colic, which radiates toward the genitalia and thighs
3. Sharp, severe pain of sudden onset
4. Dull, aching pain in the kidney
5. Nausea and vomiting, pallor, and diaphoresis during acute pain
6. Urinary frequency, with alternating retention
7. Signs of a UTI
8. Low-grade fever
9. High numbers of red blood cells, WBCs, and bacteria noted in the urinalysis report
10. Gross hematuria

D. Interventions
1. Monitor vital signs, especially temperature, for signs of infection.
2. Monitor intake and output.
3. Assess for fever, chills, and infection.
4. Monitor for nausea, vomiting, and diarrhea.
5. Encourage fluid intake up to 3000 mL/day, unless contraindicated, to facilitate the passage of the stone and prevent infection; monitor for obstruction.
6. Administer fluids intravenously as prescribed if unable to take fluids orally or in adequate amounts to increase the flow of urine and facilitate passage of the stone.
7. Provide warm baths and heat to the flank area (massage therapy should be avoided).
8. Administer analgesics at regularly scheduled intervals as prescribed to relieve pain.
9. Assess the client's response to pain medication.
10. Assist the client in performing relaxation techniques to assist in relieving pain.
11. Encourage client ambulation, if stable, to promote the passage of the stone.
12. Turn and reposition the immobilized client to promote passage of the stone.
13. Instruct the client in the diet restrictions specific to the stone composition if prescribed (Box 54-13).

BOX 54-13 Nutritional Therapy for Calculi

Note: Depending on the type of calculi, the diet is modified to decrease foods that are high in the substance that is the cause of the calculi.

Purine
- *High:* Sardines, herring, mussels, liver, kidney, goose, venison, meat soups, sweetbreads
- *Moderate:* Chicken, salmon, crab, veal, mutton, bacon, pork, beef, ham

Calcium
- *High:* Milk, cheese, ice cream, yogurt, sauces containing milk; all beans (except green beans), lentils; fish with fine bones (e.g., sardines, kippers, herring, salmon); dried fruits, nuts; cocoa powder, chocolate, cocoa

Oxalate
- *High:* Dark roughage, spinach, rhubarb, asparagus, cabbage, tomatoes, beets, nuts, celery, parsley, runner beans; chocolate, cocoa, instant coffee, cocoa powder, tea; Worcestershire sauce

* Uric acid is a waste product from purine in food.
Adapted from Lewis SL, Dirksen SR, Heitkemper MM, Bucher L, Camera IA: *Medical-surgical nursing: assessment and management of clinical problems,* ed 8, St. Louis, 2011, Mosby.

14. Prepare the client for surgical procedures if prescribed.

For the client with renal calculi, strain all urine for the presence of stones and send the stones to the laboratory for analysis.

XXI. Treatment Options for Renal Calculi (Fig. 54-6)

A. Cystoscopy
1. Cystoscopy may be done for stones in the bladder or lower ureter.
2. One or two ureteral catheters are inserted past the stone.
3. The catheters are left in place for 24 hours to drain the urine trapped proximal to the stone and to dilate the ureter.
4. A continuous chemical irrigation may be prescribed to dissolve the stone.

B. Extracorporeal shock wave lithotripsy (ESWL)
1. A noninvasive mechanical procedure for breaking up stones located in the kidney or upper ureter so that they can pass spontaneously or be removed by other methods
2. A stent may be placed to facilitate passing stone fragments.
3. Fluoroscopy is used to visualize the stone, and ultrasonic waves are delivered to the area of the stone to disintegrate it.
4. The stones are passed in the urine within a few days.

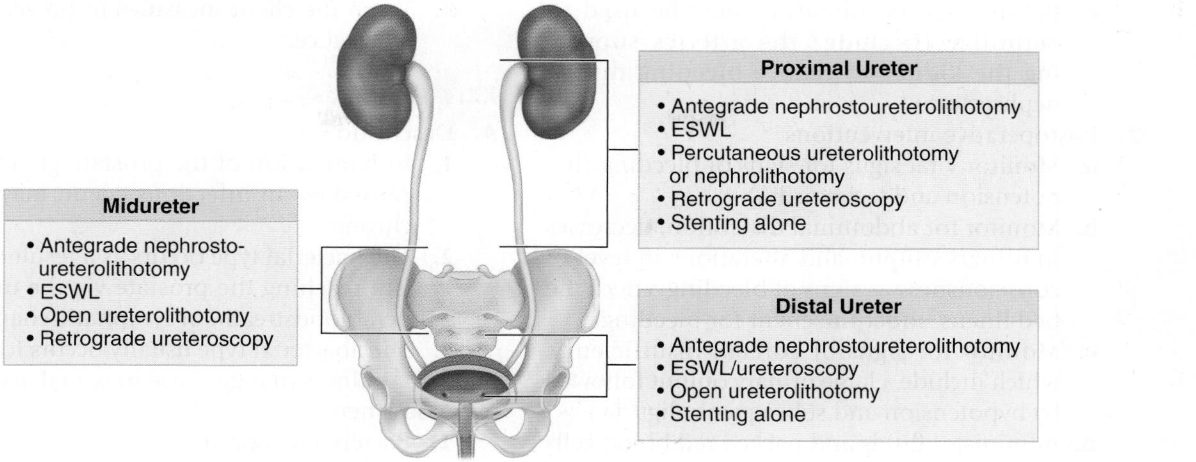

Proximal Ureter
• Antegrade nephrostoureterolithotomy
• ESWL
• Percutaneous ureterolithotomy or nephrolithotomy
• Retrograde ureteroscopy
• Stenting alone
Midureter
• Antegrade nephrosto-ureterolithotomy
• ESWL
• Open ureterolithotomy
• Retrograde ureteroscopy
Distal Ureter
• Antegrade nephrostoureterolithotomy
• ESWL/ureteroscopy
• Open ureterolithotomy
• Stenting alone

FIG. 54-6 Treatment options for ureteral stones. *ESWL*, Extracorporeal shock wave lithotripsy.

5. The client is taught to watch for signs of urinary obstruction, bleeding, or hematoma formation.
6. Instruct the client to increase fluid intake to flush out the stone fragments.

C. Percutaneous lithotripsy
1. An invasive procedure in which a guide is inserted under fluoroscopy near the area of the stone; an ultrasonic wave is aimed at the stone to break it into fragments.
2. Percutaneous lithotripsy may be performed via cystoscopy or nephroscopy (a small flank incision is needed for nephroscopy).
3. The client might have an indwelling urinary catheter.
4. A nephrostomy tube may be placed to administer chemical irrigations to break up the stone; the nephrostomy tube may remain in place for 1 to 5 days.
5. Encourage the client to drink 3000 to 4000 mL of fluid per day as prescribed following the procedure.
6. Instruct the client to monitor for complications of infection, hemorrhage, and extravasation of fluid into the retroperitoneal cavity.

D. Ureterolithotomy
1. An open surgical procedure performed if lithotripsy is not effective for removal of a stone in the ureter
2. An incision is made through the lower abdomen or flank and then into the ureter to remove the stone.
3. The client may have a drain, ureteral stent catheter, and/or indwelling bladder catheter.

E. Pyelolithotomy and nephrolithotomy
1. Pyelolithotomy is an incision into the renal pelvis to remove a stone; a large flank incision is required, and the client may have a drain and indwelling bladder catheter.
2. Nephrolithotomy is an incision into the kidney made to remove a stone; a large flank incision is required, and the client may have a nephrostomy tube and an indwelling bladder catheter.

F. Partial or total nephrectomy
1. Performed for extensive kidney damage, renal infection, severe obstruction from stones or tumors, and prevention of stone recurrence
2. Monitor the incision, particularly if a drain is in place, because it will drain large amounts of urine.
3. Protect the skin from urinary drainage, changing dressings frequently if necessary; place an ostomy pouch over the drain to protect the skin if urinary drainage is excessive.
4. Monitor the nephrostomy tube, which may be attached to a drainage bag, for a continuous flow of urine.
5. Do not irrigate the nephrostomy or bladder catheters unless specifically prescribed.
6. Encourage fluid intake to ensure a urine output of 2500 to 3000 mL/day or more as prescribed.

XXII. Kidney Tumors

A. Description
1. Kidney tumors may be benign or malignant, bilateral or unilateral.
2. Common sites of metastasis of malignant tumors include bone, lungs, liver, spleen, and the other kidney.
3. The exact cause of renal carcinoma is unknown.

B. Assessment
1. Dull flank pain
2. Palpable renal mass
3. Painless gross hematuria

C. Radical nephrectomy
1. Description
   a. Surgical removal of the entire kidney, adjacent adrenal gland, and renal artery and vein
   b. Radiation therapy and possibly chemotherapy may follow radical nephrectomy.

c. Before surgery, radiation may be used to embolize (occlude) the arteries supplying the kidney to reduce bleeding during nephrectomy.
2. Postoperative interventions
   a. Monitor vital signs for signs of bleeding (hypotension and tachycardia).
   b. Monitor for abdominal distention, decreases in urinary output, and alterations in level of consciousness as signs of bleeding; check the bed linens under the client for bleeding.
   c. Monitor for signs of adrenal insufficiency, which include a large urinary output followed by hypotension and subsequent oliguria.
   d. Administer fluids and packed red blood cells intravenously as prescribed.
   e. Monitor intake and output and daily weight.
   f. Monitor for a urinary output of 30 to 50 mL/hr to ensure adequate renal function.
   g. Maintain the client in a semi-Fowler's position.
   h. If a nephrostomy tube is in place, do not irrigate (unless specifically prescribed) or manipulate the tube.

XXIII. Epididymitis

A. Description
1. Acute or chronic inflammation of the epididymis that occurs as a result of a UTI, STI, prostatitis, or long-term use of a bladder catheter
2. The infective organism travels upward through the urethra and ejaculatory duct and along the vas deferens to the epididymis.

B. Assessment
1. Scrotal and groin pain
2. Swelling in the scrotum and groin
3. Pus and bacteria in the urine
4. Fever and chills
5. Abscess development

C. Interventions
1. Encourage fluid intake.
2. Encourage bed rest with the scrotum elevated to prevent traction on the spermatic cord, facilitate drainage, and relieve pain.
3. Instruct the client in the intermittent application of cold compresses to the scrotum.
4. Instruct the client in the use of tub or sitz baths.
5. Instruct the client in the administration of antibiotics for self and sexual partner if the cause is chlamydial or gonorrheal infection.
6. Instruct the client to avoid lifting, straining, and sexual contact until the infection subsides.
7. Instruct the client to limit the force of the urine stream, because organisms can be forced into the vas deferens and epididymis from strain or pressure during voiding.
8. Teach the client that condom use can help prevent urethritis and epididymitis.
9. Teach the client measures to prevent UTI or STI recurrence.

XXIV. Prostatitis

A. Description
1. Inflammation of the prostate gland commonly caused by an infectious agent; may be acute or chronic.
2. The bacterial type occurs as a result of the organism reaching the prostate via the urethra, bladder, bloodstream, or lymphatic channels.
3. The abacterial type usually occurs following a viral illness or a decrease in sexual activity.

B. Assessment
1. Bacterial prostatitis
   a. Client becomes acutely ill.
   b. Fever and chills
   c. Frequency and urgency of urination; dysuria
   d. Perineal and low back pain
   e. Urethral discharge
   f. Prostate is tender, indurated, and warm to the touch.
   g. Urethral discharge on palpation of prostate
   h. WBCs are found in prostatic secretions.
   i. Urine culture is usually positive for gram-negative bacteria, especially after prostate massage.
2. Abacterial prostatitis (most common form of chronic prostatitis)
   a. Backache
   b. Dysuria
   c. Perineal pain
   d. Frequency
   e. Hematuria
   f. Irregularly enlarged, firm, and tender prostate

C. Interventions
1. Encourage adequate fluid intake.
2. Instruct the client in the use of tub or sitz baths to promote comfort.
3. Administer antibiotics, analgesics, antispasmodics, and stool softeners as prescribed.
4. Inform the client of activities to drain the prostate, such as intercourse, masturbation, and prostatic massage.
5. Instruct the client to avoid spicy foods, coffee, alcohol, prolonged automobile rides, and sexual intercourse during an acute inflammation.

XXV. Benign Prostatic Hypertrophy (Hyperplasia)

A. Description
1. Benign prostatic hypertrophy (benign prostatic hyperplasia; BPH) is a slow enlargement of the prostate gland, with hypertrophy and hyperplasia of normal tissue.
2. Enlargement compresses the urethra, resulting in partial or complete obstruction.
3. Usually occurs in men older than 50 years

B. Assessment
1. Diminished size and force of urinary stream (early sign of BPH)
2. Urinary urgency and frequency
3. Nocturia
4. Inability to start (hesitancy) or continue a urinary stream
5. Feelings of incomplete bladder emptying
6. Postvoid dribbling from overflow incontinence (later sign)
7. Urinary retention and bladder distention
8. Hematuria
9. Urinary stasis and UTIs
10. Dysuria and bladder pain

C. Interventions
1. Encourage fluid intake of up to 2000 to 3000 mL/day unless contraindicated.
2. Prepare for urinary catheterization to drain the bladder and prevent distention.
3. Avoid administering medications that cause urinary retention, such as anticholinergics, antihistamines, decongestants, and antidepressants.
4. Administer medications as prescribed to shrink the prostate gland and improve urine flow.
5. Administer medications as prescribed to relax prostatic smooth muscle and improve urine flow.

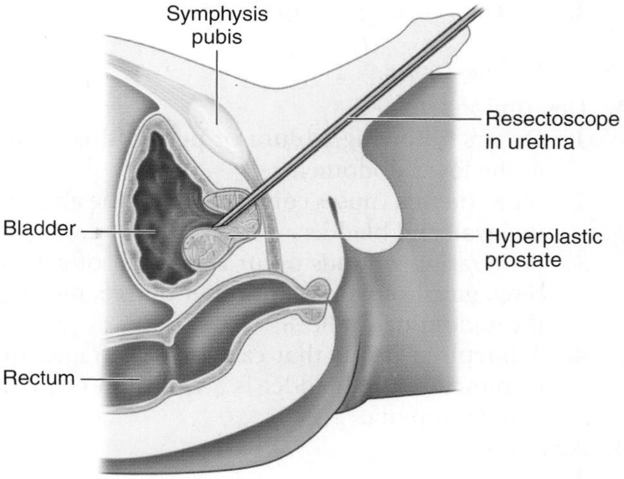

FIG. 54-7 Transurethral resection of the prostate.

6. Instruct the client to decrease intake of caffeine and artificial sweeteners and limit spicy or acidic foods.
7. Instruct the client to follow a timed voiding schedule.
8. Prepare the client for surgery or invasive procedures as prescribed (Figs. 54-7 and 54-8).

D. Surgical interventions and postoperative care (see Chapter 44)

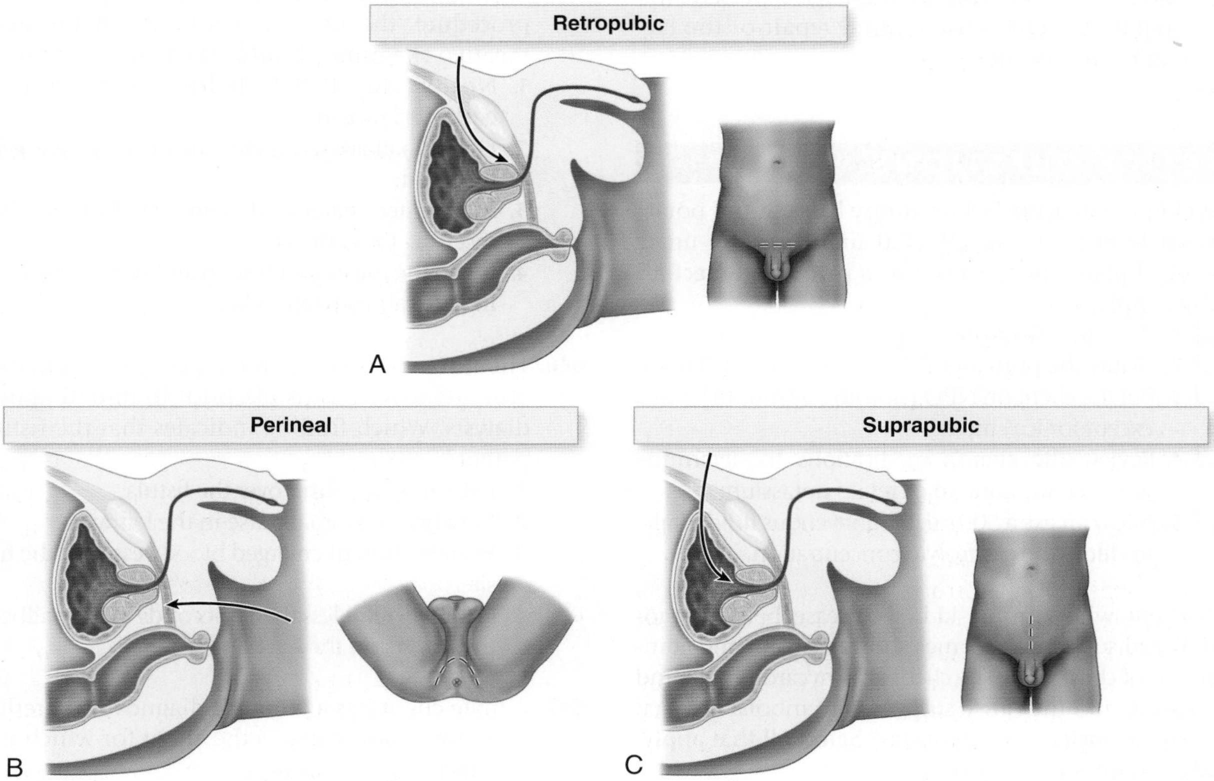

FIG. 54-8 Surgical approaches for prostatectomy. **A,** Retropubic approach involves a low abdominal incision. **B,** Perineal approach involves an incision between the scrotum and anus. **C,** Suprapubic approach involves a midline abdominal incision.

XXVI. Bladder Cancer: Refer to Chapter 44

XXVII. Bladder Trauma

A. Description
1. Occurs following a blunt or penetrating injury to the lower abdomen
2. Blunt trauma causes compression of the abdominal wall and bladder.
3. Penetrating wounds occur as a result of a stabbing, gunshot wound, or other objects piercing the abdominal wall.
4. A fractured pelvis that causes bone fragments to puncture the bladder is a common cause of bladder trauma.

B. Assessment
1. Anuria
2. Hematuria
3. Pain below the level of the umbilicus; can radiate to the shoulders
4. Nausea and vomiting

C. Interventions
1. Monitor vital signs.
2. Monitor for hematuria, bleeding, and signs of shock.
3. Maintain bed rest.
4. If blood is seen at the meatus, avoid urinary catheterization until a retrograde ureterogram can be obtained.
5. Prepare the client for insertion of a suprapubic catheter to aid in urinary drainage if prescribed.
6. Prepare the client for surgical repair of the laceration if indicated.

PRACTICE QUESTIONS

641. A client with acute kidney injury has a serum potassium level of 7.0 mEq/L (7.0 mmol/L). The nurse should plan which actions as a **priority? Select all that apply.**
- ☐ 1. Place the client on a cardiac monitor.
- ☐ 2. Notify the primary health care provider (PHCP).
- ☐ 3. Put the client on NPO (nothing by mouth) status except for ice chips.
- ☐ 4. Review the client's medications to determine whether any contain or retain potassium.
- ☐ 5. Allow an extra 500 mL of intravenous fluid intake to dilute the electrolyte concentration.

642. A client with chronic kidney disease being hemodialyzed suddenly becomes short of breath and complains of chest pain. The client is tachycardic, pale, and anxious, and the nurse suspects air embolism. What are the **priority** nursing actions? **Select all that apply.**
- ☐ 1. Administer oxygen to the client.
- ☐ 2. Continue dialysis at a slower rate after checking the lines for air.
- ☐ 3. Notify the primary health care provider (PHCP) and Rapid Response Team.
- ☐ 4. Stop dialysis, and turn the client on the left side with head lower than feet.
- ☐ 5. Bolus the client with 500 mL of normal saline to break up the air embolus.

643. A client arrives at the emergency department with complaints of low abdominal pain and hematuria. The client is afebrile. The nurse **next** assesses the client to determine a history of which condition?
1. Pyelonephritis
2. Glomerulonephritis
3. Trauma to the bladder or abdomen
4. Renal cancer in the client's family

644. The nurse discusses plans for future treatment options with a client with symptomatic polycystic kidney disease. Which treatment should be included in this discussion? **Select all that apply.**
- ☐ 1. Hemodialysis
- ☐ 2. Peritoneal dialysis
- ☐ 3. Kidney transplant
- ☐ 4. Bilateral nephrectomy
- ☐ 5. Intense immunosuppression therapy

645. A client is admitted to the emergency department following a fall from a horse, and the primary health care provider (PHCP) prescribes insertion of a urinary catheter. While preparing for the procedure, the nurse notes blood at the urinary meatus. The nurse should take which action?
1. Notify the PHCP before performing the catheterization.
2. Use a small-sized catheter and an anesthetic gel as a lubricant.
3. Administer parenteral pain medication before inserting the catheter.
4. Clean the meatus with soap and water before opening the catheterization kit.

646. The nurse is assessing the patency of a client's left arm arteriovenous fistula prior to initiating hemodialysis. Which finding indicates that the fistula is patent?
1. Palpation of a thrill over the fistula.
2. Presence of a radial pulse in the left wrist.
3. Visualization of enlarged blood vessels at the fistula site.
4. Capillary refill less than 3 seconds in the nailbeds of the fingers on the left hand.

647. A male client has a tentative diagnosis of urethritis. The nurse should assess the client for which manifestation of the disorder?
1. Hematuria and pyuria
2. Dysuria and proteinuria

3. Hematuria and urgency
4. Dysuria and penile discharge

648. The nurse is assessing a client with epididymitis. The nurse anticipates which findings on physical examination?
1. Fever, diarrhea, groin pain, and ecchymosis
2. Nausea, painful scrotal edema, and ecchymosis
3. Fever, nausea, vomiting, and painful scrotal edema
4. Diarrhea, groin pain, testicular torsion, and scrotal edema

649. A client complains of fever, perineal pain, and urinary urgency, frequency, and dysuria. To assess whether the client's problem is related to bacterial prostatitis, the nurse reviews the results of the prostate examination for which characteristic of this disorder?
1. Soft and swollen prostate gland
2. Swollen and boggy prostate gland
3. Tender and edematous prostate gland
4. Tender, indurated prostate gland that is warm to the touch

650. The nurse is collecting data from a client. Which symptom described by the client is characteristic of an **early** symptom of benign prostatic hyperplasia?
1. Nocturia
2. Scrotal edema
3. Occasional constipation
4. Decreased force in the stream of urine

651. The nurse monitoring a client receiving peritoneal dialysis notes that the client's outflow is less than the inflow. Which actions should the nurse take? **Select all that apply.**
- ☐ 1. Check the level of the drainage bag.
- ☐ 2. Reposition the client to her or his side.
- ☐ 3. Place the client in good body alignment.
- ☐ 4. Check the peritoneal dialysis system for kinks.
- ☐ 5. Contact the primary health care provider (PHCP).
- ☐ 6. Increase the flow rate of the peritoneal dialysis solution.

652. A hemodialysis client with a left arm fistula is at risk for arterial steal syndrome. The nurse should assess for which manifestations of this complication?
1. Warmth, redness, and pain in the left hand
2. Ecchymosis and audible bruit over the fistula
3. Edema and reddish discoloration of the left arm
4. Pallor, diminished pulse, and pain in the left hand

653. The nurse is reviewing a client's record and notes that the primary health care provider has documented that the client has chronic kidney disease. On review of the laboratory results, the nurse **most likely** would expect to note which finding?
1. Elevated creatinine level
2. Decreased hemoglobin level
3. Decreased red blood cell count
4. Increased number of white blood cells in the urine

654. A client with chronic kidney disease returns to the nursing unit following a hemodialysis treatment. On assessment, the nurse notes that the client's temperature is 38.5° C (101.2° F). Which nursing action is **most appropriate**?
1. Encourage fluid intake.
2. Continue to monitor vital signs.
3. Notify the primary health care provider.
4. Monitor the site of the shunt for infection.

655. The nurse is performing an assessment on a client who has returned from the dialysis unit following hemodialysis. The client is complaining of headache and nausea and is extremely restless. Which is the **priority** nursing action?
1. Monitor the client.
2. Elevate the head of the bed.
3. Assess the fistula site and dressing.
4. Notify the primary health care provider (PHCP).

656. A client with severe back pain and hematuria is found to have hydronephrosis due to urolithiasis. The nurse anticipates which treatment will be done to relieve the obstruction? **Select all that apply.**
- ☐ 1. Peritoneal dialysis
- ☐ 2. Analysis of the urinary stone
- ☐ 3. Intravenous opioid analgesics
- ☐ 4. Insertion of a nephrostomy tube
- ☐ 5. Placement of a ureteral stent with ureteroscopy

657. The nurse is instructing a client with diabetes mellitus about peritoneal dialysis. The nurse tells the client that it is important to maintain the prescribed dwell time for the dialysis because of the risk of which complication?
1. Peritonitis
2. Hyperglycemia
3. Hyperphosphatemia
4. Disequilibrium syndrome

658. A week after kidney transplantation, a client develops a temperature of 101° F (38.3° C), the blood pressure is elevated, and there is tenderness over the transplanted kidney. The serum creatinine is rising and urine output is decreased. The x-ray indicates that the transplanted kidney is enlarged. Based on these assessment findings, the nurse anticipates which treatment?
1. Antibiotic therapy
2. Peritoneal dialysis
3. Removal of the transplanted kidney
4. Increased immunosuppression therapy

659. A client is admitted to the hospital with a diagnosis of benign prostatic hyperplasia, and a transurethral resection of the prostate is performed. Four hours after surgery, the nurse takes the client's vital signs and empties the urinary drainage bag. Which assessment finding indicates the need to notify the primary health care provider (PHCP)?
1. Red, bloody urine
2. Pain rated as 2 on a 0 to 10 pain scale
3. Urinary output of 200 mL higher than intake
4. Blood pressure, 100/50 mm Hg; pulse, 130 beats per minute

660. The client newly diagnosed with chronic kidney disease recently has begun hemodialysis. Knowing that the client is at risk for disequilibrium syndrome, the nurse should assess the client during dialysis for which associated manifestations?
1. Hypertension, tachycardia, and fever
2. Hypotension, bradycardia, and hypothermia
3. Restlessness, irritability, and generalized weakness
4. Headache, deteriorating level of consciousness, and twitching

ANSWERS

641. *Answer:* 1, 2, 4
Rationale: The normal potassium level is 3.5 to 5.0 mEq/L (3.5 to 5.0 mmol/L). A potassium level of 7.0 is elevated. The client with hyperkalemia is at risk of developing cardiac dysrhythmias and cardiac arrest. Because of this, the client should be placed on a cardiac monitor. The nurse should notify the PHCP and also review medications to determine whether any contain potassium or are potassium retaining. The client does not need to be put on NPO status. Fluid intake is not increased because it contributes to fluid overload and would not affect the serum potassium level significantly.
Test-Taking Strategy: Note the strategic word, *priority.* First, note that the potassium level is significantly elevated to select options 1 and 4. Also, use the ABCs—airway, breathing, and circulation—to select option 2.
Level of Cognitive Ability: Analyzing
Client Needs: Physiological Integrity
Integrated Process: Nursing Process—Planning
Content Area: Adult Health: Renal and Urinary
Health Problem: Adult Health: Renal and Urinary: Acute kidney injury
Priority Concepts: Clinical Judgment; Fluids and Electrolytes
Reference: Ignatavicius, Workman, Rebar (2018), pp. 178-179, 192.

642. *Answer:* 1, 3, 4
Rationale: If the client experiences air embolus during hemodialysis, the nurse should terminate dialysis immediately, position the client so the air embolus is in the right side of the heart, notify the PHCP and Rapid Response Team, and administer oxygen as needed. Slowing the dialysis treatment or giving an intravenous bolus will not correct the air embolism or prevent complications.
Test-Taking Strategy: Note the strategic word, *priority.* Recall that air embolism is an emergency situation that affects the cardiopulmonary system suddenly and profoundly. Select the options that deal with the problem, supply oxygen, and get needed assistance.
Level of Cognitive Ability: Synthesizing
Client Needs: Physiological Integrity
Integrated Process: Nursing Process—Implementation
Content Area: Complex Care: Emergency Situations/Management
Health Problem: Adult Health: Renal and Urinary: Chronic kidney disease
Priority Concepts: Clinical Judgment; Gas Exchange
Reference: Ignatavicius, Workman, Rebar (2018), p. 214.

643. *Answer:* 3
Rationale: Bladder trauma or injury should be considered or suspected in the client with low abdominal pain and hematuria. Glomerulonephritis and pyelonephritis would be accompanied by fever and are thus not applicable to the client described in this question. Renal cancer would not cause pain that is felt in the low abdomen; rather, the pain would be in the flank area.
Test-Taking Strategy: Note the strategic word, *next.* Eliminate options 1 and 2 because they are comparable or alike, knowing that any inflammatory disease or infection is accompanied by fever. Because this client is afebrile, these are not possible options. Use knowledge of anatomy and pain assessment to select the correct option. Pain from renal cancer is a later finding and is localized in the flank area.
Level of Cognitive Ability: Analyzing
Client Needs: Physiological Integrity
Integrated Process: Nursing Process—Assessment
Content Area: Adult Health: Renal and Urinary
Health Problem: N/A
Priority Concepts: Clinical Judgment; Pain
Reference: Lewis et al. (2017), p. 1050.

644. *Answer:* 1, 3, 4
Rationale: Polycystic kidney disease is a genetic familial disease in which the kidneys enlarge with cysts that rupture and scar the kidney, eventually resulting in end-stage renal disease. Treatment options include hemodialysis or kidney transplant. Clients usually undergo bilateral nephrectomy to remove the large, painful, cyst-filled kidneys. Peritoneal dialysis is not a treatment option due to the cysts. The condition does not respond to immunosuppression.
Test-Taking Strategy: Focus on the subject, treatment options for polycystic kidney disease. Recall that the condition results in end-stage renal disease. This will direct you to the correct options.
Level of Cognitive Ability: Analyzing
Client Needs: Physiological Integrity
Integrated Process: Nursing Process—Planning
Content Area: Adult Health: Renal and Urinary
Health Problem: Adult Health: Renal and Urinary: Hereditary diseases

Priority Concepts: Clinical Judgment; Client Education
Reference: Ignatavicius, Workman, Rebar (2018), pp. 1381-1382.

645. *Answer:* 1
Rationale: The presence of blood at the urinary meatus may indicate urethral trauma or disruption. The nurse notifies the PHCP, knowing that the client should not be catheterized until the cause of the bleeding is determined by diagnostic testing. The other options include performing the catheterization procedure and therefore are incorrect.
Test-Taking Strategy: Focus on the subject, the complications associated with a traumatic fall. Noting the words *blood at the urinary meatus* suggests more extensive internal trauma that could be further aggravated by the catheterization.
Level of Cognitive Ability: Applying
Client Needs: Physiological Integrity
Integrated Process: Nursing Process—Implementation
Content Area: Adult Health: Renal and Urinary
Health Problem: N/A
Priority Concepts: Clinical Judgment; Safety
Reference: Ignatavicius, Workman, Rebar (2018), p. 1369.

646. *Answer:* 1
Rationale: The nurse assesses the patency of the fistula by palpating for the presence of a thrill or auscultating for a bruit. The presence of a thrill and bruit indicate patency of the fistula. Enlarged visible blood vessels at the fistula site are a normal observation but are not indicative of fistula patency. Although the presence of a radial pulse in the left wrist and capillary refill less than 3 seconds in the nailbeds of the fingers on the left hand indicate adequate circulation to the hand, they do not assess fistula patency.
Test-Taking Strategy: Eliminate options 2 and 4 first because they are comparable or alike, and assess for adequate circulation in the distal portion of the extremity (not the fistula). Enlarged blood vessels occur when the fistula is created. Select option 1, because a thrill indicates blood flow and patency of the fistula.
Level of Cognitive Ability: Analyzing
Client Needs: Physiological Integrity
Integrated Process: Nursing Process—Assessment
Content Area: Adult Health: Renal and Urinary
Health Problem: Adult Health: Renal and Urinary: Chronic kidney disease
Priority Concepts: Clinical Judgment; Clotting
Reference: Ignatavicius, Workman, Rebar (2018), p. 1415.

647. *Answer:* 4
Rationale: Urethritis in the male client often results from chlamydial infection and is characterized by dysuria, which is accompanied by a clear to mucopurulent discharge. Because this disorder often coexists with gonorrhea, diagnostic tests are done for both and include culture and rapid assays. Hematuria is not associated with urethritis. Proteinuria is associated with kidney dysfunction.
Test-Taking Strategy: Focus on the subject, manifestations of urethritis. Recalling that urethritis generally is accompanied by dysuria in the male client will assist you in eliminating options 1 and 3. Knowing that the problem originates in the urethra, not the kidneys, will assist you in eliminating option 2, because proteinuria indicates a problem with kidney function.
Level of Cognitive Ability: Analyzing
Client Needs: Physiological Integrity
Integrated Process: Nursing Process—Assessment
Content Area: Adult Health: Renal and Urinary
Health Problem: Adult Health: Renal and Urinary: Inflammation/Infections
Priority Concepts: Infection; Sexuality
Reference: Ignatavicius, Workman, Rebar (2018), pp. 1359-1361.

648. *Answer:* 3
Rationale: Typical signs and symptoms of epididymitis include scrotal pain and edema, which often are accompanied by fever, nausea and vomiting, and chills. Epididymitis most often is caused by infection, although sometimes it can be caused by trauma. The remaining options do not present all of the accurate manifestations.
Test-Taking Strategy: Any disorder that ends in *-itis* results from inflammation or infection. Therefore, an expected finding would be elevated temperature. With this in mind, eliminate options 2 and 4 because they are comparable or alike and do not contain fever as part of the option. Knowing that ecchymosis results from bleeding, which is not part of this clinical picture, directs you to the correct option.
Level of Cognitive Ability: Analyzing
Client Needs: Physiological Integrity
Integrated Process: Nursing Process—Assessment
Content Area: Adult Health: Renal and Urinary
Health Problem: Adult Health: Renal and Urinary: Inflammation/Infections
Priority Concepts: Infection; Inflammation
Reference: Lewis et al. (2017), p. 1284.

649. *Answer:* 4
Rationale: The client with bacterial prostatitis has a swollen and tender prostate gland that is also warm to the touch, firm, and indurated. Systemic symptoms include fever with chills, perineal and low back pain, and signs of urinary tract infection, which often accompany the disorder.
Test-Taking Strategy: Focus on the subject, manifestations of bacterial prostatitis. Begin to answer this question by reasoning that inflammation of the prostate gland would cause the area to be tender. This would allow you to eliminate options 1 and 2. Recalling that inflammation is accompanied by local warmth will direct you to the correct option.
Level of Cognitive Ability: Analyzing
Client Needs: Physiological Integrity
Integrated Process: Nursing Process—Assessment
Content Area: Adult Health: Renal and Urinary
Health Problem: Adult Health: Renal and Urinary: Inflammation/Infections
Priority Concepts: Infection; Inflammation
Reference: Lewis et al. (2017), p. 1282-1283.

650. *Answer:* 4
Rationale: Decreased force in the stream of urine is an early symptom of benign prostatic hyperplasia. The stream later becomes weak and dribbling. The client then may develop hematuria, frequency, urgency, urge incontinence, and nocturia. If untreated, complete obstruction and urinary retention can occur. Constipation or scrotal edema is not associated with benign prostatic hyperplasia.

Test-Taking Strategy: Note the strategic word, *early*. Also, if you know that benign prostatic hyperplasia can lead to urinary obstruction, look for the option that identifies the least severe symptom.
Level of Cognitive Ability: Analyzing
Client Needs: Physiological Integrity
Integrated Process: Nursing Process—Assessment
Content Area: Adult Health: Renal and Urinary
Health Problem: Adult Health: Renal and Urinary: Obstructive problems
Priority Concepts: Elimination; Inflammation
Reference: Ignatavicius, Workman, Rebar (2018), pp. 1474, 1476.

651. *Answer:* 1, 2, 3, 4
Rationale: If outflow drainage is inadequate, the nurse attempts to stimulate outflow by changing the client's position. Turning the client to the side or making sure that the client is in good body alignment may assist with outflow drainage. The drainage bag needs to be lower than the client's abdomen to enhance gravity drainage. The connecting tubing and peritoneal dialysis system are also checked for kinks or twisting, and the clamps on the system are checked to ensure that they are open. There is no reason to contact the PHCP. Increasing the flow rate should not be done and also is not associated with the amount of outflow solution.
Test-Taking Strategy: Focus on the subject, outflow is less than inflow, and use the principles related to gravity flow and preventing obstruction to flow to answer this question. This will assist in determining the correct interventions.
Level of Cognitive Ability: Analyzing
Client Needs: Physiological Integrity
Integrated Process: Nursing Process—Implementation
Content Area: Adult Health: Renal and Urinary
Health Problem: Adult Health: Renal and Urinary: Chronic kidney disease
Priority Concepts: Clinical Judgment; Elimination
Reference: Ignatavicius, Workman, Rebar (2018), p. 1420.

652. *Answer:* 4
Rationale: Steal syndrome results from vascular insufficiency after creation of a fistula. The client exhibits pallor and a diminished pulse distal to the fistula. The client also complains of pain distal to the fistula, caused by tissue ischemia. Warmth and redness probably would characterize a problem with infection. Ecchymosis and a bruit are normal findings for a fistula.
Test-Taking Strategy: Focus on the subject, arterial steal syndrome. Eliminate signs associated with infection or normal fistula findings. Recalling that steal syndrome results from vascular insufficiency after creation of a fistula will direct you to the correct option.
Level of Cognitive Ability: Analyzing
Client Needs: Physiological Integrity
Integrated Process: Nursing Process—Assessment
Content Area: Adult Health: Renal and Urinary
Health Problem: Adult Health: Renal and Urinary: Chronic kidney disease
Priority Concepts: Clinical Judgment; Perfusion
Reference: Ignatavicius, Workman, Rebar (2018), p. 1415.

653. *Answer:* 1
Rationale: The creatinine level is the most specific laboratory test to determine renal function. The creatinine level increases when at least 50% of renal function is lost. A decreased hemoglobin level and red blood cell count are associated with anemia or blood loss and not specifically with decreased renal function. Increased white blood cells in the urine are noted with urinary tract infection.
Test-Taking Strategy: Note the strategic words, *most likely*. Recalling the relationship between the creatinine level and renal function will direct you to the correct option.
Level of Cognitive Ability: Analyzing
Client Needs: Physiological Integrity
Integrated Process: Nursing Process—Assessment
Content Area: Adult Health: Renal and Urinary
Health Problem: Adult Health: Renal and Urinary: Chronic kidney disease
Priority Concepts: Cellular Regulation; Elimination
Reference: Ignatavicius, Workman, Rebar (2018), pp. 1331-1332.

654. *Answer:* 3
Rationale: A temperature of 101.2° F (38.5° C) is significantly elevated and may indicate infection. The nurse should notify the primary health care provider (PHCP). Dialysis clients cannot have fluid intake encouraged. Vital signs and the shunt site should be monitored, but the PHCP should be notified first.
Test-Taking Strategy: Note the strategic words, *most appropriate*. Focus on the data in the question. Note the temperature elevation. This warrants notification of the PHCP, who may prescribe diagnostic tests or medications.
Level of Cognitive Ability: Applying
Client Needs: Physiological Integrity
Integrated Process: Nursing Process—Implementation
Content Area: Adult Health: Renal and Urinary
Health Problem: Adult Health: Renal and Urinary: Chronic kidney disease
Priority Concepts: Clinical Judgment; Elimination
Reference: Ignatavicius, Workman, Rebar (2018), pp. 1415-1416.

655. *Answer:* 4
Rationale: Disequilibrium syndrome may be caused by rapid removal of solutes from the body during hemodialysis. These changes can cause cerebral edema that leads to increased intracranial pressure. The client is exhibiting early signs and symptoms of disequilibrium syndrome, and appropriate treatments with anticonvulsive medications and barbiturates may be necessary to prevent a life-threatening situation. The PHCP must be notified. Monitoring the client, elevating the head of the bed, and assessing the fistula site are correct actions, but the priority action is to notify the PHCP.
Test-Taking Strategy: Note the strategic word, *priority*, and focus on the client's signs and symptoms. Determine if an abnormality exists. Recalling the serious complications associated with hemodialysis such as disequilibrium syndrome will direct you to the correct option.
Level of Cognitive Ability: Applying
Client Needs: Physiological Integrity
Integrated Process: Nursing Process—Implementation
Content Area: Adult Health: Renal and Urinary
Health Problem: Adult Health: Renal and Urinary: Chronic kidney disease
Priority Concepts: Clinical Judgment; Intracranial Regulation
Reference: Ignatavicius, Workman, Rebar (2018), p. 1417.

656. *Answer:* 4, 5

Rationale: Urolithiasis is the condition that occurs when a stone forms in the urinary system. Hydronephrosis develops when the stone has blocked the ureter and urine backs up and dilates and damages the kidney. Priority treatment is to allow the urine to drain and relieve the obstruction in the ureter. This is accomplished by placement of a percutaneous nephrostomy tube to drain urine from the kidney and placement of a ureteral stent to keep the ureter open. Peritoneal dialysis is not needed, since the kidney is functioning. Stone analysis will be done later when the stone has been retrieved and analyzed. Opioid analgesics are necessary for pain relief but do not treat the obstruction.

Test-Taking Strategy: Focus on the subject, treatment to relieve the obstruction. Think about what each option will accomplish. Eliminate the options that do not address the obstruction.

Level of Cognitive Ability: Analyzing

Client Needs: Physiological Integrity

Integrated Process: Nursing Process—Analysis

Content Area: Adult Health: Renal and Urinary

Health Problem: Adult Health: Renal and Urinary: Obstructive problems

Priority Concepts: Clinical Judgment; Elimination

Reference: Ignatavicius, Workman, Rebar (2018), pp. 1361, 1382-1383.

657. *Answer:* 2

Rationale: An extended dwell time increases the risk of hyperglycemia in the client with diabetes mellitus as a result of absorption of glucose from the dialysate and electrolyte changes. Diabetic clients may require extra insulin when receiving peritoneal dialysis. Peritonitis is a risk associated with breaks in aseptic technique. Hyperphosphatemia is an electrolyte imbalance that occurs with renal dysfunction. Disequilibrium syndrome is a complication associated with hemodialysis.

Test-Taking Strategy: Focus on the subject, a complication associated with an extended dwell time. Noting the client's diagnosis and recalling that the dialysate solution contains glucose will direct you to the correct option.

Level of Cognitive Ability: Applying

Client Needs: Physiological Integrity

Integrated Process: Teaching and Learning

Content Area: Adult Health: Renal and Urinary

Health Problem: Adult Health: Renal and Urinary: Chronic kidney disease

Priority Concepts: Elimination; Glucose Regulation

Reference: Ignatavicius, Workman, Rebar (2018), p. 1421.

658. *Answer:* 4

Rationale: Acute rejection most often occurs within 1 week after transplantation but can occur any time post-transplantation. Clinical manifestations include fever, malaise, elevated white blood cell count, acute hypertension, graft tenderness, and manifestations of deteriorating renal function. Treatment consists of increasing immunosuppressive therapy. Antibiotics are used to treat infection. Peritoneal dialysis cannot be used with a newly transplanted kidney due to the recent surgery. Removal of the transplanted kidney is indicated with hyperacute rejection, which occurs within 48 hours of the transplant surgery.

Test-Taking Strategy: Note the words *A week after kidney transplantation.* Focus on the data in the question and the time frame and symptoms, which describe acute rejection. Recall the treatment for *acute* rejection to direct you to the correct option.

Level of Cognitive Ability: Synthesizing

Client Needs: Physiological Integrity

Integrated Process: Nursing Process—Analysis

Content Area: Adult Health: Renal and Urinary

Health Problem: Adult Health: Immune: Transplantation

Priority Concepts: Elimination; Immunity

Reference: Ignatavicius, Workman, Rebar (2018), pp. 1423-1424.

659. *Answer:* 4

Rationale: Frank bleeding (arterial or venous) may occur during the first day after surgery. Some hematuria is usual for several days after surgery. A urinary output of 200 mL more than intake is adequate. A client pain rating of 2 on a 0 to 10 scale indicates adequate pain control. A rapid pulse with a low blood pressure is a potential sign of excessive blood loss. The PHCP should be notified.

Test-Taking Strategy: Focus on the subject, the need to notify the PHCP, and determine if an abnormality exists. Think about the expected findings following this procedure and note that the vital signs are not within the normal range and could indicate excessive blood loss.

Level of Cognitive Ability: Analyzing

Client Needs: Physiological Integrity

Integrated Process: Nursing Process—Analysis

Content Area: Adult Health: Renal and Urinary

Health Problem: Adult Health: Renal and Urinary: Obstructive problems

Priority Concepts: Collaboration; Clotting

Reference: Lewis et al. (2017), pp. 1274-1275.

660. *Answer:* 4

Rationale: Disequilibrium syndrome is characterized by headache, mental confusion, decreasing level of consciousness, nausea, vomiting, twitching, and possible seizure activity. Disequilibrium syndrome is caused by rapid removal of solutes from the body during hemodialysis. At the same time, the blood–brain barrier interferes with the efficient removal of wastes from brain tissue. As a result, water goes into cerebral cells because of the osmotic gradient, causing increased intracranial pressure and onset of symptoms. The syndrome most often occurs in clients who are new to dialysis and is prevented by dialyzing for shorter times or at reduced blood flow rates. Tachycardia and fever are associated with infection. Generalized weakness is associated with low blood pressure and anemia. Restlessness and irritability are not associated with disequilibrium syndrome.

Test-Taking Strategy: Focus on the subject, disequilibrium syndrome. Think about the pathophysiology and that brain cells are responsive to changes in osmolarity. This will assist you to choose the correct option describing neurological symptoms.

Level of Cognitive Ability: Analyzing

Client Needs: Physiological Integrity

Integrated Process: Nursing Process—Assessment

Content Area: Adult Health: Renal and Urinary

Health Problem: Adult Health: Renal and Urinary: Chronic kidney disease

Priority Concepts: Elimination; Intracranial Regulation

Reference: Ignatavicius, Workman, Rebar (2018), p. 1417.

CHAPTER 55

Renal and Urinary Medications

PRIORITY CONCEPTS Elimination; Safety

I. Urinary Tract Antiseptics

A. Description
1. Urinary tract antiseptics inhibit the growth of bacteria in the urine (Box 55-1).
2. Act as disinfectants within the urinary tract
3. Used to treat acute cystitis or urinary tract infections (UTIs)
4. Urinary tract antiseptics do not achieve effective antibacterial concentrations in blood or tissues and therefore cannot be used for infections outside the urinary tract.

B. Side and adverse effects and nursing considerations
1. Fosfomycin
   a. The medication is available as granules that must be dissolved; instruct the client to mix the contents of a package in about ½ cup (120 mL) of cold water, stir well, and drink all of the liquid.
   b. Medications that increase gastrointestinal motility reduce the absorption of fosfomycin.
2. Methenamine
   a. Used to treat chronic UTIs but not recommended for acute infections
   b. Administer after meals and at bedtime to minimize gastric distress.
   c. Chronic high-dose therapy can cause bladder irritation.
   d. Methenamine can cause crystalluria and should not be used in clients with renal impairment.
   e. Decomposition of the medication generates ammonia; therefore, it should not be used for clients with liver dysfunction.
   f. Methenamine requires acidic urine with a pH of 5.5 or lower.
   g. Increasing fluid intake reduces antibacterial effects by diluting the medication and raising urine pH.
   h. Methenamine should not be combined with sulfonamides because of the risk of crystalluria and urinary tract injury.
   i. Clients taking this medication should avoid alkalinizing agents, including over-the-counter antacids containing sodium bicarbonate or sodium carbonate.
3. Nitrofurantoin
   a. Gastrointestinal effects include anorexia, nausea, vomiting, and diarrhea; administration with milk or meals minimizes gastrointestinal distress.
   b. Pulmonary reactions include dyspnea, chest pain, chills, fever, cough, and alveolar infiltrates; these resolve in 2 to 4 days following cessation of treatment.
   c. Hematological effects include agranulocytosis, leukopenia, thrombocytopenia, and megaloblastic anemia.
   d. Peripheral neuropathy effects include muscle weakness, tingling sensations, and numbness.
   e. Neurological effects include headache, vertigo, drowsiness, and nystagmus.
   f. Allergic reactions include anaphylaxis, hives, rash, and tingling sensations around the mouth.
   g. Nitrofurantoin may impart a harmless brown color to the urine.
   h. Nitrofurantoin is contraindicated in clients with renal impairment.
   i. Instruct the client in expected side and adverse effects, signs warranting notification of the primary health care provider (PHCP), and not to take nitrofurantoin with antacids.

II. Fluoroquinolones (Box 55-2)

A. Description: Suppress bacterial growth by inhibiting an enzyme necessary for DNA synthesis; active against a broad spectrum of microbes

B. Side and adverse effects and nursing considerations
1. Can cause dizziness, drowsiness, gastric distress, diarrhea, vaginitis, nausea, and vomiting
2. Adverse effects include psychoses, hallucinations, confusion, tremors, hypersensitivity, and interstitial nephritis.

BOX 55-1 Urinary Tract Antiseptics

- Amoxicillin
- Cefixime
- Fosfomycin
- Methenamine
- Nitrofurantoin

BOX 55-2 Fluoroquinolones

- Ciprofloxacin
- Delafloxacin
- Gemifloxacin
- Levofloxacin
- Moxifloxacin
- Ofloxacin
- Gatifloxacin

⚠ With fluoroquinolones, there is an increased risk for tendonitis and tendon rupture. The Achilles tendon is most often involved, but the shoulder and hand tendons can also be affected. Clients at increased risk are those over the age of 60 years, those taking corticosteroids, and clients who have undergone organ transplant.

3. Fluoroquinolones should be used with caution in clients with hepatic, renal, or central nervous system (CNS) disorders.
4. Monitor client for side and adverse effects.
5. Ciprofloxacin and ofloxacin may be taken with or without food.
6. Intravenously administered ciprofloxacin and ofloxacin are infused slowly over 60 minutes to minimize discomfort and vein irritation.
7. Advise the client to report dizziness, lightheadedness, visual disturbances, increased light sensitivity, and feelings of depression, because these signs could indicate CNS toxicity.
8. Inform the client of signs of hepatic and renal toxicity and the importance of reporting these signs to the PHCP.

⚠ Administer oral fluoroquinolones with a full glass of water and ensure that the client maintains a urine output of at least 1200 to 1500 mL daily to minimize the development of crystalluria.

III. Sulfonamides (Box 55-3)

A. Description: Suppress bacterial growth by inhibiting the synthesis of folic acid; active against a broad spectrum of microbes; used primarily to treat acute UTIs

B. Side and adverse effects and nursing considerations

1. Hypersensitivity reactions include rash, fever, and photosensitivity.

BOX 55-3 Sulfonamides

- Sulfadiazine
- Sulfasalazine
- Sulfacetamide
- Trimethoprim-sulfamethoxazole

2. Stevens-Johnson syndrome, the most severe hypersensitivity response, produces symptoms that include widespread lesions of the skin and mucous membranes, fever, malaise, and toxemia.
3. Sulfonamides can cause hemolytic anemia, agranulocytosis, leukopenia, and thrombocytopenia; instruct the client to notify the PHCP if sore throat or fever occurs.
4. Administer sulfonamides with caution in clients with renal impairment.
5. Sulfonamides are contraindicated if hypersensitivity exists to sulfonamides, sulfonylureas, or thiazide or loop diuretics.
6. Sulfonamides are contraindicated in infants younger than 2 months and in pregnant women or mothers who are breast-feeding.
7. Sulfonamides can potentiate the effects of warfarin sodium, phenytoin, and orally administered hypoglycemics (when combined with sulfonamides, hypoglycemics may require a reduction in dosage).
8. Instruct the client to take the medication on an empty stomach with a full glass of water.
9. Instruct the client to complete the entire course of the prescribed medication.
10. Instruct the client to avoid prolonged exposure to sunlight, wear protective clothing, and apply a sunscreen to exposed skin.
11. Adults should maintain a daily urine output of at least 1200 mL by consuming 8 to 10 glasses of water each day to minimize the risk of renal damage from the medication.
12. Inform the client that some combination medications of sulfonamides can cause the urine to turn dark brown or red.
13. The sulfonamide combination of trimethoprim-sulfamethoxazole is more effective than either medication alone, because it inhibits the sequential steps in bacterial folic acid synthesis.
14. Trimethoprim-sulfamethoxazole is used cautiously with clients experiencing impaired kidney function, folate deficiency, severe allergy, or bronchial asthma.
15. An intravenous (IV) dose of trimethoprim-sulfamethoxazole is administered over 60 to 90 minutes and is not mixed with other medications.

⚠ Sulfonamides should be withheld if a rash is noted. Inform the client to contact the PHCP if a rash appears.

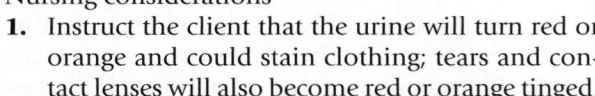

BOX 55-4 Urinary Tract Analgesics

- Pentosan polysulfate sodium
- Phenazopyridine

IV. Urinary Tract Analgesics (Box 55-4)

A. Description: A urinary tract analgesic is administered with an antibiotic because the analgesic only treats pain, not the infection.

B. Side and adverse effects
1. Nausea
2. Headache
3. Vertigo

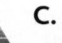

C. Nursing considerations
1. Instruct the client that the urine will turn red or orange and could stain clothing; tears and contact lenses will also become red or orange tinged.
2. A urinary tract analgesic is contraindicated in clients with renal or hepatic disease.
3. The medication interferes with accurate urine testing for glucose and ketones.

V. Anticholinergics/Antispasmodics (Box 55-5)

A. Description: Used for overactive bladder (urge incontinence)

B. Side and adverse effects
1. Anorexia, nausea, vomiting, and dry mouth
2. Blurred vision
3. Confusion in older clients
4. Constipation
5. Decreased sweating
6. Dizziness
7. Drowsiness
8. Dry eyes
9. Gastric distress
10. Headache
11. Tachycardia
12. Urinary retention

C. Nursing considerations
1. Extended-release capsules should not be split, chewed, or crushed.
2. Tolterodine should be used cautiously in clients with narrow-angle glaucoma.
3. Do not administer oxybutynin to clients with known hypersensitivity, gastrointestinal or genitourinary obstruction, glaucoma, severe colitis, or myasthenia gravis.
4. Do not administer propantheline to clients with narrow-angle glaucoma, obstructive uropathy, gastrointestinal disease, or ulcerative colitis.
5. Instruct the client to avoid hazardous activities because of the effects of dizziness and drowsiness.
6. Monitor intake and output.
7. Provide gum or hard candy for dry mouth.
8. Monitor for signs of toxicity (CNS stimulation) such as hypotension or hypertension, confusion, tachycardia, flushed or red face, signs of respiratory depression, nervousness, restlessness, hallucinations, and irritability.

BOX 55-5 Anticholinergics/Antispasmodics

- Darifenacin
- Dicyclomine
- Oxybutynin chloride
- Flavoxate
- Fesoterodine
- Mirabegron
- Propantheline
- Solifenacin
- Tolterodine
- Trospium

! Antispasmodic medications used to treat overactive bladder (urge incontinence) should not be used by clients diagnosed with open-angle glaucoma. These medications will block the flow of intraocular fluid and raise the intraocular pressure. This may cause permanent damage to the optic nerve.

VI. Cholinergics

A. Description: Bethanechol chloride is a cholinergic used to increase bladder tone and function and to treat nonobstructive urinary retention and neurogenic bladder.

B. Side and adverse effects
1. Headache
2. Hypotension
3. Flushing and sweating
4. Increased salivation
5. Nausea and vomiting
6. Abdominal cramps
7. Diarrhea
8. Urinary urgency
9. Bronchoconstriction
10. Transient complete heart block

C. Nursing considerations
1. Administer on an empty stomach, 1 hour before or 2 hours after meals to lessen nausea and vomiting.
2. Never administer by the intramuscular or IV route.
3. Monitor intake and output.
4. Monitor for increased bladder tone and function.
5. Monitor for cholinergic overdose (excessive salivation, sweating, involuntary urination and defecation, bradycardia, and severe hypotension).
6. Have atropine sulfate (antidote for cholinergic overdose) readily available for IV or subcutaneous administration.

A cholinergic such as bethanechol chloride is not given to a client who has a urinary stricture or obstruction.

VII. Medications for Preventing Organ Rejection (Box 55-6)

A. Medications include immunosuppressants, corticosteroids, cytotoxic medications, and antibodies.

B. Some medications may be used in combination to produce different actions on the immune system; combination therapy also allows for administration of the medications in lower doses, reducing the possibility of adverse effects.

C. Cyclosporine

1. Cyclosporine inhibits calcineurin and acts on T lymphocytes to suppress the production of interleukin-2, interferon-γ, and other cytokines.
2. Cyclosporine may be used to prevent rejection of allogeneic kidney, liver, and heart transplants.
3. Prednisone may be administered concurrently.
4. Oral administration of cyclosporine is preferred; IV administration is reserved for clients who cannot take the medication orally.
5. Blood levels of the medication should be measured regularly because of its nephrotoxic effects.
6. The most common adverse effects are nephrotoxicity, infection, hypertension, tremor, and hirsutism.
7. Assure the client that hirsutism is reversible; instruct on depilatory (hair removal) methods.
8. Other adverse effects include neurotoxicity, gastrointestinal effects, hyperkalemia, and hyperglycemia.
9. The risk of infection and lymphomas is increased with the use of cyclosporine.
10. Cyclosporine is contraindicated in the presence of hypersensitivity, pregnancy and breastfeeding, recent inoculation with live virus vaccines, and recent contact with an active infection such as chickenpox or herpes zoster.
11. Cyclosporine is embryotoxic, and women of childbearing age should use a mechanical form of contraception and avoid oral contraceptives.
12. The client should be informed about the possibility of renal damage and liver damage and the need for periodic liver function tests and determination of coagulation factors and blood urea nitrogen, serum creatinine, serum potassium, and blood glucose levels.
13. The client should be instructed to monitor for early signs of infection and to report these signs immediately.
14. Available in a pill form; if the client is unable to swallow the pill, instruct the client to follow the medication administration instructions exactly; dispense the oral liquid medication into a glass container using a specially calibrated pipette, mix well, and drink immediately; rinse the glass container with diluent and drink it to ensure ingestion of the complete dose; dry the outside of the pipette and return to its cover for storage.
15. To promote palatability, instruct the client to mix the liquid medication with milk, chocolate milk, or orange juice just before administration.
16. Consuming grapefruit juice is prohibited because it raises cyclosporine levels and increases the risk of toxicity.
17. Ketoconazole, erythromycin, and amphotericin B can elevate cyclosporine levels.
18. Phenytoin, phenobarbital, rifampin, and trimethoprim-sulfamethoxazole can decrease cyclosporine levels.
19. Renal damage can be intensified by the concurrent use of other nephrotoxic medications.

D. Sirolimus

1. Sirolimus is used for the prevention of renal transplant rejection by inhibiting the response of helper T lymphocytes and B lymphocytes to cytokinesis.
2. It may be used with cyclosporine or tacrolimus and corticosteroids.
3. Increases the risk of infection, increases the risk of renal injury, increases the risk of lymphocele (a complication of renal transplant surgery), and raises cholesterol and triglyceride levels
4. Side and adverse effects include rash, acne, anemia, thrombocytopenia, joint pain, diarrhea, and hypokalemia.

E. Tacrolimus

1. Tacrolimus inhibits calcineurin and thereby prevents T cells from producing interleukin-2, interferon-γ, and other cytokines.

BOX 55-6 Medications for Preventing Organ Rejection

Immunosuppressants

- Cyclosporine
- Sirolimus
- Tacrolimus

Glucocorticoid

- Prednisone

Cytotoxic Medications

- Azathioprine
- Mercaptopurine
- Mycophenolate mofetil

Antibodies

- Antithymocyte globulin, equine
- Basiliximab

2. Tacrolimus is more effective than cyclosporine but is more toxic.
3. Adverse effects are similar to those of cyclosporine and include nephrotoxicity, infection, hypertension, tremor, hirsutism, neurotoxicity, gastrointestinal effects, hyperkalemia, and hyperglycemia.
4. Tacrolimus should be used cautiously in immunosuppressed clients and those with renal, hepatic, or pancreatic impairment.
5. Tacrolimus is contraindicated for clients hypersensitive to cyclosporine.
6. Monitor blood glucose levels and administer prescribed insulin or oral hypoglycemics.

F. Prednisone
1. Prednisone is a glucocorticoid that inhibits accumulation of inflammatory cells at inflammation sites.
2. Hyperglycemia and hypokalemia can occur with prednisone use; monitor glucose and serum potassium levels.
3. See Chapter 47 for additional information about prednisone.

G. Azathioprine
1. Azathioprine suppresses cell-mediated and humoral immune responses by inhibiting the proliferation of B and T lymphocytes.
2. Can cause neutropenia and thrombocytopenia from bone marrow suppression
3. Contraindicated in pregnancy; associated with an increased incidence of neoplasms
4. Monitor hematocrit, white blood cell count, platelet count, liver enzyme levels, and coagulation factors.

H. Mycophenolate mofetil
1. Mycophenolate mofetil causes selective inhibition of B- and T-lymphocyte proliferation.
2. May be used with cyclosporine or tacrolimus and glucocorticoids for prophylaxis against organ rejection
3. Adverse effects include diarrhea, severe neutropenia, vomiting, and sepsis.
4. Mycophenolate mofetil is associated with an increased risk of infection and malignancies.
5. Absorption is decreased by the use of magnesium and aluminum antacids and by cholestyramine.
6. It is contraindicated in pregnancy and during breast-feeding.
7. Instruct the client to take the medication on an empty stomach and not to open or crush capsules.
8. Instruct the client to contact the PHCP for unusual bleeding or bruising, sore throat, mouth sores, abdominal pain, or fever.

Persons who have undergone organ transplant, such as a kidney, must take the prescribed immunosuppressant medications at the same time each day to ensure that the immune system is sufficiently suppressed to prevent organ rejection.

I. Basiliximab
1. Basiliximab binds to interleukin-2 receptors on lymphocytes, resulting in diminished cell-mediated immune reactions.
2. Used primarily as an induction agent at the time of transplantation; may be used with other immunosuppressants to prevent acute rejection of transplanted kidneys
3. Administered by the IV route; initial dose is administered within 2 hours before transplantation.
4. Side and adverse effects include headache, insomnia, dizziness, and tremors; chest pain, gastrointestinal distress, edema, shortness of breath, pain in the joints, and slow wound healing can also occur.

J. Antithymocyte globulin, equine
1. Antithymocyte globulin, equine, causes a decrease in the number and activity of thymus-derived lymphocytes and is used to suppress organ rejection following renal, liver, bone marrow, and heart transplantation.
2. It is used primarily to treat acute rejection episodes.
3. Before the first infusion, the client should undergo intradermal skin testing to determine hypersensitivity.
4. Because this product is made using equine and human blood components, it may carry a risk of transmitting infectious agents, such as viruses.
5. Monitor the platelet count and report low counts to the PHCP per agency policy.
6. Arrange for outpatient referral for repeated infusions after discharge.

VIII. Hematopoietic Growth Factors (Box 55-7)

A. Erythropoietic growth factors
1. Stimulate the production of red blood cells
2. Used to treat anemia of **chronic kidney disease**, chemotherapy-induced anemia, anemia caused by zidovudine, and anemia in clients requiring surgery
3. Initial effects can be seen within 1 to 2 weeks, and the hematocrit reaches normal levels in 2 to 3 months.

BOX 55-7 Hematopoietic Growth Factors

Erythropoietic Growth Factors
- Epoetin alfa
- Darbepoetin alfa
- Peginesatide

Leukopoietic Growth Factors
- Filgrastim
- Pegfilgrastim
- Sargramostim

4. Major adverse effect is hypertension.
5. Adverse effects can also include heart failure, thrombotic effects such as stroke or myocardial infarction, and cardiac arrest.

B. Leukopoietic growth factors
1. Stimulate the production of white blood cells (leukocytes)
2. Used for clients undergoing myelosuppressive chemotherapy or bone marrow transplantation and those with severe chronic neutropenia
3. Can cause bone pain, leukocytosis, and elevation of plasma uric acid, lactate dehydrogenase, and alkaline phosphatase levels; long-term therapy has caused splenomegaly.

C. Thrombopoietic growth factor
1. Stimulates the production of platelets
2. Used for clients undergoing myelosuppressive chemotherapy to minimize thrombocytopenia and to decrease the need for platelet transfusions
3. Adverse effects include fluid retention, cardiac dysrhythmias, conjunctival infection, visual blurring, and papilledema.

IX. Medications for Benign Prostatic Hyperplasia (Box 55-8)

A. Alpha blockers
1. Relax bladder neck muscles and muscle fibers in the prostate, allowing urine to pass more easily
2. Adverse effects include dizziness and retrograde ejaculation

B. 5a-alpha reductase inhibitors
1. Shrinks the prostate by preventing hormonal changes that result in growth of the prostate
2. May take up to 6 months to be effective
3. Adverse effects include retrograde ejaculation

BOX 55-8 Medications to Treat Benign Prostatic Hyperplasia

Alpha blockers
- Alfuzosin
- Doxazosin
- Tamsulosin
- Silodosin

5a-alpha reductase inhibitors
- Finasteride
- Dutasteride

PRACTICE QUESTIONS

661. A client who has a cold is seen in the emergency department with an inability to void. Because the client has a history of benign prostatic hyperplasia, the nurse determines that the client should be questioned about the use of which medication?
1. Diuretics
2. Antibiotics
3. Antilipemics
4. Decongestants

662. Nitrofurantoin is prescribed for a client with a urinary tract infection. The client contacts the nurse and reports a cough, chills, fever, and difficulty breathing. The nurse should make which interpretation about the client's complaints?
1. The client may have contracted the flu.
2. The client is experiencing anaphylaxis.
3. The client is experiencing expected effects of the medication.
4. The client is experiencing a pulmonary reaction requiring cessation of the medication.

663. The nurse is providing discharge instructions to a client receiving trimethoprim-sulfamethoxazole. Which instruction should be included in the list?
1. Advise that sunscreen is not needed.
2. Drink 8 to 10 glasses of water per day.
3. Decrease the dosage when symptoms are improving to prevent an allergic response.
4. If the urine turns dark brown, call the primary health care provider (PHCP) immediately.

664. Trimethoprim-sulfamethoxazole is prescribed for a client. The nurse should instruct the client to report which symptom if it develops during the course of this medication therapy?
1. Nausea
2. Diarrhea
3. Headache
4. Sore throat

665. Phenazopyridine is prescribed for a client with a urinary tract infection. The nurse evaluates that the medication is **effective** based on which observation?
1. Urine is clear amber.
2. Urination is not painful.
3. Urge incontinence is not present.
4. A reddish-orange discoloration of the urine is present.

666. Bethanechol chloride is prescribed for a client with urinary retention. Which disorder would be a contraindication to the administration of this medication?

1. Gastric atony
2. Urinary strictures
3. Neurogenic atony
4. Gastroesophageal reflux

667. The nurse, who is administering bethanechol chloride, is monitoring for cholinergic overdose associated with the medication. The nurse should check the client for which sign of overdose?
1. Dry skin
2. Dry mouth
3. Bradycardia
4. Signs of dehydration

668. Oxybutynin chloride is prescribed for a client with urge incontinence. Which sign would indicate a possible toxic effect related to this medication?
1. Pallor
2. Drowsiness
3. Bradycardia
4. Restlessness

669. Following kidney transplantation, cyclosporine is prescribed for a client. Which laboratory result would indicate an adverse effect from the use of this medication?
1. Hemoglobin level of 14.0 g/dL (140 mmol/L)
2. Creatinine level of 0.6 mg/dL (53 mcmol/L)
3. Blood urea nitrogen level of 25 mg/dL (8.8 mmol/L)
4. Fasting blood glucose level of 99 mg/dL (5.5 mmol/L)

670. The nurse is providing dietary instructions to a client who has been prescribed cyclosporine. Which food item should the nurse instruct the client to exclude from the diet?
1. Red meats
2. Orange juice
3. Grapefruit juice
4. Green, leafy vegetables

671. Tacrolimus is prescribed for a client who underwent a kidney transplant. Which instruction should the nurse include when teaching the client about this medication?
1. Eat at frequent intervals to avoid hypoglycemia.
2. Take the medication with a full glass of grapefruit juice.
3. Change positions carefully due to risk of orthostatic hypotension.
4. Take the oral medication every 12 hours at the same times every day.

672. The nurse is reviewing the laboratory results for a client receiving tacrolimus. Which laboratory result would indicate to the nurse that the client is experiencing an adverse effect of the medication?
1. Potassium level of 3.8 mEq/L (3.8 mmol/L)
2. Platelet count of 300,000 mm^3 (300×10^9/L)
3. Fasting blood glucose of 200 mg/dL (11.1 mmol/L)
4. White blood cell count of 6000 mm^3 (6.0×10^9/L)

673. The nurse receives a call from a client concerned about eliminating brown-colored urine after taking nitrofurantoin for a urinary tract infection. The nurse should make which appropriate response?
1. "Continue taking the medication; the brown urine occurs and is not harmful."
2. "Take magnesium hydroxide with your medication to lighten the urine color."
3. "Discontinue taking the medication and make an appointment for a urine culture."
4. "Decrease your medication to half the dose, because your urine is too concentrated."

674. A client with chronic kidney disease is receiving epoetin alfa. Which laboratory result would indicate a therapeutic effect of the medication?
1. Hematocrit of 33% (0.33)
2. Platelet count of 400,000 mm^3 (400×10^9/L)
3. White blood cell count of 6000 mm^3 (6.0×10^9/L)
4. Blood urea nitrogen level of 15 mg/dL (5.4 mmol/L)

675. A client with a urinary tract infection is receiving ciprofloxacin by the intravenous (IV) route. The nurse appropriately administers the medication by performing which action?
1. Infusing slowly over 60 minutes
2. Infusing in a light-protective bag
3. Infusing only through a central line
4. Infusing rapidly as a direct IV push medication

ANSWERS

661. *Answer:* 4

Rationale: In the client with benign prostatic hyperplasia, episodes of urinary retention can be triggered by certain medications, such as decongestants, anticholinergics, and antidepressants. These medications lessen the voluntary ability to contract the bladder. The client should be questioned about the use of these medications if he has urinary retention. Diuretics increase urine output. Antibiotics and antilipemics do not affect ability to urinate.

Test-Taking Strategy: Focus on the subject, medications that could exacerbate or contribute to urinary retention in the client with benign prostatic hyperplasia. Recalling that medications that contain anticholinergics may cause urinary retention will direct you to the correct option.

Level of Cognitive Ability: Analyzing

Client Needs: Physiological Integrity

Integrated Process: Nursing Process—Assessment

Content Area: Adult Health: Renal and Urinary

Health Problem: Adult Health: Renal and Urinary: Obstructive problems

Priority Concepts: Elimination; Safety

Reference: Lewis et al. (2017), p. 1273.

662. *Answer:* 4

Rationale: Nitrofurantoin can induce 2 kinds of pulmonary reactions: acute and subacute. Acute reactions, which are most common, manifest with dyspnea, chest pain, chills, fever, cough, and alveolar infiltrates. These symptoms resolve 2 to 4 days after discontinuing the medication. Acute pulmonary responses are thought to be hypersensitivity reactions. Subacute reactions are rare and occur during prolonged treatment. Symptoms (e.g., dyspnea, cough, malaise) usually regress over weeks to months following nitrofurantoin withdrawal. However, in some clients, permanent lung damage may occur. The remaining options are incorrect interpretations.

Test-Taking Strategy: Focus on the subject, interpreting the client's complaints, and the information in the question. Note the relationship of the information in the question and the words *pulmonary reaction* in the correct option.

Level of Cognitive Ability: Analyzing

Client Needs: Physiological Integrity

Integrated Process: Nursing Process—Analysis

Content Area: Pharmacology: Renal and Urinary Medications: Urinary tract antiseptics

Health Problem: Adult Health: Renal and Urinary: Inflammation/Infections

Priority Concepts: Clinical Judgment; Infection

Reference: Lilley et al. (2017), pp. 636, 638.

663. *Answer:* 2

Rationale: Each dose of trimethoprim-sulfamethoxazole should be administered with a full glass of water, and the client should maintain a high fluid intake to avoid crystalluria. The medication is more soluble in alkaline urine. The client should not be instructed to taper or discontinue the dose. Clients should be advised to use sunscreen since the skin becomes sensitive to the sun. Some forms of trimethoprim-sulfamethoxazole cause urine to turn dark brown or red. This does not indicate the need to notify the PHCP.

Test-Taking Strategy: Focus on the subject, client instructions for trimethoprim-sulfamethoxazole. Recalling that this medication is used to treat urinary tract infections will direct you to the correct option.

Level of Cognitive Ability: Applying

Client Needs: Physiological Integrity

Integrated Process: Teaching and Learning

Content Area: Pharmacology: Renal and Urinary Medications: Sulfonamides

Health Problem: Adult Health: Renal and Urinary: Inflammation/Infections

Priority Concepts: Client Teaching; Infection

Reference: Ignatavicius, Workman, Rebar (2018), p. 1360.

664. *Answer:* 4

Rationale: Clients taking trimethoprim-sulfamethoxazole should be informed about early signs and symptoms of blood disorders that can occur from this medication. These include sore throat, fever, and pallor, and the client should be instructed to notify the primary health care provider (PHCP) if these occur. The other options do not require PHCP notification.

Test-Taking Strategy: Focus on the subject, the symptoms to report. Knowledge that this medication can cause blood dyscrasias will direct you to the correct option.

Level of Cognitive Ability: Applying

Client Needs: Physiological Integrity

Integrated Process: Teaching and Learning

Content Area: Pharmacology: Renal and Urinary Medications: Sulfonamides

Health Problem: Adult Health: Renal and Urinary: Inflammation/Infections

Priority Concepts: Client Education; Infection

Reference: Hodgson, Kizior (2018), pp. 1188-1189.

665. *Answer:* 2

Rationale: Phenazopyridine is a urinary analgesic. It is effective when it eliminates pain and burning with urination. It does not eliminate the bacteria causing the infection, so it would not make the urine clear amber. It does not treat urge incontinence. It will cause the client to have reddish-orange discoloration of urine, but this is a side effect of the medication, not the desired effect.

Test-Taking Strategy: Note the strategic word, *effective*. Focus on the subject, effectiveness of phenazopyridine. Recalling the classification of this medication and that it is a urinary analgesic will direct you to the correct option.

Level of Cognitive Ability: Evaluating

Client Needs: Physiological Integrity

Integrated Process: Nursing Process—Evaluation

Content Area: Pharmacology: Renal and Urinary Medications: Urinary tract analgesics

Health Problem: Adult Health: Renal and Urinary: Inflammation/Infections

Priority Concepts: Elimination; Pain

Reference: Ignatavicius, Workman, Rebar (2018), p. 1360.

666. *Answer:* 2

Rationale: Bethanechol chloride can be hazardous to clients with urinary tract obstruction or weakness of the bladder wall. The medication has the ability to contract the bladder and thereby increase pressure within the urinary tract. Elevation of

pressure within the urinary tract could damage or rupture the bladder in clients with these conditions.
Test-Taking Strategy: Focus on the subject, a contraindication for the use of the medication. Noting that the medication is used for urinary retention may assist in directing you to the correct option.
Level of Cognitive Ability: Analyzing
Client Needs: Physiological Integrity
Integrated Process: Nursing Process—Analysis
Content Area: Pharmacology: Renal and Urinary Medications: Cholinergics
Health Problem: Adult Health: Renal and Urinary: Obstructive problems
Priority Concepts: Elimination; Safety
Reference: Skidmore-Roth (2017), pp. 141-142.

667. *Answer:* 3
Rationale: Cholinergic overdose of bethanechol chloride produces manifestations of excessive muscarinic stimulation such as salivation, sweating, involuntary urination and defecation, bradycardia, and severe hypotension. Remember that the sympathetic nervous system speeds the heart rate and the cholinergic (parasympathetic) nervous system slows the heart rate. Treatment includes supportive measures and the administration of atropine sulfate (anticholinergic) subcutaneously or intravenously.
Test-Taking Strategy: Focus on the subject, signs of cholinergic overdose. Noting that options 1, 2, and 4 are comparable or alike will assist in eliminating these options.
Level of Cognitive Ability: Analyzing
Client Needs: Physiological Integrity
Integrated Process: Nursing Process—Assessment
Content Area: Pharmacology: Renal and Urinary Medications: Cholinergics
Health Problem: N/A
Priority Concepts: Elimination; Safety
Reference: Lilley et al. (2017), pp. 327-328.

668. *Answer:* 4
Rationale: Toxicity (overdosage) of oxybutynin produces central nervous system excitation, such as nervousness, restlessness, hallucinations, and irritability. Other signs of toxicity include hypotension or hypertension, confusion, tachycardia, flushed or red face, and signs of respiratory depression. Drowsiness is a frequent side effect of the medication but does not indicate overdosage.
Test-Taking Strategy: Focus on the subject, signs of toxicity (overdosage) of oxybutynin. Remember that restlessness is a sign of toxicity.
Level of Cognitive Ability: Analyzing
Client Needs: Physiological Integrity
Integrated Process: Nursing Process—Assessment
Content Area: Pharmacology: Renal and Urinary Medications: Anticholinergics/antispasmodics
Priority Concepts: Clinical Judgment; Safety
Health Problem: N/A
Reference: Hodgson, Kizior (2018), pp. 874-875.

669. *Answer:* 3
Rationale: Cyclosporine is an immunosuppressant. Nephrotoxicity can occur from the use of cyclosporine. Nephrotoxicity is evaluated by monitoring for elevated blood urea nitrogen and serum creatinine levels. The normal blood urea nitrogen level is 10 to 20 mg/dL (3.6 to 7.1 mmol/L). The normal creatinine level for a male is 0.6 to 1.2 mg/dL (53 to 106 mcmol/L) and for a female is 0.5 to 1.1 mg/dL (44 to 97 mcmol/L). Cyclosporine can lower complete blood cell count levels. A normal hemoglobin is 14 to 18 g/dL (140 to 180 mmol/L) for a male and 12 to 16 g/dL (120 to 160 mmol/L) for a female. A normal hemoglobin is not an adverse effect. Cyclosporine does affect the glucose level. The normal fasting glucose is 70 to 99 mg/dL (3.9–5.5 mmol/L).
Test-Taking Strategy: Focus on the subject, the adverse effects of cyclosporine. Recall that cyclosporine can be nephrotoxic. The correct option is the only one that indicates an increased level of a renal function test. Also, recalling the normal laboratory reference levels will direct you to the correct option, the only abnormal level.
Level of Cognitive Ability: Analyzing
Client Needs: Physiological Integrity
Integrated Process: Nursing Process—Analysis
Content Area: Pharmacology: Renal and Urinary Medications: Organ rejection prevention
Health Problem: Adult Health: Immune: Transplantation
Priority Concepts: Immunity; Safety
Reference: Lewis et al. (2017), pp. 211, 1026.

670. *Answer:* 3
Rationale: A compound present in grapefruit juice inhibits metabolism of cyclosporine through the cytochrome P450 system. As a result, consumption of grapefruit juice can raise cyclosporine levels by 50% to 100%, thereby greatly increasing the risk of toxicity. Red meats, orange juice, and green, leafy vegetables do not interact with the cytochrome P450 system.
Test-Taking Strategy: Focus on the subject, the item to exclude from the diet. Recall that grapefruit juice is contraindicated with many medications. Use of general pharmacology guidelines will direct you to the correct option.
Level of Cognitive Ability: Applying
Client Needs: Physiological Integrity
Integrated Process: Teaching and Learning
Content Area: Pharmacology: Renal and Urinary Medications: Organ rejection prevention
Health Problem: N/A
Priority Concepts: Client Education; Safety
Reference: Lewis et al. (2017), p. 209.

671. *Answer:* 4
Rationale: Tacrolimus is a potent immunosuppressant used to prevent organ rejection in transplant clients. It is important that the medication be taken at 12-hour intervals to maintain a stable blood level to prevent organ rejection. Adverse effects include hyperglycemia and hypertension, so the client does not eat frequently to avoid hypoglycemia or use precautions to avoid orthostatic hypotension. Tacrolimus is metabolized through the cytochrome P450 system, so grapefruit juice is not allowed.
Test-Taking Strategy: Focus on the subject, teaching a transplant client regarding tacrolimus. Focus on the goal of avoiding organ rejection by maintaining a stable level of tacrolimus in the blood by taking the medication at regular intervals every day.

Level of Cognitive Ability: Applying
Client Needs: Physiological Integrity
Integrated Process: Teaching and Learning
Content Area: Pharmacology: Renal and Urinary Medications: Organ rejection prevention
Health Problem: Adult Health: Immune: Transplantation
Priority Concepts: Client Education; Immunity
Reference: Skidmore-Roth (2017), p. 1106.

672. *Answer:* 3
Rationale: A fasting blood glucose level of 200 mg/dL (11.1 mmol/L) is significantly elevated above the normal range of 70 to 99 mg/dL (3.9–5.5 mmol/L) and suggests an adverse effect. Recall that fasting blood glucose levels are sometimes based on primary health care provider preference. Other adverse effects include neurotoxicity evidenced by headache, tremor, and insomnia; gastrointestinal effects such as diarrhea, nausea, and vomiting; hypertension; and hyperkalemia. The remaining options identify normal reference levels. The normal potassium level is 3.5 to 5.0 mEq/L (3.5 to 5.0 mmol/L). The normal platelet count is 150,000 to 400,000 mm^3 (150 to 400 × 10^9/L). The normal white blood cell count is 5000 to 10,000 mm^3 (5 to 10 × 10^9/L).
Test-Taking Strategy: Focus on the subject, an adverse effect. Note that options 1, 2, and 4 are comparable or alike and represent normal values. The correct option has the only abnormal value, reflecting an elevation.
Level of Cognitive Ability: Analyzing
Client Needs: Physiological Integrity
Integrated Process: Nursing Process—Analysis
Content Area: Pharmacology: Renal and Urinary Medications: Organ rejection prevention
Health Problem: Adult Health: Immune: Transplantation
Priority Concepts: Clinical Judgment; Safety
Reference: Hodgson, Kizior (2018), p. 1112.

673. *Answer:* 1
Rationale: Nitrofurantoin imparts a harmless brown color to the urine, and the medication should not be discontinued until the prescribed dose is completed. Magnesium hydroxide will not affect urine color. In addition, antacids should be avoided because they interfere with medication effectiveness.
Test-Taking Strategy: Focus on the subject, brown-colored urine. Option 2 can be eliminated, because antacids should be avoided as a result of their interference with the effectiveness of nitrofurantoin. In addition, magnesium hydroxide will not have an effect on urine color. Next, eliminate options 3 and 4, because the nurse should not tell the client to discontinue medication or alter the dose.
Level of Cognitive Ability: Applying
Client Needs: Physiological Integrity
Integrated Process: Nursing Process—Implementation
Content Area: Pharmacology: Renal and Urinary Medications: Urinary tract antiseptics
Health Problem: Adult Health: Renal and Urinary: Inflammation/Infections
Priority Concepts: Elimination; Safety
Reference: Lewis et al. (2017), p. 1036.

674. *Answer:* 1
Rationale: Epoetin alfa is synthetic erythropoietin, which the kidneys produce to stimulate red blood cell production in the bone marrow. It is used to treat anemia associated with chronic kidney disease. The normal hematocrit level is 42% to 52% (0.42 to 0.52) for males and 37% to 47% (0.37 to 0.47) for females. Therapeutic effect is seen when the hematocrit reaches between 30% and 33% (0.30 and 0.33). The normal platelet count is 150,000 to 400,000 mm^3 (150 to 400 × 10^9/L). The normal blood urea nitrogen level is 10 to 20 mg/dL (3.6 to 7.1 mmol/L). The normal white blood cell count is 5000 to 10,000 mm^3 (5 to 10 × 10^9/L). Platelet production, white blood cell production, and blood urea nitrogen do not respond to erythropoietin.
Test-Taking Strategy: Focus on the subject, a therapeutic effect. Relate the name of the medication, epoetin alfa, to the potential action or effect of erythropoietin. The only laboratory test that would reflect the effect of this medication is a hematocrit of 33% (0.33), found in the correct option.
Level of Cognitive Ability: Evaluating
Client Needs: Physiological Integrity
Integrated Process: Nursing Process—Evaluation
Content Area: Pharmacology: Hematological Medications: Hematopoietic agents
Health Problem: Adult Health: Renal and Urinary: Chronic kidney disease
Priority Concepts: Clinical Judgment; Evidence
Reference: Skidmore-Roth (2017), p. 441.

675. *Answer:* 1
Rationale: Ciprofloxacin is prescribed for treatment of mild, moderate, severe, and complicated infections of the urinary tract, lower respiratory tract, and skin and skin structure. A single dose is administered slowly over 60 minutes to minimize discomfort and vein irritation. Ciprofloxacin is not light-sensitive, may be infused through a peripheral IV access, and is not given by IV push method.
Test-Taking Strategy: Focus on the subject, the appropriate way to administer an IV medication ciprofloxacin. Recall that this medication has adverse effects, so IV push would not be the recommended method of administration. Eliminate option 3 because of the closed-ended word, "only." Next, it is necessary that the presence of light does not affect the integrity of this medication.
Level of Cognitive Ability: Applying
Client Needs: Physiological Integrity
Integrated Process: Nursing Process—Implementation
Content Area: Pharmacology: Renal and Urinary Medications: Urinary tract antiseptics
Health Problem: Adult Health: Renal and Urinary: Inflammation/Infections
Priority Concepts: Clinical Judgment; Safety
Reference: Gahart, Nazareno, Ortega (2017), pp. 310-311.

UNIT XIV

Eye and Ear Problems of the Adult Client

Pyramid to Success

Pyramid Points focus on safety and nursing interventions for clients with impairment of sight or hearing and on the nursing care related to disorders such as cataracts, glaucoma, and retinal detachment. Communicating with clients who are visually or hearing impaired is also a priority. Emergency interventions for eye and ear disorders and injuries are a priority point. Pyramid Points also focus on client instructions related to medication administration, sensory perceptual alterations and safety issues, and available support systems.

Client Needs: Learning Objectives

Safe and Effective Care Environment

Caring for the recipient of a tissue (corneal) donation
Communicating with the interprofessional health care team
Establishing priorities
Maintaining asepsis with procedures and treatments
Maintaining standard and other precautions
Preventing accidents that can occur as a result of sensory impairments
Upholding client rights
Verifying that informed consent for invasive procedures is obtained

Health Promotion and Maintenance

Discussing changes that occur with the aging process
Discussing expected body image changes and self-care deficits
Implementing measures for the prevention and early detection of health problems and diseases related to the eye and the ear
Performing physical assessments of the eye and ear
Providing home care instructions following procedures related to the eye and ear
Providing instructions regarding activity limitations or postoperative activities
Providing instructions regarding the administration of eye and ear medications
Teaching regarding the importance of compliance with the prescribed therapy

Psychosocial Integrity

Assessing the client's ability to cope with feelings of isolation, fear, or anxiety regarding a possible change in vision and/or hearing status, and loss of independence
Discussing role changes
Identifying family support systems
Informing the client about available community resources
Monitoring for sensory perceptual alterations
Using appropriate communication techniques for impaired vision and hearing

Physiological Integrity

Monitoring for complications related to procedures
Monitoring for expected responses to therapy
Providing care for assistive devices such as eyeglasses, contact lenses, and hearing aids
Taking action in medical emergencies

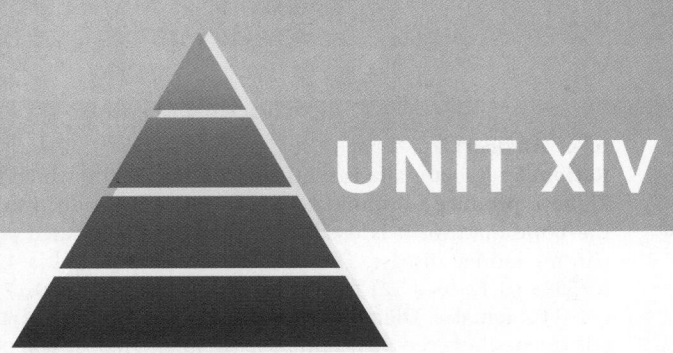

CHAPTER 56

Eye and Ear Problems

PRIORITY CONCEPTS **Safety, Sensory Perception**

I. Anatomy and Physiology of the Eye

A. The eye
  1. The eye is 1 inch (2.5 cm) in diameter and is located in the anterior portion of the orbit.
  2. The orbit is the bony structure of the skull that surrounds the eye and offers protection to the eye.

B. Layers of the eye
  1. External layer
    a. The fibrous coat that supports the eye
    b. Contains the cornea, the dense transparent outer layer
    c. Contains the sclera, the fibrous "white of the eye"
  2. Middle layer
    a. Called the *uveal tract*
    b. Consists of the choroid, ciliary body, and iris
    c. The choroid is the dark brown membrane located between the sclera and the retina that has dark pigmentation to prevent light from reflecting internally.
    d. The choroid lines most of the sclera and is attached to the retina but can detach easily from the sclera.
    e. The choroid contains many blood vessels and supplies nutrients to the retina.
    f. The ciliary body connects the choroid with the iris and secretes aqueous humor that helps give the eye its shape; the muscles of the ciliary body control the thickness of the lens.
    g. The iris is the colored portion of the eye, located in front of the lens, and it has a central circular opening called the *pupil*. The pupil controls the amount of light (darkness produces dilation and light produces constriction) admitted into the retina.
  3. Internal layer
    a. Consists of the retina, a thin, delicate structure in which the fibers of the optic nerve are distributed.
    b. The retina is bordered externally by the choroid and sclera and internally by the vitreous.
    c. The retina is the visual receptive layer of the eye in which light waves are changed into nerve impulses; it contains blood vessels and photoreceptors called *rods* and *cones*.

C. Vitreous body
  1. Contains a gelatinous substance that occupies the vitreous chamber, the space between the lens and the retina
  2. The vitreous body transmits light and gives shape to the posterior eye.

D. Vitreous
  1. Gel-like substance that maintains the shape of the eye
  2. Provides additional physical support to the retina

E. Rods and cones
  1. Rods are responsible for peripheral vision and function at reduced levels of illumination.
  2. Cones function at bright levels of illumination and are responsible for color vision and central vision.

F. Optic disc
  1. It is a creamy pink to white depressed area in the retina.
  2. The optic nerve enters and exits the eyeball at this area.
  3. This area is called the *blind spot* because it contains only nerve fibers, lacks photoreceptor cells, and is insensitive to light.

G. Macula lutea
  1. Small, oval, yellowish-pink area located laterally and temporally to the optic disc
  2. The central depressed part of the macula is the fovea centralis, the area of sharpest and keenest vision, where most acute vision occurs.
  3. Its functions include central vision, night and color vision, and motion detection.

H. Aqueous humor
  1. A clear, watery fluid that fills the anterior and posterior chambers of the eye

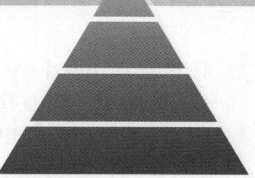

2. It is produced by the ciliary processes, and the fluid drains into the canal of Schlemm.
3. The anterior chamber lies between the cornea and the iris.
4. The posterior chamber lies between the iris and the lens.

I. Canal of Schlemm: Passageway that extends completely around the eye; it permits fluid to drain out of the eye into the systemic circulation so that a constant intraocular pressure (IOP) is maintained.

J. Lens
1. Transparent convex structure behind the iris and in front of the vitreous body
2. The lens bends rays of light so that the light falls on the retina.
3. The curve of the lens changes to focus on near or distant objects.

K. Conjunctivae: Thin, transparent mucous membranes of the eye that line the posterior surface of each eyelid, located over the sclera

L. Lacrimal gland: Produces tears that are drained through the punctum into the lacrimal duct and sac

M. Eye muscles
1. Muscles do not work independently; each muscle works with the muscle that produces the opposite movement.
2. Rectus muscles exert their pull when the eye turns temporally.
3. Oblique muscles exert their pull when the eye turns nasally.

N. Nerves
1. Cranial nerve II: Optic nerve (sight)
2. Cranial nerve III: Oculomotor (eye movement)
3. Cranial nerve IV: Trochlear (eye movement)
4. Cranial nerve VI: Abducens (eye movement)

O. Blood vessels
1. The ophthalmic artery is the major artery supplying the structures in the eye.
2. The ophthalmic veins drain the blood from the eye.

II. Assessment of Vision (see Chapter 12)

III. Diagnostic Tests for the Eye

A. Fluorescein angiography
1. Description
   a. A detailed imaging and recording of ocular circulation by a series of photographs taken after the administration of a dye
   b. Used to assess problems with retinal circulation, such as those that occur in diabetic retinopathy, retinal bleeding, and macular degeneration, or to rule out intraocular tumors
2. Preprocedure interventions
   a. Assess the client for allergies and previous reactions to dyes.
   b. An informed consent is necessary.
   c. A mydriatic medication, which causes pupil dilation, is instilled into the eye 1 hour before the test.
   d. The dye is injected into a vein of the client's arm.
   e. Inform the client that the dye may cause the skin to appear yellow for several hours after the test and is eliminated gradually through the urine. Urine may be bright green or orange for up to 2 days following the procedure.
   f. The client may experience nausea, vomiting, sneezing, paresthesia of the tongue, or pain at the injection site.
   g. If hives appear, antihistamines such as diphenhydramine are administered as prescribed.
3. Postprocedure interventions
   a. Encourage rest.
   b. Encourage fluid intake to assist in eliminating the dye.
   c. Remind the client that the yellow skin appearance will disappear.
   d. Inform the client that the urine will appear bright green or orange until the dye is excreted.
   e. Advise the client to avoid direct sunlight for a few hours after the test and to wear sunglasses, if staying indoors is not possible.
   f. Inform the client that the photophobia will continue until pupil size returns to normal.

B. Computed tomography (CT)
1. Description
   a. The test is performed to examine the eye, bony structures around the eye, and extraocular muscles.
   b. Contrast material may be used unless eye trauma is suspected.
2. Interventions
   a. No special client preparation or follow-up care is required.
   b. Instruct the client that he or she will be positioned in a confined space and will need to keep the head still during the procedure.
   c. Ask about and document allergies and/or previous exposure to contrast.

C. Slit lamp
1. Description
   a. Allows examination of the anterior ocular structures under microscopic magnification
   b. The client leans on a chin rest to stabilize the head while a narrowed beam of light is aimed so that it illuminates only a narrow segment of the eye.
2. Interventions: Advise the client about the brightness of the light and the need to look forward at a point over the examiner's ear.

D. Corneal staining
  1. Description
    a. A topical dye is instilled into the conjunctival sac to outline irregularities of the corneal surface that are not easily visible.
    b. The eye is viewed through a blue filter, and a bright green color indicates areas of a nonintact corneal epithelium.
  2. Interventions
    a. If the client wears contact lenses, the lenses must be removed.
    b. The client is instructed to blink after the dye has been applied to distribute the dye evenly across the cornea.

E. Tonometry
  1. Description: The test is used primarily to assess for an increase in IOP and potential glaucoma.
  2. Noncontact tonometry
    a. No direct contact with the client's cornea is needed, and no topical eye anesthetic is needed.
    b. A puff of air is directed at the cornea to indent the cornea, which can be unpleasant and may startle the client.
    c. It is a less accurate method of measurement compared with contact tonometry.
  3. Contact tonometry
    a. Requires a topical anesthetic
    b. A flattened cone is brought into contact with the cornea, and the amount of pressure needed to flatten the cornea is measured.
    c. The client must be instructed to avoid rubbing the eye following the examination if the eye has been anesthetized because of the potential for scratching the cornea.

Normal IOP is 10 to 21 mm Hg; IOP varies throughout the day and is normally higher in the morning (always document the time of IOP measurement).

F. Ultrasound: Procedure is similar to an ultrasound procedure done in other parts of the body and is done to detect lesions or tumors in the eye.

G. Magnetic resonance imaging (MRI): Similar to an MRI done in other parts of the body; refer to Chapter 58 for additional information on MRI.

IV. Problems of the Eye

A. Risk factors related to eye problems (Box 56-1)

BOX 56-1 Risk Factors for Eye Problems

- Aging process
- Congenital
- Diabetes mellitus
- Hereditary
- Medications
- Trauma

B. Refractive errors
  1. Description
    a. Refraction is the bending of light rays; any problem associated with eye length or refraction can lead to refractive errors.
    b. Myopia (nearsightedness): Refractive ability of the eye is too strong for the eye length; images are bent and fall in front of, not on, the retina.
    c. Hyperopia (farsightedness): Refractive ability of the eye is too weak; images are focused behind the retina.
    d. Presbyopia: Loss of lens elasticity because of aging; less able to focus the eye for close work and images fall behind the retina.
    e. Astigmatism: Occurs because of the irregular curvature of the cornea; image focuses at 2 different points on the retina.
  2. Assessment
    a. Refractive errors are diagnosed through a process called *refraction*.
    b. The client views an eye chart while various lenses of different strengths are systematically placed in front of the eye and is asked whether the lenses sharpen or worsen the vision.
  3. Nonsurgical interventions: Eyeglasses or contact lenses
  4. Surgical interventions
    a. Radial keratotomy: Incisions are made through the peripheral cornea to flatten the cornea, which allows the image to be focused closer to the retina; used to treat myopia.
    b. Photorefractive keratotomy: A laser beam is used to remove small portions of the corneal surface to reshape the cornea to focus an image properly on the retina; used to treat myopia and astigmatism.
    c. Laser-assisted in-situ keratomileusis (LASIK): The superficial layers of the cornea are lifted as a flap, a laser reshapes the deeper corneal layers, and then the corneal flap is replaced; used to treat hyperopia, myopia, and astigmatism.
    d. Corneal ring: The shape of the cornea is changed by placing a flexible ring in the outer edges of the cornea; used to treat myopia.

C. Legal blindness
  1. Description: In the client who is legally blind, the best visual acuity with corrective lenses in the better eye is 20/200 or less, or the visual field is no greater than 20 degrees in its widest diameter in the better eye.
  2. Interventions
    a. When speaking to the client who has limited sight or is blind, the nurse should use a normal tone of voice.

b. Alert the client when approaching.
c. Orient the client to the environment.
d. Use a focal point and provide further orientation to the environment from that focal point; ensure that the client has a clear pathway.
e. Allow the client to touch objects in the room.
f. Use the clock placement of foods on the meal tray to orient the client.
g. Promote independence as much as is possible.
h. Provide radios, televisions, and clocks that give the time orally, or provide a Braille watch.
i. When ambulating, allow the client to grasp the nurse's arm at the elbow; the nurse keeps her or his arm close to the body so that the client can detect the direction of movement.
j. Instruct the client to remain 1 step behind the nurse when ambulating.
k. Instruct the client in the use of the cane for the blind, which is differentiated from other canes by its straight shape and white color with red tip.
l. Instruct the client that the cane is held in the dominant hand several inches (centimeters) off the floor.
m. Instruct the client that the cane sweeps the ground where the client's foot will be placed next to determine the presence of obstacles.

D. Cataracts (Fig. 56-1)
1. Description
a. A cataract is an opacity of the lens that distorts the image projected onto the retina and that can progress to blindness.
b. Causes include the aging process (senile cataracts), heredity (congenital cataracts), and injury (traumatic cataracts); cataracts also can result from another eye disease (secondary cataracts).
c. Causes of secondary cataracts include diabetes mellitus, maternal rubella, severe myopia, ultraviolet light exposure, and medications such as corticosteroids.
d. Intervention is indicated when visual acuity has been reduced to a level that the client finds unacceptable or that adversely affects her or his lifestyle.

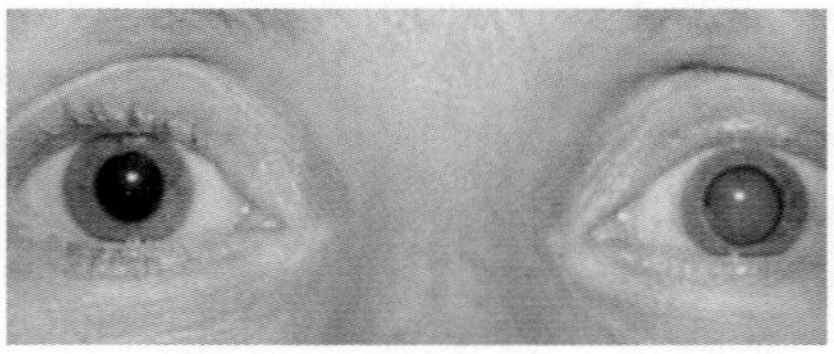

FIG. 56-1 The cloudy appearance of a lens affected by cataract. (From Patton, Thibodeau, 2010.)

2. Assessment
a. Blurred vision and decreased color perception are early signs.
b. Diplopia, reduced visual acuity, absence of the red reflex, and the presence of a white pupil are late signs. Pain or eye redness is associated with age-related cataract formation.
c. Loss of vision is gradual.
3. Interventions
a. Surgical removal of the lens, 1 eye at a time, is performed.
b. With extracapsular extraction, the lens is lifted out without removing the lens capsule; the procedure may be performed by phacoemulsification, in which the lens is broken up by ultrasonic vibrations and extracted.
c. With intracapsular extraction, the lens and capsule are removed completely.
d. A partial iridectomy may be performed with the lens extraction to prevent acute secondary glaucoma.
e. A lens implantation may be performed at the time of the surgical procedure.
4. Preoperative interventions
a. Instruct the client regarding the postoperative measures such as the importance of hand washing and measures to prevent or decrease IOP, such as bending over, coughing, straining, and rubbing the eye.
b. Stress to the client that care after surgery requires instillation of various types of eye drops several times a day for 2 to 4 weeks.
c. Administer eye medications preoperatively, including mydriatics and cycloplegics as prescribed.
5. Postoperative interventions
a. Elevate the head of the bed 30 to 45 degrees.
b. Turn the client to the back or nonoperative side.
c. Maintain an eye patch as prescribed; orient the client to the environment.
d. Position the client's personal belongings to the nonoperative side.
e. Use side rails for safety (per agency guidelines).
f. Assist with ambulation.
6. Client education (Box 56-2)

E. Glaucoma
1. Description
a. A group of ocular diseases resulting in increased IOP
b. IOP is the fluid (aqueous humor) pressure within the eye (normal IOP is 10 to 21 mm Hg).
c. Increased IOP results from inadequate drainage of aqueous humor from the canal of Schlemm or overproduction of aqueous humor.

BOX 56-2 Client Education Following Cataract Surgery

- Avoid eye straining.
- Avoid rubbing or placing pressure on the eyes.
- Avoid rapid movements, straining, sneezing, coughing, bending, vomiting, or lifting objects heavier than 5 lb (2.25 kg).
- Take measures to prevent constipation.
- Follow instructions for dressing changes and prescribed eye drops and medications.
- Wipe excess drainage or tearing with a sterile wet cotton ball from the inner to the outer canthus.
- Use an eye shield at bedtime.
- If lens implantation is not performed, accommodation is affected and glasses must be worn at all times.
- Cataract glasses act as magnifying glasses and replace central vision only, and objects will appear closer; therefore, the client needs to accommodate, judge distance, and climb stairs carefully.
- Contact lenses provide sharp visual acuity but dexterity is needed to insert them.
- Eye itching and mild discomfort are normal for a few days after the procedure.
- Contact the health care provider about any decrease in vision, severe eye pain, increase in redness, or increase in eye discharge.

d. The condition damages the optic nerve and can result in blindness.
e. The gradual loss of visual fields may go unnoticed, because central vision is unaffected.

2. Types
a. Primary open-angle glaucoma (POAG) results from obstruction to outflow of aqueous humor and is the most common type.
b. Primary angle-closure glaucoma (PACG) results from blocking the outflow of aqueous humor into the trabecular meshwork; causes include lens or pupil dilation from medications or sympathetic stimulation.

3. Assessment
a. Early signs include diminished **accommodation** and increased IOP.
b. POAG: Painless, and vision changes are slow; results in "tunnel" vision
c. PACG: Blurred vision, halos around lights, and ocular erythema

4. Interventions for acute angle-closure glaucoma

⚠ Acute angle-closure glaucoma is a medical emergency that causes sudden eye pain and possible nausea and vomiting.

a. Treat acute angle-closure glaucoma as a medical emergency.
b. Administer medications as prescribed to lower IOP.
c. Prepare the client for peripheral iridectomy, which allows aqueous humor to flow from the posterior to the anterior chamber.

5. Interventions for the client with glaucoma
a. Instruct the client on the importance of medications to constrict the pupils (**miotics**), to decrease the production of aqueous humor (carbonic anhydrase inhibitors), and to decrease the production of aqueous humor and IOP (beta blockers).
b. Instruct the client about the need for lifelong medication use, to wear a MedicAlert bracelet, to avoid anticholinergic medications to prevent increased IOP, and to contact the primary health care provider (PHCP) before taking medications, including over-the-counter medications.
c. Instruct the client to report eye pain, halos around the eyes, and changes in vision to the PHCP.
d. Instruct the client that when maximal medical therapy has failed to halt the progression of visual field loss and optic nerve damage, surgery will be recommended.
e. Prepare the client for trabeculectomy as prescribed, which allows drainage of aqueous humor into the conjunctival spaces by the creation of an opening.

F. Retinal detachment

1. Description
a. Detachment or separation of the retina from the epithelium
b. Occurs when the layers of the retina separate because of the accumulation of fluid between them, or when both retinal layers elevate away from the choroid as a result of a tumor
c. Partial detachment becomes complete if untreated.
d. When detachment becomes complete, blindness occurs.

2. Assessment
a. Flashes of light
b. Floaters or black spots (signs of bleeding)
c. Increase in blurred vision
d. Sense of a curtain being drawn over the eye
e. Loss of a portion of the visual field; painless loss of central or peripheral vision

3. Immediate interventions
a. Provide bed rest.
b. Cover both eyes with patches as prescribed to prevent further detachment.
c. Speak to the client before approaching.
d. Position the client's head as prescribed.
e. Protect the client from injury.
f. Avoid jerky head movements.
g. Minimize eye stress.

h. Prepare the client for a surgical procedure as prescribed.

4. Surgical procedures

a. Draining fluid from the subretinal space so that the retina can return to the normal position

b. Sealing retinal breaks by cryosurgery, a cold probe applied to the sclera, to stimulate an inflammatory response leading to adhesions

c. Diathermy, the use of an electrode needle and heat through the sclera, to stimulate an inflammatory response

d. Laser therapy, to stimulate an inflammatory response and seal small retinal tears before the detachment occurs

e. Scleral buckling, to hold the choroid and retina together with a splint until scar tissue forms, closing the tear (Fig. 56-2)

f. Insertion of gas or silicone oil to promote reattachment; these agents float against the retina to hold it in place until healing occurs.

5. Postoperative interventions

a. Maintain eye patches as prescribed.

b. Monitor for hemorrhage.

c. Prevent nausea and vomiting and monitor for restlessness, which can cause hemorrhage.

d. Monitor for sudden, sharp eye pain (notify the PHCP).

e. Encourage deep breathing but avoid coughing.

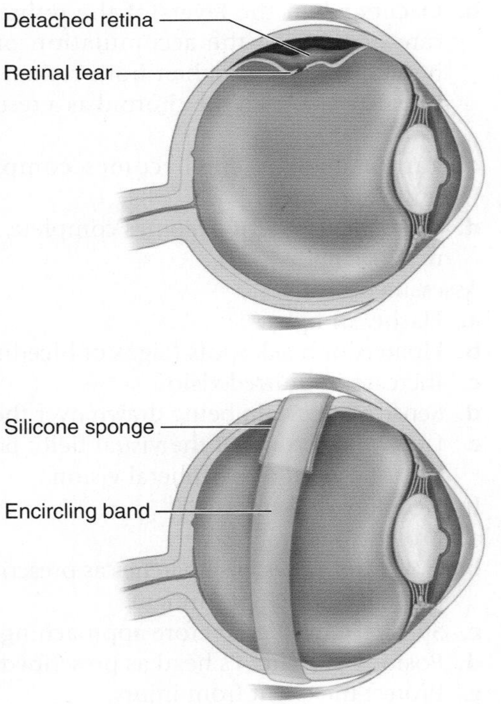

FIG. 56-2 The scleral buckling procedure for repair of retinal detachment.

f. Provide bed rest as prescribed.

g. Position the client as prescribed (positioning depends on the location of the detachment).

h. Administer eye medications as prescribed.

i. Assist the client with activities of daily living.

j. Avoid sudden head movements or anything that increases IOP.

k. Instruct the client to limit reading for 3 to 5 weeks.

l. Instruct the client to avoid squinting, straining and constipation, lifting heavy objects, and bending from the waist.

m. Instruct the client to wear dark glasses during the day and an eye patch at night.

n. Encourage follow-up care because of the danger of recurrence or occurrence in the other eye.

G. Macular degeneration

1. A deterioration of the macula, the area of central vision

2. Can be atrophic (age-related or dry) or exudative (wet)

3. Age-related: Caused by gradual blocking of retinal capillaries leading to an ischemic and necrotic macula; rod and cone photoreceptors die.

4. Exudative: Serous detachment of pigment epithelium in the macula occurs; fluid and blood collect under the macula, resulting in scar formation and visual distortion.

5. Interventions are aimed at maximizing the remaining vision.

6. Assessment

a. A decline in central vision

b. Blurred vision and distortion

7. Interventions

a. Initiate strategies to assist in maximizing remaining vision and maintaining independence.

b. Provide referrals to community organizations.

c. Laser therapy, photodynamic therapy, or other therapies may be prescribed to seal the leaking blood vessels in or near the macula.

H. Ocular melanoma

1. Most common malignant eye tumor in adults

2. Tumor is usually found in the uveal tract and can spread easily because of the rich blood supply.

3. Assessment

a. Tumor can be discovered during routine examination.

b. If the macular area is invaded, blurring of vision occurs.

c. Increased IOP is present if the canal of Schlemm is invaded.

d. Change of iris color is noted if the tumor invades the iris.

e. Ultrasonography may be performed to determine tumor size and location.

4. Interventions
 a. Surgery: Enucleation
 b. Radiation may be given via a radioactive plaque that is sutured to the sclera; the radioactive plaque remains in place until the prescribed radiation dose is delivered.

I. Enucleation and exenteration
 1. Description
  a. Enucleation is the removal of the entire eyeball.
  b. Exenteration is the removal of the eyeball and surrounding tissues and bone.
  c. The procedures are performed for the removal of ocular tumors.
  d. After the eye is removed, a ball implant is inserted to provide a firm base for a socket prosthesis and to facilitate the best cosmetic result.
  e. A prosthesis is fitted about 1 month after surgery.
 2. Preoperative interventions
  a. Provide emotional support to the client.
  b. Encourage the client to verbalize feelings related to loss.
  c. Encourage family support in care.
 3. Postoperative interventions
  a. Monitor vital signs.
  b. Assess a pressure patch or dressing as prescribed.
  c. Report changes in vital signs or the presence of bright red drainage on the pressure patch or dressing.

J. Hyphema
 1. Description: Presence of blood in the anterior chamber that occurs as a result of an injury; usually resolves in 5 to 7 days.
 2. Interventions
  a. Encourage rest in a semi-Fowler's position.
  b. Avoid sudden eye movements for 3 to 5 days to decrease the likelihood of bleeding.
  c. Administer cycloplegic eye drops as prescribed to relax the eye muscles and place the eye at rest.
  d. Instruct the client in the use of eye shields or eye patches as prescribed.
  e. Instruct the client to restrict reading and limit watching television.

K. Contusions
 1. Description
  a. Bleeding into the soft tissue as a result of an injury.
  b. A contusion causes a black eye; the discoloration disappears in about 10 days.
  c. Pain, photophobia, edema, and diplopia may occur.
 2. Interventions
  a. Place ice on the eye immediately.
  b. Instruct the client to receive a thorough eye examination.

L. Foreign bodies
 1. Description: An object such as dust or dirt that enters the eye and causes irritation
 2. Interventions
  a. Have the client look upward, expose the lower lid, wet a cotton-tipped applicator with sterile normal saline, gently twist the swab over the particle, and remove it.
  b. If the particle cannot be seen, have the client look downward, place a cotton applicator horizontally on the outer surface of the upper eye lid, grasp the lashes, and pull the upper lid outward and over the cotton applicator; if the particle is seen, gently twist a swab over it to remove.

M. Penetrating objects
 1. Description: An eye injury in which an object penetrates the eye
 2. Interventions
  a. Never remove the object, because it may be holding ocular structures in place; the object must be removed by the PHCP.
  b. Cover the eye with a cup (paper or plastic) and tape in place.
  c. Do not allow the client to bend over or lie flat; these positions may move the object.
  d. Do not place pressure on the eye.
  e. The client is to be seen by the PHCP immediately.
  f. X-rays and CT scans of the orbit are usually obtained.
  g. MRI is contraindicated because of the possibility of metal-containing projectile movement during the procedure.

N. Chemical burns
 1. Description: An eye injury in which a caustic substance enters the eye
 2. Interventions (see Priority Nursing Actions)

PRIORITY NURSING ACTIONS

Chemical Eye Injury Interventions in the Emergency Department

1. Quickly assess the client and visual acuity.
2. Check the pH of the eye.
3. Irrigate the eye continuously as prescribed, until the pH is at an acceptable level.
4. Document the event, actions taken, and the client's response.

Reference
Lewis et al. (2017), p. 371.

If a chemical splash to the eye occurs, treatment should begin immediately; immediately flush the eyes with water for at least 15 to 20 minutes at the scene of the injury, and then the client is brought to the emergency department. If possible, obtain a sample of the chemical involved.

O. Eye (tissue) donation
1. Donor eyes
a. Donor eyes are obtained from cadavers.
b. Donor eyes must be enucleated soon after death and stored in a preserving solution because of rapid endothelial cell death.
c. Storage, handling, and coordination of donor tissue with surgeons is provided by a network of state and national eye bank associations.
2. Care to the deceased client as a potential eye donor
a. The option of eye donation is discussed with the family.
b. Raise the head of the bed 30 degrees.
c. Instill antibiotic eye drops as prescribed.
d. Close the eyes and apply a small ice pack as prescribed to the closed eyes.
3. Preoperative care to the recipient of the cornea
a. The recipient may be told of the tissue (cornea) availability only several hours to 1 day before the surgery.
b. Assist in alleviating client anxiety.
c. Assess the recipient's eye for signs of infection.
d. Report the presence of any redness, watery or purulent drainage, or edema around the recipient's eye to the PHCP.
e. Instill antibiotic drops into the recipient's eye as prescribed to reduce the number of microorganisms present.
f. Administer fluids and medications intravenously as prescribed.
4. Postoperative care to the recipient
a. The eye is covered with a patch and protective shield that is left in place for 1 day.
b. Do not remove or change the dressing without a PHCP's prescription.
c. Monitor vital signs.
d. Monitor level of consciousness.
e. Assess the eye dressing.
f. Position the client with the head elevated and on the nonoperative side to reduce IOP.
g. Orient the client frequently.
h. Monitor for complications of bleeding, wound leakage, infection, and tissue rejection.
i. Instruct the client how to apply a patch and eye shield.
j. Instruct the client to wear the eye shield at night for 1 month and whenever around small children or pets.
k. Advise the client not to rub the eye.
l. Instruct the client to avoid activities that increase IOP.
5. Graft rejection (Fig. 56-3)
a. Rejection can occur at any time.
b. Inform the client of the signs of rejection.
c. Signs include *r*edness, *s*welling, decreased *v*ision, and *p*ain (RSVP).
d. The eye is treated with topical corticosteroids.

V. Anatomy and Physiology of the Ear

A. Functions
1. Hearing
2. Maintenance of balance

B. External ear (pinna)
1. It is embedded in the temporal bone bilaterally at the level of the eyes.
2. It extends from the auricle through the external canal to the tympanic membrane or eardrum and includes the mastoid process, the bony ridge located over the temporal bone.

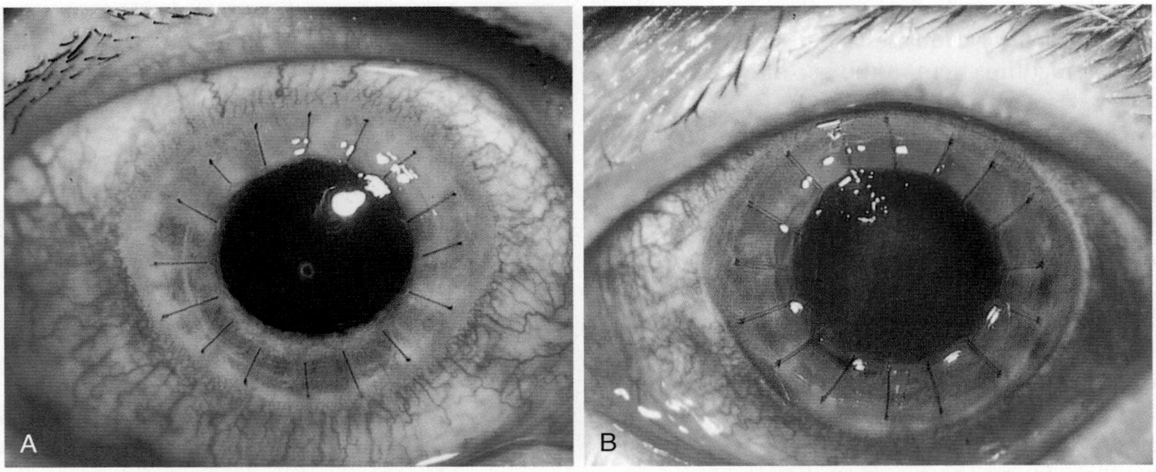

FIG. 56-3 Graft rejection. **A,** Clinical appearance of the eye after keratoplasty. **B,** Acute graft rejection. (From Black, Hawks, 2009. Courtesy Ophthalmic Photography at the University of Michigan, W.K. Kellogg Eye Center, Ann Arbor, Mich.)

C. Middle ear
1. The middle ear consists of the medial side of the tympanic membrane.
2. It contains 3 bony ossicles.
   a. Malleus
   b. Incus
   c. Stapes
3. Functions of the middle ear
   a. Conduct sound vibrations from the outer ear to the central hearing apparatus in the inner ear
   b. Protect the inner ear by reducing the amplitude of loud sounds
   c. The auditory canal (eustachian tube) allows equalization of air pressure on each side of the tympanic membrane so that the membrane does not rupture.

D. Inner ear
1. The inner ear contains the semicircular canals, cochlea, and distal end of the eighth cranial nerve.
2. The semicircular canals contain fluid and hair cells connected to sensory nerve fibers of the vestibular portion of the eighth cranial nerve.
3. The inner ear maintains the sense of balance or equilibrium.
4. The cochlea is the spiral-shaped organ of hearing.
5. The organ of Corti (within the cochlea) is the receptor and organ of hearing.
6. Eighth cranial nerve
   a. The cochlear branch of the nerve transmits neuroimpulses from the cochlea to the brain, where they are interpreted as sound.
   b. The vestibular branch maintains balance and equilibrium.

E. Hearing and equilibrium
1. The external ear conducts sound waves to the middle ear.
2. The middle ear, also called the *tympanic cavity*, conducts sound waves to the inner ear.
3. The middle ear is filled with air, which is kept at atmospheric pressure by the opening of the auditory canal.
4. The inner ear contains sensory receptors for sound and for equilibrium.
5. The receptors in the inner ear transmit sound waves and changes in body position as nerve impulses.

VI. Assessment of the Ear (see Chapter 12)

VII. Diagnostic Tests for the Ear

A. Tomography
1. Description
   a. Tomography may be performed with or without contrast medium.
   b. Tomography assesses the mastoid, middle ear, and inner ear structures and is especially helpful in the diagnosis of acoustic tumors.
   c. Multiple radiographs of the head are obtained.
2. Interventions
   a. All jewelry is removed.
   b. Lead eye shields are used to cover the cornea to diminish the radiation dose to the eyes.
   c. The client must remain still in a supine position.
   d. No follow-up care is required.
   e. If contrast is to be used, assess for allergies or previous response to contrast.

B. Audiometry
1. Description
   a. Audiometry measures hearing acuity.
   b. Audiometry uses 2 types, pure tone audiometry and speech audiometry.
   c. Pure tone audiometry is used to identify problems with hearing, speech, music, and other sounds in the environment.
   d. In speech audiometry, the client's ability to hear spoken words is measured.
   e. After testing, audiographic patterns are depicted on a graph to determine the type and level of the hearing loss.
2. Interventions
   a. Inform the client regarding the procedure.
   b. Instruct the client to identify the sounds as they are heard.

C. Electronystagmography (ENG)
1. Description
   a. ENG is a vestibular test that evaluates spontaneous and induced eye movements known as *nystagmus*.
   b. ENG is used to distinguish between normal nystagmus and medication-induced nystagmus, or nystagmus caused by a lesion in the central or peripheral vestibular pathway.
   c. ENG records changing electrical fields with the movement of the eye, as monitored by electrodes placed on the skin around the eye.
2. Interventions
   a. The client is instructed to remain NPO (nothing by mouth) for 3 hours before testing, and to avoid caffeine-containing beverages for 24 to 48 hours before the test.
   b. Unnecessary medications are withheld for 24 hours before testing.
   c. Instruct the client that this is a long and tiring procedure.
   d. The client should bring prescription eyeglasses to the examination.
   e. The client sits and is instructed to gaze at lights, focus on a moving pattern, focus on a moving point, and then close the eyes.

f. While sitting in a chair, the client may be rotated to obtain information about vestibular function.
g. In addition, the client's ears are irrigated with cool and warm water, which may cause nausea and vomiting.
h. Following the procedure, the client begins taking clear fluids slowly and cautiously because nausea and vomiting may occur.
i. Assistance with ambulation may also be necessary following the procedure.

D. MRI: Refer to Chapter 58 for information on MRI.

VIII. Problems of the Ear

A. Risk factors related to ear problems (Box 56-3)

B. **Conductive hearing loss** (Fig. 56-4)

1. Description
   a. Occurs when sound waves are blocked to the inner ear fibers because of external or middle ear problems
   b. Problems often can be corrected with no damage to hearing or minimal permanent hearing loss.

BOX 56-3 Risk Factors for Ear Problems

- Aging process
- Infection
- Medications
- Ototoxicity
- Trauma
- Tumors

2. Causes
   a. Any inflammatory process or obstruction of the external or middle ear
   b. Tumors
   c. Otosclerosis
   d. A buildup of scar tissue on the ossicles from previous middle ear surgery

C. **Sensorineural hearing** loss (see Fig. 56-4)

1. Description
   a. A pathological process of the inner ear or of the sensory fibers that lead to the cerebral cortex
   b. Sensorineural hearing loss is often permanent, and measures must be taken to reduce further damage.
2. Causes
   a. Damage to the inner ear structures
   b. Damage to the eighth cranial nerve or the brain itself
   c. Prolonged exposure to loud noise
   d. Medications
   e. Trauma
   f. Inherited problems
   g. Metabolic and circulatory problems
   h. Infections
   i. Surgery
   j. Meniere's syndrome
   k. Diabetes mellitus
   l. Myxedema

D. Mixed hearing loss (see Fig. 56-4)

1. Also known as conductive-sensorineural hearing loss

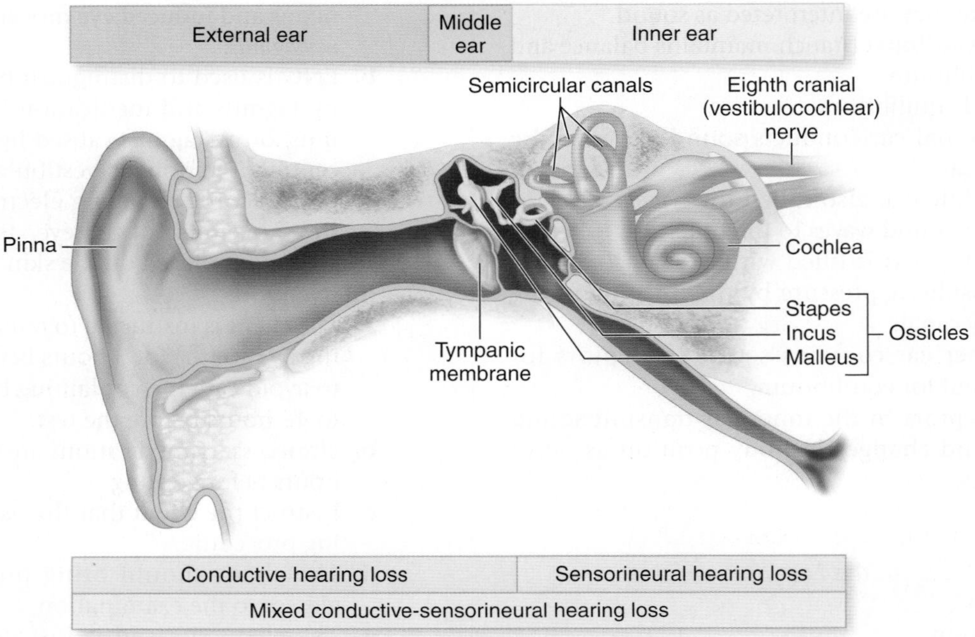

FIG. 56-4 Anatomy of hearing loss. Hearing loss can be divided into 3 types: (1) conductive (difficulty in the external or the middle ear); (2) sensorineural (difficulty in the inner ear or vestibulocochlear nerve); and (3) mixed conductive-sensorineural (a combination of the two).

2. The client has both sensorineural and conductive hearing loss.

E. Central hearing loss: Involves the inability to interpret sound, including speech, due to a problem in the brain

F. Signs of hearing loss and facilitating communication (Boxes 56-4 and 56-5)

G. Cochlear implantation
1. Cochlear implants are used for sensorineural hearing loss.
2. A small computer converts sound waves into electrical impulses.
3. Electrodes are placed by the internal ear with a computer device attached to the external ear.
4. Electronic impulses directly stimulate nerve fibers.

H. Hearing aids
1. Used for the client with conductive hearing loss
2. Have limited value for the client with sensorineural hearing loss, because they make sounds only louder, not clearer
3. A difficulty that exists in the use of hearing aids is the amplification of background noise and voices.
4. Hearing aids are costly and often not covered by insurance. Some clients can obtain hearing aids through a rehabilitation facility or through other resources.
5. Client education (Box 56-6)

I. Presbycusis
1. Description
a. A sensorineural hearing loss associated with aging
b. **Presbycusis** leads to degeneration or atrophy of the ganglion cells in the cochlea and a loss of elasticity of the basilar membranes.
c. Presbycusis leads to compromise of the vascular supply to the inner ear, with changes in several areas of the ear structure.
2. Assessment
a. Hearing loss is gradual and bilateral.
b. Client states that he or she has no problem with hearing but cannot understand what the words are.
c. Client thinks that the speaker is mumbling.

Instruct the client that cotton-tipped applicators should not be inserted into the ear canal, because their use can lead to trauma to the canal and can puncture the tympanic membrane.

BOX 56-4 Signs of Hearing Loss

- Frequently asking others to repeat statements
- Straining to hear
- Turning the head or leaning forward to favor 1 ear
- Shouting in conversation
- Ringing in the ears
- Failing to respond when not looking in the direction of the sound
- Answering questions incorrectly
- Raising the volume of the television or radio
- Avoiding large groups
- Better understanding of speech when in small groups
- Withdrawing from social interactions

BOX 56-5 Facilitating Communication

- Using written words if the client is able to see, read, and write
- Providing plenty of light in the room
- Getting the attention of the client before beginning to speak
- Facing the client when speaking
- Talking in a room without distracting noises
- Moving close to the client and speaking slowly and clearly
- Keeping hands and other objects away from the mouth when talking to the client
- Talking in normal volume and at a lower pitch because shouting is not helpful and higher frequencies are less easily heard
- Rephrasing sentences and repeating information
- Validating with the client the understanding of statements made by asking the client to repeat what was said
- Reading lips
- Encouraging the client to wear glasses when talking to someone to improve vision for lip reading
- Using sign language, which combines speech with hand movements that signify letters, words, or phrases
- Using telephone amplifiers
- Using flashing lights that are activated by ringing of the telephone or doorbell
- Using specially trained dogs to help the client be aware of sound and alert the client to potential danger

BOX 56-6 Client Education Regarding a Hearing Aid

- Begin using the hearing aid slowly to adjust to the device.
- Adjust the volume to the minimal hearing level to prevent feedback squealing.
- Concentrate on the sounds that are to be heard and to filter out background noise.
- Clean the ear mold and cannula per manufacturer's instructions.
- Keep the hearing aid dry.
- Turn the hearing aid off before removing from the ear to prevent squealing feedback; remove the battery when not in use.
- Keep extra batteries on hand.
- Keep the hearing aid in a safe place.
- Prevent hairsprays, oils, or other hair and face products from coming into contact with the receiver of the hearing aid.
- Instruct the client to keep the hearing aid in the proper environmental climate as recommended by the manufacturer in order to prolong the life of the device.

J. Otitis externa: See Chapter 34.
K. Otitis media: See Chapter 34.
   1. Myringotomy: See Chapter 34.
   2. Client education (Box 56-7)
L. Chronic otitis media
   1. Description
      a. A chronic infective, inflammatory, or allergic response involving the structure of the middle ear
      b. Frequent removal of debris from the ear canal may be required.
      c. Myringoplasty can reconstruct the tympanic membrane and ossicles and improve conductive hearing loss.
      d. Mastoidectomy may be performed if the infection has spread to involve the mastoid bone.

Monitor the client with otitis media closely for response to treatment. Otic and systemic antibiotics may be used to treat the infection, but often the organism is resistant.

   2. Preoperative interventions
      a. Administer antibiotic drops as prescribed.
      b. Clean the ear of debris as prescribed; irrigate the ear with a solution of equal parts vinegar and sterile water as prescribed to restore the normal pH of the ear.
      c. Instruct the client to avoid persons with upper respiratory infections, obtain adequate rest, eat a balanced diet, and drink adequate fluids.
      d. Instruct the client in deep breathing and coughing; forceful coughing, which increases pressure in the middle ear, is to be avoided postoperatively.
   3. Postoperative interventions

BOX 56-7 Client Education Following Myringotomy

- Avoid strenuous activities.
- Avoid rapid head movements, bouncing, or bending.
- Avoid straining on bowel movement.
- Avoid drinking through a straw.
- Avoid traveling by air.
- Avoid forceful coughing.
- Avoid contact with persons with colds.
- Avoid washing hair, showering, or getting the head wet for 1 week as prescribed.
- Use proper hand hygiene to prevent infection.
- Instruct the client that if he or she needs to blow the nose, to blow 1 side at a time with the mouth open.
- Instruct the client to keep ears dry by keeping a ball of cotton coated with petroleum jelly in the ear and to change the cotton ball daily.
- Instruct the client to report excessive ear drainage to the primary health care provider.

      a. Inform the client that initial hearing after surgery is diminished because of the packing in the ear canal; hearing improvement will occur after the ear canal packing is removed.
      b. Keep the dressing clean and dry.
      c. Keep the client flat as prescribed, with the operative ear up for at least 12 hours.
      d. Administer antibiotics as prescribed.
M. Mastoiditis
   1. Description
      a. Mastoiditis may be acute or chronic and results from untreated or inadequately treated chronic or acute otitis media.
      b. The pain is not relieved by myringotomy.
   2. Assessment
      a. Swelling behind the ear and pain with minimal movement of the head
      b. Cellulitis on the skin or external scalp over the mastoid process
      c. A reddened, dull, thick, immobile tympanic membrane, with or without perforation
      d. Tender and enlarged postauricular lymph nodes
      e. Low-grade fever
   3. Interventions
      a. Prepare the client for surgical removal of infected material.
      b. Simple or modified radical mastoidectomy with tympanoplasty is the most common treatment.
      c. Once infected tissue is removed, the tympanoplasty is performed to reconstruct the ossicles and tympanic membrane in an attempt to restore normal hearing.
   4. Complications
      a. Damage to the abducens and facial cranial nerves; exhibited by an inability to look laterally (cranial nerve VI, abducens) and a drooping of the mouth on the affected side (cranial nerve VII, facial)
      b. Meningitis
      c. Brain abscess
      d. Chronic purulent otitis media
      e. Wound infections
      f. Vertigo, if the infection spreads into the labyrinth
   5. Postoperative interventions
      a. Monitor for dizziness.
      b. Monitor for signs of meningitis, as evidenced by a stiff neck and vomiting, and for other complications.
      c. Prepare for a wound dressing change 24 hours postoperatively.
      d. Monitor the surgical incision for edema, drainage, and redness.
      e. Position the client flat with the operative side up as prescribed.

f. Restrict the client to bed with bedside commode privileges for 24 hours as prescribed.
g. Assist the client with getting out of bed to prevent falling or injuries from dizziness.
h. With reconstruction of the ossicles via a graft, take precautions to prevent dislodging of the graft.

N. Otosclerosis
1. Description
a. A genetic problem of the labyrinthine capsule of the middle ear that results in a bony overgrowth of the tissue surrounding the ossicles
b. Otosclerosis causes the development of irregular areas of new bone formation and causes the fixation of the bones.
c. Stapes fixation leads to a conductive hearing loss.
d. If the disease involves the inner ear, sensorineural hearing loss is present.
e. Bilateral involvement is common, although hearing loss may be worse in 1 ear.
f. Nonsurgical intervention promotes the improvement of hearing through amplification.
g. Surgical intervention involves removal of the bony growth causing the hearing loss.
h. A partial stapedectomy or complete stapedectomy with prosthesis (fenestration) may be performed surgically.
2. Assessment
a. Slowly progressing conductive hearing loss
b. Bilateral hearing loss
c. A ringing or roaring type of constant tinnitus
d. Loud sounds heard in the ear when chewing
e. Pinkish discoloration (Schwartze's sign) of the tympanic membrane, which indicates vascular changes within the ear

O. Fenestration
1. Description
a. Removal of the stapes, with a small hole drilled in the footplate; a prosthesis is connected between the incus and footplate.
b. Sounds cause the prosthesis to vibrate in the same manner as the stapes.
c. Complications include complete hearing loss, prolonged vertigo, infection, and facial nerve damage.
2. Preoperative interventions
a. Instruct the client in measures to prevent middle ear or external ear infections.
b. Instruct the client to avoid excessive nose blowing.
3. Postoperative interventions
a. Inform the client that hearing is initially worse after the surgical procedure because of swelling, and that no noticeable improvement in hearing may occur for as long as 6 weeks.
b. Inform the client that the Gelfoam ear packing (if used) interferes with hearing but is used to decrease bleeding.
c. Assist with ambulating during the first 1 to 2 days after surgery.
d. Administer antibiotic, antivertiginous, and pain medications as prescribed.
e. Assess for facial nerve damage, weakness, changes in tactile sensation and taste sensation, vertigo, nausea, and vomiting.
f. Instruct the client to move the head slowly when changing positions to prevent vertigo.
g. Instruct the client to avoid persons with upper respiratory infections.
h. Instruct the client to avoid showering and getting the head and wound wet.
i. Instruct the client to avoid rapid extreme changes in pressure caused by quick head movements, sneezing, nose blowing, straining, and changes in altitude.
j. Instruct the client to avoid changes in middle ear pressure, because they could dislodge the graft or prosthesis.

P. Labyrinthitis
1. Description: Infection of the labyrinth that occurs as a complication of acute or chronic otitis media
2. May result from growth of a cholesteatoma, a benign overgrowth of squamous cell epithelium in the middle ear
3. Assessment
a. Hearing loss that may be permanent on the affected side
b. Tinnitus
c. Spontaneous nystagmus to the affected side
d. Vertigo
e. Nausea and vomiting
4. Interventions
a. Monitor for signs of meningitis, the most common complication, as evidenced by headache, stiff neck, and lethargy.
b. Administer systemic antibiotics as prescribed.
c. Advise the client to rest in bed in a darkened room.
d. Administer antiemetics and antivertiginous medications as prescribed.
e. Instruct the client that the vertigo subsides as the inflammation resolves.
f. Instruct the client that balance problems that persist may require gait training through physical therapy.

Q. Meniere's syndrome
1. Description
a. Also called endolymphatic hydrops; it refers to dilation of the endolymphatic system by overproduction or decreased reabsorption of endolymphatic fluid.

b. The syndrome is characterized by tinnitus, unilateral sensorineural hearing loss, and vertigo.
c. Symptoms occur in attacks and last for several days, and the client becomes totally incapacitated during the attacks.
d. Initial hearing loss is reversible, but as the frequency of attacks increases, hearing loss becomes permanent.

A priority nursing intervention in the care of a client with Meniere's syndrome is instituting safety measures.

2. Causes
a. Any factor that increases endolymphatic secretion in the labyrinth
b. Viral and bacterial infections
c. Allergic reactions
d. Biochemical disturbances
e. Vascular disturbance, producing changes in the microcirculation in the labyrinth
f. Long-term stress may be a contributing factor.

3. Assessment
a. Feelings of fullness in the ear
b. Tinnitus, as a continuous low-pitched roar or humming sound, that is present much of the time but worsens just before and during severe attacks
c. Hearing loss that is worse during an attack
d. Vertigo; that is, a sensation of whirling that might cause the client to fall to the ground
e. Vertigo that is so intense that even while lying down, the client holds the bed or ground in an attempt to prevent the whirling
f. Nausea and vomiting
g. Nystagmus
h. Severe headaches

4. Nonsurgical interventions
a. Prevent injury during vertigo attacks.
b. Provide bed rest in a quiet environment.
c. Provide assistance with walking.
d. Instruct the client to move the head slowly to prevent worsening of the vertigo.
e. Initiate sodium and fluid restrictions as prescribed.
f. Instruct the client to stop smoking.
g. Instruct the client to avoid watching television because the flickering of lights may exacerbate symptoms.
h. Administer nicotinic acid as prescribed for its vasodilatory effect.
i. Administer antihistamines as prescribed to reduce the production of histamine and the inflammation.
j. Administer antiemetics as prescribed.
k. Administer tranquilizers and sedatives as prescribed to calm the client; allow the client to rest; and control vertigo, nausea, and vomiting.
l. Mild diuretics may be prescribed to decrease endolymph volume.
m. Inform the client about vestibular rehabilitation as prescribed.

5. Surgical interventions
a. Surgery is performed when medical therapy is ineffective and the functional level of the client has decreased significantly.
b. Endolymphatic drainage and insertion of a shunt may be an option early in the course of the disease to assist with the drainage of excess fluids.
c. A resection of the vestibular nerve or total removal of the labyrinth (i.e., a labyrinthectomy) may be performed.

6. Postoperative interventions
a. Assess packing and dressing on the ear.
b. Speak to the client on the side of the unaffected ear.
c. Perform neurological assessments.
d. Maintain safety.
e. Assist with ambulating.
f. Encourage the client to use a bedside commode rather than ambulating to the bathroom.
g. Administer antivertiginous and antiemetic medications as prescribed.

R. Acoustic neuroma
1. Description
a. A benign tumor of the vestibular or acoustic nerve
b. The tumor may cause damage to hearing and to facial movements and sensations.
c. Treatment includes surgical removal of the tumor via craniotomy.
d. Care is taken to preserve the function of the facial nerve.
e. The tumor rarely recurs after surgical removal.
f. Postoperative nursing care is similar to postoperative craniotomy care.

2. Assessment
a. Symptoms usually begin with tinnitus and progress to gradual sensorineural hearing loss.
b. As the tumor enlarges, damage to adjacent cranial nerves occurs.

S. Trauma
1. Description
a. The tympanic membrane has limited stretching ability and gives way under high pressure.
b. Foreign objects placed in the external canal may exert pressure on the tympanic membrane and cause perforation.
c. If the object continues through the canal, the bony structure of the stapes, incus, and malleus may be damaged.

d. A blunt injury to the basal skull and ear can damage the middle ear structures through fractures extending to the middle ear.
e. Excessive nose blowing and rapid changes of pressure that occur with nonpressurized air flights can increase pressure in the middle ear.
f. Depending on the damage to the ossicles, hearing loss may or may not be reversible.

2. Interventions
a. Tympanic membrane perforations usually heal within 24 hours.
b. Surgical reconstruction of the ossicles and tympanic membrane through tympanoplasty or myringoplasty may be performed to improve hearing.

T. Cerumen and foreign bodies
1. Description
a. Cerumen, or wax, is the most common cause of impacted canals.
b. Foreign bodies can include vegetables, beads, pencil erasers, insects, and other objects.
2. Assessment
a. Sensation of fullness in the ear with or without hearing loss
b. Pain, itching, or bleeding
3. Cerumen
a. Removal of wax may be done by irrigation.
b. Irrigation is contraindicated in clients with a history of tympanic membrane perforation or otitis media.
c. If prescribed to soften cerumen, glycerin or mineral oil is placed in the ear at bedtime; hydrogen peroxide may also be prescribed.
d. After several days, the ear is irrigated.
e. The maximum amount of solution that should be used for irrigation is 50 to 70 mL.

Inform the client that ear candles should never be used to remove cerumen. Their use can cause burns and a vacuum effect, causing a perforation in the tympanic membrane.

4. Foreign bodies
a. With a foreign object of vegetable matter, irrigation is used with care, because this material expands with hydration.
b. Insects are killed before removal, unless they can be coaxed out by flashlight or a humming noise; lidocaine may be placed in the ear to relieve pain.
c. Mineral oil or diluted alcohol is instilled to suffocate the insect, which then is removed using ear forceps.
d. Use a small ear forceps to remove the object; avoid pushing the object farther into the canal and damaging the tympanic membrane.

PRACTICE QUESTIONS

676. During the early postoperative period, a client who has undergone a cataract extraction complains of nausea and severe eye pain over the operative site. What should be the **initial** nursing action?
1. Call the surgeon.
2. Reassure the client that this is normal.
3. Turn the client onto her or his operative side.
4. Administer the prescribed pain medication and antiemetic.

677. The nurse is developing a teaching plan for a client with glaucoma. Which instruction should the nurse include in the plan of care?
1. Avoid overuse of the eyes.
2. Decrease the amount of salt in the diet.
3. Eye medications will need to be administered for life.
4. Decrease fluid intake to control the intraocular pressure.

678. The nurse is performing an admission assessment on a client with a diagnosis of detached retina. Which sign or symptom is associated with this eye problem?
1. Total loss of vision
2. Pain in the affected eye
3. A yellow discoloration of the sclera
4. A sense of a curtain falling across the field of vision

679. The nurse is performing an otoscopic examination on a client with mastoiditis. On examination of the tympanic membrane, which finding should the nurse expect to observe?
1. A pink-colored tympanic membrane
2. A pearly colored tympanic membrane
3. A transparent and clear tympanic membrane
4. A red, dull, thick, and immobile tympanic membrane

680. A client is diagnosed with a problem involving the inner ear. Which is the **most** common client complaint associated with a problem involving this part of the ear?
1. Pruritus
2. Tinnitus
3. Hearing loss
4. Burning in the ear

681. The nurse is performing an assessment on a client with a suspected diagnosis of cataract. Which clinical manifestation should the nurse expect to note in the **early** stages of cataract formation?
1. Diplopia
2. Eye pain
3. Floating spots
4. Blurred vision

682. A client arrives in the emergency department following an automobile crash. The client's forehead hit the steering wheel, and a hyphema is diagnosed. The nurse should place the client in which position?
1. Flat in bed
2. A semi-Fowler's position
3. Lateral on the affected side
4. Lateral on the unaffected side

683. The client sustains a contusion of the eyeball following a traumatic injury with a blunt object. Which intervention should be initiated **immediately**?
1. Apply ice to the affected eye.
2. Irrigate the eye with cool water.
3. Notify the primary health care provider (PHCP).
4. Accompany the client to the emergency department.

684. A client arrives in the emergency department with a penetrating eye injury from wood chips that occurred while cutting wood. The nurse assesses the eye and notes a piece of wood protruding from the eye. What is the **initial** nursing action?
1. Apply an eye patch.
2. Perform visual acuity tests.
3. Irrigate the eye with sterile saline.
4. Remove the piece of wood using a sterile eye clamp.

685. The nurse is caring for a client following enucleation to treat an ocular tumor and notes the presence of bright red drainage on the dressing. Which action should the nurse take at this time?
1. Document the finding.
2. Continue to monitor the drainage.
3. Notify the primary health care provider (PHCP).
4. Mark the drainage on the dressing and monitor for any increase in bleeding.

686. A woman was working in her garden. She accidentally sprayed insecticide into her right eye. She calls the emergency department, frantic and screaming for help. The nurse should instruct the woman to take which **immediate** action?
1. Irrigate the eyes with water.
2. Come to the emergency department.
3. Call the primary health care provider (PHCP).
4. Irrigate the eyes with diluted hydrogen peroxide.

687. The nurse is preparing a teaching plan for a client who had a cataract extraction with intraocular implantation. Which home care measures should the nurse include in the plan? **Select all that apply.**
- ☐ 1. Avoid activities that require bending over.
- ☐ 2. Contact the surgeon if eye scratchiness occurs.
- ☐ 3. Take acetaminophen for minor eye discomfort.
- ☐ 4. Expect episodes of sudden severe pain in the eye.
- ☐ 5. Place an eye shield on the surgical eye at bedtime.
- ☐ 6. Contact the surgeon if a decrease in visual acuity occurs.

688. Tonometry is performed on a client with a suspected diagnosis of glaucoma. The nurse looks at the documented test results and notes an intraocular pressure (IOP) value of 23. What should be the nurse's **initial** action?
1. Apply normal saline drops.
2. Note the time of day the test was done.
3. Contact the primary health care provider (PHCP).
4. Instruct the client to sleep with the head of the bed flat.

689. The nurse is caring for a client following craniotomy for removal of an acoustic neuroma. Assessment of which cranial nerve would identify a complication specifically associated with this surgery?
1. Cranial nerve I, olfactory
2. Cranial nerve IV, trochlear
3. Cranial nerve III, oculomotor
4. Cranial nerve VII, facial nerve

690. The nurse notes that the primary health care provider has documented a diagnosis of presbycusis on a client's chart. Based on this information, what action should the nurse take?
1. Speak loudly but mumble or slur the words.
2. Speak loudly and clearly while facing the client.
3. Speak at normal tone and pitch, slowly and clearly.
4. Speak loudly and directly into the client's affected ear.

691. A client with Meniere's disease is experiencing severe vertigo. Which instruction should the nurse give to the client to assist in controlling the vertigo?
1. Increase sodium in the diet.
2. Avoid sudden head movements.
3. Lie still and watch the television.
4. Increase fluid intake to 3000 mL a day.

692. The nurse is preparing to test the visual acuity of a client, using a Snellen chart. Which identifies the accurate procedure for this visual acuity test?
1. The right eye is tested, followed by the left eye, and then both eyes are tested.
2. Both eyes are assessed together, followed by an assessment of the right eye and then the left eye.
3. The client is asked to stand at a distance of 40 feet (12 meters) from the chart and to read the largest line on the chart.
4. The client is asked to stand at a distance of 40 feet (12 meters) from the chart and to read the line that can be read 200 feet (60 meters) away by an individual with unimpaired vision.

693. A client's vision is tested with a Snellen chart. The results of the tests are documented as 20/60. What action should the nurse implement based on this finding?
1. Provide the client with materials on legal blindness.
2. Instruct the client that he or she may need glasses when driving.
3. Inform the client of where he or she can purchase a white cane with a red tip.
4. Inform the client that it is best to sit near the back of the room when attending lectures.

694. The nurse is caring for a hearing-impaired client. Which approach will facilitate communication?
1. Speak loudly.
2. Speak frequently.
3. Speak at a normal volume.
4. Speak directly into the impaired ear.

ANSWERS

676. *Answer:* 1
Rationale: Severe pain or pain accompanied by nausea following a cataract extraction is an indicator of increased intraocular pressure and should be reported to the surgeon immediately. Options 2, 3, and 4 are inappropriate actions.
Test-Taking Strategy: Note the strategic word, *initial*, and the word *severe*. Eliminate option 2 because this is not a normal condition. The client should not be turned to the operative side; therefore, eliminate option 3. From the remaining options, focusing on the strategic word will direct you to the correct option.
Level of Cognitive Ability: Analyzing
Client Needs: Physiological Integrity
Integrated Process: Nursing Process—Implementation
Content Area: Complex Care: Emergency Situations/Management
Health Problem: Adult Health: Eye: Cataracts
Priority Concepts: Clinical Judgment; Pain
Reference: Ignatavicius, Workman, Rebar (2018), p. 971.

677. *Answer:* 3
Rationale: The administration of eye drops is a critical component of the treatment plan for the client with glaucoma. The client needs to be instructed that medications will need to be taken for the rest of her or his life. Options 1, 2, and 4 are not accurate instructions.
Test-Taking Strategy: Focus on the subject, client teaching for glaucoma. Recalling that medications are an integral component of the treatment plan will assist in directing you to the correct option.
Level of Cognitive Ability: Applying
Client Needs: Physiological Integrity
Integrated Process: Teaching and Learning
Content Area: Adult Health: Eye
Health Problem: Adult Health: Eye: Glaucoma
Priority Concepts: Client Education; Sensory Perception
Reference: Ignatavicius, Workman, Rebar (2018), p. 975.

678. *Answer:* 4
Rationale: A characteristic manifestation of retinal detachment described by the client is the feeling that a shadow or curtain is falling across the field of vision. No pain is associated with detachment of the retina. Options 1 and 3 are not characteristics of this problem. A retinal detachment is an ophthalmic emergency, and even more so if visual acuity is still normal.
Test-Taking Strategy: Focus on the subject, manifestations of retinal detachment. Thinking about the pathophysiology associated with this problem will direct you to the correct option.
Level of Cognitive Ability: Analyzing
Client Needs: Physiological Integrity
Integrated Process: Nursing Process—Assessment
Content Area: Adult Health: Eye
Health Problem: Adult Health: Eye: Retinal Detachment
Priority Concepts: Clinical Judgment; Sensory Perception
Reference: Ignatavicius, Workman, Rebar (2018), p. 979.

679. *Answer:* 4
Rationale: Otoscopic examination in a client with mastoiditis reveals a red, dull, thick, and immobile tympanic membrane, with or without perforation. Postauricular lymph nodes are tender and enlarged. Clients also have a low-grade fever, malaise, anorexia, swelling behind the ear, and pain with minimal movement of the head.
Test-Taking Strategy: Focus on the subject, the assessment findings in mastoiditis. Think about the pathophysiology associated with mastoiditis and remember that mastoiditis reveals a red, dull, thick, and immobile tympanic membrane.
Level of Cognitive Ability: Analyzing
Client Needs: Physiological Integrity
Integrated Process: Nursing Process—Assessment
Content Area: Adult Health: Ear
Health Problem: Adult Health: Ear: Inflammatory/Infections/Structural Problems
Priority Concepts: Infection; Inflammation
Reference: Lewis et al. (2017), pp. 384-385.

680. *Answer:* 2
Rationale: Tinnitus is the most common complaint of clients with otological problems, especially problems involving the inner ear. Symptoms of tinnitus range from mild ringing in the ear, which can go unnoticed during the day, to a loud roaring in the ear, which can interfere with the client's thinking process and attention span. Options 1, 3, and 4 are not associated specifically with problems of the inner ear.
Test-Taking Strategy: Note the strategic word, *most*. Recalling the anatomy and the function of the inner ear will direct you to the correct option.
Level of Cognitive Ability: Analyzing
Client Needs: Physiological Integrity
Integrated Process: Nursing Process—Assessment
Content Area: Adult Health: Ear

Health Problem: Adult Health: Ear: Vertigo/Tinnitus
Priority Concepts: Clinical Judgment; Sensory Perception
Reference: Ignatavicius, Workman, Rebar (2018), p. 995.

681. *Answer:* 4
Rationale: A gradual, painless blurring of central vision is the chief clinical manifestation of a cataract. Early symptoms include slightly blurred vision and a decrease in color perception. Options 1, 2, and 3 are not characteristics of a cataract.
Test-Taking Strategy: Note the strategic word, *early*. Remember the pathophysiology related to cataract development. As a cataract develops, the lens of the eye becomes opaque. This description will assist in directing you to the correct option.
Level of Cognitive Ability: Analyzing
Client Needs: Physiological Integrity
Integrated Process: Nursing Process—Assessment
Content Area: Adult Health: Eye
Health Problem: Adult Health: Eye: Cataracts
Priority Concepts: Clinical Judgment; Sensory Perception
Reference: Ignatavicius, Workman, Rebar (2018), p. 969.

682. *Answer:* 2
Rationale: A hyphema is the presence of blood in the anterior chamber. Hyphema is produced when a force is sufficient to break the integrity of the blood vessels in the eye and can be caused by direct injury, such as a penetrating injury from a BB or pellet, or indirectly, such as from striking the forehead on a steering wheel during an accident. The client is treated by bed rest in a semi-Fowler's position to assist gravity in keeping the hyphema away from the optical center of the cornea.
Test-Taking Strategy: Focus on the subject, care of the client who has sustained a hyphema. Remember that placing the client flat will produce an increase in pressure at the injured site. Also, note that the correct option is the one that identifies a position different from the other options.
Level of Cognitive Ability: Applying
Client Needs: Physiological Integrity
Integrated Process: Nursing Process—Implementation
Content Area: Complex Care: Emergency Situations/Management
Health Problem: Adult Health: Eye: Inflammation/Infections/Injuries
Priority Concepts: Safety; Tissue Integrity
Reference: Jarvis (2016), p. 321.

683. *Answer:* 1
Rationale: Treatment for a contusion begins at the time of injury. Ice is applied immediately. The client then should be seen by a PHCP and receive a thorough eye examination to rule out the presence of other eye injuries.
Test-Taking Strategy: Focus on the strategic word, *immediately*. Recalling the principles related to initial treatment of injuries and noting the type of injury sustained will direct you to the correct option.
Level of Cognitive Ability: Applying
Client Needs: Physiological Integrity
Integrated Process: Nursing Process—Implementation
Content Area: Complex Care: Emergency Situations/Management
Health Problem: Adult Health: Eye: Inflammation/Infections/Injuries
Priority Concepts: Clinical Judgment; Tissue Integrity
Reference: Ignatavicius, Workman, Rebar (2018), p. 981.

684. *Answer:* 2
Rationale: If the eye injury is the result of a penetrating object, the object may be noted protruding from the eye. This object must never be removed except by the ophthalmologist, because it may be holding ocular structures in place. Application of an eye patch or irrigation of the eye may disrupt the foreign body and cause further tearing of the cornea.
Test-Taking Strategy: Note the strategic word, *initial*, and note the word *penetrating*. This should indicate that a laceration has occurred and that interventions are directed at preventing further disruption of the integrity of the eye. The only option that will prevent further disruption is to assess visual acuity.
Level of Cognitive Ability: Applying
Client Needs: Physiological Integrity
Integrated Process: Nursing Process—Implementation
Content Area: Complex Care: Emergency Situations/Management
Health Problem: Adult Health: Eye: Inflammation/Infections/Injuries
Priority Concepts: Clinical Judgment; Tissue Integrity
Reference: Ignatavicius, Workman, Rebar (2018), p. 981.

685. *Answer:* 3
Rationale: If the nurse notes the presence of bright red drainage on the dressing, it must be reported to the PHCP, because this indicates hemorrhage. Options 1, 2, and 4 are inappropriate at this time.
Test-Taking Strategy: Determine if an abnormality exists. Note the words, *bright red*. Since an abnormality does exist, eliminate options that state to document and continue to monitor because an action is needed.
Level of Cognitive Ability: Applying
Client Needs: Physiological Integrity
Integrated Process: Nursing Process—Implementation
Content Area: Complex Care: Emergency Situations/Management
Health Problem: Adult Health: Eye: Ocular tumors, retinoblastoma
Priority Concepts: Clinical Judgment; Tissue Integrity
Reference: Lewis et al. (2017), pp. 382-383.

686. *Answer:* 1
Rationale: In this type of accident, the client is instructed to irrigate the eyes immediately with running water for at least 20 minutes, or until the emergency medical services personnel arrive. In the emergency department, the cleansing agent of choice is usually normal saline. Calling the PHCP and going to the emergency department delays necessary intervention. Hydrogen peroxide is never placed in the eyes.
Test-Taking Strategy: Note the strategic word, *immediate*. Focus on the type of injury and eliminate options 2 and 3 because they delay necessary intervention. Next, eliminate option 4 because hydrogen peroxide is never placed in the eyes.
Level of Cognitive Ability: Applying
Client Needs: Physiological Integrity
Integrated Process: Nursing Process—Implementation
Content Area: Complex Care: Emergency Situations/Management

Health Problem: Adult Health: Eye: Inflammation/Infections/Injuries
Priority Concepts: Client Education; Tissue Integrity
Reference: Lewis et al. (2017), p. 371.

687. *Answer:* 1, 3, 5, 6
Rationale: Following eye surgery, some scratchiness and mild eye discomfort may occur in the operative eye and usually is relieved by mild analgesics. If the eye pain becomes severe, the client should notify the surgeon, because this may indicate hemorrhage, infection, or increased intraocular pressure (IOP). The nurse also would instruct the client to notify the surgeon of increased purulent drainage, increased redness, or any decrease in visual acuity. The client is instructed to place an eye shield over the operative eye at bedtime to protect the eye from injury during sleep and to avoid activities that increase IOP, such as bending over.
Test-Taking Strategy: Focus on the subject, postoperative care following eye surgery. Recalling that the eye needs to be protected and that increased IOP is a concern will assist in determining the home care measures to be included in the plan.
Level of Cognitive Ability: Analyzing
Client Needs: Physiological Integrity
Integrated Process: Teaching and Learning
Content Area: Adult Health: Eye
Health Problem: Adult Health: Eye: Cataracts
Priority Concepts: Client Education; Safety
Reference: Lewis et al. (2017), p. 376.

688. *Answer:* 2
Rationale: Tonometry is a method of measuring intraocular fluid pressure. Pressures between 10 and 21 mm Hg are considered within the normal range. However, IOP is slightly higher in the morning. Therefore, the initial action is to check the time the test was performed. Normal saline drops are not a specific treatment for glaucoma. It is not necessary to contact the PHCP as an initial action. Flat positions may increase the pressure.
Test-Taking Strategy: Focus on the subject, normal IOP, and note the strategic word, *initial*. Remember that normal IOP is between 10 and 21 mm Hg and the pressure may be higher in the morning.
Level of Cognitive Ability: Analyzing
Client Needs: Physiological Integrity
Integrated Process: Nursing Process—Implementation
Content Area: Adult Health: Eye
Health Problem: Adult Health: Eye: Glaucoma
Priority Concepts: Clinical Judgment; Sensory Perception
Reference: Ignatavicius, Workman, Rebar (2018), p. 965.

689. *Answer:* 4
Rationale: An acoustic neuroma (or vestibular schwannoma) is a unilateral benign tumor that occurs where the vestibulocochlear or acoustic nerve (cranial nerve VIII) enters the internal auditory canal. It is important that an early diagnosis be made, because the tumor can compress the trigeminal and facial nerves and arteries within the internal auditory canal. Treatment for acoustic neuroma is surgical removal via a craniotomy. Assessment of the trigeminal and facial nerves is important. Extreme care is taken to preserve remaining hearing and preserve the function of the facial nerve. Acoustic neuromas rarely recur following surgical removal.
Test-Taking Strategy: Focus on the subject, a complication following surgery. Think about the anatomical location of an acoustic neuroma and the nerves that the neuroma can compress to direct you to the correct option.
Level of Cognitive Ability: Analyzing
Client Needs: Physiological Integrity
Integrated Process: Nursing Process—Assessment
Content Area: Adult Health: Ear
Health Problem: Adult Health: Ear: Hearing Loss
Priority Concepts: Clinical Judgment; Sensory Perception
Reference: Ignatavicius, Workman, Rebar (2018), pp. 951, 996.

690. *Answer:* 3
Rationale: Presbycusis is a type of hearing loss that occurs with aging. Presbycusis is a gradual sensorineural loss caused by nerve degeneration in the inner ear or auditory nerve. When communicating with a client with this condition, the nurse should speak at a normal tone and pitch, slowly and clearly. It is not appropriate to speak loudly, mumble or slur words, or speak into the client's affected ear.
Test-Taking Strategy: Focus on the subject, presbycusis and the effective method to communicate. Visualize each of the communication techniques to direct you to the correct option.
Level of Cognitive Ability: Applying
Client Needs: Physiological Integrity
Integrated Process: Nursing Process—Implementation
Content Area: Adult Health: Ear
Health Problem: Adult Health: Ear: Hearing Loss
Priority Concepts: Communication; Sensory Perception
Reference: Ignatavicius, Workman, Rebar (2018), pp. 997-998.

691. *Answer:* 2
Rationale: The nurse instructs the client to make slow head movements to prevent worsening of the vertigo. Dietary changes such as salt and fluid restrictions that reduce the amount of endolymphatic fluid are sometimes prescribed. Lying still and watching television will not control vertigo.
Test-Taking Strategy: Focus on the subject, preventing vertigo. Note the relationship between vertigo and avoiding sudden head movements in the correct option.
Level of Cognitive Ability: Applying
Client Needs: Safe and Effective Care Environment
Integrated Process: Teaching and Learning
Content Area: Adult Health: Ear
Health Problem: Adult Health: Ear: Vertigo/Tinnitus
Priority Concepts: Client Education; Safety
Reference: Ignatavicius, Workman, Rebar (2018), pp. 995-996.

692. *Answer:* 1
Rationale: Visual acuity is assessed in 1 eye at a time, and then in both eyes together, with the client comfortably standing or sitting. The right eye is tested with the left eye covered; then the left eye is tested with the right eye covered. Both eyes are then tested together. Visual acuity is measured with or without corrective lenses, and the client stands at a distance of 20 feet (6 meters) from the chart.
Test-Taking Strategy: Remember that normal visual acuity as measured by a Snellen chart is 20/20 vision. This should assist in eliminating options 3 and 4, because they are comparable

or alike in that they indicate standing at a distance of 40 feet (12 meters). From the remaining options, remember that it is best and most accurate to test each eye separately and then test both eyes together.
Level of Cognitive Ability: Applying
Client Needs: Health Promotion and Maintenance
Integrated Process: Nursing Process—Assessment
Content Area: Adult Health: Health Assessment/Physical Exam: Eye
Health Problem: N/A
Priority Concepts: Clinical Judgment; Sensory Perception
Reference: Jarvis (2016), pp. 289-290, 303.

693. ***Answer:*** **2**
Rationale: Vision that is 20/20 is normal—that is, the client is able to read from 20 feet (6 meters) what a person with normal vision can read from 20 feet (6 meters). A client with a visual acuity of 20/60 can only read at a distance of 20 feet (6 meters) what a person with normal vision can read at 60 feet (18 meters). With this vision, the client may need glasses while driving in order to read signs and to see far ahead. The client should be instructed to sit in the front of the room for lectures to aid in visualization. This is not considered to be legal blindness.
Test-Taking Strategy: Focus on the subject, interpreting a Snellen chart result. Note the test result, 20/60, and recall the associated interventions for this result. Also, eliminate options 1 and 3, as they are comparable or alike, implying that the test results indicate blindness.
Level of Cognitive Ability: Analyzing
Client Needs: Physiological Integrity
Integrated Process: Nursing Process—Implementation
Content Area: Adult Health: Health Assessment/Physical Exam: Eye
Health Problem: Adult Health: Eye: Visual problems/refractive errors
Priority Concepts: Clinical Judgment; Sensory Perception
Reference: Lewis et al. (2017), p. 356.

694. ***Answer:*** **3**
Rationale: Speaking in a normal tone to the client with impaired hearing and not shouting are important. The nurse should talk directly to the client while facing the client and speak clearly. If the client does not seem to understand what is said, the nurse should express it differently. Moving closer to the client and toward the better ear may facilitate communication, but the nurse should avoid talking directly into the impaired ear.
Test-Taking Strategy: Focus on the subject, an effective communication technique for the hearing impaired. Remember that it is important to speak in a normal tone.
Level of Cognitive Ability: Applying
Client Needs: Psychosocial Integrity
Integrated Process: Communication and Documentation
Content Area: Adult Health: Ear
Health Problem: Adult Health: Ear: Hearing Loss
Priority Concepts: Communication; Sensory Perception
Reference: Ignatavicius, Workman, Rebar (2018), p. 998.

CHAPTER 57

Eye and Ear Medications

PRIORITY CONCEPTS **Safety; Sensory Perception**

I. Ophthalmic Medication Administration

A. Guidelines for the use of eye medications
1. Eye medications are usually in the form of drops or ointments.
2. To prevent overflow of medication into the nasal and pharyngeal passages, thus reducing systemic absorption, instruct the client to apply pressure over the inner canthus next to the nose for 30 to 60 seconds following administration of the medication; instruct the client to close the eye gently to help distribute the medication (Fig. 57-1).
3. If both an eye drop and eye ointment are scheduled to be administered at the same time, administer the eye drop first.
4. Wash hands and don gloves before administering eye medications to avoid contaminating the eye or medication dropper or applicator.
5. Use a separate bottle or tube of medication for each client to avoid accidental cross-contamination.
6. Place the prescribed dose of eye medication in the lower conjunctival sac, never directly onto the cornea.
7. Avoid touching any part of the eye with the dropper or applicator.
8. Administer glucocorticoid preparations before other medications.
9. Monitor the pulse and blood pressure if the client is receiving an ophthalmic beta blocker, and instruct the client to do the same; the nurse should obtain pulse parameters from the primary health care provider (PHCP).
10. Instruct the client how to instill medication correctly and supervise instillation until the client can do it safely; adaptive devices that position the bottle of eye drops directly over the eye can also be purchased if instillation is difficult for the client.
11. Instruct the client to read the medication labels carefully to ensure administration of the correct medication and correct strength.
12. Remind the client to keep these medications out of the reach of children.
13. Instruct the client to avoid driving or operating hazardous equipment if vision is blurred.
14. Inform the client that she or he may be unable to drive home after eye examinations when a medication to dilate the pupil (**mydriatic**) or to paralyze the ciliary muscle (**cycloplegic**) is used.
15. If photophobia occurs, instruct the client to wear sunglasses and avoid bright lights.
16. Instruct the client to administer a missed dose of the eye medication as soon as it is remembered, unless the next dose is scheduled to be administered in 1 to 2 hours.
17. Inform the client with **glaucoma** that the disorder cannot be cured, only controlled.
18. Reinforce the importance of using medications to treat glaucoma as prescribed and not to discontinue these medications without consulting the PHCP.
19. Inform the client that medications used to treat glaucoma may cause pain and blurred vision, especially when therapy is begun.
20. Instruct the client to report the development of any eye irritation.
21. Inform the client using eye gel to store the gel at room temperature or in the refrigerator, but not to freeze it.
22. Instruct the client to discard unused eye gel kept at room temperature as recommended by the PHCP and/or the pharmacist.
23. Inform the client that soft contact lenses may absorb certain eye medications and that preservatives in eye medications may discolor the contact lenses.
24. Advise the client wearing contact lenses to question the PHCP carefully about special precautions to observe with eye medications.
25. Inform the parents of infants that atropine sulfate eye drops may contribute to abdominal distention.

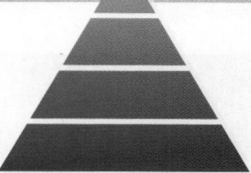

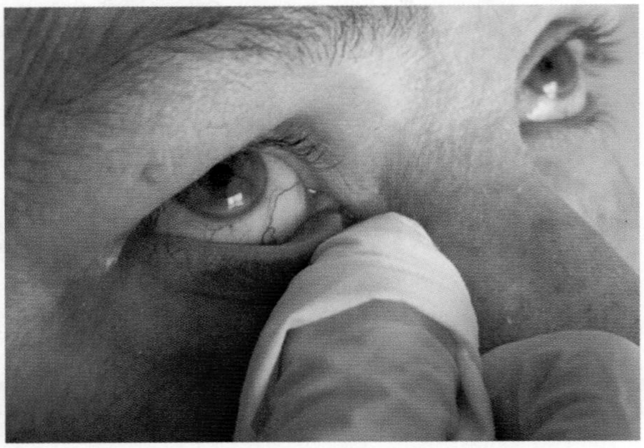

FIG. 57-1 Applying punctual occlusion to prevent systemic absorption of eye drops. (From Ignatavicius, Workman, 2013.)

26. Instruct the parents to keep a record of the infant's bowel movements if atropine sulfate eye drops are being administered.
27. Auscultate bowel sounds of the infant or child receiving atropine sulfate eye drops.

⚠ Because the timing of medication administration is critical, administer eye medications at precise intervals as prescribed; separate the instillation by 3 to 5 minutes if two medications must be administered at the same time.

B. Instillation of eye medications
1. Drops
a. Wash hands.
b. Put gloves on.
c. Check the name, strength, and expiration date of the medication.
d. Instruct the client to tilt the head backward, open the eyes, and look up.
e. Pull the lower lid down against the cheekbone.
f. Hold the bottle like a pencil, with the tip downward.
g. Holding the bottle, gently rest the wrist of the hand on the client's cheek.
h. Squeeze the bottle gently to allow the drop to fall into the conjunctival sac.
i. Instruct the client to close the eyes gently and not to squeeze the eyes shut.
j. Wait 3 to 5 minutes before instilling another drop, if more than one drop is prescribed, to promote maximal absorption of the medication.
k. Do not allow the medication bottle, dropper, or applicator to come into contact with the eyelid or conjunctival sac.
l. To prevent systemic absorption of the medication, apply gentle pressure with a clean tissue to the client's nasolacrimal duct for 30 to 60 seconds (see Fig. 57-1).

2. Ointments
a. Instruct the client to lie down or tilt the head backward and look up.
b. Hold the ointment tube near but not touching, the eye or eyelashes. This action prevents the spread of contaminants from 1 eye to the other.
c. Squeeze a thin ribbon of ointment along the lining of the lower conjunctival sac, from the inner to the outer canthus.
d. Instruct the client to close the eyes gently, rolling the eyeball in all directions (increases contact area of medication to eye).
e. Instruct the client that vision may be blurred by the ointment.
f. If possible, apply ointment just before bedtime.

II. Mydriatic, Cycloplegic, and Anticholinergic Medications (Box 57-1)

A. Description
1. Mydriatics and cycloplegics dilate the pupils (**mydriasis**) and relax the ciliary muscles (**cycloplegia**).
2. Anticholinergics block responses of the sphincter muscle in the ciliary body, producing mydriasis and cycloplegia.
3. These medications are used preoperatively or for eye examinations to produce mydriasis.
4. Mydriatics are contraindicated in glaucoma, cardiac dysrhythmias, and cerebral atherosclerosis and should be used with caution in the older client and in clients with prostatic hypertrophy, diabetes mellitus, or parkinsonism.

B. Side and adverse effects
1. Tachycardia
2. Photophobia
3. Conjunctivitis
4. Dermatitis
5. Elevated blood pressure

C. Atropine toxicity
1. Dry mouth
2. Blurred vision
3. Photophobia
4. Tachycardia

BOX 57-1 Mydriatic, Cycloplegic, and Anticholinergic Medications

- Atropine
- Cyclopentolate
- Homatropine
- Phenylephrine
- Scopolamine
- Tropicamide

5. Fever
6. Urinary retention
7. Constipation
8. Headache, brow pain
9. Worsening of **glaucoma**
10. Confusion
11. Hallucinations, delirium
12. Coma

D. Systemic reactions to anticholinergics
1. Dry mouth and skin
2. Fever
3. Thirst
4. Hyperactivity
5. Confusion

E. Interventions
1. Monitor for allergic response.
2. Assess for risk of injury.
3. Assess for constipation and urinary retention.
4. Instruct the client that a burning sensation may occur on instillation.
5. Instruct the client not to drive or perform hazardous activities for 24 hours after instillation of the medication unless otherwise directed by the PHCP.
6. Instruct the client to wear sunglasses until the effects of the medication wear off.
7. Instruct the client to notify the PHCP if blurring of vision, loss of sight, difficulty breathing, sweating, or flushing occurs.
8. Instruct the client to report eye pain to the PHCP.

⚠ Mydriatics are contraindicated in clients with glaucoma because of the risk of increased intraocular pressure.

III. Anti-infective Eye Medications (Box 57-2)

A. Description: Anti-infective medications kill or inhibit the growth of bacteria, fungi, and viruses.

B. Side and adverse effects
1. Superinfection
2. Global irritation

C. Interventions
1. Assess for risk of injury.
2. Instruct the client how to apply the eye medication; remind the client to clean exudates from the eyes before administering the medication.
3. Reinforce the importance of completing the prescribed medication regimen.
4. Instruct the client to wash the hands thoroughly and frequently.
5. Advise the client to notify the PHCP if improvement does not occur.

BOX 57-2 Anti-infective Eye Medications

Antibacterial
- Chloramphenicol
- Erythromycin
- Bacitracin

Aminoglycosides
- Gentamicin sulfate
- Tobramycin

Antifungal
- Natamycin

Antiviral
- Ganciclovir
- Trifluridine

Sulfonamide
- Sulfacetamide

IV. Antiinflammatory Eye Medications (Box 57-3)

A. Description
1. Antiinflammatory medications control inflammation, thereby reducing vision loss and scarring.
2. Antiinflammatory medications are used for uveitis, allergic conditions, and inflammation of the conjunctiva, cornea, and lids.

B. Side and adverse effects
1. **Cataracts**
2. Increased intraocular pressure
3. Impaired healing
4. Masking signs and symptoms of infection

BOX 57-3 Antiinflammatory Eye Medications

Corticosteroids
- Dexamethasone
- Difluprednate
- Fluocinolone
- Fluorometholone; sulfacetamide
- Loteprednol etabonate
- Prednisolone, gentamicin
- Rimexolone

Ophthalmic Immunosuppressant and Antiinflammatory Agent
- Cyclosporine

Nonsteroidal Antiinflammatory Agents
- Bromfenac
- Diclofenac
- Flurbiprofen sodium
- Ketorolac tromethamine
- Nepafenac

Mast Cell Stabilizers
- Azelastine hydrochloride
- Cromolyn sodium
- Epinastine
- Ketotifen fumarate
- Nedocromil sodium
- Olopatadine hydrochloride

C. Interventions
1. Interventions are the same as for anti-infective medications.
2. Note that dexamethasone should not be used for eye abrasions and wounds.

V. Topical Eye Anesthetics

A. Description
1. Topical anesthetics produce corneal anesthesia.
2. Topical anesthetics are used for anesthesia for eye examinations and surgery or to remove foreign bodies from the eye.
3. Do not use the solution if it is discolored, and store the bottle tightly closed.
4. An example is tetracaine.

B. Side and adverse effects
1. Temporary stinging or burning of the eye
2. Temporary loss of corneal reflex

C. Interventions
1. Assess for risk of injury.
2. Note that the medications should not be given to the client for home use and are not to be self-administered by the client.
3. Instruct the client not to rub or touch the eye while it is anesthetized.
4. Note that the blink reflex is lost temporarily and that the corneal epithelium needs to be protected.
5. Provide an eye patch to protect the eye from injury until the corneal reflex returns.

VI. Eye Lubricants (Box 57-4)

A. Description
1. Eye lubricants replace tears or add moisture to the eyes.
2. Eye lubricants moisten contact lenses or an artificial eye and protect the eyes during surgery or diagnostic procedures.
3. Eye lubricants are used for keratitis, during anesthesia, or for a client who is unconscious or has decreased blinking.

B. Side and adverse effects
1. Burning on instillation
2. Discomfort or pain on instillation
3. Allergic reaction

C. Interventions
1. Inform the client that burning may occur on instillation.
2. Be alert to allergic responses to the preservatives in the lubricants.

BOX 57-4 Eye Lubricants

- Carboxymethylcellulose
- Hydroxypropyl methylcellulose
- Petroleum-based ointment
- Polyvinyl alcohol

VII. Medications to Treat Glaucoma (Box 57-5)

A. Description
1. These medications reduce intraocular pressure by constricting the pupil and contracting the ciliary muscle, thereby increasing the blood flow to the retina and decreasing retinal damage and loss of vision.
2. These medications open the anterior chamber angle and increase the outflow of aqueous humor.
3. Some may be used to achieve **miosis** during eye surgery.
4. Contraindicated in clients with retinal detachment, adhesions between the iris and lens, or inflammatory diseases.
5. Use with caution in clients with asthma, hypertension, corneal abrasion, hyperthyroidism, coronary vascular disease, urinary tract obstruction, gastrointestinal obstruction, ulcer disease, parkinsonism, and bradycardia.

B. Side effects
1. **Myopia**
2. Headache
3. Eye pain
4. Decreased vision in poor light
5. Local irritation

C. Adverse effects
1. Flushing
2. Diaphoresis
3. Gastrointestinal upset and diarrhea
4. Frequent urination
5. Increased salivation
6. Muscle weakness
7. Respiratory difficulty

D. Toxicity
1. Vertigo and syncope
2. Bradycardia or other dysrhythmias
3. Hypotension

BOX 57-5 Medications to Treat Glaucoma

Miotics
- Echothiophate
- Carbachol
- Pilocarpine hydrochloride

β-Adrenergic Blocking Eye Medications
- Betaxolol hydrochloride
- Carteolol hydrochloride
- Levobunolol hydrochloride
- Metipranolol
- Timolol maleate

α-Adrenergic Agonists
- Apraclonidine
- Brimonidine

Prostaglandin Analogs
- Latanoprost
- Tafluprost
- Travoprost
- Bimatoprost

Cholinergic Agonists
- Carbachol
- Pilocarpine hydrochloride
- Echothiophate iodide

Carbonic Anhydrase Inhibitors
- Dorzolamide
- Brinzolamide

4. Tremors
5. Seizures

E. Interventions
1. Assess vital signs.
2. Assess for risk of injury.
3. Assess the client for the degree of diminished vision.
4. Monitor for side and adverse effects and toxic effects.
5. Monitor for postural hypotension, and instruct the client to change positions slowly.
6. Assess breath sounds for wheezes and rhonchi, because some medications can cause bronchospasms and increased bronchial secretions.
7. Maintain oral hygiene because of the increase in salivation.
8. Have atropine sulfate available as an antidote for pilocarpine.
9. Instruct the client or family regarding the correct administration of eye medications.
10. Instruct the client not to stop the medication suddenly.
11. Instruct the client to avoid activities such as driving while vision is impaired.

Instruct the client with glaucoma to read labels on over-the-counter medications and to avoid atropine-like medications, because atropine will increase intraocular pressure.

VIII. β-Adrenergic Blocker Eye Medications (see Box 57-5)

A. Description
1. These medications reduce intraocular pressure by decreasing sympathetic impulses and decreasing aqueous humor production without affecting **accommodation** or pupil size.
2. These medications are used to treat glaucoma.
3. These medications are contraindicated in the client with asthma or chronic obstructive pulmonary disease, because systemic absorption can cause increased airway resistance.
4. Use these medications with caution in the client receiving oral beta blockers.

B. Side and adverse effects
1. Ocular irritation
2. Visual disturbances
3. Bradycardia
4. Hypotension
5. Bronchospasm

C. Interventions
1. Monitor vital signs, especially blood pressure and pulse, before administering medication.
2. Usually if the pulse is 60 beats per minute or less or if the systolic blood pressure is less than 90 mm Hg, the medication is withheld and the PHCP is contacted. The nurse should obtain pulse parameters from the PHCP for clients receiving ophthalmic beta blockers.
3. Monitor for shortness of breath.
4. Assess for risk of injury.
5. Monitor intake and output.
6. Instruct the client to notify the PHCP if shortness of breath occurs.
7. Instruct the client not to discontinue the medication abruptly.
8. Instruct the client to change positions slowly because of the potential for orthostatic hypotension.
9. Instruct the client to avoid hazardous activities.
10. Instruct the client to avoid over-the-counter medications without the PHCP's approval.
11. Instruct clients with diabetes mellitus using β-adrenergic blockers to monitor blood glucose levels frequently.

IX. Carbonic Anhydrase Inhibitors (see Box 57-5)

A. Description
1. Carbonic anhydrase inhibitors interfere with the production of carbonic acid, which leads to decreased aqueous humor formation and decreased intraocular pressure.
2. These medications are used for the long-term treatment of glaucoma.
3. These medications are contraindicated in the client allergic to sulfonamides.
4. Use with caution for clients with severe renal or liver disease.

B. Side and adverse effects
1. Appetite loss
2. Gastrointestinal upset
3. Paresthesias in the fingers, toes, and face
4. Polyuria
5. Hypokalemia
6. Renal calculi
7. Photosensitivity
8. Lethargy and drowsiness
9. Depression

C. Interventions
1. Monitor vital signs.
2. Assess visual acuity.
3. Assess for risk of injury.
4. Monitor intake and output.
5. Monitor weight.
6. Maintain oral hygiene.
7. Monitor for side effects such as lethargy, anorexia, drowsiness, polyuria, nausea, and vomiting.
8. Monitor electrolyte levels for hypokalemia.
9. Increase fluid intake unless contraindicated.
10. Advise the client to avoid prolonged exposure to sunlight.
11. Encourage the use of artificial tears for dry eyes.
12. Instruct the client not to discontinue the medication abruptly.

13. Instruct the client to avoid hazardous activities while vision is impaired.
14. Teach the client not to wear contact lenses during or within 15 minutes of instilling these medications.

X. Ocusert System

A. Description
1. A thin eye wafer (disk) is impregnated with a time-release dose of pilocarpine.
2. The Ocusert system was devised to overcome the need for frequent instillation of pilocarpine.
3. It is placed in the upper or lower cul-de-sac of the eye.
4. The pilocarpine is released over 1 week.
5. The disk is replaced every 7 days.
6. Drawbacks of its use include sudden leakage of pilocarpine, migration of the system over the cornea, and unnoticed loss of the system.

B. Interventions
1. Assess the client's ability to insert the medication disk.
2. Store the medication in the refrigerator.
3. Instruct the client to discard damaged or contaminated disks.
4. Inform the client that temporary stinging is expected but to notify the PHCP if blurred vision or brow pain occurs.
5. Instruct the client to check for the presence of the disk in the upper or lower cul-de-sac daily at bedtime and on arising.
6. Because vision may change in the first few hours after the eye system is inserted, instruct the client to replace the disk at bedtime.

XI. Osmotic Medications

A. Description
1. Osmotic medications lower intraocular pressure; an example is mannitol.
2. They are used in emergency treatment of glaucoma and are used preoperatively and postoperatively to decrease vitreous humor volume.

B. Side and adverse effects
1. Headache
2. Nausea, vomiting, diarrhea, dehydration
3. Disorientation
4. Electrolyte imbalances

C. Interventions
1. Assess vital signs.
2. Assess visual acuity.
3. Assess for risk of injury.
4. Monitor intake and output.
5. Monitor weight.
6. Monitor for electrolyte imbalances.
7. Increase fluid intake unless contraindicated.
8. Monitor for changes in level of orientation.

XII. Medications to Treat Macular Degeneration

A. Pegaptanib, ranibizumab, bevacizumab, aflibercept, verteporfin

B. Description
1. Age-related **macular degeneration** (ARMD) can be dry ARMD (atrophic) or wet ARMD (neovascular).
2. Dry ARMD is more common; macular photoreceptors undergo gradual breakdown, leading to gradual blurring of central vision.
3. Wet ARMD progresses faster, and macular degeneration is caused by the growth of new subretinal blood vessels, which leads to fluid leakage that lifts the macula and causes permanent injury.
4. Characterized by the presence of drusen (yellow deposits under the retina).

C. Side and adverse effects
1. Endophthalmitis (eye inflammation caused by bacterial, viral, or fungal infection)
2. Blurred vision
3. Cataracts
4. Corneal edema
5. Eye discomfort and discharge
6. Conjunctival hemorrhage
7. Increased intraocular pressure
8. Reduced visual acuity

D. Interventions
1. Teach the client about administration of the medications.
2. Teach the client about the side effects and the need to notify the PHCP.

XIII. Otic Medication Administration

A. Instillation of ear drops
1. In an adult, pull the pinna up and back to straighten the external canal to instill ear drops.
2. Tilt the client's head in the opposite direction of the affected ear and apply the drops into the ear.
3. With the head tilted, gently move the head back and forth 5 times.
4. Pull the pinna down and back for infants and children younger than 3 years, up and back for older children.

B. Irrigation of the ear (Fig. 57-2)
1. Irrigation of the ear needs to be prescribed by the PHCP.
2. Ensure direct visualization of the tympanic membrane.
3. Warm the irrigating solution to 98.6° F (37.0° C), because a solution temperature that is not close to the client's body temperature will cause ear injury, nausea, vertigo, and nystagmus.
4. Irrigation must be done gently to avoid damage to the eardrum.
5. When irrigating, to prevent injury, do not direct irrigation solution directly toward the eardrum

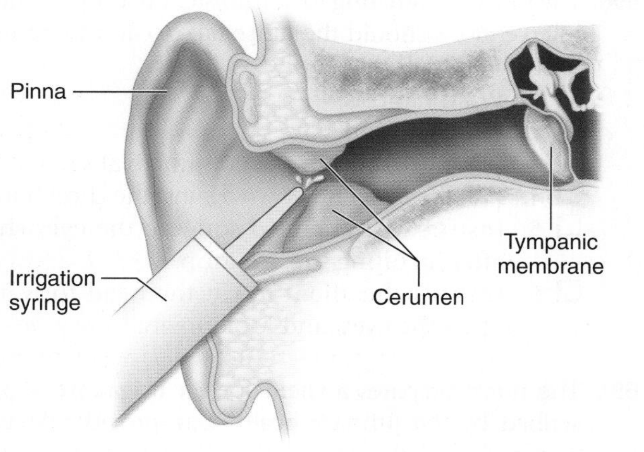

FIG. 57-2 Irrigation of the external canal. Cerumen and debris can be removed from the ear by irrigation with warm water. The stream of water is aimed above or below the impaction to allow back pressure to push it out rather than further down the canal.

but rather toward the wall of the ear canal. In addition, to remove cerumen, the solution is directed above or below the impaction toward the wall of the canal to allow back pressure to push the impaction out.

6. During irrigation, the client should be positioned with the ear to be irrigated facing up. Fall precautions should be instituted, because the client may get dizzy, and an emesis basin should be available, because vomiting can occur.

C. Systemic medications that affect hearing (Box 57-6)

If a perforation of the eardrum is suspected, do not perform ear irrigation.

BOX 57-6 Medications That Affect Hearing

Antibiotics
- Amikacin
- Chloramphenicol
- Erythromycin
- Gentamicin
- Neomycin
- Streptomycin sulfate
- Tetracycline
- Tobramycin sulfate
- Vancomycin

Diuretics
- Ethacrynic acid
- Furosemide

Others
- Cisplatin
- Bleomycin
- Chloroquine
- Nitrogen mustard
- Quinine
- Quinidine
- Sildenafil
- Aspirin
- Ibuprofen
- Naproxen

XIV. Anti-infective Ear Medications (Box 57-7)

A. Description
1. Anti-infective medications kill or inhibit the growth of bacteria and are used for otitis media or otitis externa.
2. These medications are contraindicated if a prior hypersensitivity exists.

B. Side and adverse effect: Overgrowth of nonsusceptible organisms

C. Interventions
1. Monitor vital signs.
2. Assess for allergies.
3. Assess for pain.
4. Monitor for signs of secondary infection.
5. Instruct the client to report dizziness, fatigue, fever, or sore throat, which may indicate a superimposed infection.
6. Instruct the client to complete the entire course of the medication.
7. Instruct the client to keep ear canals dry.

XV. Antihistamines and Decongestants (Box 57-8)

A. Description
1. These medications produce vasoconstriction.
2. These medications stimulate the receptors of the respiratory mucosa.
3. These medications reduce respiratory tissue hyperemia and edema to open obstructed eustachian tubes.
4. These medications are used for acute otitis media.

BOX 57-7 Anti-infective Ear Medications

- Acetic acid; aluminum acetate
- Amoxicillin
- Ampicillin
- Cefaclor
- Chloramphenicol
- Ciprofloxacin
- Clarithromycin
- Clindamycin hydrochloride
- Erythromycin
- Gentamicin sulfate otic solution
- Ofloxacin
- Penicillin V potassium
- Trimethoprim; sulfamethoxazole

BOX 57-8 Antihistamines and Decongestants

- Loratadine
- Cetirizine
- Diphenhydramine
- Fexofenadine
- Levocetirizine
- Phenylephrine
- Pseudoephedrine

B. Side and adverse effects
  1. Drowsiness
  2. Blurred vision
  3. Dry mucous membranes

C. Interventions
  1. Inform the client that drowsiness, blurred vision, and a dry mouth may occur.
  2. Instruct the client to increase fluid intake unless contraindicated and to suck on hard candy to alleviate the dry mouth.
  3. Instruct the client to avoid hazardous activities if drowsiness occurs.
  4. Instruct the client with hypertension to consult the PHCP prior to the use of these medications.

XVI. Ceruminolytic Medication

A. Carbamide peroxide

B. Description
  1. Emulsifies and loosens cerumen deposits
  2. Used to loosen and remove impacted wax from the ear canal

C. Side and adverse effects
  1. Irritation
  2. Redness or swelling of the ear canal

D. Interventions
  1. Instruct the client not to use drops more often than prescribed.
  2. Moisten a cotton plug with medication and insert the cotton plug after instilling the ear drops.
  3. Keep the container tightly closed and away from moisture.
  4. Avoid touching the ear with the dropper.
  5. Thirty minutes after instillation, gently irrigate the ear as prescribed with warm water, using a soft rubber bulb ear syringe.
  6. Irrigation may be done with hydrogen peroxide solution as prescribed to flush cerumen deposits out of the ear canal.
  7. For a chronic cerumen impaction, 1 or 2 drops of mineral oil (if prescribed) will soften the wax.
  8. Instruct the client to notify the PHCP if redness, pain, or swelling persists.

PRACTICE QUESTIONS

695. Betaxolol hydrochloride eye drops have been prescribed for a client with glaucoma. Which nursing action is **most appropriate** related to monitoring for side and adverse effects of this medication?
1. Assessing for edema
2. Monitoring temperature
3. Monitoring blood pressure
4. Assessing blood glucose level

696. The nurse is preparing to administer eye drops. Which interventions should the nurse take to administer the drops? **Select all that apply.**
- ☐ 1. Wash hands.
- ☐ 2. Put gloves on.
- ☐ 3. Place the drop in the conjunctival sac.
- ☐ 4. Pull the lower lid down against the cheekbone.
- ☐ 5. Instruct the client to squeeze the eyes shut after instilling the eye drop.
- ☐ 6. Instruct the client to tilt the head forward, open the eyes, and look down.

697. The nurse prepares a client for ear irrigation as prescribed by the primary health care provider. Which action should the nurse take when performing the procedure?
1. Warm the irrigating solution to 98.6° F (37.0° C).
2. Position the client with the affected side up following the irrigation.
3. Direct a slow, steady stream of irrigation solution toward the eardrum.
4. Assist the client to turn her or his head so that the ear to be irrigated is facing upward.

698. The nurse is providing instructions to a client who will be self-administering eye drops. To minimize systemic absorption of the eye drops, the nurse should instruct the client to take which action?
1. Eat before instilling the drops.
2. Swallow several times after instilling the drops.
3. Blink vigorously to encourage tearing after instilling the drops.
4. Occlude the nasolacrimal duct with a finger after instilling the drops.

699. A client is prescribed an eye drop and an eye ointment for the right eye. How should the nurse **best** administer the medications?
1. Administer the eye drop first, followed by the eye ointment.
2. Administer the eye ointment first, followed by the eye drop.
3. Administer the eye drop, wait 15 minutes, and administer the eye ointment.
4. Administer the eye ointment, wait 15 minutes, and administer the eye drop.

700. Which medication, if prescribed for the client with glaucoma, should the nurse question?
1. Betaxolol
2. Pilocarpine
3. Erythromycin
4. Atropine sulfate

701. A miotic medication has been prescribed for the client with glaucoma, and the client asks the nurse about the purpose of the medication. Which response should the nurse provide to the client?
1. "The medication will help dilate the eye to prevent pressure from occurring."
2. "The medication will relax the muscles of the eyes and prevent blurred vision."
3. "The medication causes the pupil to constrict and will lower the pressure in the eye."
4. "The medication will help block the responses that are sent to the muscles in the eye."

702. A client was just admitted to the hospital to rule out a gastrointestinal (GI) bleed. The client has brought several bottles of medications prescribed by different specialists. During the admission assessment, the client states, "Lately, I have been hearing some roaring sounds in my ears, especially when I am alone." Which medication would the nurse identify as the cause of the client's complaint?
1. Doxycycline
2. Atropine sulfate
3. Acetylsalicylic acid
4. Diltiazem hydrochloride

703. In preparation for cataract surgery, the nurse is to administer cyclopentolate eye drops at 9:00 a.m. for surgery that is scheduled for 9:15 a.m. What **initial** action should the nurse take in relation to the characteristics of the medication action?
1. Provide lubrication to the operative eye prior to giving the eye drops.
2. Call the surgeon, as this medication will further constrict the operative pupil.
3. Consult the surgeon, as there is not sufficient time for the dilative effects to occur.
4. Give the medication as prescribed; the surgeon needs optimal constriction of the pupil.

ANSWERS

695. ***Answer:*** 3

Rationale: Hypotension, dizziness, nausea, diaphoresis, headache, fatigue, constipation, and diarrhea are side and adverse effects of the medication. Nursing interventions include monitoring the blood pressure for hypotension and assessing the pulse for strength, weakness, irregular rate, and bradycardia. Options 1, 2, and 4 are not specifically associated with this medication.

Test-Taking Strategy: Note the strategic words, *most appropriate*. Use the ABCs—airway, breathing, and circulation—to direct you to the correct option.

Level of Cognitive Ability: Analyzing

Client Needs: Physiological Integrity

Integrated Process: Nursing Process—Implementation

Content Area: Pharmacology: Eye and Ear: Glaucoma Medications

Health Problem: Adult Health: Eye: Glaucoma

Priority Concepts: Safety; Sensory Perception

Reference: Lewis et al. (2017), p. 381.

696. ***Answer:*** 1, 2, 3, 4

Rationale: To administer eye medications, the nurse should wash hands and put gloves on. The client is instructed to tilt the head backward, open the eyes, and look up. The nurse pulls the lower lid down against the cheekbone and holds the bottle like a pencil with the tip downward. Holding the bottle, the nurse gently rests the wrist of the hand on the client's cheek and squeezes the bottle gently to allow the drop to fall into the conjunctival sac. The client is instructed to close the eyes gently and not to squeeze the eyes shut to prevent the loss of medication.

Test-Taking Strategy: Focus on the subject, the procedure for administering eye drops. Use guidelines related to standard precautions and visualize this procedure. This will assist in determining the correct interventions.

Level of Cognitive Ability: Applying

Client Needs: Physiological Integrity

Integrated Process: Nursing Process—Implementation

Content Area: Skills: Medication Administration

Health Problem: N/A

Priority Concepts: Clinical Judgment; Safety

Reference: Ignatavicius, Workman, Rebar (2018), p. 966.

697. ***Answer:*** 1

Rationale: Before ear irrigation, the nurse should inspect the tympanic membrane to ensure that it is intact. The irrigating solution should be warmed to 98.6° F (37.0° C), because a solution temperature that is not close to the client's body temperature will cause ear injury, nausea, and vertigo. The nurse should check the temperature of the solution on the inner forearm. The affected side should be down following the irrigation to assist in drainage of the fluid. When irrigating, a direct and slow steady stream of irrigation solution is directed toward the wall of the canal, not toward the eardrum. The client is positioned sitting, facing forward with the head in a natural position; if the ear is faced upward, the nurse would not be able to visualize the canal.

Test-Taking Strategy: Focus on the subject, the procedure for performing ear irrigation. Think about the purpose of this procedure and keep safety in mind. Visualizing each step and the information in the options will assist in eliminating the incorrect ones.

Level of Cognitive Ability: Applying

Client Needs: Physiological Integrity

Integrated Process: Nursing Process—Implementation

Content Area: Foundations of Care: Safety

Health Problem: N/A

Priority Concepts: Safety; Sensory Perception

Reference: Perry et al. (2018), p. 494.

698. ***Answer:*** 4

Rationale: Applying pressure on the nasolacrimal duct prevents systemic absorption of the medication. Options 1, 2, and 3 will not prevent systemic absorption.

Test-Taking Strategy: Focus on the subject, systemic effects. Eating and swallowing are comparable or alike and are not related to the systemic absorption of eye drops. Blinking vigorously to produce tearing may result in the loss of the administered medication.
Level of Cognitive Ability: Applying
Client Needs: Physiological Integrity
Integrated Process: Teaching and Learning
Content Area: Foundations of Care: Client Teaching
Health Problem: N/A
Priority Concepts: Client Education; Safety
Reference: Lilley et al. (2017), p. 130.

699. *Answer:* 1
Rationale: When an eye drop and an eye ointment are scheduled to be administered at the same time, the eye drop is administered first. The instillation of two medications is separated by 3 to 5 minutes.
Test-Taking Strategy: Note the strategic word, *best.* Focus on the subject, the guidelines for administering eye medications. Eliminate options 3 and 4 first because of the words *15 minutes*. Next, thinking about the consistency and absorption of a drop versus ointment will direct you to the correct option.
Level of Cognitive Ability: Applying
Client Needs: Physiological Integrity
Integrated Process: Nursing Process—Implementation
Content Area: Skills: Medication Administration
Health Problem: N/A
Priority Concepts: Clinical Judgment; Safety
Reference: Potter et al. (2017), p. 631.

700. *Answer:* 4
Rationale: Options 1 and 2 are miotic agents used to treat glaucoma. Option 3 is an anti-infective medication used to treat bacterial conjunctivitis. Atropine sulfate is a mydriatic and cycloplegic (also anticholinergic) medication, and its use is contraindicated in clients with glaucoma. Mydriatic medications dilate the pupil and can cause an increase in intraocular pressure in the eye.
Test-Taking Strategy: Focus on the subject, the medication that the nurse should question. Recalling the classifications of the medications identified in the options will assist in answering the question. Remember that mydriatics dilate the pupil and that these medications are contraindicated in glaucoma.
Level of Cognitive Ability: Analyzing
Client Needs: Physiological Integrity
Integrated Process: Nursing Process—Analysis
Content Area: Pharmacology: Eye and Ear: Glaucoma Medications
Health Problem: Adult Health: Eye: Glaucoma
Priority Concepts: Collaboration; Safety
Reference: Burchum, Rosenthal (2016), pp. 120, 1272-1273

701. *Answer:* 3
Rationale: Miotics cause pupillary constriction and are used to treat glaucoma. They lower the intraocular pressure, thereby increasing blood flow to the retina and decreasing retinal damage and loss of vision. Miotics cause a contraction of the ciliary muscle and a widening of the trabecular meshwork. Options 1, 2, and 4 are incorrect.
Test-Taking Strategy: Note that the client has glaucoma. Recall that prevention of increased intraocular pressure is the goal in the client with glaucoma. Options 1, 2, and 4 are comparable or alike and describe actions related to mydriatic medications, which primarily dilate the pupils and relax the ciliary muscles.
Level of Cognitive Ability: Applying
Client Needs: Physiological Integrity
Integrated Process: Nursing Process—Implementation
Content Area: Pharmacology: Eye and Ear: Glaucoma Medications
Health Problem: Adult Health: Eye: Glaucoma
Priority Concepts: Client Education; Safety
Reference: Ignatavicius, Workman, Rebar (2018), p. 976.

702. *Answer:* 3
Rationale: Aspirin (acetylsalicylic acid) is contraindicated for GI bleeding and is potentially ototoxic. The client should be advised to notify the prescribing primary health care provider so the medication can be discontinued and/or a substitute that is less toxic to the ear can be taken instead. Options 1, 2, and 4 do not have effects that are potentially associated with hearing difficulties.
Test-Taking Strategy: Focus on the subject, the medication that may be causing the client's complaint. Review the classifications and/or therapeutic effects as well as the side and adverse effects of each medication in the options. Of the medications identified, only aspirin can cause ototoxicity. In addition, it is contraindicated for GI bleed.
Level of Cognitive Ability: Analyzing
Client Needs: Physiological Integrity
Integrated Process: Nursing Process—Analysis
Content Area: Pharmacology: Pain: Nonopioid Analgesics
Health Problem: Adult Health: Ear: Vertigo/tinnitus
Priority Concepts: Safety; Sensory Perception
Reference: Hodgson, Kizior (2018), pp. 87-89.

703. *Answer:* 3
Rationale: Cyclopentolate is a rapidly acting mydriatic and cycloplegic medication. Cyclopentolate is effective in 25 to 75 minutes, and accommodation returns in 6 to 24 hours. Cyclopentolate is used for preoperative mydriasis, not pupil constriction. The nurse should consult with the surgeon about the time of administration of the eye drops, because 15 minutes is not adequate time for dilation to occur.
Test-Taking Strategy: Note the strategic word, *initial.* Options 2 and 4 are comparable or alike and are eliminated first (*miosis* refers to a constricted pupil). Note that the question identifies a client being prepared for eye surgery. The pupil would need to be dilated for the surgical procedure.
Level of Cognitive Ability: Analyzing
Client Needs: Physiological Integrity
Integrated Process: Nursing Process—Implementation
Content Area: Pharmacology: Eye and Ear Medications: Mydriatic, Cycloplegic, Anticholinergics
Health Problem: Adult Health: Eye: Cataracts
Priority Concepts: Clinical Judgment; Safety
Reference: Lilley et al. (2017), p. 916.

UNIT XV

Neurological Problems of the Adult Client

Pyramid to Success

Pyramid Points related to neurological disorders focus on nursing care and monitoring for increased intracranial pressure, assessing level of consciousness, positioning clients, head injuries, spinal cord injuries, spinal shock, autonomic dysreflexia, interventions during a seizure, stroke, Parkinson's disease, myasthenia gravis, and the edrophonium test. Focus on the points related to the psychosocial effects as a result of the neurological disorder, such as anxiety, unexpected body image changes, and the appropriate and available support services needed for the client.

Client Needs: Learning Objectives

Safe and Effective Care Environment

Acting as a client advocate
Collaborating with the interprofessional health care team
Ensuring that advance directives are in the client's medical record
Ensuring that informed consent for invasive procedures has been obtained
Establishing priorities
Initiating referrals to appropriate services
Maintaining asepsis with procedures and treatments
Maintaining confidentiality
Maintaining standard, transmission-based, and other precautions
Preventing accidents that can occur as a result of neurological deficits
Upholding client rights

Health Promotion and Maintenance

Discussing expected and unexpected body image changes resulting from neurological deficits
Performing neurological assessment using various techniques
Preventing and detecting health problems associated with neurological deficits
Providing home care instructions regarding care related to the neurological disorder
Teaching about the importance of prescribed therapy

Psychosocial Integrity

Addressing grief and loss issues
Assessing the ability to cope with feelings of isolation and loss of independence
Considering the cultural, religious, and spiritual influences of the client when planning care
Identifying sensory and perceptual alterations
Identifying support systems and encouraging the use of community resources
Mobilizing coping mechanisms

Physiological Integrity

Administering pharmacological therapy
Maintaining nutrition
Monitoring for alterations in body systems
Monitoring for complications related to procedures
Monitoring for fluid and electrolyte imbalances
Promoting normal elimination patterns
Promoting self-care measures
Providing assistive devices for mobility
Providing emergency care
Providing measures to promote comfort

CHAPTER 58

Neurological Problems

PRIORITY CONCEPTS Functional Ability; Intracranial Regulation

I. Anatomy and Physiology of the Brain and Spinal Cord

A. Cerebrum
1. The cerebrum consists of the right and left hemispheres.
2. Each hemisphere receives sensory information from the opposite side of the body and controls the skeletal muscles of the opposite side.
3. The cerebrum governs sensory and motor activity and thought and learning.

B. Cerebral cortex (Box 58-1)
1. The cerebral cortex is the outer gray layer; it is divided into 5 lobes.
2. It is responsible for the conscious activities of the cerebrum.

C. Basal ganglia: Cell bodies in white matter that help the cerebral cortex produce smooth voluntary movements

D. Diencephalon
1. Thalamus
   a. Relays sensory impulses to the cortex
   b. Provides a pain gate
   c. Part of the reticular activating system
2. Hypothalamus
   a. Regulates autonomic responses of the sympathetic and parasympathetic nervous systems
   b. Regulates the stress response, sleep, appetite, body temperature, fluid balance, and emotions
   c. Responsible for the production of hormones secreted by the pituitary gland and the hypothalamus

E. Brainstem
1. Midbrain
   a. Responsible for motor coordination
   b. Contains the visual reflex and auditory relay centers
2. Pons: Contains the respiratory centers and regulates breathing
3. Medulla oblongata
   a. Contains all afferent and efferent tracts and cardiac, respiratory, vomiting, and vasomotor centers
   b. Controls heart rate, respiration, blood vessel diameter, sneezing, swallowing, vomiting, and coughing

F. Cerebellum: Coordinates muscle movement, posture, equilibrium, and muscle tone

G. Spinal cord
1. Provides neuron and synapse networks to produce involuntary responses to sensory stimulation
2. Controls body movement and regulates visceral function
3. Carries sensory information to and motor information from the brain
4. Extends from the first cervical to the second lumbar vertebra
5. Protected by the meninges, cerebrospinal fluid (CSF), and adipose tissue
6. Horns
   a. Inner column of gray matter; contains 2 anterior and 2 posterior horns
   b. Posterior horns connect with afferent (sensory) nerve fibers.
   c. Anterior horns contain efferent (motor) nerve fibers.
7. Nerve tracts
   a. White matter contains the nerve tracts.
   b. Ascending tracts (sensory pathway)
   c. Descending tracts (motor pathway)

H. Meninges
1. The dura mater is a tough and fibrous membrane.
2. The arachnoid membrane is a delicate membrane and contains CSF.
3. The pia mater is a vascular membrane.
4. The subarachnoid space is formed by the arachnoid membrane and the pia mater.

I. CSF
1. Secreted in the ventricles; circulates in the subarachnoid space and through the ventricles to the subarachnoid space of the meninges, where it is reabsorbed
2. Acts as a protective cushion; aids in the exchange of nutrients and wastes

BOX 58-1 Cerebral Cortex

Frontal Lobe
- Broca's area for production of speech
- Morals, emotions, reasoning and judgment, concentration, and abstraction

Parietal Lobe
- Interpretation of taste, pain, touch, temperature, and pressure
- Spatial perception

Temporal Lobe
- Auditory center
- Wernicke's area for comprehension of speech

Occipital Lobe
- Visual area

Limbic System
- Emotional and visceral patterns for survival
- Learning and memory

3. Normal pressure is 50 to 175 mm H_2O.
4. Normal volume is 125 to 150 mL.

J. Ventricles
1. Four ventricles
2. The ventricles communicate between the subarachnoid spaces and produce and circulate CSF.

K. Blood supply
1. Right and left internal carotid arteries
2. Right and left vertebral arteries
3. These arteries supply the brain via an anastomosis at the base of the brain called the *circle of Willis*.

L. Neurotransmitters
1. Acetylcholine
2. Norepinephrine
3. Dopamine
4. Serotonin
5. Amino acids
6. Polypeptides

M. Neurons
1. The neuron consists of the cell body, axon, and dendrites.
2. The cell body contains the nucleus.
3. Neurons carrying impulses from the peripheral nervous system to the central nervous system (CNS) are called *sensory neurons*.
4. Neurons carrying impulses away from the CNS are called *motor neurons*.
5. Synapse is the chemical transmission of impulses from 1 neuron to another.

N. Axons and dendrites
1. The axon conducts impulses from the cell body.
2. The dendrites receive stimuli from the body and transmit them to the axon.
3. The neurons are protected and insulated by Schwann cells.
4. The Schwann cell sheath is called the *neurolemma*.
5. Neurons do not reproduce after the neonatal period.
6. If an axon or dendrite is damaged, it will die and be replaced slowly only if the neurolemma is intact and the cell body has not died.

O. Spinal nerves
1. There are 31 pairs of spinal nerves.
2. Mixed nerve fibers are formed by the joining of the anterior motor and posterior sensory roots.
3. Posterior roots contain afferent (sensory) nerve fibers.
4. Anterior roots contain efferent (motor) nerve fibers.

P. Autonomic nervous system
1. Sympathetic (adrenergic) fibers dilate pupils, increase heart rate and rhythm, contract blood vessels, and relax smooth muscles of the bronchi.
2. Parasympathetic (cholinergic) fibers produce the opposite effect.

II. Diagnostic Tests

A. Skull and spinal radiography
1. Description
   a. Radiographs of the skull reveal the size and shape of the skull bones, suture separation in infants, fractures or bony defects, erosion, and calcification.
   b. Spinal radiographs identify fractures, dislocation, compression, curvature, erosion, narrowed spinal cord, and degenerative processes.
2. Preprocedure interventions
   a. Provide nursing support for the confused, combative, or ventilator-dependent client.
   b. Maintain immobilization of the neck if a spinal fracture is suspected.
   c. Remove metal items from the client.
   d. If the client has thick and heavy hair, this should be documented because it could affect interpretation of the x-ray film.
3. Postprocedure intervention: Maintain immobilization until results are known.

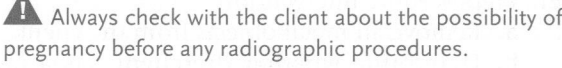

Always check with the client about the possibility of pregnancy before any radiographic procedures.

B. Computed tomography (CT)
1. Description
   a. A type of brain scanning that may or may not require injection of a dye.
   b. It is used to detect intracranial bleeding, space-occupying lesions, cerebral edema, infarctions, hydrocephalus, cerebral atrophy, and shifts of brain structures.

⚠ An informed consent is needed for any invasive procedure, including those that use a contrast medium (dye).

2. Preprocedure interventions
   a. Assess for allergies to iodine, contrast dyes, or shellfish if a dye is used.
   b. Assess renal function and verify contrast dose with the pharmacy.
   c. Instruct the client of the need to lie still and flat during the test.
   d. Instruct the client to hold her or his breath when requested.
   e. Initiate an intravenous line with the appropriate gauge size if prescribed.
   f. Remove objects from the head, such as wigs, barrettes, earrings, and hairpins.
   g. Assess for claustrophobia.
   h. Inform the client of possible mechanical noises as the scanning occurs.
   i. Inform the client that there may be a hot, flushed sensation and a metallic taste in the mouth when the dye is injected.
   j. Note that some clients may be given the dye even if they report an allergy; they may be treated with an antihistamine and corticosteroids before the injection to reduce the severity of a reaction.

⚠ Assess the need to withhold metformin if iodinated contrast dye is used for a diagnostic procedure because of the risk for metformin-induced lactic acidosis.

3. Postprocedure interventions
   a. Provide replacement fluids, because diuresis from the dye is expected.
   b. Monitor for an allergic reaction to the dye.
   c. Assess the dye injection site for bleeding or hematoma, and monitor the extremity for color, warmth, and the presence of distal pulses.

C. Magnetic resonance imaging (MRI)
1. Description
   a. A noninvasive procedure that identifies tissues, tumors, and vascular abnormalities.
   b. It is similar to CT scanning but provides more detailed pictures.
2. Preprocedure interventions
   a. Remove all metal objects from the client.
   b. Determine whether the client has a pacemaker, implanted defibrillator, or other metal implants such as a hip prosthesis or vascular clips, because these clients cannot have this test performed.
   c. Insert an intermittent infusion device (saline lock) to all intravenous accesses prior to the procedure (intravenous fluid pumps are not allowed in the MRI room).
   d. Provide precautions for the client who is attached to a pulse oximeter, because it can cause a burn during testing if coiled around the body or a body part.
   e. Provide an assessment of the client with claustrophobia (may not be necessary if an open MRI machine is used).
   f. Administer medication as prescribed for the client with claustrophobia.
   g. Determine whether a contrast agent is to be used and follow the prescription related to the administration of food, fluids, and medications. Verify allergies and renal function prior to administration.
   h. Instruct the client that she or he will need to remain still during the procedure.

⚠ An MRI is contraindicated in a pregnant woman, because the increase in amniotic fluid temperature that occurs during the procedure may be harmful to the fetus.

3. Postprocedure interventions
   a. The client may resume normal activities.
   b. Increase fluid intake and expect diuresis if a contrast agent is used.

D. Lumbar puncture
1. Description
   a. Insertion of a spinal needle through the L3–L4 interspace into the lumbar subarachnoid space to obtain CSF; measure CSF fluid or pressure; or instill air, dye, or medications
   b. The test is contraindicated in clients with **increased intracranial pressure (ICP)**, because the procedure will cause a rapid decrease in pressure in the CSF around the spinal cord, leading to brain herniation.
2. Preprocedure interventions: Have the client empty the bladder.
3. Interventions during the procedure
   a. Position the client in a lateral recumbent position and have the client draw the knees up to the abdomen and the chin onto the chest; the prone position may be required for radiologically guided punctures.
   b. Assist with the collection of specimens (label the specimens in sequence).
   c. Maintain strict asepsis.
4. Postprocedure interventions
   a. Monitor vital signs and neurological signs to check for the presence of leakage of CSF and also monitor for headache.
   b. Position the client flat as prescribed.
   c. Encourage fluids to replace CSF obtained from the specimen collection or from leakage.
   d. Monitor intake and output.

E. Cerebral angiography
1. Description: Injection of a contrast material usually through the femoral artery (or another artery) into the carotid arteries to visualize the cerebral arteries and assess for lesions
2. Preprocedure interventions
   a. Assess the client for allergies to iodine and shellfish. Assess renal function.
   b. Assess for a medication history of anticoagulation therapy; withhold the anticoagulant medication prior to the procedure as prescribed.
   c. Encourage hydration for 2 days before the test.
   d. Maintain the client on NPO (nothing by mouth) status 4 to 6 hours before the test as prescribed.
   e. Perform a neurological assessment, which will serve as a baseline for postprocedure assessments.
   f. Mark the peripheral pulses.
   g. Remove metal items from the hair.
   h. Administer premedication as prescribed.
3. Postprocedure interventions
   a. Monitor neurological status, vital signs, and neurovascular status of the affected extremity frequently until stable.
   b. Monitor for swelling in the neck and for difficulty swallowing; notify a primary health care provider (PHCP) if these symptoms occur.
   c. Maintain bed rest for 12 hours as prescribed.
   d. Elevate the head of the bed 15 to 30 degrees only if prescribed.
   e. Keep the bed flat, as prescribed, if the femoral artery is used.
   f. Assess peripheral pulses.
   g. Apply sandbags or another device to immobilize the limb and a pressure dressing to the injection site to decrease bleeding as prescribed.
   h. Place ice on the puncture site as prescribed.
   i. Encourage fluid intake.

F. Electroencephalography
1. Description: Graphic recording of the electrical activity of the superficial layers of the cerebral cortex
2. Preprocedure interventions
   a. Wash the client's hair.
   b. Inform the client that electrodes are attached to the head and that electricity does not enter the head.
   c. Withhold stimulants such as coffee, tea, and caffeine beverages; antidepressants; tranquilizers; and possibly antiseizure medications for 24 to 48 hours before the test as prescribed.
   d. Allow the client to have breakfast if prescribed.
   e. Premedicate for sedation as prescribed.
3. Postprocedure interventions
   a. Wash the client's hair.
   b. Maintain safety precautions, if the client was sedated.

G. Caloric testing (oculovestibular reflex)
1. Description: Caloric testing provides information about the function of the vestibular portion of cranial nerve VIII and aids in the diagnosis of cerebellar and brainstem lesions.
2. Procedure
   a. Patency of the external auditory canal is confirmed.
   b. The client is positioned supine with the head of the bed elevated 30 degrees.
   c. Water that is warmer or cooler than body temperature is infused into the ear.
   d. A normal response is the onset of vertigo and nystagmus (involuntary eye movements) within 20 to 30 seconds.
   e. Absent or disconjugate eye movements indicate brainstem damage.

III. Neurological Assessment (see Chapter 12 for additional information on neurological assessment)

A. Assessment of risk factors
1. Trauma
2. Hemorrhage
3. Tumors
4. Infection
5. Toxicity
6. Metabolic disorders
7. Hypoxic conditions
8. Hypertension
9. Cigarette smoking
10. Stress
11. Aging process
12. Chemicals, either ingestion or environmental exposure

B. Assessment of cranial nerves (see Chapter 12)

C. Assessment of level of consciousness (LOC) (see Chapter 12)

! Level of consciousness is the most sensitive indicator of neurological status.

D. Assessment of vital signs: Monitor for blood pressure or pulse changes, which may indicate increased ICP.

E. Assessment of respirations (Box 58-2)

F. Assessment of temperature
1. An elevated temperature increases the metabolic rate of the brain.
2. An elevation in temperature may indicate a dysfunction of the hypothalamus or brainstem.

BOX 58-2 Assessment of Respirations

Cheyne-Stokes
- Rhythmic, with periods of apnea
- Can indicate a metabolic dysfunction or dysfunction in the cerebral hemisphere or basal ganglia

Neurogenic Hyperventilation
- Regular rapid and deep sustained respirations
- Indicates a dysfunction in the low midbrain and middle pons

Apneustic
- Irregular respirations, with pauses at the end of inspiration and expiration
- Indicates a dysfunction in the middle or caudal pons

Ataxic
- Totally irregular in rhythm and depth
- Indicates a dysfunction in the medulla

Cluster
- Clusters of breaths with irregularly spaced pauses
- Indicates a dysfunction in the medulla and pons

3. A slow rise in temperature may indicate infection.

G. Assessment of pupils (Fig. 58-1)
1. Unilateral pupil dilation indicates compression of cranial nerve III.
2. Midposition fixed pupils indicate midbrain injury.
3. Pinpoint fixed pupils indicate pontine damage.

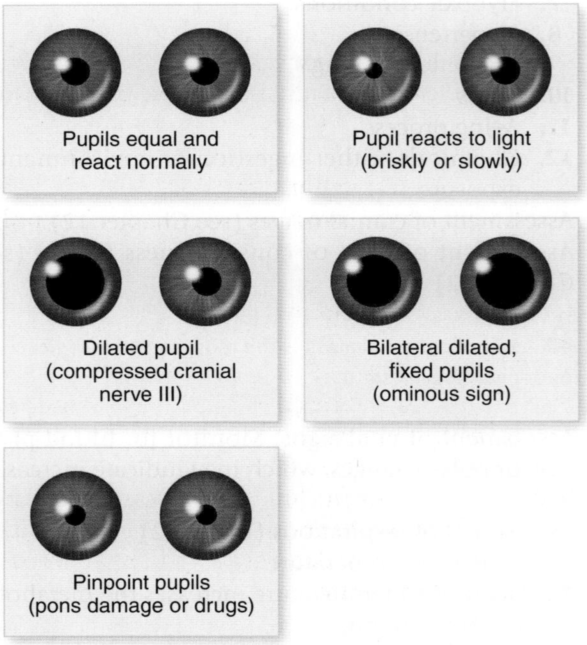

FIG. 58-1 Pupillary check for size and response.

H. Assessment for posturing (see Chapter 38, Fig. 38-3)
1. Posturing indicates a deterioration of the condition.
2. Flexor (**decorticate posturing**)
   a. Client flexes 1 or both arms on the chest and may extend the legs stiffly.
   b. Flexor posturing indicates a nonfunctioning cortex.
3. Extensor (**decerebrate posturing**)
   a. Client stiffly extends 1 or both arms and possibly the legs.
   b. Extensor posturing indicates a brainstem lesion.
4. **Flaccid posturing**: Client displays no motor response in any extremity.

I. Assessment of reflexes (Box 58-3)

J. Assessment of meningeal irritation (Box 58-4)

K. Assessment of the autonomic system
1. Sympathetic functions, adrenergic responses
   a. Increased pulse and blood pressure
   b. Dilated pupils
   c. Decreased peristalsis
   d. Increased perspiration
2. Parasympathetic function, cholinergic responses
   a. Decreased pulse and blood pressure
   b. Constricted pupils
   c. Increased salivation
   d. Increased peristalsis
   e. Dilated blood vessels
   f. Bladder contraction

L. Assessment of sensory function: Touch, pressure, pain

BOX 58-3 Assessment of Reflexes

Babinski's Reflex
- Dorsiflexion of the big toe and fanning of the other toes; elicited by firmly stroking the lateral aspect of the sole of the foot
- Is a pathological or abnormal reflex in anyone older than 2 years and represents the presence of central nervous system (CNS) disease

Corneal (Blink) Reflex
- Involuntary closure of the eyelids in response to stimulation of the cornea
- Loss of the blink reflex indicates a dysfunction of cranial nerve V.

Gag Reflex
- Contraction of pharyngeal muscle, elicited by touching the back of the throat
- Loss of the gag reflex indicates a dysfunction of cranial nerves IX and X.

BOX 58-4 Assessment of Meningeal Irritation

General Findings

- Irritability
- Nuchal rigidity
- Severe, unrelenting headaches
- Generalized muscle aches and pains
- Nausea and vomiting
- Fever and chills
- Tachycardia
- Photophobia
- Nystagmus
- Abnormal pupil reaction and eye movement

Brudzinski's Sign

- Involuntary flexion of the hip and knee when the neck is passively flexed; indicates meningeal irritation

Kernig's Sign

- Loss of the ability of a supine client to straighten the leg completely when it is fully flexed at the knee and hip; indicates meningeal irritation

Motor Response

- Hemiparesis, hemiplegia, and decreased muscle tone
- Cranial nerve dysfunction, especially cranial nerves III, IV, VI, VII, and VIII

Memory Changes

- Short attention span
- Personality and behavioral changes
- Bewilderment

BOX 58-5 Glasgow Coma Scale

Score

- The lowest possible score is 3 points (deep coma or death).
- The highest possible score is 15 points (fully awake).

Motor Response Points

- Obeys a simple response = 6
- Localizes painful stimuli = 5
- Normal flexion (withdrawal) = 4
- Abnormal flexion (decorticate posturing) = 3
- Extensor response (decerebrate posturing) = 2
- No motor response to pain = 1

Verbal Response Points

- Oriented = 5
- Confused conversation = 4
- Inappropriate words = 3
- Responds with incomprehensible sounds = 2
- No verbal response = 1

Eye-Opening Points

- Spontaneous = 4
- In response to sound = 3
- In response to pain = 2
- No response, even to painful stimuli = 1

Data from Ignatavicius D, Workman M: *Medical-surgical nursing: patient-centered collaborative care*, ed 7, St. Louis, 2013, Saunders.

M. Glasgow Coma Scale (Box 58-5)
  1. The scale is a method of assessing a client's neurological condition.
  2. The scoring system is based on a scale of 3 to 15 points.
  3. A score lower than 8 indicates that coma is present.

IV. The Unconscious Client

A. Description
  1. The unconscious client is in a state of depressed cerebral functioning with unresponsiveness to stimulation of sensory and motor function.
  2. Some causes include head trauma, cerebral toxins, shock, hemorrhage, tumor, and infection.

B. Assessment
  1. Unarousable
  2. Primitive or no response to painful stimuli
  3. Altered respirations
  4. Decreased cranial nerve and reflex activity

C. Interventions (Box 58-6)

V. Increased Intracranial Pressure (ICP)

A. Description
  1. Increased ICP may be caused by trauma, hemorrhage, growths or tumors, hydrocephalus, edema, or inflammation.
  2. Increased ICP can impede circulation to the brain, impede the absorption of CSF, affect the functioning of nerve cells, and lead to brainstem compression and death.

B. Assessment
  1. Altered level of consciousness, which is the most sensitive and earliest indication of increasing ICP.
  2. Headache
  3. Abnormal respirations (see Box 58-2)
  4. Rise in blood pressure with widening pulse pressure
  5. Slowing of pulse
  6. Elevated temperature
  7. Vomiting
  8. Pupil changes
  9. Late signs of increased ICP include increased systolic blood pressure, widened pulse pressure, and slowed heart rate.
  10. Other late signs include changes in motor function from weakness to hemiplegia, a positive **Babinski's reflex**, decorticate or decerebrate posturing, and seizures.

C. Interventions
  1. Monitor respiratory status and prevent hypoxia.
  2. Avoid the administration of morphine sulfate to prevent the occurrence of hypoxia.

BOX 58-6 Care of the Unconscious Client

- Assess patency of the airway and keep airway and emergency equipment readily available.
- Monitor blood pressure, pulse, and heart sounds.
- Assess respiratory and circulatory status.
- Do not leave the client unattended if unstable.
- Maintain a patent airway and ventilation, because a high carbon dioxide (CO_2) level increases intracranial pressure.
- Assess lung sounds for the accumulation of secretions; suction as needed.
- Assess neurological status, including level of consciousness, pupillary reactions, and motor and sensory function, using a coma scale.
- Place the client in a semi-Fowler's position.
- Change position of the client every 2 hours, avoiding injury when turning.
- Avoid Trendelenburg's position.
- Use side rails unless contraindicated or according to agency protocol.
- Assess for edema.
- Monitor for dehydration.
- Monitor intake and output and daily weight.
- Maintain NPO (nothing by mouth) status until consciousness returns.
- Maintain nutrition as prescribed (intravenous or enteral feedings), and monitor fluid and electrolyte balance (when consciousness returns, check the gag and swallow reflex before resuming a diet).
- Assess bowel sounds.
- Monitor elimination patterns.
- Monitor for constipation, impaction, and paralytic ileus.
- Maintain urinary output to prevent stasis, infection, and calculus formation.
- Monitor the status of skin integrity.
- Initiate measures to prevent skin breakdown.
- Provide frequent mouth care.
- Remove dentures and contact lenses.
- Assess the eyes for the presence of a corneal reflex and irritation, and instill artificial tears or cover the eyes with eye patches.
- Monitor drainage from the ears or nose for the presence of cerebrospinal fluid.
- Assume that the unconscious client can hear.
- Avoid restraints.
- Initiate seizure precautions if necessary.
- Provide range-of-motion exercises to prevent contractures.
- Use a footboard or high-topped sneakers to prevent footdrop.
- Use splints to prevent wrist deformities.
- Initiate physical therapy as appropriate.

3. Maintain mechanical ventilation as prescribed; maintaining the $PaCO_2$ at 30 to 35 mm Hg (30 to 35 mm Hg) will result in vasoconstriction of the cerebral blood vessels, decreased blood flow, and therefore decreased ICP.
4. Maintain body temperature.
5. Prevent shivering, which can increase ICP.
6. Decrease environmental stimuli.
7. Monitor electrolyte levels and acid–base balance.
8. Monitor intake and output.
9. Limit fluid intake to 1200 mL/day.
10. Instruct the client to avoid straining activities, such as coughing and sneezing.
11. Instruct the client to avoid Valsalva's maneuver.

⚠ For the client with increased ICP, elevate the head of the bed 30 to 40 degrees, avoid the Trendelenburg's position, and prevent flexion of the neck and hips.

D. Medications (Box 58-7)

E. Surgical intervention: Also see Chapter 38 for additional information on ventriculoperitoneal shunts (Box 58-8)

BOX 58-7 Medications for Increased Intracranial Pressure

Antiseizure

- Seizures increase metabolic requirements and cerebral blood flow and volume, thus increasing intracranial pressure (ICP).
- Medications may be given prophylactically to prevent seizures.

Antipyretics and Muscle Relaxants

- Temperature reduction decreases metabolism, cerebral blood flow, and thus ICP.
- Antipyretics prevent temperature elevations.
- Muscle relaxants prevent shivering.

Blood Pressure Medication

- Blood pressure medication may be required to maintain cerebral perfusion at a normal level.
- Notify the primary health care provider if the blood pressure range is lower than 100 or higher than 150 mm Hg systolic.

Corticosteroids

- Corticosteroids stabilize the cell membrane and reduce leakiness of the blood-brain barrier.
- Corticosteroids decrease cerebral edema.
- A histamine blocker may be administered to counteract the excess gastric secretion that occurs with the corticosteroid.
- Clients must be withdrawn slowly from corticosteroid therapy to reduce the risk of adrenal crisis.

Intravenous Fluids

- Fluids are administered intravenously via an infusion pump to control the amount administered.
- Infusions are monitored closely because of the risk of promoting additional cerebral edema and fluid overload.

Hyperosmotic Agent

- A hyperosmotic agent increases intravascular pressure by drawing fluid from the interstitial spaces and from the brain cells.
- Monitor renal function.
- Diuresis is expected.

BOX 58-8 Surgical Intervention for Chronic Increased Intracranial Pressure: Ventriculoperitoneal Shunt

Description
- A ventriculoperitoneal shunt diverts cerebrospinal fluid from the ventricles into the peritoneum.

Postprocedure Interventions
- Position the client supine and turn from the back to the nonoperative side.
- Monitor for signs of increasing intracranial pressure resulting from shunt failure.
- Monitor for signs of infection.

VI. Hyperthermia

A. Description
1. Temperature higher than 105° F (40.6° C), which increases the cerebral metabolism and increases the risk of hypoxia
2. Causes include infection, heat stroke, exposure to high environmental temperatures, and dysfunction of the thermoregulatory center.

B. Assessment
1. Temperature higher than 105° F (40.6° C)
2. Shivering
3. Nausea and vomiting

C. Interventions
1. Maintain a patent airway.
2. Initiate seizure precautions.
3. Monitor intake and output and assess the skin and mucous membranes for signs of dehydration.
4. Monitor lung sounds.
5. Monitor for dysrhythmias.
6. Assess peripheral pulses for systemic blood flow.
7. Induce normothermia with fluids, cool baths, fans, or a hypothermia blanket.

D. Inducement of normothermia
1. Prevent shivering, which will increase ICP and oxygen consumption.
2. Administer medications as prescribed to prevent shivering and to lower body temperature.
3. Monitor neurological status.
4. Monitor for infection and respiratory complications because hyperthermia may mask the signs of infection.
5. Monitor for cardiac dysrhythmias.
6. Monitor intake and output and fluid balance.
7. Prevent trauma to the skin and tissues.
8. Apply lotion to the skin frequently.
9. Inspect for frostbite if a hypothermia blanket is used.

VII. Traumatic Head Injury

A. Description
1. Head injury is trauma to the skull, resulting in mild to extensive damage to the brain.
2. Immediate complications include cerebral bleeding, hematomas, uncontrolled increased ICP, infections, and seizures.
3. Changes in personality or behavior, cranial nerve deficits, and any other residual deficits depend on the area of the brain damage and the extent of the damage.

B. Types of head injuries (Box 58-9)
1. Open
   a. Scalp lacerations
   b. Fractures in the skull
   c. Interruption of the dura mater

BOX 58-9 Types of Head Injuries

Concussion
- Concussion is a jarring of the brain within the skull; there may or may not be a loss of consciousness.

Contusion
- Contusion is a bruising type of injury to the brain tissue.
- Contusion may occur along with other neurological injuries, such as with subdural or extradural collections of blood.

Skull Fractures
- Linear
- Depressed
- Compound
- Comminuted

Epidural Hematoma
- The most serious type of hematoma, epidural hematoma forms rapidly and results from arterial bleeding.
- The hematoma forms between the dura and skull from a tear in the meningeal artery.
- It is often associated with temporary loss of consciousness, followed by a lucid period that then rapidly progresses to coma.
- Epidural hematoma is a surgical emergency.

Subdural Hematoma
- Subdural hematoma forms slowly and results from a venous bleed.
- It occurs under the dura as a result of tears in the veins crossing the subdural space.

Intracerebral Hemorrhage
- Intracerebral hemorrhage occurs when a blood vessel within the brain ruptures, allowing blood to leak inside the brain.

Subarachnoid Hemorrhage
- A subarachnoid hemorrhage is bleeding into the subarachnoid space. It may occur as a result of head trauma or spontaneously, such as from a ruptured cerebral aneurysm.

2. Closed
   a. Concussions
   b. Contusions
   c. Fractures

C. Hematoma
1. Description: A collection of blood in the tissues that can occur as a result of a subarachnoid hemorrhage or an intracerebral hemorrhage.
2. Assessment
   a. Assessment findings depend on the injury.
   b. Clinical manifestations usually result from increased ICP.
   c. Changing neurological signs in the client
   d. Changes in level of consciousness
   e. Airway and breathing pattern changes
   f. Vital signs change, reflecting increased ICP.
   g. Headache, nausea, and vomiting
   h. Visual disturbances, pupillary changes, and papilledema
   i. **Nuchal rigidity** (not tested until spinal cord injury is ruled out)
   j. CSF drainage from the ears or nose
   k. Weakness and paralysis
   l. Posturing
   m. Decreased sensation or absence of feeling
   n. Reflex activity changes
   o. Seizure activity

CSF can be distinguished from other fluids by the presence of concentric rings (bloody fluid surrounded by yellowish stain; halo sign) when the fluid is placed on a white sterile background, such as a gauze pad. CSF also tests positive for glucose when tested using a strip test.

3. Interventions
   a. Monitor respiratory status and maintain a patent airway, because increased carbon dioxide (CO_2) levels increase cerebral edema.
   b. Monitor neurological status and vital signs, including temperature.
   c. Monitor for increased ICP.
   d. Maintain head elevation to reduce venous pressure.
   e. Prevent neck flexion.
   f. Initiate normothermia measures for increased temperature.
   g. Assess cranial nerve function, reflexes, and motor and sensory function.
   h. Initiate seizure precautions.
   i. Monitor for pain and restlessness.
   j. Morphine sulfate or opioid medication may be prescribed to decrease agitation and control restlessness caused by pain for the head-injured client on a ventilator; administer with caution because it is a respiratory depressant and may increase ICP.
   k. Monitor for drainage from the nose or ears, because this fluid may be CSF.
   l. Do not attempt to clean the nose, suction, or allow the client to blow her or his nose if drainage occurs.
   m. Do not clean the ear if drainage is noted, but apply a loose, dry sterile dressing.
   n. Check drainage for the presence of CSF.
   o. Notify the PHCP if drainage from the ears or nose is noted and if the drainage tests positive for CSF.
   p. Instruct the client to avoid coughing because this increases ICP.
   q. Monitor for signs of infection.
   r. Prevent complications of immobility.
   s. Inform the client and family about the possible behavior changes that may occur, including those that are expected and those that need to be reported.

D. Craniotomy
1. Description
   a. Surgical procedure that involves an incision through the cranium to remove accumulated blood or a tumor
   b. Complications of the procedure include increased ICP from cerebral edema, hemorrhage, or obstruction of the normal flow of CSF.
   c. Additional complications include hematomas, hypovolemic shock, hydrocephalus, respiratory and neurogenic complications, pulmonary edema, and wound infections.
   d. Complications related to fluid and electrolyte imbalances include diabetes insipidus and inappropriate secretion of antidiuretic hormone.
   e. Stereotactic radiosurgery (SRS) may be an alternative to traditional surgery and is usually used to treat tumors and arteriovenous malformations.
2. Preoperative interventions
   a. Explain the procedure to the client and family.
   b. Prepare to shave the client's head as prescribed (usually done in the operating room) and cover the head with an appropriate covering.
   c. Stabilize the client before surgery.

PRIORITY NURSING ACTIONS

Autonomic Dysreflexia in a Spinal Cord Injury Client

1. Raise the head of the bed and ask that the primary health care provider (PHCP) be notified.
2. Loosen tight clothing on the client.
3. Check for bladder distention or other noxious stimulus.
4. Administer an antihypertensive medication.
5. Document the occurrence, treatment, and response.

Reference

Ignatavicius, *Workman, Rebar* (2018), p. 898.

BOX 58-10 Nursing Care Following Craniotomy

- Monitor vital signs and neurological status every 30 to 60 minutes.
- Monitor for increased intracranial pressure (ICP).
- Monitor for decreased level of consciousness, motor weakness or paralysis, aphasia, visual changes, and personality changes.
- Maintain mechanical ventilation and slight hyperventilation for the first 24 to 48 hours as prescribed to prevent increased ICP.
- Assess the primary health care provider's (PHCP's) prescription regarding client positioning.
- Avoid extreme hip or neck flexion, and maintain the head in a midline neutral position.
- Provide a quiet environment.
- Monitor the head dressing frequently for signs of drainage.
- Mark any area of drainage at least once each nursing shift for baseline comparison.
- Monitor the drain, which may be in place for 24 hours; maintain suction on the drain as prescribed.
- Measure drainage from the drain every 8 hours, and record the amount and color.
- Notify the PHCP if drainage is more than the normal amount of 30 to 50 mL per shift.
- Notify the PHCP immediately of excessive amounts of drainage or a saturated head dressing.
- Record strict measurement of hourly intake and output.
- Maintain fluid restriction at 1500 mL/day as prescribed.
- Monitor electrolyte levels.
- Monitor for dysrhythmias, which may occur as a result of fluid or electrolyte imbalance.
- Apply ice packs or cool compresses as prescribed; expect periorbital edema and ecchymosis of 1 or both eyes.
- Provide range-of-motion exercises every 8 hours.
- Place antiembolism stockings on the client as prescribed.
- Administer antiseizure medications, antacids, corticosteroids, and antibiotics as prescribed.
- Administer analgesics such as codeine sulfate or acetaminophen as prescribed for pain.

BOX 58-11 Client Positioning Following Craniotomy

- Positions prescribed following a craniotomy vary with the type of surgery and the specific postoperative primary health care provider's (PHCP's) prescription.
- Always check the PHCP's prescription regarding client positioning.
- Incorrect positioning may cause serious and possibly fatal complications.

Removal of a Bone Flap for Decompression

- To facilitate brain expansion, the client should be turned from the back to the nonoperative side, but not to the side on which the operation was performed.

Posterior Fossa Surgery

- To protect the operative site from pressure and minimize tension on the suture line, position the client on the side, with a pillow under the head for support, and not on the back.

Infratentorial Surgery

- Infratentorial surgery involves surgery below the tentorium of the brain.
- The PHCP may prescribe a flat position without head elevation or may prescribe that the head of the bed be elevated at 30 to 45 degrees.
- Do not elevate the head of the bed in the acute phase of care following surgery without an PHCP's prescription.

Supratentorial Surgery

- Supratentorial surgery involves surgery above the tentorium of the brain.
- The PHCP may prescribe that the head of the bed be elevated at 30 degrees to promote venous outflow through the jugular veins.
- Do not lower the head of the bed in the acute phase of care following surgery without a PHCP's prescription.

3. Postoperative interventions (Box 58-10)
4. Postoperative positioning (Box 58-11)

VIII. Cerebral Aneurysm

A. Description: Dilation of the walls of a weakened cerebral artery; can lead to rupture

B. Assessment
1. Headache and pain
2. Irritability
3. Visual changes
4. Tinnitus
5. Hemiparesis
6. Nuchal rigidity
7. Seizures

C. Interventions
1. Maintain a patent airway (suction only with an PHCP's prescription).
2. Administer oxygen as prescribed.
3. Monitor vital signs and for hypertension or dysrhythmias.
4. Avoid taking temperatures via the rectum.
5. Initiate aneurysm precautions (Box 58-12).

IX. Seizures

A. Description
1. Seizures are an abnormal, sudden, excessive discharge of electrical activity within the brain.

BOX 58-12 Aneurysm Precautions

- Maintain the client on bed rest in a semi-Fowler's or a side-lying position.
- Maintain a darkened room (subdued lighting and avoid direct, bright, artificial lights) without stimulation (a private room is optimal).
- Provide a quiet environment (avoid activities or startling noises); a telephone in the room is not usually allowed.
- Reading, watching television, and listening to music are permitted, provided that they do not overstimulate the client.
- Limit visitors.
- Maintain fluid restrictions.
- Provide diet as prescribed; avoid stimulants in the diet.
- Prevent any activities that initiate the Valsalva maneuver (straining at stool, coughing); provide stool softeners to prevent straining.
- Administer care gently (such as the bath, back rub, range of motion).
- Limit invasive procedures.
- Maintain normothermia.
- Prevent hypertension.
- Provide sedation.
- Provide pain control.
- Administer prophylactic antiseizure medications.
- Provide deep vein thrombosis (DVT) prophylaxis as prescribed.

2. Epilepsy is a disorder characterized by chronic seizure activity and indicates brain or CNS irritation.
3. Causes include genetic factors, trauma, tumors, circulatory or metabolic disorders, toxicity, and infections.
4. Status epilepticus involves a rapid succession of epileptic spasms without intervals of consciousness; it is a potential complication that can occur with any type of seizure, and brain damage may result.

B. Types of seizures (Box 58-13)

C. Assessment
1. Seizure history
2. Type of seizure
3. Occurrences before, during, and after the seizure
4. Prodromal signs, such as mood changes, irritability, and insomnia
5. Aura: Sensation that warns the client of the impending seizure
6. Loss of motor activity or bowel and bladder function or loss of consciousness during the seizure
7. Occurrences during the postictal state, such as headache, loss of consciousness, sleepiness, and impaired speech or thinking

D. Interventions

⚠ If the client is having a seizure, maintain a patent airway. Do not force the jaws open or place anything in the client's mouth.

1. Note the time and duration of the seizure.
2. Assess behavior at the onset of the seizure: If the client has experienced an aura, if a change in facial expression occurred, or if a sound or cry occurred from the client.
3. If the client is standing or sitting, place the client on the floor and protect the head and body.
4. Support airway, breathing, and circulation.
5. Administer oxygen.
6. Prepare to suction secretions.

BOX 58-13 Types of Seizures

Generalized Seizures

Tonic-Clonic
- Tonic-clonic seizures may begin with an aura.
- The tonic phase involves the stiffening or rigidity of the muscles of the arms and legs and usually lasts 10 to 20 seconds, followed by loss of consciousness.
- The clonic phase consists of hyperventilation and jerking of the extremities and usually lasts about 30 seconds.
- Full recovery from the seizure may take several hours.

Absence
- A brief seizure that lasts seconds, and the individual may or may not lose consciousness.
- No loss or change in muscle tone occurs.
- Seizures may occur several times during a day.
- The victim appears to be daydreaming.
- This type of seizure is more common in children.

Myoclonic
- Myoclonic seizures present as a brief generalized jerking or stiffening of extremities.
- The victim may fall from the seizure.

Atonic or Akinetic (Drop Attacks)
- An atonic seizure is a sudden momentary loss of muscle tone.
- The victim may fall as a result of the seizure.

Partial Seizures

Simple Partial
- The simple partial seizure produces sensory symptoms accompanied by motor symptoms that are localized or confined to a specific area.
- The client remains conscious and may report an aura.

Complex Partial
- The complex partial seizure is a psychomotor seizure.
- The area of the brain most usually involved is the temporal lobe.
- The seizure is characterized by periods of altered behavior of which the client is not aware.
- The client loses consciousness for a few seconds.

7. Turn the client to the side to allow secretions to drain while maintaining the airway.
8. Prevent injury during the seizure.
9. Remain with the client.
10. Do not restrain the client.
11. Loosen restrictive clothing.
12. Note the type, character, and progression of the movements during the seizure.
13. Monitor for incontinence.
14. Administer intravenous medications as prescribed to stop the seizure.
15. Document the characteristics of the seizure.
16. Provide privacy.
17. Monitor behavior following the seizure, such as the state of consciousness, motor ability, and speech ability.
18. Instruct the client about the importance of lifelong medication and the need for follow-up determination of medication blood levels.
19. Instruct the client to avoid alcohol, excessive stress, fatigue, and strobe lights.
20. Encourage the client to contact available community resources, such as the Epilepsy Foundation of America.
21. Encourage the client to wear a MedicAlert bracelet.

X. Stroke (Brain Attack)

A. Description
1. A stroke or brain attack manifests as a sudden focal neurological deficit and is caused by cerebrovascular disease.
2. Cerebral anoxia lasting longer than 10 minutes causes cerebral infarction with irreversible change.
3. Cerebral edema and congestion cause further dysfunction.
4. Diagnosis is determined by a CT scan, electroencephalography, cerebral arteriography, and MRI. In most facilities, the type of stroke needs to be determined within a certain time frame after arrival in order for timely treatment to be initiated.
5. Transient ischemic attack may be a warning sign of an impending stroke.
6. The permanent disability cannot be determined until the cerebral edema subsides.
7. The order in which function may return is facial, swallowing, lower limbs, speech, and arms.
8. Carotid endarterectomy is a surgical intervention used in stroke management; it is targeted at stroke prevention, especially in clients with symptomatic carotid stenosis.
9. The National Institutes of Health through the National Institute of Neurological Disorders and Stroke (NINDS) developed the *Know Stroke: Know the Signs. Act in Time* campaign devised to help educate the public about the symptoms of stroke and the importance of getting to the hospital quickly (http://stroke.nih.gov).

BOX 58-14 Clinical Manifestations of Stroke Based on Type

Thrombotic Stroke
- Typically, there is no decreased level of consciousness within the first 24 hours.
- Symptoms get progressively worse as the infarction and edema increase.

Embolic Stroke
- Sudden, severe symptoms
- Warning signs are less common.
- Client remains conscious and may have a headache.

Hemorrhagic Stroke
- Sudden onset of symptoms
- Symptoms progress over minutes to hours due to ongoing bleeding.

B. Causes (Box 58-14)
1. Thrombosis
2. Embolism
3. Thrombotic and embolic strokes are classified as ischemic strokes.
4. Hemorrhage from rupture of a vessel; classified as a hemorrhagic stroke
5. Manifestations of different types of stroke are similar and, therefore it is critical to determine the type of stroke occurring; the type cannot be determined solely based on manifestations, and the correct and appropriate treatment for the stroke type must be initiated.

C. Risk factors
1. Atherosclerosis
2. Hypertension
3. Anticoagulation therapy
4. Diabetes mellitus
5. Stress
6. Obesity
7. Oral contraceptives

D. Assessment (Fig. 58-2; Boxes 58-14 and 58-15)

A critical factor in the early intervention and treatment of stroke is the accurate identification of stroke manifestations and establishing the onset of the manifestations. Stroke screening scales may be used to identify stroke manifestations quickly. Identification of the type of stroke occurring is critical in determining the appropriate treatment, and this is usually done using imaging such as a CT scan.

1. Assessment findings depend on the area of the brain affected; stroke scales such as the NIH Stroke Scale (stroke.nih.gov/resources/scale.htm) may be used by the health care facility for assessment.

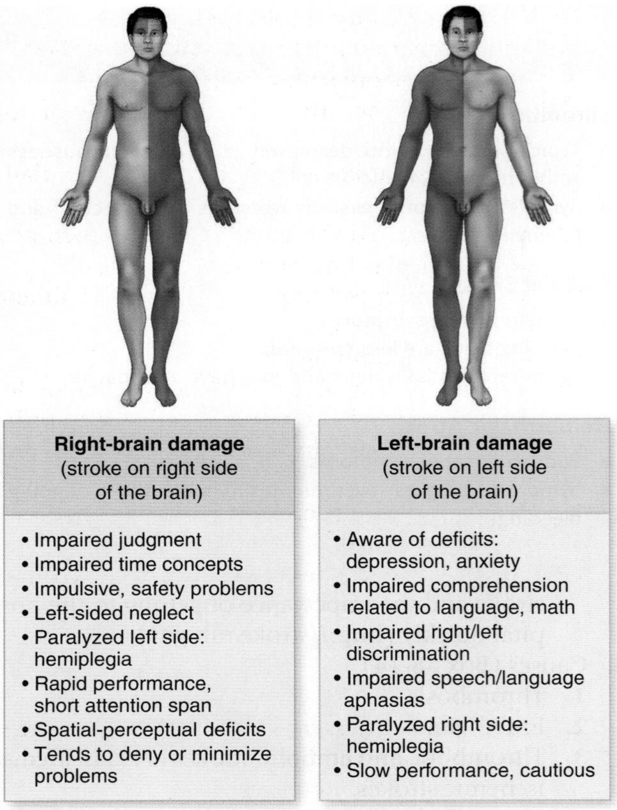
Right-brain damage
(stroke on right side of the brain)
• Impaired judgment
• Impaired time concepts
• Impulsive, safety problems
• Left-sided neglect
• Paralyzed left side: hemiplegia
• Rapid performance, short attention span
• Spatial-perceptual deficits
• Tends to deny or minimize problems
Left-brain damage
(stroke on left side of the brain)
• Aware of deficits: depression, anxiety
• Impaired comprehension related to language, math
• Impaired right/left discrimination
• Impaired speech/language aphasias
• Paralyzed right side: hemiplegia
• Slow performance, cautious

FIG. 58-2 Manifestations of right brain and left brain stroke.

BOX 58-15 Assessment Findings in a Stroke

Agnosia

- The inability to recognize familiar objects or persons

Apraxia

- Called *dyspraxia* if the condition is mild
- Characterized by loss of ability to execute or carry out skilled movements or gestures, despite having the desire and physical ability to perform them

Hemianopsia

- Blindness in half the visual field

Homonymous Hemianopsia

- Loss of half of the field of view on the same side in both eyes

Neglect Syndrome (Unilateral Neglect)

- Client unaware of the existence of her or his paralyzed side

Proprioception Alterations

- Altered position sense that places the client at increased risk of injury
- *Pyramid Point*: With visual problems, the client must turn the head to scan the complete range of vision.

Data from U.S. Department of Health and Human Services, National Institutes of Health: *Know stroke: know the signs. Act in time*, NIH Publication #10-4872. Bethesda, Md., June 2013, National Institutes of Health, http://stroke.nih.gov.

2. Lesions in the cerebral hemisphere result in manifestations on the contralateral side, which is the side of the body opposite the stroke.
3. Airway patency is always a priority.
4. Pulse (may be slow and bounding)
5. Respirations (Cheyne-Stokes)
6. Blood pressure (hypertension)
7. Headache, nausea, and vomiting
8. Facial drooping
9. Nuchal rigidity
10. Visual changes
11. Ataxia
12. Dysarthria
13. Dysphagia
14. Speech changes
15. Decreased sensation to pressure, heat, and cold
16. Bowel and bladder dysfunctions
17. Paralysis

E. Aphasia

1. Expressive
   a. Damage occurs in Broca's area of the frontal brain.
   b. The client understands what is said but is unable to communicate verbally.
2. Receptive
   a. Injury involves Wernicke's area in the temporoparietal area.
   b. The client is unable to understand the spoken and often the written word.
3. Global or mixed: Language dysfunction occurs in expression and reception.
4. Interventions for aphasia
   a. Provide repetitive directions.
   b. Break tasks down to 1 step at a time.
   c. Repeat names of objects frequently used.
   d. Allow time for the client to communicate.
   e. Use a picture board, communication board, or computer technology.

F. Interventions during the acute phase of stroke

1. Maintain a patent airway and administer oxygen as prescribed.
2. Monitor vital signs.
3. Usually a blood pressure of 150/100 mm Hg is maintained to ensure cerebral perfusion.
4. Suction secretions to prevent aspiration as prescribed, but never suction nasally or for longer than 10 seconds to prevent increased ICP.
5. Monitor for increased ICP, because the client is most at risk during the first 72 hours following the stroke.
6. Position the client on the side to prevent aspiration, with the head of the bed elevated 15 to 30 degrees as prescribed.
7. Monitor level of consciousness, pupillary response, motor and sensory response, cranial nerve function, and reflexes.
8. Maintain a quiet environment.

9. Insert a urinary catheter as prescribed.
10. Administer intravenous fluids as prescribed.
11. Maintain fluid and electrolyte balance.
12. Prepare to administer anticoagulants, antiplatelets, diuretics, antihypertensives, and antiseizure medications as prescribed depending on the type of stroke that has been diagnosed.
13. Establish a form of communication.

G. Interventions in the postacute phase of a stroke

1. Continue with interventions from the acute phase.
2. Position the client 2 hours on the unaffected side and 20 minutes on the affected side; the prone position may also be prescribed.
3. Provide skin, mouth, and eye care.
4. Perform passive range-of-motion exercises to prevent contractures.
5. Place antiembolism stockings on the client; remove daily to check skin.
6. Monitor the gag reflex and ability to swallow.
7. Provide sips of fluids and slowly advance diet to foods that are easy to chew and swallow.
8. Provide soft and semisoft foods and flavored, cool or warm, thickened fluids rather than thin liquids, because the stroke client can tolerate these types of food better; speech therapists may do swallow studies to recommend consistency of food and fluids.
9. When the client is eating, position the client sitting in a chair or sitting up in bed, with the head and neck positioned slightly forward and flexed.
10. Place food in the back of the mouth on the unaffected side to prevent trapping of food in the affected cheek.

H. Interventions in the chronic phase of stroke

1. Neglect syndrome
   a. The client is unaware of the existence of her or his paralyzed side (**unilateral neglect**), which places the client at risk for injury.
   b. Teach the client to touch and use both sides of the body.
2. **Hemianopsia**
   a. The client has blindness in half of the visual field.
   b. **Homonymous hemianopsia** is blindness in the same visual field of both eyes.
   c. Encourage the client to turn the head to scan the complete range of vision; otherwise, she or he does not see half of the visual field.
3. Approach the client from the unaffected side.
4. Place the client's personal objects within the visual field.
5. Provide eye care for visual deficits.
6. Place a patch over the affected eye if the client has diplopia.
7. Increase mobility as tolerated.
8. Encourage fluid intake and a high-fiber diet.
9. Administer stool softeners as prescribed.
10. Encourage the client to express her or his feelings.
11. Encourage independence in activities of daily living.
12. Assess the need for assistive devices such as a cane, walker, splint, or braces.
13. Teach transfer technique from bed to chair and from chair to bed.
14. Provide gait training.
15. Initiate physical and occupational therapy for assessment and the need for adaptive equipment or other supports for self-care and mobility.
16. Refer client to a speech and language pathologist as prescribed.
17. Encourage the client and family to contact available community resources.

XI. Multiple Sclerosis

A. Description

1. A chronic, progressive, noncontagious, degenerative disease of the CNS characterized by demyelinization of the neurons.
2. It usually occurs between the ages of 20 and 40 years and consists of periods of remissions and exacerbations.
3. The causes are unknown, but the disease is thought to be the result of an autoimmune response or viral infection.
4. Precipitating factors include pregnancy, fatigue, stress, infection, and trauma.
5. Electroencephalographic findings are abnormal.
6. Assessment of a lumbar puncture indicates an increased gamma globulin level, but the serum globulin level is normal.

B. Assessment

1. Fatigue and weakness
2. Ataxia and vertigo
3. Tremors and spasticity of the lower extremities
4. Paresthesias
5. Blurred vision, diplopia, and transient blindness
6. Nystagmus
7. Dysphasia
8. Decreased perception to pain, touch, and temperature
9. Bladder and bowel disturbances, including urgency, frequency, retention, and incontinence
10. Abnormal reflexes, including hyperreflexia, absent reflexes, and a positive Babinski's reflex
11. Emotional changes such as apathy, euphoria, irritability, and depression
12. Memory changes and confusion

C. Interventions
1. Provide energy conservation measures during exacerbation.
2. Protect the client from injury by providing safety measures.
3. Place an eye patch on the eye for diplopia.
4. Monitor for potential complications such as urinary tract infections, calculi, pressure ulcers, respiratory tract infections, and contractures.
5. Promote regular elimination by bladder and bowel training.
6. Encourage independence.
7. Assist the client to establish a regular exercise and rest program and to balance moderate activity with rest periods.
8. Assess the need for and provide assistive devices.
9. Initiate physical and speech therapy.
10. Instruct the client to avoid fatigue, stress, infection, overheating, and chilling.
11. Instruct the client to increase fluid intake and eat a balanced diet, including low-fat, high-fiber foods and foods high in potassium.
12. Instruct the client in safety measures related to sensory loss, such as regulating the temperature of bath water and avoiding heating pads.
13. Instruct the client in safety measures related to motor loss, such as avoiding the use of scatter rugs and using assistive devices.
14. Instruct the client in the self-administration of prescribed medications.
15. Provide information about the National Multiple Sclerosis Society.

XII. Myasthenia Gravis

A. Description
1. A neuromuscular disease characterized by considerable weakness and abnormal fatigue of the voluntary muscles
2. A defect in the transmission of nerve impulses at the myoneural junction occurs.
3. 3.Causes include insufficient secretion of acetylcholine, excessive secretion of cholinesterase, and unresponsiveness of the muscle fibers to acetylcholine.

B. Assessment
1. Weakness and fatigue
2. Difficulty chewing and swallowing
3. Dysphagia
4. Ptosis
5. Diplopia
6. Weak, hoarse voice
7. Difficulty breathing
8. Diminished breath sounds
9. Respiratory paralysis and failure

C. Interventions
1. Monitor respiratory status and ability to cough and deep-breathe adequately.
2. Monitor for respiratory failure.
3. Maintain suctioning and emergency equipment at the bedside.
4. Monitor vital signs.
5. Monitor speech and swallowing abilities to prevent aspiration.
6. Encourage the client to sit up when eating.
7. Assess muscle status.
8. Instruct the client to conserve strength.
9. Plan short activities that coincide with times of maximal muscle strength.
10. Monitor for myasthenic and cholinergic crises.
11. Administer anticholinesterase medications as prescribed.
12. Instruct the client to avoid stress, infection, fatigue, and over-the-counter medications.
13. Instruct the client to wear a MedicAlert bracelet.
14. Inform the client about services from the Myasthenia Gravis Foundation.

D. Anticholinesterase medications: Increase levels of acetylcholine at the myoneural junction (see Chapter 59)

E. Myasthenic crisis
1. Description
   a. An acute exacerbation of the disease
   b. The crisis is caused by a rapid, unrecognized progression of the disease, inadequate amount of medication, infection, fatigue, or stress.
2. Assessment
   a. Increased pulse, respirations, and blood pressure
   b. Dyspnea, anoxia, and cyanosis
   c. Bowel and bladder incontinence
   d. Decreased urine output
   e. Absent cough and swallow reflex
3. Interventions
   a. Assess for signs of myasthenic crisis.
   b. Increase anticholinesterase medication, as prescribed.

F. Cholinergic crisis
1. Description
   a. Results in depolarization of the motor end plates
   b. The crisis is caused by overmedication with anticholinesterase.
2. Assessment
   a. Abdominal cramps
   b. Nausea, vomiting, and diarrhea
   c. Blurred vision
   d. Pallor
   e. Facial muscle twitching
   f. Hypotension
   g. Pupillary miosis
3. Interventions
   a. Withhold anticholinesterase medication.
   b. Prepare to administer the antidote, atropine sulfate, if prescribed.

G. Edrophonium (Tensilon) test

Have atropine sulfate available when performing the edrophonium test.

1. Description
   a. This test is performed by the neurologist to diagnose myasthenia gravis and to differentiate between myasthenic crisis and cholinergic crisis.
   b. The test places the client at risk for ventricular fibrillation and cardiac arrest; emergency equipment needs to be available.
2. To diagnose myasthenia gravis
   a. Edrophonium injection is administered to the client.
   b. Positive for myasthenia gravis: Client shows improvement in muscle strength after the administration of edrophonium.
   c. Negative for myasthenia gravis: Client shows no improvement in muscle strength, and strength may even deteriorate after injection of edrophonium.
3. To differentiate crisis
   a. Myasthenic crisis: Edrophonium is administered and, if strength improves, the client needs more medication.
   b. Cholinergic crisis: Edrophonium is administered and, if weakness is more severe, the client is overmedicated; prepare to administer atropine sulfate, the antidote, as prescribed.

XIII. Parkinson's Disease

A. Description
1. A degenerative disease caused by the depletion of dopamine, which interferes with the inhibition of excitatory impulses, resulting in a dysfunction of the extrapyramidal system.
2. It is a slow, progressive disease that results in a crippling disability.
3. The debilitation can result in falls, self-care deficits, failure of body systems, and depression.
4. Mental deterioration occurs late in the disease.

B. Assessment
1. Bradykinesia, abnormal slowness of movement, and sluggishness of physical and mental responses
2. Akinesia
3. Monotonous speech
4. Handwriting that becomes progressively smaller
5. Tremors in hands and fingers at rest (pill rolling)
6. Tremors increasing when fatigued and decreasing with purposeful activity or sleep
7. Rigidity with jerky movements
8. Restlessness and pacing
9. Blank facial expression; mask-like faces
10. Drooling
11. Difficulty swallowing and speaking
12. Loss of coordination and balance
13. Shuffling steps, stooped position, and propulsive gait

C. Interventions
1. Assess neurological status.
2. Assess ability to swallow and chew.
3. Provide high-calorie, high-protein, high-fiber soft diet with small, frequent feedings.
4. Increase fluid intake to 2000 mL/day.
5. Monitor for constipation.
6. Promote independence along with safety measures.
7. Avoid rushing the client with activities.
8. Assist with ambulation and provide assistive devices.
9. Instruct the client to rock back and forth to initiate movement.
10. Instruct the client to wear low-heeled shoes.
11. Encourage the client to lift the feet when walking and to avoid prolonged sitting.
12. Provide a firm mattress and position the client prone, without a pillow, to facilitate proper posture.
13. Instruct in proper posture by teaching the client to hold the hands behind the back to keep the spine and neck erect.
14. Promote physical therapy and rehabilitation.
15. Administer antiparkinsonian medications to increase the level of dopamine in the CNS.
16. Instruct the client to avoid foods high in vitamin B_6, because they block the effects of antiparkinsonian medications.
17. Avoid the use of monoamine oxidase inhibitors, because they will precipitate hypertensive crisis.
18. See Chapter 59 regarding medication to treat Parkinson's disease.

XIV. Trigeminal Neuralgia

A. Description
1. A sensory disorder of the trigeminal (fifth cranial) nerve
2. It results in severe, recurrent, sharp facial pain along the trigeminal nerve.

B. Assessment
1. The client has severe pain on the lips, gums, or nose, or across the cheeks.
2. Situations that stimulate symptoms include cold, washing the face, chewing, or food or fluids of extreme temperatures.

C. Interventions
1. Instruct the client to avoid hot or cold foods and fluids.
2. Provide small feedings of liquid and soft foods.
3. Instruct the client to chew food on the unaffected side.
4. Administer medications as prescribed (see Chapter 59).

D. Surgical interventions
1. Microvascular decompression: Surgical relocation of the artery that compresses the trigeminal nerve as it enters the pons, which may relieve pain without compromising facial sensation
2. Radiofrequency waveforms: Create lesions that provide relief of pain without compromising touch or motor function
3. Rhizotomy: Resection of the root of the nerve to relieve pain
4. Glycerol injection: Destroys the myelinated fibers of the trigeminal nerve (may take up to 3 weeks for pain relief to occur)

XV. Bell's Palsy (Facial Paralysis)

A. Description
1. Caused by a lower motor neuron lesion of cranial nerve VII that may result from infection, trauma, hemorrhage, meningitis, or tumor.
2. It results in paralysis of 1 side of the face.
3. Recovery usually occurs in a few weeks, without residual effects.

B. Assessment
1. Flaccid facial muscles
2. Inability to raise the eyebrows, frown, smile, close the eyelids, or puff out the cheeks
3. Upward movement of the eye when attempting to close the eyelid
4. Loss of taste

C. Interventions
1. Encourage facial exercises to prevent the loss of muscle tone (a face sling may be prescribed to prevent stretching of weak muscles).
2. Protect the eyes from dryness and prevent injury.
3. Promote frequent oral care.
4. Instruct the client to chew on the unaffected side.

XVI. Guillain-Barré Syndrome

A. Description
1. An acute infectious neuronitis of the cranial and peripheral nerves.
2. The immune system overreacts to the infection and destroys the myelin sheath.
3. The syndrome usually is preceded by a mild upper respiratory infection or gastroenteritis.
4. The recovery is a slow process and can take years.

! The major concern in Guillain-Barré syndrome is difficulty breathing; monitor respiratory status closely.

B. Assessment
1. Paresthesias
2. Pain and/or hypersensitivity such as with the weight of bed sheets or other items touching the body
3. Weakness of lower extremities
4. Gradual progressive weakness of the upper extremities and facial muscles
5. Possible progression to respiratory failure
6. Cardiac dysrhythmias
7. CSF that reveals an elevated protein level
8. Abnormal electroencephalogram

C. Interventions
1. Care is directed toward the treatment of symptoms, including pain management.
2. Monitor respiratory status closely.
3. Provide respiratory treatments.
4. Prepare to initiate respiratory support.
5. Monitor cardiac status.
6. Assess for complications of immobility.
7. Provide the client and family with support.

XVII. Amyotrophic Lateral Sclerosis

A. Description
1. Also known as Lou Gehrig's disease
2. It is a progressive degenerative disease involving the motor system.
3. The sensory and autonomic systems are not involved, and mental status changes do not result from the disease.
4. The cause of the disease may be related to an excess of glutamate, a chemical responsible for relaying messages between the motor neurons.
5. As the disease progresses, muscle weakness and atrophy develop until a flaccid tetraplegia develops.
6. Eventually, the respiratory muscles become affected, leading to respiratory compromise, pneumonia, and death.
7. No cure is known, and the treatment is symptomatic.

B. Assessment
1. Respiratory difficulty
2. Fatigue while talking
3. Muscle weakness and atrophy
4. Tongue atrophy
5. Dysphagia
6. Weakness of the hands and arms
7. Fasciculations of the face
8. Nasal quality of speech
9. Dysarthria

C. Interventions
1. Care is directed toward the treatment of symptoms.
2. Monitor respiratory status and institute measures to prevent aspiration.
3. Provide respiratory treatments.
4. Prepare to initiate respiratory support.
5. Assess for complications of immobility.
6. Address advance directives as appropriate.
7. Provide the client and family with psychosocial support.

XVIII. Encephalitis

A. Description
1. An inflammation of the brain parenchyma and often of the meninges.

2. It affects the cerebrum, brainstem, and cerebellum.
3. It most often is caused by a viral agent, although bacteria, fungi, or parasites also may be involved.
4. Viral encephalitis is almost always preceded by a viral infection.

B. Transmission
1. Arboviruses can be transmitted to human beings through the bite of an infected mosquito or tick.
2. Echovirus, coxsackievirus, poliovirus, herpes zoster virus, and viruses that cause mumps and chickenpox are common enteroviruses associated with encephalitis.
3. Herpes simplex type 1 virus can cause viral encephalitis.
4. The organism that causes amebic meningoencephalitis can enter the nasal mucosa of persons swimming in warm fresh water, such as a pond or lake.

C. Assessment
1. Presence of cold sores, lesions, or ulcerations of the oral cavity
2. History of insect bites and swimming in fresh water
3. Exposure to infectious diseases
4. Travel to areas where the disease is prevalent
5. Fever
6. Nausea and vomiting
7. Nuchal rigidity
8. Changes in level of consciousness and mental status
9. Signs of increased ICP
10. Motor dysfunction and focal neurological deficits

D. Interventions
1. Monitor vital and neurological signs.
2. Assess level of consciousness using the Glasgow Coma Scale.
3. Assess for mental status changes and personality and behavior changes.
4. Assess for signs of increased ICP.
5. Assess for the presence of nuchal rigidity and a positive **Kernig's sign** or **Brudzinski's sign**, indicating meningeal irritation (Fig. 58-3).
6. Assist the client to turn, cough, and deep-breathe frequently.
7. Elevate the head of the bed 30 to 45 degrees.

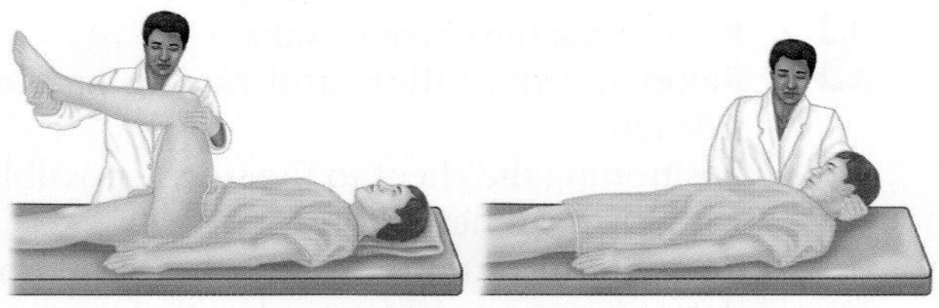

FIG. 58-3 Kernig's sign and Brudzinski's sign.

8. Assess for muscle and neurological deficits.
9. Administer acyclovir as prescribed (usually the medication of choice for herpes encephalitis).
10. Initiate rehabilitation as needed for motor dysfunction or neurological deficits.

XIX. West Nile Virus Infection

A. Description
1. A potentially serious illness that affects the CNS
2. The virus is contracted primarily by the bite of an infected mosquito (mosquitoes become carriers when they feed on infected birds).
3. Symptoms typically develop between 3 and 14 days after being bitten by the infected mosquito.
4. Neurological effects can be permanent.

B. Assessment
1. Many individuals will not experience any symptoms.
2. Mild symptoms include fever; headache and body aches; nausea; vomiting; swollen glands; or a rash on the chest, stomach, or back.
3. Severe symptoms include a high fever, headache, neck stiffness, stupor, disorientation, tremors, muscle weakness, vision loss, numbness, paralysis, seizures, or coma.

C. Interventions are supportive; there is no specific treatment for the virus.

D. Prevention
1. Use insect repellents containing DEET (diethyltoluamide) when outdoors and wear long sleeves and pants and light-colored clothing.
2. Stay indoors at dusk and dawn when mosquitoes are most active.
3. Ensure that mosquito breeding sites are eliminated, such as standing water and water in bird baths, and keep wading pools empty and on their sides when not in use.

XX. Meningitis

A. Description
1. An inflammation of the arachnoid and pia mater of the brain and spinal cord
2. It is caused by bacterial and viral organisms, although fungal and protozoan meningitis also occur.
3. Predisposing factors include skull fractures, brain or spinal surgery, sinus or upper respiratory infections, the use of nasal sprays, and a compromised immune system.
4. CSF is analyzed to determine the diagnosis and type of meningitis. In meningitis, CSF is cloudy, with increased protein, increased white blood cells, and decreased glucose counts.

B. Transmission: Transmission occurs in areas of high population density, crowded living areas such as college dormitories, and prisons.

⚠ Transmission of meningitis is by direct contact, including droplet spread.

C. Assessment (see Box 58-4)
1. Mild lethargy
2. Photophobia
3. Deterioration in the level of consciousness
4. Signs of meningeal irritation, such as nuchal rigidity and a positive Kernig's sign and Brudzinski's sign
5. Red, macular rash with meningococcal meningitis
6. Abdominal and chest pain with viral meningitis

D. Interventions
1. Monitor vital signs and neurological signs.
2. Assess for signs of increased ICP.
3. Initiate seizure precautions.
4. Monitor for seizure activity.
5. Monitor for signs of meningeal irritation.
6. Perform cranial nerve assessment.
7. Assess peripheral vascular status (septic emboli may block circulation).
8. Maintain isolation precautions as necessary with bacterial meningitis.
9. Maintain urine and stool precautions with viral meningitis.
10. Maintain respiratory isolation for the client with pneumococcal meningitis.
11. Elevate the head of the bed 30 degrees, and avoid neck flexion and extreme hip flexion.
12. Prevent stimulation and restrict visitors.
13. Administer analgesics and/or antibiotics as prescribed.

PRACTICE QUESTIONS

704. The nurse is assessing the motor and sensory function of an unconscious client who sustained a head injury. The nurse should use which technique to test the client's peripheral response to pain?
1. Sternal rub
2. Nailbed pressure
3. Pressure on the orbital rim
4. Squeezing of the sternocleidomastoid muscle

705. The nurse is caring for the client with increased intracranial pressure as a result of a head injury? The nurse would note which trend in vital signs if the intracranial pressure is rising?
1. Increasing temperature, increasing pulse, increasing respirations, decreasing blood pressure
2. Increasing temperature, decreasing pulse, decreasing respirations, increasing blood pressure
3. Decreasing temperature, decreasing pulse, increasing respirations, decreasing blood pressure
4. Decreasing temperature, increasing pulse, decreasing respirations, increasing blood pressure

706. A client recovering from a head injury is participating in care. The nurse determines that the client understands measures to prevent elevations in intracranial pressure if the nurse observes the client doing which activity?
1. Blowing the nose
2. Isometric exercises
3. Coughing vigorously
4. Exhaling during repositioning

707. A client has clear fluid leaking from the nose following a basilar skull fracture. Which finding would alert the nurse that cerebrospinal fluid is present?
1. Fluid is clear and tests negative for glucose.
2. Fluid is grossly bloody in appearance and has a pH of 6.
3. Fluid clumps together on the dressing and has a pH of 7.
4. Fluid separates into concentric rings and tests positive for glucose.

708. A client with a spinal cord injury is prone to experiencing autonomic dysreflexia. The nurse should include which measures in the plan of care to minimize the risk of occurrence? **Select all that apply.**
- ☐ 1. Keeping the linens wrinkle-free under the client
- ☐ 2. Preventing unnecessary pressure on the lower limbs
- ☐ 3. Limiting bladder catheterization to once every 12 hours
- ☐ 4. Turning and repositioning the client at least every 2 hours
- ☐ 5. Ensuring that the client has a bowel movement at least once a week

709. The nurse is evaluating the neurological signs of a client in spinal shock following spinal cord injury. Which observation indicates that spinal shock persists?
1. Hyperreflexia
2. Positive reflexes
3. Flaccid paralysis
4. Reflex emptying of the bladder

710. The nurse is caring for a client who begins to experience seizure activity while in bed. Which actions should the nurse take? **Select all that apply.**
- ☐ 1. Loosening restrictive clothing.
- ☐ 2. Restraining the client's limbs.
- ☐ 3. Removing the pillow and raising padded side rails.
- ☐ 4. Positioning the client to the side, if possible, with the head flexed forward.
- ☐ 5. Keeping the curtain around the client and the room door open so when help arrives they can quickly enter to assist.

711. The nurse is assigned to care for a client with complete right-sided hemiparesis from a stroke (brain attack). Which characteristics are associated with this condition? **Select all that apply.**

- ☐ 1. The client is aphasic.
- ☐ 2. The client has weakness on the right side of the body.
- ☐ 3. The client has complete bilateral paralysis of the arms and legs.
- ☐ 4. The client has weakness on the right side of the face and tongue.
- ☐ 5. The client has lost the ability to move the right arm but is able to walk independently.
- ☐ 6. The client has lost the ability to ambulate independently but is able to feed and bathe herself or himself without assistance.

712. The nurse has instructed the family of a client with stroke (brain attack) who has homonymous hemianopsia about measures to help the client overcome the deficit. Which statement suggests that the family understands the measures to use when caring for the client?

1. "We need to discourage him from wearing eyeglasses."
2. "We need to place objects in his impaired field of vision."
3. "We need to approach him from the impaired field of vision."
4. "We need to remind him to turn his head to scan the lost visual field."

713. The nurse is assessing the adaptation of a client to changes in functional status after a stroke (brain attack). Which observation indicates to the nurse that the client is adapting **most** successfully?

1. Gets angry with family if they interrupt a task
2. Experiences bouts of depression and irritability
3. Has difficulty with using modified feeding utensils
4. Consistently uses adaptive equipment in dressing self

714. The nurse is teaching a client with myasthenia gravis about the prevention of myasthenic and cholinergic crises. Which client activity suggests that teaching is **most effective**?

1. Taking medications as scheduled
2. Eating large, well-balanced meals
3. Doing muscle-strengthening exercises
4. Doing all chores early in the day while less fatigued

715. The nurse is instructing a client with Parkinson's disease about preventing falls. Which client statement reflects a **need for further teaching**?

1. "I can sit down to put on my pants and shoes."
2. "I try to exercise every day and rest when I'm tired."
3. "My son removed all loose rugs from my bedroom."
4. "I don't need to use my walker to get to the bathroom."

716. The nurse has given suggestions to a client with trigeminal neuralgia about strategies to minimize episodes of pain. The nurse determines that the client **needs further teaching** if the client makes which statement?

1. "I will wash my face with cotton pads."
2. "I'll have to start chewing on my unaffected side."
3. "I should rinse my mouth if toothbrushing is painful."
4. "I'll try to eat my food either very warm or very cold."

717. The client is admitted to the hospital with a diagnosis of Guillain-Barré syndrome. Which past medical history finding makes the client **most** at risk for this disease?

1. Meningitis or encephalitis during the last 5 years
2. Seizures or trauma to the brain within the last year
3. Back injury or trauma to the spinal cord during the last 2 years
4. Respiratory or gastrointestinal infection during the previous month

718. A client with Guillain-Barré syndrome has ascending paralysis and is intubated and receiving mechanical ventilation. Which strategy should the nurse incorporate in the plan of care to help the client cope with this illness?

1. Giving client full control over care decisions and restricting visitors
2. Providing positive feedback and encouraging active range of motion
3. Providing information, giving positive feedback, and encouraging relaxation
4. Providing intravenously administered sedatives, reducing distractions, and limiting visitors

719. A client has a neurological deficit involving the limbic system. On assessment, which finding is specific to this type of deficit?

1. Is disoriented to person, place, and time.
2. Affect is flat, with periods of emotional lability.
3. Cannot recall what was eaten for breakfast today.
4. Demonstrates inability to add and subtract; does not know who is the president of the United States.

720. The nurse is instituting seizure precautions for a client who is being admitted from the emergency department. Which measures should the nurse include in planning for the client's safety? **Select all that apply.**

- ☐ 1. Padding the side rails of the bed.
- ☐ 2. Placing an airway at the bedside.
- ☐ 3. Placing the bed in the high position.

❑ 4. Putting a padded tongue blade at the head of the bed.
❑ 5. Placing oxygen and suction equipment at the bedside.
❑ 6. Flushing the intravenous catheter to ensure that the site is patent.

721. The nurse is evaluating the status of a client who had a craniotomy 3 days ago. Which assessment finding would indicate that the client is developing meningitis as a complication of surgery?
1. A negative Kernig's sign
2. Absence of nuchal rigidity
3. A positive Brudzinski's sign
4. A Glasgow Coma Scale score of 15

722. The nurse has completed discharge instructions for a client with application of a halo device who sustained a cervical spinal cord injury. Which statement indicates that the client **needs further clarification** of the instructions?
1. "I will use a straw for drinking."
2. "I will drive only during the daytime."
3. "I will be careful because the device alters balance."
4. I will wash the skin daily under the lamb's wool liner of the vest."

723. The nurse is admitting a client with Guillain-Barré syndrome to the nursing unit. The client has complaints of inability to move both legs and reports a tingling sensation above the waistline. Knowing the complications of the disorder, the nurse should bring which **most essential** items into the client's room?
1. Nebulizer and pulse oximeter
2. Blood pressure cuff and flashlight
3. Nasal cannula and incentive spirometer
4. Electrocardiographic monitoring electrodes and intubation tray

ANSWERS

704. *Answer:* 2
Rationale: Nailbed pressure tests a basic motor and sensory peripheral response. Cerebral responses to pain are tested using a sternal rub, placing upward pressure on the orbital rim, or squeezing the clavicle or sternocleidomastoid muscle.
Test-Taking Strategy: Focus on the subject, testing peripheral response to pain. The nailbeds are the most distal of all options and are therefore the most peripheral. Each of the other options may elicit a generalized response, but not a localized one.
Level of Cognitive Ability: Analyzing
Client Needs: Health Promotion and Maintenance
Integrated Process: Nursing Process—Assessment
Content Area: Adult Health: Neurological
Health Problem: Adult Health: Neurological: Head injury/trauma
Priority Concepts: Intracranial Regulation; Pain
Reference: Ignatavicius, Workman, Rebar (2018), pp. 441-443.

705. *Answer:* 2
Rationale: A change in vital signs may be a late sign of increased intracranial pressure. Trends include increasing temperature and blood pressure and decreasing pulse and respirations. Respiratory irregularities also may occur.
Test-Taking Strategy: Focus on the subject, signs of increased intracranial pressure. If you remember that the temperature rises, you are able to eliminate options 3 and 4. If you know that the client becomes bradycardic, or know that the blood pressure rises, you are able to select the correct option.
Level of Cognitive Ability: Analyzing
Client Needs: Physiological Integrity
Integrated Process: Nursing Process—Assessment
Content Area: Adult Health: Neurological
Health Problem: Adult Health: Neurological: Head injury/trauma
Priority Concepts: Clinical Judgment; Intracranial Regulation
Reference: Lewis et al. (2017), pp. 1318-1319.

706. *Answer:* 4
Rationale: Activities that increase intrathoracic and intraabdominal pressures cause an indirect elevation of the intracranial pressure. Some of these activities include isometric exercises, Valsalva's maneuver, coughing, sneezing, and blowing the nose. Exhaling during activities such as repositioning or pulling up in bed opens the glottis, which prevents intrathoracic pressure from rising.
Test-Taking Strategy: Focus on the subject, preventing elevations in intracranial pressure. Evaluate each option in terms of the tension it puts on the body. Doing so will help you eliminate each incorrect option systematically.
Level of Cognitive Ability: Evaluating
Client Needs: Physiological Integrity
Integrated Process: Nursing Process—Evaluation
Content Area: Adult Health: Neurological
Health Problem: Adult Health: Neurological: Head injury/trauma
Priority Concepts: Client Education; Intracranial Regulation
Reference: Ignatavicius, Workman, Rebar (2018), pp. 936-937.

707. *Answer:* 4
Rationale: Leakage of cerebrospinal fluid (CSF) from the ears or nose may accompany basilar skull fracture. CSF can be distinguished from other body fluids, because the drainage will separate into bloody and yellow concentric rings on dressing material, called a *halo sign*. The fluid also tests positive for glucose.

Test-Taking Strategy: Focus on the subject, the characteristics of CSF. Recall that CSF contains glucose, whereas other secretions, such as mucus, do not. Knowing that CSF separates into rings also will help you answer this question.
Level of Cognitive Ability: Analyzing
Client Needs: Physiological Integrity
Integrated Process: Nursing Process—Assessment
Content Area: Adult Health: Neurological
Health Problem: Adult Health: Neurological: Head injury/trauma
Priority Concepts: Clinical Judgment; Intracranial Regulation
Reference: Ignatavicius, Workman, Rebar (2018), p. 946.

708. *Answer:* 1, 2, 4
Rationale: The most frequent cause of autonomic dysreflexia is a distended bladder. Straight catheterization should be done every 4 to 6 hours (catheterization every 12 hours is too infrequent), and urinary catheters should be checked frequently to prevent kinks in the tubing. Constipation and fecal impaction are other causes, so maintaining bowel regularity is important. Ensuring a bowel movement once a week is much too infrequent. Other causes include stimulation of the skin from tactile, thermal, or painful stimuli. The nurse administers care to minimize risk in these areas.
Test-Taking Strategy: Focus on the subject, preventing autonomic dysreflexia. Remember that autonomic dysreflexia is caused by noxious stimuli to the bowel, bladder, or skin. With this in mind, you can eliminate easily each of the incorrect options.
Level of Cognitive Ability: Analyzing
Client Needs: Physiological Integrity
Integrated Process: Nursing Process—Implementation
Content Area: Adult Health: Neurological
Health Problem: Adult Health: Neurological: Spinal cord injury
Priority Concepts: Caregiving; Intracranial Regulation
Reference: Lewis et al. (2017), p. 1431.

709. *Answer:* 3
Rationale: Resolution of spinal shock is occurring when there is return of reflexes (especially flexors to noxious cutaneous stimuli), a state of hyper-reflexia rather than flaccidity, and reflex emptying of the bladder.
Test-Taking Strategy: Recall that spinal shock is characterized by the loss of movement of skeletal muscles, loss of bowel or bladder wall function, and depressed reflex action. Return of any of these indicates that spinal shock is beginning to resolve. Note that options 1, 2, and 4 are comparable or alike, indicating the presence of reflexes.
Level of Cognitive Ability: Evaluating
Client Needs: Physiological Integrity
Integrated Process: Nursing Process—Evaluation
Content Area: Adult Health: Neurological
Health Problem: Adult Health: Neurological: Spinal cord injury
Priority Concepts: Evidence; Intracranial Regulation
Reference: Lewis et al. (2017), p. 1420.

710. *Answer:* 1, 3, 4
Rationale: Nursing actions during a seizure include providing for privacy, loosening restrictive clothing, removing the pillow and raising padded side rails in the bed, and placing the client on 1 side with the head flexed forward, if possible, to allow the tongue to fall forward and facilitate drainage. The limbs are never restrained because the strong muscle contractions could cause the client harm. If the client is not in bed when seizure activity begins, the nurse lowers the client to the floor, if possible; protects the head from injury; and moves furniture that may injure the client.
Test-Taking Strategy: Focus on the subject, interventions during a seizure. Think about ethical and legal issues to eliminate option 5. Next, evaluate this question from the perspective of causing possible harm. No harm can come to the client from any of the options except for restraining the limbs. Remember to avoid restraints.
Level of Cognitive Ability: Applying
Client Needs: Physiological Integrity
Integrated Process: Nursing Process—Implementation
Content Area: Adult Health: Neurological
Health Problem: Adult Health: Neurological: Seizure disorder/epilepsy
Priority Concepts: Intracranial Regulation; Safety
Reference: Ignatavicius, Workman, Rebar (2018), p. 878.

711. *Answer:* 1, 2, 4
Rationale: Hemiparesis is a weakness of one side of the body that may occur after a stroke. It involves weakness of the face and tongue, arm, and leg on one side. These clients are also aphasic, unable to discriminate words and letters. They are generally very cautious and get anxious when attempting a new task. Complete bilateral paralysis does not occur in hemiparesis. The client with right-sided hemiparesis has weakness of the right arm and leg and needs assistance with feeding, bathing, and ambulating.
Test-Taking Strategy: Focus on the subject, right-sided hemiparesis. Recalling that hemiparesis indicates weakness on one side of the body and focusing on the subject will direct you to the correct option. Also, noting the word *complete* in the question will assist you in answering correctly.
Level of Cognitive Ability: Analyzing
Client Needs: Physiological Integrity
Integrated Process: Nursing Process—Assessment
Content Area: Adult Health: Neurological
Health Problem: Adult Health: Neurological: Stroke
Priority Concepts: Functional Ability; Intracranial Regulation
Reference: Lewis et al. (2017), p. 1345.

712. *Answer:* 4
Rationale: Homonymous hemianopsia is loss of half of the visual field. The client with homonymous hemianopsia should have objects placed in the intact field of vision, and the nurse also should approach the client from the intact side. The nurse instructs the client to scan the environment to overcome the visual deficit and does client teaching from within the intact field of vision. The nurse encourages the use of personal eyeglasses, if they are available.
Test-Taking Strategy: Focus on the subject, homonymous hemianopsia. Eliminate options 2 and 3 first because they are comparable or alike. Recalling the definition of homonymous hemianopsia will direct you easily to the correct option.
Level of Cognitive Ability: Evaluating
Client Needs: Safe and Effective Care Environment
Integrated Process: Nursing Process—Evaluation
Content Area: Adult Health: Neurological
Health Problem: Adult Health: Neurological: Stroke

Priority Concepts: Intracranial Regulation; Safety
Reference: Lewis et al. (2017), p. 1362.

713. *Answer:* 4
Rationale: Clients are evaluated as coping successfully with lifestyle changes after a stroke if they make appropriate lifestyle alterations, use the assistance of others, and have appropriate social interactions. Options 1 and 2 are not adaptive behaviors; option 3 indicates a not yet successful attempt to adapt.
Test-Taking Strategy: Note the strategic word, *most*, and focus on the subject, indications that a client who has had a stroke is adapting most successfully. Options 1 and 2 are behaviors that may be expected in the client with a stroke, but they are not adaptive responses. Instead, they are a result of the insult to the brain. Options 3 and 4 indicate that the client is trying to adapt, but the correct option has the best outcome.
Level of Cognitive Ability: Evaluating
Client Needs: Psychosocial Integrity
Integrated Process: Nursing Process—Evaluation
Content Area: Adult Health: Neurological
Health Problem: Adult Health: Neurological: Stroke
Priority Concepts: Coping; Functional Ability
Reference: Ignatavicius, Workman, Rebar (2018), pp. 939-940.

714. *Answer:* 1
Rationale: Clients with myasthenia gravis are taught to space out activities over the day to conserve energy and restore muscle strength. Taking medications correctly to maintain blood levels that are not too low or too high is important. Muscle-strengthening exercises are not helpful and can fatigue the client. Overeating is a cause of exacerbation of symptoms, as is exposure to heat, crowds, erratic sleep habits, and emotional stress.
Test-Taking Strategy: Note the strategic words, *most effective*. Recalling that the common causes of myasthenic and cholinergic crises are undermedication and overmedication, respectively, will assist you in eliminating each of the incorrect options. No other option would prevent both of those complications.
Level of Cognitive Ability: Evaluating
Client Needs: Physiological Integrity
Integrated Process: Nursing Process—Evaluation
Content Area: Adult Health: Neurological
Health Problem: Adult Health: Neurological: Myasthenia gravis
Priority Concepts: Client Education; Safety
Reference: Ignatavicius, Workman, Rebar (2018), pp. 920, 922.

715. *Answer:* 4
Rationale: The client with Parkinson's disease should be instructed regarding safety measures in the home. The client should use her or his walker as support to get to the bathroom because of bradykinesia. The client should sit down to put on pants and shoes to prevent falling. The client should exercise every day in the morning when energy levels are highest. The client should have all loose rugs in the home removed to prevent falling.
Test-Taking Strategy: Note the strategic words, *need for further teaching*. These words indicate a negative event query and the need to select the incorrect client statement as the answer. Recall that clients with Parkinson's disease are at risk for falls.
Level of Cognitive Ability: Evaluating
Client Needs: Physiological Integrity
Integrated Process: Teaching and Learning
Content Area: Adult Health: Neurological
Health Problem: Adult Health: Neurological: Parkinson's disease
Priority Concepts: Client Education; Safety
Reference: Ignatavicius, Workman, Rebar (2018), pp. 872-873.
www.michaeljfox.org
www.parkinson.org

716. *Answer:* 4
Rationale: Facial pain can be minimized by using cotton pads to wash the face and using room temperature water. The client should chew on the unaffected side of the mouth, eat a soft diet, and take in foods and beverages at room temperature. If brushing the teeth triggers pain, an oral rinse after meals may be helpful instead.
Test-Taking Strategy: Note the strategic words, *needs further teaching*. These words indicate a negative event query and ask you to select an option that is incorrect. Recall that the pain of trigeminal neuralgia is triggered by mechanical or thermal stimuli. Very hot or cold foods are likely to trigger the pain, not relieve it.
Level of Cognitive Ability: Evaluating
Client Needs: Physiological Integrity
Integrated Process: Teaching and Learning
Content Area: Adult Health: Neurological
Health Problem: Adult Health: Neurological: Trigeminal neuralgia
Priority Concepts: Client Education; Pain
Reference: Lewis et al. (2017), pp. 1437-1438.

717. *Answer:* 4
Rationale: Guillain-Barré syndrome is a clinical syndrome of unknown origin that involves cranial and peripheral nerves. Many clients report a history of respiratory or gastrointestinal infection in the 1 to 4 weeks before the onset of neurological deficits. On occasion, the syndrome can be triggered by vaccination or surgery.
Test-Taking Strategy: Note the strategic word, *most*. Use knowledge regarding the causes related to this disorder. Remember that a recent history of respiratory or gastrointestinal infection is a predisposing factor.
Level of Cognitive Ability: Analyzing
Client Needs: Physiological Integrity
Integrated Process: Nursing Process—Assessment
Content Area: Adult Health: Neurological
Health Problem: Adult Health: Neurological: Guillain-Barré syndrome
Priority Concepts: Clinical Judgment; Infection
Reference: Lewis et al. (2017), pp. 1440-1441.

718. *Answer:* 3
Rationale: The client with Guillain-Barré syndrome experiences fear and anxiety from the ascending paralysis and sudden onset of the disorder. The nurse can alleviate these fears by providing accurate information about the client's condition, giving expert care and positive feedback to the client, and encouraging relaxation and distraction. The family can become involved with selected care activities and provide diversion for the client as well.
Test-Taking Strategy: Focus on the subject, helping a client cope with illness. Option 1 should be eliminated first, because

it is not practical to think that the client would want full control over all care decisions. The client who is paralyzed cannot participate in active range of motion, which eliminates option 2. From the remaining options, the correct option is more beneficial in helping the client cope.
Level of Cognitive Ability: Applying
Client Needs: Psychosocial Integrity
Integrated Process: Caring
Content Area: Adult Health: Neurological
Health Problem: Adult Health: Neurological: Guillain-Barré syndrome
Priority Concepts: Caregiving; Coping
Reference: Ignatavicius, Workman, Rebar (2018), pp. 916-917.

719. *Answer:* 2
Rationale: The limbic system is responsible for feelings (affect) and emotions. Calculation ability and knowledge of current events relate to function of the frontal lobe. The cerebral hemispheres, with specific regional functions, control orientation. Recall of recent events is controlled by the hippocampus.
Test-Taking Strategy: Focus on the **subject**, neurological deficit of the limbic system. It is necessary to recall that the limbic system is responsible for feelings and emotions to direct you to the correct option.
Level of Cognitive Ability: Applying
Client Needs: Psychosocial Integrity
Integrated Process: Nursing Process—Assessment
Content Area: Adult Health: Neurological
Health Problem: N/A
Priority Concepts: Clinical Judgment; Intracranial Regulation
Reference: Lewis et al. (2017), pp. 79, 1298.

720. *Answer:* 1, 2, 5, 6
Rationale: Seizure precautions may vary from agency to agency, but they generally have some common features. Usually, an airway, oxygen, and suctioning equipment are kept available at the bedside. The side rails of the bed are padded, and the bed is kept in the lowest position. The client has an intravenous access in place to have a readily accessible route if antiseizure medications must be administered, and as part of the routine assessment the nurse should be checking patency of the catheter. The use of padded tongue blades is highly controversial, and they should not be kept at the bedside. Forcing a tongue blade into the mouth during a seizure more likely will harm the client who bites down during seizure activity. Risks include blocking the airway from improper placement, chipping the client's teeth, and subsequent risk of aspirating tooth fragments. If the client has an aura before the seizure, it may give the nurse enough time to place an oral airway before seizure activity begins.
Test-Taking Strategy: Focus on the **subject**, seizure precautions. Evaluate this question from the perspective of causing possible harm. No harm can come to the client from any of the options except for placing the bed in the high position and using a tongue blade.
Level of Cognitive Ability: Analyzing
Client Needs: Safe and Effective Care Environment
Integrated Process: Nursing Process—Planning
Content Area: Adult Health: Neurological
Health Problem: Adult Health: Neurological: Seizure disorder/epilepsy
Priority Concepts: Intracranial Regulation; Safety
Reference: Lewis et al. (2017), p. 1378.

721. *Answer:* 3
Rationale: Signs of meningeal irritation compatible with meningitis include nuchal rigidity, a positive Brudzinski's sign, and positive Kernig's sign. Nuchal rigidity is characterized by a stiff neck and soreness, which is especially noticeable when the neck is flexed. Kernig's sign is positive when the client feels pain and spasm of the hamstring muscles when the leg is fully flexed at the knee and hip. Brudzinski's sign is positive when the client flexes the hips and knees in response to the nurse gently flexing the head and neck onto the chest. A Glasgow Coma Scale score of 15 is a perfect score and indicates that the client is awake and alert, with no neurological deficits.
Test-Taking Strategy: Focus on the **subject**, a client's diagnosis of meningitis. You can eliminate options 1, 2, and 4 because they are **comparable or alike** and are normal findings.
Level of Cognitive Ability: Analyzing
Client Needs: Physiological Integrity
Integrated Process: Nursing Process—Assessment
Content Area: Adult Health: Neurological
Health Problem: Adult Health: Neurological: Inflammation/infections
Priority Concepts: Clinical Judgment; Intracranial Regulation
Reference: Heuther & McCance (2017), pp. 408-409.

722. *Answer:* 2
Rationale: The halo device alters balance and can cause fatigue because of its weight. The client should cleanse the skin daily under the vest to protect the skin from ulceration and should avoid the use of powder or lotions. The liner should be changed if odor becomes a problem. The client should have food cut into small pieces to facilitate chewing and use a straw for drinking. Pin care is done as instructed. The client cannot drive at all, because the device impairs the range of vision.
Test-Taking Strategy: Note the **strategic words**, *needs further clarification*. These words indicate a **negative event query** and ask you to select an option that is incorrect. Visualize this device to answer correctly. The inability to turn the head without turning the torso would contraindicate driving. Also note the **closed-ended word** "only" in the correct option.
Level of Cognitive Ability: Evaluating
Client Needs: Physiological Integrity
Integrated Process: Teaching and Learning
Content Area: Adult Health: Neurological
Health Problem: Adult Health: Neurological: Spinal cord injury
Priority Concepts: Client Education; Safety
Reference: Lewis et al. (2017), pp. 1427-1428.

723. *Answer:* 4
Rationale: The client with Guillain-Barré syndrome is at risk for respiratory failure because of ascending paralysis. An intubation tray should be available for use. Another complication of this syndrome is cardiac dysrhythmias, which necessitates the use of electrocardiographic monitoring. Because the client is immobilized, the nurse should assess for deep vein thrombosis and pulmonary embolism routinely. Although items in the incorrect options may be used in care, they are not the most essential items from the options provided.

Test-Taking Strategy: Note the strategic words, *most essential.* With an ascending paralysis, the client is at risk for involvement of respiratory muscles and subsequent respiratory failure. The correct option is the only one that includes an intubation tray, which would be needed if the client's status deteriorated to needing intubation and mechanical ventilation. This option most directly addresses the airway.
Level of Cognitive Ability: Applying
Client Needs: Physiological Integrity
Integrated Process: Nursing Process—Implementation
Content Area: Adult Health: Neurological
Health Problem: Adult Health: Neurological: Guillain-Barré syndrome
Priority Concepts: Clinical Judgment; Safety
Reference: Lewis et al. (2017), pp. 1440-1441.

CHAPTER 59

Neurological Medications

PRIORITY CONCEPTS Intracranial Regulation; Pain

I. Antimyasthenic Medications

A. Description

1. Antimyasthenic medications, also called *anticholinesterase medications,* relieve muscle weakness associated with myasthenia gravis by blocking acetylcholine breakdown at the neuromuscular junction.

2. These are used to treat or diagnose myasthenia gravis or to distinguish cholinergic crisis from myasthenic crisis.

3. Neostigmine bromide and pyridostigmine are used to control myasthenic symptoms.

4. Edrophonium is used to diagnose myasthenia gravis and to distinguish cholinergic crisis from myasthenic crisis.

B. Medications (Box 59-1)

C. Side and adverse effects: Cholinergic crisis (Box 59-2)

D. Interventions

1. Assess neuromuscular status, including reflexes, muscle strength, and gait.

2. Monitor the client for signs and symptoms of medication overdose (cholinergic crisis) and underdose (myasthenic crisis).

3. Instruct the client to take medications on time to maintain therapeutic blood level, thus preventing weakness, because weakness can impair the client's ability to breathe and swallow.

4. Instruct the client to take the medication with a small amount of food to prevent gastrointestinal symptoms.

5. Instruct the client to eat a meal 45 to 60 minutes after taking medications to decrease the risk for aspiration.

6. Instruct the client to wear a MedicAlert bracelet.

7. Note that antimyasthenic therapy is lifelong therapy.

8. Evaluate for medication effectiveness, which is based on the improvement of neuromuscular symptoms or strength without cholinergic signs and symptoms.

9. When administering edrophonium, have emergency resuscitation equipment on hand and atropine sulfate available for cholinergic crisis.

E. Edrophonium test (may be known as the *Tensilon test*)

1. Edrophonium is injected intravenously.

2. The edrophonium test can cause bronchospasm, laryngospasm, hypotension, bradycardia, and cardiac arrest.

3. Atropine sulfate is the antidote for overdose.

4. Diagnosis of myasthenia gravis: Most myasthenic clients will show a significant improvement in muscle tone within 30 to 60 seconds after injection, and the muscle improvement lasts 4 to 5 minutes.

5. The edrophonium test is also used to diagnose cholinergic crisis (overdose with anticholinesterase) or myasthenic crisis (undermedication).

a. In cholinergic crisis, muscle tone does not improve after the administration of edrophonium, and muscle twitching may be noted around the eyes and face.

b. An edrophonium injection temporarily worsens the condition when a client is in cholinergic crisis (negative edrophonium test).

c. An edrophonium injection temporarily improves the condition when the client is in myasthenic crisis (positive edrophonium test).

II. Multiple Sclerosis Medications

A. Description

1. Medication therapy is aimed at modifying the disease, treating acute episodes or relapses, and treating symptoms.

2. Disease-modifying medications decrease the frequency and severity of relapses, reduce brain lesions, increase future functional capability, and increase overall quality of life.

3. The 2 main groups of disease-modifying medications are immunomodulators and immunosuppressants (Box 59-3).

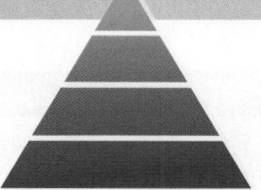

BOX 59-1 Antimyasthenic Medications

- Edrophonium chloride
- Neostigmine bromide
- Pyridostigmine

BOX 59-2 Signs of Cholinergic Crisis

- Abdominal cramps
- Nausea, vomiting, and diarrhea
- Pupillary miosis
- Hypotension and dizziness
- Increased bronchial secretions
- Increased tearing and salivation
- Increased perspiration
- Bronchospasm, wheezing, and bradycardia

BOX 59-3 Medications for Multiple Sclerosis

Immunomodulators

Interferons (β-1a, 1b, peginterferon β-1a)
Glatiramer acetate
Fingolimod
Teriflunomide
Dimethyl fumarate

Immunosuppressant

Mitoxantrone

Monoclonal antibodies

Natalizumab
Alemtuzumab
Ocrelizumab

Potassium channel blockers

Dalfampridine (used to improve walking)

4. Treating acute episodes usually consists of giving a high-dose glucocorticoid intravenously to suppress inflammation or giving gamma globulin intravenously.
5. Treating symptoms of multiple sclerosis can be done with a variety of medications, and the medication can be changed if unfavorable effects occur.
6. Box 59-4 identifies medications commonly used to treat symptoms.

B. Side and adverse effects
1. Immunomodulators: Flu-like reactions, hepatotoxicity, myelosuppression, injection site reactions, depression, and neutralizing antibodies.
2. Immunosuppressants: Myelosuppression, cardiotoxicity, fetal harm, reversible hair loss, injury to the gastrointestinal mucosa, nausea and vomiting, and menstrual irregularities.

BOX 59-4 Medications to Treat Symptoms of Multiple Sclerosis

- Bladder and bowel dysfunction: psyllium, docusate
- Fatigue: amantadine, modafinil
- Depression: fluoxetine, sertraline
- Sexual dysfunction: sildenafil, vardenafil
- Neuropathic pain: gabapentin, carbamazepine

Adapted from Burchum JR, Rosenthal LD: *Lehne's pharmacology for nursing care*, ed 9. St. Louis, 2016, Elsevier.

III. Antiparkinsonian Medications

A. Description
1. Antiparkinsonian medications restore the balance of the neurotransmitters acetylcholine and dopamine in the central nervous system (CNS), decreasing the signs and symptoms of Parkinson's disease to maximize the client's functional abilities.
2. These medications include the dopaminergics, which stimulate the dopamine receptors; the anticholinergics, which block the cholinergic receptors; and the catechol-*O*-methyltransferase inhibitors, which inhibit the metabolism of dopamine in the periphery.

B. Dopaminergic medications
1. Description
   a. Dopaminergic medications stimulate the dopamine receptors and increase the amount of dopamine available in the CNS or enhance neurotransmission of dopamine.
   b. Dopaminergic medications are contraindicated in clients with cardiac, renal, or psychiatric disorders.

⚠ Carbidopa-levodopa taken with a monoamine oxidase inhibitor antidepressant can cause a hypertensive crisis.

2. Medications (Box 59-5)
3. Side and adverse effects
   a. Dyskinesia
   b. Involuntary body movements
   c. Chest pain
   d. Nausea and vomiting
   e. Urinary retention
   f. Constipation
   g. Sleep disturbances, insomnia, or periods of sedation
   h. Orthostatic hypotension and dizziness
   i. Confusion
   j. Mood changes, especially depression
   k. Hallucinations
   l. Dry mouth
4. Interventions
   a. Assess vital signs.
   b. Assess for risk of injury.
   c. Instruct the client to take the medication with food if nausea or vomiting occurs.

BOX 59-5 Medications to Treat Parkinson's Disease

Medications Affecting the Amount of Dopamine

- Amantadine
- Apomorphine
- Bromocriptine
- Carbidopa-levodopa
- Pramipexole
- Rasagiline
- Ropinirole
- Rotigotine
- Selegiline hydrochloride

Anticholinergics

- Benztropine mesylate
- Trihexyphenidyl hydrochloride

Catechol-*O*-Methyltransferase (COMT) Inhibitors

- Carbidopa/levodopa/entacapone
- Entacapone
- Tolcapone

d. Assess for signs and symptoms of parkinsonism such as rigidity, tremors, akinesia, bradykinesia, a stooped forward posture, shuffling gait, and masked facies.
e. Monitor for signs of dyskinesia.
f. Instruct the client to report side and adverse effects and symptoms of dyskinesia.
g. Monitor the client for improvement in signs and symptoms of parkinsonism.
h. Instruct the client to change positions slowly to minimize orthostatic hypotension.
i. Instruct the client not to discontinue the medication abruptly.
j. Instruct the client to avoid alcohol.
k. Inform the client that urine or perspiration may be discolored and that this is harmless but may stain the clothing.
l. Advise the client with diabetes mellitus that glucose testing should not be done by urine testing, because the results will not be reliable.
m. Instruct the client taking carbidopa-levodopa to divide the total daily prescribed protein intake among all meals of the day; high-protein diets interfere with medication availability to the CNS.
n. When administering carbidopa-levodopa, instruct the client to avoid excessive vitamin B_6 intake to prevent medication reactions.

C. Anticholinergic medications
1. Description
a. Anticholinergic medications block the cholinergic receptors in the CNS, thereby suppressing acetylcholine activity.
b. They reduce the tremors and drooling but have a minimal effect on the bradykinesia, rigidity, and balance abnormalities.
c. They are contraindicated in clients with glaucoma.
d. The client with chronic obstructive lung disease can develop dry, thick mucous secretions.
2. Medications (see Box 59-5)
3. Side and adverse effects
a. Blurred vision
b. Dryness of the nose, mouth, throat, and respiratory secretions
c. Increased pulse rate, palpitations, and dysrhythmias
d. Constipation
e. Urinary retention
f. Restlessness, confusion, depression, and hallucinations
g. Photophobia
4. Interventions
a. Monitor vital signs.
b. Assess for risk of injury.
c. Monitor the client for improvement in signs and symptoms.
d. Assess the client's bowel and urinary function and monitor for urinary retention, constipation, and paralytic ileus.
e. Monitor for involuntary movements.
f. Encourage the client to avoid alcohol, smoking, caffeine, and acetylsalicylic acid to decrease gastric acidity.
g. Instruct the client to consult with a primary health care provider (PHCP) before taking any nonprescription medications.
h. Instruct the client to minimize dry mouth by increasing fluid intake and using ice chips, hard candy, or gum.
i. Instruct the client to prevent constipation by increasing fluids and fiber in the diet.
j. Instruct the client to use sunglasses in direct sunlight because of possible photophobia.
k. Instruct the client to have routine eye examinations to assess intraocular pressure.

If an anticholinergic medication is discontinued abruptly, the signs and symptoms of parkinsonism, such as rigidity, tremors, akinesia, bradykinesia, stooped forward posture, shuffling gait, and masked facies, may be intensified.

IV. Antiseizure Medications

A. Description
1. Antiseizure medications are used to depress abnormal neuronal discharges and prevent the spread of seizures to adjacent neurons.

2. These should be used with caution in clients taking anticoagulants, acetylsalicylic acid, sulfonamides, cimetidine, and antipsychotic medications.
3. Absorption is decreased with the use of antacids, calcium preparations, and antineoplastic medications.

B. Interventions for clients on antiseizure medications
1. Initiate seizure precautions.
2. Monitor urinary output.
3. Monitor liver and renal function tests and medication blood serum levels (Table 59-1).
4. Monitor for signs of medication toxicity, which would include CNS depression, ataxia, nausea, vomiting, drowsiness, dizziness, restlessness, and visual disturbances.
5. If a seizure occurs, assess seizure activity, including location and duration (see Chapter 58 for management of seizures).
6. Protect the client from hazards in the environment during a seizure.

C. Client education (Box 59-6)

D. Hydantoins: Fosphenytoin, phenytoin
1. Hydantoins are used to treat partial and generalized tonic-clonic seizures.
2. Phenytoin is also used to treat dysrhythmias.
3. Side and adverse effects
   a. Gingival hyperplasia (reddened gums that bleed easily)
   b. Slurred speech
   c. Confusion
   d. Sedation and drowsiness
   e. Nausea and vomiting
   f. Blurred vision and nystagmus
   g. Headaches
   h. Blood dyscrasias: Decreased platelet count and decreased white blood cell count
   i. Elevated blood glucose level
4. Interventions
   a. Alopecia or hirsutism
   b. Rash or pruritus
   c. Tube feedings may interfere with the absorption of the enteral form of phenytoin and diminish the effectiveness of the medication; therefore, feedings should be scheduled as far as possible away from the time of phenytoin administration.
   d. Monitor therapeutic serum levels to assess for toxicity.
   e. Monitor for signs of toxicity.
   f. When administering phenytoin intravenously, dilute in normal saline, because dextrose causes the medication to precipitate.
   g. When administering phenytoin intravenously, infuse with an inline filter and no faster than 25 to 50 mg/minute; otherwise, a decrease in blood pressure and cardiac dysrhythmias could occur.
   h. Assess for ataxia (staggering gait).
   i. Instruct the client to consult with the PHCP before taking other medications to ensure compatibility with anticonvulsants.

TABLE 59-1 Common Antiseizure Medications

Medication	Therapeutic Serum Range
Carbamazepine	3-14 mcg/mL (13-59 mcmol/L)
Clonazepam	20-80 ng/mL (0.02-0.08 mcg/L)
Divalproex	50-100 mcg/mL (347-693 mcmol/L)
Ethosuximide	40-100 mcg/mL (283-708 mcmol/L)
Lorazepam	50-240 ng/mL (156-746 nmol/L)
Phenobarbital	15-40 mcg/mL (65-172 mcmol/L)
Phenytoin	10-20 mcg/mL (40-79 mcmol/L)

BOX 59-6 Client Education: Antiseizure Medications

- Take the prescribed medication in the prescribed dose and frequency.
- Take with food to decrease gastrointestinal irritation, but avoid milk and antacids, which impair absorption.
- If taking liquid medication, shake well before ingesting.
- Do not discontinue the medications.
- Avoid alcohol.
- Avoid over-the-counter medications.
- Wear a MedicAlert bracelet.
- Use caution when performing activities that require alertness.
- Maintain good oral hygiene and use a soft toothbrush.
- Maintain preventive dental checkups.
- Maintain follow-up health care visits with periodic blood studies related to determining toxicity.
- Monitor serum glucose levels (diabetes mellitus).
- Urine may be a harmless pink-red or red-brown color.
- Report symptoms of sore throat, bruising, and nosebleeds, which may indicate a blood dyscrasia.
- Inform the primary health care provider if side and adverse effects occur, such as bleeding gums, nausea, vomiting, blurred vision, slurred speech, rash, or dizziness.

Phenytoin must be given slowly to prevent hypotension and cardiac dysrhythmias. Also, it may decrease the effectiveness of some birth control pills and may cause teratogenic effects, if taken during pregnancy.

E. Barbiturates: Amobarbital, phenobarbital
1. Barbiturates are used for tonic-clonic seizures and acute episodes of seizures caused by status epilepticus.
2. Barbiturates also may be used as adjuncts to anesthesia.
3. Side and adverse effects
   a. Sedation, ataxia, and dizziness during initial treatment

b. Mood changes
c. Hypotension
d. Respiratory depression
e. Tolerance to the medication

F. Benzodiazepines: Clonazepam, clorazepate, diazepam, lorazepam
1. Benzodiazepines are used to treat absence seizures.
2. Diazepam and lorazepam are used to treat status epilepticus, anxiety, and skeletal muscle spasms.
3. Clorazepate is used as adjunctive therapy for partial seizures.
4. Side and adverse effects
a. Sedation, drowsiness, dizziness, blurred vision
b. For intravenous injection, administer slowly to prevent bradycardia.
c. Medication tolerance and dependency
d. Blood dyscrasias: Decreased platelet count and decreased white blood cell count
e. Hepatotoxicity

Flumazenil reverses the effects of benzodiazepines. It should not be administered to clients with increased intracranial pressure or status epilepticus who were treated with benzodiazepines, because these problems may recur with reversal.

G. Succinimides: Ethosuximide, methsuximide
1. Succinimides are used to treat absence seizures.
2. Side and adverse effects
a. Anorexia, nausea, vomiting
b. Blood dyscrasias

H. Valproates: Valproic acid, divalproex sodium
1. Valproates are used to treat tonic-clonic, partial, and myoclonic seizures.
2. Side and adverse effects
a. Transient nausea, vomiting, and indigestion
b. Sedation, drowsiness, and dizziness
c. Pancreatitis
d. Blood dyscrasias: Decreased platelet count and decreased white blood cell count
e. Hepatotoxicity

I. Iminostilbenes
1. Iminostilbenes are used to treat seizure disorders that have not responded to other anticonvulsants (Box 59-7).
2. Iminostilbenes are also used to treat trigeminal neuralgia.
3. Side and adverse effects
a. Drowsiness
b. Dizziness
c. Nausea and vomiting, dry mouth
d. Constipation or diarrhea
e. Rash
f. Visual abnormalities
g. Blood dyscrasias, agranulocytosis
h. Headache

BOX 59-7 Other Antiseizure Medications

- Carbamazepine
- Gabapentin
- Lacosamide
- Lamotrigine
- Levetiracetam
- Oxcarbazepine
- Pregabalin
- Tiagabine
- Topiramate
- Zonisamide
- Vigabatrin

V. Central Nervous System Stimulants

A. Description
1. Amphetamines and caffeine stimulate the cerebral cortex of the brain (Box 59-8).
2. Amphetamines have a high potential for abuse.
3. Analeptics and caffeine act on the brainstem and medulla to stimulate respiration.
4. Anorexiants act on the cerebral cortex and hypothalamus to suppress appetite (Box 59-9).
5. CNS stimulants are used to treat narcolepsy and attention-deficit/hyperactivity disorders and are used as adjunctive therapy for exogenous obesity.

B. Side and adverse effects
1. Irritability
2. Restlessness
3. Tremors
4. Insomnia
5. Heart palpitations

BOX 59-8 Amphetamines

- Amphetamine sulfate
- Amphetamine/dextroamphetamine
- Atomoxetine
- Dextroamphetamine sulfate
- Dexmethylphenidate
- Lisdexamfetamine
- Methylphenidate hydrochloride

BOX 59-9 Anorexiants

- Benzphetamine hydrochloride
- Bupropion/naltrexone
- Diethylpropion
- Lorcaserin
- Orlistat
- Phendimetrazine
- Phentermine hydrochloride
- Phentermine/topiramate

6. Tachycardia and dysrhythmias
7. Hypertension
8. Dry mouth
9. Anorexia and weight loss
10. Abdominal cramping
11. Diarrhea or constipation
12. Hepatic failure
13. Psychoses
14. Impotence
15. Dependence and tolerance

C. Interventions
1. Monitor vital signs.
2. Assess mental status.
3. Document the degree of inattention, impulsivity, hyperactivity, and periods of sleepiness.
4. Assess height, weight, and growth of the child.
5. Monitor complete blood count and white blood cell and platelet counts before and during therapy.
6. Monitor for side and adverse effects.
7. Monitor sleep patterns.
8. Monitor for withdrawal symptoms such as nausea, vomiting, weakness, and headache.
9. Instruct the client to take the medication before meals.
10. Instruct the client to avoid foods and beverages containing caffeine to prevent additional stimulation.
11. Instruct the client not to chew or crush long-acting forms of the medications.
12. Instruct the client to read labels on over-the-counter products, because they may contain caffeine.
13. Instruct the client to avoid alcohol.
14. Instruct the client not to discontinue the medication abruptly (can produce extreme fatigue and depression).
15. Instruct the client to take the last daily dose of the CNS stimulant at least 6 hours before bedtime to prevent insomnia.
16. Monitor for medication dependence and abuse with amphetamines.
17. If a child is taking a CNS stimulant, instruct the parents to notify the school nurse.
18. Monitor for calming effects of CNS stimulants within 3 to 4 weeks on children with attention-deficit/hyperactivity disorder.
19. Monitor growth in the child on long-term therapy with methylphenidate or other medications to treat attention-deficit/hyperactivity disorder.

VI. Nonopioid Analgesics

A. Nonsteroidal antiinflammatory drugs (NSAIDs; Box 59-10)

BOX 59-10 Nonopioid Analgesics

Acetaminophen
- Acetaminophen

Aspirin
- Aspirin (acetylsalicylic acid; ASA)
- Aspirin (acetylsalicylic acid), buffered

Nonsteroidal Antiinflammatory Drugs
- Ibuprofen
- Naproxen

Cyclooxygenase-2 (COX-2) Inhibitor
- Celecoxib

Other Nonsteroidal Antiinflammatory Drugs
- Diclofenac
- Diflunisal
- Etodolac
- Indomethacin
- Ketoprofen
- Ketorolac
- Meclofenamate
- Mefenamic acid
- Meloxicam
- Nabumetone
- Piroxicam
- Sulindac
- Tolmetin

1. Description
a. NSAIDs are acetylsalicylic acid and acetylsalicylic acid–like medications that inhibit the synthesis of prostaglandins.
b. The medications act as an analgesic to relieve pain, an antipyretic to reduce body temperature, and an anticoagulant to inhibit platelet aggregation.
c. NSAIDs are used to relieve inflammation and pain and to treat rheumatoid arthritis, bursitis, tendinitis, osteoarthritis, and acute gout.
d. NSAIDs are contraindicated in clients with hypersensitivity or liver or renal disease.
e. Clients taking anticoagulants should not take acetylsalicylic acid or NSAIDs.
f. Acetylsalicylic acid and an NSAID should not be taken together, because aspirin decreases the blood level and effectiveness of the NSAID and can increase the risk of bleeding.
g. NSAIDs can increase the effects of warfarin, sulfonamides, cephalosporins, and phenytoin.
h. Hypoglycemia can result if ibuprofen is taken with insulin or an oral hypoglycemic medication.
i. A high risk of toxicity exists if ibuprofen is taken concurrently with calcium channel blockers.

Adolescents and children with flu symptoms, viral illnesses, and varicella should not take acetylsalicylic acid because of the risk of Reye's syndrome.

2. Side and adverse effects (Box 59-11)
3. Interventions
   a. Assess client for allergies.
   b. Obtain a medication history on the client.
   c. Assess for history of gastric upset or bleeding or liver or renal disease.
   d. Assess the client for gastrointestinal upset during medication administration.
   e. Monitor for edema.
   f. Monitor the serum salicylate (acetylsalicylic acid) level when the client is taking high doses.
   g. Monitor for signs of bleeding such as tarry stools, bleeding gums, petechiae, ecchymosis, and purpura.
   h. Instruct the client to take the medication with milk, or food.
   i. An enteric-coated or buffered form of acetylsalicylic acid can be taken to decrease gastric distress.
   j. Instruct the client that enteric-coated tablets cannot be crushed or broken.
   k. Clients taking acetylsalicylic acid should sit upright for 20 to 30 minutes after taking the dose.

BOX 59-11 Side and Adverse Effects of Acetylsalicylic Acid and Nonsteroidal Antiinflammatory Drugs

Acetylsalicylic acid
- Allergic reactions (anaphylaxis, laryngeal edema)
- Bleeding (anemia, hemolysis, increased bleeding time)
- Dizziness
- Drowsiness
- Flushing
- Gastrointestinal symptoms (distress, heartburn, nausea, vomiting)
- Headaches
- Decreased renal function
- Tinnitus
- Visual changes

Nonsteroidal Antiinflammatory Drugs
- Dysrhythmias
- Blood dyscrasias
- Cardiovascular thrombotic events
- Dizziness
- Gastric irritation
- Hepatotoxicity
- Hypotension
- Pruritus
- Decreased renal function
- Sodium and water retention
- Tinnitus

   l. Advise the client to inform other health care professionals if they are taking high doses of acetylsalicylic acid.
   m. Note that acetylsalicylic acid should be discontinued 3 to 7 days before surgery as prescribed to reduce the risk of bleeding.
   n. Instruct the client to avoid alcoholic beverages.

B. Acetaminophen
1. Description
   a. Acetaminophen inhibits prostaglandin synthesis.
   b. Used to decrease pain and fever
   c. Should not be taken if liver dysfunction exists
2. Side and adverse effects
   a. Anorexia, nausea, vomiting
   b. Rash
   c. Hypoglycemia
   d. Oliguria
   e. Hepatotoxicity
3. Interventions
   a. Monitor vital signs.
   b. Assess client for history of liver and renal dysfunction, alcoholism, and malnutrition.
   c. Monitor for hepatic damage, which includes nausea, vomiting, diarrhea, and abdominal pain.
   d. Monitor liver enzyme test results.
   e. Instruct the client that self-medication should not be used longer than 10 days for an adult and 5 days for a child.
   f. Note that the antidote for acetaminophen is acetylcysteine.
   g. Evaluate for the effectiveness of the medication.

Acetaminophen is contraindicated in clients with hepatic or renal disease, alcoholism, and/or hypersensitivity.

VII. Opioid Analgesics

A. Description
1. Opioid analgesics suppress pain impulses but can suppress respiration and coughing by acting on the respiratory and cough center in the medulla of the brainstem.
2. They can produce euphoria and sedation and can cause physical dependence.
3. Used for relief of mild, moderate, or severe pain

B. Medications (Box 59-12)
1. Codeine
   a. Codeine also is an effective cough suppressant at low doses.
   b. It can cause constipation.
2. Hydromorphone
   a. Hydromorphone can decrease respirations.
   b. It can cause constipation.

BOX 59-12 Opioid Analgesics

- Acetaminophen; hydrocodone*
- Buprenorphine
- Butorphanol tartrate
- Codeine
- Fentanyl
- Hydrocodone
- Hydromorphone
- Levorphanol
- Meperidine
- Methadone
- Morphine
- Nalbuphine
- Oxycodone
- Oxycodone; acetaminophen
- Oxymorphone
- Pentazocine
- Remifentanil
- Sufentanil
- Tapentadol
- Tramadol

* Combinations of opioids with acetaminophen or nonsteroidal antiinflammatory drug analgesics may be used.

3. Meperidine
   a. Meperidine can cause hypotension, dizziness, and urinary retention.
   b. Is not commonly prescribed but may be used for acute pain and as a preoperative medication
   c. May lead to **increased intracranial pressure (ICP)** in clients with head injuries
   d. Contraindicated in clients with head injuries and increased ICP, respiratory disorders, hypotension, shock, and severe hepatic and renal disease and in clients taking monoamine oxidase inhibitors
   e. Should not be taken with alcohol or a sedative-hypnotic, because it may increase the CNS depression
   f. Should be used cautiously in children and adults with a seizure disorder or a history of seizures, because it decreases the seizure threshold
4. Morphine
   a. Morphine can cause respiratory depression, orthostatic hypotension, and constipation.
   b. May cause nausea and vomiting because of increased vestibular sensitivity
   c. Used for acute pain caused by myocardial infarction or cancer, for dyspnea caused by pulmonary edema, for surgery, and as a preoperative medication
   d. Is contraindicated in clients with severe respiratory disorders; head injuries; increased ICP; severe renal, hepatic, or pulmonary disease; or seizure activity
   e. Morphine is used with caution in clients with blood loss or shock.

⚠ Respiratory depression is the priority concern with morphine.

5. Nalbuphine is preferable for treating the pain of a myocardial infarction because it reduces the oxygen needs of the heart without reducing blood pressure.
6. Methadone
   a. Dilute doses of oral concentrate with at least 90 mL of water.
   b. Dilute dispersible tablets in at least 120 mL of water, orange juice, or acidic fruit beverage.
   c. Methadone is used as a replacement medication for opiate dependence and to facilitate withdrawal.
7. Hydrocodone/homatropine frequently is used for cough suppression.

C. Interventions for opioid analgesics
1. Monitor vital signs.
2. Assess the client thoroughly before administering pain medication.
3. Initiate nursing measures such as massage, distraction, deep breathing and relaxation exercises, the application of heat or cold as prescribed, and providing care and comfort along with administering the opioid analgesic.
4. Administer medications 30 to 60 minutes before painful activities.
5. Monitor respiratory rate and, if the rate is less than 12 breaths per minute in an adult, withhold the medication unless ventilatory support is being provided or the client has terminal disease (as prescribed).
6. Monitor pulse and, if bradycardia develops, withhold the dose and notify the PHCP.
7. Monitor blood pressure for hypotension.
8. Auscultate breath sounds, because opioid analgesics suppress the cough reflex.
9. Encourage activities such as turning, deep breathing, and incentive spirometry to prevent atelectasis and pneumonia.
10. Monitor level of consciousness.
11. Initiate safety precautions such as a night light and supervised ambulation.
12. Monitor intake and output.
13. Assess for urinary retention.
14. Instruct the client to take oral doses with milk or a snack to reduce gastric irritation.
15. Instruct the client to avoid alcohol.
16. Instruct the client to avoid activities that require alertness.
17. Assess bowel function for constipation, abdominal distention, and decreased peristalsis.
18. Evaluate the effectiveness of medication.
19. Have an opioid antagonist, oxygen, and resuscitation equipment available.

D. Morphine
 1. Side and adverse effects
  a. Respiratory depression
  b. Orthostatic hypotension
  c. Urinary retention
  d. Nausea and vomiting
  e. Constipation
  f. Sedation, confusion, and hallucinations
  g. Cough suppression
  h. Reduction in pupillary size
  i. Miosis
 2. Interventions
  a. Have naloxone available for overdose.
  b. Assess vital signs and level of consciousness.
  c. Compare rate and depth of respirations to baseline.
  d. Withhold the medication if the respiratory rate is less than 12 breaths per minute; respirations of less than 10 breaths per minute can indicate respiratory distress.
  e. Monitor urinary output, which should be at least 30 mL/hr.
  f. Monitor bowel sounds for decreased peristalsis, because constipation can occur.
  g. Monitor for pupil changes because pinpoint pupils can indicate morphine overdose.
  h. Avoid alcohol or CNS depressants because they can cause respiratory depression.
  i. Instruct the client to report dizziness or difficulty breathing.
  j. If taking sustained-release morphine, the client may need short-acting opioid doses for breakthrough pain.
  k. To administer morphine intravenously, dilute in at least 5 mL of sterile water (per agency procedure) for injection and administer slowly over 4 to 5 minutes.
  l. Explain to the client and family about administration and the side and adverse effects of the medication.

E. Meperidine
 1. Side and adverse effects
  a. Respiratory depression
  b. Hypotension and dizziness
  c. Tachycardia
  d. Drowsiness and confusion
  e. Constipation
  f. Urinary retention
  g. Nausea and vomiting
  h. Seizures
  i. Tremors
 2. Interventions
  a. Monitor vital signs.
  b. Monitor for respiratory depression and hypotension.
  c. Have naloxone available for overdose.
  d. Monitor for urinary retention.
  e. Monitor bowel sounds and for constipation.
  f. To administer meperidine intravenously, dilute in at least 5 mL of sterile water or normal saline (per agency procedure) for injection and administer the dose over 4 to 5 minutes.

VIII. Opioid Antagonists

A. Opioid antagonists (Box 59-13) are used to treat respiratory depression from opioid overdose.

B. Interventions
 1. Monitor blood pressure, pulse, and respiratory rate every 5 minutes initially, tapering to every 15 minutes, and then every 30 minutes until the client is stable.
 2. Place the client on a cardiac monitor and monitor cardiac rhythm.
 3. Auscultate breath sounds.
 4. Have resuscitation equipment available.
 5. Do not leave the client unattended.
 6. Monitor the client closely for several hours, because when the effects of the antagonist wear off, the client may again display signs of opioid overdose.

IX. Osmotic Diuretics

A. Description
 1. Osmotic diuretics increase osmotic pressure of the glomerular filtrate, inhibiting reabsorption of water and electrolytes.
 2. They are used for oliguria and to prevent kidney failure, decrease ICP, and decrease intraocular pressure in clients with narrow-angle glaucoma.
 3. Mannitol is used with chemotherapy to induce diuresis.

B. Side and adverse effects
 1. Fluid and electrolyte imbalances
 2. Pulmonary edema from the rapid shifts of fluid
 3. Nausea and vomiting
 4. Headache
 5. Tachycardia from the rapid fluid loss
 6. Hyponatremia and dehydration

C. Interventions
 1. Monitor vital signs.
 2. Monitor weight.
 3. Monitor urine output.
 4. Monitor electrolyte levels.
 5. Monitor lungs and heart sounds for signs of pulmonary edema.

BOX 59-13 Opioid Antagonists

- Alvimopan
- Methylnaltrexone
- Naldemedine
- Naloxone
- Naltrexone
- Naloxegol

6. Monitor for signs of dehydration.
7. Monitor neurological status.
8. Monitor for increased intraocular pressure.
9. Assess for signs of decreasing ICP if appropriate.
10. Change the client's position slowly to prevent orthostatic hypotension.
11. Monitor for crystallization in the vial of mannitol before administering the medication; if crystallization is noted, do not administer the medication from that vial.

PRACTICE QUESTIONS

724. Carbidopa-levodopa is prescribed for a client with Parkinson's disease. The nurse monitors the client for side and adverse effects of the medication. Which finding indicates that the client is experiencing an adverse effect?

1. Pruritus
2. Tachycardia
3. Hypertension
4. Impaired voluntary movements

725. The home health nurse visits a client who is taking phenytoin for control of seizures. During the assessment, the nurse notes that the client is taking birth control pills. Which information should the nurse include in the teaching plan?

1. Pregnancy must be avoided while taking phenytoin.
2. The client may stop the medication if it is causing severe gastrointestinal effects.
3. There is the potential of decreased effectiveness of birth control pills while taking phenytoin.
4. There is the increased risk of thrombophlebitis while taking phenytoin and birth control pills together.

726. The nurse is caring for a client in the emergency department who has been diagnosed with Bell's palsy. The client has been taking acetaminophen, and acetaminophen overdose is suspected. Which antidote should the nurse prepare for administration if prescribed?

1. Pentostatin
2. Auranofin
3. Fludarabine
4. Acetylcysteine

727. Meperidine has been prescribed for a client to treat pain. Which side and adverse effects should the nurse monitor for? **Select all that apply.**

- ☐ 1. Diarrhea
- ☐ 2. Tremors
- ☐ 3. Drowsiness
- ☐ 4. Hypotension
- ☐ 5. Urinary frequency
- ☐ 6. Increased respiratory rate

728. A client is taking the prescribed dose of phenytoin to control seizures. Results of a phenytoin blood level study reveal a level of 35 mcg/mL (140 mcmol/L). Which finding would be expected as a result of this laboratory result?

1. Hypotension
2. Tachycardia
3. Slurred speech
4. No abnormal finding

729. The client arrives at the emergency department complaining of back spasms. The client states, "I have been taking 2 to 3 aspirin every 4 hours for the last week, and it hasn't helped my back." Since acetylsalicylic acid intoxication is suspected, the nurse should assess the client for which manifestation?

1. Tinnitus
2. Diarrhea
3. Constipation
4. Photosensitivity

730. A client with trigeminal neuralgia is being treated with carbamazepine, 400 mg orally daily. Which value indicates that the client is experiencing an adverse effect to the medication?

1. Sodium level, 140 mEq/L (140 mmol/L)
2. Uric acid level, 4.0 mg/dL (240 mcmol/L)
3. White blood cell count, 3000 mm^3 (3.0×10^9/L)
4. Blood urea nitrogen level, 10 mg/dL (3.6 mmol/L)

731. The nurse is caring for a client with chronic back pain. Codeine has been prescribed for the client. Specific to this medication, which intervention should the nurse include in the plan of care while the client is taking this medication?

1. Monitor radial pulse.
2. Monitor bowel activity.
3. Monitor apical heart rate.
4. Monitor peripheral pulses.

732. The nurse has given medication instructions to a client receiving phenytoin. Which statement indicates that the client has an adequate understanding of the instructions?

1. "Alcohol is not contraindicated while taking this medication."
2. "Good oral hygiene is needed, including brushing and flossing."
3. "The medication dose may be self-adjusted, depending on side effects."
4. "The morning dose of the medication should be taken before a serum medication level is drawn."

733. A client with myasthenia gravis has become increasingly weaker. The primary health care provider prepares to identify whether the client is reacting to an overdose of the medication (cholinergic crisis) or an

increasing severity of the disease (myasthenic crisis). An injection of edrophonium is administered. Which finding would indicate that the client is in cholinergic crisis?
1. No change in the condition
2. Complaints of muscle spasms
3. An improvement of the weakness
4. A temporary worsening of the condition

734. A client with trigeminal neuralgia tells the nurse that acetaminophen is taken daily for the relief of generalized discomfort. Which laboratory value would indicate toxicity associated with the medication?
1. Sodium level of 140 mEq/L (140 mmol/L)
2. Platelet count of 400,000 mm^3 (400×10^9/L)
3. Prothrombin time of 12 seconds (12 seconds)
4. Direct bilirubin level of 2 mg/dL (34 mcmol/L)

ANSWERS

724. *Answer:* 4
Rationale: Dyskinesia and impaired voluntary movements may occur with high carbidopa-levodopa dosages. Nausea, anorexia, dizziness, orthostatic hypotension, bradycardia, and akinesia are frequent side effects of the medication.
Test-Taking Strategy: Focus on the subject, an adverse effect. Options 2 and 3 are comparable or alike and are cardiac-related options, so these options can be eliminated first. Next, focus on the client's diagnosis and select the correct option over option 1 because it relates to the neurological system.
Level of Cognitive Ability: Analyzing
Client Needs: Physiological Integrity
Integrated Process: Nursing Process—Assessment
Content Area: Pharmacology: Neurological Medications: Antiparkinsonian
Health Problem: Adult Health: Neurological: Parkinson's disease
Priority Concepts: Clinical Judgment; Safety
Reference: Lewis et al. (2017), p. 1390.

725. *Answer:* 3
Rationale: Phenytoin enhances the rate of estrogen metabolism, which can decrease the effectiveness of some birth control pills. Options 1, 2, and 4 are inappropriate instructions. Pregnancy does not need to be "avoided" while taking phenytoin; however, because phenytoin may cause some risk to the fetus (Pregnancy Category D medication), consultation with the primary health care provider should be done if pregnancy is considered. Telling a client that there is an increased risk of thrombophlebitis is incorrect and inappropriate and could cause anxiety in the client. A client should not be instructed to stop antiseizure medication.
Test-Taking Strategy: Focus on the subject, teaching points for the client taking phenytoin. Eliminate option 1 because of the words *must be avoided*. Use general medication guidelines to eliminate option 2; the client would not be advised to stop a medication. For the remaining options, eliminate option 4, as it will cause anxiety in the client.
Level of Cognitive Ability: Applying
Client Needs: Physiological Integrity
Integrated Process: Teaching and Learning
Content Area: Pharmacology: Neurological Medications: Anticonvulsants
Health Problem: Adult Health: Neurological: Seizure disorder/epilepsy
Priority Concepts: Client Education; Safety
Reference: Burchum, Rosenthal (2016), pp. 236-237.

726. *Answer:* 4
Rationale: The antidote for acetaminophen is acetylcysteine. The normal therapeutic serum level of acetaminophen is 10 to 20 mcg/mL. A toxic level is higher than 50 mcg/mL, and levels higher than 200 mcg/mL 4 hours after ingestion indicates that there is risk for liver damage. Auranofin is a gold preparation that may be used to treat rheumatoid arthritis. Pentostatin and fludarabine are antineoplastic agents.
Test-Taking Strategy: Eliminate options 1 and 3 first because they are comparable or alike (antineoplastic agents). Recalling that auranofin is used to treat rheumatoid arthritis will direct you to the correct option.
Level of Cognitive Ability: Applying
Client Needs: Physiological Integrity
Integrated Process: Nursing Process—Planning
Content Area: Pharmacology: Pain Medications: Nonopioid analgesics
Health Problem: Adult Health: Neurological: Bell's palsy
Priority Concepts: Clinical Judgment; Safety
Reference: Hodgson, Kizior (2018), p. 11.

727. *Answer:* 2, 3, 4
Rationale: Meperidine is an opioid analgesic. Side and adverse effects include respiratory depression, drowsiness, hypotension, constipation, urinary retention, nausea, vomiting, and tremors. Meperidine is not commonly prescribed but may be used for acute pain and as a preoperative medication.
Test-Taking Strategy: Note the subject, side and adverse effects of meperidine. Recalling that this medication is an opioid analgesic and recalling the effects of an opioid analgesic will assist you in identifying the correct options.
Level of Cognitive Ability: Analyzing
Client Needs: Physiological Integrity
Integrated Process: Nursing Process—Assessment
Content Area: Pharmacology: Pain Medications: Opioid analgesics
Health Problem: Adult Health: Neurological: Pain
Priority Concepts: Pain; Safety
Reference: Lewis et al. (2017), pp. 114-115.

728. *Answer:* 3
Rationale: The therapeutic phenytoin level is 10 to 20 mcg/mL (40 to 79 mcmol/L). At a level higher than 20 mcg/mL, involuntary movements of the eyeballs (nystagmus) occur. At a level higher than 30 mcg/mL (120 mcmol/L), ataxia and slurred speech occur.
Test-Taking Strategy: Focus on the subject, a phenytoin level of 35 mcg/mL. Use knowledge regarding the therapeutic phenytoin level. From this point, you must know the symptoms

that would be noted in the client when the phenytoin level is 35 mcg/mL. Remember that ataxia and slurred speech occur with levels higher than 30 mcg/mL.
Level of Cognitive Ability: Analyzing
Client Needs: Physiological Integrity
Integrated Process: Nursing Process—Assessment
Content Area: Pharmacology: Neurological Medications: Anticonvulsants
Health Problem: Adult Health: Neurological: Seizure disorder/epilepsy
Priority Concepts: Intracranial Regulation; Safety
Reference: Hodgson, Kizior (2018), pp. 937-938.

729. *Answer:* 1
Rationale: Mild intoxication with acetylsalicylic acid is called *salicylism* and is experienced commonly when the daily dosage is higher than 4 g. Tinnitus (ringing in the ears) is the most frequent effect noted with intoxication. Hyperventilation may occur, because salicylate stimulates the respiratory center. Fever may result, because salicylate interferes with the metabolic pathways coupling oxygen consumption and heat production. Options 2, 3, and 4 are not associated specifically with toxicity.
Test-Taking Strategy: Focus on the **subject**, acetylsalicylic acid intoxication. Options 2 and 3 relate to gastrointestinal symptoms, are **comparable or alike**, and are eliminated first. From the remaining options, you must know that tinnitus occurs.
Level of Cognitive Ability: Analyzing
Client Needs: Physiological Integrity
Integrated Process: Nursing Process—Assessment
Content Area: Pharmacology: Pain Medications: Nonopioid analgesics
Health Problem: Adult Health: Neurological: Pain
Priority Concepts: Clinical Judgment; Safety
Reference: Lilley et al. (2017), pp. 696-697.

730. *Answer:* 3
Rationale: Carbamazepine, classified as an antiseizure medication, is used to treat nerve pain. Adverse effects of carbamazepine appear as blood dyscrasias, including aplastic anemia, agranulocytosis, thrombocytopenia, and leukopenia; cardiovascular disturbances, including thrombophlebitis and dysrhythmias; and dermatological effects. The low white blood cell count reflects agranulocytosis. The laboratory values in options 1, 2, and 4 are normal values.
Test-Taking Strategy: Focus on the **subject**, an adverse effect of carbamazepine. If you are familiar with normal laboratory values, you will note that the only option that indicates an abnormal value is the correct option.
Level of Cognitive Ability: Analyzing
Client Needs: Physiological Integrity
Integrated Process: Nursing Process—Analysis
Content Area: Pharmacology: Neurological Medications: Antiseizure
Health Problem: Adult Health: Neurological: Pain
Priority Concepts: Clinical Judgment; Cellular Regulation
Reference: Hodgson, Kizior (2018), p. 186.

731. *Answer:* 2
Rationale: While the client is taking codeine, the nurse would monitor vital signs and assess for hypotension. The nurse also should increase fluid intake, palpate the bladder for urinary retention, auscultate bowel sounds, and monitor the pattern of daily bowel activity and stool consistency, because the medication causes constipation. The nurse should monitor respiratory status and initiate deep breathing and coughing exercises. In addition, the nurse monitors the effectiveness of the pain medication.
Test-Taking Strategy: Focus on the **subject**, a specific nursing consideration related to codeine. Eliminate options 1, 3, and 4 because they are **comparable or alike**. In addition, relate *c*odeine with *c*onstipation.
Level of Cognitive Ability: Analyzing
Client Needs: Physiological Integrity
Integrated Process: Nursing Process—Planning
Content Area: Pharmacology: Neurological Medications: Opioid analgesics
Health Problem: Adult Health: Neurological: Pain
Priority Concepts: Clinical Judgment; Pain
Reference: Hodgson, Kizior (2018), pp. 277-279.

732. *Answer:* 2
Rationale: Typical antiseizure medication instructions include taking the prescribed daily dosage to keep the blood level of the medication constant and having a sample drawn for serum medication level determination before taking the morning dose. The client is taught not to stop the medication abruptly, to avoid alcohol, to check with a primary health care provider before taking over-the-counter medications, to avoid activities in which alertness and coordination are required until medication effects are known, to provide good oral hygiene, and to obtain regular dental care. The client should also wear a MedicAlert bracelet.
Test-Taking Strategy: Focus on the **subject**, an understanding of medication instructions for phenytoin. Using knowledge of general principles related to medication administration will assist you in eliminating options 1 and 3. From the remaining options, recall that medications generally are not taken just before determining therapeutic serum levels, because the results would be artificially high. This leaves oral hygiene as the correct option because of the risk of gingival hyperplasia.
Level of Cognitive Ability: Evaluating
Client Needs: Physiological Integrity
Integrated Process: Nursing Process—Evaluation
Content Area: Pharmacology: Neurological Medications: Anticonvulsants
Health Problem: Adult Health: Neurological Medications: Seizure disorder/epilepsy
Priority Concepts: Client Education; Safety
Reference: Hodgson, Kizior (2018), pp. 937-938.

733. *Answer:* 4
Rationale: An edrophonium injection makes the client in cholinergic crisis temporarily worse. An improvement in the weakness indicates myasthenia crisis. Muscle spasms are not associated with this test.
Test-Taking Strategy: Focus on the **subject**, results of an edrophonium test. Recalling that a cholinergic crisis indicates an overdose of medication, it seems reasonable that a worsening of the condition will occur when additional medication is administered.
Level of Cognitive Ability: Analyzing
Client Needs: Physiological Integrity
Integrated Process: Nursing Process—Analysis

Content Area: Adult Health: Neurological
Health Problem: Adult Health: Neurological: Myasthenia gravis
Priority Concepts: Clinical Judgment; Mobility
Reference: Gahart, Nazareno, Ortega (2017), pp. 494-495.

734. *Answer:* 4

Rationale: In adults, overdose of acetaminophen causes liver damage. The correct option is an indicator of liver function and is the only option that indicates an abnormal laboratory value. The normal direct bilirubin level is 0.1 to 0.3 mg/dL (1.7 to 5.1 mcmol/L). The normal sodium level is 135 to 145 mEq/L (135 to 145 mmol/L). The normal prothrombin time is 11 to 12.5 seconds (11 to 12.5 seconds). The normal platelet count is 150,000 to 400,000 mm^3 (150 to 400×10^9/L).

Test-Taking Strategy: Focus on the **subject**, acetaminophen toxicity. Knowledge that acetaminophen causes liver damage and knowledge of normal laboratory results will assist you in answering this question. The correct option is the only abnormal value. Also, of all the options, the bilirubin level is the laboratory value most directly related to liver function.
Level of Cognitive Ability: Analyzing
Client Needs: Physiological Integrity
Integrated Process: Nursing Process—Analysis
Content Area: Pharmacology: Pain Medications: Nonopioid analgesics
Health Problem: Adult Health: Neurological: Trigeminal neuralgia
Priority Concepts: Clinical Judgment; Cellular Regulation
Reference: Ignatavicius, Workman, Rebar (2018), p. 55.

UNIT XVI

Musculoskeletal Problems of the Adult Client

Pyramid to Success

The Pyramid to Success focuses on the emergency care for a client who sustains a fracture or other musculoskeletal injury, monitoring for complications, and carrying out interventions if complications occur. Nursing care related to casts and traction is emphasized. Skill related to instructing the client in the use of an assistive device such as a cane, walker, or crutches is a Pyramid Point. Pyramid Points also include postoperative care following hip surgery or amputation and care of the client with rheumatoid arthritis or osteoporosis. Focus on the points related to the psychosocial effects as a result of the musculoskeletal disorder, such as unexpected body image changes, and the appropriate and available support services needed for the client.

Client Needs: Learning Objectives

Safe and Effective Care Environment

Communicating with the interprofessional health care team
Ensuring that informed consent is obtained for treatments and procedures
Establishing priorities
Handling hazardous and infectious materials safely
Maintaining asepsis related to wounds
Maintaining confidentiality
Maintaining standard and other precautions
Preventing accidents and injuries
Providing physical therapy and occupational therapy referrals
Upholding client rights

Health Promotion and Maintenance

Performing physical assessment related to the musculoskeletal system
Preventing diseases that occur as a result of the aging process
Promoting health related to diet and activity
Providing home care instructions regarding care related to a musculoskeletal disorder
Reinforcing the importance of prescribed therapy

Psychosocial Integrity

Assessing available support systems and use of community resources
Assessing the client's ability to cope with mobility limitations and restrictions, feelings of isolation, and loss of independence
Considering cultural, religious, and spiritual influences
Discussing situational role changes as a result of the musculoskeletal disorder
Discussing unexpected body image changes as a result of injury or disease
Identifying sensory and perceptual alterations
Mobilizing coping mechanisms

Physiological Integrity

Identifying complications of procedures, injuries, or a fracture
Providing care following diagnostic testing and procedures and surgical interventions
Providing care related to casts and traction
Promoting normal elimination patterns
Promoting self-care measures
Providing emergency care for a fracture or other injury
Providing emergency care if complications following injuries or surgical interventions arise
Providing measures to promote comfort
Teaching about the use of assistive devices for mobility such as canes, walkers, and crutches
Teaching pharmacological therapy

CHAPTER 60

Musculoskeletal Problems

PRIORITY CONCEPTS Functional Ability; Mobility

I. Anatomy and Physiology

A. Skeleton
- **1.** Axial portion
  - **a.** Cranium
  - **b.** Vertebrae
  - **c.** Ribs
- **2.** Appendicular portion
  - **a.** Limbs
  - **b.** Shoulders
  - **c.** Hips

B. Types of bones: Long, short, flat, irregular
- **1.** Spongy bone
  - **a.** Spongy bone is located in the ends of long bones and the center of flat and irregular bones.
  - **b.** Spongy bone can withstand forces applied in many directions.
- **2.** Dense (compact) bone
  - **a.** Dense bone covers spongy bone.
  - **b.** Forms a cylinder around a central marrow cavity
  - **c.** Better able to withstand longitudinal forces than horizontal forces
- **3.** Characteristics of bones
  - **a.** Support and protect structures of the body
  - **b.** Provide attachments for muscles, tendons, and ligaments
  - **c.** Contain tissue in the central cavities, which aids in the formation of blood cells
  - **d.** Assist in regulating calcium and phosphate concentrations
- **4.** Bone growth
  - **a.** The length of bone growth results from ossification of the epiphyseal cartilage at the ends of bones; bone growth stops between the ages of 18 and 25 years.
  - **b.** The width of bone growth results from the activity of osteoblasts; it occurs throughout life but slows down with aging.

⚠ As aging occurs, bone resorption accelerates, decreasing bone mass and predisposing the client to injury.

C. Types of joints (Table 60-1)
- **1.** Characteristics of joints
  - **a.** Allow movement between bones
  - **b.** Formed where 2 bones join
  - **c.** Surfaces are covered with cartilage.
  - **d.** Enclosed in a capsule (synovial joints)
  - **e.** Contain a cavity filled with synovial fluid (synovial joints)
  - **f.** Ligaments hold the bone and joint in the correct position.
  - **g.** Articulation is the meeting point of 2 or more bones.
- **2.** Synovial fluid
  - **a.** Found in the synovial joint capsule
  - **b.** Formed by the synovial membrane, which lines the joint capsule
  - **c.** Lubricates the cartilage
  - **d.** Provides a cushion against shocks

D. Muscles
- **1.** Characteristics of muscles
  - **a.** Made up of bundles of muscle fibers
  - **b.** Provide the force to move bones
  - **c.** Assist in maintaining posture
  - **d.** Assist with heat production
- **2.** Process of contraction and relaxation
  - **a.** Muscle contraction and relaxation require large amounts of adenosine triphosphate.
  - **b.** Contraction also requires calcium, which functions as a catalyst.
  - **c.** Acetylcholine released by the motor end plate of the motor neuron initiates an action potential.
  - **d.** Acetylcholine is then destroyed by acetylcholinesterase.
  - **e.** Calcium is required for muscle fiber contraction and acts as a catalyst for the enzyme needed for the sliding-together action of actin and myosin.
  - **f.** Following contraction, adenosine triphosphate transports calcium out to allow actin and myosin to separate and allow the muscle to relax.

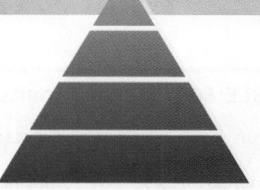

TABLE 60-1 Types of Joints

Type	Description
Amphiarthrosis	Cartilaginous joint Slightly movable
Diarthrosis	Synovial joint Ball-and-socket joint Permit free movement
Synarthrosis	Fibrous or fixed joint No movement associated with these joints

3. Skeletal muscles
   a. Skeletal muscles are attached to 2 bones by cartilaginous tendons called *enthuses* (the connective tissue between tendon or ligament and bone).
   b. The point of origin is the point of attachment that does not move.
   c. The point of insertion is the point of attachment that moves when the muscle contracts.
   d. Skeletal muscles act in groups.
   e. Prime movers contract to produce movement.
   f. Antagonists relax.
   g. Synergists contract to stabilize body movement.
   h. Nerves activate and control the muscles.

E. Bone healing
   1. Description: Bone union or healing is the process that occurs after the integrity of a bone is interrupted.
   2. Stages (Fig. 60-1)

II. Risk Factors Associated with Musculoskeletal Problems: See Box 60-1 for more information

III. Diagnostic Tests

A. Radiography and magnetic resonance imaging (MRI) (refer to Chapter 58 for information on MRI)
   1. Description: Radiography and MRI are commonly used procedures to diagnose problems of the musculoskeletal system.

BOX 60-1 Risk Factors Associated with Musculoskeletal Problems

- Autoimmune disorders
- Calcium deficiency
- Falls
- Hyperuricemia
- Infection
- Medications
- Metabolic disorders
- Neoplastic disorders
- Obesity
- Postmenopausal states
- Trauma and injury

   2. Interventions
      a. Handle injured areas carefully and support extremities above and below the joint.
      b. Administer analgesics as prescribed before the procedure, particularly if the client is in pain.
      c. Remove any radiopaque and metallic objects, such as jewelry.
      d. Ask the client if she is pregnant; MRI may be contraindicated in pregnancy.
      e. Shield the client's testes, ovaries, or pregnant abdomen.
      f. The client must lie still during a procedure.
      g. Inform the client that exposure to radiation from radiography is minimal and not dangerous.
      h. The health care provider wears a lead apron if staying in the room with the client having radiography.
      i. Complete the screening process per agency policy.

B. Arthrocentesis
   1. Description: Arthrocentesis is used to diagnose joint inflammation and infection.
      a. Arthrocentesis involves aspirating synovial fluid, blood, or pus via a needle inserted into a joint cavity.

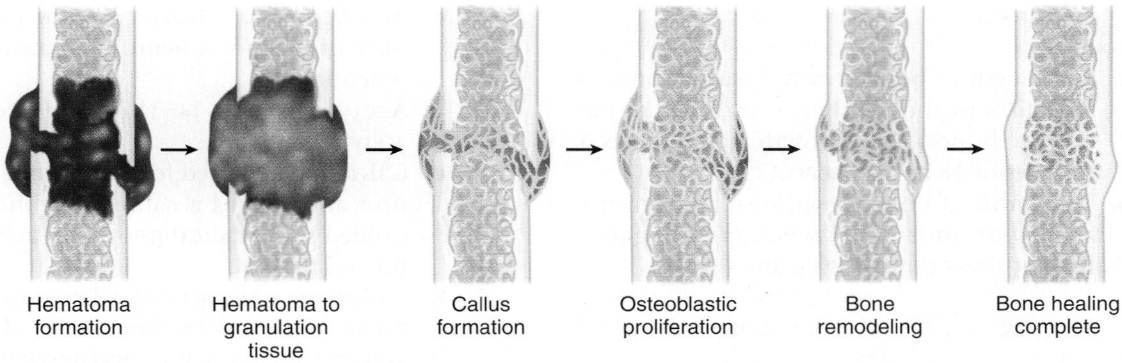

FIG. 60-1 The stages of bone healing.

b. Medication, such as corticosteroids, may be instilled into the joint if necessary to alleviate inflammation.
2. Interventions
a. Ensure that informed consent has been obtained.
b. Apply an elastic compression bandage postprocedure as prescribed.
c. Use ice to decrease pain and swelling.
d. Pain may worsen after aspirating fluid from the joint; analgesics may be prescribed.
e. Pain can continue for up to 2 days after administration of corticosteroids into a joint.
f. Instruct the client to rest the joint for 8 to 24 hours postprocedure.
g. Instruct the client to notify the primary health care provider (PHCP) if a fever or swelling of the joint occurs.

C. Arthroscopy
1. Description: Used to diagnose and treat acute and chronic problems of the joint.
a. Arthroscopy provides an endoscopic examination of various joints.
b. Articular cartilage abnormalities can be assessed, loose bodies removed, and the cartilage trimmed.
c. A biopsy may be performed during the procedure.
2. Interventions
a. Instruct the client to fast for 8 to 12 hours before the procedure.
b. Ensure that informed consent was obtained.
c. Administer pain medication as prescribed postprocedure.
d. Assess the neurovascular status of the affected extremity.
e. An elastic compression bandage should be worn postprocedure for 2 to 4 days as prescribed.
f. Instruct the client that walking with weight-bearing usually is permitted after sensation returns but to limit activity for 1 to 4 days as prescribed following the procedure.
g. Instruct the client to elevate the extremity as often as possible for 24 hours following the procedure and to place ice on the site to minimize swelling for 12 to 24 hours postprocedure.
h. Advise the client to notify the PHCP if fever or increased knee pain occurs or if edema continues for more than 3 days postprocedure.

D. Bone mineral density measurements
1. Dual-energy x-ray absorptiometry
a. Dual-energy x-ray absorptiometry measures the bone mass of the spine, wrist and hip bones, and total body.
b. Radiation exposure is minimal.
c. It is used to diagnose metabolic bone disease and to monitor changes in bone density with treatment.
d. Inform the client that the procedure is painless.
e. All metallic objects are removed before the test.
2. Quantitative ultrasound
a. Quantitative ultrasound evaluates strength, density, and elasticity of various bones, using ultrasound rather than radiation.
b. Inform the client that the procedure is painless.

E. Bone scan
1. Description: A bone scan is used to identify, evaluate, and stage bone cancer before and after treatment; it is also used to detect fractures.
a. Radioisotope is injected intravenously and will collect in areas that indicate abnormal bone metabolism and some fractures, if they exist.
b. The isotope is excreted in the urine and feces within 48 hours and is not harmful to others.
2. Interventions
a. Food and fluids may be withheld before the procedure.
b. Ensure that informed consent has been obtained.
c. Remove all jewelry and metal objects.
d. Following the injection of the radioisotope, the client must drink 32 oz of water (if not contraindicated) to promote renal filtering of the excess isotope.
e. From 1 to 3 hours after the injection, have the client void to clear excess isotope from the bladder before the scanning procedure is completed.
f. Inform the client of the need to lie supine during the procedure and that the procedure is not painful.
g. Monitor the injection site for redness and swelling.
h. Encourage oral fluid intake following the procedure.

! No special precautions are required after a bone scan, because only a minimal amount of radioactivity exists in the radioisotope used for the procedure.

F. Bone or muscle biopsy
1. Description: Biopsy may be done during surgery or through aspiration or punch or needle biopsy.
2. Interventions
a. Ensure that informed consent was obtained.
b. Monitor for bleeding, swelling, hematoma, or severe pain.

c. Elevate the site for 24 hours following the procedure to reduce edema.
d. Apply ice packs as prescribed following the procedure to prevent the development of a hematoma and to decrease site discomfort.
e. Monitor for signs of infection following the procedure.
f. Inform the client that mild to moderate discomfort is normal following the procedure.

G. Electromyography (EMG)
1. Description: EMG is used to evaluate muscle weakness.
   a. Electromyography measures electrical potential associated with skeletal muscle contractions.
   b. Needles are inserted into the muscle, and recordings of muscular electrical activity are traced on recording paper through an oscilloscope.
2. Interventions
   a. Ensure that informed consent was obtained.
   b. Instruct the client that the needle insertion is uncomfortable.
   c. Instruct the client not to take any stimulants or sedatives for 24 hours before the procedure.
   d. Inform the client that slight bruising may occur at the needle insertion sites.
   e. Mild analgesics can be used for the pain.

IV. Injuries

A. Strains
1. Strains are an excessive stretching of a muscle or tendon.
2. Management involves cold and heat applications, exercise with activity limitations, antiinflammatory medications, and muscle relaxants.
3. Surgical repair may be required for a severe strain (ruptured muscle or tendon).

B. Sprains
1. Sprains are an excessive stretching of a ligament, usually caused by a twisting motion, such as in a fall or stepping onto an uneven surface.
2. Sprains are characterized by pain and swelling.
3. Management involves rest, ice, a compression bandage, and elevation (RICE) to reduce swelling, as well as joint support. RICE is considered a first-aid treatment, rather than a cure for soft tissue injuries.
4. Casting may be required for moderate sprains to allow the tear to heal.
5. Surgery may be necessary for severe ligament damage.

C. Rotator cuff injuries
1. The musculotendinous or rotator cuff of the shoulder can sustain a tear, usually as a result of trauma.
2. Injury is characterized by shoulder pain and the inability to maintain abduction of the arm at the shoulder (drop arm test).
3. Management involves nonsteroidal antiinflammatory drugs (NSAIDs), physical therapy, sling support, and ice–heat applications.
4. Surgery may be required if medical management is unsuccessful or a complete tear is present.

V. Fractures

A. Description: A break in the continuity of the bone caused by trauma, twisting as a result of muscle spasm or indirect loss of leverage, or bone decalcification and disease that result in osteopenia.

B. Types of fractures (Box 60-2)

C. Assessment of a fracture of an extremity
1. Pain or tenderness over the involved area
2. Decrease or loss of muscular strength or function
3. Obvious deformity of the affected area
4. Crepitation, erythema, edema, or bruising
5. Muscle spasm and neurovascular impairment

D. Initial care of a fracture of an extremity
1. Immobilize the affected extremity with a cast or splint.
2. Assess the neurovascular status of the extremity.
3. Interventions for a fracture: **Reduction, fixation, traction, cast**

If a compound (open) fracture exists, splint the extremity and cover the wound with a sterile dressing.

BOX 60-2 Types of Fractures

Closed or Simple: Skin over the fractured area remains intact.
Comminuted: The bone is splintered or crushed, creating numerous fragments.
Complete: The bone is separated completely by a break into 2 parts.
Compression: A fractured bone is compressed by other bone.
Depressed: Bone fragments are driven inward.
Greenstick: One side of the bone is broken and the other is bent; these fractures occur most commonly in children.
Impacted: A part of the fractured bone is driven into another bone.
Incomplete: Fracture line does not extend through the full transverse width of the bone.
Oblique: The fracture line runs at an angle across the axis of the bone.
Open or Compound: The bone is exposed to air through a break in the skin, and soft tissue injury and infection are common.
Pathological: The fracture results from weakening of the bone structure by pathological processes such as neoplasia; also called *spontaneous fracture*.
Spiral: The break partially encircles bone.
Transverse: The bone is fractured straight across.

E. Reduction restores the bone to proper alignment.
  1. Closed reduction is a nonsurgical intervention performed by manual manipulation.
    a. Closed reduction may be performed under local or general anesthesia.
    b. A cast may be applied following reduction.
  2. Open reduction involves a surgical intervention; the fracture may be treated with internal fixation devices.

F. Fixation
  1. Internal fixation follows an open reduction (Fig. 60-2).
    a. Internal fixation involves the application of screws, plates, pins, wires, or intramedullary rods to hold the fragments in alignment.
    b. Internal fixation may involve the removal of damaged bone and replacement with a prosthesis.
    c. Internal fixation provides immediate bone stabilization.

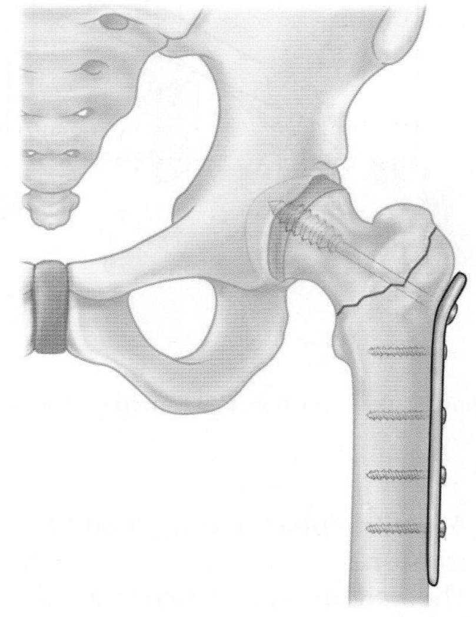

FIG. 60-2 A compression hip screw used for open reduction with internal fixation.

  2. External fixation is the use of an external frame to stabilize a fracture by attaching skeletal pins through bone fragments to a rigid external support (Fig. 60-3).
    a. External fixation provides more freedom of movement than with traction.
    b. Monitor pin stability and provide pin care to decrease infection risks.
    c. Risk of infection exists with both fixation methods.
    d. External fixation is commonly used when massive tissue trauma is present.

G. Traction (Fig. 60-4)
  1. Description
    a. Traction is the exertion of a pulling force applied in 2 directions to reduce and immobilize a fracture.
    b. It provides proper bone alignment and reduces muscle spasms.
  2. Interventions
    a. Maintain proper body alignment.
    b. Ensure that the weights hang freely and do not touch the floor.
    c. Do not remove or lift the weights without a PHCP's prescription.
    d. Ensure that pulleys are not obstructed and that ropes in the pulleys move freely.
    e. Place knots in the ropes to prevent slipping.
    f. Check the ropes for fraying.

H. Skeletal traction
  1. Description
    a. Traction is applied mechanically to the bone with pins, wires, or tongs.
    b. Typical weight for skeletal traction is 25 to 40 lb (11 to 18 kg).
  2. Interventions
    a. Monitor color, motion, and sensation of the affected extremity.
    b. Monitor the insertion sites for redness, swelling, drainage, or increased pain.
    c. Provide insertion site care as prescribed.

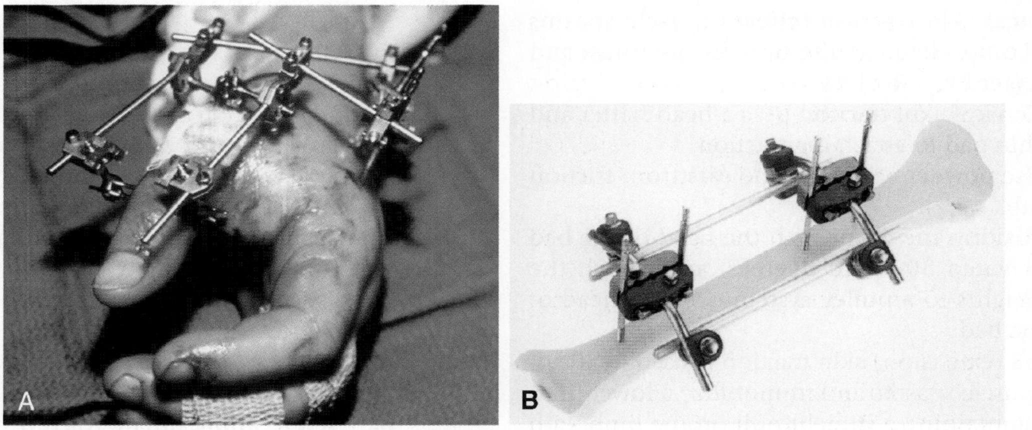

FIG. 60-3 External fixators. **A,** Mini-Hoffman system in use on hand. **B,** Hoffman II on the tibia (standard system). (From Lewis et al., 2011.)

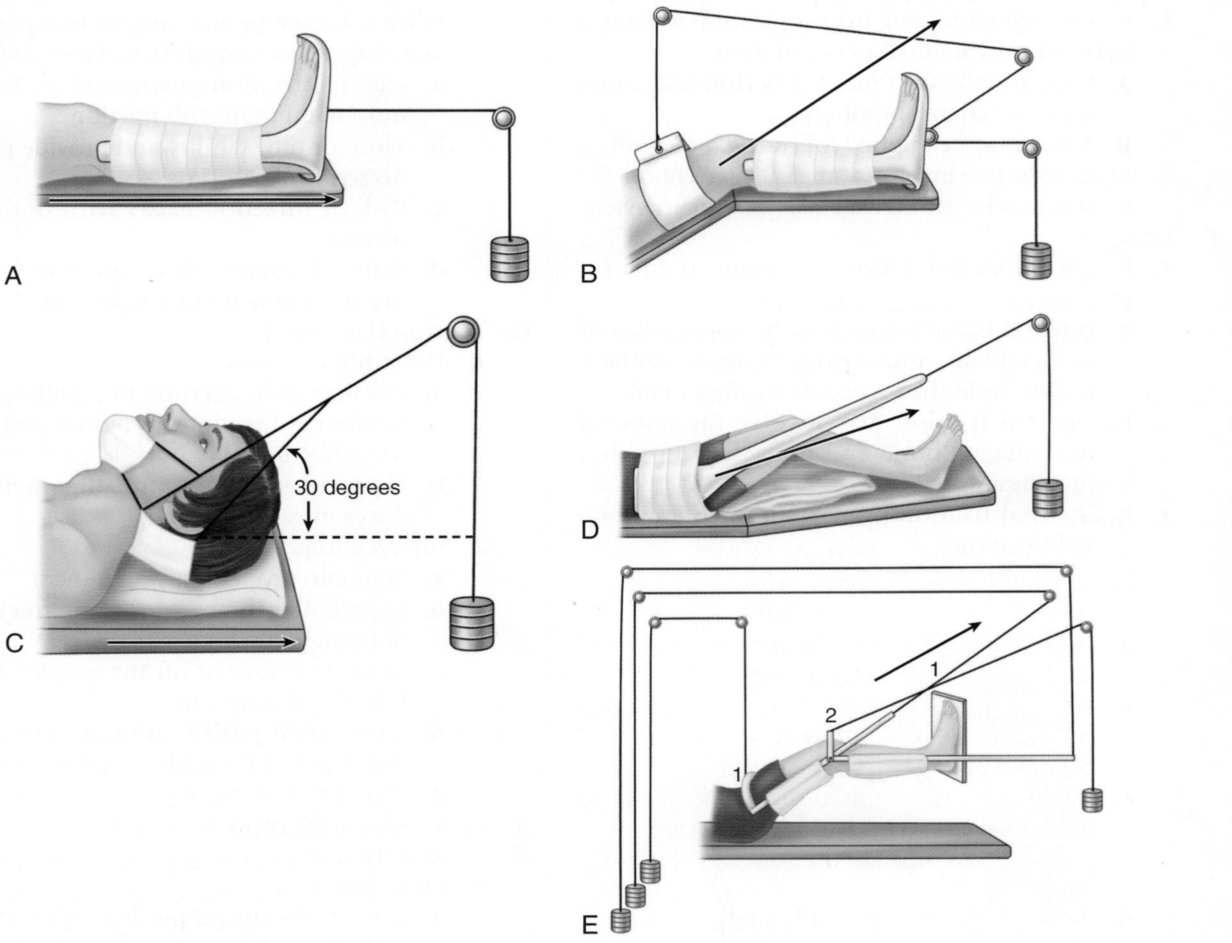

FIG. 60-4 Types of traction. **A,** Buck's traction. **B,** Russell's traction. **C,** Head halter traction. **D,** Pelvic traction. **E,** Balanced suspension traction.

3. Cervical tongs and a halo fixation device: See Chapter 58 regarding care of the client with these types of devices.

I. Skin traction
1. Description: Skin traction is applied by using elastic bandages or adhesive, foam boot, or sling.
2. Cervical skin traction relieves muscle spasms and compression in the upper extremities and neck (see Fig. 60-4).
   a. Cervical skin traction uses a head halter and chin pad to attach the traction.
   b. Use powder to protect the ears from friction rub.
   c. Position the client with the head of the bed elevated 30 to 40 degrees, and attach the weights to a pulley system over the head of the bed.
3. Buck's (extension) skin traction is used to alleviate muscle spasms and immobilize a lower limb by maintaining a straight pull on the limb with the use of weights (see Fig. 60-4).
   a. A boot appliance is applied to attach to the traction.
   b. The weights are attached to a pulley; allow the weights to hang freely over the edge of bed.
   c. Not more than 8 to 10 lb (3.5 to 4.5 kg) of weight should be applied as prescribed.
   d. Elevate the foot of the bed to provide the traction.
4. Russell's skin (sling) traction: See Fig. 60-4 and Chapter 39 regarding this type of traction.
5. Pelvic skin traction is used to relieve low back, hip, or leg pain or to reduce muscle spasm (see Fig. 60-4).
   a. Apply the traction belt snugly over the pelvis and iliac crest and attach to the weights.
   b. Use measures as prescribed to prevent the client from slipping down in bed.

J. Balanced suspension traction (see Fig. 60-4)
1. Description
   a. Balanced suspension traction is used with skin or skeletal traction.
   b. Used to approximate fractures of the femur, tibia, or fibula

c. Balanced suspension traction is produced by a counterforce other than the client.

2. Interventions
   a. Position the client in a low-Fowler's position on either the side or the back.
   b. Maintain a 20-degree angle from the thigh to the bed.
   c. Protect the skin from breakdown.
   d. Provide pin care if pins are used with skeletal traction.
   e. Clean the pin sites with sterile normal saline and hydrogen peroxide or povidone-iodine as prescribed or per agency policy.

K. Casts
1. Description: Plaster, fiberglass, or air casts are used to immobilize bones and joints into correct alignment after a fracture or injury.
2. Interventions
   a. Keep the cast and extremity elevated.
   b. Allow a wet plaster cast 24 to 72 hours to dry (synthetic casts dry in 20 minutes).
   c. Handle a wet plaster cast with the palms of the hands (not fingertips) until dry.
   d. Turn the extremity every 1 to 2 hours, unless contraindicated, to allow air circulation and promote drying of the cast.
   e. A hair dryer can be used on a cool setting to dry a plaster cast (heat cannot be used on a plaster cast, because the cast heats up and burns the skin).
   f. Monitor closely for circulatory impairment; prepare for bivalving or cutting the cast if circulatory impairment occurs.
   g. Petal the cast or apply moleskin to the edges to protect the client's skin; maintain smooth edges around the cast to prevent crumbling of the cast material.
   h. Monitor for signs of infection such as increased temperature, hot spots on the cast, foul odor, or changes in pain.
   i. If an open draining area exists on the affected extremity, the PHCP will make a cutout portion of the cast known as a *window*, for assessment and wound care purposes.
   j. Instruct the client not to stick objects inside the cast.
   k. Teach the client to keep the cast clean and dry.
   l. Instruct the client in isometric exercises to prevent muscle atrophy.

Monitor a casted extremity for circulatory impairment such as pain, swelling, discoloration, tingling, numbness, coolness, or diminished pulse. Notify the PHCP immediately if circulatory compromise occurs.

VI. Complications of Fractures (Box 60-3)

A. Fat embolism (see Priority Nursing Actions)

BOX 60-3 Complications of Fractures

- Avascular necrosis
- Compartment syndrome
- Fat embolism
- Infection and osteomyelitis
- Pulmonary embolism

PRIORITY NURSING ACTIONS

Fat Embolism in a Client Following a Fracture

1. Notify the primary health care provider (PHCP).
2. Administer oxygen.
3. Administer intravenous (IV) fluids as prescribed.
4. Monitor vital signs and respiratory status.
5. Prepare for intubation and mechanical ventilation if necessary as indicated by arterial blood gas values.
6. Follow up on results of diagnostic tests such as chest x-ray or computed tomography (CT) scan.
7. Document the event, actions taken, and the client's response.

Reference
Ignatavicius, Workman, Rebar (2018), p. 1034.

B. Pulmonary embolism
1. Description: Pulmonary embolism is caused by the movement of foreign particles (blood clot, fat, or air) into the pulmonary circulation.
2. Assessment
   a. Restlessness and apprehension
   b. Sudden onset of dyspnea and chest pain
   c. Cough, hemoptysis, hypoxemia, or crackles
3. Interventions
   a. Notify the PHCP immediately if signs of emboli are present.
   b. Administer oxygen and other prescriptions; intravenous (IV) anticoagulant therapy may be prescribed.

C. Compartment syndrome
1. Description
   a. Tough fascia surrounds muscle groups, forming compartments from which arteries, veins, and nerves enter and exit at opposite ends.
   b. Compartment syndrome occurs when pressure increases within 1 or more compartments, leading to decreased blood flow, tissue ischemia, and neurovascular impairment.
   c. Neurovascular damage may be irreversible if not treated within 4 to 6 hours after the onset of compartment syndrome.
2. Assessment
   a. Unrelieved or increased pain in the limb
   b. Tissue that is distal to the involved area becomes pale, dusky, or edematous.

c. Pain with passive movement
d. Loss of sensation (paresthesia)
e. Pulselessness (a late sign)
3. Interventions
a. Notify the PHCP immediately and prepare to assist the PHCP.
b. Place the affected extremity at heart level; elevation is contraindicated because it decreases arterial flow.
c. If severe, assist the PHCP with fasciotomy to relieve pressure and restore tissue perfusion.
d. Loosen tight dressings or bivalve restrictive cast as prescribed.

D. Infection and osteomyelitis
1. Description: Infection and osteomyelitis (inflammatory response in bone tissue) can be caused by the introduction of organisms into bones leading to localized bone infection.
2. Assessment
a. Tachycardia and fever (usually above 101° F [38.3° C]).
b. Erythema and pain in the area surrounding the infection
c. Leukocytosis and elevated erythrocyte sedimentation rate (ESR)
d. Confirmed by radiographic assessment, such as plain radiographs, MRI, or bone scan
3. Interventions
a. Notify the PHCP.
b. Prepare to initiate aggressive, long-term IV antibiotic therapy. A central venous access line will likely be required.
c. Surgery is performed for resistant osteomyelitis with sequestrectomy and/or bone grafts.
d. For unrelenting infection and osteomyelitis, hyperbaric oxygen therapy is used (if available) to promote healing.

E. Avascular necrosis
1. Description: Avascular necrosis occurs when a fracture interrupts the blood supply to a section of bone, leading to bone death.
2. Assessment
a. Pain
b. Decreased sensation
c. Confirmed by radiographic assessment, such as plain radiographs, MRI, or bone scan
3. Interventions
a. Notify the PHCP if pain or numbness occurs.
b. Prepare the client for removal of necrotic tissue, because it serves as a focus for infection.

VII. Crutch Walking

A. Description
1. An accurate measurement of the client for crutches is important, because an incorrect measurement could damage the brachial plexus.
2. The distance between the axillae and the arm pieces on the crutches should be 2 to 3 fingerwidths in the axilla space.
3. The elbows should be slightly flexed, 20 to 30 degrees, when the client is walking.
4. When ambulating with the client, stand on the affected side.
5. Instruct the client never to rest the axillae on the axillary bars.
6. Instruct the client to look up and outward when ambulating and to place the crutches 6 to 10 inches (25.5 cm) diagonally in front of the foot.
7. Instruct the client to stop ambulation if numbness or tingling in the hands or arms occurs.

B. Crutch gaits (Table 60-2)

C. Assisting the client with crutches to sit and stand
1. Place the unaffected leg against the front of the chair.
2. Move the crutches to the affected side, and grasp the arm of the chair with the hand on the unaffected side.
3. Flex the knee of the unaffected leg to lower self into the chair while placing the affected leg straight out in front.
4. Reverse the steps to move from a sitting to standing position.

TABLE 60-2 Crutch Gaits

Type of Gait	Use	Procedure
Two-point gait	Used with partial weight-bearing limitations and with bilateral lower extremity prostheses	The crutch on the affected side and the unaffected foot are advanced at the same time
Three-point gait	Used for partial weight bearing or no weight bearing on the affected leg; requires that the client have strength and balance	Both crutches and the foot of the affected extremity are advanced together, followed by the foot of the unaffected extremity
Four-point gait	Used if weight bearing is allowed and 1 foot can be placed in front of the other	The right crutch is advanced, then the left foot, then the left crutch, and then the right foot
Swing-to gait	Used when there is adequate muscle power and balance in the arms and legs	Both crutches are advanced together, then both legs are lifted and placed down on a spot behind the crutches. The feet and crutches form a tripod.
Swing-through gait	Used when there is adequate muscle power and balance in the arms and legs	Both crutches are advanced together; then both legs are lifted through and beyond the crutches and placed down again at a point in front of the crutches

Adapted from Linton AD: *Introduction to medical-surgical nursing*, ed 4, St. Louis, 2007, Saunders.

D. Going up and down stairs
 1. Up the stairs
  a. The client moves the unaffected leg up first.
  b. The client moves the affected leg and the crutches up.
 2. Down the stairs
  a. The client moves the crutches and the affected leg down.
  b. The client moves the unaffected leg down.

VIII. Canes and Walkers

A. Description: Canes and walkers are made of a lightweight material with a rubber tip at the bottom.

B. Interventions
 1. Stand at the affected side of the client when ambulating; use of a gait or transfer belt may be necessary.
 2. The handle should be at the level of the client's greater trochanter.
 3. The client's elbow should be flexed at a 15- to 30-degree angle.
 4. Instruct the client to hold the cane 4 to 6 inches (10 to 15 cm) to the side of the foot.
 5. Instruct the client to hold the cane in the hand on the unaffected side so that the cane and weaker leg can work together with each step.
 6. Instruct the client to move the cane at the same time as the affected leg.
 7. Instruct the client to inspect the rubber tips regularly for worn places.

C. Hemicanes or quadripod canes
 1. Hemicanes or quadripod canes are used for clients who have the use of only 1 upper extremity.
 2. Hemicanes provide more security than a quadripod cane; however, both types provide more security than a single-tipped cane.
 3. Position the cane at the client's unaffected side, with the straight, nonangled side adjacent to the body.
 4. Position the cane 6 inches (15 cm) from the unaffected client's side, with the hand grip level with the greater trochanter.

D. Walker
 1. Stand adjacent to the client on the affected side.
 2. Instruct the client to put all 4 points of the walker flat on the floor before putting weight on the hand pieces.
 3. Instruct the client to move the walker forward, followed by the affected or weaker foot and then the unaffected foot.

Safety is the priority concern when the client uses an assistive device such as a cane, walker, or crutches. Be sure that the client demonstrates correct use of the device.

IX. Fractured Hip

A. Types
 1. Intracapsular (femoral head is broken within the joint capsule)
  a. Femoral head and neck receive decreased blood supply and heal slowly.
  b. Skin traction is applied preoperatively to reduce the fracture and decrease muscle spasms.
  c. Treatment includes a total hip replacement or open reduction internal fixation (ORIF) with femoral head replacement.
  d. To prevent hip displacement postoperatively, avoid extreme hip flexion, and check the surgeon's prescriptions regarding positioning.
 2. Extracapsular (fracture is outside the joint capsule)
  a. Fracture can occur at the greater trochanter or can be an intertrochanteric fracture.
  b. Preoperative treatment includes balanced suspension or skin traction to relieve muscle spasms and reduce pain.
  c. Surgical treatment includes ORIF with nail plate, screws, pins, or wires.

B. Postoperative interventions
 1. Monitor for signs of delirium and institute safety measures.
 2. Maintain leg and hip in proper alignment and prevent internal or external rotation; avoid extreme hip flexion.
 3. Follow the PHCP's prescriptions regarding turning and repositioning; usually, turning to the unaffected side is allowed; protective devices may be prescribed.
 4. Elevate the head of the bed 30 to 45 degrees for meals only.
 5. Assist the client to ambulate as prescribed by the PHCP.
 6. Avoid weight bearing on the affected leg as prescribed; instruct the client in the use of a walker to avoid weight bearing.
 7. Weight bearing is often restricted after ORIF and may not be restricted after total hip arthroplasty (THA); always refer to the PHCP's prescriptions.
 8. Keep the operative leg extended, supported, and elevated (preventing hip flexion) when getting the client out of bed.
 9. Avoid hip flexion greater than 90 degrees and avoid low chairs when out of bed.
 10. Monitor for wound infection or hemorrhage.
 11. Administer antibiotics if prescribed within a specified time frame (antibiotics also may be prescribed in the preoperative period).
 12. Neurovascular assessment of affected extremity: Check color, pulses, capillary refill, movement, and sensation.
 13. Maintain the compression of the drain if present, to facilitate wound drainage.

14. Monitor and record drainage amount, which decreases consistently.
15. As prescribed, carry out postoperative blood salvage to collect, filter, and reinfuse salvaged blood into the client.
16. Use antiembolism stockings or sequential compression stockings as prescribed; encourage the client to flex and extend the feet to reduce the risk of deep vein thrombosis (DVT).
17. Instruct the client to avoid crossing the legs and activities that require bending over.
18. Physical therapy will be instituted postoperatively with progressive ambulation as prescribed by the PHCP.

X. Total Knee Replacement

A. Description: Total knee replacement is the implantation of a device to substitute for the femoral condyles and tibial joint surfaces.

B. Postoperative interventions
1. Monitor surgical incision for drainage and infection.
2. If prescribed, continuous passive motion (CPM) is started soon after the client is admitted to the postoperative unit.
3. Administer analgesics before CPM to decrease pain.
4. Prepare the client for out-of-bed activities as prescribed; have the client avoid leg dangling.
5. Weight bearing with an assistive device is prescribed as tolerated.
6. Postoperative blood salvage may be prescribed to collect, filter, and reinfuse salvaged blood into the client.
7. Administer antibiotics if prescribed within a specified time frame (antibiotics also may be prescribed in the preoperative period).

XI. Joint Dislocation and Subluxation

A. Dislocation: Injury of the ligaments surrounding a joint, which leads to displacement or separating of the articular surfaces of the joint

B. Subluxation: Incomplete displacement of joint surfaces when forces disrupt the soft tissue that surrounds the joints

C. Assessment
1. Asymmetry of the contour of affected body parts
2. Pain, tenderness, dysfunction, and swelling
3. Complications include neurovascular compromise, avascular necrosis, and open joint injuries.
4. X-rays are taken to determine joint shifting.

D. Interventions
1. Focus of treatment includes pain relief, joint support, and joint protection.
2. Immediate treatment is done to reduce the dislocation and realign the dislocated joint.
3. Open or closed reduction is done followed with a postprocedural joint immobilization device.
4. Intravenous conscious sedation, local, or general anesthesia is used during joint manipulation.
5. Initial activity restriction is followed by gentle range-of-motion activities and a gradual return of activities to normal levels while supporting the affected joint.
6. A weakened joint is prone to recurrent dislocation and may require extended activity restriction.

XII. Herniation: Intervertebral Disk

A. Description: The nucleus of the disk protrudes into the annulus, causing nerve compression.

B. Cervical disk herniation occurs at the C5 to C6 and C6 to C7 interspaces.
1. Cervical disk herniation causes pain radiation to shoulders, arms, hands, scapulae, and pectoral muscles.
2. Motor and sensory deficits can include paresthesia, numbness, and weakness of the upper extremities.
3. Interventions
   a. Conservative management is used unless the client develops signs of neurological deterioration.
   b. Bed rest is prescribed to decrease pressure, inflammation, and pain.
   c. Immobilize the cervical area with a cervical collar or brace.
   d. Apply heat to reduce muscle spasms and apply ice to reduce inflammation and swelling.
   e. Maintain head and spine alignment.
   f. Instruct the client in the use of analgesics, sedatives, antiinflammatory agents, and corticosteroids as prescribed.
   g. Prepare the client for a corticosteroid injection into the epidural space if prescribed.
   h. Assist and instruct the client in the use of a cervical collar or cervical traction as prescribed.
4. Cervical collar is used for cervical disk herniation.
   a. A cervical collar limits neck movement and holds the head in a neutral or slightly flexed position.
   b. The cervical collar may be worn intermittently or 24 hours daily.
   c. Inspect the skin under the collar for irritation.
   d. When prescribed and after pain decreases, exercises are done to strengthen the muscles.
5. Client education related to cervical disk conditions
   a. Avoid flexing, extending, and rotating the neck.
   b. Avoid the prone position and maintain the neck, spine, and hips in a neutral position while sleeping.

c. Minimize long periods of sitting.
d. Instruct the client regarding medications such as analgesics, sedatives, antiinflammatory agents, and corticosteroids.

C. Lumbar disk herniation most often occurs at the L4 to L5 or L5 to S1 interspace.
1. Herniation produces muscle weakness, sensory deficits, and diminished tendon reflexes.
2. The client experiences pain and muscle spasms in the lower back, with radiation of the pain into 1 hip and down the leg (sciatica).
3. Pain is relieved by bed rest and aggravated by movement, lifting, straining, and coughing.
4. Interventions
a. Conservative management is indicated unless neurological deterioration or bowel and bladder dysfunction occurs.
b. Apply heat to decrease muscle spasms and apply ice to decrease inflammation and swelling.
c. Instruct the client to sleep on the side, with the knees and hips flexed, and place a pillow between the legs.
d. Apply pelvic traction as prescribed to relieve muscle spasms and decrease pain.
e. Begin progressive ambulation as inflammation, edema, and pain subside.
5. Client education related to lumbar disk conditions
a. Instruct the client in the use of prescribed medications such as analgesics, muscle relaxants, antiinflammatory agents, or corticosteroids.
b. Instruct the client about application techniques for corsets or braces to maintain immobilization and proper spine alignment.
c. Instruct the client in correct posture while sitting, standing, walking, and working.
d. Instruct the client in the correct technique to use when lifting objects such as bending the knees, maintaining a straight back, and avoiding lifting objects above the elbow level.
e. Instruct in a weight control program as prescribed.
f. Instruct the client in an exercise program to strengthen back and abdominal muscles as prescribed.

D. Disk surgery is used when spinal cord compression is suspected or symptoms do not respond to conservative treatment; minimally invasive techniques may be prescribed (Box 60-4).
1. Postoperative interventions: Cervical disk
a. Monitor for respiratory difficulty from inflammation or hematoma.
b. Encourage coughing, deep breathing, and early ambulation as prescribed.

BOX 60-4 Types of Disk Surgery

Diskectomy: Removal of herniated disk tissue and related matter
Diskectomy with Fusion: Fusion of vertebrae with bone graft
Laminectomy: Excision of part of the vertebrae (lamina) to remove the disk
Laminotomy: Division of the lamina of a vertebra

c. Monitor for hoarseness and inability to cough effectively, because this may indicate laryngeal nerve damage.
d. Use throat sprays or lozenges for sore throat, avoiding anesthetic lozenges that may numb the throat and increase choking risks.
e. Assess the surgical dressing; monitor the surgical wound for infection, swelling, redness, drainage, or pain; and manage surgical drains accordingly.
f. Provide a soft diet if the client complains of dysphagia.
g. Monitor for sudden return of radicular pain, which may indicate cervical spine instability.
2. Postoperative interventions: Lumbar disk
a. Assess the surgical dressing, monitoring for wound drainage and bleeding and monitoring surgical drains accordingly.
b. Monitor lower extremities for sensation, movement, color, temperature, and paresthesia.
c. Monitor for urinary retention, paralytic ileus, and constipation, which can result from decreased movement, opioid administration, or spinal cord compression.
d. Prevent constipation by encouraging a high-fiber diet, increased fluid intake, and stool softeners as prescribed.
e. Administer opioids and sedatives as prescribed to relieve pain and anxiety.
f. Assist and instruct the client to use a prescribed back brace or corset and to wear cotton underwear to prevent skin irritation.
3. Postoperative lumbar disk positioning
a. In the immediate postoperative period, the client may be expected to lie supine or have other activity restrictions, depending on the specific surgical intervention.
b. Instruct the client to avoid spinal flexion or twisting and that the spine should be kept aligned.
c. Instruct the client to minimize sitting, which may place a strain on the surgical site.
d. When the client is lying supine, place a pillow under the neck and slightly flex the knees.
e. Avoid extreme hip flexion when lying on the side.

▲ Following disk surgery, instruct the client in correct logrolling techniques for turning and repositioning and for getting out of bed.

XIII. Amputation of a Lower Extremity

A. Description
1. Amputation (Fig. 60-5) is the surgical removal of a limb or part of the limb.
2. Complications include hemorrhage, infection, phantom limb sensation and pain, neuroma, and flexion contractures.

B. Postoperative interventions
1. Monitor for signs of complications.
2. Mark bleeding and drainage on the dressing if it occurs.
3. Evaluate for phantom limb sensation and pain; explain sensation and pain to the client, and medicate the client as prescribed.
4. To prevent hip flexion contractures, do not elevate the residual limb on a pillow.
5. First 24 hours: Elevate the foot of the bed to reduce edema; then keep the bed flat to prevent hip flexion contractures, if prescribed by the PHCP.

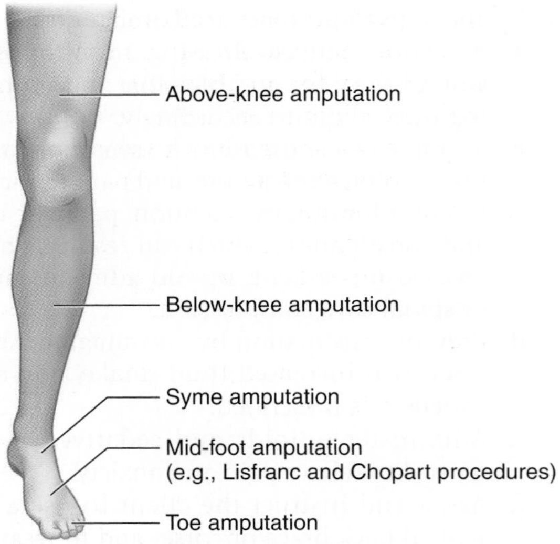

FIG. 60-5 Common levels of lower extremity amputation.

6. After 24 to 48 hours postoperatively, position the client prone to stretch the muscles and prevent hip flexion contractures, if prescribed.
7. Maintain surgical application of dressing, elastic compression wrap, or elastic stump (residual limb) shrinker as prescribed to reduce swelling, minimize pain, and mold the residual limb in preparation for prosthesis (Fig. 60-6)
8. As prescribed, wash the residual limb with mild soap and water and dry completely.
9. Massage the skin toward the suture line if prescribed, to mobilize scar tissue and prevent its adherence to underlying bone.
10. Prepare for the prosthesis and instruct the client in progressive resistive techniques by gently pushing the residual limb against pillows and progressing to firmer surfaces.
11. Encourage verbalization regarding loss of the body part, and assist the client to identify coping mechanisms to deal with the loss.

C. Interventions for below-knee amputation
1. Prevent edema.
2. Do not allow the residual limb to hang over the edge of the bed.
3. Discourage long periods of sitting to lessen complications of knee flexion.
4. Place the client in a prone position throughout the day as prescribed by the PHCP.

D. Interventions for above-knee amputation
1. Prevent internal or external rotation of the limb.
2. Place a sandbag, rolled towel, or trochanter roll along the outside of the thigh to prevent external rotation.
3. Place the client in a prone position throughout the day as prescribed by the PHCP.

E. Rehabilitation
1. Instruct the client in the use of a mobility aid such as crutches or a walker.
2. Prepare the residual limb for a prosthesis.
3. Prepare the client for fitting of the residual limb for a prosthesis.

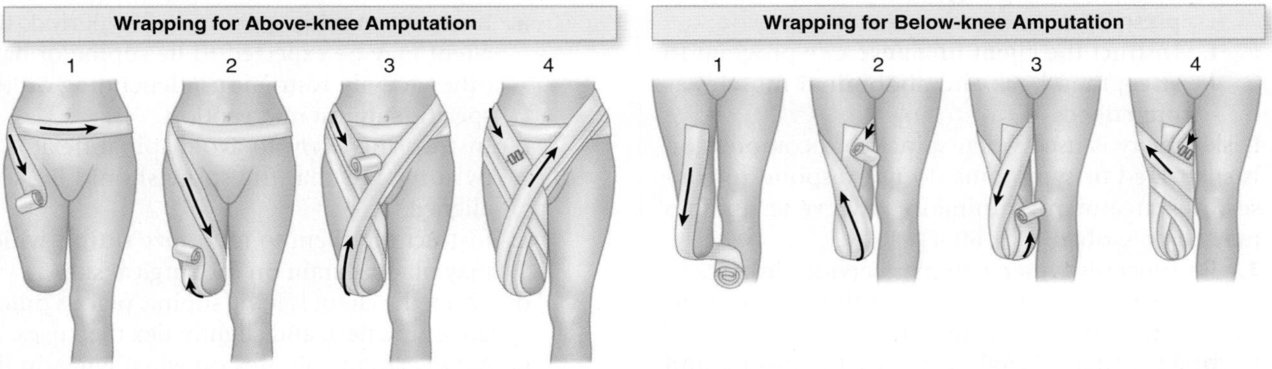

FIG. 60-6 A common method of wrapping a residual limb. *Left*, Wrapping for above-knee amputation. *Right*, Wrapping for below-knee amputation.

4. Instruct the client in exercises to maintain range of motion and upper body strengthening.
5. Provide psychosocial support to the client.

F. Traumatic amputation: Emergency care
1. Obtain emergency medical assistance (call 911).
2. Stay with the victim, check the amputation site, and apply direct pressure with gauze or cloth (do not remove applied pressure dressing to prevent dislodging of a formed clot).
3. Elevate the extremity above heart level.
4. If finger(s) were amputated, place them in a watertight, sealed plastic bag; place the bag in ice water (not directly on ice); and transport to the emergency department with the victim.

XIV. Rheumatoid Arthritis

A. Description
1. Rheumatoid arthritis is a chronic systemic inflammatory disease (immune complex disorder); the cause may be related to a combination of environmental and genetic factors.
2. Rheumatoid arthritis leads to destruction of connective tissue and synovial membrane within the joints.
3. Rheumatoid arthritis weakens the joint, leading to dislocation and permanent deformity of the joint.
4. Pannus forms at the junction of synovial tissue and articular cartilage and projects into the joint cavity, causing necrosis.
5. Exacerbations of disease manifestations occur during periods of physical or emotional stress and fatigue.
6. Vasculitis can impede blood flow, leading to organ or organ system malfunction and failure caused by tissue ischemia.

B. Assessment
1. Inflammation, tenderness, and stiffness of the joints
2. Moderate to severe pain, with morning stiffness lasting longer than 30 minutes
3. Joint deformities, muscle atrophy, and decreased range of motion in affected joints
4. Spongy, soft feeling in the joints
5. Low-grade temperature, fatigue, and weakness
6. Anorexia, weight loss, and anemia
7. Elevated ESR and positive rheumatoid factor
8. Radiographic study showing joint deterioration
9. Synovial tissue biopsy reveals inflammation

C. Rheumatoid factor
1. Blood test used to assist in diagnosing rheumatoid arthritis
2. Reference interval: Negative or less than 60 IU/mL

D. Medications: Combination of pharmacological therapies includes NSAIDs, disease-modifying antirheumatic drugs (DMARDs), and glucocorticoids

E. Physical mobility
1. Preserve joint function.
2. Provide range-of-motion exercises to maintain joint motion and muscle strengthening.
3. Balance rest and activity.
4. Splints may be used during acute inflammation to prevent deformity.
5. Prevent flexion contractures.
6. Apply heat or cold therapy as prescribed to joints.
7. Apply paraffin baths and massage as prescribed.
8. Encourage consistency with exercise program.
9. Use joint-protecting devices.
10. Avoid weight bearing on inflamed joints.

F. Self-care (Box 60-5)
1. Assess the need for assistive devices such as raised toilet seats, self-rising chairs, wheelchairs, and scooters to facilitate mobility.
2. Work with an occupational therapist or PHCP to obtain assistive or adaptive devices.
3. Instruct the client in alternative strategies for providing activities of daily living.

G. Fatigue
1. Identify factors that may contribute to fatigue.
2. Monitor for signs of anemia and administer iron, folic acid, and vitamins as prescribed.
3. Monitor for medication-related blood loss by testing the stool for occult blood.
4. Instruct the client in measures to conserve energy, such as pacing activities and obtaining assistance when possible.

H. Disturbed body image
1. Assess the client's reaction to the body change.
2. Encourage the client to verbalize feelings.
3. Assist the client with self-care activities and grooming.
4. Encourage the client to get dressed daily and to wear street clothes.

BOX 60-5 Client Education for Rheumatoid Arthritis and Degenerative Joint Disease

- Assist the client to identify and correct safety hazards in the home.
- Instruct the client in the correct use of assistive or adaptive devices.
- Instruct the client in energy conservation measures.
- Review the prescribed exercise program.
- Instruct the client to sit in a chair with a high, straight back.
- Instruct the client to use only a small pillow when lying down.
- Instruct the client in measures to protect the joints.
- Instruct the client regarding the prescribed medications.
- Stress the importance of follow-up visits with the primary health care provider.

I. Surgical interventions
1. Synovectomy: Surgical removal of the synovia to help maintain joint function
2. Arthrodesis: Bony fusion of a joint to regain some mobility
3. Joint replacement (arthroplasty): Surgical replacement of diseased joints with artificial joints; performed to restore motion to a joint and function to the muscles, ligaments, and other soft tissue structures that control a joint

XV. Osteoarthritis (Degenerative Joint Disease)

A. Description
1. Osteoarthritis is marked by progressive deterioration of the articular cartilage.
2. Osteoarthritis causes bone buildup and the loss of articular cartilage in peripheral and axial joints.
3. Osteoarthritis affects the weight-bearing joints and joints that receive the greatest stress, such as the hips, knees, lower vertebral column, and hands.
4. The cause of primary osteoarthritis is not known. Risk factors include trauma, aging, obesity, genetic changes, and smoking.

B. Assessment
1. The client experiences joint pain that diminishes after rest and intensifies after activity, noted early in the disease process.
2. As the disease progresses, pain occurs with slight motion or even at rest.
3. Symptoms are aggravated by temperature change and climate humidity.
4. Presence of Heberden's nodes or Bouchard's nodes (hands)
5. Joint swelling (may be minimal), crepitus, and limited range of motion
6. Difficulty getting up after prolonged sitting
7. Skeletal muscle disuse atrophy
8. Inability to perform activities of daily living
9. Compression of the spine as manifested by radiating pain, stiffness, and muscle spasms in 1 or both extremities

C. Pain
1. Administer medications as prescribed, such as acetaminophen or topical applications; if acetaminophen or topical agents do not relieve pain, NSAIDs may be prescribed. Muscle relaxants may also be prescribed for muscle spasms, especially those occurring in the back.
2. Prepare the client for corticosteroid injections into joints as prescribed.
3. Position joints in function position and avoid flexion of knees and hips.
4. Immobilize the affected joint with a splint or brace until inflammation subsides.
5. Avoid large pillows under the head or knees.
6. Provide a bed or foot cradle to keep linen off of feet and legs until inflammation subsides.
7. Instruct the client in the importance of moist heat, hot packs or compresses, and paraffin dips as prescribed.
8. Apply cold applications as prescribed when the joint is acutely inflamed.
9. Encourage adequate rest.

D. Nutrition
1. Encourage a well-balanced diet.
2. Maintain weight within normal range to decrease stress on the joints.

E. Physical mobility
1. Instruct the client to balance activity with rest and to participate in an exercise program that limits stressing affected joints.
2. Instruct the client that exercises should be active rather than passive and to stop exercise if pain occurs.
3. Instruct the client to limit exercise when joint inflammation is severe.

F. Surgical management
1. Osteotomy: The bone is resected to correct joint deformity, promote realignment, and reduce joint stress.
2. Total joint replacement or arthroplasty
   a. Total joint replacement is performed when all measures of pain relief have failed.
   b. Hips and knees are replaced most commonly.
   c. Total joint replacement is contraindicated in the presence of infection, advanced osteoporosis, or severe joint inflammation.

XVI. Osteoporosis

A. Description
1. Osteoporosis is a metabolic disease characterized by bone demineralization, with loss of calcium and phosphorus salts leading to fragile bones and the subsequent risk for fractures.
2. Bone resorption accelerates as bone formation slows.
3. Osteoporosis occurs most commonly in the wrist, hip, and vertebral column.
4. Osteoporosis can occur postmenopausally or as a result of a metabolic disorder or calcium deficiency.
5. The client may be asymptomatic until the bones become fragile and a minor injury or movement causes a fracture.
6. Primary osteoporosis
   a. Most often occurs in postmenopausal women; occurs in men with low testosterone levels
   b. Risk factors include decreased calcium intake, deficient estrogen, and sedentary lifestyle.
7. Secondary osteoporosis
   a. Causes include prolonged therapy with corticosteroids, thyroid-reducing medications,

BOX 60-6 Risk Factors for Osteoporosis

- Cigarette smoking
- Early menopause
- Excessive use of alcohol
- Family history
- Female gender
- Increasing age
- Insufficient intake of calcium
- Sedentary lifestyle
- Thin, small frame
- White (European descent) or Asian race

aluminum-containing antacids, or antiseizure medications.

b. Associated with immobility, alcoholism, malnutrition, or malabsorption

B. Assessment

1. Risk factors (Box 60-6)
2. Possibly asymptomatic
3. Back pain that occurs after lifting, bending, or stooping
4. Back pain that increases with palpation
5. Pelvic or hip pain, especially with weight bearing
6. Problems with balance
7. Decline in height from vertebral compression
8. Kyphosis of the dorsal spine, also known as "dowager's hump"
9. Degeneration of lower thorax and lumbar vertebrae on radiographic studies

⚠ The client with osteoporosis is at risk for pathological fractures.

C. Interventions

1. Assess risk for and prevent injury in the client's personal environment.
   a. Assist the client to identify and correct hazards in his or her environment.
   b. Position household items and furniture to ensure an unobstructed walkway.
   c. Use side rails to prevent falls.
   d. Instruct in use of assistive devices such as a cane or walker.
   e. Encourage the use of a firm mattress.
2. Provide personal care to the client to reduce injuries.
   a. Move the client gently when turning and repositioning.
   b. Assist with ambulation if the client is unsteady.
   c. Provide gentle range-of-motion exercises.
   d. Apply a back brace as prescribed during an acute phase to immobilize the spine and provide spinal column support.
3. Provide the client with instructions to promote optimal level of health and function.
   a. Instruct the client in the use of correct body mechanics.
   b. Instruct the client in exercises to strengthen abdominal and back muscles to improve posture and provide support for the spine.
   c. Instruct the client to avoid activities that can cause vertebral compression.
   d. Instruct the client to eat a diet high in protein, calcium, vitamins C and D, and iron.
   e. Instruct the client to avoid alcohol and coffee.
   f. Instruct the client to maintain an adequate fluid intake to prevent renal calculi.
4. Administer medications as prescribed to promote bone strength and decrease pain.

XVII. Gout

A. Description

1. Gout is a systemic disease in which urate crystals deposit in joints and other body tissues.
2. Gout results from abnormal amounts of uric acid in the body.
3. Primary gout results from a disorder of purine metabolism.
4. Secondary gout involves excessive uric acid in the blood, caused by another disease.

B. Phases

1. Asymptomatic: Client has no symptoms, but serum uric acid level is elevated.
2. Acute: Client has excruciating pain and inflammation of 1 or more small joints, especially the great toe.
3. Intermittent: Client has intermittent periods without symptoms between acute attacks.
4. Chronic: Results from repeated episodes of acute gout
   a. Results in deposits of urate crystals under the skin
   b. Results in deposits of urate crystals within major organs, such as the kidneys, leading to organ dysfunction

C. Assessment

1. Swelling and inflammation of the joints, leading to excruciating pain
2. Tophi: Hard, irregularly shaped nodules in the skin containing chalky deposits of sodium urate
3. Low-grade fever, malaise, and headache
4. Pruritus from urate crystals in the skin
5. Presence of renal stones from elevated uric acid levels

D. Interventions

1. Provide a low-purine diet as prescribed, avoiding foods such as organ meats, wines, and aged cheese.
2. Encourage a high fluid intake of 2000 mL/day to prevent stone formation.
3. Encourage a weight reduction diet if required.

4. Instruct the client to avoid alcohol and starvation diets, because they may precipitate a gout attack.
5. Increase urinary pH (above 6) by eating alkaline ash foods (i.e., green beans, broccoli).
6. Provide bed rest during acute attacks, with the affected extremity elevated.
7. Monitor joint range-of-motion ability and appearance of joints.
8. Position the joint in mild flexion during acute attack.
9. Protect the affected joint from excessive movement or direct contact with sheets or blankets.
10. Provide heat or cold for local treatments to affected joint as prescribed.
11. Administer medications such as analgesic, antiinflammatory, and uricosuric agents as prescribed.

PRACTICE QUESTIONS

735. The nurse is conducting health screening for osteoporosis. Which client is at greatest risk of developing this problem?
1. A 25-year-old woman who runs
2. A 36-year-old man who has asthma
3. A 70-year-old man who consumes excess alcohol
4. A sedentary 65-year-old woman who smokes cigarettes

736. The nurse has given instructions to a client returning home after knee arthroscopy. Which statement by the client indicates that the instructions are understood?
1. "I can resume regular exercise tomorrow."
2. "I can't eat food for the remainder of the day."
3. "I need to stay off the leg entirely for the rest of the day."
4. "I need to report a fever or swelling to my health care provider."

737. The nurse witnessed a vehicle hit a pedestrian. The victim is dazed and tries to get up. A leg appears fractured. Which intervention should the nurse take?
1. Try to reduce the fracture manually.
2. Assist the victim to get up and walk to the sidewalk.
3. Leave the victim for a few moments to call an ambulance.
4. Stay with the victim and encourage him or her to remain still.

738. Which cast care instructions should the nurse provide to a client who just had a plaster cast applied to the right forearm? **Select all that apply.**
- ☐ 1. Keep the cast clean and dry.
- ☐ 2. Allow the cast 24 to 72 hours to dry.
- ☐ 3. Keep the cast and extremity elevated.
- ☐ 4. Expect tingling and numbness in the extremity.
- ☐ 5. Use a hair dryer set on a warm to hot setting to dry the cast.
- ☐ 6. Use a soft, padded object that will fit under the cast to scratch the skin under the cast.

739. The nurse is evaluating a client in skeletal traction. When evaluating the pin sites, the nurse would be **most** concerned with which finding?
1. Redness around the pin sites
2. Pain on palpation at the pin sites
3. Thick, yellow drainage from the pin sites
4. Clear, watery drainage from the pin sites

740. The nurse is assessing the casted extremity of a client. Which sign is indicative of infection?
1. Dependent edema
2. Diminished distal pulse
3. Presence of a "hot spot" on the cast
4. Coolness and pallor of the extremity

741. A client has sustained a closed fracture and has just had a cast applied to the affected arm. The client is complaining of intense pain. The nurse elevates the limb, applies an ice bag, and administers an analgesic, with little relief. Which problem may be causing this pain?
1. Infection under the cast
2. The anxiety of the client
3. Impaired tissue perfusion
4. The recent occurrence of the fracture

742. The nurse is admitting a client with multiple trauma injuries to the nursing unit. The client has a leg fracture and had a plaster cast applied. Which position would be **best** for the casted leg?
1. Elevated for 3 hours, then flat for 1 hour
2. Flat for 3 hours, then elevated for 1 hour
3. Flat for 12 hours, then elevated for 12 hours
4. Elevated on pillows continuously for 24 to 48 hours

743. A client is being discharged to home after application of a plaster leg cast. Which statement indicates that the client understands proper care of the cast?
1. "I need to avoid getting the cast wet."
2. "I need to cover the casted leg with warm blankets."
3. "I need to use my fingertips to lift and move my leg."
4. "I need to use something like a padded coat hanger end to scratch under the cast if it itches."

744. A client being measured for crutches asks the nurse why the crutches cannot rest up underneath the arm for extra support. The nurse responds knowing that which would **most likely** result from this improper crutch measurement?
1. A fall and further injury
2. Injury to the brachial plexus nerves
3. Skin breakdown in the area of the axilla
4. Impaired range of motion while the client ambulates

745. The nurse has given the client instructions about crutch safety. Which statements indicate that the client understands the instructions? **Select all that apply.**
- ☐ 1. "I should not use someone else's crutches."
- ☐ 2. "I need to remove any scatter rugs at home."
- ☐ 3. "I can use crutch tips even when they are wet."
- ☐ 4. "I need to have spare crutches and tips available."
- ☐ 5. "When I'm using the crutches, my arms need to be completely straight."

746. The nurse is caring for a client being treated for fat embolus after multiple fractures. Which data would the nurse evaluate as the **most** favorable indication of resolution of the fat embolus?
1. Clear mentation
2. Minimal dyspnea
3. Oxygen saturation of 85%
4. Arterial oxygen level of 78 mm Hg

747. The nurse has conducted teaching with a client in an arm cast about the signs and symptoms of compartment syndrome. The nurse determines that the client understands the information if the client states that he or she should report which **early** symptom of compartment syndrome?
1. Cold, bluish-colored fingers
2. Numbness and tingling in the fingers
3. Pain that increases when the arm is dependent
4. Pain that is out of proportion to the severity of the fracture

748. A client with diabetes mellitus has had a right below-knee amputation. Given the client's history of diabetes mellitus, which complication is the client at **most** risk for after surgery?
1. Hemorrhage
2. Edema of the residual limb
3. Slight redness of the incision
4. Separation of the wound edges

749. The nurse is caring for a client who had an above-knee amputation 2 days ago. The residual limb was wrapped with an elastic compression bandage, which has come off. Which **immediate** action should the nurse take?
1. Apply ice to the site.
2. Call the primary health care provider (PHCP).
3. Rewrap the residual limb with an elastic compression bandage.
4. Apply a dry, sterile dressing and elevate the residual limb on 1 pillow.

750. A client is complaining of low back pain that radiates down the left posterior thigh. The nurse should ask the client if the pain is worsened or aggravated by which factor?
1. Bed rest
2. Ibuprofen
3. Bending or lifting
4. Application of heat

751. The nurse is caring for a client who has had spinal fusion, with insertion of hardware. The nurse would be **most** concerned with which assessment finding?
1. Temperature of 101.6° F (38.7° C) orally
2. Complaints of discomfort during repositioning
3. Old bloody drainage outlined on the surgical dressing
4. Discomfort during coughing and deep-breathing exercises

752. The nurse is caring for a client with a diagnosis of gout. Which laboratory value would the nurse expect to note in the client?
1. Calcium level of 9.0 mg/dL (2.25 mmol/L)
2. Uric acid level of 9.0 mg/dL (540 mcmol/L)
3. Potassium level of 4.1 mEq/L (4.1 mmol/L)
4. Phosphorus level of 3.1 mg/dL (1.0 mmol/L)

753. A client with a hip fracture asks the nurse about Buck's (extension) traction that is being applied before surgery and what is involved. The nurse should provide which information to the client?
1. Allows bony healing to begin before surgery and involves pins and screws
2. Provides rigid immobilization of the fracture site and involves pulleys and wheels
3. Lengthens the fractured leg to prevent severing of blood vessels and involves pins and screws
4. Provides comfort by reducing muscle spasms, provides fracture immobilization, and involves pulleys and wheels

ANSWERS

735. *Answer:* 4

Rationale: Risk factors for osteoporosis include female gender, being postmenopausal, advanced age, a low-calcium diet, excessive alcohol intake, being sedentary, and smoking cigarettes. Long-term use of corticosteroids, anticonvulsants, and/or furosemide also increases the risk.

Test-Taking Strategy: Focus on the subject, risk factors for osteoporosis. The 25-year-old woman who runs (exercises using the long bones) has negligible risk. The 36-year-old man with asthma is eliminated next because his only risk factor might be long-term corticosteroid use (if prescribed) to treat the asthma. Of the remaining options, the 65-year-old woman has higher risk (age, gender, postmenopausal, sedentary, smoking) than the 70-year-old man (age, alcohol consumption).

Level of Cognitive Ability: Analyzing
Client Needs: Health Promotion and Maintenance
Integrated Process: Nursing Process—Assessment
Content Area: Adult Health: Musculoskeletal
Health Problem: Adult Health: Musculoskeletal: Osteoporosis
Priority Concepts: Health Promotion; Mobility
Reference: Ignatavicius, Workman, Rebar (2018), p. 1017.

736. *Answer:* 4

Rationale: After arthroscopy, the client usually can walk carefully on the leg once sensation has returned. The client is instructed to avoid strenuous exercise for the length of time prescribed by the surgeon. The client may resume the usual diet. Signs and symptoms of infection should be reported to the primary health care provider.

Test-Taking Strategy: Focus on the subject, teaching points following knee arthroscopy. Recalling the general client teaching points related to surgical procedures and that a risk for infection exists after a surgical procedure will direct you to the correct option.

Level of Cognitive Ability: Evaluating
Client Needs: Physiological Integrity
Integrated Process: Nursing Process—Evaluation
Content Area: Adult Health: Musculoskeletal
Health Problem: N/A
Priority Concepts: Client Education; Safety
Reference: Ignatavicius, Workman, Rebar (2018), p. 1014.

737. *Answer:* 4

Rationale: With a suspected fracture, the victim is not moved unless it is dangerous to remain in that spot. The nurse should remain with the victim and have someone else call for emergency help. A fracture is not reduced at the scene. Before the victim is moved, the site of fracture is immobilized to prevent further injury.

Test-Taking Strategy: Eliminate options 1 and 2 first because they are comparable or alike in that either of these options could result in further injury to the victim. Of the remaining options, the more prudent action would be for the nurse to remain with the victim and have someone else call for emergency assistance.

Level of Cognitive Ability: Applying
Client Needs: Physiological Integrity
Integrated Process: Nursing Process—Implementation
Content Area: Adult Health: Musculoskeletal
Health Problem: Adult Health: Musculoskeletal: Skeletal Injury
Priority Concepts: Clinical Judgment; Safety
Reference: Ignatavicius, Workman, Rebar (2018), pp. 1037-1038.

738. *Answer:* 1, 2, 3

Rationale: A plaster cast takes 24 to 72 hours to dry (synthetic casts dry in 20 minutes). The cast and extremity should be elevated to reduce edema if prescribed. A wet cast is handled with the palms of the hand until it is dry, and the extremity is turned (unless contraindicated) so that all sides of the wet cast will dry. A cool setting on the hair dryer can be used to dry a plaster cast (heat cannot be used on a plaster cast because the cast heats up and burns the skin). The cast needs to be kept clean and dry, and the client is instructed not to stick anything under the cast because of the risk of breaking skin integrity. The client is instructed to monitor the extremity for circulatory impairment, such as pain, swelling, discoloration, tingling, numbness, coolness, or diminished pulse. The primary health care provider is notified immediately if circulatory impairment occurs.

Test-Taking Strategy: Focus on the subject, a plaster cast. Recalling that edema occurs following a fracture and recalling the complications associated with a cast will assist you in answering the question.

Level of Cognitive Ability: Analyzing
Client Needs: Physiological Integrity
Integrated Process: Teaching and Learning
Content Area: Adult Health: Musculoskeletal
Health Problem: Adult Health: Musculoskeletal: Skeletal Injury
Priority Concepts: Client Education; Safety
Reference: Lewis et al. (2017), pp. 1471-1472.

739. *Answer:* 3

Rationale: The nurse should monitor for signs of infection such as inflammation, purulent (thick white or yellow) drainage, and pain at the pin site. However, some degree of inflammation, pain at the pin site, and serous drainage would be expected; the nurse should correlate assessment findings with other clinical findings, such as fever, elevated white blood cell count, and changes in vital signs. Additionally, the nurse should compare any findings to baseline findings to determine if there were any changes.

Test-Taking Strategy: Note the strategic word, *most*. Determine if an abnormality exists. Recall that purulent drainage is indicative of infection, and that some degree of pain, inflammation, and serous drainage should be expected.

Level of Cognitive Ability: Evaluating
Client Needs: Physiological Integrity
Integrated Process: Nursing Process—Evaluation
Content Area: Adult Health: Musculoskeletal
Health Problem: Adult Health: Musculoskeletal: Skeletal Injury
Priority Concepts: Clinical Judgment; Tissue Integrity
Reference: Ignatavicius, Workman, Rebar (2018), pp. 1040-1041.

740. *Answer:* 3

Rationale: Signs of infection under a casted area include odor or purulent drainage from the cast or the presence of "hot spots," which are areas of the cast that are warmer than others. The primary health care provider should be notified if any of these occur. Signs of impaired circulation in the distal limb include coolness and pallor of the skin, diminished distal pulse, and edema.

Test-Taking Strategy: Focus on the subject, signs of infection. Think about what you would expect to note with infection—redness, swelling, heat, and purulent drainage. With this in mind, you can eliminate options 2 and 4 easily. From the remaining options, remember that "dependent edema" is not necessarily indicative of infection. Swelling would be continuous. The hot spot on the cast could signify infection underneath that area.

Level of Cognitive Ability: Analyzing
Client Needs: Physiological Integrity
Integrated Process: Nursing Process—Assessment
Content Area: Adult Health: Musculoskeletal
Health Problem: Adult Health: Musculoskeletal: Skeletal Injury
Priority Concepts: Infection; Tissue Integrity
Reference: Ignatavicius, Workman, Rebar (2018), p. 1039.

741. ***Answer:*** 3

Rationale: Most pain associated with fractures can be minimized with rest, elevation, application of cold, and administration of analgesics. Pain that is not relieved by these measures should be reported to the primary health care provider because pain unrelieved by medications and other measures may indicate neurovascular compromise. Because this is a new closed fracture and cast, infection would not have had time to set in. Intense pain after casting is normally not associated with anxiety or the recent occurrence of the injury. Treatment following the fracture should assist in relieving the pain associated with the injury.

Test-Taking Strategy: Focus on the subject, intense pain, and focus on the data in the question. Use of the ABCs—airway, breathing, and circulation—will direct you to the correct option.

Level of Cognitive Ability: Analyzing
Client Needs: Physiological Integrity
Integrated Process: Nursing Process—Assessment
Content Area: Adult Health: Musculoskeletal
Health Problem: Adult Health: Musculoskeletal: Skeletal Injury
Priority Concepts: Pain; Tissue Integrity
Reference: Ignatavicius, Workman, Rebar (2018), p. 1039.

742. ***Answer:*** 4

Rationale: A casted extremity is elevated continuously for the first 24 to 48 hours to minimize swelling and promote venous drainage. Options 1, 2, and 3 are incorrect.

Test-Taking Strategy: Note the strategic word, *best.* Recalling that edema is a concern following an injury and knowledge of the effects of gravity on edema will direct you to the correct option.

Level of Cognitive Ability: Applying
Client Needs: Physiological Integrity
Integrated Process: Nursing Process—Implementation
Content Area: Adult Health: Musculoskeletal
Health Problem: Adult Health: Musculoskeletal: Skeletal Injury
Priority Concepts: Perfusion; Tissue Integrity
Reference: Ignatavicius, Workman, Rebar (2018), p. 1039.

743. ***Answer:*** 1

Rationale: A plaster cast must remain dry to keep its strength. The cast should be handled with the palms of the hands, not the fingertips, until fully dry; using the fingertips results in indentations in the cast and skin pressure under the cast. Air should circulate freely around the cast to help it dry; the cast also gives off heat as it dries. The client should never scratch under the cast because of the risk of altered skin integrity; the client may use a hair dryer on the cool setting to relieve an itch.

Test-Taking Strategy: Focus on the subject, client understanding about cast care. Knowing that a wet cast can be dented with the fingertips, causing pressure underneath, helps eliminate option 3 first. Knowing that the cast needs to dry helps eliminate option 2 next. Option 4 is dangerous to skin integrity and is also eliminated. Remember that plaster casts, once they have dried after application, should not become wet.

Level of Cognitive Ability: Evaluating
Client Needs: Physiological Integrity
Integrated Process: Nursing Process—Evaluation
Content Area: Adult Health: Musculoskeletal
Health Problem: Adult Health: Musculoskeletal: Skeletal Injury
Priority Concepts: Client Education; Safety
Reference: Ignatavicius, Workman, Rebar (2018), p. 1039.

744. ***Answer:*** 2

Rationale: Crutches are measured so that the tops are 2 to 3 fingerwidths from the axillae. This ensures that the client's axillae are not resting on the crutch or bearing the weight of the crutch, which could result in injury to the nerves of the brachial plexus. Although the conditions in options 1, 3, and 4 can occur, they are not the most likely result from resting the axilla directly on the crutches.

Test-Taking Strategy: Note the strategic words, *most likely*, and focus on the data in the question. Recalling the risk associated with brachial nerve plexus injury will direct you to the correct option.

Level of Cognitive Ability: Applying
Client Needs: Physiological Integrity
Integrated Process: Teaching and Learning
Content Area: Adult Health: Musculoskeletal
Health Problem: Adult Health: Musculoskeletal: Skeletal Injury
Priority Concepts: Client Education; Safety
Reference: Potter et al. (2017), pp. 806-807.

745. ***Answer:*** 1, 2, 4

Rationale: The client should use only crutches measured for the client. When assessing for home safety, the nurse ensures that the client knows to remove any scatter rugs and does not walk on highly waxed floors. The tips should be inspected for wear, and spare crutches and tips should be available if needed. Crutch tips should remain dry. If crutch tips get wet, the client should dry them with a cloth or paper towel. When walking with crutches, both elbows need to be flexed not more than 30 degrees when the palms are on the handle.

Test-Taking Strategy: Focus on the subject, client understanding of instructions of using crutches. Visualize each option and think about the safety associated with each instruction. This will assist in answering correctly.

Level of Cognitive Ability: Evaluating
Client Needs: Safe and Effective Care Environment
Integrated Process: Nursing Process—Evaluation
Content Area: Adult Health: Musculoskeletal
Health Problem: Adult Health: Musculoskeletal: Skeletal Injury
Priority Concepts: Mobility; Safety
Reference: Potter et al. (2017), pp. 806-807.

746. *Answer:* 1

Rationale: An altered mental state is an early indication of fat emboli; therefore, clear mentation is a good indicator that a fat embolus is resolving. Eupnea, not minimal dyspnea, is a normal sign. Arterial oxygen levels should be 80 to 100 mm Hg. Oxygen saturation should be higher than 95%.

Test-Taking Strategy: Note the strategic word, *most*. Knowing that the arterial oxygen and oxygen saturation levels are below normal helps eliminate options 3 and 4. Dyspnea, even at a minimal level, is not normal, so eliminate option 2.

Level of Cognitive Ability: Evaluating
Client Needs: Physiological Integrity
Integrated Process: Nursing Process—Evaluation
Content Area: Adult Health: Musculoskeletal
Health Problem: Adult Health: Musculoskeletal: Skeletal Injury
Priority Concepts: Evidence; Perfusion
Reference: Lewis et al. (2017), p. 1480.

747. *Answer:* 2

Rationale: The earliest symptom of compartment syndrome is paresthesia (numbness and tingling in the fingers). Other symptoms include pain unrelieved by opioids, pain that increases with limb elevation, and pallor and coolness to the distal limb. Cyanosis is a late sign. Pain that is out of proportion to the severity of the fracture, along with other symptoms associated with the pain, is not an early manifestation.

Test-Taking Strategy: Note the strategic word, *early*. Knowing that compartment syndrome is characterized by insufficient circulation and ischemia caused by pressure will direct you to the correct option.

Level of Cognitive Ability: Evaluating
Client Needs: Physiological Integrity
Integrated Process: Nursing Process—Evaluation
Content Area: Adult Health: Musculoskeletal
Health Problem: Adult Health: Musculoskeletal: Skeletal Injury
Priority Concepts: Client Education; Perfusion
Reference: Lewis et al. (2017), p. 1479.

748. *Answer:* 4

Rationale: Clients with diabetes mellitus are more prone to wound infection, wound separation, and delayed wound healing because of the disease. Postoperative hemorrhage and edema of the residual limb are complications in the immediate postoperative period that apply to any client with an amputation. Slight redness of the incision is considered normal, as long as the incision is dry and intact.

Test-Taking Strategy: Note the strategic word, *most*, and focus on the subject, complications following surgery for the client with diabetes mellitus. Recalling that diabetes mellitus increases the client's chances of developing infection and delayed wound healing will direct you to the correct option.

Level of Cognitive Ability: Analyzing
Client Needs: Physiological Integrity
Integrated Process: Nursing Process—Assessment
Content Area: Adult Health: Musculoskeletal
Health Problem: Adult Health: Musculoskeletal: Amputation
Priority Concepts: Glucose Regulation; Tissue Integrity
Reference: Lewis et al. (2017), p. 1487.

749. *Answer:* 3

Rationale: If the client with an amputation has a cast or elastic compression bandage that slips off, the nurse must wrap the residual limb immediately with another elastic compression bandage. Otherwise, excessive edema will form rapidly, which could cause a significant delay in rehabilitation. If the client had a cast that slipped off, the nurse would have to call the PHCP so that a new one could be applied. Elevation on 1 pillow is not going to impede the development of edema greatly once compression is released. Ice would be of limited value in controlling edema from this cause. If the PHCP were called, the prescription likely would be to reapply the compression dressing anyway.

Test-Taking Strategy: Note the strategic word, *immediate*, and focus on the data in the question. Recalling that excessive edema can form rapidly in the residual limb will direct you to the correct option.

Level of Cognitive Ability: Analyzing
Client Needs: Physiological Integrity
Integrated Process: Nursing Process—Implementation
Content Area: Adult Health: Musculoskeletal
Health Problem: Adult Health: Musculoskeletal: Amputation
Priority Concepts: Clinical Judgment; Tissue Integrity
Reference: Lewis et al. (2017), p. 1487.

750. *Answer:* 3

Rationale: Low back pain that radiates down 1 leg (sciatica) is consistent with herniated lumbar disk. The nurse assesses the client to see whether the pain is aggravated by events that increase intraspinal pressure, such as bending, lifting, sneezing, and coughing, or by lifting the leg straight up while supine (straight leg-raising test). Bed rest, heat (or sometimes ice), and nonsteroidal antiinflammatory drugs (NSAIDs) usually relieve back pain.

Test-Taking Strategy: Focus on the subject, factors that aggravate back pain. Think about how each item in the options would relieve or exacerbate back pain. Recall that bed rest, heat (or sometimes ice), and NSAIDs usually relieve back pain, whereas bending, lifting, and straining aggravate it.

Level of Cognitive Ability: Analyzing
Client Needs: Physiological Integrity
Integrated Process: Nursing Process—Assessment
Content Area: Adult Health: Musculoskeletal
Health Problem: Adult Health: Musculoskeletal: Intervertebral Disc Herniation
Priority Concepts: Mobility; Pain
Reference: Ignatavicius, Workman, Rebar (2018), pp. 903-904.

751. *Answer:* 1

Rationale: The nursing assessment conducted after spinal surgery is similar to that done after other surgical procedures. For this specific type of surgery, the nurse assesses the neurovascular status of the lower extremities, watches for signs and symptoms of infection, and inspects the surgical site for evidence of cerebrospinal fluid leakage (drainage is clear and tests positive for glucose). A mild temperature is expected after insertion of hardware, but a temperature of 101.6° F (38.7° C) should be reported.

Test-Taking Strategy: Note the strategic word, *most*. Determine if an abnormality exists. Thus, you are looking for the option that has the greatest deviation from normal. Options 2 and 4 are expected after surgery and, although the nurse tries to minimize discomfort, the client is likely to have some discomfort, even with proper analgesic use. The words *old* and *outlined* in option 3 indicate that this is not a new occurrence. This leaves the temperature of 101.6° F (38.7° C), which is excessive and should be reported.
Level of Cognitive Ability: Analyzing
Client Needs: Physiological Integrity
Integrated Process: Nursing Process—Assessment
Content Area: Adult Health: Musculoskeletal
Health Problem: Adult Health: Musculoskeletal: Skeletal Injury
Priority Concepts: Clinical Judgment; Infection
Reference: Ignatavicius, Workman, Rebar (2018), pp. 906-908.

752. *Answer:* 2
Rationale: In addition to the presence of clinical manifestations, gout is diagnosed by the presence of persistent hyperuricemia, with a uric acid level higher than 8 mg/dL (480 mcmol/L); a normal value for a male ranges from 4.0 to 8.5 mg/dL (240–501 mcmol/L) and for a female, from 2.7 to 7.3 mg/dL (160–430 mcmol/L). Options 1, 3, and 4 indicate normal laboratory values. In addition, the presence of uric acid in an aspirated sample of synovial fluid confirms the diagnosis.
Test-Taking Strategy: Focus on the subject, manifestation of gout. Use knowledge of normal laboratory values. Recalling that increased uric acid levels occur in gout and noting that the correct option has the only abnormal value will assist you in answering the question.
Level of Cognitive Ability: Analyzing
Client Needs: Physiological Integrity
Integrated Process: Nursing Process—Assessment
Content Area: Adult Health: Musculoskeletal
Health Problem: Adult Health: Musculoskeletal: Gout
Priority Concepts: Cellular Regulation; Clinical Judgment
Reference: Lewis et al. (2017), pp. 1026, 1532-1534.

753. *Answer:* 4
Rationale: Buck's (extension) traction is a type of skin traction often applied after hip fracture before the fracture is reduced in surgery. Traction reduces muscle spasms and helps immobilize the fracture. Traction does not allow for bony healing to begin or provide rigid immobilization. Traction does not lengthen the leg for the purpose of preventing blood vessel severance. This type of traction involves pulleys and wheels, not pins and screws.
Test-Taking Strategy: Focus on the subject, use of traction following a hip fracture. Read each option carefully and note that each option has more than one part. All parts of the option need to be correct in order for the answer to be correct. Noting the words *provides comfort* and *fracture immobilization* will direct you to the correct option.
Level of Cognitive Ability: Applying
Client Needs: Physiological Integrity
Integrated Process: Nursing Process—Implementation
Content Area: Adult Health: Musculoskeletal
Health Problem: Adult Health: Musculoskeletal: Skeletal Injury
Priority Concepts: Clinical Judgment; Mobility
Reference: Lewis et al. (2017), p. 1470.

CHAPTER 61

Musculoskeletal Medications

PRIORITY CONCEPTS Inflammation; Safety

I. Skeletal Muscle Relaxants

A. Description
1. Skeletal muscle relaxants (Box 61-1) act directly on the neuromuscular junction or act indirectly on the central nervous system (CNS).
2. Centrally acting muscle relaxants depress neuron activity in the spinal cord or brain.
3. Peripherally acting muscle relaxants act directly on the skeletal muscles, interfering with calcium release from muscle tubules and thus preventing the fibers from contracting.
4. Skeletal muscle relaxants are used to prevent or relieve muscle spasms and treat spasticity associated with spinal cord disease or lesions, acute painful musculoskeletal conditions, and chronic debilitating disorders such as multiple sclerosis, stroke (brain attacks), or cerebral palsy.
5. Skeletal muscle relaxants are contraindicated in clients with severe liver, renal, or heart disease; these medications are often metabolized in the liver or excreted by the kidneys.
6. Skeletal muscle relaxants should not be taken with CNS depressants, such as barbiturates, opioids, alcohol, sedatives, hypnotics, or tricyclic antidepressants, unless specifically prescribed.

B. Side and adverse effects
1. Dizziness and hypotension
2. Drowsiness and muscle weakness
3. Dry mouth
4. Gastrointestinal upset
5. Photosensitivity
6. Liver toxicity

C. Interventions
1. Obtain a medical history and ask about current medications being taken.
2. Monitor vital signs.
3. Monitor for CNS effects.
4. Assess for risk of injury.
5. Assess involved joints and muscles for pain and mobility.
6. Monitor renal function studies.
7. Instruct the client to take the medication with food to decrease gastrointestinal upset.
8. Instruct the client to report adverse effects.
9. Instruct the client to avoid alcohol and CNS depressants.
10. Instruct the client to avoid activities requiring alertness, such as driving or operating equipment.

Monitor liver function tests when a client is taking a skeletal muscle relaxant, because hepatotoxicity can occur.

D. Nursing considerations
1. Baclofen
   a. Baclofen causes CNS effects such as drowsiness, dizziness, weakness, and fatigue and nausea, constipation, and urinary retention.
   b. Administer with caution in the client with renal or hepatic dysfunction or a seizure disorder.
   c. Baclofen can be administered by the primary health care provider (PHCP) through intrathecal infusion using an implantable pump or by direct intrathecal administration over 1 minute.
   d. Instruct the client with an implantable pump to maintain medication refill appointments to prevent the pump from emptying and experiencing sudden withdrawal symptoms, which could be life-threatening.
2. Carisoprodol
   a. Advise the client to take the medication with food to prevent gastrointestinal upset.
   b. Instruct the client to report any rash or hypersensitivity to the PHCP.
3. Chlorzoxazone
   a. Monitor the client for hypersensitivity reactions such as urticaria, redness or itching, and possibly angioedema.
   b. Chlorzoxazone may cause malaise and may cause the urine to turn orange or red.
   c. Can cause hepatitis and hepatic necrosis.

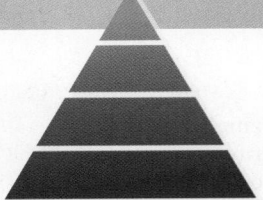

BOX 61-1 Skeletal Muscle Relaxants

- Baclofen
- Carisoprodol
- Chlorzoxazone
- Cyclobenzaprine
- Dantrolene
- Diazepam
- Metaxalone
- Methocarbamol
- Orphenadrine
- Tizanidine

4. Cyclobenzaprine
   a. Cyclobenzaprine is contraindicated in clients who have received monoamine oxidase inhibitors (MAOIs) within 14 days of initiation of cyclobenzaprine therapy and in clients with cardiac disorders.
   b. Cyclobenzaprine has significant anticholinergic (atropine-like) effects and should be used with caution in clients with a history of urinary retention, angle-closure glaucoma, or increased intraocular pressure.
   c. Cyclobenzaprine should be used only for short-term therapy (2 to 3 weeks).
5. Dantrolene
   a. Dantrolene acts directly on skeletal muscles to relieve spasticity.
   b. Liver damage is the most serious adverse effect.
   c. Liver function values should be monitored before the initiation of treatment and during treatment.
   d. Dantrolene can cause gastrointestinal bleeding, urinary frequency, impotence, photosensitivity, rash, and muscle weakness.
   e. Instruct the client to wear protective clothing when in the sun.
   f. Instruct the client to notify the PHCP if rash, bloody or tarry stools, or yellow discoloration of the skin or eyes occurs.
6. Diazepam
   a. Acts on the CNS to suppress spasticity; does not affect skeletal muscle directly
   b. Sedation commonly occurs.
7. Methocarbamol
   a. The parenteral form is contraindicated in clients with renal impairment.
   b. The parenteral form can cause hypotension, bradycardia, anaphylaxis, and seizures, especially when the medication is given too rapidly.
   c. Monitor site for extravasation, which can result in thrombophlebitis and tissue sloughing.
   d. Methocarbamol may cause the urine to turn brown, black, or green.
   e. Inform the client to notify the PHCP if blurred vision, nasal congestion, urticaria, or rash occurs.
8. Tizanidine and metaxalone: Can cause liver damage
9. Orphenadrine has significant anticholinergic (atropine-like) effects and should be used with caution in clients with a history of urinary retention, angle-closure glaucoma, or increased intraocular pressure.

Safety is a primary concern when the client is taking a skeletal muscle relaxant, because these medications cause drowsiness.

II. Antigout Medications

A. Description
1. Antigout medications (allopurinol, colchicine, probenecid) reduce uric acid production and increase uric acid excretion (uricosuric) to prevent or relieve gout or to manage hyperuricemia.
2. Nonsteroidal antiinflammatory drugs (NSAIDs) are used for their antiinflammatory effects and to relieve pain during an acute gouty attack (see Chapter 59 for information on NSAIDs).
3. Glucocorticoids may be prescribed to reduce inflammation during an acute gout attack (see Chapter 47 for information on glucocorticoids).
4. Antigout medications should be used cautiously in clients with gastrointestinal, renal, cardiac, or hepatic disease.

B. Side and adverse effects
1. Headaches
2. Nausea, vomiting, and diarrhea
3. Blood dyscrasias, such as bone marrow depression
4. Flushed skin and rash
5. Uric acid kidney stones
6. Sore gums
7. Metallic taste

C. Interventions
1. Assess serum uric acid levels.
2. Monitor intake and output.
3. Maintain a fluid intake of at least 2000 to 3000 mL/day to prevent kidney stones.
4. Monitor complete blood cell count and renal and liver function studies.
5. Instruct the client to avoid alcohol and caffeine, because these products can increase uric acid levels.
6. Encourage the client to comply with therapy to prevent elevated uric acid levels, which can trigger a gout attack.
7. Instruct the client to avoid foods high in purine as prescribed, such as wine, alcohol, organ meats, sardines, salmon, scallops, and gravy.
8. Instruct the client to take the medication with food to decrease gastric irritation.

9. Instruct the client to report adverse effects to the PHCP.
10. Caution the client not to take aspirin with these medications, because this could trigger a gout attack.

D. Nursing considerations
1. Allopurinol
   a. Can increase the effect of warfarin and oral hypoglycemic agents
   b. Instruct the client not to take large doses of vitamin C while taking allopurinol, because kidney stones may occur.
   c. Hypersensitivity syndrome (rare) can occur, characterized by rash, fever, eosinophilia, and liver and kidney alterations (medication is withheld and the PHCP is notified).
   d. Advise the client to minimize exposure to sunlight and have an annual eye examination, because visual changes can occur from prolonged use of allopurinol.
2. Colchicine
   a. Used with caution in older clients, debilitated clients, and clients with cardiac, renal, and/or gastrointestinal disease.
   b. If gastrointestinal symptoms occur (nausea, vomiting, diarrhea, and abdominal pain), the medication is withheld and the PHCP is notified.
3. Probenecid
   a. Mild gastrointestinal effects can occur and can be reduced by taking the medication with food.
   b. Aspirin and other salicylates interfere with the uricosuric action of the medication.

! The concurrent use of antigout medications and aspirin causes elevated uric acid levels; the client should be instructed to take acetaminophen if prescribed rather than aspirin.

III. Antiarthritic Medications (Box 61-2)

A. Description (Fig. 61-1)
1. Rheumatoid arthritis occurs as inflammation progresses into the synovia, cartilage, and bone; if this inflammation is not controlled, it will lead to joint destruction, thus affecting client mobility and comfort.
2. The focus of treatment is early diagnosis and aggressive treatment to preserve joint function.
3. Medication therapy includes NSAIDs, glucocorticoids, and disease-modifying antirheumatic drugs (DMARDs).
4. Gold salts: Use of gold salts has decreased, but their purpose is to reduce the progression of joint damage caused by arthritic processes. Gold toxicity, characterized by pruritus, rash, metallic taste, stomatitis, and diarrhea, can occur; if toxicity occurs, dimercaprol may be prescribed to enhance gold excretion.

B. DMARDs
1. Description
   a. DMARDs are effective antirheumatic medications that are used to slow the degenerative effects of the disorder.

BOX 61-2 Antiarthritic Medications

- Anakinra
- Adalimumab
- Azathioprine
- Cyclosporine
- Etanercept
- Hydroxychloroquine
- Infliximab
- Leflunomide
- Methotrexate
- Penicillamine
- Rituximab
- Sulfasalazine

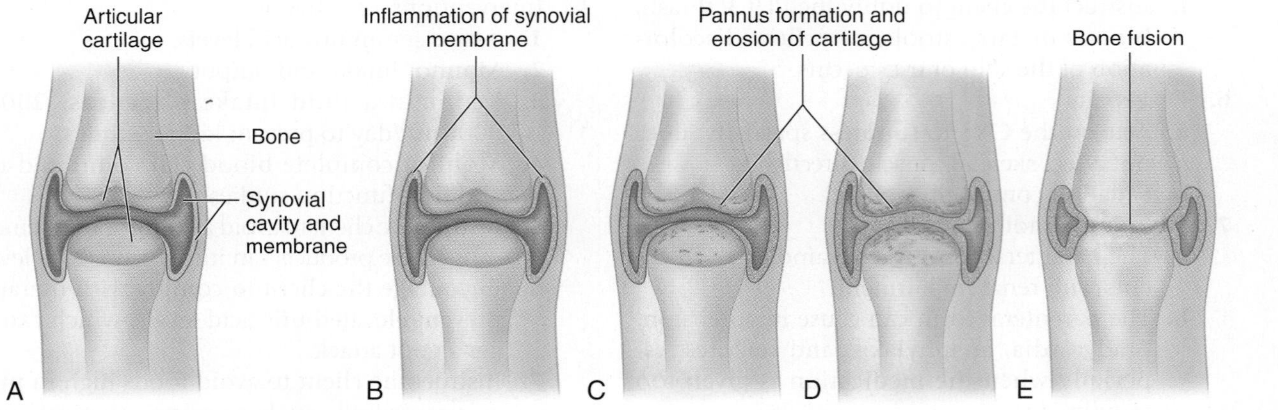

FIG. 61-1 Progressive joint degeneration in rheumatoid arthritis. **A,** Healthy joint. **B,** Inflammation of synovial membrane. **C,** Onset of pannus formation and cartilage erosion. **D,** Pannus formation progresses and cartilage deteriorates further. **E,** Complete destruction of joint cavity, together with fusion of articulating bones.

b. DMARDs are usually prescribed secondary to NSAIDs but are often the first choice in the treatment of severe arthritis.

2. Common side and adverse effects of DMARDs include injection site inflammation and pain, ecchymosis, and edema; pancytopenia and infection; fatigue, headache, nausea, vomiting, and flu-like symptoms; and allergic response.
3. Interventions
   a. Instruct the client to monitor for signs of infection and report signs to the PHCP.
   b. Monitor the injection site for signs of irritation, pain, inflammation, and swelling.
   c. Instruct the client to consult with the PHCP before receiving live vaccines and to avoid exposure to infections.
   d. Inform the client about the importance of laboratory tests for neutrophil counts, white blood cell counts, and platelet counts before initiation of treatment and during treatment.
4. Anakinra: Injection site reactions are common (pruritus, erythema, rash, pain).
5. Adalimumab
   a. Injection site reactions are common.
   b. Has been associated with neurological injury (numbness, tingling, dizziness, visual disturbances, weakness in the legs)
6. Azathioprine: Immunosuppressive and anti-inflammatory actions; toxic effects include hepatitis and blood dyscrasias.
7. Cyclosporine: Immunosuppressive actions; can cause nephrotoxicity
8. Etanercept
   a. Injection site reactions are common.
   b. Poses a risk for heart failure; has been associated with CNS demyelinating disorders and hematological disorders
9. Hydroxychloroquine: Associated with retinal damage; inform the client to contact the PHCP if visual disturbances occur.
10. Leflunomide: Side and adverse effects include diarrhea, respiratory infection, reversible alopecia, rash, and nausea; medication is hepatotoxic.
11. Methotrexate: Can cause hepatic fibrosis, bone marrow suppression, gastrointestinal ulceration, and pneumonitis
12. Penicillamine: Can cause bone marrow suppression and autoimmune disorders
13. Infliximab: Can cause infusion reactions (fever, chills, pruritus, urticaria, chest pain); medication is hepatotoxic.
14. Rituxan: Can cause increased thirst or urination, swelling of the hands or feet, or tingling of the hands or feet; the PHCP should be notified if any of these occur.
15. Sulfasalazine: Can cause gastrointestinal and dermatological reactions, bone marrow suppression, and hepatitis

C. NSAIDs may be prescribed for their antiinflammatory and analgesic effects (see Chapter 59 for information on NSAIDs).

D. Glucocorticoids may be prescribed for their anti-inflammatory effects (see Chapter 47 for information on glucocorticoids).

IV. Medications to Prevent and Treat Osteoporosis

A. Description
1. Osteoporosis is characterized by decreased bone mass and increased bone fragility.
2. Calcium and vitamin D supplementation can reduce the risk of osteoporosis; calcium maximizes bone growth early in life and maintains bone integrity later in life, and vitamin D ensures calcium absorption (see Chapter 47 for information on calcium and vitamin D supplements).
3. Treatment is aimed at reducing the occurrence of fractures by maintaining or increasing bone strength.
4. Medications that decrease bone resorption (antiresorptive) and medications that promote bone formation are used (Box 61-3).
5. Antiresorptive medications include raloxifene, calcitonin, and bisphosphonates.
6. Teriparatide promotes bone growth.

B. Interventions
1. Calcitonin-salmon
   a. Calcitonin is secreted by the thyroid gland and inhibits osteoclastic bone resorption.
   b. Instruct the client on how to administer the intranasal or subcutaneous form, depending on the route prescribed.
   c. Intranasal route: Examine the nares for irritation; alternate nostrils for doses.
   d. When calcitonin is taken, it is important to monitor for hypocalcemia.

BOX 61-3 Medications to Prevent or Treat Osteoporosis

- Calcium and vitamin D
- Alendronate
- Calcitonin-salmon
- Denosumab
- Ibandronate
- Pamidronate
- Raloxifene
- Risedronate
- Teriparatide
- Zoledronic acid

2. Bisphosphonates
   a. Bisphosphonates inhibit osteoclast-mediated bone resorption, thereby increasing total bone mass.
   b. Bisphosphonates include alendronate, risedronate, ibandronate, pamidronate, and zoledronic acid.
   c. Contraindicated for clients with esophageal disorders that can impede swallowing and for clients who cannot sit or stand for at least 30 minutes (60 minutes with ibandronate)
   d. Adverse effects include esophagitis, muscle pain, and ocular problems; the client is instructed to contact the PHCP if adverse effects occur.

⚠ Because of the risk of esophagitis, bisphosphonates must be administered in the morning before eating or drinking with a full glass of water; the client must then remain sitting or standing and postpone ingesting anything for at least 30 minutes (60 minutes with ibandronate).

3. Raloxifene
   a. Antiresorptive medication (nonbisphosphonate)
   b. Contraindicated in clients who have a history of venous thrombotic events
   c. Needs to be discontinued 72 hours prior to prolonged immobilization periods (such as with periods of extended bed rest)
   d. Instruct the client to avoid extended periods of restricted activity (such as when traveling).
4. Denosumab: A monoclonal antibody that treats osteoporosis and hypercalcemia; can also treat bone cancer and bone problems in those who have cancer.
5. Teriparatide
   a. Teriparatide stimulates new bone formation, thus increasing bone mass.
   b. Teriparatide is a portion of the human parathyroid hormone and works by increasing the action of osteoblasts.
   c. Is usually reserved for clients at high risk for fractures
   d. Has been associated with the development of bone cancer

⚠ NSAIDs such as ibuprofen, indomethacin, and naproxen are commonly used to treat musculoskeletal pain. Acetaminophen may also be used to treat this type of pain as well and are often considered first-line treatments.

PRACTICE QUESTIONS

754. A client has been on treatment for rheumatoid arthritis for 3 weeks. During the administration of etanercept, which is **most important** for the nurse to assess?
   1. The injection site for itching and edema
   2. The white blood cell counts and platelet counts
   3. Whether the client is experiencing fatigue and joint pain
   4. Whether the client is experiencing a metallic taste in the mouth and a loss of appetite

755. Allopurinol is prescribed for a client and the nurse provides medication instructions to the client. Which instruction should the nurse provide?
   1. Drink 3000 mL of fluid a day.
   2. Take the medication on an empty stomach.
   3. The effect of the medication will occur immediately.
   4. Any swelling of the lips is a normal expected response.

756. Colchicine is prescribed for a client with a diagnosis of gout. The nurse reviews the client's record, knowing that this medication would be used with caution in which disorder?
   1. Myxedema
   2. Kidney disease
   3. Hypothyroidism
   4. Diabetes mellitus

757. Alendronate is prescribed for a client with osteoporosis, and the nurse is providing instructions on administration of the medication. Which instruction should the nurse provide?
   1. Take the medication at bedtime.
   2. Take the medication in the morning with breakfast.
   3. Lie down for 30 minutes after taking the medication.
   4. Take the medication with a full glass of water after rising in the morning.

758. The nurse is preparing discharge instructions for a client who sustained a skeletal muscle injury and is receiving baclofen. Which instruction should be included in the teaching plan?
   1. Restrict fluid intake.
   2. Avoid the use of alcohol.
   3. Stop the medication if diarrhea occurs.
   4. Notify the primary health care provider (PHCP) if fatigue occurs.

759. The nurse is analyzing the laboratory studies on a client receiving dantrolene to treat muscle spasms from an injury. Which laboratory test would identify an adverse effect associated with the administration of this medication?
   1. Platelet count
   2. Creatinine level
   3. Liver function tests
   4. Blood urea nitrogen level

760. Cyclobenzaprine is prescribed for a client for muscle spasms, and the nurse is reviewing the client's record. Which disorder, if noted in the record, would indicate a need to contact the primary health care provider about the administration of this medication?
   1. Glaucoma

2. Emphysema
3. Hypothyroidism
4. Diabetes mellitus

761. In monitoring a client's response to disease-modifying antirheumatic drugs (DMARDs), which assessment findings would the nurse consider acceptable responses? **Select all that apply.**

- ☐ 1. Control of symptoms during periods of emotional stress
- ☐ 2. Normal white blood cell, platelet, and neutrophil counts
- ☐ 3. Radiological findings that show no progression of joint degeneration
- ☐ 4. An increased range of motion in the affected joints 3 months into therapy
- ☐ 5. Inflammation and irritation at the injection site 3 days after the injection is given
- ☐ 6. A low-grade temperature on rising in the morning that remains throughout the day

762. The nurse is administering an intravenous dose of methocarbamol to a client with a muscle skeletal injury. For which adverse effect should the nurse monitor?

1. Tachycardia
2. Rapid pulse
3. Bradycardia
4. Hypertension

ANSWERS

754. ***Answer:*** 2

Rationale: Infection and pancytopenia are adverse effects of etanercept. Laboratory studies are performed prior to and during medication treatment. The appearance of abnormal white blood cell counts and abnormal platelet counts can alert the nurse to a potentially life-threatening infection. Injection site itching is a common occurrence following administration. A metallic taste and loss of appetite are not common signs of adverse effects of this medication.

Test-Taking Strategy: Note the strategic words, *most important*. Option 4 can be eliminated because this is not a common adverse effect. In early treatment, residual fatigue and joint pain may still be apparent. For the remaining options, the correct option monitors for a hematological disorder, which could indicate a reason for discontinuing this medication and should be reported.

Level of Cognitive Ability: Analyzing
Client Needs: Physiological Integrity
Integrated Process: Nursing Process—Assessment
Content Area: Pharmacology: Musculoskeletal Medications: Antiarthritic Medications
Health Problem: Adult Health: Musculoskeletal: Rheumatoid arthritis and osteoarthritis
Priority Concepts: Clinical Judgment; Safety
Reference: Skidmore-Roth (2017), p. 472.

755. ***Answer:*** 1

Rationale: Clients taking allopurinol are encouraged to drink 3000 mL of fluid a day, unless otherwise contraindicated. A full therapeutic effect may take 1 week or longer. Allopurinol is to be given with, or immediately after, meals or milk. A client who develops a rash, irritation of the eyes, or swelling of the lips or mouth should contact the primary health care provider because this may indicate hypersensitivity.

Test-Taking Strategy: Focus on the subject, client instructions for allopurinol. Option 4 can be eliminated easily because it indicates hypersensitivity, which is not a normal expected response. From the remaining options, recalling that this medication is used to treat gout and recalling the pathophysiology of this disorder will direct you to the correct option.

Level of Cognitive Ability: Applying
Client Needs: Physiological Integrity
Integrated Process: Teaching and Learning
Content Area: Pharmacology: Musculoskeletal Medications: Antigout
Health Problem: Adult Health: Musculoskeletal: Gout
Priority Concepts: Client Education; Safety
Reference: Ignatavicius, Workman, Rebar (2018), pp. 331-332.

756. ***Answer:*** 2

Rationale: Colchicine is used with caution in older clients, debilitated clients, and clients with cardiac, kidney, or gastrointestinal disease. The disorders in options 1, 3, and 4 are not concerns with administration of this medication.

Test-Taking Strategy: Focus on the subject, the cautions associated with colchicine. Note that options 1, 3, and 4 are comparable or alike and are endocrine-related disorders. The correct option is different from the others.

Level of Cognitive Ability: Analyzing
Client Needs: Physiological Integrity
Integrated Process: Nursing Process—Analysis
Content Area: Pharmacology: Musculoskeletal Medications: Antigout
Health Problem: Adult Health: Musculoskeletal: Gout
Priority Concepts: Clinical Judgment; Safety
Reference: Lilley et al. (2017), pp. 701, 703.

757. ***Answer:*** 4

Rationale: Precautions need to be taken with the administration of alendronate to prevent gastrointestinal adverse effects (especially esophageal irritation) and to increase absorption of the medication. The medication needs to be taken with a full glass of water after rising in the morning. The client should not eat or drink anything for 30 minutes following administration and should not lie down after taking the medication.

Test-Taking Strategy: Focus on the subject, the administration of alendronate. Recalling that this medication can cause esophageal irritation will direct you to the correct option.

Level of Cognitive Ability: Applying
Client Needs: Physiological Integrity
Integrated Process: Teaching and Learning
Content Area: Pharmacology: Musculoskeletal Medications: Osteoporosis Medications

Health Problem: Adult Health: Musculoskeletal: Osteoporosis
Priority Concepts: Client Education; Tissue Integrity
Reference: Lilley et al. (2017), p. 542.

758. *Answer:* 2
Rationale: Baclofen is a skeletal muscle relaxant. The client should be cautioned against the use of alcohol and other central nervous system depressants, because baclofen potentiates the depressant activity of these agents. Constipation, rather than diarrhea, is a side effect. Restriction of fluids is not necessary, but the client should be warned that urinary retention can occur. Fatigue is related to a central nervous system effect that is most intense during the early phase of therapy and diminishes with continued medication use. The client does not need to notify the PHCP about fatigue.
Test-Taking Strategy: Focus on the subject, teaching points for baclofen. Recalling that baclofen is a skeletal muscle relaxant will direct you easily to the correct option. If you were unsure of the correct option, use general principles related to medication administration. Alcohol should be avoided with the use of medications.
Level of Cognitive Ability: Applying
Client Needs: Physiological Integrity
Integrated Process: Teaching and Learning
Content Area: Pharmacology: Musculoskeletal Medications: Muscle Relaxants
Health Problem: Adult Health: Musculoskeletal: Tissue or ligament injury
Priority Concepts: Client Education; Safety
Reference: Hodgson, Kizior (2018), pp. 113-114.

759. *Answer:* 3
Rationale: Dose-related liver damage is the most serious adverse effect of dantrolene. To reduce the risk of liver damage, liver function tests should be performed before treatment and throughout the treatment interval. Dantrolene is administered at the lowest effective dosage for the shortest time necessary.
Test-Taking Strategy: Eliminate options 2 and 4 because these tests assess kidney function and are comparable or alike. From the remaining options, you must recall that this medication affects liver function.
Level of Cognitive Ability: Analyzing
Client Needs: Physiological Integrity
Integrated Process: Nursing Process—Analysis
Content Area: Pharmacology: Musculoskeletal Medications: Muscle Relaxants
Health Problem: Adult Health: Musculoskeletal: Tissue or ligament injury
Priority Concepts: Cellular Regulation; Tissue Integrity
Reference: Lilley et al. (2017), p. 198.

760. *Answer:* 1
Rationale: Because cyclobenzaprine has anticholinergic effects, it should be used with caution in clients with a history of urinary retention, glaucoma, and increased intraocular pressure. Cyclobenzaprine should be used only for a short time (2 to 3 weeks). The conditions in options 2, 3, and 4 are not a concern with this medication.
Test-Taking Strategy: Focus on the subject, a contraindication to cyclobenzaprine. Recalling that this medication has anticholinergic effects will direct you to the correct option.
Level of Cognitive Ability: Analyzing
Client Needs: Physiological Integrity
Integrated Process: Nursing Process—Analysis
Content Area: Pharmacology: Musculoskeletal Medications: Muscle Relaxants
Health Problem: Adult Health: Musculoskeletal: Tissue or ligament injury
Priority Concepts: Collaboration; Safety
Reference: Skidmore-Roth (2017), pp. 300-301.

761. *Answer:* 1, 2, 3, 4
Rationale: Because emotional stress frequently exacerbates the symptoms of rheumatoid arthritis, the absence of symptoms is a positive finding. DMARDs are given to slow the progression of joint degeneration. In addition, an improvement in the range of motion after 3 months of therapy with normal blood work is a positive finding. Temperature elevation and inflammation and irritation at the medication injection site could indicate signs of infection.
Test-Taking Strategy: Focus on the subject, acceptable responses to therapy. Recalling that signs of an infection can indicate an unexpected and unwanted finding will assist in eliminating options 5 and 6.
Level of Cognitive Ability: Evaluating
Client Needs: Physiological Integrity
Integrated Process: Nursing Process—Evaluation
Content Area: Pharmacology: Musculoskeletal Medications: Antiarthritic Medications
Health Problem: Adult Health: Musculoskeletal: Rheumatoid arthritis and osteoarthritis
Priority Concepts: Clinical Judgment; Evidence
Reference: Ignatavicius, Workman, Rebar (2018), pp. 322, 370.

762. *Answer:* 3
Rationale: Intravenous administration of methocarbamol can cause hypotension and bradycardia. The nurse needs to monitor for these adverse effects. Options 1, 2, and 4 are not effects with administration of this medication.
Test-Taking Strategy: Eliminate options 1 and 2 first because they are comparable or alike. Knowledge about the specific adverse effects related to the intravenous use of this medication will direct you to the correct option. Remember that hypotension and bradycardia can occur with intravenous administration of methocarbamol.
Level of Cognitive Ability: Analyzing
Client Needs: Physiological Integrity
Integrated Process: Nursing Process—Assessment
Content Area: Pharmacology: Musculoskeletal Medications: Muscle Relaxants
Health Problem: Adult Health: Musculoskeletal: Tissue or ligament injury
Priority Concepts: Clinical Judgment; Safety
Reference: Hodgson, Kizior (2018), pp. 737-738.

UNIT XVII

Immune Problems of the Adult Client

Pyramid to Success

Pyramid Points focus on the effects of and complications associated with an immune deficiency. Specific focus relates to the nursing care related to the disorder, the impact of the treatment or disorder, and client adaptation. Human immunodeficiency virus and acquired immunodeficiency syndrome is a Pyramid focus, along with protecting the client from infection and preventing the transmission of infection to other individuals. Psychosocial issues relate to social isolation and the body image disturbances that can occur as a result of the immune disorder.

Client Needs: Learning Objectives

Safe and Effective Care Environment

Acting as an advocate related to the client's decisions
Addressing advance directives
Consulting with the interprofessional health care team
Ensuring that informed consent for treatments and procedures has been obtained
Establishing priorities
Handling hazardous and infectious materials safely
Implementing standard and other precautions
Maintaining asepsis
Maintaining confidentiality regarding diagnosis
Preventing infection
Upholding client rights

Health Promotion and Maintenance

Ensuring that the client receives recommended immunizations
Implementing health screening measures
Monitoring for expected body image changes
Performing physical assessment techniques related to the immune system
Preventing disease related to infection
Providing health promotion programs
Respecting client lifestyle choices

Psychosocial Integrity

Assisting in mobilizing appropriate support and resource systems
Assisting the client and family to cope
Assisting the client and family to adapt, and solve problems during illness or stressful events
Considering religious, spiritual, and cultural preferences
Discussing grief and loss related to death and the dying process
Promoting a positive environment to maintain optimal quality of life

Physiological Integrity

Managing medical emergencies
Managing pain
Monitoring for the expected and unexpected responses to treatments
Optimizing pharmacological treatment
Promoting nutrition
Protecting the client from infection
Providing basic care and comfort
Reviewing diagnostic test and laboratory test results

CHAPTER 62

Immune Problems

PRIORITY CONCEPTS **Immunity; Infection**

I. Functions of the Immune System (Fig. 62-1)

A. Provides protection against invasion by microorganisms from outside the body

B. Protects the body from internal threats and maintains the internal environment by removing dead or damaged cells

II. Immune Response

A. T lymphocytes and B lymphocytes

1. Lymphocytes are produced in the bone marrow and migrate to lymphoid tissue, where they remain dormant until they need to form sensitized lymphocytes for cellular immunity or antibodies for humoral immunity.
2. Some B lymphocytes lie dormant until a specific antigen enters the body, at which time they greatly increase in number and are available for defense.
3. Types of T lymphocytes include helper/inducer, suppressor, and cytotoxic/cytolytic.
4. T and B lymphocytes are necessary for a normal immune response.

B. Humoral response

1. Humoral response is immediate.
2. This type of response provides protection against acute, rapidly developing bacterial and viral infections.

C. Cellular response

1. Cellular response is delayed; this is also called *delayed hypersensitivity*.
2. This type of response is active against slowly developing bacterial infections and is involved in autoimmune responses, some allergic reactions, and rejection of foreign cells.

III. Immunity

A. Innate immunity

1. Innate immunity is also called *native* or *natural immunity*.
2. It is present at birth and includes biochemical, physical, and mechanical barriers of defense, as well as the inflammatory response.

B. Acquired immunity

1. Acquired or adaptive immunity is received passively from the mother's antibodies, animal serum, or antibodies produced in response to a disease.
2. Immunization produces active acquired immunity.

IV. Immunizations: See Chapter 18 for information about immunizations

V. Laboratory Studies

A. Antinuclear antibody (ANA) determination

1. The ANA determination is a blood test used for the differential diagnosis of rheumatic diseases and for the detection of antinucleoprotein factors and patterns associated with certain autoimmune diseases.
2. The test is negative at a 1:40 dilution, depending on the laboratory.
3. A positive result does not necessarily confirm a disease.
4. The ANA is positive in most individuals diagnosed with systemic lupus erythematosus (SLE); it may also be positive in individuals with systemic sclerosis (scleroderma) or rheumatoid arthritis.
5. An ANA result can be false positive in some individuals.

B. Anti-dsDNA antibody test

1. The anti-dsDNA (double-stranded DNA) antibody test is a blood test done specifically to identify or differentiate DNA antibodies found in SLE.
2. The test supports a diagnosis, monitors disease activity and response to therapy, and establishes a prognosis for SLE.
3. Values: negative, lower than 70 U/mL by enzyme-linked immunosorbent assay (ELISA)

C. Human immunodeficiency virus (HIV) testing

1. $CD4^+$ T cell count
   - **a.** Monitors the progression of HIV
   - **b.** As the disease progresses, usually the number of $CD4^+$ T cells decreases, with a resultant decrease in immunity.

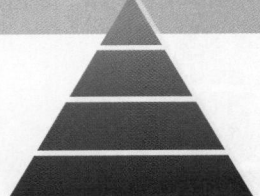

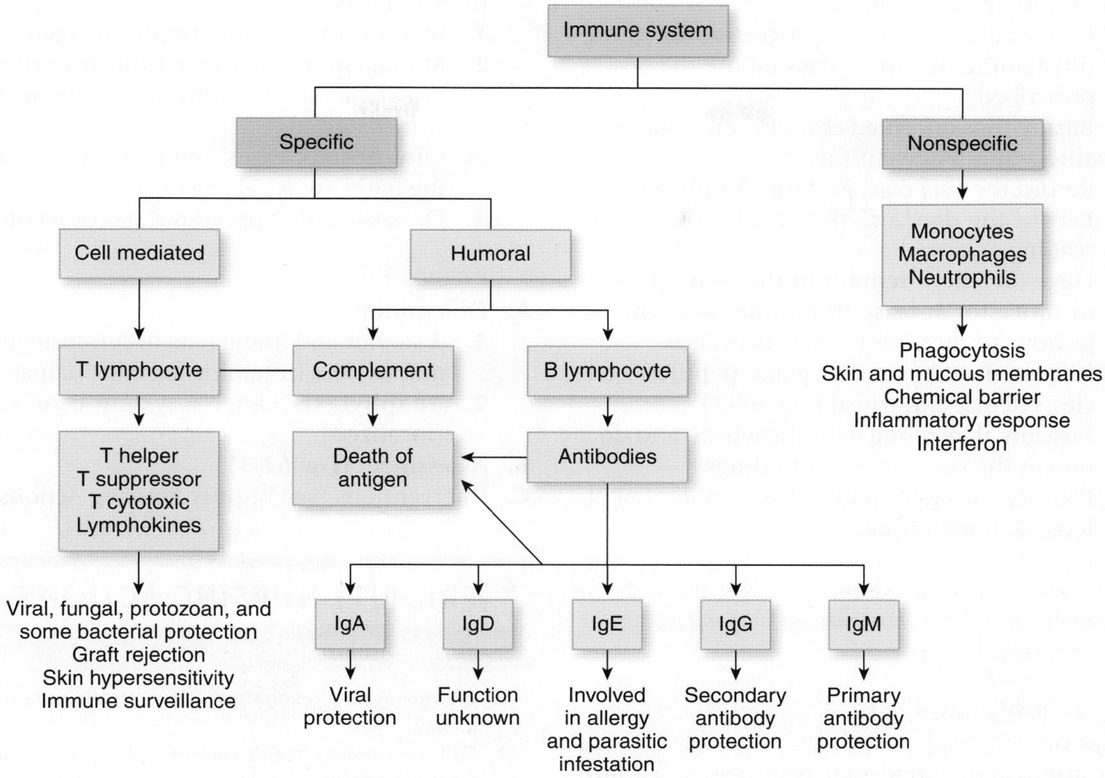

FIG. 62-1 Components of the immune system. *Ig*, Immunoglobulin.

   c. The normal $CD4^+$ T cell count is between 500 and 1600 cells/L.
   d. In general, the immune system remains healthy with $CD4^+$ T cell counts higher than 500 cells/L.
   e. Immune system problems occur when the $CD4^+$ T cell count is between 200 and 499 cells/L.
   f. Severe immune system problems occur when the $CD4^+$ T cell count is lower than 200 cells/L.
2. CD4-to-CD8 ratio
   a. Monitors progression of HIV
   b. Normal ratio is approximately 2:1.
3. Viral culture involves placing the infected client's blood cells in a culture medium and measuring the amount of reverse transcriptase activity over a specified period of time.
4. Viral load testing measures the presence of HIV viral genetic material (RNA) or another viral protein in the client's blood.
5. The p24 antigen assay quantifies the amount of HIV viral core protein in the client's serum.
6. Oral testing for HIV
   a. Uses a device that is placed against the gum and cheek for 2 minutes
   b. Fluid (not saliva) is drawn into an absorbable pad, which, in an HIV-positive individual, contains antibodies.
   c. The pad is placed in a solution, and a specified observable change is noted if the test result is positive.
   d. If the result is positive, a blood test is needed to confirm the results.
7. Home test kits for HIV
   a. In one at-home test kit, a drop of blood is placed on a test card with a special code number; the card is mailed to a laboratory for testing for HIV antibodies.
   b. The individual receives the results by calling a special telephone number and entering the special code number; test results are then given.
8. Nursing considerations
   a. Maintain issues of confidentiality surrounding HIV and acquired immunodeficiency syndrome (AIDS) testing.
   b. Follow prescribed state regulations and protocols related to reporting positive test results.

D. Skin testing
1. Description
   a. The administration of an allergen to the surface of the skin or into the dermis
   b. Administered by patch, scratch, or intradermal techniques

2. Preprocedure interventions
   a. Discontinue systemic corticosteroids or antihistamine therapy 5 days before the test as prescribed.
   b. Ensure that informed consent was obtained.
3. Postprocedure interventions
   a. Record the site, date, and time of the test.
   b. Record the date and time for follow-up site reading.
   c. Have the client remain in the waiting room or office for at least 30 minutes after the injections to monitor for adverse effects.
   d. Inspect the site for erythema, papules, vesicles, edema, and wheal (Fig. 62-2).
   e. Measure flare along with the wheal, and document the size and other findings.
   f. Provide the client with a list of potential allergens, if identified.

Have resuscitation equipment available if skin testing is performed, because the allergen may induce an anaphylactic reaction.

VI. Hypersensitivity and Allergy

A. Description
1. An abnormal, individual response to certain substances that normally do not trigger such an exaggerated reaction.
2. In some types of allergies, a reaction occurs on a second and subsequent contact with the allergen.
3. Skin testing may be done to determine the allergen.

B. Assessment
1. History of exposure to allergens
2. Itching, tearing, and burning of eyes and skin
3. Rashes
4. Nose twitching, nasal stuffiness

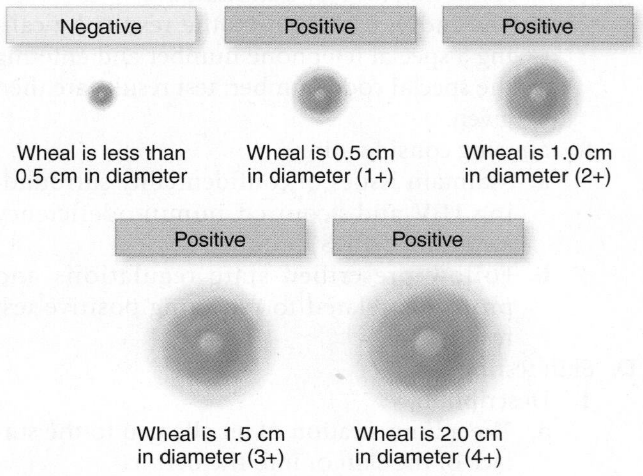

FIG. 62-2 Interpretation of intradermal test results, based on the size of the wheal after 15 to 30 minutes.

C. Interventions
1. Identification of the specific allergen
2. Management of the symptoms with antihistamines, antiinflammatory agents, and/or corticosteroids
3. Ointments, creams, wet compresses, and soothing baths for local reactions
4. Desensitization programs may be recommended.

VII. Anaphylaxis

A. Description
1. A serious and immediate hypersensitivity reaction that releases histamine from the damaged cells
2. Anaphylaxis can be systemic or cutaneous (localized).

B. Assessment (Fig. 62-3)

C. Interventions (see Priority Nursing Actions)

PRIORITY NURSING ACTIONS

Anaphylactic Reaction

1. Quickly assess respiratory status and maintain a patent airway.
2. Call the primary health care provider (PHCP) and Rapid Response Team.
3. Administer oxygen.
4. Start an intravenous (IV) line and infuse normal saline.
5. Prepare to administer diphenhydramine and epinephrine.
6. Document the event, actions taken, and the client's response.

Reference

Ignatavicius. (2018). Workman, Rebar, 364–365.

VIII. Latex Allergy

A. Description
1. Latex allergy is a hypersensitivity to latex.
2. The source of the allergic reaction is thought to be the proteins in the natural rubber latex or the various chemicals used in the manufacturing process of latex gloves.
3. Symptoms of the allergy can range from mild contact dermatitis to moderately severe symptoms of rhinitis, conjunctivitis, urticaria, and bronchospasm to severe life-threatening anaphylaxis.

B. Common routes of exposure (Box 62-1)
1. Cutaneous: Natural latex gloves and latex balloons
2. Percutaneous and parenteral: Intravenous lines and catheters; hemodialysis equipment
3. Mucosal: Use of latex condoms, catheters, airways, and nipples
4. Aerosol: Aerosolization of powder from latex gloves can occur when gloves are dispensed from the box or when gloves are removed from the hands.

C. At-risk individuals
1. Health care workers
2. Individuals who work in the rubber industry
3. Individuals having multiple surgeries
4. Individuals with spina bifida
5. Individuals who wear gloves frequently, such as food handlers, hairdressers, and auto mechanics
6. Individuals allergic to kiwis, bananas, pineapples, tropical fruits, grapes, avocados, potatoes, hazelnuts, and water chestnuts

D. Assessment
1. Anaphylaxis or type 1 hypersensitivity is a response to natural rubber latex (Fig. 62-4; also see Fig. 62-3).
2. A delayed type 4 hypersensitivity reaction can occur; symptoms of contact dermatitis include pruritus, edema, erythema, vesicles, papules, and crusting and thickening of the skin and can occur within 6 to 48 hours following exposure.

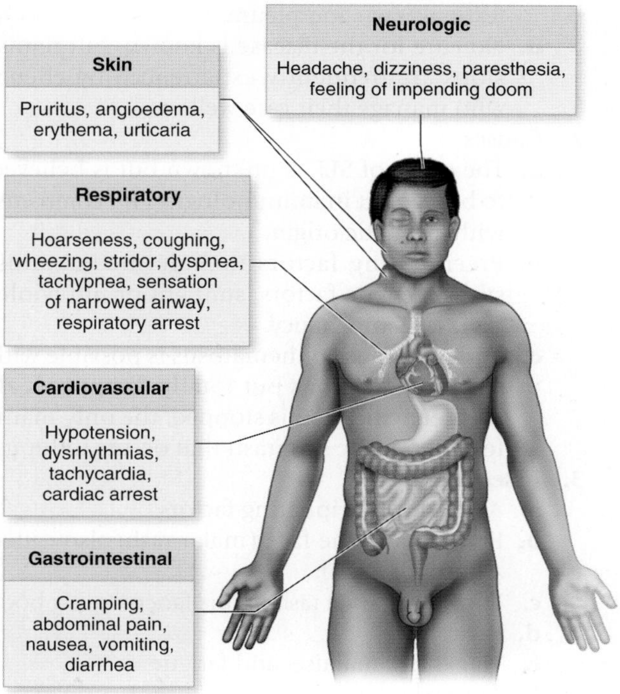
Neurologic
Headache, dizziness, paresthesia, feeling of impending doom
Skin
Pruritus, angioedema, erythema, urticaria
Respiratory
Hoarseness, coughing, wheezing, stridor, dyspnea, tachypnea, sensation of narrowed airway, respiratory arrest
Cardiovascular
Hypotension, dysrhythmias, tachycardia, cardiac arrest
Gastrointestinal
Cramping, abdominal pain, nausea, vomiting, diarrhea

FIG. 62-3 Clinical manifestations of a systemic anaphylactic reaction.

BOX 62-1 Products That May Contain Natural Rubber Latex

- ACE bandages (brown)
- Adhesive or elastic bandages
- Ambu bag
- Balloons
- Blood pressure cuff (tubing and bladder)
- Catheter leg bag straps
- Catheters
- Condoms
- Diaphragms
- Elastic pressure stockings
- Electrocardiographic pads
- Feminine hygiene pads
- Gloves
- Intravenous catheters, tubing, and rubber injection ports
- Nasogastric tubes
- Pads for crutches
- Prepackaged enema kits
- Rubber stoppers on medication vials
- Stethoscopes
- Syringes

Note: Health care agencies use as many nonlatex products as possible and have nonlatex supplies available for clients with a latex allergy.

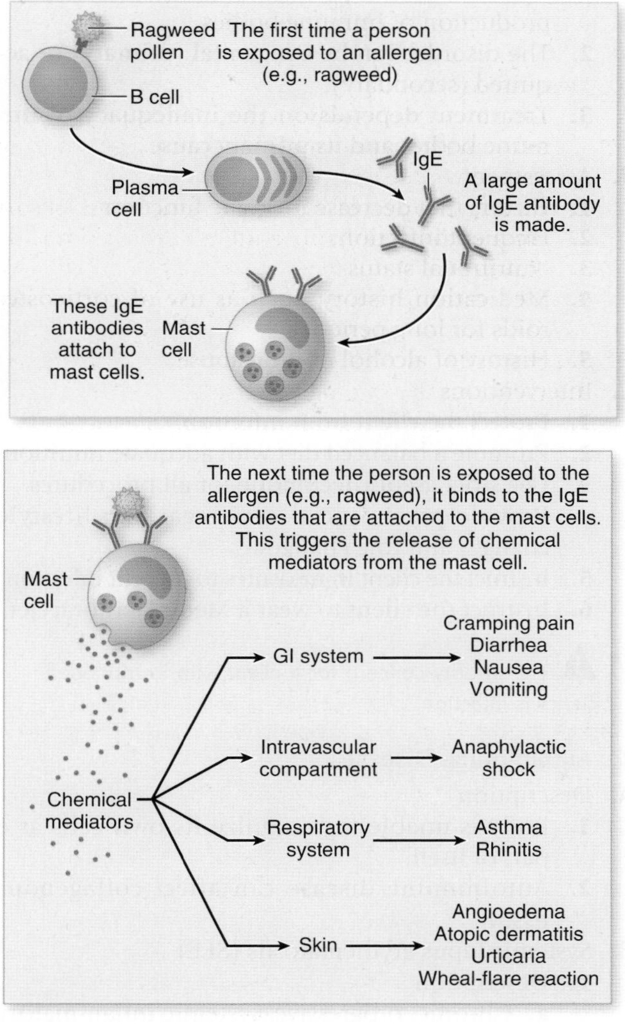
Ragweed pollen
The first time a person is exposed to an allergen (e.g., ragweed)
B cell
IgE
Plasma cell
A large amount of IgE antibody is made.
These IgE antibodies attach to mast cells.
Mast cell
The next time the person is exposed to the allergen (e.g., ragweed), it binds to the IgE antibodies that are attached to the mast cells. This triggers the release of chemical mediators from the mast cell.
Mast cell
Chemical mediators
GI system
Cramping pain
Diarrhea
Nausea
Vomiting
Intravascular compartment
Anaphylactic shock
Respiratory system
Asthma
Rhinitis
Skin
Angioedema
Atopic dermatitis
Urticaria
Wheal-flare reaction

FIG. 62-4 Steps in a type I allergic reaction. *GI*, Gastrointestinal; *IgE*, immunoglobulin E.

BOX 62-2 Interventions for the Client with a Latex Allergy

- Ask the client about a known allergy to latex when performing the initial assessment.
- Identify risk factors for a latex allergy in the client.
- Use nonlatex gloves and all latex-safe supplies.
- Keep a latex-safe supply cart near the client's room.
- Apply a cloth barrier to the client's arm under a blood pressure cuff.
- Use latex-free syringes and medication containers (glass ampules) and latex-safe intravenous equipment.
- Instruct the client to wear a MedicAlert bracelet.
- Instruct the client about the importance of informing health care providers and local and paramedic ambulance companies about the allergy.

E. Interventions (Box 62-2)

IX. Immunodeficiency

A. Description
1. **Immunodeficiency** is the absence or inadequate production of immune bodies.
2. The disorder can be congenital (primary) or acquired (secondary).
3. Treatment depends on the inadequacy of immune bodies and its primary cause.

B. Assessment
1. Factors that decrease immune function
2. Frequent infections
3. Nutritional status
4. Medication history, such as use of corticosteroids for long periods
5. History of alcohol or drug abuse

C. Interventions
1. Protect the client from infection.
2. Promote a balanced diet with adequate nutrition.
3. Use strict aseptic technique for all procedures.
4. Provide psychosocial care regarding lifestyle changes and role changes.
5. Instruct the client in measures to prevent infection.
6. Instruct the client to wear a MedicAlert bracelet.

! The priority concern for a client with immunodeficiency is infection.

X. Autoimmune Disease

A. Description
1. Body is unable to recognize its own cells as a part of itself.
2. Autoimmune disease can affect collagenous tissue.

B. Systemic lupus erythematosus (SLE)
1. Description
   - **a.** Chronic, progressive, systemic inflammatory disease that can cause major organs and systems to fail
   - **b.** Connective tissue and fibrin deposits collect in blood vessels on collagen fibers and on organs.
   - **c.** The deposits lead to necrosis and inflammation in blood vessels, lymph nodes, gastrointestinal tract, and pleura.
   - **d.** No cure for the disease is known, but remissions are frequently experienced by clients who manage their care well.
2. Causes
   - **a.** The cause of SLE is unknown but is believed to be a defect in immunological mechanisms, with a genetic origin.
   - **b.** Precipitating factors include medications, stress, genetic factors, sunlight or ultraviolet light, and pregnancy.
   - **c.** Discoid lupus erythematosus is possible with some medications but totally disappears after the medication is stopped; the only manifestation is the skin rash that occurs in lupus.
3. Assessment
   - **a.** Assess for precipitating factors.
   - **b.** Erythema of the face (malar rash; also called a butterfly rash)
   - **c.** Dry, scaly, raised rash on the face or upper body
   - **d.** Fever
   - **e.** Weakness, malaise, and fatigue
   - **f.** Anorexia
   - **g.** Weight loss
   - **h.** Photosensitivity
   - **i.** Joint pain
   - **j.** Erythema of the palms
   - **k.** Anemia
   - **l.** Positive ANA test and lupus erythematosus preparation
   - **m.** Elevated erythrocyte sedimentation rate (ESR) and C-reactive protein level
4. Interventions
   - **a.** Monitor skin integrity and provide frequent oral care.
   - **b.** Instruct the client to clean the skin with a mild soap, avoiding harsh and perfumed substances.
   - **c.** Assist with the use of ointments and creams for the rash as prescribed.
   - **d.** Identify factors contributing to fatigue.
   - **e.** Administer iron, folic acid, or vitamin supplements as prescribed if anemia occurs.
   - **f.** Provide a high-vitamin and high-iron diet.
   - **g.** Provide a high-protein diet if there is no evidence of kidney disease.
   - **h.** Instruct in measures to conserve energy, such as pacing activities and balancing rest with exercise.
   - **i.** Administer topical or systemic corticosteroids, salicylates, and nonsteroidal anti-inflammatory drugs as prescribed for pain and inflammation.

j. Administer medications to decrease the inflammatory response as prescribed.
k. Monitor intake and output, as well as daily weight for signs of fluid overload if corticosteroids are used.
l. Instruct the client to avoid exposure to sunlight and ultraviolet light.
m. Monitor for proteinuria and red cell casts in the urine.
n. Monitor for bruising, bleeding, and injury.
o. Assist with plasmapheresis as prescribed to remove autoantibodies and immune complexes from the blood before organ damage occurs.
p. Monitor for signs of organ involvement such as pleuritis, nephritis, pericarditis, coronary artery disease, hypertension, neuritis, anemia, and peritonitis.
q. Note that lupus nephritis occurs early in the disease process.
r. Provide supportive therapy as major organs become affected.
s. Provide emotional support and encourage the client to verbalize feelings.
t. Provide information regarding support groups and encourage the use of community resources.

⚠ For the client with SLE, monitor the blood urea nitrogen and creatinine levels frequently for signs of renal impairment.

C. Scleroderma (systemic sclerosis)
1. Description
a. Scleroderma is a chronic connective tissue disease, similar to SLE, that is characterized by inflammation, fibrosis, and sclerosis.
b. This disorder affects the connective tissue throughout the body.
c. It causes fibrotic changes involving the skin, synovial membranes, esophagus, heart, lungs, kidneys, and gastrointestinal tract.
d. Treatment is directed toward forcing the disease into remission and slowing its progress.
2. Assessment
a. Pain
b. Stiffness and muscle weakness
c. Pitting edema of the hands and fingers that progresses to the rest of the body
d. Taut and shiny skin that is free from wrinkles
e. Skin tissue is tight, hard, and thick; loses its elasticity; and adheres to underlying structures.
f. Dysphagia
g. Decreased range of motion
h. Joint contractures
i. Inability to perform activities of daily living
3. Interventions
a. Encourage activity as tolerated.
b. Maintain a constant room temperature.
c. Provide small frequent meals, eliminating foods that stimulate gastric secretions, such as spicy foods, caffeine, and alcohol.
d. Monitor for esophageal involvement; if present, advise the client to sit up for 1 to 2 hours after meals. Using additional pillows and raising the head of the bed on blocks may help reduce nocturnal reflux.
e. Provide supportive therapy as the major organs become affected.
f. Administer corticosteroids as prescribed for inflammation.
g. Provide emotional support and encourage the use of resources as necessary.

D. Polyarteritis nodosa
1. Description
a. Polyarteritis nodosa is a collagen disease; it is a form of systemic vasculitis that causes inflammation of the arteries in visceral organs, brain, and skin.
b. Treatment is similar to the treatment for SLE.
c. Polyarteritis nodosa affects middle-aged men.
d. The cause is unknown and the prognosis is poor.
e. Renal disorders and cardiac involvement are the most frequent causes of death.
2. Assessment
a. Malaise and weakness
b. Low-grade fever
c. Severe abdominal pain
d. Bloody diarrhea
e. Weight loss
f. Elevated ESR
3. Interventions: Refer to interventions for SLE.

E. Pemphigus
1. Description
a. Pemphigus is a rare autoimmune disease that occurs predominantly between middle age and old age.
b. The cause is unknown, and the disorder is potentially fatal.
c. Treatment is aimed at suppressing the immune response and blister formation.
2. Assessment
a. Fragile, partial-thickness lesions bleed, weep, and form crusts when bullae are disrupted.
b. Debilitation, malaise, pain, and dysphagia
c. Nikolsky's sign: Separation of the epidermis caused by rubbing the skin
d. Leukocytosis, eosinophilia, foul-smelling discharge from skin
3. Interventions
a. Provide supportive care.
b. Provide oral hygiene and increase fluid intake.

c. Soothe oral lesions.
d. Assist with soothing baths, as prescribed for relief of symptoms.
e. Administer topical or systemic antibiotics as prescribed for secondary infections.
f. Administer corticosteroids and cytotoxic agents as prescribed to bring about remission.

XI. Goodpasture's Syndrome

A. Description
1. An autoimmune disorder; autoantibodies are made against the glomerular basement membrane and alveolar basement membrane.
2. It is most common in males and young adults who smoke; the exact cause is unknown.
3. The lungs and the kidneys are affected primarily, and the disorder usually is not diagnosed until significant pulmonary or renal involvement occurs.

B. Assessment
1. Clinical manifestations indicating pulmonary and renal involvement
2. Shortness of breath
3. Hemoptysis
4. Decreased urine output
5. Edema and weight gain
6. Hypertension and tachycardia

C. Interventions
1. Focus on suppressing the autoimmune response with medications such as corticosteroids and on plasmapheresis (filtration of the plasma to remove some proteins and autoantibodies).
2. Provide supportive therapy for pulmonary and renal involvement.

XII. Lyme Disease

A. Description
1. An infection caused by the spirochete *Borrelia burgdorferi*, acquired from a tick bite (ticks live in wooded areas and survive by attaching to a host)
2. Infection with the spirochete stimulates inflammatory cytokines and autoimmune mechanisms.

B. Assessment (Box 62-3; Fig. 62-5)
1. The typical ring-shaped rash of Lyme disease does not occur in all clients. Many clients never develop a rash.
2. If a rash does occur, it can occur anywhere on the body, not only at the site of the bite.

C. Interventions
1. Gently remove the tick with tweezers, wash the skin with antiseptic, and dispose of the tick by flushing it down the toilet; the tick may also be placed in a sealed jar so that the primary health care provider can inspect it and determine its type.
2. Perform a blood test 4 to 6 weeks after a bite to detect the presence of the disease (testing before this time is not reliable).

BOX 62-3 Assessment and Stages of Lyme Disease

First Stage
- Symptoms can occur several days to months following the bite.
- A small red pimple develops that may spread into a ring-shaped rash; it may occur anywhere on the body.
- Ring-shaped rash may be large or small, or may not occur at all.
- Flu-like symptoms occur, such as headaches, stiff neck, muscle aches, and fatigue.

Second Stage
- This stage occurs several weeks following the bite.
- Joint pain occurs.
- Neurological complications occur.
- Cardiac complications occur.

Third Stage
- Large joints become involved.
- Arthritis progresses.

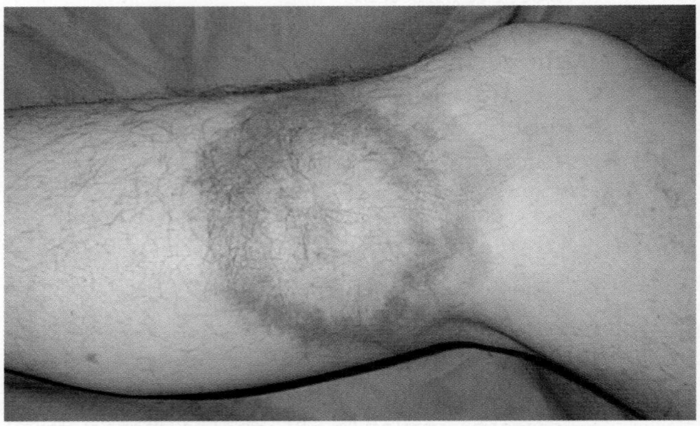

FIG. 62-5 Erythema migrans of Lyme disease. (From Swartz, 2010.)

3. Instruct the client in the administration of antibiotics as prescribed; these are initiated immediately (even before the blood testing results are known).
4. Instruct the client to avoid areas that contain ticks, such as wooded grassy areas, especially in the summer months.
5. Instruct the client to wear long-sleeved tops, long pants, closed shoes, and hats while outside.
6. Instruct the client to spray the body with tick repellent before going outside.
7. Instruct the client to examine the body when returning inside for the presence of ticks.

XIII. Immunodeficiency Syndrome

A. Acquired immunodeficiency syndrome (AIDS)
1. AIDS is a viral disease caused by HIV, which destroys T cells, thereby increasing susceptibility to infection and malignancy (Fig. 62-6).

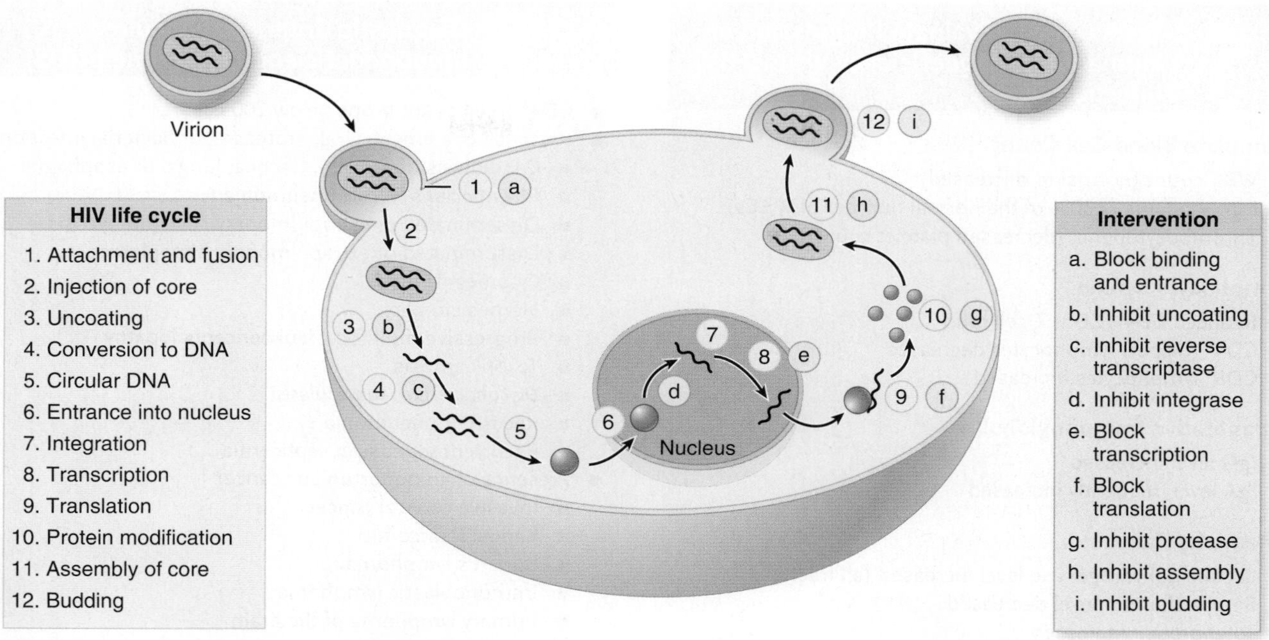

FIG. 62-6 The life cycle of human immunodeficiency virus (HIV).

2. The syndrome is manifested clinically by opportunistic infections and unusual neoplasms.
3. AIDS is considered a chronic illness.
4. The disease has a long incubation period, sometimes 10 years or longer.
5. Manifestations may not appear until late in the infection.

B. Diagnosis and monitoring of the client with AIDS
1. Refer to Box 62-4 for tests used to evaluate the progression of HIV infection.
2. Refer to Box 62-5 for information used to diagnose AIDS.

C. High-risk groups
1. Heterosexual or homosexual contact with high-risk individuals
2. Intravenous drug abusers
3. Persons receiving blood products
4. Health care workers
5. Babies born to infected mothers

D. Assessment
1. Malaise, fever, anorexia, weight loss, influenza-like symptoms
2. Lymphadenopathy for at least 3 months
3. Leukopenia
4. Diarrhea
5. Fatigue
6. Night sweats
7. Presence of opportunistic infections
8. Protozoan infections (*Pneumocystis jiroveci* pneumonia, a major source of mortality)
9. Neoplasms (Kaposi's sarcoma, manifested as purplish-red lesions of internal organs and skin, B-cell non-Hodgkin's lymphoma, cervical cancer)
10. Fungal infections (candidiasis, histoplasmosis)
11. Viral infections (cytomegalovirus, herpes simplex)
12. Bacterial infections

E. Interventions
1. Provide respiratory support.
2. Administer oxygen and respiratory treatments as prescribed.
3. Provide psychosocial support and support services as needed.
4. Maintain fluid and electrolyte balance.
5. Monitor for signs of infection and institute protective isolation precautions as necessary.
6. Prevent the spread of infection.
7. Initiate standard and other necessary precautions.
8. Provide comfort as necessary.
9. Provide meticulous skin care.
10. Provide adequate nutritional support as prescribed.

F. Kaposi's sarcoma
1. Description: Skin lesions that occur primarily in individuals with a compromised immune system
2. Assessment
   a. Kaposi's sarcoma is a slow-growing tumor that appears as raised, oblong, purplish, reddish-brown lesions; may be tender or nontender.
   b. Organ involvement includes the lymph nodes, airways or lungs, or any part of the gastrointestinal tract from the mouth to anus.

BOX 62-4 Tests Used to Evaluate Progression of Human Immunodeficiency Virus (HIV) Infection

Complete Blood Cell Count
- WBC count (normal to decreased)
- Lymphopenia (<30% of the normal number of WBCs)
- Thrombocytopenia (decreased platelet count)

Lymphocyte Screen
- Reduced $CD4^+/CD8^+$ T cell ratio
- $CD4^+$ (helper) lymphocytes decreased
- $CD8^+$ lymphocytes increased

Quantitative Immunoglobulin
- IgG level increased
- IgA level frequently increased

Chemistry Panel
- Lactate dehydrogenase level increased (all fractions)
- Serum albumin level decreased
- Total protein increased
- Cholesterol level decreased
- AST and ALT levels elevated

Anergy Panel
- Nonreactive (anergic) or poorly reactive to infectious agents or environmental materials (e.g., pokeweed, phytohemagglutinin mitogens and antigens, mumps, *Candida*)

Hepatitis B Surface Antigen Testing
- To detect the presence of hepatitis B

Blood Cultures
- To detect septicemia

Chest Radiography
- To detect *Pneumocystis jiroveci* infection or tuberculosis

Data from Copstead-Kirkhorn L, Banasik J: *Pathophysiology*, ed 5, St. Louis, 2014, Mosby.
ALT, Alanine aminotransferase; *AST*, aspartate aminotransferase; *Ig*, immunoglobulin; *WBC*, white blood cell.

3. Interventions
   a. Maintain standard precautions.
   b. Provide protective isolation if the immune system is depressed.
   c. Prepare the client for radiation therapy or chemotherapy as prescribed.
   d. Administer immunotherapy, as prescribed, to stabilize the immune system.

XIV. Posttransplantation Immunodeficiency

A. Description
   1. Secondary immunodeficiency is immunosuppression caused by therapeutic agents.
   2. The client must take immunosuppressive agents for the rest of his or her life posttransplantation to decrease rejection of the transplanted organ or tissue.

BOX 62-5 Diagnostic Criteria for Acquired Immunodeficiency Syndrome (AIDS)

- $CD4^+$ T cell count drops below 200 cells/L
- Presence of a fungal, viral, protozoal, or bacterial infection
  - Candidiasis of bronchi, trachea, lungs, or esophagus
  - *Pneumocystis jiroveci* pneumonia
  - Disseminated or extrapulmonary coccidiomycosis
  - Disseminated or extrapulmonary histoplasmosis
  - Cytomegalovirus
  - Herpes simplex
  - Progressive multifocal leukoencephalopathy
  - Toxoplasmosis
  - *Mycobacterium tuberculosis*
  - Recurrent pneumonia
  - Recurrent *salmonella* septicemia
- Presence of an opportunistic cancer
  - Invasive cervical cancer
  - Kaposi's sarcoma
  - Burkitt's lymphoma
  - Immunoblastic lymphoma
  - Primary lymphoma of the brain
- Wasting syndrome (10% or more of ideal body mass)
- AIDS dementia complex

Adapted from Lewis S, Dirksen S, Heitkemper M, Bucher L: *Medical-surgical nursing: assessment and management of clinical problems*, ed 9, St. Louis, 2014, Mosby.

B. Diagnosis and monitoring of posttransplantation clients
   1. Check renal and hepatic function.
   2. Monitor the complete cell count with differential to determine signs of infection.
   3. Assess all body secretions periodically for blood.

C. High-risk clients
   1. Clients with a history of malignancy or premalignancy have an increased susceptibility to malignancy if immunosuppressed.
   2. Clients with recent infection or exposure to tuberculosis, herpes zoster, or chickenpox have a high risk for severe generalized disease when on immunosuppressive agents.

D. Assessment
   1. Assess for signs of opportunistic infections.
   2. Assess nutritional status.
   3. Assess for signs of rejection (signs will depend on the organ or tissue transplant).

E. Interventions
   1. Strict aseptic technique is necessary.
   2. Provide teaching regarding asepsis and the signs of infection and rejection.
   3. Institute protective isolation precautions as necessary.
   4. Provide psychosocial support as needed.
   5. Provide client teaching about immunosuppressants.

PRACTICE QUESTIONS

763. The nurse prepares to give a bath and change the bed linens of a client with cutaneous Kaposi's sarcoma lesions. The lesions are open and draining a scant amount of serous fluid. Which would the nurse incorporate into the plan during the bathing of this client?
1. Wearing gloves
2. Wearing a gown and gloves
3. Wearing a gown, gloves, and a mask
4. Wearing a gown and gloves to change the bed linens, and gloves only for the bath

764. The nurse provides home care instructions to a client with systemic lupus erythematosus and tells the client about methods to manage fatigue. Which statement by the client indicates a **need for further instruction**?
1. "I should take hot baths because they are relaxing."
2. "I should sit whenever possible to conserve my energy."
3. "I should avoid long periods of rest because it causes joint stiffness."
4. "I should do some exercises, such as walking, when I am not fatigued."

765. A client develops an anaphylactic reaction after receiving morphine. The nurse should plan to institute which actions? **Select all that apply.**
- ❑ 1. Administer oxygen.
- ❑ 2. Quickly assess the client's respiratory status.
- ❑ 3. Document the event, interventions, and client's response.
- ❑ 4. Leave the client briefly to contact a primary health care provider (PHCP).
- ❑ 5. Keep the client supine regardless of the blood pressure readings.
- ❑ 6. Start an intravenous (IV) infusion of D5W and administer a 500-mL bolus.

766. The nurse is conducting a teaching session with a client on their diagnosis of pemphigus. Which statement by the client indicates that the client understands the diagnosis?
1. "My skin will have tiny red vesicles."
2. "The presence of the skin vesicles is caused by a virus."
3. "I have an autoimmune disease that causes blistering in the skin."
4. "Red, raised papules and large plaques covered by silvery scales will be present on my skin."

767. The nurse is assisting in planning care for a client with a diagnosis of immunodeficiency and should incorporate which action as a **priority** in the plan?
1. Protecting the client from infection
2. Providing emotional support to decrease fear
3. Encouraging discussion about lifestyle changes
4. Identifying factors that decreased the immune function

768. A client calls the nurse in the emergency department and states that he was just stung by a bumblebee while gardening. The client is afraid of a severe reaction because the client's neighbor experienced such a reaction just 1 week ago. Which action should the nurse take?
1. Advise the client to soak the site in hydrogen peroxide.
2. Ask the client if he ever sustained a bee sting in the past.
3. Tell the client to call an ambulance for transport to the emergency department.
4. Tell the client not to worry about the sting unless difficulty with breathing occurs.

769. The community health nurse is conducting a research study and is identifying clients in the community at risk for latex allergy. Which client population is **most** at risk for developing this type of allergy?
1. Hairdressers
2. The homeless
3. Children in day care centers
4. Individuals living in a group home

770. Which interventions apply in the care of a client at high risk for an allergic response to a latex allergy? **Select all that apply.**
- ❑ 1. Use nonlatex gloves.
- ❑ 2. Use medications from glass ampules.
- ❑ 3. Place the client in a private room only.
- ❑ 4. Keep a latex-safe supply cart available in the client's area.
- ❑ 5. Avoid the use of medication vials that have rubber stoppers.
- ❑ 6. Use a blood pressure cuff from an electronic device only to measure the blood pressure.

771. A client presents at the primary health care provider's office with complaints of a ring-like rash on his upper leg. Which question should the nurse ask **first**?
1. "Do you have any cats in your home?"
2. "Have you been camping in the last month?"
3. "Have you or close contacts had any flu-like symptoms within the last few weeks?"
4. "Have you been in physical contact with anyone who has the same type of rash?"

772. A client is diagnosed with scleroderma. Which intervention should the nurse anticipate to be prescribed?
1. Maintain bed rest as much as possible.
2. Administer corticosteroids as prescribed for inflammation.

3. Advise the client to remain supine for 1 to 2 hours after meals.
4. Keep the room temperature warm during the day and cool at night.

773. A client arrives at the health care clinic and tells the nurse that she was just bitten by a tick and would like to be tested for Lyme disease. The client tells the nurse that she removed the tick and flushed it down the toilet. Which actions are **most appropriate**? **Select all that apply.**

- ☐ 1. Tell the client that testing is not necessary unless arthralgia develops.
- ☐ 2. Tell the client to avoid any woody, grassy areas that may contain ticks.
- ☐ 3. Instruct the client to immediately start to take the antibiotics that are prescribed.
- ☐ 4. Inform the client to plan to have a blood test 4 to 6 weeks after a bite to detect the presence of the disease.
- ☐ 5. Tell the client that if this happens again, to never remove the tick but vigorously scrub the area with an antiseptic.

774. The nurse is preparing a group of Cub Scouts for an overnight camping trip and instructs the Scouts about the methods to prevent Lyme disease. Which statement by one of the Scouts indicates a **need for further instruction**?

1. "I need to bring a hat to wear during the trip."
2. "I should wear long-sleeved tops and long pants."
3. "I should not use insect repellents because it will attract the ticks."
4. "I need to wear closed shoes and socks that can be pulled up over my pants."

775. The client with acquired immunodeficiency syndrome is diagnosed with cutaneous Kaposi's sarcoma. Based on this diagnosis, the nurse understands that this has been confirmed by which finding?

1. Swelling in the genital area
2. Swelling in the lower extremities
3. Positive punch biopsy of the cutaneous lesions
4. Appearance of reddish-blue lesions noted on the skin

776. The nurse is conducting allergy skin testing on a client. Which postprocedure interventions are **most appropriate**? **Select all that apply.**

- ☐ 1. Record site, date, and time of the test.
- ☐ 2. Give the client a list of potential allergens if identified.
- ☐ 3. Estimate the size of the wheal and document the finding.
- ☐ 4. Tell the client to return to have the site inspected only if there is a reaction.
- ☐ 5. Have the client wait in the waiting room for at least 1 to 2 hours after injection.

777. The nurse is performing an assessment on a client who has been diagnosed with an allergy to latex. In determining the client's risk factors, the nurse should question the client about an allergy to which food item?

1. Eggs
2. Milk
3. Yogurt
4. Bananas

ANSWERS

763. *Answer:* 2

Rationale: Gowns and gloves are required if the nurse anticipates contact with soiled items such as those with wound drainage, or is caring for a client who is incontinent with diarrhea or a client who has an ileostomy or colostomy. Masks are not required unless droplet or airborne precautions are necessary. Regardless of the amount of wound drainage, a gown and gloves must be worn.

Test-Taking Strategy: Focus on the **subject**, the method of transmission of infection from Kaposi's sarcoma. Read the question, noting the task that is presented; in this case, it is bathing and changing linens. Eliminate option 3, because the method of transmission is not respiratory. Eliminate options 1 and 4 because neither provides adequate protection based on the method of transmission.

Level of Cognitive Ability: Applying

Client Needs: Safe and Effective Care Environment

Integrated Process: Nursing Process—Planning

Content Area: Foundations of Care: Infection Control

Health Problem: Adult Health: Immune: Immunodeficiency Syndrome

Priority Concepts: Infection; Safety

Reference: Ignatavicius, Workman, Rebar (2018), pp. 418-419.

764. *Answer:* 1

Rationale: To help reduce fatigue in the client with systemic lupus erythematosus, the nurse should instruct the client to sit whenever possible, avoid hot baths (because they exacerbate fatigue), schedule moderate low-impact exercises when not fatigued, and maintain a balanced diet. The client is instructed to avoid long periods of rest because it promotes joint stiffness.

Test-Taking Strategy: Note the **strategic words**, *need for further instruction*. These words indicate a **negative event query** and the need to select the incorrect client statement. Also, focus on the **subject**, fatigue. This will assist in directing you to the correct option as the action that would exacerbate fatigue.

Level of Cognitive Ability: Evaluating
Client Needs: Physiological Integrity
Integrated Process: Teaching and Learning
Content Area: Adult Health: Immune
Health Problem: Adult Health: Immune: Autoimmune Disease
Priority Concepts: Client Education; Immunity
Reference: Lewis et al. (2017), p. 1542.

765. *Answer:* 1, 2, 3
Rationale: An anaphylactic reaction requires immediate action, starting with quickly assessing the client's respiratory status. Although the PHCP and the Rapid Response Team must be notified immediately, the nurse must stay with the client. Oxygen is administered and an IV of normal saline is started and infused per PHCP prescription. Documentation of the event, actions taken, and client outcomes needs to be performed. The head of the bed should be elevated if the client's blood pressure is normal.
Test-Taking Strategy: Focus on the subject, interventions the nurse takes for an anaphylactic reaction. Read each option carefully and remember that this is an emergency. Think about the pathophysiology that occurs in this reaction to answer correctly.
Level of Cognitive Ability: Analyzing
Client Needs: Physiological Integrity
Integrated Process: Nursing Process—Planning
Content Area: Complex Care: Emergency Situations/ Management
Health Problem: Adult Health: Immune: Hypersensitivity Reactions and Allergy
Priority Concepts: Clinical Judgment; Immunity
Reference: Ignatavicius, Workman, Rebar (2018), p. 365.

766. *Answer:* 3
Rationale: Pemphigus is an autoimmune disease that causes blistering in the epidermis. The client has large flaccid blisters (bullae). Because the blisters are in the epidermis, they have a thin covering of skin and break easily, leaving large denuded areas of skin. On initial examination, clients may have crusting areas instead of intact blisters. Option 1 describes eczema, option 2 describes herpes zoster, and option 4 describes psoriasis.
Test-Taking Strategy: Focus on the subject, the characteristics of pemphigus. Think about the pathophysiology associated with this disorder and recall that pemphigus vulgaris is an autoimmune disorder.
Level of Cognitive Ability: Evaluating
Client Needs: Physiological Integrity
Integrated Process: Nursing Process—Evaluation
Content Area: Adult Health: Immune
Health Problem: Adult Health: Immune: Autoimmune Disease
Priority Concepts: Client Education; Immunity
Reference: Heuther & McCance (2017), p. 1065.

767. *Answer:* 1
Rationale: The client with immunodeficiency has inadequate or absence of immune bodies and is at risk for infection. The priority nursing intervention would be to protect the client from infection. Options 2, 3, and 4 may be components of care but are not the priority.
Test-Taking Strategy: Note the strategic word, *priority*. Use Maslow's Hierarchy of Needs theory to answer the question. Remember that physiological needs are the priority. This will direct you to the correct option.
Level of Cognitive Ability: Applying
Client Needs: Physiological Integrity
Integrated Process: Nursing Process—Planning
Content Area: Adult Health: Immune
Health Problem: Adult Health: Immune: Immunodeficiency syndrome
Priority Concepts: Immunity; Safety
Reference: Lewis et al. (2017), pp. 205-206.

768. *Answer:* 2
Rationale: In some types of allergies, a reaction occurs only on second and subsequent contacts with the allergen. The appropriate action, therefore, would be to ask the client if he ever experienced a bee sting in the past. Option 1 is not appropriate advice. Option 3 is unnecessary. The client should not be told "not to worry."
Test-Taking Strategy: Use the steps of the nursing process to answer the question. The correct option is the only one that addresses assessment.
Level of Cognitive Ability: Applying
Client Needs: Physiological Integrity
Integrated Process: Nursing Process—Implementation
Content Area: Adult Health: Immune
Health Problem: Adult Health: Immune: Hypersensitivity Reactions and Allergy
Priority Concepts: Clinical Judgment; Immunity
Reference: Ignatavicius, Workman, Rebar (2018), p. 140.

769. *Answer:* 1
Rationale: Individuals most at risk for developing a latex allergy include health care workers; individuals who work in the rubber industry; or those who have had multiple surgeries, have spina bifida, wear gloves frequently (such as food handlers, hairdressers, and auto mechanics), or are allergic to kiwis, bananas, pineapples, tropical fruits, grapes, avocados, potatoes, hazelnuts, or water chestnuts.
Test-Taking Strategy: Focus on the subject, a latex allergy, and note the strategic word, *most*. Recalling the sources of latex and of the allergic reaction will direct you easily to the correct option.
Level of Cognitive Ability: Analyzing
Client Needs: Health Promotion and Maintenance
Integrated Process: Nursing Process—Assessment
Content Area: Adult Health: Immune
Health Problem: Adult Health: Immune: Hypersensitivity Reactions and Allergy
Priority Concepts: Health Promotion; Immunity
Reference: Ignatavicius, Workman, Rebar (2018), pp. 234-235, 419.

770. *Answer:* 1, 2, 4, 5
Rationale: If a client is allergic to latex and is at high risk for an allergic response, the nurse would use nonlatex gloves and latex-safe supplies, and would keep a latex-safe supply cart available in the client's area. Any supplies or materials that contain latex would be avoided. These include blood pressure cuffs and medication vials with rubber stoppers that require puncture with a needle. It is not necessary to place the client in a private room.

Test-Taking Strategy: Focus on the subject, the client at high risk for an allergic response to latex. Recalling that items that contain rubber are likely to contain latex will direct you to the correct interventions. Also, noting the closed-ended word "only" in options 3 and 6 will assist in eliminating these options.
Level of Cognitive Ability: Analyzing
Client Needs: Safe and Effective Care Environment
Integrated Process: Nursing Process—Implementation
Content Area: Adult Health: Immune
Health Problem: Adult Health: Immune: Hypersensitivity Reactions and Allergy
Priority Concepts: Clinical Judgment; Immunity
Reference: Lewis et al. (2017), pp. 203-204.

771. *Answer:* 2
Rationale: The nurse should ask questions to assist in identifying a cause of Lyme disease, which is a multisystem infection that results from a bite by a tick carried by several species of deer. The rash from a tick bite can be a ring-like rash occurring 3 to 4 weeks after a bite and is commonly seen on the groin, buttocks, axillae, trunk, and upper arms or legs. Option 1 is referring to toxoplasmosis, which is caused by the inhalation of cysts from contaminated cat feces. Lyme disease cannot be transmitted from one person to another.
Test-Taking Strategy: Focus on the strategic word, *first.* Also focus on the data in the question. Eliminate options 3 and 4 because they are comparable or alike. It is important in the initial assessment for the nurse to determine the cause of the rash. If the client sustained a bite while out in the woods, Lyme disease should be suspected.
Level of Cognitive Ability: Analyzing
Client Needs: Safe and Effective Care Environment
Integrated Process: Nursing Process—Assessment
Content Area: Adult Health: Immune
Health Problem: Adult Health: Immune: Lyme Disease
Priority Concepts: Clinical Judgment; Infection
Reference: Lewis et al. (2017), pp. 1534-1535.

772. *Answer:* 2
Rationale: Scleroderma is a chronic connective tissue disease similar to systemic lupus erythematosus. Corticosteroids may be prescribed to treat inflammation. Topical agents may provide some relief from joint pain. Activity is encouraged as tolerated, and the room temperature needs to be constant. Clients need to sit up for 1 to 2 hours after meals if esophageal involvement is present.
Test-Taking Strategy: Focus on the subject, scleroderma. Think about the pathophysiology associated with this condition and read each option carefully to assist in answering correctly.
Level of Cognitive Ability: Analyzing
Client Needs: Physiological Integrity
Integrated Process: Nursing Process—Planning
Content Area: Adult Health: Immune
Health Problem: Adult Health: Immune: Autoimmune disease
Priority Concepts: Caregiving; Immunity
Reference: Ignatavicius, Workman, Rebar (2018), pp. 329-330.

773. *Answer:* 2, 3, 4
Rationale: A blood test is available to detect Lyme disease; however, the test is not reliable if performed before 4 to 6 weeks following the tick bite. Antibody formation takes place in the following manner. Immunoglobulin M is detected 3 to 4 weeks after Lyme disease onset, peaks at 6 to 8 weeks, and then gradually disappears; immunoglobulin G is detected 2 to 3 months after infection and may remain elevated for years. Areas that ticks inhabit need to be avoided. Ticks should be removed with tweezers and then the area is washed with an antiseptic. Options 1 and 5 are incorrect.
Test-Taking Strategy: Focus on the subject, measures to take if Lyme disease is suspected. Also note the strategic words, *most appropriate*. Eliminate option 1, because treatment should begin before the arthralgia develops. Eliminate option 5, because ticks need to be removed.
Level of Cognitive Ability: Analyzing
Client Needs: Physiological Integrity
Integrated Process: Nursing Process—Implementation
Content Area: Adult Health: Immune
Health Problem: Adult Health: Immune: Lyme Disease
Priority Concepts: Caregiving; Immunity
Reference: Ignatavicius, Workman, Rebar (2018), pp. 332-333.

774. *Answer:* 3
Rationale: In the prevention of Lyme disease, individuals need to be instructed to use an insect repellent on the skin and clothes when in an area where ticks are likely to be found. Long-sleeved tops and long pants, closed shoes, and a hat or cap should be worn. If possible, heavily wooded areas or areas with thick underbrush should be avoided. Socks can be pulled up and over the pant legs to prevent ticks from entering under clothing.
Test-Taking Strategy: Note the strategic words, *need for further instruction*. These words indicate a negative event query and ask you to select an option that is incorrect. Note that the correct option uses the words *should not*. Reading carefully will assist in directing you to this option.
Level of Cognitive Ability: Evaluating
Client Needs: Safe and Effective Care Environment
Integrated Process: Teaching and Learning
Content Area: Foundations of Care: Infection Control
Health Problem: Adult Health: Immune: Lyme Disease
Priority Concepts: Client Education; Infection
Reference: Ignatavicius, Workman, Rebar (2018), p. 333.

775. *Answer:* 3
Rationale: Kaposi's sarcoma lesions begin as red, dark blue, or purple macules on the lower legs that change into plaques. These large plaques ulcerate or open and drain. The lesions spread by metastasis through the upper body and then to the face and oral mucosa. They can move to the lymphatic system, lungs, and gastrointestinal tract. Late disease results in swelling and pain in the lower extremities, penis, scrotum, or face. Diagnosis is made by punch biopsy of cutaneous lesions and biopsy of pulmonary and gastrointestinal lesions.
Test-Taking Strategy: Focus on the subject, diagnosing Kaposi's sarcoma. Eliminate options 1 and 2 first, because these symptoms occur late in the development of Kaposi's sarcoma. Then, note the word *confirmed* in the question. This word will assist in directing you to the option that will confirm the diagnosis, the biopsy of the lesions.
Level of Cognitive Ability: Analyzing
Client Needs: Physiological Integrity
Integrated Process: Nursing Process—Assessment

Content Area: Adult Health: Immune
Health Problem: Adult Health: Immune: Immunodeficiency Syndrome
Priority Concepts: Evidence; Immunity
Reference: Ignatavicius, Workman, Rebar (2018), pp. 354-355.

776. *Answer:* **1, 2**
Rationale: Skin testing involves administration of an allergen to the surface of the skin or into the dermis. Site, date, and time of the test must be recorded, and the client must return at a specific date and time for a follow-up site evaluation, even if no reaction is suspected. A list of potential allergens is identified and reviewed and given to the client. For the follow-up evaluation, the size of the site has to be measured and not estimated. After injection, clients only need to be monitored for about 30 minutes to assess for any adverse effects.
Test-Taking Strategy: Note the **strategic words**, *most appropriate*. Eliminate option 3, because any results must be accurately measured and not estimated. Eliminate option 4 because of the **closed-ended word** "only." Eliminate option 5, because it is unreasonable to have the client wait 1 to 2 hours.
Level of Cognitive Ability: Analyzing
Client Needs: Physiological Integrity
Integrated Process: Nursing Process—Implementation
Content Area: Adult Health: Immune
Health Problem: Adult Health: Immune: Hypersensitivity Reactions and Allergies
Priority Concepts: Client Education; Immunity
Reference: Ignatavicius, Workman, Rebar (2018), pp. 444-445.

777. *Answer:* **4**
Rationale: Individuals who are allergic to kiwis, bananas, pineapples, tropical fruits, grapes, avocados, potatoes, hazelnuts, or water chestnuts are at risk for developing a latex allergy. This is thought to be the result of a possible cross-reaction between the food and the latex allergen. Options 1, 2, and 3 are unrelated to latex allergy.
Test-Taking Strategy: Recall knowledge regarding the food items related to a latex allergy. Eliminate options 1, 2, and 3 because they are **comparable or alike** and relate to dairy products.
Level of Cognitive Ability: Analyzing
Client Needs: Health Promotion and Maintenance
Integrated Process: Nursing Process—Assessment
Content Area: Adult Health: Immune
Health Problem: Adult Health: Immune: Immunodeficiency Syndrome
Priority Concepts: Clinical Judgment; Immunity
Reference: Ignatavicius, Workman, Rebar (2018), pp. 234-235, 419.

CHAPTER 63

Immune Medications

PRIORITY CONCEPTS Immunity; Safety

I. Human Immunodeficiency Virus (HIV) and Acquired Immunodeficiency Syndrome (AIDS)

A. Medications include nucleoside-nucleotide reverse transcriptase inhibitors (NRTIs), nonnucleoside reverse transcriptase inhibitors (NNRTIs), protease inhibitors (PIs), and fusion inhibitors (Box 63-1).

B. NRTIs and NNRTIs work by inhibiting the activity of reverse transcriptase.

C. PIs work by interfering with the activity of the enzyme protease.

D. Fusion inhibitors work by inhibiting the binding of HIV to cells.

E. Standard treatment consists of using 3 or 4 medications in regimens known as *highly active antiretroviral therapy (HAART)*; this therapy is not curative but can delay or reverse loss of immune function, preserve health, and prolong life.

F. Other medications include those that are used to treat complications or opportunistic infections that develop (see Box 63-1).

G. Nucleoside-nucleotide reverse transcriptase inhibitors (NRTIs)

1. Abacavir: Can cause nausea; monitor for hypersensitivity reaction, including fever, nausea, vomiting, diarrhea, lethargy, malaise, sore throat, shortness of breath, cough, and rash
2. Abacavir/lamivudine: In addition to the effects that can occur from abacavir and lamivudine, hypersensitivity reactions, lactic acidosis, and severe hepatomegaly can occur.
3. Didanosine: Can cause nausea, diarrhea, peripheral neuropathy, hepatotoxicity, and pancreatitis
4. Emtricitabine: Can cause headache, diarrhea, nausea, rash, hyperpigmentation of the palms and soles, lactic acidosis, and severe hepatomegaly
5. Emtricitabine/tenofovir: In addition to the effects that can occur from emtricitabine and tenofovir (see later), lactic acidosis and severe hepatomegaly can occur.
6. Lamivudine: Causes nausea and nasal congestion
7. Lamivudine/zidovudine: Can cause anemia and neutropenia and lactic acidosis with hepatomegaly
8. Lamivudine/zidovudine/abacavir: In addition to the effects that can occur from lamivudine, zidovudine (see later), and abacavir, hypersensitivity reactions, anemia, neutropenia, lactic acidosis, and severe hepatomegaly can occur.
9. Stavudine: Can cause peripheral neuropathy and pancreatitis
10. Tenofovir: Can cause nausea and vomiting
11. Zidovudine: Can cause nausea, vomiting, anemia, leukopenia, myopathy, fatigue, and headache

H. Nonnucleoside reverse transcriptase inhibitors (NNRTIs)

1. Delavirdine: Can cause rash, liver function changes, and pruritus
2. Efavirenz: Can cause rash, dizziness, confusion, difficulty concentrating, dreams, and encephalopathy
3. Etravirine: Can cause rash, gastrointestinal disturbances, headache, hypertension, and peripheral neuropathy
4. Nevirapine: Can cause rash, Stevens-Johnson syndrome, hepatitis, and increased transaminase levels
5. Rilpivirine can cause headache, nausea, stomach pain, rash, dizziness, and feeling sleepy during the daytime.

I. Protease inhibitors (PIs)

1. Atazanavir: Can cause nausea, headache, infection, vomiting, diarrhea, drowsiness, insomnia, fever, hyperglycemia, hyperlipidemia, and increased bleeding in clients with hemophilia
2. Darunavir: Can cause diarrhea, nausea, vomiting, heartburn, stomach pain, headache, rash, changes in the shape and location of body fat
3. Fosamprenavir: Can cause nausea, vomiting, headache, altered taste sensations, perioral paresthesia, rashes, and altered liver function
4. Indinavir: Can cause nausea, diarrhea, hyperbilirubinemia, nephritis, and kidney stones
5. Lopinavir/ritonavir: Can cause nausea, diarrhea, altered taste sensations, circumoral paresthesia, and hepatitis

BOX 63-1 Medications for Human Immunodeficiency Virus (HIV) and Acquired Immunodeficiency Syndrome (AIDS)

Nucleoside-Nucleotide Reverse Transcriptase Inhibitors (NRTIs)
- Abacavir
- Abacavir/lamivudine
- Didanosine
- Emtricitabine
- Emtricitabine/tenofovir
- Lamivudine
- Lamivudine/zidovudine
- Lamivudine/zidovudine/abacavir
- Stavudine
- Tenofovir
- Zidovudine

Nonnucleoside Reverse Transcriptase Inhibitors (NNRTIs)
- Delavirdine
- Efavirenz
- Etravirine
- Nevirapine
- Rilpivirine

Protease Inhibitors (PIs)
- Atazanavir
- Darunavir
- Fosamprenavir
- Indinavir
- Lopinavir/ritonavir
- Nelfinavir
- Ritonavir
- Saquinavir
- Tipranavir

Integrase Inhibitor
- Raltegravir
- Dolutegravir
- Elvitegravir

Fusion Inhibitor
- Enfuvirtide

Chemokine Receptor 5 (CCR5) Antagonist
- Maraviroc

Antiinflammatory Medication
- Sulfasalazine

Antiinfective Medications
- Atovaquone
- Metronidazole
- Pentamidine isethionate
- Sulfamethoxazole/trimethoprim

Antifungal Medications
- Amphotericin B
- Fluconazole
- Itraconazole
- Ketoconazole
- Voriconazole

Antiviral Medications
- Acyclovir
- Foscarnet
- Ganciclovir
- Valacyclovir

6. Nelfinavir: Can cause nausea, flatulence, and diarrhea
7. Ritonavir: Can cause nausea, vomiting, diarrhea, altered taste sensations, circumoral paresthesia, hepatitis, and increased triglyceride levels
8. Saquinavir: Can cause nausea, diarrhea, photosensitivity, and headache
9. Tipranavir: Hepatotoxicity (liver damage); can also cause nausea, vomiting, diarrhea, headache, and fatigue

J. Integrase inhibitors
1. Stops HIV replication and is used in combination with other antiretroviral medications
2. Can cause nausea, diarrhea, fatigue, headache, and itching; hypersensitivity and liver problems (dolutegravir)

K. Fusion inhibitor: Enfuvirtide can cause skin irritation at injection site, fatigue, nausea, insomnia, and peripheral neuropathy.

L. Chemokine receptor 5 (CCR5) antagonist: Maraviroc
1. Binds with CCR5 and blocks viral entry
2. Can cause cough, dizziness, pyrexia, rash, abdominal pain, musculoskeletal symptoms, and upper respiratory tract infections; liver injury and cardiovascular events have occurred in some clients.

M. Antiinflammatory and antiinfective medications: Used to treat opportunistic infections such as *Pneumocystis jiroveci* pneumonia; Toxoplasma encephalitis is treated with sulfamethoxazole/trimethoprim (see Box 63-1).

N. Antifungal medications: Used to treat candidiasis and cryptococcal meningitis (see Box 63-1)

O. Antiviral medications: Used to treat cytomegalovirus retinitis, herpes simplex, and varicella-zoster virus (see Box 63-1)

The client with HIV or AIDS is at high risk for the development of opportunistic infections.

II. Immunosuppressants (Box 63-2)

A. Description: Immunosuppressants are used for transplant recipients to prevent organ or tissue

BOX 63-2 Immunosuppressants

Calcineurin Inhibitors
- Cyclosporine
- Tacrolimus

Cytotoxic Medications
- Azathioprine
- Cyclophosphamide
- Methotrexate
- Mycophenolate mofetil
- Mycophenolic acid

Antibodies
- Basiliximab
- Lymphocyte immune globulin, antithymocyte globulin, Muromonab-CD3

Other
- Sirolimus
- Everolimus

Glucocorticoids
- See Chapter 47

rejection and to treat autoimmune disorders such as systemic lupus erythematosus.

B. Cyclosporine
1. Used for prevention of rejection following allogeneic organ transplantation
2. Usually administered with a glucocorticoid and another immunosuppressant
3. The most common adverse effects are nephrotoxicity, infection, hypertension, and hirsutism.

C. Tacrolimus
1. Used for prevention of rejection following liver or kidney transplantation
2. Adverse effects include nephrotoxicity, neurotoxicity, gastrointestinal effects, hypertension, hyperkalemia, hyperglycemia, hirsutism, and gum hyperplasia.

D. Azathioprine
1. Generally used with renal transplant recipients
2. Can cause neutropenia and thrombocytopenia

E. Cyclophosphamide
1. Used for its immunosuppressant action to treat autoimmune disorders
2. Can cause neutropenia and hemorrhagic cystitis

F. Methotrexate
1. Used for its immunosuppressant action to treat autoimmune disorders
2. Can cause hepatic fibrosis and cirrhosis, bone marrow suppression, ulcerative stomatitis, and renal damage

G. Mycophenolate mofetil and mycophenolic acid
1. Used to prevent rejection following kidney, heart, and liver transplantation
2. Can cause diarrhea, vomiting, neutropenia, and sepsis; increases the risk of infection and malignancies, especially lymphomas

H. Basiliximab
1. Used to prevent rejection following kidney transplantation
2. Can cause severe acute hypersensitivity reactions, including anaphylaxis

I. Lymphocyte immune globulin, antithymocyte globulin, muromonab CD3
1. Used to prevent rejection following kidney, heart, liver, and bone marrow transplantation
2. Side and adverse effects include fever, chills, leukopenia, and skin reactions.
3. Can cause anaphylactoid reactions

J. Sirolimus
1. Used to prevent renal transplant rejection
2. Increases the risk of infection; raises cholesterol and triglyceride levels; can cause renal injury
3. Can cause rash, acne, anemia, thrombocytopenia, joint pain, diarrhea, and hypokalemia.
4. Everolimus can cause mouth sores, infections, swelling and edema

Monitor the client taking an immunosuppressant closely for signs of infection.

III. Immunizations: See Chapter 18 for more information

IV. Antimicrobials (Box 63-3)

A. Inhibit the growth of bacteria

B. Include medication classifications of aminoglycosides, cephalosporins, fluoroquinolones, macrolides, lincosamides, monobactams, penicillins and penicillinase-resistant penicillins, sulfonamides, streptogramins, tetracyclines, antimycobacterials, and others (see Box 63-3)

C. Adverse effects (Table 63-1)

D. Nursing considerations
1. Assess for allergies.
2. Monitor appropriate laboratory values before therapy as appropriate and during therapy to assess for adverse effects.
3. Report adverse effects to the primary health care provider if any occur.
4. Determine the appropriate method of administration and provide instructions to the client.
5. Monitor intake and output.
6. Encourage fluid intake (unless contraindicated).
7. Initiate safety precautions because of possible central nervous system effects.
8. Teach the client about the medication and how to take it; emphasize the importance of completing the full prescribed course.

PRACTICE QUESTIONS

778. The client with acquired immunodeficiency syndrome and *Pneumocystis jiroveci* infection has been receiving pentamidine. The client develops a temperature of 101° F (38.3° C). The nurse continues to assess the client, knowing that this sign **most likely** indicates which condition?

BOX 63-3 Antimicrobials

Aminoglycosides
- Amikacin
- Gentamicin
- Neomycin
- Streptomycin
- Tobramycin

Cephalosporins
- Cefaclor
- Cefadroxil
- Cefazolin
- Cefdinir
- Cefditoren
- Cefepime
- Cefixime
- Cefotaxime
- Cefotetan
- Cefoxitin
- Cefpodoxime
- Cefprozil
- Ceftazidime
- Ceftibuten
- Ceftriaxone
- Cefuroxime
- Cephalexin

Fluoroquinolones
- Ciprofloxacin
- Gemifloxacin
- Levofloxacin
- Moxifloxacin
- Ofloxacin

Macrolides
- Azithromycin
- Clarithromycin
- Erythromycin
- Fidaxomicin

Lincosamides
- Clindamycin
- Lincomycin

Monobactam
- Aztreonam

Penicillins
- Amoxicillin
- Ampicillin
- Penicillin G
- Penicillin V
- Piperacillin

Penicillinase-Resistant Penicillins
- Dicloxacillin
- Nafcillin
- Oxacillin

Sulfonamides
- Sulfamethoxazole
- Sulfadiazine
- Sulfasalazine
- Sulfisoxazole
- Trimethoprim/sulfamethoxazole

Streptogramins
- Quinupristin/dalfopristin

Tetracyclines
- Demeclocycline
- Doxycycline
- Minocycline
- Tetracycline

Antimycobacterials
- Antituberculosis agents (see Chapter 51)
- Leprostatics: Clofazimine, Thalidomide

Antifungal Medications
- Amphotericin B
- Fluconazole
- Itraconazole
- Ketoconazole
- Posaconazole
- Voriconazole

Antiviral Medications
- Acyclovir
- Famciclovir
- Foscarnet
- Ganciclovir
- Valacyclovir

1. That the dose of the medication is too low
2. That the client is experiencing toxic effects of the medication
3. That the client has developed inadequacy of thermoregulation
4. That the client has developed another infection caused by leukopenic effects of the medication

TABLE 63-1 Antimicrobials and Their Adverse Effects

Classification	Adverse Effects
Aminoglycosides	Ototoxicity
	Confusion, disorientation
	Renal toxicity
	Gastrointestinal irritation
	Palpitations, blood pressure changes
	Hypersensitivity reactions
Cephalosporins	Gastrointestinal disturbances
	Pseudomembranous colitis
	Headache, dizziness, lethargy, paresthesias
	Nephrotoxicity
	Superinfections
Fluoroquinolones	Headache, dizziness, insomnia, depression
	Gastrointestinal effects
	Bone marrow depression
	Fever, rash, photosensitivity
Macrolides	Gastrointestinal effects
	Pseudomembranous colitis
	Confusion, abnormal thinking
	Superinfections
	Hypersensitivity reactions
Lincosamides	Gastrointestinal effects
	Pseudomembranous colitis
	Bone marrow depression
Monobactams	Gastrointestinal effects
	Hepatotoxicity
	Allergic reactions
Penicillins and penicillinase-resistant penicillins	Gastrointestinal effects, including sore mouth and furry tongue
	Superinfections
	Hypersensitivity reactions, including anaphylaxis
Sulfonamides	Gastrointestinal effects
	Hepatotoxicity
	Nephrotoxicity
	Bone marrow depression
	Dermatological effects, including hypersensitivity and photosensitivity
	Headache, dizziness, vertigo, ataxia, depression, seizures
Tetracyclines	Gastrointestinal effects
	Hepatotoxicity

TABLE 63-1 Antimicrobials and Their Adverse Effects—cont'd

Classification	Adverse Effects
	Teeth (staining) and bone damage
	Superinfections
	Dermatological reactions, including rash and photosensitivity
	Hypersensitivity reactions
Antimycobacterials, leprostatics	Gastrointestinal effects
	Neuritis, dizziness, headache, malaise, drowsiness, hallucinations
Antifungals	Gastrointestinal effects
	Headache, rash, anemia, hepatotoxicity
	Hearing loss, peripheral neuritis

779. The nurse caring for a client who is taking an aminoglycoside should monitor the client for which adverse effects of the medication? **Select all that apply.**
- ❑ 1. Seizures
- ❑ 2. Ototoxicity
- ❑ 3. Renal toxicity
- ❑ 4. Dysrhythmias
- ❑ 5. Hepatotoxicity

780. Ketoconazole is prescribed for a client with a diagnosis of candidiasis. Which interventions should the nurse include when administering this medication? **Select all that apply.**
- ❑ 1. Restrict fluid intake.
- ❑ 2. Monitor liver function studies.
- ❑ 3. Instruct the client to avoid alcohol.
- ❑ 4. Administer the medication with an antacid.
- ❑ 5. Instruct the client to avoid exposure to the sun.
- ❑ 6. Administer the medication on an empty stomach.

781. The nurse is caring for a client who has been taking a sulfonamide and should monitor for signs and symptoms of which adverse effects of the medication? **Select all that apply.**
- ❑ 1. Ototoxicity
- ❑ 2. Palpitations
- ❑ 3. Nephrotoxicity
- ❑ 4. Bone marrow suppression
- ❑ 5. Gastrointestinal (GI) effects
- ❑ 6. Increased white blood cell (WBC) count

782. The nurse is reviewing the results of serum laboratory studies drawn on a client with acquired immunodeficiency syndrome who is receiving didanosine. The nurse interprets that the client may have the medication discontinued by the health care provider if which elevated result is noted?
1. Serum protein level
2. Blood glucose level
3. Serum amylase level
4. Serum creatinine level

783. The nurse is caring for a postrenal transplantation client taking cyclosporine. The nurse notes an increase in one of the client's vital signs, and the client is complaining of a headache. What vital sign is **most likely** increased?
1. Pulse
2. Respirations
3. Blood pressure
4. Pulse oximetry

784. Amikacin is prescribed for a client with a bacterial infection. The nurse instructs the client to contact the primary health care provider (PHCP) **immediately** if which occurs?
1. Nausea
2. Lethargy
3. Hearing loss
4. Muscle aches

785. The nurse is assigned to care for a client with cytomegalovirus retinitis and acquired immunodeficiency syndrome who is receiving foscarnet, an antiviral medication. The nurse should monitor the results of which laboratory study while the client is taking this medication?
1. $CD4^+$ T cell count
2. Lymphocyte count
3. Serum albumin level
4. Serum creatinine level

786. A client who is human immunodeficiency virus seropositive has been taking stavudine. The nurse should monitor which **most** closely while the client is taking this medication?
1. Gait
2. Appetite
3. Level of consciousness
4. Gastrointestinal function

ANSWERS

778. *Answer:* 4
Rationale: Frequent adverse effects of this medication include leukopenia, thrombocytopenia, and anemia. The client should be monitored routinely for signs and symptoms of infection. Options 1, 2, and 3 are inaccurate interpretations.
Test-Taking Strategy: Note the strategic words, *most likely*. Focus on the data in the question. Noting that the temperature is elevated will direct you to the correct option.
Level of Cognitive Ability: Synthesizing
Client Needs: Physiological Integrity
Integrated Process: Nursing Process—Analysis
Content Area: Pharmacology: Immune Medications: Antimycobacterials
Health Problem: Adult Health: Respiratory: Viral, Bacterial, Fungal Infections
Priority Concepts: Infection; Immunity
Reference: Lilley et al. (2017), pp. 686-687, 690.

779. *Answer:* 2, 3, 4
Rationale: Aminoglycosides are administered to inhibit the growth of bacteria. Adverse effects of this medication include confusion, ototoxicity, renal toxicity, gastrointestinal irritation, palpitations or dysrhythmias, blood pressure changes, and hypersensitivity reactions. Therefore, the remaining options are incorrect.
Test-Taking Strategy: Focus on the subject, adverse effects of aminoglycosides. It is necessary to know the adverse effects associated with this medication to answer correctly. Remember that ototoxicity, renal toxicity, and dysrhythmias are adverse effects.
Level of Cognitive Ability: Analyzing
Client Needs: Physiological Integrity
Integrated Process: Nursing Process—Assessment
Content Area: Pharmacology: Immune Medications: Aminoglycosides
Health Problem: Adult Health: Immune: Infections
Priority Concepts: Clinical Judgment; Immunity
Reference: Lilley et al. (2017), pp. 624-626.

780. *Answer:* 2, 3, 5
Rationale: Ketoconazole is an antifungal medication. There is no reason for the client to restrict fluid intake; in fact, this could be harmful to the client. The medication is hepatotoxic, and the nurse monitors liver function. It is administered with food (not on an empty stomach), and antacids are avoided for 2 hours after taking the medication to ensure absorption. The client is also instructed to avoid alcohol. In addition, the client is instructed to avoid exposure to the sun, because the medication increases photosensitivity.
Test-Taking Strategy: Focus on the subject, administration procedures, and recall that ketoconazole is an antifungal medication. Next, use general medication guidelines to select the correct interventions. Also, remember that this medication is administered with food and that it is hepatotoxic.
Level of Cognitive Ability: Analyzing
Client Needs: Physiological Integrity
Integrated Process: Nursing Process—Implementation
Content Area: Pharmacology: Immune Medications: Antifungals
Health Problem: Adult Health: Immune: Infections
Priority Concepts: Clinical Judgment; Immunity
Reference: Burchum, Rosenthal (2016), pp. 1097-1098.

781. *Answer:* 3, 4, 5
Rationale: Adverse effects of sulfonamides include nephrotoxicity, bone marrow suppression, GI effects, hepatotoxicity, dermatological effects, and some neurological symptoms including headache, dizziness, vertigo, ataxia, depression, and seizures. Options 1, 2, and 6 are unrelated to these medications.
Test-Taking Strategy: Focus on the subject, adverse effects of sulfonamides. It is necessary to know the adverse effects associated with these medications to answer correctly. Remember that nephrotoxicity, bone marrow suppression, and GI symptoms are adverse effects of sulfonamides.
Level of Cognitive Ability: Analyzing
Client Needs: Physiological Integrity
Integrated Process: Nursing Process—Assessment
Content Area: Pharmacology: Immune Medications: Sulfonamides
Health Problem: Adult Health: Immune: Infections
Priority Concepts: Clinical Judgment; Immunity
Reference: Burchum, Rosenthal (2016), pp. 1063-1064.

782. *Answer:* 3
Rationale: Didanosine can cause pancreatitis. A serum amylase level that is increased to 1.5 to 2 times normal may signify pancreatitis in the client with acquired immunodeficiency syndrome and is potentially fatal. The medication may have to be discontinued. The medication is also hepatotoxic and can result in liver failure.
Test-Taking Strategy: Focus on the subject, adverse effects of didanosine. Recalling that this medication can cause damage to the pancreas and is hepatotoxic will direct you to the correct option.
Level of Cognitive Ability: Analyzing
Client Needs: Physiological Integrity
Integrated Process: Nursing Process—Assessment
Content Area: Pharmacology: Immune Medications: Antivirals
Health Problem: Adult Health: Immune: Immunodeficiency Syndrome
Priority Concepts: Clinical Judgment; Safety
Reference: Skidmore-Roth (2017), pp. 362-364.

783. *Answer:* 3
Rationale: Hypertension can occur in a client taking cyclosporine, and because this client is also complaining of a headache, the blood pressure is the vital sign to be monitored most closely. Other adverse effects include infection, nephrotoxicity, and hirsutism. Options 1, 2, and 4 are unrelated to the use of this medication.
Test-Taking Strategy: Note the strategic words, *most likely*. Focus on the name of the medication and recall that this medication can cause hypertension. Also, noting that the client has a headache will assist you in answering correctly.
Level of Cognitive Ability: Analyzing
Client Needs: Physiological Integrity
Integrated Process: Nursing Process—Assessment
Content Area: Pharmacology: Immune Medications: Immunosuppressants
Health Problem: Adult Health: Immune: Transplantation
Priority Concepts: Clinical Judgment; Immunity
Reference: Lewis et al. (2017), pp. 209, 211.

784. *Answer:* 3

Rationale: Amikacin is an aminoglycoside. Adverse effects of aminoglycosides include ototoxicity (hearing problems), confusion, disorientation, gastrointestinal irritation, palpitations, blood pressure changes, nephrotoxicity, and hypersensitivity. The nurse instructs the client to report hearing loss to the PHCP immediately. Lethargy and muscle aches are not associated with the use of this medication. It is not necessary to contact the PHCP immediately if nausea occurs. If nausea persists or results in vomiting, the PHCP should be notified.

Test-Taking Strategy: Note the strategic word, *immediately*. Recalling that this medication is an aminoglycoside (most aminoglycoside medication names end in *-cin*) and that aminoglycosides are ototoxic will direct you to the correct option.

Level of Cognitive Ability: Applying

Client Needs: Physiological Integrity

Integrated Process: Teaching and Learning

Content Area: Pharmacology: Immune Medications: Aminoglycosides

Health Problem: Adult Health: Immune: Infections

Priority Concepts: Client Education; Safety

Reference: Burchum, Rosenthal (2016), pp. 1052-1053.

785. *Answer:* 4

Rationale: Foscarnet is toxic to the kidneys. The serum creatinine level is monitored before therapy, two or three times per week during induction therapy, and at least weekly during maintenance therapy. Foscarnet also may cause decreased levels of calcium, magnesium, phosphorus, and potassium. Thus, these levels also are measured with the same frequency.

Test-Taking Strategy: Focus on the subject, the laboratory value to be monitored. Recalling that this medication is nephrotoxic will direct you to the correct option.

Level of Cognitive Ability: Analyzing

Client Needs: Physiological Integrity

Integrated Process: Nursing Process—Assessment

Content Area: Pharmacology: Immune Medications: Antivirals

Health Problem: Adult Health: Immune: Immunodeficiency Syndrome

Priority Concepts: Clinical Judgment; Safety

Reference: Hodgson, Kizior (2018), pp. 501-502.

786. *Answer:* 1

Rationale: Stavudine is an antiretroviral used to manage human immunodeficiency virus infection in clients who do not respond to or who cannot tolerate conventional therapy. The medication can cause peripheral neuropathy, and the nurse should monitor the client's gait closely and ask the client about paresthesia. Options 2, 3, and 4 are unrelated to this medication.

Test-Taking Strategy: Note the strategic word, *most*. Focus on the name of the medication. Recalling that this medication causes peripheral neuropathy will direct you to the correct option.

Level of Cognitive Ability: Analyzing

Client Needs: Physiological Integrity

Integrated Process: Nursing Process—Assessment

Content Area: Pharmacology: Immune Medications: Antivirals

Health Problem: Adult Health: Immune: Immunodeficiency Syndrome

Priority Concepts: Clinical Judgment; Safety

Reference: Skidmore-Roth (2017), pp. 1093-1094.

UNIT XVIII

Mental Health Problems of the Adult Client

Pyramid to Success

The Pyramid to Success focuses on the therapeutic nurse–client relationship, client rights, the ethical and legal issues related to the care of a client with a mental health problem, and grief and loss. Pyramid Points also focus on the use of restraints (security devices), seclusion, and electroconvulsive therapy. Care for a client with an addiction, such as an eating disorder, substance abuse disorder, or gambling disorder, is another focus area. Additional areas of focus include anxiety, depression, suicide, abuse and neglect, violence, rape crisis interventions, post-traumatic stress disorders, obsessive-compulsive disorders, schizophrenia, and bipolar disorders. Pyramid Points also address the use of medications prescribed for a client with a mental health problem.

Client Needs: Learning Objectives

Safe and Effective Care Environment

Ensuring client advocacy
Ensuring that informed consent related to treatments, such as restraints (security devices), seclusion, and electroconvulsive therapy, has been obtained
Implementing legal responsibilities related to reporting incidences of abuse, neglect, or violence
Maintaining confidentiality
Providing psychiatric consultations and other interprofessional referrals
Providing safety to the client and others
Upholding client rights
Using restraints (security devices) and seclusion appropriately and safely

Health Promotion and Maintenance

Identifying community resources for the client
Identifying individual lifestyle choices
Performing psychosocial assessment techniques
Providing health promotion programs related to addictions

Psychosocial Integrity

Addressing grief and loss issues
Assessing for abuse and neglect situations
Assessing for addictions
Assessing for domestic violence
Caring for the client who has been sexually abused or raped
Considering religious, cultural, and spiritual influences on health
Developing a therapeutic nurse–client relationship
Identifying coping mechanisms
Identifying support systems
Implementing behavioral interventions
Providing crisis intervention
Providing a therapeutic milieu
Teaching stress-management techniques

Physiological Integrity

Assessing for abusive and self-destructive behavior
Monitoring elimination patterns
Monitoring for alterations in body systems related to substance abuse
Monitoring for expected and untoward effects of medications
Monitoring for potential complications related to medications and treatments, such as electroconvulsive therapy
Monitoring laboratory values related to medication therapy
Monitoring rest and sleep patterns
Providing adequate nutrition
Providing personal hygiene measures

CHAPTER 64

Foundations of Mental Health Nursing

PRIORITY CONCEPTS **Caregiving; Coping**

I. Nurse–Client Relationship

A. Principles

1. Genuineness, respect, and empathic understanding are characteristics important to the development of a therapeutic nurse–client relationship.
2. The client should be cared for in a holistic manner.
3. The nurse considers the client's cultural and spiritual beliefs and values in assessing the client's response to the nurse–client relationship and her or his adaptation to stressors.
4. Appropriate limits and boundaries define and facilitate a therapeutic nurse–client relationship.
5. Honest and open communication is important for the development of trust, an underpinning of the therapeutic nurse–client relationship.
6. The nurse uses therapeutic communication techniques to encourage the client to express thoughts and feelings as they address identified problem areas.
7. The nurse respects the client's confidentiality and limits discussion of the client to the interprofessional health care team.
8. The goal of the nurse–client relationship is to assist the client to develop problem-solving abilities and **coping mechanisms**.

⚠ The nurse needs to consider the cultural, religious, and spiritual practices of the client and whether these practices may give the client hope, comfort, and support while healing.

B. Phases of a therapeutic nurse–client relationship

1. Preinteraction phase
   - **a.** Begins before the nurse's first contact with the client
   - **b.** Develops appropriate physical and interpersonal environment (seating, lighting) to promote comfort and facilitate collaboration
   - **c.** Anticipates potential client issues
   - **d.** Prepares for the client interaction
   - **e.** Determines how to initially approach client
   - **f.** The nurse should identify her or his own preconceived ideas, stereotypes, biases, and values that may impinge on the nurse–client relationship.
2. Orientation or introductory phase
   - **a.** Acceptance, rapport, trust, and boundaries are established.
   - **b.** Introduces herself or himself to the client by using first and last name and designation
   - **c.** Identifies purpose and the time frame of the relationship (establishing a contract).
   - **d.** Identifies client's strengths and needs
   - **e.** Collects data and forms basis for diagnosis and client-centered goals.
   - **f.** Termination and separation of the relationship are discussed in anticipation of the time-limited nature of the relationship.
3. Working phase
   - **a.** Exploring, focusing on, and evaluating the client's concerns and problems occur; an attitude of acceptance and active listening assists the client to express thoughts and feelings.
   - **b.** Actively problem solves with the client
   - **c.** Uses interpersonal strategies to help the client identify effective coping strategies
   - **d.** Encourages self-direction and self-management whenever possible to promote health and wellness.
4. Termination or separation phase
   - **a.** Prepares the client for termination and separation on initial contact.
   - **b.** Evaluates progress and achievement of goals.
   - **c.** Identifies responses related to termination and separation, such as anger, distancing from the relationship, a return of symptoms, and dependency.
   - **d.** Encourages the client to express feelings about termination.
   - **e.** Identifies the client's strengths and anticipated needs for follow-up care.
   - **f.** Refers the client to community resources and other support systems.

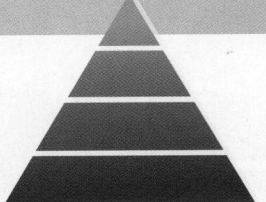

C. Family as an extension of the client
1. Family members should be viewed as collaborators in the management of a client's mental health needs (maintain confidentiality as necessary).
2. Competence and caring focused toward family members enhance the nurse's ability to identify client and family needs and to select and implement effective interventions directed toward promoting adaptive functioning.
3. Nurses have a professional obligation to be aware of and sensitive to the cultural, ethnic, religious, and spiritual factors that affect the structure and resulting needs of the client and her or his family.
4. Educating family members regarding the client's mental health problem, identification of symptoms, and effective management of maladaptive behaviors plays a vital role in the client's quality of life.

D. Impact of culture, ethnicity, religion, and spirituality on client care
1. Cultural competency allows the nurse to recognize the uniqueness of each client and the impact that culture, values, and religious and spiritual beliefs have on an individual's mental health as well as the treatment required for existing mental health problem.
2. A client's culture, ethnicity, values, and religious and spiritual belief systems can affect all aspects of mental health care, including medication therapies, and can act as either protective or risk factors when dealing with the development and/or treatment of mental health problems.
3. Nurses must be aware of the impact that their own culture, religious and spiritual beliefs, and values have on the care they provide and to avoid biases.
4. The treatment plan must be agreed upon by both client and nurse and take into consideration the needs of the client whenever possible.

II. Therapeutic Communication Process

A. Principles
1. Communication includes verbal and nonverbal expression (Fig. 64-1).
2. Successful communication includes appropriateness, efficiency, flexibility, and feedback.
3. Anxiety in the nurse or client impedes communication.
4. Communication needs to be goal-directed within a professional framework.

B. Therapeutic and nontherapeutic communication techniques (Table 64-1)

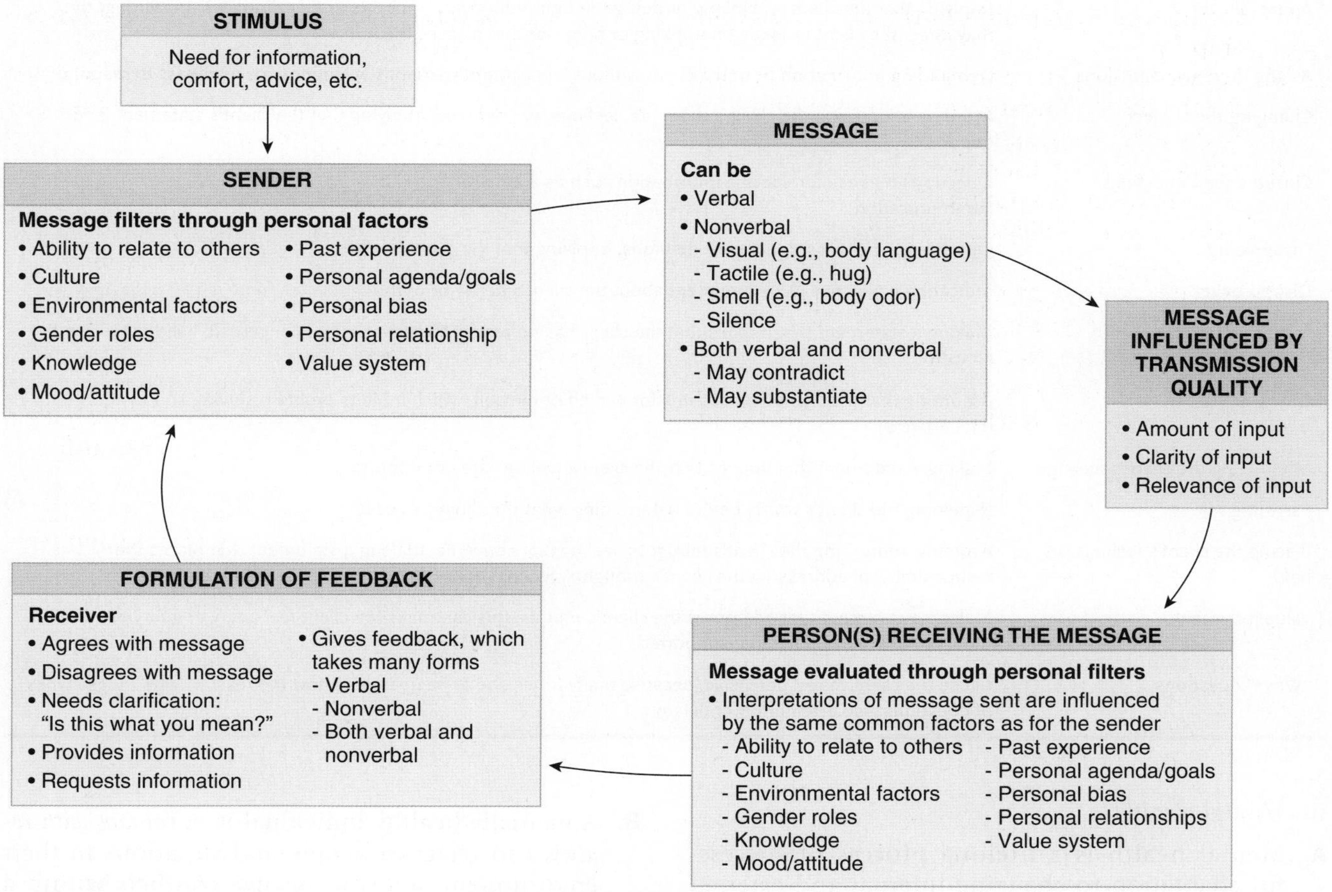

FIG. 64-1 Operational definition of communication.

TABLE 64-1 Therapeutic (Effective) and Nontherapeutic (Ineffective) Communication Techniques

Therapeutic Techniques	
Technique	**Description**
Active listening	Carefully noting what the client is saying and observing the client's nonverbal behavior
Broad openings	Encouraging the client to select topics for discussion
Clarifying	Providing a means for making the message clearer, correcting any misunderstandings, and promoting mutual understanding
Focusing	Directing the conversation on the topic being discussed
Informing	Giving information to the client
Offering self to help	Includes staying with the client, talking to the client, and offering to help the client
Open-ended questions	Encouraging conversation because these questions require more than one-word answers
Paraphrasing	Restating in different words what the client said
Reflecting	Directing the client's question or statement back to the client for consideration
Restating	Repeating what the client has said and directing the statement back to the client to provide the client the opportunity to agree or disagree or to clarify the message further
Silence	Allowing time for formulating thoughts
Summarizing	Stating briefly what was discussed during the conversation
Validating	Verifying that both the nurse and the client are interpreting the topic or message in the same way
Nontherapeutic Techniques	
Technique	**Description**
Approval	Implying that the client is thinking or doing the right thing and is not thinking or doing what is wrong; this may direct the client to focus on thinking or behavior that pleases the nurse
Asking excessive questions	Demanding information from the client without respect for the client's willingness or readiness to respond
Changing the subject	Avoiding addressing the client's thoughts, feelings, or concerns; implying that the client's statement is not important
Closed-ended questions	Questions that ask for specific information such as a "yes" or "no" answer and therefore inhibit communication
Disagreeing	Opposing the client's thinking or opinions, implying that the client is wrong
Disapproving	Indicating a negative value judgment about the client's behavior or thoughts
False reassurance	Making a statement that implies that the client has no reason to be worried or concerned; belittling a client's concerns
Giving advice	Assuming that the client cannot think for herself or himself, which inhibits problem solving and fosters dependence
Minimizing the client's feelings	Making a statement that implies that the client's feelings are not important
Parroting	Repeating the client's words before determining what the client has said
Placing the client's feelings on hold	Avoiding addressing the client's thoughts, feelings, or concerns; making a statement that places the responsibility of addressing the client's thoughts, feelings, or concerns elsewhere or on another person
Value judgments	Making a comment that addresses the client's morals; this can make the client feel angry or guilty or as though she or he is not being supported
"Why?" questions	Cause the client to feel defensive, because many times she or he does not know the reason "why"; these types of questions also often imply criticism

III. Mental Health

A. Mental health is a lifelong process of successful adaptation to changing internal and external environments.

B. A mentally healthy individual is *in contact with reality*, can relate to people and situations in their environment, and can resolve conflicts within a problem-solving framework.

C. A mentally healthy individual has psychobiological resilience.

IV. Mental Health Problem

A. Description
1. A mental health problem can cause the loss of the ability to respond to the internal and external environment in ways that are in harmony with oneself or the expectations of society.
2. It is characterized by thought or behavior patterns that impair functioning and cause distress.

B. Personality characteristics
1. Self-concept is distorted.
2. Perception of strengths and weaknesses is unrealistic.
3. Thoughts and perceptions may not be reality-based.
4. The ability to find meaning and purpose in life may be impaired.
5. Life direction and productivity may be disturbed.
6. Meeting one's own needs may be problematic.
7. Excessive reliance or preoccupation on the thoughts, opinions, and actions of self or others may be present.

C. Adaptations to stress
1. The individual's sense of self-control may be affected.
2. Perception of the environment may be distorted.
3. Coping mechanisms may not exist or may be ineffective.

D. Interpersonal relationships
1. Interpersonal relationships may be minimally existent or may be negatively affected.
2. The ability to enjoy sustained intimacy in relationships is impaired.

V. Coping and Defense Mechanisms

A. Coping mechanisms
1. Coping involves any effort to decrease anxiety.
2. Coping mechanisms can be constructive or destructive, task- or problem-oriented in relation to direct problem solving, cognitively oriented in an attempt to neutralize the meaning of the problem, or defense- or emotion-oriented, thus regulating the response to protect oneself.

B. Defense mechanisms
1. As anxiety increases, the individual copes by using defense mechanisms.
2. A defense mechanism is a coping mechanism used in an effort to protect the individual from feelings of anxiety; as anxiety increases and becomes overwhelming, the individual copes by using defense mechanisms to protect the ego and decrease anxiety (Box 64-1)

Coping mechanisms and defense mechanisms are used by the client as protection from unmanageable stress and to decrease anxiety.

BOX 64-1 Types of Defense Mechanisms

Compensation: Putting forth extra effort to counterbalance perceived deficiencies by emphasizing strengths.
Conversion: The expression of emotional conflicts through physical symptoms that have no organic cause.
Denial: Ignoring the existence of unpleasant or intolerable thoughts, feelings, needs, or impulses.
Displacement: Feelings about a person, object, or situation are directed to another less-threatening person, object, or situation.
Dissociation: The blocking of an anxiety-provoking event or period of time from the consciousness, memory, or perception to compartmentalize uncomfortable or unpleasant aspects of oneself.
Identification: The conscious or unconscious attempt to change oneself to resemble an admired person.
Insulation: Withdrawing into passivity and becoming inaccessible so as to avoid further threatening situations.
Intellectualization: Excessive reasoning of an event based solely on facts without involving feeling or emotion; the thinking is disconnected from feelings, and situations are dealt with at a cognitive level.
Introjection: A type of identification in which the individual incorporates the traits or values of another into herself or himself.
Isolation: Response in which a person blocks feelings associated with an unpleasant experience.
Projection: Transferring one's internal feelings, thoughts, and unacceptable ideas and traits to someone else.
Rationalization: An attempt to make unacceptable feelings and behaviors acceptable by justifying the behavior.
Reaction Formation: Developing conscious attitudes and behaviors and acting out behaviors opposite to what one really feels.
Regression: Returning to an earlier developmental stage and pattern of behavior to express an impulse to deal with anxiety.
Repression: An unconscious process in which the client blocks undesirable and unacceptable thoughts or ideas from conscious expression.
Sublimation: Unconscious replacement of a mature and socially acceptable need, attitude, or emotion with one more immature and unacceptable one.
Substitution: The replacement of a valued unacceptable object with an object more acceptable to the ego.
Suppression: The conscious, deliberate denial of unacceptable or painful situation, thought, idea, or feeling.

C. Interventions
1. Assist the client to identify the source of anxiety and to explore methods to reduce anxiety.
2. Assess the client's use of defense mechanisms.
3. Facilitate appropriate use of defense mechanisms.
4. Determine whether the defense mechanisms used by the client are effective for her or him or create additional distress.
5. Avoid arguing or criticizing the client's behavior and the use of defense mechanisms.

6. Do not take defense coping mechanism away until client has established more appropriate coping strategies to effectively deal with stressors.

VI. Diagnostic and Statistical Manual of Mental Health Disorders

A. The *Diagnostic and Statistical Manual of Mental Health Disorders*, published by the American Psychiatric Association, provides guidelines for health care personnel for identifying and categorizing mental health problems.

B. The manual is a system used in clinical, research, and educational settings, in which diagnostic criteria are included for each mental health problem.

C. The manual addresses culturally diverse populations and mental health problems that may be associated with a particular culture.

D. Dual diagnosis: Refers to the client who has both a mental health problem and a substance related problem simultaneously; also known as comorbidity or co-occurring problems

E. See American Psychiatric Association for updates: http://www.dsm5.org/Pages/Default.aspx.

VII. Types of Mental Health Admissions and Discharges

A. Voluntary admission
1. The client (or the client's guardian) seeks admission for care.
2. The voluntary client is free to sign out of the hospital with psychiatrist (primary health care provider [PHCP]) notification and prescription.
3. Detaining a voluntary client against her or his will is termed *false imprisonment*.
4. The client retains full civil rights (Box 64-2).

B. Right to confidentiality
1. A client has a right to confidentiality of her or his medical information; the Health Insurance Portability and Accountability Act (HIPAA) of 1996 ensures client confidentiality with regard to the release and electronic transmission of data.
2. Information sometimes must be released in life-threatening situations without the client's consent.
3. In the event of a specific threat against an identified individual, the health care professional has a legal obligation to warn the intended victim of a client's threats of harm.

Except in an emergency situation, client information can be released only with the client's informed consent, which specifies the information that can be released and the time frame for which the release is valid.

C. Involuntary admission
1. Involuntary admission may be necessary when a person is mentally ill, is a danger to self or others, or is in need of mental health treatment or physical care.
2. Involuntary admission occurs when a person is admitted or detained involuntarily for mental health treatment because of actual or imminent danger to self or others; the person's condition is deteriorating and they require hospitalization.
3. A client who is admitted involuntarily retains her or his right for informed consent.
4. The client retains the right to refuse treatments, including medications, unless a separate and specific treatment order is obtained from the court.
5. The client loses the right to refuse treatment when she or he poses an immediate danger to self or others, requiring immediate action by the interprofessional health care team.
6. Depending on the jurisdiction, an order from an external board such as a court or from the psychiatrist or PHCP is required for involuntary admissions except in the case of emergency, which allows time to obtain the necessary order from the board; in the case of all involuntary admissions, legal counsel must be provided for the client. In this situation, the client may be held for a 72-hour period until further evaluation is completed.

BOX 64-2 Client Rights

- Right to communicate with people outside the hospital through correspondence, telephone, and personal visits
- Right to keep clothing and personal effects with them in the hospital
- Right to religious freedom
- Right to be employed if possible
- Right to manage and dispose of property
- Right to execute wills
- Right to enter into contractual relationships
- Right to make purchases
- Right to education
- Right to habeas corpus
- Right to independent mental health examination
- Right to civil service status
- Right to retain licenses, privileges, or permits established by law, such as a driver's or professional license
- Right to sue or be sued
- Right to marry and divorce
- Right not to be subject to unnecessary mechanical restraints
- Right to periodic review of status
- Right to legal representation
- Right to privacy
- Right to informed consent
- Right to treatment
- Right to refuse treatment
- Right to treatment in the least restrictive setting

Note: State and province laws should always be followed.

From Stuart G: *Principles and practice of psychiatric nursing*, ed 10, St. Louis, 2013, Mosby.

7. A hearing is held by an external board within a specified time period for a client admitted involuntarily; the specific time period varies by state. The psychiatrist or PHCP may also be the person making decisions surrounding client discourse, depending on location.
8. In most states, a client can institute a hearing to seek an expedient judicial discharge (a writ of habeas corpus).
9. At the hearing, a determination is made as to whether the client may be released from the hospital or detained for further treatment and evaluation, or committed to a mental health facility for an undetermined period.
10. A client has the right to treatment in the least restrictive treatment environment; if treatment objectives can be achieved by court-ordered treatment to an outpatient facility as opposed to an inpatient facility, the client has the right to be treated in the outpatient setting.
11. A client is considered legally competent unless she or he has been declared incompetent through a legal hearing separate from the involuntary commitment hearing.
12. In the course of providing nursing care and carrying out medical prescriptions, if the nurse believes that a client lacks competency to make informed decisions, action should be initiated to determine whether a legal guardian or substitute decision-maker needs to be appointed by the court.

D. Release from the hospital

1. Description
   a. In some, but not all, jurisdictions, a client may be released voluntarily, against medical advice, or with conditions (conditional release). It is important to be familiar with the laws in the area in which you work regarding conditional release.
   b. A client who has sought voluntary admission has the right to receive release upon request.
2. Voluntary release
   a. In the absence of an act of self-harm or danger to others, a voluntary client should never be detained.
   b. If a voluntary client wishes to be discharged from treatment, but is considered potentially dangerous to self or others, the PHCP can order the client to be detained while legal proceedings for involuntary status are sought. In other areas, the PHCP places them on a 72-hour hold while further evaluation occurs.
   c. Some states provide for conditional release of involuntarily hospitalized clients; this enables the treating PHCP to prescribe continued treatment on an outpatient basis as opposed to discharging the client to follow up on her or his own initiative. Community treatment orders may also be instituted depending on the facility and on the area.
   d. Conditional release usually involves outpatient treatment for a specified period to determine the client's compliance with medication protocol, ability to meet basic needs, and ability to reintegrate into the community.
   e. An involuntary client who is released conditionally may be reinstitutionalized while the commitment is still in effect without recommencement of formal admission procedures.
3. Discharge planning and follow-up care
   a. Discharge is the termination of the client–institution relationship.
   b. The release may be prescribed by the psychiatrist, external board, or administration for involuntarily admitted clients and may be requested by voluntary clients at any time.
   c. In most states, the client can institute an external board hearing to seek an expedient judicial discharge (writ of habeas corpus).
   d. Discharge planning and follow-up care are important for the continued well-being of the client with a mental health problem.
   e. Aftercare case managers are used to facilitate the client's adaptation back into the community and to provide early referral if the treatment plan is unsuccessful.

VIII. Types of Therapy for Care

A. Milieu therapy

1. The **milieu** refers to the safe physical and social environment in which an individual is receiving treatment.
2. Safety is the most important priority in managing the milieu, and all encounters with the client have the goal of being "therapeutic."
3. All members of the interprofessional health care team contribute to the planning and functioning of the milieu and are significant and valuable to the client's successful treatment outcomes; the team generally includes a registered nurse, social worker, exercise therapist, recreational therapist, psychologist, psychiatrist, occupational therapist, and clinical nurse specialist or nurse practitioner.
4. Community meetings, activity groups, social skills groups, and physical exercise programs are included to accomplish treatment goals.
5. One-to-one relationships are used to examine client behaviors, feelings, and interactions within the context of the therapeutic group activities.

The focus of milieu therapy is to empower the client through involvement in setting her or his own goals and to develop purposeful relationships with the staff to assist in meeting these goals.

B. Interpersonal psychotherapy
1. A treatment modality that uses a therapeutic relationship to modify the client's feelings, attitudes, and behaviors and work within an agreed-upon time frame to help meet the client's goals
2. Therapeutic communication forms the foundation of the therapist–client relationship, and this relationship is used as a way for the client to examine other relationships in her or his life.
3. Supportive level of psychotherapy
    a. Brief therapy or may extend over a period of years, allowing the client to express feelings, explore alternatives, and make decisions in a safe, caring environment
    b. No plan exists to introduce new methods of coping; instead, the therapist reinforces the client's existing coping mechanisms.
4. Re-educative level of psychotherapy
    a. The client explores alternatives in a planned, systematic way; this requires a longer period of therapy than supportive therapy.
    b. The client agrees upon and specifies desired changes of behavior and learning new ways of perceiving and behaving.
    c. Techniques may include short-term psychotherapy, reality therapy, cognitive restructuring, behavior modification, and development of coping skills.
5. Reconstructive level of psychotherapy
    a. Emotional and cognitive restructuring of self takes place.
    b. Positive outcomes include a greater understanding of self and others, more emotional freedom, and the development of potential abilities.

C. Behavior therapy
1. A treatment approach that uses the principles of Skinnerian (operant conditioning) or Pavlovian (classical conditioning) behavior theory to bring about behavioral change; the belief is that most behaviors are learned.
2. *Operant conditioning* refers to the manipulation of selected reinforcers to elicit and strengthen desired behavioral responses; the *reinforcer* refers to the consequence of the behavior, which is defined as anything that increases the occurrence of a behavior (Fig. 64-2).
3. In classical conditioning (respondent conditioning), the individual responds to a stimulus but is basically a passive agent (see Fig. 64-2).
4. Desensitization is a form of behavior therapy whereby exposure to increasing increments of a feared stimulus is paired with increasing levels of relaxation, which helps reduce the intensity of fear to a more tolerable level.

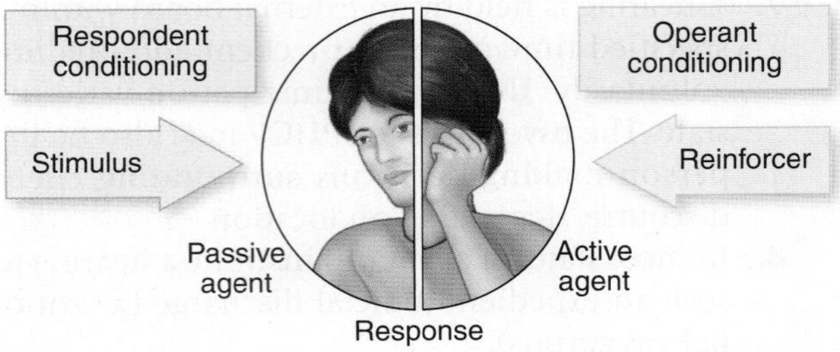

FIG. 64-2 Respondent versus operant conditioning.

5. Aversion therapy is a form of behavior therapy whereby negative reinforcement is used to change behavior; for example, a stimulus attractive to the client is paired with an unpleasant event in hopes of endowing the stimulus with negative properties, thereby dissuading the behavior.
6. Modeling is behavioral therapy whereby the therapist acts as a role model for specific identified behaviors so that the client learns through imitation.

D. Cognitive therapy
1. An active, directive, time-limited, structured approach used to treat various mental health problems, including anxiety and depressive problems
2. It is based on the principle that how individuals feel and behave is determined by how they think about the world and their place in it; their cognitions are based on the attitudes or assumptions developed from previous experiences.
3. Therapeutic techniques are designed to identify, reality-test, and correct distorted conceptualizations and the dysfunctional beliefs underlying these cognitions.
4. The therapist helps the individual change the way she or he thinks, thereby reducing symptoms.

E. Group development and group therapy
1. Involves a leader such as a therapist, nurse, or other designated health care team member and, ideally, 5 to 8 members working on their individual goals within the context of a group, which presumably increases the opportunity for feedback and support
2. Initial development of the group
    a. Involves superficial rather than open and trusting communication
    b. Members become acquainted with each other and search for similarities among themselves.
    c. Members may be unclear about the purpose or goals of the group.
    d. Group norms, roles, and responsibilities are established.
    e. The work of termination begins and is expanded upon throughout the duration of the group.

3. Working in the group
   a. The real work of the group is accomplished.
   b. Members are familiar with one another, the group leader, and the group roles and feel free to address and attempt to solve their problems.
   c. Both conflict and cooperation surface during the group's work as the members learn to work with one another.
4. Termination of the group
   a. Begins with the initial meeting
   b. Members' feelings are explored regarding their accomplishments and the impending termination of the group.
   c. The termination stage provides an opportunity for members to learn to deal more realistically and comfortably with this normal part of human experience.
5. Self-help or support groups (Box 64-3)

⚠ Support groups are based on the premise that individuals who have experienced and are insightful concerning a problem are able to help others who have a similar problem.

F. Family therapy
1. Family therapy is a specific intervention mode based on the premise that the member with the presenting symptoms signals the presence of problems in the entire family; this premise also assumes that a change in 1 member will bring about changes in other members.
2. The therapist works to assist family members to identify and express their thoughts and feelings; define family roles and rules; try new, more productive styles of relating; and restore strength to the family.

BOX 64-3 Self-Help and Support Groups

- Adult Children of Alcoholics
- Al-Anon
- Alcoholics Anonymous
- Bereavement groups
- Cancer support groups
- Co-Dependents Anonymous
- Gamblers Anonymous
- Groups to help deal with caring for family members
- Groups to help deal with unexpected body image changes, such as mastectomy or colostomy
- Mental health support groups
- Narcotics Anonymous
- Overeaters Anonymous
- Parents without Partners
- Recovery groups, such as for those who have experienced trauma
- Smoking cessation groups

PRACTICE QUESTIONS

787. A client with a diagnosis of depression who has attempted suicide says to the nurse, "I should have died. I've always been a failure. Nothing ever goes right for me." Which response by the nurse demonstrates therapeutic communication?
1. "You have everything to live for."
2. "Why do you see yourself as a failure?"
3. "Feeling like this is all part of being depressed."
4. "You've been feeling like a failure for a while?"

788. The nurse visits a client at home. The client states, "I haven't slept at all the last couple of nights." Which response by the nurse demonstrates therapeutic communication?
1. "I see."
2. "Really?"
3. "You're having difficulty sleeping?"
4. "Sometimes I have trouble sleeping too."

789. A client experiencing disturbed thought processes believes that his food is being poisoned. Which communication technique should the nurse use to encourage the client to eat?
1. Using open-ended questions and silence
2. Sharing personal preference regarding food choices
3. Documenting reasons why the client does not want to eat
4. Offering opinions about the necessity of adequate nutrition

790. The nurse should plan which goals of the termination stage of group development? **Select all that apply.**
- ❑ 1. The group evaluates the experience.
- ❑ 2. The real work of the group is accomplished.
- ❑ 3. Group interaction involves superficial conversation.
- ❑ 4. Group members become acquainted with one another.
- ❑ 5. Some structuring of group norms, roles, and responsibilities takes place.
- ❑ 6. The group explores members' feelings about the group and the impending separation.

791. A client diagnosed with terminal cancer says to the nurse, "I'm going to die, and I wish my family would stop hoping for a cure! I get so angry when they carry on like this. After all, I'm the one who's dying." Which response by the nurse is therapeutic?
1. "Have you shared your feelings with your family?"
2. "I think we should talk more about your anger with your family."
3. "You're feeling angry that your family continues to hope for you to be cured?"
4. "You are probably very depressed, which is understandable with such a diagnosis."

792. On review of the client's record, the nurse notes that the admission was voluntary. Based on this information, the nurse plans care anticipating which client behavior?

1. Fearfulness regarding treatment measures
2. Anger and aggressiveness directed toward others
3. An understanding of the pathology and symptoms of the diagnosis
4. A willingness to participate in the planning of the care and treatment plan

793. A client admitted voluntarily for treatment of an anxiety problem demands to be released from the hospital. Which action should the nurse take **initially**?

1. Contact the client's health care provider (HCP).
2. Call the client's family to arrange for transportation.
3. Attempt to persuade the client to stay "for only a few more days."
4. Tell the client that leaving would likely result in an involuntary commitment.

794. When reviewing the admission assessment, the nurse notes that a client was admitted to the mental health unit involuntarily. Based on this type of admission, the nurse should provide which intervention for this client?

1. Monitor closely for harm to self or others.
2. Assist in completing an application for admission.
3. Supply the client with written information about her or his mental health problem.
4. Provide an opportunity for the family to discuss why they felt the admission was needed.

795. When a client is admitted to an inpatient mental health unit with the diagnosis of anorexia nervosa, a cognitive behavioral approach is used as part of the treatment plan. The nurse plans care based on which purpose of this approach?

1. Providing a supportive environment
2. Examining intrapsychic conflicts and past issues
3. Emphasizing social interaction with clients who withdraw
4. Helping the client to examine dysfunctional thoughts and beliefs

796. A client is preparing to attend a Gamblers Anonymous meeting for the first time. The nurse should tell the client that which is the first step in this 12-step program?

1. Admitting to having a problem
2. Substituting other activities for gambling
3. Stating that the gambling will be stopped
4. Discontinuing relationships with people who gamble

797. The nurse employed in a mental health clinic is greeted by a neighbor in a local grocery store. The neighbor says to the nurse, "How is Carol doing? She is my best friend and is seen at your clinic every week." Which is the **most appropriate** nursing response?

1. "I cannot discuss any client situation with you."
2. "If you want to know about Carol, you need to ask her yourself."
3. "Only because you're worried about a friend, I'll tell you that she is improving."
4. "Being her friend, you know she is having a difficult time and deserves her privacy."

798. The nurse calls security and has physical restraints applied to a client who was admitted voluntarily when the client becomes verbally abusive, demanding to be discharged from the hospital. Which represents the possible legal ramifications for the nurse associated with these interventions? **Select all that apply.**

- ☐ 1. Libel
- ☐ 2. Battery
- ☐ 3. Assault
- ☐ 4. Slander
- ☐ 5. False imprisonment

799. The nurse in the mental health unit plans to use which therapeutic communication techniques when communicating with a client? **Select all that apply.**

- ☐ 1. Restating
- ☐ 2. Active listening
- ☐ 3. Asking the client "Why?"
- ☐ 4. Maintaining neutral responses
- ☐ 5. Providing acknowledgment and feedback
- ☐ 6. Giving advice and approval or disapproval

800. What is the **most appropriate** nursing action to help manage a manic client who is monopolizing a group therapy session?

1. Ask the client to leave the group for this session only.
2. Refer the client to another group that includes other manic clients.
3. Tell the client to stop monopolizing in a firm but compassionate manner.
4. Thank the client for the input, but inform the client that others now need a chance to contribute.

801. A client is participating in a therapy group and focuses on viewing all team members as equally important in helping the clients meet their goals. The nurse is implementing which therapeutic approach?

1. Milieu therapy
2. Interpersonal therapy
3. Behavior modification
4. Support group therapy

802. The nurse is working with a client who, despite making a heroic effort, was unable to rescue a neighbor trapped in a house fire. Which client-focused action should the nurse engage in during the working phase of the nurse–client relationship?

1. Exploring the client's ability to function
2. Exploring the client's potential for self-harm
3. Inquiring about the client's perception or appraisal of why the rescue was unsuccessful
4. Inquiring about and examining the client's feelings for any that may block adaptive coping

ANSWERS

787. *Answer:* 4

Rationale: Responding to the feelings expressed by a client is an effective therapeutic communication technique. The correct option is an example of the use of restating. The remaining options block communication because they minimize the client's experience and do not facilitate exploration of the client's expressed feelings. In addition, use of the word *why* is nontherapeutic because clients frequently interpret *why* questions as accusations. *Why* questions can cause resentment, insecurity and mistrust.

Test-Taking Strategy: Use therapeutic communication techniques to direct you to the option that directly addresses the client's feelings and concerns. Also, the correct option is the only one stated in the form of a question that is open-ended, which will encourage the verbalization of feelings.

Level of Cognitive Ability: Applying

Client Needs: Psychosocial Integrity

Integrated Process: Communication and Documentation

Content Area: Mental Health

Health Problem: Mental Health: Therapeutic Communication

Priority Concepts: Communication; Mood and Affect

Reference: Varcarolis (2017), pp. 97-98.

788. *Answer:* 3

Rationale: The correct option uses the therapeutic communication technique of restatement. Although restatement is a technique that has a prompting component to it, it repeats the client's major theme, which assists the nurse to obtain a more specific perception of the problem from the client. The remaining options are not therapeutic responses because none of them encourages the client to expand on the problem. Offering personal experiences moves the focus away from the client and onto the nurse.

Test-Taking Strategy: Use therapeutic communication techniques. "I see" is a general lead but does not provide the client with the opportunity to continue the discussion. "Really?" is a response that may make the client feel that she or he is not believed. Providing personal experiences focuses on the nurse's problem and thus minimizes the client's concerns. The correct option will provide information about the perception of the problem from the client's perspective.

Level of Cognitive Ability: Applying

Client Needs: Psychosocial Integrity

Integrated Process: Communication and Documentation

Content Area: Mental Health

Health Problem: Mental Health: Therapeutic Communication

Priority Concepts: Communication; Sleep

Reference: Varcarolis (2017), pp. 96-97.

789. *Answer:* 1

Rationale: Open-ended questions and silence are strategies used to encourage clients to discuss their problems. Sharing personal food preferences is not a client-centered intervention. The remaining options are not helpful to the client because they do not encourage the client to express feelings. The nurse should not offer opinions and should encourage the client to identify the reasons for the behavior.

Test-Taking Strategy: Use therapeutic communication techniques. First eliminate options that do not support the client's expression of feelings. Any option that is not client-centered should be eliminated next. Focusing on the client's feelings will direct you to the correct option.

Level of Cognitive Ability: Applying

Client Needs: Psychosocial Integrity

Integrated Process: Communication and Documentation

Content Area: Mental Health

Health Problem: Mental Health: Therapeutic Communication

Priority Concepts: Communication; Psychosis

Reference: Varcarolis (2017), pp. 92, 95.

790. *Answer:* 1, 6

Rationale: The stages of group development include the initial stage, the working stage, and the termination stage. During the initial stage, the group members become acquainted with one another, and some structuring of group norms, roles, and responsibilities takes place. During the initial stage, group interaction involves superficial conversation. During the working stage, the real work of the group is accomplished. During the termination stage, the group evaluates the experience and explores members' feelings about the group and the impending separation.

Test-Taking Strategy: Focus on the subject, the termination stage. Reading each item presented and recalling the stages of group development and the definition of termination will assist you in answering this question.

Level of Cognitive Ability: Applying

Client Needs: Psychosocial Integrity

Integrated Process: Nursing Process—Planning

Content Area: Mental Health

Health Problem: N/A

Priority Concepts: Collaboration; Communication

Reference: Varcarolis (2017), pp. 111-113.

791. *Answer:* 3

Rationale: Restating is a therapeutic communication technique in which the nurse repeats what the client says to show understanding and to review what was said. Although it is appropriate for the nurse to attempt to assess the client's ability to discuss feelings openly with family members, it does not help the client discuss the feelings causing the anger. The nurse's direct attempt to expect the client to talk more about the anger is premature. The nurse would never make a judgment regarding the reason for the client's feeling; this is nontherapeutic in the one-to-one relationship.

Test-Taking Strategy: Use therapeutic communication techniques. The correct option is the only one that identifies the

use of a therapeutic technique (restatement) and focuses on the client's feelings.
Level of Cognitive Ability: Applying
Client Needs: Psychosocial Integrity
Integrated Process: Communication and Documentation
Content Area: Mental Health
Health Problem: Mental Health: Therapeutic Communication
Priority Concepts: Communication; Family Dynamics
Reference: Varcarolis (2017), p. 96.

792. *Answer:* 4
Rationale: In general, clients seek voluntary admission. If a client seeks voluntary admission, the most likely expectation is that the client will participate in the treatment program since she or he is actively seeking help. The remaining options are not characteristics of this type of admission. Fearfulness, anger, and aggressiveness are more characteristic of an involuntary admission. Voluntary admission does not guarantee that a client understands her or his mental health problem, only the client's desire for help.
Test-Taking Strategy: Focus on the subject, voluntary admission. This should direct you to the correct option. Note the relationship between the word *voluntary* and the correct option.
Level of Cognitive Ability: Applying
Client Needs: Psychosocial Integrity
Integrated Process: Nursing Process—Planning
Content Area: Mental Health
Health Problem: Mental Health: Crisis
Priority Concepts: Adherence; Caregiving
Reference: Varcarolis (2017), p. 63.

793. *Answer:* 1
Rationale: In general, clients seek voluntary admission. Voluntary clients have the right to demand and obtain release, unless they pose an immediate danger to themselves or others, in which case the admission could become involuntary depending on the circumstances and regulations in that area and facility. The nurse needs to be familiar with the state and facility policies and procedures. The initial nursing action is to contact the PHCP, who has the authority to discuss discharge with the client. While arranging for safe transportation is appropriate, it is premature in this situation and should be done only with the client's permission. While it is appropriate to discuss why the client feels the need to leave and the possible outcomes of leaving against medical advice, attempting to get the client to agree to staying "for only a few more days" has little value and will not likely be successful. Many states require that the client submit a written release notice to the facility psychiatrist, who reevaluates the client's condition for possible conversion to involuntary status if necessary, according to criteria established by law. While this is a possibility, it should not be used as a threat with the client.
Test-Taking Strategy: Note the strategic word, *initially.* Noting the type of hospital admission will assist in directing you to the correct option while eliminating those that are unlikely to occur. Calling the family should be eliminated, based on the issues of client rights and confidentiality. To "persuade" a client to stay in the hospital is inappropriate. Threatening the client is inappropriate and illegal.
Level of Cognitive Ability: Applying
Client Needs: Psychosocial Integrity
Integrated Process: Nursing Process—Implementation
Content Area: Leadership/Management: Ethical/Legal
Health Problem: Mental Health: Crisis
Priority Concepts: Clinical Judgment; Health Care Law
Reference: Varcarolis (2017), pp. 63-64.

794. *Answer:* 1
Rationale: Involuntary admission is necessary when a person is a danger to self or others or is in need of psychiatric treatment regardless of the client's willingness to consent to the hospitalization. A written request is a component of a voluntary admission. Providing written information regarding the mental health problem, is likely premature initially. The family may have had no role to play in the client's admission.
Test-Taking Strategy: Focus on the subject, involuntary admission. Use Maslow's Hierarchy of Needs theory. Safety is the priority if a physiological need does not exist. This should direct you to the correct option. Also, note that the remaining options are not always true of an involuntary admission.
Level of Cognitive Ability: Applying
Client Needs: Psychosocial Integrity
Integrated Process: Nursing Process—Implementation
Content Area: Mental Health
Health Problem: Mental Health: Crisis
Priority Concepts: Interpersonal Violence; Safety
Reference: Varcarolis (2017), p. 63.

795. *Answer:* 4
Rationale: Cognitive behavioral therapy is used to help the client identify and examine dysfunctional thoughts and to identify and examine values and beliefs that maintain these thoughts. The remaining options, while therapeutic in certain situations, are not the focus of cognitive behavioral therapy.
Test-Taking Strategy: Focus on the subject, the purpose of a cognitive behavioral approach. Note the relationship of the word *cognitive* in the question and *thoughts* in the correct option.
Level of Cognitive Ability: Applying
Client Needs: Psychosocial Integrity
Integrated Process: Nursing Process—Planning
Content Area: Mental Health
Health Problem: Mental Health: Eating Disorders
Priority Concepts: Caregiving; Cognition
Reference: Varcarolis (2017), pp. 24, 318.

796. *Answer:* 1
Rationale: The first step in the 12-step program is to admit that a problem exists. Substituting other activities for gambling may be a strategy, but it is not the first step. The remaining options are not realistic strategies for the initial step in a 12-step program.
Test-Taking Strategy: Focus on the subject, the first step in the 12-step program. This will assist in directing you to the correct option.
Level of Cognitive Ability: Applying
Client Needs: Psychosocial Integrity
Integrated Process: Nursing Process—Implementation
Content Area: Mental Health
Health Problem: Mental Health: Addictions
Priority Concepts: Addiction; Caregiving
Reference: Varcarolis (2017), pp. 318-319.

797. *Answer:* 1
Rationale: The nurse is required to maintain confidentiality regarding the client and the client's care. Confidentiality is basic to the therapeutic relationship and is a client's right. The most appropriate response to the neighbor is the statement of that responsibility in a direct, but polite manner. A blunt statement that does not acknowledge why the nurse cannot reveal client information may be taken as disrespectful and uncaring. The remaining options identify statements that do not maintain client confidentiality.
Test-Taking Strategy: Note the strategic words, *most appropriate*. Focusing on maintaining confidentiality will direct you to the correct option. This focus will also assist you in eliminating options that inappropriately give such information without being unnecessarily blunt or rude.
Level of Cognitive Ability: Applying
Client Needs: Safe and Effective Care Environment
Integrated Process: Communication and Documentation
Content Area: Leadership/Management: Ethical/Legal
Health Problem: Mental Health: Therapeutic Communication
Priority Concepts: Ethics; Health Care Law
Reference: Potter et al. (2017), p. 306.

798. *Answer:* 2, 3, 5
Rationale: False imprisonment is an act with the intent to confine a person to a specific area. The nurse can be charged with false imprisonment if the nurse prohibits a client from leaving the hospital if the client has been admitted voluntarily and if no agency or legal policies exist for detaining the client. Assault and battery are related to the act of restraining the client in a situation that did not meet criteria for such an intervention. Libel and slander are not applicable here since the nurse did not write or verbally make untrue statements about the client.
Test-Taking Strategy: Focus on the subject, legal ramifications of nursing actions related to hospital admission. Noting the words *admitted voluntarily* will assist you in selecting the options related to inappropriately preventing the client from leaving the hospital, a right to which a voluntarily committed client is entitled. The remaining options do not relate to acts that prevent the client from leaving the hospital.
Level of Cognitive Ability: Analyzing
Client Needs: Safe and Effective Care Environment
Integrated Process: Nursing Process—Implementation
Content Area: Leadership/Management: Ethical/Legal
Health Problem: N/A
Priority Concepts: Health Care Law; Safety
Reference: Varcarolis (2017), pp. 68-69.

799. *Answer:* 1, 2, 4, 5
Rationale: Therapeutic communication techniques include listening, maintaining silence, maintaining neutral responses, using broad openings and open-ended questions, focusing and refocusing, restating, clarifying and validating, sharing perceptions, reflecting, providing acknowledgment and feedback, giving information, presenting reality, encouraging formulation of a plan of action, providing nonverbal encouragement, and summarizing. Asking "Why" is often interpreted as being accusatory by the client and should also be avoided. Providing advice or giving approval or disapproval are barriers to communication.
Test-Taking Strategy: Use therapeutic communication techniques. This will assist you in both selecting the correct answers and eliminating the examples of nontherapeutic communication.
Level of Cognitive Ability: Applying
Client Needs: Psychosocial Integrity
Integrated Process: Communication and Documentation
Content Area: Mental Health
Health Problem: Mental Health: Therapeutic Communication
Priority Concepts: Caregiving; Communication
Reference: Varcarolis (2017), pp. 95, 98.

800. *Answer:* 4
Rationale: If a client is monopolizing the group, the nurse must be direct and decisive. The best action is to thank the client and suggest that the client stop talking and try listening to others. Although telling the client to stop monopolizing in a firm but compassionate manner may be a direct response, the correct option is more specific and provides direction for the client. The remaining options are inappropriate because they are not directed toward helping the client in a therapeutic manner.
Test-Taking Strategy: Note the strategic words, *most appropriate*. Use therapeutic communication techniques to assist in directing you to the correct option. Note that the correct option is specific and provides direction for the client.
Level of Cognitive Ability: Applying
Client Needs: Psychosocial Integrity
Integrated Process: Nursing Process—Implementation
Content Area: Mental Health
Health Problem: Mental Health: Therapeutic Communication
Priority Concepts: Communication; Mood and Affect
Reference: Varcarolis (2017), pp. 30, 97-98.

801. *Answer:* 1
Rationale: All treatment team members are viewed as significant and valuable to the client's successful treatment outcomes in milieu therapy. Interpersonal therapy is based on a one-to-one or group therapy approach in which the therapist–client relationship is often used as a way for the client to examine other relationships in her or his life. Behavior modification is based on rewards and punishment. Support groups are based on the premise that individuals who have experienced and are insightful concerning a problem are able to help others who have a similar problem.
Test-Taking Strategy: Focus on the subject, characteristics of a type of therapy. Note the relationship between the words *helping the clients to meet their goals* and the correct option.
Level of Cognitive Ability: Applying
Client Needs: Psychosocial Integrity
Integrated Process: Nursing Process—Implementation
Content Area: Mental Health
Health Problem: N/A
Priority Concepts: Care Coordination; Caregiving
Reference: Varcarolis (2017), p. 86.

802. *Answer:* 4
Rationale: The client must first deal with feelings and negative responses before the client can work through the meaning of the crisis. The correct option pertains directly to the client's feelings and is client-focused. The remaining options do not directly focus on or address the client's feelings.

Test-Taking Strategy: Focus on the **subject**, the working phase of the nurse–client relationship. Also, note the words *client-focused action.* Think about the interventions that occur in this phase. Select the option that focuses on the feelings of the client.
Level of Cognitive Ability: Applying
Client Needs: Psychosocial Integrity
Integrated Process: Nursing Process: Implementation
Content Area: Mental Health
Health Problem: Mental Health: Crisis
Priority Concepts: Communication; Coping
Reference: Varcarolis (2017), pp. 109-110.

CHAPTER 65

Mental Health Problems

PRIORITY CONCEPTS Mood and Affect; Safety

I. Anxiety

A. Description
- **1.** A normal response to stress
- **2.** A subjective experience that includes feelings of apprehension, uneasiness, uncertainty, or dread
- **3.** Occurs as a result of a threat that may be misperceived or misinterpreted or a threat to identity or self-esteem
- **4.** Anxiety may result when values are threatened, or preceding new experiences.

B. Types of anxiety
- **1.** Normal: A healthy type of anxiety
- **2.** Acute: Precipitated by imminent loss or change that threatens one's sense of security
- **3.** Chronic: Anxiety that persists as a characteristic response to daily activities

C. Levels of anxiety
- **1.** Mild
  - **a.** Mild anxiety is associated with tense experiences that occur in everyday life.
  - **b.** Increased ability to grasp information
  - **c.** Sense of sight and sound are increased.
  - **d.** Perceptual field is increased.
  - **e.** Can be motivating, produce growth, enhance creativity, and increase learning
  - **f.** Physical symptoms may include restlessness, irritability, or mild tension.
- **2.** Moderate
  - **a.** The focus is on immediate concerns.
  - **b.** Narrowed perceptual field
  - **c.** Sense of sight and sound diminish as selective inattentiveness occurs.
  - **d.** Learning and problem solving still occur.
  - **e.** Physical symptoms include increased heart rate, perspiration, gastric discomfort, headache, urinary urgency, and/or mild tremors.
- **3.** Severe
  - **a.** Severe anxiety is a feeling that something bad is about to happen.
  - **b.** A significant narrowing in the perceptual field occurs.
  - **c.** Focus is on minute or scattered details.
  - **d.** All behavior is aimed at relieving the anxiety.
  - **e.** Learning and problem solving are not possible.
  - **f.** Actions are aimed at reducing or alleviating anxiety.
  - **g.** Physical symptoms are caused by stimulation of the sympathetic nervous system (e.g., headache, nausea, dizziness, sleep disturbances), increased tremors, pounding heart rate, and hyperventilation.
  - **h.** The individual needs direction to focus.
- **4.** Panic
  - **a.** Associated with dread and terror and a sense of impending doom
  - **b.** Disorganization, difficulty perceiving reality, and inability to concentrate
  - **c.** Loss of rational thoughts with distorted perception occurs.
  - **d.** The individual is unable to communicate or function effectively.
  - **e.** If prolonged, panic can lead to exhaustion and death.
  - **f.** Increased motor activity (pacing, shouting, screaming) or withdrawal
  - **g.** Impulsive and erratic behavior

D. Interventions: General nursing measures (see Priority Nursing Actions)
- **1.** Recognize the anxiety.
- **2.** Establish trust.
- **3.** Protect the client.
- **4.** Modify the environment by setting limits or limiting interaction with others.
- **5.** Do not criticize **coping mechanisms**.
- **6.** Provide creative outlets.
- **7.** Monitor for signs of impending destructive behavior.
- **8.** Promote relaxation techniques, such as breathing exercises or guided imagery.
- **9.** Monitor vital signs, and administer antianxiety medications as prescribed.
- **10.** Do not force the client into situations that provoke anxiety.

PRIORITY NURSING ACTIONS

Anxiety in a Client

1. Provide a calm environment, decrease environmental stimuli, and stay with the client.
2. Ask the client to identify what and how she or he feels.
3. Encourage the client to describe and discuss her or his feelings.
4. Help the client identify the causes of the feelings if she or he is having difficulty doing so.
5. Listen to the client for expressions of helplessness and hopelessness.
6. Document the event, significant information, actions taken and follow-up actions, and the client's response.

Reference: Varcarolis (2017), p. 134.

The immediate nursing action for a client with anxiety is to decrease stimuli in the environment and provide a calm and quiet environment.

E. Interventions: Mild to moderate levels
- **1.** Help the client identify the source of their anxiety.
- **2.** Encourage the client to talk about feelings and concerns.
- **3.** Help the client identify thoughts and feelings that occurred before the onset of anxiety.
- **4.** Encourage problem solving.
- **5.** Encourage gross motor exercise.

F. Interventions: Severe to panic levels
- **1.** Reduce the anxiety quickly.
- **2.** Use a calm manner.
- **3.** Always remain with the client.
- **4.** Minimize environmental stimuli.
- **5.** Provide clear, simple statements.
- **6.** Use a low-pitched voice.
- **7.** Attend to the physical needs of the client.
- **8.** Provide gross motor activity.
- **9.** Administer antianxiety medications as prescribed.
- **10.** Ensure safety.

II. Generalized Anxiety Disorder

A. Description (Box 65-1)
- **1.** Generalized anxiety disorder is an unrealistic anxiety about everyday worries that persists more days than not, over at least 6 months, and is not associated with another mental health or medical problem.
- **2.** Physical symptoms occur.

B. Assessment
- **1.** Restlessness and inability to relax
- **2.** Episodes of trembling and shakiness
- **3.** Chronic muscular tension
- **4.** Dizziness
- **5.** Inability to concentrate
- **6.** Chronic fatigue and sleep problems
- **7.** Inability to recognize the connection between the anxiety and physical symptoms
- **8.** Client is focused on the physical discomfort.

BOX 65-1 Criteria for General Anxiety Disorder

- Excessive anxiety and worry about several events or activities for more than 6 months
- Inability to cope with anxiety
- Anxiety associated with three (or more) of the following symptoms for more than 6 months:
  1. Feeling restless or on edge
  2. Easily tired
  3. Poor attention span
  4. Irritability
  5. Muscle tension
  6. Difficulty sleeping (insomnia, difficulty falling or staying asleep)
- Anxiety causes significant distress or impaired ability to work or maintain relationships
- No concurrent substance use or misuse
- No underlying medical cause
- Not explained by another mental health problem

From American Psychiatric Association: *Diagnostic and statistical annual of disorders*, ed 5, Washington, DC, 2013.

C. Unexpected and expected panic attacks
- **1.** Description
  - **a.** Most extreme level of anxiety resulting in disturbed behavior
  - **b.** Produces a sudden onset of feelings of intense apprehension and dread
  - **c.** Cause usually cannot be identified.
  - **d.** Severe, recurrent, intermittent anxiety attacks lasting 5 to 30 minutes occur.
- **2.** Assessment
  - **a.** Choking sensation
  - **b.** Labored breathing
  - **c.** Pounding heart
  - **d.** Chest pain
  - **e.** Dizziness
  - **f.** Nausea
  - **g.** Blurred vision
  - **h.** Numbness or tingling of the extremities
  - **i.** Sense of unreality and helplessness
  - **j.** Fear of being trapped
  - **k.** Fear of dying
- **3.** Interventions
  - **a.** Remain with the client.
  - **b.** Attend to physical symptoms.
  - **c.** Assist the client to identify the thoughts that aroused the anxiety and identify the basis for these thoughts.
  - **d.** Assist the client to change the unrealistic thoughts to more realistic thoughts.
  - **e.** Use cognitive restructuring to replace distorted thinking.
  - **f.** Administer antianxiety medications if prescribed.

III. Post-traumatic Stress Disorder

A. Description: After experiencing a psychologically traumatic event, the individual is prone to re-experience the event and have recurrent and intrusive dreams or flashbacks.

B. Diagnosis: Symptoms last at least 1 month and can occur months to years after the traumatizing events.

C. Stressors
1. Natural disaster
2. Terrorist attack
3. Combat experiences
4. Accidents
5. Rape
6. Crime or violence
7. Sexual, physical, and emotional abuse
8. Re-experiencing the event as flashbacks

D. Assessment
1. Avoidance or numbness
2. Irritability or outbursts of anger
3. Detachment
4. Depression that may involve suicidal thoughts
5. Anxiety
6. Sleep disturbances and nightmares
7. Flashbacks of event
8. Hypervigilance and exaggerated startle response
9. Guilt about surviving the event
10. Poor concentration and avoidance of activities that trigger the memory of the event

E. Interventions (Box 65-2)

BOX 65-2 Interventions for Post-traumatic Stress Disorder

- Be nonjudgmental and supportive.
- Assure the client that her or his feelings and behaviors are normal reactions.
- Assist the client to recognize the association between her or his feelings and behaviors and the trauma experience.
- Encourage the client to express her or his feelings; provide individual therapy that addresses loss of control or anger issues.
- Monitor for suicidal risk
- Teach stress management techniques.
- Assist the client to develop adaptive coping mechanisms and to use relaxation techniques.
- Encourage use of support groups.
- Facilitate a progressive review of the trauma experience (called *flooding*).
- Encourage the client to establish and re-establish relationships.
- Include the family in treatment.
- Inform the client that hypnotherapy or systematic desensitization may be recommended as a form of treatment.

Clients dealing with cancer may develop post-traumatic stress (PTS). Cancer-related PTS can occur anytime during or after treatment. The symptoms of PTS are similar to those of post-traumatic stress disorder but are generally not as severe.

IV. Specific Phobia

A. Description
1. Irrational fear of an object, activity, or situation that persists and that leads to avoidance.
2. Associated with panic-level anxiety or fear if the object, situation, or activity cannot be avoided
3. Defense mechanisms commonly used include repression and displacement.

B. Types (Box 65-3)

C. Interventions
1. Identify the basis of the anxiety.
2. Allow the client to verbalize feelings about the anxiety-producing object or situation; talking frequently about the feared object is the first step in the desensitization process.
3. Teach relaxation techniques, such as breathing exercises, muscle relaxation exercises, and visualization of pleasant situations.
4. Promote desensitization by gradually introducing the individual to the feared object or situation in small doses.

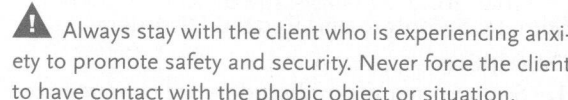

Always stay with the client who is experiencing anxiety to promote safety and security. Never force the client to have contact with the phobic object or situation.

V. Obsessive-Compulsive and Related Disorders

A. Obsessions: Preoccupation with persistently intrusive thoughts, impulses, or images and ideas

B. Compulsions: The performance of rituals or repetitive behaviors an individual is driven to perform to prevent some event, divert unacceptable thoughts, and decrease anxiety.

BOX 65-3 Some Types of Phobias

Acrophobia: Fear of heights
Agoraphobia: Fear of open spaces
Astraphobia: Fear of electrical storms
Claustrophobia: Fear of closed spaces
Hematophobia: Fear of blood
Hydrophobia: Fear of water
Monophobia: Fear of being alone
Mysophobia: Fear of dirt or germs
Nyctophobia: Fear of darkness
Pyrophobia: Fear of fires
Social Phobia: Fear of situations in which one might be embarrassed or criticized; fear of making a fool of oneself
Xenophobia: Fear of strangers
Zoophobia: Fear of animals

1. Obsessions and compulsions often occur together and can disrupt normal daily activities.
2. Anxiety occurs when one resists obsessions or compulsions and from being powerless to resist the thoughts or rituals.
3. Obsessive thoughts can involve issues of violence, aggression, sexual behavior, orderliness, or religion and uncontrollably can interrupt conscious thoughts and the ability to function.

C. Compulsive behavior patterns (behaviors or rituals)
1. Compulsive behavior patterns decrease the anxiety.
2. The patterns are associated with the obsessive thoughts.
3. The patterns neutralize the thought.
4. During stressful times, the ritualistic behavior increases.
5. Defense mechanisms include repression, displacement, and undoing.

D. Related disorders
1. Hoarding disorder
2. Excoriation (skin-picking) disorder
3. Substance- or medication-induced obsessive-compulsive and related disorder
4. Obsessive-compulsive and related disorder due to another medical condition
5. Trichotillomania (hair-pulling disorder)

E. Interventions (Box 65-4)

VI. Somatic Symptom and Related Disorders

A. Description
1. Somatic symptom disorders are characterized by a combination of persistent worry or complaints and an associated maladaptive response regarding physical illness without supportive physical findings and medical diagnosis.

BOX 65-4 Interventions for Obsessive-Compulsive and Related Disorders

- Ensure that basic needs (food, rest, hygiene) are met.
- Identify situations that precipitate compulsive behavior; encourage the client to verbalize concerns and feelings.
- Be empathetic toward the client and aware of her or his need to perform the compulsive behavior.
- Do not interrupt compulsive behaviors unless they jeopardize the safety of the client or others (provide for client safety related to the behavior).
- Allow time for the client to perform the compulsive behavior, but set limits on behaviors that may interfere with the client's physical well-being to protect the client from physical harm.
- Implement a schedule for the client that distracts from the behaviors (structure simple activities, games, or tasks for the client).
- Establish a written contract that assists the client to decrease the frequency of compulsive behaviors gradually.
- Recognize and reinforce positive nonritualistic behaviors.

2. The client focuses on the physical signs and symptoms and is unable to control the signs and symptoms.
3. The physical signs and symptoms increase with psychosocial stressors and result in a high level of functional impairment.
4. The anxiety is redirected into a somatic concern.
5. The client may unconsciously somatize for secondary gains, such as increased attention and decreased responsibilities.

B. Conversion disorder (functional neurological symptom disorder)
1. Description
   a. The sudden onset of a neurological symptom or a deficit in the absence of a neurological cause or diagnosis.
   b. Conversion disorder is an expression of a psychological conflict or need.
   c. The most common conversion symptoms are blindness, deafness, numbness, paralysis, gait disturbance, and the inability to talk.
   d. Conversion disorder has no organic cause.
   e. Symptoms are beyond the conscious control of the client and are directly related to conflict.
   f. The development of physical symptoms reduces anxiety.
2. Assessment
   a. Rule out a physiological cause for symptoms or deficits.
   b. "*La belle indifference*": Unconcerned with symptoms
   c. Physical limitation or disability
   d. Feelings of guilt, anxiety, or frustration
   e. Low self-esteem and feelings of inadequacy
   f. Unexpressed anger or conflict
   g. Secondary gain
   h. History of physical or sexual abuse

C. Interventions
1. Obtain a nursing history and assess for physical problems.
2. Explore the needs being met by the physical symptoms with the client.
3. Assist the client to identify alternative ways of meeting needs.
4. Assist the client to relate feelings and conflicts to the physical symptoms.
5. Convey understanding that the physical symptoms are real to the client.
6. Assure the client that physical illness has been ruled out.
7. Report and assess any new physical complaint.
8. Use a pain assessment scale if the client complains of pain, and implement pain reduction measures as required.
9. Explore the source of anxiety and stimulate verbalization of anxiety.

10. Assist the client in recognizing her or his own feelings and emotions.
11. Encourage the use of relaxation techniques as the anxiety increases.
12. Encourage diversional activities.
13. Provide positive feedback.
14. Administer antianxiety medications if prescribed.

For a client with a somatic symptom disorder, allow a specific time period for the client to discuss physical complaints, because the client will feel less threatened if this behavior is limited rather than stopped completely. Avoid responding with positive reinforcement about the physical complaints.

VII. Dissociative Disorder

A. Description
1. Dissociative disorder is a disruption in integrative functions of memory, consciousness, or identity.
2. It is associated with exposure to an extremely traumatic event.

B. Dissociative identity disorder (DID), formerly called *multiple personality disorder*
1. Description
a. Two or more fully developed, distinct, and unique personalities exist within the client and recurrently control behavior.
b. The host is the primary personality, and the other personalities are referred to as *alters*.
c. Alter personalities may take full control of the client, 1 at a time, and may or may not be aware of one another.
d. The alters may be aware of the host, but the host is not usually aware of the alters.
2. Assessment
a. The client may have an inability to recall important information (unrelated to ordinary forgetfulness).
b. Transition from 1 personality to the other is related to stress or a traumatic event and is sudden.
c. Dissociation is used as a method of distancing and defending one's self from anxiety and traumatizing experiences.

C. Dissociative amnesia
1. Description
a. Inability to recall important personal information often due to trauma or because it provokes anxiety
b. Memory impairment may range from partial to almost complete.
c. The client may assume a new identity in a new environment, drift from place to place, develop few relationships, and then return home unable to remember the amnesia.
2. Assessment
a. Localized: The client blocks out all memories about a specified period.
b. Selective: The client recalls some but not all memories about a specified period.
c. Generalized: The client has a loss of all memory about past life.

D. Depersonalization/derealization disorder
1. Description: An altered self-perception in which one's own reality is temporarily lost or changed
2. Assessment
a. Feelings of detachment
b. Intact reality testing

E. Interventions
1. Orient the client.
2. Develop a trusting relationship with the client.
3. Encourage verbal expression of painful experiences, anxieties, and concerns.
4. Explore methods of coping.
5. Identify sources of conflict.
6. Focus on the client's strengths and skills.
7. Provide nondemanding, simple routines.
8. Allow the client to progress at her or his own pace.
9. Implement stress reduction techniques.
10. Plan for individual, group, or family psychotherapy to integrate dissociated aspects of personality or memory and to expand self-awareness.

VIII. Mood Disorders

A. Bipolar and related disorders
1. Description (Box 65-5)
a. Bipolar disorder is characterized by extreme changes in mood, energy, and the ability to function.
b. The classifications of bipolar include Bipolar I disorder, Bipolar II disorder, cyclothymic disorder, and mixed features.
c. Bipolar I disorder: Most severe form characterized by severe mood episodes from mania to depression.
d. Bipolar II disorder: A milder form of mood elevation; there are milder episodes of hypomania that alternate with periods of severe depression.
e. Cyclothymic disorder: brief periods of hypomanic symptoms occur alternating with brief periods of depressive symptoms that are not as extensive or as long-lasting as seen in full hypomanic episodes or full depressive episodes.
f. Mixed features: the occurrence of simultaneous symptoms of opposite mood polarities during manic, hypomanic or depressive episodes. It's features are high energy, sleeplessness, and racing thoughts. At the same time, the individual may feel hopeless, despairing, irritable, and suicidal.

BOX 65-5 Assessment of Bipolar and Related Disorders

Mania
- Becomes angry quickly
- Delusional self-confidence
- Constantly pushing limits, manipulating, and finding fault
- Euphoric with intense feelings of well-being
- Demonstrates little or no inhibition
- Distracted by environmental stimuli
- Extroverted personality
- Flight of ideas
- Grandiose and persecutory delusions
- High and unstable affect
- Significant decrease in appetite
- Inability to eat or sleep because of involvement in more important things
- Unlimited energy
- Inappropriate affect
- Dress that is inappropriately bizarre, loud, and/or colorful
- Makeup is colorful and overdone
- Excessive spending
- Pressured and/or clanging speech
- Restlessness
- Sexually promiscuous
- Urgent motor activity

Depression
- Increased or decreased appetite
- Decrease in activities of daily living
- Decreased emotion and physical activity
- Easily fatigued
- Inability to make decisions
- Poor concentration
- Internalizing hostility
- Introverted personality
- Social isolation and withdrawn from groups
- Lack of energy
- Lack of initiative
- Lack of self-confidence and low self-esteem
- Lack of sexual interest
- Psychomotor retardation
- Suicidal thinking

g. The medication of choice has traditionally been lithium carbonate, which can be toxic and requires regular monitoring of serum lithium levels to help keep the medication's therapeutic index level appropriate; a stable intake of adequate dietary sodium and fluid (2 to 3 L daily) must be maintained to avoid toxicity.

h. Other medications may be prescribed both to reduce the symptoms of acute bipolar manic episodes and for maintenance therapy.

i. Antianxiety agents may be prescribed to assist in managing the psychomotor agitation characteristic of mania; these medications should be avoided in clients with a history of substance abuse.

j. Atypical antipsychotic medications may be prescribed for both their sedative and mood-stabilizing effects.

2. Assessment
- **a.** Assess and monitor whether the client is a danger to self or others.
- **b.** Assess for alcohol or substance use/misuse.
- **c.** Mood
- **d.** Behavior
- **e.** Speech (flight of ideas, tangential)
- **f.** Cognitive functioning
- **g.** Inflated self-regard (delusions of grandeur)
- **h.** Sleeping pattern
- **i.** Impulse control

3. Interventions for mania (Box 65-6)
- **a.** Remove hazardous objects from the environment (this should be done for all clients).
- **b.** Assess the client closely for fatigue.
- **c.** Provide frequent rest periods and monitor the client's sleep patterns; use comfort measures to promote sleep.
- **d.** Provide a private room if possible.
- **e.** Encourage the client to ventilate feelings.
- **f.** Use calm, slow interactions.
- **g.** Help the client focus on 1 topic during the conversation.
- **h.** Ignore or distract the client from grandiose thinking; present reality to the client.
- **i.** Do not argue with the client.
- **j.** Limit group activities and assess the client's tolerance level; solitary activities may be necessary.
- **k.** Provide high-calorie finger foods and fluids.
- **l.** Reduce environmental stimuli.
- **m.** Set limits on inappropriate behaviors.
- **n.** Provide physical activities and outlets for tension.
- **o.** Avoid competitive games.
- **p.** Provide gross motor activities such as walking.
- **q.** Provide structured activities or one-to-one activities with the nurse.
- **r.** Provide simple and direct explanations for routine procedures.
- **s.** Supervise the administration of medication.

3. Depression: See Section IX.

IX. Depressive Disorders

A. Description
1. Depression affects feelings, thoughts, and behaviors.
2. It can occur after a loss, including loss of self-esteem, the end of a significant relationship, the death of a loved one, or a traumatic event.

BOX 65-6 Dealing with Inappropriate Behaviors Associated with Bipolar Disorder

Aggressive Behavior

- Assist the client in identifying feelings of frustration and aggression.
- Encourage the client to talk out instead of acting out feelings of frustration.
- Assist the client in identifying precipitating events or situations that lead to aggressive behavior.
- Describe the consequences of the behavior for self and others.
- Assist the client in identifying previous coping mechanisms.
- Assist the client in problem-solving techniques to cope with frustration or aggression.

De-escalation Techniques

- Maintain safety for the client, other clients, and self.
- Respect personal space and use a nonaggressive posture.
- Establish verbal contact.
- Use a calm approach and communicate with a calm, clear tone of voice (be assertive, not aggressive).
- Be concise.
- Determine what the client considers to be her or his wants and feelings.
- Listen closely to what the client is saying.
- Avoid verbal struggles: agree or agree to disagree.
- Provide the client with clear options that deal with the client's behavior.
- Offer choices and optimism.
- Assist the client with problem solving and decision making regarding options.
- Debrief the client and staff.

Manipulative Behavior

- Set clear, consistent, realistic, and enforceable limits, and communicate expected behaviors.
- Be clear about consequences associated with exceeding set limits and follow through with consequences in a nonpunitive manner, if necessary.
- Discuss the client's behavior in a nonjudgmental and nonthreatening manner.
- Avoid power struggles with the client (avoid arguing with the client).
- Assist the client in developing means of setting limits on own behavior.

3. The loss is followed by grief and mourning; if this process does not resolve, depression results.
4. Depression may be mild, moderate, or severe.
5. Treatment includes counseling, antidepressant medication, and electroconvulsive therapy (ECT).
6. See Box 65-5 for general assessment findings.

B. Mild depression
1. Mild depression is triggered by an external event and follows the normal grief reaction.
2. Mild depression lasts less than 2 weeks.
3. Feeling sad
4. Feeling let down or disappointed
5. Mild alterations in sleep patterns
6. Feeling less alert
7. Irritability
8. Disinterested in spending time with others
9. Increased or decreased appetite
10. Increased use of substances such as alcohol or drugs

C. Moderate depression
1. Moderate depression persists over time.
2. The person experiences a sense of change and often seeks help.
3. Despondent and gloomy
4. Dejected
5. Low self-esteem
6. Helplessness and powerlessness
7. May experience intense anxiety and anger
8. Diurnal variation: The person may feel better at a certain time of the day.
9. Slow thought processes and difficulty in concentrating
10. Rumination: Persistent thinking about and discussion of a particular subject
11. Negative thinking and suicidal thoughts (see Chapter 67)
12. Sleep disturbances, early-morning awakening, or oversleeping
13. Social withdrawal
14. Anorexia, weight loss or gain, and fatigue
15. Somatic complaints
16. Moving or talking more slowly
17. Increased use of substances such as alcohol or drugs

D. Major depressive disorder
1. Depressed mood or loss of pleasure in activities for at least 2 weeks
2. Impaired social, occupational, and/or educational functioning
3. Mood change from person's baseline
4. Daily, experiences at least 5 of the of the following symptoms:
   a. Irritability or depressed mood most of the day, nearly every day (subjective report or observation of others)
   b. Decreased interest or pleasure in most activities
   c. Significant weight change (5%) or change in appetite
   d. Change in activity level
   e. Fatigue or loss of energy
   f. Guilt/worthlessness
   g. Diminished ability to think or concentrate, or more indecisive
   h. Thoughts of death or suicide

E. Interventions (Box 65-7)

⚠ For a client at risk for self-harm, ask the client directly, "Have you thought of hurting yourself?"

BOX 65-7 Interventions for Depressed Clients

Risk for Harm
- Assess for homicidal and suicidal ideation.
- Provide safety from suicidal actions (be certain that there are no harmful objects in the environment).
- Do not leave the client alone for extended periods.
- If the client has a suicidal plan, place on one-to-one supervision.
- Form a "no-suicide contract" with the client as appropriate.

Activities
- Use gentle encouragement to participate in activities of daily living and unit therapies.
- Do not push decision making or the making of complex choices or decisions that the client is not ready for.
- Provide achievable activities in which the client can achieve success (focus on strengths).
- Begin the client with one-to-one activities.
- Provide activities for easy mastery to increase self-esteem and help in alleviating guilt feelings and activities that do not require a great deal of concentration (simple card games, drawing).
- Engage the client in gross motor activities (walking).
- Eventually bring the client into small group activities and then into large groups.

Nutrition
- Monitor nutritional intake and weight and provide nutritional support.
- Stay with the client during meals to accurately assess intake and to assist in ensuring adequate nutritional intake.

Hygiene Care
- Monitor for general hygiene and self-care deficits; deficits may indicate worsening depression.
- Provide prompts to encourage activities of daily living.

Sleep Patterns
- Monitor sleep patterns.
- Decrease environmental stimuli at bedtime.
- Encourage relaxation techniques.
- Spend time with the client before bedtime to increase comfort and minimize feelings of loneliness and isolation.

Altered Thought Processes
- Remind the client of times when she or he felt better and was successful.
- Spend time with the client to convey the client's worth and value.
- Encourage the client to discuss losses or changes in the life situation.
- Encourage the client to express sadness or anger and allow adequate time for verbal responses.
- Respond to anger therapeutically.

X. Electroconvulsive Therapy (ECT)

A. Description
1. ECT is an effective treatment for depression (not a cure); a small amount of an electrical current is delivered through electrodes attached to the temples that cause a brief seizure within the brain; outward movement is usually a slight movement of the hands, feet, or a toe, because premedication is given to relax the muscles. In addition, a short-acting anesthetic is given.
2. The usual course is 6 to 12 treatments given every 2 to 5 days; maintenance ECT once a month may help decrease the relapse rate for a client with recurrent depression.
3. ECT is not always effective in clients with dysthymic depression, depression and personality disorders, drug dependence, or depression secondary to situational or social difficulties.
4. At-risk clients include clients with recent myocardial infarction, stroke (brain attack), or intracranial mass lesions.

B. Uses (Box 65-8)
1. Clients with severe depressive and bipolar depressive disorders, especially when psychotic symptoms are present, such as delusions of guilt, somatic delusions, and delusions of infidelity
2. Clients who have depression with marked psychomotor retardation and stupor
3. Manic clients whose conditions are resistant to lithium and antipsychotic medications and clients who are rapid cyclers (a client with a bipolar disorder who has many episodes of mood swings close together)
4. Clients with schizophrenia (especially catatonia), clients with schizoaffective syndromes, and psychotic clients

BOX 65-8 Electroconvulsive Therapy (ECT): Indications for Use

- When antidepressant medications have no effect
- When there is a need for a rapid definitive response, such as when a client is suicidal or homicidal
- When the client is in extreme agitation or stupor
- When the risks of other treatments outweigh the risk of ECT
- When the client has a history of poor medication response, a history of good ECT response, or both
- When the client prefers ECT as a treatment

C. Preprocedure
1. Explain the procedure to the client.
2. Encourage the client to discuss feelings, including myths regarding ECT.
3. Teach the client and family what to expect.
4. Informed consent must be obtained when voluntary clients are being treated.
5. For involuntary clients, when informed consent cannot be obtained, permission may be obtained from the next of kin, although in some states the permission for ECT must be obtained from the court.
6. Maintain NPO (nothing by mouth) status after midnight or at least 4 hours before treatment as prescribed.
7. Baseline vital signs are taken.
8. The client is requested to void.
9. Hairpins, contact lenses, and dentures are removed.
10. Administer preprocedure medication as prescribed.

D. During the procedure
1. As the intravenous line is inserted, electroencephalographic and electrocardiographic electrodes are attached.
2. The blood pressure, pulse, and oxygen saturation are monitored throughout the treatment.
3. A blood pressure cuff is placed around 1 ankle and inflated to block the medication from entering the foot. When the procedure begins, seizure activity can be monitored by watching for movement in that foot.
4. Medications administered may include a short-acting anesthetic and a muscle relaxant.
5. Oxygen is administered by face mask.
6. An airway or mouth guard is placed to prevent the client biting the tongue.
7. An electrical stimulus is administered; a brief seizure occurs.

E. Postprocedure
1. The client is transported to a recovery area with the blood pressure cuff and oximeter in place, where oxygen, suction, and other emergency equipment are available.
2. Client wakes about 15 minutes after procedure.
3. When the client is awake, talk to the client and take vital signs.
4. The client may be confused and disorientated for several hours; provide frequent orientation (brief, distinct, and simple) and reassurance.
5. The client returns to the nursing unit when at least a 90% oxygen saturation level is maintained, vital signs are stable, and mental status is satisfactory.
6. Assess for a gag reflex before giving the client fluids, food, or medication.

F. Potential side effects
1. Confusion, disorientation, and short-term memory loss
2. The client may be confused and disoriented on awakening.
3. Other side effects include headache, hypotension, muscle soreness, nausea, and tachycardia.
4. Memory deficits may occur, but memory usually recovers completely, although some clients have memory loss lasting 6 months.

⚠ Monitor both a depressed client and a client who has recently been prescribed an antidepressant medication closely for signs of suicidal ideation. If the client presents with increased energy, monitor closely, because it could mean that the client now has the energy to perform the suicide act.

XI. Schizophrenia

A. Description
1. Schizophrenia is a group of mental health problems characterized by psychotic features (hallucinations and delusions), disordered thought processes, and disrupted interpersonal relationships.
2. Disturbances in affect, mood, behavior, and thought processes occur.
3. Treatment with medication controls symptoms associated with the mental health problem.

B. Assessment (Fig. 65-1)
1. Physical characteristics
   a. Unkempt appearance; may neglect hygiene, eating, sleeping, and elimination
   b. Body image distortions
   c. May be preoccupied with somatic complaints
2. Motor activity (Box 65-9)
   a. Catatonic posturing: Holding bizarre postures for long periods
   b. Catatonic excitement: Moving excitedly, with no environmental stimuli present
   c. Possible total immobilization
   d. Inability to respond to commands or responding only to commands
   e. Waxy flexibility
   f. Repetitive or stereotyped movements
   g. Motor activity that may be increased, as evidenced by agitation, pacing, inability to sleep, loss of appetite and weight, and impulsiveness
   h. Possible inability to initiate activity (anergia)
3. Emotional characteristics
   a. Mistrust
   b. View of the world as threatening and unsafe
   c. Affect blunted, flat, or inappropriate
   d. May display feelings of ambivalence, helplessness, anxiety, anger, guilt, or depression in response to hallucinations or delusions or as a result of grief related to losses imposed by the illness

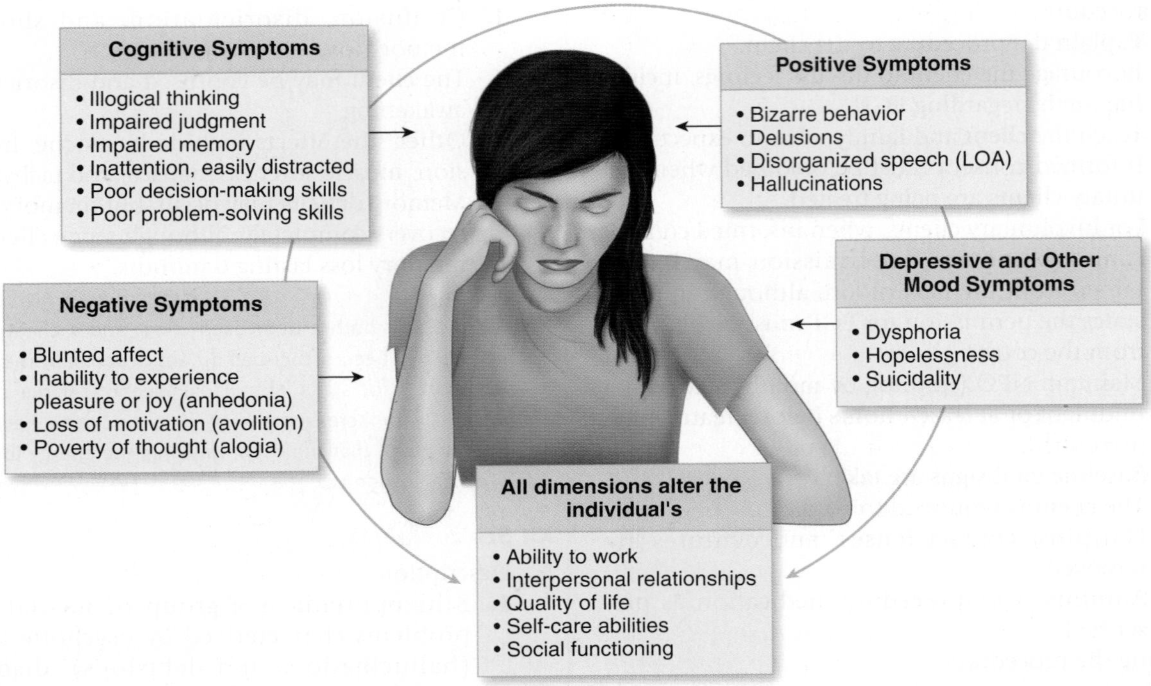

Cognitive Symptoms
• Illogical thinking
• Impaired judgment
• Impaired memory
• Inattention, easily distracted
• Poor decision-making skills
• Poor problem-solving skills
Positive Symptoms
• Bizarre behavior
• Delusions
• Disorganized speech (LOA)
• Hallucinations
Depressive and Other Mood Symptoms
• Dysphoria
• Hopelessness
• Suicidality
Negative Symptoms
• Blunted affect
• Inability to experience pleasure or joy (anhedonia)
• Loss of motivation (avolition)
• Poverty of thought (alogia)
All dimensions alter the individual's
• Ability to work
• Interpersonal relationships
• Quality of life
• Self-care abilities
• Social functioning

FIG. 65-1 Treatment-relevant dimensions of schizophrenia. *LOA*, Looseness of association.

BOX 65-9 Abnormal Motor Behaviors

Description

Abnormal motor behavior or activity displayed by a client with a mental health problem that occurs as a result of a mental health disorder

Types

Echolalia: Repeating the speech of another person

Echopraxia: Repeating the movements of another person

Waxy Flexibility: Having one's arms or legs placed in a certain position and holding that same position for hours

4. Compulsive rituals: Constant repetitive activity performed as an attempt to solve conflicting feelings
5. Overcompliance: Attempt to deny responsibility for any action by doing only what another person instructs exactly
6. Affective disturbances
   a. Flat or incongruent affect or inappropriate affect
   b. Altered thought processes
7. Abnormal thought processes (Box 65-10)
   a. Impaired reality testing
   b. Fragmentation of thoughts
   c. Thought blocking
   d. Loose associations
   e. Echolalia: Pathological repeating of another's words
   f. Distorted perception of the environment
   g. Neologisms: Made-up words that have meaning only to the client
   h. Magical thinking
   i. Inability to conceptualize meaning in words or thoughts

BOX 65-10 Abnormal Thought Processes

Description

Abnormal thought processes displayed by a client with a mental health problem that occur as a result of a mental health disorder

Types

Circumstantiality: Before getting to the point or answering a question, the client gets caught up in countless details and explanations.

Confabulation: Filling a memory gap with detailed fantasy believed by the teller; the purpose of confabulation is to maintain self-esteem; seen in organic conditions such as Korsakoff's psychosis

Flight of Ideas: Constant flow of speech in which the client jumps from 1 topic to another in rapid succession; a connection between topics exists, although it is sometimes difficult to identify; seen in manic states

Looseness of Association: Haphazard, illogical, and confused thinking and interrupted connections in thought; seen mostly in schizophrenic disorders

Neologisms: Client makes up words that have meaning only to the individual; often part of a delusional system

Thought Blocking: Sudden cessation of a thought in the middle of a sentence; client is unable to continue the train of thought; often, sudden new thoughts unrelated to the topic come up

Word Salad: Mixture of words and phrases that has no meaning

j. Inability to organize facts logically
k. Delusions associated with thought processes or content

8. Types of delusions (Box 65-11)
a. Loss of reference, in which the client believes that certain events, situations, or interactions are related directly to self
b. Delusions of persecution, in which the client believes that she or he is being harassed, threatened, or persecuted by some powerful force
c. Delusions of grandeur, in which the client attaches special significance to self in relation to others or the universe and has an exaggerated sense of self that has no basis in reality
d. Somatic delusions, in which the client believes that her or his body is changing or responding in an unusual way, which has no basis in reality

9. Perceptual distortions
a. Illusions, which may be brief experiences with a misinterpretation or misperception of reality
b. Hallucinations (5 senses) with no basis in reality (Box 65-12), such as perceiving objects, sensations, or images

10. Language and communication disturbances (Box 65-13)
a. Related to disorders in thought process
b. Inability to organize language
c. Difficulty communicating clearly
d. Inappropriate responses to a situation
e. A single word or phrase may represent the whole meaning of the conversation such that the client may feel that she or he has communicated adequately.
f. Development of a private language

BOX 65-11 Delusions

Description

A false belief held to be true, even when there is evidence to the contrary

Types

Grandeur: False belief that one is a powerful and important person
Jealousy: False belief that one's partner or mate is going out with other persons
Persecution: Thought that one is being singled out for harm by others

Interventions

- Ask the client to describe the delusion.
- Be open and honest in interactions to reduce suspiciousness.
- Focus conversation on reality-based topics, rather than on the delusion.
- Encourage the client to express feelings and focus on feelings that the delusions generate.
- If the client obsesses on the delusion, set firm limits on the amount of time spent talking about the delusion.
- Do not argue with the client or try to convince the client that the delusions are false.
- Validate if part of the delusion is real.

BOX 65-12 Hallucinations

Description

Sense perception (occurs with 1 of the 5 senses) for which no external stimuli exist; can have an organic or functional cause

Types

Auditory: Hearing voices when none are present
Gustatory: Experiencing taste in the absence of stimuli
Olfactory: Smelling smells that do not exist
Tactile: Feeling touch sensations in the absence of stimuli
Visual: Seeing things that are not there

Interventions

- Ask the client directly about the hallucination.
- Avoid reacting to the hallucination as if it were real.
- Decrease stimuli or move the client to another area.
- Do not negate the client's experience.
- Focus on reality-based topics.
- Attempt to engage the client's attention through a concrete activity.
- Respond verbally to anything real that the client talks about.
- Avoid touching the client.
- Monitor for signs of increasing anxiety or agitation, which may indicate that hallucinations are increasing.

BOX 65-13 Language and Communication Disturbances

Alogia (poverty of speech): Reduced volume or lack of spontaneous comments and overly brief responses.
Associative Looseness: Disjointed mental threads that tie thoughts logically together.
Clang Association: Repetition of words or phrases that are similar in sound but in no other way
Echolalia: Repetition of words or phrases heard from another person
Mutism: Absence of verbal speech
Neologism: A newly devised word that has special meaning only to the client
Pressured Speech: Speaking as if the words are being forced out quickly
Religiosity: Excessive preoccupation with religious ideas.
Tangentiality: Digression from one topic to another without ever completing the thought or reaching a conclusion.
Verbigeration: Purposeless repetition of words or phrases
Word Salad (Schizophasia): Form of speech in which words or phrases are connected meaninglessly

C. Interventions: Schizophrenia (Box 65-14)

D. Interventions: Active hallucinations
1. Monitor for hallucination cues and assess content of hallucinations.
2. Intervene with one-on-one contact.
3. Decrease stimuli or move the client to another area.
4. Avoid conveying to the client that others also are experiencing the hallucination.
5. Respond verbally to anything real that the client talks about.
6. Avoid touching the client.
7. Encourage the client to express feelings.
8. During a hallucination, attempt to engage the client's attention through a concrete activity.
9. Accept and do not joke about or judge the client's behavior.
10. Provide easy activities and a structured environment with routine activities of daily living.
11. Monitor for signs of increasing fear, anxiety, or agitation.
12. Decrease stimuli as needed.
13. Administer medications as prescribed.

For a client with hallucinations, safety is the first priority; ensure that the client does not have an auditory command telling him or her to harm self or others.

BOX 65-14 Interventions for Schizophrenia

- Maintain a safe environment.
- Set limits on the client's behavior if the client is unable to do so, especially when it interferes with others and becomes disruptive.
- Assess the client's physical needs.
- Initiate one-on-one interaction and progress to small groups as tolerated.
- Monitor for altered thought processes.
- Maintain ego boundaries and avoid touching the client.
- Avoid an overly warm approach; a neutral approach is less threatening.
- Do not make promises to the client that cannot be kept.
- Establish daily routines.
- Assist the client to improve grooming and accept responsibility for personal care.
- Provide brief, frequent contact with the client; limit time of interaction with the client.
- Tell the client when you are leaving.
- Tell the client when you do not understand what she or he is saying.
- Do not "go along" with the client's delusions or hallucinations.
- Provide simple, concrete activities, such as puzzles or word games.
- Reorient the client as necessary.
- Help the client establish what is real and unreal.
- Stay with the client if she or he is frightened.
- Speak to the client in a simple, direct, and concise manner.
- Reassure the client that the environment is safe.
- Remove the client from group situations if the client's behavior is too bizarre, disturbing, or dangerous to others.
- Set realistic goals.
- Initially, do not offer choices to the client; then gradually assist the client in making her or his own decisions.
- Decrease excessive stimuli in the environment.
- Monitor for suicide risk.
- Assist the client to use alternative means to express feelings, such as through music, art therapy, or writing.

E. Interventions: Delusions
1. Interact based on reality.
2. Encourage the client to express feelings.
3. Do not dispute the client or try to convince the client that delusions are false.
4. Initiate activities on a one-on-one basis.
5. Alter hospital routines as necessary, such as by using canned or packaged food or food from home.
6. Recognize accomplishments and provide positive feedback for successes.

XII. Personality Disorders

A. Description
1. Personality disorders involve the consistent expression of various inflexible maladaptive behavior patterns or traits that may impair functioning and relationships.
2. The client usually remains in touch with reality and typically has a significant lack of insight in self-identity and interpersonal behavior (empathy or intimacy).
3. Stress exacerbates manifestations of the personality disorder.
4. Not directly associated with the effects of substance misuse or a general medical condition, such as severe head injury.

B. Characteristics
1. Poor impulse control
   a. Acting out to manage internal pain
   b. Forms of acting out include physical and verbal attacks, such as yelling and swearing, and self-injurious behaviors, such as cutting own skin, banging the head, punching self, manipulation, substance abuse, promiscuous sexual behaviors, and **suicide attempts**.
   c. The client may be preoccupied with such things as self, religion, or sex.
2. Mood characteristics
   a. May experience abandonment and depression
   b. Moods may include rage, guilt, fear, and emptiness.
3. Impaired judgment
   a. Difficulty with problem solving
   b. Inability to perceive the consequences of behavior

4. Impaired reality testing: Distortion of reality and often projection of own feelings onto others
5. Impaired object relations: Rigid and inflexible, with difficulty in intimate relationships
6. Impaired self-perception: Distorted self-perception and experience of self-hate or self-idealization
7. Impaired thought processes
   a. Concrete or diffuse thinking
   b. Difficulty concentrating
   c. Impaired memory
8. Impaired stimulus barrier
   a. Inability to regulate incoming sensory stimuli
   b. Increased excitability
   c. Excessive response to noise and light
   d. Poor attention span
   e. Agitation
   f. Insomnia

C. Cluster A personality disorder types include the odd disorders—schizoid, schizotypal, and paranoid.
1. Schizoid personality disorder is characterized by an inability to form warm, close social relationships.
   a. Social detachment and lack of close relationships
   b. Interest in solitary activities
   c. Aloofness and indifference
   d. Restricted expression of emotions
   e. Lack of interest in others
2. Schizotypal personality disorder is characterized by the display of abnormal or highly unusual thoughts, perceptions, speech, and behavior patterns.
   a. Suspiciousness and paranoia
   b. Unable to understand how behaviors impact others
   c. Eccentricity
   d. Magical thinking
   e. Odd thinking and speech
   f. Relationship deficits
   g. Blunted affect
   h. Reclusiveness
3. Paranoid personality disorder is characterized by suspiciousness and mistrust of others (paranoia) (Box 65-15).
   a. May be suspicious and distrusting
   b. May be argumentative
   c. May be hostile or aloof
   d. May be rigid, critical, and controlling of others
   e. May have thoughts of grandiosity

⚠ Do not whisper or laugh in front of a client with a paranoid personality disorder, because the client will think that you are talking about or laughing at him or her; this increases the paranoia.

D. Cluster B personality disorders include the dramatic, emotional, erratic types—histrionic, narcissistic, antisocial, and borderline.

BOX 65-15 Interventions for Paranoia

- Provide a safe environment.
- Assure the client that she or he will be safe.
- Assess for suicide risk.
- Diminish suspicious behavior, such as whispering.
- Remain calm, nonthreatening, and nonjudgmental.
- Engage the client during brief but frequent interactions.
- Establish a trusting relationship.
- Maintain physical boundaries and avoid crowding the client.
- Promote increased self-esteem.
- Respond honestly to the client.
- Follow through on commitments made to the client.
- Acknowledge the client's feelings, but tell the client that you do not share her or his interpretation of an event.
- Provide a daily schedule of activities.
- Assist the client to identify diversionary activities.
- Gradually introduce the client to groups.
- Refocus conversation to reality-based topics.
- Use role playing to help the client identify thoughts and feelings.
- Provide positive reinforcement for successes.
- Do not argue with delusions.
- Do not whisper in the client's presence.
- Provide the client with the opportunity to complete small tasks.
- Monitor eating, drinking, sleeping, and elimination patterns.
- Monitor for agitation, and decrease stimuli as needed.

1. Histrionic personality disorder is characterized by overly dramatic and intensely expressive behavior.
   a. Lively and dramatic and enjoys being the center of attention
   b. Has poor and shallow interpersonal relationships
   c. May be sexually seductive or provocative
   d. Dramatizes her or his life and may appear theatrical
   e. Overly concerned with appearance
   f. Easily bored
2. Narcissistic personality disorder is characterized by an increased sense of self-importance and preoccupation with fantasies and unlimited success.
   a. Need for admiration and inflation of accomplishments
   b. Overestimation of abilities and underestimation of contributions of others
   c. Lack of empathy and sensitivity to needs of others
3. Antisocial personality disorder comprises a pattern of irresponsible and antisocial behavior, selfishness, an inability to maintain lasting relationships, poor sexual adjustment, a failure to accept social norms, and a tendency toward irritability and aggressiveness.

a. Perceives the world as hostile
b. Lack of empathy and feelings of remorse
c. Egocentrism and focused on personal gratification
d. Deceitful and manipulative
e. Irresponsible
f. Impulsive and engages in risk taking behaviors
g. Persistent or frequent feelings of anger
h. Refusal to conform to social rules and normative behavior

4. Borderline personality disorder is characterized by instability in interpersonal relationships, unstable mood and self-image, and impulsive and unpredictable behavior.
a. Poor self-regard or unstable self-image
b. Lack of self-direction
c. Unstable and intense personal relationships
d. Lack of empathy toward the needs and feelings of others
e. Extreme shifts in mood
f. Impulsive
g. Engages in risk-taking behaviors
h. Argumentative and hostile in response to perceived slights or insults
i. Depression
j. Manipulation
k. Intense feeling of anxiety in response to stress
l. Chronic feelings of emptiness and intense fear of being rejected
m. Splitting—sees others as all good or all bad; creates conflict between individuals by playing 1 person against another

E. Cluster C personality disorders include the anxious, fearful types of personality disorders—obsessive-compulsive personality, avoidant, and dependent.

1. Obsessive-compulsive personality disorder is characterized by difficulty expressing warm and tender emotions, perfectionism, stubbornness, the need to control others, and a devotion to work.
a. Perfectionist with unreasonably high expectations of self
b. Inflexible and preoccupied with details and rules
c. Sense of self derived primarily from work
d. Social and personal relationship viewed as secondary to work and productivity
e. Difficulty understanding the ideas, feelings, and behaviors of others
f. Engages in rituals

2. Avoidant personality disorder is characterized by social withdrawal and extreme sensitivity to potential rejection.
a. Feelings of inadequacy
b. Hypersensitive to reactions of others and poor reaction to criticism
c. Social isolation
d. Lack of support system

3. Dependent personality disorder is characterized by an intense lack of self-confidence, low self-esteem, and inability to function independently, such that the individual passively allows others to make decisions and assume responsibility for major areas in the person's life; the dependent client has great difficulty making decisions.

F. General interventions for a client with a personality disorder

1. Maintain safety against self-destructive behaviors.
2. Ensure health care team is consistent with information and response to the client's acting-out behaviors.
3. Allow the client to make choices and be as independent as possible.
4. Encourage the client to discuss feelings rather than act them out.
5. Encourage the client to keep a journal recording daily feelings.
6. Discuss expectations and responsibilities with the client.
7. Discuss the consequences that will follow certain behaviors.
8. Inform the client that harm to self, others, and property is unacceptable.
9. Develop a written safety or behavioral contract with the client.
10. Identify splitting behavior.
11. Assist the client to deal directly with anger.
12. Encourage the client to participate in group activities, and praise nonmanipulative behavior.
13. Set and maintain limits to decrease manipulative behavior.
14. Remove the client from group situations in which attention-seeking behaviors occur.
15. Provide realistic praise for positive behaviors in social situations.

XIII. Neurodevelopmental Disorders

A. Autism spectrum disorder: See Chapter 38.

B. Attention-deficit/hyperactivity disorder: See Chapter 38.

XIV. Neurocognitive Disorders

A. Dementia and Alzheimer's disease

1. Dementia
a. Dementia is a syndrome with progressive deterioration in intellectual functioning secondary to structural or functional changes.
b. Long-term and short-term memory loss occurs, with impairment in judgment, abstract thinking, problem-solving ability, and behavior.
c. Dementia results in a self-care deficit.

d. Dementia-like symptoms can be a result of physiological conditions, and such conditions must be ruled out initially.
e. The most common type of dementia is Alzheimer's disease.

2. Alzheimer's disease (Box 65-16)
   a. Alzheimer's disease is an irreversible form of senile dementia caused by nerve cell deterioration.
   b. Individuals with Alzheimer's disease experience cognitive deterioration and progressive loss of ability to carry out activities of daily living.
   c. The client experiences a steady decline in physical and mental functioning and usually requires long-term care in a specialized facility in the final stages of the illness.
   d. Stages and major characteristics of Alzheimer's disease: Stage 1 (mild): forgetfulness; stage 2 (moderate): confusion; stage 3 (moderate to severe): ambulatory dementia; and stage 4 (late): end stage.
3. Interventions
   a. Identify and reinforce retained skills.
   b. Provide continuity of care.
   c. Orient the client to the environment.
   d. Furnish the environment with familiar possessions.
   e. Acknowledge the client's feelings.
   f. Assist the client and family members to manage memory deficits and behavior changes.
   g. Encourage family members to express feelings about caregiving.
   h. Provide the caregiver with support and identify the resources and support groups available.
   i. Monitor the client's activities of daily living.
   j. Remind the client how to perform self-care activities.
   k. Help the client maintain independence.
   l. Provide the client with consistent routines.
   m. Provide the client with exercise, such as walking with an escort.
   n. Avoid activities that tax the memory.
   o. Allow the client plenty of time to complete a task.
   p. Use constant encouragement with the client with a simple step-by-step approach.

BOX 65-16 Alzheimer's Disease

Agnosia: Failure to recognize or identify familiar objects despite intact sensory function
Amnesia: Loss of memory caused by brain degeneration
Aphasia: Language disturbance in understanding and expressing spoken words
Apraxia: Inability to perform motor activities, despite intact motor function

   q. Provide the client with activities that distract and occupy time, such as listening to music, coloring, and watching television.
   r. Provide the client with mental stimulation with simple games or activities.
4. Wandering
   a. Provide the client with a safe environment free of clutter and hazardous items.
   b. Provide safe ambulation, including comfortably and well-fitting shoes, mobility aids.
   c. Provide close and frequent supervision.
   d. Close and secure doors.
   e. Use identification bracelets and electronic surveillance.
   f. Encourage rest periods in the afternoon, because wandering worsens at night.
   g. Provide regular supervised exercise or walking programs.
   h. Sundown syndrome (sundowning) is characterized by a pronounced increase in symptoms and problem behaviors in the evening.

Providing a safe environment is a priority in the care of a client with Alzheimer's disease.

5. Communication disorders
   a. Disorders include language disorder (expressive–receptive disorder), speech sound disorder (phonological disorder), childhood-onset fluency disorder (stuttering disorder), and social communication disorder (impaired social communication).
   b. Adapt to the communication level of the client.
   c. Pay attention to nonverbal cues.
   d. Use a firm volume and a low-pitched voice to communicate.
   e. Stand directly in front of the client and maintain eye contact.
   f. Give ample time for the client to respond.
   g. Use a calm and reassuring voice. Do not speak loudly unless the client is hearing-impaired.
   h. Use pantomime gestures if the client is unable to understand spoken words.
   i. Speak slowly and clearly, using short words and simple sentences.
   j. Ask only 1 question at a time and give 1 direction at a time.
   k. Repeat questions if necessary, but do not rephrase.
   l. Provide alternative means of communication.
   m. Minimize external noise or distractions when communicating.
6. Impaired judgment
   a. Remove throw rugs, toxic substances, and dangerous electrical appliances from the environment.
   b. Reduce hot water heater temperature.

7. Altered thought processes
   a. Call the client by name.
   b. Orient the client frequently.
   c. Use familiar objects in the room.
   d. Place a calendar and clock in a visible place.
   e. Maintain familiar routines.
   f. Allow the client to reminisce.
   g. Make tasks simple.
   h. Allow time for the client to complete a task.
   i. Provide positive reinforcement for positive behaviors.
8. Altered sleep patterns
   a. Allow the client to wander in a safe place until she or he becomes tired.
   b. Prevent shadows in the room by using indirect light.
   c. Avoid the use of hypnotics because they cause confusion and aggravate the sundown effect.
9. Agitation
   a. Assess the precipitant of the agitation.
   b. Reassure the client.
   c. Remove items that can be hazardous when the client is agitated.
   d. Approach the client slowly and calmly from the front, and speak, gesture, and move slowly.
   e. Remove the client to a less stressful environment; decrease excess stimuli.
   f. Use touch gently.
   g. Do not argue with or force the client to do something.

PRACTICE QUESTIONS

803. A client says to the nurse, "The federal guards were sent to kill me." Which is the **best** response by the nurse to the client's concern?
1. "I don't believe this is true."
2. "The guards are not out to kill you."
3. "Do you feel afraid that people are trying to hurt you?"
4. "What makes you think the guards were sent to hurt you?"

804. A client diagnosed with delirium becomes disoriented and confused at night. Which intervention should the nurse implement **initially**?
1. Move the client next to the nurses' station.
2. Use an indirect light source and turn off the television.
3. Keep the television and a soft light on during the night.
4. Play soft music during the night, and maintain a well-lit room.

805. A client is admitted to the mental health unit with a diagnosis of depression. The nurse should develop a plan of care for the client that includes which intervention?
1. Encouraging quiet reading and writing for the first few days
2. Identification of physical activities that will provide exercise
3. No socializing activities until the client asks to participate in milieu
4. A structured program of activities in which the client can participate

806. When planning the discharge of a client with chronic anxiety, which is the **most appropriate** maintenance goal?
1. Suppressing feelings of anxiety
2. Identifying anxiety-producing situations
3. Continuing contact with a crisis counselor
4. Eliminating all anxiety from daily situations

807. A client is unwilling to go to his church because his ex-girlfriend goes there and he feels that she will laugh at him if she sees him. Because of this hypersensitivity to a reaction from her, the client remains homebound. The home care nurse develops a plan of care that addresses which personality disorder?
1. Avoidant
2. Borderline
3. Schizotypal
4. Obsessive-compulsive

808. The nurse is conducting a group therapy session. During the session, a client diagnosed with mania consistently disrupts the group's interactions. Which intervention should the nurse **initially** implement?
1. Setting limits on the client's behavior
2. Asking the client to leave the group session
3. Asking another nurse to escort the client out of the group session
4. Telling the client that they will not be able to attend any future group sessions

809. A client is admitted to a medical nursing unit with a diagnosis of acute blindness after being involved in a hit-and-run accident. When diagnostic testing cannot identify any organic reason why this client cannot see, a mental health consult is prescribed. The nurse plans care based on which mental health condition?
1. Psychosis
2. Repression
3. Conversion disorder
4. Dissociative disorder

810. A manic client begins to make sexual advances toward visitors in the dayroom. When the nurse firmly states that this is inappropriate and will not be allowed, the client becomes verbally abusive and threatens physical violence to the nurse. Based on the analysis of this situation, which intervention should the nurse implement?
1. Place the client in seclusion for 30 minutes.
2. Tell the client that the behavior is inappropriate.
3. Escort the client to their room, with the assistance of other staff.
4. Tell the client that their telephone privileges are revoked for 24 hours.

811. Which nursing interventions are appropriate for a hospitalized client with mania who is exhibiting manipulative behavior? **Select all that apply.**

- ☐ 1. Communicate expected behaviors to the client.
- ☐ 2. Ensure that the client knows that they are not in charge of the nursing unit.
- ☐ 3. Assist the client in identifying ways of setting limits on personal behaviors.
- ☐ 4. Follow through about the consequences of behavior in a nonpunitive manner.
- ☐ 5. Enforce rules by informing the client that he/she will not be allowed to attend therapy groups.
- ☐ 6. Have the client state the consequences for behaving in ways that are viewed as unacceptable.

812. The nurse observes that a client is pacing, agitated, and presenting aggressive gestures. The client's speech pattern is rapid, and affect is belligerent. Based on these observations, which is the nurse's **immediate priority** of care?
1. Provide safety for the client and other clients on the unit.
2. Provide the clients on the unit with a sense of comfort and safety.
3. Assist the staff in caring for the client in a controlled environment.
4. Offer the client a less stimulating area in which to calm down and gain control.

813. The nurse is preparing a client with schizophrenia a history of command hallucinations for discharge by providing instructions on interventions for managing hallucinations and anxiety. Which statement in response to these instructions suggests to the nurse that the client has a **need for additional information**?
1. "My medications will help my anxious feelings."
2. "I'll go to support group and talk about what I am feeling."
3. "When I have command hallucinations, I'll call a friend for help."
4. "I need to get enough sleep and eat well to help prevent feeling anxious."

814. The nurse is caring for a client just admitted to the mental health unit and diagnosed with catatonic stupor. The client is lying on the bed in a fetal position. Which is the **most appropriate** nursing intervention?
1. Ask direct questions to encourage talking.
2. Leave the client alone so as to minimize external stimuli.
3. Sit beside the client in silence with simple open-ended questions.
4. Take the client into the dayroom with other clients to provide stimulation.

815. The nurse is caring for a client diagnosed with paranoid personality disorder who is experiencing disturbed thought processes. In formulating a nursing plan of care, which **best** intervention should the nurse include?
1. Increase socialization of the client with peers.
2. Avoid using a whisper voice in front of the client.
3. Begin to educate the client about social supports in the community.
4. Have the client sign a release of information to appropriate parties for assessment purposes.

816. The nurse is planning activities for a client diagnosed with bipolar disorder with aggressive social behavior. Which activity would be **most appropriate** for this client?
1. Chess
2. Writing
3. Board games
4. Group exercise

ANSWERS

803. *Answer:* 3

Rationale: It is most therapeutic for the nurse to empathize with the client's experience. The remaining options lack this connection with the client. Disagreeing with delusions may make the client more defensive, and the client may cling to the delusions even more. Encouraging discussion regarding the delusion is inappropriate.

Test-Taking Strategy: Note the strategic word, *best.* Use therapeutic communication techniques. Eliminate options that show disagreement with the client or encourage any discussion regarding the delusion.

Level of Cognitive Ability: Applying

Client Needs: Psychosocial Integrity

Integrated Process: Communication and Documentation

Content Area: Mental Health

Health Problem: Mental Health: Therapeutic Communication

Priority Concepts: Communication; Psychosis

Reference: Varcarolis (2017), pp. 257-258.

804. *Answer:* 2

Rationale: Provision of a consistent daily routine and a low-stimulating environment is important when a client is disoriented. Noise, including radio and television, may add to the confusion and disorientation. Moving the client next to the nurses' station may become necessary but is not the initial action.

Test-Taking Strategy: Note the strategic word, *initially.* Eliminate options that are inappropriate or premature actions and may increase stimulation and add to the confusion. This will direct you to the correct option.

Level of Cognitive Ability: Applying

Client Needs: Psychosocial Integrity

Integrated Process: Nursing Process—Implementation

Content Area: Mental Health

Health Problem: Mental Health: Neurocognitive Impairment

Priority Concepts: Cognition; Safety

Reference: Varcarolis (2017), pp. 275, 277.

805. *Answer:* 4

Rationale: A client with depression often is withdrawn while experiencing difficulty concentrating, loss of interest or pleasure, low energy, fatigue, and feelings of worthlessness and poor self-esteem. The plan of care needs to provide successful experiences in a stimulating yet structured environment. The remaining options are either too "restrictive" or offer little or no structure and stimulation.

Test-Taking Strategy: Focus on the subject, the plan for a client with depression. Recall that a depressed client requires a structured and stimulating program in a safe environment. The correct option is the only one that will provide a safe and effective environment.

Level of Cognitive Ability: Applying

Client Needs: Psychosocial Integrity

Integrated Process: Nursing Process—Planning

Content Area: Mental Health

Health Problem: Mental Health: Mood Disorders

Priority Concepts: Mood and Affect; Safety

Reference: Varcarolis (2017), pp. 207-208.

806. *Answer:* 2

Rationale: Recognizing situations that produce anxiety allows the client to prepare to cope with anxiety or avoid a specific stimulus. Counselors will not be available for all anxiety-producing situations, and this option does not encourage the development of internal strengths. Suppressing feelings will not resolve anxiety. Elimination of all anxiety from life is impossible.

Test-Taking Strategy: Focus on the strategic words, *most appropriate.* Eliminate any option that contains the closed-ended word "all" or suggests that feelings should be suppressed. Note that the correct option is more client-centered and helps prepare the client to deal with anxiety should it occur.

Level of Cognitive Ability: Applying

Client Needs: Safe and Effective Care Environment

Integrated Process: Nursing Process—Planning

Content Area: Mental Health

Health Problem: Mental Health: Anxiety Disorder

Priority Concepts: Anxiety; Health Promotion

Reference: Varcarolis (2017), p. 143.

807. *Answer:* 1

Rationale: The avoidant personality disorder is characterized by social withdrawal and extreme sensitivity to potential rejection. The person retreats to social isolation. Borderline personality disorder is characterized by unstable mood and self-image and impulsive and unpredictable behavior. Schizotypal personality disorder is characterized by the display of abnormal thoughts, perceptions, speech, and behaviors. Obsessive-compulsive personality disorder is characterized by perfectionism, the need to control others, and a devotion to work.

Test-Taking Strategy: Focus on the subject, a type of personality disorder. Focusing on the words *hypersensitivity to a reaction* will direct you to the correct option.

Level of Cognitive Ability: Applying

Client Needs: Psychosocial Integrity

Integrated Process: Nursing Process—Planning

Content Area: Mental Health

Health Problem: Mental Health: Personality Disorders

Priority Concepts: Anxiety; Caregiving

Reference: Varcarolis (2017), pp. 173-174.

808. *Answer:* 1

Rationale: Manic clients may be talkative and can dominate group meetings or therapy sessions by their excessive talking. If this occurs, the nurse initially would set limits on the client's behavior. Initially, asking the client to leave the session or asking another person to escort the client out of the session is inappropriate. This may agitate the client and escalate the client's behavior further. Barring the client from group sessions is also an inappropriate action because it violates the client's right to receive treatment and is a threatening action.

Test-Taking Strategy: Note the strategic word, *initially.* Eliminate options that are comparable or alike and relate to the client leaving the session. Next, eliminate the option that violates the client's right to receive treatment and is a threatening action. Remember that setting firm limits with the client initially is best.

Level of Cognitive Ability: Applying

Client Needs: Psychosocial Integrity

Integrated Process: Nursing Process—Implementation
Content Area: Mental Health
Health Problem: Mental Health: Mood Disorders
Priority Concepts: Caregiving; Psychosis
Reference: Varcarolis (2017), pp. 232-233.

809. *Answer:* 3
Rationale: A conversion disorder is the alteration or loss of a physical function that cannot be explained by any known pathophysiological mechanism. A conversion disorder is thought to be an expression of a psychological need or conflict. In this situation, the client witnessed an accident that was so psychologically painful that the client became blind. Psychosis is a state in which a person's mental capacity to recognize reality, communicate, and relate to others is impaired, interfering with the person's ability to deal with life's demands. Repression is a coping mechanism in which unacceptable feelings are kept out of awareness. A dissociative disorder is a disturbance or alteration in the normally integrative functions of identity, memory, or consciousness.
Test-Taking Strategy: Focus on the **subject**, the cause of acute blindness. The key to the correct option lies in the fact that the client presents no organic reason to account for the blindness—hence, a conversion disorder.
Level of Cognitive Ability: Applying
Client Needs: Psychosocial Integrity
Integrated Process: Nursing Process—Planning
Content Area: Mental Health
Health Problem: Mental Health: Somatization disorder
Priority Concepts: Caregiving; Psychosis
Reference: Varcarolis (2017), pp. 154-155.

810. *Answer:* 3
Rationale: The client is at risk for injury to self and others and should be escorted out of the dayroom. Seclusion is premature in this situation. Telling the client that the behavior is inappropriate has already been attempted by the nurse. Denying privileges may increase the agitation that already exists in this client.
Test-Taking Strategy: Eliminate option 2 because this intervention has already been attempted. Next, use **Maslow's Hierarchy of Needs theory** to answer the question. Remember that if a physiological need is not present, focus on safety. Look for the option that promotes safety of the client, other clients, and staff.
Level of Cognitive Ability: Applying
Client Needs: Safe and Effective Care Environment
Integrated Process: Nursing Process—Implementation
Content Area: Mental Health
Health Problem: Mental Health: Violence
Priority Concepts: Mood and Affect; Safety
Reference: Varcarolis (2017), pp. 378-379.

811. *Answer:* 1, 3, 4, 6
Rationale: Interventions for dealing with the client exhibiting manipulative behavior include setting clear, consistent, and enforceable limits on manipulative behaviors; being clear with the client regarding the consequences of exceeding the limits set; following through with the consequences in a nonpunitive manner; and assisting the client in identifying a means of setting limits on personal behaviors. Ensuring that the client knows that she or he is not in charge of the nursing unit is inappropriate; power struggles need to be avoided. Enforcing rules and informing the client that she or he will not be allowed to attend therapy groups is a violation of a client's rights.
Test-Taking Strategy: Focus on the **subject**, manipulative behavior. Recalling clients' rights and that power struggles need to be avoided will assist in selecting the correct interventions.
Level of Cognitive Ability: Analyzing
Client Needs: Psychosocial Integrity
Integrated Process: Nursing Process—Implementation
Content Area: Mental Health
Health Problem: Mental Health: Mood Disorders
Priority Concepts: Clinical Judgment; Mood and Affect
Reference: Varcarolis (2017), p. 233.

812. *Answer:* 1
Rationale: Safety of the client and other clients is the immediate priority. The correct option is the only one that addresses the safety needs of the client as well as those of the other clients.
Test-Taking Strategy: Note the **strategic words**, *immediate priority*, and use **Maslow's Hierarchy of Needs theory** to prioritize. Note the words *agitated, aggressive,* and *belligerent.* Safety is the priority focus if a physiological need does not exist. Also, the correct option is the **umbrella option** and addresses the safety of all.
Level of Cognitive Ability: Applying
Client Needs: Safe and Effective Care Environment
Integrated Process: Nursing Process—Implementation
Content Area: Mental Health
Health Problem: Mental Health: Violence
Priority Concepts: Mood and Affect; Safety
Reference: Varcarolis (2017), p. 379.

813. *Answer:* 3
Rationale: The risk for impulsive and aggressive behavior may increase if a client is receiving command hallucinations to harm self or others. If the client is experiencing a hallucination, the nurse or health care counselor, not a friend, should be contacted to discuss whether the client has intentions to hurt herself or himself or others. Talking about auditory hallucinations can interfere with subvocal muscular activity associated with a hallucination. The client statements in the remaining options will aid in wellness but are not specific interventions for hallucinations, if they occur.
Test-Taking Strategy: Note the **strategic words**, *need for additional information*. These words indicate a **negative event query** and the need to select the incorrect statement as the answer. Focus on the **subject**, managing hallucinations and anxiety. The correct option is a specific agreement to seek appropriate help. The remaining options are interventions that a client can carry out to aid wellness.
Level of Cognitive Ability: Evaluating
Client Needs: Psychosocial Integrity
Integrated Process: Nursing Process—Teaching and Learning
Content Area: Mental Health
Health Problem: Mental Health: Schizophrenia
Priority Concepts: Client Education; Safety
Reference: Varcarolis (2017), pp. 256-257.

814. *Answer:* 3

Rationale: Clients who are withdrawn may be immobile and mute and may require consistent, repeated approaches. Communication with withdrawn clients requires much patience from the nurse. Interventions include the establishment of interpersonal contact. The nurse facilitates communication with the client by sitting in silence, asking simple open-ended questions rather than direct questions, and pausing to provide opportunities for the client to respond. Although overstimulation is not appropriate, there is no therapeutic value in ignoring the client. The client's safety is not the responsibility of other clients.

Test-Taking Strategy: Note the strategic words, *most appropriate.* Eliminate options either that are nontherapeutic or could result in overstimulation. Also eliminate options that are not examples of therapeutic communication. The correct option provides for client supervision and communication as appropriate.

Level of Cognitive Ability: Applying
Client Needs: Psychosocial Integrity
Integrated Process: Nursing Process—Implementation
Content Area: Mental Health
Health Problem: Mental Health: Schizophrenia
Priority Concepts: Caregiving; Psychosis
Reference: Varcarolis (2017), p. 251.

815. *Answer:* 2

Rationale: Disturbed thought process related to paranoid personality disorder is the client's problem, and the plan of care must address this problem. The client is distrustful and suspicious of others. The members of the health care team need to establish a rapport and trust with the client. Laughing or whispering in front of the client would be counterproductive. The remaining options ask the client to trust on a multitude of levels. These options are actions that are too intrusive for a client with this disorder.

Test-Taking Strategy: Focus on the subject, interventions for paranoid personality disorder, and note the strategic word, *best.* Note that the client has paranoia; thinking about its definition will direct you to the correct option.

Level of Cognitive Ability: Applying
Client Needs: Psychosocial Integrity
Integrated Process: Nursing Process—Implementation
Content Area: Mental Health
Health Problem: Mental Health: Personality Disorders
Priority Concepts: Caregiving; Psychosis
Reference: Varcarolis (2017), pp. 252-253, 257.

816. *Answer:* 2

Rationale: Solitary activities that require a short attention span with mild physical exertion are the most appropriate activities for a client who is exhibiting aggressive behavior. Writing (journaling), walks with staff, and finger painting are activities that minimize stimuli and provide a constructive release for tension. The remaining options have a competitive element to them or are group activities and should be avoided because they can stimulate aggression and increase psychomotor activity.

Test-Taking Strategy: Note the strategic words, *most appropriate.* Eliminate options that include activities that the client cannot do alone and are competitive in nature. The correct option identifies a solitary activity.

Level of Cognitive Ability: Applying
Client Needs: Physiological Integrity
Integrated Process: Nursing Process—Planning
Content Area: Mental Health
Health Problem: Mental Health: Mood Disorders
Priority Concepts: Mood and Affect; Safety
Reference: Varcarolis (2017), p. 232.

CHAPTER 66

Addictions

PRIORITY CONCEPTS Addiction; Coping

I. Eating Disorders

A. Description: Eating disorders are characterized by unsure self-identification and grossly disturbed eating habits (Fig. 66-1).

B. Compulsive overeating
1. Compulsive overeating is binge-like overeating without purging.
2. Food consumption is out of the individual's control and occurs in a stereotyped fashion.
3. Repulsed by eating, that is, the eating relieves tension but does not produce pleasure
4. Aware that eating patterns are abnormal and feels depressed after eating
5. Eats secretly during a binge and consumes high-calorie and easily digestible food
6. Repeatedly tries to diet, but without success
7. Feels helpless and hopeless about weight
8. Responds to feelings of guilt, anger, depression, boredom, loneliness, inadequacy, or ambivalence by eating

C. Anorexia nervosa
1. Description
   a. Onset often is associated with a stressful life event.
   b. Intensely fears obesity
   c. Body image is distorted and a disturbed self-concept is common.
   d. Preoccupied with foods that prevent weight gain and has a phobia against foods that produce weight gain
   e. The eating disorder can be life-threatening.
   f. Death can occur from starvation, **suicide**, cardiomyopathies, or electrolyte imbalances.
2. Assessment
   a. Appetite loss and refusal to eat
   b. Appetite denial
   c. Feelings of lack of control
   d. Compulsive exercising
   e. Overachiever and perfectionist
   f. Physical alterations: Many occur and can include decreased temperature, pulse, and blood pressure; weight loss; gastrointestinal disturbances such as constipation; teeth and gum deterioration; esophageal varices from induced vomiting; electrolyte imbalances; dry, scaly skin; presence of lanugo on extremities; sleep disturbances; hormone deficiencies; amenorrhea for at least 3 consecutive menstrual periods; cyanosis and numbness of extremities; and bone degeneration.

D. Bulimia nervosa
1. Description
   a. Repeated episodes of excessive and uncontrollable consumption of large amounts of food (binges) followed by inappropriate compensatory actions such as self-induced vomiting, misuse of cathartics (e.g., laxatives), diuretics, and/or self-starvation
   b. Most clients remain within a normal weight range, but think that their lives are dominated by the eating-related conflict.
2. Assessment
   a. Preoccupied with body shape and weight
   b. Preoccupation with thoughts of food
   c. Extreme fear of gaining weight
   d. Consumption of high-calorie food in secret; guilt about secretive eating
   e. Binge-purge syndrome
   f. Attempts to lose weight through diets, vomiting, enemas, cathartics, and amphetamines or diuretics
   g. Assess nutritional status and the severity of any medical problems.
   h. Has a need to control, yet experiences feelings of powerlessness or loss of control
   i. Low self-esteem
   j. Poor interpersonal relationships
   k. Decreased interest, or absence of interest, in sex
   l. Mood swings
   m. Electrolyte imbalances
   n. Physical alterations: Similar to those that occur with anorexia nervosa

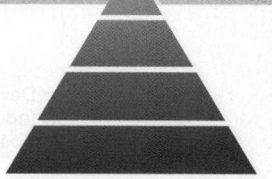

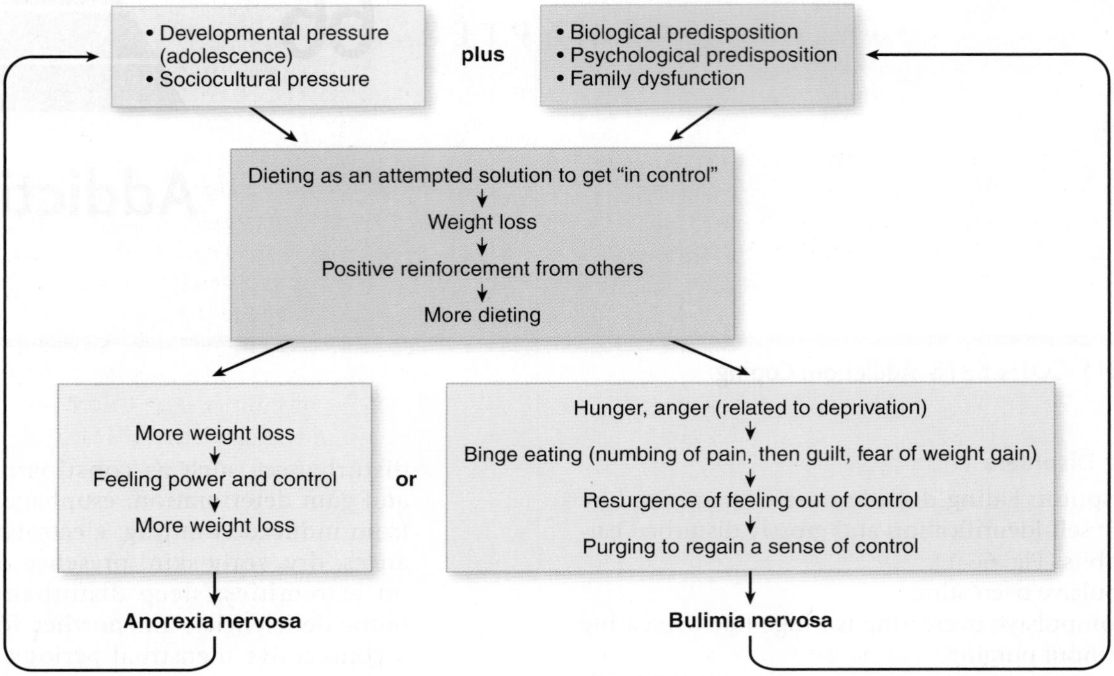

FIG. 66-1 Cycle of eating disorders.

o. Important questions to ask is about their perception of the problem and eating habits

E. Interventions: Clients with an eating disorder

1. Establish a one-to-one therapeutic relationship with the client; the nurse needs to establish trust and recognize any client reluctance to establish a relationship.

2. Establish a plan concerning the nutritional plan for the day.

3. Assist to identify precipitants to the eating disorder.

4. Encourage the client to express feelings about the eating behavior and how the client feels about her or his body.

5. Be accepting and nonjudgmental.

6. Work on exploring self-concept and establishing identity.

7. Implement behavior modification techniques.

8. Individual, group, and family therapy

9. If in a health care facility, supervise during mealtimes and for a specified period after meals and monitor intake and output; set a time limit for each meal and provide a pleasant, relaxed environment for eating.

10. Monitor for signs of physical complications related to the eating disorder.

11. When a client's weight is below 75% of ideal body weight, provide immediate medical stabilization as an inpatient.

12. Weigh daily at the same time, using the same scale, after the client voids (weighing each day may decrease anxiety in some clients); when weighing the client, ensure that the client is wearing the same clothing as when the previous weight was taken.

13. Monitor and restore fluid and electrolyte balance.

14. Monitor elimination patterns.

15. Assess and limit the client's activity level (anorexia nervosa and bulimia nervosa).

16. Encourage the client to participate in diversional activities.

17. Assess suicide potential.

18. Administer antidepressant medication if prescribed.

19. Encourage psychotherapy.

II. Substance Use Disorders

A. Description: Substance use disorders (addiction) cause behavioral and physiological changes (Box 66-1).

BOX 66-1 CAGE Screening Questionnaire

C Have you ever felt the need to *c*ut down on your drinking/drug use?

A Have you ever been *a*nnoyed at criticism of your drinking/drug use?

G Have you ever felt *g*uilty about something that you have done when you have been drinking or taking drugs?

E Have you ever had an *e*ye opener—drinking or taking drugs first thing in the morning to get going or to avoid withdrawal symptoms?

B. Substance dependence

1. Substance dependence is a pattern of repeated use of a substance, which usually results in tolerance, withdrawal symptoms, and compulsive drug-taking behavior.
2. Substances are taken in larger amounts and over longer periods than was intended.
3. There is a desire to cut down, but efforts to decrease or discontinue use are unsuccessful.
4. Daily activities revolve around the use of a substance.

Screening tools are available to assess a substance misuse disorder; some are Michigan Alcohol Screening Test (MAST), Drug Abuse Screening Test (DAST), and CAGE screening questionnaire.

C. Substance tolerance is the need for increased amounts of the substance to achieve the desired effect.

D. Substance misuse

1. Uses substances recurrently
2. Recurrent, significant harmful consequences related to the use of substances are experienced.
3. Involvement with the legal system is common; the client may have legal issues to deal with and resolve.

E. Substance withdrawal

1. Physiological and substance-specific cognitive symptoms occur.
2. Substance withdrawal occurs when an individual experiences a decrease in blood levels of a substance on which the individual is physiologically dependent.

F. Other factors to consider in a client with a substance-related disorder

1. Rebellion and peer group pressure in adolescence may contribute to the onset of substance use.
2. Substance use may become a coping mechanism used to decrease physical and emotional pain.
3. Depression may precede or occur as a result of or in association with substance use.
4. Grief and loss may be associated with substance use.

G. Dysfunctional behaviors related to substance misuse

1. Preoccupation with obtaining and using substance
2. Manipulation to avoid consequences of behavior
3. Impulsiveness
4. Anger, including physical and verbal abuse
5. Avoidance of relationships outside the family unit
6. Relationships within the family become dysfunctional as the children take on atypical roles to protect the family unit.
7. Sense of self-importance and requiring special treatment
8. Denial—blaming everything but the substance use for problems
9. Use of rationalization and projection to justify unacceptable behavior
10. Low self-esteem
11. Depression
12. Codependency issues
    - **a.** *Codependency* refers to the presence of coexisting behaviors present in a significant other, which serves to enable the addict or alcoholic to continue the irresponsible patterns of use without experiencing consequences.
    - **b.** Examples of codependency: Paying bills for which the addict or alcoholic is responsible, bailing the addict or alcoholic out of jail, and helping the addict or alcoholic call in sick to employment agency.
    - **c.** It is important to address codependency issues with the family to maximize the chance for recovery of the client with the addiction and the person with the codependent behaviors.

III. Alcohol Misuse

A. Description

1. Alcohol is a central nervous system (CNS) depressant affecting all body tissues.
2. Physical dependence is a biological need for alcohol to avoid physical withdrawal symptoms, whereas psychological dependence refers to craving for the subjective effect of alcohol.

B. Risk factors

1. Biological predisposition; genetic and familial predisposition may also be a risk factor.
2. Depressed and highly anxious characteristics
3. Low self-esteem
4. Poor self-control
5. History of rebelliousness, poor school performance, and delinquency
6. Poor parental relationships

C. Assessment

1. Slurred speech
2. Uncoordinated movements
3. Unsteady gait
4. Restlessness
5. Confusion
6. Sneaking drinks, drinking in the morning, and experiencing blackouts
7. Binge drinking
8. Arguments about drinking
9. Missing work
10. Increased tolerance to alcohol
11. Intoxication, with blood alcohol content (BAC) of 0.1% (100 mg alcohol/dL blood) or greater (legal BAC may vary state to state)

Part of the assessment should include the type of alcohol, how much, for how long, and when last consumed.

D. Psychological symptoms
1. Depression
2. Irritable, belligerent, and hostile
3. Suspiciousness
4. Rationalization
5. Isolation
6. Decrease in inhibitions
7. Decrease in self-esteem
8. Denial that a problem exists

E. Complications associated with chronic alcohol use
1. Vitamin deficiencies
   a. Vitamin B deficiency causing peripheral neuropathies
   b. Thiamine deficiency, causing Korsakoff's syndrome
2. Alcohol-induced persistent amnesic disorder, causing severe memory problems
3. Wernicke's encephalopathy, causing confusion, ataxia, and abnormal eye movements
4. Hepatitis; cirrhosis of the liver
5. Esophagitis and gastritis
6. Pancreatitis
7. Anemias
8. Immune system dysfunctions
9. Brain damage
10. Peripheral neuropathy
11. Cardiac problems

IV. Alcohol Withdrawal

A. Description
1. Early signs develop within a few hours after cessation of alcohol intake.
2. These signs peak after 24 to 48 hours and then rapidly disappear, unless the withdrawal progresses to alcohol withdrawal delirium.
3. At the onset of withdrawal (Box 66-2), follow unit or agency protocol using specified withdrawal assessment scales.
4. Chlordiazepoxide may be prescribed for acute alcohol withdrawal and is usually given orally, unless a more immediate onset is required (benzodiazepine medications would decrease the withdrawal symptoms because of cross-tolerance; see Chapter 68 for a list of benzodiazepines).
5. An intramuscular injection of vitamin B_1 (thiamine) followed by several days of oral administration is usually prescribed to prevent Wernicke's encephalopathy.

B. Withdrawal (see Box 66-2)

C. Delirium tremens: The state of delirium usually peaks 48 to 72 hours after cessation or reduction of intake (although it can occur later) and lasts 2 to 3 days (Box 66-3).

⚠ Withdrawal delirium is a medical emergency. Death can occur from myocardial infarction, fat emboli, peripheral vascular collapse, electrolyte imbalance, aspiration pneumonia, or suicide.

D. Interventions
1. Provide care in a nonjudgmental manner.
2. Check the client frequently.
3. Monitor vital signs and neurological signs (every 15 minutes) and provide one-to-one supervision.
4. Monitor serum electrolytes, including glucose and magnesium.
5. Provide a quiet, nonstimulating environment; encourage a family member (1 at a time) to stay with the client to minimize anxiety.
6. Orient frequently.
7. Explain all treatments and procedures in a quiet and simple manner.
8. Initiate seizure precautions.
9. Large amounts of benzodiazepine sedatives may be required to achieve adequate control of symptoms.
10. Provide small, frequent, high-carbohydrate foods (administer antiemetic before meals as needed).

BOX 66-2 Early Signs of Alcohol Withdrawal

- Anorexia (nausea and vomiting may occur)
- Anxiety
- Easily startled
- Hyperalertness
- Hypertension
- Insomnia
- Irritability
- Jerky movements
- Possibly experiences hallucinations, illusions, delusions, or vivid nightmares
- Possibly reports a feeling of "shaking inside"
- Seizures (usually appear 7 to 48 hours after cessation of alcohol)
- Tachycardia
- Tremors

BOX 66-3 Manifestations of Alcohol Withdrawal Delirium (Delirium Tremens)

- Agitation
- Anorexia
- Anxiety
- Delirium
- Diaphoresis
- Disorientation with fluctuating levels of consciousness
- Fever (temperature of 100° F [37.8° C] to 103° F [39.4° C])
- Hallucinations and delusions
- Insomnia
- Tachycardia and hypertension

11. Monitor intake and output.
12. Administer vitamins (multivitamin, vitamin B complex including thiamine, folic acid, and vitamin C).
13. Administer magnesium if hypomagnesia is present.
14. Assist with activities of daily living and assist with ambulation if stable.
15. Allow client to express fears.

E. Medication therapy for alcohol misuse and alcohol dependence
1. Description: Medication is prescribed only for those individuals who have stopped drinking.
2. Naltrexone: Works by blocking in the brain the "high" feeling that people experience when they drink alcohol
3. Acamprosate: Works by reducing the physical distress and emotional discomfort people usually experience when they quit drinking
4. Disulfiram: Works by causing a severe adverse reaction when someone taking the medication consumes alcohol

F. Disulfiram therapy
1. Description
   a. The client must abstain from alcohol for at least 12 hours before the initial dose is administered.
   b. Adverse effects usually begin within several minutes to 30 minutes after consuming alcohol and may last 30 minutes to 2 hours.
   c. The client must avoid drinking alcohol for 14 days after disulfiram therapy has been discontinued; otherwise, the client is at risk for a disulfiram-alcohol reaction.
2. Adverse effects
   a. Fatigue
   b. Facial flushing
   c. Sweating
   d. Throbbing headache
   e. Neck pain
   f. Nausea and vomiting
   g. Hypotension
   h. Tachycardia
   i. Respiratory distress
3. Client education
   a. Educate about the effects of the medication.
   b. Ensure agreement to abstain from alcohol and any alcohol-containing substances.
   c. Inform the client that effects of the medication may occur for several days after it is discontinued.

G. Managing the client who has a substance misuse disorder (Boxes 66-4 and 66-5)

! Instruct the client who is on disulfiram therapy to avoid the use of substances that contain alcohol, such as cough medicines, rubbing compounds, vinegar, mouthwashes, and aftershave lotions. The client needs to read the labels of all products.

BOX 66-4 Managing the Client Who Misuses Alcohol

- Direct the client's focus to the substance misuse problem.
- Identify situations that precipitate angry feelings with the client.
- Set limits on manipulative behavior and verbal and physical abuse.
- Hold the client firmly accountable to reasonable limits, consistently reinforcing rules, with reasonable consequences for breaking rules.
- Hold the client accountable for all behaviors.
- Use motivational interviewing to assist the client to explore strengths and weaknesses.
- Encourage the client to focus on strengths if the client is losing control.
- Encourage the client to participate in group therapy and support groups.

BOX 66-5 Therapies for Clients with Substance Misuse and for Their Families

- Behavior therapy (including cognitive behavioral therapy [CBT]), aversion conditioning with medication
- Hospitalization
- Psychotherapy (individual, group, family)
- 12-Step support groups such as Alcoholics Anonymous; Narcotics Anonymous; Pills Anonymous; Al-Anon, Al-a-Teen, or Narc-Anon (for family members and friends of alcoholics or addicts); and Adult Children of Alcoholics
- Transitional living programs (halfway houses)

V. Drug Dependency

A. CNS depressants
1. CNS depressants include alcohol, benzodiazepines, and barbiturates and act as a depressant, sedative, or hypnotic.
2. Intoxication (Box 66-6)
3. Overdose can produce cardiovascular or respiratory depression, coma, shock, seizures, and death.
4. Overdose: If the client is awake, vomiting is induced and activated charcoal is administered; if

BOX 66-6 Intoxication: Central Nervous System Depressants

- Drowsiness
- Hypotension
- Impairment of memory, attention, judgment, and social or occupational functioning
- Incoordination and unsteady gait
- Irritability
- Slurred speech
- Impotence

the client is comatose, establishment and maintenance of an airway and gastric lavage with activated charcoal are the priorities; seizure precautions are indicated.

5. Flumazenil intravenously may be used for benzodiazepine overdose to reverse the effects.
6. Withdrawal effects include nausea, vomiting, tachycardia, diaphoresis, irritability, tremors, insomnia, and seizures; withdrawal must be treated with a carefully titrated similar drug (abrupt withdrawal can lead to death).
7. Withdrawal from CNS depressants such as barbiturates is generally treated with a barbiturate such as phenobarbital or a long-acting benzodiazepine.

B. CNS stimulants

1. CNS stimulants include substances such as amphetamines, cocaine, and crack.
2. Intoxication (Box 66-7)
3. Overdose can produce respiratory distress, ataxia, hyperpyrexia, seizures, coma, stroke, myocardial infarction, and death.
4. Overdose is treated with antipsychotics and management of associated effects.
5. Withdrawal effects include fatigue, depression, agitation, apathy, anxiety, insomnia, disorientation, lethargy, and craving.
6. Withdrawal is treated with antidepressants, a dopamine agonist, or bromocriptine; withdrawal is primarily supportive, particularly when dealing with the severe depression and suicidal ideation that accompanies stimulant withdrawal.

C. Opioids

1. Opioids include substances such as opium, heroin, meperidine, morphine, codeine sulfate, methadone, hydromorphone, oxycodone, hydrocodone, and fentanyl.
2. Intoxication (Box 66-8)
3. Overdose can produce respiratory depression, shock, coma, seizures, and death.
4. Overdose is treated with an opioid antagonist such as naloxone.

BOX 66-7 Intoxication: Central Nervous System Stimulants

- Dilated pupils
- Euphoria
- Hypertension
- Impairment of judgment and social or occupational functioning
- Insomnia
- Nausea and vomiting
- Paranoia, delusions, hallucinations
- Potential for violence
- Tachycardia

BOX 66-8 Intoxication: Opioids

- Constricted pupils
- Decreased respirations
- Drowsiness
- Euphoria
- Hypotension
- Impairment of memory, attention, and judgment
- Psychomotor retardation
- Slurred speech

5. Withdrawal effects include yawning, insomnia, irritability, rhinorrhea, diaphoresis, cramps, nausea and vomiting, muscle aches, chills, fever, lacrimation, and diarrhea.
6. Withdrawal may be treated by methadone detoxification or tapering dosage with other opioids.
7. Clonidine, an α-adrenergic blocker, assists in reducing the severity of sympathetic nervous system–generated withdrawal discomfort.
8. Specific measures for symptom management may also be used, such as antidiarrheal agents and acetaminophen for muscle aches.

D. Hallucinogens

1. Hallucinogens include substances such as lysergic acid diethylamide (LSD), mescaline (peyote), psilocybin (mushrooms), and phencyclidine (PCP).
2. Intoxication (Box 66-9)
3. Overdose effects of LSD, peyote, and psilocybin include psychosis, brain damage, and death; effects of PCP include psychosis, hypertensive crisis, hyperthermia, seizures, and respiratory arrest.
4. Treatment (LSD, peyote, psilocybin) involves low environmental stimuli (speak slowly, clearly, and in a low voice) and medications to treat anxiety.

BOX 66-9 Intoxication: Hallucinogens

- Agitation and belligerence
- Anxiety and depression
- Bizarre behavior, regressive behavior, or violent behavior
- Blank stare
- Diaphoresis
- Dilated pupils
- Elevated vital signs, including blood pressure
- Hallucinations
- Impairment of judgment and social and occupational functioning
- Incoordination
- Muscular rigidity and chronic jerking
- Paranoia
- Seizures
- Tachycardia
- Tremors

5. Treatment (PCP) involves possible gastric lavage (if alert); treatment to acidify the urine to assist in excreting the drug; and interventions to treat behavioral disturbances, hyperthermia, hypertension, and respiratory distress.
6. Management of withdrawal is primarily supportive and may include medications to target particular problem behaviors, such as agitation.

Flashbacks, which are unexpected reexperiences of the effects of taking a hallucinogenic drug, can occur for extended periods of time after its original use. Safety during flashbacks is a priority.

E. Inhalants
1. Inhalants include gases or liquids such as butane, paint thinner, paint and wax removers, airplane glue, nail polish remover, and nitrous oxide.
2. Intoxication (Box 66-10)
3. Overdose can cause damage to the nervous system and death.
4. Management of withdrawal is mainly supportive, including the treatment of affected body systems.

F. Marijuana (*Cannabis sativa*)
1. Generally is smoked, but can be ingested; may be legally prescribed in certain states and in some states and provinces is legal without a prescription.
2. Causes euphoria, detachment, relaxation, talkativeness, slowed perception of time, anxiety, and paranoia.
3. Long-term dependence can result in lethargy, amotivation syndrome, difficulty concentrating, memory loss, and possibly chronic respiratory problems.
4. Withdrawal management is mainly supportive.

G. Other recreational and club drugs

There are many types of illegal street drugs that are harmful. The nurse needs to be knowledgeable about the physiological effects of these various drugs, be able to recognize the signs associated with their use, and be prepared to provide immediate treatment.

1. Can include methylenedioxymethamphetamine (MDMA, ecstasy), γ-hydroxybutyrate (GHB), methamphetamine (crank, meth, crystal meth), and ketamine (special K)

BOX 66-10 Intoxication: Inhalants

- Enhancement of sexual pleasure
- Euphoria
- Excitation followed by drowsiness, lightheadedness, disinhibition, and agitation
- Giggling and laughter

2. Effects include euphoria, increased energy, increased self-confidence, and increased sociability.
3. Adverse effects include hyperthermia, rhabdomyolysis, kidney failure, hepatotoxicity, depression, panic attacks, psychosis, cardiovascular collapse, and death.
4. Programs for addiction also address nicotine withdrawal and the pharmacological and psychotherapeutic interventions for this problem, such as nicotine patches, nicotine inhalers, and bupropion for the reduction of withdrawal symptoms and cravings.
5. Anabolic steroids have also gained increased attention as increasingly adverse events, including death, have become more widely publicized.

H. Interventions: Withdrawal (Box 66-11)
1. Initiate seizure precautions.
2. Hydrate the client.
3. Monitor vital signs every hour; include cardiac monitoring and diagnostic tests such as electrocardiogram and cardiac markers because of the risk of cardiac damage with certain drugs.
4. Monitor intake and output.
5. Orient the client frequently.
6. Maintain minimal stimuli.
7. Approach the client in an accepting and nonjudgmental manner.
8. Direct focus to the substance misuse problem.
9. Assist the client with identifying situations that precipitate angry feelings.
10. Assist the client to deal with emotions.
11. Limit placing blame or rationalizing to explain the substance misuse problem.
12. Assist the client to use assertive techniques rather than manipulation to meet needs.
13. Set limits on manipulative behavior and verbal and physical misuse.

BOX 66-11 Withdrawal: Nursing Care

- Obtain information regarding the type of drug and amount consumed.
- Assess vital signs.
- Remove unnecessary objects from the environment.
- Provide one-to-one supervision if necessary.
- Provide a quiet, calm environment with minimal stimuli.
- Maintain client orientation.
- Ensure the client's safety by implementing seizure precautions.
- Use security devices if necessary and as prescribed to prevent the client from harming self and others.
- Provide for physical needs.
- Provide food and fluids as tolerated.
- Administer medications as prescribed to decrease withdrawal symptoms.
- Collect blood and urine samples for drug screening.

14. Maintain firm and reasonable limits, consistently reinforcing rules, with reasonable consequences for breaking rules.
15. Hold the client accountable for all behaviors.
16. Assist the client to explore strengths and weaknesses.
17. Encourage the client to focus on strengths if the client is losing control.
18. Encourage the client to participate in unit activities.
19. Encourage the client to participate in group therapy and support groups.

I. Dual diagnoses
1. Sometimes the use of alcohol and drugs masks underlying psychiatric pathology.
2. Psychiatric pathology may also be precipitated by substance use and misuse.
3. When psychiatric disorders and substance misuse are present together, it is often referred to as *dual diagnosis*.
4. Separating psychiatric diagnosis from substance dependence can be done only over time after a sustained period of abstinence.

J. Addiction and substance misuse in health care professionals: Suspicious signs
1. Frequently reporting that drugs have been wasted without being witnessed by another nurse
2. Reporting administering maximum dosages of controlled substances to clients when other nurses do not administer the maximum dose
3. A variance in usual pain relief in the absence of a change in dosage or frequency of administration in their clients
4. Work patterns include the following: Always volunteering to carry narcotic (opioids) keys (or other opioid access devices per agency procedure); choosing shifts in which less supervision is present; choosing work areas where the use of controlled substances is high, such as critical care units, operating room, anesthesia, and trauma units
5. Nurses have a professional and ethical obligation to report impaired co-workers.
6. Most impaired nurses are able to return to work through the State Board of Nursing assistance and monitoring programs; such programs usually require strict adherence to clearly stated rules and regular reports and drug screens.

PRACTICE QUESTIONS

817. The home health nurse visits a client at home and determines that the client is dependent on drugs. During the assessment, which action should the nurse take to plan appropriate nursing care?
1. Ask the client why he started taking illegal drugs.
2. Ask the client about the amount of drug use and its effect.
3. Ask the client how long he thought that he could take drugs without someone finding out.
4. Do not ask any questions for fear that the client is in denial and will throw the nurse out of the home.

818. Which interventions are **most appropriate** for caring for a client in alcohol withdrawal? **Select all that apply.**
- ❑ 1. Monitor vital signs.
- ❑ 2. Provide a safe environment.
- ❑ 3. Address hallucinations therapeutically.
- ❑ 4. Provide stimulation in the environment.
- ❑ 5. Provide reality orientation as appropriate.
- ❑ 6. Maintain NPO (nothing by mouth) status.

819. The nurse determines that the wife of an alcoholic client is benefiting from attending an Al-Anon group if the nurse hears the wife make which statement?
1. "I no longer feel that I deserve the beatings my husband inflicts on me."
2. "My attendance at the meetings has helped me see that I provoke my husband's violence."
3. "I enjoy attending the meetings because they get me out of the house and away from my husband."
4. "I can tolerate my husband's destructive behaviors now that I know they are common among alcoholics."

820. A hospitalized client with a history of alcohol misuse tells the nurse, "I am leaving now. I have to go. I don't want any more treatment. I have things that I have to do right away." The client has not been discharged and is scheduled for an important diagnostic test to be performed in 1 hour. After the nurse discusses the client's concerns with the client, the client dresses and begins to walk out of the hospital room. What action should the nurse take?
1. Call the nursing supervisor.
2. Call security to block all exit areas.
3. Restrain the client until the primary health care provider (PHCP) can be reached.
4. Tell the client that the client cannot return to this hospital again if the client leaves now.

821. The nurse is preparing to perform an admission assessment on a client with a diagnosis of bulimia nervosa. Which assessment findings should the nurse expect to note? **Select all that apply.**
- ❑ 1. Dental decay
- ❑ 2. Moist, oily skin
- ❑ 3. Loss of tooth enamel
- ❑ 4. Electrolyte imbalances
- ❑ 5. Body weight well below ideal range

822. The nurse is caring for a female client who was admitted to the mental health unit recently for anorexia nervosa. The nurse enters the client's room and notes that the client is engaged in rigorous push-ups. Which nursing action is **most appropriate**?
1. Interrupt the client and weigh her immediately.
2. Interrupt the client and offer to take her for a walk.
3. Allow the client to complete her exercise program.
4. Tell the client that she is not allowed to exercise rigorously.

823. A client with a diagnosis of anorexia nervosa, who is in a state of starvation, is in a 2-bed room. A newly admitted client will be assigned to this client's room. Which client would be the **best** choice as a roommate for the client with anorexia nervosa?
1. A client with pneumonia
2. A client undergoing diagnostic tests
3. A client who thrives on managing others
4. A client who could benefit from the client's assistance at mealtime

824. The nurse is assessing a client who was admitted 24 hours ago for a fractured humerus. Which findings should alert the nurse to the potential for alcohol withdrawal delirium?
1. Hypotension, ataxia, hunger
2. Stupor, lethargy, muscular rigidity
3. Hypotension, coarse hand tremors, lethargy
4. Hypertension, changes in level of consciousness, hallucinations

825. The spouse of a client admitted to the mental health unit for alcohol withdrawal says to the nurse, "I should get out of this bad situation." Which is the **most** helpful response by the nurse?
1. "Why don't you tell your spouse about this?"
2. "What do you find difficult about this situation?"
3. "This is not the best time to make that decision."
4. "I agree with you. You should get out of this situation."

826. A client with anorexia nervosa is a member of a predischarge support group. The client verbalizes that she would like to buy some new clothes, but her finances are limited. Group members have brought some used clothes to the client to replace the client's old clothes. The client believes that the new clothes are much too tight and has reduced her calorie intake to 800 calories daily. How should the nurse evaluate this behavior?
1. Normal behavior
2. Evidence of the client's disturbed body image
3. Regression as the client is moving toward the community
4. Indicative of the client's ambivalence about hospital discharge

ANSWERS

817. ***Answer:*** 1, 2

Rationale: Whenever the nurse carries out an assessment for a client who is dependent on drugs, it is best for the nurse to attempt to elicit information by being nonjudgmental and direct. Option 1 is incorrect because it is judgmental and off-focus, and reflects the nurse's bias. Option 3 is incorrect because it is judgmental, insensitive, and aggressive, which is nontherapeutic. Option 4 is incorrect because it indicates passivity on the nurse's part and uses rationalization to avoid the therapeutic nursing intervention.
Test-Taking Strategy: Focus on the subject, assessment of a client dependent on drugs. Use of therapeutic communication techniques will assist in directing you to the correct option.
Level of Cognitive Ability: Applying
Client Needs: Psychosocial Integrity
Integrated Process: Nursing Process—Assessment
Content Area: Mental Health
Health Problem: Mental Health: Addictions
Priority Concepts: Addiction; Communication
Reference: Varcarolis (2017), p. 331.

818. ***Answer:*** 1, 2, 3, 5

Rationale: When the client is experiencing withdrawal from alcohol, the priority for care is to prevent the client from harming self or others. The nurse would monitor the vital signs closely and report abnormal findings. The nurse would provide a low-stimulation environment to maintain the client in as calm a state as possible. The nurse would reorient the client to reality frequently and would address hallucinations therapeutically. Adequate nutritional and fluid intake need to be maintained.
Test-Taking Strategy: Note the strategic words, *most appropriate*. Thinking about the needs of the client in alcohol withdrawal and recalling the characteristics associated with alcohol withdrawal will assist in answering correctly. Also, use therapeutic communication techniques to assist in selecting the correct interventions.
Level of Cognitive Ability: Analyzing
Client Needs: Psychosocial Integrity
Integrated Process: Nursing Process—Implementation
Content Area: Mental Health
Health Problem: Mental Health: Addictions
Priority Concepts: Addiction; Caregiving
Reference: Varcarolis (2017), p. 303.

819. ***Answer:*** 1

Rationale: Al-Anon support groups are a protected, supportive opportunity for spouses and significant others to learn what to expect and to obtain excellent pointers about successful behavioral changes. The correct option is the healthiest response because it exemplifies an understanding that the alcoholic partner is responsible for his behavior and cannot be allowed to blame family members for loss of control. Option 2 is incorrect, because the nonalcoholic partner should not feel responsible when the spouse loses control. Option 3 indicates that the group is viewed as an escape, not as a place to work on issues. Option 4 indicates that the wife remains codependent.

Test-Taking Strategy: Focus on the subject, the therapeutic effect of attending an Al-Anon group. Noting the words *benefiting from attending an Al-Anon group* will direct you to the correct option.
Level of Cognitive Ability: Evaluating
Client Needs: Psychosocial Integrity
Integrated Process: Nursing Process—Evaluation
Content Area: Mental Health
Health Problem: Mental Health: Addictions
Priority Concepts: Addiction; Family Dynamics
Reference: Varcarolis (2017), p. 319.

820. *Answer:* 1
Rationale: Most health care facilities have documents that the client is asked to sign relating to the client's responsibilities when the client leaves against medical advice. The client should be asked to wait to speak to the PHCP before leaving and to sign the "against medical advice" document before leaving. If the client refuses to do so, the nurse cannot hold the client against the client's will. Therefore, in this situation, the nurse should call the nursing supervisor. The nurse can be charged with false imprisonment if a client is made to believe wrongfully that she or he cannot leave the hospital. Restraining the client and calling security to block exits constitutes false imprisonment. All clients have a right to health care and cannot be told otherwise.
Test-Taking Strategy: Keeping the concept of false imprisonment in mind, eliminate options 2 and 3 because they are comparable or alike. Eliminate option 4, knowing that all clients have a right to health care. From the options presented, the best action is presented in the correct option.
Level of Cognitive Ability: Applying
Client Needs: Safe and Effective Care Environment
Integrated Process: Nursing Process—Implementation
Content Area: Mental Health
Health Problem: Mental Health: Addictions
Priority Concepts: Clinical Judgment; Health Care Law
Reference: Varcarolis (2017), pp. 68-69.

821. *Answer:* 1, 3, 4
Rationale: Clients with bulimia nervosa initially may not appear to be physically or emotionally ill. They are often at or slightly below ideal body weight. On further inspection, a client exhibits dental decay and loss of tooth enamel if the client has been inducing vomiting. Electrolyte imbalances are present. Dry, scaly skin (rather than moist, oily skin) is present.
Test-Taking Strategy: Focus on the subject, assessment findings in bulimia nervosa. It is necessary to recall that in anorexia nervosa the body weight is normally well below ideal body weight and that clients with bulimia nervosa are often at or slightly below ideal body weight. Also, remember that skin texture will be dry and scaly.
Level of Cognitive Ability: Analyzing
Client Needs: Psychosocial Integrity
Integrated Process: Nursing Process—Assessment
Content Area: Mental Health
Health Problem: Mental Health: Eating Disorders
Priority Concepts: Anxiety; Nutrition
Reference: Varcarolis (2017), pp. 184-185.

822. *Answer:* 2
Rationale: Clients with anorexia nervosa frequently are preoccupied with rigorous exercise and push themselves beyond normal limits to work off caloric intake. The nurse must provide for appropriate exercise and place limits on rigorous activities. The correct option stops the harmful behavior yet provides the client with an activity to decrease anxiety that is not harmful. Weighing the client immediately reinforces the client's preoccupation with weight. Allowing the client to complete the exercise program can be harmful to the client. Telling the client that she is not allowed to complete the exercise program will increase the client's anxiety.
Test-Taking Strategy: Note the strategic words, *most appropriate*, and focus on the client's diagnosis. Also, focus on the need for the nurse to maintain safety and to set firm limits with clients who have this disorder.
Level of Cognitive Ability: Applying
Client Needs: Physiological Integrity
Integrated Process: Nursing Process—Implementation
Content Area: Mental Health
Health Problem: Mental Health: Eating Disorders
Priority Concepts: Anxiety; Safety
Reference: Potter et al. (2017), p. 1060.

823. *Answer:* 2
Rationale: The client undergoing diagnostic tests is an acceptable roommate. The client with anorexia nervosa is most likely experiencing hematological complications, such as leukopenia. Having a roommate with pneumonia would place the client with anorexia nervosa at risk for infection. The client with anorexia nervosa should not be put in a situation in which the client can focus on the nutritional needs of others or be managed by others, because this may contribute to sublimation and suppression of personal hunger.
Test-Taking Strategy: Note the strategic word, *best*, and note the words *in a state of starvation* in the question. Recalling the characteristics of anorexia nervosa and that the client is immunocompromised as a result of starvation will direct you to the correct option.
Level of Cognitive Ability: Analyzing
Client Needs: Safe and Effective Care Environment
Integrated Process: Nursing Process—Planning
Content Area: Mental Health
Health Problem: Mental Health: Eating Disorders
Priority Concepts: Care Coordination; Safety
Reference: Varcarolis (2017), p. 185.

824. *Answer:* 4
Rationale: Symptoms associated with alcohol withdrawal delirium typically include anxiety, insomnia, anorexia, hypertension, disorientation, hallucinations, changes in level of consciousness, agitation, fever, and delusions.
Test-Taking Strategy: Focus on the subject, findings associated with withdrawal delirium. Review each option carefully to ensure that all symptoms in the option are correct. Eliminate options 1 and 3 first, knowing that hypertension rather than hypotension occurs. From the remaining options, recalling that the client who is stuporous is not likely to exhibit withdrawal delirium will direct you to the correct option.
Level of Cognitive Ability: Analyzing
Client Needs: Physiological Integrity

Integrated Process: Nursing Process—Assessment
Content Area: Mental Health
Health Problem: Mental Health: Addictions
Priority Concepts: Addiction; Clinical Judgment
Reference: Varcarolis (2017), p. 303.

825. *Answer:* 2
Rationale: The most helpful response is one that encourages the client to solve problems. Giving advice implies that the nurse knows what is best and can foster dependency. The nurse should not agree with the client, and the nurse should not request that the client provide explanations.
Test-Taking Strategy: Note the **strategic word**, *most.* Use **therapeutic communication techniques.** Eliminate option 1 because of the word *why,* which should be avoided in communication. Eliminate option 3, because this option places the client's feelings on hold. Eliminate option 4, because the nurse is agreeing with the client. The correct option is the only one that addresses the client's feelings.
Level of Cognitive Ability: Applying
Client Needs: Psychosocial Integrity
Integrated Process: Communication and Documentation
Content Area: Mental Health
Health Problem: Mental Health: Addictions
Priority Concepts: Caregiving; Communication
Reference: Varcarolis (2017), pp. 97-98, 302.

826. *Answer:* 2
Rationale: Disturbed body image is a concern with clients with anorexia nervosa. Although the client may struggle with ambivalence and show regressed behavior, the client's coping pattern relates to the basic issue of disturbed body image. The nurse should address this need in the support group.
Test-Taking Strategy: Note the **subject,** signs of disturbed body image. Note the relationship between the information in the question and the correct option.
Level of Cognitive Ability: Evaluating
Client Needs: Psychosocial Integrity
Integrated Process: Nursing Process—Evaluation
Content Area: Mental Health
Health Problem: Mental Health: Eating Disorders
Priority Concepts: Anxiety; Coping
Reference: Varcarolis (2017), pp. 184-185.

CHAPTER 67

Crisis Theory and Intervention

PRIORITY CONCEPTS **Coping; Interpersonal Violence**

I. Crisis Intervention

A. Description
1. **Crisis** is a temporary state of severe emotional disorganization caused by an event that presents a threat.
2. Everyone experiences crises; the outcome depends on coping mechanisms and support systems available at the time of the crisis.
3. The ability for decision making and problem solving is inadequate.
4. Treatment is aimed at assisting the client and the family through the stressful situation.

B. Phases of a crisis
1. Phase 1: External precipitating event (could be situational, developmental, cultural, or societal)
2. Phase 2
   a. Perception of the threat
   b. Increase in anxiety
   c. Client may cope or resolve the crisis.
3. Phase 3
   a. Failure of coping
   b. Increasing disorganization
   c. Emergence of physical symptoms
   d. Relationship problems
4. Phase 4
   a. Mobilization of internal and external resources
   b. Goal is to return the client to at least a precrisis level of functioning.

C. Types of crises (Box 67-1)

D. Crisis intervention
1. Treatment is immediate, supportive, and directly responsive to the immediate crisis.
2. The interprofessional health care team assists individuals in crisis to cope; interventions are goal directed.
3. Feelings of the client are acknowledged.
4. Intervention provides opportunities for expression and validation of feelings.
5. Connections are made between the meaning of the event and the crisis.
6. The client explores alternative coping mechanisms and tries out new behaviors.

II. Grief

A. Grief is a natural emotional response to loss that individuals must experience as they attempt to accept the loss.

B. Grief usually involves moving through a series of stages or tasks to help resolve the grief (Box 67-2).

C. Depending on the type of loss, feelings associated with grief include anger, frustration, loneliness, sadness, guilt, regret, and peace.

D. Healing can occur when the pain of the loss has lessened and the individual has adapted to the loss; if the grief is the result of the loss of a loved one, the individual continues to experience memories of the deceased.

E. Types of grief
1. Normal grief: Physical, emotional, cognitive, spiritual, or behavioral reactions can occur; the process of resolution can take months to years.
2. Anticipatory grief occurs before the loss of a loved one and is associated with an acute, chronic, or terminal illness.
3. Disenfranchised grief occurs when a loss of a loved one is experienced and cannot be acknowledged openly (societal norms do not define the loss as a loss within its traditional definition).
4. Dysfunctional grief occurs with prolonged emotional instability and a lack of progression to successful coping with the loss.
5. Grief in children is based on the developmental level of the child (Box 67-3).

III. Loss

A. Loss is the absence of something desired or previously thought to be available.

B. Actual loss can be identified by others and can arise in response to or in anticipation of a situation.

C. Perceived loss is experienced by one person and cannot be verified by others.

BOX 67-1 Types of Crises

Maturational

- Relates to developmental stages and associated role changes; examples include marriage, birth of a child, and retirement

Situational

- Arises from an external source, is often unanticipated, and is associated with a life event that upsets an individual's or group's psychological equilibrium; examples include loss of a job or a change in job, change in financial status, death of a loved one, divorce, abortion, addition of new family members, pregnancy, and severe physical or mental illness

Adventitious

- Relates to a crisis of disaster, is not a part of everyday life; it is unplanned and accidental. Adventitious crises may result from a natural disaster (e.g., floods, fires, tornadoes, earthquakes), a national disaster (e.g., war, riots, airplane crashes), or a crime of violence (e.g., rape, assault, murder in the workplace or school, bombings, or spousal or child abuse).

From Varcarolis E: *Essentials of psychiatric mental health nursing*, revised reprint, ed 2, Philadelphia, 2013, Saunders.

BOX 67-2 The Grief Response

Stage 1: Shock and Disbelief

- Individual may have feelings of numbness, difficulties with decision making, emotional outbursts, denial, and isolation.

Stage 2: Experiencing the Loss

- If the grief response is the result of a loss of a loved one, the individual may feel angry at the loved one who died or may feel guilt about the death.
- Bargaining or depression or both also may occur in this stage.

Stage 3: Reintegration

- Individual begins to reorganize her or his life and accepts the reality of the loss.

D. Anticipatory loss is experienced before the loss occurs.

E. Mourning

1. Mourning is the outward and social expression of loss.
2. Mourning may be dictated by cultural, spiritual, and religious beliefs.

F. Bereavement

1. Bereavement includes the inner feelings and the outward reactions of the individual experiencing the loss.
2. Bereavement includes grief and mourning.

BOX 67-3 Grief in Children

Birth to 1 Year

- Infant has no concept of death.
- Infant reacts to the loss of mother or caregiver.

1 to 2 Years

- Toddler may see death as reversible.
- Toddler may scream, withdraw, or become disinterested in the environment.
- Grief response occurs only to the death of the significant person in the toddler's life.

2 to 5 Years

- Child may see death as reversible.
- Regressive or aggressive behavior may occur.
- Child has a sense of loss and is concerned about who will provide care.

5 to 9 Years

- Child has difficulty concentrating.
- Child begins to see death as permanent.
- Child may feel responsible for the occurrence.

Preadolescent Through Adolescent

- Adolescent may regress.
- Adolescent sees death as permanent.
- Adolescent experiences a strong emotional reaction.

IV. Nurse's Role: Grief and Loss (Box 67-4)

A. Encourage the client to express feelings within a trusting, supportive, and nonjudgmental environment.

B. Allow ongoing opportunities for fully informed choices.

C. Facilitate the grief process; assess the individual's grief, and assist the individual to feel the loss and complete the tasks of the grief process.

D. Grief affects individuals physically, psychologically, socially, and spiritually; an interprofessional team approach, including a bereavement specialist, facilitates the grief process.

⚠ The nurse's role in the grief and loss process includes communicating with the client, family members, and significant other. The nurse must consider the individual's culture, spirituality, religion, family structure, life experiences, coping skills, and support systems.

V. Suicidal Behavior

A. Description

1. Suicidal clients characteristically have feelings of worthlessness, guilt, and hopelessness that are so overwhelming that they feel unable to go on with life and feel unfit to live.
2. The nurse caring for a depressed client always considers the possibility of suicide.

BOX 67-4 Communication During Grief and Loss

- Determine how much the client and family want to know about the situation.
- Determine whether there is a spokesperson for the family.
- Be aware of cultural, spiritual, and religious beliefs and how they may affect the communication process; consider personal space issues, eye contact, and touch.
- Obtain an interpreter, if necessary.
- Allow opportunity for informed choices.
- Assist with the decision-making process if asked; use problem solving to assist in decision making, and avoid interjecting personal views or opinions.
- Establish trust with the client and encourage expression of feelings, concerns, and fears within a trusting, supportive, and nonjudgmental environment.
- Be honest, and let the client and family know that you will not abandon them.
- Ask the client and family about their expectations and needs.
- Be a sensitive listener; sit in silence if necessary and appropriate.
- Extend touch and hold the client's or family member's hand if appropriate.
- Encourage reminiscing.
- If you do not know what to do in a particular situation, seek assistance.
- If you do not know what to say to a client or family who is talking about death or another loss, listen attentively and use therapeutic communication techniques, such as open-ended questions or reflection.
- Acknowledge your own feelings; let the client and family know that the topic of conversation is a difficult one and that you do not know what to say.
- Realize that it is acceptable to cry with the client and family during the grief process.

B. Individuals at risk
1. Clients with a history of previous suicide attempts
2. Family history of suicide attempts
3. Adolescents
4. Older adults
5. Disabled or terminally ill clients
6. Clients with personality disorders
7. Clients with organic brain syndrome or dementia
8. Depressed or psychotic clients (see Chapter 65 for information on depression)
9. Substance abusers
10. Those who have been consistently bullied or rejected by peers or society
11. History of child maltreatment
12. Past psychiatric hospitalizations

C. Cues (Box 67-5)

D. Assessment (Box 67-6)

BOX 67-5 Suicidal Cues

- Giving away personal, special, and prized possessions
- Canceling social engagements
- Making out or changing a will
- Taking out or changing insurance policies
- Positive or negative changes in behavior
- Poor appetite
- Sleeping difficulties
- Feelings of hopelessness
- Difficulty in concentrating
- Loss of interest in activities
- Client statements indicating an intent to attempt suicide
- Sudden calmness or improvement in a depressed client
- Client inquiries about poisons, guns, or other lethal items or objects
- Sudden deterioration in school/work performance

BOX 67-6 Suicidal Client: Assessment

Plan

- Does the client have a plan?
- Does the client have the means to carry out the plan?
- Has the client decided when she or he is going to carry out the plan?

Client History of Attempts

- What suicide attempts occurred in the past and what harm occurred?
- Was the client accidentally rescued?
- Have the past attempts and methods been the same, or have methods increased in lethality?

Psychosocial Factors

- Is the client alone or alienated from others?
- Is hostility or depression present?
- Is the client experiencing hallucinations? Type of hallucination (audio/command, visual)?
- Is substance abuse present?
- Has the client had any recent losses or physical illness?
- Has the client had any environmental or lifestyle changes?

E. Interventions
1. Assess for suicidal intent or ideation and initiate suicide precautions.
2. The client's statements, behaviors, and mood are documented every 15 minutes.
3. Remove harmful objects.
4. Do not leave the client alone.
5. Provide a nonjudgmental, caring attitude.
6. Per agency procedure and policy, develop a no-suicide contract that is written, dated, and signed and indicates alternative behavior at times when suicidal thoughts occur and that they will notify the nurse when having suicidal thoughts.

7. Encourage the client to talk about feelings and to identify positive aspects about self.
8. Encourage active participation in own care.
9. Keep the client active by assigning achievable tasks.
10. Check that visitors do not leave harmful objects in the client's room.
11. Identify support systems.
12. Do not allow the client to leave the unit unless accompanied by a staff member.
13. Continue to assess the client's suicide potential.

! Provide one-to-one supervision at all times for the client at risk for suicide.

VI. Abusive Behaviors

A. Anger
1. Anger is a feeling of annoyance that may be displaced onto an object or person.
2. Anger is used to avoid anxiety and gives a feeling of power in situations in which the person feels out of control.

B. Aggression can be harmful and destructive when not controlled.

C. Violence is physical force that is threatening to the safety of self and others.

D. Assessment
1. History of violence or self-harm
2. Poor impulse control and low tolerance of frustration
3. Defiant and argumentative
4. Raising of voice
5. Making verbal threats
6. Pacing and agitation
7. Muscle rigidity
8. Flushed face
9. Glaring at others

E. Interventions
1. Ensure a safe and low stimuli environment.
2. Use a calm approach and communicate with a calm, clear tone of voice (be assertive, not aggressive, and avoid verbal struggles).
3. Maintain a large personal space and use a nonaggressive posture (e.g., arms and hands at the side rather than folded across the chest or placed on the hips).
4. Listen actively and acknowledge the client's anger.
5. Determine what the client considers to be her or his need.
6. Provide the client with clear options that deal with the client's behavior, set limits on behavior, and make the client aware of the consequences of anger and violence.
7. Discuss the use of **restraints (security devices)** or **seclusion** if the client is unable to control angry behavior that may lead to violence.
8. Assist the client with problem solving and decision making regarding the options.

F. Restraints (security devices) and seclusion
1. Description
   a. Physical restraints: Any physical or environmental means of controlling an individual's behavior or actions that inhibits free movement
   b. Seclusion: A type of restraint in which a client is confined in a room specially designed for protection and close supervision from which they cannot freely exit.
   c. Chemical restraints: Medications given for a specific purpose of inhibiting a specific behavior or movement and that have an impact on the client's ability to relate to the environment
2. Use of restraints and seclusion
   a. Restraints and seclusion should never be used as punishment or for the convenience of the health care staff.
   b. Restraints and seclusion are used when behavior is physically harmful to the client or others and when alternative or less restrictive measures are insufficient in protecting the client or others from harm.
   c. Restraints and seclusion are used when the health care team anticipates that a controlled environment would be helpful and requests restraints or seclusion.
   d. The nurse must document the behavior leading to the use of restraints or seclusion.
   e. In most settings, a primary health care provider's prescription is required prior to the use of restraints
   f. In an emergency, a qualified nurse may place a client in restraints or seclusion and obtain a written or verbal prescription as soon as possible thereafter.
   g. Per state guidelines, within 1 hour of the initiation of restraints or seclusion, the psychiatrist must make a face-to-face assessment and evaluation of the client and must continuously reevaluate the need for continued restraints or seclusion.
   h. While in restraints or seclusion, the client must be protected from all sources of harm.
   i. The client in restraints or seclusion needs constant one-to-one supervision; physical, safety, and comfort needs must be assessed every 15 to 30 minutes, and these observations are also documented (e.g., food, fluids, bathroom needs, range-of-motion exercise, and ambulation).
   j. The nurse must always follow agency procedures and policies regarding the use of restraints and must also be familiar with their use for the older client and juveniles.

⚠ Restraints require a written prescription by a primary health care provider, which must be reviewed and renewed per agency policy; the prescription must specify the type of restraint to be used, the duration of the restraint or seclusion, and the criteria for release (agency policy and procedures need to be followed).

VII. Bullying

A. Bullying is the abuse of power by an individual toward another through repeated aggressive acts.
B. It most often occurs in children and in high school or college environments but can also occur in the workplace or other environments.
C. The bully feels power from sources such as physical strength, maturity, or a higher status within a peer group; from knowing the victim's weaknesses; or from support of others.
D. Bullying can occur in the form of physical harm, relational aggression, isolation and exclusion, and verbal harm such as slander, rumors, or threats; it is both intentionally cruel and unprovoked.
E. Cyberbullying is also a form of bullying and occurs in the form of Internet messages on social media networks, text messages, e-mails, photos being posted, and rumors.
F. The bullied person repeatedly experiences negative actions from the bully(s).
G. These bullying acts can lead to depression, low self-esteem, humiliation, isolation, and social withdrawal in the victim; they could result in self-harm such as cutting, suicide, and murder.
H. The nurse's responsibility is to observe for signs of bullying and to educate teachers, school administrators, and parents about bullying behaviors and signs that bullying may be occurring.

VIII. Family Violence

A. Description (Fig. 67-1)
1. Violence begins with threats or verbal or physical minor assaults (tension building), and the victim attempts to comply with the requests of the abuser.
2. The abuser loses control and becomes destructive and harmful (acute battering), whereas the victim attempts to protect herself or himself.
3. After the battering, the abuser becomes loving and attempts to make peace (calmness and diffusion of tension); undoing behavior is characteristic in which the abuser gives gifts and positive attention to the victim to undo the negative behavior.
4. The abuser justifies that violence is normal and the victim is responsible for the abuse.
5. Outsiders are usually unaware of what is happening in the family.
6. Family members are isolated socially and lack autonomy and trust among each other; caring and intimacy in the family are absent.
7. Family members expect other members of the family to meet their needs, but none is able to do so.
8. The abuser threatens to abandon the family.

B. Types of violence (Box 67-7)
C. The vulnerable person (victim)
1. The vulnerable person is the one in the family unit against whom violence is perpetrated.

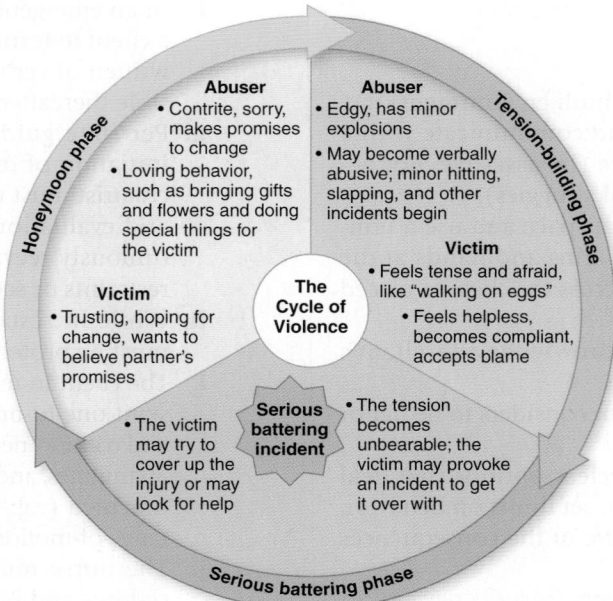

FIG. 67-1 The cycle of violence.

BOX 67-7 Types of Violence

Physical Violence: Infliction of physical pain or bodily harm
Sexual Violence: Any form of sexual contact without consent
Emotional Violence: Infliction of mental anguish
Physical Neglect: Failure to provide health care to prevent or treat physical or emotional illnesses
Developmental Neglect: Failure to provide physical and cognitive stimulation needed to prevent developmental deficits
Educational Neglect: Depriving a child of education
Economic Exploitation: Illegal or improper exploitation of money, funds, or other resources for one's personal gain

2. The most vulnerable individuals are children and older adults.
3. The perpetrator of violence and the person targeted by the violence can be male or female.
4. Battering is a crime.

D. Characteristics of abusers
1. Impaired self-esteem
2. Strong dependency needs
3. Narcissistic and suspicious
4. History of abuse during childhood
5. Perceive victims as their property and believe that they are entitled to abuse them

E. Characteristics of victims
1. Some may have a dependent personality disorder
2. Feel trapped, dependent, helpless, and powerless
3. May become depressed as they are trapped in the abusers' power and control cycle (see Fig. 67-1)
4. As victims' self-esteem becomes diminished with chronic abuse, they may blame themselves for the violence and be unable to see a way out of the situation.

F. Interventions
1. Report suspected or actual cases of child abuse or abuse of an older adult to appropriate authorities (follow state and agency guidelines).
2. Referral to appropriate sexual assault domestic violence (SADV) team or other appropriate agency team
3. Assess for evidence of physical injuries.
4. Ensure privacy and confidentiality during the assessment, and provide a nonjudgmental and empathetic approach to foster trust; reassure the victim that she or he has not done anything wrong. Box 67-8 lists sample assessment questions.
5. Assist the victim to develop self-protective and other problem-solving abilities.
6. Even if the victim is not ready to leave the situation, encourage the victim to develop a specific safety plan (a fast escape if the violence returns) and provide information on where to obtain help (hotlines, safe houses, and shelters); an abused person is usually reluctant to call the police.
7. Assess suicidal potential of the victim.
8. Assess the potential for homicide.
9. Assess for the use of drugs and alcohol.
10. Determine family coping patterns and support systems.
11. Provide support and assistance in coping with contacting the legal system.
12. Assist in resolving family dysfunction with prescribed therapies.
13. Encourage individual therapy for the victim that promotes coping with the trauma and prevents further psychological conflict.
14. Encourage individual therapy for the abuser that focuses on preventing violent behavior and repairing relationships.
15. Encourage psychotherapy, counseling, group therapy, and support groups to assist family members to develop coping strategies.
16. Assist the family to identify an access to community and personal resources.
17. Maintain accurate and thorough medical health records.

BOX 67-8 Assessment Questions for Violence and Abuse

- "Has anyone ever touched you in a way that made you uncomfortable?"
- "Are these injuries a result of someone harming you?"
- "Is anyone hurting you now?"
- "How do you and your partner deal with anger (or disagreement)?"
- "Has your partner ever hit you?"
- "Have you ever been threatened by ______?"
- "Does your partner prevent you from seeing family or friends?"
- "Does your partner ever use the children to manipulate you?"
- "Did (or does) anyone in your family deal with anger by hitting?"

IX. Child Abduction

A. Description
1. Child abduction is the kidnapping of a child (or infant) by an older person.
2. Occurrences
   a. A stranger may kidnap a child for criminal or mischievous purposes.
   b. A stranger may kidnap a child (or infant) to bring up him or her as that person's own child.
   c. A parent removes or retains a child from the other parent's care (often in the course of or after divorce proceedings).

3. Because of the increased independence that occurs in the preschool-age child, parents are less able to provide the constant protection they once did when the child reaches this age; interventions that ensure protection (including teaching the child) are necessary.
4. Questions that help reveal the potential for abuse include: "Who do you play with most often? Is there anyone you do not like playing with? Are there games you don't like playing?"

B. Interventions

1. Instruct the parents to teach a child basic guidelines about personal safety that include the following:
   - **a.** Do not go anywhere alone.
   - **b.** Always tell an adult where you are going and when you will return.
   - **c.** Say *no* if you feel uncomfortable with a situation.
   - **d.** If any adult offers you anything without asking your parent first, step away, say no, and tell someone.
   - **e.** If any adult asks for your help without asking your parent first, step away, say no, and tell someone.
   - **f.** If any adult asks you to keep a secret, say no and step away, say no, and tell someone.
   - **g.** Do not help anyone look for a lost dog or cat and do not accept candy or gifts from a stranger.
   - **h.** If lost in a store, do not wander around looking for the parent; go at once to a clerk or guard.
2. Children need to learn their full name, address, parents' names and phone numbers.
3. Watch for post-traumatic stress disorder in any child who has experienced an abduction.

X. Child Abuse

A. Description

1. Abuse is the nonaccidental physical injury or the nonaccidental act of omission of care by a parent or person responsible for a child; abuse comprises neglect and physical, sexual, and emotional maltreatment.
2. Neglect can be in the form of physical or emotional neglect and involves the deprivation of basic needs, supervision, medical care, or education and failure to meet a child's needs for attention and affection.
3. Sexual abuse can involve incest, molestation, exhibitionism, pornography, prostitution, or pedophilia; findings associated with sexual abuse may not be easily apparent in a child.
4. Shaken baby syndrome is caused by the violent shaking of an infant and results in intracranial (usually subdural hemorrhage) trauma; this can lead to cerebral edema and death.

B. Assessment (Box 67-9)

C. Interventions

1. Support the child during a thorough physical assessment.

BOX 67-9 Child Neglect and Abuse: Assessment Findings

Neglect
- Inadequate weight gain
- Poor hygiene
- Consistent hunger
- Inconsistent school attendance
- Constant fatigue
- Reports of lack of child supervision
- Delinquency

Physical Abuse
- Unexplained bruises, burns, or fractures
- Bald spots on the scalp
- Apprehensive child
- Extreme aggressiveness (typically boys) or withdrawal (typically girls)
- Fear of parents
- Lack of crying (older infant, toddler, or young preschool child) when approached by a stranger
- Spiral fractures without history of trauma from a sports injury
- Poor performance in school

Emotional Abuse
- Speech disorders
- Habit disorders such as sucking, biting, and rocking
- Psychoneurotic reactions
- Learning disorders
- Suicide attempts

Sexual Abuse
- Difficulty walking or sitting
- Torn, stained, or bloody underclothing
- Pain, swelling, or itching of genitals
- Deformities, bruises, bleeding, or lacerations in genital or anal area
- Unwillingness to change clothes or unwillingness to participate in gym activities
- Poor peer relations
- Poor performance in school

Shaken Baby Syndrome
- External signs of trauma are usually absent
- Ophthalmoscopic examination reveals retinal hemorrhages
- Full bulging fontanels and head circumference greater than expected

2. Assess injuries.
3. If shaken baby syndrome is suspected, monitor the infant for a decrease in level of consciousness, which can indicate increased intracranial pressure (ICP).
4. Report a case of suspected abuse; nurses are legally required to report all cases of suspected child abuse to the appropriate local or state agency.
5. Place the child in an environment that is safe, preventing further injury.
6. Document information related to the suspected abuse in an objective manner.
7. Assess parents' strengths and weaknesses, normal coping mechanisms, and presence or absence of support systems.
8. Assist the family in identifying stressors, support systems, and resources.
9. Refer the family to appropriate support groups.

Nurses are legally required to report all cases of suspected child abuse or elder abuse to the appropriate local or state agency; state laws and procedures may vary and are always followed.

XI. Latchkey Children

A. Description
1. Children who do not have adult supervision before or after school hours; they are left to care for themselves during these times.
2. Occurs when children are members of a single-parent family or when both parents work and need to leave the home before children are brought to school or arrive home after the children
3. This situation induces a stress-provoking environment for the children and places the children at risk for an unsafe situation, injury, and delinquent behavior.

B. Interventions
1. Identify the latchkey child.
2. Encourage the parent to teach the child about self-care and self-help skills.
3. Assist the parent to identify possible alternatives to leaving the child alone.
4. Inform the parent about available community resources such as after-school programs for children.

XII. Abuse of the Older Adult

A. Description
1. Abuse of an older adult involves physical, emotional, or sexual abuse; neglect; and economic exploitation.
2. Older adults at most risk include individuals who are dependent because of illness, immobility, or altered mental status.
3. Factors that contribute to abuse and neglect include long-standing family violence, caregiver stress, and the older adult's increasing dependence on others.
4. Victims may attempt to dismiss injuries as accidental, and abusers may prevent victims from receiving proper medical care to avoid discovery.
5. Victims often are isolated socially by their abusers.

B. Assessment
1. Physical abuse
   a. Sprains, dislocations, or fractures
   b. Abrasions, bruises, or lacerations
   c. Pressure sores
   d. Puncture wounds
   e. Burns
   f. Skin tears
2. Sexual abuse
   a. Torn or stained underclothing
   b. Discomfort or bleeding in the genital area
   c. Difficulty in walking or sitting
   d. Unexplained genital infections or disease
3. Emotional abuse
   a. Confusion
   b. Fearfulness and agitation
   c. Changes in appetite and weight
   d. Withdrawal and loss of interest in self and social activities
4. Neglect
   a. Disheveled appearance
   b. Inadequate or inappropriate dress
   c. Dehydration and malnutrition
   d. Lack of physical needs, such as glasses, hearing aids, and dentures
5. Signs of medication overdose
6. Economic exploitation
   a. Inability to pay bills and fearful when discussing finances
   b. Confusion, inaccuracy, or no knowledge of finances

C. Interventions
1. Assess for physical injuries and treat physical injuries.
2. Ask if any injury is a result of someone harming them.
3. Report cases of suspected abuse to appropriate authorities (follow state and agency guidelines).
4. Separate the older adult from the abusive environment, if possible, and contact adult protective services for assistance in placement while the abuse is being investigated.
5. Explore alternative living arrangements that are least restrictive and disruptive to the victim.
6. The older adult who has been abused may need assistance for financial or legal matters.
7. Provide referrals to emergency community resources.
8. When working with caregivers, assess the need for respite care or counseling to deal with caregiver stress (see Priority Nursing Actions).

PRIORITY NURSING ACTIONS

Physical Abuse of an Older Client

1. Assess and treat the wounds.
2. Ensure that the victim is removed from the threatening environment.
3. Adhere to mandatory abuse reporting laws.
4. Notify the caseworker of the situation.
5. Document the occurrence, findings, actions taken, and the victim's response.

Reference

Varcarolis (2017), pp. 344-345.

XIII. Rape and Sexual Assault

A. Description
   1. Rape is engaging another person in a sexual act or sexual intercourse through the use of force or coercion and without the consent of the sexual partner.
   2. The victim is not required by law to report the rape or assault.
   3. Often, the victim is blamed by others and receives no support from significant others.
   4. Acquaintance rape involves someone known to the victim.
   5. Statutory rape is the act of sexual intercourse with a person younger than the age of legal consent, even if the minor consents.
   6. Same-sex rape
      a. Females: Involves sexual touching, oral sex, or penetration with a finger or some other object
      b. Males: Same as for females; often experience stigma when seeking help
      c. See https://www.cdc.gov/violenceprevention/nisvs/index.html for more information.
   7. Marital rape
      a. The belief that marriage bestows rights to sex whenever wanted and without consent of the partner contributes to the occurrence of marital rape.
      b. Victims of marital rape describe being forced to perform acts they did not wish to perform and being physically abused during sex.

B. Assessment
   1. Female client
      a. Obtain the date of the last menstrual period.
      b. Determine the form of birth control used and the last act of intercourse before rape.
      c. Determine the duration of intercourse, orifices violated, and whether penile penetration occurred.
      d. Determine whether a condom was used by the perpetrator.

C. Shame, embarrassment, and humiliation

D. Anger and revenge

E. Afraid to tell others because of fear of not being believed

F. Males may be sexually abused as children and as adults and are the usual targeted victim of pedophiles; males may have more difficulty with disclosing their abuse.

G. Rape trauma syndrome
   1. Sleep disturbances, nightmares
   2. Loss of appetite
   3. Fears, anxiety, phobias, suspicion
   4. Decrease in activities and motivation
   5. Disruptions in relationships with partner, family, friends
   6. Self-blame, guilt, shame
   7. Lowered self-esteem, feelings of worthlessness
   8. Somatic complaints
   9. See Chapter 65 for information on post-traumatic stress disorder.

H. Interventions
   1. Perform the assessment in a quiet, private area.
   2. Referral to SADV nurse as appropriate
   3. Stay with the victim and provide client safety.
   4. Assess the client for physical injuries. Treat as appropriate.
   5. Assess the victim's stress level before performing treatments and procedures.
   6. Victim should not shower, bathe, douche (female), or change clothing until an examination is performed.
   7. Obtain written consent for the examination, photographs, laboratory tests, release of information, and laboratory samples.
   8. Assist with the female pelvic examination and obtain specimens to detect semen (the pelvic examination may trigger a flashback of the attack); a shower and fresh clothing should be made available to the client after the examination.
   9. Preserve any evidence.
   10. Treat physical injuries and provide client safety.
   11. Administer prescribed medications.
   12. Document all events in the care of the victim.
   13. Reinforce to the victim that surviving the assault is most important; if the victim survived the rape, she or he did exactly what was necessary to stay alive.
   14. Refer the victim to crisis intervention and support groups.

PRACTICE QUESTIONS

827. The nurse observes that a client with a potential for violence is agitated, pacing up and down the hallway, and making aggressive and belligerent gestures at other clients. Which statement would be **most appropriate** to make to this client?

1. "You need to stop that behavior now."
2. "You will need to be placed in seclusion."

3. "You seem restless; tell me what is happening."
4. "You will need to be restrained if you do not change your behavior."

828. The nurse is reviewing the assessment data of a client admitted to the mental health unit. The nurse notes that the admission nurse documented the client is experiencing anxiety as a result of a situational crisis. The nurse plans care for the client, determining that this type of crisis could be caused by which event?
1. Witnessing a murder
2. The death of a loved one
3. A fire that destroyed the client's home
4. A recent rape episode experienced by the client

829. The nurse is conducting an initial assessment of a client in crisis. When assessing the client's perception of the precipitating event that led to the crisis, which is the **most appropriate** question?
1. "With whom do you live?"
2. "Who is available to help you?"
3. "What leads you to seek help now?"
4. "What do you usually do to feel better?"

830. The nurse is creating a plan of care for a client in a crisis state. When developing the plan, the nurse should consider which factor?
1. A crisis state indicates that the client has a mental illness.
2. A crisis state indicates that the client has an emotional illness.
3. Presenting symptoms in a crisis situation are similar for all clients experiencing a crisis.
4. A client's response to a crisis is individualized and what constitutes a crisis for one client may not constitute a crisis for another client.

831. The nurse in the emergency department is caring for a young female victim of sexual assault. The client's physical assessment is complete, and physical evidence has been collected. The nurse notes that the client is withdrawn, distracted, tremulous, and bewildered at times. How should the nurse interpret these behaviors?
1. Signs of depression
2. Reactions to a devastating event
3. Evidence that the client is a high suicide risk
4. Indicative of the need for hospital admission

832. A depressed client on an inpatient unit says to the nurse, "My family would be better off without me." Which is the nurse's **best** response?
1. "Have you talked to your family about this?"
2. "Everyone feels this way when they are depressed."
3. "You will feel better once your medication begins to work."
4. "You sound very upset. Are you thinking of hurting yourself?"

833. The nurse has been closely observing a client who has been displaying aggressive behaviors. The nurse observes that the behavior displayed by the client is escalating. Which nursing intervention is **most** helpful to this client at this time? **Select all that apply.**
- ❑ 1. Initiate confinement measures.
- ❑ 2. Acknowledge the client's behavior.
- ❑ 3. Assist the client to an area that is quiet.
- ❑ 4. Maintain a safe distance from the client.
- ❑ 5. Allow the client to take control of the situation.

834. Which behavior observed by the nurse indicates a suspicion that a depressed adolescent client may be suicidal?
1. The adolescent gives away a DVD and a cherished autographed picture of a performer.
2. The adolescent runs out of the therapy group, swearing at the group leader, and to her room.
3. The adolescent becomes angry while speaking on the telephone and slams down the receiver.
4. The adolescent gets angry with her roommate when the roommate borrows the client's clothes without asking.

835. The police arrive at the emergency department with a client who has lacerated both wrists. Which is the **initial** nursing action?
1. Administer an antianxiety agent.
2. Assess and treat the wound sites.
3. Secure and record a detailed history.
4. Encourage and assist the client to ventilate feelings.

836. A moderately depressed client who was hospitalized 2 days ago suddenly begins smiling and reporting that the crisis is over. The client says to the nurse, "I'm finally cured." Based on the client's behavior and statement, which intervention should the nurse include in the plan?
1. Suggesting a reduction of medication
2. Allowing increased "in-room" activities
3. Increasing the level of suicide precautions
4. Allowing the client off-unit privileges as needed

837. The nurse is planning care for a client being admitted to the nursing unit who attempted suicide. Which **priority** nursing intervention should the nurse include in the plan of care?
1. One-to-one suicide precautions
2. Suicide precautions with 30-minute checks
3. Checking the whereabouts of the client every 15 minutes
4. Asking the client to report suicidal thoughts immediately

838. The emergency department nurse is caring for an adult client who is a victim of family violence. Which **priority** information should be included in the discharge instructions?
1. Information regarding shelters
2. Instructions regarding calling the police
3. Instructions regarding self-defense classes
4. Explaining the importance of leaving the violent situation

839. A female victim of a sexual assault is being seen in the crisis center. The client states that she still feels "as though the rape just happened yesterday," even though it has been a few months since the incident. Which is the **most appropriate** nursing response?
1. "You need to try to be realistic. The rape did not just occur."
2. "It will take some time to get over these feelings about your rape."
3. "Tell me more about the incident that causes you to feel like the rape just occurred."
4. "What do you think that you can do to alleviate some of your fears about being raped again?"

840. A client is admitted to the mental health unit after an attempted suicide by hanging. The nurse can **best** ensure client safety by which action?
1. Requesting that a peer remain with the client at all times.
2. Removing the client's clothing and placing the client in a hospital gown.
3. Assigning to the client a staff member who will remain with the client at all times.
4. Admitting the client to a seclusion room where all potentially dangerous articles are removed.

841. A client is admitted with a recent history of severe anxiety following a home invasion and robbery. During the initial assessment interview, which statement by the client should indicate to the nurse the possible diagnosis of post-traumatic stress disorder? **Select all that apply.**
- ☐ 1. "I'm afraid of spiders."
- ☐ 2. "I keep reliving the robbery."
- ☐ 3. "I see his face everywhere I go."
- ☐ 4. "I don't want anything to eat now."
- ☐ 5. "I might have died over a few dollars in my pocket."
- ☐ 6. "I have to wash my hands over and over again many times."

ANSWERS

827. *Answer:* 3
Rationale: The most appropriate statement is to ask the client what is causing the agitation. This will assist the client to become aware of the behavior and may assist the nurse in planning appropriate interventions for the client. Option 1 is demanding behavior that could cause increased agitation in the client. Options 2 and 4 are threats to the client and are inappropriate.
Test-Taking Strategy: Note the strategic words, *most appropriate.* Eliminate option 1 because of the demand that it places on the client. Eliminate options 2 and 4 because they indicate threats to the client.
Level of Cognitive Ability: Applying
Client Needs: Psychosocial Integrity
Integrated Process: Communication and Documentation
Content Area: Mental Health
Health Problem: Mental Health: Abusive Behaviors
Priority Concepts: Anxiety; Communication
Reference: Varcarolis (2017), pp. 140, 143.

828. *Answer:* 2
Rationale: A situational crisis arises from external rather than internal sources. External situations that could precipitate a crisis include loss or change of a job, the death of a loved one, abortion, change in financial status, divorce, addition of new family members, pregnancy, and severe illness. Options 1, 3, and 4 identify adventitious crises. An adventitious crisis refers to a crisis of disaster, is not a part of everyday life, and is unplanned and accidental. Adventitious crises may result from a natural disaster (e.g., floods, fires, tornadoes, earthquakes), a national disaster (e.g., war, riots, airplane crashes), or a crime of violence (e.g., rape, assault, murder in the workplace or school, bombings, or spousal or child abuse).
Test-Taking Strategy: Note the subject, situational crisis. Recall that this type of crisis arises from an external source, is often unanticipated, and is associated with a life event that upsets an individual's or group's psychological equilibrium. This will direct you to the correct option.
Level of Cognitive Ability: Applying
Client Needs: Psychosocial Integrity
Integrated Process: Nursing Process—Planning
Content Area: Mental Health
Health Problem: Mental Health: Anxiety Disorder
Priority Concepts: Anxiety; Coping
Reference: Varcarolis (2017), pp. 325-326.

829. *Answer:* 3
Rationale: The nurse's initial task when assessing a client in crisis is to assess the individual or family and the problem. The

more clearly the problem can be defined, the better the chance a solution can be found. The correct option would assist in determining data related to the precipitating event that led to the crisis. Options 1 and 2 assess situational supports. Option 4 assesses personal coping skills.
Test-Taking Strategy: Note the strategic words, *most appropriate*. Also note the subject, assessment techniques for the client in crisis, and note the words *precipitating event* and *led to the crisis*. Eliminate options 1 and 2, because these data would determine support systems. Eliminate option 4, because this question would be asked when determining coping skills.
Level of Cognitive Ability: Analyzing
Client Needs: Psychosocial Integrity
Integrated Process: Nursing Process—Assessment
Content Area: Mental Health
Health Problem: Mental Health: Crisis
Priority Concepts: Anxiety; Coping
Reference: Varcarolis (2017), pp. 327-329.

830. *Answer:* 4
Rationale: Although each crisis response can be described in similar terms as far as presenting symptoms are concerned, what constitutes a crisis for one client may not constitute a crisis for another client, because each is a unique individual. Being in the crisis state does not mean that the client has a mental or emotional illness.
Test-Taking Strategy: Eliminate option 3 because of the closed-ended word "all." Next, eliminate options 1 and 2, because a crisis does not indicate "illness."
Level of Cognitive Ability: Creating
Client Needs: Psychosocial Integrity
Integrated Process: Nursing Process—Planning
Content Area: Mental Health
Health Problem: Mental Health: Crisis
Priority Concepts: Caregiving; Coping
Reference: Varcarolis (2017), p. 329.

831. *Answer:* 2
Rationale: During the acute phase of the rape crisis, the client can display a wide range of emotional and somatic responses. The symptoms noted indicate an expected reaction. Options 1, 3, and 4 are incorrect interpretations.
Test-Taking Strategy: Note the subject, client response to a crisis. Use knowledge regarding client responses to devastating events and focus on the symptoms noted in the question to direct you to the correct option.
Level of Cognitive Ability: Analyzing
Client Needs: Psychosocial Integrity
Integrated Process: Nursing Process—Assessment
Content Area: Mental Health
Health Problem: Mental Health: Crisis
Priority Concepts: Caregiving; Coping
Reference: Varcarolis (2017), pp. 354-355.

832. *Answer:* 4
Rationale: Clients who are depressed may be at risk for suicide. It is critical for the nurse to assess suicidal ideation and plan. The nurse should ask the client directly whether a plan for self-harm exists. Options 1, 2, and 3 do not deal directly with the client's feelings.
Test-Taking Strategy: Note the strategic word, *best*. Recalling therapeutic communication techniques will assist in directing you to the correct option. Option 4 is the only option that deals directly with the client's feelings. In addition, clients at risk for suicide need to be assessed directly regarding the potential for self-harm.
Level of Cognitive Ability: Applying
Client Needs: Psychosocial Integrity
Integrated Process: Communication and Documentation
Content Area: Mental Health
Health Problem: Mental Health: Suicide
Priority Concepts: Clinical Judgment; Safety
Reference: Varcarolis (2017), pp. 207, 367-368.

833. *Answer:* 2, 3, 4
Rationale: During the escalation period, the client's behavior is moving toward loss of control. Nursing actions include taking control, maintaining a safe distance, acknowledging behavior, moving the client to a quiet area, and medicating the client if appropriate. To initiate confinement measures during this period is inappropriate. Initiation of confinement measures, if needed, is most appropriate during the crisis period.
Test-Taking Strategy: Focus on the strategic word, *most*, and focus on the subject, the most helpful nursing interventions. Also note the words *aggressive behaviors* and *escalating*. Recalling that, during the escalation period, the client's behavior is moving toward loss of control and that the least restrictive measures should be used will direct you to the correct options.
Level of Cognitive Ability: Analyzing
Client Needs: Psychosocial Integrity
Integrated Process: Nursing Process—Implementation
Content Area: Mental Health
Health Problem: Mental Health: Violence
Priority Concepts: Clinical Judgment; Safety
Reference: Varcarolis (2017), pp. 379-380.

834. *Answer:* 1
Rationale: A depressed suicidal client often gives away that which is of value as a way of saying goodbye and wanting to be remembered. Options 2, 3, and 4 deal with anger and acting-out behaviors that are often typical of an adolescent.
Test-Taking Strategy: Eliminate options 2, 3, and 4 because they are comparable or alike. The correct option is different and is an action that could indicate that the client may be "saying goodbye."
Level of Cognitive Ability: Analyzing
Client Needs: Psychosocial Integrity
Integrated Process: Nursing Process—Assessment
Content Area: Mental Health
Health Problem: Mental Health: Suicide
Priority Concepts: Mood and Affect; Safety
Reference: Varcarolis (2017), p. 366.

835. *Answer:* 2
Rationale: The initial nursing action is to assess and treat the self-inflicted injuries. Injuries from lacerated wrists can lead to a life-threatening situation. Other interventions, such as options 1, 3, and 4, may follow after the client has been treated medically.
Test-Taking Strategy: Note the strategic word, *initial*. Use Maslow's Hierarchy of Needs theory to prioritize.

Physiological needs come first. The correct option addresses the physiological need.
Level of Cognitive Ability: Applying
Client Needs: Physiological Integrity
Integrated Process: Nursing Process—Implementation
Content Area: Complex Care: Emergency Situations: Management
Health Problem: Mental Health—Suicide
Priority Concepts: Caregiving; Safety
Reference: Varcarolis (2017), p. 367.

836. *Answer:* 3
Rationale: A client who is moderately depressed and has only been in the hospital 2 days is unlikely to have such a dramatic cure. When a depression suddenly lifts, it is likely that the client may have made the decision to harm herself or himself. Suicide precautions are necessary to keep the client safe. The remaining options are therefore incorrect interpretations.
Test-Taking Strategy: Focus on the **subject**, suicide precautions. Options 1 and 4 support the client's notion that a cure has occurred. Option 2 allows the client to increase self-isolation and would present a threat to the client's safety. Knowing that safety is of the utmost importance will direct you to the correct option.
Level of Cognitive Ability: Analyzing
Client Needs: Safe and Effective Care Environment
Integrated Process: Nursing Process—Planning
Content Area: Mental Health
Health Problem: Mental Health: Mood Disorders
Priority Concepts: Caregiving; Safety
Reference: Varcarolis (2017), pp. 369-370.

837. *Answer:* 1
Rationale: One-to-one suicide precautions are required for a client who has attempted suicide. Options 2 and 3 may be appropriate, but not at the present time, considering the situation. Option 4 also may be an appropriate nursing intervention, but the priority is identified in the correct option. The best intervention is constant supervision so that the nurse may intervene as needed if the client attempts to harm herself or himself.
Test-Taking Strategy: Focus on the **strategic word**, *priority*, noting the words *attempted suicide*. The correct option is the only one that provides a safe environment.
Level of Cognitive Ability: Applying
Client Needs: Safe and Effective Care Environment
Integrated Process: Nursing Process—Implementation
Content Area: Complex Care: Emergency Situations: Management
Health Problem: Mental Health: Suicide
Priority Concepts: Caregiving; Safety
Reference: Varcarolis (2017), pp. 369.

838. *Answer:* 1
Rationale: Tertiary prevention of family violence includes assisting the victim after the abuse has already occurred. The nurse should provide the client with information regarding where to obtain help, including a specific plan for removing the self from the abuser and information regarding escape, hotlines, and the location of shelters. An abused person is usually reluctant to call the police. Teaching the victim to fight back is not the appropriate action for the victim when dealing with a violent person. Explaining the importance of leaving the violent situation is important, but a specific plan is necessary.
Test-Taking Strategy: Note the **strategic word**, *priority*. Focus on the **subject** of the question, which relates to providing the client with a safe environment. The correct option provides a specific plan for safety.
Level of Cognitive Ability: Applying
Client Needs: Safe and Effective Care Environment
Integrated Process: Nursing Process—Implementation
Content Area: Mental Health
Health Problem: Mental Health: Violence
Priority Concepts: Interpersonal Violence; Safety
Reference: Varcarolis (2017), pp. 330-331, 343.

839. *Answer:* 3
Rationale: The correct option allows the client to express her ideas and feelings more fully and portrays a nonhurried, nonjudgmental, supportive attitude on the part of the nurse. Clients need to be reassured that their feelings are normal and that they may express their concerns freely in a safe, caring environment. Option 1 immediately blocks communication. Option 2 places the client's feelings on hold. Option 4 places the problem solving totally on the client.
Test-Taking Strategy: Note the **strategic words**, *most appropriate*. Also, focus on the **subject**, that the client feels that the rape just happened yesterday. Use **therapeutic communication techniques**. The correct option is the only one that addresses the client's feelings. Always address the client's feelings first.
Level of Cognitive Ability: Applying
Client Needs: Psychosocial Integrity
Integrated Process: Caring
Content Area: Mental Health
Health Problem: Mental Health: Therapeutic Communication
Priority Concepts: Communication; Coping
Reference: Varcarolis (2017), p. 355.

840. *Answer:* 3
Rationale: Hanging is a serious suicide attempt. The plan of care must reflect action that ensures the client's safety. Constant observation status (one-to-one) with a staff member is the best choice. Placing the client in a hospital gown and requesting that a peer remain with the client would not ensure a safe environment. Seclusion should not be the initial intervention, and the least restrictive measure should be used.
Test-Taking Strategy: Note the **strategic word**, *best*. Focus on the **subject**, care of the client at risk for suicide. Eliminate option 4, because seclusion should not be the initial intervention. Eliminate option 1 next, because safeguarding a client is not the peer's responsibility. Eliminate option 2, because removing one's clothing would not maximize all possible safety strategies.
Level of Cognitive Ability: Applying
Client Needs: Safe and Effective Care Environment
Integrated Process: Nursing Process—Implementation
Content Area: Mental Health
Health Problem: Mental Health: Suicide
Priority Concepts: Caregiving; Safety
Reference: Varcarolis (2017), p. 367.

841. *Answer:* 2, 3, 5
Rationale: Reliving an event, experiencing emotional numbness (facing possible death), and having flashbacks of the

event (seeing the same face everywhere) are all common occurrences with post-traumatic stress disorder. The statement "I'm afraid of spiders" relates more to having a phobia. The statement "I have to wash my hands over and over again many times" describes ritual compulsive behaviors to decrease anxiety for someone with obsessive-compulsive disorder. Stating "I don't want anything to eat now" is vague and could relate to numerous conditions.

Test-Taking Strategy: Focus on the subject, post-traumatic stress disorder. There is no indication about a fear of spiders being part of the problem. There is no information in the question to support that the client has ritual behaviors. The client stating that they do not want anything to eat at the time is not relevant to this client's situation. Responses 2, 3, and 5 all indicate that the client is experiencing post-traumatic stress disorder from a recent home invasion and robbery event.

Level of Cognitive Ability: Analyzing
Client Needs: Safe and Effective Care Environment
Integrated Process: Nursing Process—Assessment
Content Area: Mental Health
Health Problem: Mental Health: Post-Traumatic Stress Disorder
Priority Concepts: Anxiety; Coping
Reference: Varcarolis (2017), p. 123.

CHAPTER 68

Psychiatric Medications

PRIORITY CONCEPTS Anxiety; Mood and Affect

I. Selective Serotonin Reuptake Inhibitors (SSRIs) (Box 68-1)

A. Description
1. Inhibit serotonin uptake and elicit an antidepressant response
2. Effective for depression with anxiety features as well as depression with psychomotor agitation
3. Relatively low side-effect profile compared with older antidepressants (tricyclics)
4. Do not create anticholinergic effects, dry mouth, blurred vision, or urinary retention
5. May interact with other medications (e.g., digoxin, warfarin).
6. The potential for medication interactions is greatest when administered with second serotonin-enhancing agent, such as a monoamine oxidase inhibitor (MAOI). A complete medication assessment must be obtained and evaluated; inquire about the use of herbal therapies, especially St. John's wort.

B. Side and adverse effects
1. Dry mouth
2. Blood pressure changes
3. Insomnia, somnolence (sleepy, drowsy), apathy
4. Nervousness
5. Weight loss or gain
6. Decreased libido
7. Apathy
8. Tremors
9. Seizure activity
10. Potential toxic effects (too high dose or interaction with other drugs)
    a. Abdominal pain, diarrhea
    b. Sweating, fever
    c. Tachycardia, elevated blood pressure
    d. Altered mental state (delirium)
    e. Myoclonus (muscle spasms), increased motor activity

C. Interventions
1. Monitor vital signs, because SSRIs can potentially lower or elevate blood pressure.
2. May cause sexual dysfunction or lack of sex drive. Inform health care provider if this occurs.
3. Initiate safety precautions and contact the PHCP if dizziness occurs.
4. Instruct the client to avoid alcohol.
5. Administer with a snack or meal to reduce the risk of dizziness and lightheadedness.
6. Monitor the suicidal client, especially during improved mood and increased energy levels.
7. Instruct the client that taking ibuprofen with SSRIs increases the risk of an upper GI bleed.
8. For the client on long-term therapy, monitor liver and renal function test results; altered values may occur, requiring dosage adjustments.
9. Monitor white blood cell and neutrophil counts; the medication may be discontinued if levels decrease below normal.
10. Instruct to change positions slowly if experiencing a hypotensive effect.
11. Educate the client to not discontinue medication abruptly. Abrupt cessation can lead to serotonin withdrawal characterized by gastrointestinal distress, movement disorders, insomnia, and sensory disturbances.
12. Be aware of the potential for serotonin syndrome, characterized by hyperactivity or restlessness, tachycardia, fever, elevated blood pressure, altered mental status (delirium), mood swings, seizures, muscle rigidity, and abdominal pain; this risk is greatly increased when SSRIs are given with MAOIs. This medication combination needs to be avoided.
13. Instruct that over-the-counter (OTC) cold medicines may increase the likelihood of serotonin syndrome.
14. In pregnancy, consultation with an obstetrician is recommended regarding taking these medications.
15. Monitor the medication response in children, adolescents, and older adults closely, because the response may be different than in an adult client.

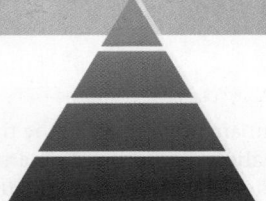

BOX 68-1 Reuptake Inhibitors

Selective Serotonin Reuptake Inhibitors
- Citalopram
- Escitalopram
- Fluoxetine
- Fluvoxamine
- Paroxetine
- Sertraline
- Vilazodone

Serotonin-Norepinephrine Reuptake Inhibitors
- Desvenlafaxine
- Duloxetine
- Levomilnacipran
- Venlafaxine

Atypical Antidepressants
- Bupropion
- Mirtazapine
- Nefazodone
- Trazodone
- Vortioxetine

16. Encourage psychotherapy.
17. Serotonin-norepinephrine reuptake inhibitors (SNRI) are similar to SSRIs, but they also work by blocking the effects of norepinephrine in addition to serotonin. Considerations are similar to that of SSRIs.

II. Tricyclic Antidepressants (Box 68-2)

A. Description
1. Block the reuptake of norepinephrine and serotonin at the presynaptic junction; used to treat depression
2. Also affect other neurotransmitters, leading to a number of side effects
3. May reduce seizure threshold
4. May reduce effectiveness of antihypertensive agents
5. Concurrent use with alcohol or antihistamines can cause CNS depression.

BOX 68-2 Tricyclic Antidepressants

- Amitriptyline
- Amoxapine
- Clomipramine
- Desipramine
- Doxepin
- Imipramine
- Nortriptyline
- Protriptyline
- Trimipramine

6. Concurrent use with MAOIs can cause hypertensive crisis.
7. Cardiac toxicity can occur, and all clients should receive an electrocardiogram (ECG) before treatment and periodically thereafter.
8. Overdose is life-threatening, necessitating immediate treatment (see Priority Nursing Actions).
9. The tricyclic antidepressant clomipramine may be used to treat obsessive-compulsive disorder.

PRIORITY NURSING ACTIONS

Tricyclic Antidepressant Overdose

1. Check airway and maintain a patent airway.
2. Administer oxygen and ventilation (as required).
3. Check vital signs and cardiac monitoring.
4. Obtain an electrocardiogram.
5. Prepare for gastric lavage with activated charcoal if within 2 hours of ingestion.
6. Administer intravenous fluids as prescribed.
7. Prepare to administer medications as prescribed to reverse the effects of the tricyclic antidepressant.
8. Document the event, actions taken, and the client's response.

Reference

Varcarolis (2017), p. 303.

B. Side and adverse effects
1. Anticholinergic effects: Dry mouth, difficulty voiding, dilated pupils and blurred vision, decreased gastrointestinal motility, constipation
2. Urinary retention
3. Cardiovascular disturbances such as tachycardia or dysrhythmias; orthostatic hypotension
4. Sedation
5. Seizures (with bupropion)
6. Weight gain or weight loss
7. Anxiety, restlessness, irritability, confusion
8. Decreased or increased libido with ejaculatory and erection disturbances
9. Symptoms of tricyclic antidepressant (TCA) toxicity
   a. Tardive dyskinesia: involuntary movement of the face and jaw
   b. Akinesia: loss of voluntary muscle movement
   c. Akathisia: state of agitation, distress, and restlessness
   d. Pseudoparkinsonism

C. Interventions
1. Monitor the suicidal client, especially during improved mood and increased energy levels.
2. Instruct the client to change positions slowly to avoid a hypotensive effect.
3. Monitor pattern of daily bowel activity.
4. Assess for urinary retention.

5. For the client on long-term therapy, monitor liver and renal function test results.
6. Administer with food or milk if gastrointestinal distress occurs.
7. Administer the entire daily oral dose preferably at bedtime because of the sedative effect. Do not split doses, such as taking half in the morning and half in the evening.
8. Instruct the client to avoid alcohol and nonprescription medications to prevent adverse medication interactions.
9. Instruct the client to avoid driving and other activities requiring alertness until the response is known; sedation is expected in early therapy and may subside with time.
10. When the medication is discontinued by the primary health care provider (PHCP), it should be tapered gradually.
11. The potential for medication interactions with OTC cold medications exists.
12. Encourage oral hygiene and the use of hard candies and mouth rinses to relieve dry mouth.
13. Encourage psychotherapy.

⚠ Inform the client that antidepressant medication may take several weeks to produce the desired effect (client response may not occur until 2 to 4 weeks after the first dose).

III. Monoamine Oxidase Inhibitors (MAOIs) (Box 68-3)

A. Description
1. Inhibit the enzyme monoamine oxidase, which is present in the brain, blood platelets, liver, spleen, and kidneys
2. Monoamine oxidase metabolizes amines (dopamine, tyramine), norepinephrine, and serotonin, so the concentration of these amines increases with MAOIs.
3. Clients who have depression and have not responded to other antidepressant therapies, including electroconvulsive therapy, may be given MAOIs. These medications are not the first choice because of other available medications and the possible serious side and adverse effects that can occur.
4. Concurrent use with amphetamines, antidepressants, dopamine, epinephrine, levodopa/carbidopa, nasal decongestants, norepinephrine, tyramine-containing foods, or vasoconstrictors may cause hypertensive crisis.
5. Concurrent use with opioid analgesics may cause hypertension or hypotension, coma, or seizures.

BOX 68-3 Monoamine Oxidase Inhibitors (MAOIs)

- Isocarboxazid
- Phenelzine (not approved for use in Canada)
- Selegiline
- Tranylcypromine

B. Side and adverse effects
1. Orthostatic hypotension
2. Changes in cardiac rate and rhythm
3. Restlessness
4. Insomnia
5. Dizziness and vertigo
6. Weakness, lethargy
7. Gastrointestinal upset or constipation
8. Urinary hesitancy
9. Dry mouth
10. Weight gain
11. Peripheral edema
12. Anticholinergic effects
13. CNS stimulation (anxiety, agitation, mania)
14. Sexual dysfunction

C. Hypertensive crisis
1. Hypertension
2. Occipital headache radiating frontally
3. Neck stiffness and soreness
4. Nausea and vomiting
5. Sweating
6. Fever and chills
7. Clammy skin
8. Dilated pupils
9. Palpitations, tachycardia, or bradycardia
10. Constricting chest pain
11. Antidote for hypertensive crisis: Phentolamine by intravenous injection

D. Interventions
1. Monitor blood pressure frequently for hypertension.
2. Monitor for signs of hypertensive crisis.
3. If palpitations or frequent headaches occur, withhold the medication and notify the PHCP.
4. Administer with food if gastrointestinal distress occurs.
5. Instruct the client that the medication effect may be noted during the first week of therapy, but maximum benefit may take 3 weeks.
6. Instruct the client to report headache, neck stiffness, or neck soreness immediately.
7. Instruct the client to change positions slowly to prevent orthostatic hypotension.
8. Instruct the client to avoid caffeine or OTC preparations such as weight-reducing pills or medications for hay fever and colds.
9. Monitor compliance with medication administration.
10. Instruct the client that she or he may take a missed dose within 3 hours of the scheduled time; otherwise, the client should skip the missed dose and take the next dose at the scheduled time.

11. Instruct the client to carry a MedicAlert card indicating that an MAOI medication is being taken.
12. Avoid administering the medication in the evening, because insomnia may result.
13. When the medication is discontinued by the PHCP, it should be discontinued gradually.
14. Instruct the client to avoid foods that require bacteria or molds for their preparation or preservation and foods that contain tyramine (Fig. 68-1; Box 68-4).

Teach the client about foods that contain tyramine. Consuming tyramine-containing foods when taking an MAOI can cause hypertensive crisis.

IV. Mood Stabilizers (Box 68-5)

A. Description: Affect cellular transport mechanism and enhance serotonin or γ-aminobutyric acid (GABA) function, or both, which are associated with mood

B. Lithium

1. Concurrent use with diuretics, fluoxetine, or nonsteroidal antiinflammatory drugs increases lithium reabsorption by the kidneys or inhibits lithium excretion, either of which increases the risk of lithium toxicity.
2. Acetazolamide, theophylline, phenothiazines, or sodium bicarbonate may increase renal excretion of lithium, reducing its effectiveness.
3. The therapeutic dose is only slightly less than the amount producing toxicity.
4. The therapeutic medication serum level of lithium is 0.6 to 1.2 mEq/L (0.6 to 1.2 mmol/L); the

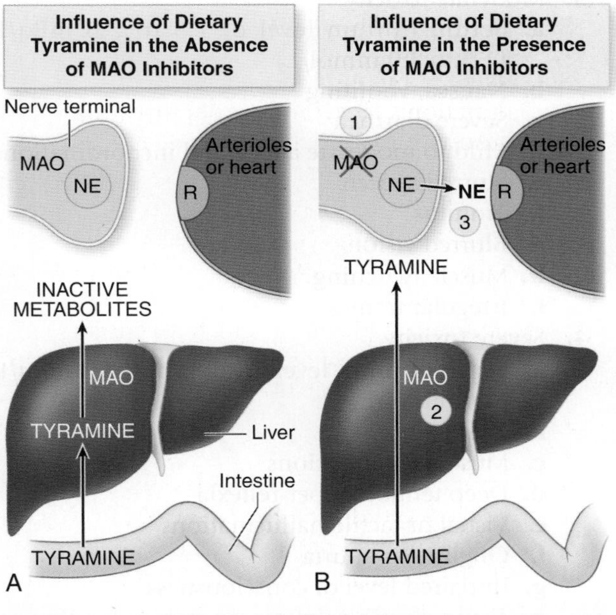

FIG. 68-1 Interaction between dietary tyramine and monoamine oxidase inhibitors (MAOIs). **A,** In the absence of MAOIs, much of the ingested tyramine is inactivated by MAO in the intestinal wall (not shown in the figure). Any dietary tyramine that is not metabolized in the intestinal wall is transported directly to the liver, where it undergoes immediate inactivation by hepatic MAO. No tyramine reaches the general circulation. **B,** Three events occur in the presence of MAOIs: (1) inhibition of neuronal MAO increases levels of norepinephrine (NE) in sympathetic nerve terminals; (2) inhibition of intestinal and hepatic MAO allows dietary tyramine to pass through the intestinal wall and liver and enter the systemic circulation intact; (3) on reaching peripheral sympathetic nerve terminals, tyramine promotes the release of accumulated NE stores, causing massive vasoconstriction and excessive stimulation of the heart. *R,* Receptor for NE.

BOX 68-4 Foods That Contain Tyramine

- Avocados
- Bananas
- Beef or chicken liver
- Brewer's yeast
- Broad beans
- Caffeine, such as in coffee, tea, or chocolate
- Cheese, especially aged, except cottage cheese
- Eggplant
- Figs
- Meat extracts and tenderizers
- Overripe fruit
- Papaya
- Pickled herring
- Raisins
- Red wine, beer, sherry
- Sauerkraut
- Sausage, bologna, pepperoni, salami
- Sour cream
- Soy sauce
- Yogurt

Note: These foods need to be avoided by the client taking an MAOI. Even a small amount of tyramine can increase the blood pressure and the force and/or rate of heart contractions.

BOX 68-5 Mood Stabilizers

Lithium Preparation

- Lithium carbonate

Other Mood Stabilizers

- Aripiprazole
- Brexpiprazole
- Carbamazepine
- Clozapine
- Gabapentin
- Lamotrigine
- Olanzapine
- Olanzapine/fluoxetine
- Oxcarbazepine
- Paliperidone
- Quetiapine
- Risperidone
- Valproate
- Ziprasidone

Mental Health

actual dose at which the therapeutic effect is achieved and the levels at which toxicity occurs are highly variable among individual clients.

5. The causes of an increase in the lithium level include decreased sodium intake; fluid and electrolyte loss associated with excessive sweating, dehydration, diarrhea, or diuretic therapy; and illness or overdose.
6. Serum lithium levels should be checked frequently after initiation of therapy and then every 1 to 2 months or whenever any behavioral change suggests an altered serum level.
7. Blood samples to check serum lithium levels should be drawn in the morning, 12 hours after the last dose was taken.
8. Lithium is classified as pregnancy category D; it crosses the placental barrier freely and has been associated with fetal toxicity.

C. Side and adverse effects

1. Polyuria
2. Polydipsia
3. Edema
4. Dysrhythmia
5. Anorexia, nausea
6. Dry mouth, mild thirst
7. Abdominal bloating
8. Soft stools or diarrhea
9. Fine hand tremors
10. Inability to concentrate
11. Muscle weakness
12. Headache
13. Hypothyroidism and goiter

D. Interventions

1. Monitor the suicidal client, especially during improved mood and increased energy levels.
2. Administer the medication with food to minimize gastrointestinal irritation.
3. Instruct the client to avoid excessive amounts of coffee, tea, or cola, which have a diuretic effect.
4. Do not administer diuretics while the client is taking lithium.
5. Instruct the client to avoid alcohol.
6. Instruct the client to avoid OTC medications.
7. Instruct the client that she or he may take a missed dose within 2 hours of the scheduled time; otherwise, the client should skip the missed dose and take the next dose at the scheduled time.
8. Instruct the client not to adjust the dosage or stop the medication without consulting the PHCP, because lithium should be tapered and not discontinued abruptly.
9. Instruct the client about the signs and symptoms of lithium toxicity.
10. Instruct the client to notify the PHCP if polyuria, prolonged vomiting, diarrhea, or fever occurs.
11. Instruct the client that the therapeutic response to the medication is noted in 1 to 3 weeks.
12. Monitor the ECG, renal function tests, and thyroid tests (ensure that these tests are performed before the start of therapy).
13. Monitor weight.

Instruct the client taking lithium to maintain a fluid intake of 6 to 8 glasses of water a day and an adequate salt intake to prevent lithium toxicity.

E. Lithium toxicity

1. Description
   a. Occurs when ingested lithium cannot be detoxified and excreted by the kidneys
   b. Symptoms of toxicity begin to appear when the serum lithium level is at 1.5 mEq/L (1.5 mmol/L).
2. Mild toxicity
   a. Serum lithium level of 1.5 mEq/L (1.5 mmol/L)
   b. Apathy
   c. Lethargy
   d. Diminished concentration
   e. Mild ataxia
   f. Coarse hand tremors
   g. Slight muscle weakness
3. Moderate toxicity
   a. Serum lithium level of 1.5 to 2.0 mEq/L (1.5 to 2.0 mmol/L)
   b. Nausea, vomiting
   c. Severe diarrhea
   d. Mild to moderate ataxia and incoordination
   e. Slurred speech
   f. Tinnitus
   g. Blurred vision
   h. Muscle twitching
   i. Irregular tremor
4. Severe toxicity
   a. Serum lithium level greater than 2.0 mEq/L (2.0 mmol/L)
   b. Nystagmus
   c. Muscle fasciculations
   d. Deep tendon hyper-reflexia
   e. Visual or tactile hallucinations
   f. Oliguria or anuria
   g. Impaired level of consciousness
   h. Tonic-clonic seizures or coma, leading to death
5. Interventions for lithium toxicity
   a. Withhold lithium and notify the PHCP.
   b. Monitor vital signs and level of consciousness.
   c. Monitor cardiac status.
   d. Prepare to obtain samples to monitor lithium, electrolyte, blood urea nitrogen, and creatinine levels and perform a complete blood cell count.
   e. Monitor for suicidal tendencies and institute suicide precautions.

V. Antianxiety or Anxiolytic Medications

A. Description
1. Antianxiety medications depress the CNS, increasing the effects of GABA, which produces relaxation and may depress the limbic system.
2. Benzodiazepines have anxiety-reducing (anxiolytic), sedative-hypnotic, muscle-relaxing, and anticonvulsant actions (Box 68-6).
3. Benzodiazepines are contraindicated in clients with acute narrow-angle glaucoma and should be used cautiously in children and older adults.
4. Benzodiazepines interact with other CNS medications, producing an additive effect, and therefore should only be considered for short-term use.
5. Abrupt withdrawal of benzodiazepines can be potentially life-threatening, and withdrawal should occur only under medical supervision.

B. Side and adverse effects
1. Daytime sedation
2. Dizziness
3. Headaches
4. Blurred or double vision
5. Hypotension
6. Tremor
7. Amnesia
8. Slurred speech
9. Constipation or diarrhea
10. Lethargy
11. Behavioral change

C. Acute toxicity
1. Somnolence
2. Confusion
3. Diminished reflexes and coma
4. Flumazenil, a benzodiazepine antagonist administered intravenously, reverses benzodiazepine intoxication in 5 minutes.
5. A client being treated for an overdose of a benzodiazepine may experience agitation, restlessness, discomfort, and anxiety.

BOX 68-6 Benzodiazepines

- Alprazolam
- Chlordiazepoxide
- Clonazepam
- Clorazepate
- Diazepam
- Lorazepam
- Midazolam
- Temazepam
- Triazolam

Nonbenzodiazepine Anxiolytic

- Buspirone

D. Interventions
1. Monitor for motor responses such as agitation, trembling, and tension.
2. Monitor for autonomic responses such as cold, clammy hands and sweating.
3. Monitor for paradoxical CNS excitement during early therapy, particularly in older adults and debilitated clients.
4. Monitor for visual disturbances, because the medications can worsen glaucoma.
5. Monitor liver and renal function test results and complete blood cell counts.
6. Reduce the medication dose as prescribed for the older adult client and for the client with impaired liver function.
7. Initiate safety precautions, because the older adult client is at risk for falling when taking the medication for sleep or anxiety.
8. Assist with ambulation if drowsiness or lightheadedness occurs.
9. Instruct the client that drowsiness usually disappears during continued therapy.
10. Instruct the client to avoid tasks that require alertness until the response to the medication is established.
11. Instruct the client to avoid alcohol.
12. Instruct the client not to take other medications without consulting the PHCP.
13. Instruct the client not to stop the medication abruptly (can result in seizure activity).

E. Withdrawal
1. To lessen withdrawal symptoms, the dosage of a benzodiazepine should be tapered gradually over 2 to 6 weeks.
2. Abrupt or too rapid withdrawal results in the following:
   a. Restlessness
   b. Irritability
   c. Insomnia
   d. Hand tremors
   e. Abdominal or muscle cramps
   f. Sweating
   g. Vomiting
   h. Seizures

VI. Barbiturates and Sedative-Hypnotics (Box 68-7)

A. Description
1. Depress the reticular activating system by promoting the inhibitory synaptic action of the neurotransmitter GABA
2. Used for short-term treatment of insomnia or for sedation to relieve anxiety, tension, and apprehension

B. Side and adverse effects
1. Dizziness and drowsiness
2. Confusion
3. Irritability

BOX 68-7 Barbiturates and Sedative-Hypnotics

Barbiturates
- Phenobarbital
- Secobarbital

Sedative-Hypnotics
- Chloral hydrate
- Eszopiclone
- Meprobamate
- Ramelteon
- Suvorexant
- Tasimelteon
- Zaleplon
- Zolpidem

4. Allergic reactions
5. Agranulocytosis
6. Thrombocytopenic purpura
7. Megaloblastic anemia

C. Overdose
1. Tachycardia
2. Hypotension
3. Cold and clammy skin
4. Dilated pupils
5. Weak and rapid pulse
6. Signs of shock
7. Depressed respirations
8. Absent reflexes
9. Coma and death may result from respiratory and cardiovascular collapse.

D. Withdrawal
1. Severe withdrawal symptoms begin within 24 hours after the medication is discontinued in an individual with severe medication dependence.
2. Gradual withdrawal is used to detoxify a dependent client.
3. Anxiety
4. Behavioral changes
5. Insomnia
6. Nightmares
7. Daytime agitation
8. Tremors
9. Delirium
10. Seizures

E. Interventions
1. Administer lower doses as prescribed for the older client.
2. Medications should be used with caution in the client who has suicidal tendencies or has a history of drug addiction.
3. Maintain safety by supervising ambulation and using side rails at night as appropriate.
4. Instruct the client to take the medication as directed.
5. Instruct the client to avoid driving or operating hazardous equipment if drowsiness, dizziness, or unsteadiness occurs.
6. Instruct the client to avoid alcohol, because this allows more medication to enter the brain, causing feelings of depression and drowsiness, dizziness, slow and difficult breathing, confusion, and coma.
7. For clients with insomnia, instruct the client to take the medication 30 minutes before bedtime; avoid taking with a large amount of food to help absorption.
8. Instruct the client that a hangover effect may occur in the morning.
9. Instruct the client not to discontinue the medication abruptly.
10. Instruct clients taking chloral hydrate to take the medication with food and a full glass of water, fruit juice, or ginger ale to prevent gastric irritation.

VII. Antipsychotic Medications (Box 68-8)

A. Description
1. Improve the thought processes and behavior of the client with psychotic symptoms, especially clients with schizophrenia
2. Affect dopamine receptors in the brain, reducing psychotic symptoms
3. Typical antipsychotics are more effective for positive symptoms of schizophrenia, such as hallucinations, aggression, and delusions; these medications also block the chemoreceptor trigger zone and vomiting center in the brain, producing an antiemetic effect.
4. Atypical antipsychotics are more effective for the negative symptoms of schizophrenia, such as avolition, apathy, and alogia.
5. The effects of antipsychotic medications are potentiated when given with other medications acting on the CNS.

B. Side and adverse effects (Box 68-9)

C. Extrapyramidal syndrome: Can include parkinsonism, dystonia, akathisia, or tardive dyskinesia (see Box 68-9)

D. Interventions
1. Monitor vital signs.
2. Monitor for symptoms of neuroleptic malignant syndrome (can occur with antipsychotic medications); refer to Section VIII.

BOX 68-8 Antipsychotic Medications

Typical Antipsychotics
- Chlorpromazine
- Fluphenazine decanoate
- Haloperidol
- Perphenazine
- Trifluoperazine

Atypical Antipsychotics
- Aripiprazole
- Asenapine
- Brexpiprazole
- Cariprazine
- Clozapine
- Lurasidone
- Olanzapine
- Paliperidone
- Pimavanserin
- Quetiapine
- Risperidone
- Ziprasidone

BOX 68-9 Side and Adverse Effects of Antipsychotic Medications

Anticholinergic Effects
- Dry mouth
- Increased heart rate
- Urinary retention
- Constipation
- Hypotension

Extrapyramidal Effects
- Parkinsonism
- Tremors
- Mask-like facies
- Rigidity
- Shuffling gait
- Dysphagia
- Drooling

Dystonias
- Abnormal or involuntary eye movements, including oculogyric crisis
- Facial grimacing
- Twisting of the torso or other muscle groups

Akathisia
- Restlessness
- Constant moving about

Tardive Dyskinesia
- Protrusion of the tongue
- Chewing motion
- Involuntary movements of the body and extremities

Other Side and Adverse Effects
- Drowsiness
- Blood dyscrasias
- Pruritus
- Photosensitivity
- Elevated blood glucose level
- Increased weight
- Impaired body temperature regulation
- Gynecomastia
- Lactation

3. Monitor urine output.
4. Monitor serum glucose level.
5. Administer the medication with food or milk to decrease gastric irritation.
6. For oral use, the liquid form might be preferred, because some clients hide tablets in their mouths to avoid taking them.
7. The absorption rate is faster with the liquid form of oral medication.
8. Avoid skin contact with the liquid concentrate to prevent contact dermatitis.
9. Protect the liquid concentrate from light.
10. Dilute the liquid concentrate with fruit juice.
11. Injectable form of risperdal consta is administered every 2 weeks for clients who have difficulty with medication adherence.
12. Inform the client that a full therapeutic effect of the medication may not be evident for 3 to 6 weeks after initiation of therapy; however, an observable therapeutic response may be apparent after 7 to 10 days.
13. Inform the client that some medications may cause a harmless change in urine color to pinkish to red-brown.
14. Instruct the client to use sunscreen, hats, and protective clothing when outdoors.
15. Instruct the client to avoid alcohol or other CNS depressants, because these substances will allow more of the medication to enter the brain, causing feelings of depression and drowsiness, dizziness, slow and difficult breathing, confusion, and coma.
16. Instruct the client to change positions slowly to avoid orthostatic hypotension.
17. Instruct the client to report signs of agranulocytosis, including sore throat, fever, and malaise.
18. Instruct the client to report signs of liver dysfunction, including jaundice, malaise, fever, and right upper abdominal pain.
19. When discontinuing antipsychotics, the medication dosage should be reduced gradually to avoid sudden recurrence of psychotic symptoms.

Monitor for extrapyramidal side and adverse effects in the client taking an antipsychotic medication.

VIII. Neuroleptic Malignant Syndrome

A. Description
1. A potentially fatal syndrome that may occur at any time during therapy with neuroleptic (antipsychotic) medications (typically with first generation antipsychotics).
2. Although rare, neuroleptic malignant syndrome more commonly occurs at the initiation of therapy, after the client has changed from one medication to another, after a dosage increase, or when a combination of medications is used.

B. Assessment
1. Dyspnea or tachypnea
2. Tachycardia or irregular pulse rate
3. Autonomic dysfunction
   a. Hyperpyrexia
   b. Hypertension
   c. Tachycardia
   d. Tachypnea
   e. Diaphoresis
   f. Drooling

4. High or low blood pressure
5. Excessive weakness or fatigue
6. Altered level of consciousness
7. Seizures
8. Severe extrapyramidal side and adverse effects
9. Skeletal muscle rigidity
10. Difficulty swallowing
11. Oculogyric crisis
12. Elevated white blood cell count, liver function results, and creatine phosphokinase level

C. Interventions
1. Notify the PHCP.
2. Monitor vital signs.
3. Initiate safety and seizure precautions.
4. Prepare to discontinue the medication.
5. Monitor level of consciousness.
6. Administer antipyretics as prescribed.
7. Use a cooling blanket to lower the body temperature.
8. Monitor electrolyte levels and administer fluids intravenously as prescribed.
9. Monitor for complications such as deep vein thrombosis (DVT) and rhabdomyolysis.

IX. Medications to Treat Attention-Deficit/Hyperactivity Disorder (Box 68-10)

A. Children with attention-deficit/hyperactivity disorder may require medication to reduce hyperactive behavior and lengthen attention span.
B. Medications that are most effective in controlling this disorder are CNS stimulants.
C. CNS stimulants, which increase agitation and activity in adults, have a calming effect on children with attention-deficit/hyperactivity disorder and increase alertness and sensitivity to stimuli.
D. Side and adverse effects
1. Tachycardia
2. Anorexia and weight loss
3. Elevated blood pressure
4. Dizziness
5. Agitation

E. Interventions
1. Monitor for CNS side and adverse effects.
2. Obtain a baseline ECG.
3. Monitor the blood pressure.
4. Instruct the child and parents that OTC medications need to be avoided.
5. Instruct the child and parents that the last dose of the day should be taken at least 6 hours before bedtime (14 hours for extended-release forms) to prevent insomnia.
6. Monitor height and weight (particularly in children).
7. Reinforce that several weeks of therapy may be necessary before the therapeutic effect is noted.
8. Instruct the client and parents that a medication-free period may be prescribed to demonstrate the continued need for the medication, and temporarily remove side effects of the medication, which commonly include sleep delay, appetite suppression, and tolerance to treatment.

BOX 68-10 Medications to Treat Attention-Deficit/Hyperactivity Disorder

- Amphetamine
- Atomoxetine
- Dexmethylphenidate
- Dextroamphetamine
- Dextroamphetamine and amphetamine
- Guanfacine
- Lisdexamfetamine
- Methylphenidate

X. Medications to Treat Alzheimer's Disease (Box 68-11)

A. Acetylcholinesterase inhibitors may be used in clients with Alzheimer's disease to improve cognitive functions in the early stages.
B. Donepezil
1. An inhibitor of acetylcholinesterase used to treat mild to moderate dementia of Alzheimer's disease
2. Side and adverse effects include nausea and diarrhea.
3. Donepezil can slow the heart rate through its vagotonic effect.

C. Galantamine
1. An inhibitor of cholinesterase used to treat mild to moderate dementia of Alzheimer's disease
2. Side and adverse effects include nausea, vomiting, diarrhea, anorexia, and weight loss.
3. Galantamine can cause bronchoconstriction; it should be used with caution in clients with asthma and chronic obstructive pulmonary disease.

D. Memantine
1. *N*-Methyl-D-aspartate (NMDA) receptor antagonist indicated for treatment of moderate to severe dementia of Alzheimer's disease
2. Side and adverse effects include dizziness, headache, confusion, and constipation.
3. Memantine should not be used in combination with other NMDA receptor antagonists such as amantadine or ketamine; such combinations produce undesirable additive effects.

BOX 68-11 Medications to Treat Alzheimer's Disease

- Donepezil
- Galantamine
- Memantine
- Rivastigmine

4. Sodium bicarbonate and other medications that alkalinize the urine can decrease renal excretion of memantine; accumulation to toxic levels can result.
5. Clearance is reduced with renal impairment; therefore, use with caution.

E. Rivastigmine
1. Cholinesterase inhibitor used to treat mild to moderate dementia of Alzheimer's disease
2. Side and adverse effects include nausea, vomiting, diarrhea, anorexia, and weight loss.
3. Should be taken with food to reduce gastrointestinal side effects.
4. Rivastigmine should be used with caution in clients with peptic ulcer disease, bradycardia, sick sinus syndrome, urinary obstruction, and lung disease because it enhances cholinergic transmission, intensifying symptoms of these disorders.

PRACTICE QUESTIONS

842. A client's medication sheet contains a prescription for sertraline. To ensure safe administration of the medication, how should the nurse administer the dose?
1. On an empty stomach
2. At the same time each evening
3. Evenly spaced around the clock
4. As needed when the client complains of depression

843. A client with schizophrenia has been started on medication therapy with clozapine. The nurse should assess the results of which laboratory study to monitor for adverse effects from this medication?
1. Platelet count
2. Blood glucose level
3. Liver function studies
4. White blood cell count

844. A client is scheduled for discharge and will be taking phenobarbital for an extended period. The nurse would place **highest priority** on teaching the client which point that directly relates to client safety?
1. Take the medication only with meals.
2. Take the medication at the same time each day.
3. Use a dose container to help prevent missed doses.
4. Avoid drinking alcohol while taking this medication.

845. The nurse is describing the medication side and adverse effects to a client who is taking amitriptyline. Which information should the nurse incorporate in the discussion?
1. Consume a low-fiber diet.
2. Increase fluids and bulk in the diet.
3. Rest if the heart begins to beat rapidly.
4. Walk if you have difficulty urinating because this is a normal side effect.

846. The nurse is administering risperidone to a client with schizophrenia who is scheduled to be discharged. Before discharge, which instruction should the nurse provide to the client?
1. Get adequate sunlight.
2. Continue driving as usual.
3. Avoid foods rich in potassium.
4. Get up slowly when changing positions.

847. The nurse is teaching a client who is being started on imipramine about the medication. The nurse should inform the client to expect maximum desired effects at which time period following initiation of the medication?
1. In 2 months
2. In 2 to 3 weeks
3. During the first week
4. During the sixth week of administration

848. A hospitalized client is started on a monoamine oxidase inhibitor (MAOI) for the treatment of depression. The nurse should instruct the client that which foods are acceptable to consume while taking this medication? **Select all that apply.**

- ☐ 1. Figs
- ☐ 2. Yogurt
- ☐ 3. Crackers
- ☐ 4. Aged cheese
- ☐ 5. Tossed salad
- ☐ 6. Oatmeal raisin cookies

849. The nurse notes that a client with schizophrenia and receiving an antipsychotic medication is moving her mouth, protruding her tongue, and grimacing as she watches television. The nurse determines that the client is experiencing which medication complication?
1. Parkinsonism
2. Tardive dyskinesia
3. Hypertensive crisis
4. Neuroleptic malignant syndrome

850. The nurse is performing a follow-up teaching session with a client discharged 1 month ago. The client is taking fluoxetine. Which information would be important for the nurse to obtain during this client visit regarding the side and adverse effects of the medication?
1. Cardiovascular symptoms
2. Gastrointestinal dysfunctions
3. Problems with mouth dryness
4. Problems with excessive sweating

851. A client who has been taking buspirone for 1 month returns to the clinic for a follow-up assessment. The nurse determines that the medication is **effective** if the absence of which manifestation has occurred?
1. Paranoid thought process

2. Rapid heartbeat or anxiety
3. Alcohol withdrawal symptoms
4. Thought broadcasting or delusions

852. A client taking lithium reports vomiting, abdominal pain, diarrhea, blurred vision, tinnitus, and tremors. The lithium level is 2.5 mEq/L (2.5 mmol/L). The nurse plans care based on which representation of this level?
1. Toxic
2. Normal
3. Slightly above normal
4. Excessively below normal

853. A client gives the home health nurse a bottle of clomipramine. The nurse notes that the medication has not been taken by the client in 2 months. Which behavior observed in the client would validate noncompliance with this medication?
1. Complaints of insomnia
2. Complaints of hunger and fatigue
3. A pulse rate less than 60 beats per minute
4. Frequent hand washing with hot, soapy water

854. A hospitalized client has begun taking bupropion as an antidepressant agent. The nurse determines that which is an adverse effect, indicating that the client is taking an excessive amount of medication?
1. Constipation
2. Seizure activity
3. Increased weight
4. Dizziness when getting upright

855. A client receiving tricyclic antidepressants arrives at the mental health clinic. Which observation would indicate that the client is following the medication plan correctly?
1. Client reports not going to work for the past week.
2. Client complains of not being able to "do anything" anymore.
3. Client arrives at the clinic neat and appropriate in appearance.
4. Client reports sleeping 12 hours per night and 3 to 4 hours during the day.

ANSWERS

842. *Answer:* 2
Rationale: Sertraline is classified as an antidepressant. Sertraline generally is administered once every 24 hours. It may be administered in the morning or evening, but evening administration may be preferable because drowsiness is a side effect. The medication may be administered without food or with food if gastrointestinal distress occurs. Sertraline is not prescribed for use as needed.
Test-Taking Strategy: Focus on the subject, administration of sertraline. Recalling that this medication is an antidepressant administered daily will direct you to the correct option.
Level of Cognitive Ability: Applying
Client Needs: Physiological Integrity
Integrated Process: Nursing Process—Implementation
Content Area: Pharmacology: Psychotherapeutics: Selective Serotonin Reuptake Inhibitors (SSRIs)
Health Problem: Mental Health: Mood Disorders
Priority Concepts: Mood and Affect; Safety
Reference: Burchum, Rosenthal (2016), pp. 346-347.

843. *Answer:* 4
Rationale: A client taking clozapine may experience agranulocytosis, which is monitored by reviewing the results of the white blood cell count. Treatment is interrupted if the white blood cell count decreases to less than 3000 mm^3 (3×10^9/L). Agranulocytosis could be fatal if undetected and untreated. The other laboratory studies are not related specifically to the use of this medication.
Test-Taking Strategy: Focus on the subject, complications associated with clozapine. It is necessary to recall that this medication causes agranulocytosis; this will direct you to the correct option.
Level of Cognitive Ability: Analyzing
Client Needs: Physiological Integrity
Integrated Process: Nursing Process—Assessment
Content Area: Pharmacology: Psychotherapeutic: Antipsychotics
Health Problem: Mental Health: Schizophrenia
Priority Concepts: Cellular Regulation; Psychosis
Reference: Varcarolis (2017), p. 48, 264.

844. *Answer:* 4
Rationale: Phenobarbital is an anticonvulsant and hypnotic agent. The client should avoid taking any other central nervous system depressants such as alcohol while taking this medication. The medication may be given without regard to meals. Taking the medication at the same time each day enhances compliance and maintains more stable blood levels of the medication. Using a dose container or "pillbox" may be helpful for some clients.
Test-Taking Strategy: Focus on the subject, client safety, and note the strategic words, *highest priority*. Eliminate option 1 because of the closed-ended word *only*. Although options 2 and 3 are correct teaching points, these are not the highest priority from the options provided. Remember that alcohol should not be consumed when a hypnotic is taken because of its adverse effects.
Level of Cognitive Ability: Applying
Client Needs: Safe and Effective Care Environment
Integrated Process: Teaching and Learning
Content Area: Pharmacology: Psychotherapeutics: Barbiturate and sedative-hypnotics
Health Problem: N/A
Priority Concepts: Client Education; Safety
Reference: Hodgson, Kizior (2018), pp. 932-933

845. *Answer:* 2
Rationale: Amitriptyline causes constipation, and the client is instructed to increase fluid intake and bulk (high fiber) in

the diet. If the heart begins to beat fast, the primary health care provider (PHCP) is notified, because this could indicate an adverse effect. Difficulty urinating is an adverse effect and indicates urinary retention; this should also be reported.
Test-Taking Strategy: Focus on the subject, side and adverse effects of amitriptyline. Recalling that constipation is a side effect of this medication will direct you to the correct option.
Level of Cognitive Ability: Applying
Client Needs: Physiological Integrity
Integrated Process: Teaching and Learning
Content Area: Pharmacology: Psychotherapeutics: Tricyclic antidepressants
Health Problem: Mental Health: Mood Disorders
Priority Concepts: Client Education; Safety
Reference: Burchum, Rosenthal (2016), p. 263.

846. *Answer:* 4
Rationale: Risperidone can cause orthostatic hypotension. Sunlight should be avoided by the client taking this medication. With any psychotropic medication, caution needs to be taken (such as with driving or other activities requiring alertness) until the individual can determine whether her or his level of alertness is affected. Food interaction is not a concern.
Test-Taking Strategy: Focus on the subject, parameters to monitor for the client taking risperidone. It is necessary to know the nursing considerations related to the administration of risperidone and that risperidone can cause orthostatic hypotension. Also, use of the ABCs—airway, breathing, circulation—will direct you to the correct option.
Level of Cognitive Ability: Applying
Client Needs: Physiological Integrity
Integrated Process: Teaching and Learning
Content Area: Pharmacology: Psychotherapeutics: Antipsychotics
Health Problem: Mental Health: Schizophrenia
Priority Concepts: Client Education; Safety
Reference: Varcarolis (2017), pp. 48, 264.

847. *Answer:* 2
Rationale: The maximum therapeutic effects of imipramine may not occur for 2 to 3 weeks after antidepressant therapy has been initiated. Options 1, 3, and 4 are incorrect time periods.
Test-Taking Strategy: Note the subject, the desired effect of this medication, and focus on the word *maximum*. Recalling that it takes 2 to 3 weeks for a maximum therapeutic effect to occur with most antidepressants will direct you to the correct option.
Level of Cognitive Ability: Applying
Client Needs: Physiological Integrity
Integrated Process: Teaching and Learning
Content Area: Pharmacology: Psychotherapeutics: Tricyclic Antidepressants
Health Problem: Mental Health: Mood Disorders
Priority Concepts: Anxiety; Client Education
Reference: Hodgson, Kizior (2018), pp. 583-584.

848. *Answer:* 3, 5
Rationale: With MAOIs, the client should avoid ingesting foods that are high in tyramine. Ingestion of these foods could trigger a potentially fatal hypertensive crisis. Foods to avoid include yogurt; aged cheeses; smoked or processed meats; red wines; and fruits such as avocados, raisins, or figs.
Test-Taking Strategy: Focus on the subject, acceptable food items while taking MAOIs. Recall that phenelzine is an MAOI and that foods high in tyramine needed to be avoided. Next, from the food items listed in the question, identify the foods that are tyramine-free.
Level of Cognitive Ability: Analyzing
Client Needs: Physiological Integrity
Integrated Process: Teaching and Learning
Content Area: Pharmacology: Psychotherapeutics: Monoamine Oxidase Inhibitors (MAOIs)
Health Problem: Mental Health: Mood Disorders
Priority Concepts: Nutrition; Safety
Reference: Varcarolis (2017), pp. 215, 218.

849. *Answer:* 2
Rationale: Tardive dyskinesia is a reaction that can occur from antipsychotic medication. It is characterized by uncontrollable involuntary movements of the body and extremities, particularly the tongue. Parkinsonism is characterized by tremors, mask-like facies, rigidity, and a shuffling gait. Hypertensive crisis can occur from the use of monoamine oxidase inhibitors and is characterized by hypertension, occipital headache radiating frontally, neck stiffness and soreness, nausea, and vomiting. Neuroleptic malignant syndrome is a potentially fatal syndrome that may occur at any time during therapy with neuroleptic (antipsychotic) medications. It is characterized by dyspnea or tachypnea, tachycardia or irregular pulse rate, fever, blood pressure changes, increased sweating, loss of bladder control, and skeletal muscle rigidity.
Test-Taking Strategy: Focus on the subject, a complication of antipsychotic medications. To direct you to the correct option, remember that tardive dyskinesia is characterized by uncontrollable involuntary movements of the body and extremities, particularly the tongue.
Level of Cognitive Ability: Analyzing
Client Needs: Physiological Integrity
Integrated Process: Nursing Process—Assessment
Content Area: Pharmacology: Psychotherapeutics: Antipsychotics
Health Problem: Mental Health: Mood Disorders
Priority Concepts: Clinical Judgment; Psychosis
Reference: Varcarolis (2017), p. 268.

850. *Answer:* 2
Rationale: The most common side and adverse effects related to fluoxetine include central nervous system and gastrointestinal system dysfunction. Fluoxetine affects the gastrointestinal system by causing nausea and vomiting, cramping, and diarrhea. Cardiovascular symptoms, dry mouth, and excessive sweating are not side and adverse effects associated with this medication.
Test-Taking Strategy: Focus on the subject, common side and adverse effects of fluoxetine. It is necessary to remember that this medication causes gastrointestinal problems. This will direct you to the correct option.
Level of Cognitive Ability: Analyzing
Client Needs: Physiological Integrity
Integrated Process: Nursing Process—Assessment
Content Area: Pharmacology: Psychotherapeutics: Selective Serotonin Reuptake Inhibitors (SSRIs)

Health Problem: Mental Health: Mood Disorders
Priority Concepts: Clinical Judgment; Safety
References: Burchum, Rosenthal (2016), pp. 360-361; Skidmore (2017), pp. 519-521.

851. *Answer:* 2
Rationale: Buspirone is not recommended for the treatment of paranoid thought disorders, drug or alcohol withdrawal, or schizophrenia. Buspirone most often is indicated for the treatment of anxiety.
Test-Taking Strategy: Note the **strategic word,** *effective*. Note the words *absence of which manifestation* in the question. Recalling that buspirone is an antianxiety medication will direct you to the correct option.
Level of Cognitive Ability: Evaluating
Client Needs: Physiological Integrity
Integrated Process: Nursing Process—Evaluation
Content Area: Pharmacology: Psychotherapeutics: Antianxiety/Anxiolytics
Health Problem: Mental Health: Anxiety Disorder
Priority Concepts: Anxiety; Evidence
Reference: Varcarolis (2017), p. 46.

852. *Answer:* 1
Rationale: Maintenance serum levels of lithium are 0.6 to 1.2 mEq/L (0.6 to 1.2 mmol/L). Symptoms of toxicity begin to appear at levels of 1.5 mEq/L (1.5 mmol/L). Lithium toxicity requires immediate medical attention and the primary health care provider is notified if symptoms of toxicity occur.
Test-Taking Strategy: Focus on the **subject,** therapeutic serum medication level of lithium. Recalling that the high end of the maintenance level is 1.2 mEq/L (1.2 mmol/L) will direct you to the correct option.
Level of Cognitive Ability: Analyzing
Client Needs: Physiological Integrity
Integrated Process: Nursing Process—Planning
Content Area: Pharmacology: Psychotherapeutics: Mood Stabilizers
Health Problem: Mental Health: Mood Disorders
Priority Concepts: Clinical Judgment; Safety
Reference: Varcarolis (2017), p. 46, 236-237.

853. *Answer:* 4
Rationale: Clomipramine is a tricyclic antidepressant used to treat obsessive-compulsive disorder. Sedation sometimes occurs. Insomnia seldom is a side effect. Weight gain and tachycardia are side and adverse effects of this medication.
Test-Taking Strategy: Focus on the **subject,** noncompliance with clomipramine. Recalling that this medication is a tricyclic antidepressant used to treat obsessive-compulsive disorder will direct you to the correct option.
Level of Cognitive Ability: Evaluating
Client Needs: Physiological Integrity
Integrated Process: Nursing Process—Evaluation
Content Area: Pharmacology: Psychotherapeutics: Tricyclic Antidepressants
Health Problem: Mental Health: OCD
Priority Concepts: Adherence; Evidence
Reference: Hodgson, Kizior (2018), pp. 262-264.

854. *Answer:* 2
Rationale: Seizure activity can occur in clients taking bupropion dosages greater than 450 mg daily. Weight gain is an occasional side effect, whereas constipation is a common side effect of this medication. This medication does not cause significant orthostatic blood pressure changes.
Test-Taking Strategy: Focus on the **subject,** signs of toxicity associated with bupropion. Note the words *excessive amount*. These words will direct you to the correct option, the one that identifies the most serious concern.
Level of Cognitive Ability: Analyzing
Client Needs: Physiological Integrity
Integrated Process: Nursing Process—Assessment
Content Area: Pharmacology: Psychotherapeutics: Atypical Antidepressant
Health Problem: Mental Health: Mood Disorders
Priority Concepts: Clinical Judgment; Safety
Reference: Hodgson, Kizior (2018), pp. 162-164.

855. *Answer:* 3
Rationale: Depressed individuals sleep for long periods, are unable to go to work, and feel as if they cannot "do anything." When these clients have had some therapeutic effect from their medication, they report resolution of many of these complaints and exhibit an improvement in their appearance. Options 1, 2, and 4 identify continued depression.
Test-Taking Strategy: The client's behaviors or reports identified in options 1, 2, and 4 are **comparable or alike** and are symptoms of depression. The improvement in appearance indicates a therapeutic response to the medication, indicating compliance with the medication regimen.
Level of Cognitive Ability: Evaluating
Client Needs: Physiological Integrity
Integrated Process: Nursing Process—Evaluation
Content Area: Pharmacology: Psychotherapeutics: Tricyclic Antidepressants
Health Problem: Mental Health: Mood Disorders
Priority Concepts: Adherence; Evidence
Reference: Varcarolis (2017), p. 44, 213.

UNIT XIX

Complex Care

Pyramid to Success

Pyramid points focus on intravenous (IV) therapies, including intravenous fluids and parenteral nutrition, administration of blood products, care of the client with a tube, and complex problems involving the integumentary, hematological, oncological, endocrine, gastrointestinal, respiratory, cardiovascular, renal and urinary, neurological, and immune systems. The different types of shock are discussed with a special focus on sepsis, systemic inflammatory response syndrome, multiple organ dysfunction syndrome, septic shock, and hemodynamic management. Sedation, agitation, and delirium are discussed. These concepts are potential topics on the NCLEX®. With regard to IV therapy, assessment of the client for allergies, including latex sensitivity, before initiation of an IV line and monitoring for complications are critical nursing responsibilities. Likewise, the procedure for administering blood components, the signs and symptoms of transfusion reaction, and the immediate interventions if a transfusion reaction occurs are a focus. Care of the client with a tube such as a gastrointestinal tube or chest tube have varying indications and associated nursing interventions. Specific problems requiring a high-level of nursing care for complex conditions are discussed in detail, as well as the associated assessment findings and nursing interventions.

Client Needs: Learning Objectives

Safe and Effective Care Environment

Applying principles of infection control
Collaborating with interprofessional health care members in the care of a client with a complex condition
Ensuring that informed consent has been obtained for invasive procedures and for the administration of blood products
Establishing priorities of assessments and interventions
Following guidelines regarding the use of invasive devices
Handing hazardous and infectious materials to prevent injury to health care personnel and others
Identifying the client with at least 2 forms of identification (e.g., name and date of birth) prior to the administration of a blood product
Maintaining confidentiality
Maintaining precautions to prevent errors, accidents, and injury
Protecting the medicated client from injury
Using equipment safely
Using standard and transmission-based precautions and asepsis procedures

Health Promotion and Maintenance

Assessing the client's ability to perform self-care
Considering lifestyle choices related to home care of the IV line
Identifying lifestyle choices related to receiving a blood transfusion
Providing client and family education regarding the administration of parenteral nutrition at home
Providing health and wellness teaching to prevent complications
Teaching the client about prescribed medications or IV therapy
Teaching the client and family about care of the IV line
Teaching the client to monitor for signs and symptoms that indicate the need to notify the primary health care provider

Psychosocial Integrity

Assessing the client and family emotional response to treatment
Discussing role changes and alterations in lifestyle related to the client's need to receive IV therapy or parenteral nutrition
Facilitating client and family coping
Identifying support systems
Identifying cultural, religious, and spiritual factors influencing health
Keeping the family informed of client progress

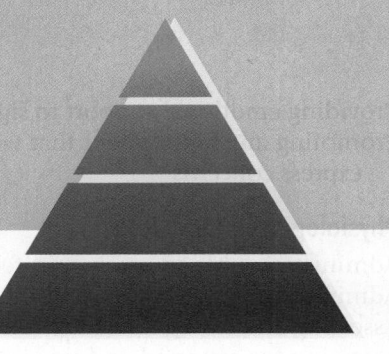

Providing emotional support to significant others
Promoting an environment that will allow the client to express concerns

Physiological Integrity

Administering blood products safely
Administering medications and IV therapy safely
Assessing and caring for central venous access devices
Assessing for expected and unexpected effects of interventions and documenting findings
Assessing the mobility and immobility level of the client
Assisting the client with activities of daily living
Documenting the client's response to complex care interventions
Handling medical emergencies
Identifying client allergies and sensitivities
Identifying the adverse effects of and contraindications to medication or IV therapy
Initiating nursing interventions when medical or surgical complications arise
Managing a client with a burn or inhalation injury
Managing a client with a cardiovascular problem
Managing a client with a gastrointestinal problem
Managing a client with a hematological or oncological problem
Managing a client with a respiratory problem
Managing a client with an endocrine problem
Managing a client with renal and urinary problem.
Managing a client with sepsis, systemic inflammatory response syndrome, multiple organ dysfunction syndrome, and septic shock
Managing a client with a neurological problem
Managing a client with an immune problem
Managing sedation, agitation, and delirium safely
Managing hemodynamic changes in a critically ill client
Managing medication emergencies if a transfusion reaction or other complication occurs
Monitoring for alterations in body systems
Monitoring of enteral feedings and the client's ability to tolerate feedings
Monitoring the client with an invasive device such as a chest tube and responding to changes in condition as necessary
Preparing for diagnostic tests to confirm accurate placement of a tube
Providing interventions compatible with the client's age, cultural, religious, spiritual and health care beliefs, education level, and language
Recognizing changes in the client's condition that indicate a potential complication and intervening appropriately
Using special and invasive monitoring equipment

CHAPTER 69

Complex Care

PRIORITY CONCEPTS Clinical Judgment, Perfusion

I. Administration of Intravenous (IV) Fluids

A. Intravenous Therapy
1. Used to sustain clients who are unable to take substances orally
2. Replaces water, electrolytes, and **nutrients** more rapidly than oral administration
3. Provides immediate access to the vascular system for the rapid delivery of specific solutions without the time required for gastrointestinal tract absorption
4. Provides a vascular route for the administration of medication or blood components

B. Types of solutions (Table 69-1)

⚠ Lactated Ringer's solution contains potassium and should not be administered to clients with acute kidney injury or chronic kidney disease.

1. Isotonic solutions
    a. Have the same osmolality as body fluids
    b. Increase extracellular fluid volume
    c. Do not enter the cells because no osmotic force exists to shift the fluids
2. Hypotonic solutions
    a. Are more dilute solutions and have a lower osmolality than body fluids
    b. Cause the movement of water into cells by osmosis
    c. Should be administered slowly to prevent cellular edema
3. Hypertonic solutions
    a. Are more concentrated solutions and have a higher osmolality than body fluids
    b. Cause movement of water from cells into the extracellular fluid by osmosis
4. Colloids
    a. Also called plasma expanders
    b. Pull fluid from the interstitial compartment into the vascular compartment
    c. Used to increase the vascular volume rapidly, such as in hemorrhage or severe hypovolemia

⚠ Administration of an intravenous (IV) solution or medication provides immediate access to the vascular system. This is a benefit of administering solutions or medications via this route, but it can also present a risk. Therefore, it is critical to ensure that the primary health care provider's (PHCP's) prescriptions are checked carefully and that the correct solution or medication is administered as prescribed. Always follow the rights for medication administration.

C. Intravenous devices
1. Butterfly sets
    a. The set is a wing-tip needle with a metal cannula, plastic or rubber wings, and a plastic catheter or hub.
    b. The needle is 0.5 to 1.5 inches in length, with needle gauge sizes from 16 to 26.
    c. **Infiltration** is more common with these devices. ⚠
    d. The butterfly infusion set is used commonly in children and older clients, whose veins are likely to be small or fragile.
2. Plastic cannulas: Used primarily for short-term therapy.

D. IV gauges
1. The gauge refers to the diameter of the lumen of the needle or cannula.
2. The smaller the gauge number, the larger the diameter of the lumen; the larger the gauge number, the smaller the diameter of the lumen.
3. The size of the gauge used depends on the solution to be administered and the diameter of the available vein.
4. Large-diameter lumens (smaller gauge numbers) allow a higher fluid rate than do smaller-diameter lumens and allow the administration of higher concentrations of solutions. ⚠
5. For rapid emergency fluid administration, blood products, or anesthetics, preoperative and postoperative clients, large-diameter lumens are used, such as an 18- or 19-gauge lumen.

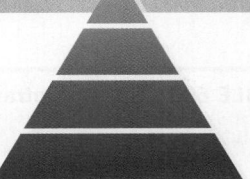

TABLE 69-1 Types of Intravenous Solutions

Solution and Type	Uses
0.9% saline (NS): Isotonic	Extracellular fluid deficits in clients with low serum levels of sodium or chloride and metabolic acid–base imbalances. Used before or after the infusion of blood products.
Ringer's lactate solution: Isotonic	Extracellular fluid deficits, such as fluid loss from burns, bleeding, and dehydration from loss of bile or diarrhea.
5% dextrose in water (D_5W): Isotonic at the time of administration; within a short time after administration, dextrose is metabolized and the tonicity decreases in proportion to the osmolarity or tonicity of the nondextrose components (electrolytes) within the water (may become hypotonic).	Replaces deficits of total body water. Not used alone to expand extracellular fluid volume because dilution of electrolytes can occur.
5% dextrose in 0.225% saline (5% D/¼ NS): Isotonic at the time of administration; within a short time after administration, dextrose is metabolized and the tonicity decreases in proportion to the osmolarity or tonicity of the nondextrose components (electrolytes) within the water (may become hypertonic).	Used as initial fluid for hydration because it provides more water than sodium. Commonly used as maintenance fluid.
5% dextrose in 0.9% saline (5% D/NS): Hypertonic	Extracellular fluid deficits in clients with low serum levels of sodium or chloride and metabolic alkalosis.
5% dextrose in 0.45% saline (5% D/½ NS): Hypertonic	Used as initial fluid for hydration because it provides more water than sodium. Commonly used as maintenance fluid.
5% dextrose in Ringer's lactate solution: Hypertonic	Extracellular fluid deficits, such as fluid loss from burns, bleeding, and dehydration from loss of bile or diarrhea.

6. For peripheral **fat emulsion (lipids)** infusions, a 20- or 21-gauge lumen or cannula is used.
7. For standard IV fluid and clear liquid IV medications, a 22- or 24-gauge lumen or cannula is used.
8. If the client has very small veins, a 24- to 25-gauge lumen or cannula is used.

A client with diabetes mellitus usually does not receive dextrose (glucose) solutions, because the solution can increase the blood glucose level.

E. IV containers
1. Container is usually plastic; some solutions are in glass containers.
2. Squeeze the plastic bag to ensure intactness and assess the glass bottle for any cracks before hanging.
3. In most agencies, the pharmacy department prepares solutions containing medication; in some situations the nurse needs to reconstitute the medication. Agency protocol and pharmacy instruction should always be followed.

Do not write on a plastic IV bag with a marking pen, because the ink may be absorbed through the plastic into the solution. Use a label and a ballpoint pen for writing on the label, placing the label onto the bag.

F. IV tubing (Fig. 69-1)
1. IV tubing contains a spike end for the bag or bottle, drip chamber, roller clamp, Y site, and adapter end for attachment to the cannula that is inserted into the client's vein.

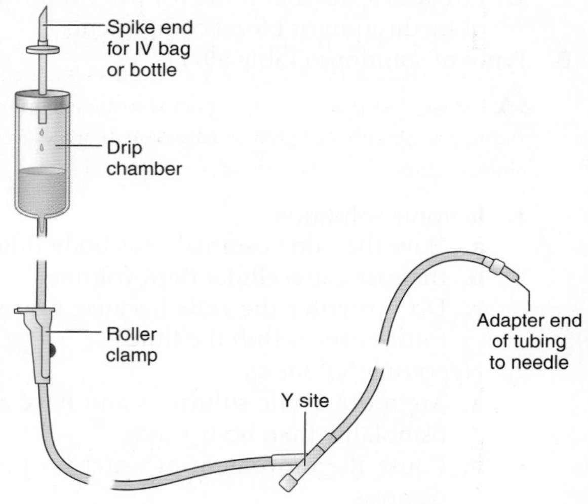

FIG. 69-1 Intravenous (IV) tubing.

2. Shorter, secondary tubing is used for piggyback solutions, connecting them to the injection sites nearest to the drip chamber (Fig. 69-2).
3. Special tubing is used for medication that absorbs into plastic (check specific medication administration guidelines when administering IV medications).
4. Vented and nonvented tubing are available.
   a. A vent allows air to enter the IV container as the fluid leaves.
   b. A vented adapter can be used to add a vent to a nonvented IV tubing system.

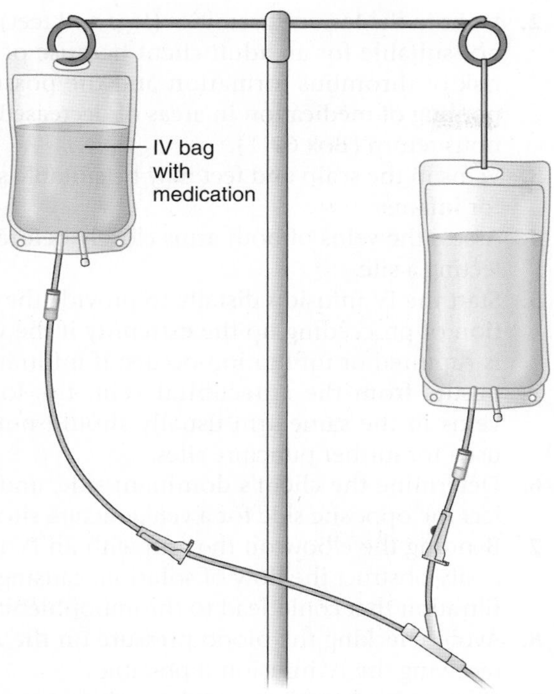

FIG. 69-2 Secondary bag with medication. *IV,* Intravenous.

c. Use nonvented tubing for flexible containers.
d. Use vented tubing for glass or rigid plastic containers to allow air to enter and displace the fluid as it leaves; fluid will not flow from a rigid IV container unless it is vented.

Extension tubing can be added to an IV tubing set to provide extra length to the tubing. Add extension tubing to the IV tubing set for children, clients who are restless, or clients who have special mobility needs.

G. Drip chambers (Fig. 69-3)
1. Macrodrip chamber
   a. The chamber is used if the solution is thick or is to be infused rapidly.
   b. The drop factor varies from 10 to 20 drops (gtt)/mL, depending on the manufacturer.

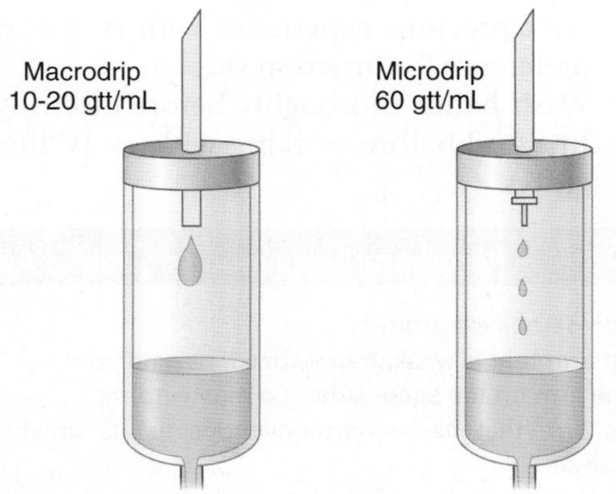

FIG. 69-3 Macrodrip and microdrip sizes.

   c. Read the tubing package to determine how many drops per milliliter are delivered (drop factor).
2. Microdrip chamber
   a. Normally, the chamber has a short vertical metal piece (stylet) where the drop forms.
   b. The chamber delivers about 60 gtt/mL.
   c. Read the tubing package to determine the drop factor (gtt/mL).
   d. Microdrip chambers are used if fluid will be infused at a slow rate (less than 50 mL/hr) or if the solution contains potent medication that needs to be titrated, such as in a critical care setting or in pediatric clients.

H. Filters
1. Filters provide protection by preventing particles from entering the client's veins.
2. They are used in IV lines to trap small particles such as undissolved substances, or medications that have precipitated in solution.
3. Check the agency policy regarding the use of filters.
4. A 0.22-μm filter is used for most solutions; a 1.2-μm filter is used for solutions containing lipids or albumin; and a special filter is used for blood components.
5. Change filters every 24 to 72 hours (depending on agency policy) to prevent bacterial growth.

I. Needleless infusion devices
1. Needleless infusion devices include recessed needles, plastic cannulas, and 1-way valves; these systems decrease the exposure to contaminated needles.
2. Do not administer parenteral nutrition or blood products through a 1-way valve.

J. Intermittent infusion devices
1. Intermittent infusion devices are used when intravascular accessibility is desired for intermittent administration of medications by IV push or IV piggyback.
2. Patency is maintained by periodic flushing with normal saline solution (*sodium chloride* and *normal saline* are interchangeable names).
3. Depending on agency policy, when administering medication, flush with 1 to 2 mL of normal saline to confirm placement of the IV cannula; administer the prescribed medication and then flush the cannula again with 1 to 2 mL of normal saline to maintain patency.

K. Electronic IV infusion devices
1. IV infusion pumps control the amount of fluid infusing and should be used with central venous lines, arterial lines, solutions containing medication, and parenteral nutrition infusions. Most agencies use IV pumps for the infusion of any IV solution.
2. A syringe pump is used when a small volume of medication is administered; the syringe that

contains the medication and solution fits into a pump and is set to deliver the medication at a controlled rate.

3. Patient-controlled analgesia (PCA)
   a. A device that allows the client to self-administer IV medication, such as an analgesic; the client can administer doses at set intervals, and the pump can be set to lock out doses that are not within the preset time frame to prevent overdose.
   b. The PCA regimen may include a basal rate of infusion along with the demand dosing, basal rate infusion alone, or demand dosing alone.
   c. A bolus dose can be given prior to any of the settings and should be set based on the PHCP's prescription.
   d. PCAs are always kept locked, and setup requires the witness of another registered nurse (RN).

Check electronic IV infusion devices frequently. Although these devices are electronic, this does not ensure that they are infusing solutions and medications accurately.

L. Latex allergy
1. Assess the client for an allergy to latex.
2. IV supplies, including IV catheters, IV tubing, IV ports (particularly IV rubber injection ports), rubber stoppers on multidose vials, and adhesive tape, may contain latex.
3. Latex-safe IV supplies need to be used for clients with a latex allergy; most agencies carry these type of supplies, but this still needs to be checked.
4. See Chapter 62 for additional information regarding latex allergy.

M. Selection of a peripheral IV site
1. Veins in the hand, forearm, and antecubital fossa are suitable sites (Fig. 69-4).
2. Veins in the lower extremities (legs and feet) are not suitable for an adult client because of the risk of thrombus formation and the possible pooling of medication in areas of decreased venous return (Box 69-1).
3. Veins in the scalp and feet may be suitable sites for infants.
4. Assess the veins of both arms closely before selecting a site.
5. Start the IV infusion distally to provide the option of proceeding up the extremity if the vein is ruptured or infiltration occurs; if infiltration occurs from the antecubital vein, the lower veins in the same arm usually should not be used for further puncture sites.
6. Determine the client's dominant side, and select the opposite side for a **venipuncture** site.
7. Bending the elbow on the arm with an IV may easily obstruct the flow of solution, causing infiltration that could lead to thrombophlebitis.
8. Avoid checking the blood pressure on the arm receiving the IV infusion if possible.
9. Do not place restraints over the venipuncture site.
10. Use an armboard as needed when the venipuncture site is located in an area of flexion.

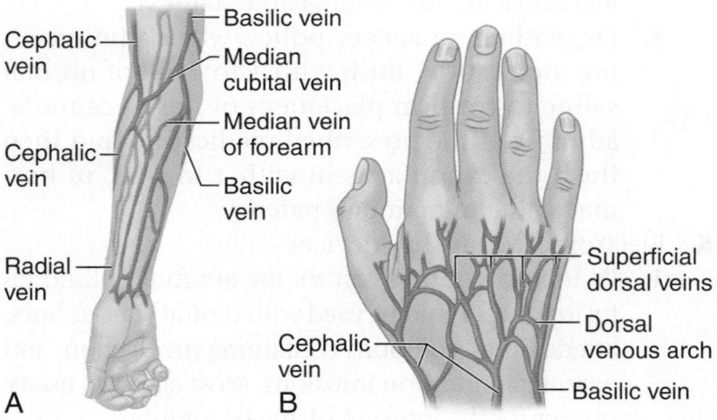

FIG. 69-4 Common intravenous sites. **A,** Inner arm. **B,** Dorsal surface of hand.

In an adult, the most frequently used sites for inserting an IV cannula or needle are the veins of the forearm, because the bones of the forearm act as a natural support and splint.

N. Initiation and administration of IV solutions
1. Check the IV solution against the PHCP's prescription for the type, amount, percentage of solution, and rate of flow; follow the rights for medication administration.
2. Assess the health status and medical disorders of the client and identify client conditions that contraindicate use of a particular IV solution or IV equipment, such as an allergy to cleansing solution, adhesive materials, or latex. Check compatibility of IV solutions as appropriate.
3. Check client's identification by 2 identifiers and explain the procedure to the client; assess client's previous experience with IV therapy and preference for insertion site.
4. Wash hands thoroughly before inserting an IV line and before working with an IV line; wear gloves.

BOX 69-1 Peripheral Intravenous Sites to Avoid

- Edematous extremity
- An arm that is weak, traumatized, or paralyzed
- The arm on the same side as a mastectomy
- An arm that has an arteriovenous fistula or shunt for dialysis
- A skin area that is infected

5. Use sterile technique when inserting an IV line and when changing the dressing over the IV site.
6. Change the venipuncture site every 72 to 96 hours in accordance with Centers for Disease Control and Prevention (CDC) recommendations and agency policy.
7. Change the IV dressing when the dressing is wet or contaminated, or as specified by the agency policy.
8. Change the IV tubing every 96 hours in accordance with CDC recommendations and agency policy or with a change of the venipuncture site.
9. Do not let an IV bag or bottle of solution hang for more than 24 hours, to diminish the potential for bacterial contamination and possibly sepsis.
10. Do not allow the IV tubing to touch the floor, to prevent potential bacterial contamination.
11. See Priority Nursing Actions for instructions on inserting an IV.
12. See Priority Nursing Actions for instructions on removing an IV.

PRIORITY NURSING ACTIONS

Inserting a Peripheral Intravenous Line

1. Check the primary health care provider's (PHCP's) prescription, determine the type and size of infusion device, and prepare intravenous (IV) tubing or extension set and solution; prime IV tubing or extension set to remove air from the system; explain procedure to the client.
2. Select the vein for insertion based on vein quality, client size, and indication of IV therapy; apply tourniquet and palpate the vein for resilience (see Fig. 69-4).
3. Clean the skin with an antimicrobial solution, using an inner to outer circular motion, or as specified by the Centers for Disease Control and Prevention (CDC) guidelines and agency policy.
4. Stabilize the vein below the insertion site and puncture the skin and vein, observing for blood in the flashback chamber; when observed, lower the catheter so that it is flush with the skin and advance the catheter into the vein (if unsuccessful, a new sterile device is used for the next attempt at insertion).
5. Remove the tourniquet. Apply pressure above the insertion site with the middle finger of the nondominant hand and retract the stylet from the catheter; connect the end of the IV tubing or extension set to the catheter tubing, secure it, and begin IV flow. Ask the client about comfort at the site and assess site for adequate flow.
6. Tape and secure insertion site with a transparent dressing as specified by agency procedure; label the tubing, dressing, and solution bags clearly, indicating the date and time.
7. Document the specifics about the procedure such as number of attempts at insertion; the insertion site, type and size of device, solution and flow rate, and time; and the client's response. In addition, follow agency procedure for documentation of procedure.

Reference

Potter et al. (2017), pp. 957, 967-969.

PRIORITY NURSING ACTIONS

Removing a Peripheral Intravenous Line

1. Check the primary health care provider's (PHCP's) prescription and explain the procedure to the client; ask the client to hold the extremity still during cannula or needle removal.
2. Turn off the intravenous (IV) tubing clamp and remove the dressing and tape covering the site, while stabilizing the catheter.
3. Apply light pressure with sterile gauze or other material as specified by agency procedure over the site and withdraw the catheter using a slow, steady movement, keeping the hub parallel to the skin.
4. Apply pressure for 2 to 3 minutes, using dry sterile gauze (apply pressure for a longer period of time if the client has a bleeding disorder or is taking anticoagulant medication).
5. Inspect the site for redness, drainage, or swelling; check the catheter for intactness.
6. Apply a dressing as needed per agency policy.
7. Document the procedure and the client's response.

Reference

Perry et al. (2018), p. 794.

O. Precautions for IV lines
1. On insertion, an IV line can cause initial pain and discomfort for the client.
2. An IV puncture provides a route of entry for microorganisms into the body.
3. Medications administered by the IV route enter the blood immediately, and any adverse reactions or allergic responses can occur immediately.
4. Fluid (circulatory) overload or electrolyte imbalances can occur from excessive or too rapid infusion of IV fluids.
5. Incompatibilities between certain solutions and medications can occur.

Clients with respiratory, cardiac, renal, or liver disease; older clients; and very young persons are at risk for circulatory overload and cannot tolerate an excessive fluid volume. Also, a client with heart failure or renal failure usually is not given a solution containing saline, because this type of fluid promotes the retention of water and would therefore exacerbate heart failure or renal failure by increasing the fluid overload.

P. Complications of intravenous therapy (Table 69-2)

Always document the occurrence of a complication, assessment findings, actions taken, and the client's response according to agency policy.

TABLE 69-2 Complications of Intravenous Therapy

Complication	Description	Signs	Prevention and Interventions
Air embolism	▪ A bolus of air enters the vein through an inadequately primed IV line, from a loose connection, during tubing change, or during removal of the IV.	▪ Tachycardia ▪ Chest pain and dyspnea ▪ Hypotension ▪ Cyanosis ▪ Decreased level of consciousness	▪ Prime tubing with fluid before use, and monitor for any air bubbles in the tubing. ▪ Secure all connections. ▪ Replace the IV fluid before the bag or bottle is empty. ▪ Monitor for signs of air embolism; if suspected, clamp the tubing, turn the client on the left side with the head of the bed lowered (Trendelenburg's position) to trap the air in the right atrium, and notify the PHCP.
Catheter embolism	▪ An obstruction that results from breakage of the catheter tip during IV line insertion or removal	▪ Decrease in blood pressure ▪ Pain along the vein Weak, rapid pulse Cyanosis of the nailbeds ▪ Loss of consciousness	▪ Remove the catheter carefully. ▪ Inspect the catheter when removed. ▪ If the catheter tip has broken off, place a tourniquet as proximally as possible to the IV site on the affected limb, notify the PHCP immediately, prepare to obtain a radiograph, and prepare the client for surgery to remove the catheter piece(s), if necessary.
Circulatory overload	▪ Also known as *fluid overload;* results from the administration of fluids too rapidly, especially in a client at risk for fluid overload.	▪ Increased blood pressure ▪ Distended jugular veins ▪ Rapid breathing Dyspnea ▪ Moist cough and crackles	▪ Identify clients at risk for circulatory overload. ▪ Calculate and monitor the drip (flow) rate frequently. ▪ Use an electronic IV infusion device and frequently check the drip rate or setting (at least every hour for an adult). ▪ If an electronic infusion device is not being used, add a time tape (label) to the IV bag or bottle next to the volume markings; mark on the tape the expected hourly decrease in volume based on the mL/hr calculation. ▪ Monitor for signs of circulatory overload. ▪ If circulatory overload occurs, decrease the flow rate to a minimum, at a keep-vein-open rate; elevate the head of the bed; keep the client warm; assess lung sounds; assess for edema; and notify the PHCP.
Electrolyte overload and imbalance	▪ An electrolyte overload leading to imbalance is caused by too rapid or excessive infusion or by use of an inappropriate IV solution.	▪ Signs depend on the specific electrolyte imbalance.	▪ Assess laboratory value reports. ▪ Verify the correct solution. ▪ Calculate and monitor the flow rate. ▪ Use an electronic IV infusion device and frequently check the drip rate or setting (at least every hour for an adult). Use a time tape label if an electronic infusion device is not being used. ▪ Per agency procedure, place a red medication sticker on the bag or bottle if a medication has been added to the IV solution. ▪ Monitor for signs of an electrolyte imbalance, and notify the PHCP if they occur.
Hematoma	▪ The collection of blood in the tissues after an unsuccessful venipuncture or after the venipuncture site is discontinued and blood continues to ooze into the tissue	▪ Ecchymosis, immediate swelling and leakage of blood at the site, and hard and painful lumps at the site	▪ When starting an IV, avoid piercing the posterior wall of the vein. ▪ Do not apply a tourniquet to the extremity immediately after an unsuccessful venipuncture. ▪ When discontinuing an IV, apply pressure to the site for 2-3 minutes and elevate the extremity; apply pressure longer for clients with a bleeding disorder or who are taking anticoagulants. ▪ If a hematoma develops, elevate the extremity and apply pressure and ice as prescribed. ▪ Document accordingly, including taking pictures of the IV site if indicated by agency policy.

TABLE 69-2 Complications of Intravenous Therapy—cont'd

Complication	Description	Signs	Prevention and Interventions
Infection	▪ Infection occurs from the entry of microorganisms into the body through the venipuncture site. ▪ Venipuncture interrupts the integrity of the skin, the first line of defense against infection. ▪ The longer the therapy continues, the greater the risk for infection. ▪ Infection can occur locally at the IV insertion site or systemically from the entry of microorganisms into the body. ▪ At-risk clients: ▪ immunocompromised clients with diseases such as cancer, human immunodeficiency virus or acquired immunodeficiency syndrome, those receiving biological modifier response medications for treatment of autoimmune conditions, or status post organ transplant are at risk for infection. ▪ Clients receiving treatments such as chemotherapy who have an altered or lowered white blood cell count are at risk for infection. ▪ Older clients, because aging alters the effectiveness of the immune system, are at risk for infection. ▪ Clients with diabetes mellitus are at risk for infection.	▪ Local—redness, swelling, and drainage at the site. ▪ Systemic—chills, fever, malaise, headache, nausea, vomiting, backache, tachycardia	▪ Assess the client for predisposition to or risk for infection. ▪ Maintain strict asepsis when caring for the IV site. ▪ Monitor for signs of local or systemic infection. ▪ Monitor white blood cell counts. ▪ Check fluid containers for cracks, leaks, cloudiness, or other evidence of contamination. ▪ Change IV tubing every 96 hours in accordance with CDC recommendations or according to agency policy; change IV site dressing when soiled or contaminated and according to agency policy. ▪ Label the IV site, bag or bottle, and tubing with the date and time to ensure that these are changed on time according to agency policy. ▪ Ensure that the IV solution is not hanging for more than 24 hours. ▪ If infection occurs, the PHCP is notified; discontinue the IV, and place the venipuncture device in a sterile container for possible culture. ▪ Prepare to obtain blood cultures as prescribed if infection occurs and document accordingly. ▪ Restart an IV in the opposite arm to differentiate sepsis (systemic infection) from local infection at the IV site. ▪ Document accordingly, including taking pictures of the IV site if indicated by agency policy.
Infiltration	▪ Infiltration is seepage of the IV fluid out of the vein and into the surrounding interstitial spaces. ▪ Infiltration occurs when an access device has become dislodged or perforates the wall of the vein or when venous backpressure occurs because of a clot or venospasm.	▪ Edema, pain, numbness, and coolness at the site; may or may not have a blood return	▪ Avoid venipuncture over an area of flexion. ▪ Anchor the cannula and a loop of tubing securely with tape. ▪ Use an armboard or splint as needed if the client is restless or active. ▪ Monitor the IV rate for a decrease or a cessation of flow. ▪ Evaluate the IV site for infiltration by occluding the vein proximal to the IV site. If the IV fluid continues to flow, the cannula is probably outside the vein (infiltrated); if the IV flow stops after occlusion of the vein, the IV device is still in the vein. ▪ Lower the IV fluid container below the IV site, and monitor for the appearance of blood in the IV tubing; if blood appears, the IV device is most likely in the vein. ▪ If infiltration has occurred, remove the IV device immediately; elevate the extremity and apply compresses (warm or cool, depending on the IV solution that was infusing and the PHCP's prescription and agency procedure) over the affected area. ▪ Do not rub an infiltrated area, which can cause hematoma. ▪ Document accordingly, including taking pictures of the IV site if indicated by agency policy.

Continued

TABLE 69-2 Complications of Intravenous Therapy—cont'd

Complication	Description	Signs	Prevention and Interventions
Phlebitis and Thrombophlebitis	▪ Phlebitis is an inflammation of the vein that can occur from mechanical or chemical (medication) trauma or from a local infection. ▪ Phlebitis can cause the development of a clot (thrombophlebitis).	▪ Phlebitis: Heat, redness, tenderness at the site; not swollen or hard; intravenous infusion sluggish Thrombophlebitis: hard and cord-like vein; heat, redness, tenderness at site; intravenous infusion sluggish.	▪ Use an IV cannula smaller than the vein, and avoid using very small veins when administering irritating solutions. ▪ Avoid using the lower extremities (legs and feet) as an access area for the IV. ▪ Avoid venipuncture over an area of flexion. ▪ Anchor the cannula and a loop of tubing securely with tape. ▪ Use an armboard or splint as needed if the client is restless or active. ▪ Change the venipuncture site every 72-96 hours in accordance with CDC recommendations and agency policy. ▪ If phlebitis occurs, remove the IV device immediately and restart it in the opposite extremity; notify the PHCP if phlebitis is suspected, and apply warm, moist compresses, as prescribed. ▪ If thrombophlebitis occurs, do not irrigate the IV catheter; remove the IV, notify the PHCP, and restart the IV in the opposite extremity. ▪ Document accordingly, including taking pictures if indicated by agency policy.
Tissue damage	▪ Tissues most commonly damaged include the skin, veins, and subcutaneous tissue. ▪ Tissue damage can be uncomfortable and can cause permanent negative effects. ▪ Extravasation is a form of tissue damage caused by the seepage of vesicant or irritant solutions into the tissues; this occurrence requires immediate PHCP notification so that treatment can be prescribed to prevent tissue necrosis.	▪ Skin color changes, sloughing of the skin, discomfort at the site	▪ Use a careful and gentle approach when applying a tourniquet. ▪ Avoid tapping the skin over the vein when starting an IV. ▪ Monitor for ecchymosis when penetrating the skin with the cannula. ▪ Assess for allergies to tape or dressing adhesives. ▪ Monitor for skin color changes, sloughing of the skin, or discomfort at the IV site. ▪ Notify the PHCP if tissue damage is suspected. ▪ Document accordingly, including taking pictures if indicated by agency policy.

Q. Central venous catheters
1. Description
   a. Central venous catheters (Fig. 69-5) are used to deliver hyperosmolar solutions, measure central venous pressure, infuse parenteral nutrition, or infuse multiple IV solutions or medications.
   b. Catheter position is determined by radiography after insertion.
   c. The catheter may have a single, double, or triple lumen.
   d. The catheter may be inserted peripherally and threaded through the basilic or cephalic vein into the superior vena cava, inserted centrally through the internal jugular or subclavian veins, or surgically tunneled through subcutaneous tissue.
   e. With multilumen catheters, more than 1 medication can be administered at the same time without incompatibility problems, and only 1 insertion site is present.

⚠ For central line insertion, tubing change, and line removal, place the client in the Trendelenburg's position if not contraindicated or in the supine position, and instruct the client to perform the Valsalva maneuver to increase pressure in the central veins when the IV system is open.

2. Tunneled central venous catheters
   a. A more permanent type of catheter, such as the Hickman, Broviac, or Groshong catheter, is used for long-term IV therapy.
   b. The catheter may be single lumen or multilumen.
   c. The catheter is inserted in the operating room, and the catheter is threaded into the lower part of the vena cava at the entrance of the right atrium (entrance site) and tunneled under the skin to the exit site where the catheter comes out of the chest; the catheter

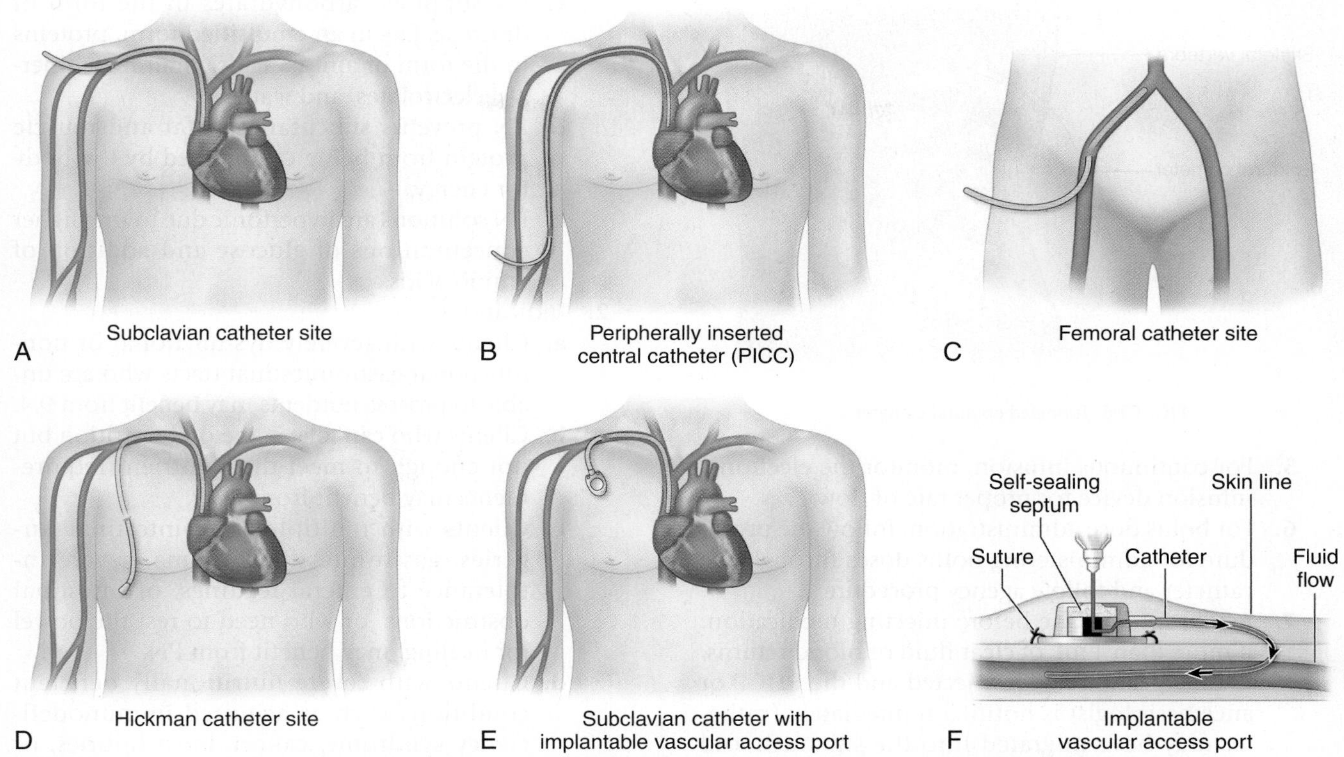

FIG. 69-5 Central venous access sites. **A,** Subclavian catheter. **B,** Peripherally inserted central catheter (PICC). **C,** Femoral catheter. **D,** Hickman catheter. **E,** Subclavian catheter with implantable vascular access port. **F,** Implantable vascular access port.

at the exit site is secured by means of a "cuff" just under the skin at the exit site.

- **d.** The catheter is fitted with an intermittent infusion device to allow access as needed and to keep the system closed and intact.
- **e.** Patency is maintained by flushing with a diluted heparin solution or normal saline solution, depending on the type of catheter, per agency policy.

3. Vascular access ports (implantable port)

- **a.** Surgically implanted under the skin, ports such as a Port-a-Cath, Mediport, or Infusaport are used for long-term administration of repeated IV therapy.
- **b.** For access, the port requires palpation and injection through the skin into the self-sealing port with a noncoring needle, such as a Huber point needle.
- **c.** Patency is maintained by periodic flushing with a diluted heparin solution as prescribed and as per agency policy.

4. Peripherally inserted central catheter (PICC) line

- **a.** The catheter is used for long-term IV therapy, frequently in the home.
- **b.** The basilic vein usually is used, but the median cubital and cephalic veins in the antecubital area also can be used.
- **c.** The catheter is threaded so that the catheter tip may terminate in the subclavian vein or superior vena cava.
- **d.** A small amount of bleeding may occur at the time of insertion and may continue for 24 hours, but bleeding thereafter is not expected.
- **e.** Phlebitis is a common complication.

R. Epidural Catheter (Fig. 69-6)

1. Catheter is placed in the epidural space for the administration of analgesics; this method of administration reduces the amount of medication needed to control pain; therefore, the client experiences fewer side effects.
2. Assess client's vital signs, level of consciousness, and motor and sensory function of the lower extremities.
3. Monitor insertion site for signs of infection and be sure that the catheter is secured to the client's skin and that all connections are taped to prevent disconnection.
4. Check PHCP's prescription regarding solution and medication administration.

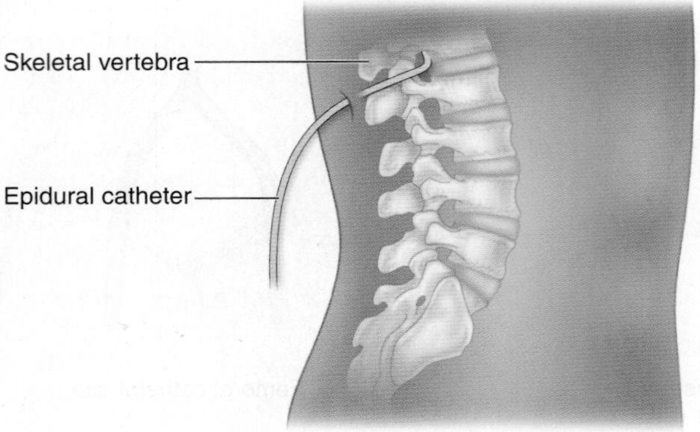

FIG. 69-6 Tunneled epidural catheter.

5. For continuous infusion, monitor the electronic infusion device for proper rate of flow.
6. For bolus dose administration, follow the procedure for administering bolus doses through the catheter and follow agency procedure.
7. Aspiration is done before injecting medication; if more than 1 mL of clear fluid or blood returns, the medication is not injected and the PHCP or anesthesiologist is notified immediately (catheter may have migrated into the subarachnoid space or a blood vessel).

⚠ Contraindications to an epidural catheter and administration of epidural analgesia include skeletal and spinal abnormalities, bleeding disorders, use of anticoagulants, history of multiple abscesses, and sepsis.

II. Administration of Parenteral Nutrition

A. Parenteral Nutrition (PN)

1. Description
   a. Parenteral nutrition supplies nutrients via the veins.
   b. PN consists of both **partial parenteral nutrition** (PPN) and **total parenteral nutrition** (TPN). The indication of the type used depends on the client's nutritional needs.
   c. PN supplies carbohydrates in the form of dextrose, fats in an emulsified form, proteins in the form of amino acids, vitamins, minerals, electrolytes, and water.
   d. PN prevents subcutaneous fat and muscle protein from being catabolized by the body for energy.
   e. PN solutions are hypertonic due to the higher concentrations of glucose and addition of amino acids.
2. Indications
   a. Clients with severely dysfunctional or nonfunctional gastrointestinal tracts who are unable to process nutrients may benefit from PN.
   b. Clients who can take some oral nutrition but not enough to meet their nutrient requirements may benefit from PN.
   c. Clients with multiple gastrointestinal surgeries, gastrointestinal trauma, severe intolerance to enteral feedings, or intestinal obstructions, or who need to rest the bowel for healing, may benefit from PN.
   d. Clients with severe nutritionally deficient conditions such as acquired immunodeficiency syndrome, cancer, burn injuries, or **malnutrition**, or clients receiving chemotherapy, may benefit from PN.

⚠ PN is a form of nutrition and is used when there is no other nutritional alternative. Administering nutrition orally or through a nasogastric tube is usually initiated first, before PN is initiated.

3. Administration of PN (Fig. 69-7).
4. PPN
   a. Usually administered through a large distal vein in the arm with a standard peripheral IV catheter or midline or through a PICC. A midline is placed in an upper arm vein such as the brachial or cephalic vein with the tip ending below the level of the axillary line.

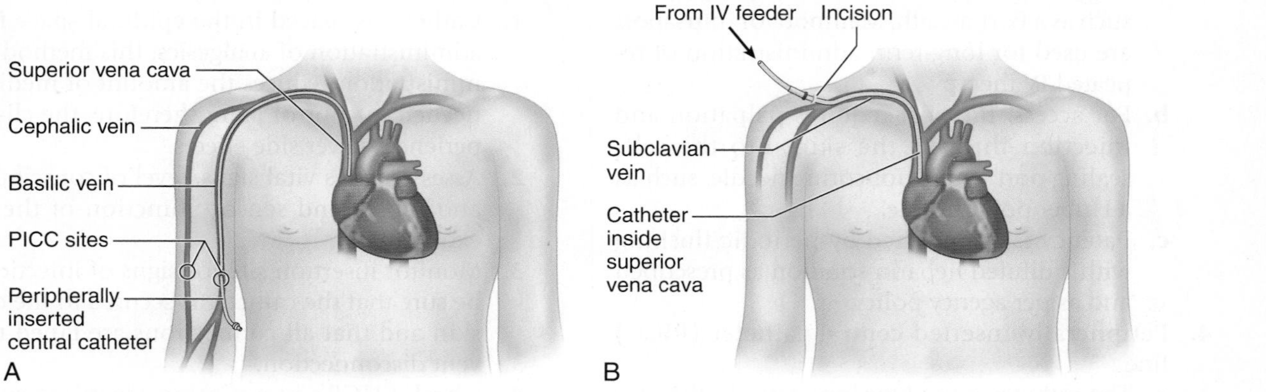

FIG. 69-7 **A,** Placement of peripherally inserted central catheter through antecubital fossa. **B,** Placement of central venous catheter inserted into subclavian vein. *IV,* Intravenous; *PICC,* peripherally inserted central catheter.

b. If a PICC cannot be established, the subclavian vein or internal or external jugular veins can be used for PPN.

5. TPN
   a. Administered through a central vein; the use of a PICC is acceptable. Other sites that can be used include the subclavian vein and the internal or external jugular veins.
   b. If the bag of intravenous solution (the TPN) is empty and the nurse is waiting for the delivery of a new bag of solution from the pharmacy, a 10% dextrose in water solution should be infused at the prescribed rate to prevent hypoglycemia; the prescribed solution should be obtained as soon as possible.

⚠ The delivery of hypertonic solutions into peripheral veins can cause sclerosis, phlebitis, or swelling. Monitor closely for these complications.

6. Components of parenteral nutrition
   a. Carbohydrates: The strength of the dextrose solution depends on the client's nutritional needs, the route of administration (central or peripheral), and agency protocols; carbohydrates typically provide 60% to 70% of calorie (energy) needs.
   b. Amino acids (protein): Concentrations range from 3.5% to 20%. Lower concentrations are most commonly used for peripheral vein administration, and higher concentrations are most often administered through a central vein; about 15% to 20% of total energy needs should come from protein.
7. **Fat emulsion (lipids)**
   a. Lipids provide up to 30% of calorie (energy) needs.
   b. Lipids provide nonprotein calories and prevent or correct fatty acid deficiency.
   c. Lipid solutions are isotonic and therefore can be administered through a peripheral or central vein; the solution may be administered through a separate IV line below the filter of the main IV administration set by a Y-connector, or as an admixture to the PN solution (3-in-1 admixture consisting of dextrose, amino acids, and lipids).
   d. Most fat emulsions are prepared from soybean or safflower oil, with egg yolk to provide emulsification; the primary components are linoleic, oleic, palmitic, linolenic, and stearic acids (assess the client for allergies).
   e. Glucose-intolerant clients or clients with diabetes mellitus may benefit from receiving a larger percentage of their PN from lipids, which helps control blood glucose levels and lower insulin requirements caused by infused dextrose.
   f. Examine the bottle for separation of emulsion into layers or fat globules or for the accumulation of froth; if observed, do not use and return the solution to the pharmacy.
   g. Additives should not be put into the fat emulsion solution.
   h. Follow agency policy regarding the filter size that should be used; usually a 1.2-μm filter or larger should be used, because the lipid particles are too large to pass through a 0.22-μm filter.
   i. Infuse solution at the flow rate prescribed—usually slowly at 1 mL/minute initially—monitor vital signs every 10 minutes, and observe for adverse reactions for the first 30 minutes of the infusion. If signs of an adverse reaction occur, stop the infusion and notify the primary health care provider (PHCP) (Box 69-2).
   j. If no adverse reaction occurs, adjust the flow rate to the prescribed rate.
   k. Monitor serum lipids 4 hours after discontinuing the infusion.

⚠ Fat emulsions (lipids) contain egg yolk phospholipids and should not be given to clients with egg allergies.

8. Other components
   a. PN solutions usually contain a standard multivitamin preparation to meet most vitamin needs and prevent deficiencies.
   b. Individual vitamin preparations can be added, as needed and as prescribed.
   c. Minerals and trace elements: Commercial mineral and trace element preparations are available in various concentrations to promote normal **metabolism**.
   d. Electrolytes: Electrolyte requirements for individuals receiving PN therapy vary, depending on body weight, presence of malnutrition or catabolism, degree of electrolyte depletion, changes in organ function, ongoing electrolyte losses, and the disease process.

BOX 69-2 Signs and Symptoms of an Adverse Reaction to Lipids

- Chest and back pain
- Chills
- Cyanosis
- Diaphoresis
- Dyspnea
- Fever
- Flushing
- Headache
- Nausea and vomiting
- Pressure over the eyes
- Thrombophlebitis
- Vertigo

e. Water: The amount of water needed in a PN solution is determined by electrolyte balance and fluid requirements.
f. Regular insulin: May be added to control the blood glucose level because of the high concentration of glucose in the PN solution.
g. Heparin: May be added to reduce the buildup of a fibrinous clot at the catheter tip.

B. Administration and discontinuation
1. Continuous PN
a. Infused continuously over 24 hours
b. Most commonly used in a hospital setting
2. Intermittent or cyclic PN
a. In general, the nutrient solution infusion regimen varies and is commonly administered overnight.
b. Allows clients requiring PN on a long-term basis to participate in activities of daily living during the day without the inconvenience of an IV bag and pump set.
c. Monitor glucose levels closely because of the risk of hypoglycemia due to lack of glucose during noninfusion times.
3. Discontinuing PN therapy
a. Evaluation of nutritional status by a nutritionist is done before PN is discontinued.
b. If discontinuation is prescribed, gradually decrease the flow rate for 1 to 2 hours while increasing oral intake (this assists in preventing hypoglycemia).
c. After removal of the IV catheter, change the dressing daily until the insertion site heals. Note that central lines should not be left in without a reason due to risk of infection, but in some situations are left in place and used for another necessary reason (venous access, medication administration).
d. Encourage oral nutrition.
e. Record oral intake, body weight, and laboratory results of serum electrolyte and glucose levels.

Abrupt discontinuation of a PN solution can result in hypoglycemia. The flow rate should be decreased gradually when the PN is discontinued.

C. Complications (Table 69-3)
1. Pneumothorax and **air embolism** are associated with central line placement; air embolism is also associated with tubing changes.
2. Other complications include infection (catheter-related), hypervolemia, and metabolic alterations such as hyperglycemia and hypoglycemia; these complications are usually caused by the PN solution itself (see Priority Nursing Actions).

PRIORITY NURSING ACTIONS

Central Venous Catheter Site with a Suspected Infection

1. Notify the primary health care provider (PHCP).
2. Prepare to remove the catheter and for possible restart at a different location.
3. Remove the tip of the catheter and send it to the laboratory for culture if prescribed by the PHCP.
4. Prepare the client for obtaining blood cultures.
5. Prepare for antibiotic administration.
6. Document the occurrence, the actions taken, and the client's response.

Reference

Ignatavicius, Workman, Rebar (2018), p. 221.

D. Additional nursing considerations
1. Check the PN solution with the PHCP's prescription to ensure that the prescribed components are contained in the solution; some health care agencies require validation of the prescription by 2 registered nurses.
2. To prevent infection and solution incompatibility, IV medications and blood are not given through the PN line.
3. Blood for testing may be drawn from the central venous access site; a port other than the port used to infuse the PN is used for blood draws after the PN has been stopped for several minutes (per agency procedure), because the PN solution can alter the results of the sample. The client with a central venous access site receiving PN should still have a venipuncture site.
4. Monitor partial thromboplastin time and prothrombin time for clients receiving anticoagulants.
5. Monitor electrolyte and albumin levels and liver and renal function studies, as well as any other prescribed laboratory studies. Blood studies for blood chemistries are normally done every other day or 3 times per week (per agency procedures) when the client is receiving PN; the results are the basis for the PHCP continuing or changing the PN solution or rate.
6. Monitor blood glucose levels as prescribed (usually every 4 hours) because of the risk for hyperglycemia from the PN solution components.
7. In severely dehydrated clients, the albumin level may drop initially after initiating PN because the treatment restores hydration.
8. With severely malnourished clients, monitor for "refeeding syndrome" (a rapid drop in **potassium, magnesium**, and phosphate serum levels).

TABLE 69-3 Complications of Parenteral Nutrition

Complication	Possible Cause	Signs or Symptoms	Intervention	Prevention
Air embolism	■ Catheter system opened or IV tubing disconnected ■ Air entry on IV tubing changes	■ Apprehension ■ Chest pain ■ Dyspnea ■ Hypotension ■ Loud churning sound heard over pericardium on auscultation ■ Rapid and weak pulse ■ Respiratory distress	■ Clamp all ports of the IV catheter. ■ Place the client in a left side-lying position with the head lower than the feet. ■ Notify the PHCP. ■ Administer oxygen.	■ Make sure all catheter connections are secure (use tape per agency protocol). ■ Clamp the catheter when not in use and when changing caps (follow agency protocol for flushing and clamping the catheter and cap changes). ■ Instruct the client in the Valsalva maneuver for tubing and cap changes. ■ For tubing and cap changes, place the client in the Trendelenburg's position (if not contraindicated) with the head turned in the opposite direction of the insertion site; client should hold breath and bear down.
Hyperglycemia	■ High concentration of dextrose in solution ■ Client receiving solution too quickly ■ Not enough insulin ■ Infection	■ Restlessness ■ Confusion ■ Weakness ■ Diaphoresis ■ Elevated blood glucose level >200 mg/dL (11.1 mmol/L) ■ Excessive thirst ■ Fatigue ■ Kussmaul respirations ■ Coma (when severe)	■ Notify the PHCP. ■ The infusion rate may need to be slowed. ■ Monitor blood glucose levels. ■ Administer regular insulin as prescribed.	■ Assess the client for a history of glucose intolerance. ■ Assess the client's medication history (corticosteroids increase blood glucose). ■ Begin infusion at a slow rate as prescribed (usually 40-60 mL/hr). ■ Monitor blood glucose levels per agency protocol. ■ Administer regular insulin as prescribed. ■ Use strict aseptic technique to prevent infection.
Hypervolemia	■ Excessive fluid administration or administration of fluid too rapidly ■ Renal dysfunction ■ Heart failure ■ Hepatic failure	■ Bounding pulse ■ Crackles on lung auscultation ■ Headache ■ Increased blood pressure ■ Jugular vein distention ■ Weight gain greater than desired	■ Slow or stop IV infusion. ■ Notify the PHCP. ■ Restrict fluids. ■ Administer diuretics as prescribed. ■ Use dialysis as prescribed (in extreme cases).	■ Assess client's history for risk for hypervolemia. ■ Administer via an electronic infusion device and ensure proper function of the device. ■ Never increase the rate of infusion of the device to "catch up" if the infusion gets behind. ■ Monitor intake and output. ■ Monitor weight daily (ideal weight gain is 1-2 lb per week).
Hypoglycemia	■ PN abruptly discontinued ■ Too much insulin being administered	■ Anxiety ■ Diaphoresis ■ Hunger ■ Low blood glucose level <70 mg/dL (<3.9 mmol/L) ■ Shakiness ■ Weakness	■ Notify the PHCP. ■ Administer IV dextrose. ■ Monitor blood glucose level.	■ Gradually decrease PN solution when discontinued. ■ Infuse 10% dextrose at same rate as the PN to prevent hypoglycemia for 1-2 hours after the PN solution is discontinued. ■ Monitor glucose levels and check the level 1 hour after discontinuing the PN.
Infection	■ Poor aseptic technique ■ Catheter contamination ■ Contamination of solution	■ Chills ■ Fever ■ Elevated white blood cell count ■ Redness or drainage at insertion site	■ Notify the PHCP. ■ Remove catheter. ■ Send catheter tip to the laboratory for culture. ■ Prepare to obtain blood cultures. ■ Prepare for antibiotic administration.	■ Use strict aseptic techniques (PN solution has a high concentration of glucose and is a medium for bacterial growth). ■ Monitor temperature (fever could indicate infection). ■ Assess IV site for signs of infection (redness, swelling, drainage). ■ Change site dressing, solution, and tubing as specified by agency policy. ■ Do not disconnect tubing unnecessarily.

Continued

TABLE 69-3 Complications of Parenteral Nutrition—cont'd

Complication	Possible Cause	Signs or Symptoms	Intervention	Prevention
Pneumothorax	■ Inexact catheter placement resulting in puncture of the pleural space	■ Chest or shoulder pain ■ Sudden shortness of breath ■ Cyanosis ■ Tachycardia ■ Absence of breath sounds on affected side	■ Notify the PHCP. ■ Prepare to obtain a chest x-ray. ■ Small pneumothorax may resolve. ■ Larger pneumothorax may require chest tube.	■ Monitor for signs of pneumothorax. ■ Obtain a chest x-ray after insertion of the catheter to ensure proper catheter placement. ■ PN is not initiated until correct catheter placement is verified and the absence of pneumothorax is confirmed.

PHCP, Primary Health care provider; *IV*, intravenous; *PN*, parenteral nutrition.
Adapted from Ignatavicius D, Workman M: *Medical-surgical nursing: patient-centered collaborative care*, ed 7, St. Louis, 2013, Saunders.

9. The electrolyte shift that occurs in "refeeding syndrome" can cause cardiovascular, respiratory, and neurological problems; monitor for shallow respirations, confusion, weakness, bleeding tendencies, and seizures. If noted, the PHCP is notified immediately.
10. Abnormal liver function values may indicate intolerance to or an excess of fat emulsion or problems with metabolism with glucose and protein.
11. Abnormal renal function tests may indicate an excess of amino acids.
12. PN solutions should be stored under refrigeration and administered within 24 hours from the time they are prepared (remove from refrigerator 0.5 to 1 hour before use).
13. PN solutions that are cloudy or darkened should not be used and should be returned to the pharmacy.
14. Additions of substances such as nutrients to PN solutions should be made in the pharmacy and not on the nursing unit.
15. Consultation with the nutritionist should be done on a regular basis (as prescribed or per agency protocol).

E. Home care instructions (Box 69-3)

BOX 69-3 Home Care Instructions for Parenteral Nutrition Therapy

- Teach the client and caregiver how to obtain, administer, and maintain parenteral nutrition fluids.
- Teach the client and caregiver how to change a sterile dressing.
- Obtain a daily weight at the same time of day in the same clothes.
- Stress that if a weight gain of more than 3 lb/week is noted, this may indicate excessive fluid intake and should be reported.
- Monitor the blood glucose level and report abnormalities immediately. Teach the client how to monitor for and manage hypoglycemia and hyperglycemia.
- Teach the client and caregiver about the signs and symptoms of side effects or adverse effects such as infection, thrombosis, air embolism, and catheter displacement.
- Teach the client and caregiver the actions to take if a complication arises and about the importance of reporting complications to the primary health care provider.
- For signs and symptoms of thrombosis, the client should report edema of the arm or at the catheter insertion site, neck pain, and jugular vein distention.
- Leaking of fluid from the insertion site or pain or discomfort as the fluids are infused may indicate displacement of the catheter; this must be reported immediately.
- Encourage the client and caregiver to contact the primary health care provider if they have questions about administration or any other questions.
- Inform the client and caregiver about the importance of follow-up care.
- Teach the client to keep electronic infusion devices fully charged in case of electrical power failure.

III. Administration of Blood Products

A. Blood products
1. Packed red blood cells (PRBCs)
   a. PBRCs are a blood product used to replace erythrocytes; infusion time for 1 unit is usually between 2 and 4 hours.
   b. Each unit increases the hemoglobin level by 1 g/dL (10 mmol/L) and hematocrit by 3% (0.03); the change in laboratory values takes 4 to 6 hours after completion of the blood transfusion.
   c. Evaluation of an effective response is based on the resolution of the symptoms of anemia and an increase in the erythrocyte, hemoglobin, and hematocrit count.
   d. Leukocyte-poor or leukocyte-depleted units are units in which leukocytes, proteins, and plasma have been reduced. They are used to restore oxygen-carrying capacity of blood and intravascular volume.

Washed red blood cells (depleted of plasma, platelets, and leukocytes) may be prescribed for a client with a history of allergic transfusion reactions or those who underwent hematopoietic stem cell transplant. Leukocyte depletion (leukoreduction) by filtration, washing, or freezing is the process used to decrease the amount of white blood cells (WBCs) in a unit of packed cells.

2. Platelet transfusion
   a. Platelets are used to treat thrombocytopenia and platelet dysfunctions.
   b. Clients receiving multiple units of platelets can become "alloimmunized" to different platelet antigens. These clients may benefit from receiving only platelets that match their specific human leukocyte antigen (HLA).
   c. Crossmatching is not required but usually is done (platelet concentrates contain few red blood cells [RBCs]).
   d. The volume in a unit of platelets may vary; always check the bag for the volume of the blood component (in milliliters).
   e. Platelets are administered immediately upon receipt from the blood bank and are given rapidly, usually over 15 to 30 minutes.
   f. Evaluation of an effective response is based on improvement in the platelet count, and platelet counts normally are evaluated 1 hour and 18 to 24 hours after the transfusion; for each unit of platelets administered, an increase of 5000 to 10,000 mm^3 (5 to 10×10^9/L) is expected.
3. Fresh-frozen plasma
   a. Fresh-frozen plasma may be used to provide clotting factors or volume expansion; it contains no platelets.
   b. Fresh-frozen plasma is infused within 2 hours of thawing, while clotting factors are still viable, and is infused over a period of 15 to 30 minutes.
   c. Rh compatibility and ABO compatibility are required for the transfusion of plasma products.
   d. Evaluation of an effective response is assessed by monitoring coagulation studies, particularly the prothrombin time and the partial thromboplastin time, and resolution of hypovolemia.
4. Cryoprecipitates
   a. Prepared from fresh-frozen plasma, cryoprecipitates can be stored for 1 year. Once thawed, the product must be used; 1 unit is administered over 15 to 30 minutes.
   b. Used to replace clotting factors, especially factor VIII and fibrinogen.
   c. Evaluation of an effective response is assessed by monitoring coagulation studies and fibrinogen levels.
5. Granulocytes
   a. May be used to treat a client with sepsis or a neutropenic client with an infection that is unresponsive to antibiotics
   b. Evaluation of an effective response is assessed by monitoring the WBC and differential counts.

Document the necessary information about the blood transfusion in the client's medical record (follow agency guidelines). Include the client's tolerance and response to the transfusion and the effectiveness of the transfusion.

B. Types of blood donations
1. Autologous
   a. A donation of the client's own blood before a scheduled procedure is an autologous donation; it reduces the risk of disease transmission and potential transfusion complications.
   b. Autologous donation is not an option for a client with leukemia or bacteremia.
   c. A donation can be made every 3 days as long as the hemoglobin remains within a safe range.
   d. Donations should begin within 5 weeks of the transfusion date and end at least 3 days before the date of transfusion.
2. Blood salvage
   a. Blood salvage is an autologous donation that involves suctioning blood from body cavities, joint spaces, or other closed body sites.
   b. Blood may need to be "washed," a special process that removes tissue debris before reinfusion.
3. Designated donor
   a. Designated donation occurs when recipients select their own compatible donors.
   b. Donation does not reduce the risk of contracting infections transmitted by the blood; however, recipients feel more comfortable identifying their donors.

C. Compatibility (Table 69-4)
1. Client (the recipient) blood samples are drawn and labeled at the client's bedside at the time the

TABLE 69-4 Compatibility Chart for Red Blood Cell Transfusions

	Recipient			
Donor	A	B	AB	O
A	X		X	
B		X	X	
AB			X	
O	X	X	X	X

The ABO type of the donor should be compatible with the recipient's. Type A can receive from type A or O; type B from type B or O; type AB can receive from type A, B, AB, or O; type O only from type O.

From Ignatavicius D, Workman ML: *Medical-surgical nursing: patient-centered collaborative care*, ed 7, Philadelphia, 2013, Saunders.

Complex Care

blood samples are drawn; the client is asked to state her or his name, which is compared with the name on the client's identification band or bracelet.
2. The recipient's ABO type and Rh type are identified.
3. An antibody screen is done to determine the presence of antibodies other than anti-A and anti-B.
4. To determine compatibility, crossmatching is done, in which donor red blood cells are combined with the recipient's serum and Coombs' serum; the crossmatch is compatible if no RBC agglutination occurs.
5. The universal RBC donor is O negative; the universal recipient is AB positive.
6. Clients with Rh-positive blood can receive RBC transfusion from an Rh-negative donor if necessary; however, an Rh-negative client should not receive Rh-positive blood.

The donor's blood and the recipient's blood must be tested for compatibility. If the blood is not compatible, a life-threatening transfusion reaction can occur.

D. Infusion pumps
1. Infusion pumps may be used to administer blood products if they are designed to function with opaque solutions; special IV tubing with a filter is used specifically for blood products to prevent hemolysis of red blood cells.
2. Always consult manufacturer guidelines for how to use the pump and compatibility for use with blood transfusions.
3. Special manual pressure cuffs designed specifically for blood product administration may be used to increase the flow rate, but it should not exceed 300 mm Hg.
4. Standard sphygmomanometer cuffs are not to be used to increase the flow rate because they do not exert uniform pressure against all parts of the bag.

E. Blood warmers
1. Blood warmers may be used to prevent hypothermia and adverse reactions when several units of blood are being administered.
2. Special warmers have been designed for this purpose, and only devices specifically approved for this use can be used.

If blood warming is necessary, use only warming devices specifically designed and approved for warming blood products. Do not warm blood products in a microwave oven or in hot water.

F. Precautions and nursing responsibilities (Box 69-4)

Check the client's identity (2 identifiers) with another licensed nurse before administering a blood product. Be sure to check the PHCP's prescription, that the client has an appropriate venous access site, that crossmatching procedures have been completed, that an informed consent has been obtained, and that the correct client is receiving the correct type of blood. Use barcode scanning systems per agency policy to ensure client safety.

G. Transfusion reactions (Box 69-5)
1. Description
a. A transfusion reaction is an adverse reaction that happens as a result of receiving a blood transfusion.
b. Types of transfusion reactions include hemolytic, allergic, febrile or bacterial reactions (septicemia), or transfusion-associated graft-versus-host disease (GVHD).
2. Signs of an immediate transfusion reaction
a. Chills and diaphoresis
b. Muscle aches, back pain, or chest pain
c. Rashes, hives, itching, and swelling
d. Rapid, thready pulse
e. Dyspnea, cough, or wheezing
f. Pallor and cyanosis
g. Apprehension
h. Tingling and numbness
i. Headache
j. Nausea, vomiting, abdominal cramping, and diarrhea
3. Signs of a transfusion reaction in an unconscious client
a. Weak pulse
b. Fever
c. Tachycardia or bradycardia
d. Hypotension
e. Visible hemoglobinuria
f. Oliguria or anuria
4. Delayed transfusion reactions
a. Reactions can occur days to years after a transfusion.
b. Signs include fever, mild jaundice, and a decreased hematocrit level.

Stay with the client for the first 15 minutes of the infusion of blood and monitor the client for signs and symptoms of a transfusion reaction; the first 15 minutes of the transfusion are the most critical, and the nurse must stay with the client. Vital signs are monitored every 30 minutes to 1 hour according to institutional protocol.

5. Interventions (see Priority Nursing Actions)

BOX 69-4 Precautions and Nursing Responsibilities for Blood Administration

General Precautions

- A large volume of refrigerated blood infused rapidly through a central venous catheter into the ventricle of the heart can cause cardiac dysrhythmias.
- No solution other than normal saline should be added to blood components.
- Medications are never added to blood components or piggybacked into a blood transfusion.
- To avoid the risk of septicemia, infusions (1 unit) should not exceed the prescribed time for administration (2 to 4 hours for packed red blood cells); follow evidence-based practice guidelines and agency procedure.
- The blood administration set should be changed with each unit of blood, or according to agency policy, to reduce the risk of septicemia.
- Check the blood bag for the date of expiration; components expire at midnight on the day marked on the bag unless otherwise specified.
- Inspect the blood bag for leaks, abnormal color, clots, and bubbles.
- Blood must be administered as soon as possible (within 20 to 30 minutes) after being received from the blood bank, because this is the maximal allowable time out of monitored storage.
- Never refrigerate blood in refrigerators other than those used in blood banks; if the blood is not administered within 20 to 30 minutes, return it to the blood bank.
- The recommended rate of infusion varies with the blood component being transfused and depends on the client's condition; generally, blood is infused as quickly as the client's condition allows (always follow agency guidelines and prescriptions).
- Components containing few red blood cells (RBCs) and platelets may be infused rapidly, but caution should be taken to avoid circulatory overload.
- The nurse should measure vital signs and assess lung sounds before the transfusion and again after the first 15 minutes and every 30 minutes to 1 hour (per agency policy) until 1 hour after the transfusion is completed.

Client Assessment

- Assess for any cultural or religious beliefs regarding blood transfusions.
- A Jehovah's Witness cannot receive blood or blood products; this group believes that receiving a blood transfusion has eternal consequences.
- Ensure that an informed consent has been obtained.
- Explain the procedure to the client and determine whether the client has ever received a blood transfusion or experienced any previous reactions to blood transfusions.
- Check the client's vital signs; assess renal, circulatory, and respiratory status and the client's ability to tolerate intravenously administered fluids.
- If the client's temperature is elevated, notify the primary health care provider (PHCP) before beginning the transfusion; a fever may be a cause for delaying the transfusion in addition to masking a possible symptom of an acute transfusion reaction.

Blood Bank Precautions

- Blood will be released from the blood bank only to personnel specified by agency policy.
- The name and identification number of the intended recipient must be provided to the blood bank, and a documented permanent record of this information must be maintained.
- Blood should be transported from the blood bank to only 1 client at a time to prevent blood delivery to the wrong client.
- Only 1 unit of blood should be transported at a time, even if the client is prescribed to have more than 1 unit transfused.

Client Identity and Compatibility

- Check the PHCP's prescription for the administration of the blood product.
- The most critical phase of the transfusion is confirming product compatibility and verifying client identity.
- Universal barcode systems for blood transfusions should be used to confirm product compatibility, client identity, and expiration (client identification requires 2 identifiers).
- Two licensed nurses (follow agency procedure) need to check the PHCP's prescription, the client's identity, and the client's identification band or bracelet and number, verifying that the name and number are identical to those on the blood component tag.
- At the bedside, the nurse asks the client to state her or his name, and the nurse compares the name with the name on the identification band or bracelet.
- The nurse checks the blood bag tag, label, and blood requisition form to ensure that ABO and Rh types are compatible. The nurse uses the barcode scanning system per agency policy.
- If the nurse notes any inconsistencies when verifying client identity and compatibility, the nurse notifies the blood bank immediately.

Administration of the Transfusion

- Maintain standard and transmission-based precautions and surgical asepsis as necessary.
- Insert an intravenous (IV) line and infuse normal saline; maintain the infusion at a keep-vein-open rate.
- An 18- or 19-gauge IV needle will be needed to achieve a maximum flow rate of blood products and to prevent damage to RBCs; if a smaller-gauge needle must be used, RBCs may be diluted with normal saline (check agency procedure).
- A central venous catheter is an acceptable venous access option for blood transfusions; for a multilumen catheter, use the largest catheter port available or check the port size to ensure that it is adequate for blood administration.
- Always check the bag for the volume of the blood component.

Continued

BOX 69-4 Precautions and Nursing Responsibilities for Blood Administration—cont'd

- Blood products should be infused through administration sets designed specifically for blood; use a Y-tubing or straight-tubing blood administration set that contains a filter designed to trap fibrin clots and other debris that accumulate during blood storage.
- Premedicate the client with acetaminophen or diphenhydramine, as prescribed, if the client has a history of adverse reactions; if prescribed, oral medications should be administered 30 minutes before the transfusion is started, and intravenously administered medications may be given immediately before the transfusion is started.
- Instruct the client to report anything unusual immediately.
- Determine the rate of infusion by the PHCP's prescription or, if not specified, by agency policy.
- Begin the transfusion slowly under close supervision; if no reaction is noted within the first 15 minutes, the flow can be increased to the prescribed rate.
- During the transfusion, monitor the client for signs and symptoms of a transfusion reaction; the first 15 minutes of the transfusion are the most critical, and the nurse must stay with the client.
- If an ABO incompatibility exists or a severe allergic reaction occurs, the reaction is usually evident within the first 50 mL of the transfusion.
- Document the client's tolerance to the administration of the blood product.
- Monitor appropriate laboratory values and document effectiveness of treatment related to the specific type of blood product.

Reactions to the Transfusion

- If a transfusion reaction occurs, stop the transfusion, change the IV tubing down to the IV site, keep the IV line open with normal saline, notify the PHCP and blood bank, and return the blood bag and tubing to the blood bank.
- Do not leave the client alone, and monitor the client's vital signs and monitor for any life-threatening signs or symptoms.
- Obtain appropriate laboratory samples, such as blood and urine samples (free hemoglobin indicates that RBCs were hemolyzed), according to agency procedures.

BOX 69-5 Complications of a Blood Transfusion

- Transfusion reactions
- Circulatory overload
- Septicemia
- Iron overload
- Disease transmission
- Hypocalcemia
- Hyperkalemia
- Citrate toxicity

PRIORITY NURSING ACTIONS

Transfusion Reaction

1. Stop the transfusion.
2. Change the intravenous (IV) tubing down to the IV site and keep the IV line open with normal saline.
3. Notify the primary health care provider (PHCP) and blood bank.
4. Stay with the client, observing signs and symptoms and monitoring vital signs as often as every 5 minutes.
5. Prepare to administer emergency medications as prescribed.
6. Obtain a urine specimen for laboratory studies (perform any other laboratory studies as prescribed).
7. Return blood bag, tubing, attached labels, and transfusion record to the blood bank.
8. Document the occurrence, actions taken, and the client's response.

Reference

Perry et al. (2018), pp. 803-805.

⚠ Stop the transfusion immediately if a blood transfusion reaction is suspected.

H. Circulatory overload
   1. Description: Caused by the infusion of blood at a rate too rapid for the client to tolerate
   2. Assessment
      a. Cough, dyspnea, chest pain, and wheezing on auscultation of the lungs
      b. Headache
      c. Hypertension
      d. Tachycardia and a bounding pulse
      e. Distended neck veins
   3. Interventions
      a. Slow the rate of infusion.
      b. Place the client in an upright position, with the feet in a dependent position.
      c. Notify the PHCP.
      d. Administer oxygen, diuretics, and morphine sulfate, as prescribed.
      e. Monitor for dysrhythmias.
      f. Phlebotomy also may be a method of prescribed treatment in a severe case.

I. Septicemia
   1. Description: Occurs with the transfusion of blood that is contaminated with microorganisms
   2. Assessment
      a. Rapid onset of chills and a high fever
      b. Vomiting
      c. Diarrhea
      d. Hypotension
      e. Shock
   3. Interventions
      a. Notify the PHCP.

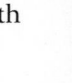

b. Obtain blood cultures and cultures of the blood bag.
c. Administer oxygen, IV fluids, antibiotics, vasopressors, and corticosteroids as prescribed.

J. Iron overload
1. Description: A delayed transfusion complication that occurs in clients who receive multiple blood transfusions, such as clients with anemia or thrombocytopenia
2. Assessment
a. Vomiting
b. Diarrhea
c. Hypotension
d. Altered hematological values
3. Interventions
a. Deferoxamine, administered intravenously or subcutaneously, removes accumulated iron via the kidneys.
b. Urine turns red as iron is excreted after the administration of deferoxamine; treatment is discontinued when serum iron levels return to normal.

Contact the PHCP immediately if a transfusion reaction or a complication of blood administration arises.

K. Disease transmission
1. The disease most commonly transmitted is hepatitis C, which is manifested by anorexia, nausea, vomiting, dark urine, and jaundice; the symptoms usually occur within 4 to 6 weeks after the transfusion.
2. Other infectious agents and diseases transmitted by blood transfusion include hepatitis B virus, human immunodeficiency virus (HIV), human herpes virus type 6, Epstein-Barr virus, human T-cell leukemia, cytomegalovirus, and malaria.
3. Donor screening has greatly reduced the risk of transmission of infectious agents; in addition, antibody testing of donors for HIV has greatly reduced the risk of transmission.

L. Hypocalcemia
1. Citrate in transfused blood binds with calcium and is excreted.
2. Assess serum calcium level before and after the transfusion.
3. Monitor for signs of hypocalcemia (hyperactive reflexes, paresthesias, tetany, muscle cramps, positive Trousseau's sign, positive Chvostek's sign).
4. Slow the transfusion and notify the PHCP if signs of hypocalcemia occur.

M. Hyperkalemia
1. Stored blood liberates potassium through hemolysis.
2. The older the blood, the greater the risk of hyperkalemia; therefore, clients at risk for hyperkalemia, such as those with renal insufficiency or renal failure, should receive fresh blood.
3. Assess the date on the blood and the serum potassium level before and after the transfusion.
4. Monitor the potassium level and for signs and symptoms of hyperkalemia (paresthesias, weakness, abdominal cramps, diarrhea, and dysrhythmias).
5. Slow the transfusion and notify the PHCP if signs of hyperkalemia occur.

N. Citrate toxicity
1. Citrate, the anticoagulant used in blood products, is metabolized by the liver.
2. Rapid administration of multiple units of stored blood may cause hypocalcemia and hypomagnesemia when citrate binds calcium and magnesium; this results in citrate toxicity, causing myocardial depression and coagulopathy.
3. Those most at risk include individuals with liver dysfunction or neonates with immature liver function.
4. Treatment includes slowing or stopping the transfusion to allow the citrate to be metabolized; hypocalcemia and hypomagnesemia are also treated with replacement therapy.

IV. Tube Care

A. Nasogastric (NG) tubes
1. These are tubes used to intubate the stomach.
2. The tube is inserted from the nose to the stomach.

B. Purpose
1. To decompress the stomach by removing fluids or gas to promote abdominal comfort
2. To allow surgical anastomoses to heal without distention
3. To decrease the risk of aspiration
4. To administer medications to clients who are unable to swallow
5. To provide nutrition by acting as a temporary feeding tube
6. To irrigate the stomach and remove toxic substances, such as in poisoning

C. Types of tubes
1. Levin tube (Fig. 69-8)
a. Single-lumen nasogastric tube
b. Used to remove gastric contents via intermittent suction or to provide tube feedings
2. Salem sump tube: A Salem sump is a double-lumen nasogastric tube with an air vent (pigtail) used for decompression with intermittent continuous suction (see Fig. 69-8).

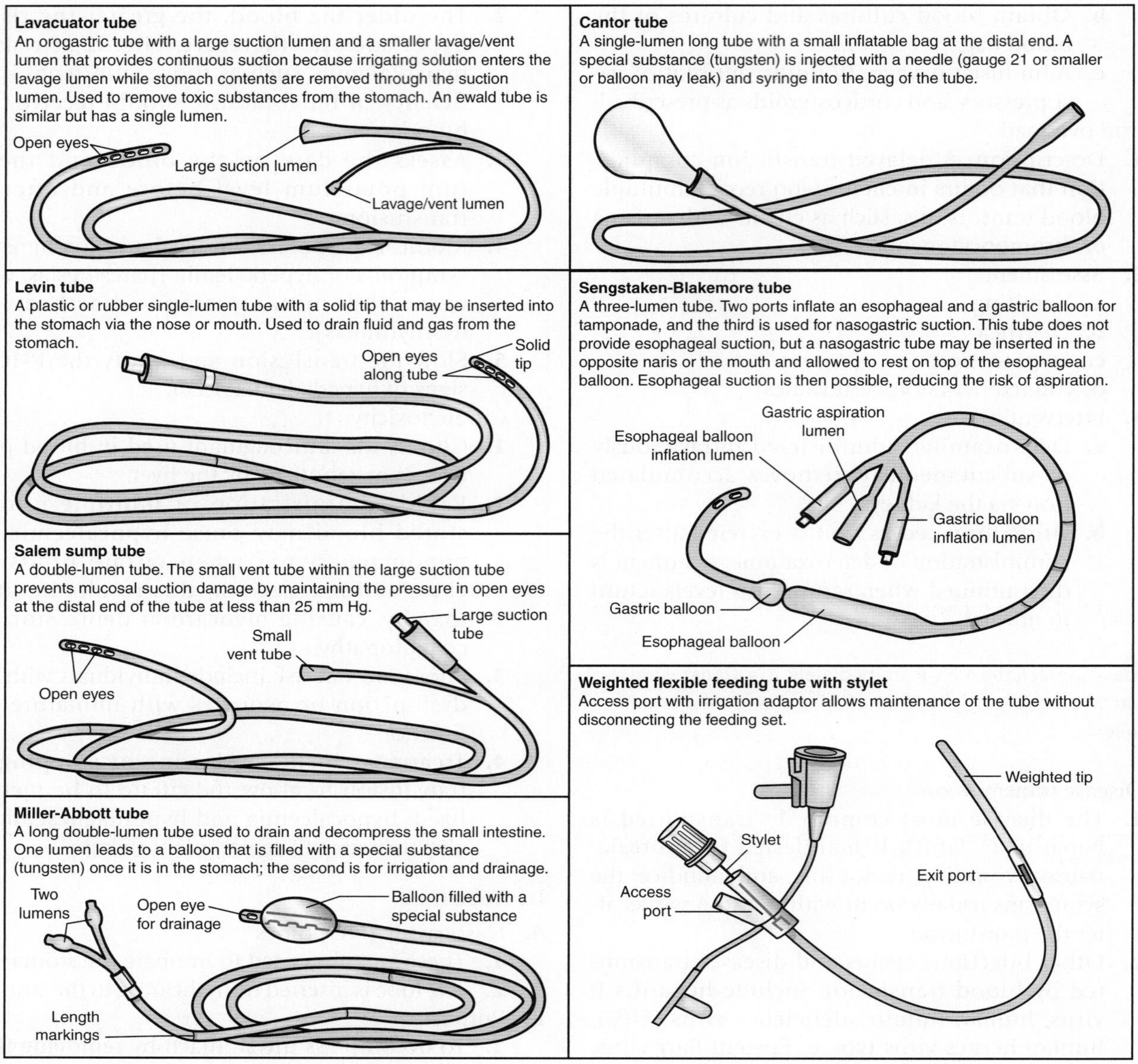
Lavacuator tube
An orogastric tube with a large suction lumen and a smaller lavage/vent lumen that provides continuous suction because irrigating solution enters the lavage lumen while stomach contents are removed through the suction lumen. Used to remove toxic substances from the stomach. An ewald tube is similar but has a single lumen.
Open eyes
Large suction lumen
Lavage/vent lumen
Cantor tube
A single-lumen long tube with a small inflatable bag at the distal end. A special substance (tungsten) is injected with a needle (gauge 21 or smaller or balloon may leak) and syringe into the bag of the tube.
Levin tube
A plastic or rubber single-lumen tube with a solid tip that may be inserted into the stomach via the nose or mouth. Used to drain fluid and gas from the stomach.
Open eyes along tube
Solid tip
Sengstaken-Blakemore tube
A three-lumen tube. Two ports inflate an esophageal and a gastric balloon for tamponade, and the third is used for nasogastric suction. This tube does not provide esophageal suction, but a nasogastric tube may be inserted in the opposite naris or the mouth and allowed to rest on top of the esophageal balloon. Esophageal suction is then possible, reducing the risk of aspiration.
Gastric aspiration lumen
Esophageal balloon inflation lumen
Gastric balloon inflation lumen
Gastric balloon
Esophageal balloon
Salem sump tube
A double-lumen tube. The small vent tube within the large suction tube prevents mucosal suction damage by maintaining the pressure in open eyes at the distal end of the tube at less than 25 mm Hg.
Large suction tube
Small vent tube
Open eyes
Weighted flexible feeding tube with stylet
Access port with irrigation adaptor allows maintenance of the tube without disconnecting the feeding set.
Weighted tip
Stylet
Exit port
Access port
Miller-Abbott tube
A long double-lumen tube used to drain and decompress the small intestine. One lumen leads to a balloon that is filled with a special substance (tungsten) once it is in the stomach; the second is for irrigation and drainage.
Two lumens
Open eye for drainage
Balloon filled with a special substance
Length markings

FIG. 69-8 Comparison of design and function of selected gastrointestinal tubes.

⚠ The air vent on a Salem sump tube is not to be clamped and is to be kept above the level of the stomach. If leakage occurs through the air vent, instill 30 mL of air into the air vent and irrigate the main lumen with normal saline (NS).

D. Intubation procedures (Box 69-6)

E. Irrigation

1. Assess placement before irrigating (see Box 69-6).
2. Perform irrigation every 4 hours to assess and maintain the patency of the tube.
3. Gently instill 30 to 50 mL of water or NS (depending on agency policy) with an irrigation syringe.
4. Pull back on the syringe plunger to withdraw the fluid to check patency; repeat if the tube flow is sluggish.

F. Removal of a nasogastric tube: Ask the client to take a deep breath and hold it; remove the tube slowly and evenly over the course of 3 to 6 seconds (coil the tube around the hand while removing it).

G. Gastrointestinal tube feedings

1. Types of tubes and anatomical placement
   - **a.** Nasogastric: Nose to stomach
   - **b.** Nasoduodenal-nasojejunal: Nose to duodenum or jejunum
   - **c.** Gastrostomy: Stomach
   - **d.** Jejunostomy: Jejunum
2. Types of administration
   - **a.** Bolus: A bolus resembles normal meal feeding patterns; formula is administrated over a 30- to 60-minute period every 3 to 6 hours; the amount of formula and frequency can

Complex Care

BOX 69-6 Nasogastric Tubes: Intubation Procedures

1. Follow agency procedures.
2. Explain the procedure and its potential discomfort to the client.
3. Position the client in a high-Fowler's position with pillows behind the shoulders.
4. Determine which nostril is more patent.
5. Measure the length of the tube from the bridge of the nose to the earlobe to the xiphoid process and indicate this length with a piece of tape on the tube (remember the abbreviation NEX, which stands for nose, earlobe, and xiphoid process).
6. If the client is conscious and alert, have him or her swallow or drink water (follow agency procedure).
7. Lubricate the tip of the tube with water-soluble lubricant.
8. Gently insert the tube into the nasopharynx and advance the tube.
9. When the tube nears the back of the throat (first black measurement on the tube), instruct the client to swallow or drink sips of water (unless contraindicated). If resistance is met, slowly rotate and aim the tube downward and toward the closer ear; in the intubated or semiconscious client, flex the head toward the chest while passing the tube.
10. Immediately withdraw the tube if any change is noted in the client's respiratory status.
11. Following insertion, obtain an abdominal x-ray study to confirm placement of the tube.
12. Connect the tube to suction, to either the intermittent or the continuous suction setting, as prescribed if the purpose of the tube is for decompression.
13. Secure the tube to the client's nose with adhesive tape and to the client's gown (follow agency procedure and check for client allergy to tape).
14. Observe the client for nausea, vomiting, abdominal fullness, or distention and monitor gastric output.
15. Check residual volumes every 4 hours, before each feeding, and before giving medications. Aspirate all stomach contents (residual) and measure the amount. Reinstill residual contents to prevent excessive fluid and electrolyte losses, unless the residual contents appear abnormal or the volume is large (greater than 250 mL). Always follow agency procedure. Withhold a feeding if the residual amount is more than 100 mL or according to agency or nutritional consult recommendations.
16. Before the instillation of any substance through the tube (i.e., irrigation solution, feeding, medications), aspirate stomach contents and test the pH (a pH of 3.5 or lower indicates that the tip of the tube is in a gastric location).
17. If irrigation is indicated, use normal saline solution (check agency procedure).
18. Observe the client for fluid and electrolyte balance.
19. Instruct the client about movement to prevent nasal irritation and dislodgment of the tube.
20. On a daily basis, remove the adhesive tape that is securing the tube to the nose and clean and dry the skin, assessing for excoriation; then reapply the tape.

Note: Gastrostomy or jejunostomy tubes are surgically inserted. A dressing is placed at the site of insertion. The dressing needs to be removed, the skin needs to be cleansed (with a solution determined by the health care provider or agency procedure), and a new sterile dressing needs to be applied every 8 hours (or as specified by agency policy). The skin at the insertion site is checked for signs of excoriation, infection, or other abnormalities, such as leakage of the feeding solution.
Adapted from Potter P, Perry A, Stockert P, Hall A: *Fundamentals of nursing,* ed 8, St. Louis, 2013, Mosby

be recommended by the dietitian and is prescribed by the PHCP.

b. Continuous: Feeding is administered continually for 24 hours; an infusion feeding pump regulates the flow.
c. Cyclical: Feeding is administered in the daytime or nighttime for approximately 8 to 16 hours (feedings at night allow for more freedom during the day).
d. An infusion feeding pump regulates the flow.

3. Administration of feedings
   a. Check the PHCP's prescription and agency policy regarding residual amounts; usually, if the residual is less than 100 mL, feeding is administered; large-volume aspirates indicate delayed gastric emptying and place the client at risk for aspiration.
   b. Assess bowel sounds; hold the feeding and notify the PHCP if bowel sounds are absent.
   c. Position the client in a high-Fowler's position; if comatose, place in high-Fowler's and on the right side.
   d. Assess tube placement by aspirating gastric contents and measuring the pH (should be 3.5 or lower) or per agency procedure.
   e. Aspirate all stomach contents (residual), measure the amount, and return the contents to the stomach to prevent electrolyte imbalances (unless the color or characteristics of the residual is abnormal or the amount is greater than 250 mL).
   f. Warm the feeding to room temperature to prevent diarrhea and cramps.
   g. Use an infusion feeding pump for continuous or cyclic feedings.
   h. For bolus feeding, maintain the client in a high-Fowler's position for 30 minutes after the feeding. Use an infusion pump or allow the feeding to infuse via gravity. Do not plunge the feeding into the stomach.
   i. For a continuous feeding, keep the client in a semi-Fowler's position at all times.

4. Precautions

Always assess the placement of a gastrointestinal tube before instilling feeding solutions, medications, or any other solution. If the tube is incorrectly placed, the client is at risk for aspiration.

   a. Change the feeding container and tubing every 24 hours or per agency policy.
   b. Do not hang more solution than is required for a 4-hour period; this prevents bacterial growth.
   c. Check the expiration date on the formula before administering.
   d. Shake the formula well before pouring it into the container (feeding bag). Some feedings require the use of a bag in which formula is added, or require the use of bottles that feeding tubing can be attached to directly. The tubing sometimes has a Y-site connection so a regular flush can be programmed using the pump rather than using a piston syringe.
   e. Always assess bowel sounds; do not administer any feedings if bowel sounds are absent.
   f. Administer the feeding at the prescribed rate or via gravity flow (intermittent bolus feedings) with a 50- to 60-mL syringe with the plunger removed.
   g. Gently flush with 30 to 50 mL of water or NS (depending on agency policy) using the irrigation syringe after the feeding.
5. Complications of feedings include aspiration, diarrhea, vomiting, a clogged tube.
6. Aspiration
   a. Verify tube placement.
   b. Do not administer the feeding if residual is more than 100 mL (check PHCP's prescription and agency policy).
   c. Keep the head of the bed elevated.
   d. If aspiration occurs, suction as needed, assess respiratory rate, auscultate lung sounds, monitor temperature for aspiration pneumonia, and prepare to obtain a chest radiograph.
7. Diarrhea
   a. Assess the client for lactose intolerance.
   b. Use fiber-containing feedings.
   c. Administer feeding slowly and at room temperature.
8. Vomiting
   a. Administer feedings slowly and, for bolus feedings, make feeding last for at least 30 minutes.
   b. Measure abdominal girth.
   c. Do not allow the feeding bag to empty.
   d. Do not allow air to enter the tubing.
   e. Administer the feeding at room temperature.
   f. Elevate the head of the bed.
   g. Administer antiemetics as prescribed.
9. Clogged tube
   a. Use liquid forms of medication, if possible.
   b. Flush the tube with 30 to 50 mL of water or NS (depending on agency policy) before and after medication administration and before and after bolus feeding.
   c. Flush with water every 4 hours for continuous feeding.

If the client vomits, stop the tube feeding and place the client in a side-lying position; suction the client as needed.

H. Administration of medications (see Priority Nursing Actions)

PRIORITY NURSING ACTIONS

Administering Medications via a Nasogastric, Gastrostomy, or Jejunostomy Tube

1. Check the primary health care provider's (PHCP's) prescription.
2. Prepare the medication for administration.
3. Ensure that the medication prescribed can be crushed or is a capsule that can be opened; use elixir forms of medications if available.
4. Dissolve crushed medication or capsule contents in 15 to 30 mL of water.
5. Verify the client's identity (2 identifiers) and explain the procedure to the client.
6. Don gloves; check tube placement and residual contents before instilling the medication; check for bowel sounds.
7. Flush with 30 to 50 mL of water or normal saline (NS), depending on agency policy.
8. Pinch off tubing and attach an irrigation syringe to the nasogastric tube and pour the medication into the syringe. Release the pinch on the tubing immediately and allow medication to infuse via gravity.
9. Flush with 30 to 50 mL of water or normal saline (NS), depending on agency policy.
10. Clamp the tube for 30 to 60 minutes, depending on medication and agency policy.
11. Document the administration of the medication and any other appropriate information.

Reference

Potter et al. (2017), pp. 636-637.

I. Intestinal tubes
1. Description
   a. The intestinal tube is passed nasally into the small intestine.
   b. It may be used to decompress the bowel or to remove accumulated intestinal secretions when other interventions to decompress the bowel are not effective.

c. The tube enters the small intestine through the pyloric sphincter because of the weight of a small bag containing tungsten at the end.

d. Types of tubes include the Cantor tube (single lumen) and the Miller-Abbott tube (double lumen) (see Fig. 69-8).

2. Interventions

a. Assess the PHCP's prescriptions and agency policy for advancement and removal of the tube and tungsten.

b. Position the client on the right side to facilitate passage of the weighted bag in the tube through the pylorus of the stomach and into the small intestine.

c. Assess the abdomen during the procedure by monitoring drainage from the tube and the abdominal girth.

d. Do not secure the tube to the face with tape until it has reached final placement (may take several hours) in the intestines.

e. If the tube becomes blocked, notify the PHCP.

f. To remove the tube, the tungsten is removed from the balloon portion of the tube with a syringe; the tube is removed gradually (6 inches [15 cm] every hour) as prescribed by the PHCP.

J. Esophageal and gastric tubes

1. Description

a. May be used to apply pressure against bleeding esophageal veins to control the bleeding when other interventions are not effective or they are contraindicated.

b. Not used if the client has ulceration or necrosis of the esophagus or has had previous esophageal surgery because of the risk of rupture.

2. Sengstaken-Blakemore tube and Minnesota tube (see Fig. 69-8)

a. The Sengstaken-Blakemore tube, used only occasionally, is a triple-lumen gastric tube with an inflatable esophageal balloon (compresses esophageal varices), an inflatable gastric balloon (applies pressure at the cardioesophageal junction), and a gastric aspiration lumen. A nasogastric tube also is inserted in the opposite naris to collect secretions that accumulate above the esophageal balloon.

b. More commonly used is the Minnesota tube, which is a modified Sengstaken-Blakemore tube with an additional lumen (a 4-lumen gastric tube) for aspirating esophagopharyngeal secretions.

c. A radiograph of the upper abdomen and chest confirms placement.

3. Interventions

a. Check patency and integrity of all balloons before insertion.

b. Label each lumen.

c. Place the client in the upright or Fowler's position for insertion.

d. Immediately after insertion, prepare for radiography to verify placement.

e. Maintain head elevation once the tube is in place.

f. Double-clamp the balloon ports to prevent air leaks.

g. Keep scissors at the bedside at all times; monitor for respiratory distress, and if it occurs, cut the tubes to deflate the balloons.

h. To prevent ulceration or necrosis of the esophagus, release esophageal pressure at intervals as prescribed and per agency policy.

i. Monitor for increased bloody drainage, which may indicate persistent bleeding and rupture of the varices.

j. Monitor for signs of esophageal rupture, which include a drop in blood pressure, increased heart rate, and back and upper abdominal pain. Esophageal rupture is an emergency, and signs of esophageal rupture must be reported to the PHCP immediately.

K. Lavage tubes

1. Used to remove toxic substances from the stomach

2. Types of tubes

a. Lavacuator: The Lavacuator is an orogastric tube with a large suction lumen and a smaller lavage–vent lumen that provides continuous suction; irrigation solution enters the lavage lumen while stomach contents are removed through the suction lumen (see Fig. 69-9).

b. Ewald tube: A single-lumen large tube used for rapid 1-time irrigation and evacuation

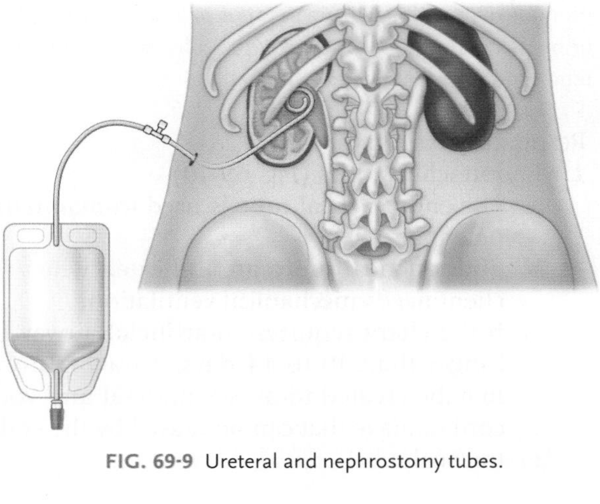

FIG. 69-9 Ureteral and nephrostomy tubes.

L. Urinary and renal tubes

1. Types of urinary catheters

a. Single lumen: Usually used for straight catheterization to empty the client's bladder, obtain sterile urine specimens, or check the residual amount of urine after the client voids

b. Double lumen: Used when an indwelling catheter is needed for continuous bladder drainage; one lumen is for drainage and the other is for balloon inflation.

c. Triple lumen: Used when bladder irrigation and drainage is necessary; 1 lumen is for instilling the bladder irrigant solution, 1 lumen is for continuous bladder drainage, and 1 lumen is for balloon inflation.

d. Strict aseptic technique is necessary for insertion and care of the catheter.

2. Routine urinary catheter care

a. Use gloves and wash the perineal area with warm soapy water.

b. With the nondominant hand, pull back the labia or foreskin to expose the meatus (in the adult male, return the foreskin to its normal position).

c. Cleanse along the catheter with soap and water.

d. Anchor the catheter to the thigh.

e. Maintain the catheter bag below the level of the bladder.

3. Ureteral and nephrostomy tubes (Fig. 69-9)

a. Never clamp the tube.

b. Maintain patency.

c. Irrigate only if prescribed by the PHCP, using strict aseptic technique; a maximum of 5 mL of sterile NS is instilled slowly and gently.

d. If patency cannot be established with the prescribed irrigation, notify the PHCP immediately.

4. Catheter insertion and removal (Box 69-7)

If the client has a ureteral or nephrostomy tube, monitor output closely; urine output of less than 30 mL/hr or lack of output for more than 15 minutes should be reported to the PHCP immediately.

M. Respiratory system tubes

1. Endotracheal tubes (Fig. 69-10)

a. The endotracheal tube is used to maintain a patent airway.

b. Endotracheal tubes are indicated when the client needs mechanical ventilation.

c. If the client requires an artificial airway for longer than 10 to 14 days, a tracheostomy may be created to avoid mucosal and vocal cord damage that can be caused by the endotracheal tube.

d. The cuff (located at the distal end of the tube), when inflated, produces a seal between the trachea and the cuff to prevent aspiration and ensure delivery of a set tidal volume when mechanical ventilation is used; an inflated cuff also prevents air from passing to the vocal cords, nose, or mouth.

e. The pilot balloon permits air to be inserted into the cuff, prevents air from escaping, and is used as a guideline for determining the presence or absence of air in the cuff.

f. The universal adapter enables attachment of the tube to mechanical ventilation tubing or other types of oxygen delivery systems.

g. Types of tubes: orotracheal and nasotracheal

2. Orotracheal tubes

a. Inserted through the mouth; allows use of a larger diameter tube and reduces the work of breathing

b. Indicated when the client has a nasal obstruction or a predisposition to epistaxis

c. Uncomfortable and can be manipulated by the tongue, causing airway obstruction; an oral airway may be needed to keep the client from biting on the tube.

3. Nasotracheal tubes

a. Inserted through a nostril; this smaller tube increases resistance and the client's work of breathing.

b. Its use is avoided in clients with bleeding disorders.

c. It is more comfortable for the client, and the client is unable to manipulate the tube with the tongue.

4. Interventions

a. Placement is confirmed by chest x-ray film (correct placement is 1 to 2 cm above the carina).

b. Assess placement by auscultating both sides of the chest while manually ventilating with a resuscitation (Ambu) bag (if breath sounds and chest wall movement are absent in the left side, the tube may be in the right main stem bronchus).

c. Perform auscultation over the stomach to rule out esophageal intubation.

d. If the tube is in the stomach, louder breath sounds will be heard over the stomach than over the chest, and abdominal distention will be present.

e. Secure the tube with adhesive tape immediately after intubation.

f. Monitor the position of the tube at the lip or nose.

g. Monitor skin and mucous membranes.

h. Suction the tube only when needed.

BOX 69-7 Urinary Catheters: Insertion and Removal Procedures

Insertion Procedure

1. Follow agency procedures.
2. Explain the procedure and its potential discomfort to the client.
3. Place the client in position for catheterization:
   Female: Assist to dorsal recumbent position (supine with knees flexed). Support legs with pillows to reduce muscle tension and promote comfort.
   Male: Assist to supine position with thighs slightly abducted.
4. Wearing clean gloves, wash perineal area with soap and water as needed; dry thoroughly. Remove and discard gloves; perform hand hygiene.
5. Open outer wrapping of the catheter kit, remembering that all components of the catheterization tray are sterile (all supplies are arranged in the box in order of sequence of use).
6. Apply waterproof sterile drape (when packed as first item in tray).
7. Urinary catheter procedure with specifics for male and female:
   a. Place a sterile drape with plastic side down under the client's buttocks.
   b. Don sterile gloves using sterile technique.
   c. Pick up fenestrated drape from tray. Allow it to unfold without touching nonsterile surface. Apply drape over perineum, exposing labia or penis.
   d. While maintaining sterility, open packet of lubricant and squeeze out on sterile field. Lubricate catheter tip by dipping it into water-soluble gel, 2.5 to 5 cm (1 to 2 inches) for women and 12.5 to 17.5 cm (5 to 7 inches) for men. Attach prefilled syringe to balloon port. Prepare cotton balls or swab sticks for cleansing perineal area.
   e. Remember with a sterile technique, the sterile field and gloved hands must be maintained above the level of the waist, the 1-inch (2.5 cm) border on the field is considered contaminated, and the nurse cannot turn her or his back to the field at any time.
   f. Catheter insertion
   Female: The female should be positioned in a dorsal recumbent position with the legs open to allow for full visualization and maintenance of the sterile field. With nondominant hand, fully expose urethral meatus by spreading labia, taking care to not allow the labia to close. Using forceps in sterile dominant hand, pick up cotton ball or swab sticks saturated with antiseptic solution, wiping from front to back (from clitoris toward anus). Using a new cotton ball or swab for each area you clean, wipe far labial fold, near labial fold, and directly over center of urethral meatus. Pick up and hold catheter 7.5 to 10 cm (3 to 4 inches) from catheter tip. Advance catheter a total of 7.5 cm (3 inches) in adult or until urine flows out of catheter end. When urine appears, advance catheter another 2.5 to 5 cm (1 to 2 inches). Do not use force to insert catheter.
   Male: Use of square sterile drape is optional; you may apply fenestrated drape with fenestrated slit resting over penis. Grasp penis at shaft just below glans. (If client is not circumcised, retract foreskin with nondominant hand.) With dominant hand, pick up antiseptic-soaked cotton ball with forceps or swab stick and clean penis. Move cotton ball or swab in circular motion from urethral meatus down to base of glans. Repeat cleaning 2 more times, using clean cotton ball/stick each time. Pick up catheter with gloved dominant hand and insert catheter by lifting penis to position perpendicular to client's body and apply light traction. Advance catheter 17.5 to 22.5 cm (7 to 9 inches) in adult or until urine flows out of catheter end. Advance an additional 2.5 to 5 cm (1 to 2 inches) after urine appears. Lower penis and hold catheter securely in nondominant hand.
8. Inflate balloon fully per manufacturer's directions and gently pull back on the catheter until resistance is felt.
9. Secure catheter tubing to inner thigh with agency-approved securing device, such as a StatLock.
10. Record type and size of catheter inserted, amount of fluid used to inflate the balloon, characteristics and amount of urine, specimen collection if appropriate, client's response to procedure, and that teaching was completed.

Removal Procedure

1. Follow agency procedures.
2. Explain the procedure and its potential discomfort to the client.
3. Position the client in the same position as during catheterization.
4. Remove the securing device and place the towel between a female client's thighs or over a male client's thighs.
5. Insert a 10-mL syringe into the balloon injection port. Slowly withdraw all of the solution to deflate the balloon totally.
6. After deflation, explain to the client that she or he may feel a burning sensation as the catheter is withdrawn. Pull the catheter out smoothly and slowly.
7. Assess the client's urinary function by noting the first voiding after catheter removal and documenting the time and amount of voiding for the next 24 hours.

Adapted from Potter P, Perry A, Stockert P, Hall A: *Fundamentals of nursing*, ed 8, St. Louis, 2013, Mosby.

i. The oral tube needs to be moved to the opposite side of the mouth daily to prevent pressure and necrosis of the lip and mouth area, prevent nerve damage, and facilitate inspection and cleaning of the mouth; moving the tube to the opposite side of the mouth should be done by 2 health care providers.

j. Prevent dislodgment and pulling or tugging on the tube; suction, coughing, and speaking attempts by the client place extra stress on the tube and can cause dislodgment.

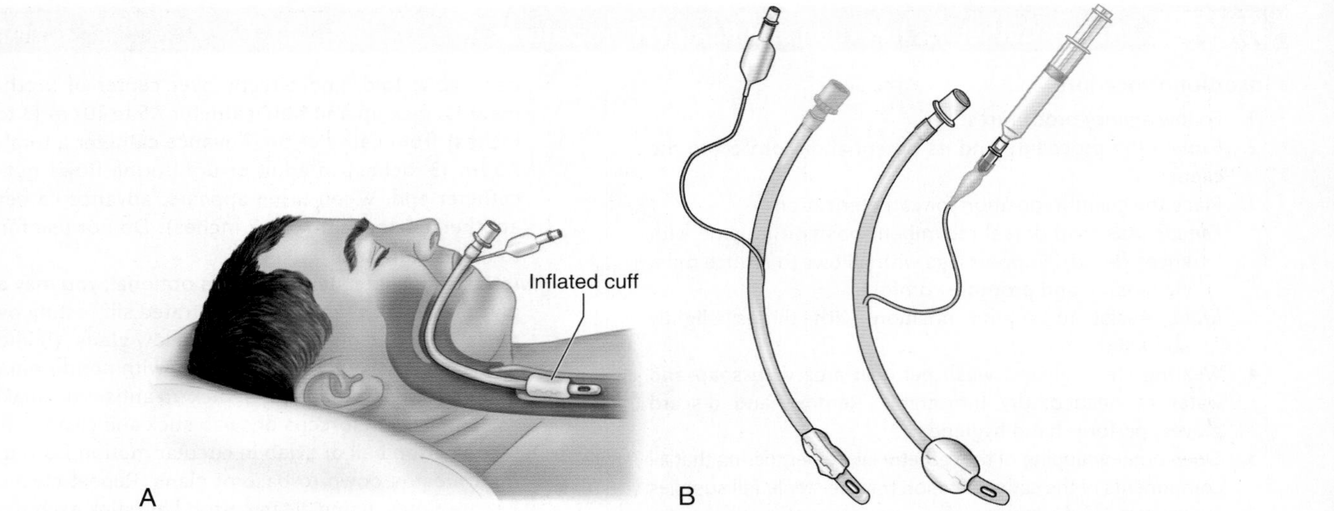

FIG. 69-10 **A,** Endotracheal (ET) tube with inflated cuff. **B,** ET tubes with uninflated and inflated cuffs and syringe for inflation.

k. Assess the pilot balloon to ensure that the cuff is inflated; maintain cuff inflation, which creates a seal and allows complete mechanical control of respiration.

l. Monitor cuff pressures at least every 8 hours per agency procedure to ensure that they do not exceed 20 mm Hg (an aneroid pressure manometer is used to measure cuff pressures); minimal leak and occlusive techniques are used for cuff inflation to check cuff pressures.

⚠ A resuscitation (Ambu) bag needs to be kept at the bedside of a client with an endotracheal tube or a tracheostomy tube at all times.

5. Minimal leak technique
- **a.** This is used for cuff inflation and checking cuff pressures for cuffs without pressure relief valves.
- **b.** Inflate the cuff until a seal is established; no harsh sound should be heard through a stethoscope placed over the trachea when the client breathes in, but a slight air leak on peak inspiration is present and can be heard.
- **c.** The client cannot make verbal sounds, and no air is felt coming out of the client's mouth.

6. Occlusive technique
- **a.** This is used for cuff inflation and checking cuff pressures for cuffs with pressure relief valves.
- **b.** Provides an adequate seal in the trachea at the lowest possible cuff pressure.
- **c.** Uses same procedure as minimal leak technique, without an air leak.

7. Extubation
- **a.** Hyperoxygenate the client and suction the endotracheal tube and the oral cavity.
- **b.** Place the client in a semi-Fowler's position.
- **c.** Deflate the cuff; have the client inhale and, at peak inspiration, remove the tube, suctioning the airway through the tube while pulling it out.
- **d.** After removal, instruct the client to cough and deep-breathe to assist in removing accumulated secretions in the throat.
- **e.** Apply oxygen therapy, as prescribed.
- **f.** Monitor for respiratory difficulty; contact the PHCP if respiratory difficulty occurs.
- **g.** Inform the client that hoarseness or a sore throat is normal and that the client should limit talking if it occurs.

N. Tracheostomy

1. A tracheostomy is an opening made surgically directly into the trachea to establish an airway; a tracheostomy tube is inserted into the opening and the tube attaches to the mechanical ventilator or another type of oxygen delivery device (Fig. 69-11).

2. Types: The tracheostomy can be temporary or permanent (Box 69-8).

3. Interventions
- **a.** Assess respirations and for bilateral breath sounds.
- **b.** Monitor arterial blood gases and pulse oximetry.
- **c.** Encourage coughing and deep breathing.
- **d.** Maintain a semi-Fowler's to high-Fowler's position.
- **e.** Monitor for bleeding, difficulty with breathing, absence of breath sounds, and crepitus (subcutaneous emphysema), which are indications of hemorrhage or pneumothorax.
- **f.** Provide respiratory treatments as prescribed.
- **g.** Suction fluids as needed; hyperoxygenate the client before suctioning (see Priority Nursing Actions).

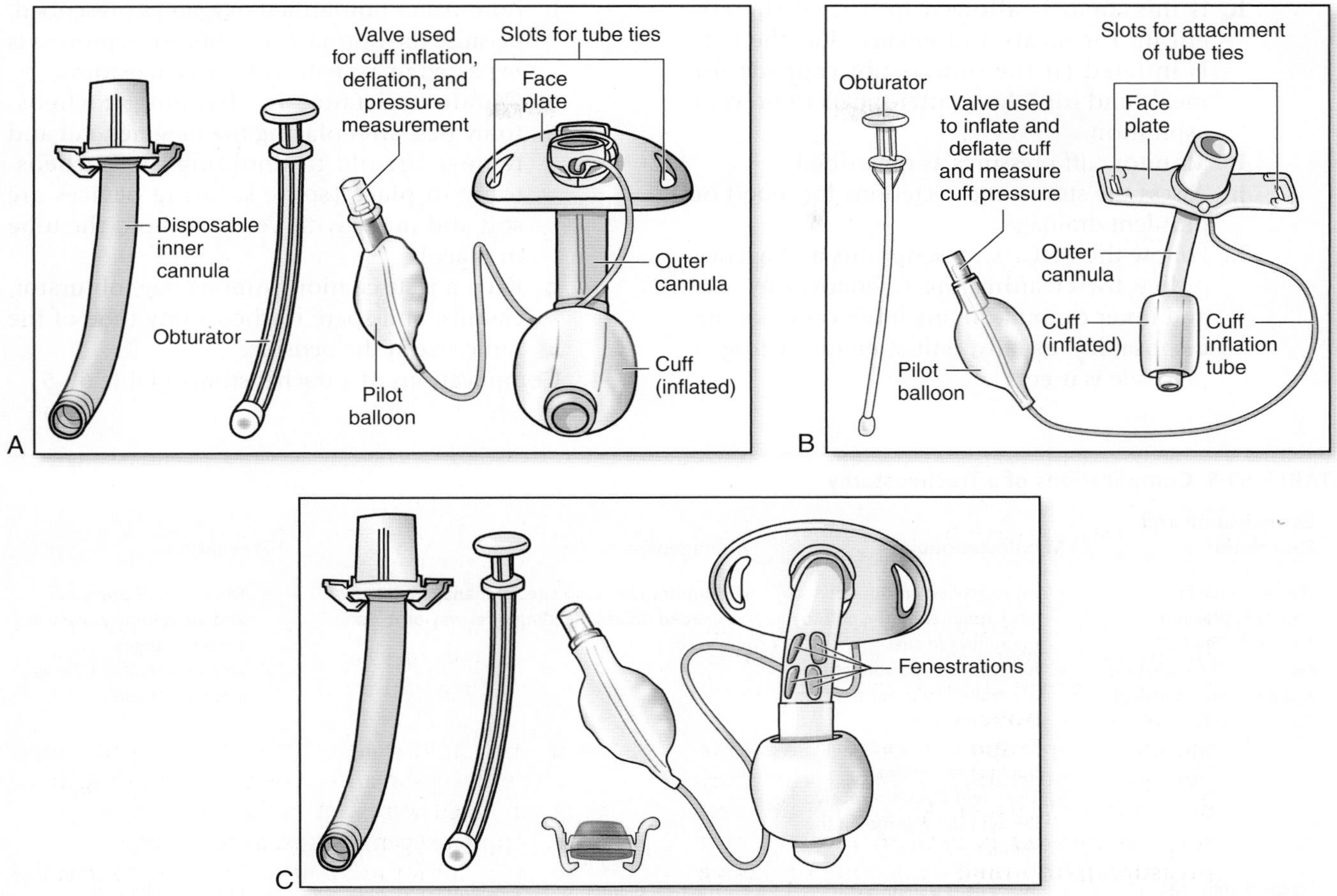

FIG. 69-11 Tracheostomy tubes. **A,** Double-lumen cuffed tracheostomy tube with disposable inner cannula. **B,** Single-lumen cannula cuffed tracheostomy tube. **C,** Double-lumen cuffed fenestrated tracheostomy tube with plug (red cap).

BOX 69-8 Some Types of Tracheostomy Tubes

Double-Lumen Tube

The double-lumen tube has the following parts:

Outer cannula—fits into the stoma and keeps the airway open. The face plate indicates the size and type of tube and has small holes on both sides for securing the tube with tracheostomy ties or another device.

Inner cannula—fits snugly into the outer cannula and locks into place. It provides the universal adaptor for use with the ventilator and other respiratory therapy equipment. Some may be removed, cleaned, and reused; others are disposable.

Obturator—a stylet with a smooth end used to facilitate the direction of the tube when inserting or changing a tracheostomy tube. The obturator is removed immediately after tube placement; an obturator is always kept with the client and at the bedside in case of accidental decannulation.

Cuff—when inflated, seals the airway. The cuffed tube is used for mechanical ventilation, preventing aspiration of oral or gastric secretions, or for the client receiving a tube feeding to prevent aspiration. A pilot balloon attached to the outside of the tube indicates the presence or absence of air in the cuff.

Single-Lumen Tube

The single-lumen tube is similar to the double-lumen tube except that there is no inner cannula. More intensive nursing care is required with this tube because there is no inner cannula to ensure a patent lumen.

Fenestrated Tube

The fenestrated tube has a precut opening (fenestration) in the upper posterior wall of the outer cannula. The tube is used to wean the client from a tracheostomy by ensuring that the client can tolerate breathing through her or his natural airway before the entire tube is removed. This tube allows the client to speak.

Cuffed Fenestrated Tube

The cuffed fenestrated tube facilitates mechanical ventilation and speech and often is used for clients with spinal cord paralysis or neuromuscular disease who do not require ventilation at all times. When not on the ventilator, the client can have the cuff deflated and the tube capped (see Fig. 69-11 for cuffed fenestrated tube with red cap) for speech. A cuffed fenestrated tube is never used in weaning from a tracheostomy, because the cuff, even fully deflated, may partially obstruct the airway.

h. If the client is allowed to eat, sit the client up for meals and ensure that the cuff is inflated (if the tube is not capped) for meals and for 1 hour after meals to prevent aspiration.
i. Monitor cuff pressures as prescribed.
j. Assess the stoma and secretions for blood or purulent drainage.
k. Follow the PHCP's prescriptions and agency policy for cleaning the tracheostomy site and inner cannula (many inner cannulas are disposable); usually, half-strength hydrogen peroxide is used.
l. Administer humidified oxygen as prescribed, because the normal humidification process is bypassed in a client with a tracheostomy.
m. Obtain assistance in changing tracheostomy ties; after placing the new ties, cut and remove the old ties holding the tracheostomy in place (some securing devices are soft and made with Velcro to hold the tube in place).
n. Keep a resuscitation (Ambu) bag, obturator, clamps, and spare tracheostomy tube of the same size at the bedside.

4. Complications of a tracheostomy (Table 69-5)

TABLE 69-5 Complications of a Tracheostomy

Complication and Description	Manifestations	Management	Prevention
Tracheomalacia: Constant pressure exerted by the cuff causes tracheal dilation and erosion of cartilage.	▪ An increased amount of air is required in the cuff to maintain the seal. ▪ A larger tracheostomy tube is required to prevent an air leak at the stoma. ▪ Food particles are seen in tracheal secretions. ▪ The client does not receive the set tidal volume on the ventilator.	▪ Monitor client; no special management is needed unless bleeding or airway problems occur	▪ Monitor cuff pressure and air volume closely to detect changes. ▪ Use an uncuffed tube as soon as possible.
Tracheal stenosis: Narrowed tracheal lumen is the result of scar formation from irritation of tracheal mucosa by the cuff.	▪ Stenosis is usually seen after the cuff is deflated or the tracheostomy tube is removed. ▪ The client has increased coughing, inability to expectorate secretions, or difficulty breathing and talking.	▪ Tracheal dilation or surgical intervention is used.	▪ Prevent pulling of and traction on the tracheostomy tube. ▪ Properly secure the tube in the midline position. ▪ Maintain cuff pressure. ▪ Minimize oronasal intubation time.
Tracheoesophageal fistula (TEF): Excessive cuff pressure causes erosion of the posterior wall of the trachea. A hole is created between the trachea and the anterior esophagus. The client at highest risk also has a nasogastric tube present.	Similar to tracheomalacia: ▪ Food particles are seen in tracheal secretions. ▪ Increased air in cuff is needed to achieve a seal. ▪ The client has increased coughing and choking while eating. ▪ The client does not receive the set tidal volume on the ventilator.	▪ Suction; manually administer oxygen by mask to prevent hypoxemia. ▪ Use a small soft feeding tube instead of a nasogastric tube for tube feedings. ▪ A gastrostomy or jejunostomy may be performed. ▪ Monitor the client with a nasogastric tube closely; assess for TEF and aspiration.	▪ Maintain cuff pressure. ▪ Monitor the amount of air needed for inflation to detect changes. ▪ Progress to a deflated or cuffless tube as soon as possible.
Trachea–innominate artery fistula: A malpositioned tube causes its distal tip to push against the lateral wall of the trachea. Continued pressure causes necrosis and erosion of the innominate artery. *This is a medical emergency.*	▪ The tracheostomy tube pulsates in synchrony with the heartbeat. ▪ There is heavy bleeding from the stoma. ▪ This is a life-threatening complication.	▪ Apply direct pressure to the innominate artery at the stoma site. ▪ The tracheostomy tube will be removed immediately. ▪ Prepare the client for immediate repair surgery.	▪ Use the correct tube size and length, and maintain the tube in midline position. ▪ Prevent pulling or tugging of the tracheostomy tube. ▪ Immediately notify the primary health care provider (PHCP) of a pulsating tube.

TABLE 69-5 Complications of a Tracheostomy—cont'd

Complication and Description	Manifestations	Management	Prevention
Tube obstruction	▪ Difficulty breathing ▪ Noisy respirations ▪ Difficulty inserting the suction catheter ▪ Thick, dry secretions ▪ Unexplained peak pressures if client is on a mechanical ventilator	▪ The PHCP repositions or replaces the tube if obstruction occurs as a result of cuff prolapse over the end of the tube.	▪ Assist the client to cough and deep-breathe. ▪ Provide humidification and suctioning. ▪ Clean the inner cannula regularly.
Tube dislodgment	▪ Difficulty breathing ▪ Noisy respirations ▪ Restlessness ▪ Excessive coughing ▪ Audible wheeze or stridor	▪ Be familiar with institutional policy regarding replacement of a tracheostomy tube as a nursing procedure. ▪ During the first 72 hours following surgical placement of the tracheostomy, the nurse manually ventilates the client by using a manual resuscitation (Ambu) bag while another nurse calls the Rapid Response Team for help. ▪ 72 hours following surgical placement of the tracheostomy: ▪ Extend the client's neck and open the tissues of the stoma to secure the airway. ▪ Grasp the retention sutures (if they are present) to spread the opening. ▪ Use a tracheal dilator (curved clamp) to hold the stoma open. ▪ Prepare to insert a tracheostomy tube; place the obturator into the tracheostomy tube, insert the tube, and remove the obturator. ▪ Maintain ventilation by resuscitation (Ambu) bag. ▪ Assess airflow and bilateral breath sounds. ▪ If unable to secure an airway, call the Rapid Response Team and the anesthesiologist.	▪ Secure the tube in place. ▪ Minimize manipulation of and traction on the tube. ▪ Ensure that the client does not pull on the tube. ▪ Ensure that a tracheostomy tube of the same type and size is at the client's bedside.

Adapted from Ignatavicius D, Workman ML: *Medical-surgical nursing: patient-centered collaborative care*, ed 7, Philadelphia, 2013, Saunders.

PRIORITY NURSING ACTIONS

Tracheal Suctioning

1. Assess the client and explain the procedure.
2. Assist the client to an upright position.
3. Perform hand hygiene and don personal protective equipment.
4. Prepare suctioning equipment and turn on the suction.
5. Hyperoxygenate the client.
6. Insert the catheter without suction applied.
7. Once inserted, apply suction intermittently while rotating and withdrawing the catheter.
8. Hyperoxygenate the client.
9. Listen to breath sounds and reassess oxygen saturation.
10. Document the procedure, client response, and effectiveness.

Reference

Lewis et al. (2017), p. 488.

⚠ Never insert a plug (cap) into a tracheostomy tube until the cuff is deflated and the inner cannula is removed; prior insertion prevents airflow to the client.

O. Chest Tube Drainage System
1. The chest tube drainage system returns negative pressure to the intrapleural space.
2. The system is used to remove abnormal accumulations of air and fluid from the pleural space (Fig. 69-12).
3. Drainage collection chamber (Fig. 69-13)
   a. The drainage collection chamber is located where the chest tube from the client connects to the system.
   b. Drainage from the tube drains into and collects in a series of calibrated columns in this chamber.
4. Water seal chamber (see Fig. 69-13)
   a. The tip of the tube is underwater, allowing fluid and air to drain from the pleural space and preventing air from entering the pleural space.

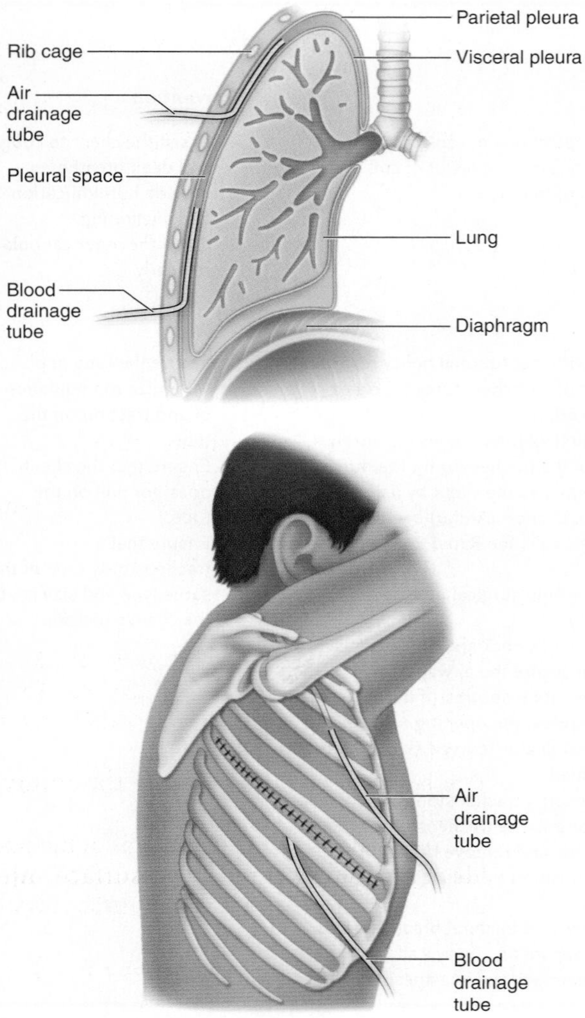

FIG. 69-12 Chest tube placement.

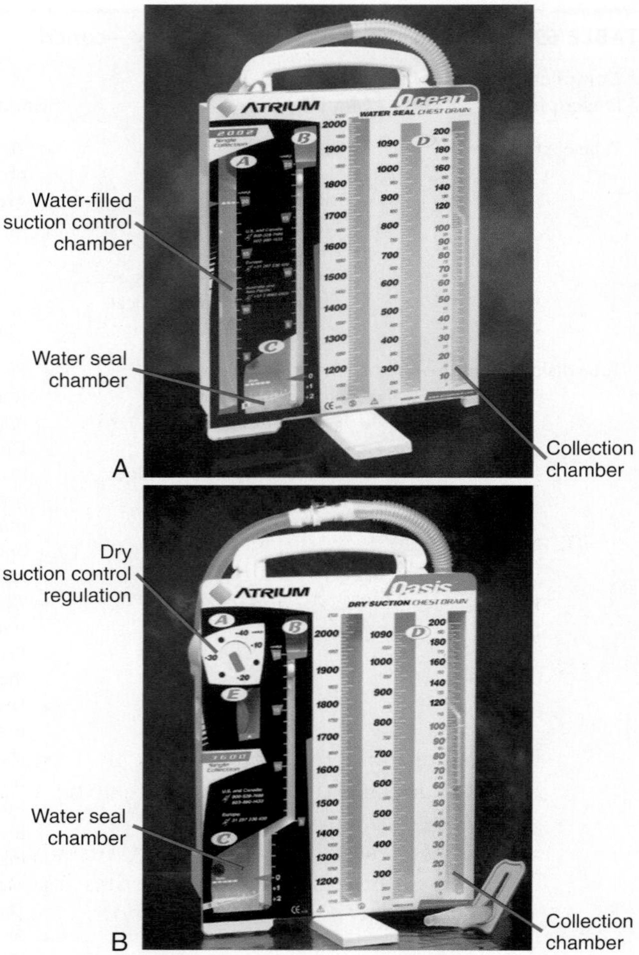

FIG. 69-13 Chest drainage system. **A,** Wet system. **B,** Dry system. (From Lewis et al., 2011. From Atrium Medical Corporation, Hudson, N.H.)

   b. Water oscillates (moves up as the client inhales and moves down as the client exhales).
   c. Excessive bubbling indicates an air leak in the chest tube system.

5. Suction control chamber (see Fig. 69-13)
   a. The suction control chamber provides the suction, which can be controlled to provide negative pressure to the chest.
   b. This chamber is filled with various levels of water to achieve the desired level of suction; without this control, lung tissue could be sucked into the chest tube.
   c. Gentle bubbling in this chamber indicates that there is suction and does not indicate that air is escaping from the pleural space.

6. Dry suction system (see Fig. 69-13)
   a. This is another type of chest drainage system. Because this is a dry suction system, absence of bubbling is noted in the suction control chamber.
   b. A knob on the collection device is used to set the prescribed amount of suction; then the wall suction source dial is turned until a small orange floater valve appears in the window on the device (when the orange floater valve is in the window, the correct amount of suction is applied).

7. Portable chest drainage system: Small and portable chest drainage systems are also available and are dry systems that use a control flutter valve to prevent the backflow of air into the client's lung. Principles of gravity and pressure, and the nursing care involved, are the same for all types of systems, and these systems allow greater ambulation and allow the client to go home with the chest tubes in place.

8. Collection chamber: Interventions
   a. Monitor drainage; notify the PHCP if drainage is more than 70 to 100 mL/hr or if drainage becomes bright red or increases suddenly.

b. Mark the chest tube drainage in the collection chamber at 1- to 4-hour intervals, using a piece of tape.
9. Water seal chamber: Interventions
a. Monitor for fluctuation of the fluid level in the water seal chamber.
b. Fluctuation in the water seal chamber stops if the tube is obstructed, if a dependent loop exists, if the suction is not working properly, or if the lung has re-expanded.
c. If the client has a known pneumothorax, intermittent bubbling in the water seal chamber is expected as air is drained from the chest, but continuous bubbling indicates an air leak in the system.
d. Notify the PHCP if there is continuous bubbling in the water seal chamber.
10. Suction control chamber: Interventions: Gentle (not vigorous) bubbling should be noted in the suction control chamber of a wet suction system.
11. Additional interventions
a. An occlusive sterile dressing is maintained at the insertion site.
b. A chest radiograph assesses the position of the tube and determines whether the lung has re-expanded.
c. Assess respiratory status and auscultate lung sounds. Assess chest tube dressing for drainage and palpate surrounding tissue for crepitus.
d. Monitor for signs of extended pneumothorax or hemothorax.
e. Keep the drainage system below the level of the chest and the tubes free of kinks, dependent loops, or other obstructions.
f. Ensure that all connections are secure.
g. Encourage coughing and deep breathing.
h. Change the client's position frequently to promote drainage and ventilation.
i. Do not strip or milk a chest tube unless specifically directed to do so by the PHCP and if agency policy allows it.
j. Keep a clamp (may be needed if the system needs to be changed) and a sterile occlusive dressing at the bedside at all times.
k. Never clamp a chest tube without a written prescription from the PHCP; also, determine agency policy for clamping a chest tube.
l. If the drainage system cracks or breaks, insert the chest tube into a bottle of sterile water, remove the cracked or broken system, and replace it with a new system.
m. Depending on the PHCP's preference, when the chest tube is removed, the client may be asked to take a deep breath and hold it, and the tube is removed. Or, the client may be asked to take a deep breath, exhale, and bear down (Valsalva maneuver). A dry sterile dressing, petroleum gauze dressing, or Telfa dressing (depending on the PHCP's preference) is taped in place after removal of the chest tube.

⚠ If the chest tube is pulled out of the chest accidentally, pinch the skin opening together, apply an occlusive sterile dressing, cover the dressing with overlapping pieces of 2-inch (5-cm) tape, and call the PHCP immediately.

V. Complex Integumentary Problems

A. Burn injuries (see Priority Nursing Actions)
1. Description: Cell destruction of the layers of the skin caused by heat, friction, electricity, radiation, or chemicals.
2. Small burns: The response of the body to injury is localized to the injured area.
3. Large or extensive burns:
a. Major or extensive burns consist of 25% or more of the total body surface area for an adult and 10% or more of the total body surface for a child.
b. The response of the body to the injury is systemic.
c. The burn affects all major systems of the body.
d. Electrical burns often have surface injury that is small, but internal injuries may be extensive.
4. Estimating the extent of injury (Fig. 69-14)

PRIORITY NURSING ACTIONS

Burn Injury: Care in the Emergency Department

1. Assess for airway patency.
2. Administer oxygen as prescribed.
3. Obtain vital signs.
4. Initiate an intravenous (IV) line and begin fluid replacement as prescribed.
5. Elevate the extremities if no fractures are obvious.
6. Keep the client warm and place the client on NPO (nothing by mouth) status.

Reference
Ignatavicius, Workman, Rebar (2018), p. 489.

B. Burn depth
1. Superficial-thickness burn
a. Involves injury to the epidermis; the blood supply to the dermis is still intact.
b. Mild to severe erythema (pink to red) is present, but no blisters.
c. Skin blanches with pressure.

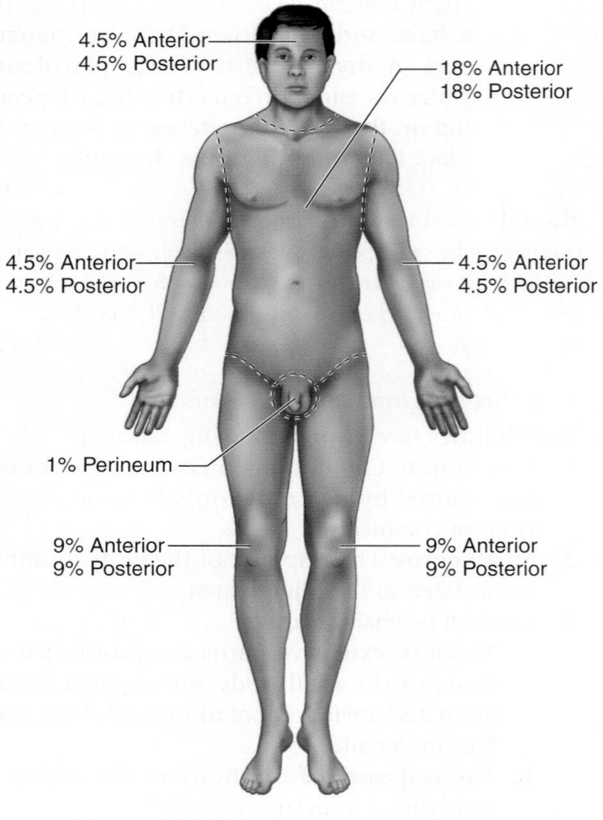

FIG. 69-14 The rule of nines for estimating burn percentage.

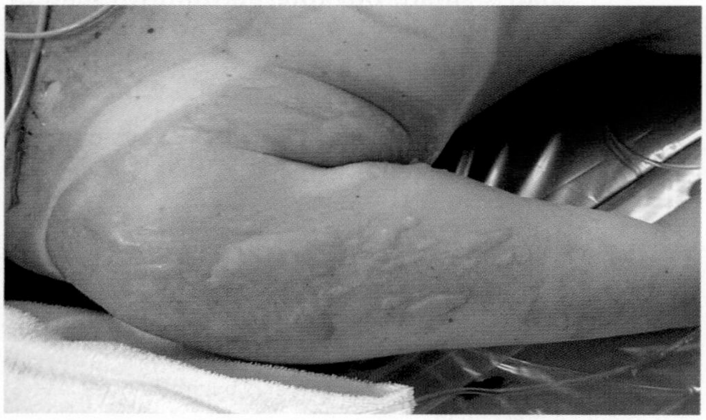

FIG. 69-15 Typical appearance of superficial partial-thickness burn injury. (From Ignatavicius, Workman, 2016.)

- **d.** Burn is painful, with tingling sensation, and the pain is eased by cooling.
- **e.** Discomfort lasts about 48 hours; healing occurs in about 3 to 6 days.
- **f.** No scarring occurs and skin grafts are not required.

2. **Superficial partial-thickness burn** (Fig. 69-15)
- **a.** Involves injury deeper into the dermis; the blood supply is reduced.
- **b.** Large blisters may cover an extensive area.
- **c.** Edema is present.

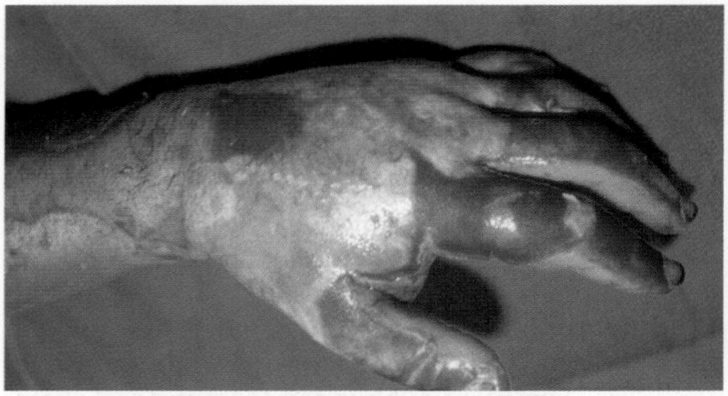

FIG. 69-16 Typical appearance of deep partial-thickness burn injury. (From Ignatavicius, Workman, 2016.)

- **d.** Mottled pink to red base and broken epidermis, with a wet, shiny, and weeping surface, are characteristic.
- **e.** Burn is painful and sensitive to cold air.
- **f.** Heals in 10 to 21 days with no scarring, but some minor pigment changes may occur.
- **g.** Grafts may be used if the healing process is prolonged.

3. **Deep partial-thickness burn** (Fig. 69-16)
- **a.** Extends deeper into the skin dermis
- **b.** Blister formation usually does not occur because the dead tissue layer is thick and sticks to underlying viable dermis.
- **c.** Wound surface is red and dry with white areas in deeper parts.
- **d.** May or may not blanch, and edema is moderate.
- **e.** Can convert to full-thickness burn if tissue damage increases with infection, hypoxia, or ischemia.
- **f.** Generally heals in 3 to 6 weeks, but scar formation results and skin grafting may be necessary.

4. **Full-thickness burn** (Fig. 69-17)
- **a.** Involves injury and destruction of the epidermis and the dermis; the wound will not heal by re-epithelialization, and grafting may be required.

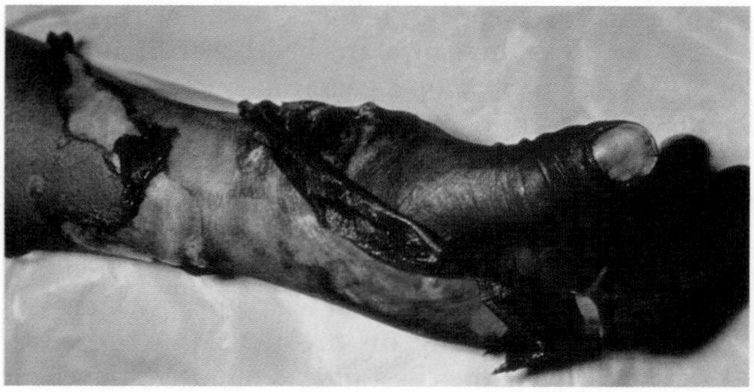

FIG. 69-17 Typical appearance of full-thickness burn injury. (From Ignatavicius, Workman, 2016.)

b. Appears as a dry, hard, leathery eschar (burn crust or dead tissue must slough off or be removed from the wound before healing can occur).
c. Appears waxy white, deep red, yellow, brown, or black.
d. Injured surface appears dry.
e. Edema is present under the eschar.
f. Sensation is reduced or absent because of nerve ending destruction.
g. Healing may take weeks to months and depends on establishing an adequate blood supply.
h. Burn requires removal of eschar and split- or full-thickness skin grafting.
i. Scarring and wound contractures are likely to develop.

5. **Deep full-thickness burn** (Fig. 69-18)
a. Injury extends beyond the skin into underlying fascia and tissues, and muscle, bone, and tendons are damaged.
b. Injured area appears black and sensation is completely absent.
c. Eschar is hard and inelastic.
d. There is lack of pain because nerve endings have been destroyed.
e. Healing takes months and grafts are required.

C. Burn location
1. Burns of the head, neck, and chest are associated with pulmonary complications.
2. Burns of the face are associated with corneal abrasion.
3. Burns of the ear are associated with auricular chondritis.
4. Hands and joints require intensive therapy to prevent disability.
5. The perineal area is prone to autocontamination by urine and feces.
6. Circumferential burns of the extremities can produce a tourniquet-like effect and lead to vascular compromise (compartment syndrome).
7. Circumferential thorax burns lead to inadequate chest wall expansion and pulmonary insufficiency.

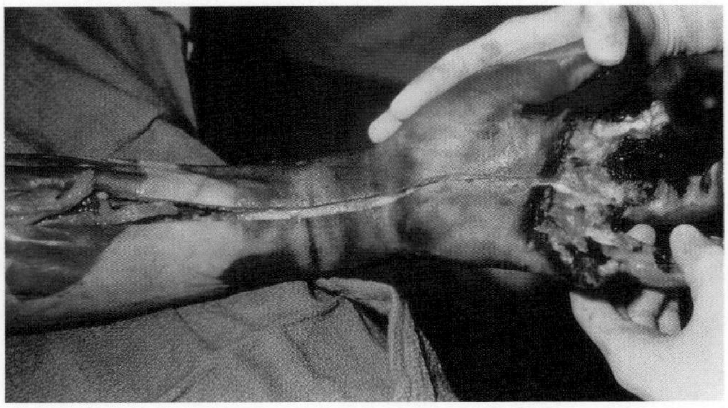

FIG. 69-18 Typical appearance of deep full-thickness burn injury. (From Ignatavicius, Workman, 2016.)

D. Age and general health
1. Mortality rates are higher for children younger than 4 years of age, particularly for children from birth to 1 year of age, and for clients older than 65 years.
2. Debilitating disorders, such as cardiac, respiratory, endocrine, and renal disorders, negatively influence the client's response to injury and treatment.
3. Mortality rate is higher when the client has a preexisting disorder at the time of the burn injury.

E. Inhalation injuries
1. **Smoke inhalation injury**
a. Respiratory injury that occurs when the victim inhales products of combustion during a fire.

⚠ The airway is a priority concern in an inhalation injury.

b. Assessment (Box 69-9)

2. **Carbon monoxide poisoning**
a. Carbon monoxide is a colorless, odorless, and tasteless gas that has an affinity for hemoglobin 200 times greater than that of oxygen.
b. Oxygen molecules are displaced and carbon monoxide reversibly binds to hemoglobin to form carboxyhemoglobin.
c. Tissue hypoxia occurs.
d. Assessment (Table 69-6)

3. Direct thermal heat injury
a. Thermal heat injury can occur to the lower airways by the inhalation of steam or explosive gases or the aspiration of scalding liquids.
b. Injury can occur to the upper airways, which appear erythematous and edematous, with mucosal blisters and ulcerations.
c. Mucosal edema can lead to upper airway obstruction, especially during the first 24 to 48 hours.
d. All clients with head or neck burns should be monitored closely for the development of airway obstruction and are considered immediately for endotracheal intubation if obstruction occurs.

BOX 69-9 Assessment Findings in a Smoke Inhalation Injury

- Facial burns
- Erythema
- Swelling of oropharynx and nasopharynx
- Singed nasal hairs
- Flaring nostrils
- Stridor, wheezing, and dyspnea
- Hoarse voice
- Sooty (carbonaceous) sputum and cough
- Tachycardia
- Agitation and anxiety

Complex Care

TABLE 69-6 Carbon Monoxide Poisoning

Blood Level (%)	Clinical Manifestations
1-10	Normal level
11-20 (mild poisoning)	Headache Flushing Decreased visual acuity Decreased cerebral functioning Slight breathlessness
21-40 (moderate poisoning)	Headache Nausea and vomiting Drowsiness Tinnitus and vertigo Confusion and stupor Pale to reddish-purple skin Decreased blood pressure Increased and irregular heart rate Depressed ST segment on electrocardiogram
41-60 (severe poisoning)	Coma Seizures Cardiopulmonary instability
61-80 (fatal poisoning)	Death

Adapted from Ignatavicius D, Workman ML: *Medical-surgical nursing: patient-centered collaborative care*, ed 8, Philadelphia, 2016, Saunders.

e. Assessment: findings include erythema and edema of the upper airways and mucosal blisters and ulcerations

F. Pathophysiology of burns

1. Following a burn, vasoactive substances are released from the injured tissue, and these substances cause an increase in capillary permeability, allowing the plasma to seep into the surrounding tissues.
2. The direct injury to the vessels increases capillary permeability (capillary permeability decreases 18 to 26 hours after the burn but does not normalize until 2 to 3 weeks following injury).
3. Extensive burns result in generalized body edema and a decrease in circulating intravascular blood volume.
4. The fluid losses result in a decrease in organ perfusion.
5. The heart rate increases, cardiac output decreases, and blood pressure drops.
6. Initially, hyponatremia and hyperkalemia occur.
7. The hematocrit level increases as a result of plasma loss; this initial increase falls to below normal by the third to fourth day after the burn as a result of red blood cell damage and loss at the time of injury.
8. Initially, the body shunts blood from the kidneys, causing oliguria; then the body begins to reabsorb fluid, and diuresis of the excess fluid occurs over the next days to weeks.
9. Blood flow to the gastrointestinal tract is diminished, leading to intestinal ileus and gastrointestinal dysfunction.
10. Immune system function is depressed, resulting in immunosuppression and thus increasing the risk of infection and sepsis.
11. Pulmonary hypertension can develop, resulting in a decrease in the arterial oxygen tension level and a decrease in lung compliance.
12. Evaporative fluid losses through the burn wound are greater than normal, and the losses continue until complete wound closure occurs.
13. If the intravascular space is not replenished with intravenously administered fluids, hypovolemic shock and ultimately death occur.

G. Management of the burn injury: Resuscitation/emergent phase (Table 69-7)

TABLE 69-7 Phases of Management of the Burn Injury

Phase	Goal
Resuscitation/Emergent Phase	
Begins at the time of injury Ends with the restoration of normal capillary permeability Duration usually 48-72 hr Includes prehospital care and emergency department care	The primary goal is to maintain a patent airway, administer intravenous fluids to prevent hypovolemic shock, and preserve vital organ functioning.
Resuscitative Phase	
Begins with the initiation of fluids Ends when capillary integrity returns to near-normal levels and large fluid shifts have decreased Amount of fluid administered is based on client's weight and extent of injury Note that most fluid replacement formulas are calculated from the time of injury and not from the time of arrival at the hospital.	The goal is to prevent shock by maintaining adequate circulating blood volume and maintaining vital organ perfusion.
Acute Phase	
Begins when the client is hemodynamically stable, capillary permeability is restored, and diuresis has begun Usually begins 48-72 hr after time of injury Focus on infection control, wound care, wound closure, nutritional support, pain management, and physical therapy	The emphasis during this phase is placed on restorative therapy, and the phase continues until wound closure is achieved.
Rehabilitative Phase	
Overlaps acute phase of care Extends beyond hospitalization	The goals of this phase are designed so that the client can gain independence and achieve maximal function.

1. Prehospital care
   a. Begins at the scene of the accident and ends when emergency care is obtained
   b. Remove the victim from the source of the burn.
   c. Assess the ABCs—airway, breathing, and circulation.
   d. Assess for associated trauma, including inhalation injury.
   e. Conserve body heat.
   f. Cover burns with sterile or clean cloths.
   g. Remove constricting jewelry and clothing.
   h. Insert IV access.
   i. Transport to the emergency department.
2. Emergency department care is a continuation of care administered at the scene of the injury.
3. Major burns
   a. Evaluate the degree and extent of the burn and treat life-threatening conditions.
   b. Ensure a patent airway and administer 100% oxygen as prescribed.
   c. Monitor for respiratory distress and assess the need for intubation.
   d. Assess the oropharynx for blisters and erythema; assess vocal quality and for singed nasal hairs and auscultate lung sounds.
   e. Monitor arterial blood gases and carboxyhemoglobin levels.
   f. For an inhalation injury, administer 100% oxygen via a tight-fitting nonrebreather face mask as prescribed until the carboxyhemoglobin level falls below 15%.
   g. Initiate peripheral IV access to nonburned skin proximal to any extremity burn, or prepare for the insertion of a central venous line as prescribed.
   h. Assess for hypovolemia and prepare to administer fluids intravenously to maintain fluid balance.
   i. Monitor vital signs closely.
   j. Insert a Foley catheter as prescribed, and manage fluid resuscitation with a goal to maintain urine output at 30 to 50 mL/hr.
   k. Maintain NPO (nothing by mouth) status.
   l. Insert a nasogastric tube as prescribed to remove gastric secretions and prevent aspiration.
   m. Administer tetanus prophylaxis as prescribed.
   n. Administer pain medication, as prescribed, by the IV route.
   o. Administer wound care and prepare the client for an escharotomy or fasciotomy as prescribed.
4. Minor burns
   a. Administer pain medication as prescribed.
   b. Instruct the client in the use of oral analgesics as prescribed.
   c. Administer tetanus prophylaxis as prescribed.
   d. Administer wound care as prescribed, which may include cleansing, debriding loose tissue, and removing any damaging agents, followed by the application of topical antimicrobial cream and a sterile dressing.
   e. Instruct the client in follow-up care, including active range-of-motion exercises and wound care treatments.

H. Management of the burn injury: Resuscitative phase (see Table 69-7)
1. Fluid resuscitation (Table 69-8)
   a. The amount of fluid administered depends on how much IV fluid per hour is required to maintain a urinary output of 30 to 50 mL/hr.
   b. Successful fluid resuscitation is evaluated by stable vital signs, an adequate urine output, palpable peripheral pulses, and intact level of consciousness and thought processes.
   c. IV fluid replacement may be titrated (adjusted) on the basis of urinary output plus serum electrolyte levels to meet the perfusion needs of the client with burns.
   d. If the hemoglobin and hematocrit levels decrease or if the urinary output exceeds 50 mL/hr, the rate of IV fluid administration may be decreased.

⚠ Urinary output is the most reliable and most sensitive noninvasive assessment parameter for cardiac output and tissue perfusion.

2. Interventions
   a. Monitor for tracheal or laryngeal edema and administer respiratory treatments as prescribed; intubation and mechanical ventilation are instituted with respiratory burns before complications develop, if needed.

TABLE 69-8 Common Fluid Resuscitation Formulas for First 24 Hours After a Burn Injury

Formula	Solution	Amount
Modified Brooke		
	5% albumin in isotonic saline	0.5 mL to 15 mL/kg/% TBSA burn
	Lactated Ringer's without dextrose	
Parkland (Baxter)		
	Crystalloid only (lactated Ringer's)	4 mL/kg/% TBSA burn
Modified Parkland		
	Crystalloid only (lactated Ringer's)	4 mL/kg/% TBSA burn + 15 mL/m^2 of TBSA

TBSA, Total body surface area.
From Ignatavicius D, Workman ML: *Medical-surgical nursing: patient-centered collaborative care*, ed 8, Philadelphia, 2016, Saunders.

b. Monitor pulse oximetry and prepare for arterial blood gases and carboxyhemoglobin levels if inhalation injury is suspected.
c. Elevate the head of the bed to 30 degrees or more for burns of the face and head.
d. Monitor for fluid overload and pulmonary edema.
e. Initiate electrocardiographic (ECG) monitoring.
f. Monitor temperature and assess for infection.
g. Initiate protective isolation techniques; maintain strict hand washing; use sterile sheets and linens when caring for the client; and use gloves, cap, masks, shoe covers, scrub clothes, and plastic aprons.
h. Clip body hair around wound margins.
i. Monitor daily weights, expecting a weight gain of 6 to 9 kilograms (15 to 20 pounds) in the first 72 hours.
j. Monitor gastric output and pH levels and for gastric discomfort and bleeding, indicating a stress ulcer.
k. Administer antacids, H2 receptor antagonists, and antiulcer medications as prescribed to prevent a stress ulcer.
l. Auscultate bowel sounds for ileus and monitor for abdominal distention and gastrointestinal dysfunction.
m. Monitor stools for occult blood.
n. Obtain urine specimen for myoglobin and hemoglobin levels.
o. Monitor IV fluids and hourly intake and output to determine the adequacy of fluid replacement therapy; notify the PHCP if urine output is less than 30 or greater than 50 mL/hr. Monitor serum laboratory results, including electrolytes and complete blood count.
p. Elevate circumferential burns of the extremities on pillows above the level of the heart to reduce dependent edema if no obvious fractures are present; diuretics increase the risk of hypovolemia and are generally avoided as a means of decreasing edema.
q. Monitor pulses and capillary refill of the affected extremities and assess perfusion of the distal extremity with a circumferential burn.
r. Prepare to obtain chest x-rays and other radiographs to rule out fractures or associated trauma.
s. Keep the room temperature warm.
t. Place the client on an air-fluidized bed or other special mattress and use a bed cradle to keep sheets off the client's skin.

3. Pain management
   a. Administer opioid analgesics as prescribed by the IV route.
   b. Avoid administering medication by the oral route because of the possibility of gastrointestinal dysfunction.
   c. Medicate the client as prescribed and before painful procedures.

⚠ Avoid the intramuscular or subcutaneous medication route for medication administration, because absorption through the soft tissue is unreliable when hypovolemia and large fluid shifts occur.

4. Nutrition
   a. Proper nutrition is essential to promote wound healing and prevent infection.
   b. The basal metabolic rate is 40 to 100 times higher than normal with a burn injury.
   c. Maintain NPO status until bowel sounds are heard, and then advance to clear liquids as prescribed.
   d. Dietary consultation may be prescribed. Nutrition may be provided via enteral tube feeding or parenteral nutrition through a central line.
   e. Provide a diet high in protein, carbohydrates, fats, and vitamins, with major burns requiring more than 5000 calories daily.
   f. Monitor calorie intake and daily weights.

I. Management of the burn injury: Acute phase (see Table 69-7)
   1. Continue with protective isolation techniques.
   2. Provide wound care as prescribed and prepare for wound closure.
   3. Provide pain management.
   4. Provide adequate nutrition as prescribed.
   5. Prepare the client for rehabilitation.

J. Circulatory compromise treatments
   1. Escharotomy
      a. A lengthwise incision is made through the burn eschar to relieve constriction and pressure and to improve circulation.
      b. Escharotomy is performed for circulatory compromise caused by circumferential burns.
      c. Escharotomy can be performed at the bedside without anesthesia, because nerve endings have been destroyed by the burn injury.
      d. Escharotomy may be necessary on the thorax to improve ventilation.
      e. Following the escharotomy, assess pulses, color, movement, and sensation of affected extremity and control any bleeding with pressure.
      f. Pack the incision gently with fine mesh gauze as prescribed after escharotomy.
      g. Apply topical antimicrobial agents to the area as prescribed.
   2. Fasciotomy
      a. An incision is made extending through the subcutaneous tissue and fascia.
      b. The procedure is performed if adequate tissue perfusion does not return following an escharotomy.

c. Fasciotomy is performed in the operating room with the client under general anesthesia.
d. Following the procedure, assess pulses, color, movement, and sensation of affected extremity and control any bleeding with pressure.
e. Apply topical antimicrobial agents and dressings to the area, as prescribed.

K. Wound care
1. Description: Cleansing, debridement, and dressing of burn wounds
2. Hydrotherapy
a. Wounds are cleansed by showering on a special table, or washing small areas of wound at the bedside.
b. Hydrotherapy occurs for 30 minutes or less to prevent increased sodium loss through the burn wound, heat loss, pain, and stress.
c. Client should be premedicated before procedure.
d. Hydrotherapy is not used for clients who are hemodynamically unstable or those with new skin grafts.
e. Care is taken to minimize bleeding and maintain body temperature during the procedure.
f. Prescribed antimicrobial agents are applied after hydrotherapy.
3. Debridement
a. Debridement is removal of eschar or necrotic tissue to prevent bacterial proliferation under the eschar and to promote wound healing.
b. Debridement may be mechanical, enzymatic, or surgical.
c. Deep partial-thickness burns or deep full-thickness burns: Wound is cleansed and debrided, and topical antimicrobial agents are applied once or twice daily.
4. Wound closure
a. Wound closure prevents infection and loss of fluid.
b. Closure promotes healing.
c. Closure prevents contractures.
d. Wound closure is performed usually on day 5 to 21 following the injury, depending on the extent of the burn.
5. Wound coverings (Box 69-10)

BOX 69-10 Wound Coverings

Biological

Amniotic Membranes
- Amniotic membrane from human placenta is used; it adheres to the wound.
- Effective as a dressing until epithelial cell regrowth occurs
- Requires frequent changes/application because it does not develop a blood supply and disintegrates in about 48 hours

Allograft or Homograft (Human Tissue)
- Donated human cadaver skin provided through a skin bank
- Monitor for wound exudate and signs of infection.
- Rejection can occur within 24 hours
- Risk of transmitting bloodborne infection exists when used.

Xenograft or Heterograft (Animal Tissue)
- Pigskin harvested after slaughter is preserved for storage and use.
- Monitor for infection and wound adherence.
- Placed over granulation tissue; replaced every 2 to 5 days until wound heals naturally or until closure with autograft is complete

Cultured Skin
- Grown in laboratory from a small specimen of epidermal cells from an unburned portion of the client's body
- Cell sheets are grafted on the client to generate permanent skin surface.
- Cell sheets are not durable; care must be taken when applying to ensure adherence and prevent sloughing.

Artificial Skin
- Consists of 2 layers—silastic epidermis and porous dermis made from bovine hide collagen and shark cartilage
- After application, fibroblasts move into the collagen part of the artificial skin and create a structure similar to normal dermis.
- Artificial dermis then dissolves; it is then replaced with normal blood vessels and connective tissue called *neodermis*.
- Neodermis supports the standard autograft placed over it when the Silastic layer is removed.

Biosynthetic
- Combination of biosynthetic and synthetic materials
- Placed in contact with the wound surface; forms an adherent bond until epithelialization occurs
- Porous substance allows exudate to pass through.
- Monitor for wound exudate and signs of infection.

Synthetic
- Applied directly to the surface of a clean or surgically prepared wound; remains in place until it falls off or is removed
- Covering is transparent or translucent; therefore, wound can be inspected without removing dressing.
- Pain at the wound site is reduced because covering prevents contact of the wound with air.

Autograft
- Skin taken from a remote unburned area of the client's own body; transplanted to cover burn wound
- Graft placed on a clean granulated bed or over surgically excised area of the burn
- Provides for permanent skin coverage

6. Autografting
   a. Autografting is the surgical removal of a thin layer of the client's own unburned skin, which then is applied to the excised burn wound.
   b. Autografting provides permanent wound coverage.
   c. Autografting is performed in the operating room under anesthesia.
   d. Monitor for bleeding following the graft procedure, because bleeding beneath an autograft can prevent adherence.
   e. If prescribed, small amounts of blood or serum can be removed by gently rolling the fluid from the center of the graft to the periphery with a sterile gauze pad, where it can be absorbed.
   f. For large accumulations of blood, the PHCP may aspirate the blood using a small-gauge needle and syringe.
   g. Autografts are immobilized following surgery for 3 to 7 days to allow time to adhere and attach to the wound bed.
   h. Position the client for immobilization and elevation of the graft site to prevent movement and shearing of the graft.
7. Care of the graft site
   a. Elevate and immobilize the graft site.
   b. Keep the site free from pressure.
   c. Avoid weight-bearing.
   d. When the graft takes, if prescribed, roll a cotton-tipped applicator over the graft to remove exudate, because exudate can lead to infection and prevent graft adherence.
   e. Monitor for foul-smelling drainage, increased temperature, increased white blood cell count, hematoma formation, and fluid accumulation.
   f. Instruct the client to avoid using fabric softeners and harsh detergents in the laundry.
   g. Instruct the client to lubricate the healing skin with prescribed agents.
   h. Instruct the client to protect the affected area from sunlight.
   i. Instruct the client to use splints and support garments as prescribed.
8. Care of the donor site
   a. Method of care varies, depending on the PHCP's preference.
   b. A nonadherent gauze dressing may be applied at the time of the surgery to maintain pressure and stop any oozing; covering the site decreases discomfort from exposed nerve endings; always check the surgeon's preference.
   c. The PHCP may prescribe site treatment with gauze impregnated with petrolatum or with a biosynthetic dressing.
   d. Keep the donor site clean, dry, and free from pressure.
   e. Prevent the client from scratching the donor site.
   f. Apply lubricating lotions to soften the area and reduce the itching after the donor site is healed.
   g. Donor site can be reused once healing has occurred (heals spontaneously within 7 to 14 days with proper care).

L. Rehabilitative phase (see Table 69-7)
1. Description: Rehabilitation is the final phase of burn care.
2. Goals
   a. Promote wound healing.
   b. Minimize deformities.
   c. Increase strength and function.
   d. Provide emotional support.

M. Physical therapy
1. An individualized program of splinting, positioning, exercises, ambulation, and activities of daily living is implemented early in the acute phase of recovery to maximize functional and cosmetic outcomes.
2. Perform range-of-motion exercises as prescribed to reduce edema and maintain strength and joint function.
3. Ambulate the client as prescribed to maintain the strength of the lower extremities.
4. Apply splints as prescribed to maintain proper joint position and prevent contractures.
   a. Static splints immobilize the joint and are applied for periods of immobilization, during sleeping, and for clients who cannot maintain proper positioning.
   b. Dynamic splints exercise the affected joint.
   c. Avoid pressure to skin areas when applying splints, which could lead to further tissue and nerve damage.
5. Scarring is controlled by elastic wraps and bandages that apply continuous pressure to the healing skin during the time in which the skin is vulnerable to shearing.
6. Anti–burn scar support garments are usually prescribed to be worn 23 hours a day until the burn scar tissue has matured, which takes 18 to 24 months.

VI. Complex Hematological and Oncological Problems

A. Oncological emergencies: include sepsis and disseminated intravascular coagulation (DIC), syndrome of inappropriate antidiuretic hormone (SIADH), spinal cord compression, hypercalcemia, and superior vena cava syndrome

B. Sepsis and DIC
1. Description: The client with cancer is at increased risk for infection, particularly gram-negative

organisms, in the bloodstream (sepsis or septicemia) and DIC, a life-threatening hematological problem frequently associated with sepsis.

2. Interventions
   a. Prevent the complication through early identification of clients at high risk for sepsis and DIC.
   b. Maintain strict aseptic technique with the immunocompromised client and monitor closely for infection and signs of bleeding.
   c. Administer antibiotics intravenously as prescribed.
   d. Administer anticoagulants as prescribed during the early phase of DIC.
   e. Administer cryoprecipitated clotting factors, as prescribed, when DIC progresses and hemorrhage is the primary problem.

⚠ Notify the PHCP immediately if signs of an oncological emergency occur.

C. SIADH
1. Description
   a. Tumors can produce, secrete, or stimulate substances that mimic antidiuretic hormone.
   b. Mild symptoms include weakness, muscle cramps, loss of appetite, and fatigue; serum sodium levels range from 115 to 120 mEq/L (115 to 120 mmol/L).
   c. More serious signs and symptoms relate to water intoxication and include weight gain, personality changes, confusion, and extreme muscle weakness.
   d. As the serum sodium level approaches 110 mEq/L (110 mmol/L), seizures, coma, and eventually death will occur, unless the condition is treated rapidly.
2. Interventions
   a. Initiate fluid restriction and increased sodium intake as prescribed.
   b. As prescribed, administer an antagonist to antidiuretic hormone.
   c. Monitor serum sodium levels.
   d. Treat the underlying cause with chemotherapy or radiation to reduce the tumor.

D. Spinal cord compression
1. Description
   a. Spinal cord compression occurs when a tumor directly enters the spinal cord or when the vertebral column collapses from tumor entry, impinging on the spinal cord.
   b. Spinal cord compression causes back pain, usually before neurological deficits occur.
   c. Neurological deficits relate to the spinal level of compression and include numbness; tingling; loss of urethral, vaginal, and rectal sensation; and muscle weakness.
2. Interventions
   a. Early recognition: Assess for back pain and neurological deficits.
   b. Administer high-dose corticosteroids to reduce swelling around the spinal cord and relieve symptoms.
   c. Prepare the client for immediate radiation and/or chemotherapy to reduce the size of the tumor and relieve compression.
   d. Surgery may need to be performed to remove the tumor and relieve the pressure on the spinal cord.
   e. Instruct the client in the use of neck or back braces if they are prescribed.

E. Hypercalcemia
1. Description
   a. Hypercalcemia is a late manifestation of extensive malignancy that occurs most often with bone metastasis, when the bone releases calcium into the bloodstream.
   b. Decreased physical mobility contributes to or worsens hypercalcemia.
   c. Early signs include fatigue, anorexia, nausea, vomiting, constipation, and polyuria.
   d. More serious signs and symptoms include severe muscle weakness, diminished deep tendon reflexes, paralytic ileus, dehydration, and changes in the electrocardiogram.
2. Interventions
   a. Monitor serum calcium level and ECG changes.
   b. Administer oral or parenteral fluids as prescribed.
   c. Administer medications that lower the calcium level and control nausea and vomiting as prescribed.
   d. Prepare the client for dialysis if the condition becomes life-threatening or is accompanied by renal impairment.
   e. Encourage walking to prevent breakdown of bone.

F. Superior vena cava syndrome
1. Description
   a. Superior vena cava (SVC) syndrome occurs when the SVC is compressed or obstructed by tumor growth (commonly associated with lung cancer and lymphoma).
   b. Signs and symptoms result from blockage of blood flow in the venous system of the head, neck, and upper trunk.
   c. Early signs and symptoms generally occur in the morning and include edema of the face, especially around the eyes, and tightness of the shirt or blouse collar (Stokes' sign).
   d. As the condition worsens, edema in the arms and hands, dyspnea, erythema of the upper body, swelling of the veins in the chest and neck, and epistaxis occur.

e. Life-threatening signs and symptoms include airway obstruction, hemorrhage, cyanosis, mental status changes, decreased cardiac output, and hypotension.

2. Interventions
   a. Assess for early signs and symptoms of SVC syndrome.
   b. Place the client in semi-Fowler's position and administer corticosteroids and diuretics as prescribed.
   c. Prepare the client for high-dose radiation therapy to the mediastinal area, and possible surgery to insert a metal stent in the vena cava.

G. Tumor lysis syndrome
1. Description
   a. Tumor lysis syndrome occurs when large quantities of tumor cells are destroyed rapidly and intracellular components such as potassium and uric acid are released into the bloodstream faster than the body can eliminate them.
   b. Tumor lysis syndrome can indicate that cancer treatment is destroying tumor cells; however, if left untreated, it can cause severe tissue damage and death.
   c. Hyperkalemia, hyperphosphatemia with resultant hypocalcemia, and hyperuricemia occur; hyperuricemia can lead to acute kidney injury.
2. Interventions
   a. Encourage oral hydration; IV hydration may be prescribed; monitor renal function and intake and output, and ensure that the client is on a renal diet low in potassium and phosphorus.
   b. Administer diuretics to increase the urine flow through the kidneys as prescribed.
   c. Administer medications that increase the excretion of purines, such as allopurinol, as prescribed.
   d. Prepare to administer IV infusion of glucose and insulin to treat hyperkalemia.
   e. Prepare the client for dialysis if hyperkalemia and hyperuricemia persist despite treatment.

VII. Complex Endocrine Problems

A. Diabetic ketoacidosis (DKA)

1. Description (Fig. 69-19)
   a. Diabetic ketoacidosis is a life-threatening complication of type 1 diabetes mellitus that develops when a severe insulin deficiency occurs.
   b. The main clinical manifestations include hyperglycemia, dehydration, ketosis, and acidosis.
2. Assessment (Table 69-9)
3. Interventions

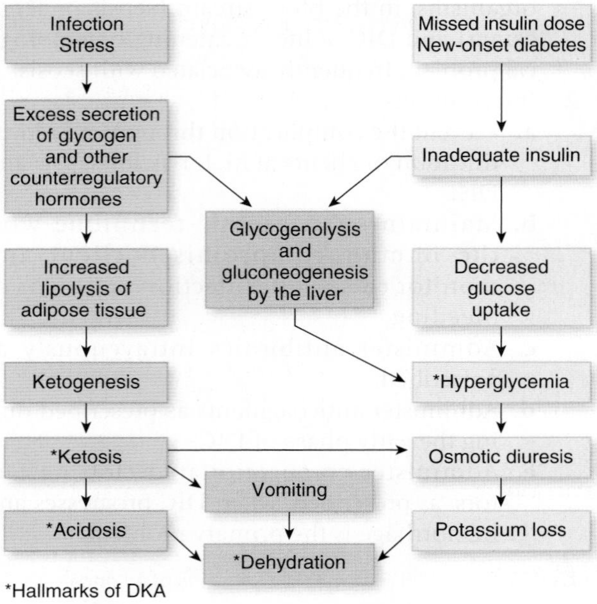

FIG. 69-19 Pathophysiology of diabetic ketoacidosis (DKA).

   a. Restore circulating blood volume and protect against cerebral, coronary, and renal hypoperfusion.
   b. Treat dehydration with rapid IV infusions of 0.9% or 0.45% NS as prescribed; dextrose is added to IV fluids when the blood glucose level reaches 250 to 300 mg/dL (14 to 17 mmol/L). Too rapid administration of IV fluids; use of the incorrect types of IV fluids, particularly hypotonic solutions; and correcting the blood glucose level too rapidly can lead to cerebral edema.
   c. Treat hyperglycemia with insulin administered intravenously as prescribed.
   d. Correct electrolyte imbalances (potassium level may be elevated as a result of dehydration and acidosis).
   e. Monitor potassium level closely, because when the client receives treatment for the dehydration and acidosis, the serum potassium level will decrease and potassium replacement may be required.
   f. Cardiac monitoring should be in place for the client with DKA due to risks associated with abnormal serum potassium levels.
4. Insulin IV administration
   a. Use short-duration insulin only.
   b. An IV bolus dose of short-duration regular U-100 insulin (usually 5 to 10 units) may be prescribed before a continuous infusion is begun.
   c. The prescribed IV dose of insulin for continuous infusion is prepared in 0.9% or 0.45% NS as prescribed.
   d. Always place the insulin infusion on an IV infusion controller.

TABLE 69-9 Differences Between Diabetic Ketoacidosis and Hyperosmolar Hyperglycemic Syndrome

	Diabetic Ketoacidosis (DKA)	Hyperosmolar Hyperglycemic Syndrome (HHS)
Onset	Sudden	Gradual
Precipitating factors	Infection	Infection
	Other stressors	Other stressors
	Inadequate insulin dose	Poor fluid intake
Manifestations	Ketosis: Kussmaul's respiration, "fruity" breath, nausea, abdominal pain	Altered central nervous system function with neurological symptoms
	Dehydration or electrolyte loss: Polyuria, polydipsia, weight loss, dry skin, sunken eyes, soft eyeballs, lethargy, coma	Dehydration or electrolyte loss: Same as for DKA
Laboratory Findings		
Serum glucose	>300 mg/dL (>17 mmol/L)	>800 mg/dL (>44.57 mmol/L)
Osmolarity	Variable	>350 mOsm/L
Serum ketones	Positive at 1:2 dilution	Negative
Serum pH	<7.35	>7.4
Serum HCO_3	<15 mEq/L <(15 mmol/L)	>20 mEq/L (>20 mmol/L)
Serum Na	Low, normal, or high	Normal or low
Serum K	Normal; elevated with acidosis, lowers following treatment	Normal or low
BUN	>20 mg/dL (>7.2 mmol/L); elevated because of dehydration	Elevated
Creatinine	>1.5 mg/dL (>132.5 mcmol/L); elevated because of dehydration	Elevated
Urine ketones	Positive	Negative

BUN, Blood urea nitrogen; *HCO_3,* bicarbonate; *K,* potassium; *Na,* sodium.
From Ignatavicius D, Workman M: *Medical-surgical nursing: patient-centered collaborative care,* ed 7, St. Louis, 2013, Saunders.

e. Insulin is infused continuously until subcutaneous administration resumes, to prevent a rebound of the blood glucose level.
f. Monitor vital signs.
g. Monitor urinary output and monitor for signs of fluid overload.
h. Monitor potassium and glucose levels and for signs of increased intracranial pressure (ICP).
i. The potassium level will fall rapidly within the first hour of treatment as the dehydration and the acidosis are treated.
j. Potassium is administered intravenously in a diluted solution as prescribed; ensure adequate renal function before administering potassium.

5. Client education (Box 69-11)

⚠ Monitor the client being treated for DKA closely for signs of increased intracranial pressure. If the blood glucose level falls too far or too fast before the brain has time to equilibrate, water is pulled from the blood to the cerebrospinal fluid and the brain, causing cerebral edema and increased ICP.

BOX 69-11 Diabetes and Client Education: Guidelines During Illness

- Take insulin or oral antidiabetic medications as prescribed.
- Determine the blood glucose level and test the urine for ketones every 3 to 4 hours.
- If the usual meal plan cannot be followed, substitute soft foods 6 to 8 times a day.
- If vomiting, diarrhea, or fever occurs, consume liquids every 30 to 60 minutes to prevent dehydration and to provide calories.
- Notify the primary health care provider (PHCP) if vomiting, diarrhea, or fever persists; if blood glucose levels are higher than 250 to 300 mg/dL (14 to 17 mmol/L); when ketonuria is present for more than 24 hours; when unable to take food or fluids for a period of 4 hours; or when illness persists for more than 2 days.

B. Hyperosmolar hyperglycemic syndrome (HHS)

1. Description
   a. Extreme hyperglycemia occurs without ketosis or acidosis.

b. The syndrome occurs most often in individuals with type 2 diabetes mellitus.
c. The major difference between HHS and DKA is that ketosis and acidosis do not occur with HHS; enough insulin is present with HHS to prevent the breakdown of fats for energy, thus preventing ketosis.
2. Assessment (see Table 69-9)
3. Interventions
a. Treatment is similar to that for DKA.
b. Treatment includes fluid replacement, correction of electrolyte imbalances, and insulin administration.
c. Fluid replacement in the older client must be done very carefully because of the potential for heart failure.
d. Insulin plays a less critical role in the treatment of HHS than it does in the treatment of DKA, because ketosis and acidosis do not occur; rehydration alone may decrease glucose levels.

VIII. Complex Gastrointestinal Problems

A. Esophageal varices
1. Description
a. Dilated and tortuous veins in the submucosa of the esophagus.
b. Caused by portal hypertension, often associated with liver **cirrhosis**; are at high risk for rupture if portal circulation pressure rises
c. Bleeding varices are an emergency.
d. The goal of treatment is to control bleeding, prevent complications, and prevent the recurrence of bleeding.
2. Assessment
a. Hematemesis
b. **Melena**
c. Ascites
d. Jaundice
e. Hepatomegaly and splenomegaly
f. Dilated abdominal veins
g. Signs of shock

Rupture and resultant hemorrhage of esophageal varices is the primary concern because it is a life-threatening situation.

3. Interventions
a. Monitor vital signs.
b. Elevate the head of the bed.
c. Monitor for orthostatic hypotension.
d. Monitor lung sounds and for the presence of respiratory distress.
e. Administer oxygen as prescribed to prevent tissue hypoxia.
f. Monitor level of consciousness.
g. Maintain NPO status.
h. Administer fluids intravenously as prescribed to restore fluid volume and electrolyte imbalances; monitor intake and output.
i. Monitor hemoglobin and hematocrit values and coagulation factors.
j. Administer blood transfusions or clotting factors as prescribed.
k. Assist in inserting an NG tube or a balloon tamponade as prescribed; balloon tamponade is not used frequently because it is very uncomfortable for the client and its use is associated with complications.
l. Prepare to assist with administering medications to induce vasoconstriction and reduce bleeding.
m. Instruct the client to avoid activities that will initiate vasovagal responses.
n. Prepare the client for endoscopic procedures or surgical procedures as prescribed.
4. Endoscopic injection (sclerotherapy)
a. The procedure involves the injection of a sclerosing agent into and around bleeding varices.
b. Complications include chest pain, pleural effusion, aspiration pneumonia, esophageal stricture, and perforation of the esophagus.
5. Endoscopic variceal ligation
a. The procedure involves ligation of the varices with an elastic rubber band.
b. Sloughing, followed by superficial ulceration, occurs in the area of ligation within 3 to 7 days.
6. Shunting procedures
a. Description: These procedures shunt blood away from the esophageal varices
b. Portacaval shunting involves anastomosis of the portal vein to the inferior vena cava, diverting blood from the portal system to the systemic circulation (Fig. 69-20).
c. Distal splenorenal shunt: The shunt involves anastomosis of the splenic vein to the left renal vein; the spleen conducts blood from the high-pressure varices to the low-pressure renal vein (see Fig. 69-20).
d. Mesocaval shunting involves a side anastomosis of the superior mesenteric vein to the proximal end of the inferior vena cava.
e. Transjugular intrahepatic portosystemic shunt (TIPS): This procedure uses the normal vascular anatomy of the liver to create a shunt with the use of a metallic stent; the shunt is between the portal and systemic venous system in the liver and is aimed at relieving portal hypertension.

B. Gastrointestinal (GI) bleeding

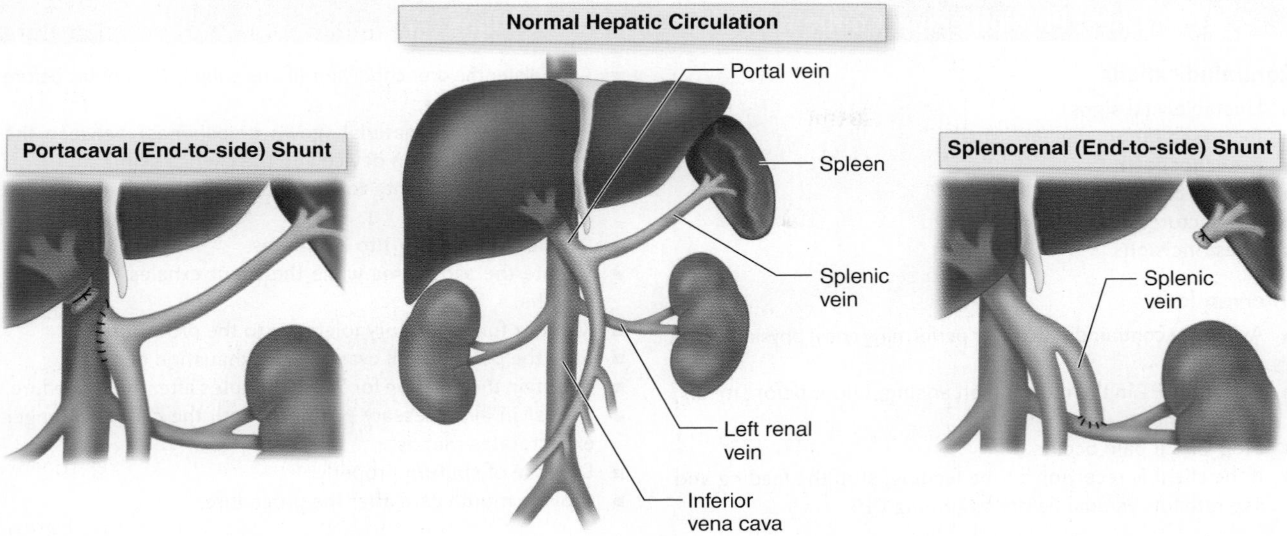

FIG. 69-20 Surgical shunting diverts portal venous blood flow from the liver to decrease portal and esophageal pressure.

1. Description: Bleeding that occurs at some area in the GI tract; classified into upper GI bleeding or lower GI bleeding.
2. Causes of upper GI bleeding include peptic ulcer disease, stress-related erosive syndrome, esophageal or gastric varices, tearing of the GI tract, esophagitis, neoplasm, aortoenteric fistula, and angiodysplasia.
3. Causes of lower GI bleeding include diverticulosis, angiodysplasia, neoplasm, inflammatory bowel disease, trauma, infectious colitis, radiation colitis, ischemia, aortoenteric fistula, and hemorrhoids.
4. GI bleeding, or hemorrhage, is a potentially life-threatening emergency condition.
5. Assessment
   a. Hematemesis
   b. Hematochezia
   c. Melena
   d. Decreased hemoglobin and hematocrit levels (may take 24 to 72 hours for the change to occur in acute blood loss)
6. Diagnosis
   a. Endoscopy once the client is hemodynamically stabilized
   b. Tagged red blood cell scanning, angiography, or both may be used to locate the source of bleeding.
7. Interventions
   a. The goal is to stop the bleeding and determine the cause of bleeding.
   b. Fluid resuscitation to achieve hemodynamic stability is necessary.
   c. Correction of hypercoagulability if indicated
   d. Therapeutic procedures to control or stop the bleeding
   e. Medications to suppress or neutralize gastric acids, including histamine-2 antagonists and proton pump inhibitors
   f. Note that these medications may place the client at risk for bacterial colonization and associated infections.
   g. Surgery may be used for a client who continues to be hemodynamically stable despite fluid resuscitation.

IX. Complex Respiratory Problems

A. Respiratory treatments
   1. Chest physiotherapy (CPT)
      a. Description: Percussion, vibration, and postural drainage techniques are performed over the thorax to loosen secretions in the affected area of the lungs and move them into more central airways.
      b. Contraindications and interventions (Box 69-12)

B. Oxygen
   1. Supplemental oxygen delivery systems (Table 69-10)
      a. Nasal cannula for low flow: Used for the client with chronic airflow limitation and for long-term oxygen use (Fig. 69-21)
      b. Nasal high-flow (NHF) respiratory therapy: Used for hypoxemic clients in mild to moderate respiratory distress (Box 69-13)
      c. Simple face mask: Used for short-term oxygen therapy or to deliver oxygen in an emergency (Fig. 69-22)
      d. Venturi mask: Used for clients at risk for or experiencing acute respiratory failure (Fig. 69-23)
      e. Partial rebreather mask: Useful when the oxygen concentration needs to be raised; not

BOX 69-12 Chest Physiotherapy: Contraindications and Interventions

Contraindications

- Unstable vital signs
- Increased intracranial pressure
- Bronchospasm
- History of pathological fractures
- Rib fractures
- Chest incisions

Interventions

- Assess for contraindications for performing chest physiotherapy (CPT)
- Perform CPT in the morning on arising, 1 hour before meals, or 2 to 3 hours after meals.
- Stop CPT if pain occurs.
- If the client is receiving a tube feeding, stop the feeding and aspirate for residual before beginning CPT.
- Administer the bronchodilator (if prescribed) 15 minutes before the procedure.
- Place a layer of material (gown or pajamas) between the hands or percussion device and the client's skin.
- Position the client for postural drainage based on assessment.
- Percuss the area for 1 to 2 minutes.
- Vibrate the same area while the client exhales 4 or 5 deep breaths.
- Monitor for respiratory tolerance to the procedure.
- Stop the procedure if cyanosis or exhaustion occurs.
- Maintain the position for 5 to 20 minutes after the procedure.
- Repeat in all necessary positions until the client no longer expectorates mucus.
- Dispose of sputum properly.
- Provide mouth care after the procedure.

TABLE 69-10 Supplemental Oxygen Delivery Systems

Device	Oxygen Delivered	Nursing Considerations
Nasal cannula (nasal prongs) (see Fig. 69-21)	▪ 1-6 L/min for oxygen concentration (FiO_2) of 24% (at 1 L/min) to 44% (at 6 L/min)	▪ Easily tolerated ▪ Can dislodge easily. Does not get in the way of eating or talking. ▪ Effective oxygen concentration can be delivered. Allows the client to breathe through the nose or mouth. ▪ Ensure that prongs are in the nares with openings facing the client. ▪ Assess nasal mucosa for irritation from drying effect of higher flow rates. ▪ Assess skin integrity, as tubing can irritate skin. ▪ Add humidification as prescribed and check water levels.
Simple face mask (see Fig. 69-22)	▪ 5-8 L/min oxygen flow for FiO_2 of 40%-60%. ▪ Minimum flow of 5 L/min needed to flush CO_2 from mask	▪ Interferes with eating and talking. ▪ Can be warm and confining. ▪ Ensure that mask fits securely over nose and mouth. ▪ Remove saliva and mucus from the mask. ▪ Provide skin care to area covered by mask. ▪ Provide emotional support to decrease anxiety in the client who feels claustrophobic. ▪ Monitor for risk of aspiration from inability of client to clear mouth (i.e., if vomiting occurs).
Venturi mask (Ventimask) (see Fig. 69-23)	▪ 4-10 L/min oxygen flow for FiO_2 of 24%-55% ▪ Delivers exact desired selected concentrations of O_2	▪ Keep the air entrapment port for the adapter open and uncovered to ensure adequate oxygen delivery. ▪ Keep mask snug on the face and ensure tubing is free of kinks, because the FiO_2 is altered if kinking occurs or if the mask fits poorly. ▪ Assess nasal mucosa for irritation; humidity or aerosol can be added to the system as needed.
Partial rebreather mask (mask with reservoir bag)	▪ 6-15 L/min oxygen flow for FiO_2 of 70%-90%	▪ The client rebreathes one-third of the exhaled tidal volume, which is high in oxygen, thus providing a high FiO_2. ▪ Adjust flow rate to keep the reservoir bag two-thirds full during inspiration. ▪ Keep mask snug on face. ▪ Make sure the reservoir bag does not twist or kink. ▪ Deflation of the bag results in decreased oxygen delivered and rebreathing of exhaled air.
Nonrebreather mask (see Fig. 69-24)	▪ FiO_2 of 60%-100% at a rate of flow that maintains the bag two-thirds full	▪ Adjust flow rate to keep the reservoir bag inflated. ▪ Remove mucus and saliva from the mask. ▪ Provide emotional support to decrease anxiety in the client who feels claustrophobic. ▪ Ensure that the valves and flaps are intact and functional during each breath (valves should open during expiration and close during inhalation). ▪ Make sure the reservoir bag does not twist or kink or that the oxygen source does not disconnect; otherwise, the client will suffocate.

TABLE 69-10 **Supplemental Oxygen Delivery Systems—cont'd**

Device	Oxygen Delivered	Nursing Considerations
Tracheostomy collar and T-bar or T-piece, endotracheal tube (face tent; face shield) (see Fig. 69-25)	▪ The tracheostomy collar can be used to deliver the desired amount of oxygen to a client with a tracheostomy. ▪ A special adaptor (T-bar or T-piece) can be used to deliver any desired FiO_2 to client with tracheostomy, laryngectomy, or endotracheal tube. ▪ The face tent provides 8-12 L/min and the FiO_2 varies due to environmental loss.	▪ Ensure that aerosol mist escapes from the vents of the delivery system during inspiration and expiration. ▪ Empty condensation from the tubing to prevent the client from being lavaged with water and to promote an adequate oxygen flow rate (remove and clean the tubing at least every 4 hr). ▪ Keep the exhalation port in the T-piece open and uncovered (if the port is occluded, the client can suffocate). ▪ Position the T-piece so that it does not pull on the tracheostomy or endotracheal tube and cause erosion of the skin at the tracheostomy insertion site.

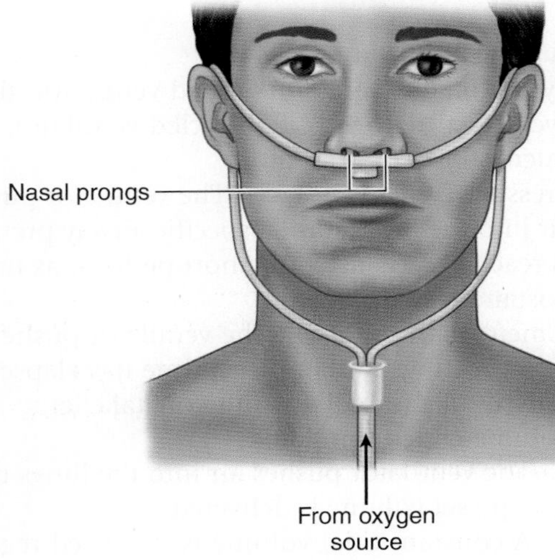

FIG. 69-21 A nasal cannula (prongs).

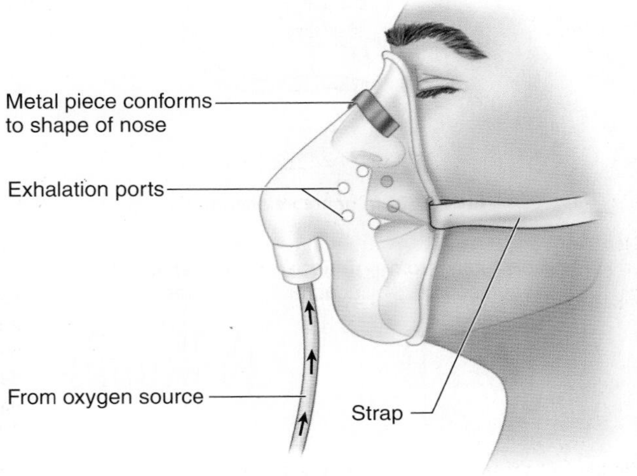

FIG. 69-22 A simple face mask used to deliver oxygen.

BOX 69-13 Nasal High-Flow (NHF) Respiratory Therapy

- Comfortably delivers high flows of heated and humidified oxygen through a wide-bore nasal cannula and humidification system
- Can deliver nasal flow rates up to 50 to 60 L/minute to deliver humidified high-flow oxygen therapy

usually prescribed for a client with chronic obstructive pulmonary disease (COPD)

f. Nonrebreather mask: Most frequently used for the client with a deteriorating respiratory status who might require intubation (Fig. 69-24)

g. Tracheostomy collar and T-bar or T-piece: Tracheostomy collar is used to deliver high humidity and the desired oxygen to the client with a tracheostomy; the T-bar or T-piece is used to deliver the desired FiO_2 to the client with a tracheostomy, laryngectomy, or endotracheal tube (Fig. 69-25).

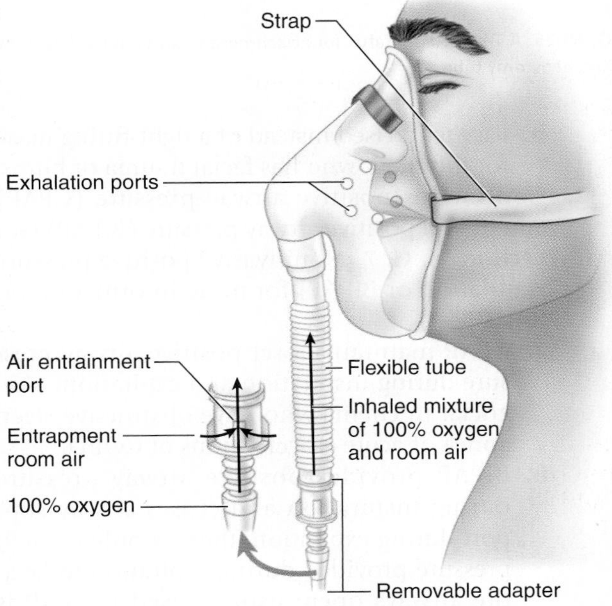

FIG. 69-23 A Venturi mask for precise oxygen delivery.

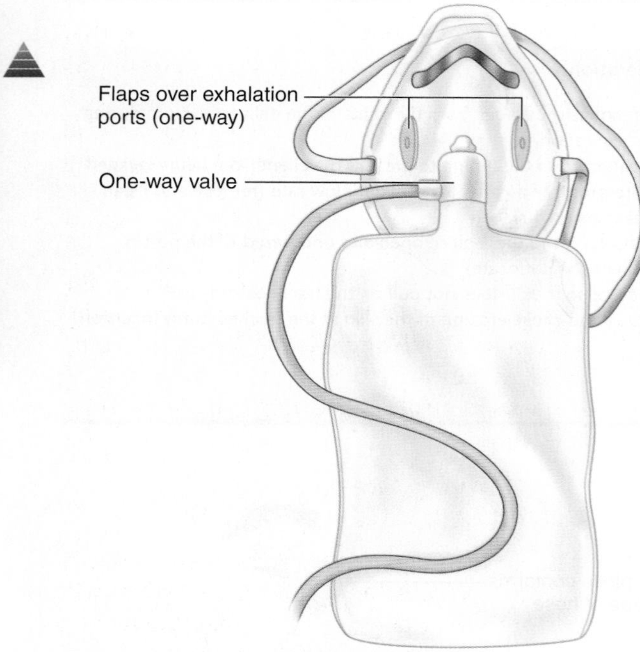

FIG. 69-24 A nonrebreather mask.

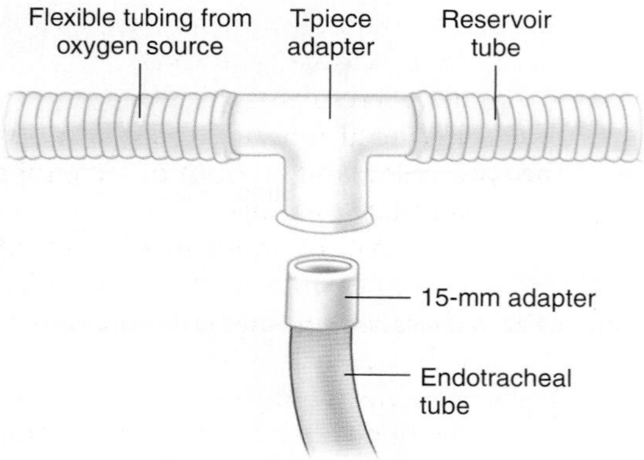

FIG. 69-25 A T-piece apparatus for attachment to an endotracheal tube or tracheostomy tube.

h. Face tent: Used instead of a tight-fitting mask for the client who has facial trauma or burns.

2. Continuous positive airway pressure (CPAP) and bilevel positive airway pressure (BiPAP) (see Section IX, C, 7 [Noninvasive positive pressure ventilation or BiPAP] for more information on BiPAP)
   a. CPAP maintains a set positive airway pressure during inspiration and expiration; beneficial in clients who have obstructive sleep apnea or acute exacerbations of COPD.
   b. BiPAP provides positive airway pressure during inspiration and ceases airway support during expiration; there is only enough pressure provided during expiration to keep the airways open; usually used if CPAP is ineffective.
   c. Both CPAP and BiPAP improve oxygenation through airway support.
3. General interventions
   a. Assess color, pulse oximetry reading, and vital signs before and during treatment.
   b. Place an *Oxygen in Use* sign at the client's bedside.
   c. Assess for the presence of chronic lung problems.
   d. Humidify the oxygen if indicated.
   e. For specific considerations for each supplemental oxygen delivery system, see Table 69-10.

A client who is hypoxemic and has chronic hypercapnia may require low levels of oxygen delivery at 1 to 2 L/minute, because a low arterial oxygen level is the client's primary drive for breathing; always check PHCP's prescriptions.

C. Mechanical ventilation

1. Types: include pressure-cycled ventilator, time-cycled ventilator, volume-cycled ventilator, and microprocessor ventilator
2. Pressure-cycled ventilator: The ventilator pushes air into the lungs until a specific airway pressure is reached; it is used for short periods, as in the postanesthesia care unit.
3. Time-cycled ventilator: The ventilator pushes air into the lungs until a preset time has elapsed; it is used for the pediatric or neonatal client.
4. Volume-cycled ventilator
   a. The ventilator pushes air into the lungs until a preset volume is delivered.
   b. A constant tidal volume is delivered regardless of the changing compliance of the lungs and chest wall or the airway resistance in the client or ventilator.
5. Microprocessor ventilator
   a. A computer or microprocessor is built into the ventilator to allow continuous monitoring of ventilatory functions, alarms, and client parameters.
   b. This type of ventilator is more responsive to clients who have severe lung disease or require prolonged weaning.
6. Modes of ventilation: include noninvasive positive pressure ventilation or BiPAP, controlled, assist-controlled, and synchronized intermittent mandatory ventilation (SIMV)
7. Noninvasive positive pressure ventilation or BiPAP (Fig. 69-26)
   a. Ventilatory support given without using an invasive artificial airway (endotracheal tube or tracheostomy tube); orofacial masks and nasal masks are used instead.
   b. An inspiratory positive airway pressure (IPAP) and an expiratory positive airway pressure (EPAP) are set on a large ventilator or a small flow generator ventilator with a

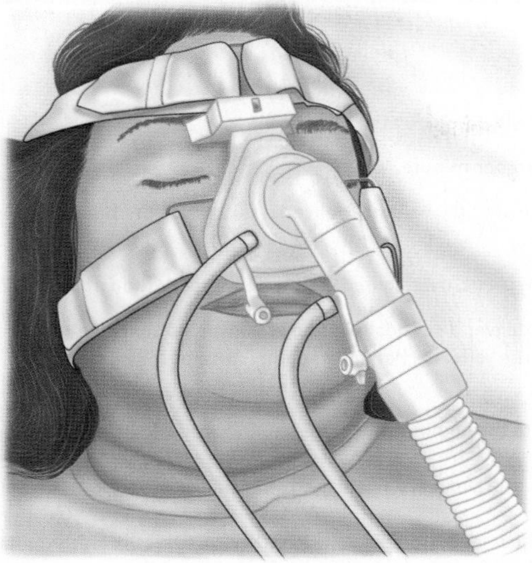

FIG. 69-26 A BiPAP (bilevel positive airway pressure) system using a nasal mask for pressure- and volume-controlled ventilation.

desired pressure support and positive end-expiratory pressure (PEEP) level. This allows more air to move into and out of the lungs without the normal muscular activity needed to do so.

c. Can be used in certain situations of COPD distress, heart failure, asthma, pulmonary edema, and hypercapnic respiratory failure.

⚠ A bag-valve resuscitation mask should be available at the bedside for all clients receiving mechanical ventilation.

8. Controlled
   a. The client receives a set tidal volume at a set rate.
   b. Used for clients who cannot initiate respiratory effort
   c. Least used mode; if the client attempts to initiate a breath, the ventilator locks out the client's inspiratory effort.
9. Assist-control
   a. Tidal volume and ventilatory rate are preset on the ventilator.
   b. The ventilator takes over the work of breathing for the client.
   c. The ventilator is programmed to respond to the client's inspiratory effort if the client does initiate a breath.
   d. The ventilator delivers the preset tidal volume when the client initiates a breath while allowing the client to control the rate of breathing.
   e. If the client's spontaneous ventilatory rate increases, the ventilator continues to deliver a preset tidal volume with each breath, which may cause hyperventilation and respiratory alkalosis.
10. SIMV
   a. Similar to assist-control ventilation in that the tidal volume and ventilatory rate are preset on the ventilator
   b. Allows the client to breathe spontaneously at her or his own rate and tidal volume between the ventilator breaths
   c. Can be used as a primary ventilatory mode or as a weaning mode
   d. When SIMV is used as a weaning mode, the number of SIMV breaths is decreased gradually, and the client gradually resumes spontaneous breathing.
11. Ventilator controls and settings (Table 69-11)
12. Interventions

⚠ For a client receiving mechanical ventilation, always assess the client first and then assess the ventilator.

   a. Assess vital signs, lung sounds, respiratory status, and breathing patterns (the client will never breathe at a rate lower than the rate set on the ventilator).
   b. Monitor skin color, particularly in the lips and nailbeds.
   c. Monitor the chest for bilateral expansion.
   d. Obtain pulse oximetry readings.
   e. Monitor ABG results.
   f. Assess the need for suctioning and observe the type, color, and amount of secretions.
   g. Assess ventilator settings.
   h. Assess the level of water in the humidifier and the temperature of the humidification system, because extremes in temperature can damage the mucosa in the airway.
   i. Ensure that the alarms are set.
   j. If a cause for an alarm cannot be determined, ventilate the client manually with a bag-valve resuscitation mask until the problem is corrected.
   k. Empty the ventilator tubing when moisture collects.
   l. Turn the client at least every 2 hours or get the client out of bed, as prescribed, to prevent complications of immobility.
   m. Have resuscitation equipment available at the bedside.
13. Causes of ventilator alarms (Box 69-14)
14. Alarm safety and alarm fatigue
   a. It is the responsibility of the nurse to be alert to the sound of an alarm, because this signals a client problem.
   b. The nurse needs to respond promptly to an alarm and immediately assess the client.
   c. According to The Joint Commission (TJC), the most common contributing factor related to alarm-related sentinel events is alarm fatigue, which results when the

TABLE 69-11 Ventilator Controls and Settings and Descriptions

Controls and Settings	Descriptions
Tidal volume	The volume of air that the client receives with each breath
Rate	The number of ventilator breaths delivered per minute
Sighs	The volumes of air that are 1.5-2 times the set tidal volume, delivered 6-10 times per hour; may be used to prevent atelectasis
Fraction of inspired oxygen (FiO_2)	The oxygen concentration delivered to the client; determined by the client's condition and ABG levels
Peak airway inspiratory pressure	The pressure needed by the ventilator to deliver a set tidal volume at a given compliance Monitoring peak airway inspiratory pressure reflects changes in compliance of the lungs and resistance in the ventilator or client.
Continuous positive airway pressure	The application of positive airway pressure throughout the entire respiratory cycle for spontaneously breathing clients Keeps the alveoli open during inspiration and prevents alveolar collapse; used primarily as a weaning modality No ventilator breaths are delivered, but the ventilator delivers oxygen and provides monitoring and an alarm system; the respiratory pattern is determined by the client's efforts.
Positive end-expiratory pressure (PEEP)	Positive pressure is exerted during the expiratory phase of ventilation, which improves oxygenation by enhancing gas exchange and preventing atelectasis. The need for PEEP indicates a severe gas exchange disturbance. Higher levels of PEEP (more than 15 cm H_2O) increase the chance of complications, such as barotrauma tension pneumothorax.
Pressure support	The application of positive pressure on inspiration that eases the workload of breathing. May be used in combination with PEEP as a weaning method. As the weaning process continues, the amount of pressure applied to inspiration is gradually decreased.

ABG, Arterial blood gas.

BOX 69-14 Causes of Ventilator Alarms

Collaborate with respiratory therapy in troubleshooting and addressing ventilator alarms.

High-Pressure Alarm

- Increased secretions are in the artificial airway or the client's own airway.
- Wheezing or bronchospasm is causing decreased airway size.
- The endotracheal tube is displaced.
- The ventilator tube is obstructed because of water or a kink in the tubing.
- Client coughs, gags, or bites on the oral endotracheal tube.
- Client is anxious or fights the ventilator.

Low-Pressure Alarm

- Disconnection or leak in the ventilator or in the client's airway cuff occurs.
- The client stops spontaneous breathing.

numerous alarms and the resulting noise tends to desensitize the nursing staff and cause them to ignore alarms or even disable them.

d. Some recommendations of TJC include establishing alarm safety as a facility policy, identifying default alarm settings, identifying the most important alarms to manage, establishing policies and procedures for managing alarms, and staff education.

e. For additional information, refer to www.pwrnewmedia.com/2013/joint_commission/medical_alarm_safety/downloads/SEA_50_alarms.pdf.

Never set ventilator alarm controls to the off position.

15. Complications
    a. Hypotension caused by the application of positive pressure, which increases intrathoracic pressure and inhibits blood return to the heart
    b. Respiratory complications such as pneumothorax or subcutaneous **emphysema** as a result of positive pressure
    c. Gastrointestinal alterations such as stress ulcers
    d. Malnutrition if nutrition is not maintained
    e. Infections
    f. Muscular deconditioning
    g. Ventilator dependence or inability to wean
    h. Bradycardia as a result of increased intrathoracic pressure or activated vagal response
16. Weaning: Process of going from ventilator dependence to spontaneous breathing; methods include SIMV, T-piece, and pressure support

17. SIMV
    a. The client breathes between the preset breaths per minute rate of the ventilator.
    b. The SIMV rate is decreased gradually until the client is breathing on her or his own without the use of the ventilator.
18. T-piece
    a. The client is taken off the ventilator and the ventilator is replaced with a T-piece or CPAP, which delivers humidified oxygen.
    b. The client is taken off the ventilator for short periods initially and allowed to breathe spontaneously.
    c. Weaning progresses as the client is able to tolerate progressively longer periods off the ventilator.
19. Pressure support
    a. Pressure support is a predetermined pressure set on the ventilator to assist the client in respiratory effort.
    b. As weaning continues, the amount of pressure is decreased gradually.
    c. With pressure support, pressure may be maintained while the preset breaths per minute of the ventilator are decreased gradually.

D. Rib fracture
1. Results from direct blunt chest trauma and causes a potential for intrathoracic injury, such as pneumothorax, hemothorax, or pulmonary contusion
2. Pain with movement, deep breathing, and coughing results in impaired ventilation and inadequate clearance of secretions.
3. Assessment
    a. Pain and tenderness at the injury site that increases with inspiration
    b. Shallow respirations
    c. Client splints chest
    d. Fractures noted on chest x-ray
4. Interventions
    a. Note that the ribs usually reunite spontaneously.
    b. Place the client in a Fowler's position.
    c. Administer pain medication as prescribed to maintain adequate ventilatory status.
    d. Monitor for increased respiratory distress.
    e. Instruct the client to self-splint with the hands, arms, or a pillow.
    f. Open reduction and internal fixation of the ribs (rib plating) may be done
    g. Prepare the client for an intercostal nerve block as prescribed if the pain is severe.

E. Flail chest
1. Occurs from blunt chest trauma associated with accidents, which may result in hemothorax and rib fractures.
2. The loose segment of the chest wall becomes paradoxical to the expansion and contraction of the rest of the chest wall.
3. Assessment
    a. Paradoxical respirations (inward movement of a segment of the thorax during inspiration with outward movement during expiration)
    b. Severe pain in the chest
    c. Dyspnea
    d. Cyanosis
    e. Tachycardia
    f. Hypotension
    g. Tachypnea, shallow respirations
    h. Diminished breath sounds
4. Interventions
    a. Maintain the client in a Fowler's position.
    b. Administer oxygen as prescribed.
    c. Monitor for increased respiratory distress.
    d. Encourage coughing and deep breathing.
    e. Administer pain medication as prescribed.
    f. Maintain bed rest and limit activity to reduce oxygen demands.
    g. Open reduction and internal fixation of the ribs (rib plating) may be done.
    h. Prepare for intubation with mechanical ventilation, with PEEP for severe flail chest associated with respiratory failure and shock.

F. Pulmonary contusion
1. Characterized by interstitial hemorrhage associated with intra-alveolar hemorrhage, resulting in decreased pulmonary compliance
2. The major complication is acute respiratory distress syndrome.
3. Assessment
    a. Dyspnea
    b. Restlessness
    c. Increased bronchial secretions
    d. Hypoxemia
    e. Hemoptysis
    f. Decreased breath sounds
    g. Crackles and wheezes
4. Interventions
    a. Maintain a patent airway and adequate ventilation.
    b. Place the client in a Fowler's position.
    c. Administer oxygen as prescribed.
    d. Monitor for increased respiratory distress.
    e. Maintain bed rest and limit activity to reduce oxygen demands.
    f. Prepare for mechanical ventilation with PEEP if required.

G. Pneumothorax (Fig. 69-27)
1. Accumulation of atmospheric air in the pleural space, which results in a rise in intrathoracic pressure and reduced vital capacity
2. The loss of negative intrapleural pressure results in collapse of the lung.

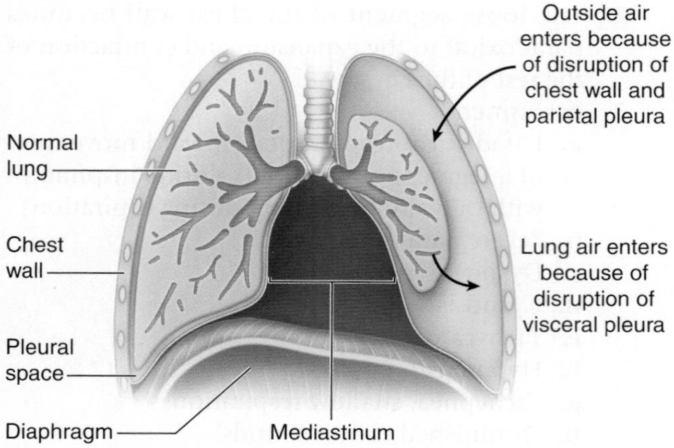

FIG. 69-27 Pneumothorax. Air in the pleural space causes the lungs to collapse around the hilus and may push the mediastinal contents (heart and great vessels) toward the other lung.

3. A spontaneous pneumothorax occurs with the rupture of a pulmonary bleb, or small air-containing spaces deep in the lung.
4. An open pneumothorax occurs when an opening through the chest wall allows the entrance of positive atmospheric air pressure into the pleural space.
5. A tension pneumothorax occurs from a blunt chest injury or from mechanical ventilation with PEEP when a buildup of positive pressure occurs in the pleural space.
6. Assessment (Box 69-15)
7. Interventions
   a. Diagnosis of pneumothorax is made by chest x-ray.
   b. Apply a nonporous dressing over an open chest wound.
   c. Administer oxygen as prescribed.
   d. Place the client in a Fowler's position.
   e. Prepare for chest tube placement, which will remain in place until the lung has expanded fully (see section IV, O, for information on chest tubes).
   f. Monitor the chest tube drainage system.
   g. Monitor for subcutaneous emphysema.

BOX 69-15 Assessment Findings: Pneumothorax

- Absent or markedly decreased breath sounds on affected side
- Cyanosis
- Decreased chest expansion unilaterally
- Dyspnea
- Hypotension
- Sharp chest pain
- Subcutaneous emphysema as evidenced by crepitus on palpation
- Sucking sound with open chest wound
- Tachycardia
- Tachypnea
- Tracheal deviation to the unaffected side with tension pneumothorax

⚠ Clients with a respiratory disorder should be positioned with the head of the bed elevated.

H. Acute respiratory failure
1. Occurs when insufficient oxygen is transported to the blood or inadequate carbon dioxide is removed from the lungs and the client's compensatory mechanisms fail
2. Causes include a mechanical abnormality of the lungs or chest wall, a defect in the respiratory control center in the brain, or an impairment in the function of the respiratory muscles.
3. In oxygenation failure, or hypoxemic respiratory failure, oxygen may reach the alveoli but cannot be absorbed or used properly, resulting in a PaO_2 lower than 60 mm Hg, arterial oxygen saturation (SaO_2) lower than 90%, or partial pressure of arterial carbon dioxide ($PaCo_2$) greater than 50 mm Hg occurring with acidemia.
4. Respiratory failure can be hypoxemic, hypercapnic, or both. Inadequate gas exchange is the mechanism behind failure. Arterial oxygen, carbon dioxide, or both are not kept at normal levels, resulting in failure.
5. Many clients experience both hypoxemic and hypercapnic respiratory failure and retained carbon dioxide in the alveoli displaces oxygen, contributing to the hypoxemia.
6. Manifestations of respiratory failure are related to the extent and rapidity of change in PaO_2 and $PaCo_2$.
7. Assessment
   a. Dyspnea
   b. Restlessness
   c. Confusion
   d. Tachycardia
   e. Hypertension
   f. Dysrhythmias
   g. Decreased level of consciousness
   h. Alterations in respirations and breath sounds
   i. Headache (less common)
8. Interventions
   a. Identify and treat the cause of the respiratory failure.
   b. Administer oxygen to maintain the PaO_2 level higher than 60 to 70 mm Hg.
   c. Place the client in a Fowler's position.
   d. Encourage deep breathing.
   e. Administer bronchodilators as prescribed.
   f. Prepare the client for mechanical ventilation if supplemental oxygen cannot maintain acceptable PaO_2 and $PaCO_2$ levels.

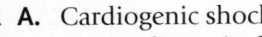

I. Acute respiratory distress syndrome
1. A form of acute respiratory failure that occurs as a complication caused by a diffuse lung injury or critical illness and leads to extravascular lung fluid.
2. The major site of injury is the alveolar capillary membrane.
3. The interstitial edema causes compression and obliteration of the terminal airways and leads to reduced lung volume and compliance.
4. The ABG levels identify respiratory acidosis and hypoxemia that do not respond to an increased percentage of oxygen.
5. The chest x-ray shows bilateral interstitial and alveolar infiltrates; interstitial edema may not be noted until there is a 30% increase in fluid content.
6. Causes include sepsis, fluid overload, shock, trauma, neurological injuries, burns, DIC, drug ingestion, aspiration, and inhalation of toxic substances.
7. Assessment
a. Tachypnea
b. Dyspnea
c. Decreased breath sounds
d. Deteriorating ABG levels
e. Hypoxemia despite high concentrations of delivered oxygen
f. Decreased pulmonary compliance
g. Pulmonary infiltrates
8. Interventions
a. Identify and treat the cause of the acute respiratory distress syndrome.
b. Administer oxygen as prescribed.
c. Place the client in a Fowler's position.
d. Restrict fluid intake as prescribed.
e. Provide respiratory treatments as prescribed.
f. Administer diuretics, anticoagulants, or corticosteroids as prescribed.
g. Prepare the client for intubation and mechanical ventilation using PEEP.

X. Complex Cardiovascular Problems

A. Cardiogenic shock
1. Cardiogenic shock is failure of the heart to pump adequately, thereby reducing cardiac output and compromising tissue perfusion.
2. Necrosis of more than 40% of the left ventricle, usually as a result of occlusion of major coronary vessels, leads to cardiogenic shock.
3. The goal of treatment is to maintain tissue oxygenation and perfusion and improve the pumping ability of the heart.
4. Assessment
a. Hypotension: BP lower than 90 mm Hg systolic or 30 mm Hg lower than the client's baseline
b. Urine output lower than 30 mL/hr
c. Cold, clammy skin
d. Poor peripheral pulses
e. Tachycardia, tachypnea
f. Pulmonary congestion
g. Disorientation, restlessness, and confusion
h. Continuing chest discomfort
5. Interventions
a. Administer oxygen as prescribed.
b. Administer morphine sulfate intravenously as prescribed to decrease pulmonary congestion and relieve chest pain.
c. Prepare for intubation and mechanical ventilation.
d. Administer diuretics and nitrates as prescribed while monitoring the BP constantly.
e. Administer vasopressors and positive inotropes as prescribed to maintain organ perfusion.
f. Prepare the client for insertion of an intra-aortic balloon pump, if prescribed, to improve coronary artery perfusion and improve cardiac output.
g. Prepare the client for immediate reperfusion procedures such as percutaneous transluminal coronary angioplasty (PTCA) or coronary artery bypass graft.
h. Monitor arterial blood gas levels and prepare to treat imbalances.
i. Monitor urinary output.
j. Assist with the insertion of a pulmonary artery (Swan-Ganz) catheter to assess degree of heart failure (Fig. 69-28).

B. Hemodynamic monitoring: includes central venous pressure (CVP), pulmonary artery pressures, and mean arterial pressure (MAP) (see Fig. 69-28)

C. Central venous pressure (CVP)
1. The CVP is the pressure within the superior vena cava; it reflects the pressure under which blood is returned to the superior vena cava and right atrium.
2. The CVP is measured with a central venous line in the superior vena cava.
3. Normal CVP pressure ranges between approximately 3 to 8 mm Hg.
4. An elevated CVP indicates an increase in blood volume as a result of sodium and water retention, excessive IV fluids, alterations in fluid balance, or kidney failure.
5. A decreased CVP indicates a decrease in circulating blood volume and may be a result of fluid imbalances, hemorrhage, or severe vasodilation, with pooling of blood in the extremities that limits venous return.

D. Measuring CVP
1. The right atrium is located at the midaxillary line at the fourth intercostal space; the zero point on the transducer needs to be at the level of the right atrium.

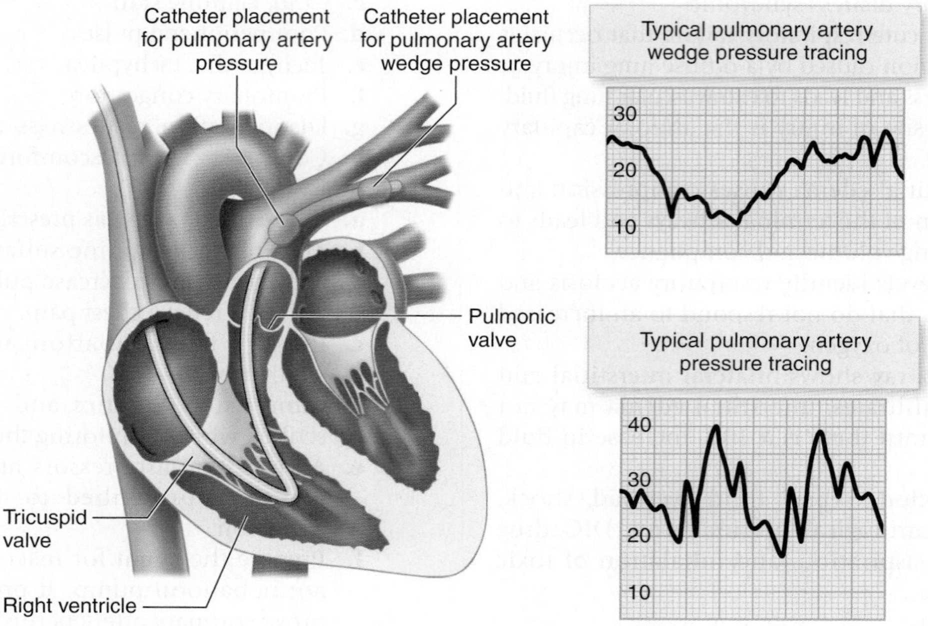

FIG. 69-28 Cardiac pressure waveforms can be visualized on the monitor.

2. The client needs to be relaxed; activity that increases intrathoracic pressure, such as coughing or straining, will cause false increases in the readings.
3. If the client is on a ventilator, the reading should be taken at the point of end-expiration.
4. To maintain patency of the central venous line, a continuous small amount of fluid is delivered under pressure.

E. Pulmonary artery pressures
1. A pulmonary artery catheter is used to measure right heart and indirect left heart pressures.
2. **Pulmonary artery wedge pressure (PAWP)** is also known as pulmonary artery occlusive pressure (PAOP) and as pulmonary capillary wedge pressure (PCWP).
3. The measurement is obtained during momentary balloon inflation of the pulmonary artery catheter and reflects left ventricular end-diastolic pressure.
4. PAWP normally ranges between approximately 4 to 12 mm Hg; elevations may indicate left ventricular failure, hypervolemia, mitral regurgitation, or intracardiac shunt, whereas decreases may indicate hypovolemia or afterload reduction.
5. Normal RA pressure ranges between approximately 2 to 6 mm Hg; increases occur with right ventricular failure, whereas decreases may indicate hypovolemia.
6. Normal pulmonary artery pressure (PAP) ranges between approximately 15 to 30 mm Hg systolic/8 to 15 mm Hg diastolic.

F. **Mean arterial pressure (MAP)**
1. An approximation of the average pressure in the systemic circulation throughout the cardiac cycle
2. MAP ranges between approximately 70 to 105 mm Hg.

G. Guidelines for performing adult CPR: refer to Chapter 52; also, refer to American Heart Association: *Guidelines for CPR and ECC*, 2015 and *Focused Updates*, 2017. Retrieved from https://eccguidelines.heart.org/index.php/circulation/cpr-ecc-guidelines-2/

H. Advanced management of pulseless rhythms
1. Initial Steps
   a. Begin CPR; attach the monitor or defibrillator.
   b. Determine whether the rhythm is shockable or nonshockable.
   c. Shockable pulseless rhythms include ventricular fibrillation and ventricular tachycardia.
   d. Nonshockable pulseless rhythms include asystole and pulseless electrical activity (PEA).
2. Shockable rhythms: ventricular fibrillation and ventricular tachycardia
   a. After beginning CPR, attaching the monitor, and determining the rhythm, shock at 100 to 200 J as an initial dose that is increased if biphasic; use 360 J if monophasic.
   b. Continue CPR and establish an IV or intraosseus (IO) access if not previously done.
   c. Analyze the rhythm; if shockable, shock again.
   d. Prepare to administer epinephrine 1 mg every 3 to 5 minutes as prescribed.
   e. An advanced airway should be considered, and capnography should be used to determine CPR quality.

f. Continue CPR, analyze the rhythm, and shock if the rhythm is shockable. If the rhythm becomes unshockable, follow the nonshockable rhythms approach.
g. As prescribed, prepare to administer amiodarone 300 mg IV/IO bolus, followed by 150 mg IV/IO if indicated at the next appropriate cycle.
h. Consider reversible causes, which include hypoxia, hypovolemia, hydrogen ions or acidosis, hyperkalemia or hypokalemia (5 Hs) and tension pneumothorax, tamponade, toxins, thrombosis (pulmonary embolus), or thrombosis (acute coronary syndrome; 5 Ts).
i. Continue to cycle through the above steps until return of spontaneous circulation (ROSC) or until CPR efforts are ceased.

3. Nonshockable rhythms: asystole and PEA
a. After beginning CPR, attaching the monitor, and determining the rhythm establish an IV or IO access if not previously done.
b. Prepare to administer epinephrine 1 mg every 3 to 5 minutes as prescribed.
c. An advanced airway should be considered and capnography should be used to determine CPR quality.
d. Continue CPR, analyze the rhythm, and follow the shockable rhythm approach if the rhythm becomes shockable.
e. Consider reversible causes, which include hypoxia, hypovolemia, hydrogen ions or acidosis, hyperkalemia or hypokalemia (5 Hs) and tension pneumothorax, tamponade, toxins, thrombosis (pulmonary embolus), or thrombosis (acute coronary syndrome; 5 Ts).
f. Continue to cycle through the above steps until return of spontaneous circulation (ROSC) or until CPR efforts are ceased.

4. Postcardiac arrest care
a. If ROSC is achieved, advanced airway placement should be done if not previously established, oxygen saturation should be maintained greater than 94%, and hyperventilation should be avoided.
b. If hypotension is present (systolic blood pressure less than 90 mm Hg), vasopressors and IV fluid boluses are needed.
c. IV fluids include 1 to 2 liters of normal saline or lactated Ringer's solution.
d. Vasopressors include epinephrine IV infusion 0.1 to 0.5 mg/kg/minute, dopamine IV infusion 5 to 10 mcg/kg/minute, or norepinephrine 0.1 to 0.5 mcg/kg/minute.
e. A 12-lead electrocardiogram should be done.
f. If the client is following commands, consider targeted temperature management to preserve neurological function, and IV fluids cooled to 4° C should be used.
g. If ST-elevation myocardial infarction (STEMI) or other form of acute MI are suspected, coronary reperfusion should be done, and the client should be managed on the critical care unit.
h. Post Cardiac Arrest Care Guidelines: Adapted from the American Heart Association. (2018). *Part 7: Advanced cardiovascular life support*. Retrieved from https://eccguidelines.heart.org/index.php/circulation/cpr-ecc-guidelines-2/part-7-adult-advanced-cardiovascular-life-support/

I. Cardiac tamponade
1. A pericardial effusion occurs when the space between the parietal and visceral layers of the pericardium fills with fluid.
2. Pericardial effusion places the client at risk for cardiac tamponade, an accumulation of fluid in the pericardial cavity.
3. Tamponade restricts ventricular filling, and cardiac output drops.

⚠ Acute cardiac tamponade can occur when small volumes (20 to 50 mL) of fluid accumulate rapidly in the pericardium.

4. Assessment
a. Pulsus paradoxus
b. Increased CVP
c. Jugular venous distention with clear lungs
d. Distant, muffled heart sounds
e. Decreased cardiac output
f. Narrowing **pulse pressure**
5. Interventions
a. The client needs to be placed in a critical care unit for hemodynamic monitoring.
b. Administer fluids intravenously as prescribed to manage decreased cardiac output.
c. Prepare the client for chest x-ray or echocardiography.
d. Prepare the client for pericardiocentesis to withdraw pericardial fluid if prescribed.
e. Monitor for recurrence of tamponade following pericardiocentesis.
f. If the client experiences recurrent tamponade or recurrent effusions or develops adhesions from chronic pericarditis, a portion (pericardial window) or all of the pericardium (pericardiectomy) may be removed to allow adequate ventricular filling and contraction.

F. Coronary artery bypass grafting
1. The occluded coronary arteries are bypassed with the client's own venous or arterial blood vessels.
2. The saphenous vein, internal mammary artery, or other arteries may be used to bypass lesions in the coronary arteries.
3. Coronary artery bypass grafting is performed when the client does not respond to medical

management of coronary artery disease or when vessels are severely occluded.

4. A minimally invasive direct coronary artery bypass (MIDCAB) may be an option for some clients who have a lesion in the LAD artery; a sternal incision is not required (usually a 2-inch [5 cm] left thoracotomy incision is done), and cardiopulmonary bypass is not required in this procedure.
5. Preoperative interventions
   - **a.** Familiarize the client and family with the cardiac surgical critical care unit.
   - **b.** Inform the client to expect a sternal incision, possible arm or leg incision(s), 1 or 2 chest tubes, a Foley catheter, and several IV fluid catheters.
   - **c.** Inform the client that an endotracheal tube will be in place for a short period of time and that she or he will be unable to speak.
   - **d.** Advise the client that she or he will be on mechanical ventilation and to breathe with the ventilator and not fight it.
   - **e.** Instruct the client that postoperative pain is expected and that pain medication will be available.
   - **f.** Instruct the client in how to splint the chest incision, cough and deep-breathe, use the incentive spirometer, and perform arm and leg exercises.
   - **g.** Encourage the client and family to discuss anxieties and fears related to surgery.
   - **h.** Note that prescribed medications may be discontinued preoperatively (usually, diuretics 2 to 3 days before surgery, digoxin 12 hours before surgery, and aspirin and anticoagulants 1 week before surgery).
   - **i.** Administer medications as prescribed, which may include potassium chloride, antihypertensives, antidysrhythmics, and antibiotics.
6. Cardiac surgical unit postoperative interventions
   - **a.** Mechanical ventilation is maintained for 6 to 24 hours as prescribed.
   - **b.** The heart rate and rhythm, pulmonary artery and arterial pressures, urinary output, and neurological status are monitored closely.
   - **c.** Mediastinal and pleural chest tubes to the water seal drainage system with prescribed suction are present; drainage exceeding 100 to 150 mL/hr is reported to the surgeon.
   - **d.** Epicardial pacing wires are covered with sterile caps or connected to a temporary pacemaker generator; all equipment in use must be properly grounded to prevent microshock.
   - **e.** Fluid and electrolyte balance is monitored closely; fluids are usually restricted to 1500 to 2000 mL because the client usually has edema.
   - **f.** The **blood pressure** is monitored closely, because hypotension can cause collapse of a vein graft; hypertension can cause increased pressure, promoting leakage from the suture line, causing bleeding.
   - **g.** Temperature is monitored, and rewarming procedures are initiated using warm or thermal blankets if the temperature drops below 96.8° F (36.0° C); rewarm the client no faster than 1.8 degrees/hr to prevent shivering, and discontinue rewarming procedures when the temperature approaches 98.6° F (37.0° C).
   - **h.** Potassium is administered intravenously as prescribed to maintain the potassium level between 4 and 5 mEq/L (4 to 5 mmol/L) to prevent dysrhythmias.
   - **i.** The client is monitored for signs of cardiac tamponade, which will include sudden cessation of previously heavy mediastinal drainage, jugular vein distention with clear lung sounds, equalization of right atrial (RA) pressure and pulmonary artery wedge pressure, and pulsus paradoxus (see Section X. I.).
   - **j.** Pain is monitored, differentiating sternotomy pain from anginal pain, which would indicate graft failure.
7. Alarm safety and alarm fatigue: Refer to Section IX, C, 14.
8. Transfer of the client from the cardiac surgical unit
   - **a.** Monitor vital signs, level of consciousness, and peripheral perfusion.
   - **b.** Monitor for dysrhythmias.
   - **c.** Auscultate lungs and assess respiratory status.
   - **d.** Encourage the client to splint the incision, cough, deep-breathe, and use the incentive spirometer to raise secretions and prevent atelectasis.
   - **e.** Monitor temperature and white blood cell count, which, if elevated after 3 to 4 days, indicate infection.
   - **f.** Provide adequate fluids and hydration as prescribed to liquefy secretions.
   - **g.** Assess suture line and chest tube insertion sites for redness, purulent discharge, and signs of infection.
   - **h.** Assess sternal suture line for instability, which may indicate infection.
   - **i.** Guide the client to gradually resume activity.
   - **j.** Assess the client for tachycardia, **postural (orthostatic) hypotension**, and fatigue before, during, and after activity.
   - **k.** Discontinue activities if the BP drops more than 10 to 20 mm Hg or if the pulse increases more than 10 beats per minute.
   - **l.** Monitor episodes of pain closely.
   - **m.** See Box 69-16 for home care instructions.

BOX 69-16 Home Care Instructions for the Client Who Has Had Cardiac Surgery

- Progressive return to activities at home
- Limiting of pushing or pulling activities for 6 weeks following discharge
- Maintenance of incisional care and reporting signs of redness, swelling, or drainage
- Sternotomy incision heals in about 6 to 8 weeks
- Avoidance of crossing legs; wearing elastic hose as prescribed until edema subsides, and elevating the surgical limb (if used to obtain the graft) when sitting in a chair
- Use of prescribed medications
- Dietary measures, including the avoidance of saturated fats and cholesterol and the use of salt
- Resumption of sexual intercourse on the advice of the health care provider after exercise tolerance is assessed (usually, if the client can walk 1 block or climb 2 flights of stairs without symptoms, she or he can resume sexual activity safely)

XI. Complex Renal and Urinary Problems

A. Urosepsis
1. Urosepsis is a gram-negative bacteremia originating in the urinary tract.
2. The most common causative organism is *Escherichia coli*.
3. In a client who is immunocompromised, a common cause is infection from an indwelling urinary catheter or an untreated urinary tract infection (UTI).
4. The major problem is the ability of this bacterium to develop resistant strains.
5. Urosepsis can lead to septic shock if not treated aggressively.
6. Assessment: Fever is the most common and earliest manifestation.
7. Interventions
   a. Obtain a urine specimen for urine culture and sensitivity before administering antibiotics.
   b. Administer antibiotics intravenously as prescribed, usually until the client has been afebrile for 3 to 5 days.
   c. Switch to oral antibiotics as prescribed after the 3- to 5-day afebrile period.

B. Continuous renal replacement therapy
1. Continuous renal replacement therapy (CRRT) provides continuous ultrafiltration of extracellular fluid and clearance of urinary toxins over a period of 8 to 24 hours; used primarily for clients in acute kidney injury (AKI) or critically ill clients with chronic kidney disease (CKD) who cannot tolerate hemodialysis.
2. Water, electrolytes, and other solutes are removed as the client's blood passes through a hemofilter.

BOX 69-17 Types of Continuous Renal Replacement Therapy

- Continuous venovenous hemofiltration (CVVH)
- Continuous arteriovenous hemofiltration (CAVH)
- Continuous venovenous hemodialysis (CVVHD)
- Continuous arteriovenous hemodialysis (CAVHD)
- Slow continuous ultrafiltration (SCUF)

3. Because rapid shifts in fluids and electrolytes typically do not occur, hemofiltration is usually better tolerated by critically ill clients.
4. There are 5 variations of CRRT (Box 69-17), some that require a hemodialysis machine and others that rely on the client's BP to power the system.
5. If CRRT does not require a hemodialysis machine, the client's mean arterial BP needs to be maintained above 60 mm Hg, and arterial and venous access sites are necessary.

XII. Complex Neurological Problems

A. Traumatic head injury
1. Head injury is trauma to the skull, resulting in mild to extensive damage to the brain.
2. Immediate complications include cerebral bleeding, hematomas, uncontrolled increased ICP, infections, and seizures.
3. Changes in personality or behavior, cranial nerve deficits, and any other residual deficits depend on the area of the brain damage and the extent of the damage.

B. Types of head injuries (Box 69-18)
1. Open
   a. Scalp lacerations
   b. Fractures in the skull
   c. Interruption of the dura mater
2. Closed
   a. Concussions
   b. Contusions
   c. Fractures

C. Hematoma
1. A collection of blood in the tissues that can occur as a result of a subarachnoid hemorrhage or an intracerebral hemorrhage.
2. Assessment
   a. Assessment findings depend on the injury.
   b. Clinical manifestations usually result from increased ICP.
   c. Changing neurological signs in the client
   d. Changes in level of consciousness
   e. Airway and breathing pattern changes
   f. Vital signs change, reflecting increased ICP (rise in blood pressure with widening pulse pressure; slowing of pulse)
   g. Headache, nausea, and vomiting

BOX 69-18 Types of Head Injuries

Concussion
- Concussion is a jarring of the brain within the skull; there may or may not be a loss of consciousness.

Contusion
- Contusion is a bruising type of injury to the brain tissue.
- Contusion may occur along with other neurological injuries, such as subdural or extradural collections of blood.

Skull Fractures
- Linear
- Depressed
- Compound
- Comminuted

Epidural Hematoma
- The most serious type of hematoma, epidural hematoma forms rapidly and results from arterial bleeding.
- The hematoma forms between the dura and the skull from a tear in the meningeal artery.
- It is often associated with temporary loss of consciousness, followed by a lucid period that then rapidly progresses to a coma.
- Epidural hematoma is a surgical emergency.

Subdural Hematoma
- Subdural hematoma forms slowly and results from a venous bleed.
- It occurs under the dura as a result of tears in the veins crossing the subdural space.

Intracerebral Hemorrhage
- Intracerebral hemorrhage occurs when a blood vessel within the brain ruptures, allowing blood to leak inside the brain.

Subarachnoid Hemorrhage
- A subarachnoid hemorrhage is bleeding into the subarachnoid space. It may occur as a result of head trauma or spontaneously, such as from a ruptured cerebral aneurysm.

h. Visual disturbances, pupillary changes, and papilledema
i. **Nuchal rigidity** (not tested until spinal cord injury is ruled out)
j. Cerebrospinal fluid (CSF) drainage from the ears or nose
k. Weakness and paralysis
l. Posturing
m. Decreased sensation or absence of feeling
n. Reflex activity changes
o. Seizure activity

CSF can be distinguished from other fluids by the presence of concentric rings (bloody fluid surrounded by yellowish stain; halo sign) when the fluid is placed on a white sterile background, such as a gauze pad. CSF also tests positive for glucose when tested using a strip test.

3. Interventions
a. Monitor respiratory status and maintain a patent airway, because increased carbon dioxide (CO_2) levels increase cerebral edema.
b. Monitor neurological status and vital signs, including temperature.
c. Monitor for increased ICP.
d. Maintain head elevation to reduce venous pressure.
e. Prevent neck flexion.
f. Initiate normothermia measures for increased temperature.
g. Assess cranial nerve function, reflexes, and motor and sensory function.
h. Initiate seizure precautions.
i. Monitor for pain and restlessness.
j. Morphine sulfate or opioid medication may be prescribed to decrease agitation and control restlessness caused by pain for the head-injured client on a ventilator; administer with caution because it is a respiratory depressant and may increase ICP.
k. Monitor for drainage from the nose or ears, because this fluid may be CSF.
l. Do not attempt to clean the nose or suction if drainage occurs; client needs to avoid blowing her or his nose.
m. Do not clean the ear if drainage is noted, but apply a loose, dry sterile dressing.
n. Check drainage for the presence of CSF.
o. Notify the PHCP if drainage from the ears or nose is noted and if the drainage tests positive for CSF.
p. Instruct the client to avoid coughing, because this increases ICP.
q. Monitor for signs of infection.
r. Prevent complications of immobility.
s. Inform the client and family about the possible behavior changes that may occur, including those that are expected and those that need to be reported.

D. Craniotomy
1. Surgical procedure that involves an incision through the cranium to remove accumulated blood or a tumor
2. Complications of the procedure include increased ICP from cerebral edema, hemorrhage, or obstruction of the normal flow of CSF.

3. Additional complications include hematomas, hypovolemic shock, hydrocephalus, respiratory and neurogenic complications, pulmonary edema, and wound infections.
4. Complications related to fluid and electrolyte imbalances include diabetes insipidus and inappropriate secretion of antidiuretic hormone.
5. Stereotactic radiosurgery (SRS) may be an alternative to traditional surgery and is usually used to treat tumors and arteriovenous malformations.
6. Preoperative interventions
   a. Explain the procedure to the client and family.
   b. Prepare to shave the client's head as prescribed (usually done in the operating room) and cover the head with an appropriate covering.
   c. Stabilize the client before surgery.
7. Postoperative interventions (Box 69-19)
8. Postoperative positioning (Box 69-20)

E. Increased ICP
1. Increased ICP may be caused by trauma, hemorrhage, growths or tumors, hydrocephalus, edema, or inflammation.
2. Increased ICP can impede circulation to the brain, impede the absorption of CSF, affect the functioning of nerve cells, and lead to brainstem compression and death.
3. Assessment
   a. Altered level of consciousness, which is the most sensitive and earliest indication of increasing ICP
   b. Headache
   c. Abnormal respirations
   d. Rise in blood pressure with widening pulse pressure
   e. Slowing of pulse

BOX 69-19 Nursing Care Following Craniotomy

- Monitor vital signs and neurological status every 30 to 60 minutes.
- Monitor for increased intracranial pressure (ICP).
- Monitor for decreased level of consciousness, motor weakness or paralysis, aphasia, visual changes, and personality changes.
- Maintain mechanical ventilation and slight hyperventilation for the first 24 to 48 hours as prescribed to prevent increased ICP.
- Assess the primary health care provider's (PHCP's) prescription regarding client positioning.
- Avoid extreme hip or neck flexion, and maintain the head in a midline neutral position.
- Provide a quiet environment.
- Monitor the head dressing frequently for signs of drainage.
- Mark any area of drainage at least once each nursing shift for baseline comparison.
- Monitor the drain, which may be in place for 24 hours; maintain suction on the drain as prescribed.
- Measure drainage from the drain every 8 hours, and record the amount and color.
- Notify the PHCP if drainage is more than the normal amount of 30 to 50 mL per shift.
- Notify the PHCP immediately of excessive amounts of drainage or a saturated head dressing.
- Record strict measurement of hourly intake and output.
- Maintain fluid restriction at 1500 mL/day as prescribed.
- Monitor electrolyte levels.
- Monitor for dysrhythmias, which may occur as a result of fluid or electrolyte imbalance.
- Apply ice packs or cool compresses as prescribed; expect periorbital edema and ecchymosis of 1 or both eyes.
- Provide range-of-motion exercises every 8 hours.
- Place antiembolism stockings on the client as prescribed.
- Administer antiseizure medications, antacids, corticosteroids, and antibiotics as prescribed.
- Administer analgesics such as codeine sulfate or acetaminophen as prescribed for pain.

BOX 69-20 Client Positioning Following Craniotomy

- Positions prescribed following a craniotomy vary with the type of surgery and the specific postoperative surgeon's prescription.
- Always check the surgeon's prescription regarding client positioning.
- Incorrect positioning may cause serious and possibly fatal complications.

Removal of a Bone Flap for Decompression

- To facilitate brain expansion, the client should be turned from the back to the nonoperative side, but not to the side on which the operation was performed.

Posterior Fossa Surgery

- To protect the operative site from pressure and minimize tension on the suture line, position the client on the side, with a pillow under the head for support, and not on the back.

Infratentorial Surgery

- Infratentorial surgery involves surgery below the tentorium of the brain.
- The surgeon may prescribe a flat position without head elevation or may prescribe that the head of the bed be elevated at 30 to 45 degrees.
- Do not elevate the head of the bed in the acute phase of care following surgery without a surgeon's prescription.

Supratentorial Surgery

- Supratentorial surgery involves surgery above the tentorium of the brain.
- The surgeon may prescribe that the head of the bed be elevated at 30 degrees to promote venous outflow through the jugular veins.
- Do not lower the head of the bed in the acute phase of care following surgery without a surgeon's prescription.

f. Elevated temperature
g. Vomiting
h. Pupil changes

4. Late signs of increased ICP include increased systolic blood pressure, widened pulse pressure, and slowed heart rate.
5. Other late signs include changes in motor function from weakness to hemiplegia, a positive **Babinski reflex**, decorticate or decerebrate posturing, and seizures.
6. Interventions
   a. Monitor respiratory status and prevent hypoxia.
   b. Avoid the administration of morphine sulfate and other opioids that depress respirations to prevent the occurrence of hypoxia.
   c. Maintain mechanical ventilation as prescribed; maintaining the $PaCO_2$ at 30 to 35 mm Hg (30 to 35 mm Hg) will result in vasoconstriction of the cerebral blood vessels, decreased blood flow, and therefore decreased ICP.
   d. Maintain body temperature.
   e. Prevent shivering, which can increase ICP.
   f. Decrease environmental stimuli.
   g. Monitor electrolyte levels and acid–base balance.
   h. Monitor intake and output.
   i. Limit fluid intake to 1200 mL/day as prescribed.
   j. Instruct the client to avoid straining activities, such as coughing and sneezing.
   k. Instruct the client to avoid Valsalva's maneuver.

⚠ For the client with increased ICP, elevate the head of the bed 30 to 40 degrees, avoid the Trendelenburg's position, and prevent flexion of the neck and hips.

7. Medications (Box 69-21)
8. Surgical intervention: Also see Chapter 38 for additional information on ventriculoperitoneal shunts (Box 69-22)

F. Spinal cord injury
1. Trauma to the spinal cord causes partial or complete disruption of the nerve tracts and neurons.
2. The injury can involve contusion, laceration, or compression of the cord.
3. Spinal cord edema develops; necrosis of the spinal cord can develop as a result of compromised capillary circulation and venous return.
4. Loss of motor function, sensation, reflex activity, and bowel and bladder control may result.
5. The most common causes include motor vehicle crashes, falls, sporting and industrial accidents, and gunshot or stab wounds.
6. Complications related to the injury include respiratory failure, **autonomic dysreflexia**, spinal shock, further cord damage, and death.

BOX 69-21 Medications for Increased Intracranial Pressure

Antiseizure
- Seizures increase metabolic requirements and cerebral blood flow and volume, thus increasing intracranial pressure (ICP).
- Medications may be given prophylactically to prevent seizures.

Antipyretics and Muscle Relaxants
- Temperature reduction decreases metabolism, cerebral blood flow, and thus ICP.
- Antipyretics prevent temperature elevations.
- Muscle relaxants prevent shivering.

Blood Pressure Medication
- Blood pressure medication may be required to maintain cerebral perfusion at a normal level.
- Notify the primary health care provider if the blood pressure range is lower than 100 or higher than 150 mm Hg systolic.

Corticosteroids
- Corticosteroids stabilize the cell membrane and reduce leakiness of the blood–brain barrier.
- Corticosteroids decrease cerebral edema.
- A histamine blocker may be administered to counteract the excess gastric secretion that occurs with the corticosteroid.
- Clients must be withdrawn slowly from corticosteroid therapy to reduce the risk of adrenal crisis.

Intravenous Fluids
- Fluids are administered intravenously; an infusion pump is always used to control the amount administered.
- Infusions are monitored closely because of the risk of promoting additional cerebral edema and fluid overload.

Hyperosmotic Agent
- A hyperosmotic agent increases intravascular pressure by drawing fluid from the interstitial spaces and from the brain cells.
- Monitor renal function.
- Diuresis is expected.

BOX 69-22 Surgical Intervention for Chronic Increased Intracranial Pressure: Ventriculoperitoneal Shunt

Description
- A ventriculoperitoneal shunt diverts cerebrospinal fluid from the ventricles into the peritoneum.

Postprocedure Interventions
- Position the client supine and turn from the back to the nonoperative side.
- Monitor for signs of increasing intracranial pressure resulting from shunt failure.
- Monitor for signs of infection.

7. Most frequently involved vertebrae
   a. Cervical—C5, C6, and C7
   b. Thoracic—T12
   c. Lumbar—L1

G. Transection of the cord
1. Complete transection of the cord: The spinal cord is severed completely, with total loss of sensation, movement, and reflex activity below the level of injury.
2. Partial transection of the cord
   a. The spinal cord is damaged or severed partially.
   b. The symptoms depend on the extent and location of the damage.
   c. If the cord has not suffered irreparable damage, early treatment is needed to prevent partial damage from developing into total and permanent damage.

H. Spinal cord syndromes in partial transection or injury (Fig. 69-29)
1. Central cord syndrome
   a. Occurs from damage in the central portion of the spinal cord
   b. Loss of motor function is more pronounced in the upper extremities, and varying degrees and patterns of sensation remain intact.
2. Anterior cord syndrome
   a. Caused by damage to the anterior portion of the gray and white matter of the spinal cord
   b. Motor function, pain, and temperature sensation are lost below the level of injury; however, the sensations of position, vibration, and touch remain intact.
3. Posterior cord syndrome
   a. Caused by damage to the posterior portion of the gray and white matter of the spinal cord
   b. Motor function remains intact, but the client experiences a loss of vibratory sense, crude touch, and position sensation.
4. Brown-Séquard syndrome
   a. Results from penetrating injuries that cause hemisection of the spinal cord or injuries that affect half of the cord
   b. Motor function, vibration, proprioception, and deep touch sensations are lost on the

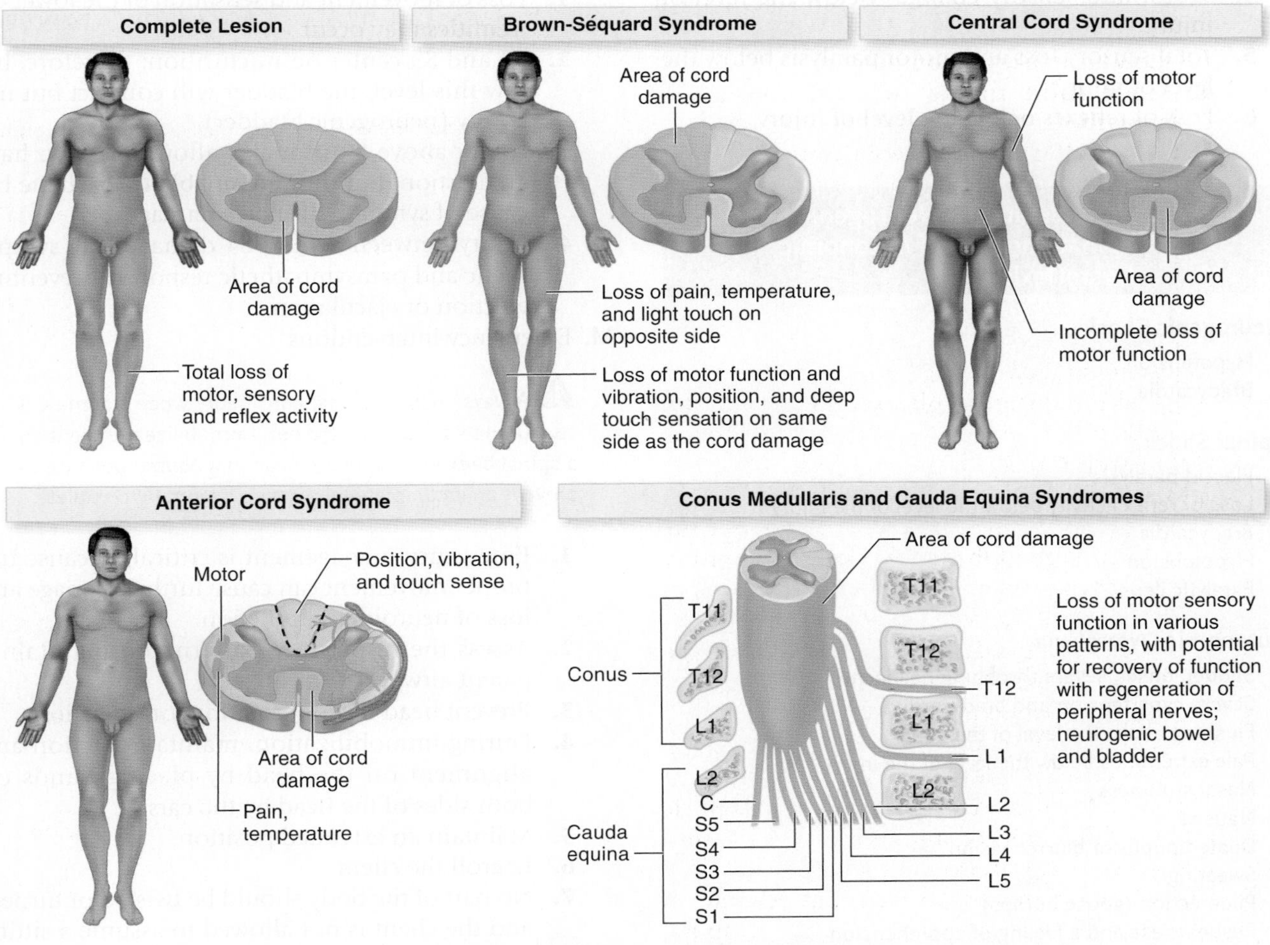

FIG. 69-29 Common spinal cord syndromes.

same side of the body (ipsilateral) as the lesion or cord damage.

c. On the opposite side of the body (contralateral) from the lesion or cord damage, the sensations of pain, temperature, and light touch are affected.

5. Conus medullaris syndrome
   a. Follows damage to the lumbar nerve roots and conus medullaris in the spinal cord
   b. The client experiences bowel and bladder areflexia and flaccid lower extremities.
   c. If damage is limited to the upper sacral segments of the spinal cord, bulbospongiosus penile (erection) and micturition reflexes will remain.
6. Cauda equina syndrome
   a. Occurs from injury to the lumbosacral nerve roots below the conus medullaris
   b. The client experiences areflexia of the bowel, bladder, and lower reflexes.

I. Assessment of spinal cord injuries (Box 69-23)
1. Dependent on the level of the cord injury
2. Level of spinal cord injury: Lowest spinal cord segment with intact motor and sensory function
3. Respiratory status changes
4. Motor and sensory changes below the level of injury
5. Total sensory loss and motor paralysis below the level of injury
6. Loss of reflexes below the level of injury

BOX 69-23 Manifestations: Neurogenic Shock, Spinal Shock, and Autonomic Dysreflexia

Neurogenic Shock
- Hypotension
- Bradycardia

Spinal Shock
- Flaccid paralysis
- Loss of reflex activity below the level of the injury
- Bradycardia
- Hypotension
- Paralytic ileus

Autonomic Dysreflexia
- Sudden onset, severe throbbing headache
- Severe hypertension and bradycardia
- Flushing above the level of the injury
- Pale extremities below the level of the injury
- Nasal stuffiness
- Nausea
- Dilated pupils or blurred vision
- Sweating
- Piloerection (goose bumps)
- Restlessness and a feeling of apprehension

7. Loss of bladder and bowel control
8. Urinary retention and bladder distention
9. Presence of sweat, which does not occur on paralyzed areas

J. Cervical injuries
1. Injury at C2 to C3 is usually fatal.
2. C4 is the major innervation to the diaphragm by the phrenic nerve.
3. Involvement above C4 causes respiratory difficulty and paralysis of all four extremities.
4. The client may have movement in the shoulder if the injury is at C5 through C8 and may also have decreased respiratory reserve.

K. Thoracic level injuries
1. Loss of movement of the chest, trunk, bowel, bladder, and legs may occur, depending on the level of injury.
2. Leg paralysis (paraplegia) may occur.
3. Autonomic dysreflexia with injuries above T6 and in cervical lesions may occur.
4. Visceral distention from noxious stimuli such as a distended bladder or an impacted rectum may cause reactions such as sweating, bradycardia, hypertension, nasal stuffiness, and goose flesh.

L. Lumbar and sacral level injuries
1. Loss of movement and sensation of the lower extremities may occur.
2. S2 and S3 center on micturition; therefore, below this level, the bladder will contract but not empty (neurogenic bladder).
3. Injury above S2 in males allows them to have an erection, but they are unable to ejaculate because of sympathetic nerve damage.
4. Injury between S2 and S4 damages the sympathetic and parasympathetic response, preventing erection or ejaculation.

M. Emergency interventions

Always suspect spinal cord injury when trauma occurs until this injury is ruled out. Immobilize the client on a spinal backboard with the head in a neutral position to prevent an incomplete injury from becoming complete.

1. Emergency management is critical, because improper movement can cause further damage and loss of neurological function.
2. Assess the respiratory pattern and maintain a patent airway.
3. Prevent head flexion, rotation, or extension.
4. During immobilization, maintain traction and alignment on the head by placing hands on both sides of the head by the ears.
5. Maintain an extended position.
6. Logroll the client.
7. No part of the body should be twisted or turned, and the client is not allowed to assume a sitting position.

8. In the emergency department, a client who has sustained a cervical fracture should be placed immediately in skeletal traction via skull tongs or halo traction to immobilize the cervical spine and reduce the fracture and dislocation.

N. Interventions during hospitalization
1. Respiratory system
   a. Assess respiratory status, because paralysis of the intercostal and abdominal muscles occurs with C4 injuries.
   b. Monitor arterial blood gas levels and maintain mechanical ventilation if prescribed to prevent respiratory arrest, especially with cervical injuries.
   c. Encourage deep breathing and the use of an incentive spirometer.
   d. Monitor for signs of infection, particularly pneumonia.
2. Cardiovascular system
   a. Monitor for cardiac dysrhythmias.
   b. Assess for signs of hemorrhage or bleeding around the fracture site.
   c. Assess for signs of shock, such as hypotension, tachycardia, and a weak and thready pulse.
   d. Assess the lower extremities for deep vein thrombosis.
   e. Measure circumferences of the calf and thigh to identify increases in size.
   f. Apply antiembolism stockings as prescribed; remove daily to assess skin integrity.
   g. Monitor for orthostatic hypotension when repositioning the client.
3. Neuromuscular system
   a. Assess neurological status.
   b. Assess motor and sensory status to determine the level of injury.
   c. Assess motor ability by testing the client's ability to squeeze hands, spread the fingers, move the toes, and turn the feet.
   d. Assess absence of sensation, hyposensation, or hypersensation by pinching the skin or pricking it with a pin, starting at the shoulders and working down the extremities.
   e. Monitor for signs of autonomic dysreflexia and spinal shock.
   f. Immobilize the client to promote healing and prevent further injury.
   g. Assess pain.
   h. Initiate measures to reduce pain.
   i. Administer analgesics as prescribed.
   j. Monitor for complications of immobility.
   k. Prepare the client for decompression laminectomy, spinal fusion, or insertion of instrumentation or rods if prescribed.
   l. Collaborate with the physical therapist and occupational therapist to determine appropriate exercise techniques, assess the need for hand and wrist splints, and develop an appropriate plan to prevent footdrop.
4. Gastrointestinal system
   a. Assess abdomen for distention and hemorrhage.
   b. Monitor bowel sounds and assess for paralytic ileus.
   c. Prevent bowel retention.
   d. Initiate a bowel control program as appropriate.
   e. Maintain adequate nutrition and a high-fiber diet.
5. Renal system
   a. Prevent urinary retention.
   b. Initiate a bladder control program as appropriate.
   c. Maintain fluid and electrolyte balance.
   d. Maintain adequate fluid intake of 2000 mL/day unless contraindicated.
   e. Monitor for urinary tract infection and calculi.
6. Integumentary system
   a. Assess skin integrity.
   b. Ensure linens under the client are wrinkle-free.
   c. Turn the client every 2 hours.
7. Psychosocial integrity
   a. Assess psychosocial status.
   b. Encourage the client to express feelings of anger, depression, and loss.
   c. Discuss the sexual concerns of the client.
   d. Promote rehabilitation with self-care measures, setting realistic goals based on the client's potential functional level.
   e. Encourage contact with appropriate community resources.

O. Spinal and neurogenic shock
1. **Spinal shock**: A complete but temporary loss of motor, sensory, reflex, and autonomic function that occurs immediately after injury as the cord's response to the injury. It usually lasts less than 48 hours but can continue for several weeks.
2. **Neurogenic shock**: Occurs most commonly in clients with injuries above T6 and usually is experienced soon after the injury. Massive vasodilation occurs, leading to pooling of the blood in blood vessels, tissue hypoperfusion, and impaired cellular metabolism.
3. Assessment (see Box 69-23)
4. Interventions
   a. Monitor for signs of shock following a spinal cord injury.
   b. Monitor for hypotension and bradycardia.
   c. Monitor for reflex activity.
   d. Assess bowel sounds.
   e. Monitor for bowel and urinary retention.
   f. Provide supportive measures as prescribed, based on the presence of symptoms.
   g. Monitor for the return of reflexes.

P. **Autonomic dysreflexia**
1. Also known as autonomic hyper-reflexia
2. It generally occurs after the period of spinal shock is resolved and occurs with lesions or injuries above T6 and in cervical lesions or injuries.
3. It is commonly caused by visceral distention from a distended bladder or impacted rectum.
4. It is a neurological emergency and must be treated immediately to prevent a hypertensive stroke.
5. Assessment (see Box 69-23)
6. Interventions (see Priority Nursing Actions)

PRIORITY NURSING ACTIONS

Anaphylactic Reaction

1. Quickly assess respiratory status and maintain a patent airway.
2. Call the primary health care provider (PHCP) and Rapid Response Team.
3. Administer oxygen.
4. Start an intravenous (IV) line and infuse normal saline.
5. Prepare to administer diphenhydramine and epinephrine, and possibly corticosteroids.
6. Document the event, actions taken, and the client's response.

Reference

Ignatavicius, Workman, Rebar (2018), p. 365.

Q. Cervical spine traction for cervical injuries
1. Skeletal traction is used to stabilize fractures or dislocations of the cervical or upper thoracic spine.
2. Two types of equipment used for cervical traction are skull (cervical) tongs and halo traction (halo fixation device).
3. Skull tongs
   a. Skull tongs are inserted into the outer aspect of the client's skull, and traction is applied.
   b. Weights are attached to the tongs, and the client is used as countertraction. The nurse should not add or remove weights.
   c. Determine the amount of weight prescribed to be added to the traction.
   d. Ensure that weights hang securely and freely at all times.
   e. Ensure that the ropes for the traction remain within the pulley.
   f. Maintain body alignment and maintain care of the client on a special bed (such as a RotoRest bed or Stryker or Foster frame) as prescribed.
   g. Turn the client every 2 hours.
   h. Assess the insertion site of the tongs for infection.
   i. Provide sterile pin site care as prescribed.
4. Halo traction
   a. Halo traction is a static traction device that consists of a headpiece with 4 pins, 2 anterior and 2 posterior, inserted into the client's skull.
   b. The metal halo ring may be attached to a vest (jacket) or cast when the spine is stable, allowing increased client mobility.
   c. Monitor the client's neurological status for changes in movement or decreased strength.
   d. Never move or turn the client by holding or pulling on the halo traction device.
   e. Assess for tightness of the jacket by ensuring that 1 finger can be placed under the jacket.
   f. Assess skin integrity to ensure that the jacket or cast is not causing pressure.
   g. Provide sterile pin site care as prescribed.
5. Client education for halo traction device (Box 69-24)
   a. Initiate interventions in support of the client's self-image.
   b. Teach the client and family pin care, care of the vest, and signs and symptoms of infection to report to her or his PHCP.

R. Interventions for thoracic, lumbar, and sacral injuries
1. Bed rest
2. Immobilization with a body cast if prescribed

BOX 69-24 Client Education for a Halo Fixation Device

- Notify the primary health care provider (PHCP) if the halo vest (jacket) or ring bolts loosen.
- Use fleece or foam inserts to relieve pressure points.
- Keep the vest lining dry.
- Clean the pin site daily.
- Notify the PHCP if redness, swelling, drainage, open areas, pain, tenderness, or a clicking sound occurs from the pin site.
- A sponge bath or tub bath is allowed; showers are not allowed.
- Assess the skin under the vest daily for breakdown, using a flashlight.
- Do not use any products other than shampoo on the hair.
- When shampooing the hair, cover the vest with plastic.
- When getting out of bed, roll onto the side and push on the mattress with the arms.
- Never use the metal frame for turning or lifting.
- Use a rolled towel or pillowcase between the back of the neck and bed or next to the cheek when lying on the side, and raise the head of the bed to increase sleep comfort.
- Adapt clothing to fit over the halo device.
- Eat foods high in protein and calcium to promote bone healing.
- Have the correct-sized wrench available at all times for an emergency (tape the wrench to the vest).
- If cardiopulmonary resuscitation is required, the anterior portion of the vest will be loosened and the posterior portion will remain in place to provide stability.

3. Assess for respiratory impairment and paralytic ileus, possible complications of the body cast.
4. Use of a brace or corset when the client is out of bed

S. Surgical interventions for thoracic, lumbar, and sacral injuries
1. Decompressive laminectomy
a. Removal of 1 or more laminae
b. Allows for cord expansion from edema; performed if conventional methods fail to prevent neurological deterioration
2. Spinal fusion
a. Spinal fusion is used for thoracic spinal injuries.
b. Bone is grafted between the vertebrae for support and to strengthen the back.
3. Postoperative interventions
a. Monitor for respiratory impairment.
b. Monitor vital signs, motor function, sensation, and circulatory status in the lower extremities.
c. Encourage breathing exercises.
d. Assess for signs of fluid and electrolyte imbalances.
e. Observe for complications of immobility.
f. Keep the client in a flat position as prescribed.
g. Provide cast care if the client is in a full body cast.
h. Turn and reposition frequently by logrolling side to back to side, using turning sheets and pillows between the legs to maintain alignment.
i. Administer pain medication as prescribed.
j. Maintain on NPO status until the client is passing flatus.
k. Monitor bowel sounds.
l. Provide the use of a fracture bedpan.
m. Monitor intake and output.
n. Maintain nutritional status.

T. Medications
1. Dexamethasone: Used for its antiinflammatory and edema-reducing effects; may interfere with healing because it suppresses the immune system
2. Dextran: Plasma expander used to increase capillary blood flow within the spinal cord and to prevent or treat hypotension
3. Baclofen: Used for clients with upper motor neuron injuries to control muscle spasticity

U. Management of sedation, agitation, and delirium
1. The Society of Critical Care Medicine (SCCM) developed guidelines for managing sedation, agitation, and delirium in critically ill clients.
a. These guidelines recommend using a standardized tool such as the Richmond Agitation-Sedation Scale (RASS) (Box 69-25) to titrate sedation medications, because not all individuals metabolize these medications at the same rate (Box 69-26).
b. Ruling out pain as a cause of agitation is an important consideration in deciding how to titrate sedation medications.
2. Sedation
a. Sedation is classified as light, moderate, deep, and general anesthesia (see Box 69-26).
b. Pharmacological sedation includes use of benzodiazepines (diazepam, lorazepam, midazolam), sedative-hypnotics (propofol),

BOX 69-25 Richmond Agitation-Sedation Scale (RASS)

−5	Unresponsive	Minimal or no response to stimuli, does not follow commands
−4	Deep sedation	No response to voice, movement or eye opening to physical stimuli
−3	Moderate sedation	Movement or eye opening to voice without eye contact
−2	Light sedation	Briefly awakens to eye contact to voice for less than 10 seconds
−1	Drowsy	Not fully alert, but with sustained awakening with eye opening and contact to voice for more than 10 seconds
0		Alert and calm
+1	Restless	Anxious without aggressive movements
+2	Agitated	Frequent movements that are nonpurposeful
+3	Very agitated	Pulls out or removes tubes, aggressive
+4	Combative	Overtly combative and violent, danger to staff

Adapted from Urden, Stacy, & Lough, (2018), p. 137.

BOX 69-26 Levels of Sedation

- Light sedation: Relieving anxiety with pharmacological measures so that the client can still respond to verbal commands (Richmond Agitation-Sedation Scale).
- Moderate sedation: Depression of the client's consciousness with pharmacological measures; known as procedural sedation.
- Deep sedation: Depression of the client's consciousness with pharmacological measures to the point that the client cannot maintain a patent airway.
- General anesthesia: Depression of the client's consciousness using multiple medications administered by an anesthesiologist or nurse anesthetist.

Adapted from Urden, Stacy, & Lough, (2018), p. 137.

and centrally acting alpha-adrenergic agonists (dexmedetomidine).

3. Propofol
   a. Propofol is contained in glass and is a white milky substance. It is a lipid emulsion substance with a short half-life that can be easily titrated because it is rapidly eliminated from the body, within 30 minutes.
   b. Opiates should be added for pain control and amnesic effects, because propofol does not produce amnesia.
   c. Propofol-related infusion syndrome causing metabolic acidosis, muscular weakness, rhabdomyolysis, myoglobinuria, acute kidney injury, and cardiac dysrhythmias has been known to occur.
   d. Propofol is conducive to bacterial growth; therefore, infusion sets should be changed every 6 to 12 hours.
4. Dexmedetomidine
   a. Dexmedetomidine is used as a short-term sedative (24 hours or less) in mechanically ventilated clients.
   b. This medication causes sedation and analgesic effects and allows for clients to be minimally interactive while sedated. It can still be used even after extubation to help with anxiety related to weaning.
   c. It is eliminated from the body within 2 hours, or dramatically longer in the case of liver failure.
5. Agitation
   a. A hyperactive state that results in movements ranging from slight restlessness to pulling out lines or tubes or physical aggression.
   b. Common causes include pain, anxiety, delirium, hypoxia, ventilator dyssychrony, neurological injury, uncomfortable position, full bladder, sleep deprivation, alcohol withdrawal, sepsis, medication reaction, and organ failure.
   c. Assessed using RASS, and the goal is to treat the cause rather than overmedicate.
   d. Haloperidol rather than benzodiazepines should be used to manage acute agitation; benzodiazepines can cause delirium.
   e. If the client is at risk for harming themselves or others, a benzodiazepine may be prescribed.
6. Delirium
   a. Global impairment of cognitive processes with a sudden onset, associated with disorientation, impaired short-term memory, hallucinations or other altered sensory patterns, abnormal thought processes, and inappropriate behavior.
   b. Common causes include acute brain dysfunction, sepsis, critical illness, or overall dysfunction of vital organs.
   c. Differentiating between agitation and delirium can be difficult but is important in targeting the cause and implementing an appropriate treatment approach.
   d. Standardized assessment tools are available that can be used in tandem with RASS; one tool is the Confusion Assessment Method for the Intensive Care Unit (CAM-ICU).
   e. Haloperidol or atypical antipsychotics can be used for hyperactive delirium.
   f. Preventive measures for delirium include spontaneous awakening for sedated clients, daily delirium monitoring using a standardized tool, mobility, and initiation of sleep protocols where nursing care is clustered to provide uninterrupted rest periods.

XIII. Complex Immune Problems

A. Anaphylaxis
   1. A serious and immediate hypersensitivity reaction that releases histamine from the damaged cells
   2. Anaphylaxis can be systemic or cutaneous (localized).
   3. Assessment (Fig. 69-30)
   4. Interventions (see Priority Nursing Actions)

PRIORITY NURSING ACTIONS

Autonomic Dysreflexia in a Spinal Cord Injury Client

1. Raise the head of the bed and ask that the primary health care provider (PHCP) be notified.
2. Loosen tight clothing on the client.
3. Check for bladder distention or other noxious stimulus.
4. Administer an antihypertensive medication.
5. Document the occurrence, treatment, and response.

Reference
Ignatavicius, Workman, Rebar (2018), p. 898.

XIV. Shock and Sepsis

A. Shock
   1. Four main types of shock: hypovolemic, cardiogenic, vasogenic (distributive), obstructive
      a. Hypovolemic shock: The most common type, defined as a shock state caused by internal or external blood or fluid loss
      b. Cardiogenic shock: Caused by heart (pump) failure resulting in diminished cardiac output
      c. Vasogenic shock: With this type, the vasculature is dilated, making it difficult for the heart to move blood and fluid to the rest of the body; types include septic shock, anaphylactic shock, and neurogenic shock.
      d. Obstructive shock: A type of shock that is caused by a physical obstruction that reduces the filling

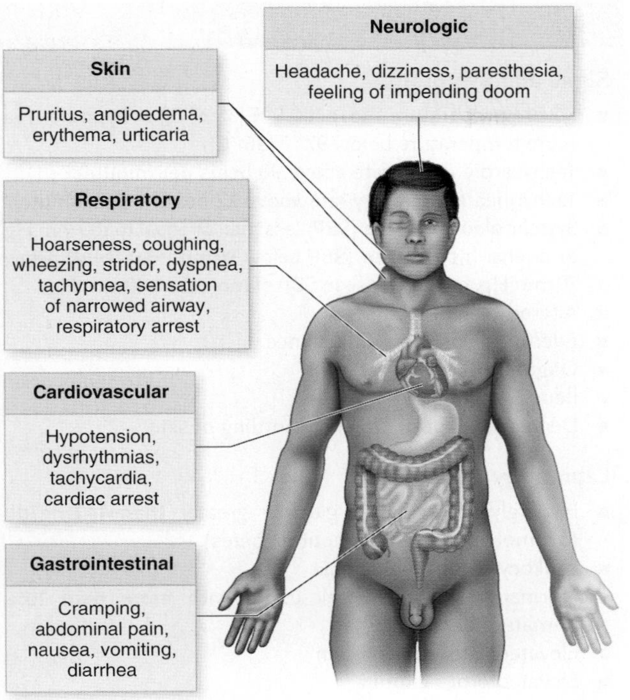

FIG. 69-30 Clinical manifestations of a systemic anaphylactic reaction.

or outflow of blood from the heart that results in a reduced cardiac output. Conditions that can contribute to this type of shock include cardiac tamponade, tension pneumothorax, superior vena cava syndrome, abdominal compartment syndrome, and pulmonary embolism.

2. Causes of vasodilation
   a. Septic shock: Massive infection leads to sepsis as a result of the release of endotoxins from bacteria; this causes vasodilation and pooling of blood.
   b. Anaphylactic shock: An allergic reaction to substances like drugs, food, and insect bites leads to anaphylactic shock, which results in an acute and life-threatening hypersensitivity reaction. This immediate reaction causes massive vasodilation, release of vasoactive mediators, and an increase in capillary permeability.
   c. Neurogenic shock: A phenomenon that occurs after spinal cord injury. The injury results in massive vasodilation without compensation as a consequence of the loss of spinal nervous system vasoconstrictor tone; this leads to a pooling of blood in the blood vessels.
3. Hemodynamic monitoring is important for assessing a client in any type of shock state and includes:
   a. Cardiac output: Reflects blood flow reaching the tissue. Normal cardiac output is 4 to 6 liters per minute.
   b. Mean arterial pressure: Amount of pressure the blood is placing on the walls of the vessels as the blood leaves the heart. Normal mean arterial pressure is between 70 mm Hg and 105 mm Hg. This measure is an important indicator of adequacy of cardiac output. Mean arterial pressure greater than 60 mm Hg is needed to maintain perfusion to vital organs.
   c. Central venous pressure: A measure of pressure in terms of right ventricular preload; measures the pressure of the blood returning from the body to the heart. The normal central venous pressure is 3 to 8 mm Hg. An elevated central venous pressure indicates right ventricular failure and volume overload. A low central venous pressure indicates hypovolemia.
   d. Cerebral perfusion pressure: A measure of perfusion to the brain, calculated by subtracting the ICP from the mean arterial pressure. The normal cerebral perfusion pressure is 70 to 100 mm Hg. A central perfusion pressure less than 50 mm Hg is associated with ischemia and tissue death. A central perfusion pressure less than 30 mm Hg is incompatible with life.
4. Stages of shock
   a. Stage 1 Initial: restlessness, increased heart rate, cool and pale skin, agitation
   b. Stage 2 Compensatory: cardiac output is less than 4 to 6 liters per minute, systolic blood pressure is less than 100 mm Hg, there is decreased urinary output, confusion, and the cerebral perfusion pressure is less than 70 mm Hg.
   c. Stage 3 Progressive: edema, excessively low blood pressure, dysrhythmias, weak and thready pulses
   d. Stage 4: This stage is unresponsive to vasopressors, there is profound hypotension, the heart rate slows, and multiple organ failure ensues. Most often, the client will not survive.

It is a priority to intervene in the early stages of shock to prevent progression to the later stages.

5. Treatments for shock
   a. Treatment depends on the cause of the shock and the type of shock.
   b. For clients in shock, central venous and pulmonary artery catheters are inserted to monitor hemodynamic status.
   c. Assessment of the central venous pressure, urine output, heart rate, and clinical and mental status is done every 5 to 15 minutes.
   d. Oxygen is administered to assist in tissue perfusion.

e. Isotonic and electrolyte intravenous solutions such as lactated Ringer's solution and normal saline are frequently used.
f. Rapid infusion of volume-expanding fluids including whole blood, plasma, and plasma substitutes such as colloid fluids
g. Whole blood is effective but is not used often as a treatment measure because of the risk of transfusion reactions.
h. Administration of medications is withheld until circulating volume has been restored.
i. The primary goal for medication therapy with shock is to improve tissue perfusion.
j. Medications used to improve perfusion in shock are administered intravenously via an infusion pump and often via a central line.
k. It is important to note that if the shock state is cardiogenic in nature, the infusion of volume-expanding fluids may result in pulmonary edema; therefore, restoration of cardiac function is the priority for this type of shock. Cardiotonic medications such as digoxin, dopamine, or norepinephrine may be administered to increase cardiac contractility and induce vasoconstriction.
l. Once improvement of perfusion is achieved, interventions are then directed toward the underlying cause of the condition.

B. Sepsis
1. A group of symptoms or syndrome in response to an infection that can include organ dysfunction related to the infection.
2. The main causative organisms are gram-negative and gram-positive bacteria; however, sepsis can also result from viral, fungal, and parasitic infections.
3. Sepsis diagnostic criteria (Box 69-27)

C. Septic shock
1. Signs and symptoms include persistent hypotension despite adequate fluid resuscitation requiring vasopressors, along with decreased tissue perfusion that progresses to tissue hypoxia.
2. In both sepsis and septic shock, the body's immune response to an invading microorganism is exaggerated, resulting in the activation of proinflammatory and antiinflammatory responses and coagulation abnormalities.
a. Increased coagulation and decreased fibrinolysis results in platelet and neutrophil aggregation with adherence to endothelium, and endothelial damage related to the formation of microthrombi in the microvasculature.
b. Endotoxins released from the invading organism's cell wall result in release of the body's cytokines (such as tumor necrosis factor [TNF] and interleukin-1 [IL-1]), which cause vasodilation and increased capillary permeability, which contributes to hypotension.

BOX 69-27 Sepsis Diagnostic Criteria

Signs and Symptoms
- Fever (temperature above 100.9° F [38.3° C]) or hypothermia (core temperature below 97° F [36° C])
- Tachycardia (heart rate above 90 beats per minute)
- Tachypnea (respiratory rate above 22 breaths per minute)
- Systolic blood pressure (SBP) less than or equal to 100 mm Hg or arterial hypotension (SBP below 90 mm Hg), MAP below 70 mm Hg, or a decrease in SBP of more than 40 mm Hg
- Altered mental status
- Edema or positive fluid balance
- Oliguria
- Ileus (absent bowel sounds)
- Decreased capillary refill or mottling of skin

Laboratory Values
- Hyperglycemia (blood glucose greater than 140 mg/dL (8 mmol/L) in client without diabetes)
- Leukocytosis or leukopenia
- Normal white blood cell count with more than 10% immature bands
- Elevated C-reactive protein
- Elevated procalcitonin
- Serum creatinine increase
- Coagulation abnormalities (INR above 1.5 [1.5] or PTT above 60 seconds [for more than 60 seconds])
- Thrombocytopenia (platelets below 100,000/mm^3 (100 × 10^9/L))
- Hyperbilirubinemia (total bilirubin above 4 mg/dL [68 mcmol/L])
- Hyperlactatemia (above 1 mmol/L)

Adapted from Lewis et al. (2017), p. 1592.

3. Three major effects septic shock has on the body include vasodilation, maldistribution of blood flow, and myocardial depression.
a. Vasodilation causes relative hypovolemia and hypotension in euvolemic clients.
b. Decreased microcirculation causes tissue hypoxia.
c. Perfusion is further impaired by a decrease in ejection fraction, in which the ventricles dilate to compensate.
d. Clients who develop septic shock are at risk for the development of respiratory failure and acute respiratory distress syndrome.
4. Nursing interventions
a. Fluid replacement: 30 to 50 mL/kg fluid resuscitation with isotonic crystalloids; albumin may also be administered.
b. Vasopressor therapy to increase cardiac output
c. Intravenous corticosteroids may be administered in clients with inadequate blood pressure readings despite fluid resuscitation and vasopressor therapy.
d. IV antibiotics should be started within the first hour of sepsis or septic shock; cultures

should be obtained before the initiation of antibiotic therapy.

e. Glucose levels should be maintained below 180 mg/dL (10.02 mmol/L).

f. Administer stress ulcer prophylaxis and venous thromboembolism prophylaxis.

g. Monitor level of consciousness, cardiovascular status, pulse oximetry, rate and depth of respirations, urine output, bowel sounds, gastric secretions and stools for occult blood, and temperature and skin changes, because the client is at risk for skin breakdown due to decreased tissue perfusion.

D. Systemic Inflammatory Response Syndrome (SIRS)

1. Defined as a systemic inflammatory response that is characterized by generalized inflammation in organs separate from the initial affected area; it is a serious condition and may be caused by a severe bacterial infection (sepsis), trauma, or pancreatitis.

2. SIRS can also be triggered by a variety of different mechanisms: mechanical tissue trauma (burns, crush injuries, surgical procedures); abscess formation; ischemic or necrotic tissue; microbial invasion; endotoxin release from invading micro-organisms; global perfusion deficits including postcardiac resuscitation or states of shock; and regional perfusion deficits.

E. Multiple Organ Dysfunction Syndrome (MODS)

1. A complication of sepsis; the failure of two or more organ systems as a result of SIRS, in which homeostasis cannot be maintained without intervention.

2. Prognosis is poor once three or more organ systems fail.

3. Clinical manifestations and management of SIRS and MODS (Table 69-12).

4. Nursing interventions for SIRS and MODS include early identification of sepsis; preventing and treating infections; maintenance of tissue oxygenation; promoting nutrition to meet metabolic needs; and support of failing organ systems.

TABLE 69-12 Clinical Manifestations and Interventions of SIRS and MODS

Manifestations	Interventions
Respiratory System	
▪ Development of acute respiratory distress syndrome (ARDS)	▪ Maximize oxygen delivery and decrease oxygen consumption ▪ Mechanical ventilation
Cardiovascular System	
▪ Myocardial depression ▪ Systemic vasodilation ▪ Systolic/diastolic dysfunction ▪ Biventricular failure ▪ Decreased systemic vascular resistance, BP, and MAP ▪ Increased cardiac output (CO) related to increased HR and stroke volume (SV)	▪ Central venous or PA catheter or minimally invasive hemodynamic monitoring/arterial pressure monitoring ▪ Volume replacement to increase preload ▪ Maintain MAP >65 mm Hg ▪ Vasopressors ▪ $S_{CV}O_2$ or S_VO_2 monitoring ▪ Balance O_2 supply and demand ▪ ECG monitoring ▪ Circulatory assist devices ▪ Venous thromboembolism prophylaxis
Central Nervous System	
▪ Acute change in mentation ▪ Fever ▪ Hepatic encephalopathy ▪ Seizures ▪ Confusion, delirium, disorientation	▪ Optimize cerebral blood flow and decrease O_2 requirements ▪ Administration of calcium channel blockers to prevent cerebral vasospasm
Endocrine System	
▪ Hyperglycemia and hypoglycemia	▪ Continuous infusion of insulin and glucose to maintain blood glucose levels of 140-180 mg/dL (7.8 -10.02 mmol/L)
Renal System	
▪ Prerenal/renal hypoperfusion ▪ Intrarenal: Acute tubular necrosis	▪ Prerenal: Administration of loop diuretics ▪ Intrarenal: Continuous renal replacement therapy
Gastrointestinal System	
▪ Mucosal ischemia, which can cause decreased pH, translocation of gut bacteria, and abdominal compartment syndrome ▪ Hypoperfusion, which can cause decreased peristalsis, paralytic ileus ▪ Mucosal ulceration ▪ GI bleeding	▪ Stress ulcer prophylaxis (antacids, proton pump inhibitors) ▪ Assess for abdominal distention ▪ Dietary consultation ▪ Enteral feedings ▪ Stimulate mucosal activity ▪ Provide essential nutrients and calories

Continued

TABLE 69-12 Clinical Manifestations and Interventions of SIRS and MODS—cont'd

Manifestations	Interventions
Hepatic System	
▪ Bilirubin >2 mg/dL (34 mcmol/L) ▪ Elevated AST, ALT, gamma-glutamyl transferase (GGT) ▪ Elevated serum ammonia ▪ Decreased serum albumin, prealbumin, and transferrin ▪ Jaundice ▪ Hepatic encephalopathy	▪ Maintain adequate tissue perfusion ▪ Provide nutritional support ▪ Avoid hepatotoxic drugs
Hematological System	
▪ Increased coagulation studies including increased PTT and increased PT ▪ Thrombocytopenia ▪ Increased D-dimer ▪ Increased fibrin split products	▪ Observe for obvious and occult bleeding ▪ Replace factors being lost via prescribed blood products ▪ Minimize traumatic interventions such as venipunctures and intramuscular injections

Adapted from Lewis et al., 2017

PRACTICE QUESTIONS

856. A client had a 1000-mL bag of 5% dextrose in 0.9% sodium chloride hung at 1500. The nurse making rounds at 1545 finds that the client is complaining of a pounding headache and is dyspneic, experiencing chills, and apprehensive, with an increased pulse rate. The intravenous (IV) bag has 400 mL remaining. The nurse should take which action **first?**

1. Slow the IV infusion.
2. Sit the client up in bed.
3. Remove the IV catheter.
4. Call the primary health care provider (PHCP).

857. Packed red blood cells have been prescribed for a female client with anemia who has a hemoglobin level of 7.6 g/dL (76 mmol/L) and a hematocrit level of 30% (0.30). The nurse takes the client's temperature before hanging the blood transfusion and records 100.6° F (38.1° C) orally. Which action should the nurse take?

1. Begin the transfusion as prescribed.
2. Administer an antihistamine and begin the transfusion.
3. Administer 2 tablets of acetaminophen and begin the transfusion.
4. Delay hanging the blood and notify the primary health care provider (PHCP).

858. The nurse is caring for a client experiencing acute lower gastrointestinal bleeding. In developing the plan of care, which **priority** problem should the nurse assign to this client?

1. Deficient fluid volume related to acute blood loss
2. Risk for aspiration related to acute bleeding in the GI tract
3. Risk for infection related to acute disease process and medications
4. Imbalanced nutrition, less than body requirements, related to lack of nutrients and increased metabolism

859. The nurse is assessing the functioning of a chest tube drainage system in a client with a chest injury who has just returned from the recovery room following a thoracotomy with wedge resection. Which are the expected assessment findings? **Select all that apply.**

- ☐ 1. Excessive bubbling in the water seal chamber
- ☐ 2. Vigorous bubbling in the suction control chamber
- ☐ 3. Drainage system maintained below the client's chest
- ☐ 4. 50 mL of drainage in the drainage collection chamber
- ☐ 5. Occlusive dressing in place over the chest tube insertion site
- ☐ 6. Fluctuation of water in the tube in the water seal chamber during inhalation and exhalation

860. A client is brought to the emergency department with partial-thickness burns to his face, neck, arms, and chest after trying to put out a car fire. The nurse should implement which nursing actions for this client? **Select all that apply.**

- ☐ 1. Restrict fluids.
- ☐ 2. Assess for airway patency.
- ☐ 3. Administer oxygen as prescribed.
- ☐ 4. Place a cooling blanket on the client.
- ☐ 5. Elevate extremities if no fractures are present.
- ☐ 6. Prepare to give oral pain medication as prescribed.

861. A client is admitted to a hospital with a diagnosis of diabetic ketoacidosis (DKA). The initial blood glucose level is 950 mg/dL (52.9 mmol/L). A continuous intravenous (IV) infusion of short-acting insulin is initiated, along with IV rehydration with normal saline. The serum glucose level is now decreased to 240 mg/dL (13.37 mmol/L). The nurse would **next** prepare to administer which medication?

1. An ampule of 50% dextrose
2. NPH insulin subcutaneously
3. IV fluids containing dextrose
4. Phenytoin for the prevention of seizures

862. The nurse is assessing a client with multiple trauma who is at risk for developing acute respiratory distress syndrome. The nurse should assess for which **earliest** sign of acute respiratory distress syndrome?

1. Bilateral wheezing
2. Inspiratory crackles
3. Intercostal retractions
4. Increased respiratory rate

863. A client is admitted to the emergency department with chest pain that is consistent with myocardial infarction based on elevated troponin levels. Heart sounds are normal. The nurse should alert the primary health care provider because the vital sign changes and client assessment are **most** consistent with which complication? **Refer to chart.**

Client's Chart

Time:	11:00 a.m.	11:15 a.m.	11:30 a.m.	11:45 a.m.
Pulse:	92 beats/min	96 beats/min	104 beats/min	118 beats/min
Respiratory rate:	24 breaths/min	26 breaths/min	28 breaths/min	32 breaths/min
Blood pressure:	140/88 mm Hg	128/82 mm Hg	104/68 mm Hg	88/58 mm Hg

1. Cardiogenic shock
2. Cardiac tamponade
3. Pulmonary embolism
4. Dissecting thoracic aortic aneurysm

864. The nurse is caring for a client with chronic kidney disease on continuous replacement renal therapy (CRRT) without the use of a hemodialysis machine. The nurse determines that which parameter is **most important** in ensuring success of this treatment?

1. Mean arterial pressure (MAP)
2. Systolic blood pressure (SBP)
3. Diastolic blood pressure (DBP)
4. Central venous pressure (CVP)

865. The nurse is monitoring a client with a head injury for signs of increased intracranial pressure. The nurse would note which trend in vital signs if the intracranial pressure is rising?

1. Increasing temperature, increasing pulse, increasing respirations, decreasing blood pressure
2. Increasing temperature, decreasing pulse, decreasing respirations, increasing blood pressure
3. Decreasing temperature, decreasing pulse, increasing respirations, decreasing blood pressure
4. Decreasing temperature, increasing pulse, decreasing respirations, increasing blood pressure

866. A client develops an anaphylactic reaction after receiving morphine. The nurse should plan to institute which actions? **Select all that apply.**

- ☐ 1. Administer oxygen.
- ☐ 2. Quickly assess the client's respiratory status.
- ☐ 3. Document the event, interventions, and client's response.
- ☐ 4. Keep the client supine regardless of the blood pressure readings.
- ☐ 5. Leave the client briefly to contact a primary health care provider (PHCP).
- ☐ 6. Start an intravenous (IV) infusion of D5W and administer a 500-mL bolus.

867. A client in shock develops a central venous pressure (CVP) of 2 mm Hg and mean arterial pressure (MAP) of 60 mm Hg. Which prescribed intervention should the nurse implement **first**?

1. Increase the rate of O_2 flow
2. Obtain arterial blood gas results
3. Insert an indwelling urinary catheter
4. Increase the rate of intravenous (IV) fluids

868. A client at risk for shock secondary to pneumonia develops restlessness and is agitated and confused. Urinary output has decreased and the blood pressure is 92/68 mm Hg. The nurse minimally suspects which stage of shock based on this data?

1. Stage 1
2. Stage 2
3. Stage 3
4. Stage 4

869. The nurse is caring for a client hospitalized for heart failure exacerbation and suspects the client may be entering a state of shock. The nurse knows that which intervention is the **priority** for this client?

1. Administration of digoxin
2. Administration of whole blood
3. Administration of intravenous fluids
4. Administration of packed red blood cells

870. Which clinical findings are consistent with sepsis diagnostic criteria? **Select all that apply.**

- ☐ 1. Urine output 50 mL/hr
- ☐ 2. Hypoactive bowel sounds
- ☐ 3. Temperature of 102° F (38.9° C)
- ☐ 4. Heart rate of 96 beats per minute
- ☐ 5. Mean arterial pressure 65 mm Hg
- ☐ 6. Systolic blood pressure 110 mm Hg

ANSWERS

856. *Answer:* 1

Rationale: The client's symptoms are compatible with circulatory overload. This may be verified by noting that 600 mL has infused in the course of 45 minutes. The first action of the nurse is to slow the infusion. Other actions may follow in rapid sequence. The nurse may elevate the head of the bed to aid the client's breathing, if necessary. The nurse also notifies the PHCP. The IV catheter is not removed; it may be needed for the administration of medications to resolve the complication.
Test-Taking Strategy: Note the strategic word, *first*. This tells you that more than 1 or all of the options are likely to be correct actions and that the nurse needs to prioritize them according to a time sequence. You must be able to recognize the signs of circulatory overload. From this point, select the option that provides the intervention specific to circulatory overload.
Level of Cognitive Ability: Analyzing
Client Needs: Physiological Integrity
Integrated Process: Nursing Process—Implementation
Content Area: Complex Care: Intravenous Therapy
Health Problem: N/A
Priority Concepts: Fluid and Electrolytes; Perfusion
Reference: Ignatavicius, Workman, Rebar (2018), p. 219.

857. *Answer:* 4

Rationale: If the client has a temperature higher than 100° F (37.8° C), the unit of blood should not be hung until the primary PHCP is notified and has the opportunity to give further prescriptions. The PHCP likely will prescribe that the blood be administered regardless of the temperature, or may instruct the nurse to administer prescribed acetaminophen and wait until the temperature has decreased before administration, but the decision is not within the nurse's scope of practice to make. The nurse needs a PHCP's prescription to administer medications to the client.
Test-Taking Strategy: Eliminate all options that indicate to begin the transfusion, noting that they are comparable or alike. In addition, the options including antihistamine and acetaminophen indicate administering medication to the client, which is not done without a PHCP's prescription.
Level of Cognitive Ability: Synthesizing
Client Needs: Physiological Integrity
Integrated Process: Nursing Process—Implementation
Content Area: Complex Care: Blood Administration
Health Problem: Adult Health: Hematological: Anemias
Priority Concepts: Clinical Judgment; Safety
Reference: Lewis et al. (2017), p. 649.

858. *Answer:* 1

Rationale: The priority problem for the client with acute gastrointestinal bleeding among these options is deficient fluid volume related to acute blood less. This state can result in decreased cardiac output and hypovolemic shock. Although nutrition is a problem, fluid volume deficit is more of a priority. The client is at risk for aspiration and infection, but these are not actual problems at this point in time.
Test-Taking Strategy: Note the strategic word *priority*. Recalling that maintaining fluid balance is important for vital bodily functions will assist in directing you to this option. Additionally, note the word *risk* in options 2 and 3.
Level of Cognitive Ability: Analyzing
Client Needs: Physiological Integrity
Integrated Process: Nursing Process—Analysis
Content Area: Complex Care: Emergency Situations/Management
Health Problem: Adult Health: Gastrointestinal: Lower GI Disorders
Reference: Urden et al. (2018). p. 685.

859. *Answer:* 3, 4, 5, 6

Rationale: The bubbling of water in the water seal chamber indicates air drainage from the client and usually is seen when intrathoracic pressure is higher than atmospheric pressure; it may occur during exhalation, coughing, or sneezing. Excessive bubbling in the water seal chamber may indicate an air leak, an unexpected finding. Fluctuation of water in the tube in the water seal chamber during inhalation and exhalation is expected. An absence of fluctuation may indicate that the chest tube is obstructed or that the lung has re-expanded and that no more air is leaking into the pleural space. Gentle (not vigorous) bubbling should be noted in the suction control chamber. A total of 50 mL of drainage is not excessive in a client returning to the nursing unit from the recovery room. Drainage that is more than 70 to 100 mL/hr is considered excessive and requires notification of the surgeon. The chest tube insertion site is covered with an occlusive (airtight) dressing to prevent air from entering the pleural space. Positioning the drainage system below the client's chest allows gravity to drain the pleural space.
Test-Taking Strategy: Focus on the subject, expected findings associated with chest tube drainage systems. Thinking about the physiology associated with the functioning of a chest tube drainage system will assist in answering this question. The words *excessive bubbling* and *vigorous bubbling* will assist in eliminating these options.
Level of Cognitive Ability: Analyzing
Client Needs: Physiological Integrity
Integrated Process: Nursing Process—Assessment
Content Area: Complex Care: Invasive Devices
Health Problem: Adult Health: Respiratory: Chest Injuries
Priority Concepts: Clinical Judgment; Gas Exchange
Reference: Lewis et al. (2017), p. 525.

860. *Answer:* 2, 3, 5

Rationale: The primary goal for a burn injury is to maintain a patent airway, administer intravenous (IV) fluids to prevent hypovolemic shock, and preserve vital organ functioning. Therefore, the priority actions are to assess for airway patency and maintain a patent airway. The nurse then prepares to administer oxygen. Oxygen is necessary to perfuse vital tissues and organs. An IV line should be obtained and fluid resuscitation started. The extremities are elevated to assist in preventing shock and decrease fluid moving to the extremities, especially in the burn-injured upper extremities. The client is kept warm, because the loss of skin integrity causes heat loss. The client is placed on NPO (nothing by mouth) status because of the altered gastrointestinal function that occurs as a result of a burn injury.
Test-Taking Strategy: Focus on the subject, actions in a burn injury. Think about the pathophysiology that occurs and how the body reacts to a major burn injury. This assists in eliminating options 1, 4, and 6.

Level of Cognitive Ability: Synthesizing
Client Needs: Physiological Integrity
Integrated Process: Nursing Process—Analysis
Content Area: Complex Care: Emergency Situations/ Management
Health Problem: Adult Health: Integumentary: Burns
Priority Concepts: Clinical Judgment; Tissue Integrity
Reference: Ignatavicius, Workman, Rebar (2018), p. 489.

861. *Answer:* 3
Rationale: Emergency management of DKA focuses on correcting fluid and electrolyte imbalances and normalizing the serum glucose level. If the corrections occur too quickly, serious consequences, including hypoglycemia and cerebral edema, can occur. During management of DKA, when the blood glucose level falls to 250 to 300 mg/dL (13.9 to 16.7 mmol/L), the IV infusion rate is reduced and a dextrose solution is added to maintain a blood glucose level of about 250 mg/dL (13.9 mmol/L), or until the client recovers from ketosis. Fifty percent dextrose is used to treat hypoglycemia. NPH insulin is not used to treat DKA. Phenytoin is not a usual treatment measure for DKA.
Test-Taking Strategy: Note the strategic word, *next.* Focus on the subject, management of DKA. Eliminate option 2 first, knowing that short-duration (rapid-acting) insulin is used in the management of DKA. Eliminate option 1 next, knowing that this is the treatment for hypoglycemia. Note the words *the serum glucose level is now decreased to 240 mg/dL (13.7 mmol/L).* This should indicate that the IV solution containing dextrose is the next step in the management of care.
Level of Cognitive Ability: Synthesizing
Client Needs: Physiological Integrity
Integrated Process: Nursing Process—Planning
Content Area: Complex Care: Emergency Situations/ Management
Health Problem: Adult Health: Endocrine: Diabetes Mellitus
Priority Concepts: Clinical Judgment; Glucose Regulation
Reference: Ignatavicius, Workman, Rebar (2018), pp. 1312-1313.

862. *Answer:* 4
Rationale: The earliest detectable sign of acute respiratory distress syndrome is an increased respiratory rate, which can begin from 1 to 96 hours after the initial insult to the body. This is followed by increasing dyspnea, air hunger, retraction of accessory muscles, and cyanosis. Breath sounds may be clear or consist of fine inspiratory crackles or diffuse coarse crackles.
Test-Taking Strategy: Note the strategic word, *earliest.* Eliminate option 3 first because intercostal retraction is a later sign of respiratory distress. Of the remaining options, recall that adventitious breath sounds (options 1 and 2) would occur later than an increased respiratory rate.
Level of Cognitive Ability: Analyzing
Client Needs: Physiological Integrity
Integrated Process: Nursing Process—Assessment
Content Area: Complex Care: Acute Respiratory Failure
Health Problem: Adult Health: Respiratory: Acute Respiratory Distress Syndrome/Failure
Priority Concepts: Gas Exchange; Perfusion
Reference: Lewis et al. (2017), pp. 1622-1623.

863. *Answer:* 1
Rationale: Cardiogenic shock occurs with severe damage (more than 40%) to the left ventricle. Classic signs include hypotension; a rapid pulse that becomes weaker; decreased urine output; and cool, clammy skin. Respiratory rate increases as the body develops metabolic acidosis from shock. Cardiac tamponade is accompanied by distant, muffled heart sounds and prominent neck vessels. Pulmonary embolism presents suddenly with severe dyspnea accompanying the chest pain. Dissecting aortic aneurysms usually are accompanied by back pain.
Test-Taking Strategy: Note the strategic word, *most.* Recalling that the early serious complications of myocardial infarction include dysrhythmias, cardiogenic shock, and sudden death will direct you to the correct option. No information in the question is associated with the remaining options.
Level of Cognitive Ability: Synthesizing
Client Needs: Physiological Integrity
Integrated Process: Nursing Process—Analysis
Content Area: Complex Care: Shock
Health Problem: Adult Health: Cardiovascular: Shock
Priority Concepts: Clinical Judgment; Perfusion
Reference: Ignatavicius, Workman (2016), p. 741.

864. *Answer:* 1
Rationale: Continuous renal replacement therapy (CRRT) provides continuous ultrafiltration of extracellular fluid and clearance of urinary toxins over a period of 8 to 24 hours; it is used primarily for clients with acute kidney injury (AKI) or critically ill clients with chronic kidney disease (CKD) who cannot tolerate hemodialysis. Water, electrolytes, and other solutes are removed as the client's blood passes through a hemofilter. If CRRT does not require a hemodialysis machine, the client's MAP needs to be maintained above 60 mm Hg, and arterial and venous access sites are necessary. The SBP, DBP, and CVP may be monitored but each of these measures a component of the cardiovascular status rather than the complete cardiac cycle.
Test-Taking Strategy: Note the strategic words, *most important.* Recall that the mean arterial pressure is a measure that takes into account the complete cardiac cycle and is therefore the umbrella option that encompasses all other options.
Level of Cognitive Ability: Analyzing
Client Needs: Physiological Integrity
Integrated Process: Nursing Process—Assessment
Content Area: Complex Care: Emergency Situations/ Management
Health Problem: Adult Health: Renal and Urinary: Chronic Kidney Disease
Reference: Lewis et al. (2017), pp. 1091-1092.

865. *Answer:* 2
Rationale: A change in vital signs may be a late sign of increased intracranial pressure. Trends include increasing temperature and blood pressure and decreasing pulse and respirations. Respiratory irregularities also may occur.
Test-Taking Strategy: Focus on the subject, signs of increased intracranial pressure. If you remember that the temperature rises, you are able to eliminate options 3 and 4. If you know that the client becomes bradycardic, or know that the blood pressure rises, you are able to select the correct option.

Level of Cognitive Ability: Analyzing
Client Needs: Physiological Integrity
Integrated Process: Nursing Process—Assessment
Content Area: Complex Care: Emergency Situations/Management
Health Problem: Adult Health: Neurological: Head Injury/Trauma
Priority Concepts: Clinical Judgment; Intracranial Regulation
Reference: Lewis et al. (2017), pp. 1318-1319.

866. *Answer:* 1, 2, 3
Rationale: An anaphylactic reaction requires immediate action, starting with quickly assessing the client's respiratory status. Although the PHCP and the Rapid Response Team must be notified immediately, the nurse must stay with the client. Oxygen is administered and an IV of normal saline is started and infused per PHCP prescription. Documentation of the event, actions taken, and client outcomes needs to be done. The head of the bed should be elevated if the client's blood pressure is normal.
Test-Taking Strategy: Focus on the subject, interventions the nurse takes for an anaphylactic reaction. Read each option carefully and remember that this is an emergency. Think about the pathophysiology that occurs in this reaction to answer correctly.
Level of Cognitive Ability: Analyzing
Client Needs: Physiological Integrity
Integrated Process: Nursing Process—Implementation
Content Area: Complex Care: Emergency Situations/Management
Health Problem: Adult Health: Immune: Hypersensitivity Reactions and Allergy
Priority Concepts: Clinical Judgment; Immunity
Reference: Ignatavicius, Workman, Rebar (2018), p. 365.

867. *Answer:* 4
Rationale: The MAP and CVP are both low for this client, indicating a shock state. Shock is the result of inadequate tissue perfusion. Fluid volume should be immediately restored first to provide adequate perfusion for the client in a shock state. Although increasing the rate of O_2 flow may be a necessary intervention, perfusion is the first priority. Obtaining arterial blood gas results and inserting an indwelling urinary catheter may be necessary interventions to monitor the client's response to prescribed therapy, but these are not the priority.
Test-Taking Strategy: Note the strategic word, *first.* Although all interventions are appropriate for the client in a shock state, focus on the client's diagnosis and think about the pathophysiology that occurs in shock, and recall that adequate perfusion is the priority.
Level of Cognitive Ability: Analyzing
Client Needs: Physiological Integrity
Integrated Process: Nursing Process—Assessment
Content Area: Complex Care: Shock
Health Problem: Adult Health: Cardiovascular: Shock
Priority Concepts: Clinical Judgment; Perfusion
Reference: Urden et al. (2018), pp. 624, 803.

868. *Answer:* 2
Rationale: Shock is categorized by 4 stages. Stage 1 is characterized by restlessness, increased heart rate, cool and pale skin, and agitation. Stage 2 is characterized by a cardiac output that is less than 4 to 6 liters per minute, systolic blood pressure less than 100 mm Hg, decreased urinary output, confusion, and cerebral perfusion pressure that is less than 70 mm Hg. Stage 3 is characterized by edema, excessively low blood pressure, dysrhythmias, and weak and thready pulses. Stage 4 is characterized as unresponsiveness to vasopressors, profound hypotension, slowed heart rate, and multiple organ failure. Most often, the client will not survive.
Test-Taking Strategy: Note the data in the question, and note the word *minimally.* Think about the stages of shock. Noting the signs of restlessness, agitation and confusion, as well as the low blood pressure and decreased urinary output, will direct you to Stage 2 as the correct answer.
Level of Cognitive Ability: Analyzing
Client Needs: Physiological Integrity
Integrated Process: Nursing Process—Assessment
Content Area: Complex Care: Shock
Health Problem: Adult Health: Cardiovascular: Shock
Priority Concepts: Clinical Judgment; Perfusion
Reference: Lewis et al. (2017), pp. 1594-1595.

869. *Answer:* 1
Rationale: The client in this question is likely experiencing cardiogenic shock secondary to heart failure exacerbation. It is important to note that if the shock state is cardiogenic in nature, the infusion of volume-expanding fluids may result in pulmonary edema; therefore, restoration of cardiac function is the priority for this type of shock. Cardiotonic medications such as digoxin, dopamine, or norepinephrine may be administered to increase cardiac contractility and induce vasoconstriction. Whole blood, intravenous fluids, and packed red blood cells are volume-expanding fluids and may further complicate the client's clinical status; therefore, they should be avoided.
Test-Taking Strategy: Note the strategic word, *priority,* and focus on the subject, suspected shock in a client hospitalized for heart failure exacerbation. Recalling that this client is at risk for fluid volume overload will direct you to the correct option. Also, note that options 2, 3, and 4 are comparable or alike and involve the administration of intravenous solutions.
Level of Cognitive Ability: Analyzing
Client Needs: Physiological Integrity
Integrated Process: Nursing Process—Assessment
Content Area: Complex Care: Shock
Health Problem: Adult Health: Cardiovascular: Shock
Priority Concepts: Clinical Judgment; Perfusion
Reference: Ignatavicius, Workman, Rebar (2018), p. 700.

870. *Answer:* 3, 4, 5
Rationale: Sepsis diagnostic criteria with regard to signs and symptoms include the following: Fever (temperature higher than 100.9° F [38.3° C]) or hypothermia (core temperature lower than 97° F [36° C]), tachycardia (heart rate above 90 beats per minute), tachypnea (respiratory rate above 22 breaths per minute), systolic blood pressure (SBP) less than or equal to 100 mm Hg or arterial hypotension (SBP below 90 mm Hg), MAP less than 70 mm Hg, or a decrease in SBP of more than 40 mm Hg, altered mental status, edema or positive fluid balance, oliguria, ileus (absent bowel sounds), and decreased capillary refill or mottling of skin.

Test-Taking Strategy: Note the **subject**, clinical findings consistent with sepsis diagnostic criteria. Recalling that a minimum of 30 mL/hr of urine is adequate will assist in eliminating this option. Noting that hypoactive bowel sounds are not suggestive of an ileus eliminates this option. Lastly, recalling that an SBP of 110 mm Hg does not fit the criteria will assist in eliminating this option.

Level of Cognitive Ability: Analyzing
Client Needs: Physiological Integrity
Integrated Process: Nursing Process—Assessment
Content Area: Complex Care: Sepsis
Health Problem: Adult Health: Cardiovascular: Shock
Priority Concepts: Clinical Judgment; Perfusion
Reference: Lewis et al. (2017), p. 1592.

UNIT XX

Comprehensive Test

PRACTICE QUESTIONS

871. The emergency department nurse is caring for a client who has been identified as a victim of physical abuse. In planning care for the client, which is the **priority** nursing action?
1. Adhering to the mandatory abuse-reporting laws
2. Notifying the caseworker of the family situation
3. Removing the client from any immediate danger
4. Obtaining treatment for the abusing family member

872. The nurse assesses a client with the admitting diagnosis of bipolar affective disorder, mania. Which client symptoms require the nurse's **immediate** action?
1. Incessant talking and sexual innuendoes
2. Grandiose delusions and poor concentration
3. Outlandish behaviors and inappropriate dress
4. Nonstop physical activity and poor nutritional intake

873. The nurse is caring for a client who was involuntarily hospitalized to a mental health unit and is scheduled for electroconvulsive therapy. The nurse notes that an informed consent has not been obtained for the procedure. Based on this information, what is the nurse's **best** determination in planning care?
1. The informed consent does not need to be obtained.
2. The informed consent should be obtained from the family.
3. The informed consent needs to be obtained from the client.
4. The health care provider will provide the informed consent.

874. A client newly diagnosed with diabetes mellitus is instructed by the primary health care provider to obtain glucagon for emergency home use. The client asks a home care nurse about the purpose of the medication. What is the nurse's **best** response to the client's question?
1. "It will boost the cells in your pancreas if you have insufficient insulin."
2. "It will help promote insulin absorption when your glucose levels are high."
3. "It is for the times when your blood glucose is too low from too much insulin."
4. "It will help prevent lipoatrophy from the multiple insulin injections over the years."

875. The nurse is providing care to a Puerto Rican–American client who is terminally ill. Numerous family members are present most of the time, and many of the family members are very emotional. What is the **most appropriate** nursing action for this client?
1. Restrict the number of family members visiting at one time.
2. Inform the family that emotional outbursts are to be avoided.
3. Make the necessary arrangements so that family members can visit.
4. Contact the primary health care provider to speak to the family regarding their behaviors.

876. A client presents to the emergency department with upper gastrointestinal bleeding and is in moderate distress. In planning care, what is the **priority** nursing action for this client?
1. Assessment of vital signs
2. Completion of abdominal examination
3. Insertion of the prescribed nasogastric tube
4. Thorough investigation of precipitating events

877. The nurse is performing an assessment on a client with dementia. Which piece of data gathered during the assessment indicates a manifestation associated with dementia?
1. Use of confabulation
2. Improvement in sleeping
3. Absence of sundown syndrome
4. Presence of personal hygienic care

878. The nurse is caring for a client with anorexia nervosa. Which behavior is characteristic of this disorder and reflects anxiety management?
1. Engaging in immoral acts
2. Always reinforcing self-approval
3. Observing rigid rules and regulations
4. Having the need always to make the right decision

879. The nurse provides instructions to a malnourished pregnant client regarding iron supplementation. Which client statement indicates an understanding of the instructions?
1. "Iron supplements will give me diarrhea."
2. "Meat does not provide iron and should be avoided."
3. "The iron is best absorbed if taken on an empty stomach."
4. "On the days that I eat green leafy vegetables or calf liver I can omit taking the iron supplement."

880. Levothyroxine is prescribed for a client diagnosed with hypothyroidism. Upon review of the client's record, the nurse notes that the client is taking warfarin. Which modification to the plan of care should the nurse review with the client's primary health care provider?
1. A decreased dosage of levothyroxine
2. An increased dosage of levothyroxine
3. A decreased dosage of warfarin sodium
4. An increased dosage of warfarin sodium

881. The nurse is teaching a client with emphysema about positions that help breathing during dyspneic episodes. The nurse instructs the client that which positions alleviate dyspnea? **Select all that apply.**
- ☐ 1. Sitting up and leaning on a table
- ☐ 2. Standing and leaning against a wall
- ☐ 3. Lying supine with the feet elevated
- ☐ 4. Sitting up with the elbows resting on knees
- ☐ 5. Lying on the back in a low-Fowler's position

882. A client is about to undergo a lumbar puncture. The nurse describes to the client that which position will be used during the procedure?
1. Side-lying with a pillow under the hip
2. Prone with a pillow under the abdomen
3. Prone in slight Trendelenburg's position
4. Side-lying with the legs pulled up and the head bent down onto the chest

883. The nurse recognizes that which interventions are likely to facilitate effective communication between a dying client and family? **Select all that apply.**
- ☐ 1. The nurse encourages the client and family to identify and discuss feelings openly.
- ☐ 2. The nurse assists the client and family in carrying out spiritually meaningful practices.
- ☐ 3. The nurse removes autonomy from the client to alleviate any unnecessary stress for the client.
- ☐ 4. The nurse makes decisions for the client and family to relieve them of unnecessary demands.
- ☐ 5. The nurse maintains a calm attitude and one of acceptance when the family or client expresses anger.

884. A depressed client verbalizes feelings of low self-esteem and self-worth typified by statements such as "I'm such a failure. I can't do anything right." How should the nurse plan to respond to the client's statement?
1. Reassure the client that things will get better.
2. Tell the client that this is not true and that we all have a purpose in life.
3. Identify recent behaviors or accomplishments that demonstrate the client's skills.
4. Remain with the client and sit in silence; this will encourage the client to verbalize feelings.

885. The nurse has just admitted to the nursing unit a client with a basilar skull fracture who is at risk for increased intracranial pressure. Pending specific primary health care provider prescriptions, the nurse should safely place the client in which positions? **Select all that apply.**
- ☐ 1. Head midline
- ☐ 2. Neck in neutral position
- ☐ 3. Head of bed elevated 30 to 45 degrees
- ☐ 4. Head turned to the side when flat in bed
- ☐ 5. Neck and jaw flexed forward when opening the mouth

886. The nurse reviews the arterial blood gas results of a client with emphysema and notes that the laboratory report indicates a pH of 7.30, $PaCO_2$ of 58 mm Hg, PaO_2 of 80 mm Hg, and HCO_3 of 27 mEq/L (27 mmol/L). The nurse interprets that the client has which acid–base disturbance?
1. Metabolic acidosis
2. Metabolic alkalosis
3. Respiratory acidosis
4. Respiratory alkalosis

887. The nurse has admitted a client to the clinical nursing unit after undergoing a right mastectomy. The nurse should plan to place the right arm in which position?
1. Elevated on a pillow
2. Level with the right atrium
3. Dependent to the right atrium
4. Elevated above shoulder level

888. On the second postpartum day, a client complains of burning on urination, urgency, and frequency of urination. A urinalysis indicates the presence of a urinary tract infection. The nurse instructs the client regarding measures to take for the treatment of the infection. Which client statement indicates to the nurse the **need for further instruction**?
1. "I need to urinate frequently throughout the day."
2. "The prescribed medication must be taken until it is finished."
3. "My fluid intake should be increased to at least 3000 mL daily."
4. "Foods and fluids that will increase urine alkalinity should be consumed."

889. A client received 20 units of Humulin N insulin subcutaneously at 08:00. At what time should the nurse plan to assess the client for a hypoglycemic reaction?
1. 10:00
2. 11:00
3. 17:00
4. 24:00

890. The nurse is the first responder after a tornado has destroyed many homes in the community. Which victim should the nurse attend to **first**?
1. A pregnant woman who exclaims, "My baby is not moving."
2. A woman who is complaining, "My leg is bleeding so bad, I am afraid it is going to fall off!"
3. A young child standing next to an adult family member who is screaming, "I want my mommy!"
4. An older victim who is sitting next to her husband sobbing, "My husband is dead. My husband is dead."

891. A pregnant client at 10 weeks' gestation calls the prenatal clinic to report a recent exposure to a child with rubella. The nurse reviews the client's chart. What is the nurse's **best** response to the client? **Refer to chart.**

History and Physical	Laboratory and Diagnostic Results	Medications
Gravida, Term Births, Preterm Births, Abortions, Living Children (GTPAL) 1,0,0,0,0	Venereal Disease Research Laboratory (VDRL) nonreactive	Prenatal vitamins
Weight 135 lb (61 kg)	Rubella immune	
Positive Goodell and Chadwick	Rh positive, type O	

1. "You should avoid all school-age children during pregnancy."
2. "There is no need to be concerned if you don't have a fever or rash within the next 2 days."
3. "You were wise to call. Your rubella titer indicates that you are immune and your baby is not at risk."
4. "Be sure to tell the primary health care provider in 2 weeks, as additional screening will be prescribed during your second trimester."

892. A breast-feeding mother of an infant with lactose intolerance asks the nurse about dietary measures. What foods should the nurse tell the mother are acceptable to consume while breast-feeding? **Select all that apply.**
- ❑ 1. 1% milk
- ❑ 2. Egg yolk
- ❑ 3. Dried beans
- ❑ 4. Hard cheeses
- ❑ 5. Green leafy vegetables

893. A client with diabetes mellitus is told that amputation of the leg is necessary to sustain life. The client is very upset and tells the nurse, "This is all my primary health care provider's fault. I have done everything I've been asked to do!" Which nursing interpretation is **best** for this situation?
1. An expected coping mechanism
2. An ineffective defense mechanism
3. A need to notify the hospital lawyer
4. An expression of guilt on the part of the client

894. A client with terminal cancer arrives at the emergency department dead on arrival (DOA). After an autopsy is prescribed, the client's family requests that no autopsy be performed. Which response to the family is **most appropriate**?
1. "The decision is made by the medical examiner."
2. "An autopsy is mandatory for any client who is DOA."
3. "I will contact the medical examiner regarding your request."
4. "It is required by federal law. Tell me why you don't want the autopsy done."

895. A client who is positive for human immunodeficiency virus (HIV) delivers a newborn infant. The nurse provides instructions to help the client with care of her infant. Which client statement indicates the **need for further instruction**?
1. "I will be sure to wash my hands before and after bathroom use."
2. "I need to breast-feed, especially for the first 6 weeks postpartum."
3. "Support groups are available to assist me with understanding my diagnosis of HIV."
4. "My newborn infant should be on antiviral medications for the first 6 weeks after delivery."

896. An adolescent client is diagnosed with conjunctivitis, and the nurse provides information to the client about the use of contact lenses. Which client statement indicates the **need for further information**?
1. "I should obtain new contact lenses."
2. "I should not wear my contact lenses."
3. "My old contact lenses should be discarded."
4. "My contact lenses can be worn if they are cleaned as directed."

897. The nurse teaches a client newly diagnosed with type 1 diabetes about storing Humulin N insulin. Which statement indicates to the nurse that the client understood the discharge teaching?
1. "I should keep the insulin in the cabinet during the day only."
2. "I know I have to keep my insulin in the refrigerator at all times."
3. "I can store the open insulin bottle in the kitchen cabinet for 1 month."
4. "The best place for my insulin is on the windowsill, but in the cupboard is just as good."

898. The nurse is caring for a client scheduled for a transsphenoidal hypophysectomy. The preoperative teaching instructions should include which statement?
1. "Your hair will need to be shaved."
2. "You will receive spinal anesthesia."
3. "You will need to ambulate after surgery."
4. "Brushing your teeth needs to be avoided for at least 2 weeks after surgery."

899. During a routine prenatal visit, a client complains of gums that bleed easily with brushing. The nurse performs an assessment and teaches the client about proper nutrition to minimize this problem. Which client statement indicates an understanding of the proper nutrition to minimize this problem?
1. "I will drink 8 oz of water with each meal."
2. "I will eat 3 servings of cracked wheat bread each day."
3. "I will eat 2 saltine crackers before I get up each morning."
4. "I will eat fresh fruits and vegetables for snacks and for dessert each day."

900. A 6-year-old child has just been diagnosed with localized Hodgkin's disease, and chemotherapy is planned to begin immediately. The mother of the child asks the nurse why radiation therapy was not prescribed as a part of the treatment. What is the nurse's **best** response?
1. "It's very costly, and chemotherapy works just as well."
2. "I'm not sure. I'll discuss it with the primary health care provider."
3. "Sometimes age has to do with the decision for radiation therapy."
4. "The primary health care provider would prefer that you discuss treatment options with the oncologist."

901. An infant born with an imperforate anus returns from surgery after requiring a colostomy. The nurse assesses the stoma and notes that it is red and edematous. Based on this finding, which action should the nurse take?
1. Elevate the buttocks.
2. Document the findings.
3. Apply ice immediately.
4. Call the primary health care provider.

902. The nurse is performing an initial assessment on a newborn infant. When assessing the infant's head, the nurse notes that the ears are low-set. Which nursing action is **most appropriate**?
1. Document the findings.
2. Arrange for hearing testing.
3. Notify the pediatrician.
4. Cover the ears with gauze pads.

903. The clinic nurse is assessing jaundice in a child with hepatitis. Which anatomical area would provide the **best** data regarding the presence of jaundice?
1. The nail beds
2. The skin in the sacral area
3. The skin in the abdominal area
4. The membranes in the ear canal

904. The nurse is assigned to care for a client in traction. The nurse creates a plan of care for the client and should include which action in the plan?
1. Ensure that the knots are at the pulleys.
2. Check the weights to ensure that they are off of the floor.
3. Ensure that the head of the bed is kept at a 45- to 90-degree angle.
4. Monitor the weights to ensure that they are resting on a firm surface.

905. The nurse is setting up the physical environment for an interview with a client and plans to obtain subjective data regarding the client's health. Which interventions are appropriate? **Select all that apply.**
- ☐ 1. Set the room temperature at a comfortable level.
- ☐ 2. Remove distracting objects from the interviewing area.
- ☐ 3. Place a chair for the client across from the nurse's desk.
- ☐ 4. Ensure comfortable seating at eye level for the client and nurse.
- ☐ 5. Provide seating for the client so that the client faces a strong light.
- ☐ 6. Ensure that the distance between the client and nurse is at least 7 feet (2.1 meters).

906. The nurse is caring for an older adult who has been placed in Buck's extension traction after a hip fracture. On assessment of the client, the nurse notes that the client is disoriented. What is the **best** nursing action based on this information?
1. Apply restraints to the client.
2. Ask the family to stay with the client.
3. Place a clock and calendar in the client's room.
4. Ask the laboratory to perform electrolyte studies.

907. The nurse is creating a plan of care for a client in skin traction. The nurse should monitor for which **priority** finding in this client?
1. Urinary incontinence
2. Signs of skin breakdown
3. The presence of bowel sounds
4. Signs of infection around the pin sites

908. The home care nurse is visiting a client who is in a body cast. While performing an assessment, the nurse plans to evaluate the psychosocial adjustment of the client to the cast. What is the **most appropriate** assessment for this client?
1. The need for sensory stimulation
2. The amount of home care support available
3. The ability to perform activities of daily living
4. The type of transportation available for follow-up care

909. What action should the nurse consider when counseling a client of the Amish tradition?
1. Speak only to the husband.
2. Use complex medical terminology.
3. Avoid using scientific or medical jargon.
4. Stand close to the client and speak loudly.

910. A client has refused to eat more than a few spoonfuls of breakfast. The primary health care provider has prescribed that tube feedings be initiated if the client fails to eat at least half of a meal because the client has lost a significant amount of weight during the previous 2 months. The nurse enters the room, looks at the tray, and states, "If you don't eat any more than that, I'm going to have to put a tube down your throat and get a feeding in that way." The client begins crying and tries to eat more. Based on the nurse's actions, the nurse may be accused of which violation?
1. Assault
2. Battery
3. Slander
4. Invasion of privacy

911. When creating an assignment for a team consisting of a registered nurse (RN), 1 licensed practical nurse (LPN), and 2 assistive personnel (AP), which is the **best** client for the LPN?
1. A client requiring frequent temperature checks
2. A client requiring assistance with ambulation every 4 hours
3. A client on a mechanical ventilator requiring frequent assessment and suctioning
4. A client with a spinal cord injury requiring urinary catheterization every 6 hours

912. To perform cardiopulmonary resuscitation (CPR), the nurse should use the method pictured to open the airway in which situation? **Refer to figure.**

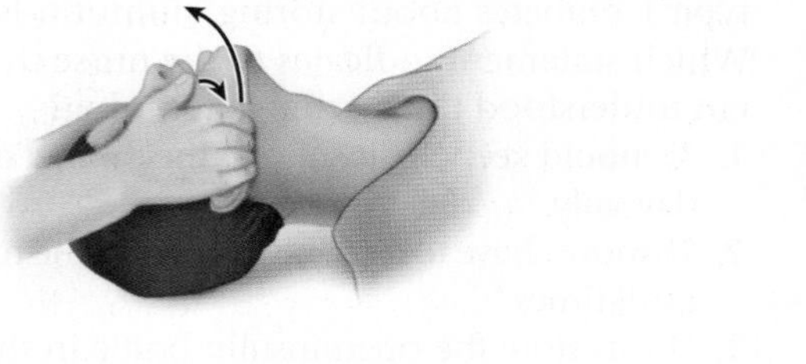

1. If neck trauma is suspected
2. In all situations requiring CPR
3. If the client has a history of seizures
4. If the client has a history of headaches

913. The nurse teaches skin care to a client receiving external radiation therapy. Which client statement indicates the **need for further instruction**?
1. "I will handle the area gently."
2. "I will wear loose-fitting clothing."
3. "I will avoid the use of deodorants."
4. "I will limit sun exposure to 1 hour daily."

914. The primary health care provider's prescription reads levothyroxine, 150 mcg orally daily. The medication label reads levothyroxine, 0.1 mg per tablet. The nurse should administer how many tablet(s) to the client? **Fill in the blank.**

Answer: _____ tablet(s)

915. Metformin is prescribed for a client with type 2 diabetes mellitus. What is the **most** common side effect that the nurse should include in the client's teaching plan?
1. Weight gain
2. Hypoglycemia
3. Flushing and palpitations
4. Gastrointestinal disturbances

916. Which nursing actions apply to the care of a child who is having a seizure? **Select all that apply.**
- ☐ 1. Time the seizure.
- ☐ 2. Restrain the child.
- ☐ 3. Stay with the child.
- ☐ 4. Insert an oral airway.
- ☐ 5. Loosen clothing around the child's neck.
- ☐ 6. Place the child in a lateral side-lying position.

917. The nurse is conducting an interview of an older client and is concerned about the possibility of benign prostatic hyperplasia (BPH). Which are characteristics of this disorder? **Select all that apply.**
- ☐ 1. Nocturia
- ☐ 2. Incontinence
- ☐ 3. Enlarged prostate
- ☐ 4. Nocturnal emissions
- ☐ 5. Decreased desire for sexual intercourse

918. The nursing instructor asks a nursing student to identify the priorities of care for an assigned client. Which statement indicates that the student correctly identifies the **priority** client needs?
1. Actual or life-threatening concerns
2. Completing care in a reasonable time frame
3. Time constraints related to the client's needs
4. Obtaining needed supplies to care for the client

919. A client arrives at the clinic complaining of fatigue, lack of energy, constipation, and depression. Hypothyroidism is diagnosed, and levothyroxine is prescribed. What is an expected outcome of the medication?
1. Alleviate depression
2. Increase energy levels
3. Increase blood glucose levels
4. Achieve normal thyroid hormone levels

920. The community health nurse is creating a poster for an educational session for a group of women and will be discussing the risk factors associated with breast cancer. Which risk factors for breast cancer should the nurse list on the poster? **Select all that apply.**
- ☐ 1. Multiparity
- ☐ 2. Early menarche
- ☐ 3. Early menopause
- ☐ 4. Family history of breast cancer
- ☐ 5. High-dose radiation exposure to chest
- ☐ 6. Previous cancer of the breast, uterus, or ovaries

921. The nurse is caring for a client with acute pancreatitis and is monitoring the client for paralytic ileus. Which piece of assessment data should alert the nurse to this occurrence?
1. Inability to pass flatus
2. Loss of anal sphincter control
3. Severe, constant pain with rapid onset
4. Firm, nontender mass palpable at the lower right costal margin

922. The nurse inspects the color of the drainage from a nasogastric tube on a postoperative client approximately 24 hours after gastric surgery. Which finding indicates the need to notify the primary health care provider (PHCP)?
1. Dark red drainage
2. Dark brown drainage
3. Green-tinged drainage
4. Light yellowish-brown drainage

923. The nurse is preparing to discontinue a client's nasogastric tube. The client is positioned properly, and the tube has been flushed with 15 mL of air to clear secretions. Before removing the tube, the nurse should make which statement to the client?
1. "Take a deep breath when I tell you, and hold it while I remove the tube."
2. "Take a deep breath when I tell you, and bear down while I remove the tube."
3. "Take a deep breath when I tell you, and slowly exhale while I remove the tube."
4. "Take a deep breath when I tell you, and breathe normally while I remove the tube."

924. A client with a history of lung disease is at risk for developing respiratory acidosis. The nurse should assess the client for which signs and symptoms characteristic of this disorder?
1. Bradycardia and hyperactivity
2. Decreased respiratory rate and depth
3. Headache, restlessness, and confusion
4. Bradypnea, dizziness, and paresthesias

925. The nurse is caring for a client with a resolved intestinal obstruction who has a nasogastric tube in place. The primary health care provider has now prescribed that the nasogastric tube be removed. What is the **priority** nursing assessment prior to removing the tube?
1. Checking for normal serum electrolyte levels
2. Checking for normal pH of the gastric aspirate
3. Checking for proper nasogastric tube placement
4. Checking for the presence of bowel sounds in all 4 quadrants

926. The nurse has reviewed with the preoperative client the procedure for the administration of an enema. Which statement by the client would indicate the **need for further instruction?**
1. "The enema will be given while I am sitting on the toilet."
2. "I should try and hold the fluid as long as possible after it is run in."
3. "I know that there will be some cramping after the enema solution is run in."
4. "I should tell the nurse if cramping occurs when the fluid is running in."

927. A client experiencing a great deal of stress and anxiety is being taught to use self-control therapy. Which statement by the client indicates a **need for further teaching** about the therapy?
1. "This form of therapy can be applied to new situations."

2. "An advantage of this technique is that change is likely to last."
3. "Talking to oneself is a basic component of this form of therapy."
4. "This form of therapy provides a negative reinforcement when the stimulus is produced."

928. The nurse is preparing a list of home care instructions regarding stoma and laryngectomy care for a client with laryngeal cancer who had a laryngectomy. Which instructions should be included in the list? **Select all that apply.**

- ☐ 1. Restrict fluid intake.
- ☐ 2. Obtain a MedicAlert bracelet.
- ☐ 3. Keep the humidity in the home low.
- ☐ 4. Prevent debris from entering the stoma.
- ☐ 5. Avoid exposure to people with infections.
- ☐ 6. Avoid swimming and use care when showering.

929. The primary health care provider prescribes 2000 mL of 5% dextrose and half-normal saline to infuse over 24 hours. The drop factor is 15 drops (gtt)/mL. The nurse should set the flow rate at how many drops per minute? **Fill in the blank. Record your answer to the nearest whole number.**

Answer: _____ gtt/minute

930. A client is returned to the nursing unit after thoracic surgery with chest tubes in place. During the first few hours postoperatively, what type of drainage should the nurse expect?

1. Serous
2. Bloody
3. Serosanguineous
4. Bloody, with frequent small clots

931. A client has had radical neck dissection and begins to hemorrhage at the incision site. The nurse should take which actions in this situation? **Select all that apply.**

- ☐ 1. Monitor vital signs.
- ☐ 2. Monitor the client's airway.
- ☐ 3. Apply manual pressure over the site.
- ☐ 4. Lower the head of the bed to a flat position.
- ☐ 5. Call the primary health care provider (PHCP) immediately.

932. A sexually active young adult client has developed viral hepatitis. Which client statement indicates the **need for further teaching**?

1. "I should avoid drinking alcohol."
2. "I can go back to work right away."
3. "My partner should get the vaccine."
4. "A condom should be used for sexual intercourse."

933. The nurse should include which interventions in the plan of care for a client with hypothyroidism? **Select all that apply.**

- ☐ 1. Provide a cool environment for the client.
- ☐ 2. Instruct the client to consume a high-fat diet.
- ☐ 3. Instruct the client about thyroid replacement therapy.
- ☐ 4. Encourage the client to consume fluids and high-fiber foods in the diet.
- ☐ 5. Inform the client that iodine preparations will be prescribed to treat the disorder.
- ☐ 6. Instruct the client to contact the primary health care provider (PHCP) if episodes of chest pain occur.

934. The nurse is preparing to care for a client who will be weaned from a cuffed tracheostomy tube. The nurse is planning to use a tracheostomy plug and plans to insert it into the opening in the outer cannula. Which nursing action is required before plugging the tube?

1. Deflate the cuff on the tube.
2. Place the inner cannula into the tube.
3. Ensure that the client is able to speak.
4. Ensure that the client is able to swallow.

935. A client is diagnosed with glaucoma. Which piece of nursing assessment data identifies a risk factor associated with this eye disorder?

1. Cardiovascular disease
2. Frequent urinary tract infections
3. A history of migraine headaches
4. Frequent upper respiratory infections

936. A client with retinal detachment is admitted to the nursing unit in preparation for a repair procedure. Which prescription should the nurse anticipate?

1. Allowing bathroom privileges only
2. Elevating the head of the bed to 45 degrees
3. Wearing dark glasses to read or watch television
4. Placing an eye patch over the client's affected eye

937. The nurse is caring for a client who is on strict bed rest and creates a plan of care with goals related to the prevention of deep vein thrombosis and pulmonary emboli. Which nursing action is **most** helpful in preventing these disorders from developing?

1. Restricting fluids
2. Placing a pillow under the knees
3. Encouraging active range-of-motion exercises
4. Applying a heating pad to the lower extremities

938. The nurse is caring for a client who is at risk for suicide. What is the **priority** nursing action for this client?
1. Provide authority, action, and participation.
2. Display an attitude of detachment, confrontation, and efficiency.
3. Demonstrate confidence in the client's ability to deal with stressors.
4. Provide hope and reassurance that the problems will resolve themselves.

939. A client with tuberculosis whose status is being monitored in an ambulatory care clinic asks the nurse when it is permissible to return to work. What factor should the nurse include when responding to the client?
1. Five blood cultures are negative.
2. Three sputum cultures are negative.
3. A blood culture and a chest x-ray are negative.
4. A sputum culture and a tuberculin skin test are negative.

940. A client comes to the emergency department after an assault and is extremely agitated, trembling, and hyperventilating. What is the **priority** nursing action for this client?
1. Begin to teach relaxation techniques.
2. Encourage the client to discuss the assault.
3. Remain with the client until the anxiety decreases.
4. Place the client in a quiet room alone to decrease stimulation.

941. The nurse is caring for a client admitted to the hospital with a suspected diagnosis of acute appendicitis. Which laboratory result should the nurse expect to note if the client does have appendicitis?
1. Leukopenia with a shift to the left
2. Leukocytosis with a shift to the left
3. Leukopenia with a shift to the right
4. Leukocytosis with a shift to the right

942. The nurse is creating a plan of care for a client who was experiencing anxiety after the loss of a job. The client is now verbalizing concerns regarding the ability to meet role expectations and financial obligations. What is the **priority** nursing problem for this client?
1. Anxiety
2. Unrealistic outlook
3. Lack of ability to cope effectively
4. Disturbances in thoughts and ideas

943. The nurse is monitoring the chest tube drainage system in a client with a chest tube. The nurse notes intermittent bubbling in the water seal chamber. Which is the **most appropriate** nursing action?
1. Check for an air leak.
2. Document the findings.
3. Notify the primary health care provider.
4. Change the chest tube drainage system.

944. After performing an initial abdominal assessment on a client with nausea and vomiting, the nurse should expect to note which finding?
1. Waves of loud gurgles auscultated in all 4 quadrants
2. Low-pitched swishing auscultated in 1 or 2 quadrants
3. Relatively high-pitched clicks or gurgles auscultated in all 4 quadrants
4. Very high-pitched, loud rushes auscultated especially in 1 or 2 quadrants

945. The primary health care provider prescribes erythromycin suspension 800 mg by mouth. After reconstitution, how many milliliters should the nurse pour into the medicine cup to deliver the prescribed dose? **Refer to figure. Fill in the blank.**

Answer: _____ mL

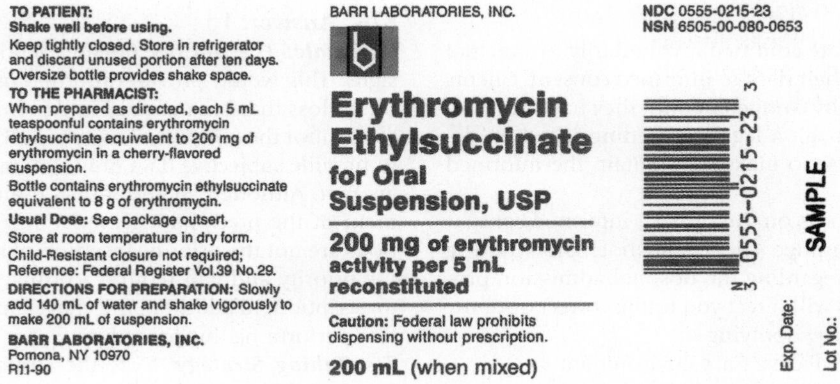
TO PATIENT:
Shake well before using.
Keep tightly closed. Store in refrigerator and discard unused portion after ten days. Oversize bottle provides shake space.
TO THE PHARMACIST:
When prepared as directed, each 5 mL teaspoonful contains erythromycin ethylsuccinate equivalent to 200 mg of erythromycin in a cherry-flavored suspension.
Bottle contains erythromycin ethylsuccinate equivalent to 8 g of erythromycin.
Usual Dose: See package outsert.
Store at room temperature in dry form.
Child-Resistant closure not required; Reference: Federal Register Vol.39 No.29.
DIRECTIONS FOR PREPARATION: Slowly add 140 mL of water and shake vigorously to make 200 mL of suspension.
BARR LABORATORIES, INC.
Pomona, NY 10970
R11-90
BARR LABORATORIES, INC.
Erythromycin Ethylsuccinate
for Oral Suspension, USP
200 mg of erythromycin activity per 5 mL reconstituted
Caution: Federal law prohibits dispensing without prescription.
200 mL (when mixed)
NDC 0555-0215-23
NSN 6505-00-080-0653
N 3 0555-0215-23 3
SAMPLE
Exp. Date:
Lot No.:
(Brown, Mulholland, 2012.)

ANSWERS

871. *Answer:* 3
Rationale: Whenever an abused client remains in the abusive environment, priority must be placed on ascertaining whether the client is in any immediate danger. If so, emergency action must be taken to remove the client from the abusing situation. Options 1, 2, and 4 may be appropriate interventions but are not the priority.
Test-Taking Strategy: Note the strategic word, *priority.* Use Maslow's Hierarchy of Needs theory, remembering that if a physiological need is not present, safety is the priority. This will direct you to the correct option, the only one that directly addresses client safety.
Level of Cognitive Ability: Applying
Client Needs: Safe and Effective Care Environment
Integrated Process: Nursing Process—Planning
Content Area: Mental Health
Health Problem: Mental Health: Abusive behaviors
Priority Concepts: Interpersonal Violence; Safety
Reference: Varcarolis (2017), p. 343.

872. *Answer:* 4
Rationale: Mania is a mood characterized by excitement, euphoria, hyperactivity, excessive energy, decreased need for sleep, and impaired ability to concentrate or complete a single train of thought. The client's mood is predominantly elevated, expansive, or irritable. All of the options reflect a client's possible symptoms. However, the correct option clearly presents a problem that compromises physiological integrity and needs to be addressed immediately.
Test-Taking Strategy: Note the strategic word, *immediate,* and use Maslow's Hierarchy of Needs theory to assist you in answering the question. The correct option is the only one that reflects a physiological need.
Level of Cognitive Ability: Analyzing
Client Needs: Physiological Integrity
Integrated Process: Nursing Process—Assessment
Content Area: Mental Health
Health Problem: Mental Health: Mood disorders
Priority Concepts: Psychosis; Safety
Reference: Varcarolis (2017), pp. 227, 229.

873. *Answer:* 3
Rationale: Clients who are admitted involuntarily to a mental health unit do not lose their right to informed consent. Clients must be considered legally competent until they have been declared incompetent through a legal proceeding. The best determination for the nurse to make is to obtain the informed consent from the client.
Test-Taking Strategy: Focus on the subject, informed consent for an involuntarily admitted client, and note the strategic word, *best.* Knowledge regarding the hospital admission processes and client's rights will direct you to the correct option.
Level of Cognitive Ability: Applying
Client Needs: Safe and Effective Care Environment
Integrated Process: Nursing Process—Planning
Content Area: Leadership/Management: Ethical/Legal
Health Problem: Mental Health: Mood disorders
Priority Concepts: Ethics; Health Care Law
Reference: Varcarolis (2017), p. 63.

874. *Answer:* 3
Rationale: Glucagon is used to treat hypoglycemia resulting from insulin overdose. The family of the client is instructed in how to administer the medication. In an unconscious client, arousal usually occurs within 20 minutes of glucagon injection. When consciousness has been regained, oral carbohydrates should be given. Lipoatrophy and lipohypertrophy result from insulin injections.
Test-Taking Strategy: Focus on the subject, the purpose of glucagon. Also note the strategic word, *best.* Noting the word glucagon will assist you in determining that the medication contains some form of glucose. This relationship will direct you to the correct option.
Level of Cognitive Ability: Applying
Client Needs: Physiological Integrity
Integrated Process: Teaching and Learning
Content Area: Adult Health: Endocrine
Health Problem: Adult Health: Endocrine: Diabetes mellitus
Priority Concepts: Client Education; Glucose Regulation
Reference: Ignatavicius, Workman, Rebar (2018), pp. 1281, 1310.

875. *Answer:* 3
Rationale: In the Puerto Rican–American culture, loud crying and other physical manifestations of grief are considered socially acceptable. Of the options provided, the correct option is the only one that identifies a culturally sensitive approach on the part of the nurse. Options 1, 2, and 4 are inappropriate nursing interventions.
Test-Taking Strategy: Note the strategic words, *most appropriate.* Focus on the clients of the question, the family members. Use therapeutic nursing interventions, recalling the characteristics of the culture and the importance of cultural sensitivity. This will direct you to the correct option.
Level of Cognitive Ability: Applying
Client Needs: Psychosocial Integrity
Integrated Process: Culture and Spirituality
Content Area: Foundations of Care: Spirituality, culture, ethnicity
Health Problem: Mental Health: Grief/Loss
Priority Concepts: Culture; Family Dynamics
Reference: Lewis et al. (2017), pp. 25, 30.

876. *Answer:* 1
Rationale: The priority nursing action is to assess the vital signs. This would provide information about the amount of blood loss that has occurred and provide a baseline by which to monitor the progress of treatment. The client may be unable to provide subjective data until the immediate physical needs are met. Although an abdominal examination and an assessment of the precipitating events may be necessary, these actions are not the priority. Insertion of a nasogastric tube is not the priority and will require a primary health care provider's prescription; in addition, the vital signs should be checked before performing this procedure.
Test-Taking Strategy: Note the strategic word, *priority,* and use the ABCs—airway, breathing, circulation. This will direct you to the correct option.
Level of Cognitive Ability: Analyzing
Client Needs: Physiological Integrity
Integrated Process: Nursing Process—Implementation

Content Area: Complex Care: Emergency Situations/Management
Health Problem: Adult Health: Gastrointestinal: Upper GI disorders
Priority Concepts: Care Coordination; Clinical Judgment
Reference: Lewis et al. (2017), p. 924.

877. *Answer:* 1
Rationale: The clinical picture of dementia ranges from mild cognitive deficits to severe, life-threatening alterations in neurological functioning. For the client to use confabulation or the fabrication of events or experiences to fill in memory gaps is not unusual. Often, lack of inhibitions on the part of the client may constitute the first indication of something being "wrong" to the client's significant others (e.g., the client may undress in front of others, or the formerly well-mannered client may exhibit slovenly table manners). As the dementia progresses, the client will have difficulty sleeping and episodes of wandering or sundowning.
Test-Taking Strategy: Focus on the client's diagnosis and note the subject, a manifestation of dementia. Think about the characteristics of dementia to direct you to the correct option.
Level of Cognitive Ability: Analyzing
Client Needs: Psychosocial Integrity
Integrated Process: Nursing Process—Assessment
Content Area: Mental Health
Health Problem: Mental Health: Neurocognitive impairment
Priority Concepts: Cognition; Coping
Reference: Ignatavicius, Workman, Rebar (2018), pp. 860-861.

878. *Answer:* 3
Rationale: Clients with anorexia nervosa have the desire to please others. Their need to be correct or perfect interferes with rational decision-making processes. These clients are moralistic. Rules and rituals help these clients manage their anxiety.
Test-Taking Strategy: Focus on the subject, managing anxiety. Eliminate options 2 and 4 because of the closed-ended word "always." Option 1 is not characteristic of a client with anorexia.
Level of Cognitive Ability: Analyzing
Client Needs: Psychosocial Integrity
Integrated Process: Nursing Process—Assessment
Content Area: Mental Health
Health Problem: Mental Health: Eating disorders
Priority Concepts: Anxiety; Coping
Reference: Lewis et al. (2017), pp. 871-872.

879. *Answer:* 3
Rationale: Iron is needed to allow for transfer of adequate iron to the fetus and to permit expansion of the maternal red blood cell mass. During pregnancy, the relative excess of plasma causes a decrease in the hemoglobin concentration and hematocrit, known as *physiological anemia of pregnancy*. This is a normal adaptation during pregnancy. Iron is best absorbed if taken on an empty stomach. Taking it with a fluid high in ascorbic acid such as tomato juice enhances absorption. Iron supplements usually cause constipation. Meats are an excellent source of iron. The client needs to take the iron supplements regardless of food intake.
Test-Taking Strategy: Note the subject, iron supplementation during pregnancy. Focus on the words *understanding of the instructions*. Knowledge of basic principles related to nutrition during pregnancy will assist in eliminating options 2 and 4. From the remaining options, remember that iron causes constipation.
Level of Cognitive Ability: Evaluating
Client Needs: Physiological Integrity
Integrated Process: Nursing Process—Evaluation
Content Area: Maternity: Antepartum
Health Problem: Adult Health: Gastrointestinal: Nutrition Problems
Priority Concepts: Client Education; Nutrition
Reference: McKinney et al. (2018), p. 266.

880. *Answer:* 3
Rationale: Levothyroxine accelerates the degradation of vitamin K–dependent clotting factors. As a result, the effects of warfarin are enhanced. If thyroid hormone replacement therapy is instituted in a client who has been taking warfarin, the dosage of warfarin should be reduced.
Test-Taking Strategy: Focus on the subject, the use of levothyroxine concurrently with warfarin. Recalling that levothyroxine enhances the effects of warfarin will direct you to the correct option.
Level of Cognitive Ability: Analyzing
Client Needs: Physiological Integrity
Integrated Process: Nursing Process—Analysis
Content Area: Pharmacology: Endocrine Medications: Thyroid hormones
Health Problem: Adult Health: Endocrine: Thyroid disorders
Priority Concepts: Collaboration; Safety
Reference: Hodgson, Kizior (2018), pp. 674-675.

881. *Answer:* 1, 2, 4
Rationale: The client should use the positions outlined in options 1, 2, and 4. These allow for maximal chest expansion. The client should not lie on the back because this reduces movement of a large area of the client's chest wall. Sitting is better than standing, whenever possible. If no chair is available, leaning against a wall while standing allows accessory muscles to be used for breathing and not posture control.
Test-Taking Strategy: Focus on the subject, the positions that could alleviate dyspnea. Remember that upright positions are best. Also, note that options 1, 2, and 4 are comparable or alike in that they all address upright positions.
Level of Cognitive Ability: Applying
Client Needs: Physiological Integrity
Integrated Process: Teaching and Learning
Content Area: Adult Health: Respiratory
Health Problem: Adult Health: Respiratory: Obstructive pulmonary disease
Priority Concepts: Client Education; Gas Exchange
Reference: Ignatavicius, Workman, Rebar (2018), pp. 546, 578.

882. *Answer:* 4
Rationale: A client undergoing lumbar puncture is positioned lying on the side, with the legs pulled up to the abdomen and the head bent down onto the chest. This position helps open the spaces between the vertebrae and allows for easier needle insertion by the primary health care provider. The nurse remains with the client during the procedure to help the client maintain this position. The other options identify incorrect positions for this procedure.

Test-Taking Strategy: Focus on the subject, lumbar puncture. Recalling that a lumbar puncture is the introduction of a needle into the subarachnoid space will direct you to the correct option. It is reasonable that the position of the client must facilitate this, and the correct option is the only position that flexes the vertebrae and widens the spaces between them.
Level of Cognitive Ability: Applying
Client Needs: Physiological Integrity
Integrated Process: Nursing Process—Implementation
Content Area: Foundations of Care: Diagnostic Tests
Health Problem: N/A
Priority Concepts: Intracranial Regulation; Safety
Reference: Ignatavicius, Workman, Rebar (2018), p. 855.

883. *Answer:* 1, 2, 5
Rationale: Maintaining effective and open communication among family members affected by death and grief is of the greatest importance. Option 1 describes encouraging discussion of feelings and is likely to enhance communication. Option 2 is also an effective intervention because spiritual practices give meaning to life and have an impact on how people react to crisis. Option 5 is also an effective technique because the client and family need to know that someone will be there who is supportive and nonjudgmental. The remaining options describe the nurse removing autonomy and decision making from the client and family, who are already experiencing feelings of loss of control in that they cannot change the process of dying. These are ineffective interventions that could impair communication further.
Test-Taking Strategy: Focus on the subject, the interventions that will facilitate effective communication. Use of therapeutic communication techniques and focusing on the subject will assist you in answering correctly. The incorrect options remove control from the client and family.
Level of Cognitive Ability: Applying
Client Needs: Psychosocial Integrity
Integrated Process: Caring
Content Area: Developmental Stages: End-of-Life Care
Health Problem: Mental Health: Grief/Loss
Priority Concepts: Caregiving; Family Dynamics
Reference: Potter et al. (2017), pp. 763-764.

884. *Answer:* 3
Rationale: Feelings of low self-esteem and worthlessness are common symptoms of a depressed client. An effective plan of care to enhance the client's personal self-esteem is to provide experiences for the client that are challenging but that will not be met with failure. Reminders of the client's past accomplishments or personal successes are ways to interrupt the client's negative self-talk and distorted cognitive view of self. Options 1 and 2 give advice and devalue the client's feelings. Silence may be interpreted as agreement.
Test-Taking Strategy: Use therapeutic communication techniques and focus on the client's diagnosis. You can eliminate options 1 and 2 easily because they are nontherapeutic. From the remaining options, focusing on the client's diagnosis will direct you to the correct option.
Level of Cognitive Ability: Applying
Client Needs: Psychosocial Integrity
Integrated Process: Nursing Process—Implementation
Content Area: Mental Health
Health Problem: Mental Health: Mood disorders
Priority Concepts: Caregiving; Mood and Affect
Reference: Varcarolis (2017), pp. 207-208.

885. *Answer:* 1, 2, 3
Rationale: Use of proper positions promotes venous drainage from the cranium to keep intracranial pressure from elevating. The head of the client at risk for or with increased intracranial pressure should be positioned so that it is in a neutral, midline position. The head of the bed should be raised to 30 to 45 degrees. The nurse should avoid flexing or extending the client's neck or turning the client's head from side to side.
Test-Taking Strategy: Focus on the subject, care of the client with increased intracranial pressure. Visualize each of the positions identified in the options and identify those that will promote venous drainage from the cranium.
Level of Cognitive Ability: Analyzing
Client Needs: Physiological Integrity
Integrated Process: Nursing Process—Implementation
Content Area: Adult Health: Neurological
Health Problem: Adult Health: Neurological: Head injury/trauma
Priority Concepts: Intracranial Regulation; Safety
Reference: Ignatavicius, Workman, Rebar (2018), p. 947.

886. *Answer:* 3
Rationale: The normal pH is 7.35 to 7.45. Normal $PaCO_2$ is 35 to 45 mm Hg. In respiratory acidosis, the pH is low and $PaCO_2$ is elevated. Options 1, 2, and 4 are incorrect interpretations of the values identified in the question.
Test-Taking Strategy: Focus on the subject, interpretation of arterial blood gas levels. Remember that in a respiratory imbalance you will find an opposite response between the pH and $PaCO_2$. Also, remember that the pH is low in an acidotic condition. Recalling this information will allow you to eliminate each of the incorrect options.
Level of Cognitive Ability: Analyzing
Client Needs: Physiological Integrity
Integrated Process: Nursing Process—Analysis
Content Area: Foundations of Care: Acid–base
Health Problem: Adult Health: Respiratory: Obstructive Pulmonary Disease
Priority Concepts: Acid–base Balance; Clinical Judgment
Reference: Lewis et al. (2017), pp. 291, 457.

887. *Answer:* 1
Rationale: The client's operative arm should be positioned so that it is elevated on a pillow and not exceeding shoulder elevation. This position promotes optimal drainage from the limb, without impairing the circulation to the arm. If the arm is positioned flat (option 2) or dependent (option 3), this could increase the edema in the arm, which is contraindicated because of lymphatic disruption caused by surgery.
Test-Taking Strategy: Focus on the subject, care of the client following mastectomy. Read each option carefully and attempt to visualize the position identified in the option. Using the principles of circulation and gravity will direct you to the correct option. The correct option avoids the two extremes of height (dependent, above shoulder level) in positioning the limb affected by surgery.
Level of Cognitive Ability: Applying
Client Needs: Physiological Integrity

Integrated Process: Nursing Process—Planning
Content Area: Adult Health: Oncology
Health Problem: Adult Health: Cancer: Breast
Priority Concepts: Perfusion; Tissue Integrity
Reference: Ignatavicius, Workman, Rebar (2018), pp. 1453-1454.

888. *Answer:* 4
Rationale: A client with a urinary tract infection must be encouraged to take the prescribed medication for the entire time it is prescribed. The client should also be instructed to drink at least 3000 mL of fluid each day to flush the infection from the bladder and to urinate frequently throughout the day. Foods and fluids that acidify the urine need to be encouraged.
Test-Taking Strategy: Note the strategic words, *need for further instruction*. These words indicate a negative event query and ask you to select an option that is incorrect. Recall that foods and fluids that acidify the urine should be consumed, rather than foods and fluids that cause urine alkalinity.
Level of Cognitive Ability: Evaluating
Client Needs: Physiological Integrity
Integrated Process: Teaching and Learning
Content Area: Maternity: Postpartum
Health Problem: Adult Health: Renal and Urinary: Inflammation/Infections
Priority Concepts: Client Education; Infection
Reference: McKinney et al. (2018), p. 611.

889. *Answer:* 3
Rationale: Humulin N is an intermediate-acting insulin. The onset of action is 60 to 120 minutes, it peaks in 6 to 14 hours, and the duration of action is 16 to 24 hours. Hypoglycemic reactions most likely occur during peak time.
Test-Taking Strategy: Focus on the subject, characteristics of Humulin N insulin, and use knowledge regarding the onset, peak, and duration of action. Recalling that it is an intermediate-acting insulin and recalling that peak action is between 6 and 14 hours will direct you to the correct option.
Level of Cognitive Ability: Applying
Client Needs: Physiological Integrity
Integrated Process: Nursing Process—Planning
Content Area: Pharmacology: Endocrine Medications: Insulin
Health Problem: Adult Health: Endocrine: Diabetes mellitus
Priority Concepts: Glucose Regulation; Safety
Reference: Lewis et al. (2017), p. 1126.

890. *Answer:* 2
Rationale: Priority nursing care in disaster situations needs to be delivered to the living and not the dead. The victim who is bleeding badly is the priority. The bleeding could be from an arterial vessel; if the bleeding is not stopped, the victim is at risk for shock and death. The pregnant client is the next priority, but the absence of fetal movement may or may not be indicative of fetal demise. The young child is with a family member and is safe at this time. The older victim will need comfort measures; there is no information indicating she is physically hurt.
Test-Taking Strategy: Note the strategic word, *first*. Use Maslow's Hierarchy of Needs theory when answering this question. Remember that physical needs should be addressed before psychosocial needs and use the ABCs—airway, breathing, and circulation. Bleeding is the priority.
Level of Cognitive Ability: Synthesizing
Client Needs: Physiological Integrity
Integrated Process: Nursing Process—Assessment
Content Area: Leadership/Management: Mass Causality Preparedness and Response
Health Problem: Adult Health: Cardiovascular: Shock
Priority Concepts: Care Coordination; Clinical Judgment
Reference: Lewis et al. (2017), pp. 1631-1632.

891. *Answer:* 3
Rationale: Rubella virus is spread by aerosol droplet transmission through the upper respiratory tract and has an incubation period of 14 to 21 days. The risks of maternal and subsequent fetal infection during the second trimester include hearing loss and congenital anomalies; these risks decrease after the first 12 weeks of pregnancy. Rubella titer determination is a standard prenatal test for pregnant women during their initial screening and entry into the health care delivery system. As noted in this client's chart, she is immune to rubella. The correct option is the only option that helps clarify maternal concerns with accurate information.
Test-Taking Strategy: Note the strategic word, *best*, and recall knowledge regarding the transmission of rubella virus to the fetus. Also, use of therapeutic communication techniques will direct you to the correct option. The correct option addresses the client's concerns.
Level of Cognitive Ability: Applying
Client Needs: Psychosocial Integrity
Integrated Process: Caring
Content Area: Maternity: Antepartum
Health Problem: Maternity: Infections/Inflammations
Priority Concepts: Immunity; Safety
Reference: Lowdermilk et al. (2016), p. 166.

892. *Answer:* 2, 3, 5
Rationale: Breast-feeding mothers with lactose-intolerant infants need to be encouraged to limit dairy products. Milk and cheese are dairy products. Alternative calcium sources that can be consumed by the mother include egg yolk, dried beans, green leafy vegetables, cauliflower, and molasses.
Test-Taking Strategy: Focus on the subject, foods acceptable for a breast-feeding mother with a lactose-intolerant infant. Recall that lactose is the sugar found in dairy products. Also note that options 1 and 4 are comparable or alike and are dairy products.
Level of Cognitive Ability: Applying
Client Needs: Physiological Integrity
Integrated Process: Teaching and Learning
Content Area: Foundations of Care: Nutrition
Health Problem: Newborn: Newborn feeding
Priority Concepts: Client Education; Nutrition
Reference: Lowdermilk et al. (2016), pp. 352–353.

893. *Answer:* 1
Rationale: The nurse needs to be aware of the effective and ineffective coping mechanisms that can occur in a client when loss is anticipated. The expression of anger is known to be a normal response to impending loss, and the anger may be directed toward the self, God or other spiritual being, or caregivers. Notifying the hospital lawyer is inappropriate. Guilt may or may not be a component of the client's feelings, and the data in the question do not indicate that guilt is present.

Test-Taking Strategy: Note the subject, psychosocial care of a client needing amputation. Also note the strategic word, *best*. Note that the correct option and option 2 address coping and defense mechanisms. This provides you with the clue that one of these options may be the correct response. In addition, knowledge of the stages of grief associated with loss will direct you to the correct option.
Level of Cognitive Ability: Analyzing
Client Needs: Psychosocial Integrity
Integrated Process: Nursing Process—Assessment
Content Area: Mental Health
Health Problem: Mental Health: Coping
Priority Concepts: Anxiety; Coping
Reference: Lewis et al. (2017), p. 133.

894. *Answer:* 3
Rationale: An autopsy is required by state law in certain circumstances, including the sudden death of a client and a death that occurs under suspicious circumstances. A client may have provided oral or written instructions regarding an autopsy after death. If an autopsy is not required by law, these oral or written requests will be granted. If no oral or written instructions were provided, state law determines who has the authority to consent for an autopsy. Most often, the decision rests with the surviving relative or next of kin.
Test-Taking Strategy: Note the strategic words, *most appropriate*. Use knowledge regarding the laws and issues surrounding autopsy and therapeutic communication techniques to answer the question. Eliminate options 2 and 4 because these statements are not completely accurate and are not therapeutic in this situation. From the remaining options, the correct option is the therapeutic and appropriate response to the family.
Level of Cognitive Ability: Applying
Client Needs: Psychosocial Integrity
Integrated Process: Caring
Content Area: Developmental Stages: End-of-Life Care
Health Problem: Mental Health: Grief/Loss
Priority Concepts: Health Care Law; Professional Identity
Reference: Potter et al. (2017), pp. 307, 765-766.

895. *Answer:* 2
Rationale: The mode of perinatal transmission of HIV to the fetus or neonate of an HIV-positive woman can occur during the prenatal, intrapartal, or postpartum period. HIV transmission can occur during breast-feeding. In the United States and most developed countries, HIV-positive clients are encouraged to bottle-feed their infants (the primary health care provider's prescription is always followed). Frequent hand washing is encouraged. Support groups and community agencies can be identified to assist the parents with the newborn infant's home care, the impact of the diagnosis of HIV infection, and available financial resources. It is recommended that infants of HIV-positive clients receive antiviral medications for the first 6 weeks of life.
Test-Taking Strategy: Note the strategic words, *need for further instruction*. These words indicate a negative event query and ask you to select an option that is incorrect. Recalling the methods of transmission of HIV and that breast-feeding is discouraged in the HIV-positive woman will direct you to the correct option.
Level of Cognitive Ability: Evaluating
Client Needs: Safe and Effective Care Environment
Integrated Process: Teaching and Learning
Content Area: Maternity: Newborn
Health Problem: Newborn: Newborn of a mother with HIV/AIDS
Priority Concepts: Client Education; Infection
Reference: McKinney et al. (2018), pp. 568-569, 940.

896. *Answer:* 4
Rationale: If the adolescent wears contact lenses, the adolescent should be instructed to discontinue wearing them until the infection has cleared completely. Obtaining new contact lenses would eliminate the chance of reinfection from contaminated contact lenses and would lessen the risk of a corneal ulceration.
Test-Taking Strategy: Note the strategic words, *need for further information*. These words indicate a negative event query and ask you to select an option that is incorrect. Options 1, 2, and 3 are comparable or alike in that they relate to avoiding the use of contact lenses during infection.
Level of Cognitive Ability: Evaluating
Client Needs: Safe and Effective Care Environment
Integrated Process: Teaching and Learning
Content Area: Pediatrics: Eye/Ear
Health Problem: Pediatric-Specific: Conjunctivitis
Priority Concepts: Client Education; Infection
Reference: McKinney et al. (2018), p. 1363.

897. *Answer:* 3
Rationale: An insulin vial in current use can be kept at room temperature for 1 month without significant loss of activity. Direct sunlight and heat must be avoided. Therefore, options 1, 2, and 4 are incorrect.
Test-Taking Strategy: Note the subject, client understanding of discharge instructions related to storage of insulin. Noting the closed-ended words "only" in option 1 and *all* in option 2 will assist you in eliminating these options. Recalling that direct sunlight and heat need to be avoided will assist you in eliminating option 4.
Level of Cognitive Ability: Evaluating
Client Needs: Physiological Integrity
Integrated Process: Nursing Process—Evaluation
Content Area: Pharmacology: Endocrine Medications: Insulin
Health Problem: Adult Health: Endocrine: Diabetes mellitus
Priority Concepts: Client Education; Glucose Regulation
Reference: Ignatavicius, Workman, Rebar (2018), p. 1297.

898. *Answer:* 4
Rationale: A trans-sphenoidal hypophysectomy is a surgical approach that uses the nasal sinuses and nose for access to the pituitary gland. Based on the location of the surgical procedure, spinal anesthesia would not be used. In addition, the hair would not be shaved. Although ambulating is important, specific to this procedure is avoiding brushing the teeth to prevent disruption of the surgical site.
Test-Taking Strategy: Focus on the subject, a preoperative instruction. Consider the anatomical location and the surgical procedure itself to eliminate options 1 and 2. Although you may be tempted to select option 3, note the location of the surgery to direct you to the correct option.
Level of Cognitive Ability: Analyzing

Client Needs: Physiological Integrity
Integrated Process: Teaching and Learning
Content Area: Adult Health: Endocrine
Health Problem: Adult Health: Endocrine: Pituitary disorders
Priority Concepts: Safety; Tissue Integrity
Reference: Ignatavicius, Workman, Rebar (2018), p. 1249.

899. *Answer:* 4
Rationale: Fresh fruits and vegetables provide vitamins and minerals needed for healthy gums. Drinking water with meals has no direct effect on gums. Cracked wheat bread may abrade the tender gums. Eating saltine crackers can also abrade the tender gums.
Test-Taking Strategy: Focus on the **subject**, dental health during pregnancy. Eliminate options 2 and 3 first because these measures could irritate fragile gums. From the remaining options, eliminate option 1 by remembering that drinking water with meals has no direct effect on gums and does not provide needed vitamins and minerals.
Level of Cognitive Ability: Evaluating
Client Needs: Physiological Integrity
Integrated Process: Nursing Process—Evaluation
Content Area: Maternity: Antepartum
Health Problem: Adult Health: Hematological: Bleeding/clotting disorders
Priority Concepts: Client Education; Nutrition
Reference: Lowdermilk et al. (2016), p. 320.

900. *Answer:* 3
Rationale: Radiation therapy is usually delayed until a child is 8 years old, whenever possible, to prevent retardation of bone growth and soft tissue development. Options 1, 2, and 4 are inappropriate responses to the mother and place the mother's question on hold.
Test-Taking Strategy: Note the **strategic word**, *best*. Also, note the **subject**, effects of radiation therapy, and the age of the child. In addition, use **therapeutic communication techniques** and knowledge regarding the effects of radiation to answer this question. Options 1, 2, and 4 are nontherapeutic and place the mother's inquiry on hold. Also use the child's age as a guide in directing you to the correct option.
Level of Cognitive Ability: Applying
Client Needs: Physiological Integrity
Integrated Process: Nursing Process—Implementation
Content Area: Pediatrics: Oncological
Health Problem: Pediatric-Specific: Cancers
Priority Concepts: Development; Safety
Reference: McKinney et al. (2018), pp. 1146-1147.

901. *Answer:* 2
Rationale: A fresh colostomy stoma would be red and edematous, but this would decrease with time. The colostomy site then becomes pink without evidence of abnormal drainage, swelling, or skin breakdown. The nurse should document these findings, because this is a normal expectation. Options 1, 3, and 4 are inappropriate and unnecessary interventions.
Test-Taking Strategy: Focus on the **subject**, postoperative colostomy assessment. Note the words *returns from surgery*. The nurse should expect redness and edema at this time.
Level of Cognitive Ability: Applying
Client Needs: Physiological Integrity
Integrated Process: Nursing Process—Implementation
Content Area: Pediatrics: Gastrointestinal
Health Problem: Pediatric-Specific: Gastrointestinal and Rectal problems
Priority Concepts: Clinical Judgment; Tissue Integrity
Reference: Perry et al. (2018), pp. 933, 938.

902. *Answer:* 3
Rationale: Low or oddly placed ears are associated with various congenital defects and should be reported immediately. Although the findings should be documented, the most appropriate action would be to notify the primary health care provider. Options 2 and 4 are inaccurate and inappropriate nursing actions.
Test-Taking Strategy: Note the **strategic words**, *most appropriate*. Focus on the **subject**, normal assessment findings in a newborn. Use knowledge regarding the normal assessment findings in a newborn infant to answer this question. Recalling that low-set ears are an abnormal finding will direct you to the correct option.
Level of Cognitive Ability: Applying
Client Needs: Physiological Integrity
Integrated Process: Nursing Process—Implementation
Content Area: Maternity: Newborn
Health Problem: Pediatric-Specific: Disorders of prenatal development
Priority Concepts: Clinical Judgment; Development
Reference: McKinney et al. (2018), p. 437.

903. *Answer:* 1
Rationale: Jaundice, if present, is best assessed in the sclera, nail beds, and mucous membranes. Generalized jaundice appears in the skin throughout the body. Option 4 is an inappropriate area to assess for the presence of jaundice.
Test-Taking Strategy: Note the **strategic word**, *best*. Options 2 and 3 can be eliminated first, because jaundice present in the skin is known as generalized jaundice. From the remaining options, recalling that skin discoloration can best be assessed in the nail beds will direct you to the correct option.
Level of Cognitive Ability: Analyzing
Client Needs: Health Promotion and Maintenance
Integrated Process: Nursing Process—Assessment
Content Area: Pediatrics: Gastrointestinal
Health Problem: Pediatric-Specific: Hepatitis
Priority Concepts: Clinical Judgment; Development
Reference: Hockenberry, Wilson, Rodgers (2017), pp. 89, 719.

904. *Answer:* 2
Rationale: To achieve proper traction, weights need to be free-hanging, with knots kept away from the pulleys. Weights should not be kept resting on a firm surface. The head of the bed is usually kept low to provide countertraction.
Test-Taking Strategy: Focus on the **subject**, care for a client in traction. Attempt to visualize the traction, recalling that there must be weight to exert the pull from the traction setup. This concept will assist in eliminating options 1 and 4. Recalling that countertraction is needed will assist in eliminating option 3.
Level of Cognitive Ability: Creating
Client Needs: Physiological Integrity
Integrated Process: Nursing Process—Planning
Content Area: Adult Health: Musculoskeletal
Health Problem: Adult Health: Musculoskeletal: Skeletal injury

Priority Concepts: Mobility; Safety
Reference: Ignatavicius, Workman, Rebar (2018), pp. 1040-1041.

905. *Answer:* 1, 2, 4
Rationale: When preparing the physical environment for an interview, the nurse should set the room temperature at a comfortable level. The nurse should provide sufficient lighting for the client and nurse to see each other. The nurse should avoid having the client face a strong light because the client would have to squint into the full light. Distracting objects and equipment should be removed from the interview area. The nurse should arrange seating so that the nurse and client are seated comfortably at eye level, and the nurse avoids facing the client across a desk or table, because this creates a barrier. The distance between the nurse and the client should be set by the nurse at 4 to 5 feet (1.2 to 1.5 meters). If the nurse places the client any closer, the nurse will be invading the client's private space and may create anxiety in the client. If the nurse places the client farther away, the nurse may be seen as distant and aloof by the client.
Test-Taking Strategy: Focus on the subject, interviewing techniques. Read each intervention carefully and think about a conducive environment. Use the guidelines for preparing the physical environment for conducting an interview to select the appropriate interventions.
Level of Cognitive Ability: Analyzing
Client Needs: Health Promotion and Maintenance
Integrated Process: Nursing Process: Planning
Content Area: Health Assessment/Physical Exam: Health History
Health Problem: N/A
Priority Concepts: Communication; Health Promotion
Reference: Jarvis (2016), pp. 29–30.

906. *Answer:* 3
Rationale: An inactive older adult may become disoriented because of lack of sensory stimulation. The most appropriate nursing intervention would be to reorient the client frequently and to place objects such as a clock and a calendar in the client's room to maintain orientation. Restraints may cause further disorientation and should not be applied unless specifically prescribed; agency policies and procedures should be followed before the application of restraints. The family can assist with orientation of the client, but it is inappropriate to ask the family to stay with the client. It is not within the scope of nursing practice to prescribe laboratory studies.
Test-Taking Strategy: Note the strategic word, *best*, and eliminate option 4 first because it is not within the realm of nursing practice to prescribe laboratory studies. Next, eliminate option 1 because restraints may add to the disorientation that the client is experiencing. It is inappropriate to place the responsibility of the client on the family, so eliminate option 2. Also, note the relationship between the words *disoriented* in the question and the implications of reorientation in the correct option.
Level of Cognitive Ability: Applying
Client Needs: Psychosocial Integrity
Integrated Process: Nursing Process—Implementation
Content Area: Adult Health: Musculoskeletal
Health Problem: Adult Health: Musculoskeletal: Skeletal injury
Priority Concepts: Cognition; Sensory Perception
Reference: Ignatavicius, Workman, Rebar (2018), pp. 26, 864-865.

907. *Answer:* 2
Rationale: Skin traction is achieved by Ace wraps, boots, or slings that apply a direct force on the client's skin. Traction is maintained with 5 to 8 lb (2.3 to 3.6 kg) of weight, and this type of traction can cause skin breakdown. Urinary incontinence is not related to the use of skin traction. Although constipation can occur as a result of immobility and monitoring bowel sounds may be a component of the assessment, this intervention is not the priority assessment. There are no pin sites with skin traction.
Test-Taking Strategy: Note the strategic word, *priority*. Eliminate option 4 first because there are no pin sites with skin traction. Visualizing the traction setup and knowledge of the complications associated with this type of traction will direct you to the correct option.
Level of Cognitive Ability: Creating
Client Needs: Physiological Integrity
Integrated Process: Nursing Process—Assessment
Content Area: Adult Health: Musculoskeletal
Health Problem: Adult Health: Musculoskeletal: Skeletal injury
Priority Concepts: Mobility; Tissue Integrity
Reference: Lewis et al. (2017), pp. 1470-1471.

908. *Answer:* 1
Rationale: A psychosocial assessment of a client who is immobilized would most appropriately include the need for sensory stimulation. This assessment should also include such factors as body image, past and present coping skills, and coping methods used during the period of immobilization. Although home care support, the ability to perform activities of daily living, and transportation are components of an assessment, they are not as specifically related to psychosocial adjustment as is the need for sensory stimulation.
Test-Taking Strategy: Focus on the strategic words, *most appropriate*, and note the subject, psychosocial adjustment. Option 3 can be eliminated first because it relates to physiological integrity rather than psychosocial integrity. Next, eliminate options 2 and 4 because they are most closely related to physical supports, rather than psychosocial needs of the client.
Level of Cognitive Ability: Applying
Client Needs: Psychosocial Integrity
Integrated Process: Nursing Process—Assessment
Content Area: Adult Health: Musculoskeletal
Health Problem: Adult Health: Musculoskeletal: Skeletal Injury
Priority Concepts: Mobility; Sensory Perception
Reference: Lewis et al. (2017), pp. 1430, 1477.

909. *Answer:* 3
Rationale: Complex scientific or medical terminology should be avoided when counseling an Amish client (or any client). When counseling a female Amish client, most often the husband and wife will want to discuss health care options together. Standing close and speaking loudly is inappropriate in most counseling situations.
Test-Taking Strategy: Use knowledge of the Amish society and therapeutic communication techniques to answer this question. Options 2 and 4 can be eliminated first because option 4 is inappropriate and option 2 is not a therapeutic intervention. In addition, note that options 2 and 3 are opposite, which may indicate that one of these options is correct. Option 1 can be eliminated because of Amish cultural habits.

Level of Cognitive Ability: Applying
Client Needs: Psychosocial Integrity
Integrated Process: Culture and Spirituality
Content Area: Foundations of Care: Spirituality, Culture, and Ethnicity
Health Problem: N/A
Priority Concepts: Communication; Culture
Reference: Lewis et al. (2017), p. 26.

910. *Answer:* 1

Rationale: Assault occurs when a person puts another person in fear of harmful or offensive contact and the victim fears and believes that harm will result from the threat. In this situation, the nurse could be accused of the tort of assault. Battery is the intentional touching of another's body without the person's consent. Slander is verbal communication that is false and harms the reputation of another. Invasion of privacy is committed when the nurse intrudes into the client's personal affairs or violates confidentiality.
Test-Taking Strategy: Note the subject, legal implications for nursing care. Focusing on the words used by the nurse and noting that the nurse threatens the client will direct you to the correct option.
Level of Cognitive Ability: Applying
Client Needs: Safe and Effective Care Environment
Integrated Process: Nursing Process—Implementation
Content Area: Leadership/Management: Ethical/Legal
Health Problem: N/A
Priority Concepts: Ethics; Health Care Law
Reference: Potter et al. (2017), p. 308.

911. *Answer:* 4

Rationale: When creating nursing assignments, the nurse needs to consider the skills and educational level of the nursing staff. Frequent temperature checks and ambulation can most appropriately be provided by the AP, considering the clients identified in each option. The client on the mechanical ventilator requiring frequent assessment and suctioning should most appropriately be cared for by the RN. The LPN is skilled in urinary catheterization, so the client in option 4 would be assigned to this staff member.
Test-Taking Strategy: Note the strategic word, *best;* focus on the subject, the principles related to delegation and assignments; and consider the education and job position as described by the Nurse Practice Act and employee guidelines. Note the word *assessment* in option 3. This should alert you that this client should be assigned to the RN. Options 1 and 2 can be eliminated because an AP can perform these tasks.
Level of Cognitive Ability: Creating
Client Needs: Safe and Effective Care Environment
Integrated Process: Nursing Process—Planning
Content Area: Leadership/Management: Delegating/Supervising
Health Problem: N/A
Priority Concepts: Care Coordination; Safety
Reference: Lewis et al. (2017), pp. 11-12.

912. *Answer:* 1

Rationale: The jaw thrust without the head tilt maneuver is used when head or neck trauma is suspected. This maneuver opens the airway while maintaining proper head and neck alignment, reducing the risk of further damage to the neck. Options 2, 3, and 4 are incorrect. In addition, it is unlikely that the nurse would be able to obtain data about the client's history.
Test-Taking Strategy: Focus on the figure and note that it is a jaw thrust maneuver. Eliminate option 2 because of the closed-ended word "all." Noting that the client requires CPR and that the figure illustrates that the client's neck remains stable will assist in eliminating options 3 and 4.
Level of Cognitive Ability: Analyzing
Client Needs: Physiological Integrity
Integrated Process: Nursing Process—Implementation
Content Area: Complex Care: Basic Life Support/Cardiopulmonary Resuscitation/Cardiac Arrest
Health Problem: N/A
Priority Concepts: Gas Exchange; Safety
Reference: Lewis et al. (2017), pp. 1630, 1650-1651.

913. *Answer:* 4

Rationale: The client needs to be instructed to avoid exposure to the sun. Because of the risk of altered skin integrity, options 1, 2, and 3 are accurate measures in the care of a client receiving external radiation therapy.
Test-Taking Strategy: Note the strategic words, *need for further instruction.* These words indicate a negative event query and ask you to select an option that is an incorrect statement. Eliminate option 1 because of the word *gently* and option 2 because of the word *loose.* From the remaining options, recalling that sun exposure is to be avoided will assist in answering the question.
Level of Cognitive Ability: Evaluating
Client Needs: Physiological Integrity
Integrated Process: Teaching and Learning
Content Area: Adult Health: Oncology
Health Problem: N/A
Priority Concepts: Client Education; Tissue Integrity
Reference: Ignatavicius, Workman, Rebar (2018), p. 390.

914. *Answer:* 1.5

Rationale: It is necessary to convert 150 mcg to mg. In the metric system, to convert smaller to larger, divide by 1000 or move the decimal 3 places to the left: 150 mcg = 0.15 mg. Next, use the formula to calculate the correct dose.
Formula:

$$\frac{\text{Desired}}{\text{Available}} \times \text{Quantity} = \text{tablet(s)}$$

$$\frac{0.15\,\text{mg}}{0.1\,\text{mg}} \times 1\ \text{tablet} = 1.5\ \text{tablets}$$

Test-Taking Strategy: Focus on the subject, a medication calculation problem. In this medication calculation problem, it is necessary first to convert micrograms to milligrams. Next, use the formula to calculate the correct dose. Recheck your work using a calculator, and make sure that the answer makes sense.
Level of Cognitive Ability: Applying
Client Needs: Physiological Integrity
Integrated Process: Nursing Process—Implementation
Content Area: Skills: Dosage Calculations
Health Problem: Adult Health: Endocrine: Thyroid Disorders

Priority Concepts: Clinical Judgment; Safety
Reference: Potter et al. (2017), pp. 327-329.

915. *Answer:* 4
Rationale: The most common side effect of metformin is gastrointestinal disturbances, including decreased appetite, nausea, and diarrhea. These generally subside over time. This medication does not cause weight gain; clients lose an average of 7 to 8 lb (3.2 to 3.6 kg) because the medication causes nausea and decreased appetite. Although hypoglycemia can occur, it is not the most common side effect. Flushing and palpitations are not specifically associated with this medication.
Test-Taking Strategy: Note the strategic word, *most*. To answer correctly, it is necessary to recall that the most common side effect of metformin is gastrointestinal disturbances.
Level of Cognitive Ability: Applying
Client Needs: Physiological Integrity
Integrated Process: Teaching and Learning
Content Area: Pharmacology: Endocrine Medications: Oral hypoglycemics
Health Problem: Adult Health: Endocrine: Diabetes mellitus
Priority Concepts: Client Education; Glucose Regulation
Reference: Hodgson, Kizior (2018), p. 734.

916. *Answer:* 1, 3, 5, 6
Rationale: During a seizure, the nurse should stay with the child to reduce the risk of injury and allow for observation and timing of the seizure. The child is not restrained, because this could cause injury to the child. The child is placed on his or her side in a lateral position. Nothing is placed in the child's mouth during a seizure because this could injure the child's mouth, gums, or teeth. Positioning on the side prevents aspiration, because saliva drains out of the corner of the child's mouth. The nurse should loosen clothing around the child's neck and ensure a patent airway.
Test-Taking Strategy: Focus on the subject, care of the child experiencing seizures, and visualize this clinical situation. Recalling that airway patency and safety are the priorities will assist in determining the correct interventions.
Level of Cognitive Ability: Analyzing
Client Needs: Physiological Integrity
Integrated Process: Nursing Process—Implementation
Content Area: Pediatrics: Neurological
Health Problem: Pediatric-Specific: Seizures
Priority Concepts: Intracranial Regulation; Safety
Reference: McKinney et al. (2018), pp. 1299, 1301.

917. *Answer:* 1, 2, 3
Rationale: Nocturia, incontinence, and an enlarged prostate are characteristics of BPH and need to be assessed for in all male clients over 50 years of age. Nocturnal emissions are commonly associated with prepubescent males. Low testosterone levels (not BPH) may be associated with a decreased desire for sexual intercourse.
Test-Taking Strategy: Focus on the subject, characteristics of BPH. Thinking about the pathophysiology associated with this disorder will assist you in answering correctly.
Level of Cognitive Ability: Analyzing
Client Needs: Physiological Integrity
Integrated Process: Nursing Process—Assessment
Content Area: Adult Health: Renal and Urinary
Health Problem: Adult Health: Renal and Urinary: Obstructive problems
Priority Concepts: Clinical Judgment; Elimination
Reference: Lewis et al. (2017), p. 1269.

918. *Answer:* 1
Rationale: Setting priorities means deciding which client needs or problems require immediate action and which can be delayed until a later time because they are not urgent. Client problems that involve actual or life-threatening concerns are always considered first. Although completing care in a reasonable time frame, time constraints, and obtaining needed supplies are components of time management, these items are not the priority in planning care for the client, based on the options provided.
Test-Taking Strategy: Note the strategic word, *priority*. Recall the principles related to prioritizing to answer the question. Noting the words *life-threatening* in the correct option will assist in directing you to this option.
Level of Cognitive Ability: Evaluating
Client Needs: Safe and Effective Care Environment
Integrated Process: Teaching and Learning
Content Area: Leadership/Management: Prioritizing
Health Problem: N/A
Priority Concepts: Care Coordination; Clinical Judgment
Reference: Potter et al. (2017), pp. 241, 284-285.

919. *Answer:* 4
Rationale: Laboratory determinations of the serum thyroid-stimulating hormone (TSH) level are an important means of evaluation. Successful therapy causes elevated TSH levels to decline. These levels begin their decline within hours of the onset of therapy and continue to decrease as plasma levels of thyroid hormone build up. If an adequate dosage is administered, TSH levels remain suppressed for the duration of therapy. Although energy levels may increase and the client's mood may improve following effective treatment, these are not noted until normal thyroid hormone levels are achieved with medication therapy. An increase in the blood glucose level is not associated with this condition.
Test-Taking Strategy: Focus on the subject, therapeutic effects of this medication. Note the words *expected outcome*. Relate the diagnosis of hypothyroidism with thyroid hormone levels in the correct option.
Level of Cognitive Ability: Evaluation
Client Needs: Physiological Integrity
Integrated Process: Nursing Process—Evaluation
Content Area: Pharmacology: Endocrine Medications: Thyroid hormones
Health Problem: Adult Health: Endocrine: Thyroid disorders
Priority Concepts: Cellular Regulation; Evidence
Reference: Lewis et al. (2017), pp. 1168-1169.

920. *Answer:* 2, 4, 5, 6
Rationale: Risk factors for breast cancer include nulliparity or first child born after age 30 years; early menarche; late menopause; family history of breast cancer; high-dose radiation exposure to the chest; and previous cancer of the breast, uterus, or ovaries. In addition, specific inherited mutations in BReast CAncer (*BRCA*)*1* and *BRCA2* increase the risk of female breast

cancer; these mutations are also associated with an increased risk for ovarian cancer.
Test-Taking Strategy: Focus on the subject, the risk factors associated with breast cancer. Thinking about the physiology associated with the reproductive system and the most common causes of cancer will assist in answering the question.
Level of Cognitive Ability: Analyzing
Client Needs: Health Promotion and Maintenance
Integrated Process: Nursing Process—Assessment
Content Area: Adult Health: Oncology
Health Problem: Adult Health: Cancer: Breast
Priority Concepts: Cellular Regulation; Client Education
Reference: Ignatavicius, Workman, Rebar (2018), p. 1442.

921. *Answer:* 1
Rationale: An inflammatory reaction such as acute pancreatitis can cause paralytic ileus, the most common form of nonmechanical obstruction. Inability to pass flatus is a clinical manifestation of paralytic ileus. Loss of sphincter control is not a sign of paralytic ileus. Pain is associated with paralytic ileus, but the pain usually manifests as a more constant generalized discomfort. Option 4 is the description of the physical finding of liver enlargement. The liver may be enlarged in cases of cirrhosis or hepatitis. Although this client may have an enlarged liver, an enlarged liver is not a sign of paralytic ileus or intestinal obstruction.
Test-Taking Strategy: Focus on the subject, clinical manifestations of paralytic ileus. Noting the word *paralytic* will assist in directing you to the correct option.
Level of Cognitive Ability: Analyzing
Client Needs: Physiological Integrity
Integrated Process: Nursing Process—Assessment
Content Area: Adult Health: Gastrointestinal
Health Problem: Adult Health: Gastrointestinal: GI Accessory organs
Priority Concepts: Elimination; Inflammation
Reference: Lewis et al. (2017), pp. 950-951.

922. *Answer:* 1
Rationale: For the first 12 hours after gastric surgery, the nasogastric tube drainage may be dark brown to dark red. Later, the drainage should change to a light yellowish-brown color. The presence of bile may cause a green tinge. The PHCP should be notified if dark red drainage, a sign of hemorrhage, is noted 24 hours postoperatively.
Test-Taking Strategy: Focus on the subject, the need to notify the PHCP. Recall that bleeding is a concern in the postoperative client. This concept will direct you to the correct option.
Level of Cognitive Ability: Analyzing
Client Needs: Physiological Integrity
Integrated Process: Nursing Process—Analysis
Content Area: Adult Health: Gastrointestinal
Health Problem: Adult Health: Gastrointestinal: Upper GI Disorders
Priority Concepts: Clinical Judgment; Collaboration
Reference: Lewis et al. (2017), p. 344.

923. *Answer:* 1
Rationale: The client should take a deep breath, because the client's airway will be temporarily obstructed during tube removal. The client is then told to hold the breath and the tube is withdrawn slowly and evenly over the course of 3 to 6 seconds (coil the tube around the hand while removing it) while the breath is held. Bearing down could inhibit the removal of the tube. Exhaling is not possible during removal because the airway is temporarily obstructed during removal. Breathing normally could result in aspiration of gastric secretions during inhalation.
Test-Taking Strategy: Focus on the subject, the procedure for removal of a nasogastric tube, and attempt to visualize the process of tube removal to direct you to the correct option. Remember, holding the breath facilitates the process of removal.
Level of Cognitive Ability: Applying
Client Needs: Physiological Integrity
Integrated Process: Nursing Process—Implementation
Content Area: Skills: Tube Care
Health Problem: N/A
Priority Concepts: Gas Exchange; Safety
Reference: Potter et al. (2017), p. 1178.

924. *Answer:* 3
Rationale: When a client is experiencing respiratory acidosis, the respiratory rate and depth increase in an attempt to compensate. The client also experiences headache; restlessness; mental status changes, such as drowsiness and confusion; visual disturbances; diaphoresis; cyanosis as the hypoxia becomes more acute; hyperkalemia; rapid, irregular pulse; and dysrhythmias. Options 1, 2, and 4 are not specifically associated with this disorder.
Test-Taking Strategy: Focus on the subject, clinical manifestations associated with respiratory acidosis, and use knowledge of the signs and symptoms of respiratory acidosis to answer this question. Eliminate options 2 and 4 first because they are comparable or alike and address a decreased respiratory rate. Remember that headache, restlessness, and confusion occur in respiratory acidosis.
Level of Cognitive Ability: Analyzing
Client Needs: Physiological Integrity
Integrated Process: Nursing Process—Assessment
Content Area: Foundations of Care: Acid–Base
Health Problem: Adult Health: Respiratory: Obstructive Pulmonary Disease
Priority Concepts: Acid–Base Balance; Clinical Judgment
Reference: Ignatavicius, Workman, Rebar (2018), pp. 192-193.

925. *Answer:* 4
Rationale: Distention, vomiting, and abdominal pain are a few of the symptoms associated with intestinal obstruction. Nasogastric tubes may be used to remove gas and fluid from the stomach, relieving distention and vomiting. Bowel sounds return to normal as the obstruction is resolved and normal bowel function is restored. Discontinuing the nasogastric tube before normal bowel function may result in a return of the symptoms, necessitating reinsertion of the nasogastric tube. Serum electrolyte levels, pH of the gastric aspirate, and tube placement are important assessments for the client with a nasogastric tube in place but would not assist in determining the readiness for removing the nasogastric tube.
Test-Taking Strategy: Eliminate options 2 and 3 first because they are comparable or alike. Assessing the pH of the gastric

aspirate is one method of assessing tube placement. Also, note the strategic word, *priority*. Focus on the client's diagnosis to direct you to the correct option.
Level of Cognitive Ability: Analyzing
Client Needs: Physiological Integrity
Integrated Process: Nursing Process—Assessment
Content Area: Adult Health: Gastrointestinal
Health Problem: Adult Health: Gastrointestinal: Lower GI disorders
Priority Concepts: Clinical Judgment; Safety
Reference: Potter et al. (2017), pp. 1177-1178.

926. *Answer:* 1
Rationale: The enema is never administered while on a toilet due to safety. The enema is administered while the client is in a left side-lying (Sims') position with the right knee flexed. This allows enema solution to flow downward by gravity along the natural curve of the sigmoid colon and rectum. It is important for the client to retain the fluid for as long as possible to promote peristalsis and defecation. If the client complains of fullness or pain, the flow is stopped for 30 seconds and restarted at a slower rate. The higher the solution container is held above the rectum, the faster the flow and the greater the force in the rectum; this could increase cramping.
Test-Taking Strategy: Note the strategic words, *need for further instruction*. This indicates a negative event query, and the need to select the option that is incorrect. Eliminate options 3 and 4 first because they are comparable or alike. From the remaining options, focusing on the subject, safety, will direct you to the correct option.
Level of Cognitive Ability: Evaluating
Client Needs: Physiological Integrity
Integrated Process: Teaching and Learning
Content Area: Skills: Elimination
Health Problem: N/A
Priority Concepts: Client Education; Elimination
Reference: Potter et al. (2017), pp. 1165, 1170-1171.

927. *Answer:* 4
Rationale: Negative reinforcement when the stimulus is produced is descriptive of aversion therapy. Options 1, 2, and 3 are characteristics of self-control therapy.
Test-Taking Strategy: Note the strategic words, *need for further teaching*. These words indicate a negative event query and ask you to select an option that is incorrect. Think about the subject, self-control. This subject will assist you in answering correctly.
Level of Cognitive Ability: Evaluating
Client Needs: Psychosocial Integrity
Integrated Process: Teaching and Learning
Content Area: Mental Health
Health Problem: Mental Health: Coping
Priority Concepts: Anxiety; Stress
Reference: Varcarolis (2017), p. 23.

928. *Answer:* 2, 4,5, 6
Rationale: The nurse should teach the client how to care for the stoma, depending on the type of laryngectomy performed. Most interventions focus on protection of the stoma and the prevention of infection. Interventions include obtaining a MedicAlert bracelet, preventing debris from entering the stoma, avoiding exposure to people with infections, and avoiding swimming and using care when showering. Additional interventions include wearing a stoma guard or high-collared clothing to protect the stoma, increasing the humidity in the home, and increasing fluid intake to 3000 mL/day to keep the secretions thin.
Test-Taking Strategy: Focus on the subject, client instructions regarding stoma care. Recalling that most interventions focus on protection of the stoma and the prevention of infection will assist in identifying the client instructions for home care.
Level of Cognitive Ability: Analyzing
Client Needs: Physiological Integrity
Integrated Process: Teaching and Learning
Content Area: Adult Health: Oncology
Health Problem: Adult Health: Cancer: Laryngeal and lung
Priority Concepts: Client Education; Gas Exchange
Reference: Lewis et al. (2017), p. 495.

929. *Answer:* 21
Rationale: Use the intravenous flow rate formula.
Formula:

$$\frac{\text{Total volume prescribed} \times \text{Drop factor}}{\text{Time in minutes}} = \text{gtt / minute}$$

$$\frac{2000\text{ mL} \times 15\text{ gtt / mL}}{1440\text{ minutes}} = 20.8\text{ gtt / minute} = 21\text{ gtt / minute}$$

Test-Taking Strategy: Focus on the subject, a medication calculation. Use the formula for calculating intravenous flow rates when answering the question. Verify the answer using a calculator, and be sure to round the answer to the nearest whole number.
Level of Cognitive Ability: Applying
Client Needs: Physiological Integrity
Integrated Process: Nursing Process—Implementation
Content Area: Skills: Dosage Calculations
Health Problems: N/A
Priority Concepts: Clinical Judgment; Safety
Reference: Potter et al. (2017), pp. 978-979.

930. *Answer:* 2
Rationale: In the first few hours after surgery, the drainage from the chest tube is bloody. After several hours, it becomes serosanguineous. The client should not experience frequent clotting. Proper chest tube function should allow for drainage of blood before it has the chance to clot in the chest or the tubing.
Test-Taking Strategy: Focus on the subject, expected findings after thoracic surgery. Recall that after thoracic surgery, there may be considerable capillary oozing for hours in the postoperative period. This will lead you to choose the bloody drainage option over the serous or serosanguineous drainage options. Knowing that patent chest tubes do not allow blood to collect in the pleural space eliminates the option of blood with clots.
Level of Cognitive Ability: Analyzing
Client Needs: Physiological Integrity
Integrated Process: Nursing Process—Assessment
Content Area: Adult Health: Respiratory
Health Problem: N/A
Priority Concepts: Clinical Judgment; Gas Exchange
Reference: Lewis et al. (2017), pp. 524-525.

931. *Answer:* 1, 2, 3, 5

Rationale: If the client begins to hemorrhage from the surgical site after radical neck dissection, the nurse elevates the head of the bed to maintain airway patency and prevent aspiration. The nurse applies pressure over the bleeding site and calls the surgeon immediately. The nurse also monitors the client's airway and vital signs.

Test-Taking Strategy: Focus on the subject, nursing actions for hemorrhage, and on the client situation. Use the ABCs—airway, breathing, and circulation—to assist you in answering the question. Note that lowering the head of the bed to a flat position increases the client's risk for aspiration.

Level of Cognitive Ability: Analyzing
Client Needs: Physiological Integrity
Integrated Process: Nursing Process—Implementation
Content Area: Complex Care: Emergency Situations/Management
Health Problem: Adult Health: Cancer: Laryngeal and lung
Priority Concepts: Clinical Judgment; Gas Exchange
Reference: Lewis et al. (2017), pp. 494-495.

932. *Answer:* 2

Rationale: To prevent transmission of hepatitis, vaccination of the partner is advised. In addition, a condom is advised during sexual intercourse. Alcohol should be avoided because it is detoxified in the liver and may interfere with recovery. Rest is especially important until laboratory studies show that liver function has returned to normal. The client's activity is increased gradually, and the client should not return to work right away.

Test-Taking Strategy: Focus on the strategic words, *need for further teaching*. These words indicate a negative event query and ask you to select an option that is incorrect. Think about the pathophysiology associated with hepatitis to direct you to the incorrect client statement. Remember that rest is needed for the liver to heal.

Level of Cognitive Ability: Evaluating
Client Needs: Physiological Integrity
Integrated Process: Teaching and Learning
Content Area: Adult Health: Gastrointestinal
Health Problem: Adult Health: Gastrointestinal: GI Accessory organs
Priority Concepts: Client Education; Infection
Reference: Ignatavicius, Workman, Rebar (2018), pp. 1182-1183.

933. *Answer:* 3, 4, 6

Rationale: The clinical manifestations of hypothyroidism are the result of decreased metabolism from low levels of thyroid hormone. Interventions are aimed at replacement of the hormone and providing measures to support the signs and symptoms related to decreased metabolism. The client often has cold intolerance and requires a warm environment. The nurse encourages the client to consume a well-balanced diet that is low in fat for weight reduction and high in fluids and high-fiber foods to prevent constipation. Iodine preparations may be used to treat hyperthyroidism. Iodine preparations decrease blood flow through the thyroid gland and reduce the production and release of thyroid hormone; they are not used to treat hypothyroidism. The client is instructed to notify the PHCP if chest pain occurs because it could be an indication of over-replacement of thyroid hormone.

Test-Taking Strategy: Focus on the subject, hypothyroidism. Recalling the manifestations of this disorder and that in this disorder the client has a decreased metabolic rate will assist in determining the appropriate interventions.

Level of Cognitive Ability: Analyzing
Client Needs: Physiological Integrity
Integrated Process: Nursing Process—Implementation
Content Area: Adult Health: Endocrine
Health Problem: Adult Health: Endocrine: Thyroid disorders
Priority Concepts: Caregiving; Thermoregulation
Reference: Lewis et al. (2017), pp. 1168-1169.

934. *Answer:* 1

Rationale: Plugging a tracheostomy tube is usually done by inserting the tracheostomy plug (decannulation stopper) into the opening of the outer cannula. This closes off the tracheostomy, and airflow and respiration occur normally through the nose and mouth. When plugging a cuffed tracheostomy tube, the cuff must be deflated. If it remains inflated, ventilation cannot occur, and respiratory arrest could result. A tracheostomy plug could not be placed in a tracheostomy if an inner cannula was in place. The ability to swallow or speak is unrelated to weaning and plugging the tube.

Test-Taking Strategy: Focus on the subject, care of the client with a tracheostomy, and note the word *required* in the question. Think about the structure and function of a tracheostomy tube. Recalling that an inflated cuff would cause airway obstruction will assist in directing you to the option that addresses a priority physiological need.

Level of Cognitive Ability: Analyzing
Client Needs: Physiological Integrity
Integrated Process: Nursing Process—Implementation
Content Area: Skills: Tube care
Health Problem: N/A
Priority Concepts: Gas Exchange; Safety
Reference: Lewis et al. (2017), pp. 487-488.

935. *Answer:* 1

Rationale: Hypertension, cardiovascular disease, diabetes mellitus, and obesity are associated with the development of glaucoma. Options 2, 3, and 4 do not identify risk factors associated with this eye disorder.

Test-Taking Strategy: Focus on the subject, a risk factor associated with glaucoma. Recall that glaucoma is associated with increased pressure in the eye. This will assist to direct you to the correct option.

Level of Cognitive Ability: Analyzing
Client Needs: Physiological Integrity
Integrated Process: Nursing Process—Assessment
Content Area: Adult Health: Eye
Health Problem: Adult Health: Eye: Glaucoma
Priority Concepts: Health Promotion; Sensory Perception
Reference: Ignatavicius, Workman, Rebar (2018), p. 972.

936. *Answer:* 4

Rationale: The nurse places an eye patch over the client's affected eye to reduce eye movement. Some clients may need bilateral patching. Depending on the location and size of the retinal break, activity restrictions may be needed immediately. These restrictions are necessary to prevent further tearing or detachment and to promote drainage of any subretinal fluid.

Therefore, reading and watching television are not allowed. The client's position is prescribed by the primary health care provider; normally, the prescription is to lie flat.
Test-Taking Strategy: Focus on the subject, retinal detachment. Remember that the eye needs to be protected and rested. This should direct you to the correct option.
Level of Cognitive Ability: Analyzing
Client Needs: Physiological Integrity
Integrated Process: Nursing Process—Planning
Content Area: Adult Health: Eye
Health Problem: Adult Health: Eye: Retinal detachment
Priority Concepts: Sensory Perception; Safety
Reference: Ignatavicius, Workman, Rebar (2018), p. 980.

937. *Answer:* 3
Rationale: Clients at greatest risk for deep vein thrombosis and pulmonary emboli are immobilized clients. Basic preventive measures include early ambulation, leg elevation, active leg exercises, elastic stockings, and intermittent pneumatic calf compression. Keeping the client well hydrated is essential because dehydration predisposes to clotting. A pillow under the knees may cause venous stasis. Heat should not be applied without a primary health care provider's prescription.
Test-Taking Strategy: Note the strategic word, *most.* Focus on the subject, measures to prevent deep vein thrombosis and pulmonary emboli. Use basic principles related to the care of the immobile client to answer this question.
Level of Cognitive Ability: Creating
Client Needs: Physiological Integrity
Integrated Process: Nursing Process—Planning
Content Area: Adult Health: Cardiovascular
Health Problem: Adult Health: Cardiovascular: Vascular disorders
Priority Concepts: Clinical Judgment; Clotting
Reference: Ignatavicius, Workman, Rebar (2018), p. 742.

938. *Answer:* 1
Rationale: A crisis is an acute, time-limited state of disequilibrium resulting from situational, developmental, or societal sources of stress. A person in this state is temporarily unable to cope with or adapt to the stressor by using previous coping mechanisms. The person who intervenes in this situation (the nurse) "takes over" for the client (authority) who is not in control and devises a plan (action) to secure and maintain the client's safety. When this has occurred, the nurse works collaboratively with the client (participates) in developing new coping and problem-solving strategies.
Test-Taking Strategy: Note the strategic word, *priority.* A client who experiences a suicidal crisis is in a state of acute disequilibrium. Remember that in a crisis an authority figure must emerge to take action.
Level of Cognitive Ability: Applying
Client Needs: Psychosocial Integrity
Integrated Process: Nursing Process—Implementation
Content Area: Mental Health
Health Problem: Mental Health: Suicide
Priority Concepts: Mood and Affect; Safety
Reference: Varcarolis (2017), pp. 367, 369.

939. *Answer:* 2
Rationale: The client with tuberculosis must have sputum cultures performed every 2 to 4 weeks after initiation of antituberculosis medication therapy. The client may return to work when the results of three sputum cultures are negative, because the client is considered noninfectious at that point. Options 1, 3, and 4 are not reliable determinants of a noninfectious status.
Test-Taking Strategy: Focus on the subject, concepts related to tuberculosis. Knowing that a positive tuberculin skin test never reverts to negative helps you eliminate option 4. From the remaining options, think about the mode of transmission of tuberculosis to direct you to the correct option. Remember, three negative sputum cultures are required.
Level of Cognitive Ability: Applying
Client Needs: Safe and Effective Care Environment
Integrated Process: Teaching and Learning
Content Area: Foundations of Care: Infection Control
Health Problem: Adult Health: Respiratory: Tuberculosis
Priority Concepts: Infection; Safety
Reference: Ignatavicius, Workman, Rebar (2018), p. 609.

940. *Answer:* 3
Rationale: This client is in a severe state of anxiety. When a client is in a severe or panic state of anxiety, it is crucial for the nurse to remain with the client. The client in a severe state of anxiety would be unable to learn relaxation techniques. Discussing the assault at this point would increase the client's level of anxiety further. Placing the client in a quiet room alone may also increase the anxiety level.
Test-Taking Strategy: Note the strategic word, *priority.* The priority action in this situation is to remain with the client.
Level of Cognitive Ability: Applying
Client Needs: Safe and Effective Care Environment
Integrated Process: Nursing Process—Implementation
Content Area: Mental Health
Health Problem: Mental Health: Anxiety disorder
Priority Concepts: Anxiety; Caregiving
Reference: Varcarolis (2017), p. 134.

941. *Answer:* 2
Rationale: Laboratory findings do not establish the diagnosis of appendicitis, but there is often an elevation of the white blood cell count (leukocytosis) with a shift to the left (an increased number of immature white blood cells). Options 1, 3, and 4 are incorrect because they are not associated findings in acute appendicitis.
Test-Taking Strategy: Focus on the subject, appendicitis. Knowledge that an inflammatory process causes an increase in the white blood cell count will assist you in eliminating options 1 and 3. From the remaining options, it is necessary to understand the significance of a shift to the left.
Level of Cognitive Ability: Analyzing
Client Needs: Physiological Integrity
Integrated Process: Nursing Process—Assessment
Content Area: Adult Health: Gastrointestinal
Health Problem: Adult Health: Gastrointestinal: GI Accessory organs
Priority Concepts: Cellular Regulation; Inflammation
Reference: Ignatavicius, Workman, Rebar (2018), pp. 1147-1148.

942. *Answer:* 3
Rationale: Lack of ability to cope effectively may be evidenced by a client's inability to meet basic needs, inability to meet

role expectations, alteration in social participation, use of inappropriate defense mechanisms, or impairment of usual patterns of communication. Anxiety is a broad description and can occur as a result of many triggers; although the client was experiencing anxiety, the client's concern now is the ability to meet role expectations and financial obligations. There is no information in the question that indicates an unrealistic outlook or disturbances in thoughts and ideas.
Test-Taking Strategy: Note the strategic word, *priority.* Focus on the subject, concerns regarding the ability to meet role expectations and financial obligations. Option 1 can be eliminated because the client was previously experiencing anxiety. Eliminate options 2 and 4 because there are no data in the question that address these problems.
Level of Cognitive Ability: Creating
Client Needs: Psychosocial Integrity
Integrated Process: Nursing Process—Planning
Content Area: Mental Health
Health Problem: Mental Health: Anxiety disorders
Priority Concepts: Anxiety; Coping
Reference: Varcarolis (2017), pp. 142-143.

943. *Answer:* 2
Rationale: Bubbling in the water seal chamber is caused by air passing out of the pleural space into the fluid in the chamber. Intermittent (not constant) bubbling is normal. It indicates that the system is accomplishing one of its purposes, removing air from the pleural space. Continuous bubbling during inspiration and expiration indicates that an air leak exists. If this occurs, it must be corrected. Notifying the primary health care provider and changing the chest tube drainage system are not indicated at this time.
Test-Taking Strategy: Note the strategic words, *most appropriate.* Note the subject, chest tube drainage systems, and focus on the words *intermittent bubbling* and *water seal chamber*. Recalling that intermittent (not constant) bubbling is normal in this chamber will direct you to the correct option.
Level of Cognitive Ability: Applying
Client Needs: Physiological Integrity
Integrated Process: Nursing Process—Implementation
Content Area: Skills: Tube care
Health Problem: N/A
Priority Concepts: Clinical Judgment; Gas Exchange
Reference: Lewis et al. (2017), p. 525.

944. *Answer:* 1
Rationale: Although frequency and intensity of bowel sounds vary depending on the phase of digestion, normal bowel sounds are relatively high-pitched clicks or gurgles. Loud gurgles (borborygmi) indicate hyperperistalsis and are commonly associated with nausea and vomiting. A swishing or buzzing sound represents turbulent blood flow associated with a bruit. Bruits are not normal sounds. Bowel sounds are very high-pitched and loud (hyper-resonance) when the intestines are under tension, such as in intestinal obstruction. Therefore, options 2, 3, and 4 are incorrect.
Test-Taking Strategy: Note the subject, techniques for abdominal assessment. Normally, bowel sounds are audible in all four quadrants, so options 2 and 4 can be eliminated. From the remaining options, focus on the data in the question and note that the client has nausea and vomiting; this will direct you to the correct option.
Level of Cognitive Ability: Analyzing
Client Needs: Physiological Integrity
Integrated Process: Nursing Process—Assessment
Content Area: Health Assessment/Physical Exam: Abdomen
Health Problem: Adult Health: Gastrointestinal: Upper GI disorders
Priority Concepts: Elimination; Health Promotion
Reference: Jarvis (2016), pp. 548–549, 572.

945. *Answer:* 20
Rationale: Use the medication calculation formula.
Formula:

$$\frac{\text{Prescribed}}{\text{Available}} \times \text{Quantity} = \text{mL / dose}$$

$$\frac{800\text{ mg}}{200\text{ mg}} \times 5\text{ mL} = 20\text{ mL}$$

Test-Taking Strategy: Note the subject, medication calculations. Review the label for the correct reconstitution, which states 200 mg in 5 mL. Calculate the prescribed number of milligrams per milliliter. Use a calculator to verify the answer and make sure that the answer makes sense.
Level of Cognitive Ability: Applying
Client Needs: Physiological Integrity
Integrated Process: Nursing Process—Implementation
Content Area: Skills: Dosage Calculations
Health Problem: N/A
Priority Concepts: Clinical Judgment; Safety
Reference: Potter et al. (2017), pp. 978-979.

References

American Academy of Dermatology Association (n.d.). *Isotretinoin: Treatment for acne.* Retrieved from https://www.aad.org/public/diseases/acne-and-rosacea/isotretinoin-treatment-for-severe-acne

American Academy of Pediatrics. (n.d.). *Healthy foster care America.* Retrieved from https://www.aap.org/en-us/advocacy-and-policy/aap-health-initiatives/healthy-foster-care-america/Documents/HFCAJudgesToolkit.pdf

American Academy of Pediatrics. (2014). *Policy statement: Screening for nonviral sexually transmitted infections in adolescents and young adults.* Retrieved from http://pediatrics.aappublications.org/content/early/2014/06/25/peds.2014-1024.

American Cancer Society. (2014). *Signs and symptoms of cancer.* Retrieved from https://www.cancer.org/cancer/cancer-basics/signs-and-symptoms-of-cancer.html.

American Cancer Society. (2015). *Tools to help measure distress.* Retrieved from https://www.cancer.org/treatment/treatments-and-side-effects/emotional-side-effects/distress/tools-to-measure-distress.html.

American College of Rheumatology. (2017). *Juvenile Arthritis: Fast Facts.* Retrieved from https://www.rheumatology.org/I-Am-A/Patient-Caregiver/Diseases-Conditions/Juvenile-Arthritis.

American Heart Association. (2017). *Highlights of the 2017 American Heart Association focused updated on adult and pediatric basic life support and cardiopulmonary pulmonary quality.* Retrieved from https://eccguidelines.heart.org/wp-content/uploads/2017/11/2017-Focused-Updates_Highlights.pdf.

American Nurses Association (n.d.) *Code of Ethics for Nurses.* Retrieved from https://www.nursingworld.org/practice-policy/nursing-excellence/ethics/.

American Nurses Association (n.d.). Social networking privacy toolkit. Retrieved from https://www.nursingworld.org/practice-policy/nursing-excellence/social-networking-Principles/

Ard, K. L. (n.d.). *Improving the health care of lesbian, gay, bisexual, and transgender people: Understanding and eliminating health disparities.* Retrieved from https://www.lgbthealtheducation.org/wp-content/uploads/Improving-the-Health-of-LGBT-People.pdf.

Benjamin, R. M. (2010). Multiple chronic conditions: A public health challenge. *Public Health Repository, 125*(5), 626–627.

Bohn, D. K., & Holz, K. A. (1996). Sequelae of abuse: Health effects of childhood sexual abuse, domestic battering, and rape. *Journal of Midwifery & Women's Health, 41*(6), 442–456.

Burchum, J., & Rosenthal, L. (2016). *Lehne's pharmacology for nursing care* (9th ed.). St. Louis: Elsevier.

Campinha-Bacote, C. (1999). A model and instrument for addressing cultural competence in health care. *Journal of Nursing Education, 38*(5), 203–207.

Centers for Disease Control and Prevention. (2019). *Conjunctivitis (Pink Eye).* Retrieved from https://www.cdc.gov/conjunctivitis/index.html.

Centers for Disease Control and Prevention. (2018). *Ebola (Ebola Virus Disease).* Retrieved from https://www.cdc.gov/vhf/ebola/index.html.

Centers for Disease Control and Prevention. (2018). *Guidance on personal protective equipment (PPE) to be used by healthcare workers during management of patients with confirmed ebola or persons under investigation (PUIs) for Ebola who are clinically unstable or have bleeding, vomiting, or diarrhea in U.S. hospitals, including procedures for donning and doffing PPE.* Retrieved from https://www.cdc.gov/vhf/ebola/healthcare-us/ppe/guidance.html.

Centers for Disease Control and Prevention. (2018). *Hand hygiene in healthcare settings.* Retrieved from https://www.cdc.gov/handhygiene/.

Centers for Disease Control and Prevention. (2016). *Identify, isolate, inform: Emergency department evaluation and management for patients under investigation (PUIs) for Ebola Virus Disease (EVD).* Retrieved from https://www.cdc.gov/vhf/ebola/clinicians/emergency-services/emergency-departments.html.

Centers for Disease Control and Prevention. (2018). *Interim guidance for environmental infection control in hospitals for Ebola virus.* Retrieved from https://www.cdc.gov/vhf/ebola/clinicians/cleaning/hospitals.html.

De Hert, M., Correll, C. U., Bobes, J., & Leucht, S. (2011). Physical illness in patients with severe mental disorders. Prevalence, impact of medications and disparities in healthcare. *World Psychiatry, 10*(1), 52–77.

Frich, L. M. (2003). Nursing interventions for patients with chronic conditions. *Journal of Advanced Nursing, 44*(2), 135–154.

Gahart, B., Nazareno, A., & Ortega, M. (2019). *2019 Intravenous medications* (35th ed.). St. Louis: Mosby.

Gahart, B., Nazareno, A., & Ortega, M. (2017). *2017 Intravenous medications* (33rd ed.). St. Louis: Mosby.

Global Citizen. (2018). *The 7 biggest challenges facing refugees and immigrants in the U.S.* Retrieved from https://www.globalcitizen.org/en/content/the-7-biggest-challenges-facing-refugees-and-immig/.

Guttmacher Institute. (2018). *Guttmacher Policy Review.* Retrieved from https://www.guttmacher.org/gpr?volume=21&language=en.

Henry, J., & Kaiser Family Foundation. (2017). *Key facts about the uninsured population.* Retrieved from https://www.kff.org/uninsured/fact-sheet/key-facts-about-the-uninsured-population/.

Heuther, S., & McCance, K. (2017). *Understanding Pathophysiology* (6th ed.). St. Louis: Elsevier.

Hockenberry, M., Wilson, D., & Rodgers, C. (2017). *Wong's essentials of pediatric nursing* (10th ed.). St. Louis: Mosby.

Hodgson, B., & Kizior, R. (2019). *Saunders nursing drug handbook 2019.* St. Louis: Saunders.

Hodgson, B., & Kizior, R. (2018). *Saunders nursing drug handbook 2018.* St. Louis: Saunders.

Huber, D. (2018). *Leadership and nursing care management* (6th ed.). St. Louis: Saunders.

iPLEDGE® program update. (2016). Retrieved from https://www.ipledgeprogram.com/iPledgeUI/home.u.

Issues in Science and Technology. (n.d.). *Correctional health is community health.* Retrieved from http://issues.org/32-1/correctional-health-is-community-health/.

Ignatavicius, D., Workman, M., & Rebar, C. (2018). *Concepts for interprofessional collaborative care* (9th ed.). St. Louis: Saunders.

International Council of Nurses. (2012). *The INC Code of Ethics for Nurses.* Retrieved from https://www.icn.ch/sites/default/files/inlinefiles/2012_ICN_Codeofethicsfornurses_%20eng.pdf.

Jarvis, C. (2020). *Physical examination and health assessment* (8th ed.). St. Louis: Saunders.

Jarvis, C. (2016). *Physical examination and health assessment* (7th ed.). St. Louis: Saunders.

Joyful Heart Foundation. (2018). *Effects of domestic violence*. Retrieved from http://www.joyfulheartfoundation.org/learn/domestic-violence/effects-domestic-violence.

Lewis, S., Bucher, L., Heitkemper, M., & Harding, M. (2017). *Medical-surgical nursing: Assessment and management of clinical problems* (10th ed.). St. Louis: Mosby.

Lilley, L., Rainforth Collins, S., & Snyder, J. (2020). *Pharmacology and the nursing process* (9th ed.). St. Louis: Mosby.

Lilley, L., Rainforth Collins, S., & Snyder, J. (2017). *Pharmacology and the nursing process* (8th ed.). St. Louis: Mosby.

Lowdermilk, D., Perry, S., Cashion, K., & Alden, K. (2016). *Maternity & Women's Health Care* (11th ed.). St. Louis: Elsevier.

Maness, D. L., & Khan, M. (2014). Care of the homeless: An overview. *American Family Physician, 89*(8), 634–640.

May, M. E., & Kennedy, C. H. (2010). Health and problem behavior among people with intellectual disabilities. *Behavioral Annals of Practice, 3*(2), 4–12.

McIntosh, J. (2015). *Single mothers at risk of poorer health later in life, study suggests*. Retrieved from https://www.medicalnewstoday.com/articles/293887.php.

McKinney, E., James, S., Murray, S., Nelson, K., & Ashwill, J. (2018). *Maternal-child nursing* (4th ed.). St. Louis: Elsevier.

Dictionary, Mosby's Medical (2017). 10th ed. St. Louis: Elsevier.

Mehta, S. (2016). *The health toll of single motherhood*. Retrieved from https://www.healthify.us/healthify-insights/the-health-toll-of-single-motherhood.

National Council of State Boards of Nursing: *2019 NCLEX-RN® detailed test plan*, Chicago, 2018, National Council of State Boards of Nursing. Retrieved from http://www.ncsbn.org

National Health Care for the Homeless. (2018). *Federal issues and priorities*. Retrieved from https://www.nhchc.org/policy-advocacy/issue/.

Nix, S. (2017). *Williams' basic nutrition and diet therapy* (15th ed.). St. Louis: Mosby.

Olenick, M., Flowers, M., & Diaz, V. J. (2015). US veterans and their unique issues: Enhancing health care professional awareness. *Advanced Medical Education Practice, 6*, 635–639.

Pagana, K., Pagana, T., & Pagana, T. N. (2019). *Mosby's diagnostic and laboratory tests reference* (14th ed.). St. Louis: Mosby.

Pagana, K., Pagana, T., & Pagana, T. N. (2017). *Mosby's diagnostic and laboratory tests reference* (13th ed.). St. Louis: Mosby.

Pamper, F. C., Krueger, P. M., & Denney, J. T. (2010). Socioeconomic disparities in health behaviors. *Annual Review of Sociology, 36*, 349–370.

Perry, A., Potter, P., & Ostendorf, W. (2018). *Clinical nursing skills & techniques* (9th ed.). St. Louis: Mosby.

Potter, P., Perry, A., Stockert, P., & Hall, A. (2019). *Essentials for Nursing Practice* (9th ed.). St. Louis: Elsevier.

Potter, P., Perry, A. G., Stockert, P. A., & Hall, A. M. (2017). *Fundamentals of nursing* (9th ed.). St. Louis: Mosby.

ProEdit. (2019). *Understanding Bloom's (and Anderson and Krathwohl's) Taxonomy*. Retrieved from http://www.proedit.com/understanding-blooms-and-anderson-and-krathwohls-taxonomy/.

Rosenthal, L., & Burcham, J. (2018). *Lehne's Pharmacotherapeutics for Advanced Practice Providers*. St. Louis: Elsevier.

Russell, L. (2010). *Fact sheet: Health disparities by race and ethnicity*. Retrieved from https://cdn.americanprogress.org/wp-content/uploads/issues/2010/12/pdf/disparities_factsheet.pdf.

Skidmore-Roth, L. (2017). *Mosby's nursing drug reference* (30th ed.). St. Louis: Mosby.

Swain, G. R. (2017). How does economic and social disadvantage affect health? *Institute for Research on Poverty, 33*(1), 1–6.

Swearingen, P. (2016). *All-in-one care planning resource: Medical-surgical, pediatric, maternity, & psychiatric nursing care plans* (4th ed.). St. Louis: Mosby.

Szilagyi, M. A., Rosin, D. S., Rubin, D., & Zlotnik, S. (2015). Health care issues for children and adolescents in foster care and kinship care. *Pediatrics, 136*(4), e1142–e1146.

The Joint Commission. (2018). *Facts about the official "do not use" list of abbreviations*. Retrieved from https://www.jointcommission.org/facts_about_do_not_use_list/.

The Joint Commission. (2018). *Hospital national patient safety goals*. Retrieved from https://www.jointcommission.org/assets/1/6/2018_HAP_NPSG_goals_final.pdf.

The Joint Commission. (2018). *National patient safety goals*. Retrieved from https://www.jointcommission.org/assets/1/6/NPSG_Chapter_HAP_Jan2018.pdf.

Thomas, C., & Siela, D. (2011). The impaired nurse: What would you do if you suspected substance abuse? *American Nurse Today, 6*(8). Retrieved from https://www.americannursetoday.com/the-impaired-nurse-would-you-know-what-to-do-if-you-suspected-substance-abuse/.

Touhy, T., & Jett, K. (2018). *Ebersole and Hess' gerontological nursing & health aging* (5th ed.). St. Louis: Mosby.

Trehearne, B., Fishman, P., & Lin, E. (2014). Role of the nurse in chronic illness management: Making the medical home more effective. *Nursing Economic$, 32*(4), 178–184.

Urden, L., Stacy, K., & Lough, M. (2020). *Priorities in critical care nursing* (8th ed.). St. Louis: Elsevier.

Urden, L., Stacy, K., & Lough, M. (2018). *Priorities in critical care nursing* (8th ed.). St. Louis: Elsevier.

U.S. National Library of Medicine. (2017). *Veterans and military health*. Retrieved from https://medlineplus.gov/veteransandmilitaryhealth.html.

U.S. Department of Health and Human Services Office (n.d.). *Health information privacy*. Retrieved from https://www.hhs.gov/hipaa/index.html

Varcarolis, E. (2017). *Essentials of Psychiatric Mental Health Nursing: A communication approach to evidence-based care* (3rd ed.). St. Louis: Saunders.

World Health Organization. (2018). *Migration and health: Key issues*. Retrieved from http://www.euro.who.int/en/health-topics/health-determinants/migration-and-health/migrant-health-in-the-european-region/migration-and-health-key-issues.

World Health Organization. (2005). *Chronic diseases and their common risk factors*. Retrieved from http://www.who.int/chp/chronic_disease_report/media/Factsheet1.pdf.

Yoder-Wise, P. (2015). *Leading and managing in nursing* (6th ed.). St. Louis: Elsevier.

Zerwekh, J., & Zerwekh Garneau, A. (2018). *Nursing Today: Transition and trends* (9th ed.). St. Louis: Elsevier.

Index

Note: Page numbers followed by *f* indicate figures, *t* indicate tables, and *b* indicate boxes.

B

C

D

G

J

O

P

S

W

X

Y

Z

United States (U.S.) Top 100 Prescription Medications (by Generic Name)*

Acetaminophen
Acetaminophen; Hydrocodone Bitartrate
Albuterol
Alendronate Sodium
Allopurinol
Alprazolam
Amitriptyline
Amlodipine Besylate
Amoxicillin
Aspirin
Atenolol
Atorvastatin
Azithromycin
Bacitracin; Neomycin; Polymyxin B
Budesonide; Formoterol
Bupropion
Buspirone Hydrochloride
Carvedilol
Cetirizine Hydrochloride
Citalopram
Clonazepam
Clonidine
Clopidogrel Bisulfate
Cyclobenzaprine
Dextroamphetamine Saccharate
Diclofenac
Diltiazem Hydrochloride
Donepezil Hydrochloride
Duloxetine
Enalapril Maleate
Ergocalciferol
Escitalopram Oxalate
Esomeprazole
Estradiol
Ethinyl Estradiol; Norethindrone
Ethinyl Estradiol; Norgestimate
Fenofibrate
Ferrous Sulfate
Finasteride
Fluoxetine Hydrochloride
Fluticasone
Folic Acid
Furosemide
Gabapentin
Glimepiride
Fluticasone Propionate; Salmeterol Xinafoate
Glipizide
Hydrochlorothiazide
Hydrochlorothiazide; Lisinopril
Hydrochlorothiazide; Losartan Potassium
Hydrochlorothiazide; Triamterene
Hydroxyzine
Ibuprofen
Insulin Aspart
Insulin Glargine
Insulin Human
Insulin Lispro
Lamotrigine
Latanoprost
Levetiracetam
Levothyroxine
Lisdexamfetamine Dimesylate
Lisinopril
Loratadine
Lorazepam
Losartan Potassium
Lovastatin
Meloxicam
Metformin hydrochloride
Methylphenidate
Metoprolol
Metronidazole
Montelukast
Naproxen
Omeprazole
Ondansetron
Oxycodone
Pantoprazole Sodium
Paroxetine
Potassium
Pravastatin Sodium
Prednisone
Pregabalin
Propranolol Hydrochloride
Quetiapine Fumarate
Ranitidine
Rosuvastatin Calcium
Sertraline Hydrochloride
Simvastatin
Sitagliptin Phosphate
Spironolactone
Tamsulosin Hydrochloride
Tiotropium
Topiramate
Tramadol Hydrochloride
Trazodone Hydrochloride
Valsartan
Venlafaxine Hydrochloride
Warfarin
Zolpidem Tartrate

*The list is based off total prescriptions issued in the most recent data made available by the U.S. Government. There is always a lag time with this date, so these statistics are considered to be the 2019 list, but the rankings are from data from January to December 2017.

Prepared by: James Guibault, Jr., BS, PharmD

Information Sources:

Note: The data source (MEPS prescribed medicines file) is released annually by the U.S. Government. This data release represents survey data from two years prior. The ClinCalc DrugStats Database sanitizes and standardizes this data, and is typically released within a few months of the MEPS release. There is an inherent delay in collecting the survey data (eg, in the 2017 calendar year), MEPS releasing the data from patients (August 2019), and the ClinCalc DrugStats release (a few months later, classified as the 2020 drug list). https://clincalc.com/DrugStats/Top200Drugs.aspx